Lists adverse reactions by body system

Details dosage adjustments needed for specific populations

Adjust-a-dose: For adults with a creatinine clearance of 10 to 30 ml/minute, give 1 to 2 g; then give 50% of the usual dose at usual interval. If clearance is less than 10 ml/minute, give 500 mg to 2 g; then give 25% of the usual dose at usual interval. For ... s, add 12½% of the initial ... ance doses after each hemo-

Easy-to-spot black box warnings

ADVERSE REACTIONS

CNS: fatigue, lethargy, fever, vivid dreams, hallucinations, mental depression, light-headedness, dizziness, insomnia.
CV: hypotension, *bradycardia, heart failure, intensification of AV block,* intermittent claudication.
GI: abdominal cramping, constipation, diarrhea, nausea, vomiting.
Hematologic: *agranulocytosis.*
Respiratory: *bronchospasm.*
Skin: rash.

INTERACTIONS

Drug-drug. *Aminophylline:* May antagonize beta-blocking effects of propranolol. Use together cautiously.
Amiodarone, diltiazem, verapamil: May cause hypotension, bradycardia, and increased depressant effect on myocardium. Use together cautiously.
Cardiac glycosides: May reduce the positive inotrope effect of the glycoside. Monitor patient for clinical effect.
Cimetidine, fluoxetine: May inhibit metabolism of propranolol. Watch for increased beta-blocking effect.
Phenothiazines (chlorpromazine, thioridazine): May increase risk of serious adverse reactions of either drug. Use with thioridazine is contraindicated. If chlorpromazine must be used, monitor patient's pulse and blood pressure; decrease propranolol dose as needed.
Propafenone, quinidine: May increase propranolol level. Monitor cardiac function, and adjust propranolol dose as needed.
Drug-herb. *Betel palm:* May decrease temperature-elevating effects and enhanced CNS effects. Discourage use together.
Ma huang: May decrease antihypertensive effects. Discourage use together.
Drug-lifestyle. *Alcohol:* May increase propranolol level. Discourage alcohol use.
Cocaine use: May increase angina-inducing potential of cocaine. Inform patient of this interaction.

Lists potential interactions with other drugs, herbs, and lifestyle factors

EFFECTS ON LAB TEST RESULTS

• May increase T_4, BUN, transaminase, alkaline phosphatase, potassium, and LDH levels. May decrease T_3 level.
• May decrease granulocyte count.

Lists how results may be affected by taking drug

CONTRAINDICATIONS & CAUTIONS

Black Box Warning Abrupt withdrawal of drug may cause exacerbation of angina or myocardial infarction. To discontinue drug, gradually reduce dosage over a few weeks. Because coronary artery disease may be unrecognized, don't discontinue drug abruptly, even when taken for other indications. ▮
• Contraindicated in patients with known hypersensitivity to drug, bronchial asthma, sinus bradycardia and heart block greater than ... and ... over ... un-... th-mia ...
• U... c or rena... ite syndrome, nonallergic bronchospastic diseases, or hepatic disease and in those taking other antihypertensives.
• Elderly patients may experience enhanced adverse reactions and may need dosage adjustment.
• Use cautiously in pregnant women because drug may be associated with small placenta and congenital anomalies.
⚠**Overdose S&S:** Bradycardia, cardiac failure, hypotension, bronchospasm.

Identifies known signs and symptoms of overdose

NURSING CONSIDERATIONS

• Drug masks common signs and symptoms of shock and hypoglycemia.
• Monitor black patients for expected therapeutic effects; dosage adjustments may be necessary.
❶ **Alert:** Don't stop drug before surgery for pheochromocytoma. Before any surgical procedure, tell anesthesiologist that patient is receiving propranolol.
• **Look alike–sound alike:** Don't confuse propranolol with Pravachol. Don't confuse Inderal with Inderide, Isordil, Adderall, or Imuran.

Points out critical information that can't be overlooked

Identifies drugs with similar appearance or name

PATIENT TEACHING

• Caution patient to continue taking this drug as prescribed, even when he's feeling well.
• Instruct patient to take drug with food.
❶ **Alert:** Tell patient not to stop drug suddenly because this can worsen chest pain and trigger a heart attack.

Lists most important information patients should know

P

35th Edition

Nursing2015

DRUG HANDBOOK®

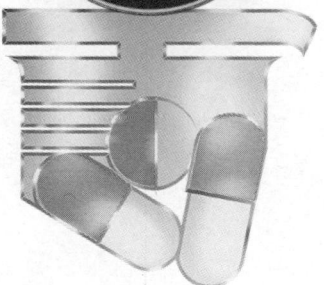

35th Anniversary

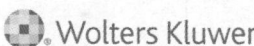
Wolters Kluwer

Philadelphia · Baltimore · New York · London
Buenos Aires · Hong Kong · Sydney · Tokyo

Staff

Publisher
Jay Abramovitz

Chief Nurse
Judith A. Schilling McCann, RN, MSN

Clinical Director
Joan M. Robinson, RN, MSN

Senior Clinical Editor
Lorraine Hallowell, RN, BSN, RVS

Clinical Editors
Lisa Morris Bonsall, RN, CRNP, MSN
Janet Rader, RN, BSN
Dorothy Terry, RN

Product Director
David Moreau

Senior Product Manager
Diane Labus

Editor
Karen C. Comerford

Copy Editor
Mary T. Durkin

Editorial Assistants
Jeri O'Shea, Linda K. Ruhf

Art Director
Elaine Kasmer

Designer
Joseph John Clark

Senior Production Project Manager
Cynthia Rudy

Manufacturing Manager
Kathleen Brown

Production Services
Aptara, Inc.

Printed in China.

NDH35-010514

ISSN 0273-320X
ISBN-13: 978-1-4698-3744-4
ISBN-10: 1-4698-3744-7

Contents

Contributors and consultants

Janine Barnaby, BS, RPh, BCOP
Clinical Pharmacy Specialist
Lehigh Valley Hospital
Allentown, PA

Lawrence Carey, PharmD
Clinical Associate Professor
Temple University School of Pharmacy
Philadelphia, PA

Jason C. Cooper, PharmD
Clinical Pharmacist
Medical University of South Carolina Drug
    Information Center
Charleston

Michele A. Danish, BS, PharmD, FASHP
Director of Performance Improvement/
    Quality Assurance
St. Joseph Health Services/CharterCARE
North Providence, RI

Abimbola Farinde, PharmD, MS
Clinical Pharmacist Specialist
Clear Lake Regional Medical Center
Webster, TX

Glen Edward Farr, PharmD
Professor of Clinical Pharmacy and Associate
    Dean
University of Tennessee College of Pharmacy
Knoxville

Jennifer Faulkner, PharmD, BCPP
Director of Education, Pharmacy Service
Central Texas Veterans Health Care System
Temple

Lauren F. Hazelton, PharmD
Pharmacy Manager
Walgreens Pharmacy
Westmont, NJ

AnhThu Hoang, PharmD
Pharmacist
Express Scripts, Inc.
Mississauga, Ontario, Canada

Rebecca Hoover, PharmD
Drug Information Resident
Idaho State University
Pocatello

James Allen Koestner, BS, PharmD
Clinical Pharmacist
Vanderbilt University Medical Center
Nashville, TN

Hannah J. Livengood, PharmD
Pharmacy Resident
MedStar Washington Hospital Center
Washington, DC

Kristy H. Lucas, PharmD
Professor, Pharmacy Practice Department
University of Charleston School of Pharmacy
Charleston, WV

Michael A. Mancano, RPh, PharmD
Professor of Clinical Pharmacy Practice
Chair, Department of Pharmacy Practice
Temple University School of Pharmacy
Philadelphia, PA

Chijioke Okafor, PharmD
Associate Director, Medical Affairs
Otsuka America Pharmaceutical, Inc.
Princeton, NJ

Priti N. Patel, PharmD, BCPS
Associate Clinical Professor
St. John's University
Queens, NY

Janet S. Rader, RN, BSN
Pre-Award Specialist, Network Office of
    Research and Innovation
Lehigh Valley Health Network
Allentown, PA

Melissa Rinaldi, RPh, PharmD
Clinical Pharmacist
Independence Blue Cross
Philadelphia, PA

Kerry A. Rinato, PharmD
Director of Clinical Applications
Mountain View Hospital
Las Vegas, NV

Joseph F. Steiner, PharmD
Dean
University of Wyoming, College of Health
    Sciences
Laramie

Joanne O'Connell Whitney, PhD, PharmD
Associate Clinical Professor
School of Pharmacy, Department of Clinical
    Pharmacy
University of California
San Francisco

How to use *Nursing2015 Drug Handbook*®

The best-selling nursing drug guide for more than 35 years, *Nursing Drug Handbook* is meticulously reviewed and updated annually by pharmacists and nurses to include the most current, relevant information that practicing nurses and students need to know to administer medications safely in any health care setting. As in previous editions, *Nursing2015 Drug Handbook* emphasizes nursing and safety aspects of drug administration without attempting to replace detailed pharmacology texts. Only the most essential information is included, and helpful graphic symbols, logos, and highlighting draw special attention to critical details that can't be overlooked. Recently redesigned, this new edition ensures easy readability and quick access to content that busy nurses need on the go.

New and outstanding features

This 35th edition provides the newest drugs in the quickest time, right at your fingertips:
- Alphabetical format—complete generic drug entries (monographs) arranged A to Z, with tabbed pages for quick retrieval of information
- Thoroughly updated text with more than 3,250 generic, brand, and combination drugs, 775 comprehensive drug monographs, and 24 generic drugs newly approved by the FDA—roughly 3,000 clinical changes in all
- Drug safety always #1—includes a special chapter with new sections on preventing and treating I.V. vesicant extravasation injury and preventing hazardous drug exposure. Additionally, there are six appendices devoted to drug safety, covering safety guidelines, dosage alerts, best practices to avoid medication errors, pediatric drugs commonly involved in drug errors, and elder care medication tips
- Three new appendices covering nutritional supplements, antacids, and laxatives
- Easy-to-spot logos and icons (such as black box warnings and alerts) and specially highlighted I.V. information
- Expanded color Photoguide insert, with actual-sized images of more than 450 tablets and capsules.

Introductory chapters

Chapter 1, "Drug actions, interactions, and reactions," explains how drugs work in the body. It provides a general overview of drug properties (absorption, distribution, metabolism, and excretion) and other significant factors affecting drug action (including protein binding, patient's age, underlying disease, dosage form, and route and timing of administration). Also discussed are drug interactions, adverse reactions, and toxic reactions. Chapter 2, "Drug therapy across the lifespan," discusses the danger associated with indiscriminate use of drugs during pregnancy and breast-feeding and the special precautions women should take when medications are necessary. This chapter also covers the unique challenges of giving drugs to children and elderly patients and offers practical suggestions on how to minimize problems with these special populations. Chapter 3, "Safe drug administration," explores the ongoing involvement of governmental and nongovernmental organizations weighing in on drug safety issues and the necessary measures nurses must take to prevent medication errors from occurring.

Chapter 4, "Selected drug classifications," summarizes the indications, actions, and contraindications and cautions of more than 60 drug classes represented in *Nursing2015 Drug Handbook*. Generic drugs within each class are also listed, allowing nurses to quickly identify and compare similar drugs when patients can't tolerate or don't respond to a particular drug.

Drug monographs

Each generic drug monograph in *Nursing 2015 Drug Handbook* includes the most pertinent clinical information nurses must know to administer medications safely, monitor for potential interactions and adverse effects, implement necessary care measures, and provide appropriate patient teaching. Entries are arranged alphabetically, with the generic drug name prominently displayed—along with its "tall man" lettering (if applicable), pronunciation, corresponding brand (or trade) names, therapeutic class, pharmacologic class, and pregnancy risk category—on a shaded background for quick and easy identification. Banners or symbols to identify new FDA-approved drugs, drugs that warrant a special safety alert, or drugs that appear in the color photoguide are also included in this highlighted area.

Specific information for each drug is then systematically organized under the headings below. Special icons and logos may be used throughout, as warranted, to point out the drug's safety concerns. For example, a clinical alert logo (❸) provides important advice about life-threatening effects associated with the drug or its administration; a black box warning (**Black Box Warning**) represents a specific warning issued by the FDA. *(See Anatomy of a drug monograph*, on the inside book cover, for a visual guide to the various symbols that may appear within a drug entry.)

Available forms
This section lists the preparations available for each drug (for example, tablets, capsules, solutions for injection) and specifies available dosage forms and strengths. Dosage strengths specifically available in Canada are designated with a dagger (†). Preparations that may be obtained over the counter, without a prescription, are marked with an open diamond (◊).

Indications & dosages
General dosage information for adults and children is found in this section. Dosage instructions reflect current trends in therapeutics and can't be considered absolute or universal. For individual patients, dosage instructions must be considered in light of the patient's condition.

Indications and dosages that aren't approved by the FDA are followed by a closed diamond (◆). It should be noted that only highly evidence-based off-label uses are included in this edition. An "Adjust-a-dose" logo appearing within this section indicates the need for a special dosage adjustment for certain patients, such as

elderly patients or those with renal or hepatic impairment. In some cases, a dosage adjustment may apply to all patient populations for all of the indications listed; this is marked accordingly.

Administration
Here, readers will find guidelines for safely administering drugs by all applicable routes, including P.O., I.V., I.M., subcutaneous, ophthalmic, inhalational, topical, rectal, vaginal, transdermal, and buccal. A special screened background highlights I.V. administration guidelines (including specific instructions on how to reconstitute, mix, and store I.V. medications) and potential I.V. incompatibilities.

Action
This section succinctly describes the mechanism of action—that is, how the drug provides its therapeutic effect. For example, although all antihypertensives lower blood pressure, they don't all do so by the same process. Also included, in table form, are the onset, peak (described in terms of effect or peak blood level), and duration of drug action for each route of administration, if data are available or applicable. Values listed are for patients with normal renal function unless otherwise specified. The drug's half-life is also provided when known.

Adverse reactions
In this section, adverse reactions to each drug are listed according to body system. Life-threatening reactions appear in ***bold italic*** type.

Interactions
Within this section, readers can find each drug's confirmed, clinically significant interactions with other drugs (additive effects, potentiated effects, and antagonistic effects), herbs, foods, beverages, and lifestyle behaviors (such as alcohol use, sun exposure, or smoking). Interactions with a rapid onset are highlighted in color; interactions with a delayed onset are in bold type.

Drug interactions are listed under the drug that's adversely affected. For example, because magnesium trisilicate, an antacid ingredient, interacts with tetracycline to decrease tetracycline's absorption, this interaction is listed under tetracycline. To check on the possible effects of using two or more drugs simultaneously, refer to the interaction section for each drug.

Effects on lab test results
This section lists increased and decreased levels, counts, and other values in laboratory test results that may be caused by the drug's systemic effects. It also indicates false-positive, false-negative, and otherwise altered results of laboratory tests a drug may cause.

Contraindications & cautions
This section outlines any conditions or special circumstances (such as diseases, pregnancy, breast-feeding) in which use of the drug is undesirable or for which the drug should be given with caution. When applicable, specific signs and symptoms of drug overdose are listed as the last bulleted item under this heading and highlighted by a special logo (**▲Overdose S&S:**) for easy identification.

Nursing considerations
Within this section, readers will find practical information on patient monitoring techniques and suggestions for the prevention and treatment of adverse reactions as well as helpful tips on promoting patient comfort.

Patient teaching
Concise guidelines for explaining the drug's purpose, encouraging compliance, ensuring proper use and storage, and preventing or minimizing adverse reactions are included in this section.

Appendices and other helpful aids
Nursing2015 Drug Handbook includes 21 appendices that provide nurses and students with hands-on access to a wealth of supportive data and clinical information. You'll find three new appendices in this edition—"Nutritional supplements: Indications and dosages," "Antacids: Indications and dosages," and "Laxatives: Indications and dosages."

"Additional new drugs: Indications and dosages" introduces brand-new FDA-approved drugs that couldn't be included in time for publication of this edition.

A handy visual "Quick guide to special symbols, logos, and highlighted terms" and "Guide to abbreviations" immediately follow this "How to use" piece.

Photoguide to tablets and capsules
To enhance patient safety and help make drug identification easier, *Nursing2015 Drug Handbook* offers a 32-page full-color photoguide to the most commonly prescribed tablets and capsules. Shown in actual size, the drugs are arranged alphabetically by generic name for quick reference followed by the brand names and their most common dosage strengths. Below the name of each drug is a cross-reference to where information on the drug can be found in the book. Brand names of drugs that appear in the photoguide are shown in text with a special capsule symbol (𝓔). Page references to the drug photos appear in boldface type in the index (for example, **C12**).

Photos for certain brands were provided by the following companies for use in this book: Forest Pharmaceuticals, Inc. (Campral); Novartis Pharmaceuticals (Enablex); Sepracor, Inc. (Lunesta); Teva Pharmaceuticals (Azilect); and Pfizer (Sutent). Additional photos were provided by Jeff Sigler of SFI Medical Publishing.

Online Toolkit
A Toolkit containing a wide array of drug-related materials that practicing nurses and students can use on the job and for study—covering safety issues, pharmacology, drug therapy guidelines, patient populations, and a host of other drug-specialty areas—can be found online at **NDHnow.com**. Included are a dosage calculator, drug safety and administration videos, pharmacology animations, English-Spanish translator, audio

drug pronunciation guide, a 325-question NCLEX®-style test, and access to free and discounted CE tests. Monthly FDA drug updates, drug warnings, and newsworthy drug information can also be accessed through this site.

Quick guide to special symbols, logos, and highlighted terms

The following symbols or highlighted features appear throughout drug monographs and select appendices in this edition.

Special symbols and logos	Usage or meaning
✳ *NEW DRUG*	New FDA-approved drug
SAFETY ALERT!	Drug that presents a heightened avoidable danger
buPROPion	"Tall man" lettering for FDA-designated generic drug names prone to mix-ups
➤	Indication for drug
✳ *NEW INDICATION:*	New indication for drug
Adjust-a-dose:	Dosage adjustment needed for certain populations
Adjust-a-dose (for all indications):	Dosage adjustment needed for all indications
☙ *Alert:*	Clinical alert
†	Available in Canada
◇	Over-the-counter (OTC)
◆	Off-label use
✐	Appears in Photoguide
*	Liquid contains alcohol
• *Look alike–sound alike:*	Drugs with easily confused names
Black Box Warning	FDA black box warning
⚠ *Overdose S&S:*	Overdose signs & symptoms
Highlighted reactions and interactions	
life-threatening	Life-threatening reaction
rapid onset	Causes interaction with rapid onset
delayed onset	Causes interaction with delayed onset

Guide to abbreviations

ACE	angiotensin-converting enzyme	g	gram	NSAID	nonsteroidal anti-inflammatory drug
ADH	antidiuretic hormone	G	gauge	OTC	over-the-counter
ADHD	attention deficit hyperactivity disorder	GABA	gamma-aminobutyric acid	oz	ounce
AEDs	antiepileptic drugs	GERD	gastroesophageal reflux disease	PABA	para-aminobenzoic acid
AIDS	acquired immunodeficiency syndrome	GFR	glomerular filtration rate	PCA	patient-controlled analgesia
ALT	alanine transaminase	GGT	gamma-glutamyltransferase	PDE5	phosphodiesterase type 5
ANA	antinuclear antibody	GI	gastrointestinal	PE	pulmonary embolus
ANC	absolute neutrophil count	gtt	drops	P.O.	by mouth
ARB	angiotensin receptor blocker	GU	genitourinary	P.R.	by rectum
AST	aspartate transaminase	G6PD	glucose-6-phosphate dehydrogenase	p.r.n.	as needed
AV	atrioventricular	H_1	histamine$_1$	PT	prothrombin time
b.i.d.	twice daily	H_2	histamine$_2$	PTT	partial thromboplastin time
BPH	benign prostatic hypertrophy	HDL	high-density lipoprotein	PVC	premature ventricular contraction
BSA	body surface area	HIV	human immunodeficiency virus	q.i.d.	four times daily
BUN	blood urea nitrogen	HMG-	3-hydroxy-3-methyl-	RBC	red blood cell
CABG	coronary artery bypass graft	CoA	glutaryl coenzyme A	RDA	recommended daily allowance
cAMP	cyclic 3′, 5′ adenosine monophosphate	I.D.	intradermal	REM	rapid eye movement
		I.M.	intramuscular	RNA	ribonucleic acid
CBC	complete blood count	INR	International Normalized Ratio	RSV	respiratory syncytial virus
CK	creatine kinase				
CMV	cytomegalovirus	IPPB	intermittent positive-pressure breathing	SA	sinoatrial
CNS	central nervous system	I.V.	intravenous	sec	second
COPD	chronic obstructive pulmonary disease	kg	kilogram	SIADH	syndrome of inappropriate antidiuretic hormone
CrCl	creatinine clearance	L	liter		
CSF	cerebrospinal fluid	lb	pound	S.L.	sublingual
CV	cardiovascular	LDH	lactate dehydrogenase	SSNRI	selective serotonin and norepinephrine reuptake inhibitor
D_5W	dextrose 5% in water	LDL	low-density lipoprotein		
DEHP	di(2-ethylhexyl) phthalate	LFTs	liver function tests	SSRI	selective serotonin reuptake inhibitor
		LVEF	left ventricular ejection fraction		
DIC	disseminated intravascular coagulation	M	molar	Subcut.	subcutaneous
dL	deciliter	m^2	square meter	T_3	triiodothyronine
DNA	deoxyribonucleic acid	MAO	monoamine oxidase	T_4	thyroxine
DPP-4	dipeptidyl peptidase-4	mcg	microgram	TCA	tricyclic antidepressant
DVT	deep vein thrombosis	mEq	milliequivalent		
ECG	electrocardiogram	mg	milligram	t.i.d.	three times daily
EEG	electroencephalogram	MI	myocardial infarction	TNF	tumor necrosis factor
EENT	eyes, ears, nose, throat	min	minute	tsp	teaspoon
		mL	milliliter	USP	United States Pharmacopeia
ESRD	end-stage renal disease	mm^3	cubic millimeter		
		mo	month	UTI	urinary tract infection
FDA	Food and Drug Administration	MS	multiple sclerosis	WBC	white blood cell
		msec	millisecond	wk	week
5-FU	fluorouracil	NNRTI	non-nucleoside reverse transcriptase inhibitor		

1

Drug actions, interactions, and reactions

Any drug a patient takes causes a series of physical and chemical events in his body. The first event, when a drug combines with cellular drug receptors, is the *drug action*. What happens next is the *drug effect*. Depending on the type of cellular drug receptors affected by a given drug, an effect can be local, systemic, or both. A systemic drug effect can follow a local effect. For example, when you apply a drug to the skin, it causes a local effect. But transdermal absorption of that drug can then produce a systemic effect. A local effect can also follow systemic absorption. For example, the peptic ulcer drug cimetidine produces a local effect after it's swallowed by blocking histamine receptors in the stomach's parietal cells. Diphenhydramine, on the other hand, causes a systemic effect by blocking histamine receptors throughout the body.

Drug properties

Drug absorption, distribution, metabolism, and excretion make up a drug's pharmacokinetics. These processes determine a drug's onset of action, peak level, duration of action, and bioavailability.

Absorption

Before a drug can act in the body, it must be absorbed into the bloodstream—usually after oral administration, the most common route. Before an oral drug can be absorbed, it must disintegrate into particles small enough to dissolve in gastric juices. Only after dissolving can the drug be absorbed. Most absorption of orally given drugs occurs in the small intestine because the mucosal villi provide extensive surface area. Once absorbed and circulated in the bloodstream, the drug is *bioavailable,* or ready to produce a drug effect. The speed of absorption and whether absorption is complete or partial depend on the drug's effects, dosage form, administration route, interactions with other substances in the GI tract, and various patient characteristics. Oral solutions and elixirs bypass the need

for disintegration and dissolution and are usually absorbed faster. Some tablets have enteric coatings to prevent disintegration in the acidic environment of the stomach; others have coatings of varying thickness that simply delay release of the drug.

Drugs given I.M. must first be absorbed through the muscle into the bloodstream. Rectal suppositories must dissolve to be absorbed through the rectal mucosa. Drugs given I.V. are injected directly into the bloodstream and are bioavailable completely and immediately.

Distribution

After absorption, a drug moves from the bloodstream into the fluids and tissues in the body, a movement known as *distribution*. All of the area to which a drug is distributed is known as the *volume of distribution*. Individual patient variations can change the amount of drug distributed throughout the body. For example, in an edematous patient, a given dose must be distributed to a larger volume than in a nonedematous patient. Occasionally, a dose is increased to account for this difference. In this case, the dose should be decreased after the edema is corrected. Conversely, a dose given to a dehydrated patient must be decreased to allow for its distribution to a much smaller volume. Patients who are very obese may present another problem when considering drug distribution. Some drugs—such as digoxin, gentamicin, and tobramycin—aren't well-distributed to fatty tissue. Sometimes, doses based on actual body weight may lead to overdose and serious toxicity. In these cases, doses must be based on lean body weight, or adjusted body weight, which may be estimated from actuarial tables that give average weight range for height.

Metabolism

Most drugs are metabolized in the liver. Hepatic diseases may affect the liver's metabolic functions and may increase or decrease a drug's usual metabolism. Closely monitor all patients with hepatic disease for drug effect and toxicity.

The rate at which a drug is metabolized varies from person to person. Some patients metabolize drugs so quickly that the drug levels in their blood and tissues prove therapeutically inadequate. In other patients, the rate of metabolism is so slow that ordinary doses can produce toxicity.

Excretion

The body eliminates drugs by metabolism (usually hepatic) and excretion (usually renal). *Drug excretion* is the movement of a drug or its metabolites from the tissues back into circulation and from the circulation into the organs of excretion, where they're removed from the body. Most drugs are excreted by the kidneys, but some can be eliminated through the lungs, exocrine glands (sweat, salivary, or mammary), liver, skin, or intestinal tract. Drugs also may be removed artificially by direct mechanical intervention, such as peritoneal dialysis or hemodialysis.

Other modifying factors

One important factor influencing a drug's action and effect is its tendency to bind to plasma proteins, especially albumin, and other tissue components. Because only a free, unbound drug can act in the body, protein binding greatly influences the amount and duration of a drug's effect. Malnutrition, renal failure, and the presence of other protein-bound drugs can influence protein binding. When protein binding changes, the drug dose may need to be changed also.

The patient's age is another important factor. Elderly patients usually have decreased hepatic function, less muscle mass, diminished renal function, and lower albumin levels. These patients need lower doses and sometimes longer dosage intervals to avoid toxicity. Neonates have underdeveloped metabolic enzyme systems and inadequate renal function, so they need highly individualized dosages and careful monitoring.

Underlying disease also may affect drug action and effect. For example, acidosis may cause insulin resistance. Genetic diseases, such as G6PD deficiency and hepatic porphyria, may turn drugs into toxins, with serious consequences. Patients with G6PD deficiency may develop hemolytic anemia when given certain drugs, such as sulfonamides. A genetically susceptible patient can develop acute porphyria if given a barbiturate. A patient with a highly active hepatic enzyme system, such as a rapid acetylator, can develop hepatitis when treated with isoniazid because of the quick intrahepatic buildup of a toxic metabolite.

Drug administration issues

How a drug is given can also influence a drug's action in the body. The dosage form of a drug is important. Some tablets and capsules are too large to be easily swallowed by sick patients. An oral solution may be substituted, but it will produce higher drug levels than a tablet because the liquid is more easily and completely absorbed. When a potentially toxic drug (such as digoxin) is given in the liquid form, its increased absorption can cause toxicity. Sometimes a change in dosage form also requires a change in dosage.

Routes of administration aren't interchangeable. For example, diazepam is readily absorbed P.O. but is slowly and erratically absorbed I.M. On the other hand, gentamicin must be given parenterally because oral administration results in drug levels too low for systemic infections.

Improper storage can alter a drug's potency. Store most drugs in tight containers protected from direct sunlight and extremes in temperature and humidity that can cause them to deteriorate. Some drugs require special storage conditions, such as refrigeration. Caution patients not to store drugs in a bathroom because of the constantly changing environment.

The timing of drug administration can be important. Sometimes, giving an oral drug during or shortly after a meal decreases the amount of drug absorbed. In most cases, this isn't significant and may even be desirable with irritating drugs such as aspirin. But penicillins and tetracyclines shouldn't be taken at mealtimes because certain foods can inactivate them. If in doubt about the effect of food on a certain drug, check with a pharmacist.

Consider the patient's age, height, and weight. The prescriber will need this information when calculating the dosage for many drugs. Record all information accurately on the patient's chart. The chart should also include all current laboratory data, especially results of renal and liver function studies, so the prescriber can adjust the dosage as needed.

Watch for metabolic changes and physiologic changes (depressed respiratory function, acidosis, or alkalosis) that might alter drug effect.

Know the patient's medical history. Whenever possible, obtain a comprehensive family history from the patient or his family. Ask about past reactions to drugs, possible genetic traits that might affect drug response, and the current use of other prescription, OTC, and illicit drugs; herbal remedies; and vitamin supplements. Multiple drug therapies can cause serious and fatal drug interactions and dramatically change many drugs' effects.

Drug interactions

A *drug interaction* occurs when a drug given with or shortly after another drug alters the effect of either or both drugs. Usually the effect of one drug is increased or decreased. For instance, one drug may inhibit or stimulate the metabolism or excretion of the other or free it for further action by releasing the drug from protein-binding sites.

Combination therapy is based on drug interactions. One drug may be given to complement the effects of another. Probenecid, which blocks the excretion of penicillin, is sometimes given with penicillin to maintain an adequate level of penicillin for a longer time. In many cases, two drugs with similar actions are given together precisely because of the additive effect. For instance, acetaminophen and codeine are commonly given in combination because together they provide greater pain relief than if either is given alone.

Drug interactions are sometimes used to prevent or antagonize certain adverse reactions. The diuretics hydrochlorothiazide and spironolactone are often given together because the former is potassium-depleting and the latter potassium-sparing.

Not all drug interactions are beneficial: many drugs interact and decrease efficacy or increase toxicity. An example of decreased efficacy occurs when a tetracycline is given with drugs or foods that contain calcium or magnesium (such as antacids or milk). These bind with tetracycline in the GI tract and cause inadequate drug absorption. An example of increased toxicity can be seen in a patient taking a diuretic and lithium. The diuretic may increase the lithium level, causing lithium toxicity. This drug effect is known as *antagonism*. Avoid drug combinations that produce these effects, if possible.

Sometimes drug interactions occur after a drug that may inhibit or increase the metabolism of another drug has been discontinued. After the drug is discontinued, the other drug's levels may increase or decrease.

Adverse reactions

Drugs cause adverse *effects*; patients have adverse *reactions*. An adverse reaction may be tolerated to obtain a therapeutic effect, or it may be hazardous and unacceptable. Some adverse reactions subside with continued use. For example, the drowsiness caused by paroxetine and the orthostatic hypotension caused by prazosin usually subside after several days when the patient develops tolerance. But many adverse reactions are dosage related and lessen or disappear only if the dosage is reduced. Most adverse reactions aren't therapeutically desirable, but a few can be put to clinical use. An outstanding example of this is the drowsiness caused by diphenhydramine, which makes it useful as a mild sedative.

Drug hypersensitivity, or drug allergy, is the result of an antigen–antibody immune reaction that occurs in the body when a drug is given to a susceptible patient. Signs and symptoms of a drug allergy may include rash, itching, angioedema, and shortness of breath. One of the most dangerous of all drug hypersensitivities is penicillin allergy. In its most severe form, penicillin anaphylaxis can rapidly become fatal.

Rarely, idiosyncratic reactions occur. These reactions are highly unpredictable and unusual. One of the best-known idiosyncratic adverse reactions is aplastic anemia caused by the antibiotic chloramphenicol. This reaction may appear in only 1 of 24,000 patients, but when it does occur, it can be fatal. A more common idiosyncratic reaction is extreme sensitivity to very low doses of a drug or insensitivity to higher-than-normal doses.

To deal with adverse reactions correctly, you need to be alert to even minor changes in the patient's clinical status. Such minor changes may be an early warning of pending toxicity. Listen to the patient's complaints about his reactions to a drug, and consider each objectively. You may be able to reduce adverse reactions in several ways. Obviously, dosage reduction can help. But, in many cases, so does a simple rescheduling of the dose. For example, pseudoephedrine may produce stimulation that will be no problem if it's given early in the day. Similarly, drowsiness from antihistamines or tranquilizers can be less important if these drugs are given at bedtime. Most important, your patient needs to be told which adverse reactions to expect so that he won't become worried or even stop taking the drug on his own. Always advise the patient to report adverse reactions to the prescriber immediately.

Your ability to recognize signs and symptoms of drug allergies or serious idiosyncratic reactions may save your patient's life. Ask each patient about the drugs he's taking currently or has taken in the past and whether he experienced any unusual reactions from taking them. If a patient claims to be allergic to a drug, ask him to tell you exactly what happens when he takes it. He may be calling a harmless adverse reaction, such as upset stomach, an allergic reaction, or he may have a true tendency toward anaphylaxis. In either case, you and the prescriber need to know this. Of course, you must record and report clinical changes throughout the patient's course of treatment. If you suspect a severe adverse reaction, withhold the drug until you can check with the pharmacist and the prescriber.

Toxic reactions

Chronic drug toxicities are usually caused by the cumulative effect and resulting buildup of the drug in the body. These effects may be extensions of the desired therapeutic effect.

For example, normal doses of glyburide normalize the glucose level, but higher doses can produce hypoglycemia.

Drug toxicities occur when a drug level rises as a result of impaired metabolism or excretion. For example, hepatic dysfunction impairs the metabolism of theophylline, raising its levels. Similarly, renal dysfunction may cause digoxin toxicity because this drug is eliminated from the body by the kidneys. Of course, excessive dosage can cause toxic levels also. For instance, tinnitus is usually a sign that the safe dose of aspirin has been exceeded.

Most drug toxicities are predictable, dosage-related, and reversible upon dosage adjustment. So, monitor patients carefully for physiologic changes that might alter drug effect. Watch especially for hepatic and renal impairment. Warn the patient about signs of pending toxicity, and tell him what to do if a toxic reaction occurs. Also, make sure to emphasize the importance of taking a drug exactly as prescribed. Warn the patient that serious problems could arise if he changes the dose or schedule or stops taking the drug without his prescriber's knowledge.

Pharmacogenetics

As a rule, prescribers typically follow a "trial and error" approach to prescribing drugs, often operating under the assumption that one size fits all. Although decisions are made with evidence-based approaches and the best of intentions, some result in the development of adverse drug reactions. It would be helpful to accurately predict which patients will (and which will not) have a response when prescribed a certain drug. Pharmacogenetics—the study of how varied responses to a drug can be caused by genetic differences between individuals—attempts to do just this.

The first pharmacogenetic detection occurred when Pythagoras recognized the dangers of ingesting fava beans in 510 B.C., eventually leading to the discovery of glucose-6-phosphate deficiency (G6PD) in 1956. Shortly after (in 1957), the term *pharmacogenetics* was coined and later defined as the study of variability in drug response due to heredity. The goals of pharmacogenetics include identification of innovative drug targets, accounting for DNA sequence variation on drug effects, development of new agents, and optimization of drug efficacy while minimizing drug toxicity via a genetic basis.

Pharmacogenetics revolves around the existence of polymorphisms, which are defined as genetic variations that occur in 1% or more of the population. If clinicians are able to predict which patients may express polymorphisms, they can provide targeted therapy. Researchers have learned that many polymorphisms involve cytochrome P450 (CYP450) isoenzymes.

Polymorphisms play a significant role in determining whether a drug will be appropriately metabolized. Patients fall into one of four classes of metabolizers: extensive, ultrarapid, intermediate, and poor. Patients considered "extensive metabolizers" possess an overwhelming capacity to metabolize certain drugs and may exhibit therapeutic failure, whereas patients who are "poor metabolizers," such as those with G6PD, exhibit toxicities due to their inability to metabolize certain drugs. Ethnicity may also play a role in determining how patients are classified in regard to metabolism.

It's vital to recognize the importance of the CYP450 system. Approximately 60 CYP enzymes are found in humans, and many genes that encode for these enzymes are polymorphic. Polymorphism associated with CYP enzymes may be expressed via amino acid substitution (thereby reducing enzymatic activity) or by amplification or duplication of activity (thereby increasing enzymatic activity). It's thought that approximately one-third of all medications prescribed today are metabolized by CYP450, including tricyclic antidepressants, antiarrhythmics, beta-receptor antagonists, codeine, warfarin, phenytoin, and nicotine.

In addition, enzymes that metabolize cancer chemotherapy drugs, such as thiopurine S-methyltransferase, dihydropyrimidine dehydrogenase, and UDP-glucuronosyl transferase, can have therapeutic implications; for example, polymorphisms affecting these enzymes can result in serious adverse reactions, such as anemia and neurotoxicity. Finally, miscellaneous polymorphisms affecting drug transport proteins such as P-glycoprotein may affect drug response; this protein acts as a safety mechanism to remove toxins from cells and has a role in the distribution of cancer chemotherapy drugs, digoxin, cyclosporine, and protease inhibitors.

As a nurse, you need to be aware of the clinical ramifications of pharmacogenetics—having an effective knowledge of which drugs, diseases, or ethnic groups are affected by these variations can help you anticipate issues that may arise with patients under your care. For example, some Asian patients have a significant reduction in enzyme activity secondary to amino acid substitution and, therefore, exhibit slower metabolism of certain drugs compared to patients of other ethnic groups. The effect of this on clinical practice is seen in the dosing of rosuvastatin: patients of Asian descent are typically started at 5 mg/day P.O., whereas other non-Asian patients are started at 10 mg/day. Giving a lower dosage helps limit the development of serious adverse reactions in Asian patients.

Another example of how drug metabolism is affected by genetic polymorphism involves the drug warfarin. Studies have shown that CYP2C9, which is the primary enzyme responsible for warfarin metabolism, has two genetic variants. These variants are associated with up to an 80% decrease in enzymatic activity that can affect approximately 7% to 11% of patients. Patients with these variant genotypes had a 2.4 times increase in the risk of serious or life-threatening bleeding after normal doses of warfarin. Consequently, patients with these variants become hypercoagulated at a faster rate and need significantly lower maintenance dosages.

Fortunately, genetic testing for polymorphisms is available when issues such as these arise. Although testing isn't done for every patient, it can be helpful for those who seem to be refractory or overly sensitive to the effects of certain necessary drugs (such as warfarin) or who meet other criteria (such as ethnicity).

2

Drug therapy across the lifespan

Drug therapy is a fact of life for millions of people of all ages, and certain aspects of a patient's life, such as age, growth, and development, can affect drug therapy.

Drugs and pregnancy

Drug administration during pregnancy has been a source of serious medical concern and controversy since the thalidomide tragedy of the late 1950s, when thousands of malformed infants were born after their mothers were given this mild sedative–hypnotic while pregnant. To identify drugs that may cause such teratogenic effects, preclinical drug studies always include tests on pregnant laboratory animals. These studies may reveal gross teratogenicity but don't establish absolute safety. This is because different animal species react to drugs in different ways. Consequently, animal studies can't reveal all possible teratogenic effects in humans. For example, the preliminary studies on thalidomide gave no warning of teratogenic effects, and it was subsequently released for general use in Europe.

What about the placental barrier? Once thought to protect the fetus from drug effects, the placenta isn't much of a barrier at all. Almost every drug a pregnant woman takes crosses the placenta and enters the fetal circulation, except for drugs with exceptionally large molecular structure, such as heparin, the injectable anticoagulant. By this standard, heparin could be used in a pregnant woman without fear of harming the fetus, but even heparin carries a warning for cautious use during pregnancy. Conversely, just because a drug crosses the placenta doesn't necessarily mean it's harmful to the fetus. The relative risk to the fetus is expressed by the drug's pregnancy risk category.

Actually, only one factor—stage of fetal development—seems clearly related to greater risk during pregnancy. During the first and third trimesters of pregnancy, the fetus is especially vulnerable to damage from maternal use of drugs. During these times, give *all* drugs with extreme caution.

Organogenesis—when fetal organs differentiate—occurs in the first trimester. This is the most sensitive period for drug-induced fetal malformation. Withhold all drugs except those in category A or B during this time, unless this would jeopardize the mother's health. Strongly advise your patient to avoid *all* self-prescribed drugs during early pregnancy.

Fetal sensitivity to drugs is also of special concern during the last trimester. At birth, when separated from his mother, the neonate must rely on his own metabolism to eliminate any remaining drug. Because his detoxifying systems aren't fully developed, any residual drug may take a long time to be metabolized and thus may induce prolonged toxic reactions. For this reason, discourage pregnant patients from taking drugs except when absolutely necessary and advised by their prescriber during the last 3 months of pregnancy.

Of course, in many circumstances, pregnant women must continue to take certain drugs. For example, a woman with a seizure disorder that is well-controlled with an anticonvulsant should keep taking the drug during pregnancy. Similarly, a pregnant woman with a bacterial infection must receive antibiotics. In such cases, the potential risk to the fetus is outweighed by the mother's medical needs.

Complying with these general guidelines can prevent indiscriminate and harmful use of drugs in pregnancy:
• Before a drug is prescribed for a woman of childbearing age, ask the date of her last menstrual period and whether she may be pregnant. If a drug is a known teratogen (for example, isotretinoin), some manufacturers may recommend special precautions to ensure that the drug isn't given to a woman of childbearing age until pregnancy is ruled out and that contraceptives are used throughout the course of therapy.

• Caution a pregnant woman to avoid all drugs except those essential to maintain her pregnancy or health—especially during the first and third trimesters.

• Topical drugs are subject to the same warning against use during pregnancy. Many topically applied drugs can be absorbed in large enough amounts to be harmful to the fetus.

• When a pregnant woman needs a drug, use the safest drug in the lowest possible dose to minimize harm to the fetus.

• Instruct a pregnant woman to check with her prescriber before taking any drug.

Drugs and breast-feeding

Most drugs a breast-feeding mother takes appear in breast milk. Drug levels in breast milk tend to be high when drug levels in maternal blood are high, especially right after each dose. Advise the mother to breast-feed *before* taking each drug dose, not *after*. Also, in general, drugs with short half-lives are preferred because they peak quickly and are then eliminated and are less likely to be excreted in breast milk.

A mother who wants to breast-feed usually may continue to do so with her prescriber's advice. However, breast-feeding should be temporarily interrupted and replaced with bottle-feeding when the mother must take tetracycline, chloramphenicol, a sulfonamide (during the first 2 weeks postpartum), an oral anticoagulant, a drug that contains iodine, or an antineoplastic.

Caution the breast-feeding patient to protect her infant by not taking drugs indiscriminately. Instruct the mother to first check with her prescriber to be sure she's taking the safest drug at the lowest dose. Also instruct her to give her prescriber a list of all drugs and herbs she's currently taking.

Drug therapy in children

Providing drug therapy to infants, children, and adolescents is challenging. Physiologic differences between children and adults, including those involving vital organ maturity and body composition, significantly influence a drug's effectiveness.

Physiologic changes affecting drug action

A child's absorption, distribution (including drug binding to plasma proteins), metabolism, and excretion processes undergo profound changes that affect drug dosage. To ensure optimal drug effect and minimal toxicity, consider these factors when giving drugs to a child.

Absorption

Drug absorption in children depends on the form of the drug, its physical properties, simultaneous ingestion of other drugs or food, physiologic changes, and concurrent disease.

The pH of neonatal gastric fluid is neutral or slightly acidic; it becomes more acidic as the infant matures, which affects drug absorption. For example, nafcillin and penicillin G are better absorbed in an infant than in an adult because of low gastric acidity.

Various infant formulas or milk products may increase gastric pH and impede absorption of acidic drugs. If possible, give a child oral drugs on an empty stomach.

Gastric emptying time and transit time through the small intestine—which takes longer in children than in adults—can affect absorption. Also, intestinal hypermotility (as occurs in patients with diarrhea) can diminish the drug's absorption.

A child's comparatively thin epidermis allows increased absorption of topical drugs.

Distribution

As with absorption, changes in body weight and physiology during childhood can significantly influence a drug's distribution and effects. In a premature infant, body fluid makes up about 85% of total body weight; in a full-term infant, it makes up 55% to 70%; in an adult, 50% to 55%. Extracellular fluid (mostly blood) constitutes 40% of a neonate's body weight, compared with 20% in an adult. Intracellular fluid remains fairly constant throughout life and has little effect on drug dosage.

Extracellular fluid volume influences a water-soluble drug's concentration and effect because most drugs travel through extracellular fluid to reach their receptors. Compared with adults, distribution area in children is proportionately greater because their fluid-to-solid body weight proportion is larger.

Because the proportion of fat to lean body mass increases with age, the distribution of fat-soluble drugs is more limited in children than in adults. As a result, a drug's fat or water solubility affects the dosage for a child.

Plasma protein binding
A decrease in albumin level or intermolecular attraction between drug and plasma protein causes many drugs to be less bound to plasma proteins in infants than in adults.

Strongly protein-bound drugs may displace endogenous compounds, such as bilirubin or free fatty acids. Displacement of bound bilirubin can increase unbound bilirubin, which can lead to increased risk of kernicterus at normal bilirubin levels. Conversely, an endogenous compound may displace a weakly bound drug.

Because only an unbound (free) drug has a pharmacologic effect, a change in the ratio of a protein-bound to an unbound active drug can greatly influence the drug's effect.

Several diseases and disorders, such as nephrotic syndrome and malnutrition, can decrease plasma protein level and increase the level of an unbound drug, which can either intensify the drug's effect or produce toxicity.

Metabolism
A neonate's ability to metabolize a drug depends on the integrity of the hepatic enzyme system, intrauterine exposure to the drug, and the nature of the drug itself.

Certain metabolic mechanisms are underdeveloped in neonates. Glucuronidation is a metabolic process that renders most drugs more water soluble, facilitating renal excretion. This process isn't developed enough to permit full pediatric doses of most drugs until the infant is age 1 month. The use of chloramphenicol in a neonate may cause gray baby syndrome because the infant's immature liver can't metabolize the drug and toxic levels accumulate in the blood. Reduce dosage in a neonate and periodically monitor his drug levels.

Conversely, intrauterine exposure to drugs may induce precocious development of hepatic enzyme mechanisms, increasing the infant's capacity to metabolize potentially harmful substances.

Older children can metabolize some drugs (theophylline, for example) more rapidly than adults. This ability may come from their increased hepatic metabolic activity. Doses larger than those recommended for adults may be required.

Also, more than one drug given to a child simultaneously may change hepatic metabolism and initiate production of hepatic enzymes. Phenobarbital, for example, accelerates the metabolism of drugs taken with it and causes hepatic enzyme production.

Excretion
Renal excretion of a drug is the net result of glomerular filtration, active tubular secretion, and passive tubular reabsorption. Many drugs are excreted in the urine. The degree of renal development or presence of renal disease can greatly affect a child's dosage requirements because if a child can't excrete a drug renally, the drug may accumulate to toxic levels.

Physiologically, an infant's kidneys differ from an adult's because infants have a high resistance to blood flow and their kidneys receive a smaller proportion of cardiac output. Infants have incomplete glomerular and tubular development and short, incomplete loops of Henle. (A child's GFR reaches an adult value between ages 2½ and 5 months; his tubular secretion rate may reach an adult value between ages 7 and 12 months.) Infants also are less able to concentrate urine or reabsorb certain filtered compounds. The proximal tubules in infants also are less able to secrete organic acids.

Children and adults have diurnal variations in urine pH that correlate with sleep patterns.

Special administration considerations
Biochemically, a drug displays the same mechanisms of action in all people. But the response to a drug can be affected by a child's age and size, as well as by the

maturity of the target organ. To ensure optimal drug effect and minimal toxicity, consider the following factors when giving drugs to children.

Adjusting dosages for children

When calculating children's dosages, don't use formulas that just modify adult dosages. Base pediatric dosages on either body weight (mg/kg) or body surface area (mg/m^2). A child isn't a scaled-down version of an adult.

Reevaluate dosages at regular intervals to ensure needed adjustments as the child develops. Although body surface area provides a useful standard for adults and older children, use the body weight method instead in premature or full-term infants. Don't exceed the maximum adult dosage when calculating amounts per kilogram of body weight (except with certain drugs such as theophylline, if indicated).

Obtain an accurate maternal drug history, including prescription and nonprescription drugs, vitamins, herbs, or other health foods taken during pregnancy. Drugs passed into breast milk can have adverse effects on the breast-feeding infant. Before giving a drug to a breast-feeding mother, investigate its potential effects on the infant.

For example, a sulfonamide given to a breast-feeding mother for a UTI appears in breast milk and may cause kernicterus in an infant with low levels of unconjugated bilirubin. Also, high levels of isoniazid appear in the breast milk of a mother taking this drug. Because this drug is metabolized by the liver, the infant's immature hepatic enzyme mechanisms can't metabolize the drug, and he may develop CNS toxicity.

Giving oral drugs

Remember the following when giving oral drugs to a child:

If the patient is an infant, give drugs in liquid form, if possible. For accuracy, measure and give the preparation by oral syringe, never a parenteral syringe. It's very important to remove the syringe cap to keep the infant from aspirating it. Be sure to instruct parents to do the same. Never use a vial or cup. Lift the patient's head to prevent aspiration of the drug, and press down on

his chin to prevent choking. You may also place the drug in a nipple and allow the infant to suck the contents.

If the patient is a toddler, explain how you're going to give him the drug. If possible, have the parents enlist the child's cooperation. Don't mix the drug with food or call it "candy," even if it has a pleasant taste. Let the child drink a liquid drug from a calibrated medication cup rather than a spoon. It's easier and more accurate. If the preparation is available only in tablet form, crush and mix it with an appropriate buffer, such as jelly or applesauce. (First, verify with the pharmacist that the tablet can be crushed without compromising its effectiveness.)

If the patient is an older child who can swallow a tablet or capsule by himself, have him place the drug on the back of his tongue and swallow it with water or nonacidic fruit juice, because milk and milk products may interfere with drug absorption.

Giving I.V. infusions

For I.V. infusions in infants, use a peripheral vein or a scalp vein in the temporal region. The scalp vein is safe because the needle isn't likely to dislodge. However, the hair must be clipped around the site, and the needle and infiltrated fluids may cause temporary disfigurement. For these reasons, scalp veins aren't used as commonly today as they were in the past.

The arms and legs are the most accessible insertion sites, but because children tend to move about, take these precautions:
● Protect the insertion site to keep the catheter or needle from being dislodged.
● Use a padded arm board to reduce the risk of dislodgment. Remove the arm board during range-of-motion exercises.
● Place the clamp out of the child's reach. If extension tubing is used to allow the child greater mobility, securely tape the connection.
● Explain in simple terms to the child why he must be restrained while asleep, to alleviate anxiety and maintain trust.

During an infusion, monitor flow rates and check the child's condition and insertion site at least every hour. Titrate the flow rate only while the patient is composed;

crying and emotional upset can constrict blood vessels. Flow rate may vary if a pump isn't used. Flow should be adequate because some drugs (calcium, for example) can be irritating at low flow rates. Infants, small children, and children with compromised cardiopulmonary status are especially vulnerable to fluid overload with I.V. drug administration. To prevent this problem and help ensure that a limited amount of fluid is infused in a controlled manner, use a volume-control device in the I.V. tubing and an infusion pump or a syringe. Don't place more than 2 hours of I.V. fluid in the volume-control set at a time.

Giving I.M. injections
I.M. injections are preferred when a drug can't be given by other parenteral routes and rapid absorption is needed.

The vastus lateralis muscle is the preferred injection site in children younger than age 2. The ventrogluteal area or gluteus medius muscle can be used in older children. To select the correct needle size, consider the patient's age, muscle mass, nutritional status, and drug viscosity.

Record and rotate injection sites. Explain to the patient that the injection will hurt but that the drug will help him. Restrain him during the injection, if needed, and comfort him afterward.

Giving topical drugs and inhalants
When you give a child a topical drug or inhalant, consider the following:

Use eardrops warmed to room temperature. Cold drops can cause pain and vertigo. To give drops, turn the patient on his side, with the affected ear up. If he's younger than age 3, pull the pinna down and back; if age 3 or older, pull the pinna up and back.

Avoid using inhalants in young children because it's difficult to get them to cooperate. Before you try to give a drug to an older child through a metered-dose inhaler, explain the inhaler to him. Then have him hold the inhaler upside down and close his lips around the mouthpiece. Have him exhale and pinch his nostrils shut. When he starts to inhale, release one dose of the drug into his mouth. Tell the patient to continue inhaling until his lungs feel full; then he

can breathe normally and unpinch his nostrils. Most inhaled drugs aren't useful if the drug remains in the mouth or throat—if you doubt the patient's ability to use the inhalant correctly, don't use it. Such devices as spacers or assist devices may help. Check with a pharmacist, the prescriber, or a respiratory therapist.

Use topical corticosteroids cautiously because prolonged use in children may delay growth. When you apply topical corticosteroids to the diaper area of infants, don't cover the area with plastic or rubber pants, which act as an occlusive dressing and may enhance systemic absorption.

Giving parenteral nutrition
Give I.V. nutrition to patients who can't or won't take adequate food orally and to patients with hypermetabolic conditions who need supplementation. The latter group includes premature infants and children with burns or other major trauma, intractable diarrhea, malabsorption syndromes, GI abnormalities, emotional disorders (such as anorexia nervosa), and congenital abnormalities.

Before giving fat emulsions to infants and children, weigh the potential benefits against any possible risks. Fats—supplied as 10% or 20% emulsions—are given both peripherally and centrally. Their use is limited by the child's ability to metabolize them. For example, an infant or child with a diseased liver can't efficiently metabolize fats.

Some fats, however, must be supplied both to prevent essential fatty acid deficiency and to permit normal growth and development. A minimum of calories (2% to 4%) must be supplied as linoleic acid—an essential fatty acid found in lipids. In infants, fats are essential for normal neurologic development.

Nevertheless, fat solutions may decrease oxygen perfusion and may adversely affect children with pulmonary disease. This risk can be minimized by supplying only the minimum fat needed for essential fatty acid requirements and not the usual intake of 40% to 50% of the child's total calories.

Fatty acids can also displace bilirubin bound to albumin, causing a rise in free, unconjugated bilirubin and an increased risk of kernicterus. But fat solutions may interfere with some bilirubin assays and cause falsely elevated bilirubin levels. To avoid this complication, draw a blood sample 4 hours after infusion of the lipid emulsion; or if the emulsion is introduced over 24 hours, be sure the laboratory is aware so they can centrifuge the blood sample before the assay is performed.

Drug therapy in elderly patients

If you're giving drugs to elderly patients, you'll need to understand the physiologic and pharmacokinetic changes in this population that may affect drug dosage, cause common adverse reactions, or create compliance problems.

Physiologic changes affecting drug action

As a person ages, gradual physiologic changes occur. Some of these age-related changes may alter the therapeutic and toxic effects of drugs.

Body composition

Proportions of fat, lean tissue, and water in the body change with age. Total body mass and lean body mass tend to decrease, but the proportion of body fat tends to increase.

Body composition varies from person to person, and these changes in body composition affect the relationship between a drug's concentration and distribution in the body.

For example, a water-soluble drug such as gentamicin isn't distributed to fat. Because there's relatively less lean tissue in an elderly person, more drug remains in the blood. Fat-soluble drugs tend to accumulate in older patients, resulting in prolonged half-lives and more pronounced effects.

Gastrointestinal function

In elderly patients, decreases in gastric acid secretion and GI motility slow the emptying of stomach contents and movement through the entire intestinal tract. Also, research suggests that elderly patients may have more difficulty absorbing drugs than younger patients. This is an especially significant problem with drugs that have a narrow therapeutic range, such as digoxin, in which any change in absorption can be crucial.

Hepatic function

The liver's ability to metabolize certain drugs decreases with age. This decrease is caused by diminished blood flow to the liver, which results from an age-related decrease in cardiac output, and from the lessened activity of certain liver enzymes. When an elderly patient takes a sleep medication such as flurazepam, for example, the liver's reduced ability to metabolize the drug and the lipophilic property of the drug can produce a hangover effect the next morning.

Decreased hepatic function may result in more intense drug effects caused by higher levels, longer-lasting drug effects because of prolonged levels, and a greater risk of drug toxicity.

Renal function

An elderly person's renal function is usually sufficient to eliminate excess body fluid and waste, but the ability to eliminate some drugs may be reduced by 50% or more.

Many drugs commonly used by elderly patients, such as digoxin, are excreted primarily through the kidneys. If the kidneys' ability to excrete the drug is decreased, high blood levels may result. Digoxin toxicity can be relatively common in elderly patients who don't receive a reduced digoxin dosage to accommodate decreased renal function.

Drug dosages can be modified to compensate for age-related decreases in renal function. Aided by results of laboratory tests, such as BUN and creatinine levels, adjust drug dosages so the patient receives therapeutic benefits without the risk of toxicity. It is important to remember that serum creatinine is a function of muscle mass and that most elderly people lose muscle mass as they age. An elderly patient can have significant renal impairment even with a serum creatinine level in the normal range. Also, observe the patient for signs and symptoms of toxicity. A patient taking digoxin, for example, may experience anorexia, nausea, vomiting, or confusion.

Special administration considerations

Aging is usually accompanied by a decline in organ function that can affect drug distribution and clearance. This physiologic decline is likely to be worsened by a disease or a chronic disorder. Together, these factors can significantly increase the risk of adverse reactions and drug toxicity, as well as noncompliance.

Adverse reactions

Compared with younger people, elderly patients experience twice as many adverse drug reactions, mostly from greater drug use, poor compliance, and physiologic changes.

Signs and symptoms of adverse drug reactions—confusion, weakness, agitation, and lethargy—are often mistakenly attributed to senility or disease. If the adverse reaction isn't identified, the patient may continue to receive the drug. He may receive other, unnecessary drugs to treat complications caused by the original drug. This regimen can sometimes result in a pattern of inappropriate and excessive drug use.

Any drug can cause adverse reactions, but most of the serious reactions in the elderly are caused by relatively few drugs. Be particularly alert for toxicities resulting from diuretics, antihypertensives, digoxin, corticosteroids, anticoagulants, sleeping aids, and OTC drugs.

Diuretic toxicity

Because total body water content decreases with age, a normal dosage of a potassium-wasting diuretic, such as hydrochlorothiazide or furosemide, may result in fluid loss and even dehydration in an elderly patient.

These diuretics may deplete a patient's potassium level, making him feel weak, and they may raise blood uric acid and glucose levels, complicating gout and diabetes mellitus.

Antihypertensive toxicity

Many elderly patients experience lightheadedness or fainting when taking antihypertensives, partly in response to atherosclerosis and decreased elasticity of the blood vessels. Antihypertensives can lower blood pressure too rapidly, resulting in insufficient blood flow to the brain, which can cause dizziness, fainting, or even a stroke.

Consequently, dosages of antihypertensives must be carefully individualized. In elderly patients, aggressive treatment of high blood pressure may be harmful. Treatment goals should be reasonable. Blood pressure needs to be reduced more slowly in elderly patients.

Digoxin toxicity

As the body's renal function and rate of excretion decline, the digoxin level in the blood of an elderly patient may increase to the point of causing nausea, vomiting, diarrhea and, most seriously, cardiac arrhythmias. Monitor the patient's digoxin level and observe him for early signs and symptoms of inotropic toxicity, such as appetite loss, confusion, or depression.

Corticosteroid toxicity

Elderly patients taking a corticosteroid may experience short-term effects, including fluid retention and psychological effects ranging from mild euphoria to acute psychotic reactions. Long-term toxic effects, such as osteoporosis, can be especially severe in elderly patients who have been taking prednisone or related steroidal compounds for months or even years. To prevent serious toxicity, carefully monitor patients on long-term regimens. Observe them for subtle changes in appearance, mood, and mobility; for impaired healing; and for fluid and electrolyte disturbances.

Anticoagulant effects

Elderly patients taking an anticoagulant have an increased risk of bleeding, especially when they take NSAIDs at the same time, which is common. They're also at increased risk of bleeding and bruising because they are more likely to fall. Observe the patient's INR carefully, and monitor him for bruising and other signs of bleeding.

Sleeping aid toxicity

Sedatives and sleeping aids such as flurazepam may cause excessive sedation or drowsiness. Keep in mind that consuming alcohol may increase depressant effects, even if the sleeping aid was taken the previous evening. Use these drugs sparingly in elderly patients.

Over-the-counter drug toxicity

Prolonged ingestion of aspirin, aspirin-containing analgesics, and other OTC NSAIDs (such as ibuprofen, ketoprofen, and naproxen) may cause GI irritation—even ulcers—and gradual blood loss resulting in severe anemia. Prescription NSAIDs may cause similar problems. Both OTC and prescription NSAIDs can cause renal toxicity in older adults. Anemia from prolonged aspirin consumption can affect all age groups, but elderly patients may be less able to compensate because of their already reduced iron stores. These drugs should be used very carefully and at the lowest effective doses.

Laxatives may cause diarrhea in elderly patients, who are extremely sensitive to drugs such as bisacodyl. Long-term oral use of mineral oil as a lubricating laxative may result in lipid pneumonia from aspiration of small residual oil droplets in the patient's mouth.

Antihistamines such as diphenhydramine have anticholinergic effects and can cause confusion and mental status changes; they are also more likely to cause dizziness, sedation, and hypotension in elderly patients. OTC decongestants can have systemic effects, such as hypertension, anxiety, insomnia, and agitation.

Noncompliance

Poor compliance can be a problem with patients of any age. Many hospitalizations result from noncompliance with a medical regimen. In elderly patients, factors linked to aging, such as diminished visual acuity, hearing loss, forgetfulness, the need for multiple drug therapy, and socioeconomic factors, can combine to make compliance a special problem. About one-third of elderly patients fail to comply with their prescribed drug therapy. They may fail to take prescribed doses or to follow the correct schedule. They may take drugs prescribed for previous disorders, stop drugs prematurely, or indiscriminately use drugs that are to be taken as needed. Elderly patients may also have multiple prescriptions for the same drug and inadvertently take an overdose.

Review the patient's drug regimen with him. Make sure he understands the dose amount, the time and frequency of doses, and why he's taking the drug. Also, explain in detail if a drug is to be taken with food, with water, or separate from other drugs. To verify the patient's understanding, ask him to repeat the instructions back to you.

Help the patient avoid drug therapy problems by suggesting that he use drug calendars, pill sorters, or other aids to help him comply. Refer him to the prescriber, a pharmacist, or social services if he needs further information or assistance with his drug therapy.

3

Safe drug administration

Medication therapy is the primary intervention for many illnesses. It greatly benefits many patients and yet is involved in many instances of harm to patients and health care workers from either unintended consequences of therapy (adverse drug reactions or exposure to hazardous drugs) or medication-related errors (adverse drug events). (See *Preventing and treating I.V. vesicant extravasation injury*, page 15.) Medication errors are a significant cause of patient morbidity and mortality in the United States. In 1999, the Institute of Medicine (IOM) published its first Quality Chasm report, "To Err is Human: Building a Safer Health System," which reported that errors related to medications accounted for approximately 1 out of 131 outpatient deaths, 1 out of 854 inpatient deaths, and more than 7,000 deaths annually. Of all sentinel events reviewed since 2004 by The Joint Commission (a nonprofit organization that seeks to improve public health care through the voluntary accreditation of health care institutions), approximately 5% have been attributed to medication errors.

Many governmental and nongovernmental organizations are dedicated to improving the safety of drug administration. One mission of the FDA, for example, is to protect the public health by assuring the safety, effectiveness, and security of human drugs, vaccines, and medical devices. In 2007, the Food and Drug Administration Amendments Act expanded the FDA's authority regarding assessing and communicating risks associated with drugs. One of the new provisions of the law granted the FDA authority to require drug manufacturers to submit Risk Evaluation and Mitigation Strategies. (See *Risk Evaluation and Mitigation Strategies*, page 16.) The U.S. Pharmacopeia (USP), a nonprofit, nongovernmental public health organization, sets official public standards for drugs and other health care products manufactured or sold in the United States. It also sets standards for the quality, purity, and strength of food ingredients and dietary supplements.

In 2005, The Patient Safety and Quality Improvement Act authorized the creation of patient safety organizations (PSOs) to improve the quality and safety of U.S. health care delivery. One of these PSOs, the Institute for Safe Medication Practices (ISMP), is a nonprofit organization entirely dedicated to preventing medication errors and using medications safely. In addition, The Joint Commission has established National Patient Safety Goals and standards to improve the safe use of medications in its accredited facilities.

Causes of medication errors

The National Coordinating Council for Medication Error Reporting and Prevention (www.nccmerp.org) defines a medication error as "any preventable event that may cause or lead to inappropriate medication use or patient harm while the medication is in the control of the health care professional, patient, or consumer. Such events may be related to professional practice, health care products, procedures, and systems, including prescribing; order communication; product labeling, packaging, and nomenclature; compounding; dispensing; distribution; administration; education; monitoring; and use."

Medication errors were once thought to be caused by lapses in an individual nurse's practice. Traditionally, teaching nurses to administer drugs safely focused on the individual nurse's practice and the application of the "rights" of safe medication administration. (See *The eight "rights" of medication administration*, page 17.)

Although individual nursing practice is still an extremely important part of safe drug administration, the focus has widened. After medication errors had been systematically studied by numerous organizations who shared data, it became apparent that medication errors are complex events with multiple factors, and are most often caused by failures within systems. As a result of these findings, research has shifted to

Preventing and treating I.V. vesicant extravasation injury

Extravasation injuries occur when *vesicant* I.V. solutions or drugs—those with the potential to cause significant tissue injury (such as certain chemotherapy drugs, antibiotics, electrolyte solutions, vasopressors, and antiemetics)—accidentally escape from blood vessels into surrounding tissue (extravasate) during administration. Drugs or solutions that produce inflammation rather than serious or lasting tissue injury from extravasation are considered *irritants*. Extravasation injuries may occur when vesicants are given centrally or peripherally. Such injury can cause significant harm, including necrotic ulcers that may require surgical intervention, infection, loss of limb function, and complex regional pain syndrome.

Signs and symptoms of peripheral extravasation include:
- changes in I.V. site appearance (blanching, bruising) or temperature (coolness, erythema)
- pain, tightness, or itching at or surrounding the insertion site
- I.V. site fluid leakage
- numbness or tingling, diminished capillary refill, or decreased motor function in the extremity.

Signs and symptoms of central venous access device (CVAD) extravasation include:
- discomfort at the insertion site or along the CVAD path
- fluid leakage from the insertion site
- increased resistance to solution injection
- shoulder, neck, or chest edema.

Preventing extravasation

Use the following measures to prevent extravasation injuries:
- Know facility policy for administering vesicant drugs and solutions. Make sure you've been properly trained in prevention measures and extravasation recognition and management.
- When administering vesicants, know the specific antidote for the drug being given, and make sure that the antidote and equipment needed to manage extravasation are on hand. (Some antidotes for vesicants and solutions include sodium thiosulfate for alkylating agents, hyaluronidase for electrolytes and antibiotics (nafcillin, vancomycin [Vancocin]), and phentolamine for vasopressors (dopamine, norepinephrine).
- Ensure that the I.V. access site or CVAD is patent before giving the drug. Make sure the insertion site is visible, and use an appropriate catheter stabilization device.
- Make sure the drug is given by the proper route according to facility policy. Most vesicants administered by continuous infusion should be given utilizing a CVAD. Know when an I.V. infusion pump device should and shouldn't be used.
- Frequently monitor the patient for extravasation signs and symptoms and teach patient to immediately report them.

Treating extravasation

- Stop the drug and aspirate any residual drug and blood from the I.V. catheter or CVAD.
- Estimate the amount of solution extravasated and notify the practitioner.
- If an antidote exists, prepare for administration through the existing I.V. catheter or CVAD. After administration, remove the peripheral I.V. catheter, but avoid pressure to the site.
- For extravasation from a CVAD, prepare the patient for a computed tomography scan to assess catheter placement and fluid collection.
- For peripheral extravasation, prepare for subcutaneous injections of drug-specific antidote.
- Elevate arm.
- Apply hot (for vasoconstrictors) or cold (for alkylating drugs) compresses, if ordered.
- Use a skin marker or photo for serial documentation of extravasation according to facility policy.
- Monitor the site for pain, erythema progression, induration, tissue necrosis, and possible compartment syndrome. Note that symptom development may be delayed for 48 hours.
- Document the date and time of the infusion, time when signs and symptoms were first noted, extravasation signs and symptoms, type and size of venous access device, estimated extravasation solution amount, treatment instituted, practitioner notification, and the patient's response to treatment. Patients with significant tissue damage may need surgery.

Risk Evaluation and Mitigation Strategies

Risk Evaluation and Mitigation Strategies (REMS) is a risk management program that goes beyond the drug's package insert and is used when necessary to make certain that a drug's benefits outweigh its risks. The Food and Drug Administration (FDA) can require a REMS at any stage of a drug's lifecycle (as part of a drug's New Drug Application or after approval as new safety information becomes available), and manufacturers who fail to comply with REMS requirements can face substantial monetary penalties.

When evaluating the necessity of REMS, the FDA takes into consideration such factors as:
- the number of patients most likely to use the drug
- the seriousness of the patient's disease
- the drug's benefit
- the projected duration of treatment
- the severity of known or potential adverse events.

The FDA has issued an outline of specific components that manufacturers should use to develop a REMS proposal. These include the development of specific REMS goals and elements to ensure a drug's safe and appropriate use. The REMS must also describe how the manufacturer plans to evaluate whether the REMS goal is being met and the timetable for periodic assessments and reassessments. The results of the evaluations must be reported to the FDA, and the FDA may require that the REMS be modified or determine if additional actions must be taken.

REMS may contain one or all of the following components:
- **Medication guide:** written safety information for patients that must be distributed by the pharmacist to each patient receiving the drug
- **Communication plan:** plan that includes the tools to teach health care professionals how to use the drug safely and appropriately
- **Elements to Assure Safe Use (EASU):** specific requirements and elements to ensure safe use of the drug, including requirements that each patient be enrolled in a registry, that essential laboratory monitoring be performed, that the drug may only be prescribed by a prescriber with a specific certification, and that the drug may only be distributed by a specialty pharmacy.
- **Implementation plan:** plan that describes how the EASUs will be put into action.

preventing medication errors by identifying their root causes and then developing and validating evidence-based prevention strategies. Organizational processes, management decisions, inadequate medication administration protocols, staffing shortages, environmental conditions, poor communication, inadequate drug knowledge and resources, and individual mistakes or protocol violations may all contribute to drug errors.

The medication administration process

Medication errors can occur from medication administration process problems within any one or more than one of the five stages of the process. Because up to 40% of a nurse's time may be spent in medication administration and nursing practice intersects multiple stages, nurses may often be involved in medication errors. Here are some of the types of errors that have been reported in each stage.

Stage 1: Ordering and prescribing
- Prescriber orders are incomplete or illegible.
- Contraindicated drugs (such as drugs to which the patient is allergic) are prescribed.
- The prescriber specifies the wrong drug, dose, route, frequency, or duration, or fails to specify the indication.
- Drugs are prescribed using inappropriate or inadequate verbal orders.

Stage 2: Transcribing and verifying
- An incorrect drug, dose, route, time, or frequency is transcribed into the medication administration record (MAR) by the pharmacist or nurse.
- Drug verification and documentation in the MAR by the pharmacist or nurse are inadequate.

The eight "rights" of medication administration

Traditionally, nurses have been taught the "five rights" of medication administration. These are broadly stated goals and practices to help individual nurses administer drugs safely.
1. The *right drug:* Check the drug label and verify that the drug and form to be given is the drug that was prescribed.
2. The *right patient:* Confirm the patient's identity by checking two patient identifiers.
3. The *right dose:* Verify that the dose and form to be given is appropriate for the patient, and check the drug label with the prescriber's order.
4. The *right time:* Ensure that the drug is administered at the correct time and frequency.
5. The *right route:* Verify that the route by which the drug is to be given is specified by the prescriber and is appropriate for the patient.

In addition to the traditional "five rights" of individual practice, best-practice researchers have added three additional "rights":
6. The *right reason:* Verify that the drug prescribed is appropriate to treat the patient's condition.
7. The *right response:* Monitor the patient's response to the drug administered.
8. The *right documentation:* Completely and accurately document in the patient's medical record the drug administered; the monitoring of the patient, including his response; and other nursing interventions.

Stage 3: Dispensing and delivery
• The prescribed drug is filled incorrectly.
• Failure to deliver the right drug to the right place for the right patient occurs.

Stage 4: Administering
• The wrong drug is given to the wrong patient by the nurse or other licensed professional.
• The wrong dose is calculated and given or infused by the nurse or other licensed professional.
• The right drug is incorrectly prepared (such as crushing a drug that shouldn't be crushed) and is given by the nurse or other licensed professional.
• The correct drug is administered by the wrong route (such as an oral drug that is injected I.V.) by the nurse or other licensed professional.
• The correct drug is given at the wrong time or frequency by the nurse or other licensed professional.

Stage 5: Monitoring and reporting
• Monitoring of the patient by the nurse before and after medication administration is inadequate.
• Documentation and reporting of the patient's condition by the nurse before and after medication administration are inadequate.

• Hand-off communication between licensed professionals is inadequate.
• Reporting of medication errors is inadequate.

Elements contributing to safer drug administration

Ensuring the safe delivery of medication involves a system-wide approach, and research has shown that improvements in communication, education, and prevention of hazardous drug exposure can facilitate the safe delivery of medication.

Communication improvements

Communication issues have been implicated in approximately 60% of reported medication errors. Communication can be improved in many ways throughout the medication administration process. The traditional nursing process "rights" of safe drug administration are still important components of safe drug administration, but even when protocols are followed exactly, some medication errors still occur. For example, a nurse who's exactly following the eight "rights" might administer a drug to which a patient is allergic if his allergy information is incomplete or undocumented or hasn't been communicated effectively. Appropriate communication among all members of the health care team, including nurses, is vitally important.

Many health care facilities have instituted measures to help standardize and organize appropriate communication. One tool commonly used is SBAR (Situation, Background, Assessment, and Recommendation); its purpose is to logically organize information to optimize proper communication among health care providers.

Each institution must have tools and policies in place for the documentation of medication administration. Each prescribed medication order must be clearly written, and verbal orders must be used and documented appropriately according to facility policy. Each verbal order should be read back and verified with the prescriber before the drug is administered. The patient's condition must be monitored after each medication is given, and the patient's response and any nursing interventions must be documented appropriately. Clear communication through documentation is essential to safe practice.

The Joint Commission has developed goals and standards regarding medication reconciliation—the process of comparing a patient's medication regimen at every transition in his care (for example, on admission, upon discharge, and between care settings and levels). Medication reconciliation helps ensure that essential information about the patient's medication regimen is communicated to the health care team. Medication reconciliation helps prevent the inadvertent omission of needed medications, prevents medication duplication, and helps identify medications with potentially harmful interactions.

Education improvements
Lack of knowledge has been implicated in many medication errors; therefore, education about medications is essential to their safe administration. All health care team members involved in the process of medication administration, including the prescriber, pharmacist, and nurse, must have access to accurate information about each drug's indications, appropriate dosing regimen, appropriate route, appropriate frequency, possible drug interactions, appropriate monitoring, any cautions, and possible adverse effects. Each facility should have processes

in place to educate staff and communicate important drug information.

Governmental and nongovernmental agencies are doing their part toward educating facilities, prescribers, and nurses. In 1995, the FDA established the black box warning system to alert prescribers to drugs with increased risks to patients. These boxed warnings are the strongest labeling requirements for drugs that can have serious reactions. The Joint Commission requires accredited health care facilities to develop a list of abbreviations to avoid in all medication communications. The ISMP maintains a list of high-alert medications that may cause significant patient harm when given. (Each facility should have protocols in place for administering high-alert medications with safeguards built into the process.) The FDA and ISMP have developed a list of drugs with similar names that can be easily confused. Dissimilarities in each drug's name are highlighted with tall letters (so each name has mixed-case letters), making each drug less prone to mix-ups.

Patient education
Patients and their families should be active participants in the patient's care and should understand the patient's plan of care, including the purpose of newly prescribed medications. The patient and family need to be taught what to watch for, how the patient's condition will be monitored, and what signs and symptoms to report, and to report anything that doesn't seem right, including unfamiliar medications. Before administering a medication, the nurse needs to verify with the patient medication allergies or unusual past reactions to medications.

The following general teaching guidelines will help ensure that the patient receives the maximum therapeutic benefit from his medication regimen and help him avoid adverse reactions, accidental overdose, and harmful changes in effectiveness.
● Instruct the patient to learn the brand names, generic name, and dosages of all drugs and supplements (such as herbs and vitamins) that he's taking.
● Tell the patient to notify the pharmacist and prescriber about everything he takes, including prescription drugs, OTC drugs,

and herbal or other supplements, and about any drug allergies.

● Advise the patient to always read the label before taking a drug, to take it exactly as prescribed, and never to share prescription drugs.

● Warn the patient not to change brands of a drug without consulting the prescriber, to avoid harmful changes in effectiveness. For example, certain generic preparations aren't equivalent in effect to brand-name preparations of the same drug.

● Tell the patient to check the expiration date before taking a drug.

● Show the patient how to safely discard drugs that are outdated or no longer needed.

● Caution the patient to keep all drugs safely out of the reach of children and pets.

● Advise the patient to store drugs in their original container, at the proper temperature, and in areas where they won't be exposed to sunlight or excessive heat or humidity. Sunlight, heat, and humidity can cause drug deterioration and reduce a drug's effectiveness.

● Encourage the patient to report adverse or unusual reactions to the prescriber, and teach him proper techniques to monitor his condition (for example, how to obtain a resting heart rate before taking digoxin).

● Suggest that the patient have all prescriptions filled at the same pharmacy so that the pharmacist can warn against potentially harmful drug interactions.

● Tell the patient to report his complete medication history to all health care providers he sees, including his dentist.

● Instruct the patient to call the prescriber, poison control center, or pharmacist immediately and to seek immediate medical attention if he or someone else has taken an overdose. The National Poison Control Center phone number is 1-800-222-1222. Tell the patient to keep this and other emergency numbers handy at all times.

● Advise the patient to make sure he has a sufficient supply of drugs when traveling. He should carry them with him in their original containers and not pack them in luggage. Also, recommend that he carry a letter from his prescriber authorizing the use of a drug, especially if the drug is a controlled substance.

● Encourage the patient to keep a wallet card that lists all his medications, including the dose, route, frequency, and indication.

Improvements in preventing hazardous drug exposure

The Centers for Disease Control and Prevention estimates that 8 million U.S. health care workers are potentially exposed to hazardous drugs in the workplace. Hazardous drugs, as defined by the American Society of Health-System Pharmacists and the National Institute for Occupational Safety and Health (NIOSH), have one or more of the following characteristics:

● carcinogenicity (cause cancer)

● teratogenicity (cause defects in the developing fetus) or cause other developmental toxicities

● reproductive toxicity

● organ toxicity at low doses

● genotoxicity (cause damage to DNA)

● a structure and toxicity profile that mimics that of existing hazardous drugs.

The NIOSH list of antineoplastics and other hazardous drugs can be found at www.cdc.gov/niosh/topics/hazdrug/.

Health care workers can be exposed to hazardous drugs through inhalation, ingestion, skin contact/absorption, or injection; exposure is most likely from skin contact/absorption or inhalation. Potential exposure can occur in many ways, such as:

● preparing drugs for administration (reconstituting powdered drugs, crushing tablets for oral liquids, compounding powders, or counting out oral doses from multidose bottles)

● administering hazardous drugs I.M., I.V., or subcutaneously

● directly contacting drugs on the contaminated exteriors of drug vials, on drug-contaminated work surfaces, and on I.V. tubing and syringes

● handling body fluids or drug-contaminated dressings, linens, or waste

● transporting hazardous drugs

● removing and disposing of personal protective equipment (PPE)

● cleaning contaminated work spaces and spills.

Protecting workers and minimizing exposure

Protecting health care workers and minimizing their exposure to hazardous drugs can be achieved through engineering and administrative controls and use of appropriate PPE.

Engineering controls include:
- class II or III biological safety cabinets (also known as *vertical flow hoods* or *ventilated cabinets*) for hazardous drug preparation
- closed-system drug transfer devices
- needleless systems.

Administrative controls include:
- implementing training, retraining, and testing programs to educate and monitor staff about best practices to prevent hazardous drug exposure
- developing and implementing management policies and protocols to reduce staff risk
- using monitoring programs to identify hazardous drugs and staff exposure or development of early disease.

Appropriate use of PPE includes:
- making sure PPE fits and is used and disposed of properly, following facility policies and protocols
- selecting PPE based on assessment of the potential for hazardous drug exposure:
– Gloves: Select gloves appropriate for the potential exposure. Double gloving may be necessary depending on the potential exposure. Polyvinyl chloride exam gloves offer little hazardous drug protection. Look for test information provided by the glove manufacturer showing resistance to specific hazardous drugs.
– Gowns: These should be long-sleeved, with tight-fitting cuffs. Disposable gowns coated with laminate materials provide better protection than noncoated gowns. Refer to the manufacturer for permeation information. Don't reuse gowns; change gowns immediately after a spill or splash.
– Respirators: A properly fit-tested certified N-95 respirator or surgical N-95 respirator provides protection from most airborne particles. Other types of respirators may be necessary to protect from airborne gases. Surgical masks don't provide adequate respiratory protection from drug exposure.

– Face shields: Using face shields with goggles protects against splashes to the face and eyes. Full-face respirators also provide protection. Face shields or eye glasses with side shields don't provide full eye and face protection.
– Sleeve, hair, and shoe covers: These covers help provide additional protection. They may be required in certain environments such as drug-compounding areas.

Strategies for reducing error rates

In addition to improvements in communication and education, other strategies that have helped reduce medication administration error rates include:
- providing adequate nurse-to-patient staffing ratios
- designing drug preparation areas as safety zones that promote making correct choices during the medication administration process according to importance, frequency of use, and sequence of use
- improving the medication administration environment (reduce noise to 50 dB, improve lighting to at least 100 foot-candles, obtain nonglare computer screens)
- developing and using protocols that reduce distractions for nursing staff directly involved in administering medications
- dispensing medications in unit-dose or unit-of-use packaging
- restricting high-alert drugs and administration routes (limiting their number, variety, and concentration in patient care areas). For example, remove all neuromuscular blockers from units where patients aren't normally intubated. Remove highly concentrated electrolytes from unit stock in patient care units. Remove concentrated oral opioids from unit stock and dispensing cabinets. Apply additional strong warnings to drug labels. Make sure emergency equipment is always available.
- switching from I.V. to oral or subcutaneous forms as soon as possible
- dispensing I.V. and epidural infusions only from the pharmacy
- labeling all medications both on and off the sterile field
- posting drug information in patient care units and having drug information available

for all health care providers at the point of care; using infusion rate and dosing charts in patient care areas

● avoiding unapproved abbreviations
● using leading zeros; for example, use "0.5 mg" rather than ".5 mg"
● avoiding trailing zeros; for example, use "5 mg" rather than "5.0 mg"
● requiring that medication orders be prescribed by metric weight, not by volume (for example, in mg/kg not mL)
● establishing protocols and checklists to double-check and document unusual drugs, dosages, or regimens
● always recalculating doses before giving drugs to children or neonates. Make sure that the dose formula is included for calculating the dose. Have a second clinician (preferably a pharmacist) double-check the calculations.
● making sure each patient is monitored appropriately before and after drug administration. Have appropriate monitoring equipment (cardiac monitors, capnography, pulse oximetry) available as needed.

Using technology to promote safety

Technology is becoming an increasingly important part of providing safer drug administration. The goal of medication administration technology is to enhance individual practice and help build safeguards into the medication administration process.

Computerized provider order entry

In computerized provider order entry (CPOE), the prescriber enters the medication orders into a computerized record, thus eliminating errors due to illegible handwriting. Such safeguards as immediate order checking for errors (such as incorrect dosing or routes of administration) and drug interactions, allergy checks, and administration protocols can be built into the system. Orders can be immediately transmitted to the appropriate department and can also be linked to drug information databases. CPOE can be used to monitor how drugs are utilized and can provide data for quality improvement.

Bar codes

Bar-code technology is widely used and was initially developed to help control and track inventory for industry. The use of this technology for safer drug administration, dispensing, inventory control, and drug storage and preparation has been endorsed by the IOM, Joint Commission, Agency for Healthcare Research and Quality, and ISMP. With this technology, the patient wears a bar-code identifier on a wristband; the medication also has a bar code that uses the medication's own unique National Drug Code to identify the name, dose, manufacturer, and type of packaging. The nurse scans the bar code using an optical scanner, verifying the patient's identity and medication. The system supports but does not replace the traditional "rights" of safe medication.

Bar-code systems have been shown to reduce medication errors, but they aren't without disadvantages. For example, they don't save time in the medication administration process. Problems with the technology can cause delays in treatment. Wristbands can become unreadable due to wear, and scanners can malfunction. These problems may tempt nurses to develop dangerous shortcuts, such as attaching patients' wristbands to clipboards or giving the patient the medication first and then scanning his wristband

Automated dispensing cabinets

Automated dispensing cabinets (ADCs) are computer-controlled medication distribution systems in the patient care unit or ancillary department that are used to store, track, and dispense medications. ADCs can provide nurses with near-total access to medications needed in their patient care area and promote the control and security of medications. They electronically track the use of drugs such as controlled substances. They may have bar-code capabilities for restocking and correct medication selection, and can be programmed to provide safeguards such as drug safety alerts. ADCs can be linked with external databases and billing systems to increase the efficiency of drug dispensing and billing.

"Smart" pumps

From 2005 through 2009, the FDA received 56,000 reports of adverse events and 500 deaths linked to infusion pumps. Currently, there are initiatives to improve infusion systems and technology. "Smart" I.V. pumps can have such features as programmable drug libraries and dosage limits, can perform automatic calculations, and can be programmed to signal dosage alerts. They can be integrated with bar-code and CPOE technologies and can be wireless. Smart pumps can help alert nurses when incorrect dosages have been selected or to dosages that may exceed recommended levels.

Smart pumps can't detect all problems with I.V. drug infusions, however. For example, an incorrect drug can be selected from the library database and, with some pumps, it's possible to override safety alerts. Other infusion pump problems include software defects and failure of built-in safety alarms. Some pumps have ambiguous on-screen directions that can lead to dosing errors. The FDA recommends reporting all infusion-related adverse events, planning ahead in case a pump fails, labeling the channels and tubing to prevent errors, checking all settings, and monitoring patients for signs and symptoms of infusion problems. Nurses should perform independent calculation of all doses and infusion rates and not rely solely on the pump. It's essential to double-check each dose calculation. Nurses shouldn't bypass pump alarms, and must verify that the pump is functioning properly before beginning an infusion.

Other technologies

Using only oral syringes that don't have luer-locks to administer oral or enteral medications helps prevent oral or enteral medications from being administered via the wrong route. (The ISMP has reported cases in which oral medications were drawn into parenteral syringes and inadvertently injected into I.V. lines, resulting in patient deaths.) Utilizing special tubing for epidural medication administration that doesn't have side ports prevents an inadvertent injection of an incorrect drug into the epidural catheter.

Reporting medication errors

Clearly, medication errors are a major threat to patient safety. Only by sharing and analyzing data and performing more research can evidence-based quality improvements be developed and validated. Several agencies and organizations provide voluntary reporting systems to study the causes and prevalence of medication errors. The FDA has its Adverse Event Reporting System, which is part of the MedWatch program. The USP maintains MEDMARX (a national database utilized to lower the incidence of hospital medication errors) and the Medication Errors Reporting Program. In addition, the USP works with the ISMP to compile voluntary reports of medication errors. The reports are analyzed by these watchdog agencies, and information is published about their findings. Nurses should be encouraged to report medication errors and "near misses" and to help identify problems within systems.

4

Selected therapeutic drug classifications

Alkylating drugs
bendamustine hydrochloride
busulfan
carboplatin
carmustine
chlorambucil
cisplatin
cyclophosphamide
dacarbazine
ifosfamide
lomustine
melphalan
oxaliplatin
temozolomide
thiotepa

INDICATIONS
➤ **Various tumors, especially those with large volume and slow cell-turnover rate**

ACTION
Alkylating drugs appear to act independently of a specific cell-cycle phase. These polyfunctional compounds can be divided chemically into five groups: nitrogen mustards, ethylene amines, alkyl sulfonates, triazines, and nitrosoureas. Highly reactive, they primarily target nucleic acids and form links with the nuclei of different molecules. This allows the drugs to cross-link double-stranded DNA and to prevent strands from separating for replication, which may contribute to these drugs' ability to destroy cells.

ADVERSE REACTIONS
The most common adverse reactions are bone marrow depression, chills, diarrhea, fever, flank pain, hair loss, leukopenia, nausea, redness or pain at the injection site, sore throat, swelling of the feet or lower legs, thrombocytopenia, secondary leukemia, infertility, and vomiting.

CONTRAINDICATIONS & CAUTIONS
Black Box Warning Refer to individual drug monographs for black box warnings. ∎

• Contraindicated in patients hypersensitive to these drugs.
• Use cautiously in patients receiving other cell-destroying drugs or radiation.
• In pregnant women, use only when potential benefits to the mother outweigh known risks to the fetus. Breast-feeding women should stop breast-feeding during therapy because drugs are found in breast milk. In children, safety and effectiveness of many alkylating drugs haven't been established. Elderly patients are at increased risk for adverse reactions; monitor closely.

Alpha blockers (peripherally acting)
alfuzosin hydrochloride
doxazosin mesylate
phentolamine mesylate
prazosin hydrochloride
tamsulosin hydrochloride
terazosin hydrochloride

INDICATIONS
➤ **Hypertension, or mild to moderate urinary obstruction in men with BPH**

ACTION
Selective alpha blockers decrease vascular resistance and increase vein capacity, thereby lowering blood pressure and causing nasal and scleroconjunctival congestion, ptosis, orthostatic and exercise hypotension, mild to moderate miosis, interference with ejaculation, and pink, warm skin. They also relax nonvascular smooth muscle, especially in the prostate capsule, which reduces urinary problems in men with BPH. Because alpha$_1$ blockers don't block alpha$_2$ receptors, they don't cause transmitter overflow.

Nonselective alpha blockers antagonize both alpha$_1$ and alpha$_2$ receptors. Generally, alpha blockade results in tachycardia, palpitations, and increased renin secretion because of abnormally large amounts of norepinephrine (from transmitter overflow) released from adrenergic nerve endings as a result of the blockade of alpha$_1$ and alpha$_2$ receptors. Norepinephrine's effects are counterproductive to the major uses of nonselective alpha blockers.

ADVERSE REACTIONS
Alpha blockers may cause severe orthostatic hypotension and syncope, especially with the first few doses, an effect commonly called the *first-dose effect*. The most common adverse effects of alpha$_1$ blockade are dizziness, headache, drowsiness, somnolence, and malaise. These drugs also may cause tachycardia, palpitations, fluid retention (from excess renin secretion), nasal and ocular congestion, and aggravation of respiratory tract infection.

CONTRAINDICATIONS & CAUTIONS
● Contraindicated in patients with MI, coronary insufficiency, or angina or with hypersensitivity to these drugs or any of their components. Also contraindicated in combination therapy with PDE5 inhibitors (sildenafil, tadalafil, vardenafil), although tadalafil may be taken with tamsulosin 0.4 mg daily.
● In pregnant or breast-feeding women, use cautiously. In children, the safety and effectiveness of many alpha blockers haven't been established; use cautiously. In elderly patients, hypotensive effects may be more pronounced.

Alzheimer disease drugs
donepezil hydrochloride
galantamine hydrobromide
memantine hydrochloride
rivastigmine tartrate

INDICATIONS
➤ **Treatment of mild to moderate dementia of the Alzheimer type**

ACTION
Current theories attribute signs and symptoms of Alzheimer disease to a deficiency of cholinergic neurotransmission. It's suggested that these drugs improve cholinergic function by increasing acetylcholine levels through reversible inhibition of its hydrol-

ysis by cholinesterase. Memantine is an N-methyl-D-aspartate (NMDA) receptor antagonist. Persistent activation of the NMDA receptors is thought to contribute to symptoms of Alzheimer disease. No evidence indicates that these drugs alter the course of the underlying disease process.

ADVERSE REACTIONS
Weight loss, diarrhea, anorexia, nausea, vomiting, dizziness, headache, bradyarrhythmias; hypertension and constipation (memantine).

CONTRAINDICATIONS & CAUTIONS
● Contraindicated in patients hypersensitive to any of the drug components.
● May exaggerate neuromuscular blocking effects of succinylcholine-type and similar neuromuscular blocking agents used during anesthesia.
● Use cautiously with concomitant drugs that slow heart rate. There is an increased risk for heart block.
● Use cautiously with NSAIDs because the drug increases gastric acid secretion. There is increased risk of developing ulcers and active or occult GI bleeding.
● Use cautiously in patients with moderate hepatic or renal impairment. The drugs are not recommended in severe hepatic impairment or severe renal impairment (CrCl less than 9 mL/minute).
● Use cautiously in patients with a history of asthma or COPD.

Aminoglycosides
amikacin sulfate
gentamicin sulfate
neomycin sulfate
tobramycin sulfate

INDICATIONS
➤ **Septicemia; postoperative, pulmonary, intra-abdominal, and urinary tract infections; skin, soft-tissue, bone, and joint infections; aerobic gram-negative bacillary meningitis not susceptible to other antibiotics; serious staphylococcal, *Pseudomonas aeruginosa*, and *Klebsiella* infections; enterococcal infections; nosocomial pneumonia; anaerobic**

infections involving *Bacteroides fragilis*; tuberculosis; initial empirical therapy in febrile, leukopenic patients

ACTION

Aminoglycosides are bactericidal. They bind directly and irreversibly to 30S ribosomal subunits, inhibiting bacterial protein synthesis. They're active against many aerobic gram-negative and some aerobic gram-positive organisms and can be used in combination with other antibiotics for short courses of therapy.

ADVERSE REACTIONS

Ototoxicity and nephrotoxicity are the most serious complications. Neuromuscular blockade also may occur. Oral forms most commonly cause diarrhea, nausea, and vomiting. Parenteral drugs may cause vein irritation, phlebitis, and sterile abscess.

CONTRAINDICATIONS & CAUTIONS

Black Box Warning Refer to individual drug monographs for black box warnings. ▪
• Contraindicated in patients hypersensitive to these drugs.
Black Box Warning Aminoglycosides are associated with significant nephrotoxicity and ototoxicity. Toxicity may develop even with conventional doses, particularly in patients with prerenal azotemia or impaired renal function. Evidence of renal function impairment or ototoxicity requires drug discontinuation or appropriate dosage adjustments. When possible, monitor serum drug concentrations. Avoid use with other ototoxic, neurotoxic, or nephrotoxic drugs. Aminoglycosides can cause fetal harm when administered to pregnant women. ▪
• Use cautiously in patients with a neuromuscular disorder and in those taking neuromuscular blockers.
• Use at lower dosages in patients with renal impairment.
• In pregnant women, use cautiously. In breast-feeding women, safety hasn't been established. In neonates and premature infants, the half-life of aminoglycosides is prolonged because of immature renal systems. In infants and children, dosage adjustment may be needed. Elderly patients have an increased risk of nephrotoxicity and

commonly need a lower dose and longer dosage intervals; they're also susceptible to ototoxicity and superinfection.

Angiotensin-converting enzyme inhibitors

benazepril hydrochloride
captopril
enalaprilat
enalapril maleate
fosinopril sodium
lisinopril
moexipril hydrochloride
perindopril erbumine
quinapril hydrochloride
ramipril
trandolapril

INDICATIONS

➤ **Hypertension, heart failure, left ventricular dysfunction (LVD), MI (ramipril and lisinopril), and diabetic nephropathy (captopril)**

ACTION

ACE inhibitors prevent conversion of angiotensin I to angiotensin II, a potent vasoconstrictor. Besides decreasing vasoconstriction and thus reducing peripheral arterial resistance, inhibiting angiotensin II decreases adrenocortical secretion of aldosterone. This reduces sodium and water retention and extracellular fluid volume. ACE inhibition also causes increased levels of bradykinin, which results in vasodilation. This decreases heart rate and systemic vascular resistance.

ADVERSE REACTIONS

The most common adverse effects of therapeutic doses are angioedema of the face and limbs, dry cough, dysgeusia, fatigue, headache, hyperkalemia, hypotension, proteinuria, rash, and tachycardia. Severe hypotension may occur at toxic drug levels.

CONTRAINDICATIONS & CAUTIONS

• Contraindicated in patients hypersensitive to these drugs.

Black Box Warning When pregnancy is detected, discontinue drug as soon as possible. Drugs that act directly on the renin-angiotensin system can cause fetal injury and death. ■

• Use cautiously in patients with impaired renal function or serious autoimmune disease and in those taking other drugs known to decrease WBC count or immune response.

• Women of childbearing potential taking ACE inhibitors should report suspected pregnancy immediately to prescriber. High risks of fetal morbidity and mortality are linked to ACE inhibitors, especially in the second and third trimesters. Some ACE inhibitors appear in breast milk. To avoid adverse effects in infants, instruct patient to stop breast-feeding during therapy. In children, safety and effectiveness haven't been established; give drug only if potential benefits outweigh risks. Elderly patients may need lower doses because of impaired drug clearance.

Antacids
aluminum hydroxide
calcium carbonate
magnesium hydroxide
magnesium oxide
sodium bicarbonate

INDICATIONS
➤ Hyperacidity; hyperphosphatemia (aluminum hydroxide); hypomagnesemia (magnesium oxide); postmenopausal hypocalcemia (calcium carbonate)

ACTION
Antacids reduce the total acid load in the GI tract and elevate gastric pH to reduce pepsin activity. They also strengthen the gastric mucosal barrier and increase esophageal sphincter tone.

ADVERSE REACTIONS
Antacids containing aluminum may cause aluminum intoxication, constipation, hypophosphatemia, intestinal obstruction, and osteomalacia. Antacids containing magnesium may cause diarrhea or hypermagnesemia (in renal failure). Calcium carbonate, magnesium oxide, and sodium bicarbonate may cause constipation, milk-alkali syndrome, or rebound hyperacidity.

CONTRAINDICATIONS & CAUTIONS
• Calcium carbonate and magnesium oxide are contraindicated in patients with severe renal disease. Sodium bicarbonate is contraindicated in patients with hypertension, renal disease, or edema; in those who are vomiting; in those receiving diuretics or continuous GI suction; and in those on sodium-restricted diets.

• In patients with mild renal impairment, give magnesium oxide cautiously.

• Give aluminum preparations and calcium carbonate cautiously in elderly patients; in those receiving antidiarrheals, antispasmodics, or anticholinergics; and in those with dehydration, fluid restriction, chronic renal disease, or suspected intestinal absorption problems.

• Pregnant women should consult their prescriber before using antacids. Breast-feeding women may take antacids.
Serious adverse effects are more likely in infants from changes in fluid and electrolyte balance; monitor them closely. Elderly patients have an increased risk of adverse reactions; monitor them closely; also, give aluminum preparations, calcium carbonate, and magnesium oxide cautiously to these patients.

Antianginals
ranolazine

Beta blockers
atenolol
bisoprolol fumarate
metoprolol
nadolol
propranolol hydrochloride

Calcium channel blockers
amlodipine besylate
diltiazem hydrochloride
niCARdipine hydrochloride
NIFEdipine
verapamil hydrochloride

Nitrates
isosorbide dinitrate
isosorbide mononltrate
nitroglycerin

INDICATIONS
➤ Moderate to severe angina (beta
blockers); classic, effort-induced angina
and Prinzmetal angina (calcium channel
blockers); recurrent angina (long-acting
nitrates and topical, transdermal, transmucosal, and oral extended-release
nitroglycerin); acute angina (S.L.
nitroglycerin and S.L. or chewable
isosorbide dinitrate); unstable angina
(I.V. nitroglycerin); chronic angina
(ranolazine)

ACTION
The mechanism of action of ranolazine's
antianginal effects hasn't been determined.
Beta blockers decrease catecholamine-
induced increases in heart rate, blood
pressure, and myocardial contraction.
Calcium channel blockers inhibit the flow of
calcium through muscle cells, which dilates
coronary arteries and decreases systemic
vascular resistance, known as *afterload*.
Nitrates decrease afterload and left ventricular end-diastolic pressure, or *preload*,
and increase blood flow through collateral
coronary vessels.

ADVERSE REACTIONS
Ranolazine may cause QT-interval prolongation, dizziness, constipation, and nausea. Beta blockers may cause bradycardia,
cough, diarrhea, disturbing dreams, dizziness, dyspnea, fatigue, fever, heart failure,
hypotension, lethargy, nausea, peripheral
edema, and wheezing. Calcium channel
blockers may cause bradycardia, confusion, constipation, depression, diarrhea,
dizziness, dyspepsia, edema, elevated liver
enzyme levels (transient), fatigue, flushing,
headache, hypotension, insomnia, nervousness, and rash. Nitrates may cause flushing,
headache, orthostatic hypotension, reflex
tachycardia, rash, syncope, and vomiting.

CONTRAINDICATIONS & CAUTIONS
● Contraindicated in patients hypersensitive
to these drugs.
Black Box Warning Abrupt discontinuation
of beta blocker therapy has been associated
with angina exacerbation and, in some
cases, MI and ventricular arrhythmias.
When discontinuation of beta blockers is
planned, gradually reduce dosage over at
least a few weeks. ■
● Ranolazine is contraindicated in patients
taking strong inhibitors of CYP3A or inducers of CYP3A and in those with clinically
significant hepatic impairment. Beta blockers are contraindicated in patients with
cardiogenic shock, sinus bradycardia, heart
block greater than first degree, or bronchial
asthma. Calcium channel blockers are contraindicated in patients with severe hypotension or heart block greater than first degree
(except with functioning pacemaker).
Nitrates are contraindicated in patients with
severe anemia, cerebral hemorrhage, head
trauma, glaucoma, or hyperthyroidism or in
patients using PDE5 inhibitors (sildenafil,
tadalafil, vardenafil).
● Use beta blockers cautiously in patients
with nonallergic bronchospastic disorders,
diabetes mellitus, or impaired hepatic or
renal function. Use calcium channel blockers cautiously in those with hepatic or renal
impairment, bradycardia, heart failure, or
cardiogenic shock. Use nitrates cautiously in
those with hypotension or recent MI.
● In pregnant women, use beta blockers cautiously. Recommendations for

breast-feeding vary by drug; use beta blockers and calcium channel blockers cautiously. In children, safety and effectiveness haven't been established. Check with prescriber before giving these drugs to children. Elderly patients have an increased risk of adverse reactions; use cautiously.

Antiarrhythmics
adenosine
dronedarone

Class IA
disopyramide
procainamide hydrochloride
quinidine gluconate
quinidine sulfate

Class IB
lidocaine hydrochloride
mexiletine hydrochloride

Class IC
flecainide acetate
propafenone hydrochloride

Class II (beta blockers)
esmolol hydrochloride

Class III
amiodarone hydrochloride
dofetilide
ibutilide fumarate
sotalol hydrochloride

Class IV (calcium channel blocker)
verapamil hydrochloride

INDICATIONS
➤ Atrial and ventricular arrhythmias

ACTION
Class I drugs reduce the inward current carried by sodium ions, which stabilizes neuronal cardiac membranes. Class IA drugs depress phase 0, prolong the action potential, and stabilize cardiac membranes. Class IB drugs depress phase 0, shorten the action potential, and stabilize cardiac membranes. Class IC drugs block the transport of sodium ions, which decreases conduction velocity but not repolarization rate. Class II drugs decrease the heart rate, myocardial contractility, blood pressure, and AV node conduction. Class III drugs prolong the repolarization phase. Class IV drugs decrease myocardial contractility and oxygen demand by inhibiting calcium ion influx; they also dilate coronary arteries and arterioles.

ADVERSE REACTIONS
Most antiarrhythmics can aggravate existing arrhythmias or cause new ones. They also may produce CNS disturbances, such as dizziness or fatigue; GI problems, such as nausea, vomiting, or altered bowel elimination; hypersensitivity reactions; and hypotension. Some antiarrhythmics may worsen heart failure. Class II drugs may cause bronchoconstriction.

CONTRAINDICATIONS & CAUTIONS
Black Box Warning Refer to individual drug monographs for black box warnings. ∎
• Contraindicated in patients hypersensitive to these drugs.
• Many antiarrhythmics are contraindicated or require cautious use in patients with cardiogenic shock, digitalis toxicity, and second- or third-degree heart block (unless patient has a pacemaker or implantable cardioverter defibrillator).
• In pregnant women, use only if potential benefits to the mother outweigh risks to the fetus. In breast-feeding women, use cautiously; many antiarrhythmics appear in breast milk. In children, monitor closely because they have an increased risk of adverse reactions. Use cautiously in elderly patients, who may exhibit physiologic alterations in CV system.

Antibiotic antineoplastics
bleomycin sulfate
DAUNOrubicin hydrochloride
DOXOrubicin hydrochloride
epirubicin hydrochloride
idarubicin hydrochloride
mitomycin

INDICATIONS
➤ Various tumors

ACTION

Although classified as antibiotics, these drugs destroy cells, thus ruling out their use as antimicrobials alone. They interfere with proliferation of malignant cells in several ways. Their action may be specific to cell-cycle phase, not specific to cell-cycle phase, or both. Some of these drugs act like alkylating drugs or antimetabolites. By binding to or creating complexes with DNA, antibiotic antineoplastics directly or indirectly inhibit DNA, RNA, and protein synthesis.

ADVERSE REACTIONS

The most common adverse reactions include anxiety, bone marrow depression, chills, confusion, diarrhea, fever, flank or joint pain, hair loss, nausea, redness or pain at the injection site, sore throat, swelling of the feet or lower legs, vomiting, and cardiomyopathy.

CONTRAINDICATIONS & CAUTIONS

Black Box Warning Refer to individual drug monographs for black box warnings. ■

• Contraindicated in patients hypersensitive to these drugs.

• In pregnant women, avoid antineoplastics. Breast-feeding during therapy isn't recommended. In children, safety and effectiveness of some drugs haven't been established; use cautiously. In elderly patients, use cautiously because of their increased risk of adverse reactions.

Anticholinergics

atropine sulfate
benztropine mesylate
dicyclomine hydrochloride
scopolamine

INDICATIONS

➤ Prevention of motion sickness, preoperative reduction of secretions and blockage of cardiac reflexes, adjunct treatment of peptic ulcers and other GI disorders, blockage of cholinomimetic effects of cholinesterase inhibitors or other drugs, and (for benztropine) various spastic conditions, including acute dystonic reactions, muscle rigidity, parkinsonism, and extrapyramidal disorders

ACTION

Anticholinergics competitively antagonize the actions of acetylcholine and other cholinergic agonists at muscarinic receptors.

ADVERSE REACTIONS

Therapeutic doses commonly cause blurred vision, constipation, cycloplegia, decreased sweating or anhidrosis, dry mouth, headache, mydriasis, palpitations, tachycardia, urinary hesitancy, and urine retention. These reactions usually disappear when therapy stops. Toxicity can cause signs and symptoms resembling psychosis (disorientation, confusion, hallucinations, delusions, anxiety, agitation, and restlessness); dilated, nonreactive pupils; blurred vision; hot, dry, flushed skin; dry mucous membranes; dysphagia; decreased or absent bowel sounds; urine retention; hyperthermia; tachycardia; hypertension; and increased respirations.

CONTRAINDICATIONS & CAUTIONS

• Contraindicated in patients hypersensitive to these drugs and in those with angle-closure glaucoma, renal or GI obstructive disease, reflux esophagitis, or myasthenia gravis.

• Use cautiously in patients with heart disease, GI infection, open-angle glaucoma, prostatic hypertrophy, hypertension, hyperthyroidism, ulcerative colitis, autonomic neuropathy, or hiatal hernia with reflux esophagitis.

• In pregnant women, safe use hasn't been established. In breast-feeding women, avoid anticholinergics because they may decrease milk production; some may appear in breast milk and cause infant toxicity. In children, safety and effectiveness haven't been established. Patients older than age 40 may be more sensitive to these drugs. In elderly patients, use cautiously and give a reduced dosage, as indicated.

Anticoagulants

Coumarin derivative
warfarin sodium

Heparin derivative
heparin sodium

Low-molecular-weight heparins
dalteparin sodium
enoxaparin sodium

Selective factor Xa inhibitors
apixaban
fondaparinux sodium
rivaroxaban

Thrombin inhibitors
argatroban
bivalirudin
dabigatran etexilate mesylate
desirudin

INDICATIONS
➤ **Pulmonary emboli, deep vein thrombosis, thrombus, blood clotting, DIC, unstable angina, MI, atrial fibrillation, heparin-induced thrombocytopenia, heparin-induced thrombosis-thrombocytopenia syndrome**

ACTION
Heparin derivatives accelerate formation of an antithrombin III–thrombin complex. They inactivate thrombin and prevent conversion of fibrinogen to fibrin. The coumarin derivative warfarin inhibits vitamin K–dependent activation of clotting factors II, VII, IX, and X, which are formed in the liver. Thrombin inhibitors directly bind to thrombin and inhibit its action. Selective factor Xa inhibitors bind to antithrombin III, which in turn initiates the neutralization of factor Xa.

ADVERSE REACTIONS
Anticoagulants commonly cause bleeding and may cause hypersensitivity reactions. Warfarin may cause agranulocytosis, alopecia (long-term use), anorexia, dermatitis, fever, nausea, tissue necrosis or gangrene, urticaria, and vomiting. Heparin derivatives may cause thrombocytopenia and may increase liver enzyme levels. Nonhemorrhagic adverse reactions associated with thrombin inhibitors may include back pain, bradycardia, and hypotension.

CONTRAINDICATIONS & CAUTIONS
Black Box Warning Refer to individual drug monographs for black box warnings. ∎
• Contraindicated in patients hypersensitive to these drugs or any of their components; in patients with aneurysm, active bleeding, CV hemorrhage, hemorrhagic blood dyscrasias, hemophilia, severe hypertension, pericardial effusions, or pericarditis; and in patients undergoing major surgery, neurosurgery, neuraxial anesthesia, spinal puncture, or ophthalmic surgery.
• Use cautiously in patients with severe diabetes, renal impairment, severe trauma, ulcerations, or vasculitis.
• Most anticoagulants (except warfarin) may be used in pregnancy only if the potential benefit to the mother outweighs the potential risk to the fetus. In pregnant women and those who have just had a threatened or complete spontaneous abortion, warfarin is contraindicated. Women should avoid breast-feeding during therapy. Infants, especially neonates, may be more susceptible to anticoagulants because of vitamin K deficiency. Elderly patients are at greater risk for hemorrhage because of altered hemostatic mechanisms or age-related deterioration of hepatic and renal functions.

Anticonvulsants
carbamazepine
clobazam
clonazepam
diazepam
ezogabine
felbamate
fosphenytoin sodium
gabapentin
lacosamide
lamotrigine
levetiracetam
magnesium sulfate
oxcarbazepine
phenytoin sodium
phenytoin sodium (extended)
primidone
rufinamide
tiagabine hydrochloride
topiramate
valproate sodium
valproic acid
vigabatrin
zonisamide

INDICATIONS
➤ **Seizure disorders; acute, isolated seizures not caused by seizure disorders; status epilepticus; prevention of seizures after trauma or craniotomy; neuropathic pain**

ACTION
Anticonvulsants include six classes of drugs: selected hydantoin derivatives, barbiturates, benzodiazepines, succinimides, iminostilbene derivatives (carbamazepine), and carboxylic acid derivatives. Magnesium sulfate is a miscellaneous anticonvulsant. Some hydantoin derivatives and carbamazepine inhibit the spread of seizure activity in the motor cortex. Some barbiturates and succinimides limit seizure activity by increasing the threshold for motor cortex stimuli. Selected benzodiazepines and carboxylic acid derivatives may increase inhibition of GABA in brain neurons. Magnesium sulfate interferes with the release of acetylcholine at the myoneural junction.

ADVERSE REACTIONS
Anticonvulsants can cause adverse CNS effects, such as ataxia, confusion, somnolence, and tremor. Many anticonvulsants also cause CV disorders, such as arrhythmias and hypotension; GI effects, such as vomiting; and hematologic disorders, such as agranulocytosis, bone marrow depression, leukopenia, and thrombocytopenia. Stevens-Johnson syndrome, other severe rashes, and abnormal liver function test results may also occur.

CONTRAINDICATIONS & CAUTIONS
Black Box Warning Refer to individual drug monographs for black box warnings. ∎
• Contraindicated in patients hypersensitive to these drugs.
• Carbamazepine is contraindicated within 14 days of MAO inhibitor use.
• Use cautiously in patients with blood dyscrasias. Also, use barbiturates cautiously in patients with suicidal ideation.
• In pregnant women, therapy usually continues despite the fetal risks caused by some anticonvulsants (barbiturates, phenytoin). In breast-feeding women, the safety of many anticonvulsants hasn't been established. Children, especially young ones, are sensitive to the CNS depression of some anticonvulsants; use cautiously. Elderly patients are sensitive to CNS effects and may require lower doses. Also, some anticonvulsants may take longer to be eliminated because of decreased renal function, and parenteral use is more likely to cause apnea, hypotension, bradycardia, and cardiac arrest.

Antidepressants, tricyclic
amitriptyline hydrochloride
clomiPRAMINE hydrochloride
desipramine hydrochloride
doxepin hydrochloride
imipramine hydrochloride
imipramine pamoate
nortriptyline hydrochloride
protriptyline hydrochloride

INDICATIONS
➤ **Depression, anxiety (doxepin), obsessive-compulsive disorder**

(clomipramine), enuresis in children
older than age 6 (imipramine), neuropathic pain

ACTION ▨▨▨▨▨▨

Tricyclic antidepressants may inhibit reuptake of norepinephrine and serotonin
in CNS nerve terminals (presynaptic neurons), thus enhancing the concentration and
activity of neurotransmitters in the synaptic
cleft. TCAs also exert antihistaminic,
sedative, anticholinergic, vasodilatory,
and quinidine-like effects.

ADVERSE REACTIONS

Adverse reactions include anticholinergic effects, orthostatic hypotension, and
sedation. The tertiary amines (amitriptyline, doxepin, and imipramine) exert the
strongest sedative effects; tolerance usually
develops in a few weeks. TCAs may cause
CV effects such as T-wave abnormalities,
conduction disturbances, and arrhythmias.

CONTRAINDICATIONS & CAUTIONS

Black Box Warning Antidepressants can
increase the risk of suicidal thinking and
behavior. Appropriately monitor patients of
all ages who are started on antidepressant
therapy, and observe closely for clinical
worsening, suicidality, or unusual changes
in behavior. Advise families and caregivers
of the need for close observation and communication with the prescriber. ▌

• Contraindicated in patients hypersensitive
to these drugs and in patients with urine
retention or angle-closure glaucoma.

• TCAs are contraindicated within 2 weeks
of MAO inhibitor therapy.

• Use cautiously in patients with suicidal
tendencies, schizophrenia, paranoia, seizure
disorders, CV disease, or impaired hepatic
function.

• In pregnant and breast-feeding women,
safety hasn't been established; use cautiously. In children younger than age 12,
TCAs aren't recommended. Elderly patients are more sensitive to therapeutic and
adverse effects; they need lower dosages.

Antidiabetics

acarbose
glimepiride
glipiZIDE
glyBURIDE
linagliptin
metformin hydrochloride
miglitol
nateglinide
pioglitazone hydrochloride
pramlintide acetate
repaglinide
rosiglitazone maleate
sitagliptin phosphate

INDICATIONS

➤ **Mild to moderately severe, stable,
nonketotic, type 2 diabetes mellitus that
can't be controlled by diet alone**

ACTION ▨▨▨▨▨▨

Oral antidiabetics come in several types.
Sulfonylureas are sulfonamide derivatives
that aren't antibacterial. They lower glucose
levels by stimulating insulin release from
the pancreas. These drugs work only in the
presence of functioning beta cells in the
islet tissue of the pancreas. After prolonged
administration, they produce hypoglycemia
by acting outside of the pancreas, resulting
in effects that include reduced glucose production by the liver and enhanced peripheral
sensitivity to insulin. The latter may result
from an increased number of insulin receptors or from changes after insulin binding.

Meglitinides, such as nateglinide and
repaglinide, are nonsulfonylurea antidiabetics that stimulate the release of insulin from
the pancreas.

Metformin decreases hepatic glucose
production, reduces intestinal glucose absorption, and improves insulin sensitivity
by increasing peripheral glucose uptake and
utilization. With metformin therapy, insulin
secretion remains unchanged, and fasting
insulin levels and all-day insulin response
may decrease.

Alpha-glucosidase inhibitors, such as
acarbose and miglitol, delay digestion of
carbohydrates, resulting in a smaller rise in
glucose levels. Pramlintide, a human amylin
analogue, slows the rate at which food

leaves the stomach, decreasing postprandial increase in glucose level, and reduces appetite.

Rosiglitazone and pioglitazone are thiazolidinediones, which lower glucose levels by improving insulin sensitivity. They are potent and highly selective agonists for receptors found in insulin-sensitive tissues, such as adipose tissue, skeletal muscle, and liver.

Sitagliptin increases insulin release by inhibiting the enzyme DPP-4.

ADVERSE REACTIONS
Sulfonylureas cause dose-related reactions that usually respond to decreased dosage: anorexia, headache, heartburn, nausea, paresthesia, vomiting, and weakness. Hypoglycemia may follow excessive dosage, increased exercise, decreased food intake, or alcohol use.

The most serious adverse reaction linked to metformin is lactic acidosis. It's a rare effect and is most likely to occur in patients with renal dysfunction. Other reactions to metformin include dermatitis, GI upset, megaloblastic anemia, rash, and unpleasant or metallic taste.

Thiazolidinediones may cause fluid retention leading to or exacerbating heart failure. Alpha-glucosidase inhibitors can cause abdominal pain, diarrhea, and flatulence.

CONTRAINDICATIONS & CAUTIONS
Black Box Warning Refer to individual drug monographs for black box warnings. ∎
• Contraindicated in patients hypersensitive to these drugs and in patients with diabetic ketoacidosis with or without coma. Metformin is also contraindicated in patients with renal disease or metabolic acidosis and generally should be avoided in patients with hepatic disease.
• Use sulfonylureas cautiously in patients with renal or hepatic disease. Use metformin cautiously in patients with adrenal or pituitary insufficiency and in debilitated and malnourished patients. Alpha-glucosidase inhibitors should be used cautiously in patients with mild to moderate renal insufficiency. Thiazolidinediones aren't recommended in patients with edema, heart failure, or liver disease.

• In pregnant or breast-feeding women, use is contraindicated. Oral antidiabetics appear in small amounts in breast milk and may cause hypoglycemia in the infant. In children, oral antidiabetics aren't effective in type 1 diabetes mellitus. Elderly patients may be more sensitive to these drugs, usually need lower dosages, and are more likely to develop neurologic symptoms of hypoglycemia; monitor these patients closely. In elderly patients, avoid chlorpropamide use because of its long duration of action.

Antidiarrheals
bismuth subsalicylate
diphenoxylate hydrochloride–
    atropine sulfate
loperamide
octreotide acetate

INDICATIONS
➤ **Mild, acute, or chronic diarrhea; certain cancers that cause diarrhea (octreotide acetate)**

ACTION
Bismuth preparations may have a mild water-binding capacity, may absorb toxins, and provide a protective coating for the intestinal mucosa.

ADVERSE REACTIONS
Bismuth preparations may cause salicylism (with high doses) or temporary darkening of tongue and stools.

CONTRAINDICATIONS & CAUTIONS
• Contraindicated in patients hypersensitive to these drugs.
• Some antidiarrheals may appear in breast milk; check individual drugs for specific recommendations. For children or teenagers recovering from flu or chickenpox, consult prescriber before giving bismuth subsalicylate. For elderly patients, use caution when giving antidiarrheal drugs.

Antiemetics
aprepitant
dimenhyDRINATE
dolasetron mesylate
dronabinol
granisetron hydrochloride
meclizine hydrochloride
metoclopramide hydrochloride
ondansetron hydrochloride
palonosetron hydrochloride
prochlorperazine
scopolamine
scopolamine hydrobromide
trimethobenzamide hydrochloride

INDICATIONS
➤ **Nausea, vomiting, motion sickness, and vertigo**

ACTION
For antihistamines (dimenhydrinate, meclizine hydrochloride, trimethobenzamide), the mechanism of action is unclear. Phenothiazines (prochlorperazine) work by blocking the dopaminergic receptors in the chemoreceptor trigger zone of the brain. Serotonin-receptor antagonists (dolasetron, granisetron, ondansetron) block serotonin stimulation centrally in the chemoreceptor trigger zone and peripherally in vagal nerve terminals.

ADVERSE REACTIONS
Antiemetics may cause asthenia, fatigue, dizziness, headache, insomnia, abdominal pain, anorexia, constipation, diarrhea, epigastric discomfort, gastritis, heartburn, nausea, vomiting, neutropenia, hiccups, tinnitus, dehydration, and fever. Metoclopramide may cause tardive dyskinesia.

CONTRAINDICATIONS & CAUTIONS
Black Box Warning Refer to individual drug monographs for black box warnings. ■
• Contraindicated in patients hypersensitive to any of the drug components.
• Contraindicated in severe vomiting until etiology of vomiting is established.
• Use cautiously in patients with tartrazine and sulfite sensitivities. Antiemetics may cause allergic-type reactions, including

hives, itching, wheezing, asthma, and anaphylaxis.

Antifungals
amphotericin B lipid complex
amphotericin B liposomal
anidulafungin
caspofungin acetate
fluconazole
itraconazole
ketoconazole
micafungin sodium
miconazole nitrate
nystatin
posaconazole
terbinafine hydrochloride
voriconazole

INDICATIONS
➤ **Various fungal infections**

ACTION
The amphotericin products bind to sterols in the fungal cell membrane, altering permeability and allowing intracellular components to leak out. These drugs usually inhibit fungal growth and multiplication, but if the level is high enough, the drugs can destroy fungi. The azole class of drugs includes fluconazole, itraconazole, keto-conazole, and voriconazole. Fluconazole inhibits fungal cytochrome P450, which weakens fungal cell walls. Itraconazole and voriconazole interfere with fungal wall synthesis by inhibiting ergosterol formation and increasing cell wall permeability and osmotic instability. Ketoconazole interferes with sterol synthesis in fungal cells, damaging cell membranes and increasing permeability. Caspofungin inhibits the synthesis of an integral component of fungal cell walls. Nystatin binds to sterols in fungal cell membranes and alters membrane permeability. Terbinafine inhibits fungal cell growth by inhibiting an enzyme responsible for the manufacture of ergosterol.

ADVERSE REACTIONS
Fluconazole may cause transient elevations of liver enzymes, alkaline phosphatase, and bilirubin levels, as well as dizziness, nausea, vomiting, abdominal pain, diarrhea, rash,

headache, hypokalemia, and elevated BUN and creatinine levels. Adverse reactions to itraconazole include headache and nausea. The most common adverse reactions to ketoconazole are nausea and vomiting. Adverse reactions to voriconazole are uncommon. However, the drug may alter renal function and cause vision changes. Common adverse reactions to caspofungin include paresthesia, tachycardia, anorexia, anemia, pain, myalgia, tachypnea, chills, and sweating. Reactions to nystatin seldom occur, but may include diarrhea, nausea, vomiting, and abdominal pain. Terbinafine may cause abdominal pain, jaundice, diarrhea, flatulence, nausea, anaphylaxis, headache, rash, and vision disturbances.

CONTRAINDICATIONS & CAUTIONS
Black Box Warning Refer to individual drug monographs for black box warnings. ■
● Contraindicated in patients hypersensitive to any of the drug components.
● Administer I.V. amphotericin under close clinical observation. Acute infusion reactions can occur, including fever, shaking chills, hypotension, anorexia, nausea, vomiting, and tachypnea.
● Caspofungin is contraindicated with concomitant use of cyclosporine because of the possibility of elevated liver enzymes.
● Amphotericin drugs aren't interchangeable and are each prescribed differently.

Antihistamines

cetirizine hydrochloride
chlorpheniramine maleate
desloratadine
diphenhydraMINE hydrochloride
fexofenadine hydrochloride
levocetirizine
loratadine
promethazine hydrochloride

INDICATIONS
➤ **Allergic rhinitis, urticaria, pruritus, vertigo, motion sickness, nausea and vomiting, sedation, dyskinesia, parkinsonism**

ACTION
Antihistamines are structurally related chemicals that compete with histamine for histamine H_1-receptor sites on smooth muscle of bronchi, GI tract, and large blood vessels, binding to cellular receptors and preventing access to and subsequent activity of histamine. They don't directly alter histamine or prevent its release.

ADVERSE REACTIONS
Most antihistamines cause drowsiness and impaired motor function early in therapy. They also can cause blurred vision, constipation, and dry mouth and throat. Some antihistamines, such as promethazine, may cause cholestatic jaundice, which may be a hypersensitivity reaction, and may predispose patients to photosensitivity. Promethazine may also cause extrapyramidal reactions with high doses.

CONTRAINDICATIONS & CAUTIONS
Black Box Warning Refer to individual drug monographs for black box warnings. ■
● Contraindicated in patients hypersensitive to these drugs and in those with angle-closure glaucoma, stenosing peptic ulcer, pyloroduodenal obstruction, or bladder neck obstruction. Also contraindicated in those taking MAO inhibitors.
● In pregnant women, safe use hasn't been established. During breast-feeding, antihistamines shouldn't be used because many of these drugs appear in breast milk and may cause unusual excitability in the infant. Neonates, especially premature infants, may experience seizures. Children, especially those younger than age 6, may experience paradoxical hyperexcitability with restlessness, insomnia, nervousness, euphoria, tremors, and seizures; give cautiously. Elderly patients usually are more sensitive to the adverse effects of antihistamines, especially dizziness, sedation, hypotension, and urine retention; use cautiously and monitor these patients closely.

Antihypertensives

Angiotensin-converting enzyme inhibitors
benazepril hydrochloride
captopril
enalaprilat
enalapril maleate
fosinopril sodium
lisinopril
moexipril hydrochloride
perindopril erbumine
quinapril hydrochloride
ramipril
trandolapril

Angiotensin II receptor blockers
candesartan cilexetil
eprosartan mesylate
irbesartan
losartan potassium
olmesartan medoxomil
telmisartan
valsartan

Beta blockers
atenolol
bisoprolol fumarate
carvedilol
labetalol hydrochloride
metoprolol succinate
metoprolol tartrate
nadolol
propranolol hydrochloride

Calcium channel blockers
amlodipine besylate
diltiazem hydrochloride
felodipine
niCARdipine hydrochloride
NIFEdipine
nisoldipine
verapamil hydrochloride

Centrally acting alpha blockers (sympatholytics)
clonidine hydrochloride
guanfacine hydrochloride
methyldopa

Direct renin inhibitor
aliskiren

Peripherally acting alpha blockers
doxazosin mesylate
prazosin hydrochloride
terazosin hydrochloride

Vasodilators
hydralAZINE hydrochloride
nitroglycerin
nitroprusside sodium

INDICATIONS
➤ Essential and secondary hypertension

ACTION
For information on the action of ACE inhibitors, alpha blockers, ARBs, beta blockers, calcium channel blockers, and diuretics, see their individual drug class entries. Centrally acting sympatholytics stimulate central alpha-adrenergic receptors, reducing cerebral sympathetic outflow, thereby decreasing peripheral vascular resistance and blood pressure. Vasodilators act directly on smooth muscle to reduce blood pressure.

ADVERSE REACTIONS
Antihypertensives commonly cause orthostatic changes in heart rate, headache, hypotension, nausea, and vomiting. Other reactions vary greatly among different drug types. Centrally acting sympatholytics may cause constipation, depression, dizziness, drowsiness, dry mouth, headache, palpitations, severe rebound hypertension, and sexual dysfunction; methyldopa also may cause aplastic anemia and thrombocytopenia. Vasodilators may cause ECG changes, diarrhea, dizziness, heart failure, palpitations, pruritus, and rash.

CONTRAINDICATIONS & CAUTIONS
Black Box Warning When pregnancy is detected in patients receivingACE inhibitors, ARBs, or direct renin inhibitors, discontinue therapy as soon as possible. Drugs that act directly on the renin-angiotensin system can cause fetal injury and death. ■
Black Box Warning Abrupt discontinuation of beta blocker therapy has been associated with angina exacerbation and, in some cases, MI and ventricular arrhythmias,

When discontinuation of beta blockers is planned, gradually reduce dosage over at least a few weeks. ■

Black Box Warning Refer to individual drug monographs for additional black box warnings. ■

• Contraindicated in patients hypersensitive to these drugs and in those with hypotension.

• Use cautiously in patients with hepatic or renal dysfunction.

• In pregnant women, use cautiously when potential benefits to the mother outweigh risks to the fetus. Check each drug because some are safe only in the first trimester. In breast-feeding women, use cautiously; some antihypertensives appear in breast milk. In children, safety and effectiveness of many antihypertensives haven't been established; give these drugs cautiously and monitor children closely. Elderly patients are more susceptible to adverse reactions and may need lower maintenance doses; monitor these patients closely.

Antilipemics

atorvastatin calcium
cholestyramine
colesevelam hydrochloride
ezetimibe
fenofibrate
fluvastatin sodium
gemfibrozil
lovastatin
pitavastatin
pravastatin sodium
rosuvastatin calcium
simvastatin

INDICATIONS
➤ Hyperlipidemia, hypercholesterolemia

ACTION
Antilipemics lower elevated lipid levels. Bile-sequestering drugs (cholestyramine, colesevelam) lower LDL level by forming insoluble complexes with bile salts, triggering cholesterol to leave the bloodstream and other storage areas to make new bile acids. Fibric acid derivatives (gemfibrozil) reduce cholesterol formation, increase sterol excretion, and decrease lipoprotein and triglyceride synthesis. HMG-CoA reductase inhibitors (atorvastatin, fluvastatin, lovastatin, pravastatin, rosuvastatin, simvastatin) interfere with the activity of enzymes that generate cholesterol in the liver. Selective cholesterol absorption inhibitors (ezetimibe) inhibit cholesterol absorption by the small intestine, reducing hepatic cholesterol stores and increasing cholesterol clearance from the blood.

ADVERSE REACTIONS
Antilipemics commonly cause GI upset. Bile-sequestering drugs may cause bloating, cholelithiasis, constipation, and steatorrhea. Fibric acid derivatives may cause cholelithiasis and have other GI or CNS effects. Use of gemfibrozil with lovastatin may cause myopathy. HMG-CoA reductase inhibitors may affect liver function or cause rash, pruritus, increased CK levels, rhabdomyolysis, and myopathy.

CONTRAINDICATIONS & CAUTIONS
• Contraindicated in patients hypersensitive to these drugs. Also, bile-sequestering drugs are contraindicated in patients with complete biliary obstruction. Fibric acid derivatives are contraindicated in patients with primary biliary cirrhosis or significant hepatic or renal dysfunction. HMG-CoA reductase inhibitors and cholesterol absorption inhibitors are contraindicated in patients with active liver disease or persistently elevated transaminase levels.

• Use bile-sequestering drugs cautiously in constipated patients. Use fibric acid derivatives cautiously in patients with peptic ulcer. Use HMG-CoA inhibitors cautiously in patients who consume large amounts of alcohol or who have a history of liver or renal disease.

• In pregnant women, use bile-sequestering drugs and fibric acid derivatives cautiously and avoid using HMG-CoA inhibitors. In breast-feeding women, avoid using fibric acid derivatives and HMG-CoA inhibitors; give bile-sequestering drugs cautiously. In children ages 10 to 17, certain antilipemics have been approved to treat heterozygous familial hypercholesterolemia. Elderly patients have an increased risk of severe constipation; use bile-sequestering drugs cautiously and monitor patients closely.

Antimetabolite antineoplastics

capecitabine
cytarabine
fludarabine phosphate
fluorouracil
gemcitabine
hydroxyurea
mercaptopurine
methotrexate
pemetrexed

INDICATIONS
➤ **Various tumors and hematologic conditions**

ACTION
Antimetabolites are structurally similar to naturally occurring metabolites and can be divided into three subcategories: purine, pyrimidine, and folinic acid analogues. Most of these drugs interrupt cell reproduction at a specific phase of the cell cycle. Purine analogues are incorporated into DNA and RNA, interfering with nucleic acid synthesis (by miscoding) and replication. They also may inhibit synthesis of purine bases through pseudofeedback mechanisms. Pyrimidine analogues inhibit enzymes in metabolic pathways that interfere with biosynthesis of uridine and thymine. Folic acid antagonists prevent conversion of folic acid to tetrahydrofolate by inhibiting the enzyme dihydrofolic acid reductase.

ADVERSE REACTIONS
The most common adverse effects include anxiety, bone marrow depression (anemia, leukopenia, thrombocytopenia), chills, diarrhea, fever, flank or joint pain, hair loss, nausea, redness or pain at injection site, stomatitis, swelling of the feet or lower legs, and vomiting.

CONTRAINDICATIONS & CAUTIONS
Black Box Warning Refer to individual drug monographs for black box warnings. ■
• Contraindicated in patients hypersensitive to these drugs.
• Pregnant women should be informed of the risks to the fetus. Breast-feeding isn't recommended for women taking these drugs. In children, safety and effectiveness of some drugs haven't been established; use cautiously. Elderly patients have an increased risk of adverse reactions; monitor them closely.

Antimigraine drugs

almotriptan malate
eletriptan hydrobromide
frovatriptan succinate
naratriptan hydrochloride
rizatriptan benzoate
sumatriptan succinate
zolmitriptan

INDICATIONS
➤ **Migraines with or without aura**

ACTION
The antimigraine drugs are serotonin 5-HT$_1$ agonists. These drugs constrict cranial vessels, inhibit neuropeptide release, and reduce transmission in the trigeminal nerve pathway.

ADVERSE REACTIONS
These drugs have a wide range of adverse reactions. These include tingling, warmth or hot sensations, flushing, nasal discomfort, visual disturbances, paresthesias, dizziness, fatigue, somnolence, chest pain, weakness, dry mouth, dyspepsia, nausea, sweating, injection-site reactions, and neck, throat, or jaw pain. Intranasal sumatriptan can cause nasal or throat discomfort and taste disturbances.

CONTRAINDICATIONS & CAUTIONS
• Contraindicated in patients hypersensitive to any of the drug components.
• Contraindicated in patients with ischemic heart disease, angina, previous MI, uncontrolled hypertension or other significant underlying CV conditions, cerebrovascular disease, peripheral vascular disease, and ischemic bowel disease.

Antiparkinsonians
amantadine hydrochloride
apomorphine hydrochloride
benztropine mesylate
bromocriptine mesylate
diphenhydrAMINE hydrochloride
entacapone
levodopa–carbidopa
levodopa–carbidopa–entacapone
pramipexole dihydrochloride
rasagiline mesylate
rOPINIRole hydrochloride
selegiline hydrochloride
tolcapone

INDICATIONS
➤ **Signs and symptoms of Parkinson disease and drug-induced extrapyramidal reactions**

ACTION
Antiparkinsonians include synthetic anticholinergics, dopaminergics, and the antiviral amantadine. Anticholinergics probably prolong the action of dopamine by blocking its reuptake into presynaptic neurons and by suppressing central cholinergic activity. Dopaminergics act in the brain by increasing dopamine availability, thus improving motor function. Entacapone is a reversible inhibitor of peripheral catechol-*O*-methyltransferase (commonly known as COMT), which is responsible for elimination of various catecholamines, including dopamine. Blocking this pathway when giving levodopa–carbidopa should result in higher levels of levodopa, thereby allowing greater dopaminergic stimulation in the CNS and leading to a greater effect in treating parkinsonian symptoms. Amantadine is thought to increase dopamine release in the substantia nigra.

ADVERSE REACTIONS
Anticholinergics may cause blurred vision, cycloplegia, constipation, decreased sweating or anhidrosis, dry mouth, headache, mydriasis, palpitations, tachycardia, and urinary hesitancy and urine retention. Dopaminergics may cause arrhythmias, confusion, disturbing dreams, dystonias, hallucinations, headache, muscle cramps, nausea, orthostatic hypotension, and vomiting. Amantadine also causes irritability, insomnia, and livedo reticularis (with prolonged use).

CONTRAINDICATIONS & CAUTIONS
Black Box Warning Refer to individual drug monographs for black box warnings. ∎
● Contraindicated in patients hypersensitive to these drugs.
● Use cautiously in patients with prostatic hyperplasia or tardive dyskinesia and in debilitated patients.
● Neuroleptic malignant-like syndrome involving muscle rigidity, increased body temperature, and mental status changes may occur with abrupt withdrawal of antiparkinsonians.
● In pregnant women, safe use hasn't been established. Antiparkinsonians may appear in breast milk; a decision should be made to stop the drug or stop breast-feeding, taking into account the importance of the drug to the mother. In children, safety and effectiveness haven't been established. Elderly patients have an increased risk for adverse reactions; monitor them closely.

Antiplatelet drugs
abciximab
cilostazol
clopidogrel bisulfate
dipyridamole
eptifibatide
prasugrel
ticagrelor
ticlopidine hydrochloride
tirofiban hydrochloride

INDICATIONS
➤ **Reduction of thrombolytic events by reducing platelet aggregation; adjunct to percutaneous coronary intervention (PCI), prevention of cardiac ischemic complications, or treatment of unstable angina not responding to conventional therapy when PCI is planned within 24 hours (abciximab); acute coronary syndrome and PCI (eptifibatide); acute coronary syndrome (tirofiban); non-ST-segment elevation acute coronary syndrome and ST-segment elevation MI,**

recent MI, recent stroke or peripheral vascular disease (clopidogrel and ticlopidine)

ACTION
The I.V. drugs abciximab, eptifibatide, and tirofiban antagonize the glycoprotein (GP)IIb/IIIa receptors located on platelets, which are involved in platelet aggregation. Clopidogrel and ticagrelor are inhibitors of platelet aggregation that inhibit the binding of adenosine diphosphate (ADP) to its platelet receptor and the subsequent ADP-mediated activation of the GPIIb/IIIa complex. Ticlopidine inhibits the binding of fibrinogen to platelets.

ADVERSE REACTIONS
The I.V. drugs can cause serious bleeding, thrombocytopenia, and anaphylaxis. The most common adverse reactions to the oral agents include anaphylaxis, rash, stomach pain, nausea, and headache. Ticlopidine may cause neutropenia and elevated alkaline phosphatase and serum transaminase levels.

CONTRAINDICATIONS & CAUTIONS
Black Box Warning Refer to individual drug monographs for black box warnings. ■
• Contraindicated in patients hypersensitive to any of the drug components.
• Contraindicated in active bleeding, bleeding disorders, intracranial neoplasm, AV malformation or aneurysm, cerebrovascular accident (within 2 years), recent major surgery or trauma, severe uncontrolled hypertension, or thrombocytopenia.
• Ticagrelor is contraindicated in patients with severe hepatic impairment.

Antipsychotics

First generation
chlorproMAZINE hydrochloride
fluphenazine decanoate
fluphenazine hydrochloride
haloperidol
haloperidol decanoate
haloperidol lactate
loxapine hydrochloride
loxapine succinate
molindone hydrochloride
perphenazine
pimozide
prochlorperazine edisylate
prochlorperazine maleate
thioridazine hydrochloride
thiothixene hydrochloride
trifluoperazine hydrochloride

Second generation
aripiprazole
asenapine maleate
clozapine
iloperidone
lurasidone hydrochloride
olanzapine
olanzapine pamoate
paliperidone
paliperidone palmitate
quetiapine fumarate
risperiDONE
ziprasidone hydrochloride
ziprasidone mesylate

INDICATIONS
➤ Schizophrenia (all but pimozide); schizoaffective disorder (paliperidone); psychosis, acute agitation, depression, or mania in bipolar I disorder; depression, hiccups (chlorpromazine); autism irritability (aripiprazole, risperidone); child hyperactivity and severe behavioral problems (chlorpromazine, haloperidol); acute intermittent porphyria (chlorpromazine); nausea, vomiting, anxiety, tetanus (chlorpromazine); Tourette syndrome (haloperidol, pimozide)

ACTION
Antipsychotics block several neurotransmitters, particularly dopamine. The exact mechanism of action and ideal combination of targeted neurotransmitters remain unknown.

ADVERSE REACTIONS
First-generation antipsychotics may cause cardiac arrhythmias, cardiac arrest, hypotension, tachycardia, agitation, akathisia, seizures, dizziness, sedation, dystonia, headache, insomnia, neuroleptic malignant syndrome (NMS), extrapyramidal symptoms, tardive dyskinesia, photosensitivity, pruritus, anorexia, constipation, dry mouth,

nausea, weight gain, amenorrhea, galac-torrhea, gynecomastia, impotence, urine retention, blurred vision, and hyperther-mia/hyperpyrexia.

Second-generation antipsychotics may cause akathisia, dizziness, drowsiness, extrapyramidal symptoms, headache, con-stipation, nausea, weight gain, hyperpro-lactinemia, dyslipidemia, hyperglycemia, and hyperthermia/hyperpyrexia.

CONTRAINDICATIONS & CAUTIONS

Black Box Warning Elderly patients with dementia-related psychosis treated with antipsychotics are at increased risk for death. Antipsychotics aren't approved for treatment of patients with dementia-related psychosis. ∎

Black Box Warning Refer to individual drug monographs for additional black box warnings. ∎

• Contraindicated in patients hypersensitive to drug.

• Use cautiously and observe for tardive dyskinesia, which may be irreversible

• Use cautiously and watch for signs and symptoms of NMS (muscle rigidity, fever, delirium), especially with first-generation injectable antipsychotics.

• Use cautiously in depressed or agitated patients.

• Use cautiously with lithium because of risk of encephalopathic syndrome (weak-ness, lethargy, fever, confusion).

• Use cautiously in patients with MI, ischemic heart disease, heart failure, con-duction abnormalities, or cerebrovascular disease, and in those at risk for hypotension.

• Use cautiously in patients with dyslipi-demia or diabetes mellitus, particularly with second-generation antipsychotics.

• Use cautiously in patients with respiratory infections or chronic disorders because of increased pneumonia risk.

• Use cautiously in patients with blood dyscrasias.

• Use cautiously in patients with history of seizures.

• Use cautiously in patients with Parkinson disease or dementia with Lewy bodies.

• Use cautiously in patients with renal impairment; lower the dosage or discontinue drug if BUN level is abnormal.

• Risk in pregnancy is unknown; use only if benefit outweighs risk.

• Patients taking antipsychotics should use caution when driving or performing hazardous work due to drowsiness.

Antirheumatics
abatacept
adalimumab
auranofin
infliximab
leflunomide

INDICATIONS
➤ **Rheumatoid arthritis, ankylosing spondylitis, Crohn disease, psoriatic arthritis**

ACTION
Inhibits T-cell activation by binding to CD80 and CD86, thereby blocking interac-tion with CD28. Activated T lymphocytes are found in the synovium of patients with rheumatoid arthritis. Some drugs bind to tumor necrosis factor (TNF) so it can't bind to a receptor and exert an effect. TNF plays an important role in pathologic inflamma-tion and joint destruction.

ADVERSE REACTIONS
The most serious adverse reactions in-clude serious infections and malignan-cies in patients treated with abatacept and adalimumab. The most common adverse reactions include rash, pruritus, hair loss, urticaria, nausea, vomiting, anorexia, flat-ulence, dyspepsia, anemia, leukopenia, thrombocytopenia, elevated liver enzymes, stomatitis, hypertension, headache, and hematuria. Serious adverse reactions from gold therapy include anaphylactic shock, bradycardia, and angioneurotic edema. The most common adverse reactions from gold therapy include dermatitis, pruritus, and stomatitis.

CONTRAINDICATIONS & CAUTIONS
Black Box Warning Refer to individual drug monographs for black box warnings. ∎

• Contraindicated in patients hypersensitive to any of the drug components.

• Use cautiously in patients receiving two antirheumatics with similar mechanisms of action.
• Use with caution in patients with a history of recurrent infections, COPD, CNS disorders, demyelinating disorders, heart failure, and immunosuppression.

Antituberculotics
cycloserine
ethambutol hydrochloride
isoniazid
pyrazinamide
rifabutin
rifampin
rifapentine

INDICATIONS
➤ Acute pulmonary and extrapulmonary tuberculosis, acute UTIs

ACTION
Inhibits cell wall synthesis in susceptible strains of gram-positive and gram-negative bacteria and if *Mycobacterium tuberculosis* is identified.

ADVERSE REACTIONS
Adverse reactions primarily affect the GI tract, peripheral nervous system, and hepatic system. Isoniazid may precipitate seizures in patients with a seizure disorder and produce optic or peripheral neuritis, as well as elevated liver enzymes. Optic neuritis is the only significant reaction to ethambutol. Rifampin may cause epigastric pain, nausea, vomiting, flatulence, abdominal cramps, anorexia, and diarrhea. Cycloserine can cause seizures, confusion, dizziness, headache, and somnolence.

CONTRAINDICATIONS & CAUTIONS
• Contraindicated in patients hypersensitive to any of the drug components.
• Drugs should be discontinued or dosage reduced if patients develop signs of CNS toxicity, including convulsions, psychosis, somnolence, depression, confusion, hyperreflexia, headache, tremor, vertigo, paresis, or dysarthria.

Benzodiazepines
alprazolam
chlordiazepoxide hydrochloride
diazepam
lorazepam
midazolam hydrochloride
oxazepam
temazepam
triazolam

INDICATIONS
➤ Seizure disorders (diazepam, midazolam, parenteral lorazepam); anxiety, tension, and insomnia (chlordiazepoxide, diazepam, lorazepam, oxazepam, temazepam, triazolam); conscious sedation or amnesia in surgery (diazepam, lorazepam, midazolam); skeletal muscle spasm and tremor (oral forms of chlordiazepoxide and diazepam); delirium

ACTION
Benzodiazepines act selectively on polysynaptic neuronal pathways throughout the CNS. Precise sites and mechanisms of action aren't fully known. However, benzodiazepines enhance or facilitate the action of GABA, an inhibitory neurotransmitter in the CNS. These drugs appear to act at the limbic, thalamic, and hypothalamic levels of the CNS to produce anxiolytic, sedative, hypnotic, skeletal muscle relaxant, and anticonvulsant effects.

ADVERSE REACTIONS
Therapeutic dose may cause drowsiness, impaired motor function, constipation, diarrhea, vomiting, altered appetite, urinary changes, visual disturbances, and CV irregularities. Toxic dose may cause continuing problems with short-term memory, confusion, severe depression, shakiness, vertigo, slurred speech, staggering, bradycardia, shortness of breath, difficulty breathing, or severe weakness. Prolonged or frequent use can cause physical dependency and withdrawal syndrome when drug is stopped.

CONTRAINDICATIONS & CAUTIONS
Black Box Warning Refer to individual drug monographs for black box warnings. ∎

• Contraindicated in patients hypersensitive to these drugs, in those with acute angle-closure glaucoma, and in those with depressive neuroses or psychotic reactions in which anxiety isn't prominent.

• Avoid use in patients with suicidal tendencies and patients with a history of drug abuse.

• Use cautiously in patients with chronic pulmonary insufficiency or sleep apnea and in those with hepatic or renal insufficiency.

• In pregnant patients, benzodiazepines increase the risk of congenital malformation if taken in the first trimester. Use during labor may cause neonatal flaccidity. A neonate whose mother took a benzodiazepine during pregnancy may have withdrawal symptoms. In breast-feeding women, benzodiazepines may cause sedation, feeding difficulties, and weight loss in the infant. In children, use caution; they're especially sensitive to CNS depressant effects. In elderly patients, benzodiazepine elimination may be prolonged; consider a lower dosage or use of a shorter-acting agent.

Beta blockers

Beta₁ blockers
atenolol
betaxolol
bisoprolol fumarate
esmolol hydrochloride
metoprolol tartrate

Beta₁ and beta₂ blockers
carvedilol
labetalol hydrochloride
nadolol
propranolol hydrochloride
sotalol hydrochloride

INDICATIONS
➤ **Hypertension (most drugs), angina pectoris (atenolol, metoprolol, nadolol, and propranolol), arrhythmias (esmolol, propranolol, and sotalol), glaucoma (betaxolol), prevention of MI (atenolol, metoprolol, and propranolol), prevention of recurrent migraine and other vascular headaches (propranolol), pheochromocytomas or essential tremors (selected**

drugs), heart failure (atenolol, carvedilol, and metoprolol)

ACTION
Beta blockers compete with beta agonists for available beta receptors; individual drugs differ in their ability to affect beta receptors. Some drugs are nonselective: they block beta₁ receptors in cardiac muscle and beta₂ receptors in bronchial and vascular smooth muscle. Several drugs are cardioselective and, in lower doses, inhibit mainly beta₁ receptors. Some beta blockers have intrinsic sympathomimetic activity and stimulate and block beta receptors, and thereby have less effect on slowing heart rate. Others stabilize cardiac membranes, which affects cardiac action potential.

ADVERSE REACTIONS
Therapeutic dose may cause bradycardia, dizziness, fatigue, and erectile dysfunction; some may cause other CNS disturbances, such as depression, hallucinations, memory loss, and nightmares. Toxic dose can produce severe hypotension, bradycardia, heart failure, or bronchospasm.

CONTRAINDICATIONS & CAUTIONS
Black Box Warning Abrupt discontinuation of beta blocker therapy has been associated with angina exacerbation and, in some cases, MI and ventricular arrhythmias. When discontinuation of beta blockers is planned, gradually reduce dosage over at least a few weeks. ∎

Black Box Warning Refer to individual drug monographs for additional black box warnings. ∎

• Contraindicated in patients hypersensitive to these drugs and in those with cardiogenic shock, sinus bradycardia, heart block greater than first degree, or bronchial asthma.

• Beta blockers may mask signs and symptoms of hypoglycemia (palpitations, tachycardia, tremor.)

• Use cautiously in patients with nonallergic bronchospastic disorders, diabetes mellitus, impaired hepatic or renal function, and congestive heart failure.

● Use caution in discontinuing drug; dose should be tapered. Suddenly stopping can worsen angina or precipitate MI.

● In pregnant women, use cautiously. Drugs appear in breast milk. In children, safety and effectiveness haven't been established; use only if the benefits outweigh the risks. In elderly patients, use cautiously; patients may need reduced maintenance doses because of increased bioavailability, delayed metabolism, and increased adverse effects.

Calcium channel blockers

amlodipine besylate
clevidipine butyrate
diltiazem hydrochloride
felodipine
niCARdipine hydrochloride
NIFEdipine
nisoldipine
verapamil hydrochloride

INDICATIONS
➤ **Prinzmetal variant angina, chronic stable angina, unstable angina, mild-to-moderate hypertension, arrhythmias**

ACTION
The main physiologic action of calcium channel blockers is to inhibit calcium influx across the slow channels of myocardial and vascular smooth muscle cells. By inhibiting calcium flow into these cells, calcium channel blockers reduce intracellular calcium levels. This, in turn, dilates coronary arteries, peripheral arteries, and arterioles and slows cardiac conduction.

When used to treat Prinzmetal variant angina, calcium channel blockers inhibit coronary spasm, which then increases oxygen delivery to the heart. Peripheral artery dilation reduces afterload, which decreases myocardial oxygen use. Inhibiting calcium flow into specialized cardiac conduction cells in the SA and AV nodes slows conduction through the heart. Verapamil and diltiazem have the greatest effect on the AV node, which slows the ventricular rate in atrial fibrillation or flutter and converts supraventricular tachycardia to a normal sinus rhythm.

ADVERSE REACTIONS
Verapamil may cause bradycardia, hypotension, various degrees of heart block, and worsening of heart failure after rapid I.V. delivery. Prolonged oral verapamil therapy may cause constipation. Nifedipine may cause flushing, headache, heartburn, hypotension, light-headedness, and peripheral edema. The most common adverse reactions to diltiazem are anorexia and nausea; it also may induce bradycardia, heart failure, peripheral edema, and various degrees of heart block.

CONTRAINDICATIONS & CAUTIONS
● Contraindicated in patients hypersensitive to these drugs and in those with second- or third-degree heart block (except those with a pacemaker) and cardiogenic shock. Use diltiazem and verapamil cautiously in patients with heart failure.

● In pregnant women, use cautiously. Calcium channel blockers may appear in breast milk; instruct patient to stop breast-feeding during therapy. In neonates and infants, adverse hemodynamic effects of parenteral verapamil are possible, but safety and effectiveness of other calcium channel blockers haven't been established; avoid use, if possible. In elderly patients, the half-life of calcium channel blockers may be increased as a result of decreased clearance.

Cephalosporins

First generation
cefadroxil
cefazolin sodium
cephalexin

Second generation
cefoxitin sodium
cefprozil
cefuroxime axetil
cefuroxime sodium

Third generation
cefdinir
cefotaxime sodium
cefpodoxime proxetil
ceftazidime
ceftriaxone sodium

Fourth generation
cefepime hydrochloride

Fifth generation
ceftaroline fosamil

INDICATIONS
➤ Infections of the lungs, skin, soft tissue, bones, joints, urinary and respiratory tracts, blood, abdomen, and heart; CNS infections caused by susceptible strains of *Neisseria meningitidis, Haemophilus influenzae,* and *Streptococcus pneumoniae;* meningitis caused by *Escherichia coli* or *Klebsiella;* infections that develop after surgical procedures classified as contaminated or potentially contaminated; penicillinase-producing *Neisseria gonorrhoeae;* otitis media and ampicillin-resistant middle ear infection caused by *H. influenzae*

ACTION
Cephalosporins are chemically and pharmacologically similar to penicillin; they act by inhibiting bacterial cell wall synthesis, causing rapid cell destruction. Their sites of action are enzymes known as penicillin-binding proteins. The affinity of certain cephalosporins for these proteins in various microorganisms helps explain the differing actions of these drugs. They are bactericidal: they act against many aerobic gram-positive and gram-negative bacteria and some anaerobic bacteria but don't kill fungi or viruses.

First-generation cephalosporins act against many gram-positive cocci, including penicillinase-producing *Staphylococcus aureus* and *S. epidermidis, S. pneumoniae,* group B streptococci, and group A beta-hemolytic streptococci. Susceptible gram-negative organisms include *Klebsiella pneumoniae, E. coli, Proteus mirabilis,* and *Shigella.*

Second-generation cephalosporins are effective against all organisms attacked by first-generation drugs and have additional activity against *Moraxella catarrhalis, H. influenzae, Enterobacter, Citrobacter, Providencia, Acinetobacter, Serratia,* and *Neisseria. Bacteroides fragilis* are susceptible to cefoxitin.

Third-generation cephalosporins are less active than first- and second-generation drugs against gram-positive bacteria but are more active against gram-negative organisms, including those resistant to first- and second-generation drugs. They have the greatest stability against beta-lactamases produced by gram-negative bacteria. Susceptible gram-negative organisms include *E. coli, Klebsiella, Enterobacter, Providencia, Acinetobacter, Serratia, Proteus, Morganella,* and *Neisseria.* Some third-generation drugs are active against *B. fragilis* and *Pseudomonas.*

The fourth-generation cephalosporin (cefepime hydrochloride) shows activity against a wide range of gram-positive and gram-negative bacteria. Cefepime exhibits resistance to beta-lactamases. Susceptible gram-negative bacteria include *Enterobacter, E. coli, K. pneumoniae, P. mirabilis,* and *Pseudomonas aeruginosa.* Susceptible gram-positive bacteria include *S. aureus, S. pneumoniae,* and *Streptococcus pyogenes.*

The fifth-generation cephalosporin (ceftaroline fosamil) has antimicrobial activity against gram-negative bacteria similar to third-generation cephalosporins. It is also active against gram-positive bacteria such as methicillin-resistant *S. aureus, S. pneumoniae,* and *Enterococcus faecalis.*

ADVERSE REACTIONS

Many cephalosporins have similar adverse effects. Hypersensitivity reactions range from mild rashes, fever, and eosinophilia to fatal anaphylaxis and are more common in patients with penicillin allergy. Adverse GI reactions include abdominal pain, diarrhea, dyspepsia, glossitis, nausea, tenesmus, and vomiting. Hematologic reactions include positive direct and indirect antiglobulin on Coombs test, thrombocytopenia or thrombocythemia, transient neutropenia, and reversible leukopenia. Minimal elevation of liver function test results occurs occasionally. Adverse renal effects may occur with any cephalosporin; they are most common in older patients, those with decreased renal function, and those taking other nephrotoxic drugs.

Local venous pain and irritation are common after I.M. injection; these reactions occur more often with higher doses and long-term therapy. Bacterial and fungal superinfections may result from suppression of normal flora.

CONTRAINDICATIONS & CAUTIONS

● Contraindicated in patients hypersensitive to cephalosporins and related antibiotics.
● Use cautiously in patients with renal or hepatic impairment, history of GI disease, or allergy to penicillins.
● In pregnant women, use cautiously; safety hasn't been definitively established. In breast-feeding women, use cautiously because drugs appear in breast milk. In neonates and infants, half-life is prolonged; use cautiously. Elderly patients are susceptible to superinfection and coagulopathies, commonly have renal impairment, and may need a lower dosage; use cautiously.

CNS stimulants
armodafinil
doxapram hydrochloride
modafinil
phentermine hydrochloride

INDICATIONS

➤ **Stimulation of respiration in patients with drug-induced postanesthesia respiratory depression or CNS depression caused by overdose and as temporary** measure in acute respiratory insufficiency **(doxapram and modafinil); obesity (phentermine); narcolepsy (armodafinil and modafinil); shift-work sleep disorder (armodafinil and modafinil)**

ACTION

Doxapram and modafinil produce respiratory stimulation through the peripheral carotid chemoreceptors. The exact mechanism of action of armodafinil isn't known. Phentermine is a sympathomimetic amine. The exact mechanism of action in treating obesity isn't established.

ADVERSE REACTIONS

Phentermine's adverse reactions are related to its stimulatory effect and include hypertension, palpitations, tachyarrhythmias, urticaria, constipation, diarrhea, dizziness, excitement, insomnia, tremor, and restlessness. Armodafinil and modafinil may cause severe rash, including Stevens-Johnson syndrome.

CONTRAINDICATIONS & CAUTIONS

● Contraindicated in patients hypersensitive to any of the drug components.
● Use armodafinil cautiously in patients with a psychiatric illness.
● Doxapram and modafinil are contraindicated in epilepsy, seizure disorders, mechanical disorders of ventilation such as muscle paresis, flail chest, pneumothorax, asthma, pulmonary fibrosis, head injury, stroke, cerebral edema, uncompensated congestive heart failure, severe coronary disease, and severe hypertension.
● Delay administration of doxapram and modafinil in patients who have received general anesthesia utilizing a volatile agent until the volatile agent has been excreted. This will lessen the chance for arrhythmias, including ventricular tachycardia or ventricular fibrillation.
● Administer doxapram and modafinil cautiously in patients taking MAO inhibitors or sympathomimetics because an added pressor effect may occur.
● Administer doxapram and modafinil cautiously in patients taking aminophylline or theophylline because agitation and hyperactivity may occur.

• Phentermine is contraindicated in agitated states, CV disease, history of drug abuse, severe hypertension, hyperthyroidism, glaucoma, and during or within 14 days after use of MAO inhibitors.

Corticosteroids

beclomethasone dipropionate
betamethasone
budesonide
ciclesonide
dexamethasone
dexamethasone sodium phosphate
fludrocortisone acetate
flunisolide
fluticasone propionate
hydrocortisone
hydrocortisone acetate
hydrocortisone butyrate
hydrocortisone cypionate
hydrocortisone probutate
hydrocortisone sodium succinate
hydrocortisone valerate
methylPREDNISolone
methylPREDNISolone acetate
methylPREDNISolone sodium
  succinate
prednisoLONE
prednisoLONE acetate
prednisoLONE sodium phosphate
predniSONE
triamcinolone

INDICATIONS
➤ Hypersensitivity; inflammation, particularly of eye, nose, and respiratory tract; to initiate immunosuppression; replacement therapy in adrenocortical insufficiency, dermatologic diseases, respiratory disorders, and rheumatic disorders

ACTION
Corticosteroids suppress cell-mediated and humoral immunity by reducing levels of leukocytes, monocytes, and eosinophils; by decreasing immunoglobulin binding to cell-surface receptors; and by inhibiting interleukin synthesis. They reduce inflammation by preventing hydrolytic enzyme release into the cells, preventing plasma exudation, suppressing polymorphonuclear leukocyte migration, and disrupting other inflammatory processes.

ADVERSE REACTIONS
Systemic corticosteroid therapy may suppress the hypothalamic-pituitary-adrenal (HPA) axis. Excessive use may cause cushingoid symptoms and various systemic disorders, such as diabetes and osteoporosis. Other effects may include dermatologic disorders, edema, euphoria, fluid and electrolyte imbalances, gastritis or GI irritation, hypertension, immunosuppression, increased appetite, insomnia, psychosis, and weight gain.

CONTRAINDICATIONS & CAUTIONS
• Contraindicated in patients hypersensitive to these drugs or any of their components and in those with systemic fungal infection.
• Use cautiously in patients with GI ulceration, renal disease, hypertension, osteoporosis, varicella, vaccinia, exanthema, diabetes mellitus, hypothyroidism, thromboembolic disorder, seizures, myasthenia gravis, heart failure, tuberculosis, ocular herpes simplex, hypoalbuminemia, emotional instability, or psychosis.
• In pregnant women, avoid use, if possible, because of risk to the fetus. Women should stop breast-feeding because these drugs appear in breast milk and could cause serious adverse effects in infants. In children, long-term use should be avoided whenever possible because stunted growth may result. Elderly patients may have an increased risk of adverse reactions; monitor them closely.

Diuretics, loop

bumetanide
ethacrynate sodium
ethacrynic acid
furosemide
torsemide

INDICATIONS
➤ Edema from heart failure, hepatic cirrhosis, or nephrotic syndrome; mild-to-moderate hypertension; adjunct treatment in acute pulmonary edema or hypertensive crisis

ACTION

Loop diuretics inhibit sodium and chloride reabsorption in the ascending loop of Henle, thus increasing excretion of sodium, chloride, and water. Like thiazide diuretics, loop diuretics increase excretion of potassium. Loop diuretics produce more diuresis and electrolyte loss than thiazide diuretics.

ADVERSE REACTIONS

Therapeutic dose commonly causes metabolic and electrolyte disturbances, particularly potassium depletion. It also may cause hyperglycemia, hyperuricemia, hypochloremic alkalosis, and hypomagnesemia. Rapid parenteral administration may cause hearing loss (including deafness) and tinnitus. High doses can produce profound diuresis, leading to hypovolemia and CV collapse. Photosensitivity also may occur.

CONTRAINDICATIONS & CAUTIONS

Black Box Warning Refer to individual drug monographs for black box warnings. ■
● Contraindicated in patients hypersensitive to these drugs and in patients with anuria, hepatic coma, or severe electrolyte depletion.
● Use cautiously in patients with severe renal disease. Also use cautiously in patients with severe hypersensitivity to sulfonamides because allergic reaction may occur.
● In pregnant women, use cautiously. In breast-feeding women, don't use. In neonates, use cautiously; the usual pediatric dose can be used, but dosage intervals should be extended. In elderly patients, use a lower dose, if needed, and monitor patient closely; these patients are more susceptible to drug-induced diuresis.

Diuretics, potassium-sparing
amiloride hydrochloride
spironolactone
triamterene

INDICATIONS

➤ **Edema from hepatic cirrhosis, nephrotic syndrome, and heart failure; mild or moderate hypertension; diagnosis of primary hyperaldosteronism; metabolic alkalosis produced by thiazide and other kaliuretic diuretics; recurrent calcium nephrolithiasis; polyuria secondary to lithium-induced nephrogenic diabetes insipidus; aid in the treatment of hypokalemia; prophylaxis of hypokalemia in patients taking cardiac glycosides; precocious puberty and female hirsutism; adjunct to treatment of myasthenia gravis and familial periodic paralysis**

ACTION

Spironolactone competitively inhibits aldosterone at the distal renal tubules, also promoting sodium excretion and potassium retention.

ADVERSE REACTIONS

Hyperkalemia is the most serious adverse reaction; it could lead to arrhythmias. Other adverse reactions include nausea, vomiting, headache, weakness, fatigue, bowel disturbances, cough, and dyspnea.

CONTRAINDICATIONS & CAUTIONS

Black Box Warning Refer to individual drug monographs for black box warnings. ■
● Contraindicated in patients hypersensitive to spironolactone, those with a potassium level above 5.5 mEq/L, those taking other potassium-sparing diuretics or potassium supplements, and those with anuria, acute or chronic renal insufficiency, or diabetic nephropathy.
● Use cautiously in patients with severe hepatic insufficiency because electrolyte imbalance may lead to hepatic encephalopathy, and in patients with diabetes, who are at increased risk for hyperkalemia.
● In pregnant women, no controlled studies exist. Women who wish to breast-feed should consult prescriber because drug may appear in breast milk. In children, use cautiously; they're more susceptible to hyperkalemia. In elderly and debilitated patients, observe closely and reduce dosage, if needed; they're more susceptible to drug-induced diuresis and hyperkalemia.

Diuretics, thiazide and thiazide-like

Thiazide
hydrochlorothiazide

Thiazide-like
indapamide
metolazone

INDICATIONS
➤ **Edema from right-sided heart failure, mild-to-moderate left-sided heart failure, or nephrotic syndrome; edema and ascites caused by hepatic cirrhosis; hypertension; diabetes insipidus, particularly nephrogenic diabetes insipidus**

ACTION
Thiazide and thiazide-like diuretics interfere with sodium transport across the tubules of the cortical diluting segment in the nephron, thereby increasing renal excretion of sodium, chloride, water, potassium, and calcium.

Thiazide diuretics also exert an antihypertensive effect. Although the exact mechanism is unknown, direct arteriolar dilation may be partially responsible. In diabetes insipidus, thiazides cause a paradoxical decrease in urine volume and an increase in renal concentration of urine, possibly because of sodium depletion and decreased plasma volume. This increases water and sodium reabsorption in the kidneys.

ADVERSE REACTIONS
Therapeutic doses cause electrolyte and metabolic disturbances, most commonly potassium depletion. Other abnormalities include elevated cholesterol levels, hypercalcemia, hyperglycemia, hyperuricemia, hypochloremic alkalosis, hypomagnesemia, hyponatremia, and photosensitivity.

CONTRAINDICATIONS & CAUTIONS
Black Box Warning Refer to individual drug monographs for black box warnings. ■
• Contraindicated in patients hypersensitive to these drugs and in those with anuria.
• Use cautiously in patients with severe renal disease, impaired hepatic function, or progressive liver disease.

• In pregnant women, use cautiously. In breast-feeding women, thiazides are contraindicated because they appear in breast milk. In children, safety and effectiveness haven't been established. In elderly patients, reduce dosage, if needed, and monitor patient closely; these patients are more susceptible to drug-induced diuresis.

Estrogens
esterified estrogens
estradiol
estradiol cypionate
estradiol hemihydrate
estradiol valerate
estrogens (conjugated)
estropipate

INDICATIONS
➤ **Prevention of moderate to severe vasomotor symptoms linked to menopause, such as hot flushes and dizziness; stimulation of vaginal tissue development, cornification, and secretory activity; inhibition of hormone-sensitive cancer growth; female hypogonadism; female castration; primary ovulation failure; ovulation control; prevention of conception**

ACTION
Estrogens promote the development and maintenance of the female reproductive system and secondary sexual characteristics. They inhibit the release of pituitary gonadotropins and have various metabolic effects, including retention of fluid and electrolytes, retention and deposition in bone of calcium and phosphorus, and mild anabolic activity. Of the six naturally occurring estrogens in humans, estradiol, estrone, and estriol are present in significant quantities.

Estrogens and estrogenic substances given as drugs have effects related to endogenous estrogen's mechanism of action. They can mimic the action of endogenous estrogen when used as replacement therapy and can inhibit ovulation or the growth of certain hormone-sensitive cancers. Conjugated estrogens and estrogenic substances are normally obtained from the urine of pregnant mares. Other estrogens are manufactured synthetically.

ADVERSE REACTIONS

Acute adverse reactions include abdominal cramps; bloating caused by fluid and electrolyte retention; breast swelling and tenderness; changes in menstrual bleeding patterns, such as spotting and prolongation or absence of bleeding; headache; loss of appetite; loss of libido; nausea; photosensitivity; swollen feet or ankles; and weight gain.

Long-term effects include benign hepatomas, cholestatic jaundice, elevated blood pressure (sometimes into the hypertensive range), endometrial carcinoma (rare), and thromboembolic disease (risk increases greatly with cigarette smoking, especially in women older than age 35).

CONTRAINDICATIONS & CAUTIONS

Black Box Warning Refer to individual drug monographs for black box warnings. ■
• Contraindicated in women with thrombophlebitis or thromboembolic disorders, unexplained abnormal genital bleeding, or estrogen-dependent neoplasia.
• Use cautiously in patients with hypertension; metabolic bone disease; migraines; seizures; asthma; cardiac, renal, or hepatic impairment; blood dyscrasia; diabetes; family history of breast cancer; or fibrocystic disease.
• Contraindicated in pregnant or breast-feeding women. In adolescents whose bone growth isn't complete, use cautiously because of effects on epiphyseal closure. Postmenopausal women with a history of long-term estrogen use are at increased risk for endometrial cancer and stroke. Postmenopausal women also have increased risk for breast cancer, MI, stroke, and blood clots with long-term use of estrogen plus progestin.

Fluoroquinolones

ciprofloxacin
gatifloxacin
gemifloxacin mesylate
levofloxacin
moxifloxacin hydrochloride
ofloxacin

INDICATIONS

➤ **Bone and joint infection, bacterial bronchitis, endocervical and urethral** chlamydial infection, bacterial gastroenteritis, endocervical and urethral gonorrhea, intra-abdominal infection, empirical therapy for febrile neutropenia, pelvic inflammatory disease, bacterial pneumonia, bacterial prostatitis, acute sinusitis, skin and soft-tissue infection, typhoid fever, bacterial UTI (prevention and treatment), chancroid, meningococcal carriers, and bacterial septicemia caused by susceptible organisms; bacterial conjunctivitis (gatifloxacin)

ACTION

Fluoroquinolones produce a bactericidal effect by inhibiting intracellular DNA topoisomerase II (DNA gyrase), which prevents DNA replication. These enzymes are essential catalysts in the duplication, transcription, and repair of bacterial DNA.

Fluoroquinolones are broad-spectrum, systemic antibacterial drugs active against a wide range of aerobic gram-positive and gram-negative organisms. Gram-positive aerobic bacteria include *Staphylococcus aureus, S. epidermidis, S. hemolyticus, S. saprophyticus;* penicillinase- and non–penicillinase-producing staphylococci and some methicillin-resistant strains; *Streptococcus pneumoniae;* group A (beta) hemolytic streptococci *(S. pyogenes);* group B streptococci *(S. agalactiae);* viridans streptococci; groups C, F, and G streptococci and nonenterococcal group D streptococci; and *Enterococcus faecalis.* These drugs are active against gram-positive aerobic bacilli, including *Corynebacterium* species, *Listeria monocytogenes,* and *Nocardia asteroides.*

Fluoroquinolones are also effective against gram-negative aerobic bacteria, including, but not limited to, *Neisseria meningitidis* and most strains of penicillinase- and non–penicillinase-producing *Haemophilus ducreyi, H. influenzae, H. parainfluenzae, Moraxella catarrhalis, N. gonorrhoeae,* most clinically important *Enterobacteriaceae,* and *Vibrio parahaemolyticus.* Certain fluoroquinolones are active against *Chlamydia trachomatis, Legionella pneumophila, Mycobacterium avium-intracellulare, Mycoplasma hominis,*

M. pneumoniae, and *Pseudomonas aeruginosa.*

ADVERSE REACTIONS
Adverse reactions that are rare but need medical attention include CNS stimulation (acute psychosis, agitation, hallucinations, tremors), hepatotoxicity, hypersensitivity reactions, interstitial nephritis, phlebitis, pseudomembranous colitis, and tendinitis or tendon rupture. Adverse reactions that need no medical attention unless they persist or become intolerable include CNS effects (dizziness, headache, nervousness, drowsiness, insomnia), GI reactions, and photosensitivity.

CONTRAINDICATIONS & CAUTIONS
Black Box Warning Fluoroquinolones are associated with increased risk of tendinitis and tendon rupture in all age-groups. The risk further increases in older patients (usually older than age 60), in patients taking corticosteroids, and in patients who have received kidney, heart, or lung transplants. ■
Black Box Warning Fluoroquinolones may exacerbate muscle weakness in persons with myasthenia gravis. Avoid use in patients with known history of myasthenia gravis. ■
• Contraindicated in patients hypersensitive to fluoroquinolones because serious, possibly fatal, reactions can occur.
• Avoid use in patients with a known history of myasthenia gravis.
• Use cautiously in patients with known or suspected CNS disorders that predispose them to seizures or lower the seizure threshold, cerebral ischemia, severe hepatic dysfunction, or renal insufficiency.
• In pregnant women, these drugs cross the placenta and may cause arthropathies. Breast-feeding isn't recommended because these drugs may cause arthropathies in newborns and infants, although it isn't known if all fluoroquinolones appear in breast milk. In children, fluoroquinolones aren't recommended because they can cause joint problems. In elderly patients, reduce dosage, if needed, because these patients are more likely to have reduced renal function.

Hematopoietic agents
darbepoetin alfa
epoetin alfa
peginesatide acetate

INDICATIONS
➤ Anemia associated with chronic renal failure, zidovudine therapy in patients with HIV, and cancer patients on chemotherapy; to reduce the need for allogeneic blood transfusions in surgical patients (epoetin alfa and related products)

ACTION
Epoetin and darbepoetin stimulate RBC production in the bone marrow.

ADVERSE REACTIONS
Hematopoietics may cause fatigue, headache, weakness, chest pain, hypertension, tachycardia, nausea, vomiting, diarrhea, constipation, mucositis, stomatitis, anorexia, myalgias, neutropenic fever, dyspnea, cough, sore throat, alopecia, rash, urticaria, and stinging at injection site.

CONTRAINDICATIONS & CAUTIONS
Black Box Warning Refer to individual drug monographs for black box warnings. ■
• Contraindicated in patients hypersensitive to any of the drug components or human albumin.
• Contraindicated in uncontrolled hypertension.
• Darbepoetin alfa and epoetin alfa shouldn't be used in patients with breast, non–small-cell lung, head and neck, lymphoid, and cervical cancers, or for the treatment of cancers with curative potential.
• Use cautiously in patients with cardiac disease, seizures, and porphyria.

Histamine₂-receptor antagonists
cimetidine
famotidine
ranitidine hydrochloride

INDICATIONS
➤ Acute duodenal or gastric ulcer, Zollinger-Ellison syndrome, gastroesophageal reflux

ACTION

All H$_2$-receptor antagonists inhibit the action of H$_2$ receptors in gastric parietal cells, reducing gastric acid output and concentration, regardless of stimulants, such as histamine, food, insulin, and caffeine, or basal conditions.

ADVERSE REACTIONS

H$_2$-receptor antagonists rarely cause adverse reactions. Cardiac arrhythmias, dizziness, fatigue, gynecomastia, headache, mild and transient diarrhea, and thrombocytopenia are possible.

CONTRAINDICATIONS & CAUTIONS

• Contraindicated in patients hypersensitive to these drugs.
• Use cautiously in patients with impaired renal or hepatic function.
• In pregnant women, use cautiously. In breast-feeding women, H$_2$-receptor antagonists are contraindicated because they may appear in breast milk. In children, safety and effectiveness haven't been established. Elderly patients have increased risk of adverse reactions, particularly those affecting the CNS; use cautiously.

Immunosuppressants
alefacept
anakinra
azathioprine
basiliximab
belimumab
certolizumab pegol
cycloSPORINE
etanercept
fingolimod
glatiramer acetate
infliximab
lymphocyte immune globulin
muromonab-CD3
mycophenolate mofetil
sirolimus
tacrolimus

INDICATIONS

➤ Prevention of rejection in organ transplants and in the management of severe rheumatoid arthritis, multiple sclerosis, psoriasis, systemic lupus erythematosus

ACTION

The exact mechanism of action is not fully known. Immunosuppressants act by suppressing cell-mediated hypersensitivity reactions and produce various alterations in antibody production, blocking the activity of interleukin, inhibiting helper T cells and suppressor T cells, and antagonizing the metabolism of purine, therefore inhibiting RNA and DNA structure and synthesis.

ADVERSE REACTIONS

Immunosuppressants may cause albuminuria, hematuria, proteinuria, renal failure, hepatotoxicity, oral *Candida* infections, gingival hyperplasia, tremors, and headache. The most serious reactions include leukopenia, thrombocytopenia, and risk of secondary infection.

CONTRAINDICATIONS & CAUTIONS

Black Box Warning Refer to individual drug monographs for black box warnings. ∎
• Contraindicated in patients hypersensitive to any of the drug components.
• Use cautiously in patients with severe renal disease, severe hepatic disease, or pregnancy.

Inotropics
digoxin
milrinone

INDICATIONS

➤ Heart failure and supraventricular arrhythmias, including supraventricular tachycardia, atrial fibrillation, and atrial flutter (digoxin); short-term heart failure and patients awaiting heart transplantation (milrinone)

ACTION

Inotropics help move calcium into the cells, which increases cardiac output by strengthening contractility. Digoxin also acts on the central nervous system to slow heart rate. Milrinone relaxes vascular smooth muscle, decreasing peripheral vascular resistance (afterload) and the amount of blood returning to the heart (preload).

ADVERSE REACTIONS

Inotropics may cause arrhythmias, nausea, vomiting, diarrhea, headache, fever, mental disturbances, visual changes, and chest pain. Milrinone may cause thrombocytopenia, hypotension, hypokalemia, and elevated liver enzymes.

CONTRAINDICATIONS & CAUTIONS

• Contraindicated in patients hypersensitive to any of the drug components.
• Digoxin is contraindicated in ventricular fibrillation.
• Use digoxin cautiously in patients with renal insufficiency because of the potential for digoxin toxicity. Use digoxin cautiously in patients with sinus node disease or AV block because of the potential for advanced heart block.

Laxatives

Bulk-forming
calcium polycarbophil
psyllium

Emollient
docusate calcium
docusate sodium

Hyperosmolar
glycerin
lactulose
lubiprostone
magnesium citrate
magnesium hydroxide
magnesium sulfate
polyethylene glycol
sodium phosphates

Stimulant
bisacodyl

INDICATIONS
➤ Constipation, irritable bowel syndrome, diverticulosis

ACTION
Laxatives promote movement of intestinal contents through the colon and rectum in several ways: bulk-forming, emollient, hyperosmolar, and stimulant.

ADVERSE REACTIONS

All laxatives may cause flatulence, diarrhea, and abdominal disturbances. Bulk-forming laxatives may cause intestinal obstruction, impaction, or (rarely) esophageal obstruction. Emollient laxatives may irritate the throat. Hyperosmolar laxatives may cause fluid and electrolyte imbalances. Stimulant laxatives may cause urine discoloration, malabsorption, and weight loss.

CONTRAINDICATIONS & CAUTIONS

• Contraindicated in patients with GI obstruction or perforation, toxic colitis, megacolon, nausea and vomiting, or acute surgical abdomen.
• Use cautiously in patients with rectal or anal conditions such as rectal bleeding or large hemorrhoids.
• For pregnant women and breast-feeding women, recommendations vary for individual drugs. Infants and children have an increased risk of fluid and electrolyte disturbances; use cautiously. In elderly patients, dependence is more likely to develop because of age-related changes in GI function. Monitor these patients closely.

Macrolide anti-infectives
azithromycin
clarithromycin
erythromycin ethylsuccinate
erythromycin lactobionate
erythromycin stearate
fidaxomicin

INDICATIONS
➤ Various common infections

ACTION
Inhibit RNA-dependent protein synthesis by acting on a small portion of the 50S ribosomal unit. They're active against *Staphylococcus aureus, Streptococcus pneumoniae, Streptococcus pyogenes, Streptococcus agalactiae, Moraxella catarrhalis, Chlamydia trachomatis, Mycoplasma pneumoniae, Haemophilus influenzae,* and *Neisseria gonorrhoeae.*

ADVERSE REACTIONS

These drugs may cause cardiac effects (prolonged QT interval, arrhythmias, torsades de pointes), nausea, vomiting, diarrhea, abdominal pain, palpitations, chest pain, vaginal candidiasis, nephritis, dizziness, headache, vertigo, somnolence, rash, and photosensitivity.

CONTRAINDICATIONS & CAUTIONS

● Contraindicated in patients hypersensitive to any of the drug components.
● Contraindicated in patients with concomitant use of terfenadine, astemizole, or cisapride due to the potential for cardiac arrhythmias. These drugs may also cause many other drug interactions when given with other drugs; screen carefully.

Neuromuscular blockers
atracurium besylate
cisatracurium besylate
pancuronium bromide
succinylcholine chloride

INDICATIONS

➤ Relax skeletal muscle during surgery, reduce the intensity of muscle spasms in drug-induced or electrically induced seizures, and manage patients who are fighting mechanical ventilation

ACTION

Nondepolarizing blockers (atracurium, cisatracurium, pancuronium) compete with acetylcholine at cholinergic receptor sites on the skeletal muscle membrane. This action blocks acetylcholine's neurotransmitter actions, preventing muscle contraction. Succinylcholine is a depolarizing blocker. This drug isn't inactivated by cholinesterase, thereby preventing repolarization of the motor endplate and causing muscle paralysis.

ADVERSE REACTIONS

Neuromuscular blockers may cause apnea, hypotension, hypertension, arrhythmias, tachycardia, bronchospasm, excessive bronchial or salivary secretions, and skin reactions.

CONTRAINDICATIONS & CAUTIONS

Black Box Warning Refer to individual drug monographs for black box warnings. ■
● Contraindicated in patients hypersensitive to any of the drug components.
● The drugs should be used only by personnel skilled in airway management and respiratory support.

Nonsteroidal anti-inflammatory drugs
aspirin
celecoxib
diclofenac epolamine
diclofenac potassium
diclofenac sodium
diflunisal
etodolac
ibuprofen
indomethacin
indomethacin sodium trihydrate
ketoprofen
ketorolac tromethamine
nabumetone
naproxen
naproxen sodium

INDICATIONS

➤ Mild-to-moderate pain, inflammation, stiffness, swelling, or tenderness caused by headache, arthralgia, myalgia, neuralgia, dysmenorrhea, rheumatoid arthritis, juvenile arthritis, osteoarthritis, dental or surgical procedures, or patent ductus arteriosus

ACTION

The analgesic effect of NSAIDs may result from interference with the prostaglandins involved in pain. Prostaglandins appear to sensitize pain receptors to mechanical stimulation or to other chemical mediators. NSAIDs inhibit synthesis of prostaglandins peripherally and possibly centrally.

Like salicylates, NSAIDs exert an anti-inflammatory effect that may result in part from inhibition of prostaglandin synthesis and release during inflammation. The exact mechanism isn't clear.

ADVERSE REACTIONS

Adverse reactions chiefly involve the GI tract, particularly erosion of the gastric mucosa. The most common symptoms are abdominal pain, dyspepsia, epigastric distress, heartburn, and nausea. CNS and skin reactions also may occur. Flank pain with other evidence of nephrotoxicity occurs occasionally. Fluid retention may aggravate hypertension or heart failure.

CONTRAINDICATIONS & CAUTIONS

Black Box Warning Refer to individual drug monographs for black box warnings. ∎
- Contraindicated in patients with GI lesions or GI bleeding and in patients hypersensitive to these drugs.
- Use cautiously in patients with heart failure, hypertension, risk of MI (except low-dose aspirin), fluid retention, renal insufficiency, or coagulation defects.
- In pregnant women, use cautiously in the first and second trimesters; don't use in the third trimester. For breast-feeding women, NSAIDs aren't recommended. In children younger than age 14, safety of long-term therapy hasn't been established. Patients older than age 60 may be more susceptible to toxic effects of NSAIDs because of decreased renal function.

Nucleoside reverse transcriptase inhibitors
abacavir sulfate
didanosine
emtricitabine
lamivudine
stavudine
tenofovir disoproxil fumarate
zidovudine

INDICATIONS

➤ **HIV infection, AIDS, prevention of maternal-fetal HIV transmission, prevention of HIV infection after occupational exposure (as by needle stick) or nonoccupational exposure to blood, genital secretions, or other potentially infectious body fluids of an HIV-infected person when there's substantial risk of transmission**

ACTION

Nucleoside reverse transcriptase inhibitors (NRTIs) suppress HIV replication by inhibiting HIV DNA polymerase. Competitive inhibition of nucleoside reverse transcriptase inhibits DNA viral replication by chain termination, competitive inhibition of reverse transcriptase, or both.

ADVERSE REACTIONS

Because of the complexity of HIV infection, it's often difficult to distinguish between disease-related symptoms and adverse drug reactions. The most frequently reported adverse effects of NRTIs are anemia, leukopenia, and neutropenia. Thrombocytopenia is less common. Rare adverse effects of NRTIs are hepatotoxicity, myopathy, and neurotoxicity. Any of these adverse effects requires prompt medical attention.

Adverse effects that don't need medical attention unless they persist or are bothersome include headache, insomnia, myalgias, nausea, or hyperpigmentation of nails.

CONTRAINDICATIONS & CAUTIONS

Black Box Warning Refer to individual drug monographs for black box warnings. ∎
- Contraindicated in patients hypersensitive to these drugs and patients with moderate to severe hepatic impairment (abacavir) or pancreatitis (didanosine).
- Use cautiously in patients with mild hepatic impairment or risk factors for liver impairment, risk for pancreatitis (didanosine), or compromised bone marrow function (zidovudine).
- In pregnant women, use drug only if benefits outweigh risks. To reduce the risk of transmitting the virus, HIV-infected mothers shouldn't breast-feed. It isn't known if NRTIs appear in breast milk. The pharmacokinetic and safety profile of NRTIs is similar in children and adults. NRTIs may be used in children age 3 months and older, but the half-life may be prolonged in neonates. In elderly patients, elimination half-life may be prolonged.

Opioids
codeine phosphate
codeine sulfate
fentanyl citrate
hydromorphone hydrochloride
meperidine hydrochloride
methadone hydrochloride
morphine sulfate
nalbuphine hydrochloride
oxycodone hydrochloride
oxymorphone hydrochloride
pentazocine lactate

INDICATIONS
➤ **Moderate-to-severe pain from acute and some chronic disorders; diarrhea; dry, nonproductive cough; management of opioid dependence; anesthesia support; sedation**

ACTION
Opioids act as agonists at specific opioid-receptor binding sites in the CNS and other tissues, altering perception of pain.

ADVERSE REACTIONS
Respiratory and circulatory depression (including orthostatic hypotension) are the major hazards of opioids. Other adverse CNS effects include agitation, coma, depression, dizziness, dysphoria, euphoria, faintness, mental clouding, nervousness, restlessness, sedation, seizures, visual disturbances, and weakness. Adverse GI effects include biliary colic, constipation, nausea, and vomiting. Urine retention or hypersensitivity also may occur. Drug tolerance and psychological or physical dependence may follow prolonged use.

CONTRAINDICATIONS & CAUTIONS
Black Box Warning Refer to individual drug monographs for black box warnings. ∎
• Contraindicated in patients hypersensitive to these drugs and in those who have recently taken an MAO inhibitor. Also contraindicated in those with acute or severe bronchial asthma or respiratory depression.
• Use cautiously in patients with head injury, increased intracranial or intraocular pressure, hepatic or renal dysfunction,
mental illness, emotional disturbances, or drug-seeking behaviors.
• In pregnant or breast-feeding women, use cautiously; codeine, meperidine, methadone, and morphine appear in breast milk. Breast-feeding infants of women taking methadone may develop physical dependence. In children, safety and effectiveness of some opioids haven't been established; use cautiously. Elderly patients may be more sensitive to opioids, and lower doses are usually given.

Penicillins

Natural penicillins
penicillin G benzathine
penicillin G potassium
penicillin G procaine
penicillin G sodium
penicillin V potassium

Aminopenicillins
amoxicillin–clavulanate potassium
ampicillin
ampicillin sodium–sulbactam
  sodium
ampicillin trihydrate

Extended-spectrum penicillins
piperacillin sodium–tazobactam
  sodium
ticarcillin disodium–clavulanate
  potassium

Penicillinase-resistant penicillins
nafcillin sodium

INDICATIONS
➤ **Streptococcal pneumonia; enterococcal and nonenterococcal group D endocarditis; diphtheria; anthrax; meningitis; tetanus; botulism; actinomycosis; syphilis; relapsing fever; Lyme disease; pneumococcal infections; rheumatic fever; bacterial endocarditis; neonatal group B streptococcal disease; septicemia; gynecologic infections; infections of urinary, respiratory, and GI tracts; infections of skin, soft tissue, bones, and joints**

ACTION

Generally bactericidal, penicillins inhibit synthesis of the bacterial cell wall, causing rapid cell destruction. They're most effective against fast-growing susceptible bacteria. Their sites of action are enzymes known as *penicillin-binding proteins* (PBPs). The affinity of certain penicillins for PBPs in various microorganisms helps explain the different activities of these drugs.

Susceptible aerobic gram-positive cocci include *Staphylococcus aureus;* nonenterococcal group D streptococci; groups A, B, D, G, H, K, L, and M streptococci; *Streptococcus viridans;* and *Enterococcus* (usually with an aminoglycoside). Susceptible aerobic gram-negative cocci include *Neisseria meningitidis* and non–penicillinase-producing *N. gonorrhoeae.*

Susceptible aerobic gram-positive bacilli include *Corynebacterium, Listeria,* and *Bacillus anthracis.* Susceptible anaerobes include *Peptococcus, Peptostreptococcus, Actinomyces, Clostridium, Fusobacterium, Veillonella,* and non–beta-lactamase–producing strains of *Streptococcus pneumoniae.* Susceptible spirochetes include *Treponema pallidum, T. pertenue, Leptospira, Borrelia recurrentis* and, possibly, *B. burgdorferi.*

Aminopenicillins have uses against more organisms, including many gram-negative organisms. Like natural penicillins, aminopenicillins are vulnerable to inactivation by penicillinase. Susceptible organisms include *Escherichia coli, Proteus mirabilis, Shigella, Salmonella, S. pneumoniae, N. gonorrhoeae, Haemophilus influenzae, S. aureus, S. epidermidis* (non–penicillinase-producing *Staphylococcus*), and *Listeria monocytogenes.*

Penicillinase-resistant penicillins are semisynthetic penicillins designed to remain stable against hydrolysis by most staphylococcal penicillinases and thus are the drugs of choice against susceptible penicillinase-producing staphylococci. They also act against most organisms susceptible to natural penicillins.

Extended-spectrum penicillins offer a wider range of bactericidal action than the other three classes and usually are given in combination with aminoglycosides.

Susceptible strains include *Enterobacter, Klebsiella, Citrobacter, Serratia, Bacteroides fragilis, Pseudomonas aeruginosa, Proteus vulgaris, Providencia rettgeri,* and *Morganella morganii.* These penicillins are also vulnerable to beta-lactamase and penicillinases.

ADVERSE REACTIONS

With all penicillins, hypersensitivity reactions range from mild rash, fever, and eosinophilia to fatal anaphylaxis. Hematologic reactions include hemolytic anemia, leukopenia, thrombocytopenia, and transient neutropenia. Certain adverse reactions are more common with specific classes. For example, bleeding episodes are usually seen with high doses of extended-spectrum penicillins, whereas GI adverse effects are most common with ampicillin. In patients with renal disease, high doses (especially of penicillin G) irritate the CNS, causing confusion, twitching, lethargy, dysphagia, seizures, and coma. Hepatotoxicity may occur with penicillinase-resistant penicillins, and hyperkalemia and hypernatremia have been reported with extended-spectrum penicillins. Local irritation from parenteral therapy may be severe enough to warrant administration by subclavian or centrally placed catheter or stopping therapy.

CONTRAINDICATIONS & CAUTIONS

Black Box Warning Refer to individual drug monographs for black box warnings. ∎
- Contraindicated in patients hypersensitive to these drugs.
- Use cautiously in patients with history of asthma or drug allergy, mononucleosis, renal impairment, CV diseases, hemorrhagic condition, or electrolyte imbalance.
- In pregnant women, use cautiously. For breast-feeding patients, recommendations vary depending on the drug. For children, dosage recommendations have been established for most penicillins. Elderly patients are susceptible to superinfection and renal impairment, which decreases excretion of penicillins; use cautiously and at a lower dosage.

Phenothiazines

chlorproMAZINE hydrochloride
fluphenazine decanoate
perphenazine
prochlorperazine maleate
promethazine hydrochloride
thioridazine hydrochloride
thiothixene
trifluoperazine hydrochloride

INDICATIONS

➤ **Agitated psychotic states, hallucinations, manic-depressive illness, excessive motor and autonomic activity, nausea and vomiting, moderate anxiety, behavioral problems caused by chronic organic mental syndrome, tetanus, acute intermittent porphyria, intractable hiccups, itching, symptomatic rhinitis**

ACTION

Phenothiazines are believed to function as dopamine antagonists by blocking postsynaptic dopamine receptors in various parts of the CNS. Their antiemetic effects result from blockage of the chemoreceptor trigger zone. They also produce varying degrees of anticholinergic effects and alpha-adrenergic–receptor blocking.

ADVERSE REACTIONS

Phenothiazines may produce extrapyramidal symptoms, such as dystonic movements, torticollis, oculogyric crises, and parkinsonian symptoms ranging from akathisia during early treatment to tardive dyskinesia after long-term use. A neuroleptic malignant syndrome resembling severe parkinsonism may occur, most often in young men taking fluphenazine.

Other adverse reactions include abdominal pain, agitation, anorexia, arrhythmias, confusion, constipation, dizziness, dry mouth, endocrine effects, fainting, hallucinations, hematologic disorders, local gastric irritation, nausea, orthostatic hypotension with reflex tachycardia, photosensitivity, seizures, skin eruptions, urine retention, visual disturbances, and vomiting. Promethazine injection can cause severe chemical irritation and tissue damage with such reactions as burning, pain, thrombophlebitis, tissue necrosis, and gangrene.

CONTRAINDICATIONS & CAUTIONS

Black Box Warning Refer to individual drug monographs for black box warnings. ∎
● Contraindicated in patients with CNS depression, bone marrow suppression, heart failure, circulatory collapse, coronary artery or cerebrovascular disorders, subcortical damage, or coma. Also contraindicated in patients receiving spinal and epidural anesthetics and adrenergic blockers.
● Use cautiously in debilitated patients and in those with hepatic, renal, or CV disease; respiratory disorders; hypocalcemia; seizure disorders; suspected brain tumor or intestinal obstruction; glaucoma; and prostatic hyperplasia.
● In pregnant women, use only if clearly necessary; safety hasn't been established. Women shouldn't breast-feed during therapy because most phenothiazines appear in breast milk and directly affect prolactin levels. For children younger than age 12, phenothiazines aren't recommended unless otherwise specified; use cautiously for nausea and vomiting. Acutely ill children, such as those with chickenpox, measles, CNS infections, or dehydration have a greatly increased risk of dystonic reactions. Elderly patients are more sensitive to therapeutic and adverse effects, especially cardiac toxicity, tardive dyskinesia, and other extrapyramidal effects; use cautiously and give reduced doses, adjusting dosage to patient response.

Progestins

medroxyPROGESTERone acetate
norethindrone
norethindrone acetate

INDICATIONS

➤ **Amenorrhea, endometrial hyperplasia, abnormal uterine bleeding, endometriosis, contraception**

ACTION

Progestins transform proliferative endometrium into secretory endometrium.

ADVERSE REACTIONS

Progestins may cause amenorrhea, break-through bleeding, spotting, changes in menstrual flow, breast enlargement and tenderness, alterations in weight, and mood changes.

CONTRAINDICATIONS & CAUTIONS

Black Box Warning Refer to individual drug monographs for black box warnings. ■
• Contraindicated in patients with impaired liver function or liver disease; known or suspected breast cancer; active deep vein thrombosis, pulmonary embolism, or history of these conditions; active or recent arterial thromboembolic disease; and undiagnosed vaginal bleeding. Also contraindicated in patients hypersensitive to the drug components.
• Use cautiously in patients with depression, epilepsy, migraine headaches, asthma, cardiac dysfunction, or renal dysfunction.
• In pregnant women, use is contraindicated. Use cautiously in breast-feeding women because detectable amounts of progestins have been identified in the breast milk of mothers receiving these drugs. Progestins aren't indicated in children.

Protease inhibitors

atazanavir sulfate
darunavir
fosamprenavir calcium
indinavir sulfate
lopinavir–ritonavir
nelfinavir mesylate
ritonavir
saquinavir mesylate
tipranavir

INDICATIONS

➤ HIV infection and AIDS

ACTION

Protease inhibitors bind to the protease active site and inhibit HIV protease activity. This enzyme is required for the proteolysis of viral polyprotein precursors into individual functional proteins found in infectious HIV. The net effect is formation of noninfectious, immature viral particles.

ADVERSE REACTIONS

The most common adverse effects, which require immediate medical attention, include kidney stones, pancreatitis, diabetes or hyperglycemia, ketoacidosis, and paresthesia.
    Common adverse effects that don't need medical attention unless they persist or are bothersome include generalized weakness, GI disturbances, headache, insomnia, and taste disturbance. Less common adverse effects include dizziness and somnolence.

CONTRAINDICATIONS & CAUTIONS

Black Box Warning Refer to individual drug monographs for black box warnings. ■
• Contraindicated in patients hypersensitive to these drugs or their components and in patients taking a drug highly dependent on CYP3A4 for metabolism.
• Use cautiously in patients with impaired hepatic or renal function and those with diabetes mellitus or hemophilia.
• In pregnant women, use drug only if benefits outweigh risks. Contact the Antiretroviral Pregnancy Registry at 1-800-258-4263 or www.apregistry.com to report pregnant women on therapy. To reduce the risk of transmitting HIV to the infant, HIV-infected mothers shouldn't breast-feed.

Proton pump inhibitors

dexlansoprazole
esomeprazole
lansoprazole
omeprazole
pantoprazole
rabeprazole

INDICATIONS

➤ Duodenal ulcers, gastric ulcers, erosive esophagitis, and GERD (all proton pump inhibitors); hypersecretory conditions (Zollinger-Ellison syndrome) (lansoprazole, omeprazole, pantoprazole, rabeprazole)

ACTION

The drugs reduce stomach acid production by combining with hydrogen, potassium, and adenosine triphosphate in parietal cells of the stomach to block the last step in gastric acid secretion.

ADVERSE REACTIONS
Proton pump inhibitors may cause abdominal pain, diarrhea, constipation, flatulence, nausea, dry mouth, headache, asthenia, cough, abnormal liver function test results, and hyperglycemia.

CONTRAINDICATIONS & CAUTIONS
• Contraindicated in patients hypersensitive to the drug components.

Selective serotonin reuptake inhibitors

citalopram hydrobromide
escitalopram oxalate
fluoxetine hydrochloride
fluvoxamine maleate
paroxetine hydrochloride
sertraline hydrochloride

INDICATIONS
➤ **Major depression, obsessive-compulsive disorder, bulimia nervosa, premenstrual dysphoric disorders, panic disorders, posttraumatic stress disorder (sertraline)**

ACTION
SSRIs selectively inhibit the reuptake of serotonin with little or no effects on other neurotransmitters such as norepinephrine or dopamine in the CNS.

ADVERSE REACTIONS
Common adverse effects include headache, tremor, dizziness, sleep disturbances, GI disturbances, and sexual dysfunction. Less common adverse effects include bleeding (ecchymoses, epistaxis), akathisia, breast tenderness or enlargement, extrapyramidal effects, dystonia, fever, hyponatremia, mania or hypomania, palpitations, serotonin syndrome, weight gain or loss, rash, urticaria, or pruritus.

CONTRAINDICATIONS & CAUTIONS
Black Box Warning Antidepressants can increase risk of suicidal thinking and behavior. Appropriately monitor patients of all ages who are started on antidepressant therapy; observe closely for clinical worsening, suicidality, or unusual behavior changes. Advise families and caregivers of the need for close observation and communication with the prescriber. ■
• Contraindicated in patients hypersensitive to these drugs or their components.
• Use cautiously in patients with hepatic, renal, or cardiac insufficiency.
• In pregnant women, use drug only if benefits outweigh risks; use of certain SSRIs in the first trimester may cause birth defects. Neonates born to women who took an SSRI during the third trimester may develop complications that warrant prolonged hospitalization, respiratory support, and tube feeding. In breast-feeding women, use isn't recommended. SSRIs appear in breast milk and may cause diarrhea and sleep disturbance in neonates. However, risks and benefits to both the woman and infant must be considered. Children and adolescents may be more susceptible to increased suicidal tendencies when taking SSRIs or other antidepressants. Elderly patients may be more sensitive to the insomniac effects of SSRIs.

Skeletal muscle relaxants
baclofen
carisoprodol
cyclobenzaprine hydrochloride
dantrolene sodium
tizanidine hydrochloride

INDICATIONS
➤ **Painful musculoskeletal disorders, spasticity caused by multiple sclerosis**

ACTION
Baclofen may reduce impulse transmission from the spinal cord to skeletal muscle. Carisoprodol, cyclobenzaprine, and tizanidine's mechanism of action is unclear. Dantrolene acts directly on skeletal muscle to decrease excitation and reduce muscle strength by interfering with intracellular calcium movement.

ADVERSE REACTIONS

Skeletal muscle relaxants may cause ataxia, confusion, depressed mood, dizziness, drowsiness, dry mouth, hallucinations, headache, hypotension, nervousness, tachycardia, tremor, and vertigo. Baclofen also may cause seizures.

CONTRAINDICATIONS & CAUTIONS

Black Box Warning Refer to individual drug monographs for black box warnings. ■
• Contraindicated in patients hypersensitive to these drugs.
• Use cautiously in patients with impaired renal or hepatic function.
• In pregnant women and breast-feeding women, use only when potential benefits to the patient outweigh risks to the fetus or infant. In children, recommendations vary. Elderly patients have an increased risk of adverse reactions; monitor them carefully.

Sulfonamides

sulfADIAZINE
sulfamethoxazole–trimethoprim

INDICATIONS

➤ **Bacterial infections, nocardiosis, toxoplasmosis, chloroquine-resistant** *Plasmodium falciparum* **malaria**

ACTION

Sulfonamides are bacteriostatic. They inhibit biosynthesis of tetrahydrofolic acid, which is needed for bacterial cell growth. They're active against some strains of staphylococci, streptococci, *Nocardia asteroides* and *N. brasiliensis, Clostridium tetani* and *C. perfringens, Bacillus anthracis, Escherichia coli,* and *Neisseria gonorrhoeae* and *N. meningitidis.* Sulfonamides are also active against organisms that cause UTIs, such as *E. coli, Proteus mirabilis* and *P. vulgaris, Klebsiella, Enterobacter,* and *Staphylococcus aureus,* and genital lesions caused by *Haemophilus ducreyi* (chancroid).

ADVERSE REACTIONS

Many adverse reactions stem from hypersensitivity, including bronchospasm, conjunctivitis, erythema multiforme, erythema nodosum, exfoliative dermatitis, fever, joint pain, pruritus, leukopenia, Lyell syndrome, photosensitivity, rash, Stevens-Johnson syndrome, and toxic epidermal necrolysis. GI reactions include anorexia, diarrhea, folic acid malabsorption, nausea, pancreatitis, stomatitis, and vomiting. Hematologic reactions include agranulocytosis, granulocytopenia, hypoprothrombinemia, thrombocytopenia and, in G6PD deficiency, hemolytic anemia. Renal effects usually result from crystalluria caused by precipitation of sulfonamide in the renal system.

CONTRAINDICATIONS & CAUTIONS

• Contraindicated in patients hypersensitive to these drugs.
• Use cautiously in patients with renal or hepatic impairment, bronchial asthma, severe allergy, or G6PD deficiency.
• In pregnant women at term and in breast-feeding women, use is contraindicated; sulfonamides appear in breast milk. In infants younger than age 2 months, sulfonamides are contraindicated unless there's no therapeutic alternative. In children with fragile X chromosome and mental retardation, use cautiously. Elderly patients are susceptible to bacterial and fungal superinfection and have an increased risk of folate deficiency anemia and adverse renal and hematologic effects.

Tetracyclines

doxycycline
doxycycline hyclate
doxycycline monohydrate
minocycline hydrochloride
tetracycline hydrochloride
tigecycline

INDICATIONS

➤ **Bacterial, protozoal, rickettsial, and fungal infections**

ACTION

Tetracyclines are bacteriostatic but may be bactericidal against certain organisms. They bind reversibly to 30S and 50S ribosomal subunits, which inhibits bacterial protein synthesis.

Susceptible gram-positive organisms include *Bacillus anthracis, Actinomyces*

israelii, Clostridium perfringens and
C. tetani, Listeria monocytogenes, and
Nocardia.

Susceptible gram-negative organisms
include *Neisseria meningitidis, Pasteurella
multocida, Legionella pneumophila,
Brucella, Vibrio cholerae, Yersinia ente-
rocolitica, Yersinia pestis, Bordetella pertussis, Haemophilus influenzae, H. ducreyi,
Campylobacter fetus, Shigella,* and many
other common pathogens.

Other susceptible organisms include
Rickettsia akari, R. typhi, R. prowazekii,
and *R. tsutsugamushi; Coxiella burnetii;
Chlamydia trachomatis* and *C. psittaci;
Mycoplasma pneumoniae* and *M. hominis;
Leptospira; Treponema pallidum* and
T. pertenue; and *Borrelia recurrentis.*

ADVERSE REACTIONS
The most common adverse effects involve
the GI tract and are dose related; they
include abdominal discomfort; anorexia;
bulky, loose stools; colitis; epigastric
burning; flatulence; nausea; and vomiting.
Superinfections also are common.

Photosensitivity reactions may be severe.
Renal failure may be caused by Fanconi
syndrome after use of outdated tetracycline.
Permanent discoloration of teeth occurs
if drug is given during tooth formation in
children younger than age 8.

CONTRAINDICATIONS & CAUTIONS
• Contraindicated in patients hypersensitive
to these drugs.
• Use cautiously in patients with renal or
hepatic impairment.
• In pregnant or breast-feeding women, use
is contraindicated; tetracyclines appear in
breast milk. Children younger than age 8
shouldn't take tetracyclines; these drugs
can cause permanent tooth discoloration,
enamel hypoplasia, and a reversible decrease in bone calcification. Elderly patients
may have decreased esophageal motility;
use these drugs cautiously, and monitor patients for local irritation from slow passage
of oral forms. Elderly patients also are more
susceptible to superinfection.

Thrombolytics
alteplase
reteplase
tenecteplase

INDICATIONS
➤ To dissolve a preexisting clot or
thrombus, often in acute or emergency
situations
➤ Acute MI, acute ischemic stroke,
pulmonary embolism, and peripheral
vascular occlusion; restore patency to
clotted grafts and I.V. access devices
(alteplase); acute MI (reteplase and
tenecteplase)

ACTION
Thrombolytics convert plasminogen to
plasmin, which lyses thrombi; fibrinogen;
and other plasma proteins.

ADVERSE REACTIONS
The most common adverse reactions are
bleeding and allergic responses. Other adverse reactions common to all are flushing,
headache, musculoskeletal pain, nausea, and
hypotension.

CONTRAINDICATIONS & CAUTIONS
• Contraindicated in patients hypersensitive
to any of the drug components.
• Contraindicated in active bleeding,
history of stroke, recent intracranial or
intraspinal surgery or trauma, intracranial
neoplasm, arteriovenous malformation or
aneurysm, bleeding diathesis, or severe
uncontrolled hypertension.

Vasopressors
DOBUTamine hydrochloride
DOPamine hydrochloride
ephedrine sulfate
norepinephrine bitartrate

INDICATIONS
➤ Correction of hemodynamic imbalances present in cardiogenic shock due
to MI, trauma, septicemia, cardiac
surgical procedures, spinal anesthesia,

drug reactions, renal failure, and heart failure
➤ Stokes-Adams syndrome with complete heart block, narcolepsy, and myasthenia gravis (ephedrine sulfate)

ACTION
Dobutamine is a direct-acting inotrope whose primary activity results from stimulation of the beta receptors of the heart while producing mild chronotropic, hypertensive, arrhythmogenic, and vasodilatory effects. Dobutamine increases cardiac output by decreasing peripheral vascular resistance, reducing ventricular filling pressure, and increasing AV node conduction. Dopamine is a natural catecholamine, a precursor to norephinephrine in noradrenergic nerves, and a neurotransmitter in certain areas of the central nervous system. It produces positive chronotropic and inotropic effects on the myocardium, resulting in increased heart rate and cardiac contractility. This is accomplished by directly exerting an agonist action on beta-adrenoreceptors.

ADVERSE REACTIONS
Adverse reactions to vasopressors may include ventricular arrhythmias, tachycardia, angina, palpitations, cardiac conduction abnormalities, widened QRS complex, bradycardia, hypotension, hypertension, vasoconstriction, headache, anxiety, azotemia, dyspnea, phlebitis, peripheral cyanosis, and gangrene of extremities. Difficult or painful urination can be seen with ephedrine. Less common are hypotension, thrombocytopenia, hypokalemia, nausea, and shortness of breath.

CONTRAINDICATIONS & CAUTIONS
Black Box Warning Refer to individual drug monographs for black box warnings. ∎
• Contraindicated in patients hypersensitive to any of the drug components.
• Contraindicated in patients with pheochromocytoma, uncorrected tachyarrhythmias, or ventricular fibrillation.
• Dobutamine is contraindicated in idiopathic hypertropic subaortic stenosis.
• Before treatment, hypovolemia should be corrected.

• Some vasopressors must be used cautiously in patients with a sulfite allergy, particularly asthmatic patients. Allergic-type reactions, including anaphylactic symptoms and severe asthmatic episodes, can occur.
• Infusion should be given into a large vein to prevent extravasation into surrounding tissue because this can cause tissue necrosis.
• Patients taking MAO inhibitors or who have been treated with MAO inhibitors 2 to 3 weeks before infusion will require substantially reduced dosage of dopamine.
• Norephinephrine bitartrate shouldn't be used during cyclopropane and halothane anesthesia because of the risk of ventricular tachycardia or fibrillation.
• Use cautiously in patients with hyperthyroidism, bradycardia, partial heart block, myocardial disease, or severe arteriosclerosis.
• Give these drugs to pregnant women only if clearly indicated. Use caution when giving these drugs to breast-feeding women. Safety and effectiveness in children haven't been established.

Xanthine derivatives
theophylline

INDICATIONS
➤ Asthma and bronchospasm from emphysema and chronic bronchitis

ACTION
Xanthine derivatives are structurally related; they directly relax smooth muscle, stimulate the CNS, induce diuresis, increase gastric acid secretion, inhibit uterine contractions, and exert weak inotropic and chronotropic effects on the heart. Of these drugs, theophylline exerts the greatest effect on smooth muscle.

The action of xanthine derivatives isn't completely caused by inhibition of phosphodiesterase. Current data suggest that inhibition of adenosine receptors or unidentified mechanisms may be responsible for therapeutic effects. By relaxing smooth muscle of the respiratory tract, they increase airflow and vital capacity. They also slow onset of diaphragmatic fatigue and stimulate the respiratory center in the CNS.

ADVERSE REACTIONS

Adverse effects, except for hypersensitivity, are dose related and can be controlled by dosage adjustment. Common reactions include arrhythmias, headache, hypotension, irritability, nausea, palpitations, restlessness, urine retention, and vomiting.

CONTRAINDICATIONS & CAUTIONS

● Contraindicated in patients hypersensitive to these drugs.

● Use cautiously in patients with arrhythmias, cardiac or circulatory impairment, cor pulmonale, hepatic or renal disease, active peptic ulcers, hyperthyroidism, or diabetes mellitus.

● In pregnant women, use cautiously. In breast-feeding women, avoid these drugs because they appear in breast milk, and infants may have serious adverse reactions. Small children may have excessive CNS stimulation; monitor them closely. In elderly patients, use cautiously.

abacavir sulfate
ah-BAK-ah-veer

Ziagen

Therapeutic class: Antiretrovirals
Pharmacologic class: Nucleoside
and nucleotide reverse transcriptase
inhibitors
Pregnancy risk category: C

AVAILABLE FORMS
Oral solution: 20 mg/mL
Tablets: 300 mg

INDICATIONS & DOSAGES
➤ **HIV-1 infection**
Adults: 300 mg P.O. b.i.d. or 600 mg P.O.
daily with other antiretrovirals.
Children ages 3 months to 16 years: Give
8 mg/kg P.O. b.i.d., up to maximum of
300 mg P.O. b.i.d., with other antiretrovirals.
Adjust-a-dose: In patients with mild hepatic
impairment (Child-Pugh score 5 to 6), give
200 mg (oral solution) P.O. b.i.d. Don't use
in patients with moderate to severe hepatic
impairment.

ADMINISTRATION
P.O.
• Always give drug with other antiretrovi-
rals, never alone.
• Patient may take drug with or without food.

ACTION
Converted intracellularly to the active
metabolite carbovir triphosphate, which
inhibits activity of HIV-1 reverse transcriptase, terminating viral DNA growth.

Route	Onset	Peak	Duration
P.O.	Unknown	Unknown	Unknown

Half-life: 1 to 2 hours.

ADVERSE REACTIONS
CNS: fever, headache, insomnia and sleep
disorders, anxiety, depressive disorders,
malaise, fatigue, dizziness.
EENT: ear, nose, and throat infections.
GI: anorexia, diarrhea, nausea, vomiting.
Hepatic: *lactic acidosis.*
Skin: rash.

Other: *hypersensitivity reaction,* redistri-
bution/accumulation of body fat.

INTERACTIONS
Drug-lifestyle. *Alcohol use:* May decrease
elimination of drug, increasing overall
exposure. Monitor alcohol consumption.
Discourage use together.

EFFECTS ON LAB TEST RESULTS
• May increase ALT, AST, glucose, and
triglyceride levels.

CONTRAINDICATIONS & CAUTIONS
Black Box Warning Patients who carry
the HLA-B*5701 allele are at high risk for
hypersensitivity reactions; patients should
be screened prior to beginning therapy. ∎
• Contraindicated in patients hypersensitive
to drug or its components.
• Contraindicated in patients with moderate
to severe hepatic impairment.
Black Box Warning Due to increased risk
of hepatotoxicity, use cautiously when
giving drug to patients at risk for liver
disease. Lactic acidosis and severe hepatomegaly with steatosis, including fatal cases,
have been reported with the use of nucleoside analogues alone or in combination, including abacavir and other antiretrovirals.
Stop treatment with drug if events occur. ∎
• Use cautiously in pregnant women because the effects are unknown. Use during
pregnancy only if the potential benefits outweigh the risk. Register pregnant women
with the Antiretroviral Pregnancy Registry
at 1-800-258-4263.

NURSING CONSIDERATIONS
• Women are more likely than men to
experience lactic acidosis and severe
hepatomegaly with steatosis. Obesity and
prolonged nucleoside exposure may be risk
factors.
Black Box Warning Drug can cause fatal
hypersensitivity reactions; if patient develops signs or symptoms of hypersensitivity
(such as fever, rash, fatigue, achiness, generalized malaise, nausea, vomiting, diarrhea, abdominal pain, cough, dyspnea, or
pharyngitis), stop drug and notify prescriber
immediately. ∎

Black Box Warning Don't restart drug or any abacavir-containing product after a hypersensitivity reaction because severe signs and symptoms will recur within hours and may include life-threatening hypotension and death. To facilitate reporting of hypersensitivity reactions, register patients with the Abacavir Hypersensitivity Registry at 1-800-270-0425. ∎

• Because of a high rate of early virologic resistance, triple antiretroviral therapy with abacavir, lamivudine, and tenofovir shouldn't be used as a new treatment regimen for treatment-naive or pretreated patients. Monitor patients currently controlled with this combination and those who use this combination in addition to other antiretrovirals, and consider modification of therapy.

• Drug may mildly elevate glucose level.

• *Look alike–sound alike:* Don't confuse abacavir with amprenavir.

PATIENT TEACHING

• Inform patient that drug can cause a life-threatening hypersensitivity reaction. Warn patient who develops signs or symptoms of hypersensitivity (such as fever, rash, severe tiredness, achiness, a generally ill feeling, nausea, vomiting, diarrhea, stomach pain, cough, shortness of breath, or sore throat) to stop taking drug and notify prescriber immediately.

• Include information leaflet about drug with each new prescription and refill. Patient also should receive, and be instructed to carry, a warning card summarizing signs and symptoms of hypersensitivity.

• Inform patient that this drug doesn't cure HIV infection. Tell patient that drug doesn't reduce the risk of transmission of HIV to others through sexual contact or blood contamination and that its long-term effects are unknown.

• Tell patient to take drug exactly as prescribed with or without food.

abatacept
uh-BAY-tuh-sept

Orencia

Therapeutic class: Antiarthritics
Pharmacologic class: Immunomodulators
Pregnancy risk category: C

AVAILABLE FORMS
Lyophilized powder for injection: 250 mg single-use vial (25 mg/mL when reconstituted)
Solution for subcutaneous administration: 125 mg/mL

INDICATIONS & DOSAGES
➤ **To reduce signs and symptoms, induce major clinical response, inhibit disease progression and structural damage, and improve physical function in patients with moderate to severe rheumatoid arthritis whose response to one or more disease-modifying antirheumatic drugs (DMARDs) has been inadequate. Used alone or with other DMARDs (except TNF antagonists and anakinra)**
Adults weighing more than 100 kg (220 lb): 1 g I.V. over 30 minutes. Repeat 2 and 4 weeks after initial infusion and then every 4 weeks thereafter.
Adults weighing 60 to 100 kg (132 to 220 lb): 750 mg I.V. over 30 minutes. Repeat 2 and 4 weeks after initial infusion and then every 4 weeks thereafter.
Adults weighing less than 60 kg: 500 mg I.V. over 30 minutes. Repeat 2 and 4 weeks after initial infusion and then every 4 weeks thereafter.
Adults (subcutaneous): Give a single I.V. loading dose based on weight. Then give 125 mg subcutaneously within a day, followed by 125 mg subcutaneously once weekly. Patients unable to receive infusion may start weekly subcutaneous dosing without I.V. loading dose. Patients transferring from I.V. to subcutaneous form should receive the first subcutaneous dose instead of the next scheduled I.V. dose.

Reactions in bold italics are *life-threatening*. Interactions may have a *rapid onset* or a *delayed onset*.

➤ As monotherapy or with methotrexate to reduce signs and symptoms of moderately to severely active juvenile idiopathic arthritis

Children ages 6 to 17 weighing less than 75 kg (165 lb): 10 mg/kg I.V. over 30 minutes. Repeat 2 and 4 weeks after initial infusion and then every 4 weeks thereafter. Maximum dose is 1,000 mg.

Children ages 6 to 17 weighing 75 kg or more: Utilize adult dosing.

ADMINISTRATION

I.V.

▼ Reconstitute vial with 10 mL of sterile water for injection, using only the silicone-free disposable syringe provided, to yield 25 mg/mL. Use an 18G to 21G needle for preparation.

▼ Gently swirl contents until completely dissolved. Avoid vigorous shaking.

▼ Vent the vial with a needle to clear away foam.

▼ The solution should be clear and colorless to pale yellow.

▼ Further dilute the solution to 100 mL with normal saline solution. Infuse over 30 minutes using an infusion set and a sterile, nonpyrogenic, low–protein-binding filter.

▼ Store diluted solution at room temperature or refrigerate at 36° to 46° F (2° to 8° C). Complete infusion within 24 hours of reconstituting.

▼ **Incompatibilities:** Don't infuse in the same line with other I.V. drugs.

Subcutaneous

● Abatacept 125-mg/mL syringe isn't intended for I.V. administration.

● Abatacept should be clear and colorless to pale yellow; don't use if you observe particulate matter or discoloration.

● Rotate injection sites.

● Never inject into tender, bruised, or hard areas.

ACTION

Inhibits T-cell activation, decreases T-cell proliferation, and inhibits production of TNF-alpha, interferon-gamma, and interleukin-2.

Route	Onset	Peak	Duration
I.V., subcut.	Unknown	Unknown	Unknown

Half-life: I.V., 13 days; subcutaneous, 14.3 days.

ADVERSE REACTIONS

CNS: headache, dizziness.
CV: hypertension.
EENT: nasopharyngitis, rhinitis, sinusitis.
GI: nausea, diverticulitis, dyspepsia.
GU: acute pyelonephritis, UTI.
Musculoskeletal: back pain, limb pain.
Respiratory: upper respiratory tract infection, bronchitis, cough, pneumonia.
Skin: cellulitis, rash.
Other: infections, *malignancies,* herpes simplex, influenza, infusion reactions, injection-site reaction.

INTERACTIONS

Drug-drug. *Anakinra, TNF antagonists:* May increase risk of infection. Don't use together.
Live-virus vaccines: May decrease effectiveness of vaccine. Avoid giving vaccines during or for 3 months after abatacept therapy.

EFFECTS ON LAB TEST RESULTS

● GDH-PQQ (glucose dehydrogenase pyrroloquinoline quinone)–based glucose monitoring systems may react with maltose present in abatacept, causing falsely elevated blood glucose readings on the day of infusion (I.V. form only).

CONTRAINDICATIONS & CAUTIONS

● Contraindicated in patients hypersensitive to drug or its components.

● Don't use in patients taking a TNF antagonist or anakinra.

● Use cautiously in patients with active infection, history of chronic infections, scheduled elective surgery, or COPD.

● Patients should be screened for viral hepatitis before starting therapy. Antirheumatic treatment may cause reactivation of hepatitis B.

● Patients who test positive for tuberculosis should be treated before receiving drug.

NURSING CONSIDERATIONS

● Make sure patient has been screened for tuberculosis before giving.
● Monitor patient, especially an older adult, carefully for infections and malignancies.
● If patient develops a severe infection, notify prescriber; therapy may need to be stopped.
❸ *Alert:* If patient has COPD, watch for worsening.
● Drug may cause serious adverse reactions in a breast-fed infant and may affect his developing immune system.
● Ensure the availability of appropriate supportive measures to treat possible hypersensitivity reactions.
● *Look alike–sound alike:* Don't confuse Orencia with Oracea.

PATIENT TEACHING

● Instruct patient to have tuberculosis screening before therapy.
● Tell patient to continue taking prescribed arthritis drugs. Caution against taking TNF antagonists, such as etanercept, infliximab, and adalimumab, or anakinra.
● Tell patient to avoid exposure to infections.
● Tell patient to immediately report signs and symptoms of infection, swollen face or tongue, and difficulty breathing.
● Tell patient with COPD to report worsening signs and symptoms.
● Advise patient to avoid live-virus vaccines during and for 3 months after therapy.
● Advise woman to consult prescriber if she becomes pregnant or plans to breast-feed.
● Advise patient to contact prescriber before taking any other drugs or herbal supplements.
● Remind patient to contact prescriber before scheduling surgery.

SAFETY ALERT!

abciximab
ab-SIX-ah-mab

ReoPro

Therapeutic class: Antiplatelet drugs
Pharmacologic class: Glycoprotein IIb/IIIa inhibitors
Pregnancy risk category: C

AVAILABLE FORMS
Injection: 2 mg/mL

INDICATIONS & DOSAGES

➤ **Adjunct to percutaneous coronary intervention (PCI) to prevent acute cardiac ischemic complications**
Adults: 0.25 mg/kg as an I.V. bolus given 10 to 60 minutes before start of PCI; then, a continuous I.V. infusion of 0.125 mcg/kg/minute to maximum 10 mcg/minute for 12 hours.
➤ **Unstable angina not responding to conventional medical therapy in patients scheduled for PCI within 24 hours**
Adults: 0.25 mg/kg as an I.V. bolus; then an 18- to 24-hour infusion of 10 mcg/minute concluding 1 hour after PCI.
➤ **Before PCI in patients with ST-segment elevation MI ◆**
Adults: 0.25 mg/kg as an I.V. bolus 10 to 60 minutes before start of PCI; then, a continuous I.V. infusion of 0.125 mcg/kg/minute to maximum of 10 mcg/minute for 12 hours.

ADMINISTRATION
I.V.
▼ Give drug in a separate I.V. line. Don't add other drugs to infusion solution.
▼ Inspect solution for particulate matter before administration. If opaque particles are visible, discard solution and obtain new vial.
▼ For bolus, withdraw needed amount of drug through a low–protein-binding 0.2- or 5-micron syringe filter.
▼ Give bolus 10 to 60 minutes before procedure.
▼ For continuous infusion, filter drug either by withdrawing needed amount

---

Reactions in bold italics are *life-threatening*. Interactions may have a *rapid onset* or a *delayed onset*.

of drug through a low–protein-binding 0.2- or 5-micron syringe filter into a syringe or by infusing with a continuous infusion set equipped with a low–protein-binding 0.2 or 0.22-micron in-line filter. Use normal saline solution or D_5W.

▼ Infuse at 0.125 mcg/kg/minute (maximum, 10 mcg/minute) for 12 hours via a continuous infusion pump.

▼ Discard unused portion after 12-hour infusion.

▼ **Incompatibilities:** None reported.

ACTION

Binds to the glycoprotein IIb/IIIa receptor of human platelets and inhibits platelet aggregation.

Route	Onset	Peak	Duration
I.V.	Immediate	Immediate	48 hr

Half-life: 10 to 30 minutes.

ADVERSE REACTIONS

CNS: headache, pain, dizziness, anxiety, abnormal thinking.
CV: hypotension, *bradycardia,* chest pain, peripheral edema, *ventricular tachycardia.*
GI: nausea, abdominal pain, vomiting, dyspepsia, diarrhea.
Hematologic: *bleeding, thrombocytopenia,* anemia.
Musculoskeletal: back pain.
Skin: increased sweating.

INTERACTIONS

Drug-drug. *Antiplatelet drugs, dipyridamole, heparin, NSAIDs, other anticoagulants, thrombolytics, ticlopidine:* May increase risk of bleeding. Monitor patient closely.
Direct factor Xa inhibitors (rivaroxaban), thrombin inhibitors (dabigatran, desirudin): May increase bleeding risk. Don't use together.

EFFECTS ON LAB TEST RESULTS

● May decrease hemoglobin level.
● May decrease platelet count.

CONTRAINDICATIONS & CAUTIONS

● Contraindicated in patients hypersensitive to drug, its ingredients, or murine proteins.

● Contraindicated in those with active internal bleeding, significant GI or GU bleeding within 6 weeks, stroke within past 2 years, or significant residual neurologic deficit, bleeding diathesis, thrombocytopenia (platelet count lower than $100,000/mm^3$), major surgery or trauma within 6 weeks, intracranial neoplasm, intracranial arteriovenous malformation, intracranial aneurysm, severe uncontrolled hypertension, or history of vasculitis.

● Contraindicated when oral anticoagulants have been given within past 7 days unless PT is 1.2 times control or less, or when I.V. dextran is used before or during PCI.

● Use with caution in patients at increased risk for bleeding, including those who weigh less than 75 kg (165 lb) or who are older than age 65, those who have a history of GI disease, and those who are receiving thrombolytics. Conditions that increase patient's risk of bleeding include PCI within 12 hours of onset of symptoms for acute MI, prolonged PCI (lasting longer than 70 minutes), or failed PCI. Heparin use may also increase the risk of bleeding.

NURSING CONSIDERATIONS

● The risk of bleeding is reduced by using low-dose, weight-adjusted heparin; early sheath removal; and careful maintenance of access site immobility.

● Drug is intended for use with aspirin and heparin; review and monitor other drugs patient is taking.

● **Alert:** Keep epinephrine, dopamine, theophylline, antihistamines, and corticosteroids readily available in case of anaphylaxis.

● Monitor patient closely for bleeding at the arterial access site used for cardiac catheterization and internal bleeding involving the GI or GU tract or retroperitoneal sites.

● Institute bleeding precautions. Keep patient on bed rest for 6 to 8 hours after sheath removal or end of drug infusion, whichever is later. Minimize arterial and venous punctures, I.M. injections, urinary catheters, nasogastric tubes, automatic blood pressure cuffs, and nasotracheal intubation; avoid, if possible.

● During infusion, remove sheath only after heparin has been stopped and its effects largely reversed.

• Before treatment, obtain platelet count, PT, activated clotting time, and activated PTT.

• Monitor platelet count closely. Obtain levels 2 to 4 hours after bolus dose, and 24 hours after bolus dose or before discharge, whichever is first.

• Anticipate stopping drug and giving platelets for severe bleeding or thrombocytopenia.

• *Look alike–sound alike:* Don't confuse abciximab with infliximab.

PATIENT TEACHING

• Explain use and administration of drug to patient and family.

• Instruct patient to report adverse reactions immediately.

SAFETY ALERT!

abiraterone acetate
a-by-RAY-ter-own

Zytiga

Therapeutic class: Antineoplastics
Pharmacologic class: Androgen biosynthesis inhibitors
Pregnancy risk category: X

AVAILABLE FORMS
Tablets: 250 mg

INDICATIONS & DOSAGES
➤ **Metastatic, castration-resistant prostate cancer in combination with prednisone**
Adult men: 1,000 mg P.O. once daily. Use in combination with 5 mg prednisone P.O. b.i.d.
Adjust-a-dose: For patients with baseline moderate hepatic impairment (Child-Pugh class B), reduce starting dosage to 250 mg P.O. once daily. If ALT or AST level increases to more than 5 times the upper limit of normal (ULN) or total bilirubin level increases to more than 3 times ULN, discontinue drug and don't restart. If hepatotoxicity develops during treatment (ALT or AST level greater than 5 times ULN or total bilirubin level greater than 3 times ULN), stop drug. Restart at 750 mg once

daily after LFTs have shown a return to patient's baseline or the AST or ALT level is 2.5 times ULN or lower and total bilirubin level is 1.5 times ULN or lower. If hepatotoxicity recurs at a dosage of 750 mg once daily, stop drug and restart at 500 mg once daily using liver function guidelines above. Discontinue drug if hepatotoxicity recurs at the 500-mg once-daily dosage. Monitor liver function at least every 2 weeks for 3 months and monthly thereafter. Safety of abiraterone retreatment in patients who develop an AST or ALT level 20 times ULN or more or bilirubin level 10 times ULN or more is unknown.

ADMINISTRATION
P.O.
• Give tablets on an empty stomach; patient shouldn't eat for 2 hours before or 1 hour after receiving drug.

• Patient should swallow tablets whole with water.

• Store tablets at room temperature.

• Women who are pregnant or may become pregnant should wear gloves when handling tablets.

ACTION
Inhibits biosynthesis of androgen production and increases mineralocorticoid production by the adrenal glands.

Route	Onset	Peak	Duration
P.O.	Rapid	2 hr	Unknown

Half-life: 12 hours.

ADVERSE REACTIONS
CV: edema, hot flushes, hypertension, *arrhythmias,* chest pain, *cardiac failure.*
GI: diarrhea, dyspepsia.
GU: UTI, urinary frequency, nocturia.
Hepatic: *hepatotoxicity.*
Metabolic: *hypokalemia, hypophosphatemia.*
Musculoskeletal: joint swelling, joint discomfort, muscle discomfort.
Respiratory: upper respiratory tract infection, cough.

INTERACTIONS
Drug-drug. *Dextromethorphan, thioridazine, other CYP2D6 substrates:* May

---

Reactions in bold italics are *life-threatening*. Interactions may have a *rapid onset* or a *delayed onset*.

inhibit metabolism of these drugs, causing higher levels. Avoid using together. If drugs must be used together, consider reducing dosage of CYP2D6 substrate drug.

Strong CYP3A4 inducers (such as carbamazepine, phenobarbital, phenytoin, rifabutin, rifampin, rifapentine) or inhibitors (such as atazanavir, clarithromycin, indinavir, itraconazole, ketoconazole, nefazodone, nelfinavir, ritonavir, saquinavir, telithromycin, voriconazole): Use together hasn't been studied. Avoid concomitant use if possible. If drugs must be used together, administer with caution and monitor patient closely.

EFFECTS ON LAB TEST RESULTS
• May increase ALT, AST, bilirubin, and triglyceride levels.
• May decrease potassium, phosphate, and serum testosterone and other androgen levels.

CONTRAINDICATIONS & CAUTIONS
• Contraindicated in patients hypersensitive to drug or its components and in those with baseline severe hepatic impairment (Child-Pugh class C).
• Use cautiously in patients with a history of CV disease (congestive heart failure, recent MI, ventricular arrhythmias) or liver disease.
• Safety in patients with left ventricular ejection fraction of less than 50% or New York Heart Association Class III or IV heart failure hasn't been established.
• Because drug may harm a developing fetus, women who are pregnant or may become pregnant shouldn't handle drug without protection (gloves). It isn't known if drug or its metabolites are present in semen.

NURSING CONSIDERATIONS
• Monitor ALT, AST, and bilirubin levels in all patients at baseline, every 2 weeks for first 3 months, then monthly thereafter. For patients with moderate hepatic impairment, measure at baseline, every week during first month of treatment, every 2 weeks for next 2 months, and monthly thereafter.
• Monitor LFTs frequently for elevated results and signs and symptoms of hepato-toxicity (malaise, jaundice, abdominal pain, nausea, and vomiting).
• Monitor patient with a history of CV disease at least monthly for hypertension, hypokalemia, and fluid retention. Control hypertension and correct hypokalemia before and during treatment.
• Monitor patient for signs and symptoms of adrenocortical insufficiency (chronic fatigue, loss of appetite, muscle weakness, weight loss, nausea, and vomiting). Patient may need an increased corticosteroid dosage before, during, and after stressful situations.
• *Look alike–sound alike:* Don't confuse Zytiga with Jevtana, Xgeva, Xtandi, or Zometa.

PATIENT TEACHING
• Teach patient to take drug on an empty stomach 2 hours before or 1 hour after a meal and to swallow tablets whole with water.
• Instruct patient that abiraterone and prednisone must be used together.
• Warn patient not to stop abiraterone, prednisone, or other chemotherapy drugs without consulting prescriber.
• Advise patient that if he misses a single dose of abiraterone or prednisone, he should take the regular dose the next day. If he misses more than one dose, he should inform his prescriber.
• Teach patient that periodic blood tests will be needed to monitor tolerance to therapy.
• Warn patient, female caregivers, and female sexual partners about risk of fetal harm from abiraterone therapy. Teach women who are pregnant or may become pregnant to wear gloves while handling drug.
• Teach patient and female sexual partners the importance of using condoms. Patient should use a condom and another effective birth control method if his partner is pregnant or of childbearing potential. Inform patient that these protective measures are required during treatment and for 1 week after treatment has ended.

acamprosate calcium
a-kam-PRO-sate

Campral◆

Therapeutic class: Alcohol deterrents
Pharmacologic class: Synthetic amino acid neurotransmitter analogues
Pregnancy risk category: C

AVAILABLE FORMS
Tablets (delayed-release): 333 mg

INDICATIONS & DOSAGES
➤ **Adjunct to management of alcohol abstinence**
Adults: 666 mg P.O. t.i.d.
Adjust-a-dose: In patients with CrCl of 30 to 50 mL/minute, give 333 mg t.i.d. Do not use in patients with severe renal impairment (CrCl 30 mL/minute or less).

ADMINISTRATION
P.O.
• Don't crush or break tablets.
• Give drug without regard for food.

ACTION
Restores the balance of neuronal excitation and inhibition, probably by interacting with glutamate and GABA neurotransmitter systems, thus reducing alcohol dependence.

Route	Onset	Peak	Duration
P.O.	Unknown	3–8 hr	Unknown

Half-life: 20 to 33 hours.

ADVERSE REACTIONS
CNS: abnormal thinking, amnesia, anxiety, asthenia, depression, dizziness, headache, insomnia, paresthesia, somnolence, *suicidal thoughts,* syncope, tremor, pain.
CV: hypertension, palpitations, peripheral edema, vasodilation.
EENT: abnormal vision, pharyngitis, rhinitis.
GI: abdominal pain, anorexia, constipation, diarrhea, dry mouth, dyspepsia, flatulence, increased appetite, nausea, taste disturbance, vomiting.
GU: erectile dysfunction.

Metabolic: weight gain.
Musculoskeletal: arthralgia, back pain, chest pain, myalgia.
Respiratory: bronchitis, dyspnea, increased cough.
Skin: increased sweating, pruritus, rash.
Other: accidental injury, chills, decreased libido, flulike symptoms, infection.

INTERACTIONS
None significant.

EFFECTS ON LAB TEST RESULTS
• May increase ALT, AST, bilirubin, blood glucose, and uric acid levels. May decrease hemoglobin level and hematocrit.
• May decrease platelet count.

CONTRAINDICATIONS & CAUTIONS
• Contraindicated in patients allergic to drug or its components and in those with CrCl of 30 mL/minute or less.
• Use cautiously in pregnant or breast-feeding women, elderly patients, patients with moderate renal impairment, and patients with a history of depression and suicidal thoughts or attempts.
⚠ **Overdose S&S:** Diarrhea, hypercalcemia in chronic overdose.

NURSING CONSIDERATIONS
• Use only after the patient successfully becomes abstinent from drinking.
• Drug doesn't eliminate or reduce withdrawal symptoms.
• Monitor patient for development of depression or suicidal thoughts.
• Drug doesn't cause alcohol aversion or a disulfiram-like reaction if used with alcohol.

PATIENT TEACHING
• Tell patient to continue the alcohol abstinence program, including counseling and support.
• Advise patient to notify his prescriber if he develops depression, anxiety, thoughts of suicide, or severe diarrhea.
• Caution patient's family or caregiver to watch for signs of depression or suicidal ideation.
• Tell patient that drug may be taken without regard to meals, but that taking it with meals may help him remember it.

Reactions in bold italics are *life-threatening*. Interactions may have a *rapid onset* or a *delayed onset*.

• Tell patient not to crush, break, or chew the tablets but to swallow them whole.
• Advise women to use effective contraception while taking this drug. Tell patient to contact her prescriber if she becomes pregnant or plans to become pregnant.
• Explain that this drug may impair judgment, thinking, or motor skills. Urge patient to use caution when driving or performing hazardous activities until drug's effects are known.
• Tell patient to continue taking acamprosate and to contact his prescriber if he resumes drinking alcohol.

SAFETY ALERT!

acarbose
a-KAR-boz

Glucobay†, Precose

Therapeutic class: Antidiabetics
Pharmacologic class: Alpha-glucosidase inhibitors
Pregnancy risk category: B

AVAILABLE FORMS
Tablets: 25 mg, 50 mg, 100 mg

INDICATIONS & DOSAGES
➤ **Adjunct to diet and exercise or, with a sulfonylurea, metformin, or insulin, to lower glucose level in patients with type 2 diabetes**
Adults: Individualized. Initially, 25 mg P.O. t.i.d. with first bite of each main meal. Adjust dosage every 4 to 8 weeks, based on 1-hour postprandial glucose level or glycosylated hemoglobin levels and tolerance. Maintenance dosage is 50 to 100 mg P.O. t.i.d. To minimize GI adverse effects, may initiate treatment at 25 mg P.O. once daily and increase to 25 mg P.O. t.i.d. For patients who weigh less than 60 kg (132 lb), don't exceed 50 mg P.O. t.i.d. For patients who weigh more than 60 kg, don't exceed 100 mg P.O. t.i.d.

ADMINISTRATION
P.O.
• Give dose with first bite of each main meal.

ACTION
Delays digestion of carbohydrates, resulting in a smaller increase in glucose level after meals.

Route	Onset	Peak	Duration
P.O.	Unknown	1 hr	2–4 hr

Half-life: 2 hours.

ADVERSE REACTIONS
GI: abdominal pain, diarrhea, flatulence.

INTERACTIONS
Drug-drug. *Calcium channel blockers, corticosteroids, estrogens, fosphenytoin, hormonal contraceptives, isoniazid, nicotinic acid, phenothiazine, phenytoin, sympathomimetics, thiazides and other diuretics, thyroid products:* May lead to loss of glucose control or cause hypoglycemia when withdrawn. Monitor glucose level.
Digestive enzyme preparations containing carbohydrate-splitting enzymes (such as amylase, pancreatin), intestinal adsorbents (such as activated charcoal): May reduce effect of acarbose. Avoid using together.
Digoxin: May reduce digoxin level. Monitor digoxin level.

EFFECTS ON LAB TEST RESULTS
• May increase ALT and AST levels.
May decrease calcium, vitamin B_6, and hematocrit.

CONTRAINDICATIONS & CAUTIONS
• Contraindicated in patients hypersensitive to drug and in those with diabetic ketoacidosis, cirrhosis, inflammatory bowel disease, colonic ulceration, renal impairment, partial intestinal obstruction, predisposition to intestinal obstruction, chronic intestinal disease with marked disorder of digestion or absorption, or conditions that may deteriorate because of increased intestinal gas formation.
• Contraindicated in pregnant or breastfeeding women and those with creatinine level greater than 2 mg/dL.
• Use cautiously in patients receiving a sulfonylurea or insulin.
• Safety and effectiveness of drug haven't been established in children.

⚠ *Overdose S&S:* Transient increases in flatulence, diarrhea, and abdominal discomfort.

NURSING CONSIDERATIONS

• Closely monitor patients receiving a sulfonylurea or insulin; drug may increase risk of hypoglycemia. If hypoglycemia occurs, give oral glucose (dextrose). Severe hypoglycemia may require I.V. glucose infusion or glucagon administration. Because dosage adjustments may be needed to prevent further hypoglycemia, report hypoglycemia and treatment required to prescriber.

• Insulin therapy may be needed during increased stress (infection, fever, surgery, or trauma). Monitor patient closely for hyperglycemia.

• Monitor patient's 1-hour postprandial glucose level to determine therapeutic effectiveness of drug and to identify appropriate dose. Report hyperglycemia to prescriber. Thereafter, measure glycosylated hemoglobin level every 3 months.

• Monitor transaminase level every 3 months in first year of therapy and periodically thereafter in patients receiving more than 50 mg t.i.d. Report abnormalities; dosage adjustment or drug withdrawal may be needed.

PATIENT TEACHING

• Tell patient to take drug daily with first bite of each of three main meals.

• Explain that therapy relieves symptoms but doesn't cure disease.

• Stress importance of adhering to therapeutic regimen, specific diet, weight reduction, exercise, and hygiene programs. Show patient how to monitor glucose level and to recognize and treat hyperglycemia.

• Teach patient taking a sulfonylurea how to recognize hypoglycemia. Advise treating symptoms with a form of dextrose rather than with a product containing table sugar.

• Urge patient to wear or carry medical identification at all times.

• Advise patient that adverse reactions usually occur in the first few weeks of therapy and diminish over time.

acetaminophen
(APAP, paracetamol)
a-seet-a-MIN-a-fen

Abenol† ◊, Acephen ◊, ACET† ◊, Aminofen ◊, APAP ◊, Aphen ◊, Aspirin Free Anacin ◊, Atasol† ◊, Cetafen ◊, Ed-APAP Children's ◊, ElixSure ◊, Feverall ◊, Genapap ◊, Infantaire ◊, Mapap ◊, Masophen ◊, Neopap ◊, Nortemp Children's Pain and Fever ◊, Ofirmev, Pediatrix† ◊, Pharbetol, Q-PAP ◊, Quick Melts ◊, Silapap ◊, Tylenol ◊, Valorin ◊

Therapeutic class: Analgesics
Pharmacologic class: Para-aminophenol derivatives
Pregnancy risk category: B

AVAILABLE FORMS
Caplets: 500 mg ◊
Caplets (extended-release): 650 mg ◊
Capsules: 325 mg ◊, 500 mg ◊
Elixir: 80 mg/2.5 mL, 160 mg/5 mL ◊*
Gelcaps: 500 mg ◊
Injection: 10 mg/mL
Oral liquid: 160 mg/5 mL ◊, 167 mg/ 5 mL ◊, 500 mg/5 mL ◊, 500 mg/15 mL ◊
Oral solution: 100 mg/mL ◊
Oral suspension: 80 mg/0.8 mL ◊, 80 mg/mL† ◊, 160 mg/5 mL ◊
Oral syrup: 32 mg/mL† ◊, 80 mg/5 mL† ◊
Suppositories: 80 mg ◊, 120 mg ◊, 325 mg ◊, 650 mg ◊
Tablets: 160 mg ◊, 325 mg ◊, 500 mg ◊, 650 mg ◊
Tablets (chewable): 80 mg ◊, 160 mg ◊, 500 mg ◊
Tablets (dispersible): 80 mg ◊, 160 mg ◊

INDICATIONS & DOSAGES
➤ **Mild pain or fever**
Adults: 325 to 650 mg P.O. every 4 to 6 hours. Or, two extended-release caplets P.O. every 8 hours. Maximum, 4 g daily (immediate-release) or 3 g daily (500-mg strength) or 3.9 g daily (650-mg strength). For long-term therapy, don't exceed 2.6 g daily unless prescribed and monitored closely by health care provider.

Children older than age 12: 325 to 650 mg P.O. every 4 to 6 hours or 1,300 mg P.O. every 8 hours (extended-release) p.r.n.
Children age 12: 640 mg P.O. every 4 to 6 hours p.r.n.
Children age 11 weighing 33 to 43 kg (72 to 95 lb): 480 mg P.O. every 4 to 6 hours p.r.n.
Children ages 9 to 10 weighing 27 to 32 kg (60 to 71 lb): 400 mg P.O. every 4 to 6 hours p.r.n.
Children ages 6 to 8 weighing 22 to 26.8 kg (48 to 59 lb): 320 mg P.O. every 4 to 6 hours p.r.n.
Children ages 4 to 5 weighing 16 to 21 kg (36 to 47 lb): 240 mg P.O. every 4 to 6 hours p.r.n.
Children ages 2 to 3 weighing 11 to 15.9 kg (24 to 35 lb): 160 mg P.O. every 4 to 6 hours p.r.n.

➤ **Arthritis**
Adults: 650 mg P.O. every 8 hours (extended-release). Maximum dose is 3.9 g in 24 hours.

➤ **Mild to moderate pain; mild to moderate pain with adjunctive opioid analgesics; fever**
Adults and children age 13 and older weighing 50 kg (110 lb) or more: 1,000 mg I.V. every 6 hours or 650 mg I.V. every 4 hours. Maximum dose is 1,000 mg as a single dose and 4,000 mg/day.
Adults and children age 13 and older weighing less than 50 kg: 15 mg/kg I.V. every 6 hours or 12.5 mg/kg I.V. every 4 hours. Maximum dose is 15 mg/kg (up to 750 mg) as a single dose and 75 mg/kg (up to 3,750 mg)/day.
Children ages 2 to 12: 15 mg/kg I.V. every 6 hours or 12.5 mg/kg I.V. every 4 hours. Maximum dose is 15 mg/kg as a single dose and 75 mg/kg/day.
Adjust-a-dose: Longer dosing intervals and a reduced total daily dose may be warranted in patients with CrCl of 30 mL/minute or less.

➤ **Mild pain or fever** ◆
P.O.
Children ages 12 to 23 months weighing 8 to 10.5 kg (18 to 23 lb): 120 mg P.O. every 4 to 6 hours p.r.n.
Children ages 4 to 11 months weighing 5.5 to 7.7 kg (12 to 17 lb): 80 mg P.O. every 4 to 6 hours p.r.n.

Children up to age 3 months weighing 2.7 to 5 kg (6 to 11 lb): 40 mg P.O. every 4 to 6 hours p.r.n. Or, 10 to 15 mg/kg/dose every 4 hours p.r.n. Don't exceed five doses in 24 hours.

Rectal
Adults and children older than age 12: 650 mg P.R. every 4 to 6 hours p.r.n. Maximum, 4 g daily. For long-term therapy, don't exceed 2.6 g daily unless prescribed and monitored closely by health care provider.
Children ages 6 to 12: 325 mg P.R. every 4 to 6 hours p.r.n. Maximum dose is 1,950 mg in 24 hours.
Children ages 3 to 6: 120 mg P.R. every 4 to 6 hours p.r.n. Maximum dose is 720 mg in 24 hours.
Children ages 1 to 3: 80 mg P.R. every 4 hours p.r.n. Maximum dose is 480 mg in 24 hours.
Children ages 3 to 11 months: 80 mg P.R. every 6 hours p.r.n.

➤ **Prevention of adverse reactions with diphtheria, tetanus toxoids, and pertussis vaccination** ◆
Children ages 2 months to 6 years: 10 to 15 mg/kg P.O. given with or prior to vaccination and continued for several doses after vaccination.

ADMINISTRATION
P.O.
● Use liquid form for children and patients who have difficulty swallowing.
● Give drug without regard for food.
● Dispersible tablet should be allowed to dissolve in the mouth or should be chewed before swallowing.

I.V.
▼ Examine vial; don't use if particulate matter or discoloration is observed.
▼ For 1,000-mg dose, give by inserting a vented I.V. set through the septum of 100-mL vial.
▼ For doses less than 1,000 mg, withdraw appropriate dose and place into separate container before administration.
▼ Place small-volume pediatric doses of up to 60 mL in a syringe and use a syringe-pump.
▼ May administer without further dilution.
▼ Give over 15 minutes.

▼ Entire 100-mL vial isn't for use in patients weighing less than 50 kg.

▼ Monitor end of infusion to prevent possibility of air embolism.

▼ **Incompatibilities:** Diazepam, chlorpromazine hydrochloride.

Rectal

• If suppository is too soft, refrigerate for 15 minutes or run under cold water in wrapper.

ACTION

Thought to produce analgesia by inhibiting prostaglandin and other substances that sensitize pain receptors. Drug may relieve fever through central action in the hypothalamic heat-regulating center.

Route	Onset	Peak	Duration
P.O., I.V., P.R.	Unknown	½–2 hr	3–4 hr

Half-life: P.O., P.R., 1 to 4 hours; I.V., 2.4 to 7 hours.

ADVERSE REACTIONS

CNS: anxiety, fatigue, headache, insomnia (I.V.).

CV: hypertension, hypotension (I.V.).

GI: nausea, vomiting (I.V.).

Hematologic: hemolytic anemia, *leukopenia, neutropenia, pancytopenia.*

Hepatic: jaundice.

Metabolic: *hypoglycemia; hypokalemia* (I.V.).

Respiratory: abnormal breath sounds, dyspnea (I.V.).

Skin: rash, urticaria; infusion-site pain (I.V.).

INTERACTIONS

Drug-drug. *Barbiturates, carbamazepine, hydantoins, rifampin, sulfinpyrazone:* High doses or long-term use of these drugs may reduce therapeutic effects and enhance hepatotoxic effects of acetaminophen. Avoid using together.

Lamotrigine: May decrease lamotrigine level. Monitor patient for therapeutic effects.

Warfarin: May increase hypoprothrombinemic effects with long-term use with high doses of acetaminophen. Monitor INR closely.

Zidovudine: May decrease zidovudine effect. Monitor patient closely.

Drug-herb. *Watercress:* May inhibit oxidative metabolism of acetaminophen. Discourage use together.

Drug-food. *Caffeine:* May enhance analgesic effects of acetaminophen. Products may combine caffeine and acetaminophen for therapeutic advantage.

Drug-lifestyle. *Alcohol use:* May increase risk of hepatic damage. Discourage use together.

EFFECTS ON LAB TEST RESULTS

• May decrease glucose and hemoglobin levels and hematocrit.

• May decrease neutrophil, WBC, RBC, and platelet counts.

• May cause false-positive test result for urinary 5-hydroxyindoleacetic acid. May falsely decrease glucose level in home monitoring systems.

CONTRAINDICATIONS & CAUTIONS

❸ *Alert:* Drug can cause acute liver failure, which may require a liver transplant or cause death. Most cases of liver injury are associated with drug doses exceeding 4,000 mg/day and often involve more than one acetaminophen-containing product.

❸ *Alert:* May cause serious, potentially fatal skin reactions, including Stevens-Johnson syndrome, toxic epidermal necrolysis, and acute generalized exanthematous pustulosis. Reaction may occur with first or subsequent use when acetaminophen is used as monotherapy or when it is one component of combination drug therapy. Monitor for reddening of the skin, rash, blisters, and detachment of the upper surface of the skin. Stop drug immediately if skin reaction is suspected.

• Contraindicated in patients hypersensitive to drug. I.V. form is contraindicated in patients with severe hepatic impairment or severe active liver disease.

• Use cautiously in patients with any type of liver disease and in patients with long-term alcohol use because therapeutic doses cause hepatotoxicity in these patients. Chronic alcoholics shouldn't take more than 2 g of acetaminophen every 24 hours.

⚠ *Overdose S&S:* Stage 1 (up to 24 hours)—abdominal pain, diaphoresis, nausea, vomiting, malaise, pallor; stage 2 (24 to 36 hours)—right upper quadrant pain, elevated LFT results and PT; stage 3 (72 to 96 hours)—hepatic failure, encephalopathy, coma.

Reactions in bold italics are *life-threatening*. Interactions may have a *rapid onset* or a *delayed onset*.

NURSING CONSIDERATIONS

۞ Alert: Many OTC and prescription products contain acetaminophen; be aware of this when calculating total daily dose.

• In children, don't exceed five doses in 24 hours.

PATIENT TEACHING

• Tell parents to consult prescriber before giving drug to children younger than age 2.

• Advise parents that drug is only for short-term use; urge them to consult prescriber if giving to children for longer than 5 days or adults for longer than 10 days.

۞ Alert: Advise patient or caregiver that many OTC products contain acetaminophen and should be counted when calculating total daily dose.

• Tell patient not to use for marked fever (temperature higher than 103.1° F [39.5° C]), fever persisting longer than 3 days, or recurrent fever unless directed by prescriber.

۞ Alert: Warn patient that high doses or unsupervised long-term use can cause liver damage. Excessive alcohol use may increase the risk of liver damage. Caution long-term alcoholics to limit drug to 2 g/day or less.

• Tell breast-feeding women that drug appears in breast milk in low levels (less than 1% of dose). Drug may be used safely if therapy is short-term and doesn't exceed recommended doses.

۞ Alert: Warn patient to stop drug and seek medical attention immediately if skin rash or reaction occurs while using acetaminophen.

---

acetaZOLAMIDE
ah-set-a-ZOLE-ah-mide

Acetazolam†, Diamox

acetaZOLAMIDE sodium

Therapeutic class: Diuretics
Pharmacologic class: Carbonic anhydrase inhibitors
Pregnancy risk category: C

AVAILABLE FORMS
acetazolamide
Capsules (extended-release): 500 mg
Tablets: 125 mg, 250 mg

acetazolamide sodium
Powder for injection: 500-mg vial

INDICATIONS & DOSAGES

➤ **Secondary glaucoma; preoperative treatment of acute angle-closure glaucoma**
Adults: 250 mg P.O. every 4 hours or 250 mg P.O. b.i.d. for short-term therapy. In acute cases, 500 mg P.O.; then 125 to 250 mg P.O. every 4 hours. Or, for extended-release capsules, 500 mg P.O. b.i.d. To rapidly lower intraocular pressure (IOP), initially, 500 mg I.V.; may repeat in 2 to 4 hours, if needed, followed by 125 to 250 mg P.O. every 4 to 6 hours.

➤ **Chronic open-angle glaucoma**
Adults: 250 mg to 1 g P.O. daily in divided doses q.i.d., or 250 mg I.V. every 4 hours, or 500 mg extended-release P.O. b.i.d.

➤ **To prevent or treat acute mountain sickness (high-altitude sickness)**
Adults and children age 12 and older: 500 mg to 1 g (regular or extended-release) P.O. daily in divided doses every 12 hours. Start 24 to 48 hours before ascent and continue for 48 hours while at high altitude. When rapid ascent is required, start with 1,000 mg P.O. daily.

➤ **Adjunct for epilepsy and myoclonic, refractory, generalized tonic-clonic, absence, or mixed seizures**
Adults: 8 to 30 mg/kg P.O. or I.V. daily in divided doses; 375 mg to 1 g daily is ideal. If given with other anticonvulsants, start at 250 mg P.O. or I.V. once daily, and increase to 375 mg to 1 g daily.

➤ **Edema caused by heart failure; drug-induced edema**
Adults: 250 to 375 mg (5 mg/kg) P.O. daily in the morning. For best results, use every other day or 2 days on followed by 1 to 2 days off. Or, 250 to 375 mg I.V. once daily for 1 or 2 days, alternating with a day of rest.

ADMINISTRATION
P.O.
• Give drug with food to minimize GI upset.
• Don't crush or open extended-release capsules.
• If patient can't swallow oral form, pharmacist may make a suspension using crushed tablets in a highly flavored syrup,

---

such as cherry, raspberry, or chocolate, to mask the bitter flavor. Although concentrations up to 500 mg/5 mL are possible, concentrations of 250 mg/5 mL are more palatable.

• Refrigeration improves palatability but doesn't improve stability. Suspensions are stable for 1 week.

I.V.

▼ Reconstitute drug in 500-mg vial with at least 5 mL of sterile water for injection. Use within 12 hours of reconstitution.

▼ Inject 100 to 500 mg/minute into a large vein using a 21G or 23G needle.

▼ Direct I.V. injection is the preferred route.

▼ Intermittent and continuous infusions aren't recommended.

▼ **Incompatibilities:** Multivitamins.

ACTION

Promotes renal excretion of sodium, potassium, bicarbonate, and water. As anticonvulsant, drug normalizes neuronal discharge. In mountain sickness, drug stimulates ventilation and increases cerebral blood flow. In glaucoma, drug reduces IOP.

Route	Onset	Peak	Duration
P.O.	60–90 min	1–4 hr	8–12 hr
P.O. (extended-release)	2 hr	3–6 hr	18–24 hr
I.V.	2 min	15 min	4–5 hr

Half-life: 10 to 15 hours.

ADVERSE REACTIONS

CNS: *seizures,* drowsiness, paresthesia, confusion, depression, weakness, ataxia, headache.

EENT: transient myopia, hearing dysfunction, tinnitus.

GI: nausea, vomiting, anorexia, metallic taste, diarrhea, black tarry stools, constipation.

GU: polyuria, hematuria, crystalluria, glycosuria, phosphaturia, renal calculus.

Hematologic: *aplastic anemia, leukopenia, thrombocytopenia,* hemolytic anemia.

Metabolic: hypokalemia, asymptomatic hyperuricemia, hyperchloremic acidosis.

Skin: pain at injection site, *Stevens-Johnson syndrome,* rash, urticaria.

Other: sterile abscesses.

INTERACTIONS

Drug-drug. *Amphetamines, anticholinergics, mecamylamine, procainamide, quinidine:* May decrease renal clearance of these drugs, increasing toxicity. Monitor patient for toxicity.

Beta blockers: May cause severe mixed acidosis in patients with respiratory disorders. Use with caution. If acidosis occurs, discontinue one or both drugs.

Cyclosporine: May increase cyclosporine level, causing nephrotoxicity and neurotoxicity. Monitor patient for toxicity.

Diflunisal: May increase acetazolamide adverse effects; may significantly decrease IOP. Use together cautiously.

Lithium: May increase lithium excretion, decreasing its effect. Monitor lithium level.

Methenamine: May reduce methenamine effect. Avoid using together.

Primidone: May decrease serum and urine primidone levels. Monitor patient closely.

Black Box Warning *Salicylates:* May cause accumulation and toxicity of acetazolamide, resulting in CNS depression, metabolic acidosis, anorexia, and death. Administer with caution and monitor patient for toxicity. ▮

Drug-lifestyle. *Sun exposure:* May increase risk of photosensitivity reactions. Advise patient to avoid excessive sunlight exposure.

EFFECTS ON LAB TEST RESULTS

• May increase uric acid level. May decrease potassium and hemoglobin levels and hematocrit.

• May decrease WBC and platelet counts.

• May decrease iodine uptake by the thyroid in hyperthyroid and euthyroid patients. May cause false-positive urine protein test result.

CONTRAINDICATIONS & CAUTIONS

Black Box Warning Fatalities have occurred due to severe reactions to sulfonamides, including Stevens-Johnson syndrome, toxic epidermal necrolysis, fulminant hepatic necrosis, agranulocytosis, aplastic anemia, and other blood dyscrasias. Sensitizations may recur when a sulfonamide is readministered, irrespective of the route of administration. If signs and symptoms of hypersensitivity or other serious reaction occur, discontinue drug. ▮

Reactions in bold italics are *life-threatening.* Interactions may have a *rapid onset* or a *delayed onset.*

• Contraindicated in patients hypersensitive to drug and in those with hyponatremia or hypokalemia, renal or hepatic disease or dysfunction, renal calculi, adrenal gland failure, hyperchloremic acidosis, or severe pulmonary obstruction.
• Contraindicated in those receiving long-term treatment for chronic noncongestive angle-closure glaucoma.
• Use cautiously in patients receiving other diuretics and in those with respiratory acidosis or COPD.

⚠ **Overdose S&S:** Electrolyte imbalance, acidotic state, CNS effects.

NURSING CONSIDERATIONS

• Cross-sensitivity between antibacterial sulfonamides and sulfonamide-derivative diuretics such as acetazolamide has been reported.
• Monitor fluid intake and output, glucose, and electrolytes, especially potassium, bicarbonate, and chloride. When drug is used in diuretic therapy, consult prescriber and dietitian about providing a high-potassium diet.
• Monitor elderly patients closely because they are especially susceptible to excessive diuresis.
• Weigh patient daily. Rapid or excessive fluid loss may cause weight loss and hypotension.
• Diuretic effect decreases when acidosis occurs but can be reestablished by using intermittent administration schedules.
• Monitor patient for signs of hemolytic anemia (pallor, weakness, and palpitations).
• Drug may increase glucose level and cause glycosuria.
• **Look alike–sound alike:** Don't confuse acetazolamide with acetaminophen or acyclovir. Don't confuse Diamox with Diabinese.

PATIENT TEACHING

• Tell patient to take oral form with food to minimize GI upset.
• Tell patient not to crush, chew, or open capsules.
• Caution patient not to perform hazardous activities if adverse CNS reactions occur.

• Instruct patient to avoid prolonged exposure to sunlight because drug may cause phototoxicity.
• Instruct patient to notify prescriber of any unusual bleeding, bruising, tingling, or tremors.

acetylcysteine
a-se-teel-SIS-tay-een

Acetadote, Mucomyst†

Therapeutic class: Mucolytics
Pharmacologic class: L-cysteine derivatives
Pregnancy risk category: B

AVAILABLE FORMS
I.V. injection: 200 mg/mL
Solution: 10%, 20%

INDICATIONS & DOSAGES
➤ **Adjunct therapy for abnormal viscid or thickened mucous secretions in patients with pneumonia, bronchitis, bronchiectasis, primary amyloidosis of the lung, tuberculosis, cystic fibrosis, emphysema, atelectasis, pulmonary complications of thoracic surgery, or CV surgery**
Adults and children: 1 to 2 mL 10% or 20% solution by direct instillation into trachea as often as every hour. Or, 1 to 10 mL of 20% solution or 2 to 20 mL of 10% solution by nebulization every 2 to 6 hours, p.r.n.
➤ **Acetaminophen toxicity**
P.O.
Adults and children: Initially, 140 mg/kg P.O.; then 70 mg/kg P.O. every 4 hours for 17 doses (total).
I.V.
Adults and children weighing 41 to 100 kg (90 to 220 lb): 150 mg/kg in 200 mL of diluent I.V. over 1 hour. Then, 50 mg/kg in 500 mL of diluent I.V. over 4 hours. Then, 100 mg/kg in 1,000 mL of diluent I.V. over 16 hours.
Adults and children weighing 21 to 40 kg (46 to 88 lb): 150 mg/kg in 100 mL of diluent I.V. over 1 hour. Then, 50 mg/kg in 250 mL of diluent I.V. over 4 hours.

Then, 100 mg/kg in 500 mL diluent I.V. over 16 hours.

Adults and childrens weighing 5 to 20 kg (11 to 44 lb): 150 mg/kg in 3 mL/kg diluent I.V. over 1 hour. Then, 50 mg/kg in 7 mL/kg diluent I.V. over 4 hours. Then, 100 mg/kg in 14 mL/kg diluent I.V. over 16 hours.

Adjust-a-dose: Refer to manufacturer's instruction for dosing in patients weighing less than 40 kg (88 lb) and requiring fluid restriction.

➤ **Complex regional pain syndrome ◆**
Adults: 600 mg P.O. t.i.d. for 17 weeks in combination with analgesics.

ADMINISTRATION
P.O.

• Dilute oral dose (used for acetaminophen overdose) with diet cola, cola, fruit juice, or water. Dilute 20% solution to 5% (add 3 mL of diluent to each milliliter of drug). If patient vomits within 1 hour of receiving loading or maintenance dose, repeat dose. Use diluted solution within 1 hour.

• Drug smells strongly of sulfur. Mixing oral form with juice or cola improves its taste.

• Drug delivered through nasogastric tube may be diluted with water.

• Store opened, undiluted oral solution in the refrigerator for up to 96 hours.

I.V.

▼ Drug may turn from a colorless liquid to a slight pink or purple color once the stopper is punctured. This color change doesn't affect the drug.

▼ Drug is hyperosmolar and is compatible with D_5W, half-normal saline, and sterile water for injection.

▼ Adjust total volume given for patients who weigh less than 40 kg (88 lb) or who are fluid restricted.

▼ For patients who weigh 40 kg or more, dilute loading dose in 200 mL of D_5W, second dose in 500 mL, and third dose in 1,000 mL.

▼ For patients who weigh 25 to less than 40 kg (55 to 88 lb), dilute loading dose in 100 mL, second dose in 250 mL, and third dose in 500 mL.

▼ For patients who weigh between 20 and 25 kg (44 to 55 lb), dilute loading dose in

60 mL, second dose in 140 mL, and third dose in 280 mL.

▼ For patients who weigh between 15 and 20 kg (33 to 44 lb), dilute loading dose in 45 mL, second dose in 105 mL, and third dose in 210 mL.

▼ For patients who weigh 10 to 15 kg (22 to 33 lb), dilute loading dose in 30 mL, second dose in 70 mL, and third dose in 140 mL.

▼ Reconstituted solution is stable for 24 hours at room temperature.

▼ Vials contain no preservatives; discard after opening.

▼ **Incompatibilities:** Incompatible with rubber and metals, especially iron, copper, and nickel.

Inhalational

• Use plastic, glass, stainless steel, or another nonreactive metal when giving by nebulization. Hand-bulb nebulizers aren't recommended because output is too small and particle size too large.

• **Incompatibilities:** Physically or chemically incompatible with inhaled tetracyclines, erythromycin lactobionate, amphotericin B, and ampicillin sodium. If given by aerosol inhalation, nebulize these drugs separately. Iodized oil, trypsin, and hydrogen peroxide are physically incompatible with acetylcysteine; don't add to nebulizer.

ACTION

Reduces the viscosity of pulmonary secretions by splitting disulfide linkages between mucoprotein molecular complexes. Also, restores liver stores of glutathione to treat acetaminophen toxicity.

Route	Onset	Peak	Duration
P.O., I.V., inhalation	Unknown	Unknown	Unknown

Half-life: 6¼ hours.

ADVERSE REACTIONS

CNS: abnormal thinking, fever, drowsiness, gait disturbances.
CV: chest tightness, flushing, hypertension, hypotension, tachycardia.
EENT: rhinorrhea, ear pain, eye pain, pharyngitis, throat tightness.
GI: nausea, stomatitis, vomiting.

Reactions in bold italics are *life-threatening*. Interactions may have a *rapid onset* or a *delayed onset*.

Respiratory: *bronchospasm,* cough, dyspnea, rhonchi.
Skin: clamminess, diaphoresis, pruritus, rash, urticaria.
Other: *anaphylactoid reaction, angioedema,* chills.

INTERACTIONS
Drug-drug. *Activated charcoal:* May limit acetylcysteine's effectiveness. Avoid using activated charcoal before or with acetylcysteine.

EFFECTS ON LAB TEST RESULTS
None reported.

CONTRAINDICATIONS & CAUTIONS
• Contraindicated in patients hypersensitive to drug.
• Use cautiously in elderly or debilitated patients with severe respiratory insufficiency. Use I.V. form cautiously in patients with asthma or a history of bronchospasm.

NURSING CONSIDERATIONS
• Monitor cough type and frequency.
❸ **Alert:** Monitor patient for bronchospasm, especially if he has asthma.
• Ingestion of more than 150 mg/kg of acetaminophen may cause liver toxicity. Measure acetaminophen level 4 hours after ingestion to determine risk of liver toxicity.
❸ **Alert:** Drug is used for acetaminophen overdose within 24 hours of ingestion. Start drug immediately; don't wait for results of acetaminophen level. Give within 10 hours of acetaminophen ingestion to minimize hepatic injury.
• If you suspect acetaminophen overdose, obtain baseline AST, ALT, bilirubin, PT, BUN, creatinine, glucose, and electrolyte levels.
❸ **Alert:** Monitor patient receiving I.V. form for anaphylactoid reactions. If anaphylactoid reaction occurs, stop infusion and treat anaphylaxis. Once anaphylaxis treatment starts, restart infusion. If anaphylactoid symptoms return, stop drug. Contact the Poison Control Center at (800) 222-1222 for more information.
• Facial erythema may occur within 30 to 60 minutes of start of I.V. infusion and usually resolves without stopping infusion.

• When acetaminophen level is below toxic level according to nomogram, stop therapy.
• The vial stopper doesn't contain natural rubber latex, dry natural rubber, or blends of natural rubber.
• *Look alike–sound alike:* Don't confuse acetylcysteine with acetylcholine. Don't confuse Mucomyst with Mucinex.

PATIENT TEACHING
• Warn patient that drug may have a foul taste or smell that may be distressing.
• For maximum effect, instruct patient to cough to clear his airway before aerosol administration.

acyclovir
ay-SYE-kloe-ver

Zovirax

acyclovir sodium
Zovirax

Therapeutic class: Antivirals
Pharmacologic class: Nucleosides and nucleotides
Pregnancy risk category: B

AVAILABLE FORMS
Capsules: 200 mg
Cream: 5%
Injection: 500 mg/vial, 1 g/vial
Ointment: 5%
Solution (I.V.): 50 mg/mL
Suspension: 200 mg/5 mL
Tablets: 400 mg, 800 mg

INDICATIONS & DOSAGES
Adjust-a-dose (for all indications): For patients receiving the I.V. form, if CrCl is 25 to 50 mL/minute, give 100% of dose every 12 hours; if CrCl is 10 to 24 mL/minute, give 100% of dose every 24 hours; if CrCl is less than 10 mL/minute, give 50% of dose every 24 hours.

For patients receiving the P.O. form, if normal dose is 200 mg every 4 hours five times daily and CrCl is less than 10 mL/minute, give 200 mg P.O. every 12 hours. If normal dose is 400 mg every 12 hours and CrCl is less than 10 mL/minute, give

200 mg every 12 hours. If normal dose is 800 mg every 4 hours five times daily and CrCl is 10 to 25 mL/minute, give 800 mg every 8 hours; if CrCl is less than 10 mL/minute, give 800 mg every 12 hours.

For patients who require hemodialysis, give additional dose after each dialysis.

➤ **First and recurrent episodes of mucocutaneous herpes simplex virus (HSV-1 and HSV-2) infections in immunocompromised patients; severe first episodes of genital herpes in patients who aren't immunocompromised**
Adults and children age 12 and older: 5 mg/kg given I.V. over 1 hour every 8 hours for 7 days. Give for 5 to 7 days for severe first episode of genital herpes.
Children younger than age 12: 10 mg/kg I.V. over 1 hour every 8 hours for 7 days.

➤ **First genital herpes episode**
Adults: 200 mg P.O. every 4 hours while awake, five times daily. Continue for 10 days.

➤ **Initial genital herpes; limited, non-life-threatening mucocutaneous HSV infections in immunocompromised patients**
Adults and children age 12 and older: Cover all lesions every 3 hours six times daily for 7 days. Although dosage varies depending on total lesion area, use about ½-inch (1.3-cm) ribbon of ointment on each 4-inch (10-cm) square of surface area.

➤ **Intermittent therapy for recurrent genital herpes**
Adults: 200 mg P.O. every 4 hours while awake, five times daily. Continue for 5 days. Begin therapy at first sign of recurrence.

➤ **Long-term suppressive therapy for recurrent genital herpes**
Adults: 400 mg P.O. b.i.d. for up to 12 months. Or, 200 mg P.O. three to five times daily for up to 12 months.

➤ **Varicella zoster infections in immunocompromised patients**
Adults and children age 12 and older: 10 mg/kg I.V. over 1 hour every 8 hours for 7 days. Dosage for obese patients is 10 mg/kg based on ideal body weight every 8 hours for 7 days. Don't exceed maximum dosage equivalent of 20 mg/kg every 8 hours.

Children younger than age 12: 20 mg/kg I.V. over 1 hour every 8 hours for 7 days.

➤ **Varicella (chickenpox) infection in immunocompetent patients**
Adults and children weighing more than 40 kg (88 lb): 800 mg P.O. q.i.d. for 5 days.
Children age 2 and older weighing less than 40 kg: 20 mg/kg (maximum 800 mg/ dose) P.O. q.i.d. for 5 days. Start therapy as soon as symptoms appear.

➤ **Acute herpes zoster infection in immunocompetent patients**
Adults and children age 12 and older: 800 mg P.O. every 4 hours five times daily for 7 to 10 days.

➤ **Herpes simplex encephalitis**
Adults and children age 12 and older: 10 mg/kg I.V. over 1 hour every 8 hours for 10 days.
Children ages 3 months to 12 years: 20 mg/kg I.V. over 1 hour every 8 hours for 10 days.

➤ **Neonatal HSV infection**
Neonates to 3 months old: 10 mg/kg I.V. over 1 hour every 8 hours for 10 days.

➤ **Recurrent herpes labialis**
Adults and children age 12 and older: Apply cream five times daily for 4 days. Start therapy as early as possible after signs and symptoms occur.

➤ **Prevention of recurrent ocular herpes infection ♦**
Adults and children age 12 and older: 600 to 800 mg P.O. daily for 8 to 12 months.

➤ **Episodic therapy of genital herpes in HIV-positive patients ♦**
Adults: 400 mg P.O. t.i.d. for 5 to 10 days.

➤ **Infection prophylaxis in neutropenia ♦**
HSV-seropositive adolescents and adults weighing 40 kg (88 lb) or more undergoing hematopoietic stem cell transplant (HSCT): For prevention of early reactivation regardless of donor HSV status, give 400 to 800 mg P.O. b.i.d. or 250 mg/m^2 I.V. every 12 hours. Start prophylaxis at beginning of conditioning and continue until engraftment or resolution of mucositis, whichever occurs last. For prevention of late reactivation in HSCT patients, give 800 mg P.O. b.i.d. Continue until 1 year after HSCT.
HSV-seropositive children weighing less than 40 kg undergoing HSCT: 250 mg/m^2 I.V. every 8 hours or 125 mg/m^2 I.V. every

---

Reactions in bold italics are *life-threatening*. Interactions may have a *rapid onset* or a *delayed onset*.

6 hours (not to exceed 80 mg/kg/day). Start prophylaxis at beginning of conditioning and continue until engraftment or resolution of mucositis, whichever occurs last. For prevention of late reactivation in HSCT patients, give 60 to 90 mg/kg/day P.O. divided into two to three doses (not to exceed 800 mg b.i.d.). Continue until 1 year after HSCT.

HSV-seropositive adolescents and adults weighing 40 kg or more with acute leukemia undergoing induction or reinduction: 400 mg P.O. b.i.d. was used in one small trial in this patient population. The Infectious Diseases Society of America recommends beginning prophylaxis at start of induction and continuing until WBC recovery or resolution of mucositis, whichever occurs last. Prophylaxis may be extended for patients with frequent HSV infection recurrences. No published data are available for children weighing less than 40 kg.

Varicella zoster virus (VZV) reactivation prophylaxis for adolescents and adults weighing 40 kg or more undergoing allogenic and autologous HSCT: 800 mg P.O. b.i.d. for 1 year. Prophylaxis may be continued beyond 1 year in allogenic HSCT patients with chronic graft-versus-host disease (GVHD) and in those receiving systemic immunosuppressants.

VZV reactivation prophylaxis for children weighing less than 40 kg undergoing allogenic and autologous HSCT: 60 to 80 mg/kg/day P.O. divided into two to three doses. Prophylaxis may be continued beyond 1 year in allogenic HSCT patients with chronic GVHD and in those receiving systemic immunosuppressants.

➤ **Suppressive therapy of genital herpes in HIV-positive patients ◆**
Adults: 400 to 800 mg P.O. b.i.d. to t.i.d. on long-term basis. Suppressive therapy with acyclovir for up to 6 years has been documented. Treatment for 1 year or longer may be appropriate in patients with frequent recurrences.

ADMINISTRATION
P.O.
● Give drug without regard for meals, but give with food if stomach irritation occurs.

● Patient should take drug as prescribed, even after he feels better.

I.V.
▼ Solutions concentrated at 7 mg/mL or more may cause a higher risk of phlebitis.
▼ Encourage fluid intake because patient must be adequately hydrated during infusion.
▼ Bolus injection, dehydration (decreased urine output), renal disease, and use with other nephrotoxic drugs increase the risk of renal toxicity. Don't give by bolus injection.
▼ Give I.V. infusion over at least 1 hour to prevent renal tubular damage.
▼ Monitor intake and output, especially during the first 2 hours after administration.
🕁 *Alert:* Don't give I.M. or subcutaneously.
▼ **Incompatibilities:** Amifostine, aztreonam, biological or colloidal solutions, cefepime, cisatracurium besylate, diltiazem hydrochloride, dobutamine hydrochloride, dopamine hydrochloride, fludarabine phosphate, foscarnet sodium, gemcitabine hydrochloride, idarubicin hydrochloride, levofloxacin, meperidine hydrochloride, meropenem, morphine sulfate, ondansetron hydrochloride, parabens, piperacillin sodium–tazobactam sodium, sargramostim, tacrolimus, vinorelbine tartrate.

Topical
● Apply with finger cot or rubber glove to prevent autoinoculation of other body sites and transmission of infection to others.
● Thoroughly cover all lesions.
● Topical form is for cutaneous use only; don't apply to eyes.

ACTION
Interferes with DNA synthesis and inhibits viral multiplication.

Route	Onset	Peak	Duration
P.O.	Unknown	2½ hr	Unknown
I.V.	Immediate	Immediate	Unknown
Topical	Unknown	Unknown	Unknown

Half-life: 2 to 3½ hours with normal renal function; up to 19 hours with renal impairment.

ADVERSE REACTIONS

CNS: headache, malaise, *encephalopathic changes (including lethargy, obtundation, tremor, confusion, hallucinations, agitation, seizures, coma).*
GI: nausea, vomiting, diarrhea.
GU: *acute renal failure,* hematuria.
Hematologic: *leukopenia, thrombocytopenia,* thrombocytosis.
Skin: inflammation or phlebitis at injection site, rash, urticaria; eczema, rash, dryness, pruritus, contact dermatitis, application-site reaction, mild pain, burning, or stinging (topical form).
Other: *angioedema, anaphylaxis.*

INTERACTIONS

Drug-drug. *Interferon:* May have synergistic effect. Monitor patient closely.
Probenecid: May increase acyclovir level. Monitor patient for possible toxicity.
Zidovudine: May cause drowsiness or lethargy. Use together cautiously.

EFFECTS ON LAB TEST RESULTS

● May increase BUN and creatinine levels.
● May decrease WBC count. May increase or decrease platelet count.

CONTRAINDICATIONS & CAUTIONS

● Contraindicated in patients hypersensitive to drug.
● Use cautiously in patients with neurologic problems, renal disease, or dehydration, and in those receiving other nephrotoxic drugs.
● Adequate studies haven't been done in pregnant women; use only if potential benefits outweigh risks to fetus.
● Women with active herpetic lesions near or on the breasts should avoid breast-feeding.
⚠ Overdose S&S: Agitation, coma, seizures, lethargy, elevated BUN and creatinine levels, renal failure.

NURSING CONSIDERATIONS

● Start therapy as early as possible after signs or symptoms occur.
● Drug isn't a cure for herpes, but it helps improve signs and symptoms.
۞ Alert: Long-term acyclovir use may result in nephrotoxicity. In patients with renal disease or dehydration and in those taking other nephrotoxic drugs, monitor renal function.
۞ Alert: If signs and symptoms of extravasation occur, stop I.V. infusion immediately and notify prescriber. Hyaluronidase may need to be injected subcutaneously at extravasation site as an antidote.
● Encephalopathic changes are more likely to occur in patients with neurologic disorders and in those who have had neurologic reactions to cytotoxic drugs.
● **Look alike–sound alike:** Don't confuse acyclovir sodium (Zovirax) with acetazolamide sodium (Diamox) vials, which may look alike. Don't confuse Zovirax with Zyvox.

PATIENT TEACHING

● Tell patient to take drug as prescribed, even after he feels better.
● Tell patient drug is effective in managing herpes infection but doesn't eliminate or cure it. Warn patient that drug won't prevent spread of infection to others.
● Tell patient to avoid sexual contact while visible lesions are present. Virus transmission can occur during treatment.
● Teach patient about early signs and symptoms of herpes infection (such as tingling, itching, or pain). Tell him to notify prescriber and get a prescription for drug before the infection fully develops. Early treatment is most effective.

---

adalimumab
ay-da-LIM-yoo-mab

Humira

Therapeutic class: Antiarthritics
Pharmacologic class: TNF blockers
Pregnancy risk category: B

AVAILABLE FORMS

Injection: 20 mg/0.4 mL, 40 mg/0.8 mL as prefilled syringes or pens

INDICATIONS & DOSAGES

➤ **Rheumatoid arthritis (RA); psoriatic arthritis; ankylosing spondylitis**
Adults: 40 mg subcutaneously every other week. Patient may continue to take methotrexate, steroids, NSAIDs, salicylates,

---

Reactions in bold italics are *life-threatening*. Interactions may have a *rapid onset* or a *delayed onset*.

analgesics or other disease-modifying antirheumatic drugs (known as DMARDs) during therapy. Patients with RA who aren't also taking methotrexate may have the dose increased to 40 mg weekly, if needed.

➤ **Moderate to severe Crohn disease when response to conventional therapy is inadequate or when response to infliximab is lost or patient can't tolerate the drug; moderate to severe active ulcerative colitis when response to immunosuppressants (such as corticosteroids, azathioprine, or 6-mercaptopurine) is inadequate**

Adults: Initially, 160 mg subcutaneously on day 1 given as four 40-mg injections in 1 day or as two 40-mg injections per day for 2 consecutive days; then 80 mg 2 weeks later (day 15), followed by a maintenance dose of 40 mg every other week starting at week 4 (day 29). For ulcerative colitis, only continue in patients who have shown evidence of clinical remission by 8 weeks (day 57) of therapy.

➤ **To reduce the signs and symptoms of moderately to severely active polyarticular juvenile idiopathic arthritis**

Children ages 4 to 17 weighing between 15 and 30 kg (33 to 66 lb): 20 mg subcutaneously every other week.

Children ages 4 to 17 weighing 30 kg or more: 40 mg subcutaneously every other week.

➤ **Moderate to severe chronic plaque psoriasis**

Adults: 80 mg subcutaneously, followed by 40 mg subcutaneously every other week starting 1 week after the initial dose. Treatment beyond 1 year has not been studied.

➤ **Uveitis ◆**

Adults: 40 mg subcutaneously every other week for up to 24 months with or without corticosteroids and other immunosuppressants. For relapse, give 40 mg subcutaneously every week.

ADMINISTRATION

Subcutaneous

- Inject subcutaneously into abdomen or thigh.
- Rotate injection sites.
- Don't give in an area that is bruised, tender, red, or hard.

ACTION

A recombinant human immunoglobulin G_1 monoclonal antibody that blocks human TNF-alpha. TNF-alpha participates in normal inflammatory and immune responses and in the inflammation and joint destruction of RA.

Route	Onset	Peak	Duration
Subcut.	Variable	Variable	Unknown

Half-life: 10 to 20 days.

ADVERSE REACTIONS

CNS: headache.
CV: *hemorrhage,* hypertension.
EENT: sinusitis.
GI: abdominal pain, nausea.
GU: hematuria, UTI.
Hematologic: *leukopenia, pancytopenia, thrombocytopenia.*
Metabolic: hypercholesterolemia, hyperlipidemia.
Musculoskeletal: back pain.
Respiratory: upper respiratory tract infection, bronchitis.
Skin: rash, injection-site reactions (erythema, itching, pain, swelling).
Other: accidental injury, *anaphylaxis, malignancy,* allergic reactions, flulike syndrome.

INTERACTIONS

Drug-drug. *Abatacept, anakinra, tocilizumab:* May increase risk of serious infections and neutropenia. Don't use together.
Live-virus vaccines: No data are available on secondary transmission of infection from live-virus vaccines. Avoid using together.
Methotrexate: May decrease clearance of adalimumab. Dosage adjustment isn't necessary.

EFFECTS ON LAB TEST RESULTS

- May increase alkaline phosphatase and cholesterol levels.

CONTRAINDICATIONS & CAUTIONS

- Contraindicated in patients hypersensitive to drug or its components, immunosuppressed patients, and those with an active chronic or localized infection.

Black Box Warning Patients taking TNF-alpha blockers are at increased risk for developing serious *Legionella* and *Listeria* infections. ■

● Use cautiously in patients with demyelinating disorders, a history of recurrent infection, those with underlying conditions that predispose them to infections, those who have lived in areas where tuberculosis and histoplasmosis are endemic, and in the elderly.

● Use cautiously and monitor closely in heart failure patients.

● Don't give to pregnant women unless benefits outweigh risks. Because of the risk of serious adverse reactions, the patient should stop breast-feeding or stop using the drug.

NURSING CONSIDERATIONS

● Give first dose under supervision of prescriber.

Black Box Warning Patient should be evaluated, and treated if necessary, for latent tuberculosis before starting adalimumab therapy. Closely monitor patient for possible development of tuberculosis even if he has tested negative before initiating therapy. ■

Black Box Warning Serious infections and sepsis, including tuberculosis and invasive fungal infections, may occur. If patient develops new infection during treatment, monitor him closely; if infection becomes serious, stop drug. ■

Black Box Warning Lymphoma and other malignancies, some fatal, have been reported in children and adolescents treated with TNF blockers, including adalimumab. ■

Black Box Warning Hepatosplenic T-cell lymphoma, a rare type of T-cell lymphoma, has occurred in adolescents and young adults with inflammatory bowel disease treated with TNF blockers, including adalimumab. ■

● *Alert:* Drug may increase the risk of malignancy. Patients with highly active RA may be at an increased risk for lymphoma.

● *Alert:* If patient develops anaphylaxis, a severe infection, other serious allergic reaction, or evidence of a lupuslike syndrome, stop drug.

● Drug may cause reactivation of hepatitis B virus in chronic carriers.

● *Alert:* The needle cover contains latex and shouldn't be handled by those with latex sensitivity.

● *Look alike–sound alike:* Don't confuse Humira with Humulin or Humalog.

PATIENT TEACHING

● Tell patient to report evidence of tuberculosis or infection.

● Teach patient or caregiver how to give drug.

● *Alert:* Warn patient to seek immediate medical attention for symptoms of blood dyscrasias or infection, including fever, bruising, bleeding, and pallor.

● Tell patient to rotate injection sites and to avoid tender, bruised, red, or hard skin.

● Teach patient to dispose of used vials, needles, and syringes properly and not in the household trash or recyclables.

● Tell patient to refrigerate drug in its original container before use.

---

adefovir dipivoxil
ah-DEF-oh-veer

Hepsera

Therapeutic class: Antivirals
Pharmacologic class: Nucleosides and nucleotides
Pregnancy risk category: C

AVAILABLE FORMS
Tablets: 10 mg

INDICATIONS & DOSAGES
➤ **Chronic hepatitis B infection**
Adults and children age 12 and older:
10 mg P.O. once daily.
Adjust-a-dose: In patients with CrCl of 30 to 49 mL/minute, give 10 mg P.O. every 48 hours. In patients with CrCl of 10 to 29 mL/minute, give 10 mg P.O. every 72 hours. In patients receiving hemodialysis, give 10 mg P.O. every 7 days, after dialysis session.

ADMINISTRATION
P.O.
● Give drug without regard for meals.

Reactions in bold italics are *life-threatening*. Interactions may have a *rapid onset* or a *delayed onset*.

ACTION
An acyclic nucleotide analogue that inhibits hepatitis B virus reverse transcription via viral DNA chain termination.

Route	Onset	Peak	Duration
P.O.	Unknown	1–4 hr	Unknown

Half-life: 7½ hours.

ADVERSE REACTIONS
CNS: asthenia, fever, headache.
GI: abdominal pain, diarrhea, dyspepsia, flatulence, nausea, vomiting.
GU: *renal failure, renal insufficiency.*
Hepatic: *hepatic failure,* hepatomegaly with steatosis.
Metabolic: *lactic acidosis.*
Skin: pruritus, rash.

INTERACTIONS
Drug-drug. *Ibuprofen:* May increase adefovir bioavailability. Monitor patient for adverse effects.
Nephrotoxic drugs (aminoglycosides, cyclosporine, NSAIDs, tacrolimus, vancomycin): May increase risk of nephrotoxicity. Use together cautiously.

EFFECTS ON LAB TEST RESULTS
● May increase ALT, amylase, AST, CK, creatinine, and lactate levels.

CONTRAINDICATIONS & CAUTIONS
● Contraindicated in patients hypersensitive to components of drug.
● Use cautiously in patients with renal dysfunction, in those receiving nephrotoxic drugs, and in those with known risk factors for hepatic disease.
● In elderly patients, use cautiously because they're more likely to have decreased renal and cardiac function.
● Safety and effectiveness in children younger than age 12 haven't been established.
⚠ **Overdose S&S:** GI adverse reactions.

NURSING CONSIDERATIONS
Black Box Warning Due to increased risk of nephrotoxicity, monitor renal function, especially in patients with renal dysfunction or those taking nephrotoxic drugs. ▪

Black Box Warning Patients may develop lactic acidosis and severe hepatomegaly with steatosis during treatment. Women, obese patients, and those taking antiretrovirals are at higher risk. Monitor hepatic function. Stop drug, if needed. ▪
Black Box Warning Stopping adefovir may cause severe worsening of hepatitis. Monitor hepatic function closely in patients who stop antihepatitis B therapy. ▪
● The ideal length of treatment hasn't been established.
Black Box Warning Offer patients HIV antibody testing; drug may promote resistance to antiretrovirals in chronic hepatitis B patients with unrecognized or untreated HIV infection. ▪
● For pregnant women, call the Antiretroviral Pregnancy Registry at 1-800-258-4263 to monitor fetal outcome.

PATIENT TEACHING
● Inform the patient that drug may be taken without regard to meals.
● Tell patient to immediately report weakness, muscle pain, trouble breathing, stomach pain with nausea and vomiting, dizziness, light-headedness, fast or irregular heartbeat, and feeling cold, especially in arms and legs.
● Warn patient not to stop taking this drug unless directed because it could cause hepatitis to become worse.
● Instruct woman to tell her prescriber if she becomes pregnant or is breast-feeding. It's unknown if drug appears in breast milk. Use cautiously in breast-feeding women.

SAFETY ALERT!

adenosine
a-DEN-oh-seen

Adenocard, Adenoscan

Therapeutic class: Antiarrhythmics
Pharmacologic class: Nucleosides
Pregnancy risk category: C

AVAILABLE FORMS
Injection: 3 mg/mL

INDICATIONS & DOSAGES

➤ **To convert paroxysmal supraventricular tachycardia (PSVT) to sinus rhythm**
Adults and children weighing 50 kg (110 lb) or more: 6 mg I.V. by rapid bolus injection over 1 to 2 seconds. If PSVT isn't eliminated in 1 to 2 minutes, give 12 mg by rapid I.V. push and repeat, if needed.
Children weighing less than 50 kg: Initially, 0.05 to 0.1 mg/kg I.V. by rapid bolus injection followed by a saline flush. If PSVT isn't eliminated in 1 to 2 minutes, give additional bolus injections, increasing the amount given by 0.05- to 0.1-mg/kg increments, followed by a saline flush. Continue, as needed, until conversion or a maximum single dose of 0.3 mg/kg (up to 12 mg) is given.

ADMINISTRATION

I.V.
▼ Don't give single doses exceeding 12 mg.
▼ In adults, avoid giving drug through a central line because more prolonged asystole may occur.
▼ Give by rapid I.V. injection to ensure drug action.
▼ Give directly into a vein, if possible. When giving through an I.V. line, use the port closest to the patient.
▼ Flush immediately and rapidly with normal saline solution to ensure that drug quickly reaches the systemic circulation.
▼ **Incompatibilities:** Other I.V. drugs.

ACTION

Naturally occurring nucleoside that acts on the AV node to slow conduction and inhibit reentry pathways. Drug is also useful in treating PSVTs, including those with accessory bypass tracts (Wolff-Parkinson-White syndrome).

Route	Onset	Peak	Duration
I.V.	Immediate	Immediate	Unknown

Half-life: Less than 10 seconds.

ADVERSE REACTIONS

CNS: dizziness, light-headedness, numbness, tingling in arms, headache.
CV: chest pressure, facial flushing.
GI: nausea.
Respiratory: dyspnea.

INTERACTIONS

Drug-drug. *Carbamazepine:* May cause high-level heart block. Use together cautiously.
Digoxin, verapamil: May cause ventricular fibrillation. Monitor ECG closely.
Dipyridamole: May increase adenosine's effects. Adenosine dose may need to be reduced. Use together cautiously.
Methylxanthines (caffeine, theophylline): May decrease adenosine's effects. Adenosine dose may need to be increased or patients may not respond to adenosine therapy.
Drug-herb. *Guarana:* May decrease patient's response to drug. Monitor patient.

EFFECTS ON LAB TEST RESULTS

None reported.

CONTRAINDICATIONS & CAUTIONS

● Contraindicated in patients hypersensitive to drug.
● Contraindicated in those with second- or third-degree heart block or sinus node disease (such as sick sinus syndrome and symptomatic bradycardia), except those with a pacemaker.
● Use cautiously in patients with asthma, emphysema, or bronchitis because bronchoconstriction may occur.

NURSING CONSIDERATIONS

🟊 *Alert:* By decreasing conduction through the AV node, drug may produce first-, second-, or third-degree heart block. Patients who develop high-level heart block after a single dose shouldn't receive additional doses.
🟊 *Alert:* New arrhythmias, including heart block and transient asystole, may develop; monitor cardiac rhythm and treat as indicated.
● If solution is cold, crystals may form; gently warm solution to room temperature. Don't use solutions that aren't clear.
● Drug lacks preservatives. Discard unused portion. Don't refrigerate.
🟊 *Alert:* Don't confuse adenosine with adenosine phosphate.

Reactions in bold italics are *life-threatening*. Interactions may have a *rapid onset* or a *delayed onset*.

PATIENT TEACHING
● Instruct patient to report adverse reactions promptly.
● Tell patient to report discomfort at I.V. site.
● Inform patient that he may experience flushing or chest pain lasting 1 to 2 minutes.

SAFETY ALERT!
✱ NEW DRUG

ado-trastuzumab emtansine
ADD-oh tras-TOOZ-oo-mab em-TAN-seen

Kadcyla

Therapeutic class: Antineoplastics
Pharmacologic class: Antibody drug conjugates
Pregnancy risk category: D

AVAILABLE FORMS
Injection (lyophilized powder for solution): 100 mg, 160 mg in single-use vials

INDICATIONS & DOSAGES
➤ **HER2-positive, metastatic breast cancer in patients who previously received trastuzumab and a taxane, separately or in combination. Patients should have either received previous treatment for metastatic disease or developed recurrence during or within 6 months of completing adjuvant treatment**
Adults: 3.6 mg/kg I.V. every 21 days until disease progression or unacceptable toxicity occurs. Maximum dose is 3.6 mg/kg.
Adjust-a-dose: If dosage reductions are necessary for adverse events, the first dosage reduction is to 3 mg/kg; the second dosage reduction is to 2.4 mg/kg. If further reduction is necessary, discontinue drug. Don't reescalate after dosage reduction is made.

For increased serum transaminase levels (AST/ALT) of more than 5 to less than 20 times the upper limit of normal (ULN) (Grade 3), withhold dose until levels return to 5 times ULN or less (Grade 2); then reduce by one dosage level. For AST or ALT of more than 20 times ULN, permanently discontinue drug.

For increased total bilirubin level of more than 1.5 to 3 times ULN (Grade 2), withhold dose until total bilirubin level returns to less than 1.5 times ULN (Grade 1); then treat at same dosage level. For increased total bilirubin level of more than 3 to 10 times ULN, withhold dose until level returns to Grade 1; then reduce by one dosage level. For total bilirubin level of more than 10 times ULN, permanently discontinue drug.

For serum transaminase levels greater than 3 times ULN concomitant with total bilirubin level greater than 2 times ULN, discontinue drug.

For left ventricular dysfunction with LVEF of less than 40%, withhold drug and repeat LVEF assessment within 3 weeks. If LVEF remains less than 40%, discontinue drug. For LVEF of 40% to 45% and LVEF decrease is 10% or more from baseline, withhold drug and repeat LVEF assessment within 3 weeks. If LVEF hasn't recovered to within 10% of baseline, discontinue drug. For LVEF of 40% to 45% and the decrease is less than 10% from baseline, continue treatment and repeat LVEF assessment within 3 weeks. For LVEF of more than 45%, continue treatment. Discontinue drug for symptomatic heart failure.

For platelet count of 25,000/mm^3 to less than 50,000/mm^3 (Grade 3), withhold drug until platelet count recovers to 75,000/mm^3 or more (Grade 1); then continue at same dosage level. For platelet count of less than 25,000/mm^3 (Grade 4), withhold drug until platelet count returns to 75,000/mm^3 or more (Grade 1); then reduce by one dosage level.

For grade 3 or 4 peripheral neuropathy, temporarily withhold drug until recovery to Grade 2 or less.

ADMINISTRATION
I.V.
Black Box Warning Don't confuse this drug with trastuzumab (Herceptin). These drugs aren't interchangeable. ∎
❸ Alert: The manufacturer recommends that the trade name be used and clearly recorded in the patient record to avoid confusion.

▼ To reconstitute, slowly inject 5 mL sterile water for injection into 100-mg vial or 8 mL sterile water for injection into 160-mg vial to yield concentration of 20 mg/mL.

▼ Swirl gently until dissolved. Don't shake. Solution should be colorless to pale brown.

▼ Add reconstituted dose to 250 mL of normal saline solution in infusion bag and administer immediately through I.V. line containing 0.22-micron in-line nonprotein adsorptive polyethersulfone filter.

▼ Administer initial infusion over 90 minutes. Don't administer as I.V. push or bolus. Monitor patient for infusion-related reactions during administration and for 90 minutes after completion. Slow or interrupt infusion for infusion-related events. Discontinue drug if life-threatening infusion-related reactions occur.

▼ May administer subsequent infusions over 30 minutes if initial infusion was uneventful. Monitor patient during infusion and for 30 minutes after completion.

▼ Observe for subcutaneous infiltration during infusion.

▼ Give at dosage and rate patient tolerated at most recent infusion.

▼ If dose is delayed or missed, give as soon as possible; don't wait for next planned cycle.

▼ Reconstituted vials can be stored in refrigerator for 4 hours at 36° to 46° F (2° to 8° C). Don't freeze.

▼ **Incompatibilities:** Dextrose solution, other drugs.

ACTION

Drug contains both trastuzumab and DM1 (a microtubule inhibitor), linked by a covalent bond, and targets the HER2 receptor by combined mechanisms of trastuzumab and DM1. The recombinant monoclonal antibody, trastuzumab, binds to the HER2 receptor and intracellular lysosomal degradation releases the cytotoxic component, DM1, resulting in microtubule disruption and cell death.

Route	Onset	Peak	Duration
I.V.	Unknown	End of infusion	Unknown

Half-life: 4 days.

ADVERSE REACTIONS

CNS: fatigue, headache, fever, asthenia, dizziness, peripheral neuropathy, insomnia.
CV: left ventricular dysfunction, edema, hypertension.
EENT: dry eyes, blurred vision, conjunctivitis, increased lacrimation, epistaxis.
GI: nausea, constipation, stomatitis, abdominal pain, vomiting, diarrhea, dyspepsia, dry mouth, taste perversion.
GU: UTI.
Hematologic: *thrombocytopenia, neutropenia,* anemia.
Hepatic: elevated transaminase levels, increased alkaline phosphatase level.
Metabolic: *hypokalemia.*
Musculoskeletal: musculoskeletal pain, arthralgia, myalgia.
Respiratory: pneumonitis, dyspnea, cough.
Skin: pruritus, rash.
Other: chills, hypersensitivity reactions, infusion reaction.

INTERACTIONS

Drug-drug. *Strong CYP3A4 inhibitors (atazanavir, clarithromycin, indinavir, itraconazole, ketoconazole, nefazodone, nelfinavir, ritonavir, saquinavir, telithromycin, voriconazole):* May increase ado-trastuzumab level and potential toxicity. Avoid use together. If use together is necessary, stop inhibitor and delay treatment until inhibitor clears from patient's circulation, or monitor patient carefully for adverse effects.

EFFECTS ON LAB TEST RESULTS

● May increase bilirubin, AST, and ALT levels. May decrease potassium level.
● May decrease hemoglobin level and platelet and neutrophil counts.

CONTRAINDICATIONS & CAUTIONS

Black Box Warning Contraindicated in pregnant women and women of childbearing potential who aren't using reliable contraception. Advise women of potential hazard to fetus (birth defects, fetal death). ∎
● Contraindicated in patients hypersensitive to drug or its components.
● Contraindicated in breast-feeding women. It isn't known if drug appears in breast milk. Patient should discontinue breast-feeding or discontinue drug.

• Use cautiously in patients with liver failure, risk of hepatotoxicity, symptomatic congestive heart failure, serious cardiac arrhythmia, history of MI, or unstable angina.

• Avoid use in patients with history of trastuzumab hypersensitivity or infusion-related events.

• Discontinue drug in patients diagnosed with interstitial lung disease or pneumonitis.

• Patients with shortness of breath at rest due to advanced malignancy and comorbidities may be at increased risk for pulmonary toxicity.

• Use cautiously in patients taking anticoagulants and in those with preexisting thrombocytopenia.

⚠ **Overdose S&S:** Thrombocytopenia, death.

NURSING CONSIDERATIONS

• Confirm HER2 testing with FDA-approved test by established laboratory. Only patients with HER2 protein overexpression should receive drug because these are the only patients studied for whom benefit has been shown.

• Infusion-related reactions, including hypersensitivity reactions, may occur. Closely monitor patient during and for 90 minutes after infusion for fever, chills, flushing, dyspnea, hypotension, wheezing, bronchospasm, or tachycardia. Slow or interrupt infusion as necessary. In most patients, these reactions resolve over the course of several hours to a day after the infusion is terminated.

• Monitor patient for extravasation, which may cause redness, tenderness, skin irritation, pain, or swelling at infusion site.

Black Box Warning Severe liver injury (including fatal liver damage, liver failure, and death) has been reported. Monitor serum transaminase and bilirubin levels before starting drug and before each dose. Dosage modifications or discontinuation of therapy may be necessary. ∎

Black Box Warning Drug may significantly reduce LVEF. Assess LVEF before starting drug and every 3 months during treatment. Withhold or discontinue drug as clinically indicated. ∎

🕓 **Alert:** Permanently discontinue drug in patients diagnosed with interstitial lung disease or pneumonitis.

• Monitor platelet count before treatment and before each dose.

• Discontinue drug in patients diagnosed with nodular regenerative hyperplasia of the liver.

🕓 **Alert:** Asian patients may have increased incidence and severity of thrombocytopenia.

PATIENT TEACHING

• Inform patient that drug may cause severe liver damage that may be life-threatening.

• Tell patient to report unexplained nausea, vomiting, abdominal pain, jaundice, dark urine, generalized itchiness, or anorexia.

• Caution patient that drug may cause heart problems, with or without symptoms. Instruct patient to report new-onset or worsening of shortness of breath, cough, swelling of the ankles or legs, palpitations, weight gain of more than 5 pounds in 24 hours, fatigue, dizziness, or loss of consciousness.

• Advise patient that drug may cause lung problems. Tell patient to report trouble breathing, cough, or tiredness.

• Alert patient that drug may cause low platelet count. Instruct patient to contact prescriber if excessive bleeding occurs.

• Warn patient that drug may cause nerve damage. Instruct patient to report numbness or tingling, burning or sharp pain, sensitivity to touch, lack of coordination, or muscle weakness or loss of muscle function.

Black Box Warning Inform patient that drug may cause birth defects and fetal death. Advise woman of childbearing potential to use effective contraception during treatment and for 6 months after last dose. ∎

🕓 **Alert:** Advise patient to immediately inform her physician if she suspects or confirms pregnancy. Encourage patient participation in MotHER Pregnancy Registry by contacting 1–800–690–6720.

• Inform breast-feeding patient that it isn't known if drug appears in breast milk and that she must discontinue either breast-feeding or drug.

albuterol sulfate
al-BYOO-ter-ole

AccuNeb, ProAir HFA, Proventil-HFA, Salbutamol†, Ventolin HFA, VoSpire ER

Therapeutic class: Bronchodilators
Pharmacologic class: Adrenergics
Pregnancy risk category: C

AVAILABLE FORMS
Inhalation aerosol: 108 mcg/actuation
Solution for inhalation: 0.083% (2.5 mg/3 mL), 0.5% (5 mg/mL), 0.042% (1.25 mg/3 mL), 0.021% (0.63 mg/3 mL)
Syrup: 2 mg/5 mL
Tablets: 2 mg, 4 mg
Tablets (extended-release): 4 mg, 8 mg

INDICATIONS & DOSAGES
➤ **To prevent or treat bronchospasm in patients with reversible obstructive airway disease**
Tablets (extended-release)
Adults and children age 12 and older: 4 to 8 mg P.O. every 12 hours. Maximum, 32 mg daily.
Children ages 6 to 11: 4 mg P.O. every 12 hours. Maximum, 24 mg daily.
Tablets
Adults and children age 13 and older: 2 to 4 mg P.O. t.i.d. or q.i.d. Maximum, 32 mg daily.
Children ages 6 to 12: 2 mg P.O. t.i.d. or q.i.d. Maximum, 24 mg daily.
Solution for inhalation
Adults and children age 13 and older: 2.5 mg t.i.d. or q.i.d. by nebulizer, given over 5 to 15 minutes. To prepare solution, use 0.5 mL of 0.5% solution diluted with 2.5 mL of normal saline solution. Or, use 3 mL of 0.083% solution.
Children ages 2 to 12 weighing more than 15 kg (33 lb): 2.5 mg by nebulizer given over 5 to 15 minutes t.i.d. or q.i.d., with subsequent doses adjusted to response. Don't exceed 2.5 mg t.i.d. or q.i.d.
Children ages 2 to 12 weighing 15 kg or less: 0.63 mg or 1.25 mg by nebulizer given over 5 to 15 minutes t.i.d. or q.i.d. with

subsequent doses adjusted to response. Don't exceed 2.5 mg t.i.d. or q.i.d.
Syrup
Adults and children age 15 and older: 2 to 4 mg (1 to 2 tsp) P.O. t.i.d. or q.i.d. Maximum, 32 mg daily.
Children ages 6 to 14: 2 mg (1 tsp) P.O. t.i.d. or q.i.d. Maximum, 24 mg daily.
Children ages 2 to 5: Initially, 0.1 mg/kg P.O. t.i.d. Starting dose shouldn't exceed 2 mg (1 tsp) t.i.d. Maximum, 12 mg daily.
Inhalation aerosol
Adults and children age 4 and older: 1 to 2 inhalations every 4 to 6 hours as needed. Regular use for maintenance therapy to control asthma symptoms isn't recommended.
Adjust-a-dose: For elderly patients and those sensitive to sympathomimetic amines, 2 mg P.O. t.i.d. or q.i.d. as oral tablets or syrup. Maximum, 32 mg daily.
➤ **To prevent exercise-induced bronchospasm**
Adults and children age 4 and older: 2 inhalations using the inhalation aerosol 15 minutes before exercise; up to 12 inhalations may be taken in 24 hours.
➤ **Hyperkalemia** ◆
Adults: 10 to 20 mg by nebulizer over 15 minutes, given with other recommended therapy.
➤ **Asthma** ◆
Children younger than age 4: For asthma exacerbation, 180 to 600 mcg metered-dose inhaler every 20 minutes for a maximum of five to six doses. For intermittent or persistent asthma, 2 inhalations albuterol (HFA) every 4 to 6 hours p.r.n.

ADMINISTRATION
P.O.
● When switching patient from regular to extended-release tablets, remember that a regular 2-mg tablet every 6 hours is equivalent to an extended-release 4-mg tablet every 12 hours.
● Give drug whole; don't break or crush extended-release tablets or mix them with food.
Inhalational
● If more than 1 inhalation is ordered, wait at least 2 minutes between inhalations.

Reactions in bold italics are *life-threatening*. Interactions may have a *rapid onset* or a *delayed onset*.

- Use spacer device to improve drug delivery, if appropriate.
- Shake the inhaler before use.

ACTION
Relaxes bronchial, uterine, and vascular smooth muscle by stimulating beta$_2$ receptors.

Route	Onset	Peak	Duration
P.O.	15–30 min	2–3 hr	4–8 hr
P.O. (extended)	Unknown	6 hr	12 hr
Inhalation	5–15 min	30–120 min	2–6 hr

Half-life: Inhalation, about 4 hours; oral, 5 to 6 hours.

ADVERSE REACTIONS
CNS: tremor, nervousness, headache, hyperactivity, insomnia, dizziness, weakness, CNS stimulation, malaise.
CV: tachycardia, palpitations, hypertension.
EENT: dry and irritated nose and throat with inhaled form, nasal congestion, epistaxis, hoarseness, conjunctivitis.
GI: nausea, vomiting, heartburn, anorexia, altered taste, increased appetite.
Metabolic: hypokalemia.
Musculoskeletal: muscle cramps.
Respiratory: *bronchospasm,* cough, wheezing, dyspnea, bronchitis, increased sputum.
Other: hypersensitivity reactions.

INTERACTIONS
Drug-drug. *Antiarrhythmics (amiodarone, bretylium, disopyramide, dofetilide, procainamide, quinidine, sotalol), arsenic trioxide, chlorpromazine, dolasetron, droperidol, mefloquine, mesoridazine, moxifloxacin, pentamidine, pimozide, tacrolimus, thioridazine, ziprasidone:* May prolong QT interval and increase risk of life-threatening arrhythmias, including torsades de pointes. Monitor QT interval and patient.
CNS stimulants: May increase CNS stimulation. Avoid using together.
Digoxin: May decrease digoxin level. Monitor digoxin level closely.
Diuretics (furosemide, thiazides): May cause ECG changes and hypokalemia. Monitor potassium level. Use caution when administered with non-potassium-sparing diuretics.

Linezolid, MAO inhibitors, TCAs: May increase adverse CV effects. Monitor patient closely.
Propranolol and other beta blockers: May cause mutual antagonism. Monitor patient carefully.
Theophyllines: May decrease theophylline plasma concentration. Adjust dosage as needed and monitor patient.

EFFECTS ON LAB TEST RESULTS
- May decrease potassium level.

CONTRAINDICATIONS & CAUTIONS
- Contraindicated in patients hypersensitive to drug or its ingredients.
- Use cautiously in patients with CV disorders (including coronary insufficiency and hypertension), hyperthyroidism, or diabetes mellitus and in those who are unusually responsive to adrenergics.
- Use extended-release tablets cautiously in patients with GI narrowing.
- **⚠ *Overdose S&S:*** Exaggeration of adverse reactions, seizures, angina, hypotension, hypertension, tachycardia, arrhythmias, nervousness, headache, tremor, dry mouth, palpitations, nausea, dizziness, fatigue, malaise, sleeplessness, hypokalemia, cardiac arrest.

NURSING CONSIDERATIONS
- Drug may decrease sensitivity of spirometry used for diagnosis of asthma.
- Syrup contains no alcohol or sugar and may be taken by children as young as age 2.
- In children, syrup may rarely cause erythema multiforme or Stevens-Johnson syndrome.
- **❸ *Alert:*** Patient may use tablets and aerosol together. Monitor these patients closely for signs and symptoms of toxicity.
- ***Look alike–sound alike:*** Don't confuse albuterol with atenolol or Albutein. Don't confuse Salbutamol with salmeterol.

PATIENT TEACHING
- Warn patient about risk of paradoxical bronchospasm and to stop drug immediately if it occurs.

• Teach patient to perform oral inhalation correctly. Give the following instructions for using the metered-dose inhaler (MDI):
– Prime before first use, if not used for 2 weeks, or if MDI has been dropped.
– Shake the inhaler.
– Clear nasal passages and throat.
– Breathe out, expelling as much air from lungs as possible.
– Place mouthpiece well into mouth, seal lips around mouthpiece, and inhale deeply as you release a dose from inhaler. Or, hold inhaler about 1 inch (two fingerwidths) from open mouth; inhale while dose is released.
– Hold breath for several seconds, remove mouthpiece, and exhale slowly.
• If prescriber orders more than 1 inhalation, tell patient to wait at least 2 minutes before repeating procedure.
• Tell patient that use of a spacer device may improve drug delivery to lungs.
• If patient is also using a corticosteroid inhaler, instruct him to use the bronchodilator first and then to wait about 5 minutes before using the corticosteroid. This lets the bronchodilator open the air passages for maximal effectiveness of the corticosteroid.
• Tell patient to remove canister and wash inhaler with warm, soapy water at least once a week.
• Advise patient not to use more frequently than prescribed and not to increase dose or frequency without consulting physician.
• Advise patient not to chew or crush extended-release tablets or mix them with food.

alefacept
ALE-fuh-sept

Amevive

Therapeutic class: Antipsoriatics
Pharmacologic class:
Immunosuppressants
Pregnancy risk category: B

AVAILABLE FORMS
Powder for injection: 15-mg single-dose vials

INDICATIONS & DOSAGES
➤ **Moderate to severe chronic plaque psoriasis in candidates for systemic therapy or phototherapy**
Adults: 15 mg I.M. once weekly for 12 weeks. Another 12-week course may be given if CD4$^+$ T-lymphocyte count is normal and at least 12 weeks have passed since the previous treatment.
Adjust-a-dose: Withhold dose if CD4$^+$ T-lymphocyte count is below 250 cells/mm^3. Stop drug if CD4$^+$ count remains below 250 cells/mm^3 for 1 month.

ADMINISTRATION
I.M.
• Reconstitute 15-mg vial of alefacept with 0.6 mL of supplied diluent. Keep the needle pointed at the side wall of the vial and slowly inject the diluent.
• Don't shake or vigorously agitate; swirl gently. Some foaming will occur, which is normal.
• Rotate I.M. injection sites so that the new injection is given at least 1 inch (2.5 cm) away from the old site, and not in an area that is bruised, tender, or hard.
• After reconstitution, use product immediately or within 4 hours.

ACTION
An immunosuppressive protein that interferes with lymphocyte activation and reduces subsets of CD2$^+$ T lymphocytes, which reduces circulating total CD4$^+$ and CD8$^+$ T-lymphocyte counts.

Route	Onset	Peak	Duration
I.M.	Unknown	Unknown	Unknown

Half-life: About 11 days.

ADVERSE REACTIONS
CNS: dizziness.
EENT: pharyngitis.
GI: nausea.
Hematologic: *lymphopenia.*
Musculoskeletal: myalgia.
Respiratory: cough.
Skin: pruritus; injection-site pain, inflammation, bleeding, edema, or mass.
Other: *infection,* chills, *malignancy,* hypersensitivity reaction, accidental injury, antibody formation.

INTERACTIONS

Drug-drug. *Immunosuppressants, phototherapy:* May increase risk of excessive immunosuppression. Avoid using together.

EFFECTS ON LAB TEST RESULTS

- May decrease CD4$^+$ and CD8$^+$ T-lymphocyte counts.
- May increase AST and ALT levels.

CONTRAINDICATIONS & CAUTIONS

- Contraindicated in patients hypersensitive to drug or its components, in breast-feeding women, and in patients with HIV, a history of systemic malignancy, or serious infection.
- Use cautiously in patients at high risk for malignancy, patients with chronic or recurrent infections, and pregnant women.
- Use cautiously in elderly patients because of their increased rate of infection and malignancies.
- Safety and effectiveness in children haven't been established.

⚠ Overdose S&S: Chills, headache, arthralgia, sinusitis.

NURSING CONSIDERATIONS

- Ensure that CD4$^+$ T-lymphocyte count is normal before therapy. Monitor CD4$^+$ T-lymphocyte count weekly for the 12-week course.
- Monitor patient carefully for evidence of infection or malignancy, and stop drug if it appears.
- Because effects on fetal development aren't known, give drug only if clearly needed.

PATIENT TEACHING

- Tell patient about potential adverse reactions.
- Urge patient to report evidence of infection immediately.
- Tell patient that blood tests will be done regularly to monitor WBC counts.
- Tell patient to notify prescriber if she is or could be pregnant within 8 weeks of receiving drug.
- Advise patient to either stop breast-feeding or stop using the drug because of the risk of serious adverse reactions in the infant.

alendronate sodium
ah-LEN-dro-nate

Binosto, Fosamax*◢*, Fosamax Plus D

Therapeutic class: Antiosteoporotics
Pharmacologic class: Bisphosphonates
Pregnancy risk category: C

AVAILABLE FORMS

Oral solution: 70 mg/75 mL
Tablets: 5 mg, 10 mg, 35 mg, 40 mg, 70 mg, 70 mg plus 2,800 international units vitamin D$_3$, 70 mg plus 5,600 international units vitamin D$_3$
Tablets (effervescent): 70 mg

INDICATIONS & DOSAGES

➤ **Osteoporosis in postmenopausal women; to increase bone mass in men with osteoporosis**
Adults: 10 mg P.O. daily or 70-mg tablet or solution P.O. once weekly.

➤ **Paget disease of bone (osteitis deformans) (excluding Binosto)**
Adults: 40 mg P.O. daily for 6 months.

➤ **To prevent osteoporosis in postmenopausal women (excluding Binosto)**
Adults: 5 mg P.O. daily or 35-mg tablet P.O. once weekly.

➤ **Glucocorticoid-induced osteoporosis in patients receiving glucocorticoids in a daily dose equivalent to 7.5 mg or more of prednisone and who have low bone mineral density (excluding Binosto)**
Adults: 5 mg P.O. daily. For postmenopausal women not receiving estrogen, recommended dose is 10 mg P.O. daily.

➤ **Osteogenesis imperfecta ◆**
Adults: 10 mg P.O. once daily or 70 mg P.O. once weekly.
Children and adolescents ages 2 to 18 weighing more than 30 kg (66 lb): 10 mg P.O. once daily.
Children and adolescents ages 2 to 18 weighing 30 kg or less: 5 mg P.O. once daily.

➤ **Postoperative knee arthroplasty ◆**
Adults: 10 mg P.O. once daily beginning after knee arthroplasty.

ADMINISTRATION
P.O.
- Give drug with 6 to 8 ounces of water at least 30 minutes before patient's first food or drink of the day to facilitate delivery to the stomach.
- Dissolve effervescent tablet in 4 ounces of plain room-temperature water.
- Give at least 2 ounces of water after oral solution.
- Don't allow patient to lie down for 30 minutes after taking drug and until after first food of the day.

ACTION
Suppresses osteoclast activity on newly formed resorption surfaces, which reduces bone turnover. Bone formation exceeds resorption at remodeling sites, leading to progressive gains in bone mass.

Route	Onset	Peak	Duration
P.O.	Unknown	Unknown	Unknown

Half-life: More than 10 years.

ADVERSE REACTIONS
CNS: headache.
GI: abdominal pain, nausea, dyspepsia, constipation, diarrhea, flatulence, acid regurgitation, esophageal ulcer, vomiting, dysphagia, abdominal distention, gastritis, taste perversion.
Musculoskeletal: pain.

INTERACTIONS
Drug-drug. *Antacids, calcium supplements, many oral drugs:* May interfere with absorption of alendronate. Instruct patient to wait at least 30 minutes after taking alendronate before taking other drug orally.
Aspirin, NSAIDs: May increase risk of upper GI adverse reactions with drug doses greater than 10 mg daily. Monitor patient closely.
Ranitidine (I.V. form): May increase availability of alendronate. Reduce dosage as needed.
Drug-food. *Any food:* May decrease absorption of drug. Advise patient to take with full glass of water at least 30 minutes before food, beverages, or ingestion of other drugs.

EFFECTS ON LAB TEST RESULTS
- May decrease calcium and phosphate levels.

CONTRAINDICATIONS & CAUTIONS
- Contraindicated in patients hypersensitive to drug and in those with hypocalcemia, severe renal insufficiency (CrCl of less than 35 mL/minute), or abnormalities of the esophagus that delay esophageal emptying.
- **Alert:** There may be an increased risk of atypical fractures of the thigh in patients treated with bisphosphonates.
- Contraindicated in patients unable to stand or sit upright for at least 30 minutes.
- Use cautiously in patients with active upper GI problems (dysphagia, symptomatic esophageal diseases, gastritis, duodenitis, ulcers) or mild to moderate renal insufficiency.
- Use cautiously in patients with known risk factors for osteonecrosis of the jaw (diagnosis of cancer; concomitant treatment with chemotherapy, radiotherapy, corticosteroids; poor oral hygiene, and comorbid disorders, such as preexisting dental disease, anemia, coagulopathy, or infection.
- **Overdose S&S:** Hypocalcemia, hypophosphatemia, upset stomach, heartburn, esophagitis, gastritis, ulcer.

NURSING CONSIDERATIONS
- Correct hypocalcemia and other disturbances of mineral metabolism (such as vitamin D deficiency) before therapy begins.
- When used to treat osteoporosis, disease may be confirmed by findings of low bone mass on diagnostic studies or by history of osteoporotic fracture.
- The recommended daily intake of vitamin D is 400 to 800 international units. Fosamax Plus D provides 400 international units daily when taken once weekly. Patients at risk for vitamin D deficiency, such as those who are chronically ill, who are nursing home bound, who have a GI malabsorption syndrome, or who are older than age 70, may require additional supplementation.
- In Paget disease, drug is indicated for patients with alkaline phosphatase level at least two times upper limit of normal, for those who are symptomatic, and for those

at risk for future complications from the disease.

• Monitor patient's calcium and phosphate levels throughout therapy.

• Severe musculoskeletal pain has been associated with bisphosphonate use and may occur within days, months, or years of start of therapy. When drug is stopped, symptoms may resolve partially or completely.

• Patients who develop osteonecrosis of the jaw should receive care by an oral surgeon.

• *Look alike–sound alike:* Don't confuse Fosamax with Flomax.

PATIENT TEACHING

• Stress importance of taking tablet only with 6 to 8 ounces of water at least 30 minutes before ingesting anything else, including food, beverages, and other drugs. Tell patient that waiting longer than 30 minutes improves absorption.

• Warn patient not to lie down for at least 30 minutes after taking drug to facilitate delivery to stomach and to reduce risk of esophageal irritation.

• Tell patient who misses a once-weekly dose to take one dose on the morning after she remembers and then return to weekly dosing on the chosen day as originally scheduled.

• Advise patient to report adverse effects immediately, especially chest pain or difficulty swallowing.

• Advise patient to take supplemental calcium and vitamin D if dietary intake is inadequate.

• Tell patient about benefits of weight-bearing exercises in increasing bone mass. If applicable, explain importance of reducing or eliminating cigarette smoking and alcohol use.

alfuzosin hydrochloride
al-foo-ZOE-sin

Uroxatral✔, Xatral†

Therapeutic class: BPH drugs
Pharmacologic class: Alpha₁ blockers
Pregnancy risk category: B

AVAILABLE FORMS
Tablets (extended-release): 10 mg

INDICATIONS & DOSAGES
➤ BPH
Men: 10 mg P.O. immediately after same meal each day.

ADMINISTRATION
P.O.
• Give drug after same meal each day.
• Don't crush tablets.

ACTION
Selectively blocks alpha₁ receptors in the prostate, which relaxes the smooth muscles in the bladder neck and prostate, improving urine flow and reducing symptoms of BPH.

Route	Onset	Peak	Duration
P.O.	Unknown	8 hr	Unknown

Half-life: 10 hours.

ADVERSE REACTIONS
CNS: dizziness, fatigue, headache, pain.
EENT: pharyngitis, sinusitis.
GI: abdominal pain, constipation, dyspepsia, nausea.
GU: erectile dysfunction.
Respiratory: bronchitis, upper respiratory tract infection.

INTERACTIONS
Drug-drug. *Amiodarone:* May increase alfuzosin plasma level and pharmacologic effects. Use with caution and monitor patient.
Antihypertensives (diltiazem): May cause hypotension. Monitor blood pressure and use together cautiously.
Beta blockers (atenolol): May cause hypotension and reduce heart rate. Monitor blood pressure and heart rate for these effects.
Cimetidine: May increase alfuzosin level. Use together cautiously.
Moderate CYP3A4 inhibitors (diltiazem, verapamil): May increase alfuzosin level. Use cautiously together and monitor patient for adverse reactions.
Potent CYP3A4 inhibitors (itraconazole, ketoconazole, ritonavir): May inhibit hepatic metabolism of alfuzosin. Use together is contraindicated.
Drug-lifestyle. *Alcohol use:* May increase risk of hypotension. Don't use together.

EFFECTS ON LAB TEST RESULTS
None reported.

CONTRAINDICATIONS & CAUTIONS
• Contraindicated in patients with moderate hepatic impairment (Child-Pugh class B or C) and those hypersensitive to alfuzosin or its ingredients.
• Use cautiously in patients with severe renal insufficiency, congenital or acquired QT-interval prolongation, or symptomatic hypotension and hypotensive responses to other drugs.
⚠ *Overdose S&S:* Hypotension.

NURSING CONSIDERATIONS
• Don't use drug to treat hypertension.
• Asymptomatic orthostatic hypotension may develop within a few hours.
• Symptoms of BPH and prostate cancer are similar; rule out prostate cancer before therapy.
• If angina pectoris develops or worsens, stop drug.
• Current or previous use of an alpha blocker may predispose the patient to intraoperative floppy iris syndrome during cataract surgery.

PATIENT TEACHING
• Tell patient to take drug just after the same meal each day.
• At start of therapy, warn patient about possible hypotension and explain that the drug may cause dizziness. Caution patient against performing hazardous activities until he knows how the drug affects him.
• Tell patient to avoid situations in which he could be injured if he became light-headed or fainted.
• Warn patient not to crush or chew the tablets.
• Advise patient planning cataract surgery to alert his ophthalmologist about this drug and current or previous alpha blocker therapy.

aliskiren hemifumarate
a-LIS-ke-ren

Rasilez†, Tekturna

Therapeutic class: Antihypertensives
Pharmacologic class: Renin inhibitors
Pregnancy risk category: C for 1st trimester; D for 2nd and 3rd trimesters

AVAILABLE FORMS
Tablets: 150 mg, 300 mg

INDICATIONS & DOSAGES
➤ **Hypertension, alone or with other antihypertensives**
Adults: 150 mg P.O. daily; may increase to 300 mg P.O. daily.

ADMINISTRATION
P.O.
• Don't give drug with high-fat meal because this may decrease the drug's effectiveness.

ACTION
Inhibits conversion of angiotensin to angiotensin I, decreasing vasoconstriction and lowering blood pressure.

Route	Onset	Peak	Duration
P.O.	Unknown	1–3 hr	Unknown

Half-life: Unknown.

ADVERSE REACTIONS
CNS: headache, dizziness, fatigue, *seizures.*
CV: hypotension.
EENT: nasopharyngitis.
GI: abdominal pain, diarrhea, dyspepsia, gastroesophageal reflux.
Metabolic: hyperuricemia, *hyperkalemia.*
Musculoskeletal: back pain.
Respiratory: cough, upper respiratory tract infection.
Skin: rash.
Other: *angioedema.*

INTERACTIONS
Drug-drug. ❸ *Alert: ACE inhibitors (benazepril, captopril, lisinopril, moexipril, perindopril, quinapril, ramipril, trandolapril), ARBs (azilsartan, candesartan,*

Reactions in bold italics are *life-threatening*. Interactions may have a *rapid onset* or a *delayed onset*.

eprosartan, irbesartan, losartan, olmesartan, telmisartan, valsartan): May increase risk of renal impairment, hypotension, and hyperkalemia in diabetic patients and those with moderate to severe renal impairment (GFR <60 mL/minute). Concomitant use is contraindicated in diabetic patients. Avoid concomitant use in those with renal impairment.

Atorvastatin: May increase aliskiren levels. Use cautiously together.

CYP3A4/P-glycoprotein inhibitors (cyclosporine, itraconazole, ketoconazole, verapamil): May increase aliskiren concentration and risk of adverse reactions. Use with caution. Avoid concurrent use with cyclosporine or itraconazole.

Furosemide: May reduce furosemide peak levels. Monitor patient for effectiveness.

Irbesartan: May decrease aliskiren levels. Monitor patient for effectiveness.

NSAIDs, potassium-sparing diuretics, potassium supplements: May increase risk of hyperkalemia. Use cautiously together.

Rifampin: May decrease aliskiren plasma concentration. Larger aliskiren doses may be needed.

Thiazide diuretics: May increase serum uric acid level. Use with caution, especially in patients at risk for hyperuricemia.

Drug-food. *Grapefruit:* May decrease aliskiren plasma level. Advise patient to avoid grapefruit products.

High-fat meals: May substantially decrease plasma levels of drug. Monitor patient for effectiveness.

EFFECTS ON LAB TEST RESULTS
● May increase potassium, CK, BUN, uric acid, and serum creatinine levels.

CONTRAINDICATIONS & CAUTIONS
● Contraindicated in patients hypersensitive to drug or its components.

Black Box Warning Contraindicated in pregnant women. Because of risk of fetal toxicity or death, stop drug as soon as possible if patient becomes pregnant. ∎

● Contraindicated in breast-feeding patients and patients taking cyclosporine.

● Use cautiously in patients with history of angioedema, severe renal dysfunction (creatinine of 1.7 mg/dL in women and

2 mg/dL in men, or GFR of less than 30 mL/minute), history of dialysis, nephrotic syndrome, or renovascular hypertension.

⚠ *Overdose S&S:* Hypotension.

NURSING CONSIDERATIONS
● Monitor blood pressure for hypotension, especially if used in combination with other antihypertensives.

● Monitor potassium levels, especially in patients also taking ACE inhibitors.

● *Alert:* Rarely, angioedema may occur at any time during treatment. Supportive measures may include antihistamines, steroids, and epinephrine.

● Monitor renal function. It's unknown how patients with significant renal disorders will respond to the use of this drug.

● Effect of any dose is usually seen within 2 weeks.

● *Look alike–sound alike:* Don't confuse Tekturna with Valturna.

PATIENT TEACHING
● Instruct patient not to take drug with a high-fat meal because this may decrease the drug's effectiveness.

● Instruct patient to monitor blood pressure daily, if possible, and to report low readings, dizziness, and headaches to prescriber.

● Tell patient to immediately report swelling of the face or neck or difficulty breathing.

● Advise patient of need for regular laboratory tests to monitor for adverse effects.

allopurinol
al-oh-PURE-i-nole

Lopurin, Zyloprim

allopurinol sodium
Aloprim

Therapeutic class: Antigout drugs
Pharmacologic class: Xanthine oxidase inhibitors
Pregnancy risk category: C

AVAILABLE FORMS
allopurinol
Tablets (scored): 100 mg, 300 mg
allopurinol sodium
Injection: 500 mg/30-mL vial

INDICATIONS & DOSAGES

Adjust-a-dose (for all indications): If CrCl is 10 to 20 mL/minute, give 200 mg P.O. or I.V. daily; if CrCl is less than 10 mL/minute, give 100 mg P.O. or I.V. daily; if CrCl is less than 3 mL/minute, give a maximum of 100 mg P.O. or I.V. at extended intervals. If patient is receiving hemodialysis, give a 50% supplemental dose after dialysis.

➤ **Gout or hyperuricemia**

Adults: Mild gout, 200 to 300 mg P.O. daily; severe gout with large tophi, 400 to 600 mg P.O. daily. Maximum 800 mg daily. Dosage varies with severity of disease; can be given as single dose or divided, but doses greater than 300 mg should be divided.

➤ **Hyperuricemia caused by malignancies**

Adults and children older than age 10: 200 to 400 mg/m^2 daily I.V. as a single infusion or in equally divided doses every 6, 8, or 12 hours beginning 24 to 48 hours before initiation of chemotherapy. Maximum 600 mg daily.

Children age 10 and younger: Initially, 200 mg/m^2 daily I.V. as single infusion or in equally divided doses every 6, 8, or 12 hours beginning 24 to 48 hours before initiation of chemotherapy. Then titrate according to uric acid levels. For children ages 6 to 10, give 300 mg P.O. daily or in three divided doses; for children younger than age 6, give 150 mg P.O. daily.

➤ **To prevent uric acid nephropathy during cancer chemotherapy**

Adults: 600 to 800 mg P.O. daily for 2 to 3 days, with high fluid intake.

➤ **Recurrent calcium oxalate calculi**

Adults: 200 to 300 mg P.O. daily in single or divided doses.

ADMINISTRATION

P.O.

● Give drug with or immediately after meals to minimize GI upset.

I.V.

▼ When possible, initiate therapy 24 to 48 hours before the start of chemotherapy known to cause tumor lysis.

▼ Dissolve contents of each 30-mL vial in 25 mL of sterile water for injection.

▼ Dilute solution to desired concentration (no greater than 6 mg/mL) with normal saline solution for injection or D$_5$W.

▼ Store solution at 68° to 77° F (20° to 25° C) and use within 10 hours. Don't use solution if it contains particulates or is discolored.

▼ **Incompatibilities:** Amikacin, amphotericin B, carmustine, cefotaxime, chlorpromazine, cimetidine, clindamycin phosphate, cytarabine, dacarbazine, daunorubicin, diphenhydramine, doxorubicin, doxycycline hyclate, droperidol, floxuridine, gentamicin, haloperidol lactate, hydroxyzine, idarubicin, imipenem–cilastatin sodium, mechlorethamine, meperidine, methylprednisolone sodium succinate, metoclopramide, minocycline, nalbuphine, netilmicin, ondansetron, prochlorperazine edisylate, promethazine, sodium bicarbonate (or solutions containing sodium bicarbonate), streptozocin, tobramycin sulfate, vinorelbine.

ACTION

Reduces uric acid production by inhibiting xanthine oxidase.

Route	Onset	Peak	Duration
P.O.	Unknown	30–120 hr	1–2 wk
I.V.	Unknown	30 min	Unknown

Half-life: Allopurinol, 1 to 2 hours; oxypurinol, about 15 hours.

ADVERSE REACTIONS

GI: nausea, vomiting, abdominal pain, diarrhea.

GU: *renal failure.*

Musculoskeletal: acute gout attack.

Skin: rash, maculopapular rash.

INTERACTIONS

Drug-drug. *Amoxicillin, ampicillin:* May increase possibility of rash. Avoid using together.

Anticoagulants: May increase anticoagulant effect. Dosage may need to be adjusted.

Antineoplastics: May increase potential for bone marrow suppression. Monitor patient carefully.

Azathioprine, mercaptopurine: May increase levels of these drugs. Concomitant administration of 300 to 600 mg of oral allopurinol per day requires dosage reduction to ⅓ to ¼ of usual dose of azathioprine or mercaptopurine. Make subsequent dosage

---

Reactions in bold italics are *life-threatening*. Interactions may have a *rapid onset* or a *delayed onset*.

adjustments based on therapeutic response and appearance of toxic effects.

Chlorpropamide: May increase hypoglycemic effect. Avoid using together.

Ethacrynic acid, thiazide diuretics: May increase risk of allopurinol toxicity. Reduce allopurinol dosage, and monitor renal function closely.

Uricosurics: May have additive effect. May be used to therapeutic advantage.

Urine-acidifying drugs (ammonium chloride, ascorbic acid, potassium or sodium phosphate): May increase possibility of kidney stone formation. Monitor patient carefully.

Xanthines: May increase theophylline level. Adjust dosage of theophylline as needed.

Drug-lifestyle. *Alcohol use:* May increase uric acid level. Discourage use together.

EFFECTS ON LAB TEST RESULTS

● May increase alkaline phosphatase, ALT, and AST levels.
● May decrease hemoglobin level and hematocrit.
● May increase eosinophil count.
● May decrease granulocyte and platelet counts.
● May increase or decrease WBC count.

CONTRAINDICATIONS & CAUTIONS

● Contraindicated in patients hypersensitive to drug and in those with idiopathic hemochromatosis.

NURSING CONSIDERATIONS

❸ Alert: Discontinue drug at first sign of rash or allergic reaction.
● Monitor uric acid level to evaluate drug's effectiveness.
● Monitor fluid intake and output; daily urine output of at least 2 L and maintenance of neutral or slightly alkaline urine are desirable.
● Periodically monitor CBC and hepatic and renal function, especially at start of therapy.
● Optimal benefits may need 2 to 6 weeks of therapy. Because acute gout attacks may occur during this time, concurrent use of colchicine may be prescribed prophylactically.
● Don't restart drug in patients who have a severe reaction.

● *Look alike–sound alike:* Don't confuse Zyloprim with ZORprin.

PATIENT TEACHING

● To minimize GI adverse reactions, tell patient to take drug with or immediately after meals.
● Encourage patient to drink plenty of fluids while taking drug unless otherwise contraindicated.
● Drug may cause drowsiness; tell patient not to drive or perform hazardous tasks requiring mental alertness until CNS effects of drug are known.
● If patient is taking drug for recurrent calcium oxalate stones, advise him also to reduce his dietary intake of animal protein, sodium, refined sugars, oxalate-rich foods, and calcium.
● Tell patient to stop drug at first sign of rash, which may precede severe hypersensitivity or other adverse reactions. Rash is more common in patients taking diuretics and in those with renal disorders. Tell patient to report all adverse reactions.
● Advise patient to avoid alcohol during therapy.
● Teach patient importance of continuing drug even if asymptomatic.

almotriptan malate
al-moh-I RIP-tan

Axert

Therapeutic class: Antimigraine drugs
Pharmacologic class: Serotonin 5-HT₁ receptor agonists
Pregnancy risk category: C

AVAILABLE FORMS
Tablets: 6.25 mg, 12.5 mg

INDICATIONS & DOSAGES
➤ **Acute migraine with or without aura**
Adults and adolescents ages 12 to 17: 6.25-mg or 12.5-mg tablet P.O., with one additional dose after 2 hours if headache is unresolved or recurs. Maximum, two doses (total of 25 mg) within 24 hours.

Adjust-a-dose: For patients with hepatic or renal impairment, initially 6.25 mg, with maximum daily dose of 12.5 mg.

ADMINISTRATION
P.O.
- Give drug without regard for food.
- Give only one repeat dose within 24 hours, no sooner than 2 hours after first dose.

ACTION
May act as an agonist at serotonin receptors on extracerebral intracranial blood vessels, which constricts the affected vessels, inhibits neuropeptide release, and reduces pain transmission in the trigeminal pathways.

Route	Onset	Peak	Duration
P.O.	1–3 hr	1–3 hr	3–4 hr

Half-life: 3 to 4 hours.

ADVERSE REACTIONS
CNS: paresthesia, headache, dizziness, somnolence.
CV: *coronary artery vasospasm, transient myocardial ischemia, MI, ventricular tachycardia, ventricular fibrillation.*
GI: nausea, vomiting, dry mouth.

INTERACTIONS
Drug-drug. *CYP3A4 inhibitors (such as ketoconazole):* May increase almotriptan level. Monitor patient for potential adverse reaction. May need to reduce dosage. Avoid concomitant use in patients with renal or hepatic impairment.
Ergot-containing drugs, serotonin 5-HT$_{1B/1D}$ agonists: May cause additive effects. Avoid using within 24 hours of almotriptan.
MAO inhibitors, verapamil: May increase almotriptan level. No dose adjustment is necessary.
SSNRIs, SSRIs: May cause additive serotonin effects, resulting in weakness, hyperreflexia, or incoordination. Monitor patient closely if given together.

EFFECTS ON LAB TEST RESULTS
None reported.

CONTRAINDICATIONS & CAUTIONS
- Contraindicated in patients hypersensitive to drug.
- Contraindicated in those with angina pectoris, history of MI, silent ischemia, coronary artery vasospasm, Prinzmetal variant angina, or other CV disease; uncontrolled hypertension; and hemiplegic or basilar migraine.
- Don't give within 24 hours after treatment with other 5-HT$_{1B/1D}$ agonists or ergot derivatives.
- Use cautiously in patients with renal or hepatic impairment and in those with cataracts because of the potential for corneal opacities.
- Use cautiously in patients with risk factors for coronary artery disease (CAD), such as obesity, diabetes, and family history of CAD.
⚠ ***Overdose S&S:*** Hypertension, more serious CV symptoms.

NURSING CONSIDERATIONS
- Patients with renal or hepatic impairment should receive a reduced dosage.
- Repeat dose after 2 hours, if needed, and don't give more than two doses (or 25 mg) in 24 hours.
🖊 **Alert:** Combining triptans with SSRIs or SSNRIs may cause serotonin syndrome. Signs and symptoms include restlessness, hallucinations, loss of coordination, rapid heartbeat, rapid changes in blood pressure, increased body temperature, overactive reflexes, nausea, vomiting, and diarrhea. Serotonin syndrome occurs more often when starting or increasing the dose of a triptan, SSRI, or SSNRI.
- **Look alike–sound alike:** Don't confuse Axert with Antivert.

PATIENT TEACHING
- Tell patient that drug can be taken with or without food.
- Advise patient to take drug only when he's having a migraine; explain that drug isn't taken on a regular schedule.
- Advise patient to use only one repeat dose within 24 hours, no sooner than 2 hours after first dose.
- Advise patient that other commonly prescribed migraine drugs can interact with almotriptan.

Reactions in bold italics are *life-threatening*. Interactions may have a *rapid onset* or a *delayed onset*.

• Advise patient to report chest or throat tightness, pain, or heaviness.
• Teach patient to avoid possible migraine triggers, such as cheese, chocolate, citrus fruits, caffeine, and alcohol.

SAFETY ALERT!
✳ NEW DRUG

alogliptin benzoate
AL-oh-GLIP-tin

Nesina

Therapeutic class: Antidiabetics
Pharmacologic class: Dipeptidyl peptidase-4 inhibitors
Pregnancy risk category: B

AVAILABLE FORMS
Tablets: 6.25 mg, 12.5 mg, 25 mg

INDICATIONS & DOSAGES
➤ **Adjunct to diet and exercise to improve glycemic control in adults with type 2 diabetes**
Adults: 25 mg P.O. daily.
Adjust-a-dose: For patients with moderate renal impairment (CrCl of 30 to less than 60 mL/minute), give 12.5 mg P.O. daily. For patients with severe renal impairment (CrCl of 15 to less than 30 mL/minute) and for those with ESRD (CrCl of less than 15 mL/minute) or requiring hemodialysis, give 6.25 mg P.O. daily.

ADMINISTRATION
P.O.
• Give without regard for food.
• Store at room temperature.

ACTION
Slows inactivation of incretin, which increases blood concentrations of incretin and reduces fasting or postprandial glucose in patients with type 2 diabetes.

Route	Onset	Peak	Duration
P.O.	Unknown	1–2 hr	Unknown

Half-life: 21 hours.

ADVERSE REACTIONS
CNS: headache.
EENT: nasopharyngitis.

Metabolic: *hypoglycemia.*
Respiratory: upper respiratory tract infection.

INTERACTIONS
Drug-drug. *Insulin, sulfonylureas:* May enhance hypoglycemic activity. Adjust dosage of insulin or sulfonylurea.

EFFECTS ON LAB TEST RESULTS
• May decrease glucose level.

CONTRAINDICATIONS & CAUTIONS
• Contraindicated in patients hypersensitive to drug or its components and in those with type 1 diabetes mellitus or ketoacidosis.
• Use cautiously in patients with liver disease or injury, history of pancreatitis, gallstones, history of alcoholism, renal disease, or history of angioedema with another dipeptidyl peptidase-4 inhibitor.
• Use cautiously in pregnant and breast-feeding women and only when clearly needed.

NURSING CONSIDERATIONS
• Assess renal function at baseline and periodically during treatment.
• Monitor patient for hypersensitivity reactions, including Stevens-Johnson syndrome (rare). Stop drug immediately if hypersensitivity is suspected.
• Monitor patient for signs and symptoms (rare) of acute pancreatitis (severe abdominal pain that may radiate to the back, with or without vomiting).
• Assess LFTs before treatment. If liver injury (rare) is suspected during treatment (fatigue, anorexia, abdominal discomfort, dark urine, jaundice), obtain LFTs. If elevated LFT values are present, persist, or worsen, withhold drug and determine probable cause. Restart drug only if cause isn't alogliptin-related.
• Monitor blood glucose level if patient is receiving concurrent hypoglycemic medications; adjust dosages of these medications if needed.

PATIENT TEACHING
• Instruct patient to monitor blood glucose level carefully.

• Advise patient to report respiratory symptoms to prescriber.

• Caution patient to seek medical attention for signs and symptoms of pancreatitis (severe abdominal pain that may radiate to the back, with or without vomiting) or liver injury (fatigue, anorexia, abdominal discomfort, dark urine, or jaundice).

alosetron hydrochloride
ah-LOSS-e-tron

Lotronex

Therapeutic class: Anti-IBS drugs
Pharmacologic class: Selective 5-HT$_3$ receptor antagonists
Pregnancy risk category: B

AVAILABLE FORMS
Tablets: 0.5 mg, 1 mg

INDICATIONS & DOSAGES
➤ **Severe diarrhea-predominant irritable bowel syndrome (IBS)**
Women: 0.5 mg P.O. b.i.d. If, after 4 weeks, drug is well tolerated but doesn't adequately control IBS symptoms, increase to 1 mg b.i.d. After 4 weeks at this dosage, if symptoms aren't controlled, stop drug.

ADMINISTRATION
P.O.
• Give drug without regard for food.

ACTION
Selectively inhibits 5-HT$_3$ receptors in the GI tract, which blocks neuronal depolarization, resulting in less visceral pain, a longer colonic transit, and GI secretions.

Route	Onset	Peak	Duration
P.O.	Unknown	1 hr	Variable

Half-life: 1½ hours.

ADVERSE REACTIONS
CNS: headache.
GI: constipation, nausea, GI discomfort and pain, abdominal discomfort and pain, abdominal distention, hemorrhoids, regurgitation, reflux, *ileus perforation, ischemic colitis, small-bowel mesenteric ischemia,* impaction, obstruction.
Skin: rash.

INTERACTIONS
Drug-drug. *CYP1A2 inhibitors (such as cimetidine, quinolones):* May increase alosetron level. Avoid use together.
CYP3A4 inhibitors (such as ciprofloxacin, clarithromycin, ketoconazole): May decrease alosetron metabolism. Use cautiously together.
Fluvoxamine: May increase alosetron level. Coadministration is contraindicated.
Hydralazine, isoniazid, procainamide: May cause slower metabolism of these drugs because of *N*-acetyltransferase inhibition. Monitor patient for toxicity.

EFFECTS ON LAB TEST RESULTS
• May increase ALT level.

CONTRAINDICATIONS & CAUTIONS
• Contraindicated in patients hypersensitive to drug or its components, and in those with a history of or current chronic or severe constipation, sequelae from constipation, severe hepatic impairment, intestinal obstruction, stricture, toxic megacolon, GI perforation, GI adhesions, ischemic colitis, impaired intestinal circulation, thrombophlebitis, or hypercoagulable state.
• Contraindicated in patients with a history of or current Crohn disease, ulcerative colitis, or diverticulitis and in those who are unable to understand or comply with the Patient-Physician Agreement.
• Don't use drug if predominant symptom is constipation.
• Use cautiously in patients with mild to moderate liver impairment; contraindicated in patients with severe liver impairment.
• Use cautiously in women who are pregnant, breast-feeding, or planning to become pregnant.
• Use in children younger than age 18 hasn't been studied.
⚠ *Overdose S&S:* Inhibited metabolic elimination, reduced elimination of other drugs.

Reactions in bold italics are *life-threatening*. Interactions may have a *rapid onset* or a *delayed onset*.

NURSING CONSIDERATIONS

Black Box Warning Drug is only appropriate for women who experience symptoms for at least 6 months, have no anatomic or biochemical GI tract abnormalities, and haven't responded to other therapies. ∎

• Diarrhea-predominant IBS is considered severe if one or more of the following accompanies the diarrhea:

− frequent and severe abdominal pain or discomfort

− frequent bowel urgency or fecal incontinence

− disability or restriction of daily activities.

Black Box Warning Patients taking drug have developed ischemic colitis and serious complications of constipation, resulting in death. If patient develops ischemic colitis (acute colitis, rectal bleeding, or sudden worsening of abdominal pain) while taking drug, stop therapy. If patient taking drug develops constipation, stop drug until symptoms subside. ∎

Black Box Warning Only providers who are enrolled in the manufacturer's Prescribing Program should prescribe this drug. Prescribers can register by calling 1-888-423-5227. ∎

• Drug is approved for use only in women with IBS. This drug isn't indicated for use in men.

• Elderly women may be at greater risk for complications of constipation.

• **Look alike–sound alike:** Don't confuse Lotronex with Lovenox.

PATIENT TEACHING

Black Box Warning Have patient sign a Patient Acknowledgement form before starting therapy. ∎

• Urge patient to read the Medication Guide before starting drug and each time she refills the prescription.

• Tell patient that this drug won't cure but may alleviate some IBS symptoms.

• Inform patient that most women notice their symptoms improving after about 1 week of therapy, but some may take up to 4 weeks to get relief from abdominal pain, discomfort, and diarrhea. Let patient know that symptoms usually return within 1 week after stopping the drug.

• Advise patient that drug may be taken with or without food.

Black Box Warning If constipation or signs of ischemic colitis occur (rectal bleeding, bloody diarrhea, or worsened abdominal pain or cramping), tell patient to stop the drug and consult prescriber immediately. Patients with resolved constipation should resume the drug only on the advice of their health care provider. ∎

• Inform patient not to share drug with other people having similar symptoms. This drug hasn't been shown to be safe or effective for men.

• Tell woman to notify the prescriber immediately if she becomes pregnant.

SAFETY ALERT!

alprazolam

al-PRAH-zoo lam

Apo-Alpraz†, Apo-Alpraz TS†, Niravam, Novo-Alprazol†, Nu-Alpraz†, Xanax℘, Xanax XR

Therapeutic class: Anxiolytics
Pharmacologic class: Benzodiazepines
Pregnancy risk category: D
Controlled substance schedule: IV

AVAILABLE FORMS

Oral solution. 1 mg/mL (concentrate)
Orally disintegrating tablets (ODTs):
0.25 mg, 0.5 mg, 1 mg, 2 mg
Tablets: 0.25 mg, 0.5 mg, 1 mg, 2 mg
Tablets (extended-release): 0.5 mg, 1 mg, 2 mg, 3 mg

INDICATIONS & DOSAGES

Adjust-a-dose (for all indications): For debilitated patients or those with advanced hepatic disease, usual first dose is 0.25 mg P.O. b.i.d. or t.i.d. For extended-release tablets, 0.5 mg P.O. once daily.

➤ **Anxiety**

Adults: Usual first dose, 0.25 to 0.5 mg (immediate-release) P.O. t.i.d. Maximum, 4 mg daily in divided doses.

Elderly patients: Usual first dose, 0.25 mg P.O. b.i.d. or t.i.d. Maximum, 4 mg daily in divided doses. For extended-release tablets,

0.5 mg P.O. once daily. May increase gradually as needed and tolerated.
➤ **Panic disorders**
Adults: 0.5 mg P.O. t.i.d., increased at intervals of 3 to 4 days in increments of no more than 1 mg. Maximum, 10 mg daily in divided doses. If using extended-release tablets, start with 0.5 to 1 mg P.O. once daily. Increase by no more than 1 mg every 3 to 4 days. Maximum daily dose is 10 mg.
Elderly patients: Usual first dose, 0.25 mg (immediate-release) P.O. b.i.d. or t.i.d. Maximum, 4 mg daily in divided doses.

ADMINISTRATION
P.O.
● Don't break or crush extended-release tablets.
● Mix oral solution with liquids or semisolid food, such as water, juices, carbonated beverages, applesauce, and puddings. Use only calibrated dropper provided with this product.
● Use dry hands to remove ODTs from bottle. Discard cotton from inside bottle.
● Discard unused portion if breaking scored ODT.
● Patients treated with divided doses of immediate-release tablets can be switched to extended-release tablets at same total daily dose.

ACTION
Unknown. Probably potentiates the effects of GABA, depresses the CNS, and suppresses the spread of seizure activity.

Route	Onset	Peak	Duration
P.O.	Unknown	1–2 hr	Unknown
P.O. (extended-release)	Unknown	Unknown	Unknown

Half-life: Immediate-release, 12 to 15 hours; extended-release, 11 to 16 hours.

ADVERSE REACTIONS
CNS: insomnia, irritability, dizziness, headache, anxiety, confusion, drowsiness, light-headedness, sedation, somnolence, difficulty speaking, impaired coordination, memory impairment, fatigue, depression, *suicide,* mental impairment, ataxia, paresthesia, dyskinesia, hypoesthesia, lethargy, vertigo, malaise, tremor, nervousness, restlessness, agitation, nightmare, syncope, akathisia, mania.
CV: palpitations, chest pain, hypotension.
EENT: allergic rhinitis, blurred vision, nasal congestion.
GI: diarrhea, dry mouth, constipation, nausea, increased or decreased appetite, anorexia, vomiting, dyspepsia, abdominal pain.
GU: dysmenorrhea, sexual dysfunction, premenstrual syndrome, difficulty urinating.
Metabolic: increased or decreased weight.
Musculoskeletal: arthralgia, myalgia, arm or leg pain, back pain, muscle rigidity, muscle cramps, muscle twitch.
Respiratory: upper respiratory tract infection, dyspnea, hyperventilation.
Skin: pruritus, increased sweating, dermatitis.
Other: influenza, injury, emergence of anxiety between doses, dependence, feeling warm, increased or decreased libido.

INTERACTIONS
Drug-drug. *Anticonvulsants, antidepressants, antihistamines, barbiturates, benzodiazepines, general anesthetics, narcotics, phenothiazines:* May increase CNS depressant effects. Avoid using together.
Azole antifungals (including fluconazole, itraconazole, ketoconazole, miconazole): May increase and prolong alprazolam level, CNS depression, and psychomotor impairment. Avoid using together.
Carbamazepine: May induce alprazolam metabolism and may reduce therapeutic effects. May need to increase dose.
Cimetidine, fluoxetine, fluvoxamine, hormonal contraceptives, nefazodone: May increase alprazolam level. Use cautiously together, and consider alprazolam dosage reduction.
TCAs: May increase levels of these drugs. Monitor patient closely.
Drug-herb. *Kava, valerian root:* May increase sedation. Discourage use together.
St. John's wort: May decrease drug level. Discourage use together.
Drug-food. *Grapefruit juice:* May increase drug level. Discourage use together.
Drug-lifestyle. *Alcohol use:* May cause additive CNS effects. Discourage use together.

Smoking: May decrease effectiveness of drug. Monitor patient closely.

EFFECTS ON LAB TEST RESULTS
• May increase ALT and AST levels.

CONTRAINDICATIONS & CAUTIONS
• Contraindicated in patients hypersensitive to drug or other benzodiazepines and in those with acute angle-closure glaucoma.
• Use cautiously in patients with hepatic, renal, or pulmonary disease or history of substance abuse.
⚠ Overdose S&S: Somnolence, confusion, impaired coordination, diminished reflexes, coma.

NURSING CONSIDERATIONS
• The optimum duration of therapy is unknown.
🕃 Alert: Don't withdraw drug abruptly; withdrawal symptoms, including seizures, may occur. Gradually reduce dosage. Abuse or addiction is possible.
• Monitor hepatic, renal, and hematopoietic function periodically in patients receiving repeated or prolonged therapy.
• Closely monitor addiction-prone patients.
• **Look alike–sound alike:** Don't confuse alprazolam with alprostadil or lorazepam. Don't confuse Xanax with Zantac, Xopenex, or Tenex.

PATIENT TEACHING
• Warn patient to avoid hazardous activities that require alertness and good coordination until effects of drug are known.
• Tell patient to avoid use of alcohol while taking drug.
• Advise patient that smoking may decrease drug's effectiveness.
• Warn patient not to stop drug abruptly because withdrawal symptoms or seizures may occur.
• Tell patient to swallow extended-release tablets whole.
• Tell patient using ODT to remove it from bottle using dry hands and to immediately place it on his tongue where it will dissolve and can be swallowed with saliva.
• Tell patient taking half a scored ODT to discard the unused half.

• Advise patient to discard the cotton from the bottle of ODTs and keep it tightly sealed to prevent moisture from dissolving the tablets.
• Warn women to avoid use during pregnancy and breast-feeding.

SAFETY ALERT!

alprostadil (injection)
al-PROSS-ta-dil

Prostin VR Pediatric

Therapeutic class: Prostaglandins
Pharmacologic class: Prostaglandins
Pregnancy risk category: NR

AVAILABLE FORMS
Injection: 500 mcg/mL

INDICATIONS & DOSAGES
➤ **Palliative therapy for temporary maintenance of patency of ductus arteriosus until surgery can be performed**
Neonates: 0.05 to 0.1 mcg/kg/minute by I.V. infusion. When therapeutic response is achieved, reduce infusion rate to lowest dose that will maintain response. Maximum dose is 0.4 mcg/kg/minute. Or, give drug through umbilical artery catheter placed at ductal opening.
➤ **Raynaud phenomenon ◆**
Adults: 20 mcg/hour I.V. over 3 hours for 5 days followed by two maintenance doses once every 30 days.

ADMINISTRATION
I.V.
▼ Dilute drug before giving. Prepare fresh solution daily; discard solution after 24 hours.
▼ For infusion, dilute 1 mL of concentrate labeled as containing 500 mcg in normal saline solution or D_5W injection to yield a solution containing 2 to 20 mcg/mL.
▼ When using a device with a volumetric infusion chamber, add appropriate volume of diluent to the chamber; then add 1 mL of alprostadil concentrate.
▼ During dilution, avoid direct contact between concentrate and wall of plastic volumetric infusion chamber because

solution may become hazy. If this occurs, discard solution.

▼ Don't use diluents that contain benzyl alcohol. Fatal toxic syndrome may occur.

▼ Drug isn't recommended for direct injection or intermittent infusion. Give by continuous infusion using an infusion pump. Infuse through a large peripheral or central vein or through an umbilical artery catheter placed at the level of the ductus arteriosus. If flushing from peripheral vasodilation occurs, reposition catheter.

▼ Reduce infusion rate if patient develops fever or significant hypotension.

▼ **Incompatibilities:** None reported.

ACTION

Relaxes smooth muscle of ductus arteriosus.

Route	Onset	Peak	Duration
I.V.	20 min	1–2 hr	Length of infusion

Half-life: About 5 to 10 minutes.

ADVERSE REACTIONS

CNS: fever, *seizures.*
CV: flushing, *bradycardia, cardiac arrest,* edema, hypotension, tachycardia.
GI: diarrhea.
Hematologic: *DIC.*
Metabolic: hypokalemia.
Respiratory: *apnea.*
Other: *sepsis.*

INTERACTIONS

None significant.

EFFECTS ON LAB TEST RESULTS

● May decrease potassium level.

CONTRAINDICATIONS & CAUTIONS

● Contraindicated in neonates before making differential diagnosis between respiratory distress syndrome and cyanotic heart disease; also contraindicated in those with respiratory distress syndrome.

● Use cautiously in neonates with bleeding tendencies because drug inhibits platelet aggregation.

⚠ *Overdose S&S:* Apnea, bradycardia, pyrexia, hypotension, flushing.

NURSING CONSIDERATIONS

Black Box Warning Apnea is most often seen in neonates weighing less than 2 kg (4.5 lb) at birth and usually appears during the first hour of drug infusion. Monitor respiratory status and keep emergency ventilatory support available. ∎

● In infants with restricted pulmonary blood flow, measure drug's effectiveness by monitoring blood oxygenation. In infants with restricted systemic blood flow, measure drug's effectiveness by monitoring systemic blood pressure and blood pH.

● Monitor arterial pressure by umbilical artery catheter, auscultation, or Doppler transducer. If arterial pressure falls significantly, slow infusion rate.

● Carefully monitor neonates receiving drug at recommended doses for longer than 120 hours for gastric outlet obstruction and antral hyperplasia.

⊙ *Alert:* CV and CNS adverse reactions occur more often in infants weighing less than 2 kg and in those receiving infusions for longer than 48 hours.

⊙ *Alert:* Stop infusion immediately if overdose is suspected.

● *Look alike–sound alike:* Don't confuse alprostadil with alprazolam.

PATIENT TEACHING

● Tell parents why this drug is needed, and explain its use.

● Encourage parents to ask questions and express concerns.

SAFETY ALERT!

alteplase (tissue plasminogen activator, recombinant; t-PA)

al-ti-PLAZE

Activase, Cathflo Activase

Therapeutic class: Thrombolytics
Pharmacologic class: Enzymes
Pregnancy risk category: C

AVAILABLE FORMS

Cathflo Activase injection: 2-mg single-patient vials

Reactions in bold italics are *life-threatening*. Interactions may have a *rapid onset* or a *delayed onset.*

Injection: 50-mg (29 million international units) vials, 100-mg (58 million international units) vials

INDICATIONS & DOSAGES
➤ **Lysis of thrombi obstructing coronary arteries in acute MI (Activase)**
3-hour infusion
Adults weighing 65 kg (143 lb) or more:
100 mg by I.V. infusion over 3 hours, as follows: 60 mg in first hour, 6 to 10 mg of which is given as a bolus over first 1 to 2 minutes. Then 20 mg/hour infused for 2 hours.
Adults weighing less than 65 kg:
1.25 mg/kg in a similar fashion: 60% in first hour, 10% of which is given as a bolus; then 20% of total dose per hour for 2 hours. Don't exceed total dose of 100 mg.
Accelerated infusion
Adults weighing more than 67 kg (147 lb):
100 mg maximum total dose. Give 15 mg I.V. bolus over 1 to 2 minutes, followed by 50 mg infused over the next 30 minutes; then 35 mg infused over the next hour. Don't exceed total dose of 100 mg.
Adults weighing 67 kg or less: 15 mg I.V. bolus over 1 to 2 minutes, followed by 0.75 mg/kg (not to exceed 50 mg) infused over the next 30 minutes; then 0.5 mg/kg (not to exceed 35 mg) infused over the next hour. Don't exceed total dose of 100 mg.
➤ **To manage acute massive pulmonary embolism (PE) (Activase)**
Adults: 100 mg by I.V. infusion over 2 hours. Begin heparin at end of infusion when PTT or thrombin time returns to twice normal or less. Don't exceed 100-mg dose. Higher doses may increase risk of intracranial bleeding.
➤ **Acute ischemic stroke (Activase)**
Adults: 0.9 mg/kg by I.V. infusion over 1 hour with 10% of total dose given as an initial I.V. bolus over 1 minute. Maximum total dose is 90 mg.
➤ **To restore function to central venous access devices (Cathflo Activase)**
Adults and children older than age 2:
For patients weighing more than 30 kg (66 lb), instill 2 mg in 2 mL sterile water into catheter. For patients weighing between 10 and 30 kg (22 to 66 lb), instill 110% of the internal lumen volume of the catheter,

not to exceed 2 mg in 2 mL sterile water. After 30 minutes of dwell time, assess catheter function by aspirating blood. If function is restored, aspirate 4 to 5 mL of blood in patients weighing 10 kg or 3 mL in patients weighing less than 10 kg to remove drug and residual clot, and gently irrigate the catheter with normal saline solution. If catheter function isn't restored after 120 minutes, instill a second dose.

ADMINISTRATION
I.V.
▼ Immediately before use, reconstitute solution with unpreserved sterile water for injection. Check manufacturer's labeling for specific information.
▼ Don't use 50-mg vial if vacuum isn't present; 100-mg vials don't have a vacuum.
▼ Using an 18G needle, direct stream of sterile water at lyophilized cake. Don't shake.
▼ Slight foaming is common. Let it settle before giving drug. Solution should be colorless or pale yellow.
▼ Drug may be given reconstituted (at 1 mg/mL) or diluted with an equal volume of normal saline solution or D_5W to yield 0.5 mg/mL.
▼ Give drug using a controlled infusion device.
▼ Discard any unused drug after 8 hours.
Cathflo Activase
▼ Assess the cause of catheter dysfunction before using drug. Possible causes of occlusion include catheter malposition, mechanical failure, constriction by a suture, and lipid deposits or drug precipitates in the catheter lumen. Don't try to suction the catheter because you risk damaging the vessel wall or collapsing a soft-walled catheter.
▼ Reconstitute Cathflo Activase with 2.2 mL sterile water to yield 1 mg/mL. Dissolve completely to produce a colorless to pale yellow solution. Don't shake.
▼ Don't use excessive pressure while instilling drug into catheter; doing so could rupture the catheter or expel a clot into circulation.
▼ Solution is stable up to 8 hours at room temperature.

▼ **Incompatibilities:** None reported, but don't mix with other drugs.

ACTION
Converts plasminogen to plasmin by directly cleaving peptide bonds at two sites, causing fibrinolysis.

Route	Onset	Peak	Duration
I.V.	Unknown	Unknown	Unknown

Half-life: Less than 10 minutes.

ADVERSE REACTIONS
CNS: *cerebral hemorrhage,* fever.
CV: *arrhythmias,* hypotension, edema, *cholesterol embolization, venous thrombosis.*
GI: *bleeding (Cathflo Activase),* nausea, vomiting.
GU: *bleeding.*
Hematologic: *spontaneous bleeding.*
Skin: ecchymosis.
Other: *anaphylaxis, sepsis (Cathflo Activase),* bleeding at puncture sites, hypersensitivity reactions.

INTERACTIONS
Drug-drug. *Aspirin, clopidogrel, dipyridamole, drugs affecting platelet activity (abciximab), heparin, warfarin, anticoagulants:* May increase risk of bleeding. Monitor patient carefully.
Nitroglycerin: May decrease alteplase antigen level. Avoid using together. If use together is unavoidable, use the lowest effective dose of nitroglycerin.

EFFECTS ON LAB TEST RESULTS
● May alter coagulation and fibrinolytic test results.

CONTRAINDICATIONS & CAUTIONS
● Activase therapy for acute MI or PE is contraindicated in patients with active internal bleeding; history of stroke; recent intracranial or intraspinal surgery or trauma; intracranial neoplasm, AV malformation, or aneurysm; known bleeding diathesis; or severe uncontrolled hypertension.
● Activase therapy for acute ischemic stroke is contraindicated in patients with evidence of intracranial hemorrhage; suspected subarachnoid hemorrhage; recent (within

3 months) intracranial or intraspinal surgery; serious head trauma or previous stroke; history of intracranial hemorrhage; uncontrolled hypertension (blood pressure greater than 185 mm Hg systolic or 110 mm Hg diastolic) at time of treatment; seizure at onset of stroke; active internal bleeding; intracranial neoplasm, AV malformation, or aneurysm; bleeding diathesis (which may include current use of oral anticoagulants, INR greater than 1.7, PT greater than 15 seconds, platelet count less than 100,000/mm^3, or a patient who has received heparin within the previous 48 hours and who at presentation has an elevated aPTT).
● In patients with acute ischemic stroke, Activase may be initiated before available coagulation study results. The infusion should be discontinued if either a pretreatment INR is greater than 1.7 or an elevated aPTT is identified.
● Patients with severe neurologic deficits (National Institutes of Health Stroke Scale greater than 22) or who have major early infarct signs on a CT scan may have increased risk of bleeding.
● Use cautiously in patients having major surgery within 10 days (when bleeding is difficult to control because of its location); previous puncture of a noncompressible vessel; concomitant oral anticoagulant therapy; organ biopsy; trauma (including cardiopulmonary resuscitation); GI or GU bleeding; cerebrovascular disease; systolic pressure of 175 mm Hg or higher or diastolic pressure of 110 mm Hg or higher; mitral stenosis, atrial fibrillation, or other conditions that may lead to left heart thrombus; acute pericarditis or subacute bacterial endocarditis; hemostatic defects caused by hepatic or renal impairment; septic thrombophlebitis; or diabetic hemorrhagic retinopathy.
● Use cautiously in patients receiving anticoagulants, in patients age 75 and older, and during pregnancy and the first 10 days postpartum.

NURSING CONSIDERATIONS
❸ *Alert:* When used for acute ischemic stroke, give drug within 3 hours after symptoms occur and only when intracranial bleeding has been ruled out.

• Drug may be given to menstruating women.

• To recannulize occluded coronary arteries and improve heart function, begin treatment as soon as possible after symptoms start.

• Anticoagulant and antiplatelet therapy is commonly started during or after treatment, to decrease risk of another thrombosis.

• Monitor vital signs and neurologic status carefully. Keep patient on strict bed rest.

• Coronary thrombolysis is linked with arrhythmias caused by reperfusion of ischemic myocardium. Such arrhythmias don't differ from those commonly linked with MI. Have antiarrhythmics readily available, and carefully monitor ECG.

• Avoid invasive procedures, I.M. injections, and nonessential handling of the patient during thrombolytic therapy. Perform essential venipunctures carefully. Closely monitor patient for signs of internal bleeding, and frequently check all puncture sites. Bleeding is the most common adverse effect and may occur internally and at external puncture sites.

• If an arterial puncture is necessary during Activase infusion, use an arm vessel that can be manually compressed. Apply pressure for at least 30 minutes followed by a pressure dressing. Check the site regularly for bleeding.

• If uncontrollable bleeding occurs, stop infusion (and heparin) and notify prescriber.

• *Look alike–sound alike:* Don't confuse alteplase with Altace or Activase with TNKase.

PATIENT TEACHING
• Explain use and administration of drug to patient and family.
• Tell patient to report adverse reactions promptly.

alvimopan
al-VIM-oh-pan

Entereg

Therapeutic class: Bowel restorative drugs
Pharmacologic class: Peripherally acting mu-opioid receptor antagonists
Pregnancy risk category: B

AVAILABLE FORMS
Capsules: 12 mg

INDICATIONS & DOSAGES
➤ **Acceleration of recovery after partial large- or small-bowel resection surgery with primary anastomosis**
Adults: 12 mg P.O. 30 minutes to 5 hours before surgery, followed by 12 mg P.O. b.i.d. beginning day after surgery, for maximum of 15 doses (180 mg).

ADMINISTRATION
P.O.
• May give with or without food.

ACTION
Competitively and selectively binds to mu-opioid receptors in GI tract, preventing peripheral effects of opioids on GI motility and secretion and thereby shortening recovery time after surgery.

Route	Onset	Peak	Duration
P.O.	Rapid	2 hr	Unknown

Half-life: 10 to 18 hours.

ADVERSE REACTIONS
GI: constipation, dyspepsia, flatulence.
GU: urine retention.
Hematologic: anemia.
Metabolic: hypokalemia.
Musculoskeletal: back pain.

INTERACTIONS
None.

EFFECTS ON LAB TEST RESULTS
None.

CONTRAINDICATIONS & CAUTIONS

Black Box Warning Alvimopan is available only for short-term (15 doses) use in hospitalized patients. Only hospitals that have registered in and met all of requirements for the Entereg Access Support and Education (E.A.S.E.) program may use alvimopan. ■

• Contraindicated in patients who have taken opioids for more than 7 days immediately before taking this drug. Avoid use in patients with severe renal or hepatic impairment.

• Use cautiously in patients with history of recent opioid use.

• Use in pregnancy only if benefit to mother outweighs risk to fetus. It isn't known if drug appears in breast milk. Use cautiously.

NURSING CONSIDERATIONS

• Drug is available only to hospitals that enroll in the E.A.S.E. program (1-866-423-6567). Hospitals that enroll must educate staff about limiting use to inpatients for maximum of 15 doses.

• Monitor GI status closely.

• Closely monitor patients with history of opioid use for chronic pain; drug is associated with increased incidence of MI in these patients.

• To avoid increasing sensitivity, take careful drug history to rule out recent opioid use. Signs and symptoms of increased sensitivity include abdominal pain, nausea, vomiting, and diarrhea.

• *Look alike–sound alike:* Don't confuse alvimopan with almotriptan.

PATIENT TEACHING

• Tell patient to report previous use of opioids, including in the week before surgery.

• Instruct patient to report adverse effects, such as diarrhea, abdominal pain, nausea, and vomiting.

• Explain that drug is to be used only while in the hospital, for no more than 7 days after surgery.

amantadine hydrochloride
a-MAN-ta-deen

Therapeutic class: Antivirals
Pharmacologic class: Synthetic cyclic primary amines
Pregnancy risk category: C

AVAILABLE FORMS
Capsules: 100 mg
Syrup: 50 mg/5 mL
Tablets: 100 mg

INDICATIONS & DOSAGES

Adjust-a-dose (for all indications): For patients with CrCl of 30 to 50 mL/minute, 200 mg the first day and 100 mg thereafter; if CrCl is 15 to 29 mL/minute, 200 mg the first day and then 100 mg on alternate days; if CrCl is less than 15 mL/minute or if patient is receiving hemodialysis, 200 mg every 7 days.

➤ **Parkinson disease**

Adults: Initially, if used as monotherapy, 100 mg P.O. b.i.d. In patients with serious illness or in those already receiving high doses of other antiparkinsonians, begin dose at 100 mg P.O. once daily. Increase to 100 mg b.i.d. if needed after at least 1 week. Some patients may benefit from 400 mg daily in divided doses.

➤ **To prevent or treat symptoms of influenza type A virus and respiratory tract illnesses**

Children age 13 and older and adults up to age 65: 200 mg P.O. daily as a single dose or 100 mg P.O. b.i.d.

Children ages 9 to 12: 100 mg P.O. b.i.d.

Children ages 1 to 8: 4.4 to 8.8 mg/kg P.O. as a total daily dose given once daily or in two equally divided doses. Maximum daily dose is 150 mg.

Elderly patients: 100 mg P.O. once daily in patients older than age 65 with normal renal function.

Begin treatment within 24 to 48 hours after symptoms appear and continue for 24 to 48 hours after symptoms disappear (usually 2 to 7 days). Start prophylaxis as soon as possible after exposure and continue for at least 10 days after exposure. May continue prophylactic treatment up to

90 days for repeated or suspected exposures if influenza vaccine is unavailable. If used with influenza vaccine, continue dose for 2 to 3 weeks until antibody response to vaccine has developed.

➤ **Drug-induced extrapyramidal reactions**

Adults: 100 mg P.O. b.i.d. May increase to 300 mg daily in divided doses.

ADMINISTRATION

P.O.

● Give without regard for food.

ACTION

May exert its antiparkinsonian effect by causing the release of dopamine in the substantia nigra. As an antiviral, may prevent release of viral nucleic acid into the host cell, reducing duration of fever and other systemic symptoms.

Route	Onset	Peak	Duration
P.O.	Unknown	1–4 hr	Unknown

Half-life: About 24 hours; with renal dysfunction, as long as 10 days.

ADVERSE REACTIONS

CNS: dizziness, insomnia, irritability, lightheadedness, depression, fatigue, confusion, hallucinations, anxiety, ataxia, headache, nervousness, dream abnormalities, agitation.
CV: *heart failure,* peripheral edema, orthostatic hypotension.
EENT: blurred vision.
GI: nausea, anorexia, constipation, vomiting, dry mouth.
Skin: livedo reticularis.

INTERACTIONS

Drug-drug. *Anticholinergics:* May increase anticholinergic effects. Use together cautiously; reduce dosage of anticholinergic before starting amantadine.
CNS stimulants: May increase CNS stimulation. Use together cautiously.
Quinidine, sulfamethoxazole–trimethoprim, thiazide diuretics, triamterene: May increase amantadine level, increasing the risk of toxicity. Use together cautiously.
Thioridazine: May worsen Parkinson disease tremor. Monitor patient closely.

Drug-herb. *Jimsonweed:* May adversely affect CV function. Discourage use together.
Drug-lifestyle. *Alcohol use:* May increase CNS effects, including dizziness, confusion, and orthostatic hypotension. Discourage use together.

EFFECTS ON LAB TEST RESULTS

● May increase CK, BUN, creatinine, alkaline phosphatase, LDH, bilirubin, GGT, AST, and ALT levels.

CONTRAINDICATIONS & CAUTIONS

● Contraindicated in patients hypersensitive to drug.
● Use cautiously in elderly patients and in patients with seizure disorders, heart failure, peripheral edema, hepatic disease, mental illness, eczematoid rash, renal impairment, orthostatic hypotension, and CV disease. Monitor renal and liver function tests.

⚠ *Overdose S&S:* Arrhythmia, hypertension, tachycardia, pulmonary edema, respiratory distress, increased BUN level, decreased creatinine clearance, renal insufficiency, insomnia, anxiety, aggressive behavior, hypertonia, hyperkinesia, tremor, confusion, disorientation, depersonalization, fear, delirium, hallucinations, psychotic reactions, lethargy, somnolence, coma, seizures, hyperthermia.

NURSING CONSIDERATIONS

● Patients with Parkinson disease who don't respond to anticholinergics may respond to this drug.
● *Alert:* Elderly patients are more susceptible to adverse neurologic effects. Monitor patient for mental status changes.
● *Alert:* Suicidal ideation and attempts may occur in any patient, regardless of psychiatric history.
● *Alert:* Sporadic cases of neuroleptic malignant syndrome have been reported with dosage reduction or drug withdrawal. Observe patient carefully when dosage is abruptly reduced or drug is discontinued.
● Drug can worsen mental problems in patients with a history of psychiatric disorders or substance abuse.
● *Look alike–sound alike:* Don't confuse amantadine with rimantadine or ranitidine.

PATIENT TEACHING
🔄 *Alert:* Tell patient to take drug exactly as prescribed because not doing so may result in serious adverse reactions or death.
• If insomnia occurs, tell patient to take drug several hours before bedtime.
• If patient gets dizzy when he stands up, instruct him not to stand or change positions too quickly.
• Instruct patient to notify prescriber of adverse reactions, especially dizziness, depression, anxiety, nausea, and urine retention.
• Caution patient to avoid activities that require mental alertness until effects of drug are known.
• Encourage patient with Parkinson disease to gradually increase his physical activity as his symptoms improve.
• Advise patient to avoid alcohol while taking drug.

SAFETY ALERT!

ambrisentan
am-bree-SEN-tan

Letairis, Volibris†

Therapeutic class: Antihypertensives
Pharmacologic class: Endothelin-receptor antagonists
Pregnancy risk category: X

AVAILABLE FORMS
Tablets: 5 mg, 10 mg

INDICATIONS & DOSAGES
➤ **Pulmonary arterial hypertension in patients with World Health Organization class II (with significant exertion) or III (with mild exertion) symptoms to improve exercise tolerance and decrease rate of clinical worsening**
Adults: 5 mg P.O. once daily; may increase to 10 mg P.O. once daily if tolerated.

ADMINISTRATION
P.O.
• Give without regard for food.
• Give whole; don't crush or split tablets.

ACTION
Blocks endothelin-1 receptors on vascular endothelin and smooth muscle. Stimulation of these receptors in smooth muscle cells is associated with vasoconstriction and pulmonary artery hypertension.

Route	Onset	Peak	Duration
P.O.	Rapid	2 hr	Unknown

Half-life: 9 hours.

ADVERSE REACTIONS
CNS: asthenia, dizziness, fatigue.
CV: peripheral edema, flushing, *heart failure.*
EENT: nasal congestion, sinusitis.
GI: nausea, vomiting.
Hematologic: anemia.
Hepatic: hepatic impairment.
Respiratory: *pulmonary arterial hypertension.*
Other: hypersensitivity reaction (*angioedema,* rash).

INTERACTIONS
Drug-drug. *Cyclosporine:* May increase ambrisentan levels. Use together cautiously. Limit ambrisentan dosage to 5 mg daily.
Rifampin: May increase ambrisentan area under the curve. Use together cautiously.

EFFECTS ON LAB TEST RESULTS
• May increase AST, ALT, and bilirubin levels.
• May decrease hemoglobin level and hematocrit.

CONTRAINDICATIONS & CAUTIONS
• Contraindicated in patients hypersensitive to drug or its components and in those with idiopathic pulmonary fibrosis, including patients with pulmonary hypertension (WHO group 3).
Black Box Warning Contraindicated in pregnant women because it may harm the fetus. Don't begin drug until pregnancy has been excluded. ∎
• Use cautiously in those with mild hepatic impairment.
• Use cautiously in those with renal impairment; drug hasn't been studied in those with severe renal impairment.

◐ Alert: Patients who develop acute pulmonary edema during initial treatment may have pulmonary veno-occlusive disease. Discontinue drug if pulmonary veno-occlusive disease is confirmed.

⚠ Overdose S&S: Headache, flushing, dizziness, nausea, nasal congestion, hypotension.

NURSING CONSIDERATIONS

Black Box Warning Because of risk of birth defects, ambrisentan is available only through the Letairis Education and Access Program (LEAP). Only registered prescribers and pharmacies may prescribe and dispense ambrisentan and only to patients enrolled in and meeting all the conditions of LEAP (1-866-664-5327). ∎

Black Box Warning Women of childbearing potential must use acceptable methods of contraception during and for 1 month following treatment. Obtain monthly pregnancy tests during treatment and 1 month after therapy discontinuation. ∎

• Treat women of childbearing age only after negative pregnancy tests.

PATIENT TEACHING

Black Box Warning Inform female patient that she'll need to have a pregnancy test done monthly and to report suspected pregnancy to her prescriber immediately. ∎

Black Box Warning Teach woman of childbearing age to use two reliable birth control methods unless she has had tubal sterilization or has a Copper T 380A intrauterine device (IUD) or an LNg 20 IUD inserted. ∎

• Tell patient that monthly blood tests will be done to monitor for adverse effects.

• Advise patient to take the pill whole and not to split, crush, or chew the tablet.

◐ Alert: Teach patient to notify prescriber immediately of signs or symptoms of liver injury, including anorexia, nausea, vomiting, fever, malaise, fatigue, right upper quadrant abdominal discomfort, itching, and jaundice.

• Tell the patient to report edema and weight gain.

• Inform male patients of the potential for decreased sperm count.

amikacin sulfate
am-i-KAY-sin

Therapeutic class: Antibiotics
Pharmacologic class: Aminoglycosides
Pregnancy risk category: D

AVAILABLE FORMS

Injection: 50-mg/mL (pediatric) vial, 250-mg/mL vial, 250-mg/mL disposable syringe

INDICATIONS & DOSAGES

Adjust-a-dose (for all indications): For adults with impaired renal function, initially, 7.5 mg/kg I.M. or I.V. Subsequent doses and frequency determined by amikacin levels and renal function studies. For adults receiving hemodialysis, give supplemental doses of 50% of initial loading dose at end of each dialysis session. Monitor drug levels and adjust dosage accordingly.

➤ **Serious infections caused by sensitive strains of *Pseudomonas aeruginosa, Escherichia coli, Proteus, Klebsiella,* or *Staphylococcus***

Adults and children: Maximum dosage is 15 mg/kg/day I.M. or I.V. infusion, in divided doses every 8 to 12 hours for 7 to 10 days.

Neonates: Initially, loading dose of 10 mg/kg I.V.; then 7.5 mg/kg every 12 hours for 7 to 10 days.

➤ **Uncomplicated UTI caused by organisms not susceptible to less toxic drugs**

Adults: 250 mg I.M. or I.V. b.i.d.

➤ **Active tuberculosis, with other antituberculotics ♦**

Adults and children age 15 and older: 15 mg/kg (up to 1 g) I.M. or I.V. once daily five to seven times per week for 2 to 4 months or until culture conversion. Then reduce dose to 15 mg/kg daily given two or three times weekly depending on other drugs in regimen. Patients older than age 59 may receive a reduced dose of 10 mg/kg (up to 750 mg) daily.

ADMINISTRATION

I.V.

▼ Obtain specimen for culture and sensitivity tests before giving first dose. Begin therapy while awaiting results.

▼ For adults, dilute I.V. drug in 100 to 200 mL of D_5W or normal saline solution. For children, the amount of fluid will depend on the ordered dose.

▼ In adults and children, infuse over 30 to 60 minutes. In infants, infuse over 1 to 2 hours.

▼ After infusion, flush line with normal saline solution or D_5W.

▼ **Incompatibilities:** Allopurinol, aminophylline, amphotericin B, ampicillin, azithromycin, bacitracin, cefazolin, ceftazidime, chlorothiazide sodium, cisplatin, heparin sodium, hetastarch in 0.9% sodium chloride, oxacillin, phenytoin, propofol, thiopental, vancomycin, vitamin B complex with vitamin C.

I.M.

• Obtain specimen for culture and sensitivity tests before giving first dose. Begin therapy while awaiting results.

• Obtain blood for peak level 1 hour after I.M. injection and 30 minutes to 1 hour after I.V. infusion ends; for trough levels, draw blood just before next dose. Don't collect blood in a heparinized tube; heparin is incompatible with aminoglycosides.

ACTION

Inhibits protein synthesis by binding directly to the 30S ribosomal subunit; bactericidal.

Route	Onset	Peak	Duration
I.V.	Immediate	30 min	8–12 hr
I.M.	Unknown	1 hr	8–12 hr

Half-life: Adults, 2 to 3 hours. Patients with severe renal damage, 30 to 86 hours.

ADVERSE REACTIONS

CNS: *neuromuscular blockade.*
EENT: ototoxicity.
GU: azotemia, *nephrotoxicity,* increase in urinary excretion of casts.
Respiratory: *apnea.*

INTERACTIONS

Drug-drug. Black Box Warning *Acyclovir, amphotericin B, bacitracin, cephalosporins,* *cidofovir, cisplatin, methoxyflurane, vancomycin, other aminoglycosides:* May increase nephrotoxicity. Use together cautiously, and monitor renal function test results. ▪

Atracurium, pancuronium, rocuronium, vecuronium: May increase effects of nondepolarizing muscle relaxants, including prolonged respiratory depression. Use together only when necessary, and expect to reduce dosage of nondepolarizing muscle relaxant.

Dimenhydrinate: May mask ototoxicity symptoms. Monitor patient's hearing.

General anesthetics: May increase neuromuscular blockade. Monitor patient for increased effects.

Indomethacin: May increase trough and peak amikacin levels. Monitor amikacin level.

Black Box Warning *I.V. loop diuretics (ethacrynic acid, furosemide):* May increase ototoxicity. Use together cautiously, and monitor patient's hearing. ▪

NSAIDs: May increase amikacin level. Avoid administering together.

Parenteral penicillins: May inactivate amikacin in vitro. Don't mix.

EFFECTS ON LAB TEST RESULTS

• May increase BUN, creatinine, nonprotein nitrogen, and urine urea levels.

CONTRAINDICATIONS & CAUTIONS

• Contraindicated in patients hypersensitive to drug or other aminoglycosides.

• Use cautiously in patients with impaired renal function or neuromuscular disorders, in neonates and infants, and in elderly patients.

⚠ *Overdose S&S:* Nephrotoxicity, ototoxicity, neurotoxicity.

NURSING CONSIDERATIONS

Black Box Warning Due to increased risk of ototoxicity, evaluate patient's hearing before and during therapy if he'll be receiving the drug for longer than 2 weeks. Notify prescriber if patient has tinnitus, vertigo, or hearing loss. ▪

• Weigh patient and review renal function studies before therapy begins.

• Correct dehydration before therapy because of increased risk of toxicity.

Reactions in bold italics are *life-threatening*. Interactions may have a *rapid onset* or a *delayed onset*.

- Peak drug levels greater than 35 mcg/mL and trough levels greater than 10 mcg/mL may be linked to a higher risk of toxicity.

Black Box Warning Due to increased risk of nephrotoxicity, monitor renal function: urine output, specific gravity, urinalysis, BUN and creatinine levels, and CrCl. Report evidence of declining renal function to prescriber. ∎

- Watch for signs and symptoms of superinfection (especially of upper respiratory tract), such as continued fever, chills, and increased pulse rate.

Black Box Warning Neuromuscular blockage and respiratory paralysis have been reported after aminoglycoside administration. Monitor patient closely. ∎

- Therapy usually continues for 7 to 10 days. If no response occurs after 3 to 5 days, stop therapy and obtain new specimens for culture and sensitivity testing.
- *Look alike–sound alike:* Don't confuse amikacin with anakinra.

PATIENT TEACHING

- Instruct patient to promptly report adverse reactions to prescriber.
- Encourage patient to maintain adequate fluid intake.

amiloride hydrochloride
a-MILL-oh-ride

Midamor

Therapeutic class: Diuretics
Pharmacologic class: Potassium-sparing diuretics
Pregnancy risk category: B

AVAILABLE FORMS
Tablets: 5 mg

INDICATIONS & DOSAGES

➤ **Hypertension; hypokalemia; edema of heart failure, usually in patients also taking thiazide or other potassium-wasting diuretics**
Adults: 5 mg P.O. daily, increased to 10 mg daily if needed. If hypokalemia persists with 10 mg, dosage can be increased to 15 mg, then 20 mg with careful monitoring of electrolyte levels.

➤ **Hypokalemia unrelated to potassium-wasting diuretics** ◆
Adults: 10 mg P.O. daily, increased by 10 mg at weekly intervals p.r.n. up to 40 mg daily.

ADMINISTRATION
P.O.
- Give with food to minimize GI upset.

ACTION
Inhibits sodium reabsorption and potassium excretion in the distal tubules.

Route	Onset	Peak	Duration
P.O.	2 hr	6–10 hr	24 hr

Half-life: 6 to 9 hours.

ADVERSE REACTIONS
CNS: dizziness, fatigue, headache, weakness, *encephalopathy.*
GI: abdominal pain, anorexia, appetite changes, constipation, diarrhea, nausea, vomiting.
GU: erectile dysfunction.
Metabolic: hyperkalemia.
Musculoskeletal: muscle cramps.
Respiratory: cough, dyspnea.

INTERACTIONS
Drug-drug. *ACE inhibitors, indomethacin, other potassium-sparing diuretics, potassium supplements:* May cause severe hyperkalemia. Avoid use together if possible. Monitor potassium level closely if using together.
Digoxin: May decrease digoxin clearance and decrease inotropic effects. Monitor digoxin level.
Lithium: May decrease lithium clearance, increasing risk of lithium toxicity. Monitor lithium level.
NSAIDs: May decrease diuretic effectiveness. Avoid use together.
Drug-food. *Foods high in potassium (such as bananas, oranges), salt substitutes containing potassium:* May cause hyperkalemia. Advise patient to choose diet carefully and to use low-potassium salt substitutes.

EFFECTS ON LAB TEST RESULTS

• May increase BUN and potassium levels. May decrease pH, hemoglobin, and liver enzyme and sodium levels.
• May decrease neutrophil count.

CONTRAINDICATIONS & CAUTIONS

• Contraindicated in patients hypersensitive to drug, in those with potassium level greater than 5.5 mEq/L, and in those with anuria, acute or chronic renal insufficiency, or diabetic nephropathy.
• Contraindicated in patients receiving potassium supplementation or other potassium-sparing diuretics, such as spironolactone and triamterene.
• Use cautiously in patients with diabetes mellitus, cardiopulmonary disease, or severe hepatic insufficiency.
• Use cautiously in elderly or debilitated patients.
• Use during pregnancy only if clearly needed. It's not known whether drug appears in breast milk. Consider having patient discontinue either drug or breast-feeding.
• Safety and effectiveness in children haven't been established.
⚠ **Overdose S&S:** Dehydration, electrolyte imbalance.

NURSING CONSIDERATIONS

• To prevent nausea, give with meals.
Black Box Warning Carefully monitor potassium level because of the risk of hyperkalemia. Monitor potassium level when drug is initiated, when diuretic dosages are adjusted, and during an illness that could affect renal function. Alert prescriber immediately if potassium level exceeds 5.5 mEq/L; expect to stop drug. ∎
• Drug may cause severe hyperkalemia after glucose tolerance testing in patients with diabetes; stop drug at least 3 days before testing.
• **Look alike–sound alike:** Don't confuse amiloride with amiodarone or amlodipine.

PATIENT TEACHING

• Instruct patient to take drug with food to minimize GI upset.

• Advise patient to avoid sudden posture changes and to rise slowly to avoid dizziness.
• Caution patient not to perform hazardous activities if adverse CNS reactions occur.
• To prevent serious hyperkalemia, warn patient to avoid eating potassium-rich foods, potassium-containing salt substitutes, and potassium supplements.
• Advise patient to reports signs of hyperkalemia, such as tingling, muscle weakness, muscle cramps, fatigue, and limb paralysis.
• Instruct patient to check with prescriber before taking new prescriptions or OTC drugs.

SAFETY ALERT!

amiodarone hydrochloride
am-ee-OH-dah-rohn

Cordarone, Nexterone, Pacerone

Therapeutic class: Antiarrhythmics
Pharmacologic class: Benzofuran derivatives
Pregnancy risk category: D

AVAILABLE FORMS

Injection: 50 mg/mL, 150 mg/100 mL, 360 mg/200 mL
Tablets: 100 mg, 200 mg, 400 mg

INDICATIONS & DOSAGES

Black Box Warning Amiodarone is intended for use only in patients with life-threatening recurrent ventricular fibrillation or recurrent hemodynamically unstable ventricular tachycardia unresponsive to adequate doses of other antiarrhythmics or when alternative drugs can't be tolerated. ∎
Adults: Give loading dose of 800 to 1,600 mg P.O. daily or divided into two equal doses daily for 1 to 3 weeks until first therapeutic response occurs; then 600 to 800 mg P.O. daily for 1 month, followed by maintenance dose of 400 mg P.O. daily or, for patients with severe GI intolerance, 200 mg P.O. b.i.d.
  Or, give loading dose of 150 mg I.V. over 10 minutes (15 mg/minute); then 360 mg I.V. over next 6 hours (1 mg/minute), followed by 540 mg I.V. over next 18 hours (0.5 mg/minute). After first 24 hours,

continue with maintenance I.V. infusion of 720 mg/24 hours (0.5 mg/minute).

Maintenance infusion can continue cautiously for 2 to 3 weeks. To convert to oral form from I.V.: If I.V. infusion has been for less than 1 week, initial dose is 800 to 1,600 mg P.O. daily; if I.V. infusion has been from 1 to 3 weeks, initial dose is 600 to 800 mg P.O. daily; if I.V. infusion has been more than 3 weeks, initial dose is 400 mg P.O. daily.

If breakthrough episodes of ventricular fibrillation or hemodynamically unstable ventricular tachycardia occur, may give supplemental infusions of 150 mg I.V. over 10 minutes.

➤ **Conversion of atrial fibrillation to sinus rhythm** ◆

Adults: 5 to 7 mg/kg I.V. over 30 to 60 minutes; then 1.2 to 1.8 g/day as a continuous I.V. infusion or in divided oral doses until a total of 10 g has been given; then 200 to 400 mg/day P.O. daily as maintenance therapy.

ADMINISTRATION

P.O.

● Divide oral loading dose into two or three equal doses and give with meals to decrease GI intolerance. Give maintenance dose once daily or divide into two doses with meals to decrease GI intolerance.

I.V.

▼ Give drug I.V. only if continuous ECG and electrophysiologic monitoring are available.

▼ Mix first dose of 150 mg in 100 mL of D₅W solution.

▼ If infusion will last 2 hours or longer, mix solution in glass or polyolefin bottles.

▼ If concentration is 2 mg/mL or more, give drug through a central line. If possible, use a dedicated line.

▼ Use an in-line filter.

▼ Continuously monitor patient's cardiac status. If hypotension occurs, reduce infusion rate.

▼ I.V. amiodarone leaches out plasticizers from I.V. tubing and adsorbs to polyvinyl chloride (PVC) tubing, which can adversely affect male reproductive tract development in fetuses, infants, and tod-

dlers when used at concentrations or flow rates outside of recommendations.

▼ **Incompatibilities:** Aminophylline, ampicillin sodium–sulbactam sodium, bivalirudin, cefazolin sodium, ceftazidime, digoxin, furosemide, heparin sodium, imipenem–cilastatin sodium, magnesium sulfate, normal saline solution, piperacillin sodium, piperacillin–tazobactam sodium, quinidine gluconate, sodium bicarbonate, sodium nitroprusside, sodium phosphates.

ACTION

Effects result from blockade of potassium chloride, leading to a prolongation of action potential duration.

Route	Onset	Peak	Duration
P.O.	Variable	3–7 hr	Variable
I.V.	Unknown	Unknown	Variable

Half-life: 25 to 110 days (usually 40 to 50 days).

ADVERSE REACTIONS

CNS: fatigue, malaise, tremor, peripheral neuropathy, ataxia, paresthesia, insomnia, sleep disturbances, headache.
CV: hypotension, *bradycardia, arrhythmias, heart failure, heart block, sinus arrest,* edema.
EENT: asymptomatic corneal microdeposits, visual disturbances, optic neuropathy or neuritis resulting in visual impairment, abnormal smell.
GI: nausea, vomiting, abnormal taste, anorexia, constipation, abdominal pain.
Hematologic: *coagulation abnormalities.*
Hepatic: *hepatic failure,* hepatic dysfunction.
Metabolic: hypothyroidism, hyperthyroidism.
Respiratory: *acute respiratory distress syndrome, severe pulmonary toxicity.*
Skin: photosensitivity, solar dermatitis, blue-gray skin.

INTERACTIONS

Drug-drug. *Antiarrhythmics:* May reduce hepatic or renal clearance of certain antiarrhythmics, especially flecainide, procainamide, and quinidine. Use of amiodarone with other antiarrhythmics, especially mexiletine, propafenone, disopyramide, and procainamide, may induce torsades de pointes. Avoid using together.

Azole antifungals, disopyramide, pimozide: May increase the risk of arrhythmias, including torsades de pointes. Avoid using together.

Beta blockers, calcium channel blockers: May potentiate bradycardia, sinus arrest, and AV block; may increase hypotensive effect. Use together cautiously.

Cimetidine: May increase amiodarone level. Use together cautiously.

Cyclosporine: May increase cyclosporine level, resulting in an increase in the serum creatinine level and renal toxicity. Monitor cyclosporine levels and renal function tests.

Dabigatran: May increase bleeding risk. Monitor patient closely.

Digoxin: May increase digoxin level 70% to 100%. Monitor digoxin level closely, and reduce digoxin dosage by half or stop drug completely when starting amiodarone therapy.

Fentanyl: May cause hypotension, bradycardia, and decreased cardiac output. Monitor patient closely.

Fluoroquinolones: May increase risk of arrhythmias, including torsades de pointes. Avoid using together.

HMG-CoA reductase inhibitors (such as simvastatin): May cause myopathy or rhabdomyolysis. Monitor patient carefully.

Loratadine, trazodone: May cause prolonged QT interval and torsades de pointes. Monitor closely.

Macrolide antibiotics (azithromycin, clarithromycin, erythromycin, telithromycin): May cause additive prolongation of the QT interval. Use with caution. Avoid use with telithromycin.

Methotrexate: May impair methotrexate metabolism, causing toxicity. Use together cautiously.

Phenytoin: May decrease phenytoin metabolism and amiodarone level. Monitor phenytoin level and adjust dosages of drugs if needed.

Protease inhibitors (amprenavir, atazanavir, indinavir, lopinavir–ritonavir, nelfinavir, ritonavir, saquinavir): May increase the risk of amiodarone toxicity. Use of ritonavir or nelfinavir with amiodarone is con-

traindicated. Use other protease inhibitors cautiously.

Quinidine: May increase quinidine level, causing life-threatening cardiac arrhythmias. Avoid using together, or monitor quinidine level closely if use together can't be avoided. Adjust quinidine dosage as needed.

Rifamycins: May decrease amiodarone level. Monitor patient closely.

Simvastatin: May cause myopathy and rhabdomyolysis with concomitant use. Simvastatin dosage shouldn't exceed 20 mg daily.

Theophylline: May increase theophylline level and cause toxicity. Monitor theophylline level.

Warfarin: May increase anticoagulant response, with the potential for serious or fatal bleeding. Decrease warfarin dosage 33% to 50% when starting amiodarone. Monitor patient closely.

Drug-herb. *Pennyroyal:* May change rate of formation of toxic metabolites of pennyroyal. Discourage use together.

St. John's wort: May decrease amiodarone levels. Discourage use together.

Drug-food. *Grapefruit juice:* May inhibit CYP3A4 metabolism of drug in the intestinal mucosa, causing increased levels and risk of toxicity. Discourage use together.

Drug-lifestyle. *Sun exposure:* May cause photosensitivity reaction. Advise patient to avoid excessive sunlight exposure and to take precautions while in the sun.

EFFECTS ON LAB TEST RESULTS
● May increase alkaline phosphatase, ALT, AST, GGT, reverse T_3, and T_4 levels. May decrease T_3 level.
● May increase total cholesterol and serum lipid levels.
● May increase PT and INR.

CONTRAINDICATIONS & CAUTIONS
● Contraindicated in patients hypersensitive to drug or to iodine.
● Contraindicated in those with cardiogenic shock, second- or third-degree AV block, severe SA node disease resulting in bradycardia unless an artificial pacemaker is present, and in those for whom bradycardia has caused syncope.

Reactions in bold italics are *life-threatening*. Interactions may have a *rapid onset* or a *delayed onset*.

• Use cautiously in patients receiving other antiarrhythmics.

• Use cautiously in patients with pulmonary, hepatic, or thyroid disease.

⚠ *Overdose S&S:* AV block, bradycardia, hypotension, cardiogenic shock, hepatotoxicity.

NURSING CONSIDERATIONS

• Be aware of the high risk of adverse reactions.

• Obtain baseline pulmonary, liver, and thyroid function test results and baseline chest X-ray.

Black Box Warning Give loading doses in a hospital setting and with continuous ECG monitoring because of the slow onset of antiarrhythmic effect and the risk of life-threatening arrhythmias. ▮

Black Box Warning Drug may pose life-threatening management problems in patients at risk for sudden death. Use only in patients with life-threatening, recurrent ventricular arrhythmias unresponsive to or intolerant of other antiarrhythmics or alternative drugs. Amiodarone can cause fatal toxicities, including hepatic and pulmonary toxicity. ▮

Black Box Warning Drug is highly toxic. Watch carefully for pulmonary toxicity. Risk increases in patients receiving doses over 400 mg/day. ▮

• Watch for evidence of pneumonitis, exertional dyspnea, nonproductive cough, and pleuritic chest pain. Monitor pulmonary function tests and chest X-ray.

• Monitor liver and thyroid function test results and electrolyte levels, particularly potassium and magnesium.

• Monitor PT and INR if patient takes warfarin and digoxin level if he takes digoxin.

• Instill methylcellulose ophthalmic solution during amiodarone therapy to minimize corneal microdeposits. About 1 to 4 months after starting amiodarone, most patients develop corneal microdeposits, although 10% or less have vision disturbances. Regular ophthalmic examinations are advised.

• Monitor blood pressure and heart rate and rhythm frequently. Perform continuous ECG monitoring when starting or changing dosage. Notify prescriber of significant change in assessment results.

• Safety and effectiveness in children haven't been established. Life-threatening gasping syndrome may occur in neonates given I.V. solutions containing benzyl alcohol.

• During or after treatment with I.V. form, patient may be transferred to oral therapy.

• *Look alike–sound alike:* Don't confuse amiodarone with amiloride. Don't confuse Cordarone with Cardura.

PATIENT TEACHING

• Advise patient to wear sunscreen or protective clothing to prevent sensitivity reaction to the sun. Monitor patient for skin burning or tingling, followed by redness and blistering. Exposed skin may turn blue-gray.

• Advise patient to keep follow-up appointments, including eye exams and blood tests.

• Tell patient to contact prescriber if he has vision changes, weakness, "pins and needles" or numbness, poor coordination, weight change, heat or cold intolerance, or neck swelling.

• Tell patient to take oral drug with food if GI reactions occur.

• Inform patient that adverse effects of drug are more common at high doses and become more frequent with treatment lasting longer than 6 months, but are generally reversible when drug is stopped. Resolution of adverse reactions may take up to 4 months.

• Tell patient not to stop taking this medication without consulting with prescriber.

amitriptyline hydrochloride
a-mee-TRIP-ti-leen

Elavil†, Levate†

Therapeutic class: Antidepressants
Pharmacologic class: Tricyclic antidepressants
Pregnancy risk category: C

AVAILABLE FORMS
Tablets: 10 mg, 25 mg, 50 mg, 75 mg, 100 mg, 150 mg

INDICATIONS & DOSAGES
➤ **Depression (outpatients)**
Adults: 75 mg P.O. daily in divided doses. May increase by 25 to 50 mg, as needed,

to a total of 150 mg/day. Make increases preferably in late afternoon or at bedtime. Continue for at least 3 months. Maintenance, 40 to 100 mg daily.
Elderly patients and adolescents: 10 mg P.O. t.i.d. and 20 mg at bedtime daily.
➤ **Depression (hospitalized patients)**
Adults: Initially, 100 mg P.O. daily. If necessary, gradually increase to 200 to 300 mg daily. Maintenance dose is 40 to 100 mg daily. Continue for at least 3 months.
➤ **Postherpetic neuralgia ◆**
Adults: 65 to 100 mg P.O. daily for at least 3 weeks.
➤ **Prevention of chronic headache ◆**
Adults: 20 to 100 mg P.O. daily.
➤ **Prevention of migraine ◆**
Adults: 10 to 100 mg P.O. daily.
➤ **Fibromyalgia ◆**
Adults: 10 to 50 mg P.O. at bedtime.
➤ **Irritable bowel syndrome ◆**
Adults: 10 to 50 mg P.O. daily.
Black Box Warning Drug isn't approved for use in children. ∎

ADMINISTRATION
P.O.
● Give drug without regard for food.

ACTION
Unknown. A TCA that increases the amount of norepinephrine, serotonin, or both in the CNS by blocking their reuptake by the presynaptic neurons.

Route	Onset	Peak	Duration
P.O.	Unknown	2–12 hr	Unknown

Half-life: 10 to 50 hours.

ADVERSE REACTIONS
CNS: *stroke, seizures, coma,* ataxia, tremor, peripheral neuropathy, anxiety, insomnia, restlessness, drowsiness, dizziness, weakness, fatigue, headache, extrapyramidal reactions, hallucinations, delusions, disorientation.
CV: orthostatic hypotension, tachycardia, *heart block, arrhythmias, MI,* ECG changes, hypertension, edema.
EENT: blurred vision, tinnitus, mydriasis, increased intraocular pressure (IOP).

GI: dry mouth, nausea, vomiting, anorexia, epigastric pain, diarrhea, constipation, paralytic ileus.
GU: urine retention, altered libido, erectile dysfunction.
Hematologic: *agranulocytosis, thrombocytopenia, leukopenia,* eosinophilia.
Metabolic: *hypoglycemia,* hyperglycemia.
Skin: rash, urticaria, photosensitivity reactions, diaphoresis.
Other: hypersensitivity reactions.

INTERACTIONS
Drug-drug. *Barbiturates, CNS depressants:* May enhance CNS depression. Avoid using together.
Cimetidine, **fluoxetine, fluvoxamine,** *hormonal contraceptives,* **paroxetine, sertraline:** May increase TCA level. Monitor drug levels and patient for signs of toxicity.
Clonidine: May cause life-threatening hypertension. Avoid using together.
Disulfiram: May increase pharmacologic effects of amitriptyline. May cause acute organic brain syndrome. Monitor patient. Stop amitriptyline or decrease amitriptyline dosage if an interaction is suspected.
Epinephrine, norepinephrine: May increase hypertensive effect. Use together cautiously.
Linezolid, methylene blue: May cause serotonin syndrome. Use extreme caution and monitor closely.
MAO inhibitors: May cause severe excitation, hyperpyrexia, or seizures, usually with high doses. Avoid using within 14 days of MAO inhibitor therapy.
Quinolones: May increase the risk of life-threatening arrhythmias. Avoid using together.
Drug-herb. *Evening primrose:* May cause additive or synergistic effect, resulting in lower seizure threshold and increasing the risk of seizures. Discourage use together.
St. John's wort, SAM-e, yohimbe: May cause serotonin syndrome and decrease amitriptyline level. Discourage use together.
Drug-lifestyle. *Alcohol use:* May enhance CNS depression. Discourage use together.
Smoking: May lower drug level. Watch for lack of effect.

Sun exposure: May increase risk of photosensitivity reactions. Advise patient to avoid excessive sunlight exposure.

EFFECTS ON LAB TEST RESULTS
• May increase or decrease glucose level.
• May increase eosinophil count and LFT values. May decrease granulocyte, platelet, and WBC counts.

CONTRAINDICATIONS & CAUTIONS
• Contraindicated in patients hypersensitive to drug and in those who have received an MAO inhibitor within the past 14 days.
❸ *Alert:* Concomitant use with linezolid or methylene blue can cause serotonin syndrome (fever, mental status changes, muscle twitching, excessive sweating, shivering or shaking, diarrhea, loss of coordination). Use drug with linezolid or methylene blue only for life-threatening or urgent conditions when the potential benefits outweigh the risks of toxicity.
• Contraindicated during acute recovery phase of MI.
• Use cautiously in patients with history of seizures, urine retention, angle-closure glaucoma, or increased IOP; in those with hyperthyroidism, CV disease, diabetes, or impaired liver function; and in those receiving thyroid drugs.
• Use cautiously in elderly patients and in patients with suicidal ideation.
• Use cautiously in those receiving electroconvulsive therapy.
⚠ *Overdose S&S:* Cardiac arrhythmias, severe hypotension, seizures, CNS depression, impaired myocardial contractility, confusion, disturbed concentration, transient visual hallucinations, dilated pupils, disorders of ocular motility, agitation, hyperactive reflexes, polyradiculoneuropathy, stupor, drowsiness, muscle rigidity, vomiting, hypothermia.

NURSING CONSIDERATIONS
Black Box Warning Drug may increase the risk of suicidal thinking and behavior in children, adolescents, and young adults with major depressive disorder or other psychiatric disorder. Don't use in children younger than age 12. ∎

❸ *Alert:* If linezolid or methylene blue must be given, amitriptyline must be stopped and the patient should be monitored for serotonin toxicity for 2 weeks, or until 24 hours after the last dose of methylene blue or linezolid, whichever comes first. Treatment with amitriptyline may be resumed 24 hours after last dose of methylene blue or linezolid.
• Amitriptyline has strong anticholinergic effects and is one of the most sedating TCAs. Anticholinergic effects have rapid onset even though therapeutic effect is delayed for weeks.
• Elderly patients may have an increased sensitivity to anticholinergic effects of drug; sedating effects of drug may increase the risk of falls in this population.
• If signs or symptoms of psychosis occur or increase, expect prescriber to reduce dosage. Record mood changes. Monitor patient for suicidal tendencies and allow only minimum supply of drug.
• Because patients using TCAs may suffer hypertensive episodes during surgery, stop drug gradually several days before surgery.
• Monitor glucose level.
• Watch for nausea, headache, and malaise after abrupt withdrawal of long-term therapy; these symptoms don't indicate addiction.
• Don't withdraw drug abruptly.
• *Look alike–sound alike:* Don't confuse amitriptyline with nortriptyline or aminophylline. Don't confuse Elavil with Eldepryl or enalapril.

PATIENT TEACHING
Black Box Warning Advise families and caregivers to closely observe patient for increased suicidal thinking and behavior. ∎
❸ *Alert:* Teach patient to recognize and immediately report symptoms of serotonin toxicity (fever, mental status changes, muscle twitching, excessive sweating, shivering or shaking, diarrhea, loss of coordination).
• Whenever possible, advise patient to take full dose at bedtime, but warn him of possible morning orthostatic hypotension.
• Tell patient to avoid alcohol during drug therapy.
• Advise patient to consult prescriber before taking other drugs.

• Warn patient to avoid activities that require alertness and good psychomotor coordination until CNS effects of drug are known. Drowsiness and dizziness usually subside after a few weeks.
• Inform patient that dry mouth may be relieved with sugarless hard candy or gum. Saliva substitutes may be useful.
• To prevent photosensitivity reactions, advise patient to use a sunblock, wear protective clothing, and avoid prolonged exposure to strong sunlight.
• Warn patient not to stop drug abruptly.
• Advise patient that it may take as long as 30 days to achieve full therapeutic effect.

amlodipine besylate
am-LOE-di-peen

Norvasc↺

Therapeutic class: Antihypertensives
Pharmacologic class: Calcium channel blockers
Pregnancy risk category: C

AVAILABLE FORMS
Tablets: 2.5 mg, 5 mg, 10 mg

INDICATIONS & DOSAGES
➤ **Chronic stable angina, vasospastic angina (Prinzmetal or variant angina); to reduce risk of hospitalization because of angina; to reduce risk of coronary revascularization procedure in patients with recently documented coronary artery disease (CAD) by angiography and without heart failure or with ejection fraction less than 40%**
Adults: Initially, 5 to 10 mg P.O. daily. Most patients need 10 mg daily.
Elderly patients: Initially, 5 mg P.O. daily.
Adjust-a-dose: For patients who are small or frail or have hepatic insufficiency, initially, 5 mg P.O. daily.
➤ **Hypertension**
Adults: Initially, 5 mg P.O. daily. Dosage adjusted according to patient response and tolerance. Titration should occur over 7 to 14 days. Maximum daily dose is 10 mg.

Children ages 6 to 17: 2.5 to 5 mg P.O. once daily. Maximum dosage is 5 mg daily.
Elderly patients: Initially, 2.5 mg P.O. daily.
Adjust-a-dose: For patients who are small or frail, are taking other antihypertensives, or have hepatic insufficiency, initially, 2.5 mg P.O. daily.

ADMINISTRATION
P.O.
• Give drug without regard for food.

ACTION
Inhibits calcium ion influx across cardiac and smooth-muscle cells, dilates coronary arteries and arterioles, and decreases blood pressure and myocardial oxygen demand.

Route	Onset	Peak	Duration
P.O.	Unknown	6–12 hr	24 hr

Half-life: 30 to 50 hours.

ADVERSE REACTIONS
CNS: headache, somnolence, fatigue, dizziness.
CV: edema, flushing, palpitations.
GI: nausea, abdominal pain.

INTERACTIONS
Conivaptan, CYP3A4 strong inhibitors (itraconazole, ketoconazole, ritonavir): May increase amlodipine plasma concentration. Monitor patient for hypotension and edema.
Cyclosporine: May increase cyclosporine level. Monitor level and patient.
Simvastatin: May increase risk of myopathy, including rhabdomyolysis. Simvastatin dosage shouldn't exceed 20 mg daily.

EFFECTS ON LAB TEST RESULTS
None reported.

CONTRAINDICATIONS & CAUTIONS
• Contraindicated in patients hypersensitive to drug.
• Use cautiously in patients receiving other peripheral vasodilators, especially those with severe aortic stenosis, and in those with heart failure. Because drug is metabolized by the liver, use cautiously and in reduced dosage in patients with severe hepatic disease.

Reactions in bold italics are *life-threatening*. Interactions may have a *rapid onset* or a *delayed onset*.

⚠ *Overdose S&S:* Marked peripheral vasodilation with hypotension and possibly reflex tachycardia.

NURSING CONSIDERATIONS
☀ *Alert:* Monitor patient carefully. Some patients, especially those with severe obstructive CAD, have developed increased frequency, duration, or severity of angina or acute MI after initiation of calcium channel blocker therapy or at time of dosage increase.
• Monitor blood pressure frequently during initiation of therapy. Because drug-induced vasodilation has a gradual onset, acute hypotension is rare.
• Notify prescriber if signs of heart failure occur, such as swelling of hands and feet or shortness of breath.
☀ *Alert:* Abrupt withdrawal of drug may increase frequency and duration of chest pain. Taper dose gradually under medical supervision.
• *Look alike–sound alike:* Don't confuse amlodipine with amiloride.

PATIENT TEACHING
• Caution patient to continue taking drug, even when he feels better.
• Tell patient S.L. nitroglycerin may be taken as needed when angina symptoms are acute. If patient continues nitrate therapy during adjustment of amlodipine dosage, urge continued compliance.

---

amoxicillin
a-mox-i-SILL-in

Amox†, Apo-Amoxi†, Moxatag, Novamoxin†, Nu-Amoxi†

Therapeutic class: Antibiotics
Pharmacologic class: Aminopenicillins
Pregnancy risk category: B

AVAILABLE FORMS
Capsules: 250 mg, 500 mg
Oral suspension: 50 mg/mL (pediatric drops), 125 mg/5 mL, 200 mg/5 mL, 250 mg/5 mL, 400 mg/5 mL (after reconstitution)
Tablets (chewable): 125 mg, 200 mg, 250 mg, 400 mg

Tablets (extended-release): 775 mg
Tablets (film-coated): 500 mg, 875 mg
Tablets for oral suspension: 200 mg, 400 mg, 600 mg

INDICATIONS & DOSAGES
Adjust-a-dose (for all indications): Adults with GFR of less than 30 mL/minute shouldn't receive the 875-mg tablet. Adults with GFR of 10 to 30 mL/minute should receive 250 or 500 mg every 12 hours depending on the infection. Adults with GFR of less than 10 mL/minute should receive 250 or 500 mg every 24 hours depending on the severity of infection. Adults on hemodialysis should receive 250 or 500 mg every 24 hours with an extra dose both during and at the end of dialysis.
➤ **Mild to moderate infections of the ear, nose, and throat; skin and skin structure; or GU tract**
Adults and children weighing 40 kg (88 lb) or more: 500 mg P.O. every 12 hours or 250 mg P.O. every 8 hours.
Children older than age 3 months weighing less than 40 kg: 25 mg/kg/day P.O. divided every 12 hours or 20 mg/kg/day P.O. divided every 8 hours.
Neonates and infants up to age 3 months: Up to 30 mg/kg/day P.O. divided every 12 hours.
➤ **Mild to severe infections of the lower respiratory tract and severe infections of the ear, nose, and throat; skin and skin structure; or GU tract**
Adults and children weighing 40 kg (88 lb) or more: 875 mg P.O. every 12 hours or 500 mg P.O. every 8 hours.
Children older than age 3 months weighing less than 40 kg: 45 mg/kg/day P.O. divided every 12 hours or 40 mg/kg/day P.O. divided every 8 hours.
Neonates and infants up to age 3 months: Up to 30 mg/kg/day P.O. divided every 12 hours.
➤ **Pharyngitis, tonsillitis, or both secondary to *Streptococcus pyogenes* infection**
Adults and children age 12 and older: 775-mg extended-release tablet P.O. once daily with a meal for 10 days.

➤ **Uncomplicated gonorrhea**
Adults and children weighing more than 45 kg (99 lb): 3 g P.O. with 1 g probenecid given as a single dose.
Children age 2 and older weighing less than 45 kg: 50 mg/kg to a maximum of 3 g P.O. with 25 mg/kg of probenecid, to a maximum of 1 g, as a single dose. Don't give probenecid to children younger than age 2.
➤ *Helicobacter pylori* **eradication to reduce risk of duodenal ulcer recurrence**
Adults: Amoxicillin 1 g with lansoprazole 30 mg P.O. every 8 hours for 14 days (dual therapy). Or, amoxicillin 1 g, clarithromycin 500 mg, and lansoprazole 30 mg, all given P.O. every 12 hours for 14 days (triple therapy).
➤ **Lyme neuroborreliosis ◆**
Adults: 500 mg P.O. t.i.d. for 14 days.
Children: 50 mg/kg/day P.O. in three divided doses (maximum, 500 mg/dose) for 14 days.
➤ **Acute otitis media ◆**
Children age 6 and older with mild to moderate infection: 80 to 90 mg/kg P.O. daily for 5 to 7 days.
Children younger than age 6 and those with severe infection: 80 to 90 mg/kg P.O. daily for 10 days.

ADMINISTRATION
P.O.
● Before giving, ask patient about allergic reactions to penicillin. A negative history of penicillin allergy is no guarantee against allergic reaction.
● Obtain specimen for culture and sensitivity tests before giving first dose. Begin therapy while awaiting results.
● Give drug with or without food, except for extended-release tablets, which are given with a meal.
● Don't crush or split extended-release tablets.
● For a child, place drops directly on child's tongue for swallowing or add to formula, milk, fruit juice, water, ginger ale, or other cold drink for immediate and complete consumption.
● Store reconstituted oral suspension in refrigerator, if possible. Be sure to check individual product labels for storage information.

ACTION
Inhibits cell-wall synthesis during bacterial multiplication.

Route	Onset	Peak	Duration
P.O.	Unknown	1–2 hr	6–8 hr

Half-life: 1 to 1½ hours (7½ hours in severe renal impairment).

ADVERSE REACTIONS
CNS: *seizures,* anxiety, confusion, agitation, dizziness, reversible hyperactivity, anxiety, insomnia, behavioral changes.
GI: diarrhea, nausea, *pseudomembranous colitis,* vomiting.
GU: interstitial nephritis, nephropathy.
Hematologic: *agranulocytosis, leukopenia, thrombocytopenia, thrombocytopenic purpura,* anemia, eosinophilia, hemolytic anemia.
Other: *anaphylaxis,* hypersensitivity reactions, overgrowth of nonsusceptible organisms.

INTERACTIONS
Drug-drug. *Beta blockers:* May potentiate anaphylactic reactions. Monitor patient.
Hormonal contraceptives: May decrease contraceptive effectiveness. Advise use of additional form of contraception during penicillin therapy.
Live-virus vaccines: May decrease effectiveness of live-virus vaccines. Concurrent use isn't recommended.
Methotrexate: May increase methotrexate serum concentration. Monitor patient closely for toxicity.
Probenecid: May increase levels of amoxicillin and other penicillins. Probenecid may be used for this purpose.
Drug-herb. *Khat:* May decrease antimicrobial effect of certain penicillins. Discourage herb use, or tell patient to take drug 2 hours after herb use.

EFFECTS ON LAB TEST RESULTS
● May increase AST and ALT levels.
● May decrease hemoglobin level.

● May increase eosinophil count. May decrease granulocyte, platelet, and WBC counts.
● May falsely decrease aminoglycoside level. May alter results of urine glucose tests that use cupric sulfate, such as Benedict's reagent and Clinitest.

CONTRAINDICATIONS & CAUTIONS
● Contraindicated in patients hypersensitive to drug or other penicillins.
● Use cautiously in patients with other drug allergies (especially to cephalosporins) because of possible cross-sensitivity.
● Use cautiously in those with mononucleosis because of high risk of maculopapular rash.
⚠ *Overdose S&S:* Oliguric renal failure.

NURSING CONSIDERATIONS
● If large doses are given or if therapy is prolonged, bacterial or fungal superinfection may occur, especially in elderly, debilitated, or immunosuppressed patients.
● *Clostridium difficile*–associated diarrhea, ranging from mild diarrhea to fatal colitis, has been reported with nearly all antibacterial agents, including amoxicillin. Evaluate patient if diarrhea occurs.
● Amoxicillin usually causes fewer cases of diarrhea than ampicillin.
● *Look alike–sound alike:* Don't confuse amoxicillin with amoxapine.

PATIENT TEACHING
● Tell patient to take entire quantity of drug exactly as prescribed, even after he feels better.
● Instruct patient to take drug with or without food, except extended-release tablets, which are taken with a meal.
● Tell patient to swallow extended-release tablets whole and not to chew, crush, or split them.
● Tell patient to notify prescriber if rash, fever, or chills develop. A rash is the most common allergic reaction, especially if allopurinol is also being taken.
● Tell parent to place drops directly on child's tongue for swallowing or add to formula, milk, fruit juice, water, ginger ale, or other cold drink for immediate and complete consumption.

amoxicillin–clavulanate potassium (amoxycillin–clavulanate potassium)
a-mox-i-SILL-in

Apo-Amoxi Clav†, Augmentin, Augmentin XR, Clavulin†

Therapeutic class: Antibiotics
Pharmacologic class: Aminopenicillins–beta-lactamase inhibitors
Pregnancy risk category: B

AVAILABLE FORMS
Oral suspension: 125 mg amoxicillin trihydrate, 31.25 mg clavulanic acid/5 mL (after reconstitution); 200 mg amoxicillin trihydrate, 28.5 mg clavulanic acid/5 mL (after reconstitution); 250 mg amoxicillin trihydrate, 62.5 mg clavulanic acid/5 mL (after reconstitution); 400 mg amoxicillin trihydrate, 57 mg clavulanic acid/5 mL (after reconstitution); 600 mg amoxicillin trihydrate, 42.9 mg clavulanic acid/5 mL (after reconstitution)
Tablets (chewable): 200 mg amoxicillin trihydrate, 28.5 mg clavulanic acid; 250 mg amoxicillin trihydrate, 62.5 mg clavulanic acid; 400 mg amoxicillin trihydrate, 57 mg clavulanic acid
Tablets (extended-release): 1,000 mg amoxicillin trihydrate, 62.5 mg clavulanic acid
Tablets (film-coated): 250 mg amoxicillin trihydrate, 125 mg clavulanic acid; 500 mg amoxicillin trihydrate, 125 mg clavulanic acid; 875 mg amoxicillin trihydrate, 125 mg clavulanic acid

INDICATIONS & DOSAGES
➤ **Recurrent or persistent acute otitis media caused by** *Streptococcus pneumoniae, Haemophilus influenzae,* **or** *Moraxella catarrhalis* **in patients exposed to antibiotics within the previous 3 months, who are age 2 or younger or in day care facilities**
Children age 3 months and older: 90 mg/kg/day (600 mg amoxicillin/42.9 mg clavulanic acid/5 mL) P.O., based on amoxicillin component, every 12 hours for 10 days.

➤ **Lower respiratory tract infections, otitis media, sinusitis, skin and skin-structure infections, and UTIs caused by susceptible strains of gram-positive and gram-negative organisms**

Adults and children weighing 40 kg (88 lb) or more: 250 mg P.O., based on amoxicillin component, every 8 hours; or 500 mg every 12 hours. For more severe infections, 500 mg every 8 hours or 875 mg every 12 hours.

Children age 3 months and older and weighing less than 40 kg: 20 to 45 mg/kg P.O., based on amoxicillin component and severity of infection, daily in divided doses every 8 to 12 hours.

Children younger than age 3 months: 30 mg/kg/day P.O., based on amoxicillin component of the 125-mg/5-mL oral suspension, in divided doses every 12 hours.

Adjust-a-dose: Don't give the 875-mg tablet to patients with CrCl of less than 30 mL/minute. If CrCl is 10 to 30 mL/minute, give 250 to 500 mg P.O. every 12 hours. If CrCl is less than 10 mL/minute, give 250 to 500 mg P.O. every 24 hours. Give hemodialysis patients 250 to 500 mg P.O. every 24 hours with an additional dose both during and after dialysis.

➤ **Community-acquired pneumonia or acute bacterial sinusitis caused by *H. influenzae, M. catarrhalis, H. parainfluenzae, Klebsiella pneumoniae,* methicillin-susceptible *Staphylococcus aureus,* or *S. pneumoniae* with reduced susceptibility to penicillin**

Adults and children age 16 and older: 2,000 mg/125 mg Augmentin XR tablets every 12 hours for 7 to 10 days for pneumonia; 10 days for sinusitis.

Adjust-a-dose: In patients with CrCl less than 30 mL/minute and patients receiving hemodialysis, don't use Augmentin XR.

ADMINISTRATION

P.O.

● Before giving drug, ask patient about allergic reactions to penicillin. A negative history of penicillin allergy is no guarantee against an allergic reaction.

● Obtain specimen for culture and sensitivity tests before giving first dose. Begin therapy while awaiting results.

● Give drug at the start of a meal to enhance absorption.

● Give drug at least 1 hour before a bacteriostatic antibiotic.

● Avoid use of 250-mg tablet in children weighing less than 40 kg (88 lb). Use chewable form instead.

● After reconstitution, refrigerate the oral suspension; discard after 10 days.

ACTION

Prevents bacterial cell-wall synthesis during replication. Increases amoxicillin's effectiveness by inactivating beta-lactamases, which destroy amoxicillin.

Route	Onset	Peak	Duration
P.O.	Unknown	1–2½ hr	6–8 hr
P.O. (600 mg amoxicillin/ 42.9 mg clavulanic acid)	Unknown	1–4 hr	Unknown
P.O. (Augmentin XR)	Unknown	1–6 hr	Unknown

Half-life: 1 to 1½ hours. For patients with severe renal impairment, 7½ hours for amoxicillin and 4½ hours for clavulanate.

ADVERSE REACTIONS

CNS: agitation, anxiety, behavioral changes, confusion, dizziness, insomnia, headache.

GI: nausea, vomiting, diarrhea, indigestion, gastritis, stomatitis, glossitis, black hairy tongue, enterocolitis, *pseudomembranous colitis,* mucocutaneous candidiasis, abdominal pain.

GU: vaginal candidiasis, vaginitis.

Hematologic: anemia, *thrombocytopenia, thrombocytopenic purpura,* eosinophilia, *leukopenia, agranulocytosis.*

Other: hypersensitivity reactions, *anaphylaxis,* pruritus, rash, urticaria, *angioedema,* overgrowth of nonsusceptible organisms, serum sickness–like reaction.

INTERACTIONS

Drug-drug. *Allopurinol:* May increase risk of rash. Monitor patient for rash.

Hormonal contraceptives: May decrease hormonal contraceptive effectiveness. Advise use of additional form of contraception during penicillin therapy.

Reactions in bold italics are *life-threatening*. Interactions may have a *rapid onset* or a *delayed onset*.

Methotrexate: May increase risk of methotrexate toxicity. Monitor methotrexate levels.

Probenecid: May increase levels of amoxicillin and other penicillins. Probenecid may be used for this purpose.

Tetracyclines: May reduce therapeutic action of penicillins. Avoid administering together.

Drug-herb. *Khat:* May decrease antimicrobial effect of certain penicillins. Discourage khat chewing, or tell patient to take amoxicillin 2 hours after khat chewing.

EFFECTS ON LAB TEST RESULTS

• May increase eosinophil count.
• May falsely decrease aminoglycoside level. May alter results of urine glucose tests that use cupric sulfate, such as Benedict's reagent and Clinitest.

CONTRAINDICATIONS & CAUTIONS

• Contraindicated in patients hypersensitive to drug or other penicillins and in those with a history of amoxicillin-related cholestatic jaundice or hepatic dysfunction.
• Augmentin XR is contraindicated in patients receiving hemodialysis and those with CrCl of less than 30 mL/minute.
• Use cautiously in patients with other drug allergies (especially to cephalosporins) because of possible cross-sensitivity and in those with mononucleosis because of high risk of maculopapular rash.
• Use cautiously in breast-feeding women; it's unknown if drug appears in breast milk.
• Use cautiously in hepatically impaired patients, and monitor the hepatic function of these patients.
• Don't give ampicillin-class antibiotics to patients with mononucleosis due to high incidence of erythematous rash.
⚠ Overdose S&S: Crystalluria, oliguric renal failure, GI symptoms, rash, hyperactivity or drowsiness.

NURSING CONSIDERATIONS

• Each Augmentin XR tablet contains 29.3 mg (1.27 mEq) of sodium.
• Augmentin XR isn't indicated for treating infections caused by *S. pneumoniae* with penicillin minimum inhibitory concentration, or MIC, of 4 mcg/mL or greater.

• If large doses are given or therapy is prolonged, bacterial or fungal superinfection may occur, especially in elderly, debilitated, or immunosuppressed patients.
⚠ Alert: Don't interchange the oral suspensions because of varying clavulanic acid contents.
• 600 mg amoxicillin/42.9 mg clavulanic acid/5 mL is intended only for children ages 3 months to 12 years with persistent or recurrent acute otitis media.
⚠ Alert: Both 250- and 500-mg film-coated tablets contain the same amount of clavulanic acid (125 mg). Therefore, two 250-mg tablets aren't equivalent to one 500-mg tablet. Regular tablets aren't equivalent to Augmentin XR.
• This drug combination is particularly useful in clinical settings with a high prevalence of amoxicillin-resistant organisms.
• *Look alike–sound alike:* Don't confuse amoxicillin with amoxapine or Azulfidine.

PATIENT TEACHING

• Tell patient to take entire quantity of drug exactly as prescribed, even after feeling better.
• Instruct patient to take drug with food to prevent GI upset. If he's taking the oral suspension, tell him to keep drug refrigerated, to shake it well before taking it, and to discard remaining drug after 10 days.
• Tell patient to call prescriber if a rash occurs because rash is a sign of an allergic reaction.

SAFETY ALERT!

amphotericin B lipid complex
am-foe-TER-i-sin

Abelcet

Therapeutic class: Antifungals
Pharmacologic class: Polyene antibiotics
Pregnancy risk category: B

AVAILABLE FORMS

Suspension for injection: 100 mg/20-mL vial

INDICATIONS & DOSAGES
➤ **Invasive fungal infections, including** *Aspergillus* **and** *Candida* **species, in patients refractory to or intolerant of conventional amphotericin B therapy**
Adults and children: 5 mg/kg daily I.V. as a single infusion given at rate of 2.5 mg/kg/hour.
Adjust-a-dose: For patients with CrCl of less than 10 mL/minute, give 5 mg/kg every 24 to 36 hours.

ADMINISTRATION
I.V.
▼ To prepare, shake vial gently until there's no yellow sediment. Using aseptic technique, withdraw calculated dose into one or more 20-mL syringes using an 18G needle. More than one vial will be needed.
▼ Attach a 5-micron filter needle to syringe and inject dose into I.V. bag of D₅W. Volume of D₅W should be sufficient to yield 1 mg/mL (2 mg/mL for pediatric and cardiovascular patients). One filter needle can be used for up to four vials of amphotericin B lipid complex.
▼ Don't use an in-line filter.
▼ If infusing through an existing I.V. line, flush first with D₅W.
▼ Use an infusion pump, and give by continuous infusion at 2.5 mg/kg/hour.
▼ If infusion time exceeds 2 hours, mix contents by shaking infusion bag every 2 hours.
▼ Monitor vital signs closely. Fever, shaking chills, and hypotension may appear within 2 hours of starting infusion. Slowing infusion rate may decrease risk of infusion-related reactions.
▼ If severe respiratory distress occurs, stop infusion, provide supportive therapy for anaphylaxis, and notify prescriber. Don't restart drug.
▼ Reconstituted drug is stable up to 48 hours if refrigerated (36° to 46° F [2° to 8° C]) and up to 6 hours at room temperature.
▼ Discard any unused drug because it contains no preservative.
▼ **Incompatibilities:** Electrolytes, other I.V. drugs, saline solutions.

ACTION
Binds to sterols of fungal cell membranes, altering cell permeability and causing cell death.

Route	Onset	Peak	Duration
I.V.	Unknown	Unknown	Unknown

Half-life: About 1 week.

ADVERSE REACTIONS
CNS: fever, headache, pain.
CV: *cardiac arrest,* chest pain, hypertension, hypotension.
GI: *GI hemorrhage,* abdominal pain, diarrhea, nausea, vomiting.
GU: *renal failure.*
Hematologic: *leukopenia, thrombocytopenia,* anemia.
Hepatic: bilirubinemia.
Metabolic: hypokalemia.
Respiratory: *respiratory failure,* dyspnea, respiratory disorder.
Skin: rash.
Other: *multiple organ failure,* chills, *sepsis,* infection.

INTERACTIONS
Drug-drug. *Antineoplastics:* May increase risk of renal toxicity, bronchospasm, and hypotension. Use together cautiously.
Cardiac glycosides: May increase risk of digitalis toxicity from amphotericin B–induced hypokalemia. Monitor potassium level closely.
Clotrimazole, fluconazole, itraconazole, ketoconazole, miconazole: May counteract effects of amphotericin B by inducing fungal resistance. Monitor patient closely.
Corticosteroids, corticotropin: May enhance hypokalemia, which could lead to cardiac toxicity. Monitor electrolyte levels and cardiac function.
Cyclosporine: May increase renal toxicity. Monitor renal function test results closely.
Flucytosine: May increase risk of flucytosine toxicity from increased cellular uptake or impaired renal excretion. Use together cautiously.
Leukocyte transfusions: May increase risk of pulmonary reactions, such as acute dyspnea, tachypnea, hypoxemia, hemoptysis, and interstitial infiltrates. Use together with

caution; separate doses as much as possible, and monitor pulmonary function.

Nephrotoxic drugs (such as aminoglycosides, pentamidine): May increase risk of renal toxicity. Use together cautiously and monitor renal function closely.

Skeletal muscle relaxants: May enhance skeletal muscle relaxant effects of amphotericin B–induced hypokalemia. Monitor potassium level closely.

Zidovudine: May increase myelotoxicity and nephrotoxicity. Monitor renal and hematologic function.

EFFECTS ON LAB TEST RESULTS

• May increase alkaline phosphatase, ALT, AST, bilirubin, BUN, creatinine, GGT, and LDH levels. May decrease hemoglobin and magnesium and potassium levels.
• May decrease platelet and WBC counts.

CONTRAINDICATIONS & CAUTIONS

• Contraindicated in patients hypersensitive to amphotericin B or its components.
• Use cautiously in patients with renal impairment. Adjust dosage based on patient's overall condition. Renal toxicity is more common at higher dosages.
• It's unknown if drug appears in breast milk. Encourage patient to stop either breast-feeding or treatment.
⚠ Overdose S&S: Cardiorespiratory arrest.

NURSING CONSIDERATIONS

❸ Alert: Different amphotericin B preparations aren't interchangeable, so dosages will vary. Confusing the preparations may cause permanent damage or death.
• Hydrate before infusion to reduce risk of nephrotoxicity.
• Monitor creatinine and electrolyte levels (especially magnesium and potassium), liver function, and CBC during therapy.
• Acute infusion reactions, including fever and chills, may occur 1 to 2 hours after start of infusion and are more common with first few doses. Infusion has rarely been associated with arrhythmias, hypotension, and shock.
❸ Alert: Immediately stop infusion if severe respiratory distress occurs. Patient shouldn't receive further infusions.

PATIENT TEACHING

• Inform patient that he may develop fever, chills, nausea, and vomiting during infusion, but that these symptoms usually subside with subsequent doses.
• Instruct patient to report any redness or pain at infusion site.
• Teach patient to recognize and report to prescriber signs and symptoms of acute hypersensitivity, such as respiratory distress.
• Warn patient that therapy may take several months.
• Tell patient to expect frequent laboratory testing to monitor kidney and liver function.

SAFETY ALERT!

amphotericin B liposomal
am-foe-TER-i-sin

AmBisome

Therapeutic class: Antifungals
Pharmacologic class: Polyene antibiotics
Pregnancy risk category: B

AVAILABLE FORMS
Powder for injection: 50-mg vial

INDICATIONS & DOSAGES

Adjust-a-dose (for all indications): For patients with CrCl of less than 10 mL/minute, give 3 mg/kg I.V. every 24 hours. For adults receiving standard intermittent hemodialysis or continuous renal replacement therapy, give 3 to 5 mg/kg I.V. every 24 hours and after the dialysis session.

➤ **Empirical therapy for presumed fungal infection in febrile, neutropenic patients**
Adults and children: 3 mg/kg I.V. infusion over 2 hours daily.

➤ **Systemic fungal infections caused by *Aspergillus* species, *Candida* species, or *Cryptococcus* species refractory to conventional amphotericin B therapy in patients for whom renal impairment or unacceptable toxicity precludes use of conventional amphotericin B therapy**
Adults and children: 3 to 5 mg/kg I.V. infusion over 2 hours daily.

➤ **Visceral leishmaniasis in immunocompetent patients**
Adults and children: 3 mg/kg I.V. infusion over 2 hours daily on days 1 to 5, day 14, and day 21. A repeat course of therapy may be beneficial if initial treatment fails to clear parasites.

➤ **Visceral leishmaniasis in immunocompromised patients**
Adults and children: 4 mg/kg I.V. infusion over 2 hours on days 1 to 5, day 10, day 17, day 24, day 31, and day 38.

➤ **Cryptococcal meningitis in patients with HIV infection**
Adults and children: 6 mg/kg/day I.V. infusion over 2 hours. Reduce infusion time to 1 hour if treatment is well tolerated, and increase infusion time if discomfort occurs.

ADMINISTRATION

I.V.
▼ Don't reconstitute with bacteriostatic water for injection, and don't allow bacteriostatic product in solution.
▼ Don't reconstitute with saline solution, add saline solution to reconstituted concentration, or mix with other drugs.
▼ Reconstitute each 50-mg vial with 12 mL of sterile water for injection to yield 4 mg/mL. A yellow, translucent suspension will form.
▼ After reconstitution, shake vial vigorously for 30 seconds or until particulate matter disperses.
▼ Dilute to 1 to 2 mg/mL by withdrawing calculated amount of reconstituted solution into a sterile syringe and injecting it through a 5-micron filter into D_5W. Use only one filter needle per vial. Concentrations of 0.2 to 0.5 mg/mL may provide sufficient volume of infusion for children.
▼ Flush existing I.V. line with D_5W before infusing drug. If this isn't possible, give drug through a separate line.
▼ Use a controlled infusion device and an in-line filter with a mean pore diameter of 1 micron or larger.
▼ Initially, infuse drug over at least 2 hours. If drug is tolerated well, reduce infusion time to 1 hour. If discomfort occurs, increase infusion time.

▼ Store unopened vial at 36° to 46° F (2° to 8° C). Store reconstituted drug for up to 24 hours at 36° to 46° F. Use within 6 hours of dilution with D_5W. Don't freeze.
▼ **Incompatibilities:** Other I.V. drugs, saline solutions.

ACTION

Binds to sterols of fungal cell membranes, altering cell permeability and causing cell death.

Route	Onset	Peak	Duration
I.V.	Unknown	Unknown	Unknown

Half-life: About 4 to 6 days.

ADVERSE REACTIONS

CNS: fever, anxiety, confusion, headache, insomnia, asthenia, pain.
CV: chest pain, hypotension, tachycardia, hypertension, edema, flushing.
EENT: epistaxis, rhinitis.
GI: nausea, vomiting, abdominal pain, diarrhea, *GI hemorrhage.*
GU: hematuria, *renal failure.*
Hematologic: anemia, thrombocytopenia.
Hepatic: bilirubinemia, *hepatotoxicity.*
Metabolic: hyperglycemia, hypernatremia, hypocalcemia, hypokalemia, *hypomagnesemia.*
Musculoskeletal: back pain.
Respiratory: increased cough, dyspnea, hypoxia, pleural effusion, lung disorder, hyperventilation.
Skin: pruritus, rash, sweating.
Other: chills, infection, *anaphylaxis, sepsis,* blood product infusion reaction.

INTERACTIONS

Drug-drug. *Antineoplastics:* May enhance potential for renal toxicity, bronchospasm, and hypotension. Use together cautiously.
Cardiac glycosides: May increase risk of digitalis toxicity caused by amphotericin B–induced hypokalemia. Monitor potassium level closely.
Clotrimazole, fluconazole, ketoconazole, miconazole: May induce fungal resistance to amphotericin B. Use together cautiously.
Corticosteroids, corticotropin: May increase potassium depletion, which could cause cardiac dysfunction. Monitor electrolyte levels and cardiac function.

Reactions in bold italics are *life-threatening*. Interactions may have a *rapid onset* or a *delayed onset.*

Flucytosine: May increase flucytosine toxicity by increasing cellular reuptake or impairing renal excretion of flucytosine. Use together cautiously.

Leukocyte transfusions: Increases risk of pulmonary toxicity. Don't use together.

Other nephrotoxic drugs, such as antibiotics and antineoplastics: May cause additive nephrotoxicity. Use together cautiously; monitor renal function closely.

Skeletal muscle relaxants: May enhance effects of skeletal muscle relaxants resulting from amphotericin B–induced hypokalemia. Monitor potassium level.

EFFECTS ON LAB TEST RESULTS
● May increase alkaline phosphatase, ALT, AST, bilirubin, BUN, creatinine, GGT, glucose, LDH, and sodium levels. May decrease calcium, magnesium, and potassium levels.
● May decrease hemoglobin and platelet count.

CONTRAINDICATIONS & CAUTIONS
● Contraindicated in patients hypersensitive to drug or its components.
● Use cautiously in patients with impaired renal function, in elderly patients, and in pregnant women.
● It's unknown if drug appears in breast milk. Because of risk of serious adverse reactions in breast-fed infants, encourage patient to stop either breast-feeding or therapy, taking into account importance of drug.
⚠ *Overdose S&S:* Cardiorespiratory arrest.

NURSING CONSIDERATIONS
● Patients also receiving chemotherapy or bone marrow transplantation are at greater risk for additional adverse reactions, including seizures, arrhythmias, and thrombocytopenia.
🔆 *Alert:* Different amphotericin B preparations aren't interchangeable, so dosages will vary. Confusing the preparations may cause permanent damage or death.
● Premedicate patient with antipyretics, antihistamines, antiemetics, or corticosteroids.
● Hydrate before infusion to reduce the risk of nephrotoxicity.

● Monitor BUN, creatinine, and electrolyte levels (particularly magnesium and potassium), liver function, and CBC.
● Watch for signs and symptoms of hypokalemia (ECG changes, muscle weakness, cramping, drowsiness).
● Patients treated with this drug have a lower risk of chills, elevated BUN level, hypokalemia, hypertension, and vomiting than patients treated with conventional amphotericin B.
● Therapy may take several weeks or months.
● Observe patient closely for adverse reactions during infusion. If anaphylaxis occurs, stop infusion immediately, provide supportive therapy, and notify prescriber.

PATIENT TEACHING
● Teach patient signs and symptoms of hypersensitivity, and stress importance of reporting them immediately.
● Warn patient that therapy may take several months; teach personal hygiene and other measures to prevent spread and recurrence of lesions.
● Instruct patient to report any adverse reactions that occur while receiving drug.
● Tell patient to watch for and report signs and symptoms of low levels of potassium in the blood (muscle weakness, cramping, drowsiness).
● Advise patient that frequent laboratory testing will be needed.

ampicillin
am-pi-SILL-in

Apo-Ampi†, Novo-Ampicillin†

ampicillin sodium

Therapeutic class: Antibiotics
Pharmacologic class: Aminopenicillins
Pregnancy risk category: B

AVAILABLE FORMS
Capsules: 250 mg, 500 mg
Injection: 125 mg, 250 mg, 500 mg, 1 g, 2 g, 10 g
Oral suspension: 125 mg/5 mL, 250 mg/ 5 mL

INDICATIONS & DOSAGES

Adjust-a-dose (for all indications): When giving I.V. to patients with impaired renal function, use the following schedule: If CrCl is 10 to 50 mL/minute, give dose every 6 to 12 hours. If CrCl is less than 10 mL/minute, give dose every 12 to 16 hours. If patient is receiving intermittent hemodialysis three times a week, give 1 to 2 g every 12 to 24 hours. If the dose is given every 24 hours, administer after dialysis.

➤ **Respiratory tract infections**
Adults and children weighing more than 20 kg (44 lb): 250 mg P.O. every 6 hours.
Children weighing 20 kg or less:
50 mg/kg/day P.O. in equally divided doses every 6 to 8 hours.

➤ **GI infections or GU infections (excluding gonorrhea)**
Adults and children weighing 20 kg or more: 500 mg P.O. every 6 hours. For severe infections, larger doses may be needed.
Children weighing less than 20 kg: 100 mg/kg/day P.O. in equally divided doses every 6 hours.

➤ **Uncomplicated gonorrhea**
Adults and children weighing more than 20 kg: 3.5 g P.O. with 1 g probenecid given as a single dose.

➤ **Bacterial meningitis or septicemia**
Adults: 150 to 200 mg/kg/day I.V. in divided doses every 3 to 4 hours. May be given I.M. after 3 days of I.V. therapy. Maximum recommended daily dose is 14 g.
Children: 150 to 200 mg/kg I.V. daily in divided doses every 3 to 4 hours. Give I.V. for 3 days; then give I.M.

➤ **GI infections and GU tract infections (including gonorrhea in females)**
Adults and children weighing 40 kg (88 lb) or more: 500 mg I.V. or I.M. every 6 hours.
Adults and children weighing less than 40 kg: 50 mg/kg/day I.V. or I.M. in equally divided doses every 6 to 8 hours.

➤ **Respiratory tract and soft-tissue infections**
Adults and children weighing 40 kg (88 lb) or more: 250 to 500 mg I.V. or I.M. every 6 hours.
Adults and children weighing less than 40 kg: 25 to 50 mg/kg/day I.V. or I.M. in equally divided doses every 6 to 8 hours.

➤ **Urethritis in males due to gonorrhea**
Adult men: Two doses of 500 mg each I.V. or I.M. at 8- to 12-hour intervals. May repeat or extend treatment if necessary.

ADMINISTRATION
P.O.
● Before giving drug, ask patient about allergic reactions to penicillin. A negative history of penicillin allergy is no guarantee against a future allergic reaction.
● Obtain specimen for culture and sensitivity tests before giving. Begin therapy while awaiting results.
● Give drug 1 to 2 hours before or 2 to 3 hours after meals. When given orally, drug may cause GI disturbances. Food may interfere with absorption.
● Give drug I.M. or I.V. if infection is severe or if patient can't take oral dose.

I.V.
▼ Before giving drug, ask patient about allergic reactions to penicillin. A negative history of penicillin allergy is no guarantee against a future allergic reaction.
▼ Obtain specimen for culture and sensitivity tests before giving. Begin therapy while awaiting results.
▼ Give drug I.M. or I.V. only if infection is severe or if patient can't take oral dose.
▼ Give drug intermittently to prevent vein irritation. Change site every 48 hours.
▼ For direct injection, reconstitute with bacteriostatic water for injection. Use 5 mL for 250-mg or 500-mg vials, 7.4 mL for 1-g vials, and 14.8 mL for 2-g vials. Give drug over 10 to 15 minutes to avoid seizures. Don't exceed 100 mg/minute.
▼ For intermittent infusion, dilute in 50 to 100 mL of normal saline solution for injection. Give drug over 15 to 30 minutes.
▼ Use first dilution within 1 hour. Follow manufacturer's directions for stability data when drug is further diluted for I.V. infusion.
▼ **Incompatibilities:** Amikacin, amino acid solutions, chlorpromazine, dextran solutions, dextrose solutions, dopamine, erythromycin lactobionate, 10% fat emulsions, fructose, gentamicin, heparin sodium, hetastarch, hydrocortisone sodium

---

Reactions in bold italics are *life-threatening*. Interactions may have a *rapid onset* or a *delayed onset*.

succinate, hydromorphone, kanamycin, lidocaine, lincomycin, polymyxin B, prochlorperazine edisylate, sodium bicarbonate, streptomycin, tobramycin.

I.M.

• Before giving drug, ask patient about allergic reactions to penicillin. A negative history of penicillin allergy is no guarantee against a future allergic reaction.

• Obtain specimen for culture and sensitivity tests before giving. Begin therapy while awaiting results.

• Give drug I.M. or I.V. only if infection is severe or if patient can't take oral dose.

ACTION

Inhibits cell-wall synthesis during bacterial multiplication.

Route	Onset	Peak	Duration
P.O.	Unknown	2 hr	6–8 hr
I.V.	Immediate	Immediate	Unknown
I.M.	Unknown	1 hr	Unknown

Half-life: 1 to 1½ hours (10 to 24 hours in severe renal impairment).

ADVERSE REACTIONS

GI: diarrhea, nausea, *pseudomembranous colitis,* abdominal pain, black hairy tongue, enterocolitis, gastritis, glossitis, stomatitis, vomiting.

Hematologic: *leukopenia, thrombocytopenia, thrombocytopenic purpura,* anemia, eosinophilia, hemolytic anemia, *agranulocytosis.*

Other: hypersensitivity reactions, overgrowth of nonsusceptible organisms.

INTERACTIONS

Drug-drug. *Allopurinol:* May increase risk of rash. Monitor patient for rash.

H_2 antagonists, proton pump inhibitors: May decrease ampicillin absorption and level. Separate administration times. Monitor patient for continued antibiotic effectiveness.

Hormonal contraceptives: May decrease hormonal contraceptive effectiveness. Advise use of another form of contraception during therapy.

Live-virus vaccines: May decrease effectiveness of live-virus vaccines. Concurrent use isn't recommended.

Oral anticoagulants: May increase risk of bleeding. Monitor PT and INR.

Probenecid: May increase levels of ampicillin and other penicillins. Probenecid may be used for this purpose.

EFFECTS ON LAB TEST RESULTS

• May decrease hemoglobin level.

• May increase eosinophil count. May decrease granulocyte, platelet, and WBC counts.

• May falsely decrease aminoglycoside level. May alter results of urine glucose tests that use cupric sulfate, such as Benedict reagent and Clinitest.

CONTRAINDICATIONS & CAUTIONS

• Contraindicated in patients hypersensitive to drug or other penicillins.

• Use cautiously in patients with other drug allergies (especially to cephalosporins) because of possible cross-sensitivity, and in those with mononucleosis because of high risk of maculopapular rash.

• May cause *Clostridium difficile*–associated diarrhea, which can be fatal. Antibiotic may need to be stopped and other treatment begun.

NURSING CONSIDERATIONS

• Monitor sodium level because each gram of ampicillin contains 2.9 mEq of sodium.

• If large doses are given or if therapy is prolonged, bacterial or fungal superinfection may occur, especially in elderly, debilitated, or immunosuppressed patients.

• Watch for signs and symptoms of hypersensitivity, such as erythematous maculopapular rash, urticaria, and anaphylaxis.

• In patients with impaired renal function, decrease dosage.

• In pediatric meningitis, drug may be given with parenteral chloramphenicol for 24 hours, pending cultures.

PATIENT TEACHING

• Tell patient to take entire quantity of drug exactly as prescribed, even after he feels better.

• Instruct patient to take oral form on an empty stomach 1 hour before or 2 hours after meals.

• Inform patient to notify prescriber if rash, fever, or chills develop. A rash is the most common allergic reaction, especially if allopurinol is also being taken.

• Instruct patient to report diarrhea.

ampicillin sodium–sulbactam sodium
am-pi-SILL-in

Unasyn

Therapeutic class: Antibiotics
Pharmacologic class: Aminopenicillins–beta-lactamase inhibitors
Pregnancy risk category: B

AVAILABLE FORMS
Injection: Vials and piggyback vials containing 1.5 g (1 g ampicillin sodium and 0.5 g sulbactam sodium), 3 g (2 g ampicillin sodium and 1 g sulbactam sodium)

INDICATIONS & DOSAGES
Adjust-a-dose (for all indications): If CrCl in adults is 15 to 29 mL/minute, give 1.5 to 3 g every 12 hours; if clearance is 5 to 14 mL/minute, give 1.5 to 3 g every 24 hours. Give dose after hemodialysis.

➤ **Intra-abdominal, gynecologic, and skin-structure infections caused by susceptible strains**
Adults: 1.5 to 3 g I.M. or I.V. every 6 hours. Don't exceed 4 g/day of sulbactam.
Children age 1 or older weighing 40 kg (88 lb) or more (skin and skin-structure infections only): 1.5 to 3 g I.V. or I.M. every 6 hours. Don't exceed 4 g/day sulbactam.
Children age 1 or older weighing less than 40 kg (skin and skin-structure infections only): 300 mg/kg/day I.V. in divided doses every 6 hours for no longer than 14 days.

➤ **Community-acquired pneumonia ◆**
Adults: 3 g I.V. every 12 hours with either azithromycin or a fluoroquinolone for at least 5 days.

➤ **Hospital-acquired pneumonia ◆**
Adults: 1.5 to 3 g I.V. every 6 hours for 7 to 8 days.

➤ **Infective endocarditis ◆**
Adults: 12 g/day I.V. in four equally divided doses. Duration depends on causative agent.
Children: 300 mg/kg/day I.V. in four or six equally divided doses. Duration depends on causative agent.

➤ **Pelvic inflammatory disease ◆**
Adults and adolescents: 3 g I.V. every 6 hours given with doxycycline. Continue for 24 hours after clinical improvement. Oral doxycycline should be continued for total of 14 days.

ADMINISTRATION
I.V.

▼ Before giving drug, ask patient about allergic reactions to penicillin. A negative history of penicillin allergy is no guarantee against future allergic reaction.

▼ Obtain specimen for culture and sensitivity tests. Begin therapy while awaiting results.

▼ Reconstitute powder with one of these diluents: normal saline solution, sterile water for injection, D_5W, lactated Ringer's injection, M/6 sodium lactate, dextrose 5% in half-normal saline solution for injection, or 10% invert sugar.

▼ After reconstitution, let vials stand for a few minutes so foam can dissipate. Inspect solution for particles.

▼ Give drug at least 1 hour before giving a bacteriostatic antibiotic.

▼ For infusion, dilute in 50 to 100 mL of compatible diluent and infuse over 15 to 30 minutes.

▼ Stability varies with diluent, temperature, and concentration of solution.

▼ **Incompatibilities:** Amikacin, amino acid solutions, amiodarone, amphotericin B, chlorpromazine, ciprofloxacin, dextran solutions, dopamine, erythromycin lactobionate, 10% fat emulsions, fructose, gentamicin, heparin sodium, hetastarch, hydrocortisone sodium succinate, idarubicin, kanamycin, lidocaine, lincomycin, netilmicin, polymyxin B, nicardipine, ondansetron, prochlorperazine edisylate, sargramostim, sodium bicarbonate, streptomycin, tobramycin.

I.M.

• Before giving drug, ask patient about allergic reactions to penicillin. A negative

---

history of penicillin allergy is no guarantee against future allergic reaction.
• Obtain specimen for culture and sensitivity tests. Begin therapy while awaiting results.
• For I.M. injection, reconstitute with sterile water for injection or 0.5% or 2% lidocaine hydrochloride injection. Add 3.2 mL to a 1.5-g vial (or 6.4 mL to a 3-g vial) to yield 375 mg/mL. Give deep into muscle.
• I.M. injection may cause pain at injection site.
• In children, don't use I.M. route.

ACTION

Inhibits cell-wall synthesis during bacterial multiplication.

Route	Onset	Peak	Duration
I.V.	Immediate	15 min	Unknown
I.M.	Unknown	30–52 min	Unknown

Half-life: 1 to 1½ hours (10 to 24 hours in severe renal impairment).

ADVERSE REACTIONS

GI: diarrhea, nausea, *pseudomembranous colitis,* black hairy tongue, enterocolitis, gastritis, glossitis, stomatitis, vomiting.
Hematologic: *agranulocytosis, leukopenia, thrombocytopenia, thrombocytopenic purpura,* anemia, eosinophilia.
Skin: pain at injection site, thrombophlebitis.
Other: hypersensitivity reactions, *anaphylaxis,* overgrowth of nonsusceptible organisms.

INTERACTIONS

Drug-drug. *Allopurinol:* May increase risk of rash. Monitor patient for rash.
Hormonal contraceptives: May decrease hormonal contraceptive effectiveness. Strongly advise use of another contraceptive during therapy.
Live-virus vaccines: May decrease effectiveness of live-virus vaccines. Use together isn't recommended.
Oral anticoagulants: May increase risk of bleeding. Monitor PT and INR.
Probenecid: May increase ampicillin level. Probenecid may be used for this purpose.

EFFECTS ON LAB TEST RESULTS

• May increase alkaline phosphatase, ALT, AST, bilirubin, BUN, CK, creatinine, GGT, and LDH levels. May decrease hemoglobin level. May transiently decrease conjugated estriol, conjugated estrone, estradiol, and estriol glucuronide levels in pregnant women.
• May increase eosinophil count. May decrease granulocyte, platelet, and WBC counts.
• May alter results of urine glucose tests that use cupric sulfate, such as Benedict's reagent and Clinitest.

CONTRAINDICATIONS & CAUTIONS

• Contraindicated in patients hypersensitive to drug or other penicillins.
• Use cautiously in patients with other drug allergies (especially to cephalosporins) because of possible cross-sensitivity, and in those with mononucleosis because of high risk of maculopapular rash.
⚠ **Overdose S&S:** Neuromuscular hyperexcitability, seizures.

NURSING CONSIDERATIONS

• Dosage is expressed as total drug. Each 1.5-g vial contains 1 g ampicillin sodium and 0.5 g sulbactam sodium.
• In patients with impaired renal function, decrease dosage.
• Monitor LFT results during therapy, especially in patients with impaired liver function.
• If large doses are given or if therapy is prolonged, bacterial or fungal superinfection may occur, especially in elderly, debilitated, or immunosuppressed patients.

PATIENT TEACHING

• Tell patient to report rash, fever, or chills. A rash is the most common allergic reaction.
• Warn patient that I.M. injection may cause pain at injection site.

anakinra

ann-ACK-in-rah

Kineret

Therapeutic class: Immune response modifiers
Pharmacologic class: Interleukin-1 receptor antagonists
Pregnancy risk category: B

AVAILABLE FORMS
Injection: 100 mg/0.67 mL in a prefilled glass syringe

INDICATIONS & DOSAGES
Adjust-a-dose (for all indications): In severe renal insufficiency or ESRD (CrCl less than 30 mL/minute), consider every-other-day dosing.

✳ *NEW INDICATION:* Neonatal-onset multisystem inflammatory disease
Adults and children: Initially, 1 to 2 mg/kg subcutaneously once daily. May increase in 0.5- to 1-mg increments to maximum dosage of 8 mg/kg daily for adults or 7.6 mg/kg daily for children. Maintenance dosage is 3 to 4 mg/kg daily. May divide total daily dosage into two equal doses and give b.i.d.

➤ **To reduce signs and symptoms and slow progression of structural damage in moderately to severely active rheumatoid arthritis (RA) after one or more failures with disease-modifying antirheumatic drugs (DMARDs), alone or combined with DMARDs other than TNF blockers**
Adults: 100 mg subcutaneously daily at the same time each day.

ADMINISTRATION
Subcutaneous
● Inject entire contents of prefilled syringe.
● Store drug in the refrigerator at 35° to 46° F (2° to 8° C). Don't freeze or shake.
● Protect drug from light.

ACTION
A recombinant, nonglycosylated form of the human interleukin-1 receptor antagonist (IL-1Ra). The level of naturally occurring IL-1Ra in synovium and synovial fluid from patients with RA isn't enough to compete with the elevated level of locally produced IL-1. Anakinra blocks the biological activity of IL-1 by competitively inhibiting IL-1 from binding to the interleukin-1 receptor, which is expressed in various tissues and organs.

Route	Onset	Peak	Duration
Subcut.	Unknown	3–7 hr	Unknown

Half-life: 4 to 6 hours.

ADVERSE REACTIONS
CNS: headache, fever.
EENT: sinusitis, nasopharyngitis.
GI: abdominal pain, diarrhea, nausea, vomiting.
Hematologic: *neutropenia.*
Musculoskeletal: worsening of RA, arthralgia.
Respiratory: upper respiratory tract infection.
Skin: ecchymosis, injection-site reactions (erythema, inflammation, pain).
Other: infection (cellulitis, pneumonia, bone and joint), flulike symptoms.

INTERACTIONS
Drug-drug. *Etanercept, other TNF blockers:* May increase risk of severe infection. Use together isn't recommended.
Vaccines: May decrease effectiveness of vaccines or may increase risk of secondary transmission of infection with live-virus vaccines. Avoid using together.

EFFECTS ON LAB TEST RESULTS
● May increase eosinophil count. May decrease neutrophil, platelet, and WBC counts.

CONTRAINDICATIONS & CAUTIONS
● Contraindicated in patients hypersensitive to *Escherichia coli*–derived proteins or any components of the product, or in patients with active infections.
● Use drug cautiously in immunosuppressed patients, those with a chronic infection, the elderly, and breast-feeding women.
● Safety and effectiveness in patients with juvenile RA haven't been established.

Reactions in bold italics are *life-threatening*. Interactions may have a *rapid onset* or a *delayed onset*.

NURSING CONSIDERATIONS
• Don't start treatment if patient has active infection.
• Obtain neutrophil count before treatment, monthly for the first 3 months of treatment, and then quarterly for up to 1 year.
• Monitor patient for infections and injection-site reactions.
• Stop drug if a serious infection develops.
• Monitor patient for possible anaphylactic reaction.
• **Look alike–sound alike:** Don't confuse anakinra with amikacin.

PATIENT TEACHING
• Tell patient to store drug in refrigerator and not to freeze or expose to excessive heat. Advise letting drug come to room temperature before giving dose.
• Tell patient not to shake drug.
• Teach patient proper dosage, administration, and needle and syringe disposal.
• Urge patient to rotate injection sites.
• Review signs and symptoms of allergic and other adverse reactions, especially signs of serious infections. Urge patient to contact prescriber if they arise.
• Inform patient that injection-site reactions are common, usually mild, and typically last 14 to 28 days.
• Tell patient to avoid live-virus vaccines during therapy.

SAFETY ALERT!

anastrozole
an-AHS-troh-zol

Arimidex⁄

Therapeutic class: Antineoplastics
Pharmacologic class: Aromatase inhibitors
Pregnancy risk category: X

AVAILABLE FORMS
Tablets: 1 mg

INDICATIONS & DOSAGES
➤ First-line treatment of postmenopausal women with hormone receptor–positive or hormone receptor–unknown locally advanced or metastatic breast cancer; advanced breast cancer in postmenopausal women with disease progression after tamoxifen therapy; adjunctive treatment of postmenopausal women with hormone receptor–positive early breast cancer
Adults: 1 mg P.O. daily.

ADMINISTRATION
P.O.
• Drug is a potential teratogen. Follow safe handling procedures when preparing, administering, or dispensing.
• Give drug without regard for meals.

ACTION
A selective nonsteroidal aromatase inhibitor that significantly lowers estradiol levels, which inhibits breast cancer cell growth in postmenopausal women.

Route	Onset	Peak	Duration
P.O.	<24 hr	Unknown	<7 days

Half-life: 50 hours.

ADVERSE REACTIONS
CNS: headache, asthenia, pain, dizziness, depression, paresthesia, anxiety, *insomnia.*
CV: hot flashes, *thromboembolic disease,* chest pain, peripheral edema, hypertension, vasodilation.
EENT: pharyngitis, cataracts.
GI: nausea, vomiting, diarrhea, constipation, abdominal pain, anorexia, dry mouth, dyspepsia.
GU: vaginal dryness, pelvic pain.
Metabolic: weight gain, increased appetite.
Musculoskeletal: bone pain, back pain, arthritis, arthralgia, osteoporosis, fractures.
Respiratory: dyspnea, increased cough.
Skin: rash, sweating.
Other: lymphedema.

INTERACTIONS
Estrogen: May decrease pharmacologic action of anastrozole. Use together isn't recommended.
Tamoxifen: May reduce anastrozole plasma level. Don't use together.

EFFECTS ON LAB TEST RESULTS
• May increase liver enzyme and cholesterol levels.

CONTRAINDICATIONS & CAUTIONS
- Don't use in women who are or may be pregnant.
- Use cautiously in breast-feeding women.

NURSING CONSIDERATIONS
- Give drug under supervision of a prescriber experienced in use of antineoplastics.
- Patients with hormone receptor–negative disease and patients who didn't respond to previous tamoxifen therapy rarely respond to anastrozole.
- For patients with advanced breast cancer, continue anastrozole until tumor progresses.
- Monitor bone mineral density as indicated.
- Use drug only in postmenopausal women.
- Rule out pregnancy before starting drug.

PATIENT TEACHING
- Instruct patient to report adverse reactions, especially difficulty breathing, chest pain, or skin lesions or blisters.
- Tell patient to take medication at the same time each day.
- Stress need for follow-up care.
- Counsel women about risks of pregnancy during therapy.
- Tell patient that drug lowers estrogen level, which may lead to decreased bone strength and increased risk of fractures.

anidulafungin
an-ah-DOO-lah-fun-gin

Eraxis

Therapeutic class: Antifungals
Pharmacologic class: Echinocandins
Pregnancy risk category: C

AVAILABLE FORMS
Powder for injection: 50-mg/vial, 100-mg/vial with companion diluent

INDICATIONS & DOSAGES
➤ **Candidemia and other *Candida* infections (intra-abdominal abscess, peritonitis)**
Adults: A single 200-mg loading dose given by I.V. infusion at no more than 1.1 mg/ minute on day 1; then 100 mg daily for at least 14 days after last positive culture result.
➤ **Esophageal candidiasis**
Adults: A single 100-mg loading dose given by I.V. infusion at no more than 1.1 mg/minute on day 1; then 50 mg daily for at least 14 days and for at least 7 days after symptoms resolve.
➤ **Catheter-related bloodstream infections caused by *Candida* species ◆**
Adolescents and children age 2 and older: 1.5 mg/kg/day I.V. Maximum daily dosage is 100 mg.

ADMINISTRATION
I.V.
▼ Obtain specimens for culture and sensitivity tests and baseline laboratory tests before starting therapy.
▼ Reconstitute each 50-mg vial with 15 mL of supplied diluent. Reconstitute each 100-mg vial with 30 mL of supplied diluent.
▼ Further dilute with D₅W or normal saline solution.
▼ Add 50-mg dose (in 15 mL) to 100 mL of D₅W or normal saline solution. Resulting volume is 115 mL and concentration is 0.43 mg/mL. Add 100-mg dose (in 30 mL) to 250 mL of D₅W or normal saline solution. Resulting volume is 280 mL and concentration is 0.36 mg/mL. Add 200-mg dose (in 60 mL) to 500 mL of D₅W or normal saline solution. Resulting volume is 560 mL and concentration is 0.36 mg/mL.
▼ Don't infuse faster than 1.1 mg/minute.
▼ Store at room temperature; don't freeze. Use reconstituted solution within 24 hours of preparation.
▼ **Incompatibilities:** Unknown. Only use supplied diluent to reconstitute and D₅W or normal saline solution to further dilute.

ACTION
Inhibits glucan synthase, which in turn inhibits formation of 1,3-β-D-glucan, an essential component of fungal cell walls.

Route	Onset	Peak	Duration
I.V.	<24 hr	Unknown	Unknown

Half-life: 40 to 50 hours.

ADVERSE REACTIONS

CNS: headache.
CV: *deep vein thrombosis,* hypotension.
GI: nausea, diarrhea.
Hematologic: *leukopenia, neutropenia.*
Metabolic: hypokalemia.
Skin: rash.
Other: histamine-mediated symptoms (bronchospasm, dyspnea, flushing, hypotension, pruritus, rash, urticaria).

INTERACTIONS

None reported.

EFFECTS ON LAB TEST RESULTS

● May increase AST, ALT, alkaline phosphatase, GGT, amylase, lipase, bilirubin, CK, creatinine, urea, calcium, glucose, potassium, and sodium levels. May decrease potassium and magnesium levels.
● May increase PT. May decrease neutrophil and WBC counts. May increase or decrease platelet count.

CONTRAINDICATIONS & CAUTIONS

● Contraindicated in patients hypersensitive to drug, other echinocandins, or any component of the drug.
● Use cautiously in patients with liver impairment and in pregnant or breast-feeding women.
● Safety and effectiveness in children haven't been established.

NURSING CONSIDERATIONS

● Use only the supplied diluent to reconstitute powder.
● To avoid histamine-mediated symptoms, such as rash, urticaria, flushing, itching, dyspnea, and hypotension, don't infuse faster than 1.1 mg/minute.
● Monitor patient closely for changes in liver function and blood cell counts during therapy.
● Notify prescriber about signs or symptoms of liver toxicity, such as dark urine, jaundice, abdominal pain, and fatigue.
● Patients with esophageal candidiasis who are HIV positive may need suppressive antifungal therapy after drug to prevent relapse.

PATIENT TEACHING

● Tell patient to call the nurse if he develops a rash, itching, trouble breathing, or other adverse effects during infusion.
● Explain that blood tests will be needed to monitor the drug's effects.

SAFETY ALERT!
✱ NEW DRUG

apixaban
a-PIX-a-ban

Eliquis

Therapeutic class: Anticoagulants
Pharmacologic class: Factor Xa inhibitors
Pregnancy risk category: B

AVAILABLE FORMS

Tablets: 2.5 mg, 5 mg

INDICATIONS & DOSAGES

➤ **Reduction of risk of stroke and systemic embolism in patients with nonvalvular atrial fibrillation**
Adults: 5 mg P.O. b.i.d.
Adjust-a-dose: Reduce dosage to 2.5 mg b.i.d. in patients with any two of the following characteristics: age 80 or older, body weight 60 kg (132 lb) or less, serum creatinine 1.5 mg/dL or greater.

ADMINISTRATION

P.O.
● May give without regard for food.
● If patient doesn't take dose at the scheduled time, he should take the dose as soon as possible on the same day, then resume twice-daily administration. Patient shouldn't double the dose to make up for a missed dose.
● Store at room temperature.

ACTION

Selectively inhibits factor Xa, decreasing thrombin generation and thrombus development.

Route	Onset	Peak	Duration
P.O.	Unknown	3–4 hr	Unknown

Half-life: 12 hours.

ADVERSE REACTIONS

CNS: syncope.
Hematologic: *major bleeding.*
Other: hypersensitivity reaction.

INTERACTIONS

Drug-drug. *Aspirin and other antiplatelet agents/anticoagulants, heparin, NSAIDs, SNRIs, SSRIs, thrombolytics:* May increase bleeding risk. Avoid use together.
Enoxaparin, naproxen: May increase anti-factor Xa activity. Avoid use together.
Strong dual inducers of CYP3A4 and P-glycoprotein (P-gp) (carbamazepine, phenytoin, rifampin): May decrease apixaban concentration. Avoid use together.
Strong dual inhibitors of CYP3A4 and P-gp (clarithromycin, itraconazole, ketoconazole, ritonavir): May increase apixaban concentration. Recommended dosage is 2.5 mg b.i.d.; avoid use together in patients already taking 2.5 mg b.i.d..
Drug-herb. *St. John's wort:* May decrease apixaban concentration. Discourage use together.

EFFECTS ON LAB TEST RESULTS

• May increase PT, INR, and activated partial thromboplastin time.

CONTRAINDICATIONS & CAUTIONS

• Contraindicated in patients hypersensitive to drug or its components, in those with active pathological bleeding, and in breast-feeding women.
• Use cautiously in patients at risk for severe bleeding (especially those concomitantly taking drugs that affect hemostasis).
Black Box Warning Discontinuing drug increases risk of thrombotic events. If anticoagulation with apixaban must be discontinued for a reason other than pathological bleeding, strongly consider coverage with another anticoagulant. ∎
⊕ Alert: Discontinue apixaban at least 48 hours before elective surgery or invasive procedures with a moderate or high risk of unacceptable or clinically significant bleeding.
⊕ Alert: Discontinue apixaban at least 24 hours before elective surgery or invasive procedures with a low risk of bleeding

or when the bleeding would be noncritical in location and easily controlled.
• Drug isn't recommended for patients with severe hepatic impairment or prosthetic heart valves.
• Use cautiously in pregnant women. Drug may increase risk of hemorrhage during pregnancy and delivery; use only if benefit outweighs risk.
• It isn't known if drug appears in breast milk. Patient should discontinue breast-feeding or discontinue therapy, taking into account the importance of the drug to the mother.

NURSING CONSIDERATIONS

• Monitor patient for bleeding. Discontinue drug if acute pathological bleeding occurs.
⊕ Alert: Promptly evaluate signs and symptom of blood loss. Drug can cause serious, potentially fatal bleeding.
• Keep in mind that protamine sulfate and vitamin K have no effect on the activity of apixaban.
• When switching from warfarin to apixaban, discontinue warfarin and start apixaban when INR is below 2.0.
• If switching from apixaban to warfarin, discontinue apixaban and begin both a parenteral anticoagulant and warfarin at the time the next dose of apixaban would have been taken. Discontinue the parenteral anticoagulant when INR reaches an acceptable range.
• If switching between apixaban and anticoagulants other than warfarin, discontinue drug being taken and begin other drug at next scheduled dose.

PATIENT TEACHING

• Warn patient not to discontinue drug without first talking to prescriber, because of risk of clot formation and stroke.
• Caution patient that bruising or bleeding may occur more easily.
• Advise patient to report unusual bleeding.
• Instruct patient to inform all health care providers (including dentists) about taking this drug as well as other products known to affect bleeding (including non-prescription products, such as aspirin or NSAIDs) before scheduling surgery or

---

Reactions in bold italics are *life-threatening*. Interactions may have a *rapid onset* or a *delayed onset*.

medical or dental procedure and before taking any new drug.

• Tell female patient to inform practitioner if she is pregnant, plans to become pregnant, is breast-feeding, or intends to breast-feed during treatment.

aprepitant
ah-PRE-pit-ant

Emend

fosaprepitant dimeglumine
Emend

Therapeutic class: Antiemetics
Pharmacologic class: Substance P and neurokinin-1 receptor antagonists
Pregnancy risk category: B

AVAILABLE FORMS
Capsules: 40 mg, 80 mg, 125 mg
Injection: 115 mg, 150 mg

INDICATIONS & DOSAGES
➤ **To prevent nausea and vomiting after highly emetogenic chemotherapy (including cisplatin) and moderately emetogenic chemotherapy, with a 5-HT$_3$ antagonist and a corticosteroid**
Adults: On day 1 of chemotherapy, 125 mg P.O. 1 hour before treatment, or 115 mg by I.V. infusion over 15 minutes, given 30 minutes before treatment; on days 2 and 3, give 80 mg P.O. every morning. Or, a single dose of 150 mg I.V. over 20 to 30 minutes, given 30 minutes before treatment.
➤ **To prevent postoperative nausea and vomiting**
Adults: 40 mg P.O. within 3 hours before induction of anesthesia.

ADMINISTRATION
P.O.
• Give drug without regard for food.
• Drug may be given with other antiemetics.
I.V.
▼ Reconstitute with 5 mL of normal saline solution. Add the saline along the vial wall to prevent foaming. Swirl gently and avoid shaking.

▼ Add entire volume to infusion bag containing 110 mL of saline solution. Total volume will be 115 mL and final concentration is 1 mg/mL. If using the 150-mg vial, add the reconstituted volume to 145 mL. Total volume will be 150 mL and concentration will be 1 mg/mL.
▼ Gently invert the bag two to three times.
▼ Administer 115-mg dose over 15 minutes by I.V. infusion.
▼ Administer 150-mg dose over 20 to 30 minutes by I.V. infusion.
▼ Final solution is stable for 24 hours at ambient room temperature.
▼ **Incompatibilities:** Any solutions containing divalent cations (e.g., Ca^{2+}, Mg^{2+}), including lactated Ringer's solution and Hartmann's solution.

ACTION
Inhibits emesis by selectively antagonizing substance P and neurokinin-1 receptors in the brain; appears to be synergistic with 5-HT$_3$ antagonists and corticosteroids.

Route	Onset	Peak	Duration
P.O.	Unknown	4 hr	Unknown
I.V.	Unknown	Less than 30 min	Unknown

Half-life: 9 to 13 hours.

ADVERSE REACTIONS
CNS: asthenia, fatigue, dizziness, fever, headache, insomnia.
CV: *bradycardia,* hypertension, hypotension.
EENT: mucous membrane disorder, tinnitus.
GI: anorexia, constipation, diarrhea, nausea, abdominal pain, epigastric pain, flatulence, gastritis, heartburn, vomiting.
GU: UTI.
Hematologic: *neutropenia,* anemia.
Respiratory: hiccups.
Skin: pruritus, infusion-site pain, infusion-site induration.
Other: dehydration.

INTERACTIONS
Drug-drug. *Alprazolam, midazolam, triazolam:* May increase levels of these drugs. Watch for CNS effects, such as increased

sedation. Decrease benzodiazepine dose by 50%.

Carbamazepine, phenytoin, rifampin, other CYP3A4 inducers: May decrease aprepitant level. Watch for decreased antiemetic effect.

Clarithromycin, diltiazem, erythromycin, itraconazole, ketoconazole, nefazodone, nelfinavir, ritonavir, troleandomycin, other CYP3A4 inhibitors: May increase aprepitant level and risk of toxicity. Use together cautiously.

Dexamethasone, methylprednisolone: May increase levels of these drugs and risk of toxicity. Decrease P.O. corticosteroid dose by 50%; decrease I.V. methylprednisolone dose by 25%.

Diltiazem: May increase diltiazem level. Monitor heart rate and blood pressure. Avoid using together.

Docetaxel, etoposide, ifosfamide, imatinib, irinotecan, paclitaxel, vinorelbine, vinblastine, vincristine: May increase levels and risk of toxicity of these drugs. Use together cautiously.

Hormonal contraceptives: May decrease contraceptive effectiveness. Tell women to use additional birth control method during therapy.

Paroxetine: May decrease paroxetine and aprepitant effects. Monitor patient for effectiveness.

Phenytoin: May decrease phenytoin level. Monitor level carefully. Avoid using together. Increase phenytoin dose as needed during therapy.

Pimozide: May increase pimozide level. Avoid using together.

Tolbutamide: May decrease tolbutamide effects. Monitor glucose level.

Warfarin: May decrease warfarin effectiveness. Monitor INR carefully for 2 weeks after each aprepitant treatment.

Drug-herb. *St. John's wort:* May decrease antiemetic effects by inducing CYP3A4. Discourage use together.

Drug-food. *Grapefruit juice:* May increase drug level and risk of toxicity. Discourage use together.

EFFECTS ON LAB TEST RESULTS

● May increase alkaline phosphatase, AST, ALT, BUN, creatinine, glucose, and urine protein levels. May decrease sodium level.

● May increase RBC and WBC counts. May decrease neutrophil count.

CONTRAINDICATIONS & CAUTIONS

● Contraindicated in patients hypersensitive to fosaprepitant, aprepitant, or its components.

● Use cautiously in patients receiving chemotherapy drugs metabolized mainly via CYP3A4 and in those with severe hepatic disease.

● Use in pregnant women only when drug's benefits clearly outweigh its risks.

● Don't use in breast-feeding women; it's unknown if drug appears in breast milk.

● Safety and effectiveness haven't been established in children.

⚠ *Overdose S&S:* Drowsiness, headache.

NURSING CONSIDERATIONS

● Avoid giving drug for more than 3 days per chemotherapy cycle.

☙ *Alert:* Fosaprepitant is given I.V. on day 1 only of a 3-day regimen.

☙ *Alert:* Before giving drug, screen patient carefully for possible drug and herb interactions.

● Don't give drug for existing nausea or vomiting.

● Expect to give drug with other antiemetics to treat breakthrough emesis.

● Monitor CBC, LFT results, and creatinine level periodically during therapy.

● *Look alike–sound alike:* Don't confuse aprepitant (oral form) with fosaprepitant (I.V. form).

PATIENT TEACHING

● If nausea or vomiting occurs, instruct patient to take breakthrough antiemetics rather than more aprepitant.

● Urge patient to report use of any other drugs or herbs.

● Caution patient against taking drug with grapefruit juice.

● Advise woman who takes a hormonal contraceptive to use an additional form of birth control.

● Tell patient who takes warfarin that PT and INR will be monitored closely for 2 weeks after therapy starts.

Reactions in bold italics are *life-threatening*. Interactions may have a *rapid onset* or a *delayed onset*.

• Teach patient to take drug 1 hour before chemotherapy, then daily in the morning or as directed.

arformoterol tartrate
arr-fohr-MOH-tur-ahl

Brovana

Therapeutic class: Bronchodilators
Pharmacologic class: Long-acting selective beta$_2$ agonists
Pregnancy risk category: C

AVAILABLE FORMS
Solution for inhalation: 15 mcg/2-mL vials

INDICATIONS & DOSAGES
➤ **Long-term maintenance treatment of bronchoconstriction in patients with COPD, including chronic bronchitis and emphysema**
Adults: 15 mcg, inhaled b.i.d. (morning and evening) via nebulizer. Maximum dose is 30 mcg daily.

ADMINISTRATION
Inhalational
• Use only the recommended nebulizer and compressor for treatment.
• Don't mix with other drugs or solutions in the nebulizer.
• Store vials in the foil pouches in the refrigerator and use immediately after opening.

ACTION
Relaxes bronchial and cardiac smooth muscle by acting on beta$_2$-adrenergic receptors; stimulates the enzyme adenyl cyclase, which catalyzes the conversion from ATP to cAMP. This further relaxes bronchial smooth muscle and inhibits release of mediators (like histamine and leukotrienes) from mast cells.

Route	Onset	Peak	Duration
Inhalation	Rapid	30 min	Unknown

Half-life: 26 hours.

ADVERSE REACTIONS
CNS: pain.
CV: chest pain, *AV block,* atrial flutter, *heart failure, MI, prolonged QT interval, supraventricular tachycardia,* inverted T wave, peripheral edema.
EENT: sinusitis.
GI: diarrhea.
Metabolic: *hypoglycemia,* hypokalemia.
Musculoskeletal: back pain, leg cramps.
Respiratory: dyspnea, pulmonary or chest congestion, *bronchospasm.*
Skin: rash.
Other: hypersensitivity reaction, flu syndrome.

INTERACTIONS
Drug-drug. *Aminophylline, corticosteroids (such as dexamethasone, prednisone), theophylline:* May increase the risk of hypokalemia. Monitor patient's potassium level.
Beta blockers (such as metoprolol, atenolol): May decrease effectiveness of arformoterol and increase risk of bronchospasm. Avoid using together, if possible; otherwise, use with extreme caution.
Non–potassium-sparing diuretics (such as furosemide, hydrochlorothiazide): May increase the risk of hypokalemia and ECG changes. Use cautiously together and monitor patient's ECG and potassium level.
Other beta$_2$ adrenergics (such as albuterol, formoterol): May cause additive effects. Avoid using together.
QT interval-prolonging drugs (such as MAO inhibitors, TCAs): May increase risk of ventricular arrhythmias. Use cautiously together.

EFFECTS ON LAB TEST RESULTS
• May increase prostate specific antigen levels. May decrease potassium levels. May increase or decrease glucose levels.

CONTRAINDICATIONS & CAUTIONS
• Contraindicated in patients hypersensitive to drug, formoterol, or any other components of this drug.
Black Box Warning Safe and effective use of arformoterol in patients with asthma hasn't been established. Arformoterol is contraindicated in patients with asthma who

aren't using a long-term asthma control medication. ∎

• Don't use in patients with acutely deteriorating COPD.

• Use cautiously in patients with seizure disorder; thyrotoxicosis; hepatic insufficiency; preexisting CV disease, including coronary insufficiency, arrhythmias, and hypertension; or in those unresponsive to sympathomimetic amines.

⚠ **Overdose S&S:** Exaggeration of adverse reactions, hyperglycemia, hypertension, hypotension, metabolic acidosis, cardiac arrest.

NURSING CONSIDERATIONS

Black Box Warning Drug may increase the risk of asthma-related death. ∎

• Drug is twice as potent as formoterol inhaler.

☉ Alert: Make sure patient has a rescue inhaler, such as albuterol, to treat an acute asthma attack or bronchospasm.

☉ Alert: Notify prescriber if patient experiences decreasing control of symptoms or begins using his short-acting beta₂ agonist more often.

• If paradoxical bronchospasm occurs, stop drug immediately.

• Monitor blood pressure, pulse, and ECG, as indicated.

• **Look alike–sound alike:** Don't confuse Brovana (arformoterol tartrate) with Boniva (ibandronate sodium).

PATIENT TEACHING

• Tell patient to store vials in the foil pouches in the refrigerator and use immediately after opening.

• Tell patient to use only the recommended nebulizer and compressor for treatment and not to mix drug with other inhaled drugs or solutions.

☉ Alert: Warn patient that drug is for maintenance treatment only and shouldn't be used to stop an asthma attack or bronchospasm. For emergency treatment, use a short-acting rescue inhaler such as albuterol.

• Educate patient using a short-acting bronchodilator on a scheduled basis, to stop scheduled use and use only for rescue therapy.

☉ Alert: Warn patient that serious adverse effects, including death, can occur at higher than recommended doses and not to take more inhalations than prescribed.

• Tell patient to stop drug immediately and obtain medical help if life-threatening bronchospasm, severe rash, or swelling in throat occurs.

• Inform patient that he may experience palpitations, chest pain, rapid heartbeat, tremors, or nervousness.

• Tell patient not to swallow the inhalation solution.

• Caution patient to notify prescriber if he notices a decrease in symptom control or more frequent use of his rescue inhaler.

SAFETY ALERT!

argatroban
ahr-GAH-troh-ban

Therapeutic class: Anticoagulants
Pharmacologic class: Direct thrombin inhibitors
Pregnancy risk category: B

AVAILABLE FORMS
Injection: 1 mg/mL, 100 mg/mL

INDICATIONS & DOSAGES
➤ **To prevent or treat thrombosis in patients with heparin-induced thrombocytopenia**
Adults without hepatic impairment: 2 mcg/kg/minute, given as a continuous I.V. infusion; adjust dose until the steady-state activated PTT (aPTT) is 1½ to 3 times the initial baseline value, not to exceed 100 seconds; maximum dose 10 mcg/kg/minute. See current manufacturer's label for recommended doses and infusion rates.
Children: 0.75 mcg/kg/minute by I.V. infusion. Check aPTT after 2 hours and adjust dosage in 0.1- to 0.25-mcg/kg/minute increments to achieve target aPTT of 1½ to 3 times the baseline value, not to exceed 100 seconds.
Adjust-a-dose: For adults with moderate hepatic impairment, reduce first dose to 0.5 mcg/kg/minute, given as a continuous infusion. Monitor aPTT closely and adjust dosage as needed. For children

with hepatic impairment, initial dose is 0.2 mcg/kg/minute. Adjust dosage in 0.05-mcg/kg/minute or lower increments. Monitor aPTT after 2 hours and adjust dosage as needed to achieve target aPTT.

➤ **Anticoagulation in patients with or at risk for heparin-induced thrombocytopenia during percutaneous coronary intervention (PCI)**

Adults: 350 mcg/kg I.V. bolus over 3 to 5 minutes. Start a continuous I.V. infusion at 25 mcg/kg/minute. Check activated clotting time (ACT) 5 to 10 minutes after the bolus dose is completed.

Adjust-a-dose: Use the following table to adjust the dosage.

Activated clotting time	Additional I.V. bolus	Continuous I.V. infusion
<300 sec	150 mcg/kg	30 mcg/kg/min*
>450 sec	None needed	15 mcg/kg/min*

*Check ACT again after 5 to 10 minutes.

Once a therapeutic ACT (300 to 450 sec) has been achieved, continue this dose for the duration of the procedure. In case of dissection, impending abrupt closure, thrombus formation during the procedure, or inability to achieve or maintain an ACT exceeding 300 seconds, give an additional bolus of 150 mcg/kg and increase infusion rate to 40 mcg/kg/minute. Check ACT again after 5 to 10 minutes.

ADMINISTRATION

I.V.

▼ Before starting therapy, obtain a complete list of patient's prescription and OTC drugs and supplements, including herbs.

▼ Stop all parenteral anticoagulants before giving drug. Giving with antiplatelets, thrombolytics, and other anticoagulants may increase risk of bleeding.

▼ Before starting drug, get results of baseline coagulation tests, platelet count, hemoglobin level, and hematocrit, and report any abnormalities to prescriber.

▼ Dilute in normal saline solution, D_5W, or lactated Ringer's injection to a final concentration of 1 mg/mL.

▼ Dilute each 2.5-mL vial 100-fold by mixing it with 250 mL of diluent.

▼ Mix the solution by repeated inversion of the diluent bag for 1 minute.

▼ Don't expose solution to direct sunlight.

▼ Prepared solutions are stable for up to 24 hours at 77° F (25° C).

▼ **Incompatibilities:** Other I.V. drugs.

ACTION

Reversibly binds to the thrombin-active site and inhibits thrombin-catalyzed or -induced reactions: fibrin formation; coagulation factor V, VIII, and XIII activation; protein C activation; and platelet aggregation. May inhibit the action of free and clot-associated thrombin.

Route	Onset	Peak	Duration
I.V.	Rapid	1–3 hr	Duration of infusion

Half-life: 39 to 51 minutes.

ADVERSE REACTIONS

CNS: *cerebrovascular disorder, hemorrhage,* fever, pain.

CV: *atrial fibrillation, cardiac arrest,* hypotension, *ventricular tachycardia.*

GI: abdominal pain, diarrhea, *GI bleeding,* nausea, vomiting.

GU: abnormal renal function, groin bleeding, hematuria, UTI.

Hematologic: anemia, *bleeding.*

Respiratory: cough, dyspnea, pneumonia, hemoptysis.

Other: allergic reactions, brachial bleeding, infection, *sepsis.*

INTERACTIONS

Drug-drug. *Antiplatelet drugs (clopidogrel, NSAIDs, salicylates), heparin, thrombolytics:* May increase risk of intracranial bleeding. Avoid using together.

Oral anticoagulants: May prolong PT and INR and may increase risk of bleeding. Monitor patient closely.

Drug-herb. *Angelica (dong quai), boldo, bromelains, capsicum, chamomile, dandelion, danshen, devil's claw, fenugreek, feverfew, garlic, ginger, ginkgo, ginseng, horse chestnut, licorice, meadowsweet, onion, passion flower, red clover, willow:* May increase risk of bleeding. Discourage use together.

EFFECTS ON LAB TEST RESULTS
• May decrease hemoglobin level and hematocrit.

CONTRAINDICATIONS & CAUTIONS
• Contraindicated in patients who have overt major bleeding or who are hypersensitive to drug or any of its components.
• Use cautiously in patients with hepatic disease or conditions that increase the risk of hemorrhage, such as severe hypertension.
• Use cautiously in patients who have just had lumbar puncture, spinal anesthesia, or major surgery, especially of the brain, spinal cord, or eye; patients with hematologic conditions causing increased bleeding tendencies, such as congenital or acquired bleeding disorders; and patients with GI ulcers or other lesions.
⚠ *Overdose S&S:* Excessive anticoagulation, with or without bleeding.

NURSING CONSIDERATIONS
• Check aPTT 2 hours after giving drug; dose adjustments may be required to get a targeted aPTT of 1.5 to 3 times the baseline, no longer than 100 seconds. Steady state is achieved 1 to 3 hours after starting drug.
• Draw blood for additional ACT about every 20 to 30 minutes during prolonged PCI.
❸ *Alert:* Patients can hemorrhage from any site in the body. Any unexplained decrease in hematocrit or blood pressure or any other unexplained symptoms may signify a hemorrhagic event.
• To convert to oral anticoagulant therapy, give warfarin P.O. with argatroban at up to 2 mcg/kg/minute until the INR exceeds 4 on combined therapy. After argatroban is stopped, repeat the INR in 4 to 6 hours. If the repeat INR is less than the desired therapeutic range, resume the I.V. argatroban infusion. Repeat the procedure daily until the desired therapeutic range on warfarin alone is reached.
• Use cautiously in breast-feeding women; it's unknown if drug appears in breast milk.
• *Look alike–sound alike:* Don't confuse argatroban with Aggrastat.

PATIENT TEACHING
• Tell patient that this drug can cause bleeding, and ask him to report any unusual bruising or bleeding (nosebleeds, bleeding gums) or tarry stools to the prescriber immediately.
• Advise patient to avoid activities that carry a risk of injury, and to use a soft toothbrush and an electric razor during therapy.
• Advise patient to consult with prescriber before initiating any herbal therapy; many herbs have anticoagulant, antiplatelet, and fibrinolytic properties.
• Instruct patient to notify prescriber if he has wheezing, trouble breathing, or skin rash.
• Instruct woman who is pregnant, has recently delivered, or is breast-feeding to notify her prescriber.
• Tell patient to notify prescriber if he has GI ulcers or liver disease, or has had recent surgery, radiation treatment, falling episodes, or injury.

---

aripiprazole
air-eh-PIP-rah-zole

Abilify❖, Abilify Discmelt, Abilify Maintena

Therapeutic class: Antipsychotics
Pharmacologic class: Quinolinone derivatives
Pregnancy risk category: C

AVAILABLE FORMS
Injection: 9.75 mg/1.3 mL (7.5 mg/mL) single-dose vial
Oral solution: 1 mg/mL
Orally disintegrating tablets (ODTs): 10 mg, 15 mg
Suspension for I.M. use: 300 mg, 400 mg
Tablets: 2 mg, 5 mg, 10 mg, 15 mg, 20 mg, 30 mg

INDICATIONS & DOSAGES
Adjust-a-dose (for all indications): When using with CYP3A4 inhibitors, such as ketoconazole or clarithromycin, or CYP2D6 inhibitors, such as quinidine, fluoxetine, or paroxetine, give half the aripiprazole dose. When using with CYP3A4 inducers such as carbamazepine, double the aripiprazole

---

dose. Return to original dosing after the other drugs are stopped.

➤ **Schizophrenia**

Adults: Initially, 10 to 15 mg P.O. daily; increase to maximum daily dose of 30 mg, if needed, after at least 2 weeks. Responding patients should be continued on the lowest dosage needed to maintain remission. Patients should be periodically reassessed to determine the need for maintenance treatment.

Or, 400 mg (extended-release suspension) I.M. monthly. Maintenance dosage is 400 mg I.M. monthly, no sooner than 26 days after previous injection. If adverse reactions occur or for patients who are poor metabolizers of CYP2D6, give 300 mg I.M. monthly. If second or third doses are missed and more than 4 but less than 5 weeks have elapsed since last injection, give dose as soon as possible. If more than 5 weeks have elapsed, restart concomitant oral aripiprazole for 14 days with next scheduled injection. If fourth or subsequent doses are missed and more than 4 but less than 6 weeks have elapsed since last injection, give dose as soon as possible. If more than 6 weeks have elapsed, restart concomitant oral aripiprazole for 14 days with next scheduled injection.

Adjust-a-dose (for extended-release suspension): For patients who are poor metabolizers of CYP2D6 and who are taking concomitant CYP3A4 inhibitors, dose is 200 mg. For patients taking 400-mg I.M. dose who are taking strong CYP2D6 or CYP3A4 inhibitors for more than 14 days, dose is 300 mg. For patients taking 400-mg I.M. dose who are taking CYP2D6 and CYP3A4 inhibitors for more than 14 days, dose is 200 mg. For patients taking 400-mg I.M. dose who are taking CYP3A4 inducers for more than 14 days, avoid use. For patients taking 300-mg I.M. dose who are taking strong CYP2D6 or CYP3A4 inhibitors for more than 14 days, adjusted dosage is 200 mg. For patients taking 300-mg I.M. dose who are taking CYP2D6 and CYP3A4 inhibitors for more than 14 days, dose is 160 mg. Avoid use in patients taking CYP3A4 inducers for more than 14 days. If CYP2D6 or CYP3A4 inhibitor is withdrawn, dosage may need to be increased.

Adolescents ages 13 to 17: Initially, 2 mg P.O. daily; increase to 5 mg after 2 days, then to recommended dose of 10 mg in 2 more days. May titrate to maximum daily dose of 30 mg in 5-mg increments. Responding patients should be continued on the lowest dosage needed to maintain remission. Patients should be periodically reassessed to determine the need for maintenance treatment.

➤ **Bipolar mania, including manic and mixed episodes, with or without psychotic features; adjunctive therapy to either lithium or valproate for treatment of manic and mixed episodes associated with bipolar I disorder with or without psychotic features**

Adults: Initially, 15 mg P.O. once daily as monotherapy or 10 to 15 mg P.O. once daily as adjunctive therapy with lithium or valproate. Target dose is 15 mg/day as monotherapy or adjunctive therapy. Dose can be increased to maximum of 30 mg/day based on clinical response. For maintenance, responding patients on monotherapy should be continued on the lowest dose needed to maintain remission. Patients should be periodically reassessed to determine the long-term usefulness of maintenance treatment.

Children ages 10 to 17: Initially, 2 mg P.O. daily; increase to 5 mg P.O. daily after 2 days, then to recommended dose of 10 mg in 2 more days. May titrate to maximum daily dose of 30 mg in 5-mg increments every 5 days. For maintenance, responding patients on monotherapy should be continued on the lowest dose needed to maintain remission. Patients should be periodically reassessed to determine the need for maintenance treatment.

➤ **Adjunctive treatment of major depressive disorder**

Adults: Initially, 2 to 5 mg P.O. daily. Dose range is 2 to 15 mg/day. Dosage adjustments of up to 5 mg/day should occur gradually, at intervals of no less than 1 week.

➤ **Agitation associated with schizophrenia or bipolar I disorder, mixed or manic**

Adults: 5.25 to 15 mg by deep I.M. injection. Recommended dose is 9.75 mg. May give a second dose after 2 hours, if needed. Safety of giving more frequently than every

2 hours or a total daily dose more than 30 mg isn't known. Switch to oral form as soon as possible.

➤ **Irritability associated with autistic disorder**
Children ages 6 to 17: Initially, 2 mg P.O. daily. Increase dosage to 5 mg/day, with subsequent increases to 10 or 15 mg/day if needed. Dosage adjustments of up to 5 mg/day should occur gradually, at intervals of no less than 1 week.

ADMINISTRATION
P.O.
- Give drug without regard for food.
- Substitute the oral solution on a milligram-by-milligram basis for the 5-, 10-, 15-, or 20-mg tablets, up to 25 mg. Give patients taking 30-mg tablets 25 mg of solution.
- Keep ODTs in blister package until ready to use. Use dry hands to carefully peel open the foil backing and remove the tablet. Don't split tablet.
- Store oral solution in refrigerator; it can be used up to 6 months after opening.
I.M.
- Inject slowly and deep into the muscle mass.
- Don't give I.V. or subcutaneously.
- Don't confuse I.M. formulations. They aren't interchangeable.

ACTION
Thought to exert partial agonist activity at dopamine 2 and 5-HT$_{1A}$ receptors and antagonist activity at 5-HT$_{2A}$ receptors.

Route	Onset	Peak	Duration
P.O.	Unknown	3–5 hr	Unknown
I.M.	Unknown	1–3 hr	Unknown

Half-life: About 75 hours in patients with normal metabolism; about 6 days in those who can't metabolize the drug through CYP2D6.

ADVERSE REACTIONS
CNS: headache, anxiety, insomnia, lightheadedness, somnolence, akathisia, *increased suicide risk, neuroleptic malignant syndrome, seizures, suicidal thoughts,* extrapyramidal disorder (children), tremor, asthenia, depression, fatigue, dizziness, nervousness, hostility, manic behavior, confusion, abnormal gait, cogwheel rigidity, fever, tardive dyskinesia, restlessness.
CV: peripheral edema, chest pain, hypertension, tachycardia, orthostatic hypotension, *bradycardia.*
EENT: rhinitis, blurred vision, increased salivation, conjunctivitis, ear pain.
GI: nausea, vomiting, constipation, anorexia, dry mouth, dyspepsia, diarrhea, abdominal pain, esophageal dysmotility.
GU: urinary incontinence.
Hematologic: ecchymosis, anemia.
Metabolic: weight gain, weight loss, hyperglycemia, hypercholesterolemia.
Musculoskeletal: neck pain, neck stiffness, muscle cramps.
Respiratory: dyspnea, pneumonia, cough.
Skin: rash, dry skin, pruritus, sweating, ulcer.
Other: flulike syndrome.

INTERACTIONS
Drug-drug. *Antihypertensives:* May enhance antihypertensive effects. Monitor blood pressure.
Benzodiazepines: May cause excessive sedation and orthostatic hypotension. Monitor patient closely (I.M. form).
Carbamazepine and other CYP3A4 inducers: May decrease levels and effectiveness of aripiprazole. Double the usual dose of aripiprazole, and monitor the patient closely.
CNS depressants: May lead to enhanced CNS depression. Use together with caution.
Ketoconazole and other CYP3A4 inhibitors: May increase risk of serious toxic effects. Start treatment with half the usual dose of aripiprazole, and monitor patient closely.
Metoclopramide: May increase risk of extrapyramidal reactions. Use together is contraindicated.
Potential CYP2D6 inhibitors (fluoxetine, paroxetine, quinidine): May increase levels and toxicity of aripiprazole. Give half the usual dose of aripiprazole (P.O.) or 25% the usual dose (I.M.).
Drug-food. *Grapefruit juice:* May increase drug level. Tell patient not to take drug with grapefruit juice.
Drug-lifestyle. *Alcohol use:* May increase CNS effects. Discourage use together.

Reactions in bold italics are *life-threatening*. Interactions may have a *rapid onset* or a *delayed onset*.

EFFECTS ON LAB TEST RESULTS
● May increase CK and glucose levels.

CONTRAINDICATIONS & CAUTIONS
● Contraindicated in patients hypersensitive to drug.
● Use cautiously in patients with CV disease, cerebrovascular disease, or conditions that could predispose the patient to hypotension, such as dehydration or hypovolemia.
● Use cautiously in patients with history of seizures or with conditions that lower the seizure threshold.
● Use cautiously in patients who engage in strenuous exercise, are exposed to extreme heat, take anticholinergics, or are susceptible to dehydration.
● Use cautiously in patients at risk for aspiration pneumonia, such as those with Alzheimer disease.
۞ Alert: Neonates exposed to antipsychotics during the third trimester of pregnancy are at risk for developing extrapyramidal signs and symptoms (repetitive muscle movements of the face and body) and withdrawal signs and symptoms (agitation, abnormally increased or decreased muscle tone, tremors, sleepiness, severe difficulty breathing, and difficulty feeding) after delivery. Use in pregnant women only if the potential benefit to the mother justifies the risk to the fetus.
● Use cautiously in breast-feeding women.
Black Box Warning Abilify isn't approved for use in children with depression. ▮
Black Box Warning Elderly patients with dementia-related psychosis treated with atypical antipsychotics are at an increased risk for death. Abilify isn't approved for the treatment of patients with dementia-related psychosis. ▮
⚠ Overdose S&S: Somnolence, tremor, vomiting, acidosis, aggression, atrial fibrillation, bradycardia, coma, confusion, seizures, depressed level of consciousness, hypertension, hypokalemia, hypotension, increased AST and blood CK levels, lethargy, loss of consciousness, aspiration pneumonia, prolonged QRS complex, prolonged QT interval, respiratory arrest, status epilepticus, tachycardia.

NURSING CONSIDERATIONS
۞ Alert: Neuroleptic malignant syndrome may occur. Monitor patient for hyperpyrexia, muscle rigidity, altered mental status, irregular pulse or blood pressure, tachycardia, diaphoresis, and cardiac arrhythmias.
● If signs and symptoms of neuroleptic malignant syndrome occur, immediately stop drug and notify prescriber.
● Monitor patient for signs and symptoms of tardive dyskinesia. Elderly patients, especially women, are at highest risk of developing this adverse effect.
۞ Alert: Fatal cerebrovascular adverse events (stroke, transient ischemic attack) may occur in elderly patients with dementia. Drug isn't safe or effective in these patients.
Black Box Warning Drug may increase the risk of suicidal thinking and behavior in children, adolescents, and young adults ages 18 to 24 during the first 2 months of treatment, especially in those with major depressive or other psychiatric disorder. ▮
۞ Alert: Hyperglycemia may occur. Monitor patient with diabetes regularly. Patient with risk factors for diabetes should undergo fasting blood glucose testing at baseline and periodically. Monitor all patients for symptoms of hyperglycemia, including increased hunger, thirst, frequent urination, and weakness. Hyperglycemia may resolve when patient stops taking drug.
۞ Alert: Monitor patient for symptoms of metabolic syndrome (significant weight gain and increased body mass index, hypertension, hyperglycemia, hypercholesterolemia, and hypertriglyceridemia).
● Treat patient with the smallest dose for the shortest time, and periodically reevaluate for need to continue.
● Give prescriptions only for small quantities of drug, to reduce risk of overdose.
● **Look alike–sound alike:** Don't confuse aripiprazole with rabeprazole, omeprazole, or pantoprazole.

PATIENT TEACHING
Black Box Warning Advise families and caregivers to closely observe patient for clinical worsening, suicidality, or unusual changes in behavior. ▮

• Tell patient to use caution while driving or operating hazardous machinery because psychoactive drugs may impair judgment, thinking, or motor skills.
• Tell patient that drug may be taken without regard to meals.
• Advise patients that grapefruit juice may interact with aripiprazole and to limit or avoid its use.
• Advise patient that gradual improvement in symptoms should occur over several weeks rather than immediately.
• Tell patients to avoid alcohol use while taking drug.
• Advise patients to limit strenuous activity while taking drug to avoid dehydration.
• Tell patient to keep ODT in blister package until ready to use. Using dry hands, he should carefully peel open the foil backing and place tablet on the tongue. Tell him not to split tablet.
• Tell patient to store oral solution in refrigerator, and that the solution can be used for up to 6 months after opening.

---

armodafinil
are-moe-DAFF-ih-nihl

Nuvigil

Therapeutic class: Stimulants
Pharmacologic class: CNS stimulants
Pregnancy risk category: C
Controlled substance schedule: IV

AVAILABLE FORMS
Tablets: 50 mg, 150 mg, 250 mg

INDICATIONS & DOSAGES
➤ **To improve wakefulness in patients with excessive sleepiness caused by narcolepsy, obstructive sleep apnea-hypoapnea syndrome (OSAHS), or shift-work sleep disorder**
Adults: 150 or 250 mg P.O. daily in the morning. For OSAHS, doses exceeding 150 mg daily may not be more effective. For shift-work sleep disorder, 150 mg P.O. daily, 1 hour before start of shift.
Adjust-a-dose: Reduce dosage in patients with severe hepatic impairment, with or without cirrhosis.

ADMINISTRATION
P.O.
• Give drug consistently with or without food at same time each day. Food may delay effect of drug.

ACTION
Unknown. May be similar to sympathomimetics, such as amphetamine and methylphenidate. Also may inhibit dopamine reuptake.

Route	Onset	Peak	Duration
P.O.	Unknown	2 hr	Unknown

Half-life: 15 hours.

ADVERSE REACTIONS
CNS: agitation, anxiety, depression, dizziness, fatigue, headache, insomnia, migraine, nervousness, pain, paresthesia, pyrexia, tremor.
CV: increased blood pressure, increased pulse, palpitations.
GI: abdominal pain, anorexia, constipation, diarrhea, dry mouth, dyspepsia, loose stools, nausea, vomiting.
Respiratory: dyspnea.
Skin: contact dermatitis, hyperhydrosis, rash, *Stevens-Johnson syndrome.*
Other: allergic reactions, flulike illness, thirst.

INTERACTIONS
Drug-drug. *CNS stimulants (amphetamine, methylphenidate):* May produce additive effects. Use cautiously together.
Drugs metabolized by CYP2C19 (diazepam, omeprazole, phenytoin, propranolol): May increase levels of these drugs. Monitor patient and reduce doses as needed.
Drugs metabolized by CYP3A (cyclosporine, ethinyl estradiol, midazolam, triazolam): May decrease levels of these drugs. Adjust doses as needed.
Drugs that induce CYP3A (carbamazepine, phenobarbital, rifampin): May decrease armodafinil level. Check drug level and adjust dose as needed.
Drugs that inhibit CYP3A (erythromycin, ketoconazole): May increase armodafinil level. Monitor patient carefully and decrease dose as needed.

Reactions in bold italics are *life-threatening*. Interactions may have a *rapid onset* or a *delayed onset*.

Drug-food. *Any food:* May delay onset of action by several hours. Monitor effect and give drug consistently with or without food, at the same time daily.

Drug-lifestyle. *Alcohol use:* May counteract armodafinil's effect. Discourage use together.

EFFECTS ON LAB TEST RESULTS
● May increase GGT and alkaline phosphatase levels.

CONTRAINDICATIONS & CAUTIONS
● Contraindicated in patients younger than age 17.
● Contraindicated in patients hypersensitive to modafinil, armodafinil, or their inactive ingredients.
● Contraindicated in patients with left ventricular hypertrophy and in those who have experienced mitral valve prolapse when drug is given with other CNS stimulants.
● Use cautiously in breast-feeding or elderly patients.
● Use in pregnant patient only when benefit to mother outweighs risk to fetus.
● Use cautiously in those with a history of drug abuse or dependence.
⊕ Alert: Use cautiously in patients with a psychiatric illness; drug may increase the risk of mania, delusion, hallucinations, and suicidal ideation.
● Use cautiously in patients with cardiac disease, multiorgan hypersensitivity, or rash, including Stevens-Johnson syndrome and severe hepatic impairment.
⚠ Overdose S&S: Excitation or agitation, insomnia, slight or moderate elevations in hemodynamic parameters, restlessness, disorientation, confusion, hallucinations, nausea, diarrhea, tachycardia, bradycardia, hypertension, chest pain.

NURSING CONSIDERATIONS
● Obtain a thorough medication history to avoid potentially dangerous drug interactions.
● Obtain a complete cardiac history. Monitor patient for increased blood pressure and pulse rate, ECG changes, chest pain, and arrhythmias.
● Monitor patient carefully for evidence of allergic reaction. If rash or other symptoms appear, stop drug immediately, notify prescriber, and monitor carefully.

● Monitor patients for signs and symptoms of misuse or abuse, especially those with a history of drug or stimulant abuse.
● Assess patient for abnormal level of sleepiness. Don't allow patient to engage in dangerous activities, such as driving, until effect of medication is known.
● Patients receiving continuous positive airway pressure therapy for OSAHS should continue its use regardless of armodafinil therapy.

PATIENT TEACHING
⊕ Alert: Instruct patient to stop taking drug and notify prescriber if rash, hives, mouth sores, blister, peeling skin, trouble swallowing or breathing, or other symptoms of allergic reaction occur.
● Tell patient not to perform hazardous tasks, such as driving, if he feels excessive sleepiness or until effects of drug are known.
● Tell patient to notify prescriber of all drugs he takes to avoid potentially dangerous drug interactions.
● Tell patient to take drug at the same time, with or without food, every day.
● Advise patient that taking drug with food may delay its effects.
● Urge patient to notify prescriber right away if she becomes pregnant or plans to breast-feed.

asenapine
a-SEN-uh-peen

Saphris

Therapeutic class: Antipsychotics
Pharmacologic class: Dopamine–serotonin antagonists
Pregnancy risk category: C

AVAILABLE FORMS
Tablets (sublingual): 5 mg, 10 mg

INDICATIONS & DOSAGES
➤ **Acute schizophrenia**
Adults: 5 mg S.L. b.i.d. May increase up to 10 mg b.i.d. after 1 week based on tolerability.

➤ **Acute manic or mixed episodes associated with bipolar I disorder as monotherapy or as adjunctive therapy with either lithium or valproate**
Adults: For monotherapy, 10 mg S.L. b.i.d. For adjunctive therapy, 5 mg S.L. b.i.d. Dosage may be increased to a maximum of 10 mg S.L. b.i.d.
Adjust-a-dose: If adverse effects occur, reduce dosage to 5 mg b.i.d.

ADMINISTRATION
P.O.
● Obtain blood pressure before starting drug and monitor pressure regularly. Watch for orthostatic hypotension.
● Peel back colored tab on tablet pack, gently remove tablet, place under patient's tongue, and allow to dissolve completely.
● Advise patient not to eat or drink for 10 minutes after taking drug.

ACTION
Unknown. May block dopamine and 5-HT$_2$ receptors.

Route	Onset	Peak	Duration
S.L.	Immediate	1 hr	Unknown

Half-life: 24 hours.

ADVERSE REACTIONS
CNS: akathisia, anxiety, depression, dizziness, extrapyramidal symptoms, fatigue, headache, insomnia, irritability, somnolence.
CV: hypertension, *prolonged QTc interval.*
EENT: dry mouth, oral hypoesthesia, salivary hypersecretion, toothache.
GI: constipation, dyspepsia, increased appetite, stomach discomfort, taste perversion, vomiting.
Metabolic: weight gain.
Musculoskeletal: arthralgia, extremity pain.

INTERACTIONS
Drug-drug. *Alpha$_1$ blockers (such as doxazosin, terazosin):* May increase risk of hypotension. Use together cautiously.
Antiarrhythmics, class IA (procainamide, quinidine) and class III (amiodarone, sotalol); antibiotics (gatifloxacin, moxifloxacin); antipsychotics (chlorpromazine,

thioridazine, ziprasidone); citalopram: May prolong QTc interval, leading to lethal arrhythmias such as torsades de pointes. Avoid use together.
Antidepressants (fluvoxamine, imipramine, paroxetine): May increase asenapine level. Use together cautiously.
CNS agents (opioids): May enhance CNS depression. Use with caution.
Dextromethorphan, paroxetine: May increase dextromethorphan and paroxetine levels. Use together cautiously.
Metoclopramide: May increase risk of extrapyramidal reactions. Avoid administering together.
Drug-lifestyle. *Alcohol use:* May increase CNS effects. Discourage use together.

EFFECTS ON LAB TEST RESULTS
● May increase glucose, cholesterol, ALT, AST, and prolactin levels.
● May decrease WBC and neutrophil counts.

CONTRAINDICATIONS & CAUTIONS
Black Box Warning Elderly patients with dementia-related psychosis treated with atypical or conventional antipsychotics are at increased risk for death. Antipsychotics aren't approved for the treatment of dementia-related psychosis. ▮
☼ Alert: Don't administer drug to patients with a known hypersensitivity. Hypersensitivity reactions may occur as early as the first dose. Monitor patient for serious allergic reactions (anaphylaxis, angioedema, hypotension, difficulty breathing, wheezing, swollen tongue, rash).
☼ Alert: Watch for signs and symptoms of neuroleptic malignant syndrome (extrapyramidal effects, hyperthermia, autonomic disturbance), which are rare but can be fatal.
☼ Alert: Avoid use in patients with conditions that may increase risk of torsades de pointes and in those taking other drugs that prolong QTc interval.
☼ Alert: Neonates exposed to antipsychotics during the third trimester of pregnancy are at risk for developing extrapyramidal signs and symptoms (repetitive muscle movements of the face and body) and withdrawal signs and symptoms (agitation, abnormally increased or decreased muscle tone, tremors, sleepiness, severe difficulty

breathing, and difficulty feeding) after de-livery. Use in pregnant women only if the potential benefit to the mother justifies the risk to the fetus.
• It isn't known if drug appears in breast milk. Because of risk of adverse effects, an alternative method of feeding the baby is recommended.
• Safety and effectiveness in children haven't been established.
⚠ **Overdose S&S:** Agitation, confusion, hypotension, circulatory collapse.

NURSING CONSIDERATIONS
• Monitor ECG before and regularly during treatment for prolongation of QTc interval.
• Monitor patient for tardive dyskinesia, which may occur after prolonged use. It may disappear spontaneously or persist for life, despite stopping drug.
• Drug may alter glucose control in diabet-ics. Monitor glucose levels closely.
• Monitor CBC frequently during first few months of therapy in those with history of leukopenia or neutropenia. If WBC count decreases, monitor patient for signs and symptoms of infection; if infection occurs, discontinue drug in the absence of another cause.
• Obtain blood pressure before starting drug, and monitor pressure regularly. Watch for orthostatic hypotension.
• Monitor patient for dysphagia, which can lead to aspiration and aspiration pneumonia.
• Dispense lowest appropriate quantity of drug, to reduce risk of overdose.
• Monitor patient for abnormal body tem-perature regulation, especially if he ex-ercises, is exposed to extreme heat, takes anticholinergics, or is dehydrated.

PATIENT TEACHING
• Instruct patient to peel back colored tab on tablet pack, gently remove tablet, place under the tongue, and allow to dissolve completely. Advise patient not to eat or drink for 10 minutes after taking drug.
• Warn patient to avoid activities that re-quire mental alertness, such as operating hazardous machinery or operating a motor vehicle, until drug's effects are known.
• Advise patient to contact prescriber if palpitations or rapid heartbeat occurs.

• Advise patient not to stand up quickly but to get up slowly from a sitting position to avoid dizziness.
• Inform patient that weight gain may occur.
• Warn patient against exposure to extreme heat because drug may impair body's ability to reduce temperature.
• Advise patient to avoid alcohol.

aspirin (acetylsalicylic acid, ASA)
ASS-pir-in

Asaphen† ◊, Asatab† ◊, Aspir-Low ◊, Aspir-81 ◊, Bayer ◊, Ecotrin ◊, Empirin ◊, Entrophen† ◊, Halfprin ◊, Norwich ◊, Novasen† ◊, St. Joseph ◊, ZORprin ◊

Therapeutic class: NSAIDs
Pharmacologic class: Salicylates
Pregnancy risk category: C; D if used full dose in 3rd trimester

AVAILABLE FORMS
Suppositories: 120 mg ◊, 200 mg ◊, 300 mg ◊, 600 mg ◊
Tablets: 325 mg ◊, 500 mg ◊
Tablets (chewable): 81 mg ◊
Tablets (controlled-release): 800 mg
Tablets (enteric-coated): 81 mg ◊, 162 mg ◊, 325 mg ◊, 500 mg ◊, 650 mg ◊
Tablets (extended-release): 650 mg ◊

INDICATIONS & DOSAGES
➤ **Rheumatoid arthritis, osteoarthritis, or other polyarthritic or inflammatory conditions**
Adults: Initially, 3 g P.O. daily in di-vided doses. Increase as needed, with target plasma salicylate levels of 150 to 300 mcg/mL.
➤ **Juvenile rheumatoid arthritis**
Children: 90 to 130 mg/kg/day in di-vided doses. Increase as needed, with target plasma salicylate levels of 150 to 300 mcg/mL.
➤ **Mild pain or fever**
Adults and children older than age 12: 324 to 1,000 mg P.O. or P.R. every 4 hours p.r.n. Or, for controlled-, extended-, or delayed-release products, 1,300 mg followed by 650

to 1,300 mg every 8 hours. Maximum dose is 4,000 mg in 24 hours.
Children ages 2 to 11: 10 to 15 mg/kg/dose P.O. or P.R. every 4 hours up to 80 mg/kg daily.

➤ **Suspected acute MI**
Adults: Initial dose of 160 to 325 mg P.O. as soon as MI is suspected. Continue maintenance dose of 160 to 325 mg P.O. daily for 30 days after infarction. After 30 days, consider further therapy for prevention of MI.

➤ **To reduce risk of MI in patients with previous MI, unstable angina, and chronic stable angina pectoris**
Adults: 75 to 325 mg P.O. daily.

➤ **To reduce risk of recurrent transient ischemic attacks and stroke or death in patients at risk**
Adults: 50 to 325 mg P.O. daily.

➤ **Acute ischemic stroke**
Adults: 50 to 325 mg P.O. daily, started within 48 hours of stroke onset and continued for up to 2 to 4 weeks.

➤ **CABG**
Adults: 325 mg P.O. daily starting 6 hours postprocedure.

➤ **Percutaneous transluminal coronary angioplasty**
Adults: Initial dose of 325 mg P.O. 2 hours presurgery and then 160 to 325 mg P.O. daily.

➤ **Carotid endarterectomy**
Adults: 80 mg P.O. daily to 650 mg P.O. b.i.d. starting before surgery.

➤ **Kawasaki disease ◆**
Children: 80 to 100 mg/kg P.O. daily, in four divided doses with immune globulin I.V. After the fever subsides, reduce dosage to 1 to 5 mg/kg once daily. Aspirin therapy usually continues for 6 to 8 weeks.

➤ **Polycythemia vera ◆**
Adults: 75 or 100 mg P.O. daily. Pregnant women should take 75 mg P.O. daily throughout pregnancy and for 6 weeks after delivery.

ADMINISTRATION
P.O.
● For patient with swallowing difficulties, crush non–enteric-coated aspirin and dissolve in soft food or liquid. Give liquid

immediately after mixing because drug will break down rapidly.
● Give drug with food, milk, antacid, or large glass of water to reduce GI effects.
● Give sustained-release or enteric-coated forms whole; don't crush or break these tablets.
● For acute MI, have patient chew tablet.
Rectal
● Refrigerate suppositories.

ACTION
Thought to produce analgesia and exert its anti-inflammatory effect by inhibiting prostaglandin and other substances that sensitize pain receptors. Drug may relieve fever through central action in the hypothalamic heat-regulating center. In low doses, drug also appears to interfere with clotting by keeping a platelet-aggregating substance from forming.

Route	Onset	Peak	Duration
P.O. (buffered)	5–30 min	1–2 hr	1–4 hr
P.O. (enteric-coated)	5–30 min	Variable	1–4 hr
P.O. (extended-release)	5–30 min	1–4 hr	1–4 hr
P.O. (solution)	5–30 min	15–40 min	1–4 hr
P.O. (tablet)	5–30 min	25–40 min	1–4 hr
P.R.	Unknown	3–4 hr	Unknown

Half-life: 15 to 20 minutes.

ADVERSE REACTIONS
CNS: agitation, *cerebral edema, coma,* confusion, dizziness, headache, lethargy, *seizures, subdural or intracranial hemorrhage.*
CV: *arrhythmias,* hypotension, tachycardia.
EENT: tinnitus, hearing loss.
GI: nausea, *GI bleeding,* dyspepsia, GI distress, occult bleeding, *pancreatitis,* vomiting.
GU: *antepartum and postpartum bleeding,* interstitial nephritis, lower-birth weight infants, papillary necrosis, prolonged pregnancy and labor, proteinuria, renal insufficiency, renal failure, stillbirths.
Hematologic: prolonged bleeding time, *leukopenia, thrombocytopenia,* coagulopathy, *DIC.*
Hepatic: *hepatitis.*

Reactions in bold italics are *life-threatening*. Interactions may have a *rapid onset* or a *delayed onset*.

Metabolic: dehydration, *hyperkalemia, metabolic acidosis,* respiratory alkalosis.
Skin: rash, bruising, urticaria, hives.
Other: *angioedema, Reye syndrome,* hypersensitivity reactions.

INTERACTIONS

Drug-drug. *ACE inhibitors:* May decrease antihypertensive effects. Monitor blood pressure closely.
Ammonium chloride and other urine acidifiers: May increase levels of aspirin products. Watch for aspirin toxicity.
Antacids in high doses and other urine alkalinizers: May decrease levels of aspirin products. Watch for decreased aspirin effect.
Anticoagulants: May increase risk of bleeding. Use with extreme caution if must be used together.
Beta blockers: May decrease antihypertensive effect. Avoid long-term aspirin use if patient is taking antihypertensives.
Corticosteroids: May enhance salicylate elimination and decrease drug level. Watch for decreased aspirin effect.
Heparin: May increase risk of bleeding. Monitor coagulation studies and patient closely if used together.
Ibuprofen, other NSAIDs: May negate the antiplatelet effect of low-dose aspirin therapy. Patients using immediate-release aspirin (not enteric-coated) should take ibuprofen at least 30 minutes after or more than 8 hours before aspirin. Occasional use of ibuprofen is unlikely to have a negative effect.
Influenza virus vaccine, live: Increases risk of Reye syndrome. Use together is contraindicated in children and adolescents.
Methotrexate: May increase risk of methotrexate toxicity. Avoid using together.
Nizatidine: May increase risk of salicylate toxicity in patients receiving high doses of aspirin. Monitor patient closely.
Oral antidiabetics: May increase hypoglycemic effect. Monitor patient closely.
Probenecid, sulfinpyrazone: May decrease uricosuric effect. Avoid using together.
Valproic acid: May increase valproic acid level. Avoid using together.
Drug-herb. *Dong quai, feverfew, ginkgo, horse chestnut, kelpware, red clover:* May increase risk of bleeding. Monitor patient

closely for increased effects. Discourage use together.
White willow: May increase risk of adverse effects. Discourage use together.
Drug-food. *Caffeine:* May increase drug absorption. Watch for increased effects.
Drug-lifestyle. *Alcohol use:* May increase risk of GI bleeding. Discourage use together.

EFFECTS ON LAB TEST RESULTS

● May increase LFT values, BUN, creatinine, and potassium levels.
● May decrease platelet and WBC counts.
● May falsely increase protein-bound iodine level.
● May interfere with urine glucose analysis with Diastix, Chemstrip uG, Clinitest, and Benedict solution; with urinary 5-hydroxyindoleacetic acid and vanillylmandelic acid tests; and with Gerhardt test for urine acetoacetic acid.

CONTRAINDICATIONS & CAUTIONS

● Contraindicated in patients hypersensitive to drug and in those with NSAID-induced sensitivity reactions, G6PD deficiency, or bleeding disorders, such as hemophilia, von Willebrand disease, or telangiectasia.
● Use cautiously in patients with GI lesions, impaired renal function, hypoprothrombinemia, vitamin K deficiency, thrombocytopenia, thrombotic thrombocytopenic purpura, or severe hepatic impairment.
🛈 *Alert:* Oral and rectal OTC products containing aspirin and nonaspirin salicylates shouldn't be given to children or teenagers who have or are recovering from chickenpox or flulike symptoms with or without fever because of the risk of Reye syndrome.
⚠ *Overdose S&S:* Severe acid-base and electrolyte disturbance, hyperthermia, dehydration, tinnitus, vertigo, headache, confusion, drowsiness, diaphoresis, hyperventilation, vomiting, diarrhea.

NURSING CONSIDERATIONS

● For inflammatory conditions, rheumatic fever, and thrombosis, give aspirin on a schedule rather than as needed.
● Because enteric-coated and sustained-release tablets are slowly absorbed, they aren't suitable for rapid relief of acute pain,

fever, or inflammation. They cause less GI bleeding and may be better suited for long-term therapy, such as for arthritis.

• For patients who can't tolerate oral drugs, ask prescriber about using aspirin rectal suppositories. Watch for rectal mucosal irritation or bleeding.

• Febrile, dehydrated children can develop toxicity rapidly.

• Monitor elderly patients closely because they may be more susceptible to aspirin's toxic effects.

• Monitor salicylate level. Therapeutic salicylate level for arthritis is 150 to 300 mcg/mL. Tinnitus may occur at levels above 200 mcg/mL, but this isn't a reliable indicator of toxicity, especially in very young patients and those older than age 60. With long-term therapy, severe toxic effects may occur with levels exceeding 400 mcg/mL.

• During prolonged therapy, assess hematocrit, hemoglobin level, PT, INR, and renal function periodically.

• Drug irreversibly inhibits platelet aggregation. Stop drug 5 to 7 days before elective surgery to allow time for production and release of new platelets.

• Monitor patient for hypersensitivity reactions, such as anaphylaxis and asthma.

• *Look alike–sound alike:* Don't confuse aspirin with Asendin or Afrin.

PATIENT TEACHING

• Tell patient who's allergic to tartrazine to avoid aspirin.

• Advise patient on a low-salt diet that 1 tablet of buffered aspirin contains 553 mg of sodium.

• Advise patient to take drug with food, milk, antacid, or large glass of water to reduce GI reactions.

• Tell patient not to crush or chew sustained-release or enteric-coated forms but to swallow them whole.

• Instruct patient to discard aspirin tablets that have a strong vinegar-like odor.

• Tell patient to consult prescriber if giving drug to children for longer than 5 days or adults for longer than 10 days.

• Advise patient receiving prolonged treatment with large doses of aspirin to watch for small, round, red pinprick spots,

bleeding gums, and signs of GI bleeding, and to drink plenty of fluids. Encourage use of a soft-bristled toothbrush.

• Because of the many drug interactions with aspirin, warn patient taking prescription drugs to check with prescriber or pharmacist before taking aspirin or OTC products containing aspirin.

• Ibuprofen can interfere with the antiplatelet effect of low-dose aspirin therapy, negating its effect. Tell patient how to safely use ibuprofen in relation to aspirin therapy.

• Urge pregnant women to avoid aspirin during last trimester of pregnancy unless specifically directed by prescriber.

• Drug is a leading cause of poisoning in children. Caution parents to keep drug out of reach of children. Encourage use of child-resistant containers.

atazanavir sulfate
ah-TAZ-ah-nah-veer

Reyataz◆

Therapeutic class: Antiretrovirals
Pharmacologic class: Protease inhibitors
Pregnancy risk category: B

AVAILABLE FORMS
Capsules: 100 mg, 150 mg, 200 mg, 300 mg

INDICATIONS & DOSAGES
Adjust-a-dose (for all indications): In patients with Child-Pugh class B hepatic insufficiency who haven't experienced prior virologic failure, reduce dosage to 300 mg P.O. once daily. Treatment-naive patients with ESRD who are on hemodialysis should receive atazanavir 300 mg with ritonavir 100 mg. Don't give to treatment-experienced patients on hemodialysis.
➤ **HIV-1 infection, with other antiretrovirals**
Adults: Give antiretroviral-experienced patients 300 mg (as one 300-mg capsule or two 150-mg capsules) once daily, plus 100 mg ritonavir once daily with food. Give antiretroviral-naive patients 400 mg (as two 200-mg capsules) once daily with food. When drug is given with efavirenz in antiretroviral-naive patients, give atazanavir

300 mg and ritonavir 100 mg as a single daily dose with food and efavirenz on an empty stomach, preferably at bedtime. Dosage recommendations for efavirenz and atazanavir in treatment-experienced patients haven't been established.

Adolescents at least age 13 and weighing at least 40 kg (88 lb) who are treatment-naive and unable to tolerate ritonavir: 400 mg P.O. once daily with food.

Children and adolescents ages 6 to 17 who are treatment-naive or treatment-experienced and receiving ritonavir: For patients weighing 40 kg or more, give 300 mg with ritonavir 100 mg P.O. once daily. For patients weighing 20 to 39 kg (44 to 86 lb), give 200 mg with ritonavir 100 mg P.O. once daily. For patients weighing 15 to 19 kg (33 to 42 lb), give 150 mg with ritonavir 100 mg P.O. once daily.

ADMINISTRATION
P.O.
- Give drug with food.
- Give drug to pregnant woman only if potential benefit justifies fetal risk.
- Don't open capsules.

ACTION
Inhibits viral maturation in HIV-1–infected cells, resulting in the formation of immature noninfectious viral particles.

Route	Onset	Peak	Duration
P.O.	Unknown	2½ hr	Unknown

Half-life: About 7 hours.

ADVERSE REACTIONS
CNS: headache, depression, dizziness, fatigue, fever, insomnia, pain, peripheral neurologic symptoms.
CV: prolonged PR interval.
EENT: scleral yellowing.
GI: abdominal pain, diarrhea, nausea, vomiting.
Hepatic: hyperbilirubinemia, jaundice.
Metabolic: lipodystrophy.
Musculoskeletal: arthralgia, back pain.
Respiratory: increased cough.
Skin: rash.

INTERACTIONS
Drug-drug. *Alfuzosin:* May increase alfuzosin plasma concentration, increasing risk of hypotension. Use together is contraindicated.

Antacids, buffered medications (didanosine buffered preparation): May reduce atazanavir plasma concentration. Administer atazanavir 2 hours before or 1 hour after these medications.

Antiarrhythmics (amiodarone, bepridil, systemic lidocaine, quinidine): May produce serious or life-threatening adverse reactions. Use cautiously. Monitor antiarrhythmic therapeutic concentration.

Anticoagulants (warfarin): May cause serious or life-threatening bleeding. Monitor INR.

Antifungals (itraconazole, ketoconazole, posaconazole, voriconazole): May increase risk of toxicity of both antifungal and atazanavir. Use cautiously when high doses of ketoconazole or itraconazole are administered with atazanavir and ritonavir. Administration of voriconazole with atazanavir and ritonavir isn't recommended.

Aripiprazole: May increase aripiprazole plasma concentration. Monitor patient and adjust aripiprazole dosage as needed when atazanavir is started or stopped.

Benzodiazepines (midazolam, triazolam): May increase plasma concentrations of these drugs. Oral midazolam and triazolam are contraindicated because of the potential for serious or life-threatening events, such as prolonged or increased sedation or respiratory depression. Use I.V. midazolam with caution and close monitoring.

Boceprevir: May decrease plasma concentrations of ritonavir-boosted atazanavir and boceprevir. Use together isn't recommended because of potential loss in virologic response.

Bosentan: May decrease atazanavir plasma concentration when administered without ritonavir; coadministration of atazanavir and bosentan without ritonavir isn't recommended. May increase bosentan plasma concentration. For patients who have been receiving atazanavir and ritonavir for at least 10 days, start bosentan at 62.5 mg once daily or every other day based on individual tolerability. For patients taking bosentan, discontinue bosentan at least 36 hours before starting atazanavir and ritonavir. At least 10 days after starting atazanavir and ritonavir, resume bosentan at 62.5 mg once daily or every other day based on individual tolerability.

Brentuximab: May increase brentuximab plasma concentration. Close monitoring is warranted. Adjust brentuximab dosage as needed.

Cabazitaxel: May increase cabazitaxel plasma concentration. Avoid administering together.

Calcium channel blockers (amlodipine, diltiazem, felodipine, nicardipine, nifedipine, verapamil): May prolong PR interval in some patients; use caution. Consider reducing diltiazem dosage by 50% and titrating dosages of other calcium channel blockers. Monitor ECG.

Carbamazepine: May increase carbamazepine level. May decrease atazanavir level, resulting in antiretroviral treatment failure. If coadministration can't be avoided, monitor patient closely. Consider alternative therapy for carbamazepine.

Cilostazol: May increase cilostazol plasma concentration. Consider reducing cilostazol dosage.

Clarithromycin: May prolong QTc interval; reduce clarithromycin dosage by 50%. Significantly reduces concentration of active metabolite (14-OH clarithromycin); consider alternative therapy for indications other than *Mycobacterium avium* complex.

Colchicine: May increase plasma concentrations of colchicine. Don't give colchicine and atazanavir together to patients with hepatic or renal impairment. For treatment of gout flares, give colchicine 0.6 mg followed by 0.3 mg 1 hour later. Repeat dose in no earlier than 3 days. For prophylaxis of gout flares, if original colchicine regimen was colchicine 0.6 mg b.i.d., adjust dosage to 0.3 mg once a day. If original colchicine dosage was 0.6 mg once daily, adjust regimen to colchicine 0.3 mg every other day. For treatment of familial Mediterranean fever, give colchicine at maximum daily dosage of 0.3 mg b.i.d.

Corticosteroids (fluticasone, prednisone): May increase corticosteroid plasma concentration. Monitor patient for signs and symptoms of adrenal insufficiency. Consider alternatives to fluticasone for long-term use.

Crizotinib, docetaxel, dronedarone, ixabepilone, ticagrelor, toremifene: May increase plasma concentration of these drugs. Avoid administering together.

Delavirdine: May increase atazanavir plasma concentration and decrease delavirdine plasma concentration. Atazanavir dosage reduction may be needed during coadministration of delavirdine. Delavirdine dosage increases may be required when administered with atazanavir. Closely monitor patient and adjust therapy as needed.

Didanosine (buffered): May decrease atazanavir concentration. Give atazanavir 2 hours before or 1 hour after buffered formulation of didanosine. Coadministration of enteric-coated didanosine capsules and atazanavir decreases didanosine exposure. Separate atazanavir and didanosine administration times.

Digoxin: May prolong PR interval. Use with caution.

Eletriptan: May increase eletriptan plasma concentration. Don't use eletriptan within 72 hours of atazanavir.

Eplerenone: May increase eplerenone plasma concentration. Monitor patient closely and adjust eplerenone dosage as needed.

Ergot derivatives (dihydroergotamine, ergonovine, ergotamine, methylergonovine): May cause serious or life-threatening events such as acute ergot toxicity (peripheral vasospasm, ischemia of the extremities). Coadministration is contraindicated.

Erlotinib: May increase erlotinib plasma concentration. Monitor clinical response and watch for adverse reactions. Adjust erlotinib dosage as needed.

Erythromycin: May increase erythromycin plasma concentration, increasing risk of sudden death from cardiac causes. Avoid concurrent use.

Eszopiclone: May increase eszopiclone plasma concentration. Monitor patient closely. Consider reducing eszopiclone dosage when administered with atazanavir.

Fluoxetine: May increase plasma concentrations of both drugs. Closely monitor patient for adverse reactions, including serotonin syndrome. Fluoxetine or atazanavir dosage reduction may be needed.

H₂-receptor antagonists (famotidine): May decrease atazanavir plasma concentration, possibly causing development of resistance. Monitor patient.

HMG-CoA reductase inhibitors (atorvastatin, lovastatin, rosuvastatin, simvastatin): May increase serum concentrations of these drugs, possibly increasing their toxicity, including rhabdomyolysis. Administration with simvastatin or lovastatin is contraindicated. If using atorvastatin or rosuvastatin, start with lowest possible dosage with careful monitoring. Consider pravastatin or fluvastatin in combination with atazanavir.

Hormonal contraceptives (ethinyl estradiol, norethindrone, norgestimate): Unboosted atazanavir may increase hormonal contraceptive plasma concentration. Ritonavir-boosted atazanavir may decrease hormonal contraceptive plasma concentration. Alternative methods of nonhormonal contraception are recommended.

Iloperidone: May increase iloperidone plasma concentration. Reduce iloperidone dosage by one-half when administering with atazanavir. If atazanavir is discontinued, increase iloperidone dosage to original dosage.

Immunosuppressants (cyclosporine, sirolimus, tacrolimus): May increase levels of these drugs. Monitor immunosuppressant concentrations.

Irinotecan: May interfere with irinotecan metabolism, resulting in increased toxicity. Coadministration is contraindicated.

Lurasidone: May increase lurasidone plasma concentration. Coadministration is contraindicated.

Maraviroc: May increase maraviroc plasma concentration. Monitor patient response and adjust maraviroc dosage as needed.

mTOR inhibitors (everolimus, temsirolimus): May increase plasma concentrations of these drugs. If coadministration can't be avoided, monitor clinical response and adjust mTOR inhibitor dosage as needed.

Muscarinic receptor antagonists (darifenacin, fesoterodine, solifenacin, tolterodine): May increase plasma concentrations of these drugs. When atazanavir is coadministered, don't exceed the following dosages: darifenacin 7.5 mg daily, fesoterodine 4 mg daily, solifenacin 5 mg daily, and tolterodine 2 mg daily.

Nilotinib: May increase nilotinib plasma concentration. Avoid coadministration. If atazanavir must be given with nilotinib, consider interrupting nilotinib therapy. Consult manufacturer's instructions for specific recommendations.

NNRTIs (efavirenz, nevirapine): May decrease atazanavir plasma level. In treatment-naive patients, administer atazanavir 400 mg and ritonavir 100 mg with efavirenz 600 mg. Don't administer atazanavir with efavirenz in treatment-experienced patients. Nevirapine may decrease atazanavir exposure; coadministration may increase nevirapine exposure. Coadministration isn't recommended.

Opioid analgesics (buprenorphine, fentanyl, oxycodone, sufentanil): May increase plasma concentration and half-life of opioid; reduced opioid dosage may be needed. Closely monitor respiratory function during opioid administration and for a longer period than usual after stopping opioid. Atazanavir without ritonavir shouldn't be administered with buprenorphine.

PDE5 inhibitors (sildenafil, tadalafil, vardenafil): Coadministration of atazanavir and sildenafil for pulmonary arterial hypertension is contraindicated; coadministration may result in an increase in PDE5 inhibitor–associated adverse reactions, including hypotension, visual changes, and priapism. In patients with pulmonary arterial hypertension who have received atazanavir for at least 1 week, start tadalafil at 20 mg once daily. May increase tadalafil dosage to 40 mg once daily based on individual tolerability. In patients with pulmonary hypertension already taking tadalafil, avoid tadalafil during initiation of atazanavir. Stop tadalafil at least 24 hours before starting atazanavir. After at least 1 week after starting atazanavir, resume tadalafil at 20 mg once daily. May increase tadalafil dosage to 40 mg once daily based on individual tolerability. For treatment of erectile dysfunction, use cautiously at reduced dosages and increase monitoring for adverse events: Limit sildenafil dosage to 25 mg every 48 hours, tadalafil dosage to 10 mg every 72 hours, or vardenafil dosage to no more than 2.5 mg every 24 hours. Use vardenafil with atazanavir and ritonavir cautiously at reduced dosages of no more than 2.5 mg every 72 hours.

Pimozide: May cause serious or life-threatening reactions (cardiac arrhythmias). Use is contraindicated.

Protease inhibitors (amprenavir, darunavir, fosamprenavir, indinavir, nelfinavir, ritonavir, saquinavir, tipranavir): If atazanavir is administered with ritonavir, decrease atazanavir dosage to 300 mg once daily with ritonavir 100 mg once daily. Administration of atazanavir with other protease inhibitors may increase exposure to the other protease inhibitor; coadministration isn't recommended. Coadministration of atazanavir and indinavir is contraindicated because both drugs are associated with indirect (unconjugated) hyperbilirubinemia. Saquinavir 1,200 mg administered with atazanavir 400 mg and tenofovir 300 mg plus NRTIs don't provide adequate efficacy.

Proton pump inhibitors (omeprazole): Substantially decreases atazanavir plasma concentration, possibly causing development of resistance. In treatment-naive patients, administer proton pump inhibitors 12 hours before atazanavir dose. Don't use proton pump inhibitors in treatment-experienced patients receiving atazanavir.

Quetiapine: May increase quetiapine plasma concentration. Administer cautiously; closely monitor clinical response. Adjust quetiapine dosage as needed.

Raltegravir: May increase raltegravir plasma concentration. Closely monitor clinical response. Adjust raltegravir dosage as needed.

Ranolazine: Increases risk of dose-related QTc-interval prolongation, torsades de pointes–type arrhythmias, and sudden death. Use together is contraindicated.

Rifabutin: May increase blood levels of rifabutin. Rifabutin dosage reduction of up to 75% (150 mg every other day or three times/week) is recommended.

Rifampin: May decrease atazanavir plasma concentration, possibly causing development of resistance. Use together is contraindicated.

Risperidone: May increase risperidone plasma concentration. Closely monitor clinical response. Adjust risperidone dosage as needed.

Romidepsin: May increase romidepsin plasma concentration, increasing risk of adverse reactions, including QT-interval prolongation. If coadministration can't be avoided, closely monitor clinical, laboratory, and ECG results. Adjust romidepsin dosage as needed.

Salmeterol: May increase salmeterol concentration, increasing risk of CV events, including QT-interval prolongation, palpitations, and sinus tachycardia. Use together isn't recommended.

Saxagliptin: May increase saxagliptin plasma concentration. Limit saxagliptin dosage to 2.5 mg daily.

Tenofovir: May decrease atazanavir area under the curve and minimum (trough) concentration. Don't administer atazanavir with tenofovir unless also administering ritonavir; administer as atazanavir 300 mg, ritonavir 100 mg, and tenofovir 300 mg. Atazanavir increases tenofovir concentration; watch for tenofovir-associated adverse reactions.

Tetracyclines (minocycline): May reduce atazanavir plasma concentration. Closely monitor atazanavir concentration and clinical response. Adjust atazanavir dosage as needed.

Trazodone: May increase trazodone plasma concentration. Use cautiously and reduce trazodone dosage.

Tricyclic antidepressants (amitriptyline): May cause serious or life-threatening adverse reactions. Monitor concentration of tricyclic antidepressant.

Tyrosine kinase inhibitors (dasatinib, lapatinib, pazopanib, sorafenib, sunitinib): May increase protein-tyrosine kinase inhibitor plasma concentrations. If coadministration can't be avoided, closely monitor clinical response and adjust protein-tyrosine kinase inhibitor dosage as needed.

Reactions in bold italics are *life-threatening*. Interactions may have a *rapid onset* or a *delayed onset*.

Vasopressin receptor antagonists (conivaptan, tolvaptan): May increase plasma concentration of these drugs. Coadministration is contraindicated.

Vemurafenib: May increase vemurafenib plasma concentration. Use cautiously and closely monitor clinical and laboratory results. Adjust vemurafenib dosage as needed.

Vilazodone: May increase vilazodone plasma concentration. Reduce vilazodone dosage to 20 mg in patients receiving atazanavir.

Vinca alkaloids (vinblastine, vincristine): May increase pharmacologic effects of these drugs and risk of toxicity (characterized by profound neutropenia or severe neuropathy). Consider temporarily suspending atazanavir in patients experiencing hematologic or GI toxicity during administration of atazanavir and vinca alkaloids. Or, reducing vinca alkaloid dosage may decrease toxicity.

Drug-herb. *Cat's claw:* May increase risk of toxicity. Discourage concomitant use.

St. John's wort: May decrease drug level, reducing therapeutic effect and causing drug resistance. Discourage use together.

Drug-food. *Any food:* May increase bioavailability of drug. Tell patient to take drug with food.

EFFECTS ON LAB TEST RESULTS
• May increase ALT, amylase, AST, bilirubin, and lipase levels. May decrease hemoglobin level.
• May decrease neutrophil count.

CONTRAINDICATIONS & CAUTIONS
• Contraindicated in patients hypersensitive to drug or its ingredients.
• Contraindicated in patients taking drugs cleared mainly by CYP3A4 or drugs that can cause serious or life-threatening reactions at high levels (alfuzosin, dihydroergotamine, ergonovine, ergotamine, indinavir, irinotecan, lovastatin, methylergonovine, midazolam (P.O.), pimozide, rifampin, sildanefil (Revatio), St. John's wort, simvastatin, triazolam).
• Don't use in patients with Child-Pugh class C hepatic insufficiency.
• Use cautiously in patients with conduction system disease or hepatic impairment.

• Use cautiously in elderly patients because of the increased likelihood of other disease, additional drug therapy, and decreased hepatic, renal, or cardiac function.

⚠ **Overdose S&S:** Asymptomatic bifascicular block, PR-interval prolongation, jaundice.

NURSING CONSIDERATIONS
◑ **Alert:** Drug may prolong the PR interval.
• Monitor the patient for hyperglycemia and new-onset diabetes or worsened diabetes. Insulin and oral antidiabetic dosages may need adjustment.
• Monitor a patient with hepatitis B or C for elevated liver enzymes or hepatic decompensation.
• Watch for life-threatening lactic acidosis syndrome and symptomatic hyperlactatemia, especially in women and obese patients.
• If the patient has hemophilia, watch for bleeding.
• Monitor patient for renal colic; drug may cause nephrolithiasis.
• Most patients have an asymptomatic increase in indirect bilirubin, possibly with yellowed skin or sclerae. This hyperbilirubinemia will resolve when therapy stops.
• Although cross-resistance occurs among protease inhibitors, resistance to drug doesn't preclude use of other protease inhibitors.
• Register pregnant women for monitoring of maternal-fetal outcomes by calling the Antiretroviral Pregnancy Registry at 1-800-258-4263.

PATIENT TEACHING
• Urge patient to take drug with food every day and to take other antiretrovirals as prescribed.
• Explain that drug doesn't cure HIV infection and that the patient may develop opportunistic infections and other complications of HIV disease.
• Caution patient that drug doesn't reduce the risk of transmitting HIV to others.
• Tell patient that drug may cause altered or increased body fat, central obesity, buffalo hump, peripheral wasting, facial wasting, breast enlargement, and a cushingoid appearance.

• Tell patient to report yellowed skin or eyes, dizziness, or light-headedness.
• Caution patient not to take other prescriptions or OTC or herbal medicines without first consulting his prescriber.

SAFETY ALERT!

atenolol
a-TEN-o-loll

Tenormin✐

Therapeutic class: Antihypertensives
Pharmacologic class: Beta blockers
Pregnancy risk category: D

AVAILABLE FORMS
Tablets: 25 mg, 50 mg, 100 mg

INDICATIONS & DOSAGES
Adjust-a-dose (for all indications): If CrCl is 15 to 35 mL/minute, maximum dose is 50 mg daily; if CrCl is below 15 mL/minute, maximum dose is 25 mg daily. Hemodialysis patients need 25 to 50 mg after each dialysis session. For elderly patients, initial dose is 25 mg P.O. daily.
➤ **Hypertension**
Adults: Initially, 50 mg P.O. daily alone or in combination with a diuretic as a single dose, increased to 100 mg once daily after 7 to 14 days. Dosages of more than 100 mg daily are unlikely to produce further benefit.
➤ **Angina pectoris**
Adults: 50 mg P.O. once daily, increased as needed to 100 mg daily after 7 days for optimal effect. Maximum, 200 mg daily.
➤ **Cardiac risk reduction during surgery** ◆
Adults: 50 mg P.O. daily. Titrate according to heart rate. Start therapy well before planned procedure and continue for 7 to 30 days after procedure.
➤ **Unstable angina** ◆
Adults: 50 to 200 mg P.O. daily.

ADMINISTRATION
P.O.
• Check apical pulse before giving drug; if slower than 60 beats/minute, withhold drug and call prescriber.

• Give drug exactly as prescribed, at the same time each day.

ACTION
Selectively blocks beta$_1$-adrenergic receptors, decreases cardiac output and cardiac oxygen consumption, and depresses renin secretion.

Route	Onset	Peak	Duration
P.O.	1 hr	2–4 hr	24 hr

Half-life: 6 to 7 hours.

ADVERSE REACTIONS
CNS: dizziness, fatigue, lethargy, vertigo, drowsiness, fever.
CV: hypotension, ***bradycardia, heart failure,*** intermittent claudication.
GI: nausea, diarrhea.
Musculoskeletal: leg pain.
Respiratory: ***bronchospasm,*** dyspnea.
Skin: rash.

INTERACTIONS
Drug-drug. *Aluminum salts:* May reduce bioavailability of atenolol. Separate doses by at least 2 hours.
Amiodarone: May increase risk of bradycardia, AV block, and myocardial depression. Monitor ECG and vital signs.
Antihypertensives: May increase hypotensive effect. Use together cautiously.
Calcium channel blockers, hydralazine, methyldopa: May cause additive hypotension and bradycardia. Adjust dosage as needed.
Cardiac glycosides, diltiazem, verapamil: May cause excessive bradycardia and increased depressant effect on myocardium. Use together cautiously.
Clonidine: May exacerbate rebound hypertension if clonidine is withdrawn. Atenolol should be withdrawn before clonidine by several days or added several days after clonidine is stopped.
Dolasetron: May decrease clearance of dolasetron and increase risk of toxicity. Monitor patient for toxicity.
Insulin, oral antidiabetics: May alter dosage requirements in previously stabilized diabetic patient. Observe patient carefully.
I.V. lidocaine: May reduce hepatic metabolism of lidocaine, increasing risk of toxicity. Give bolus doses of lidocaine

---

Reactions in bold italics are ***life-threatening***. Interactions may have a *rapid onset* or a *delayed onset*.

at a slower rate and monitor lidocaine level closely.
NSAIDs: May decrease antihypertensive effects. Monitor blood pressure.
Penicillins: May reduce bioavailability of atenolol. Monitor blood pressure closely.
Prazosin: May increase the risk of orthostatic hypotension in the early phases of use together. Help patient stand slowly until effects are known.
Reserpine: May cause hypotension or marked bradycardia. Use together cautiously.
Rifamycins: May reduce effects of atenolol. Monitor blood pressure.
Salicylates: May reduce effects of atenolol. Consider lowering salicylate dosage or changing to a nonsalicylate antiplatelet agent.

EFFECTS ON LAB TEST RESULTS
● May increase alkaline phosphatase, BUN, creatinine, glucose, LDH, potassium, AST, ALT, and uric acid levels. May decrease glucose level.
● May increase platelet count.

CONTRAINDICATIONS & CAUTIONS
● Contraindicated in patients with sinus bradycardia, heart block greater than first degree, overt cardiac failure, untreated pheochromocytoma, or cardiogenic shock.
● Use cautiously in patients at risk for heart failure and in those with bronchospastic disease, diabetes, hyperthyroidism, and impaired renal or hepatic function.
⚠ *Overdose S&S:* Lethargy, decreased respiratory drive, wheezing, sinus pause, bradycardia.

NURSING CONSIDERATIONS
● Monitor patient's blood pressure.
● Monitor hemodialysis patients closely because of hypotension risk.
● Beta blockers may mask tachycardia caused by hyperthyroidism. In patients with suspected thyrotoxicosis, withdraw beta blocker gradually to avoid thyroid storm.
● Drug may mask signs and symptoms of hypoglycemia in diabetic patients.
● Drug may cause changes in exercise tolerance and ECG.

Black Box Warning Avoid abrupt discontinuation of therapy. Withdraw drug gradually to avoid serious adverse reactions, such as severe exacerbations of angina, MI, and ventricular arrhythmias even in patients treated only for hypertension. ■
● *Look alike–sound alike:* Don't confuse atenolol with timolol or albuterol.

PATIENT TEACHING
● Instruct patient to take drug exactly as prescribed, at the same time every day.
● Caution patient not to stop drug suddenly, but to notify prescriber if unpleasant adverse reactions occur.
● Teach patient how to take his pulse. Tell him to withhold drug and call prescriber if pulse rate is below 60 beats/minute.
● Tell woman of childbearing age to notify prescriber about planned, suspected, or known pregnancy. Drug will need to be stopped.
● Advise breast-feeding mother to contact prescriber; drug isn't recommended for breast-feeding women.

atomoxetine hydrochloride
at-oh-MOX-ah-teen

Strattera✐

Therapeutic class: ADHD drugs
Pharmacologic class: Selective norepinephrine reuptake inhibitors
Pregnancy risk category: C

AVAILABLE FORMS
Capsules: 10 mg, 18 mg, 25 mg, 40 mg, 60 mg, 80 mg, 100 mg

INDICATIONS & DOSAGES
➤ **ADHD**
Adults, children older than age 6, and adolescents weighing more than 70 kg (154 lb): Initially, 40 mg P.O. daily; increase after at least 3 days to a total of 80 mg/day P.O., as a single dose in the morning or two evenly divided doses in the morning and late afternoon or early evening. After 2 to 4 weeks, increase total dose to a maximum of 100 mg, if needed.

Children older than age 6 weighing 70 kg or less: Initially, 0.5 mg/kg P.O. daily; increase after a minimum of 3 days to a target total daily dose of 1.2 mg/kg P.O. as a single dose in the morning or two evenly divided doses in the morning and late afternoon or early evening. Don't exceed 1.4 mg/kg or 100 mg daily, whichever is less.

Adjust-a-dose: In patients with moderate hepatic impairment, reduce to 50% of the normal dose; in those with severe hepatic impairment, reduce to 25% of the normal dose. Poor metabolizers of CYP2D6 or concomitant administration with strong CYP2D6 inhibitors may require a reduced dose. In children weighing less than 70 kg, adjust dosage to 0.5 mg/kg daily and increase to 1.2 mg/kg daily if symptoms don't improve after 4 weeks and if first dose is tolerated. In children and adults weighing more than 70 kg, start at 40 mg daily and increase to 80 mg daily if symptoms don't improve after 4 weeks and if first dose is tolerated.

➤ **Nocturnal enuresis** ◆
Children: 1.5 mg/kg P.O. daily in two divided doses for 12 weeks.

ADMINISTRATION
P.O.
- Give drug without regard for meals.
- Capsules should be swallowed whole and not opened.

ACTION
May be related to selective inhibition of the presynaptic norepinephrine transporter.

Route	Onset	Peak	Duration
P.O.	Rapid	1–2 hr	Unknown

Half-life: 21½ hours.

ADVERSE REACTIONS
CNS: headache, insomnia, dizziness, somnolence, crying, irritability, mood swings, pyrexia, fatigue, sedation, depression, tremor, early-morning awakening, paresthesia, abnormal dreams, sleep disorder.
CV: orthostatic hypotension, tachycardia, hypertension, palpitations, hot flashes.
EENT: mydriasis.
GI: abdominal pain, constipation, dyspepsia, nausea, vomiting, decreased appetite, dry mouth.

GU: urine retention, urinary hesitation, ejaculatory problems, difficulty in micturition, dysmenorrhea, erectile disturbance, erectile dysfunction, delayed menses, menstrual disorder, prostatitis.
Respiratory: cough, upper respiratory tract infection.
Skin: dermatitis, pruritus, increased sweating, rash.
Other: decreased libido, chills.

INTERACTIONS
Drug-drug. *Albuterol:* May increase CV effects. Use together cautiously.
MAO inhibitors: May cause hyperthermia, rigidity, myoclonus, autonomic instability with possible rapid fluctuations of vital signs, and mental status changes. Avoid use within 2 weeks of MAO inhibitor.
Pressor agents: May increase blood pressure. Use together cautiously.
Strong CYP2D6 inhibitors (paroxetine, fluoxetine, quinidine): May increase atomoxetine level. Reduce first dose. Increase to the usual target dose of 80 mg only if signs and symptoms fail to improve after 4 weeks and the initial dose is well tolerated.

EFFECTS ON LAB TEST RESULTS
None reported.

CONTRAINDICATIONS & CAUTIONS
- Contraindicated in patients hypersensitive to drug and its components, in those with serious heart problems, in those who are intolerant of increased blood pressure or heart rate, in those who have taken an MAO inhibitor within the past 2 weeks, and in those with angle-closure glaucoma.
- Use cautiously in patients with hypertension, tachycardia, or CV or cerebrovascular disease, and in pregnant or breast-feeding women.
- Safety and effectiveness haven't been established in patients younger than age 6.
⚠ *Overdose S&S:* Somnolence, agitation, hyperactivity, abnormal behavior, GI symptoms, mydriasis, tachycardia, dry mouth, prolonged QT interval, disorientation, hallucinations, seizures.

NURSING CONSIDERATIONS

● Use drug as part of a total treatment program for ADHD, including psychological, educational, and social intervention.

● Monitor patient for the appearance or worsening of aggressive behavior or hostility, especially when treatment is initiated. **Black Box Warning** Monitor children and adolescents closely for worsening of condition, agitation, irritability, suicidal thinking or behaviors, and unusual changes in behavior, especially the first few months of therapy or when the dosage is increased or decreased. ■

● Periodically monitor patient for changes in heart rate or blood pressure.

● Patients taking drug for extended periods must be reevaluated periodically to determine drug's usefulness.

● Monitor growth during treatment. If growth or weight gain is unsatisfactory, consider interrupting therapy.

● **Alert:** Severe liver injury may occur and progress to liver failure. Notify prescriber of any sign of liver injury: yellowing of the skin or the sclera of the eyes, pruritus, dark urine, upper right-sided tenderness, or unexplained flulike syndrome.

● Monitor blood pressure and pulse at baseline, after each dose increase, and during treatment periodically.

● Monitor for urinary hesitancy or urine retention and sexual dysfunction.

● Patient can stop drug without tapering off.

PATIENT TEACHING

Black Box Warning Advise parents to call prescriber immediately about unusual behavior or suicidal thoughts. ■

● Instruct patient to immediately report chest pain, shortness of breath, or fainting.

● Tell pregnant women, women planning to become pregnant, and breast-feeding women to consult prescriber before taking atomoxetine.

● Tell patient to use caution when operating a vehicle or machinery until the effects of drug are known.

● Warn male patient to seek prompt medical attention for an erection that lasts more than 4 hours.

atorvastatin calcium
ah-TOR-va-stah-tin

Lipitor🔊

Therapeutic class: Antilipemics
Pharmacologic class: HMG-CoA reductase inhibitors
Pregnancy risk category: X

AVAILABLE FORMS
Tablets: 10 mg, 20 mg, 40 mg, 80 mg

INDICATIONS & DOSAGES
➤ **In patients with clinically evident coronary artery disease (CAD), to reduce the risk of nonfatal MI, fatal and nonfatal strokes, angina, heart failure, and revascularization procedures**
Adults: Initially, 10 to 20 mg P.O. daily. May increase based on patient response and tolerance; usual dosage, 10 to 80 mg P.O. daily.
➤ **To reduce the risk of MI, stroke, angina, or revascularization procedures in patients with multiple risk factors for CAD but who don't yet have the disease**
Adults: 10 to 80 mg P.O. daily.
➤ **To reduce the risk of MI or stroke in patients with type 2 diabetes and multiple risk factors for CAD but who don't yet have the disease**
Adults: 10 to 80 mg P.O. daily.
➤ **Adjunct to diet to reduce LDL, total cholesterol, apolipoprotein B, and triglyceride levels and to increase HDL levels in patients with primary hypercholesterolemia (heterozygous familial and nonfamilial) and mixed dyslipidemia (Fredrickson types IIa and IIb); adjunct to diet to reduce triglyceride level (Fredrickson type IV); primary dysbetalipoproteinemia (Fredrickson type III) in patients who don't respond adequately to diet**
Adults: Initially, 10 or 20 mg P.O. once daily. Patient who requires a reduction of more than 45% in LDL level may be started at 40 mg once daily. Increase dose, as needed, to maximum of 80 mg daily as single dose. Dosage based on lipid levels drawn within

2 to 4 weeks of starting therapy and after dosage adjustment.

➤ **Alone or as an adjunct to lipid-lowering treatments, such as LDL apheresis, to reduce total and LDL cholesterol in patients with homozygous familial hypercholesterolemia**

Adults: 10 to 80 mg P.O. once daily.

➤ **Heterozygous familial hypercholesterolemia**

Children ages 10 to 17 (girls should be 1 year postmenarche): Initially, 10 mg P.O. once daily. Adjustment intervals should be at least 4 weeks. Maximum daily dose is 20 mg.

ADMINISTRATION
P.O.
● Give drug without regard for meals.

ACTION
Inhibits HMG-CoA reductase, an early (and rate-limiting) step in cholesterol biosynthesis.

Route	Onset	Peak	Duration
P.O.	Unknown	1–2 hr	Unknown

Half-life: 14 hours.

ADVERSE REACTIONS
CNS: headache, asthenia, insomnia.
CV: peripheral edema.
EENT: pharyngitis, rhinitis, sinusitis, nasopharyngitis.
GI: abdominal pain, constipation, diarrhea, dyspepsia, flatulence, nausea.
GU: UTI.
Musculoskeletal: *rhabdomyolysis,* arthritis, arthralgia, myalgia, extremity pain.
Respiratory: bronchitis.
Skin: rash.
Other: allergic reactions, flulike syndrome, infection.

INTERACTIONS
Drug-drug. *Amiodarone:* May increase risk of severe myopathy or rhabdomyolysis. Avoid use together or decrease atorvastatin dose.
Antacids, cholestyramine, colestipol: May decrease atorvastatin level. Separate administration times.

Cyclosporine, diltiazem, fibric acid derivatives, macrolides (azithromycin, clarithromycin, erythromycin, telithromycin), nefazodone, niacin, protease inhibitors, tacrolimus, verapamil: May decrease metabolism of HMG-CoA reductase inhibitors, increasing toxicity. Monitor patient for adverse effects and report unexplained muscle pain.
Darunavir and ritonavir, fosamprenavir, fosamprenavir and ritonavir, saquinavir and ritonavir: May increase atorvastatin level and risk of myopathy and rhabdomyolysis. Atorvastatin dosage shouldn't exceed 20 mg daily.
Digoxin: May increase digoxin level. Monitor digoxin level and patient for evidence of toxicity.
Fluconazole, itraconazole, ketoconazole, voriconazole: May increase atorvastatin level and adverse effects. Avoid using together or, if unavoidable, reduce dose of atorvastatin.
Hormonal contraceptives: May increase norethindrone and ethinyl estradiol levels. Consider increased drug levels when selecting an oral contraceptive.
Lopinavir and ritonavir: May increase statin level and risk of myopathy and rhabdomyolysis. Use together cautiously and at lowest atorvastatin dosage necessary.
Nelfinavir: May increase statin level and risk of myopathy and rhabdomyolysis. Atorvastatin dosage shouldn't exceed 40 mg daily.
Telaprevir, tipranavir and ritonavir: May increase statin level and risk of myopathy and rhabdomyolysis. Avoid use together.
Drug-herb. *Eucalyptus, jin bu huan, kava:* May increase risk of hepatotoxicity. Discourage use together.
Red yeast rice: May increase risk of adverse reactions because herb contains compounds similar to those in drug. Discourage use together.
Drug-food. *Grapefruit juice:* May increase drug levels, increasing risk of adverse reactions. Discourage use together.

EFFECTS ON LAB TEST RESULTS
● May increase ALT, AST, and CK levels.

CONTRAINDICATIONS & CAUTIONS
• Contraindicated in patients hypersensitive to drug and in those with active liver disease or unexplained persistent elevations of transaminase levels.
• Contraindicated in pregnant and breast-feeding women and in women of childbearing age.
• Use cautiously in patients with hepatic impairment or heavy alcohol use.
• Withhold or stop drug in patients at risk for renal failure caused by rhabdomyolysis resulting from trauma; in serious, acute conditions that suggest myopathy; and in major surgery, severe acute infection, hypotension, uncontrolled seizures, or severe metabolic, endocrine, or electrolyte disorders.
• Limit use in children to those older than age 9 with homozygous familial hypercholesterolemia.

NURSING CONSIDERATIONS
• Patient should follow a standard cholesterol-lowering diet before and during therapy.
• Before treatment, assess patient for underlying causes for hypercholesterolemia and obtain a baseline lipid profile. Obtain periodic LFT results and lipid levels before starting treatment and at 6 and 12 weeks after initiation, or after an increase in dosage and periodically thereafter.
• Watch for signs of myositis.
• *Look alike–sound alike:* Don't confuse Lipitor with Levatol.

PATIENT TEACHING
• Teach patient about proper dietary management, weight control, and exercise. Explain their importance in controlling high fat levels.
• Warn patient to avoid alcohol.
• Tell patient to inform prescriber of adverse reactions, such as muscle pain, malaise, and fever.
• Advise patient that drug can be taken at any time of day, without regard for meals.
• *Alert:* Tell woman to stop drug and notify prescriber immediately if she is or may be pregnant or if she's breast-feeding.

atovaquone
a-TOE-va-kwon

Mepron

Therapeutic class: Antiprotozoals
Pharmacologic class: Ubiquinone analogues
Pregnancy risk category: C

AVAILABLE FORMS
Suspension: 750 mg/5 mL

INDICATIONS & DOSAGES
➤ **Acute, mild to moderate *Pneumocystis jiroveci (carinii)* pneumonia in patients who can't tolerate sulfamethoxazole–trimethoprim**
Adults and adolescents ages 13 to 16: Give 750 mg (5 mL) P.O. b.i.d. with food for 21 days.
➤ **To prevent *P. jiroveci (carinii)* pneumonia in patients who are unable to tolerate sulfamethoxazole–trimethoprim**
Adults and adolescents ages 13 to 16: Give 1,500 mg (10 mL) P.O. daily with food.

ADMINISTRATION
P.O.
• Taking with meals enhances absorption.
• Shake bottle gently before using.

ACTION
May interfere with electron transport in protozoal mitochondria, inhibiting enzymes needed to synthesize nucleic acids and adenosine triphosphate.

Route	Onset	Peak	Duration
P.O.	Unknown	Unknown	Unknown

Half-life: 2 to 3 days.

ADVERSE REACTIONS
CNS: headache, insomnia, fever, pain, asthenia, anxiety, dizziness.
CV: hypotension.
EENT: sinusitis, rhinitis.
GI: abdominal pain, nausea, diarrhea, oral candidiasis, vomiting, constipation, anorexia, dyspepsia, taste perversion.
Hematologic: *neutropenia,* anemia.
Metabolic: *hypoglycemia,* hyponatremia.

Respiratory: cough.
Skin: rash, diaphoresis, pruritus.

INTERACTIONS
Drug-drug. *Metoclopramide:* May decrease atovaquone bioavailability. Use another antiemetic.
Rifabutin, rifampin: May decrease atovaquone's steady-state level. Avoid using together.
Tetracycline: May decrease atovaquone level. Monitor parasitemia.
Zidovudine: May elevate zidovudine level and lead to toxicity. Monitor closely.

EFFECTS ON LAB TEST RESULTS
● May increase alkaline phosphatase, ALT, and AST levels. May decrease glucose, hemoglobin, and sodium levels.
● May decrease neutrophil count.

CONTRAINDICATIONS & CAUTIONS
● Contraindicated in patients hypersensitive to drug.
● Use cautiously in patients with hepatic impairment.
● Use cautiously in breast-feeding patients; it's unknown if drug appears in breast milk.
● Use cautiously with other highly protein-bound drugs; if used together, assess patient for toxicity.
⚠ *Overdose S&S:* Methemoglobinemia, rash.

NURSING CONSIDERATIONS
۞ *Alert:* Monitor patient closely during therapy because of risk of pulmonary infection.
● Monitor patients with hepatic impairment closely.

PATIENT TEACHING
● Instruct patient to take drug with meals; food significantly enhances absorption.

atovaquone–proguanil hydrochloride
a-TOE-va-kwon

Malarone, Malarone Pediatric

Therapeutic class: Antimalarials
Pharmacologic class: Hydroxynaphthoquinone and biguanide derivatives
Pregnancy risk category: C

AVAILABLE FORMS
Tablets (adult-strength): 250 mg atovaquone and 100 mg proguanil hydrochloride
Tablets (pediatric-strength): 62.5 mg atovaquone and 25 mg proguanil hydrochloride

INDICATIONS & DOSAGES
➤ To prevent *Plasmodium falciparum* malaria, including in areas where chloroquine resistance has been reported
Adults and children weighing more than 40 kg (88 lb): 1 adult-strength tablet P.O. once daily with food or milk, beginning 1 or 2 days before entering a malaria-endemic area. Continue prophylactic treatment during stay and for 7 days after return.
Children weighing 31 to 40 kg (68 to 88 lb): 3 pediatric-strength tablets P.O. once daily with food or milk, beginning 1 or 2 days before entering endemic area. Continue prophylactic treatment during stay and for 7 days after return.
Children weighing 21 to 30 kg (46 to 66 lb): 2 pediatric-strength tablets P.O. once daily with food or milk, beginning 1 or 2 days before entering endemic area. Continue prophylactic treatment during stay and for 7 days after return.
Children weighing 11 to 20 kg (24 to 44 lb): 1 pediatric-strength tablet P.O. daily with food or milk, beginning 1 or 2 days before entering endemic area. Continue prophylactic treatment during stay and for 7 days after return.
Adjust-a-dose: Don't use for malaria prophylaxis in patients with severe renal impairment (CrCl less than 30 mL/minute).

➤ **Acute, uncomplicated** *P. falciparum* **malaria**
Adults and children weighing more than 40 kg (88 lb): 4 adult-strength tablets P.O. once daily, with food or milk, for 3 consecutive days.
Children weighing 31 to 40 kg (68 to 88 lb): 3 adult-strength tablets P.O. once daily, with food or milk, for 3 consecutive days.
Children weighing 21 to 30 kg (46 to 66 lb): 2 adult-strength tablets P.O. once daily, with food or milk, for 3 consecutive days.
Children weighing 11 to 20 kg (24 to 44 lb): 1 adult-strength tablet P.O. once daily, with food or milk, for 3 consecutive days.
Children weighing 9 to 10 kg (20 to 22 lb): 3 pediatric-strength tablets P.O. once daily, with food or milk, for 3 consecutive days.
Children weighing 5 to 8 kg (11 to 18 lb): 2 pediatric-strength tablets P.O. once daily, with food or milk, for 3 consecutive days.

ADMINISTRATION
P.O.
● Give dose at same time each day, with food or milk.
● If child has difficulty swallowing tablets, parents may crush tablet and mix it in condensed milk.
● Store tablets at controlled room temperature of 59° to 86° F (15° to 30° C).

ACTION
Thought to interfere with nucleic acid replication in the malarial parasite. Atovaquone selectively inhibits mitochondrial electron transport in the parasite. Cycloguanil, an active metabolite of proguanil hydrochloride, inhibits dihydrofolate reductase. Atovaquone and cycloguanil are active against the erythrocytic and exoerythrocytic stages of *Plasmodium* species.

Route	Onset	Peak	Duration
P.O.	Unknown	Unknown	Unknown

Half-life: Atovaquone: 2 to 3 days in adults; proguanil: 12 to 21 hours in adults and children.

ADVERSE REACTIONS
CNS: headache, asthenia, dizziness, dreams, insomnia.

GI: abdominal pain, nausea, vomiting, diarrhea, anorexia, dyspepsia, gastritis, oral ulcers.
Skin: pruritus.

INTERACTIONS
Drug-drug. *Metoclopramide:* May decrease atovaquone bioavailability. Use another antiemetic.
Rifampin, rifabutin: May decrease atovaquone level by about 50%. Avoid using together.
Tetracycline: May decrease atovaquone level by about 40%. Monitor patient with parasitemia closely.

EFFECTS ON LAB TEST RESULTS
● May increase alkaline phosphatase, ALT, and AST levels. May decrease hemoglobin level and hematocrit.
● May decrease WBC count.

CONTRAINDICATIONS & CAUTIONS
● Contraindicated in patients hypersensitive to atovaquone, proguanil hydrochloride, or any component of the drug.
● Use cautiously in patients with severe renal impairment and in those who are vomiting.
● Use cautiously in elderly patients because they have a greater frequency of decreased renal, hepatic, and cardiac function.
● It isn't known if atovaquone appears in breast milk, but proguanil does in small amounts. Use cautiously in breast-feeding women.
● Safety and effectiveness haven't been established for prevention in children who weigh less than 11 kg (24 lb) or for treatment in children who weigh less than 5 kg (11 lb).
⚠ *Overdose S&S:* Rash, methemoglobinemia (atovaquone); epigastric discomfort, vomiting, reversible hair loss, scaling of the skin on the palms or soles, reversible aphthous ulceration, hematologic adverse effects (proguanil).

NURSING CONSIDERATIONS
● Persistent diarrhea or vomiting may decrease drug absorption. Patients with these symptoms may need a different antimalarial.

PATIENT TEACHING
● Tell patient to take dose at the same time each day with food or milk.
● Tell parents that if child has difficulty swallowing tablets, to crush and mix in condensed milk.
● Tell patient to repeat dose if he vomits within 1 hour.
● Advise patient to notify prescriber if he can't complete the course of therapy as prescribed.
● Instruct patient to supplement preventive antimalarial with use of protective clothing, bed nets, and insect repellents.

SAFETY ALERT!

atracurium besylate
at-truh-KYOO-ree-um

Therapeutic class: Skeletal muscle relaxants
Pharmacologic class: Nondepolarizing neuromuscular blockers
Pregnancy risk category: C

AVAILABLE FORMS
Injection: 10 mg/mL

INDICATIONS & DOSAGES
➤ **Adjunct to general anesthesia to facilitate endotracheal intubation and relax skeletal muscles during surgery or mechanical ventilation**
Adults and children age 2 and older: 0.4 to 0.5 mg/kg by I.V. bolus. Give maintenance dose of 0.08 to 0.1 mg/kg within 20 to 45 minutes during prolonged surgery. Give maintenance doses every 15 to 25 minutes in patients receiving balanced anesthesia. For prolonged procedures, use a constant infusion at an initial rate of 9 to 10 mcg/kg/minute; then reduce to 5 to 9 mcg/kg/minute. For infusion in the intensive care unit, an infusion rate of 11 to 13 mcg/kg/minute should provide adequate neuromuscular blockade.
Children ages 1 month to 2 years: First dose, 0.3 to 0.4 mg/kg I.V. for children under halothane anesthesia. Frequent maintenance doses may be needed.

Adjust-a-dose: In adults, adolescents, children, or infants with significant CV disease or history suggesting a greater risk of histamine release (anaphylactic reaction, asthma), give initial dose of 0.3 to 0.4 mg/kg slowly or in divided doses over 1 minute. In adults receiving enflurane or isoflurane at the same time, reduce initial atracurium dose by 33% (0.25 to 0.35 mg/kg). In adults receiving atracurium following succinylcholine, initial dose is 0.3 to 0.4 mg/kg.

ADMINISTRATION
I.V.
▼ Use drug only under direct supervision by medical staff skilled in using neuromuscular blockers and maintaining patent airway. Keep available emergency respiratory support (endotracheal equipment, ventilator, oxygen, atropine, edrophonium, neostigmine, and epinephrine).
▼ Give sedatives or general anesthetics before neuromuscular blockers, which don't reduce consciousness or alter pain threshold.
▼ Drug usually is given by rapid I.V. bolus injection but may be given by intermittent infusion or continuous infusion.
▼ Don't give by I.M. injection.
▼ At concentrations of 0.2 to 0.5 mg/mL, drug is compatible in D_5W, normal saline solution for injection, or dextrose 5% in normal saline solution for injection for 24 hours (at room temperature or refrigerated).
▼ Stable if undiluted for 6 weeks.
▼ Store in refrigerator. Don't freeze. Once removed from refrigeration, use within 14 days, even if re-refrigerated.
▼ **Incompatibilities:** Alkaline solutions (such as barbiturates), lactated Ringer's solution.

ACTION
Prevents acetylcholine from binding to receptors on motor end plate, thus blocking neuromuscular transmission.

Route	Onset	Peak	Duration
I.V.	2 min	3–5 min	35–70 min

Half-life: 20 minutes.

Reactions in bold italics are *life-threatening*. Interactions may have a *rapid onset* or a *delayed onset*.

ADVERSE REACTIONS
CV: *bradycardia,* hypotension, tachycardia.
Respiratory: *prolonged, dose-related apnea; bronchospasm; laryngospasm;* wheezing; increased bronchial secretions; dyspnea.
Skin: flushing.
Other: *anaphylaxis.*

INTERACTIONS
Drug-drug. *Amikacin, gentamicin, neomycin, streptomycin, tobramycin:* May increase the effects of atracurium, including prolonged respiratory depression. Use together cautiously. May reduce atracurium dose.
Carbamazepine, phenytoin, theophylline: May reverse, or cause resistance to, neuromuscular blockade. May need to increase atracurium dose.
Clindamycin, general anesthetics (enflurane, halothane, isoflurane), kanamycin, polymyxin antibiotics (colistin, polymyxin B sulfate), procainamide, quinidine, quinine, thiazide and loop diuretics, trimethaphan, verapamil: May enhance neuromuscular blockade, increasing skeletal muscle relaxation and prolonging effect of atracurium. Use together cautiously during and after surgery.
Corticosteroids: May cause prolonged weakness. Monitor patient closely.
Edrophonium, neostigmine, pyridostigmine: May inhibit drug and reverse neuromuscular block. Monitor patient closely.
Lithium, magnesium salts, opioid analgesics: May enhance neuromuscular blockade, increasing skeletal muscle relaxation and possibly causing respiratory paralysis. Reduce atracurium dosage.
Succinylcholine: May cause quicker onset of atracurium; may increase depth of neuromuscular blockade. Monitor patient.

EFFECTS ON LAB TEST RESULTS
None reported.

CONTRAINDICATIONS & CAUTIONS
● Contraindicated in patients hypersensitive to drug.

● Use cautiously in elderly or debilitated patients and in those with CV disease; severe electrolyte disorder; bronchogenic carcinoma; hepatic, renal, or pulmonary impairment; neuromuscular disease; or myasthenia gravis.
⚠ Overdose S&S: Hypotension, prolonged neuromuscular blockade.

NURSING CONSIDERATIONS
● Dosage depends on anesthetic used, individual needs, and response. Recommended dosages must be individually adjusted.
● Resistance may develop in burn patients; increase dosage if needed.
● Give analgesics for pain. Patient may have pain but may be unable to express it.
● Once spontaneous recovery starts, reverse atracurium-induced neuromuscular blockade with an anticholinesterase (such as neostigmine or edrophonium), usually given with an anticholinergic such as atropine. Complete reversal of neuromuscular blockade is usually achieved within 8 to 10 minutes after using an anticholinesterase.
● Monitor respirations and vital signs closely until patient has fully recovered from neuromuscular blockade, as indicated by tests of muscle strength (hand grip, head lift, and ability to cough).
● A nerve stimulator and train-of-four monitoring are recommended to confirm antagonism of neuromuscular blockade and recovery of muscle strength. Make sure spontaneous recovery is evident before attempting reversal with neostigmine.
● Prior use of succinylcholine doesn't prolong duration of action but quickens onset and may deepen neuromuscular blockade.
● Drug contains benzyl alcohol as a preservative.
⊙ Alert: Careful dosage calculation is essential. Always verify dosage with another health care professional.

PATIENT TEACHING
● Explain all events and procedures to patient because he can still hear.

atropine sulfate
AT-troe-peen

AtroPen, Sal-Tropine

Therapeutic class: Antiarrhythmics
Pharmacologic class: Anticholinergics–
belladonna alkaloids
Pregnancy risk category: C

AVAILABLE FORMS
Injection: 0.05 mg/mL, 0.1 mg/mL,
0.4 mg/mL, 0.8 mg/mL, 1 mg/mL
Prefilled auto-injectors: 0.25 mg, 0.5 mg,
1 mg, 2 mg
Tablets: 0.4 mg

INDICATIONS & DOSAGES
➤ **Bradyarrhythmias**
Adults: Usually 0.4 to 1 mg I.V. push, repeated
every 1 to 2 hours to maximum of 2 mg.
Children and adolescents: 0.01 to
0.03 mg/kg I.V.
➤ **Poisoning**
*Adults and children weighing more than
41 kg (90 lb):* For anticholinesterase poisoning, give at least 2 to 3 mg parenterally;
repeat until signs of atropine intoxication
appear. For muscarinic mushroom poisoning, give in doses sufficient to control
parasympathetic signs before coma and CV
collapse occur. When using the AtroPen,
2 mg I.M. is typically used for patients
weighing more than 41 kg. More than one
AtroPen may be needed until atropinization
occurs. No more than three AtroPens should
be used unless given under the supervision
of a trained medical provider.
Children weighing 18 to 41 kg (40 to 90 lb):
AtroPen 1 mg I.M. per dose for one to three
doses.
Children weighing 7 to 18 kg (15 to 40 lb):
AtroPen 0.5 mg I.M. per dose for one to
three doses.
Infants weighing less than 7 kg (15 lb):
AtroPen 0.25 mg I.M. per dose for one to
three doses.
➤ **Preoperatively to diminish secretions
and block cardiac vagal reflexes**
*Adults and children weighing 20 kg
(44 lb) or more:* 0.4 to 0.6 mg I.V., I.M.,

or subcutaneously 30 to 60 minutes before
anesthesia.
Children weighing less than 20 kg:
0.01 mg/kg I.V., I.M., or subcutaneously
up to maximum dose of 0.4 mg 30 to
60 minutes before anesthesia. May repeat
every 4 to 6 hours p.r.n.
Infants weighing more than 5 kg (11 lb):
0.03 mg/kg I.V. or I.M. every 4 to 6 hours
p.r.n.
Infants weighing 5 kg or less: 0.04 mg/kg
I.V. or I.M. every 4 to 6 hours p.r.n.
➤ **Antimuscarinic**
*Adults and children weighing more than
41 kg (90 lb):* 0.4 to 0.6 mg I.V., I.M., or
subcutaneously.
Children weighing 29.5 kg (65 lb) to 41 kg:
0.4 mg I.V., I.M., or subcutaneously.
*Children weighing 18 kg (40 lb) to less
than 29.5 kg:* 0.3 mg I.V., I.M., or subcuta-
neously.
*Children weighing 11 kg (24 lb) to less than
18 kg:* 0.2 mg I.V., I.M., or subcutaneously.
*Children weighing 7 kg (16 lb) to less than
11 kg:* 0.15 mg I.V., I.M., or subcutaneously.
*Children weighing 3 kg (7 lb) to less than
7 kg:* 0.1 mg I.V., I.M., or subcutaneously.
➤ **Hypotonic radiography**
Adults: 1 mg I.M.
➤ **Antispasmodic; to reduce salivation
and bronchial secretions**
*Adults and children weighing 41 kg (90 lb)
or more:* 0.4 mg P.O. every 4 to 6 hours as
needed.
*Children weighing 29.5 kg (65 lb) to
41 kg:* 0.4 mg P.O. Recommended maximum dosage is 0.4 mg/day.
*Children weighing 18 kg (40 lb) to less
than 29.5 kg:* 0.3 mg P.O. Recommended
maximum dosage is 0.4 mg/day.
*Children weighing 11 kg (24 lb) to less
than 18 kg:* 0.2 mg P.O. Recommended
maximum dosage is 0.4 mg/day.
*Children weighing 7 kg (16 lb) to less than
11 kg:* 0.15 mg P.O. Recommended maximum dosage is 0.4 mg/day.
Children weighing 3 kg (7 lb) to 7 kg:
0.1 mg P.O. Recommended maximum
dosage is 0.4 mg/day.

Reactions in bold italics are *life-threatening*. Interactions may have a *rapid onset* or a *delayed onset*.

ADMINISTRATION
P.O.
● Give drug without regard for food.
I.V.
▼ Give into a large vein or into I.V. tubing over at least 1 minute.
▼ Slow delivery may cause slowing of the heart rate.
▼ **Incompatibilities:** Alkalies, bromides, iodides, isoproterenol, methohexital, norepinephrine, pentobarbital sodium, sodium bicarbonate.
Subcutaneous
● Document administration site.
I.M.
● Auto-injection may be given through clothing.
● Firmly jab tip into outer thigh at 90-degree angle.
● Hold auto-injector in place for at least 10 seconds to allow time for complete administration.
● Make sure needle is visible after removing auto-injector. If needle didn't engage, repeat injection, jabbing more firmly.
● Massage injection site for several seconds after removing auto-injector.
● In very thin or young patients, pinch the skin on the thigh together before injection.

ACTION
Inhibits acetylcholine at parasympathetic neuroeffector junction, blocking vagal effects on SA and AV nodes, enhancing conduction through AV node and increasing heart rate.

Route	Onset	Peak	Duration
P.O.	30–120 min	1–2 hr	4 hr
I.V.	Immediate	2–4 min	4 hr
I.M.	5–40 min	20–60 min	4 hr
Subcut.	Unknown	Unknown	Unknown

Half-life: Initial, 2 hours; second phase, 12½ hours.

ADVERSE REACTIONS
CNS: headache, restlessness, insomnia, dizziness, ataxia, disorientation, hallucinations, delirium, excitement, agitation, confusion.
CV: *bradycardia,* palpitations, tachycardia.

EENT: blurred vision, mydriasis, photophobia, cycloplegia, increased intraocular pressure.
GI: dry mouth, constipation, thirst, nausea, vomiting.
GU: urine retention, erectile dysfunction.
Other: *anaphylaxis.*

INTERACTIONS
Drug-drug. *Antacids:* May decrease absorption of oral anticholinergics. Separate doses by at least 1 hour.
Anticholinergics, drugs with anticholinergic effects (amantadine, antiarrhythmics, antiparkinsonians, glutethimide, meperidine, phenothiazines, tricyclic antidepressants): May increase anticholinergic effects. Use together cautiously.
Ketoconazole, levodopa: May decrease absorption of these drugs. Separate doses by at least 2 hours, and monitor patient for clinical effect.
Potassium chloride wax-matrix tablets: May increase risk of mucosal lesions. Use together cautiously.
Drug-herb. *Jaborandi tree, pill-bearing spurge:* May decrease effectiveness of drug. Discourage use together.
Jimsonweed: May adversely affect CV function. Discourage use together.
Squaw vine: Tannic acid may decrease metabolic breakdown of drug. Monitor patient.

EFFECTS ON LAB TEST RESULTS
None reported.

CONTRAINDICATIONS & CAUTIONS
● Contraindicated in patients hypersensitive to drug.
● Contraindicated in those with acute angle-closure glaucoma, obstructive uropathy, obstructive disease of GI tract, paralytic ileus, toxic megacolon, intestinal atony, unstable CV status in acute hemorrhage, tachycardia, myocardial ischemia, asthma, or myasthenia gravis.
● Use cautiously in patients with Down syndrome because they may be more sensitive to drug.
⚠ **Overdose S&S:** Delirium, seizures, coma, tachycardia, fever, mydriasis, decreased

salivation and sweating, urine retention, hypertension, vasodilation, hyperthermia.

NURSING CONSIDERATIONS
● In adults, avoid doses less than 0.5 mg because of risk of paradoxical bradycardia.
❸ **Alert:** Watch for tachycardia in cardiac patients because it may lead to ventricular fibrillation.
● Many adverse reactions (such as dry mouth and constipation) vary with dose.
● Monitor fluid intake and urine output. Drug causes urine retention and urinary hesitancy.

PATIENT TEACHING
● Teach patient receiving oral form of drug how to handle distressing anticholinergic effects such as dry mouth.
● Instruct patient to report serious or persistent adverse reactions promptly.
● Tell patient about potential for sensitivity of the eyes to the sun and suggest use of sunglasses.
● Tell patient to protect the AtroPen from light and not to freeze it.

avanafil
a-VAN-ah-fill

Stendra

Therapeutic class: Erectile dysfunction drugs
Pharmacologic class: PDE5 inhibitors
Pregnancy risk category: C

AVAILABLE FORMS
Tablets: 50 mg, 100 mg, 200 mg

INDICATIONS & DOSAGES
➤ **Erectile dysfunction**
Adults: 100 mg P.O. daily as needed 30 minutes before sexual activity. May increase to a maximum of 200 mg daily or decrease to 50 mg daily. Use lowest effective dosage.
Adjust-a-dose: In patients taking moderate CYP3A4 inhibitors, maximum dosage is 50 mg P.O. daily. In patients taking a stable dose of alpha blocker, initially give 50 mg P.O. daily; adjust as needed and tolerated.

ADMINISTRATION
P.O.
● May give without regard for food.
● Store at controlled room temperature; protect from light.

ACTION
Increases cyclic guanosine monophosphate level, prolongs smooth-muscle relaxation, and promotes blood flow into the corpus cavernosum.

Route	Onset	Peak	Duration
P.O.	Rapid	30–45 min	Unknown

Half-life: 5 hours.

ADVERSE REACTIONS
CNS: headache, dizziness.
CV: hypertension, flushing.
EENT: nasal congestion, nasopharyngitis, sinusitis, sinus congestion.
GI: dyspepsia, nausea, constipation, diarrhea.
Musculoskeletal: back pain, arthralgia.
Respiratory: upper respiratory tract infection, bronchitis.
Skin: rash.
Other: influenza.

INTERACTIONS
Drug-drug. *Alpha blockers, antihypertensives:* May cause additive hypotensive effect. Use cautiously together.
CYP450 inducers: Use together hasn't been evaluated and isn't recommended.
Moderate CYP3A4 inhibitors (amprenavir, aprepitant, diltiazem, erythromycin, fluconazole, fosamprenavir, verapamil): May increase avanafil concentration. Use cautiously together at maximum avanafil daily dosage of 50 mg.
Nitrates: May increase hypotensive effects. Use together is contraindicated. If nitrate administration is deemed medically necessary in a life-threatening situation, at least 12 hours should elapse after last dose of avanafil before nitrate administration.
PDE5 inhibitors (sildenafil, tadalafil): May cause additive hypotensive effects. Use together is contraindicated.
Strong CYP3A4 inhibitors (atazanavir, clarithromycin, indinavir, itraconazole, ketoconazole, nefazodone, nelfinavir, ritonavir,

saquinavir, telithromycin): May increase avanafil concentration. Use together is contraindicated.

Drug-food. *Grapefruit juice:* May increase avanafil serum level. Don't use together.

Drug-lifestyle. *Alcohol use:* May increase risk of hypotension, including orthostatic hypotension (increased heart rate, dizziness, headache). Discourage use together.

Street drug "poppers" (amyl nitrate, butyl nitrate): May increase risk of severe hypotensive effects. Discourage use together.

EFFECTS ON LAB TEST RESULTS
None reported.

CONTRAINDICATIONS & CAUTIONS
• Contraindicated in patients hypersensitive to drug or its components and in patients taking nitrates.
• Drug hasn't been studied in patients with severe renal disease, those on dialysis, or patients with severe hepatic disease. Don't use in these patients.
• Contraindicated in patients with MI, stroke, life-threatening arrhythmia, or coronary revascularization within the past 6 months; resting hypotension or hypertension; unstable angina; angina with sexual intercourse; New York Heart Association Class 2 or greater heart failure; or conditions in which sexual activity is not advised.
• Use cautiously in patients with anatomic deformities of the penis, including angulation, cavernosal fibrosis, and Peyronie disease, and in patients with conditions that may predispose them to priapism (such as sickle cell anemia, multiple myeloma, and leukemia).

NURSING CONSIDERATIONS
• Drug isn't for use in women.
• Assess patients with preexisting CV disease to determine if they're healthy enough for sexual activity.

PATIENT TEACHING
• Teach patient that drug is only to be taken once daily.
• Caution patient to take drug only as prescribed.
• Advise patient that drug shouldn't be used with nitrates under any circumstances.

Instruct patient who experiences chest pain after taking avanafil to seek immediate medical attention.
• Discuss with patient who has preexisting heart disease the potential cardiac risk of sexual activity; advise patient to seek immediate medical help if cardiac signs and symptoms occur upon initiation of sexual activity.
• Counsel patient to stop drug and seek prompt medical assistance if sudden loss of vision in one or both eyes or sudden decrease in or loss of hearing occurs.
• Advise patient to seek emergency medical attention for an erection lasting longer than 4 hours, whether painful or not.
• Tell patient that drug doesn't protect against sexually transmitted diseases, including HIV.
• Instruct patient to take drug approximately 30 minutes before sexual activity and that sexual stimulation is required for an erection to occur.

SAFETY ALERT!

axitinib
ax-I-ti-nib

Inlyta

Therapeutic class: Antineoplastics
Pharmacologic class: Kinase inhibitors
Pregnancy risk category: D

AVAILABLE FORMS
Tablets: 1 mg, 5 mg

INDICATIONS & DOSAGES
➤ **Advanced renal cell carcinoma after failure of one prior systemic therapy**
Adults: 5 mg P.O. b.i.d. approximately 12 hours apart. If patient tolerates drug for at least 2 consecutive weeks with adverse reactions no greater than Grade 2 CTCAE guidelines, is normotensive, and isn't receiving antihypertensives, may increase dosage to 7 mg b.i.d., then 10 mg b.i.d.
Adjust-a-dose: Base dosage adjustment on individual safety and tolerability. Management of adverse reactions may require temporary interruption or permanent discontinuation. If dosage reduction from

5 mg b.i.d. is needed, recommended dosage is 2 or 3 mg b.i.d. If a strong CYP3A4/5 inhibitor must be coadministered, decrease axitinib dosage by approximately half; may increase or decrease subsequent doses based on individual safety and tolerability. If strong CYP3A4/5 inhibitor is discontinued, return axitinib dosage to that used before initiation after inhibitor is out of system (3 to 5 half-life periods of the strong inhibitor). Reduce axitinib starting dose by approximately half in patients with baseline moderate hepatic impairment (Child-Pugh class B); may increase or decrease subsequent doses based on individual safety and tolerability.

ADMINISTRATION
P.O.
● May give without regard for food.
● Have patient swallow tablets whole with a glass of water. Don't crush, break, or allow patient to chew tablets.
● If a dose is missed or patient vomits, don't give an additional dose; give next prescribed dose at usual time.
● Store at room temperature.

ACTION
Inhibits receptor tyrosine kinases, which decreases cell proliferation, tumor growth, angiogenesis, and cancer progression.

Route	Onset	Peak	Duration
P.O.	Unknown	2½–4 hr	Unknown

Half-life: 2.5 to 6.1 hours.

ADVERSE REACTIONS
CNS: asthenia, fatigue, headache, dizziness, transient ischemic attack, *reversible posterior leukoencephalopathy syndrome (RPLS).*
CV: hypertension, *deep vein thrombosis.*
EENT: dysphonia, mucosal inflammation, stomatitis, dysgeusia, epistaxis, tinnitus, retinal-vein occlusion thrombosis.
GI: diarrhea, nausea, vomiting, constipation, abdominal pain, upper abdominal pain, dyspepsia, hemorrhoids, *rectal hemorrhage, hemoptysis.*
GU: hematuria, proteinuria.
Hematologic: anemia, *polycythemia.*

Metabolic: decreased appetite, decreased weight, hypothyroidism, dehydration.
Musculoskeletal: arthralgia, extremity pain, myalgia.
Respiratory: cough, dyspnea, *pulmonary embolism.*
Skin: alopecia, hand-foot syndrome, rash, dry skin, pruritus, erythema.

INTERACTIONS
Drug-drug. *Moderate CYP3A4/5 inducers (bosentan, efavirenz, etravirine, modafinil, nafcillin), strong CYP3A4/5 inducers (such as carbamazepine, dexamethasone, phenobarbital, phenytoin, rifabutin, rifampin, rifapentine):* May reduce axitinib level. Avoid concurrent use.
Strong CYP3A4/5 inhibitors (such as atazanavir, clarithromycin, indinavir, itraconazole, ketoconazole, nefazodone, nelfinavir, ritonavir, saquinavir, telithromycin, voriconazole): May increase axitinib level. Avoid concurrent use; if strong CYP3A4/5 inhibitor is absolutely necessary, reduce axitinib dosage.
Drug-herb. *St. John's wort:* May decrease axitinib plasma concentration. Discourage concurrent use.
Drug-food. *Grapefruit, grapefruit juice:* May increase axitinib plasma concentration. Discourage concurrent use.

EFFECTS ON LAB TEST RESULTS
● May increase potassium, amylase, lipase, alkaline phosphatase, ALT, AST, bilirubin, and creatinine levels. May decrease bicarbonate, calcium, albumin, phosphate, and thyroid hormone levels.
● May decrease hemoglobin level and lymphocyte, neutrophil, and platelet counts.
● May increase or decrease glucose, sodium, and thyroid-stimulating hormone levels.

CONTRAINDICATIONS & CAUTIONS
● Contraindicated in patients hypersensitive to drug and in patients with brain metastases or recent GI bleed.
● Contraindicated in pregnant or breast-feeding women.
● Use cautiously in patients with hypertension; in those at risk for GI perforation, fistula formation, thyroid dysfunction, or

arterial or venous thromboembolic events; and in patients with moderate hepatic impairment (Child-Pugh class B) or ESRD (CrCl less than 15 mL/minute). Drug hasn't been studied in patients with Child-Pugh class C hepatic impairment.

⚠ *Overdose S&S:* Dizziness, hypertension, seizures, possible fatal hemoptysis.

NURSING CONSIDERATIONS
● Hypertension should be well controlled before start of therapy. Monitor patient for increased blood pressure; treat as indicated. If hypertension persists despite antihypertensive use, decrease axitinib dosage, as ordered.
● Watch for hypotension if drug is withheld for any reason and patient continues antihypertensive use.
● Monitor patient for signs and symptoms of hematologic or neurologic disease, thromboembolic events, and GI disorders.
● Monitor patient for bleeding or hemorrhagic event. Temporarily interrupt treatment if bleeding occurs.
● Counsel both male and female patients in the effective use of contraceptives during treatment.
● Monitor use of all prescription drugs, OTC medications, grapefruit or grapefruit juice, and supplements.
● Obtain liver and renal function tests before and periodically during therapy.
● Stop drug at least 24 hours before surgery; resume based on clinical judgment of wound healing. Monitor wound healing carefully.
● Monitor patient for signs and symptoms of RPLS (headache, seizures, lethargy, confusion, blindness, and other visual disturbances) and other neurologic signs and symptoms. Discontinue drug if these occur.
● Monitor patient for proteinuria before and during therapy. Decrease dosage or temporarily interrupt therapy if signs and symptoms occur. Stop drug if proteinuria becomes moderate or severe. Monitor thyroid function before and periodically during therapy.

PATIENT TEACHING
● Counsel both male and female patients to use effective birth control during treatment.
● Instruct patient that drug may be taken without regard to meals and to swallow capsules whole with a glass of water.
● Tell patient to avoid grapefruit and grapefruit juice while taking this drug.
● Caution patient that if a dose is missed, to wait until next scheduled dose and never to take two doses at the same time to make up for a missed dose.
● Advise patient to alert prescriber if stomach pain, bruising, bleeding, delayed wound healing, fatigue, high blood pressure, or neurologic signs and symptoms (headache, seizures, lethargy, confusion, blindness, other visual changes) occur.
● Teach patient to consult prescriber before starting new drugs or supplements.
● Instruct patient to keep lab test appointments as requested by prescriber, to monitor drug's safety and effectiveness.

SAFETY ALERT!

azacitidine
az-uh-SIT-uh-deen

Vidaza

Therapeutic class: Antineoplastics
Pharmacologic class: Pyrimidine nucleoside analogues
Pregnancy risk category: D

AVAILABLE FORMS
Powder for injection: 100-mg vials

INDICATIONS & DOSAGES
➤ **Myelodysplastic syndrome, including refractory anemia, refractory anemia with ringed sideroblasts (if patient has neutropenia or thrombocytopenia, or needs transfusions), refractory anemia with excess blasts, refractory anemia with excess blasts in transformation, or chronic myelomonocytic leukemia**
Adults: Initially, 75 mg/m^2 subcutaneously or I.V. daily for 7 days; repeat cycle every 4 weeks. May increase to 100 mg/m^2 if no response after two treatment cycles and nausea and vomiting are the only toxic reactions. Four to six treatment cycles are recommended.

Adjust-a-dose: If bicarbonate level is less than 20 mEq/L, reduce next dose by 50%. If BUN or creatinine levels rise during treatment, delay the next cycle until they are normal; then give 50% of previous dose.

For patients with baseline WBC greater than or equal to 3×10^9/L, ANC greater than or equal to 1.5×10^9/L, and platelet count greater than or equal to 75×10^9/L, adjust the dose based on nadir counts as follows: If ANC is less than 0.5×10^9/L and platelet count is less than 25×10^9/L, give 50% of dose. If ANC is 0.5 to 1.5×10^9/L and platelet count is 25 to 50×10^9/L, give 67% of dose

For patients with baseline WBC less than 3×10^9/L, ANC less than 1.5×10^9/L, or platelet count less than 75×10^9/L, adjust dosage as shown in the table below.

▼ Give the infusion over 10 to 40 minutes. Infusion must be completed within 1 hour of reconstitution.

▼ **Incompatibilities:** Dextrose 5%, hespan, bicarbonate.

Subcutaneous

● Dilute using aseptic and hazardous substances techniques.

● Reconstitute with 4 mL sterile water for injection. Vigorously shake or roll the vial until a uniform suspension forms. The resulting cloudy suspension will be 25 mg/mL.

● Draw up suspension into syringes for injection (no more than 4 mL per syringe).

● Just before giving drug, resuspend drug by vigorously rolling the syringe between the palms for 30 seconds. Divide doses greater than 4 mL into two syringes and inject into two separate sites.

Azacitidine dosage adjustments based on nadir counts and bone marrow biopsy cellularity

	Bone marrow biopsy cellularity at time of nadir		
WBC or platelet nadir % decrease in counts from baseline	30%–60%	15%–30%	<15%
		% dose in the next course	
50%–75%	100%	50%	33%
> 75%	75%	50%	33%

If a nadir, as defined in the table, has occurred, the next course of treatment should be given 28 days after the start of the preceding course, provided that both the WBC and platelet counts are greater than 25% above the nadir and rising. If an increase greater than 25% above nadir isn't seen by day 28, counts should be reassessed every 7 days. If a 25% increase isn't seen by day 42, patient should be treated with 50% of scheduled dose. Adjust further dosages during therapy based on hematologic or renal toxicities.

ADMINISTRATION

I.V.

▼ Reconstitute drug with 10 mL of sterile water for injection.

▼ Vigorously shake or roll the vial until powder is dissolved. The resulting solution will be 10 mg/mL.

▼ Use only clear solution.

▼ Withdraw proper dose and mix in a total volume of 50 to 100 mL of normal saline solution or lactated Ringer's solution.

● Give new injections at least 1 inch (2.5 cm) from previous site, and never into tender, bruised, red, or hardened skin.

● Reconstituted drug is stable 1 hour at room temperature and 8 hours refrigerated (36° to 46° F [2° to 8° C]). After refrigeration, suspension may be allowed to warm for 30 minutes at room temperature.

ACTION

Causes hypomethylation of DNA and is toxic to abnormal hematopoietic cells in bone marrow. Hypomethylation may restore normal function to genes needed for proliferation and differentiation. Drug has little effect on nonproliferating cells.

Route	Onset	Peak	Duration
I.V.	Unknown	Unknown	Unknown
Subcut.	Unknown	30 min	Unknown

Half-life: About 40 minutes after subcutaneous injection; unknown after I.V.

ADVERSE REACTIONS
CNS: anxiety, dizziness, fatigue, headache, insomnia, malaise, pain, weakness, lethargy.
CV: chest pain, edema, hypotension, peripheral swelling.
EENT: nasopharyngitis, pharyngitis, rhinitis, nasal congestion.
GI: abdominal pain and tenderness, anorexia, constipation, diarrhea, nausea, vomiting, abdominal distention, dyspepsia, gingival bleeding, loose stools, mouth hemorrhage, stomatitis.
GU: UTI.
Hematologic: anemia, *febrile neutropenia, leukopenia, neutropenia, thrombocytopenia,* hematoma, postprocedural hemorrhage.
Metabolic: decreased weight.
Musculoskeletal: arthralgia, bone pain, limb pain, myalgia.
Respiratory: dyspnea, pneumonia, upper respiratory tract infection.
Skin: ecchymosis, erythema (including erythema at injection site), pain, pallor, petechiae, pitting edema, rash, cellulitis, dry skin, granuloma, pigmentation, pruritus at injection site, skin nodules, swelling at injection site, urticaria.
Other: pyrexia, rigors.

INTERACTIONS
None reported.

EFFECTS ON LAB TEST RESULTS
• May increase BUN and creatinine levels. May decrease bicarbonate and potassium levels.
• May decrease neutrophil, platelet, and WBC counts.

CONTRAINDICATIONS & CAUTIONS
• Contraindicated in patients hypersensitive to azacitidine or mannitol and in patients with advanced malignant hepatic tumors.
• Use cautiously in patients with hepatic and renal disease.
⚠ **Overdose S&S:** Diarrhea, nausea, vomiting.

NURSING CONSIDERATIONS
• Check LFT results and creatinine level before therapy starts.
• Obtain CBC before each cycle or more often.

• Premedicate patient for nausea and vomiting.
• Monitor renal function closely in elderly patients and in renally impaired patients receiving drug because renal impairment may increase toxicity.
• Store unreconstituted vials at room temperature (59° to 86° F [15° to 30° C]).

PATIENT TEACHING
• Inform patient that blood counts may decrease with febrile neutropenia, thrombocytopenia, and anemia.
• Advise men and women to use birth control during therapy.

azathioprine
ay-za-THYE-oh-preen

Azasan, Imuran

Therapeutic class: Immunosuppressants
Pharmacologic class: Purine antagonists
Pregnancy risk category: D

AVAILABLE FORMS
Powder for injection: 100 mg
Tablets: 25 mg, 50 mg, 75 mg, 100 mg

INDICATIONS & DOSAGES
➤ **Immunosuppression in kidney transplantation**
Adults: Initially, 3 to 5 mg/kg P.O. or I.V. daily, usually beginning on day of transplantation. Maintained at 1 to 3 mg/kg daily based on patient response and tolerance.
Adjust-a-dose: Give drug in lower doses to patients with oliguria in the posttransplant period and in those with impaired renal function. In patients receiving allopurinol, decrease azathioprine dose to one-fourth to one-third of the usual dose.
➤ **Severe, refractory rheumatoid arthritis (RA)**
Adults: Initially, 1 mg/kg P.O. as single dose or divided into two doses. Usual dose is 50 to 100 mg. If patient response isn't satisfactory after 6 to 8 weeks, dosage may be increased by 0.5 mg/kg daily to maximum of 2.5 mg/kg daily at 4-week intervals. Maintenance therapy should be at lowest

effective dose. Attempt gradual dose reduction once the patient is stable. Reduce dosage by 0.5 mg/kg (about 25 mg daily) every 4 weeks.

➤ **Multiple sclerosis** ◆
Adults: 2 to 3 mg/kg P.O. daily alone or with other immunosuppressants.

➤ **Psoriasis** ◆
Adults: Initially, 0.5 mg/kg P.O. daily. May increase by 0.5 mg/kg/day after 6 to 8 weeks if cytopenia doesn't occur. Further increase can be made by 0.5 mg/kg/day every 4 weeks. Usual dosage is 75 to 150 mg/day. Dosages up to 300 mg daily have been used in a limited number of patients.

➤ **Idiopathic thrombocytopenic purpura** ◆
Adults: 1 to 2 mg/kg P.O. daily for at least 3 to 6 months. Maximum is 150 mg daily.

➤ **Lupus nephritis (maintenance phase)** ◆
Adults and children older than age 12: 2 mg/kg/day P.O. with or without low-dose daily glucocorticoid therapy.

ADMINISTRATION
P.O.
• Give drug after meals to minimize adverse GI effects.
• Drug is a potential teratogen and mutagen. Use safe handling procedures.

I.V.
▼ Drug is a potential teratogen and mutagen. Use safe handling procedures.
▼ Use only in patients who can't tolerate oral drugs.
▼ Reconstitute drug in 100-mg vial with 10 mL of sterile water for injection.
▼ Inspect for particles before use.
▼ Give by direct I.V. injection, or further dilute in normal saline solution for injection or D₅W solution and infuse over 30 to 60 minutes.
▼ **Incompatibilities:** None reported.

ACTION
May alter antibody production and suppress T-cell effects.

Route	Onset	Peak	Duration
P.O., I.V.	Unknown	1–2 hr	Unknown

Half-life: About 5 hours.

ADVERSE REACTIONS
CNS: fever.
GI: nausea, vomiting, anorexia, *pancreatitis,* steatorrhea, diarrhea, abdominal pain.
Hematologic: *leukopenia, myelosuppression,* macrocytic anemia, anemia, *pancytopenia, thrombocytopenia, immunosuppression.*
Hepatic: *hepatotoxicity.*
Musculoskeletal: arthralgia, myalgia.
Skin: rash, alopecia.
Other: infections, *increased risk of neoplasia.*

INTERACTIONS
Drug-drug. *ACE inhibitors:* May cause severe leukopenia and increase risk of anemia. Monitor patient closely.
Allopurinol: May impair inactivation of azathioprine. Avoid using if possible; decrease azathioprine to one-third to one-fourth usual dose.
Anticoagulants: May decrease action of anticoagulants. Monitor patient. Adjust warfarin dosage as needed.
Cyclosporine: May decrease cyclosporine level. Monitor cyclosporine level closely.
Febuxostat: May increase risk of toxicity. Concomitant use is contraindicated.
Live-virus vaccines: May reduce effectiveness of live-virus vaccines. Immunocompromised patients may be at increased risk for vaccine-induced infection. Defer live-virus vaccines until immune function improves.
Mercaptopurine: May increase risk of myelosuppression, including pancytopenia. Avoid concomitant use.
Nondepolarizing neuromuscular blockers: May decrease or reverse pharmacologic action of neuromuscular blockers. Monitor respiratory function; dosage requirements for nondepolarizing muscle relaxants may need to be increased.
Ribavirin: May increase risk of severe pancytopenia and azathioprine-related myelotoxicity. Monitor CBC, including platelet count.
Sulfamethoxazole–trimethoprim and other drugs that interfere with myelopoiesis: May cause severe leukopenia, especially in renal transplant patients. Use together cautiously.

Reactions in bold italics are *life-threatening*. Interactions may have a *rapid onset* or a *delayed onset*.

EFFECTS ON LAB TEST RESULTS
● May increase alkaline phosphatase, ALT, AST, and bilirubin levels. May decrease hemoglobin and uric acid levels.
● May decrease platelet, RBC, and WBC counts.

CONTRAINDICATIONS & CAUTIONS
● Contraindicated in patients hypersensitive to drug or its components and in pregnant women.
● Use cautiously in patients with hepatic or renal dysfunction.
● Benefits must be weighed against risk when giving to patient with systemic viral infection, such as chickenpox or herpes zoster.
● Patients with RA previously treated with alkylating drugs, such as cyclophosphamide, chlorambucil, or melphalan, may be at risk for tumor development if treated with this drug.
⚠ Overdose S&S: Nausea, vomiting, diarrhea, abnormal liver function, leukopenia.

NURSING CONSIDERATIONS
Black Box Warning Chronic immunosuppression with this drug increases the risk of neoplasia. Physicians using this drug should be very familiar with its risks, the mutagenic potential to both men and women, and possible hematologic toxicities. ■
● Consider genotype or phenotype testing for thiopurine S-methyltransferase. Patients with low or absent levels are at increased risk for hematologic effects of drug.
● To prevent bleeding, avoid all I.M. injections when platelet count is below 100,000/mm³.
● Monitor CBC and platelet counts weekly for 1 month and then twice monthly. Notify prescriber if counts drop suddenly or become dangerously low. Drug may need to be temporarily withheld.
● Watch for early signs and symptoms of hepatotoxicity (such as clay-colored stools, dark urine, pruritus, and yellow skin and sclera) and for increased alkaline phosphatase, bilirubin, AST, and ALT levels.
● Therapeutic response usually occurs within 8 weeks. Patients not improved after 12 weeks can be considered refractory to treatment.

● **Look alike–sound alike:** Don't confuse azathioprine with Azulfidine. Don't confuse Imuran with Inderal.

PATIENT TEACHING
Black Box Warning Warn patient of the risk of malignancy. ■
● Warn patient to report even mild infections (colds, fever, sore throat, malaise), because drug is a potent immunosuppressant.
● Instruct patient to avoid conception during therapy and for 4 months after therapy stops.
● Warn patient that some hair thinning is possible.
● Tell patient taking drug for refractory RA that it may take up to 12 weeks to be effective.
● Advise patient to report unusual bleeding or bruising.
● Tell patient that drug may be taken with food to decrease nausea.
● Advise patient to use soft toothbrush and perform oral care cautiously.

azelastine hydrochloride
ah-ZELL-ass-teen

Optivar

Therapeutic class: Antihistamines
Pharmacologic class: H₁-receptor antagonists
Pregnancy risk category: C

AVAILABLE FORMS
Ophthalmic solution: 0.05%

INDICATIONS & DOSAGES
➤ **Pruritus from allergic conjunctivitis**
Adults and children age 3 and older: Instill 1 drop into affected eye b.i.d.

ADMINISTRATION
Ophthalmic
● Keep bottle tightly closed when not in use.
● Don't touch tip of dropper to any surface.

ACTION

Inhibits the release of histamine and other mediators from cells involved in the allergic response.

Route	Onset	Peak	Duration
Ophthalmic	3 min	Unknown	8 hr

Half-life: 22 hours.

ADVERSE REACTIONS
CNS: headache, fatigue.
EENT: bitter taste, transient eye burning or stinging, conjunctivitis, eye pain, pharyngitis, rhinitis, temporary blurring.
Respiratory: *asthma,* dyspnea.
Skin: pruritus.
Other: flulike syndrome.

INTERACTIONS
None reported.

EFFECTS ON LAB TEST RESULTS
None reported.

CONTRAINDICATIONS & CAUTIONS
• Contraindicated in patients hypersensitive to any of drug's components.

NURSING CONSIDERATIONS
• Drug is for ophthalmic use only. Don't inject or give orally.
• Don't use for irritation caused by contact lenses.

PATIENT TEACHING
• Instruct patient not to touch any surface, eyelid, or surrounding areas with tip of dropper.
• Tell patient to keep bottle tightly closed when not in use.
• Advise patient not to wear contact lens if eye is red.
• Warn patient that soft contact lenses may absorb the preservative benzalkonium.
• Instruct patient who wears soft contact lenses and whose eyes aren't red to wait at least 10 minutes after instilling drug before inserting contact lenses.

azelastine hydrochloride–fluticasone propionate
ah-ZELL-ass-teen/floo-TIK-a-sone

Dymista

Therapeutic class: Antihistamines–corticosteroids
Pharmacologic class: H_1-receptor antagonists–corticosteroids
Pregnancy risk category: C

AVAILABLE FORMS
Nasal spray: 137 mcg azelastine hydrochloride and 50 mcg fluticasone propionate/spray

INDICATIONS & DOSAGES
➤ **Symptoms of seasonal allergic rhinitis**
Adults and children age 12 and older:
1 spray/nostril b.i.d.

ADMINISTRATION
Intranasal
• Shake gently before each use.
• Prime the spray before initial use; spray six times or until a fine mist appears. If the spray hasn't been used within the past 14 days, prime the spray again with 1 spray or until a fine mist appears.
• Store upright at room temperature with dust cap in place. Don't freeze or refrigerate.
• Protect from light.

ACTION
Azelastine inhibits release of histamine and other mediators from cells involved in the allergic response. Fluticasone may decrease inflammation by inhibiting mast cells, macrophages, and mediators such as leukotrienes.

Route	Onset	Peak	Duration
Intranasal	Rapid	½ hr (azelastine), 1 hr (fluticasone)	Unknown

Half-life: Azelastine, 25 hours; fluticasone, unknown.

ADVERSE REACTIONS
CNS: headache, fever, pain.
EENT: epistaxis, nasal congestion, rhinitis, pharyngitis.
GI: diarrhea, dysgeusia.

Reactions in bold italics are *life-threatening*. Interactions may have a *rapid onset* or a *delayed onset*.

Respiratory: cough, upper respiratory tract infection.
Other: viral infection.

INTERACTIONS
Drug-drug. *CNS depressants:* May increase risk of drowsiness. Use together cautiously.
CYP4503A4 inhibitors (fluconazole, keto-conazole): May increase fluticasone plasma level. Use together cautiously.
Ritonavir: May increase fluticasone plasma level and risk of systemic corticosteroid effects, including Cushing syndrome and adrenal suppression. Avoid use together.
Drug-lifestyle. *Alcohol use:* May increase risk of somnolence and CNS impairment. Discourage use together.

EFFECTS ON LAB TEST RESULTS
None reported.

CONTRAINDICATIONS & CAUTIONS
• Contraindicated in patients hypersensitive to either drug or its components and in those with current nasal ulcers, nasal trauma, or nasal surgery until healing occurs.
• Use cautiously in patients with glaucoma, cataracts, ongoing infection, or history of adrenal suppression.
• Use cautiously in pregnant and breast-feeding women and only if benefits outweigh risks.

NURSING CONSIDERATIONS
• Monitor patient for fungal, bacterial, or viral infections.
• Monitor patient for localized nasopha-ryngeal *Candida albicans* infection with prolonged use.
• Ensure patient receives regular eye exams to screen for cataracts and glaucoma with long-term use.
• Monitor growth rate in children using the spray long-term.
• Monitor patient for adrenal insufficiency (tiredness, weakness, nausea, vomiting, hypotension).

PATIENT TEACHING
• Instruct patient to shake bottle gently before each use and to prime the spray un-til a fine mist appears before initial use or if the spray hasn't been used in the past

14 days. Advise patient to follow full pack-age directions for use.
• Caution patient to avoid spraying into eyes and, if exposure occurs, to flush eyes with water for 10 minutes.
• Warn patient to watch for changes in vision, which can indicate serious eye prob-lems, such as glaucoma or cataracts. Advise patient to have regular eye exams while taking drug.
• Tell patient to watch for nasal problems, such as nose bleeds and nasal septal perfora-tion.
• Advise patient that drug can decrease the body's ability to heal or fight infection. Tell patient to report fever, aches or pains, chills, fatigue, or exposure to chickenpox or measles. Caution patient to avoid exposure to communicable diseases.
• Warn patient that drug can cause drowsi-ness. Instruct patient to avoid alcohol and other drugs that cause drowsiness while taking this medication.
• Advise patient to avoid driving or tasks that require alertness until drug's effects are known.
• Instruct patient to notify prescriber if she is pregnant, thinking of becoming pregnant, or breast-feeding.

azilsartan medoxomil
ay-zil-SAH-tan

Edarbi

Therapeutic class: Antihypertensives
Pharmacologic class: ARBs
Pregnancy risk category: C in 1st trimester; D in 2nd and 3rd trimesters

AVAILABLE FORMS
Tablets: 40 mg, 80 mg

INDICATIONS & DOSAGES
➤ **Hypertension (alone or in combination with other antihypertensives)**
Adults: 80 mg P.O. once daily.
Adjust-a-dose: For patients treated with high doses of diuretics, consider initiating therapy at 40 mg P.O. daily.

ADMINISTRATION
P.O.
• Give drug with or without food.
• Store at room temperature in original container.
• Protect from moisture and light.

ACTION
Blocks vasoconstricting and aldosterone-secreting effects of angiotensin II by preventing angiotensin II from binding to angiotensin I receptors on vascular smooth muscle and the adrenal glands.

Route	Onset	Peak	Duration
P.O.	Rapid	1½–3 hr	Unknown

Half-life: 11 hours.

ADVERSE REACTIONS
CNS: asthenia, dizziness, fatigue.
GI: diarrhea, nausea.
Musculoskeletal: muscle spasm.
Respiratory: cough.

INTERACTIONS
Drug-drug. *Aliskiren:* May increase risk of renal impairment, hypotension, and hyperkalemia in diabetic patients and those with moderate to severe renal impairment (GFR less than 60 mL/minute). Concomitant use is contraindicated in diabetic patients. Avoid concomitant use in those with moderate to severe renal impairment.
NSAIDs: May decrease renal function and azilsartan effectiveness. Monitor renal function and blood pressure periodically.

EFFECTS ON LAB TEST RESULTS
• May increase serum creatinine level.
• May increase or decrease platelet and WBC counts.
• May decrease hemoglobin level, hematocrit, and RBC count.

CONTRAINDICATIONS & CAUTIONS
• Contraindicated in patients hypersensitive to drug or its components and in breast-feeding women.
Black Box Warning Contraindicated in pregnant women because drug can cause injury or death to the developing fetus, especially during the second and third trimesters.

If pregnancy occurs, stop drug as soon as possible. ■
• Use cautiously in patients with volume or salt depletion (such as those taking high-dose diuretics) because of the risk of symptomatic hypotension. Correct the cause before start of therapy or initiate drug at 40 mg P.O. daily.

NURSING CONSIDERATIONS
• Monitor blood pressure closely. If blood pressure isn't controlled with azilsartan alone, consider adding additional antihypertensives.
• If hypotension occurs, place patient in the supine position, and administer volume expanders if necessary.
• Monitor renal function periodically. Drug may cause oliguria or progressive azotemia and (rarely) acute renal failure or death in patients whose renal function may depend on the activity of the renin-angiotensin-aldosterone system (such as those with congestive heart failure).

PATIENT TEACHING
• Advise female patients who plan to become pregnant to notify their provider so other treatment options can be considered.
• Instruct female patients to report suspected pregnancy to prescriber immediately to prevent potential fetal harm.
• Advise breast-feeding women to stop either drug or breast-feeding because of possible harm to the infant.
• Tell patient to notify his provider if dizziness occurs, especially upon standing. If patient experiences dizziness, caution him to lie down, rise slowly from a lying to standing position, and to climb stairs slowly.
• Teach patient that azilsartan may be prescribed alone or with other antihypertensives to control blood pressure.
• Inform patient that azilsartan may be taken with or without food.
• Warn patient to store drug in its original container and to protect it from light and moisture.
• Advise patient that routine blood work will be needed to monitor renal function and drug tolerance.

Reactions in bold italics are *life-threatening*. Interactions may have a *rapid onset* or a *delayed onset*.

azithromycin
ay-zi-thro-MY-sin

Zithromax&, Zmax

Therapeutic class: Antibiotics
Pharmacologic class: Macrolides
Pregnancy risk category: B

AVAILABLE FORMS
Injection: 500 mg
Oral suspension (extended-release): 2 g
Powder for oral suspension: 100 mg/5 mL,
200 mg/5 mL; 1,000 mg/packet
Tablets: 250 mg, 500 mg, 600 mg

INDICATIONS & DOSAGES
➤ **Acute bacterial worsening of COPD
caused by** *Haemophilus influenzae,
Moraxella catarrhalis,* **or** *Streptococcus pneumoniae;* **uncomplicated skin
and skin-structure infections caused by**
*Staphylococcus aureus, Streptococcus
pyogenes,* **or** *Streptococcus agalactiae;*
**second-line therapy for pharyngitis
or tonsillitis caused by** *Staphylococcus
pyogenes*
Adults and adolescents age 16 and older:
Initially, 500 mg P.O. as a single dose on
day 1, followed by 250 mg daily on days 2
through 5. Total cumulative dose is 1.5 g.
Or, for worsening COPD, 500 mg P.O. daily
for 3 days.
➤ **Community-acquired pneumonia
from** *Chlamydia pneumoniae, H. influenzae, Mycoplasma pneumoniae,* **or**
S. pneumoniae; **or caused by** *Legionella
pneumophila, M. catarrhalis,* **or** *S. aureus*
Adults and adolescents age 16 and older:
For mild infections, give 500 mg P.O. as a
single dose on day 1; then 250 mg P.O. daily
on days 2 through 5. Total dose is 1.5 g. For
more severe infections or those caused by
S. aureus, give 500 mg I.V. as a single daily
dose for 2 days; then 500 mg P.O. as a single
daily dose to complete a 7- to 10-day course
of therapy. Switch from I.V. to P.O. therapy
based on patient response.
➤ **Community-acquired pneumonia
caused by** *C. pneumoniae, H. influenzae,
M. pneumoniae,* **or** *S. pneumoniae*

Children age 6 months and older: 10 mg/kg
oral suspension P.O. (maximum of 500 mg)
as a single dose on day 1, followed by
5 mg/kg (maximum of 250 mg) daily on
days 2 through 5. Or, a single dose of Zmax
60 mg/kg.
➤ **Single-dose treatment for mild to
moderate acute bacterial sinusitis caused
by** *H. influenzae, M. catarrhalis,* **or**
S. pneumoniae; **or community-acquired
pneumonia caused by** *C. pneumoniae,
H. influenzae, M. pneumoniae,* **or**
S. pneumoniae
Adults: 2 g Zmax P.O. as a single dose taken
1 hour before or 2 hours after a meal.
➤ **Acute bacterial sinusitis caused by**
H. influenzae, M. catarrhalis, **or**
S. pneumoniae
Adults: 500 mg P.O. daily for 3 days.
Children age 6 months and older: 10 mg/kg
oral suspension P.O. once daily for 3 days.
➤ **Chancroid**
Adults: 1 g P.O. as a single dose.
➤ **Nongonococcal urethritis or cervicitis
caused by** *Chlamydia trachomatis*
Adults and adolescents age 16 and older:
1 g P.O. as a single dose.
➤ **To prevent disseminated** *Mycobacterium avium* **complex in patients with
advanced HIV infection**
Adults and adolescents: 1.2 g P.O. once
weekly alone or with rifabutin.
➤ *M. avium* **complex in patients with
advanced HIV infection**
Adults: 600 mg P.O. daily with ethambutol
15 mg/kg daily.
➤ **Urethritis and cervicitis caused by**
Neisseria gonorrhoeae
Adults: 2 g P.O. as a single dose.
➤ **Pelvic inflammatory disease caused
by** *C. trachomatis, N. gonorrhoeae,* **or**
Mycoplasma hominis **in patients who need
initial I.V. therapy**
Adults and adolescents age 16 and older:
500 mg I.V. as a single daily dose for 1 to
2 days; then 250 mg P.O. daily to complete a
7-day course of therapy. Switch from I.V. to
P.O. therapy based on patient response.
➤ **Otitis media**
Children older than age 6 months: 30 mg/kg
oral suspension P.O. as a single dose; or
10 mg/kg P.O. once daily for 3 days; or

---

10 mg/kg P.O. on day 1 and then 5 mg/kg once daily on days 2 to 5.

➤ **Pharyngitis, tonsillitis**
Children age 2 and older: 12 mg/kg oral suspension (maximum, 500 mg) P.O. daily for 5 days.

➤ **Traveler's diarrhea ◆**
Adults: 1,000 mg P.O. as a single dose.

ADMINISTRATION
P.O.
● Obtain specimen for culture and sensitivity tests before giving first dose. Begin therapy while awaiting results.
● Reconstitute Zmax with 60 mL of water. Shake well. Patient should consume within 12 hours of reconstitution.
● Give Zmax 1 hour before or 2 hours after a meal. Tablets and single-dose packets for oral suspension can be taken with or without food. Don't give with antacids.
● Reconstitute suspension packet with 2 ounces (60 mL) water. After taking, rinse glass with additional 2 ounces water and have patient drink it to ensure he has taken entire dose. Packets aren't for children.

I.V.
▼ Reconstitute drug in 500-mg vial with 4.8 mL of sterile water for injection to yield 100 mg/mL.
▼ Shake well until all drug is dissolved.
▼ Further dilute in 250- or 500-mL normal saline solution, half-normal saline solution, D_5W, or lactated Ringer's solution to yield a final concentration of 1 or 2 mg/mL, respectively.
▼ Infuse a 500-mg dose of azithromycin I.V. over 1 hour or longer. Never give it as a bolus or I.M. injection.
▼ Reconstituted solution and diluted solution are stable for 24 hours when stored below 86° F (30° C). Diluted solution is stable for 7 days when refrigerated at 41° F (5° C).
▼ **Incompatibilities:** Amikacin sulfate, aztreonam, cefotaxime, ceftazidime, ceftriaxone sodium, cefuroxime, ciprofloxacin, clindamycin phosphate, famotidine, fentanyl citrate, furosemide, gentamicin sulfate, imipenem–cilastatin sodium, ketorolac tromethamine, levofloxacin, morphine sulfate, piperacillin–tazobactam sodium, potassium chloride, ticarcillin disodium–clavulanate potassium, tobramycin sulfate.

ACTION
Binds to the 50S subunit of bacterial ribosomes, blocking protein synthesis; bacteriostatic or bactericidal, depending on concentration.

Route	Onset	Peak	Duration
P.O.	Unknown	2–5 hr	Unknown
I.V.	Unknown	Unknown	Unknown

Half-life: About 3 days.

ADVERSE REACTIONS
CNS: fatigue, headache, somnolence.
CV: chest pain, palpitations.
GI: abdominal pain, anorexia, diarrhea, nausea, vomiting, ***pseudomembranous colitis,*** dyspepsia, flatulence, melena.
GU: candidiasis, nephritis, vaginitis.
Hepatic: cholestatic jaundice.
Skin: photosensitivity reactions, rash, pain at injection site, pruritus.
Other: *angioedema.*

INTERACTIONS
Drug-drug. *Antacids containing aluminum and magnesium:* May lower peak azithromycin level (immediate-release form). Separate doses by at least 2 hours.
Antiarrhythmics (amiodarone, quinidine): May increase risk of life-threatening arrhythmias, including torsades de pointes. Monitor ECG rhythm carefully.
Carbamazepine, phenytoin: May increase levels of these drugs. Monitor drug levels.
Cyclosporine: May elevate cyclosporine concentrations with increased risk of nephrotoxicity and neurotoxicity. Monitor cyclosporine levels and renal function.
Digoxin: May increase digoxin level. Monitor digoxin level.
Drugs that prolong QT interval (fluoroquinolones, lithium, methadone, paliperidone, perflutren): May prolong QT interval. Coadminister with caution and monitor patient.
Ergotamine: May cause acute ergotamine toxicity. Monitor patient closely.
HMG-CoA reductase inhibitors (atorvastatin, lovastatin): May increase HMG-CoA reductase inhibitor levels, resulting in

---

Reactions in bold italics are *life-threatening*. Interactions may have a *rapid onset* or a *delayed onset*.

severe myopathy or rhabdomyolysis. Consider alternative therapy.

Nelfinavir: May increase azithromycin level. Monitor for liver enzyme abnormalities and hearing impairment.

Pimozide: May prolong QT interval and cause ventricular tachycardia. Concurrent use is contraindicated.

Theophylline: May increase theophylline level. Monitor theophylline level carefully.

Triazolam: May decrease triazolam clearance. Monitor patient closely.

Warfarin: May increase INR. Monitor INR carefully.

Drug-food. *Any food:* May decrease absorption of multidose oral suspension form. Advise patient to take drug on empty stomach.

Drug-lifestyle. *Sun exposure:* May cause photosensitivity reactions. Advise patient to avoid excessive sunlight exposure.

EFFECTS ON LAB TEST RESULTS
• May increase ALT, AST, creatinine, LDH, and bilirubin levels.

CONTRAINDICATIONS & CAUTIONS
• Contraindicated in patients hypersensitive to erythromycin or other macrolide or ketolide antibiotics.
• Use cautiously in patients with impaired hepatic function.
⚠ **Alert:** Use cautiously in patients at increased risk for torsades de pointes and fatal arrhythmias, including those with known prolonged QT interval, history of torsades de pointes, congenital long QT syndrome, bradyarrhythmias, uncompensated heart failure, uncorrected hypokalemia or hypomagnesemia, clinically significant bradycardia, or concomitant use of drugs known to prolong the QT interval or class IA (procainamide, quinidine) or class III (amiodarone, dofetilide, sotalol) antiarrhythmics.
⚠ **Alert:** Elderly patients may be at increased risk for drug-associated QT-interval effects.

NURSING CONSIDERATIONS
• Monitor patient for superinfection. Drug may cause overgrowth of nonsusceptible bacteria or fungi.

• If patient vomits within 60 minutes of taking Zmax, notify prescriber; additional or different therapy may be needed.
⚠ **Alert:** Monitor patient for *Clostridium difficile* infection, which may range in severity from mild diarrhea to fatal colitis.
⚠ **Alert:** Consider full risk profile when choosing appropriate antibiotic therapy. Alternative macrolide or fluoroquinolone class drugs also have the potential to cause QT-interval prolongation and other significant adverse effects.

PATIENT TEACHING
• Tell patient to take drug as prescribed, even after he feels better.
• Advise patient to avoid excessive sunlight and to wear protective clothing and use sunscreen when outside.
• Tell patient to report adverse reactions promptly.
⚠ **Alert:** Warn patient to seek immediate medical care for irregular heartbeat, shortness of breath, dizziness, or fainting.
• Advise patient not to stop taking drug without first contacting the health care provider.
• Tell patient to take Zmax at least 1 hour before or 2 hours after a meal.
• Teach patient to reconstitute Zmax and to shake well before use.
• Tell patient that immediate-release tablets and suspension can be taken with or without food. Food may reduce GI upset.

aztreonam
AZ-tree-oh-nam

Azactam, Cayston

Therapeutic class: Antibiotics
Pharmacologic class: Monobactams
Pregnancy risk category: B

AVAILABLE FORMS
Inhalation: 75-mg ampule
Injection: 1-g vials, 2-g vials

INDICATIONS & DOSAGES

➤ **UTI; septicemia; infections of lower respiratory tract, skin, and skin structures; intra-abdominal infections, surgical infections, and gynecologic infections caused by susceptible *Escherichia coli, Klebsiella pneumoniae, Proteus mirabilis, Pseudomonas aeruginosa, Enterobacter cloacae, Klebsiella oxytoca, Citrobacter* species, and *Serratia marcescens;* respiratory infections caused by *Haemophilus influenzae***

Adults: 500 mg to 2 g I.V. or I.M. every 8 to 12 hours. For severe systemic or life-threatening infections, 2 g every 6 to 8 hours. Maximum dose is 8 g daily.

Children ages 9 months and older: 30 mg/kg I.V. every 6 to 8 hours. Maximum dose is 120 mg/kg/day.

Adjust-a-dose: For adults with CrCl of 10 to 30 mL/minute, give 1 to 2 g; then give 50% of the usual dose at usual interval. If CrCl is less than 10 mL/minute, give 500 mg to 2 g; then give 25% of the usual dose at usual interval. For serious infections, add one-eighth of the initial dose to maintenance doses after each hemodialysis session.

➤ **To improve respiratory symptoms in cystic fibrosis patients with *P. aeruginosa* infection**

Adults and children age 7 and older: 75 mg inhalation t.i.d. for 28 days, followed by 28 days off.

➤ **Surgical prophylaxis ◆**

Adults: 1 to 2 g I.V. over 20 to 60 minutes 1 hour before incision. Redosing may be necessary every 3 to 5 hours, with discontinuation within 24 hours after operation.

ADMINISTRATION

Inhalation

● Give bronchodilator before administering aztreonam.

● Give short-acting bronchodilators 15 minutes to 4 hours before each dose or long-acting bronchodilators 30 minutes to 12 hours before each dose.

● Space doses at least 4 hours apart.

● Treatment order for patients on multiple therapies is bronchodilator, mucolytics, then aztreonam.

● Don't reconstitute until ready to give dose.

● Add one ampule of diluent to one amber glass vial of aztreonam. Replace rubber stopper on vial and gently swirl until contents have completely dissolved. Administer immediately.

● Don't use diluent or reconstituted drug if it's cloudy or if there are particles in the solution.

● Use only Altera Nebulizer System to administer drug.

● Never mix with other drugs in nebulizer.

● Administration usually takes 2 to 3 minutes.

I.V.

▼ Obtain specimen for culture and sensitivity tests before giving first dose. Begin therapy while awaiting results.

▼ For direct injection, reconstitute with 6 to 10 mL of sterile water for injection and immediately shake vial vigorously. Constituted solutions aren't for multiple-dose use. Discard unused solution.

▼ To give a bolus, inject drug over 3 to 5 minutes, directly into I.V. tubing.

▼ For infusion, reconstitute with a compatible I.V. solution to yield 20 mg/mL or less.

▼ Give infusions over 20 minutes to 1 hour.

▼ Give thawed solutions only by I.V. infusion.

▼ **Incompatibilities:** Acyclovir, amphotericin B, ampicillin sodium, azithromycin, chlorpromazine, daunorubicin, ganciclovir, lorazepam, metronidazole, mitomycin, mitoxantrone, nafcillin, prochlorperazine, streptozocin, vancomycin.

I.M.

● To prepare I.M. injection, add at least 3 mL of one of the following solutions per gram of aztreonam: sterile water for injection, bacteriostatic water for injection, normal saline solution, or bacteriostatic normal saline solution.

● Give I.M. injections deep into a large muscle, such as the upper outer quadrant of the gluteus maximus or the side of the thigh. Give doses more than 1 g by I.V. route.

❸ *Alert:* Don't give I.M. injection to children.

● Pain and swelling may occur at injection site.

Reactions in bold italics are ***life-threatening***. Interactions may have a ***rapid onset*** or a ***delayed onset***.

ACTION

Inhibits bacterial cell-wall synthesis, ultimately causing cell-wall destruction; bactericidal.

Route	Onset	Peak	Duration
I.V.	Unknown	Immediate	Unknown
I.M.	Unknown	<1 hr	Unknown
Inhalation	Unknown	1 hr	Unknown

Half-life: 2 hours.

ADVERSE REACTIONS

CNS: *seizures,* confusion, headache, insomnia, pyrexia.
CV: hypotension, thrombophlebitis, chest discomfort.
EENT: nasal congestion, sore throat.
GI: *pseudomembranous colitis,* diarrhea, abdominal pain, nausea, vomiting.
Hematologic: *neutropenia, pancytopenia, thrombocytopenia,* anemia, leukocytosis, thrombocytosis.
Respiratory: bronchospasm, cough.
Skin: discomfort and swelling at I.M. injection site, rash.
Other: hypersensitivity reactions.

INTERACTIONS

Drug-drug. *Aminoglycosides:* May have synergistic nephrotoxic effects. Monitor renal function.
Cefoxitin, imipenem: May have antagonistic effect. Avoid using together.
Furosemide: May increase aztreonam level. Avoid using together.
Probenecid: May increase aztreonam level. Avoid using together.

EFFECTS ON LAB TEST RESULTS

• May increase ALT, AST, BUN, creatinine, and LDH levels. May decrease hemoglobin level.
• May increase PT, PTT, and INR. May decrease neutrophil and RBC counts. May increase or decrease platelet and WBC counts.
• May cause false-positive Coombs test result. May alter urine glucose determinations using cupric sulfate (Clinitest or Benedict reagent).

CONTRAINDICATIONS & CAUTIONS

• Contraindicated in patients hypersensitive to drug or its components.
• Use cautiously in elderly patients and in those with impaired renal or hepatic function. Dosage adjustment may be needed. Monitor renal function test results.
• Use during pregnancy only if clearly needed. Because aztreonam is excreted in breast milk, consider advising breast-feeding women to temporarily discontinue breast-feeding.

NURSING CONSIDERATIONS

• Observe patient for signs and symptoms of superinfection.
❸ *Alert:* Because drug is ineffective against gram-positive and anaerobic organisms, combine it with other antibiotics for immediate treatment of life-threatening illnesses.
❸ *Alert:* Patients allergic to penicillins or cephalosporins may not be allergic to this drug. Monitor closely those who have had an immediate hypersensitivity reaction to these antibiotics, especially to ceftazidime.
• Antibiotics may promote overgrowth of nonsusceptible organisms. Monitor patient for signs of superinfection.
• Dosage of Cayston isn't based on weight or adjusted for age.

PATIENT TEACHING

• Warn patient receiving I.M. drug that pain and swelling may occur at injection site.
• Tell patient to report discomfort at I.V. insertion site.
• Instruct patient to report adverse reactions and signs and symptoms of superinfection promptly.
• Instruct patient or caregiver in proper administration of drug by nebulizer.
• Teach patient or caregiver to use bronchodilator before using Cayston.

baclofen
BAK-loe-fen

Gablofen, Lioresal Intrathecal

Therapeutic class: Skeletal muscle relaxants
Pharmacologic class: Gamma-aminobutyric acid derivatives
Pregnancy risk category: C

AVAILABLE FORMS
Intrathecal injection: 50 mcg/mL, 500 mcg/mL, 1,000 mcg/mL, 2,000 mcg/mL
Tablets: 10 mg, 20 mg

INDICATIONS & DOSAGES
Adjust-a-dose (for all indications): For patients with impaired renal function, decrease oral and intrathecal doses.
➤ **Spasticity in multiple sclerosis; spinal cord injury**
Adults and children age 12 and older:
Initially, 5 mg P.O. t.i.d. for 3 days; then 10 mg t.i.d. for 3 days, 15 mg t.i.d. for 3 days, 20 mg t.i.d. for 3 days. Increase daily dosage, based on response, to maximum of 80 mg.
Adjust-a-dose: For patients with psychiatric or brain disorders and for elderly patients, increase dose gradually.
➤ **To manage severe spasticity in patients who don't respond to or can't tolerate oral baclofen therapy**
Adults: For screening phase, after test dose to check responsiveness, give drug via implantable infusion pump. Give test dose of 1 mL of 50-mcg/mL dilution into intrathecal space by barbotage over 1 minute or longer. Significantly decreased severity or frequency of muscle spasm or reduced muscle tone should appear within 4 to 8 hours. If response is inadequate, give second test dose of 75 mcg/1.5 mL 24 hours after the first. If response is still inadequate, give final test dose of 100 mcg/2 mL after 24 hours. Patients unresponsive to the 100-mcg dose shouldn't be considered candidates for implantable pump.
Children: Initial test dose is the same as that for adults (50 mcg); for very small children, initial dose is 25 mcg.

For maintenance therapy: Adjust first dose based on screening dose that elicited an adequate response. Double this effective dose and give over 24 hours. However, if screening dose effectiveness was maintained for 12 hours or longer, don't double the dose. After the first 24 hours, increase dose slowly as needed and tolerated by 10% to 30% increments at 24-hour intervals in spasticity of spinal cord origin. In children with spasticity of spinal cord origin and adults and children with spasticity of cerebral origin, increase by 5% to 15% increments at 24-hour intervals. During prolonged maintenance therapy, increase daily dose by 10% to 40% in spasticity of spinal cord origin, or increase daily dose by 5% to 15% in spasticity of cerebral origin, if needed; if patient experiences adverse effects, decrease dose by 10% to 20%. Maintenance dosages range from 12 to 2,000 mcg daily, but experience with dosages of more than 1,000 mcg daily is limited. Most patients need 300 to 800 mcg daily.
➤ **Hiccups that are intractable and unresponsive to other therapies** ◆
Adults: Initially, 5 to 10 mg P.O. t.i.d. Higher doses (up to 30 mg P.O. t.i.d.) may be needed.
➤ **Migraine prevention** ◆
Adults: 15 to 30 mg P.O. t.i.d.
➤ **Trigeminal neuralgia** ◆
Adults: 30 to 80 mg/day P.O. in three to four divided doses. Initial dose is typically 5 to 10 mg P.O. daily and then titrated (10 mg every other day) over 1 to 2 weeks.
➤ **Tourette syndrome** ◆
Children and adolescents: 10 to 15 mg P.O. daily in three to four divided doses. Titrate to 60 to 80 mg daily for up to 4 weeks.

ADMINISTRATION
P.O.
● Give drug with meals or milk to prevent GI distress.
Intrathecal
Black Box Warning Don't discontinue abruptly. This can result in high fever, altered mental status, exaggerated rebound spasticity, and muscle rigidity, which in rare cases, has led to rhabdomyolysis, multiple organ-system failure, and death. ∎

Reactions in bold italics are *life-threatening*. Interactions may have a *rapid onset* or a *delayed onset*.

● Don't give intrathecal injection by I.V., I.M., subcutaneous, or epidural route.
● If patient suddenly requires a large intrathecal dose increase, check for a catheter complication, such as kinking or dislodgment.
● With long-term intrathecal use, about 5% of patients may develop tolerance to drug. In some cases, this may be treated by hospitalizing patient and slowly withdrawing drug over a 2-week period.

ACTION

Hyperpolarizes fibers to reduce impulse transmission. Appears to reduce transmission of impulses from the spinal cord to skeletal muscle, thus decreasing the frequency and amplitude of muscle spasms in patients with spinal cord lesions.

Route	Onset	Peak	Duration
P.O.	Unknown	2–3 hr	Unknown
Intrathecal	30 min–1 hr	4 hr	4–8 hr

Half-life: 2½ to 4 hours.

ADVERSE REACTIONS

CNS: drowsiness, dizziness, headache, weakness, fatigue, hypotonia, confusion, insomnia, *seizures with intrathecal use.*
CV: hypotension.
EENT: nasal congestion.
GI: nausea, constipation.
GU: urinary frequency.
Metabolic: hyperglycemia, weight gain.
Musculoskeletal: muscle rigidity or spasticity, *rhabdomyolysis,* muscle weakness.
Respiratory: dyspnea.
Skin: rash, pruritus, excessive sweating.
Other: *multiple organ-system failure.*

INTERACTIONS

Drug-drug. *CNS depressants:* May increase CNS depression. Avoid using together.
Drug-lifestyle. *Alcohol use:* May increase CNS depression. Discourage use together.

EFFECTS ON LAB TEST RESULTS

● May increase alkaline phosphatase, AST, CK, and glucose levels.

CONTRAINDICATIONS & CAUTIONS

● Contraindicated in patients hypersensitive to drug.
● Use cautiously in patients with impaired renal function or seizure disorder or when spasticity is used to maintain motor function.
● Use cautiously in patients with psychotic disorders, schizophrenia, or confusional states. Exacerbations of these conditions have occurred.
⚠ **Overdose S&S:** Coma, dizziness, lightheadedness, diminished reflexes, vomiting, hypotonia, increased salivation, drowsiness, vision changes, respiratory depression, seizures.

NURSING CONSIDERATIONS

❂ **Alert:** Don't use oral drug to treat muscle spasm caused by rheumatic disorders, cerebral palsy, Parkinson disease, or stroke because drug's effectiveness for these indications hasn't been established.
● Watch for sensitivity reactions, such as fever, skin eruptions, and respiratory distress.
● Expect an increased risk of seizures in patients with seizure disorder.
● The amount of relief determines whether dosage (and drowsiness) can be reduced.
Black Box Warning Don't withdraw intrathecal drug abruptly after long-term use unless severe adverse reactions demand it; doing so may precipitate seizures, high fever, hallucinations, or rebound spasticity. ▮
● *Look alike–sound alike:* Don't confuse baclofen with Bactroban.

PATIENT TEACHING

Black Box Warning Advise patient and caregivers of risks associated with abrupt discontinuation of intrathecal form. Tell them to keep scheduled refill visits and teach them the signs and symptoms of baclofen withdrawal. ▮
● Instruct patient to take oral form with meals or milk.
● Tell patient to avoid activities that require alertness until CNS effects of drug are known. Drowsiness usually is transient.

- Tell patient to avoid alcohol and OTC antihistamines while taking drug.
- Advise patient to follow prescriber's orders regarding rest and physical therapy.
- Teach patient and caregivers about the signs and symptoms of overdose and what to do if an overdose occurs.
- Teach patient and caregivers proper home care of pump and insertion site.

basiliximab
ba-sil-IK-si-mab

Simulect

Therapeutic class: Immunosuppressants
Pharmacologic class: Monoclonal antibodies
Pregnancy risk category: B

AVAILABLE FORMS
Injection: 10-mg, 20-mg vials

INDICATIONS & DOSAGES
➤ **To prevent acute organ rejection in patients receiving renal transplantation when used as part of an immunosuppressive regimen that includes cyclosporine and corticosteroids**
Adults and children weighing 35 kg (77 lb) or more: 20 mg I.V. given within 2 hours before transplant surgery and 20 mg I.V. given 4 days after transplantation.
Children weighing less than 35 kg: 10 mg I.V. given within 2 hours before transplant surgery and 10 mg I.V. given 4 days after transplantation.

ADMINISTRATION
I.V.
▼ Reconstitute 10-mg vial with 2.5 mL sterile water for injection. Reconstitute 20-mg vial with 5 mL sterile water for injection. Shake gently to dissolve powder.
▼ Use reconstituted solution immediately.
▼ Dilute reconstituted solution to 25 mL (10-mg vial) or 50 mL (20-mg vial) with normal saline solution or D₅W for infusion.
▼ When mixing solution, invert bag gently to avoid foaming. Don't shake.
▼ Infuse over 20 to 30 minutes.

▼ Drug may be given as a bolus injection, but doing so may cause nausea, vomiting, pain, and local reactions.
▼ Reconstituted solution may be refrigerated at 36° to 46° F (2° to 8° C) for up to 24 hours or kept at room temperature for 4 hours.
▼ **Incompatibilities:** Don't add or infuse other drugs simultaneously through same I.V. line.

ACTION
Binds specifically to and blocks the interleukin (IL)-2 receptor alpha chain on the surface of activated T lymphocytes, inhibiting IL-2–mediated activation of lymphocytes, a critical pathway in the cellular immune response involved in allograft rejection.

Route	Onset	Peak	Duration
I.V.	Unknown	Immediate	Unknown

Half-life: About 7¼ days in adults, 9½ days in children, 9 days in adolescents.

ADVERSE REACTIONS
CNS: fever, headache, insomnia, tremor, agitation, anxiety, asthenia, depression, dizziness, hypoesthesia, neuropathy, paresthesia, fatigue.
CV: hypertension, leg or peripheral edema, *arrhythmias, heart failure,* angina pectoris, atrial fibrillation, chest pain, abnormal heart sounds, aggravated hypertension, hypotension, tachycardia, generalized edema.
EENT: pharyngitis, rhinitis, abnormal vision, cataract, conjunctivitis, sinusitis.
GI: abdominal pain, candidiasis, constipation, diarrhea, dyspepsia, nausea, vomiting, *GI hemorrhage,* esophagitis, enlarged abdomen, flatulence, gastroenteritis, GI disorder, gum hyperplasia, melena, ulcerative stomatitis.
GU: UTI, abnormal renal function, albuminuria, bladder disorder, dysuria, frequent micturition, genital edema, hematuria, increased nonprotein nitrogen, oliguria, *renal tubular necrosis,* ureteral disorder, urine retention, erectile dysfunction.
Hematologic: anemia, *hemorrhage, thrombocytopenia,* hematoma, polycythemia, purpura, thrombosis.

Reactions in bold italics are *life-threatening*. Interactions may have a *rapid onset* or a *delayed onset*.

B

Metabolic: hypercholesterolemia, hyperglycemia, hyperkalemia, hyperuricemia, hypokalemia, hypophosphatemia, acidosis, dehydration, *diabetes mellitus,* fluid overload, hypercalcemia, hyperlipidemia, hypertriglyceridemia, hypocalcemia, *hypomagnesemia,* hypoproteinemia, weight gain.

Musculoskeletal: arthralgia, arthropathy, back pain, bone fracture, cramps, hernia, leg pain, myalgia.

Respiratory: dyspnea, upper respiratory tract infection, *bronchospasm, pulmonary edema,* abnormal chest sounds, bronchitis, cough, pneumonia, pulmonary disorder.

Skin: acne, cyst, hypertrichosis, pruritus, rash, skin disorder or ulceration.

Other: surgical wound complications, viral infection, *hypersensitivity reactions, sepsis,* accidental trauma, infection, herpes zoster, herpes simplex.

INTERACTIONS
None significant.

EFFECTS ON LAB TEST RESULTS
• May increase calcium, cholesterol, glucose, lipid, and uric acid levels. May decrease hemoglobin, magnesium, phosphorus, and protein levels. May increase or decrease potassium level.
• May increase RBC count. May decrease platelet count.

CONTRAINDICATIONS & CAUTIONS
• Contraindicated in patients hypersensitive to drug or its components.
Black Box Warning Use cautiously and only under supervision of prescriber qualified and experienced in immunosuppressive therapy and organ transplantation. Patients should be managed in facilities equipped with adequate laboratory and supportive medical services. ∎
• Use cautiously in elderly patients.

NURSING CONSIDERATIONS
• Severe acute hypersensitivity reactions can occur within 24 hours after administration. Make sure drugs for treating hypersensitivity reactions are readily available; withhold second dose if hypersensitivity reactions occur.

• Check for electrolyte imbalances and acidosis during drug therapy.
• Monitor patient's intake and output, vital signs, hemoglobin level, and hematocrit during therapy.
• Be alert for signs and symptoms of opportunistic infections during drug therapy.

PATIENT TEACHING
• Inform patient of potential benefits of and risks related to immunosuppressive therapy, including decreased risk of graft loss or acute rejection.
• Advise patient that immunosuppressive therapy increases risk of developing infection. Tell him to report signs and symptoms of infection promptly.
• Inform women of childbearing age to use effective contraception before therapy starts and for 4 months after therapy ends.
• Instruct patient to report adverse effects immediately.
• Explain that drug is used with cyclosporine and corticosteroids.

beclomethasone dipropionate (inhalation)
be-kloe-METH-a-sone

QVAR 40, QVAR 80

Therapeutic class: Corticosteroids
Pharmacologic class: Corticosteroids
Pregnancy risk category: C

AVAILABLE FORMS
Oral inhalation aerosol: 40 mcg/metered spray, 80 mcg/metered spray

INDICATIONS & DOSAGES
➤ **Chronic asthma**
Adults and children age 12 and older: Starting dose, 40 to 80 mcg b.i.d. when previously used bronchodilators alone, or 40 to 160 mcg b.i.d. when previously used inhaled corticosteroids. Maximum, 320 mcg b.i.d.
Children ages 5 to 11: 40 mcg b.i.d., up to 80 mcg b.i.d.

➤ **Asthma** ◆
Children younger than age 5: 200 to
400 mcg inhaled nebulized suspension
b.i.d. for up to 6 months.

ADMINISTRATION
Inhalational
● Prime the inhaler before first use by depressing canister twice into the air.
● Allow 1 minute to elapse between inhalations.

ACTION
May decrease inflammation by decreasing
the number and activity of inflammatory
cells, inhibiting bronchoconstrictor mechanisms producing direct smooth-muscle
relaxation, and decreasing airway hyperresponsiveness.

Route	Onset	Peak	Duration
Inhalation	1–4 wk	Unknown	Unknown

Half-life: 2.8 hours.

ADVERSE REACTIONS
CNS: headache.
EENT: hoarseness, throat irritation, fungal
infection of throat, pharyngitis, rhinitis,
sinusitis.
GI: fungal infection of mouth, dry mouth.
Musculoskeletal: back pain.
Respiratory: cough, upper respiratory
tract infection, exacerbation of asthma,
wheezing.
Other: *angioedema,* facial edema, hypersensitivity reactions, *adrenal insufficiency,*
suppression of hypothalamic-pituitary-
adrenal function.

INTERACTIONS
None significant.

EFFECTS ON LAB TEST RESULTS
None reported.

CONTRAINDICATIONS & CAUTIONS
● Contraindicated in patients hypersensitive
to drug or its ingredients and in those with
status asthmaticus, nonasthmatic bronchial
diseases, or asthma controlled by bronchodilators or other noncorticosteroids
alone.

● Use cautiously, if at all, in patients with
tuberculosis, fungal or bacterial infections,
ocular herpes simplex, or systemic viral
infections.
● Use cautiously in patients receiving systemic corticosteroid therapy.

NURSING CONSIDERATIONS
● Check mucous membranes frequently for
signs and symptoms of fungal infection.
● During times of stress (trauma, surgery,
or infection), systemic corticosteroids may
be needed to prevent adrenal insufficiency
in previously corticosteroid-dependent
patients.
● Periodic measurement of growth and
development may be needed during high-
dose or prolonged therapy in children.
❸ *Alert:* Taper oral corticosteroid therapy
slowly. Acute adrenal insufficiency and
death may occur in patients with asthma
who change abruptly from oral corticosteroids to beclomethasone.
❸ *Alert:* Bronchospasm may occur after
dosing and should be treated immediately
with a short-acting inhaled bronchodilator.

PATIENT TEACHING
● Tell patient to prime the inhaler before
first use, or after 10 days of not using it, by
depressing canister twice into the air.
● Inform patient that drug doesn't relieve
acute asthma attacks.
● Tell patient who needs a bronchodilator to
use it several minutes before beclomethasone.
● Instruct patient to carry or wear medical
identification indicating his need for supplemental systemic corticosteroids during
stress.
● Advise patient to allow 1 minute to elapse
between inhalations of drug and to hold his
breath for a few seconds to enhance drug
action.
● Tell patient it may take up to 4 weeks to
feel the full benefit of the drug.
● Tell patient to keep inhaler clean by wiping it weekly with a dry tissue or cloth; don't
get it wet.
● Advise patient to prevent oral fungal
infections by gargling or rinsing his mouth
with water after each use. Caution him not
to swallow the water.

Reactions in bold italics are *life-threatening*. Interactions may have a *rapid onset* or a *delayed onset*.

• Tell patient to report evidence of corticosteroid withdrawal, including fatigue, weakness, arthralgia, orthostatic hypotension, and dyspnea.
• Instruct patient to store drug at 77° F (25° C). Advise patient to ensure delivery of proper dose by gently warming canister to room temperature before using.

beclomethasone dipropionate (intranasal)
be-kloe-METH-a-sone

Beconase AQ, Qnasl

Therapeutic class: Corticosteroids
Pharmacologic class: Corticosteroids
Pregnancy risk category: C

AVAILABLE FORMS
Nasal aerosol solution: 80 mcg/actuation
Nasal spray: 42 mcg/metered spray

INDICATIONS & DOSAGES
➤ **To relieve symptoms of seasonal or perennial rhinitis and nonallergic (vasomotor) rhinitis; to prevent nasal polyp recurrence after surgical removal (Beconase AQ)**
Adults and children age 12 and older: 1 or 2 sprays in each nostril b.i.d.
Children ages 6 to 12: Initially, 1 spray in each nostril b.i.d. May increase to 2 sprays in each nostril b.i.d. Once adequate control is achieved, decrease to 1 spray in each nostril b.i.d.
➤ **To relieve symptoms of seasonal or perennial rhinitis (Qnasl)**
Adults and children age 12 and older: 320 mcg/day administered as 2 nasal aerosol sprays in each nostril once daily.

ADMINISTRATION
Intranasal
• Pump nasal spray six times until a fine mist is produced before first use.
• Shake before use; pump once or twice before first use each day.

ACTION
May reduce nasal inflammation by inhibiting mediators of inflammation.

Route	Onset	Peak	Duration
Intranasal	5–7 days	3 wk	Unknown

Half-life: 15 hours.

ADVERSE REACTIONS
CNS: headache, light-headedness.
EENT: mild, transient nasal burning and stinging; dryness, epistaxis, nasal congestion, nasopharyngeal fungal infections, rhinorrhea, sneezing, watery eyes.
GI: nausea.
Metabolic: growth velocity reduction in children and adolescents.

INTERACTIONS
None significant.

EFFECTS ON LAB TEST RESULTS
None reported.

CONTRAINDICATIONS & CAUTIONS
• Contraindicated in patients hypersensitive to drug and in those with untreated localized infection involving the nasal mucosa.
• Not recommended for children younger than age 6.
• Use cautiously, if at all, in patients with active or quiescent respiratory tract tuberculous infections or untreated fungal, bacterial, or systemic viral or ocular herpes simplex infections.
• Use cautiously in patients who have recently had nasal septal ulcers, nasal surgery, or trauma until wound healing occurs.
⚠ **Overdose S&S:** Hypercorticism, adrenal suppression.

NURSING CONSIDERATIONS
• Observe patient for fungal infections.
• Drug isn't effective for acute exacerbations of rhinitis. Decongestants or antihistamines may be needed.
• Stop drug if no significant symptom improvement occurs after 3 weeks.

PATIENT TEACHING
• Advise patient or parent to read package insert for instructions on drug use.

• Advise patient to pump nasal spray six times until a fine mist is produced before first use. If nasal spray pump hasn't been used for 7 or more days, it should be reprimed.

• To instill, instruct patient to blow nose to clear nasal passages, shake container, tilt head slightly forward, and insert nozzle into nostril, pointing away from septum. Tell him to hold other nostril closed and inhale gently while spraying, hold breath for a few seconds, and exhale through the mouth. Next, have him shake container and repeat in other nostril.

• Tell patient to pump nasal spray once or twice before first use each day. He should clean the cap and nosepiece of the activator in warm water every day, and then allow them to air-dry.

• Advise patient to use drug regularly, as prescribed, because its effectiveness depends on regular use.

• Explain that unlike decongestants, drug doesn't work right away. Most patients notice improvement within a few days, but some may need 2 to 3 weeks.

• Warn patient not to exceed recommended dosage because of risk of hypothalamic-pituitary-adrenal axis suppression.

• Tell patient to notify prescriber if signs and symptoms don't improve within 3 weeks or if nasal irritation persists.

• Teach patient good nasal and oral hygiene.

✳ NEW DRUG

bedaquiline fumarate
bed-AK-wi-leen

Sirturo

Therapeutic class: Antituberculotics
Pharmacologic class: Diarylquinolines
Pregnancy risk category: B

AVAILABLE FORMS
Tablets: 100 mg

INDICATIONS & DOSAGES
Black Box Warning Drug should be reserved for use when an effective treatment regimen can't otherwise be provided. ∎

➤ **Pulmonary multidrug-resistant tuberculosis (TB) as part of combination therapy**
Adults: Weeks 1 and 2, give 400 mg P.O. once daily. Weeks 3 to 24, give 200 mg P.O. three times a week (48 hours between doses) for a total of 600 mg/week.
Adjust-a-dose: In first 2 weeks, if a dose is missed, don't make it up but continue the dosing schedule. From 3 weeks on, if a dose is missed, have patient take dose as soon as possible, then resume the three-times-a-week schedule.

ADMINISTRATION
P.O.
• Administer by directly observed therapy (DOT).
• Give with food.
• Give tablets whole with water. Don't crush, split, or allow patient to chew tablets.
• Allow a minimum of 48 hours between doses after initial 2 weeks of therapy.
• Store tablets at room temperature in a light-resistant container with an expiration of not more than 3 months if transferred from the original container.

ACTION
Inhibits mycobacterial adenosine 5′-triphosphate synthase, an enzyme essential for the generation of energy in *Mycobacterium tuberculosis*.

Route	Onset	Peak	Duration
P.O.	Unknown	5 hr	Unknown

Half-life: 5 months.

ADVERSE REACTIONS
CNS: headache.
CV: chest pain, *QTc-interval prolongation.*
GI: nausea, anorexia.
Musculoskeletal: arthralgia.
Respiratory: hemoptysis.
Skin: rash.

INTERACTIONS
Drug-drug. **Black Box Warning** *Drugs that prolong QT interval (clofazimine, fluoroquinolones, macrolides):* May increase risk of prolonged QT interval. Monitor ECG frequently. ∎

Reactions in bold italics are *life-threatening*. Interactions may have a *rapid onset* or a *delayed onset*.

Lopinavir–ritonavir: May increase bedaquiline level and risk of adverse reactions. Use together only if benefits outweigh risk.
Strong CYP3A4 inducers (rifabutin, rifampin, rifapentine): May decrease bedaquiline level. Avoid use together.
Strong CYP3A4 inhibitors (ketoconazole): May increase bedaquiline level. Avoid concomitant use for more than 14 consecutive days. Monitor patient for adverse reactions.
Drug-lifestyle. *Alcohol use:* May increase risk of liver injury. Discourage use together.

EFFECTS ON LAB TEST RESULTS
• May increase transaminase and amylase levels.

CONTRAINDICATIONS & CAUTIONS
Black Box Warning Drug's use increased risk of death compared to placebo. Only use when an effective treatment regimen can't otherwise be provided. ∎
Black Box Warning QT-interval prolongation can occur. Use of bedaquiline with drugs that prolong QT interval may cause additive QT-interval prolongation. ∎
• Contraindicated in patients hypersensitive to drug or its components and in those with latent, extrapulmonary, or drug-sensitive TB.
• Use cautiously in patients with severe renal impairment, history of torsades de pointes, congenital long QT syndrome, hypothyroidism, bradyarrhythmia, uncompensated heart failure, hypocalcemia, hypomagnesemia, or hypokalemia.
• Use in severe hepatic dysfunction hasn't been study. Use only if benefits outweigh risk.
• Use in pregnant women hasn't been studied. Use only if benefits outweigh risk.
• It's unknown if drug appears in breast milk. Patient should discontinue drug or discontinue breast-feeding.

NURSING CONSIDERATIONS
• There is a risk of treatment failure if patient is noncompliant. Drug must be given by DOT.
• Monitor LFTs at baseline and monthly as needed. Repeat within 48 hours if elevation of more than 3 times the upper limit of normal (ULN) occurs. Test for viral hepatitis and discontinue all hepatotoxic drugs.
• Discontinue drug if transaminase levels are more than 8 times ULN, persist for more than 2 weeks, or occur with total bilirubin level elevation of more than 2 times ULN.
• Monitor patient for hepatic dysfunction (fatigue, anorexia, nausea, jaundice, dark urine, liver tenderness, hepatomegaly).
• Monitor ECG before therapy and at 2, 12, and 24 weeks after start of therapy.
• Discontinue drug if clinically significant ventricular arrhythmia occurs or QTc interval is more than 500 ms. Continue to monitor ECG to confirm QTc interval returns to baseline.
• Assess ECG for QT-interval prolongation with syncopal episode.
• Monitor potassium, calcium, and magnesium levels before therapy and correct if abnormal. Assess electrolyte levels if QT-interval prolongation is detected.

PATIENT TEACHING
• Inform patient that drug will be given as part of DOT.
• Advise patient that tablet must be swallowed whole and not dissolved, crushed, or chewed.
• Caution patient to take bedaquiline with the other medications prescribed for TB.
• Advise patient not to miss doses and to complete full course of therapy for treatment to be effective and to decrease risk of untreatable TB.
• Instruct patient to keep all follow-up appointments to monitor for drug's side effects.
• Warn patient to avoid alcohol and hepatotoxic drugs or herbal supplements while taking bedaquiline, to decrease risk of liver complications.
• Advise patient to consult practitioner if there is a personal or family history of congenital QT-interval prolongation or heart failure.

belimumab

beh-LIH-moo-mab

Benlysta

Therapeutic class: Immunosuppressants
Pharmacologic class: Human mono-clonal antibodies
Pregnancy risk category: C

AVAILABLE FORMS
Injection: 120-mg, 400-mg single-use vials

INDICATIONS & DOSAGES
➤ **Active, autoantibody-positive systemic lupus erythematosus**
Adults: 10 mg/kg I.V. infusion every 2 weeks for first three doses, then every 4 weeks thereafter.

ADMINISTRATION
I.V.
▼ Premedicate for prophylaxis against infusion or hypersensitivity reactions.
▼ Store unopened vials in refrigerator.
▼ Once vial has been at room temperature for 10 to 15 minutes, reconstitute with sterile water: 1.5 mL for 120-mg vial and 4.8 mL for 400-mg vial.
▼ Direct stream of sterile water toward side of vial to minimize foaming. Gently swirl for 60 seconds every 5 minutes until dissolved. Don't shake. Protect solution from light while dissolving.
▼ Solution should be opalescent and color-less to pale yellow.
▼ Dilute in 250 mL normal saline solution only.
▼ From the 250-mL normal saline solution bag, withdraw a volume of saline solution equal to the amount of medication to be added so total volume remains at 250 mL. Add the medication to the 250-mL saline bag and discard any unused drug solution.
▼ Protect unused reconstituted solution from light and store in refrigerator. So-lutions in normal saline may be stored in refrigerator or at room temperature.
▼ Administer as an I.V. infusion over 1 hour.
▼ Complete infusion within 8 hours of reconstitution.

▼ **Incompatibilities:** Dextrose solution, other I.V. drugs.

ACTION
Inhibits survival of B cells, including au-toreactive B cells, and reduces their differ-entiation into immunoglobulin-producing plasma cells.

Route	Onset	Peak	Duration
I.V.	Unknown	Unknown	Unknown

Half-life: 19.4 days.

ADVERSE REACTIONS
CNS: insomnia, migraine, depression.
EENT: nasopharyngitis, pharyngitis.
GI: nausea, diarrhea, viral gastroenteritis.
GU: cystitis.
Hematologic: *leukopenia.*
Musculoskeletal: extremity pain.
Respiratory: bronchitis.
Other: infection, antibody detection, pyrexia, hypersensitivity reactions, infu-sion reactions.

INTERACTIONS
Drug-drug. *I.V. cyclophosphamide, other biological agents:* Use together hasn't been studied. Don't use together.
Live-virus vaccines: May impair response to vaccines. Don't give live-virus vaccines for 30 days before or concurrently with belimumab.

EFFECTS ON LAB TEST RESULTS
● May decrease leukocyte count.

CONTRAINDICATIONS & CAUTIONS
● Contraindicated in patients with a history of anaphylaxis to belimumab.
● Use cautiously in patients with a history of chronic infection, hypersensitivity re-actions, infusion reactions, depression, or malignancies.
● More deaths occurred with belimumab than with placebo during the controlled period of the main clinical trials. No single cause of death predominated, but possible causes included infection, CV disease, and suicide.

• Use cautiously in pregnant women and only if the potential benefit outweighs the risk to the fetus. A pregnancy registry to monitor maternal-fetal outcomes of exposure to belimumab has been established. Health care providers or pregnant women should call 1-877-681-6296 to enroll.

• Use cautiously in breast-feeding women after considering the risk to the infant and the importance of the drug to the mother.

• Safety and effectiveness in children haven't been established.

NURSING CONSIDERATIONS

• Patient shouldn't receive live-virus vaccines for 30 days before or concurrently with drug.

• Premedication is recommended to avoid or minimize allergic reactions.

• Drug should be administered only by a health care professional prepared to manage anaphylaxis.

• Monitor patient for infection. Serious and sometimes fatal infections have occurred in patients receiving immunosuppressants.

• Monitor patient for depression, suicidal ideation, malignancies, allergic reactions, and infusion reactions.

PATIENT TEACHING

• Inform patient that drug will be given in the doctor's office or hospital.

• Warn patient not to skip appointments to ensure drug is given on schedule to improve effectiveness of treatment.

• Tell patient to immediately report signs and symptoms of an allergic reaction (such as itching, hives, shortness of breath, swelling of the face, and throat closure).

• Teach patient infection-prevention measures.

• Instruct patient to immediately report signs and symptoms of infection (such as fever, body aches, cough, and sore throat).

• Tell patient to report history of cancer to health care provider.

• Instruct patient not to receive live-virus vaccines while taking drug.

• Counsel women of childbearing age to use adequate contraception during treatment and for at least 4 months after final dose.

• Advise women to tell their health care provider if they are pregnant or breast-feeding.

benazepril hydrochloride

B

ben-A-za-pril

Lotensin*

Therapeutic class: Antihypertensives
Pharmacologic class: ACE inhibitors
Pregnancy risk category: D

AVAILABLE FORMS

Tablets: 5 mg, 10 mg, 20 mg, 40 mg

INDICATIONS & DOSAGES

Adjust-a-dose (for all indications): If CrCl is below 30 mL/minute, give 5 mg P.O. daily. Daily dose may be adjusted up to 40 mg.

➤ **Hypertension**

Adults: For patients not receiving a diuretic, 10 mg P.O. daily initially. Adjust dosage as needed and tolerated; usually 20 to 40 mg daily in one or two divided doses. For patients receiving a diuretic, 5 mg P.O. daily initially.

Children age 6 and older: 0.2 mg/kg (between 0.1 and 0.6 mg/kg) P.O. daily. Adjust as needed up to 0.6 mg/kg (maximum 40 mg) P.O. daily.

➤ **Nephropathy (nondiabetic)** ◆

Adults: 10 to 20 mg P.O. daily.

➤ **Heart failure; prevention of recurrent stroke** ◆

Adults: 10 mg P.O. daily. May increase monthly. Maintenance dosage is generally between 20 and 40 mg/day. Evaluate patient for potential hypotension within 2 weeks of dosage changes.

ADMINISTRATION

P.O.

• Protect tablets from moisture.

ACTION

Inhibits ACE, preventing conversion of angiotensin I to angiotensin II, a potent vasoconstrictor. Less angiotensin II decreases peripheral arterial resistance, decreasing aldosterone secretion, which reduces sodium and water retention and lowers blood pressure. Drug also acts as antihypertensive in patients with low-renin hypertension.

Route	Onset	Peak	Duration
P.O.	1 hr	2–4 hr	24 hr

Half-life: 10 to 11 hours.

ADVERSE REACTIONS
CNS: headache, dizziness, somnolence.
CV: symptomatic hypotension.

INTERACTIONS
Drug-drug. *Aliskiren:* May increase risk of renal impairment, hypotension, and hyperkalemia in diabetic patients and those with moderate to severe renal impairment (GFR less than 60 mL/minute). Concomitant use is contraindicated in diabetic patients. Avoid concomitant use in those with moderate to severe renal impairment.
Angiotensin II receptor antagonists (telmisartan): May increase risk of renal dysfunction. Use with caution and monitor renal function.
Antidiabetics, insulin: May increase risk of hypoglycemia. Monitor patient carefully.
Azathioprine: May increase risk of anemia or leukopenia. Monitor hematologic study results if used together.
Diuretics, other antihypertensives: May cause excessive hypotension. Stop diuretic or lower dosage of benazepril, as needed.
Everolimus: May increase risk of angioedema. Discontinue one or both agents if an interaction is suspected.
Gold salts: May increase risk of nitritoid reaction. Carefully monitor patients.
Iron salts (parenteral): May increase risk of adverse reactions to iron salts. Monitor patient closely.
Lithium: May increase lithium level and toxicity. Use together cautiously; monitor lithium level.
Nesiritide: May increase risk of hypotension. Monitor blood pressure.
NSAIDs: May decrease antihypertensive effects. Monitor blood pressure.
Pergolide, phenothiazines (chlorpromazine): May cause profound hypotension. Use with caution and monitor blood pressure.
Potassium-sparing diuretics, potassium supplements: May cause hyperkalemia. Monitor potassium level and renal function.
Salicylates: May decrease hypotensive effects of benazepril. Consider increasing benazepril dosage or decreasing or stopping salicylate.
Thiazide diuretics: May attenuate potassium loss. Also may increase risk of renal failure. Monitor serum potassium level and renal function.
Trimethoprim: May increase risk of hyperkalemia. Monitor serum potassium level and clinical response.
Drug-herb. *Capsaicin:* May cause cough. Discourage use together.
Ma huang: May decrease antihypertensive effects. Discourage use together.
Drug-food. *Salt substitutes containing potassium:* May cause hyperkalemia. Monitor potassium level and renal function.

EFFECTS ON LAB TEST RESULTS
● May increase BUN, creatinine, and potassium levels.

CONTRAINDICATIONS & CAUTIONS
● Contraindicated in patients hypersensitive to ACE inhibitors and in those with a history of angioedema regardless of prior ACE inhibitor use.
Black Box Warning ACE inhibitors can cause injury and even death to the developing fetus when used during the second and third trimesters. When pregnancy is detected, discontinue drug as soon as possible. ■
● Use cautiously in patients with impaired hepatic or renal function.
⚠ *Overdose S&S:* Hypotension.

NURSING CONSIDERATIONS
● Monitor patient for hypotension. Excessive hypotension can occur when drug is given with diuretics. If possible, diuretic therapy should be stopped 2 to 3 days before starting benazepril to decrease potential for excessive hypotensive response. If drug doesn't adequately control blood pressure, diuretic may be cautiously reinstituted.
● Although ACE inhibitors reduce blood pressure in all races, they reduce it less in blacks taking the ACE inhibitor alone. Black patients should take drug with a thiazide diuretic for a more favorable response.
● Drug may increase risk of angioedema in black patients.

Reactions in bold italics are ***life-threatening***. Interactions may have a ***rapid onset*** or a ***delayed onset***.

• Measure blood pressure when drug level is at peak (2 to 6 hours after administration) and at trough (just before a dose) to verify adequate blood pressure control.

• Assess renal and hepatic function before and periodically during therapy. Monitor potassium level.

• Monitor patient for excessive cough. Therapy may need to be changed if cough is intolerable.

• **Look alike–sound alike:** Don't confuse benazepril with Benadryl or Lotensin with lovastatin.

PATIENT TEACHING

• Instruct patient to avoid salt substitutes because they may contain potassium, which can cause high potassium level in patients taking drug.

• Inform patient that light-headedness can occur, especially during first few days of therapy. Tell him to rise slowly to minimize this effect and to report dizziness to prescriber. If fainting occurs, he should stop drug and call prescriber immediately.

• Warn patient to use caution in hot weather and during exercise. Inadequate fluid intake, vomiting, diarrhea, and excessive perspiration can lead to light-headedness and fainting.

• Advise patient to report signs of infection, such as fever and sore throat. Tell him to call prescriber if he develops easy bruising or bleeding; swelling of tongue, lips, face, eyes, mucous membranes, or extremities; difficulty swallowing or breathing; or hoarseness.

• Tell woman of childbearing age to notify prescriber if she becomes pregnant. Drug will need to be stopped.

• Tell patient to contact physician if intolerable cough develops.

SAFETY ALERT!

B

bendamustine hydrochloride
ben-dah-MOO-steen

Treanda

Therapeutic class: Antineoplastics
Pharmacologic class: Mechlorethamine derivatives
Pregnancy risk category: D

AVAILABLE FORMS
Lyophilized powder for injection: 25 mg, 100 mg in single-use vials

INDICATIONS & DOSAGES

➤ **Chronic lymphocytic leukemia (CLL)**
Adults: 100 mg/m^2 I.V. over 30 minutes on days 1 and 2 of a 28-day cycle, given for up to six cycles.

Adjust-a-dose: For patients with grade 4 hematologic toxicity or clinically significant grade 2, 3, or 4 nonhematologic toxicity, delay treatment. Resume treatment when nonhematologic toxicity has improved to grade 1 or ANC is 1×10^9/L or higher and platelet count is 75×10^9/L or higher. In those with grade 3 or greater hematologic toxicity, give 50 mg/m^2 on days 1 and 2 of each cycle; if grade 3 or greater toxicity recurs, reduce dose to 25 mg/m^2 on days 1 and 2 of each cycle. In patients with clinically significant grade 3 nonhematologic toxicity or greater, give 50 mg/m^2 on days 1 and 2 of each cycle. Increase dose in subsequent cycles, as tolerated.

➤ **Indolent B-cell non-Hodgkin lymphoma that has progressed during or within 6 months of treatment with rituximab or a rituximab-containing regimen**
Adults: 120 mg/m^2 I.V. over 60 minutes on days 1 and 2 of a 21-day cycle, given in up to eight cycles.

Adjust-a-dose: For patients with grade 4 hematologic toxicity or clinically significant grade 2, 3, or 4 nonhematologic toxicity, delay treatment. Resume treatment when nonhematologic toxicity has improved to grade 1 or ANC is 1×10^9/L or higher and platelet count is 75×10^9/L or higher. In patients with grade 4 or greater hematologic toxicity, reduce dosage to 90 mg/m² on days 1 and 2 of each cycle; if grade 4 hematologic toxicity recurs, reduce the dose to 60 mg/m² on days 1 and 2 of each cycle. In patients with grade 3 or greater nonhematologic toxicity, reduce dosage to 90 mg/m² on days 1 and 2 of each cycle; if grade 3 or greater nonhematologic toxicity recurs, give 60 mg/m² on days 1 and 2 of each cycle.

ADMINISTRATION

I.V.

▼ Preparation and administration of parenteral form of drug may be mutagenic, teratogenic, or carcinogenic to staff. Follow institutional policy to reduce risks.

▼ Reconstitute powder using sterile water for injection. Add 20 mL to a 100-mg vial. Drug should dissolve within 5 minutes. Inspect vial for particulate matter and discoloration; discard if present.

▼ Reconstituted solutions must be further diluted within 30 minutes using 500 mL of normal saline solution; 500 mL of dextrose 2.5%/sodium chloride 0.45% may also be used. Discard cloudy or discolored solution (solution should be clear and colorless to slightly yellow).

▼ Reconstituted solution is stable for 24 hours when refrigerated, or 3 hours at room temperature.

▼ **Incompatibilities:** Compatibility with solutions other than normal saline and sterile water for injection hasn't been established.

ACTION

Exact mechanism unknown. Mechlorethamine splits into electrophilic alkyl groups, which covalently bond with electron-rich nucleophilic moieties, possibly leading to cell death.

Route	Onset	Peak	Duration
I.V.	Rapid	30 min	Unknown

Half-life: About 3½ hours.

ADVERSE REACTIONS

CNS: asthenia, fatigue, chills, anxiety, depression, dizziness, headache, insomnia.
CV: hypotension, tachycardia.
EENT: nasopharyngitis, sinusitis, nasal congestion.

GI: nausea, vomiting, diarrhea, abdominal pain, constipation, dyspepsia, gastroesophageal reflux, stomatitis.
GU: UTI.
Hematologic: *neutropenia, thrombocytopenia,* anemia, *leukopenia,* lymphopenia.
Metabolic: weight loss, hyperuricemia, *tumor lysis syndrome.*
Musculoskeletal: arthralgia, back pain, bone pain, extremity pain.
Respiratory: cough, dyspnea, pneumonia, upper respiratory tract infection, wheezing.
Skin: rash, pruritus.
Other: pyrexia, hypersensitivity, infection, herpes simplex, herpes zoster, *infusion reactions.*

INTERACTIONS

Drug-drug. *CYP1A2 inducers (omeprazole):* May decrease drug levels. Use together cautiously.
CYP1A2 inhibitors (fluvoxamine, ciprofloxacin): May increase drug levels. Use together cautiously.
Live-virus vaccines: May increase risk of vaccine-induced adverse reactions. Avoid concomitant use.
Drug-lifestyle. *Smoking:* May decrease drug levels. Discourage smoking.

EFFECTS ON LAB TEST RESULTS

● May increase uric acid, bilirubin, AST, ALT, and creatinine levels.
● May decrease neutrophil, platelet, RBC, leukocyte, hemoglobin, and lymphocyte counts.

CONTRAINDICATIONS & CAUTIONS

● Contraindicated in patients hypersensitive to bendamustine or mannitol.
● Use cautiously in patients with mild to moderate renal impairment or mild hepatic impairment. Avoid use in patients with CrCl less than 40 mL/minute. Avoid use in those with moderate to severe hepatic impairment.
● Don't use in breast-feeding women.
● Safety and effectiveness in children haven't been established.
⚠ *Overdose S&S:* QT-interval prolongation, sinus tachycardia, ST and T-wave deviations, left anterior fascicular block.

Reactions in bold italics are *life-threatening.* Interactions may have a *rapid onset* or a *delayed onset.*

NURSING CONSIDERATIONS
● Give through a separate I.V. line using an infusion pump.
● Routinely monitor BUN, creatinine and uric acid levels, LFTs, and complete blood count.
● Monitor closely for signs of allergic reaction, including chills, rash, and pruritus.
● Administer antipyretics, corticosteroids, and antihistamines, as prescribed.
● Monitor for signs of infection (fever, chills, malaise).
● Monitor fluid intake and output closely, and maintain adequate hydration.
● Allopurinol may be necessary during the first 2 weeks of treatment to combat elevated uric acid levels associated with tumor lysis syndrome.

PATIENT TEACHING
● Advise patient to avoid exposure to people with infections.
● Instruct patient to watch for signs and symptoms of infection (fever, sore throat, malaise) or bleeding.
● Advise patient to report immediately any signs of allergic reaction (rash, facial swelling, or difficulty breathing) during or soon after infusion.
● Caution women of childbearing age to avoid pregnancy throughout treatment and for 3 months after therapy.
● Advise male patients to use reliable contraception during treatment and for 3 months after therapy.
● Advise women to stop breast-feeding during therapy because of toxicity risk to infant.
● Tell patient that drug may cause tiredness and to avoid driving or operating dangerous tools or machinery until the effects of drug are known.
● Advise patient to report nausea, vomiting, or diarrhea.

benzonatate
ben-ZOE-na-tate

Tessalon

Therapeutic class: Antitussives
Pharmacologic class: Local anesthetics
Pregnancy risk category: C

AVAILABLE FORMS
Capsules: 100 mg, 200 mg

INDICATIONS & DOSAGES
➤ **Symptomatic relief of cough**
Adults and children older than age 10:
100 to 200 mg P.O. t.i.d.; up to 600 mg daily.

ADMINISTRATION
P.O.
● Protect drug from light and moisture.
● Give without regard to meals but give with food or milk if GI upset occurs.

ACTION
Chemical relative of tetracaine that suppresses the cough reflex by direct action on the cough center in the medulla and through an anesthetic action on stretch receptors of vagal afferent fibers in the respiratory passages, lungs, and pleura.

Route	Onset	Peak	Duration
P.O.	15–20 min	Unknown	3–8 hr

Half-life: Unknown.

ADVERSE REACTIONS
CNS: dizziness, headache, sedation, mental confusion, visual hallucinations.
EENT: nasal congestion, burning sensation in eyes.
GI: nausea, constipation, GI upset.
Skin: pruritus, skin eruptions.
Other: chills, hypersensitivity reactions.

INTERACTIONS
None significant.

EFFECTS ON LAB TEST RESULTS
None reported.

CONTRAINDICATIONS & CAUTIONS

• Contraindicated in patients hypersensitive to drug or related compounds.

• Use cautiously in patients hypersensitive to PABA anesthetics (procaine, tetracaine) because cross-sensitivity reactions may occur.

🕄 *Alert:* Use of drug in children has been approved only for children age 10 and older. Overdose and death have occurred in younger children after accidental ingestion. Drug has a candylike appearance and should be kept in childproof containers and out of the reach of children.

⚠ *Overdose S&S:* Restlessness, tremors, clonic seizures, profound CNS depression.

NURSING CONSIDERATIONS

• Don't use drug when cough is a valuable diagnostic sign or is beneficial (such as after thoracic surgery).

• Monitor cough type and frequency.

PATIENT TEACHING

• Warn patient not to chew capsules or dissolve in mouth, which produces either local anesthesia that may result in aspiration, or CNS stimulation that may cause restlessness, tremor, and seizures.

• Instruct patient to report adverse reactions.

• Instruct patient to protect drug from light and moisture.

• Tell patient to contact prescriber if cough lasts longer than 1 week, recurs frequently, or is accompanied by high fever, rash, or severe headache.

benztropine mesylate
BENZ-troe-peen

Cogentin

Therapeutic class: Antiparkinsonians
Pharmacologic class: Anticholinergics
Pregnancy risk category: C

AVAILABLE FORMS

Injection: 1 mg/mL in 2-mL ampules
Tablets: 0.5 mg, 1 mg, 2 mg

INDICATIONS & DOSAGES

➤ **Drug-induced extrapyramidal disorders (except tardive dyskinesia)**

Adults: 1 to 4 mg P.O. or I.M. once daily or b.i.d.

➤ **Transient extrapyramidal disorders**

Adults: 1 to 2 mg P.O. or I.M. b.i.d. or t. i. d. After 1 or 2 weeks, withdraw drug to determine continued need.

➤ **Acute dystonic reaction**

Adults: 1 to 2 mg I.V. or I.M.; then 1 to 2 mg P.O. b.i.d. to prevent recurrence.

➤ **Parkinsonism**

Adults: 0.5 to 6 mg P.O. or I.M. daily. First dosage is 0.5 to 1 mg, increased by 0.5 mg every 5 to 6 days. Adjust dosage to meet individual requirements. Maximum, 6 mg daily.

➤ **Postencephalitic parkinsonism**

Adults: 2 mg P.O. or I.M. daily in one or more doses. In highly sensitive patients, therapy may be initiated with 0.5 mg P.O. or I.M. at bedtime, and increased as needed. Maximum, 6 mg daily.

ADMINISTRATION

P.O.

• Drug may be given before or after meals depending on patient reaction. If patient is prone to excessive salivation, give drug after meals. If his mouth dries excessively, give drug before meals unless it causes nausea.

I.V.

▼ Reserve I.V. delivery for emergencies, such as acute dystonic reactions.

▼ The I.V. form is seldom used because no significant difference exists between it and the I.M. form.

▼ **Incompatibilities:** Haloperidol lactate.

I.M.

• Use filtered needle to draw up solution from ampule.

ACTION

Unknown. May block central cholinergic receptors, helping to balance cholinergic activity in the basal ganglia.

Route	Onset	Peak	Duration
P.O.	1–2 hr	Unknown	24 hr
I.V., I.M.	15 min	Unknown	24 hr

Half-life: Unknown.

Reactions in bold italics are *life-threatening*. Interactions may have a *rapid onset* or a *delayed onset*.

ADVERSE REACTIONS

CNS: confusion, memory impairment, nervousness, depression, disorientation, hallucinations, toxic psychosis, fever.
CV: tachycardia.
EENT: dilated pupils, blurred vision.
GI: dry mouth, constipation, nausea, vomiting, paralytic ileus.
GU: urine retention, dysuria.
Musculoskeletal: muscle weakness.
Skin: decreased sweating.
Other: heat stroke.

INTERACTIONS

Drug-drug. *Amantadine, phenothiazines, TCAs:* May cause additive anticholinergic adverse reactions, such as confusion and hallucinations. Reduce dosage before giving.
Cholinergics (donepezil, galantamine, rivastigmine, tacrine): May antagonize the therapeutic effects of these drugs. If used together, monitor patient for therapeutic effect.

EFFECTS ON LAB TEST RESULTS

None reported.

CONTRAINDICATIONS & CAUTIONS

• Contraindicated in patients hypersensitive to drug or its components, in those with angle-closure glaucoma, and in children younger than age 3.
• Drug isn't recommended for use in patients with tardive dyskinesia.
• Drug may produce anhidrosis. Use cautiously in hot weather, in patients with mental disorders, in elderly patients, and in children age 3 and older.
• Use cautiously in patients with prostatic hyperplasia, arrhythmias, or seizure disorders.
⚠ *Overdose S&S:* CNS depression preceded or followed by stimulation; confusion, nervousness, listlessness, intensification of mental symptoms or toxic psychosis (in patients with mental illness being treated with neuroleptic drugs), hallucinations, dizziness, muscle weakness, ataxia, dry mouth, mydriasis, blurred vision, palpitations, tachycardia, hypertension, nausea, vomiting, dysuria, numbness of fingers, dysphagia, allergic reactions, headache,

delirium, coma, shock, seizures, respiratory arrest, anhidrosis, hyperthermia, glaucoma, constipation; hot, dry, flushed skin.

NURSING CONSIDERATIONS

• Monitor vital signs carefully. Watch closely for adverse reactions, especially in elderly or debilitated patients. Call prescriber promptly if adverse reactions occur.
• At certain doses, drug produces atropine-like toxicity, which may aggravate tardive dyskinesia.
• Watch for intermittent constipation and abdominal distention and pain, which may indicate onset of paralytic ileus.
• Monitor elderly patients closely as they are more prone to severe adverse effects.
❸ *Alert:* Never stop drug abruptly. Reduce dosage gradually.
• *Look alike–sound alike:* Don't confuse benztropine with bromocriptine.

PATIENT TEACHING

• Warn patient to avoid activities that require alertness until CNS effects of drug are known.
• If patient takes a single daily dose, tell him to do so at bedtime.
• Advise patient to report signs and symptoms of urinary hesitancy or urine retention.
• Tell patient to relieve dry mouth with cool drinks, ice chips, sugarless gum, or hard candy.
• Advise patient to limit hot weather activities because drug-induced lack of sweating may cause overheating.

bepotastine besilate
beh-POT-uh-steen

Bepreve

Therapeutic class: Antihistamines (ophthalmic)
Pharmacologic class: Histamine₁-receptor antagonists
Pregnancy risk category: C

AVAILABLE FORMS

Ophthalmic solution: 1.5%

INDICATIONS & DOSAGES
➤ **Itching associated with conjunctivitis**
Adults and children age 2 and older: Instill
1 drop into affected eye(s) b.i.d.

ADMINISTRATION
Ophthalmic
● To minimize contamination of dropper
tip and solution, avoid touching patient's
eyelids or surrounding areas with dropper
tip of bottle. Keep bottle tightly closed when
not in use.

ACTION
Inhibits release of histamine from mast cells
by blocking histamine₁ receptors.

Route	Onset	Peak	Duration
Ophthalmic	Unknown	1–2 hr	Unknown

Half-life: Unknown.

ADVERSE REACTIONS
CNS: headache.
EENT: eye irritation, mild taste, na-
sopharyngitis.

INTERACTIONS
None known.

EFFECTS ON LAB TEST RESULTS
None known.

CONTRAINDICATIONS & CAUTIONS
● Drug hasn't been studied in pregnant
women. Use during pregnancy only if potential benefit justifies risk to fetus.
● It isn't known if drug appears in breast
milk. Use cautiously in breast-feeding
women.

NURSING CONSIDERATIONS
● Don't use drug for irritation caused by
contact lenses.
● Remove contact lenses before instilling
drops because preservative in bepotastine,
benzalkonium chloride, may be absorbed by
soft contact lenses.

PATIENT TEACHING
● Advise patient not to use drug while
wearing contact lenses. Lenses may be
reinserted 10 minutes after administration.

● Instruct patient to avoid wearing contact
lenses if eye redness occurs.
● Advise patient to avoid touching eyelids
or surrounding areas with dropper tip of bottle, to minimize contamination of dropper
tip and solution, and to keep bottle tightly
closed when not in use.

besifloxacin
beh-sih-FLOX-ah-sin

Besivance

Therapeutic class: Antibiotics
Pharmacologic class: Fluoroquinolones
Pregnancy risk category: C

AVAILABLE FORMS
Ophthalmic suspension: 0.6%

INDICATIONS & DOSAGES
➤ **Conjunctivitis caused by CDC coryne-
form group G,** *Aerococcus viridans,*
Corynebacterium pseudodiphtheriticum,
Corynebacterium striatum, Haemophilus
influenzae, Moraxella catarrhalis,
Moraxella lacunata, Pseudomonas
aeruginosa, Staphylococcus aureus,
Staphylococcus epidermidis, Staphylococ-
cus hominis, Staphylococcus lugdunensis,
Staphylococcus warneri, Streptococcus
mitis group, Streptococcus oralis, Strep-
tococcus pneumoniae, Streptococcus
salivarius
Adults and children age 1 and older: Instill
1 drop into affected eye t.i.d., 4 to 12 hours
apart, for 7 days.

ADMINISTRATION
Ophthalmic
● Invert bottle and shake once before use.
Remove cap with bottle in inverted position.
♻ *Alert:* Don't inject into eye or introduce
into anterior chamber of eye.

ACTION
Inhibits DNA gyrase and topoisomerase,
preventing cell replication and division.

Route	Onset	Peak	Duration
Ophthalmic	Unknown	Unknown	Unknown

Half-life: 7 hours.

Reactions in bold italics are *life-threatening*. Interactions may have a *rapid onset* or a *delayed onset*.

ADVERSE REACTIONS
CNS: headache.
EENT: blurred vision, conjunctival erythema, eye irritation, eye pain, eye pruritus.

INTERACTIONS
None reported.

EFFECTS ON LAB TEST RESULTS
None reported.

CONTRAINDICATIONS & CAUTIONS
• Although drug isn't intended for systemic administration, hypersensitivity reactions have been reported with systemic administration of quinolones. Discontinue drug at first sign of allergic reaction or rash.
• Use cautiously in pregnant or breastfeeding women.
• Safety and effectiveness in infants younger than age 1 haven't been established.

NURSING CONSIDERATIONS
• Be aware that prolonged use may lead to growth of resistant organisms.

PATIENT TEACHING
• Instruct patient to wash his hands before and after instilling the drug.
• Teach patient how to instill drug correctly. Remind him not to touch the tip of the bottle with his hands and not to let the tip touch the eye or surrounding tissue.
• Advise patient to avoid wearing contact lenses if he has signs and symptoms of conjunctivitis while taking the drug.
• Remind patient not to share washcloths or towels with other family members to avoid spreading infection.
• Tell patient to take drug exactly as prescribed for as long as prescribed, even if he's feeling better.
• Instruct patient to stop the drug and notify his prescriber if rash or allergic reaction occurs.

B

betamethasone dipropionate
bay-ta-METH-a-sone

Diprolene, Diprolene AF

betamethasone valerate
Beta-Val, Dermabet, Luxiq, Valnac

Therapeutic class: Corticosteroids
Pharmacologic class: Corticosteroids
Pregnancy risk category: C

AVAILABLE FORMS
betamethasone dipropionate
Cream: 0.05%
Gel: 0.05%
Lotion: 0.05%
Ointment: 0.05%
betamethasone valerate
Cream: 0.1%
Foam: 0.12%
Lotion: 0.1%
Ointment: 0.1%

INDICATIONS & DOSAGES
➤ **Inflammation and pruritus from corticosteroid-responsive dermatoses**
Adults and children older than age 12:
Clean area; apply cream, ointment, lotion, or gel sparingly. Give dipropionate products once daily to b.i.d.; give valerate 0.1% solution b.i.d., or valerate 0.1% cream or ointment once daily to t.i.d. Maximum dosage of augmented betamethasone dipropionate 0.05% ointment, cream, gel, or lotion is 45 g, 50 g, 45 g, or 50 mL per week, respectively. Therapy with augmented formulations shouldn't exceed 2 weeks.
➤ **Inflammation and pruritus from corticosteroid-responsive dermatoses of scalp (valerate only)**
Adults: Gently massage small amounts of foam into affected scalp areas b.i.d., morning and evening, until control is achieved. If no improvement is seen in 2 weeks, reassess diagnosis.

ADMINISTRATION
Topical
● Shake well before use and protect from light.
● Gently wash skin before applying. To prevent skin damage, rub in gently, leaving a thin coat. When treating hairy sites, part hair and apply directly to lesions.
● Decrease dosing frequency to once daily if clinical improvement is seen.
● Avoid applying near eyes or mucous membranes or in ear canal, groin area, or armpit.
● Don't dispense foam directly into warm hands because foam will begin to melt on contact.
● For patients with eczematous dermatitis whose skin may be irritated by adhesive material, hold dressing in place with gauze, elastic bandages, stockings, or stockinette.
🕔 *Alert:*Product is flammable. Avoid fire, flame, or smoking during use. Don't expose to heat.
🕔 *Alert:*Don't use occlusive dressings.
● Continue drug for a few days after lesions clear.

ACTION
Unclear. Is diffused across cell membranes to form complexes with receptors. Has anti-inflammatory, antipruritic, vasoconstrictive, and antiproliferative activity. Considered a medium-potency to very-high-potency drug (depending on product), according to vasoconstrictive properties.

Route	Onset	Peak	Duration
Topical	Unknown	Unknown	Unknown

Half-life: Unknown.

ADVERSE REACTIONS
GU: glycosuria (with dipropionate).
Metabolic: hyperglycemia.
Skin: burning, pruritus, irritation, dryness, erythema, folliculitis, striae, acneiform eruptions, perioral dermatitis, hypopigmentation, hypertrichosis, allergic contact dermatitis, secondary infection, maceration, atrophy, miliaria with occlusive dressings.
Other: *hypothalamic-pituitary-adrenal (HPA) axis suppression,* Cushing syndrome.

INTERACTIONS
None significant.

EFFECTS ON LAB TEST RESULTS
● May increase glucose level.

CONTRAINDICATIONS & CAUTIONS
● Contraindicated in patients hypersensitive to corticosteroids.
● Don't use as monotherapy in primary bacterial infections (impetigo, paronychia, erysipelas, cellulitis, angular cheilitis), rosacea, perioral dermatitis, or acne.
● Don't use augmented betamethasone dipropionate 0.05% ointment; betamethasone dipropionate 0.05% gel, cream, and ointment; or betamethasone valerate 0.1% ointment on the face, groin, or axilla.
● Use cautiously in pregnant or breast-feeding women.
⚠ *Overdose S&S:*Systemic effects.

NURSING CONSIDERATIONS
● Drug isn't for ophthalmic use.
● Because of alcohol content of vehicle, gel products may cause mild, transient stinging, especially when used on or near excoriated skin.
● If antifungal or antibiotic combined with corticosteroid fails to provide prompt improvement, stop corticosteroid until infection is controlled.
● Systemic absorption is likely with prolonged or extensive body surface treatment. Watch for symptoms of HPA axis suppression, manifestations of Cushing syndrome, hyperglycemia, and glycosuria. If HPA axis suppression occurs, attempt to withdraw drug or substitute a less potent steroid.
● Evaluate patient for HPA axis suppression by using the urinary free cortisol and corticotropin stimulation tests.
🕔 *Alert:*Children may demonstrate greater susceptibility to HPA axis suppression and Cushing syndrome.
● Avoid using plastic pants or tight-fitting diapers on treated areas in young children. Children may absorb larger amounts of drug and be more susceptible to systemic toxicity.
🕔 *Alert:*Diprolene and Diprolene AF may not be replaced with generics because other products have different potencies.

PATIENT TEACHING
● Teach patient how to apply drug.
● Emphasize that drug is for external use only.
● Tell patient to wash hands after application.
● Tell patient to stop drug and report signs of systemic absorption, skin irritation or ulceration, hypersensitivity, or infection.
● Instruct patient not to use occlusive dressings.
● Discuss personal hygiene measures to reduce chance of infection.

betaxolol hydrochloride
beh-TAX-oh-lol

Betoptic, Betoptic S

Therapeutic class: Antiglaucoma drugs
Pharmacologic class: Beta blockers
Pregnancy risk category: C

AVAILABLE FORMS
Ophthalmic solution: 0.5%
Ophthalmic suspension: 0.25%

INDICATIONS & DOSAGES
➤ **Chronic open-angle glaucoma, ocular hypertension**
Adults: Instill 1 or 2 drops in the affected eye(s) b.i.d.

ADMINISTRATION
Ophthalmic
● Shake suspension well.
● Apply light finger pressure on lacrimal sac for 1 minute after instilling drug.
● Don't touch tip of dropper to eye or surrounding tissue.

ACTION
Unknown. Reduces aqueous formation and may increase outflow of aqueous humor.

Route	Onset	Peak	Duration
Ophthalmic	30–60 min	2 hr	>12 hr

Half-life: Unknown.

ADVERSE REACTIONS
CNS: insomnia, depression, dizziness, headache.

CV: *arrhythmias, heart block, heart failure,* palpitations.
EENT: eye stinging on instillation causing brief discomfort, erythema, itching, keratitis, occasional tearing, photophobia.
Respiratory: *bronchospasm, asthma.*

INTERACTIONS
Drug-drug. *Calcium channel blockers:* May cause AV conduction disturbances, ventricular failure, and hypotension if significant systemic absorption occurs. Monitor patient closely.
Cardiac glycosides: May cause excessive bradycardia if significant systemic absorption occurs. Patient may need ECG monitoring.
Dipivefrin, ophthalmic epinephrine: May produce mydriasis. Use together cautiously.
Inhaled hydrocarbon anesthetics: May prolong severe hypotension if significant systemic absorption occurs. Tell anesthesiologist that patient is receiving ophthalmic betaxolol.
Insulin, oral antidiabetics: May cause hypoglycemia or hyperglycemia if significant systemic absorption occurs. May need to adjust dosage of antidiabetics.
Phenothiazines: May have additive hypotensive effects; may increase risk of adverse effects if significant systemic absorption occurs. Monitor patient closely.
Prazosin: May increase risk of orthostatic hypotension in early phases of use together. Help patient stand slowly until effects are known.
Reserpine: May cause excessive beta blockade. Monitor patient closely.
Systemic beta blockers: May have additive effects. Monitor patient closely.
Verapamil: May increase effects of both drugs. Monitor cardiac function closely and decrease dosages as necessary.
Drug-lifestyle. *Sun exposure:* May cause photophobia. Advise patient to wear sunglasses.

EFFECTS ON LAB TEST RESULTS
None reported.

CONTRAINDICATIONS & CAUTIONS
● Contraindicated in patients hypersensitive to drug and in those with sinus bradycardia,

greater than first-degree AV block, cardiogenic shock, or overt heart failure.
• Use cautiously in patients with restricted pulmonary function, diabetes mellitus, hyperthyroidism, or history of heart failure.

NURSING CONSIDERATIONS
• Stabilization of intraocular pressure (IOP)–lowering response may take a few weeks. Determine IOP after 4 weeks of treatment.

PATIENT TEACHING
• Teach patient how to instill drug. Advise him to wash hands before and after instillation and to apply light finger pressure on lacrimal sac for 1 minute after instilling drug. Warn him not to touch tip of dropper to eye or surrounding tissue. Tell him to shake suspension well before instilling.
• Encourage patient to comply with twice-daily regimen.
• Tell patient to remove contact lenses before instilling drug. Lenses may be reinserted about 15 minutes after using drops.
• Advise patient to ease sun sensitivity by wearing sunglasses.

---

bethanechol chloride
be-THAN-e-kole

Duvoid, Urecholine

Therapeutic class: Urinary stimulants
Pharmacologic class: Cholinergic agonists
Pregnancy risk category: C

AVAILABLE FORMS
Tablets: 5 mg, 10 mg, 25 mg, 50 mg

INDICATIONS & DOSAGES
➤ **Acute postoperative and postpartum nonobstructive (functional) urine retention, neurogenic atony of urinary bladder with urine retention**
Adults: 10 to 50 mg P.O. t.i.d. to q.i.d. Determine minimum effective dose by giving 5 or 10 mg and repeating same amount at hourly intervals until satisfactory response or maximum of 50 mg has been given.

➤ **GERD** ◆
Adults: 25 mg P.O. q.i.d.

ADMINISTRATION
P.O.
• Give drug 1 hour before or 2 hours after meals because drug may cause nausea and vomiting if taken soon after eating.

ACTION
Directly stimulates muscarinic cholinergic receptors, mimicking acetylcholine action, increasing GI tract tone and peristalsis and contraction of the detrusor muscle of the urinary bladder.

Route	Onset	Peak	Duration
P.O.	30–90 min	1 hr	6 hr

Half-life: Unknown.

ADVERSE REACTIONS
CNS: headache, malaise.
CV: *bradycardia,* profound hypotension with reflexive tachycardia, flushing.
EENT: lacrimation, miosis.
GI: abdominal cramps, diarrhea, excessive salivation, nausea, belching, borborygmus.
GU: urinary urgency.
Respiratory: *bronchoconstriction, asthma attack.*
Skin: diaphoresis.

INTERACTIONS
Drug-drug. *Anticholinergics, atropine, belladonna alkaloids, procainamide, quinidine:* May reverse cholinergic effects. Observe patient for lack of drug effect.
Cholinesterase inhibitors (donepezil), cholinergic agonists: May cause additive effects or increase toxicity. Avoid using together.
Ganglionic blockers: May cause critical drop in blood pressure, usually preceded by severe abdominal pain. Avoid using together.

EFFECTS ON LAB TEST RESULTS
• May increase amylase, lipase, and liver enzyme levels.

CONTRAINDICATIONS & CAUTIONS

• Contraindicated in patients hypersensitive to drug or its components and in those with uncertain strength or integrity of bladder wall, mechanical obstruction of GI or urinary tract, hyperthyroidism, peptic ulceration, latent or active bronchial asthma, obstructive pulmonary disease, pronounced bradycardia or hypotension, vasomotor instability, cardiac or coronary artery disease, AV conduction defects, hypertension, seizure disorder, Parkinson disease, spastic GI disturbances, acute inflammatory lesions of the GI tract, peritonitis, or marked vagotonia.

• Use cautiously in pregnant or breast-feeding women.

⚠ **Overdose S&S:** Abdominal discomfort, excessive salivation, flushing, hot feeling, sweating, nausea, vomiting.

NURSING CONSIDERATIONS

• Adverse effects are rare with oral use.
• Monitor vital signs frequently, especially respirations. Always have atropine injection available, and be prepared to give 0.6 mg subcutaneously or by slow I.V. push. Provide respiratory support, if needed.
• Monitor patient for orthostatic hypotension.
• Watch closely for adverse reactions that may indicate drug toxicity.

PATIENT TEACHING

• Tell patient to take drug on an empty stomach and at regular intervals.
• Inform patient that drug is usually effective 30 to 90 minutes after use.

bevacizumab
beh-vah-SIZZ-yoo-mab

Avastin

Therapeutic class: Antineoplastics
Pharmacologic class: Monoclonal antibodies
Pregnancy risk category: C

AVAILABLE FORMS
Solution: 25 mg/mL in 4-mL and 16-mL vials

INDICATIONS & DOSAGES
✳ *NEW INDICATION:* **Metastatic colorectal cancer with fluoropyrimidine-irinotecan–based or fluoropyrimidine-oxaliplatin–based chemotherapy for second-line treatment after progression on a first-line bevacizumab-containing regimen**
Adults: 5 mg/kg I.V. every 2 weeks or 7.5 mg/kg I.V. every 3 weeks.
➤ **First- or second-line treatment, with 5-FU-based chemotherapy, for metastatic colon or rectal cancer**
Adults: If used with bolus irinotecan, 5-FU, and leucovorin (IFL) regimen, give 5 mg/kg I.V. every 14 days. If used with oxaliplatin, 5-FU, and leucovorin (known as FOLFOX 4) regimen, give 10 mg/kg I.V. every 14 days. Infusion rate varies by patient tolerance and number of infusions.
➤ **With carboplatin and paclitaxel as first-line treatment of unresectable, locally advanced, recurrent, or metastatic nonsquamous, non–small-cell lung cancer**
Adults: 15 mg/kg I.V. infusion once every 3 weeks.
➤ **With interferon alfa for metastatic renal cell carcinoma; as single agent for progressive glioblastoma following prior therapy**
Adults: 10 mg/kg I.V. every 14 days.

ADMINISTRATION
I.V.
▼ Don't freeze or shake vials.
▼ Dilute drug using aseptic technique. Withdraw proper dose and mix in a total

volume of 100 mL normal saline solution in an I.V. bag.

▼ Don't give by I.V. push or bolus.

▼ Give the first infusion over 90 minutes and, if tolerated, the second infusion over 60 minutes. Later infusions can be given over 30 minutes if previous infusions were tolerated.

▼ Discard unused portion; drug is preservative-free.

▼ Drug is stable 8 hours if refrigerated at 36° to 46° F (2° to 8° C) and protected from light.

▼ **Incompatibilities:** Dextrose solutions.

ACTION

A recombinant humanized vascular endothelial growth factor inhibitor.

Route	Onset	Peak	Duration
I.V.	Unknown	Unknown	Unknown

Half-life: About 20 days.

ADVERSE REACTIONS

CNS: asthenia, dizziness, headache, abnormal gait, confusion, pain, syncope.

CV: *intra-abdominal thrombosis,* hypertension, *thromboembolism, deep vein thrombosis,* heart failure, hypotension.

EENT: epistaxis, excess lacrimation, gum bleeding, taste disorder, voice alteration.

GI: anorexia, constipation, diarrhea, dyspepsia, flatulence, stomatitis, vomiting, *GI hemorrhage,* abdominal pain, colitis, dry mouth, nausea.

GU: *vaginal hemorrhage,* proteinuria, urinary urgency.

Hematologic: *leukopenia, neutropenia, thrombocytopenia.*

Metabolic: hypokalemia, weight loss, bilirubinemia.

Musculoskeletal: back pain, myalgia.

Respiratory: *hemoptysis,* dyspnea, upper respiratory tract infection.

Skin: alopecia, dermatitis, discoloration, dry skin, exfoliative dermatitis, nail disorder, skin ulcer.

Other: decreased wound healing, hypersensitivity.

INTERACTIONS

None reported.

EFFECTS ON LAB TEST RESULTS

● May increase bilirubin and urine protein levels. May decrease potassium level.

● May decrease neutrophil, platelet, and WBC counts.

CONTRAINDICATIONS & CAUTIONS

● Contraindicated in patients with recent hemoptysis or within 28 days after major surgery.

● Use cautiously in patients hypersensitive to drug or its components, in those who need surgery, are taking anticoagulants, or have significant CV disease.

● *Alert:* May increase risk of ovarian failure and may impair fertility. Long-term effects on fertility are unknown.

⚠ *Overdose S&S:* Headache.

NURSING CONSIDERATIONS

● *Alert:* Reversible posterior leukoencephalopathy syndrome (RPLS)-associated symptoms (hypertension, headache, visual disturbances, altered mental function, and seizures) may occur 16 hours to 1 year after starting the drug. Monitor patient closely. If syndrome occurs, stop drug and provide supportive care.

● RPLS can be confirmed only by magnetic resonance imaging.

● Hypersensitivity reactions can occur during infusion. Monitor the patient closely.

● In patients who develop nephrotic syndrome, severe hypertension, hypertensive crisis, serious hemorrhage, GI perforation, or wound dehiscence that needs intervention, stop drug.

● *Alert:* Discontinue drug at least 28 days before elective surgery. Don't initiate for at least 28 days after surgery or until wound is fully healed.

● *Alert:* Drug may increase risk of serious arterial thromboembolic events, including MI, transient ischemic attacks, stroke, and angina. Those patients at highest risk are age 65 or older, have a history of arterial thromboembolism, and have taken the drug before. If patient has an arterial thrombotic event, permanently stop drug.

Black Box Warning Drug may cause fatal GI perforation. Monitor patient closely. ∎

Reactions in bold italics are *life-threatening*. Interactions may have a *rapid onset* or a *delayed onset*.

Black Box Warning Bevacizumab can result in life-threatening wound dehiscence. Permanently discontinue bevacizumab therapy in patients who experience wound dehiscence that requires medical intervention. Discontinue drug at least 28 days before elective surgery and don't restart drug for at least 28 days after surgery and until the surgical wound is fully healed. ■

Black Box Warning Drug increases risk of severe or fatal hemorrhage, hemoptysis, GI bleeding, CNS hemorrhage, and vaginal bleeding. Don't give to patients with serious hemorrhage or recent hemoptysis. ■

• Monitor urinalysis for worsening proteinuria. Patients with 2+ or greater urine dipstick test should undergo 24-hour urine collection. Discontinue use in patients with nephrotic syndrome.

• Monitor patient's blood pressure every 2 to 3 weeks.

• It's unknown whether drug appears in breast milk. Women shouldn't breast-feed during therapy and for about 3 weeks after therapy ends.

• Adverse reactions occur more often in older patients.

PATIENT TEACHING

• Inform patient about potential adverse reactions.

• Tell patient to report adverse reactions immediately, especially abdominal pain, constipation, and vomiting.

• Advise patient that blood pressure and urinalysis will be monitored during treatment.

• Caution women of childbearing age to avoid pregnancy during treatment.

۞ Alert: Inform women of the potential for ovarian failure and impaired fertility before starting treatment.

• Urge patient to alert other health care providers about treatment and to avoid elective surgery during treatment.

bimatoprost
by-MAT-oh-prost

Latisse, Lumigan

Therapeutic class: Antiglaucoma drugs
Pharmacologic class: Prostaglandin analogues
Pregnancy risk category: C

AVAILABLE FORMS
Ophthalmic solution: 0.01%, 0.03%
Topical solution: 0.03%

INDICATIONS & DOSAGES
➤ **Increased intraocular pressure (IOP) in patients with open-angle glaucoma or ocular hypertension**
Adults: Instill 1 drop in conjunctival sac of affected eye once daily in the evening.
➤ **Hypotrichosis of the eyelashes**
Adults: Apply 1 drop nightly directly to skin of upper eyelid margin at base of eyelashes with single-use applicator.

ADMINISTRATION
Ophthalmic
• Don't touch tip of dropper to eye or surrounding tissue.
• If more than one ophthalmic drug is being used, give drugs at least 5 minutes apart.
• Store drug in original container between 59° and 77° F (15° and 25° C).
Topical
• Before application, ensure face is clean and makeup and contact lenses are removed.
• Use new applicator for each eye; never reuse. Don't use any other brush or applicator.
• Blot excess solution from beyond eyelid margin.

ACTION
Has ocular hypotensive activity, which selectively mimics the effects of naturally occurring prostaglandins. Drug may also increase outflow of aqueous humor. Mechanism in treating hypotrichosis is unknown.

Route	Onset	Peak	Duration
Ophthalmic	4 hr	10 min	Unknown
Topical	Unknown	Unknown	Unknown

Half-life: 45 minutes.

ADVERSE REACTIONS

CNS: headache, asthenia.
EENT: conjunctival hyperemia, growth of eyelashes, ocular pruritus, allergic conjunctivitis, asthenopia, blepharitis, cataract, conjunctival edema; eye discharge, tearing, and pain; eyelash darkening, eyelid erythema, foreign body sensation, increase in iris pigmentation; ocular burning, dryness, and irritation; photophobia, superficial punctate keratitis, visual disturbance.
Respiratory: upper respiratory tract infection.
Skin: hirsutism, hyperpigmentation of periocular skin.
Other: infection.

INTERACTIONS

Drug-drug. *Latanoprost:* May decrease IOP-lowering effect. Use cautiously with either ophthalmic or topical form.

EFFECTS ON LAB TEST RESULTS

● May cause abnormal LFT values.

CONTRAINDICATIONS & CAUTIONS

● Contraindicated in patients hypersensitive to bimatoprost, benzalkonium chloride, or other ingredients in product.
● Drug hasn't been approved for use in patients with angle-closure glaucoma or inflammatory or neovascular glaucoma.
● Use cautiously in patients with renal or hepatic impairment.
● Use cautiously in patients with active intraocular inflammation (iritis, uveitis), aphakic patients, pseudophakic patients with torn posterior lens capsule, and patients at risk for macular edema.

NURSING CONSIDERATIONS

● Temporary or permanent increased pigmentation of iris and eyelid, as well as increased pigmentation and growth of eyelashes, may occur.
● Patient should remove contact lenses before using solution. Lenses may be reinserted 15 minutes after administration.

PATIENT TEACHING

● Tell patient receiving treatment in only one eye about potential for increased brown pigmentation of iris, eyelid skin darkening, and increased length, thickness, pigmentation, or number of lashes in treated eye.
● Teach patient how to instill drops, and advise him to wash hands before and after instilling solution. Warn him not to touch tip of dropper to eye or surrounding tissue.
● If eye trauma or infection occurs or if eye surgery is needed, tell patient to seek medical advice before continuing to use multidose container.
● Advise patient to immediately report eye inflammation or lid reactions.
● Advise patient to apply light pressure on lacrimal sac for 1 minute after instillation of drops to minimize systemic absorption of drug.
● Tell patient to remove contact lenses before using solution and that lenses may be reinserted 15 minutes after administration.
● Teach patient that Latisse applicators are for single use only. Instruct patient to wash face and remove makeup and contact lenses before applicator use.
● Tell patient that effects of Latisse are gradual in onset and may not be significant for 2 months. Results last only as long as treatment is continued.
● Instruct patient to blot excess solution from beyond eyelid margin.
● If patient is using more than one ophthalmic drug, tell him to apply them at least 5 minutes apart.
● Stress importance of compliance with recommended therapy.

Reactions in bold italics are *life-threatening*. Interactions may have a *rapid onset* or a *delayed onset*.

B

bismuth subsalicylate
BIS-mith

Bismatrol ◊, Kaopectate ◊,
Kao-Tin ◊, Maalox Total Stomach
Relief Liquid ◊, Peptic Relief ◊,
Pepto-Bismol ◊, Pink Bismuth ◊

Therapeutic class: Antidiarrheals
Pharmacologic class: Adsorbents
Pregnancy risk category: C

AVAILABLE FORMS
Caplets: 262 mg ◊
Oral suspension: 262 mg/15 mL (regular strength), 525 mg/15 mL (maximum strength)
Tablets (chewable): 262 mg ◊

INDICATIONS & DOSAGES
➤ **Mild, nonspecific diarrhea**
Adults and children age 12 and older:
30 mL or 2 tablets P.O. every 30 minutes to 1 hour, up to maximum of eight doses (regular strength) or four doses (maximum strength) and for no longer than 2 days.
Children ages 9 to 11: 15 mL or 1 chewable tablet every 30 minutes to 1 hour, up to maximum of eight doses (regular strength) or four doses (maximum strength) and for no longer than 2 days.
Children ages 6 to 8: 10 mL or ⅔ of a chewable tablet P.O. every 30 minutes to 1 hour, up to maximum of eight doses (regular strength) or four doses (maximum strength) and for no longer than 2 days.
Children ages 3 to 5: 5 mL or ⅓ of a chewable tablet P.O. every 30 minutes to 1 hour, up to maximum of eight doses (regular strength) or four doses (maximum strength) and for no longer than 2 days.
➤ **Traveler's diarrhea ♦**
Adults: 30 mL P.O. every 30 minutes for eight doses/day (regular strength) or four doses/day (maximum strength).

ADMINISTRATION
P.O.
● Shake liquid well before administration.
● Have patient chew or dissolve chewable tablets in mouth.
● Make sure patient swallows caplets whole.

ACTION
May have antisecretory, antimicrobial, and anti-inflammatory effects against bacterial and viral enteropathogens.

Route	Onset	Peak	Duration
P.O.	1 hr	Unknown	Unknown

Half-life: Unknown.

ADVERSE REACTIONS
GI: temporary darkening of tongue and stools.
Other: salicylism with high doses.

INTERACTIONS
Drug-drug. *Aspirin, other salicylates:* May cause salicylate toxicity. Monitor patient.
Oral anticoagulants, oral antidiabetics: May increase effects of these drugs after high doses of bismuth subsalicylate. Monitor patient closely.
Tetracycline: May decrease tetracycline absorption. Separate doses by at least 2 hours.

EFFECTS ON LAB TEST RESULTS
None reported.

CONTRAINDICATIONS & CAUTIONS
● Contraindicated in patients hypersensitive to salicylates.
● Use cautiously in patients taking aspirin. Stop therapy if tinnitus occurs.
● Use cautiously in children and in patients with bleeding disorders or salicylate sensitivity.
● Avoid use in children or teenagers who have or who are recovering from influenza or chickenpox.
● Use cautiously in infants and debilitated patients because of increased risk of constipation with impaction.

NURSING CONSIDERATIONS
● Avoid use before GI radiologic procedures because drug is radiopaque and may interfere with X-rays.
● Liquid form is preferred for children, to give more accurate dosing.

PATIENT TEACHING
● Advise patient that drug contains salicylate. Each tablet has 102 mg salicylate.

Regular-strength liquid has 130 mg/15 mL. Extra-strength liquid has 230 mg/15 mL.

• Instruct patient to shake liquid before measuring dose and to chew chewable tablets well before swallowing.

• Tell patient to call prescriber if diarrhea lasts longer than 2 days or is accompanied by high fever.

• Advise patient to drink plenty of clear fluids to help prevent dehydration, which may accompany diarrhea.

• Tell patient that tongue and stools may temporarily turn gray-black.

• Urge patient to consult with prescriber before giving drug to children or teenagers during or after recovery from the flu or chickenpox.

• Inform patient that all forms of drug are effective against traveler's diarrhea. Tablets and caplets may be more convenient to carry.

• Tell patient to watch for hives, ringing in the ears, and rectal bleeding.

bisoprolol fumarate
BIS-oh-PROE-lol

Zebeta

Therapeutic class: Antihypertensives
Pharmacologic class: Selective beta blockers
Pregnancy risk category: C

AVAILABLE FORMS
Tablets: 5 mg, 10 mg

INDICATIONS & DOSAGES
➤ **Hypertension**
Adults: Initially, 5 mg P.O. daily alone or with other antihypertensives. May increase to 10 mg daily, then to 20 mg once daily if needed.
Adjust-a-dose: In patients with bronchospastic disease or hepatic or renal insufficiency (CrCl less than 40 mL/minute), initially give 2.5 mg; then titrate with caution.
➤ **Stable heart failure due to reduced LVEF** ◆
Adults: Initially, 1.25 mg P.O. once daily, up to a maximum dosage of 10 mg once daily.

➤ **Cardiac risk reduction during surgery** ◆
Adults: Initially, 2.5 mg/day in patients with a resting heart rate of at least 50 beats/minute. Initiate therapy well before a planned procedure. Titrate according to heart rate in increments of 1.25 or 2.5 mg/day. Maximum dosage is 10 mg/day. Continue for 7 to 30 days after procedure.

ADMINISTRATION
P.O.
• May give without regard to meals.
• Store at room temperature. Protect from moisture.

ACTION
Selectively blocks cardiac adrenoceptors, reducing resting and exercise heart rate, decreasing cardiac output, depressing renin secretion, and decreasing tonic sympathetic outflow from the vasomotor centers in the brain.

Route	Onset	Peak	Duration
P.O.	Unknown	2–4 hr	Unknown

Half-life: 9 to 12 hours.

ADVERSE REACTIONS
CNS: headache, dizziness, hypoesthesia, insomnia, asthenia, fatigue.
CV: chest pain, peripheral edema, bradycardia.
EENT: dry mouth, pharyngitis, rhinitis, sinusitis.
GI: diarrhea, nausea, vomiting.
Musculoskeletal: arthralgia.
Respiratory: cough, dyspnea, upper respiratory tract infection.
Skin: sweating.

INTERACTIONS
Drug-drug. *Antiarrhythmics (such as disopyramide), calcium channel blockers (such as diltiazem, verapamil):* May increase myocardial depression or conduction delay. Use cautiously together.
Beta blockers: May increase beta blocker effects to unsafe level. Use together is contraindicated.
Catecholamine-depleting drugs (such as guanethidine, reserpine): May cause

hypotension or bradycardia. Monitor patient closely.

Clonidine: May cause rebound hypertension if clonidine is discontinued. Stop bisoprolol for several days before discontinuing clonidine.

Digoxin: May increase risk of slow AV conduction and bradycardia. Use together cautiously.

Insulin, oral antidiabetics: May mask signs and symptoms of hypoglycemia, particularly tachycardia. Use together cautiously.

Rifampin: May increase bisoprolol metabolism. Monitor patient for decreased bisoprolol effects.

EFFECTS ON LAB TEST RESULTS
• May increase serum triglyceride, AST, ALT, uric acid, creatinine, BUN, potassium, glucose, and phosphorus levels.
• May decrease WBC and platelet counts.
• May cause ANA conversion.

CONTRAINDICATIONS & CAUTIONS
• Contraindicated in patients hypersensitive to drug and in those with cardiogenic shock, overt cardiac failure, second- or third-degree AV block, or marked sinus bradycardia.
• Use cautiously in patients with hepatic or renal insufficiency, hypothyroidism, congestive heart failure, arterial insufficiency, peripheral vascular disease, or diabetes.
• Use cautiously in patients with a history of severe anaphylactic reaction to a variety of allergens. Patients may be more sensitive if allergen is reintroduced; usual epinephrine doses may not be effective.
• Use cautiously in patients with bronchospastic disease who don't tolerate or respond to other antihypertensive treatment. Patients should have a bronchodilator on hand in the event of an episode.
• Use cautiously in pregnant and breast-feeding women and only if benefits outweigh risks.

NURSING CONSIDERATIONS
• Monitor blood pressure closely.
• Avoid use in patients with acute congestive heart failure because of worsening of disease. If bisoprolol administration is necessary, monitor patient closely.
• Use cautiously in patients with known compensated heart failure. In patients with-

out a history of heart failure, drug may precipitate signs and symptoms of new heart failure. Consider stopping drug at first indication of new heart failure. Drug may be continued while heart failure is being treated with other drugs.
• Drug interruption or abrupt discontinuation may exacerbate angina pectoris, MI, or ventricular arrhythmia and may exacerbate the signs and symptoms of hyperthyroidism, possibly leading to thyroid storm. If drug is to be discontinued, taper over approximately 1 week while monitoring patient. If withdrawal signs and symptoms occur, restart drug at least temporarily.
• A long-term bisoprolol regimen shouldn't be discontinued before major surgery. However, the impaired ability of the heart to respond to reflex adrenergic stimuli may increase the risks of general anesthesia and surgical procedures.
• Drug may mask tachycardia caused by hyperthyroidism. In patients with suspected thyrotoxicosis, withdraw drug gradually to avoid thyroid storm.
• Drug may mask signs and symptoms of hypoglycemia in diabetic patients.

PATIENT TEACHING
• Tell patient to report slowed heartbeat, difficulty breathing, or other signs of heart failure.
• Caution patient not to discontinue bisoprolol without first consulting health care provider.
• Warn diabetic patient that bisoprolol may mask the signs and symptoms of hypoglycemia (such as tachycardia, dizziness, and weakness).
• Urge patient to use caution when operating automobiles and machinery or performing activities requiring alertness.

bivalirudin
bye-VAL-ih-roo-din

Angiomax

Therapeutic class: Anticoagulants
Pharmacologic class: Direct thrombin inhibitors
Pregnancy risk category: B

AVAILABLE FORMS
Injection: 250-mg vial

INDICATIONS & DOSAGES
Adjust-a-dose (for all indications): For patients with CrCl of 30 mL/minute or less, decrease infusion rate to 1 mg/kg/hour. For patients on hemodialysis, reduce infusion rate to 0.25 mg/kg/hour. No reduction of bolus dose is needed.
➤ **Anticoagulation in patients with unstable angina undergoing percutaneous transluminal coronary angioplasty (PTCA); anticoagulation in patients with unstable angina undergoing percutaneous coronary intervention (PCI), with provisional use of a platelet glycoprotein (GP) IIb/IIIa inhibitor**
Adults: 0.75 mg/kg I.V. bolus followed by a continuous infusion of 1.75 mg/kg/hour during the procedure. Check activated clotting time 5 minutes after bolus dose is given. May give additional 0.3 mg/kg bolus dose if needed. Infusion may continue for up to 4 hours after procedure. After 4-hour infusion, may give an additional infusion of 0.2 mg/kg/hour for up to 20 hours, if needed. Use with 300 to 325 mg aspirin.
➤ **Patients undergoing PCI who have or are at risk for heparin-induced thrombocytopenia (HIT) or heparin-induced thrombocytopenia and thrombosis syndrome (HITTS)**
Adults: 0.75 mg/kg I.V. bolus, followed by a continuous infusion of 1.75 mg/kg/hour throughout the procedure. Infusion up to 4 hours after procedure is optional. After 4 hours, may give an additional infusion of 0.2 mg/kg/hour for up to 20 hours. Use with 300 to 325 mg aspirin.

ADMINISTRATION
I.V.
▼ Reconstitute each 250-mg vial with 5 mL of sterile water for injection. Gently swirl until all material is dissolved.
▼ Dilute each reconstituted vial in 50 mL D_5W or normal saline solution to yield a final concentration of 5 mg/mL.
▼ To prepare low-rate infusion, further dilute each reconstituted vial in 500 mL D_5W or normal saline solution to yield a final concentration of 0.5 mg/mL.
▼ Solutions with concentrations of 0.5 to 5 mg/mL are stable at room temperature for 24 hours.
▼ **Incompatibilities:** Alteplase, amiodarone, amphotericin B, chlorpromazine, diazepam, prochlorperazine, reteplase, streptokinase, vancomycin. *Note:* Compatible with dobutamine at concentrations up to 4 mg/mL, but incompatible at concentration of 12.5 mg/mL.

ACTION
Binds specifically and rapidly to thrombin to produce an anticoagulant effect.

Route	Onset	Peak	Duration
I.V.	Rapid	Immediate	1–2 hr

Half-life: 25 minutes in patients with normal renal function.

ADVERSE REACTIONS
CNS: anxiety, headache, insomnia, nervousness, fever, pain.
CV: *bradycardia,* hypertension, hypotension.
GI: abdominal pain, dyspepsia, nausea, vomiting.
GU: urine retention.
Hematologic: *severe, spontaneous bleeding (cerebral, retroperitoneal, GU, GI).*
Musculoskeletal: back pain, pelvic pain.
Skin: pain at injection site.

INTERACTIONS
Drug-drug. *GPIIb/IIIa inhibitors, heparin, thrombolytics, warfarin:* May increase risk of hemorrhage. Use together cautiously.
Drug-herb. *Angelica (dong quai), boldo, bromelains, capsicum, chamomile, dandelion, danshen, devil's claw, fenugreek, feverfew, garlic, ginger, ginkgo, ginseng,*

Reactions in bold italics are *life-threatening*. Interactions may have a *rapid onset* or a *delayed onset*.

horse chestnut, licorice, meadowsweet, onion, passion flower, red clover, willow: May increase risk of bleeding. Discourage use together.

EFFECTS ON LAB TEST RESULTS
None reported.

CONTRAINDICATIONS & CAUTIONS
• Contraindicated in patients hypersensitive to drug or its components and in those with active major bleeding. Avoid using in patients with unstable angina who aren't undergoing PTCA or PCI or in patients with other acute coronary syndromes.
• Use cautiously in patients with HIT or HITTS and in those with diseases linked to increased risk of bleeding.
• Use cautiously in breast-feeding women; it's unknown if drug appears in breast milk.

NURSING CONSIDERATIONS
• Monitor coagulation test results, hemoglobin level, and hematocrit before starting therapy and periodically thereafter.
• Circumstances for provisional use of a glycoprotein inhibitor during PCI include decreased Thrombolysis in Myocardial Infarction (TIMI) score 0–2 flow, slow reflow, dissection with decreased flow, new or suspected thrombus, persistent residual stenosis, distal embolization, unplanned stent, suboptimal stenting, side-branch closure, abrupt closure, instability, and prolonged ischemia.
• Obtain a complete list of patient's pre-scription and OTC drugs and supplements, including herbs.
🕭 *Alert:* Hemorrhage can occur at any site in the body. If patient has unexplained de-crease in hematocrit, decrease in blood pressure, or other unexplained symptoms, suspect hemorrhage.
• Monitor venipuncture sites for bleeding, hematoma, or inflammation.
• Puncture-site hemorrhage and catheterization-site hematoma may occur in patients age 65 and older more often than in younger patients.
• Don't give drug I.M.

PATIENT TEACHING
• Advise patient that drug can cause bleed-ing, and tell him to report unusual bruising or bleeding (nosebleeds, bleeding gums) or tarry stools immediately.
• Counsel patient that drug is given with aspirin, and caution him to avoid other aspirin-containing drugs or NSAIDs while receiving this drug.
• Advise patient to consult with prescriber before initiating any herbal therapy; many herbs have anticoagulant, antiplatelet, and fibrinolytic properties.
• Advise patient to avoid activities that carry a risk of injury, and instruct him to use a soft toothbrush and electric razor while on drug.

SAFETY ALERT!

bleomycin sulfate
blee-oh-MYE-sin

Therapeutic class: Antineoplastics
Pharmacologic class: Cytotoxic glycopeptide antibiotics
Pregnancy risk category: D

AVAILABLE FORMS
Injection: 15-unit vials, 30-unit vials

INDICATIONS & DOSAGES
Adjust-a-dose (for all indications): For pa-tients with CrCl of 40 to 50 mL/minute, give 70% of dose; for CrCl of 30 to 39 mL/minute, give 60% of dose; for CrCl of 20 to 29 mL/minute, give 55% of dose; for CrCl of 10 to 19 mL/minute, give 45% of dose; and for CrCl of 5 to 9 mL/minute, give 40% of dose.
➤ **Squamous cell carcinoma (head, neck, skin, penis, cervix, and vulva), non-Hodgkin lymphoma, testicular carcinoma**
Adults: 2 units or less of bleomycin for in-jection for the first two doses. If no acute reaction occurs, then 0.25 to 0.5 units/kg (10 to 20 units/m^2) I.V., I.M., or subcuta-neously once or twice weekly to total of 400 units.
➤ **Hodgkin lymphoma**
Adults: 2 units or less of bleomycin for injection for the first two doses. If no acute reaction occurs, then 0.25 to

0.5 units/kg (10 to 20 units/m^2) I.V., I.M., or subcutaneously one or two times weekly. After 50% response, maintenance dose is 1 unit I.V. or I.M. daily or 5 units I.V. or I.M. weekly. Total cumulative dose is 400 units.

➤ **Malignant pleural effusion**
Adults: 60 units given as single-dose bolus intrapleural injection.

➤ **Malignant pericardial effusion ♦**
Adults: Dissolve bleomycin 5 to 20 units in 10 to 20 mL of normal saline solution and instill via catheter into pericardial space after pericardiocentesis. Clamp catheter for up to 6 hours. Continue drainage of effusion until volume is less than 20 to 30 mL/day. Repeat if needed to reach desired drainage level.

➤ **Malignant peritoneal effusion ♦**
Adults: 30 to 60 units in 100 mL of normal saline solution administered by intraperitoneal infusion.

➤ **Warts ♦**
Adults: Reconstitute with normal saline solution to 0.5 to 1 unit/mL. Give 0.1 to 2 units intralesionally.

ADMINISTRATION
I.V.
▼ Preparing and giving parenteral form of drug may be mutagenic, teratogenic, and carcinogenic. Follow facility policy to reduce risks.
▼ Drug may adsorb to plastic I.V. bags. For prolonged infusions, use glass containers.
▼ Reconstitute drug with 5 or 10 mL of normal saline solution for injection to equal 3 units/mL solution.
▼ Administer slowly over 10 minutes.
▼ Use reconstituted solution within 24 hours.
▼ Refrigerate unopened vials containing dry powder.
▼ **Incompatibilities:** Amino acids; aminophylline; ascorbic acid injection; cefazolin; diazepam; drugs containing sulfhydryl groups; fluids containing dextrose; furosemide; hydrocortisone; methotrexate; mitomycin; nafcillin; penicillin G; riboflavin; solutions containing divalent and trivalent cations, especially calcium salts and copper; terbutaline sulfate.

I.M.
● Dilute 15 unit-vial in 1 to 5 mL or 30 unit-vial in 2 to 10 mL of sterile water for injection, bacteriostatic water for injection, or normal saline solution for injection.
● Monitor injection site for irritation.
Subcutaneous
● Dilute 15 unit-vial in 1 to 5 mL or 30 unit-vial in 2 to 10 mL of sterile water for injection, bacteriostatic water for injection, or normal saline solution for injection.
● Monitor injection site for irritation.
Intrapleural
● For intrapleural use, dilute 60 units of drug in 50 to 100 mL normal saline solution for injection; give drug through a thoracotomy tube.
● If patient's condition requires sclerosis, instill drug when chest tube drainage is 100 to 300 mL/24 hours; ideally, drainage should be less than 100 mL. After instillation, clamp thoracotomy tube and move patient from his back to his left then right side for the next 4 hours. Remove clamp and reestablish suction. Amount of time chest tube is left in place after sclerosis depends on patient's condition.
● Don't use adhesive dressings.

ACTION
May inhibit DNA synthesis and cause scission of single- and double-stranded DNA; also inhibits RNA and protein synthesis.

Route	Onset	Peak	Duration
I.V., subcut.	Unknown	30–60 min	Unknown
I.M.	Unknown	30–60 min	Unknown

Half-life: 2 hours.

ADVERSE REACTIONS
CNS: fever.
GI: stomatitis, anorexia, nausea, vomiting, diarrhea.
Metabolic: weight loss, hyperuricemia.
Respiratory: *pneumonitis, pulmonary fibrosis.*
Skin: erythema, hyperpigmentation, acne, rash, striae, skin tenderness, pruritus, reversible alopecia, hyperkeratosis, nail changes.
Other: chills, *anaphylactoid reactions.*

INTERACTIONS

Drug-drug. *Anesthesia:* May increase oxygen requirements. Monitor patient closely.
Brentuximab: May increase risk of pulmonary toxicity. Use together is contraindicated.
Cardiac glycosides: May decrease digoxin level. Monitor digoxin level closely.
Cisplatin: May decrease bleomycin elimination. Monitor renal function and adjust bleomycin dosage as needed.
Fosphenytoin, phenytoin: May decrease phenytoin and fosphenytoin levels. Monitor drug levels closely.
Live-virus vaccines: May increase risk of vaccine-induced adverse reactions. Avoid concomitant use.

EFFECTS ON LAB TEST RESULTS

● May increase uric acid level.

CONTRAINDICATIONS & CAUTIONS

● Contraindicated in patients hypersensitive to drug.
● Use cautiously in patients with renal or pulmonary impairment.

NURSING CONSIDERATIONS

Black Box Warning Drug should be administered under the supervision of a physician experienced in the use of cancer chemotherapeutic agents. ■
● Obtain pulmonary function tests. If tests show a marked decline, stop drug.
Black Box Warning Fatal pulmonary fibrosis may occur, especially when cumulative dose exceeds 400 units. ■
Black Box Warning Monitor lymphoma patient for idiosyncratic reaction (hypotension, confusion, fever, and wheezing) after receiving drug. ■
● *Alert:* Adverse pulmonary reactions are more common in patients older than age 70. Also, in patients receiving radiation therapy, patients with lung disease, and patients who need oxygen therapy, pulmonary toxic adverse effects may be increased.
● Monitor chest X-ray and listen to lungs regularly.
● Watch for fever, which may be treated with antipyretics. Fever usually occurs within 3 to 6 hours of administration.

● *Alert:* Watch for hypersensitivity reactions, which may be delayed for several hours, especially in patients with lymphoma. (Give test dose of 1 to 2 units before first two doses in these patients. If no reaction occurs, follow regular dosage schedule.)

PATIENT TEACHING

● Warn patient that hair loss may occur but is usually reversible.
● Tell patient to report adverse reactions promptly and to take infection-control and bleeding precautions.
● For patient who is to receive anesthesia, tell him to inform anesthesiologist that he has taken this drug. High oxygen levels inhaled during surgery may enhance pulmonary toxicity of drug.

boceprevir
boe-SEH-pre-veer

Victrelis

Therapeutic class: Antivirals
Pharmacologic class: Protease inhibitors
Pregnancy risk category: X when used with ribavirin and peginterferon alfa

AVAILABLE FORMS
Capsules: 200 mg

INDICATIONS & DOSAGES

Adjust-a-dose (for all indications): Discontinue drug if hepatitis C virus (HCV)-RNA level is 100 international units/mL or more at treatment week 12, or if HCV-RNA level is confirmed detectable at treatment week 24.
➤ **Chronic HCV genotype 1 infection, in combination with ribavirin and peginterferon alfa, in patients with compensated liver disease, including cirrhosis**
Adults age 18 and older: Initiate treatment with 4 weeks of peginterferon alfa and ribavirin therapy; then add boceprevir 800 mg P.O. t.i.d. (every 7 to 9 hours) for 44 weeks.
➤ **Chronic HCV genotype 1 infection, in combination with ribavirin and peginterferon alfa, in patients without cirrhosis**

who were previously untreated or who failed or were partial responders to previous interferon and ribavirin therapy
Adults age 18 and older: Initiate treatment with 4 weeks of peginterferon alfa and ribavirin therapy; then add boceprevir 800 mg P.O. t.i.d. (every 7 to 9 hours).
Adjust-a-dose: Duration of treatment in noncirrhotic patients is based on HCV-RNA results. For previously untreated patients, if HCV-RNA level is undetectable at weeks 8 and 24, continue three-drug regimen through treatment week 28. If HCV-RNA level is detectable at week 8 and undetectable at week 24, continue all three drugs until treatment week 36; then give peginterferon alfa and ribavirin through week 48. For previous partial responders or relapsers, if HCV-RNA level is undetectable at weeks 8 and 24, continue three-drug regimen through treatment week 36. If HCV-RNA level is detectable at week 8 and undetectable at week 24, continue all three drugs until treatment week 36; then give peginterferon alfa and ribavirin through week 48.

ADMINISTRATION
P.O.
- Give drug with a meal or light snack.
- Drug is dispensed in single, daily-use bottles.
- Capsules must be refrigerated until dispensed from pharmacy.
- Capsules can be left at room temperature (up to 77° F [25° C]) for 3 months after dispensed from pharmacy.
- Don't give drug as monotherapy; always administer as part of a ribavirin and peginterferon alfa regimen.

ACTION
Inhibits certain proteases that enable HCV polyproteins to mature, resulting in inhibition of viral replication.

Route	Onset	Peak	Duration
P.O.	Unknown	2 hr	Unknown

Half-life: 3.4 hours.

ADVERSE REACTIONS
CNS: dizziness, fatigue, asthenia, insomnia, headache, irritability.

GI: nausea, dysgeusia, diarrhea, vomiting, dry mouth, decreased appetite.
Hematologic: anemia, *neutropenia, thrombocytopenia.*
Musculoskeletal: arthralgia.
Respiratory: exertional dyspnea.
Skin: alopecia, dry skin, rash.
Other: chills.

INTERACTIONS
Drug-drug. *Alfuzosin, drospirenone, ergot derivatives, lovastatin, midazolam (oral), pimozide, rifampin, simvastatin, triazolam:* May increase levels of these drugs and cause severe adverse effects. Don't use together.
Alprazolam, amiodarone, azole antifungals, bepridil, bosentan, clarithromycin, cyclosporine, desipramine, digoxin, dihydropyridine calcium channel blockers, flecainide, midazolam (I.V.), propafenone, quinidine, ritonavir, salmeterol, sirolimus, tacrolimus, trazodone: May increase levels of these drugs. Use together cautiously; monitor drug levels and adjust dosages when appropriate.
Atorvastatin: May increase atorvastatin level. Don't exceed 40 mg daily when given with boceprevir.
Buprenorphine, methadone: May increase or decrease levels of these drugs. Use together cautiously.
Carbamazepine, phenobarbital, phenytoin: May cause loss of virologic response to boceprevir. Don't use together.
Colchicine: May significantly increase colchicine level; decrease colchicine dosage. Administration with boceprevir is contraindicated in patients with renal or hepatic impairment.
Combination drug lopinavir–ritonavir, ritonavir-boosted HIV protease inhibitors (atazanavir, darunavir): May reduce effectiveness of these medications, allowing viral load of HIV or HCV to increase. Use together is contraindicated.
Dexamethasone, efavirenz, ritonavir: May decrease boceprevir levels. Use together cautiously.
Inhaled corticosteroids (budesonide, fluticasone): May increase serum levels of these drugs. Avoid use together if possible, especially for extended periods of time.

Reactions in bold italics are *life-threatening*. Interactions may have a *rapid onset* or a *delayed onset*.

Lovastatin, simvastatin: May increase statin level and risk of myopathy and rhabdomyolysis. Use together is contraindicated.

Oral hormonal contraceptives (ethinyl estradiol): May decrease effectiveness of these drugs. Patient should use two alternative effective methods of contraception (such as intrauterine device [IUD] and barrier method) during combination therapy with ribavirin.

Rifabutin: May increase rifabutin level and decrease exposure of boceprevir. Not recommended for use together.

Sildenafil, tadalafil (when used for pulmonary arterial hypertension): May increase levels of these drugs and increase adverse events. Don't use together.

Sildenafil, tadalafil, vardenafil (when used for erectile dysfunction): May increase levels of these drugs. Limit dosage of sildenafil to 25 mg every 48 hours, tadalafil to 10 mg every 72 hours, or vardenafil to 2.5 mg every 24 hours.

Warfarin: May increase or decrease warfarin level. Monitor INR carefully.

Drug-herb. *St. John's wort:* May lead to loss of antiviral response. Use is contraindicated.

EFFECTS ON LAB TEST RESULTS
● May decrease hemoglobin level and neutrophil and platelet counts.

CONTRAINDICATIONS & CAUTIONS
● All contraindications to peginterferon alfa and ribavirin apply because boceprevir must be administered with peginterferon alfa and ribavirin. Consult prescribing information for peginterferon alfa and ribavirin.
● Contraindicated in pregnant women and in men whose partners are pregnant because of the risk of birth defects and fetal death associated with ribavirin.
● Use cautiously in patients receiving peginterferon alfa and ribavirin who are anemic or neutropenic at baseline, and in those who are at risk for anemia or neutropenia; severe anemia or neutropenia may occur.
● It's unknown if drug appears in breast milk. Use in breast-feeding women only if benefits to mother outweigh risk to infant.

NURSING CONSIDERATIONS
● Always give drug with concurrent ribavirin and peginterferon alfa therapy.
● Monitor CBC with differential at baseline; at treatment weeks 4, 8, and 12; and periodically thereafter as clinically needed. If hemoglobin level is less than 10 mg/dL, decrease or interrupt ribavirin therapy; if hemoglobin level is less than 8.5 mg/dL, discontinue ribavirin.
● Monitor HCV-RNA at treatment weeks 4, 8, 12, and 24; at the end of treatment; during treatment follow-up; and as clinically indicated.
● Women of childbearing potential and men with sexual partners of childbearing potential must use two effective forms of nonhormonal contraception (such as an IUD and a barrier method) during treatment and for at least 6 months after end of treatment because of risk associated with concomitant ribavirin therapy.
● Patient should perform monthly pregnancy tests while on therapy and for 6 months after therapy ends. Patient should notify prescriber immediately if pregnancy occurs.
● Don't start ribavirin unless baseline negative pregnancy test is obtained immediately before therapy initiation.

PATIENT TEACHING
● Advise patient to take drug with food for better absorption.
● Inform patient that drug must be taken in combination with peginterferon alfa and ribavirin therapy.
● Warn male patients with partners of childbearing potential and female patients of childbearing potential to use two forms of contraception (such as an IUD and a barrier method) during and for 6 months after therapy. Advise patients that frequent pregnancy tests must be obtained as directed.
● Advise female patient to notify prescriber immediately if pregnancy occurs. Pregnant women exposed to boceprevir in combination with ribavirin should register with Ribavirin Pregnancy Registry at 1-800-593-2214.
● Caution patient to obtain blood work as directed.

- Instruct patient to inform prescriber of drugs, vitamins, or supplements he is taking or starts to take during treatment.
- Advise patient to contact prescriber if medical conditions change or if side effects occur.
- Warn patient to continue to take precautions against transmitting hepatitis C; it isn't known how drug affects transmission.

SAFETY ALERT!

bortezomib
bore-TEZ-uh-mib

Velcade

Therapeutic class: Antineoplastics
Pharmacologic class: Proteosome inhibitors
Pregnancy risk category: D

AVAILABLE FORMS
Powder for injection: 3.5 mg

INDICATIONS & DOSAGES
➤ **Previously untreated multiple myeloma**
Adults: 1.3 mg/m^2 I.V. over 3 to 5 seconds or subcutaneously in combination with oral melphalan and oral prednisone for nine 6-week treatment cycles. In cycles 1 to 4, bortezomib is given twice weekly (days 1, 4, 8, 11, 22, 25, 29, and 32). In cycles 5 to 9, bortezomib is given once weekly (days 1, 8, 22, and 29). Separate consecutive doses of drug by at least 72 hours. Prior to initiating any cycle, platelet count should be 70 × 10^9/L or greater, ANC should be 1 × 10^9/L or greater, and nonhematologic toxicities should have resolved to grade 1 or baseline.
Adjust-a-dose: If prolonged grade 4 neutropenia or thrombocytopenia, or thrombocytopenia with bleeding in previous cycle, consider reducing dose by 25% for next cycle. If platelet count is less than or equal to 30 × 10^9/L or ANC is 0.75 × 10^9/L or less on a day other than day 1, withhold dose. If several doses in consecutive cycles are withheld due to toxicity, reduce dose by one dose level (from 1.3 mg/m^2 to 1 mg/m^2, or from 1 mg/m^2 to 0.7 mg/m^2). For grade 3 nonhematologic toxicities, withhold drug

until symptoms are grade 1 or baseline, then restart with one dose level reduction. If patient has neuropathic pain, peripheral neuropathy, or both, see table.

If patient has moderate to severe hepatic dysfunction with bilirubin level greater than 1.5 to 3 times upper limit of normal, reduce dose of first cycle to 0.7 mg/m^2. If patient tolerates this dose, may increase to 1 mg/m^2 in subsequent cycles. Based on tolerability, dose may be reduced to 0.5 mg/m^2.

➤ **Multiple myeloma or mantle cell lymphoma that still progresses after at least one therapy**
Adults: 1.3 mg/m^2 by I.V. bolus or subcutaneously twice weekly for 2 weeks (days 1, 4, 8, and 11), followed by a 10-day rest period (days 12 through 21). This 3-week period is a treatment cycle. For therapy longer than eight cycles, may adjust dosage schedule to once weekly for 4 weeks on days 1, 8, 15, and 22, followed by a rest period on days 23 through 35. Separate consecutive doses of drug by at least 72 hours.
Adjust-a-dose: If grade 3 nonhematologic or grade 4 hematologic toxicity (excluding neuropathy) develops, withhold drug. When toxicity has resolved, restart at a 25% reduced dose. If patient has neuropathic pain, peripheral neuropathy, or both, see table.

If patient has moderate to severe hepatic dysfunction with bilirubin level greater than 1.5 to 3 times upper limit of normal, reduce dose of first cycle to 0.7 mg/m^2. If patient tolerates this dose, may increase to 1 mg/m^2 in subsequent cycles. Based on tolerability, dose may be reduced to 0.5 mg/m^2.

Severity of neuropathy	Dosage
Grade 1 (paresthesia, loss of reflexes, or both) without pain or loss of function	No change.
Grade 1 with pain or grade 2 (function altered but not activities of daily living)	Reduce to 1 mg/m^2.
Grade 2 with pain or grade 3 (interference with activities of daily living)	Hold drug until toxicity resolves; then start at 0.7 mg/m^2 once weekly.
Grade 4 (permanent sensory loss that interferes with function)	Stop drug.

ADMINISTRATION

I.V.

▼ Use caution and aseptic technique when preparing and handling drug. Wear gloves and protective clothing to prevent skin contact.

▼ Reconstitute with 3.5 mL of normal saline solution and give by I.V. bolus over 3 to 5 seconds.

▼ Inspect solution before administration. Don't give if discolored or if particles are seen.

▼ Reconstituted drug may be stored in a syringe at 59° to 86° F (15° to 30° C); total storage time must not exceed 8 hours.

▼ Store unopened vial at a controlled room temperature, in original packaging, protected from light.

▼ **Incompatibilities:** None reported.

Subcutaneous

● Give at concentration of 2.5 mg/mL.

● Rotate injection sites. New injections should be given at least 1 inch from an old site and never in areas that are tender, bruised, erythematous, or indurated.

● If injection-site reactions occur, a less concentrated solution (1 mg/mL) may be used.

ACTION

Disrupts intracellular homeostatic mechanisms by inhibiting the 26S proteosome, which regulates intracellular levels of certain proteins, causing cells to die.

Route	Onset	Peak	Duration
I.V.	Unknown	Unknown	Unknown

Half-life: 40 to 193 hours (1-mg/m^2 dose); 76 to 108 hours (1.3-mg/m^2 dose).

ADVERSE REACTIONS

CNS: anxiety, asthenia, dizziness, dysesthesia, fatigue, fever, headache, insomnia, paresthesia, peripheral neuropathy, rigors.
CV: edema, hypotension.
EENT: blurred vision.
GI: abdominal pain, constipation, decreased appetite, diarrhea, dysgeusia, dyspepsia, nausea, vomiting.
Hematologic: *neutropenia, thrombocytopenia,* anemia, leukopenia, lymphopenia.

Hepatic: *acute liver failure, hepatitis,* hyperbilirubinemia, increased liver enzyme levels.
Metabolic: anorexia.
Musculoskeletal: arthralgia, back pain, bone pain, limb pain, muscle cramps, myalgia.
Respiratory: cough, dyspnea, pneumonia, upper respiratory tract infection.
Skin: pruritus, rash.
Other: dehydration, herpes zoster, pyrexia.

INTERACTIONS

Drug-drug. *Antihypertensives:* May cause hypotension. Monitor patient's blood pressure closely.
Cyclosporine: May enhance neurotoxic effects of cyclosporine. Closely monitor patient. Adjust cyclosporine dosage as needed.
Drugs linked to peripheral neuropathy, such as amiodarone, antivirals, isoniazid, nitrofurantoin, statins: May worsen neuropathy. Use together cautiously.
Inhibitors or inducers of CYP3A4: May increase risk of toxicity or may reduce drug's effects. Monitor patient closely.
Oral antidiabetics: May cause hypoglycemia or hyperglycemia. Monitor glucose level closely.
Drug-herb. *St. John's wort:* May decrease bortezomib exposure. Avoid concomitant use.

EFFECTS ON LAB TEST RESULTS

● May decrease hemoglobin level.
● May increase liver enzyme levels.
● May increase or decrease glucose level.
● May decrease neutrophil and platelet counts.

CONTRAINDICATIONS & CAUTIONS

● Contraindicated in patients hypersensitive to bortezomib, boron, or mannitol. Intrathecal administration is contraindicated.

● Use cautiously in patients with hepatic or renal impairment or with a history of syncope and in those who are dehydrated or receiving other drugs known to cause hypotension.

● Safety and effectiveness haven't been established for pregnant women or children.

⚠ **Overdose S&S:** Symptomatic hypotension, thrombocytopenia.

NURSING CONSIDERATIONS

• Monitor for evidence of neuropathy, such as a burning sensation, hyperesthesia, hypoesthesia, paresthesia, discomfort, or neuropathic pain.

• Consider subcutaneous administration for patients at high risk for or with preexisting peripheral neuropathy.

• Monitor for signs and symptoms of tumor lysis syndrome (hyperuricemia, hyperkalemia, hyperphosphatemia, hypocalcemia, and acute renal failure).

• Watch carefully for adverse effects, especially in the elderly.

• Be sure patient has an order for an antiemetic, antidiarrheal, or both to treat drug-induced nausea, vomiting, or diarrhea.

• Provide fluid and electrolyte replacement to prevent dehydration.

• To manage orthostatic hypotension, adjust antihypertensive dosage, maintain hydration status, and give mineralocorticoids.

• Dialysis may reduce drug level; give after dialysis.

❸ **Alert:** Because thrombocytopenia is common, monitor patient's CBC and platelet counts carefully during treatment, before each dose, and especially on day 11.

PATIENT TEACHING

• Tell patient to notify prescriber about new or worsening peripheral neuropathy.

• Urge women to use effective contraception and not to breast-feed during treatment.

• Teach patient how to avoid dehydration, and stress the need to tell prescriber about dizziness, light-headedness, or fainting spells.

• Tell patient to use caution when driving or performing other hazardous activities because drug may cause fatigue, dizziness, faintness, light-headedness, and doubled or blurred vision.

bosentan
bow-SEN-tan

Tracleer

Therapeutic class: Vasodilators
Pharmacologic class: Endothelin-receptor antagonists
Pregnancy risk category: X

AVAILABLE FORMS
Tablets: 62.5 mg, 125 mg

INDICATIONS & DOSAGES

Black Box Warning Only prescribers and pharmacies registered with the Tracleer Access Program (call 1-866-228-3546) may prescribe and distribute bosentan. ∎

➤ **Pulmonary arterial hypertension in patients with World Health Organization class III (with mild exertion) or IV (at rest) symptoms, to improve exercise ability and decrease rate of clinical worsening**

Adults: 62.5 mg P.O. b.i.d. in the morning and evening for 4 weeks. If patient weighs 40 kg (88 lb) or more, increase to maintenance dosage of 125 mg P.O. b.i.d. in the morning and evening. If patient weighs less than 40 kg, maintenance dosage is 62.5 mg P.O. b.i.d.

Adjust-a-dose: For patients who develop ALT and AST abnormalities, dosage may need to be decreased or therapy stopped until ALT and AST levels return to normal. If therapy is resumed, begin with initial dose. Test levels within 3 days; then give using the following table. If liver function abnormalities are accompanied by symptoms of liver injury or if bilirubin level is at least twice the upper limit of normal (ULN), stop treatment and don't restart. In patients who weigh less than 40 kg (88 lb), the initial and maintenance dosage is 62.5 mg b.i.d.

Reactions in bold italics are *life-threatening*. Interactions may have a *rapid onset* or a *delayed onset*.

ALT and AST levels	Treatment and monitoring recommendations
>3 and ≤5 times ULN	Confirm with repeat test; if confirmed, reduce dose to 62.5 mg b.i.d. or interrupt treatment and retest every 2 wk. Once ALT and AST levels return to pretreatment levels, continue or reintroduce treatment at starting dose.
>5 and ≤8 times ULN	Confirm with repeat test; if confirmed, stop treatment and retest at least every 2 wk. Once levels return to pretreatment levels, consider reintroduction of treatment.
>8 times ULN	Stop treatment; don't consider restarting drug.

Discontinue bosentan at least 36 hours before starting ritonavir. After at least 10 days following the initiation of ritonavir, resume bosentan at 62.5 mg P.O. once daily or every other day.

➤ **Raynaud phenomenon ◆**
Adults: 62.5 mg P.O. b.i.d. for 4 weeks; then 125 mg P.O. b.i.d. for up to 72 weeks.

ADMINISTRATION
P.O.
• Give drug in morning and evening without regard for meals.

ACTION
Specific and competitive antagonist for endothelin-1 (ET-1). ET-1 levels are elevated in patients with pulmonary arterial hypertension, suggesting a pathogenic role for ET-1 in this disease.

Route	Onset	Peak	Duration
P.O.	Unknown	3–5 hr	Unknown

Half-life: About 5 hours.

ADVERSE REACTIONS
CNS: headache, fatigue, syncope.
CV: edema, flushing, hypotension, palpitations, chest pain.
EENT: sinusitis.
Hematologic: anemia.
Hepatic: *hepatotoxicity.*
Musculoskeletal: arthralgia.
Respiratory: respiratory tract infection.

INTERACTIONS
Drug-drug. *Clarithromycin:* May increase risk of bosentan hepatotoxicity. Monitor patient closely. Stop one or both drugs if an interaction is suspected.
Cyclosporine A: May increase bosentan level and decrease cyclosporine level. Use together is contraindicated.
Glyburide: May increase risk of elevated LFT values and decrease levels of both drugs. Use together is contraindicated.
Hormonal contraceptives: May cause contraceptive failure. Advise use of an additional method of birth control.
Ketoconazole: May increase bosentan effect. Watch for adverse effects.
PDE5 inhibitors (sildenafil): May increase bosentan level. Use together with caution.
Rifampin: May alter bosentan level. Monitor hepatic function weekly for 4 weeks followed by routine monitoring.
Ritonavir: May increase risk of bosentan toxicity. Dosage adjustment may be needed.
Simvastatin, other statins: May decrease levels of these drugs. Monitor cholesterol levels to assess need to adjust statin dose.
Tacrolimus: May increase bosentan levels. Use together cautiously.
Warfarin: May decrease warfarin level. Monitor coagulation tests and adjust warfarin dosage as needed.

EFFECTS ON LAB TEST RESULTS
Black Box Warning May increase AST, ALT, and bilirubin levels. ∎
• May decrease hemoglobin level and hematocrit.

CONTRAINDICATIONS & CAUTIONS
• Contraindicated in patients hypersensitive to drug and in those taking cyclosporine A or glyburide.
Black Box Warning Generally avoid using in patients with moderate to severe hepatic impairment or in those with elevated aminotransferase levels greater than 3 times the ULN. ∎
Black Box Warning Contraindicated in pregnant women. Exclude pregnancy before giving drug. ∎
• Use cautiously in patients with mild hepatic impairment.

• Because it's unknown whether drug appears in breast milk, drug isn't recommended for breast-feeding women.
• Safety and effectiveness in children haven't been established.
⚠ **Overdose S&S:** Headache, nausea, vomiting, hypotension, dizziness, blurred vision.

NURSING CONSIDERATIONS
Black Box Warning Use of this drug can cause serious liver injury. AST and ALT level elevations may be dose dependent and reversible, so measure these levels before treatment and monthly thereafter, adjusting dosage accordingly. If elevations are accompanied by symptoms of liver injury (nausea, vomiting, fever, abdominal pain, jaundice, or unusual lethargy or fatigue) or if bilirubin level increases by greater than twice the ULN, notify prescriber immediately. ■
• Fluid retention and heart failure may occur. Patient may require diuretics, fluid management, or hospitalization for decompensating heart failure.
• Monitor hemoglobin level after 1 and 3 months of therapy; then every 3 months.
• Gradually reduce dose before stopping drug.

PATIENT TEACHING
• Advise patient to take doses in the morning and evening, with or without food.
Black Box Warning Warn patient to avoid becoming pregnant while taking this drug. Hormonal contraceptives, including oral, implantable, and injectable methods, may not be effective when used with this drug. Advise patient to use a backup method of contraception. A monthly pregnancy test must be performed. ■
• Tell women who have had tubal ligation or have Copper T 380A IUD or levonorgestrol 20 IUS that they can use those contraceptive methods alone.
• Inform male patients of risk of low sperm count.
• Advise patient to have LFTs and blood counts performed regularly.

SAFETY ALERT!

brentuximab vedotin
bren-TUX-eh-mab

Adcetris

Therapeutic class: Antineoplastics
Pharmacologic class: Antibodies
Pregnancy risk category: D

AVAILABLE FORMS
Powder for injection: 50-mg single-use vial

INDICATIONS & DOSAGES
Adjust-a-dose (for all indications): In patients with peripheral neuropathy, delay dose as necessary, and reduce dosage to 1.2 mg/kg. In patients with new or worsening grade 2 or 3 neuropathy, withhold dose until neuropathy improves to grade 1 or baseline; then restart at 1.2 mg/kg. For patients with grade 4 neuropathy, discontinue drug. For patients with grade 3 or 4 neutropenia, withhold dose until resolution to baseline or grade 2 or lower. Consider the use of growth factor for subsequent cycles in patients with grade 3 or 4 neutropenia. For recurrent grade 4 neutropenia despite the use of growth factors, discontinue drug or reduce dosage to 1.2 mg/kg.
➤ **Hodgkin lymphoma after failure of autologous stem cell transplant (ASCT) or after failure of at least two prior multiagent chemotherapy regimens in patients who aren't ASCT candidates, or systemic anaplastic large cell lymphoma after failure of at least one prior multiagent chemotherapy regimen**
Adults: 1.8 mg/kg I.V. infusion over 30 minutes every 3 weeks for a maximum of 16 cycles, or until patient exhibits signs of disease progression or toxicities. Calculate dosage for patients weighing more than 100 kg (220 lb) based on a weight of 100 kg.

ADMINISTRATION
I.V.
▼ Use proper handling and disposal of this anticancer drug.
▼ Reconstitute each 50-mg vial with 10.5 mL sterile water for injection to yield a single-use solution containing 5 mg/mL.

▼ Gently swirl contents; don't shake vial. Inspect for particulates and discoloration.
▼ Dilute further to yield 0.4 to 1.8 mg/mL in infusion bag of normal saline injection, 5% dextrose injection, or lactated Ringer injection. Gently mix by inverting bag.
▼ After reconstitution, infuse immediately or store at 36° to 46° F (2° to 8° C) and use within 24 hours of reconstitution. Don't freeze. Discard unused portion left in vial.
▼ Administer drug only by I.V. infusion over 30 minutes; don't give by I.V. push or bolus.
▼ **Incompatibilities:** Don't mix or administer drug with other medications or fluids.

ACTION

Disrupts microtubule network of the cancer cell, which induces cell-cycle arrest and apoptotic death of the cells.

Route	Onset	Peak	Duration
I.V.	Rapid	1–3 days	Unknown

Half-life: 4 to 6 days.

ADVERSE REACTIONS

CNS: peripheral neuropathy, headache, dizziness, fatigue, pyrexia, chills, insomnia, anxiety, pain.
CV: peripheral edema, *pulmonary embolism, supraventricular arrhythmia,* lymphadenopathy.
EENT: oropharyngeal pain.
GI: nausea, diarrhea, abdominal pain, vomiting, constipation, decreased appetite.
GU: pyelonephritis, UTI.
Hematologic: *neutropenia,* anemia, *thrombocytopenia.*
Metabolic: decreased weight.
Musculoskeletal: arthralgia, myalgia, back pain, extremity pain, muscle spasms.
Respiratory: upper respiratory tract infection, cough, dyspnea, pneumonitis, pneumothorax.
Skin: rash, pruritus, alopecia, night sweats, dry skin.
Other: *septic shock, anaphylaxis,* immunogenicity.

INTERACTIONS

Drug-drug. *Bleomycin:* May increase risk of pulmonary toxicity. Concomitant use is contraindicated.
Strong CYP3A4 inducers (such as rifampin): May decrease brentuximab level. Monitor patient for brentuximab effectiveness.
Strong CYP3A4 inhibitors (such as ketoconazole): May increase brentuximab level. Monitor patient for increased adverse effects.

EFFECTS ON LAB TEST RESULTS

• May decrease RBC, WBC, platelet, and neutrophil counts.

CONTRAINDICATIONS & CAUTIONS

Black Box Warning JC virus infection resulting in progressive multifocal leukoencephalopathy (PML) and death can occur in patients receiving brentuximab. ∎
• Contraindicated in patients hypersensitive to drug and in breast-feeding women.
• Use cautiously in women of childbearing age.

NURSING CONSIDERATIONS

• Drug may cause severe peripheral neuropathy. Monitor patient for new or worsening signs and symptoms.
• Monitor patient closely for infusion-related adverse effects; interrupt therapy and treat as necessary. Premedicate patient with history of infusion-related reactions with acetaminophen, an antihistamine, and a corticosteroid. If anaphylaxis occurs, permanently stop drug.
• Monitor patient for signs and symptoms of neutropenia. Monitor CBC before each dose, and more frequently if patient exhibits grade 3 or 4 neutropenia. Delay or reduce dose, or discontinue drug as required.
• Monitor patient for tumor lysis syndrome, characterized by changes in electrolytes and kidney damage.
• Monitor patient for skin reactions, especially Stevens-Johnson syndrome. Discontinue drug if reactions occur.
• Monitor patient for vision loss, impaired speech, muscle weakness or paralysis, and cognitive deterioration, which may indicate PML.

PATIENT TEACHING
• Tell patient to report muscle weakness or numbness or tingling of the hands or feet.
• Advise patient to report signs or symptoms of possible infection, including temperature of 100.5° F (38° C) or greater, chills, cough, or pain on urination.
• Warn patient to report signs or symptoms of possible infusion-related reactions, including fever, chills, rash, or breathing problems.
• Warn women of childbearing age about risk of fetal harm. Caution women to avoid becoming pregnant and to avoid breastfeeding while taking drug. Instruct women to report possible pregnancy immediately.

brimonidine tartrate
bri-MOE-ni-deen

Alphagan P

Therapeutic class: Antiglaucoma drugs
Pharmacologic class: Selective alpha$_2$ agonists
Pregnancy risk category: B

AVAILABLE FORMS
Ophthalmic solution: 0.1%, 0.15%, 0.2%

INDICATIONS & DOSAGES
➤ **To reduce intraocular pressure (IOP) in open-angle glaucoma or ocular hypertension**
Adults and children age 2 and older: 1 drop in affected eye t.i.d., about 8 hours apart.

ADMINISTRATION
Ophthalmic
• Don't touch tip of dropper to eye or surrounding tissue.
• If more than one ophthalmic product is being used, give them at least 5 minutes apart.

ACTION
Reduces aqueous humor production and increases uveoscleral outflow.

Route	Onset	Peak	Duration
Ophthalmic	Unknown	30 min–2½ hr	Unknown

Half-life: 2 hours.

ADVERSE REACTIONS
CNS: asthenia, dizziness, headache, fatigue, somnolence.
CV: hypertension, hypotension.
EENT: allergic conjunctivitis, ocular hyperemia, pruritus, abnormal vision, allergic reaction, blepharitis, burning, conjunctival edema, hemorrhage, or inflammation, dryness, eyelid edema or erythema, follicular conjunctivitis, foreign body sensation, increased tearing, pain, pharyngitis, photophobia, rhinitis, sinus infection or inflammation, stinging, superficial punctate keratopathy, visual disturbances, visual field defect, vitreous floaters, worsened visual acuity.
GI: dyspepsia, oral dryness.
Metabolic: diabetes mellitus.
Musculoskeletal: arthralgia, arthritis, joint disorder, osteoporosis.
Respiratory: bronchitis, cough, dyspnea.
Skin: rash.
Other: flulike syndrome.

INTERACTIONS
Drug-drug. *Antihypertensives, beta blockers, cardiac glycosides:* May further decrease blood pressure or pulse. Monitor vital signs.
Apraclonidine, dorzolamide, pilocarpine, timolol: May have additive IOP-lowering effects. Use cautiously together.
CNS depressants: May increase effects. Use cautiously together.
Linezolid, MAO inhibitors: May increase effects. Avoid using together.
TCAs: May interfere with brimonidine's effect. Use cautiously together.
Drug-lifestyle. *Alcohol use:* May increase CNS-depressant effect. Urge patient to avoid alcohol.

EFFECTS ON LAB TEST RESULTS
• May increase cholesterol level.

CONTRAINDICATIONS & CAUTIONS
• Contraindicated in patients hypersensitive to drug or its components and in those taking MAO inhibitors.
• Use cautiously in patients with CV disease, cerebral or coronary insufficiency, hepatic or renal impairment, depression,

Raynaud phenomenon, orthostatic hypotension, or thromboangiitis obliterans.

⚠ **Overdose S&S:** Hypotension.

NURSING CONSIDERATIONS
• Monitor IOP because drug effect may reverse after first month of therapy.

PATIENT TEACHING
• Tell patient to wait at least 15 minutes after instilling drug before wearing soft contact lenses.
• Caution patient to avoid hazardous activities because of risk of decreased mental alertness, fatigue, or drowsiness.
• Advise patient to avoid alcohol.
• If patient is using more than one ophthalmic drug, tell him to apply them at least 5 minutes apart.

bromfenac
BROM-fen-ak

Bromday, Prolensa

Therapeutic class: Anti-inflammatory drugs (ophthalmic)
Pharmacologic class: NSAIDs
Pregnancy risk category: C

AVAILABLE FORMS
Ophthalmic solution: 0.07%, 0.09%

INDICATIONS & DOSAGES
➤ **Inflammation and pain after cataract surgery**
Adults: For generic solution, 1 drop in each eye b.i.d., starting 24 hours after surgery and continuing for 2 weeks. Or, for Bromday or Prolensa, 1 drop in affected eye(s) once daily beginning 1 day before surgery, continued on the day of surgery and for the first 14 days after surgery.

ADMINISTRATION
Ophthalmic
• Begin treatment at least 24 hours after surgery and continue for 2 weeks. Starting treatment less than 24 hours after surgery or giving for longer than 14 days increases risk of ocular adverse effects.

• After giving drop, have patient close his eyes and apply gentle pressure to lacrimal sac for 1 to 2 minutes.

ACTION
Blocks prostaglandin synthesis by inhibiting cyclooxygenase 1 and 2.

Route	Onset	Peak	Duration
Ophthalmic	Unknown	Unknown	Unknown

Half-life: Unknown.

ADVERSE REACTIONS
CNS: headache (Bromday).
EENT: abnormal sensation in the eye, burning, conjunctival hyperemia, eye irritation, eye pain, eye pruritus, eye redness, iritis, keratitis, stinging (Bromday); anterior chamber inflammation, foreign body sensation, eye pain, photophobia, blurred vision (Prolensa).

INTERACTIONS
None reported.

EFFECTS ON LAB TEST RESULTS
• May increase bleeding time.

CONTRAINDICATIONS & CAUTIONS
• Contraindicated in patients hypersensitive to drug or its components. Drug contains sulfite, which may cause allergic-type reactions, including anaphylaxis and life-threatening or less severe asthmatic episodes in patients sensitive to sulfites.
• Use cautiously in patients with bleeding tendencies, those taking anticoagulants, and those sensitive to aspirin products, phenylacetic acid derivatives, and other NSAIDs.
• Use cautiously in patients who have had complicated or repeat ocular surgeries or those with corneal denervation, corneal epithelial defects, diabetes mellitus, ocular surface diseases (such as dry-eye syndrome), or rheumatoid arthritis because of the increased risk of corneal adverse effects, which may threaten sight.
• Use in pregnant women only if potential benefit justifies risk; avoid use late in pregnancy because NSAIDs may cause premature closure of the ductus arteriosus, a necessary structure of fetal circulation.
• Use cautiously in breast-feeding women.

NURSING CONSIDERATIONS

- Ask patient if he's sensitive to sulfites, aspirin, or other NSAIDs before treatment. Drug contains sulfite, which may cause allergic-type reactions, including anaphylaxis and life-threatening or less severe asthmatic episodes, in patients sensitive to sulfites.
- Sulfite sensitivity is more common in patients with asthma than in those without asthma. If patient has asthma, monitor closely.
- If patient takes an anticoagulant, watch closely for increased bleeding.

PATIENT TEACHING

- Teach patient how to instill the drops.
- Instruct patient to start therapy 24 hours after surgery and to continue for 14 days.
- Tell patient not to use for longer than 2 weeks after surgery or to save unused amount for other conditions.
- Tell patient the signs and symptoms of adverse effects. If bothersome or serious adverse effects occur, advise patient to stop therapy and contact prescriber.
- Tell patient to store drug at room temperature.
- Advise patient not to use while wearing contact lenses.

bromocriptine mesylate

broe-moe-KRIP-teen

Cycloset, Parlodel

Therapeutic class: Antiparkinsonians
Pharmacologic class: Dopamine receptor agonists
Pregnancy risk category: B

AVAILABLE FORMS

Capsules: 5 mg (Parlodel)
Tablets: 0.8 mg (Cycloset), 2.5 mg (Parlodel)

INDICATIONS & DOSAGES

➤ **Parkinson disease (not Cycloset)**
Adults: 1.25 mg P.O. b.i.d. with meals. Increase dosage by 2.5 mg/day every 14 to 28 days, up to 100 mg daily. Usual dose is 20 to 30 mg daily.

➤ **Amenorrhea and galactorrhea from hyperprolactinemia; hypogonadism; infertility (not Cycloset)**
Adults and adolescents age 16 and older: 1.25 to 2.5 mg P.O. daily, increased by 2.5 mg daily at 2- to 7-day intervals until desired effect occurs. Therapeutic daily dose is 2.5 to 15 mg.
Children ages 11 to 15: 1.25 to 2.5 mg P.O. daily. May increase as tolerated until therapeutic response is achieved. Range, 2.5 to 10 mg daily in children with prolactin-secreting pituitary adenomas.

➤ **Acromegaly (not Cycloset)**
Adults: 1.25 to 2.5 mg P.O. with bedtime snack for 3 days. Another 1.25 to 2.5 mg may be added every 3 to 7 days until therapeutic benefit occurs. Maximum, 100 mg daily.

➤ **Type 2 diabetes mellitus (Cycloset only)**
Adults: Initially, 0.8 mg P.O. daily. May increase by 0.8 mg weekly until maximum tolerated dosage of 1.6 to 4.8 mg daily is achieved.

➤ **Traumatic brain injury ◆**
Adults: 2.5 mg P.O. daily. Continue longterm if response is adequate.

ADMINISTRATION

P.O.
- Give drug in the evening with food to minimize adverse reactions.
- For treatment of type 2 diabetes mellitus, give Cycloset within 2 hours of patient's waking in the morning.

ACTION

Inhibits secretion of prolactin and acts as a dopamine receptor agonist by activating postsynaptic dopamine receptors; improves glycemic control.

Route	Onset	Peak	Duration
P.O.	2 hr	8 hr	24 hr

Half-life: 15 hours.

ADVERSE REACTIONS

CNS: dizziness, headache, fatigue, *seizures, stroke,* mania, light-headedness, drowsiness, delusions, hallucinations, nervousness, insomnia, depression.
CV: orthostatic hypotension, *acute MI.*
EENT: nasal congestion, rhinitis, blurred vision.

Reactions in bold italics are *life-threatening*. Interactions may have a *rapid onset* or a *delayed onset*.

GI: nausea, abdominal cramps, constipation, diarrhea, vomiting, anorexia.
GU: urine retention, urinary frequency.
Skin: coolness and pallor of fingers and toes.

INTERACTIONS

Drug-drug. *Amitriptyline, haloperidol, imipramine, loxapine, MAO inhibitors, methyldopa, phenothiazines, reserpine:* May interfere with bromocriptine's effects. Bromocriptine dosage may need to be increased.
Antihypertensives: May increase hypotensive effects. Adjust dosage of antihypertensive.
Chloramphenicol, probenecid, salicylates, sulfonamides: May increase unbound fraction of other highly protein-bound drugs. Monitor patient for increased adverse reactions.
CYP3A4 inhibitors or inducers: May increase or decrease circulating levels of Cycloset, respectively. Use together with caution.
Dopamine receptor agonists (butyrophenones, phenothiazines, thioxanthenes): May diminish effects of Cycloset. Concurrent use isn't recommended.
Ergot-related drugs: May increase occurrence of ergot-related adverse effects and reduce effectiveness of these therapies. Avoid concomitant use.
Estrogens, hormonal contraceptives, progestins: May interfere with effects of bromocriptine. Avoid using together.
Levodopa: May have additive effects. Adjust dosage of levodopa, if needed.
Macrolides (erythromycin): May increase bromocriptine level and risk of adverse reactions. Use together cautiously.
Triptans (sumatriptan): May have additive vasoconstrictive effects. Concomitant use is contraindicated; don't use within 24 hours of one another.
Drug-lifestyle. *Alcohol use:* May cause disulfiram-like reaction. Discourage use together.

EFFECTS ON LAB TEST RESULTS

● May increase alkaline phosphatase, ALT, AST, BUN, CK, and uric acid levels.

CONTRAINDICATIONS & CAUTIONS

● Contraindicated in patients hypersensitive to ergot derivatives and in those with uncontrolled hypertension, toxemia of pregnancy, severe ischemic heart disease, hereditary galactose intolerance, lactase deficiency, glucose-galactose malabsorption, or peripheral vascular disease.
● Cycloset is contraindicated in patients with syncopal migraines or severe psychotic disorders and in breast-feeding women.
● Use cautiously in patients with impaired renal or hepatic function and in those with a history of MI with residual arrhythmias.
● Use cautiously in patients taking antihypertensives.
⚠ Overdose S&S: Nausea, vomiting, constipation, diaphoresis, dizziness, pallor, severe hypotension, malaise, confusion, lethargy, drowsiness, delusions, hallucinations, repetitive yawning.

NURSING CONSIDERATIONS

● For Parkinson disease, bromocriptine usually is given with levodopa or levodopa–carbidopa. The levodopa–carbidopa dosage may need to be reduced.
☉ Alert: Monitor patient for adverse reactions, which occur in 68% of patients, particularly at start of therapy. Most reactions are mild to moderate; nausea is most common. Minimize adverse reactions by gradually adjusting dosages to effective levels. Adverse reactions are more common when drug is used for Parkinson disease.
● Baseline and periodic evaluations of cardiac, hepatic, renal, and hematopoietic function are recommended during prolonged therapy.
● Drug may lead to early postpartum conception. After menses resumes, test for pregnancy every 4 weeks or as soon as a period is missed.
● Drug can cause orthostatic hypotension and syncope, particularly at start of therapy or when dosage is increased. Assess orthostatic vital signs before initiation of therapy and periodically thereafter.
● *Look alike–sound alike:* Don't confuse bromocriptine with benztropine or brimonidine. Don't confuse Parlodel with pindolol.

PATIENT TEACHING

● Instruct patient to take drug with meals.

● Tell patient to take Cycloset within 2 hours of waking in the morning.

● Advise patient to use contraceptive methods other than oral contraceptives or subdermal implants during treatment.

● Instruct patient to avoid dizziness and fainting by rising slowly to an upright position and avoiding sudden position changes.

● Inform patient that it may take 8 weeks or longer for menses to resume and excess production of milk to slow down.

● Advise patient to avoid alcohol while taking drug.

● Advise patients not to operate heavy machinery if somnolence occurs while taking Cycloset.

budesonide (inhalation; intranasal)

byoo-DES-oh-nide

Pulmicort Flexhaler, Pulmicort Respules, Pulmicort Turbuhaler†, Rhinocort Aqua

Therapeutic class: Corticosteroids
Pharmacologic class: Corticosteroids
Pregnancy risk category: B

AVAILABLE FORMS

Dry powder inhaler: 90 mcg/dose, 180 mcg/dose, 200 mcg/dose†
Inhalation suspension: 0.25 mg, 0.5 mg, 1 mg
Nasal spray: 32 mcg/metered spray

INDICATIONS & DOSAGES

➤ **As a preventative in maintenance of asthma**

All patients: Use lowest effective dose after stabilizing asthma.

Respules

Children ages 1 to 8 previously taking bronchodilator alone: 0.5 mg daily or 0.25 mg b.i.d. suspension via jet nebulizer. Maximum dose is 0.5 mg daily.

Children ages 1 to 8 previously taking inhaled corticosteroid: 0.5 mg daily or 0.25 mg b.i.d. suspension via jet nebulizer to maximum dose of 0.5 mg b.i.d.

Children ages 1 to 8 previously taking oral corticosteroid: 1 mg daily or 0.5 mg b.i.d. via jet nebulizer. Maximum dose is 1 mg/day.

Adjust-a-dose: Symptomatic children not responding to nonsteroidal therapy may require starting dose of 0.25 mg daily.

Flexhaler

Adults: Initially, inhaled dose of 360 mcg b.i.d. to maximum of 720 mcg b.i.d.

Children ages 6 to 17: Initially, inhaled dose of 180 mcg b.i.d. to maximum of 360 mcg b.i.d.

Turbuhaler†

Adults previously taking bronchodilator alone: Initially, inhaled dose of 200 to 400 mcg b.i.d. to maximum of 400 mcg b.i.d.

Adults previously taking inhaled corticosteroid: Initially, inhaled dose of 200 to 400 mcg b.i.d. to maximum of 800 mcg b.i.d.

Adults previously taking oral corticosteroid: Initially, inhaled dose of 400 to 800 mcg b.i.d. to maximum of 800 mcg b.i.d.

Children older than age 6 previously taking bronchodilator alone or inhaled corticosteroid: Initially, inhaled dose of 200 mcg b.i.d. to maximum of 400 mcg b.i.d.

Children older than age 6 previously taking oral corticosteroid: 400 mcg b.i.d., maximum.

➤ **Symptoms of seasonal or perennial allergic rhinitis**

Adults and children age 6 and older: 1 spray in each nostril once daily. Maximum dose is 4 sprays per nostril once daily (256 mcg/day) for adults and children older than age 12 and 2 sprays per nostril once daily (128 mcg/day) for children age 6 to less than age 12.

ADMINISTRATION

Inhalation

● Give inhalation suspension at regular intervals once or twice a day, as directed.

● Give suspension with a jet nebulizer connected to a compressor with adequate airflow. Make sure that it's equipped with a mouthpiece or suitable face mask.

● Total daily dose may be increased or given as a divided dose to improve control if needed. Titrate dosage downward again after asthma is stabilized.

• When aluminum foil envelope has been opened, the shelf-life of unused ampules is 2 weeks when protected from light.

• Prime inhaler before first use.

Intranasal

• Prime pump by actuating eight times before first use. Reprime pump if not used for 2 or more days. Discard bottle after 120 sprays.

• Shake before each actuation.

ACTION

Exhibits potent glucocorticoid activity and weak mineralocorticoid activity. Drug inhibits mast cells, macrophages, and mediators (such as leukotrienes) involved in inflammation.

Route	Onset	Peak	Duration
Inhalation, powder	24 hr	1–2 wk	Unknown
Inhalation, Respules	2–8 days	4–6 wk	Unknown
Intranasal	10 hr	2 wk	Unknown

Half-life: 2 to 3 hours (inhalation); unknown (intranasal).

ADVERSE REACTIONS

CNS: headache, asthenia, fever, hypertonia, insomnia, pain, syncope.

EENT: sinusitis, pharyngitis, rhinitis, otitis media, voice alteration; epistaxis and nasal irritation (intranasal).

GI: abdominal pain, dry mouth, dyspepsia, diarrhea, gastroenteritis, nausea, oral candidiasis, taste perversion, vomiting.

Metabolic: weight gain.

Musculoskeletal: back pain, fractures, myalgia.

Respiratory: respiratory tract infection, *bronchospasm,* increased cough.

Skin: ecchymoses.

Other: flulike symptoms, hypersensitivity reactions, viral infection.

INTERACTIONS

Drug-drug. *Ketoconazole, other strong CYP3A4 inhibitors (atazanavir, clarithromycin, indinavir, itraconazole, nefazodone, nelfinavir, ritonavir, saquinavir, telithromycin):* May inhibit metabolism and increase level of budesonide. Monitor patient for adverse reactions and adjust dosage as needed.

EFFECTS ON LAB TEST RESULTS

None reported.

CONTRAINDICATIONS & CAUTIONS

• Contraindicated in patients hypersensitive to drug, in those with severe hypersensitivity to milk proteins (powder for inhalation), and in those with status asthmaticus or other acute asthma episodes.

• Nasal formula is contraindicated in patients with septal ulcers, nasal surgery, nasal trauma, or untreated localized nasal mucosa infections.

• Use cautiously, if at all, in patients with active or inactive tuberculosis, ocular herpes simplex, or untreated systemic fungal, bacterial, viral, or parasitic infections.

⚠ Overdose S&S: Hyperadrenocorticism.

NURSING CONSIDERATIONS

🛈 *Alert:* When transferring from systemic corticosteroid to inhalation drug, use caution and gradually decrease corticosteroid dose to prevent adrenal insufficiency.

• Inhalation drug doesn't remove the need for systemic corticosteroid therapy in some situations.

• Systemic effects of corticosteroid therapy may occur if recommended daily dosage is exceeded.

• If bronchospasm occurs after inhalation use, stop therapy and treat with a bronchodilator.

• Lung function may improve within 24 hours of starting therapy, but maximum benefit may not be achieved for 1 to 2 weeks or longer.

• For Pulmicort Respules, lung function improves in 2 to 8 days, but maximum benefit may not be seen for 4 to 6 weeks.

• Watch for *Candida* infections of the mouth or pharynx.

🛈 *Alert:* Corticosteroids may increase risk of developing serious or fatal infections in patients exposed to viral illnesses, such as chickenpox or measles.

• In rare cases, inhaled corticosteroids have been linked to increased intraocular pressure and cataract development. Stop drug if local irritation occurs.

PATIENT TEACHING

● Tell patient that budesonide inhaler isn't a bronchodilator and isn't intended to treat acute episodes of asthma.

● Instruct patient to use the inhaler at regular intervals because effectiveness depends on twice-daily use on a regular basis, by following these instructions:

– Keep Pulmicort Turbuhaler upright (mouthpiece on top) during loading, to provide the correct dose.

– Prime Turbuhaler when using it for the first time. To prime, hold unit upright and turn brown grip fully to the right, then fully to the left until it clicks. Repeat priming.

– Load first dose by holding unit upright and turning brown grip to the right and then to the left until it clicks.

– Turn your head away from the inhaler and breathe out.

– During inhalation, Turbuhaler must be in the upright or horizontal position.

– Don't shake inhaler.

– Place mouthpiece between lips and inhale forcefully and deeply.

– You may not taste the drug or sense it entering your lungs, but this doesn't mean it isn't effective.

– Don't exhale through the Turbuhaler. If more than one dose is required, repeat steps.

– Rinse your mouth with water and then spit out the water after each dose to decrease the risk of developing oral candidiasis.

– When 20 doses remain in the Turbuhaler, a red mark appears in the indicator window. When red mark reaches the bottom, the unit is empty.

– Don't use Turbuhaler with a spacer device and don't chew or bite the mouthpiece.

– Replace mouthpiece cover after use and always keep it clean and dry.

● Pulmicort Flexhaler must be primed before use. Refer to patient information guide for complete administration instructions.

● Tell patient that improvement in asthma control may be seen within 24 hours, although the maximum benefit may not appear for 1 to 2 weeks. If signs or symptoms worsen during this time, instruct patient to contact prescriber.

● Advise patient to avoid exposure to chickenpox or measles and to contact prescriber if exposure occurs.

● Instruct patient using inhaler to carry or wear medical identification indicating need for supplementary corticosteroids during periods of stress or an asthma attack.

● Advise patient that unused Respules are good for 2 weeks after the foil envelope has been opened; however, unused Respules should be returned to the envelope to protect them from light.

● Tell patient to read and follow the patient information leaflet contained in the package.

● To instill intranasal drug, instruct patient to shake container before use, blow nose to clear nasal passages, tilt head slightly forward, and insert nozzle into nostril, pointing away from septum. Tell him to hold other nostril closed and inhale gently while spraying. Next, have him shake container and repeat in other nostril.

● Advise patient to store nasal canister with valve upward and away from extreme heat or cold. Caution him not to incinerate or break canister because contents are under pressure.

● Tell patient to use nasal drug within 6 months of opening the protective aluminum pouch.

● Advise patient using nasal formula to notify prescriber if signs or symptoms don't improve or if they worsen in 3 weeks.

● Teach patient good nasal and oral hygiene and not to share drug because this could spread infection.

budesonide (oral)
byoo-DES-oh-nide

Entocort EC, Uceris

Therapeutic class: Corticosteroids
Pharmacologic class: Glucocorticoids
Pregnancy risk category: C

AVAILABLE FORMS
Capsules: 3 mg
Tablets (24-hour): 9 mg

INDICATIONS & DOSAGES
Adjust-a-dose (for all indications): In patients with moderate to severe liver disease who have increased signs or symptoms of hypercorticism, reduce dose.

Reactions in bold italics are *life-threatening*. Interactions may have a *rapid onset* or a *delayed onset*.

➤ **Mild to moderate active Crohn disease involving the ileum, ascending colon, or both (capsules)**
Adults: 9 mg P.O. once daily in morning for up to 8 weeks. For recurrent episodes of active Crohn disease, a repeat 8-week course may be given.

➤ **To maintain remission in mild to moderate Crohn disease that involves the ileum or ascending colon**
Adults: 6 mg P.O. daily for up to 3 months. If symptom control is maintained at 3 months, taper dose to stop therapy. Therapy for longer than 3 months doesn't have added benefit.

➤ **Induction of remission in active mild to moderate ulcerative colitis (tablets)**
Adults: 9 mg P.O. once daily in the morning for up to 8 weeks.

➤ **Eosinophilic esophagitis ♦**
Children older than age 10: Initially, 1 mg P.O. b.i.d. Usual dosage is 1 to 2 mg as a viscous slurry each day, divided into two doses, for 3 to 4 months before repeat endoscopy.
Children younger than age 10: 500 mcg P.O. b.i.d. May increase to 1 mg b.i.d. if no response.

ADMINISTRATION
P.O.
● Give drug whole; don't break or crush capsule or tablet.

ACTION
Significant glucocorticoid effects caused by drug's high affinity for glucocorticoid receptors.

Route	Onset	Peak	Duration
P.O.	Unknown	½–10 hr	Unknown

Half-life: About 2 hours.

ADVERSE REACTIONS
CNS: headache, dizziness, asthenia, hyperkinesia, paresthesia, tremor, vertigo, fatigue, malaise, agitation, confusion, insomnia, nervousness, somnolence, pain.
CV: chest pain, hypertension, palpitations, tachycardia, flushing.
EENT: facial edema, ear infection, eye abnormality, abnormal vision, sinusitis.

GI: nausea, diarrhea, dyspepsia, abdominal pain, flatulence, vomiting, anal disorder, aggravated Crohn disease, enteritis, epigastric pain, fistula, glossitis, hemorrhoids, intestinal obstruction, tongue edema, tooth disorder, increased appetite.
GU: dysuria, micturition frequency, nocturia, intermenstrual bleeding, menstrual disorder, hematuria, pyuria.
Hematologic: leukocytosis, anemia.
Metabolic: hypercorticism, dependent edema, hypokalemia, increased weight.
Musculoskeletal: back pain, aggravated arthritis, cramps, arthralgia, myalgia.
Respiratory: respiratory tract infection, bronchitis, dyspnea.
Skin: acne, alopecia, dermatitis, eczema, skin disorder, increased sweating.
Other: flulike disorder, sleep disorder, candidiasis, viral infection.

INTERACTIONS
Drug-drug. *CYP inhibitors (erythromycin, indinavir, itraconazole, ketoconazole, ritonavir, saquinavir):* May increase effects of budesonide. If use together is unavoidable, reduce budesonide dosage.
Drug-food. *Grapefruit juice:* May increase drug effects. Discourage use together.

EFFECTS ON LAB TEST RESULTS
● May increase alkaline phosphatase and C-reactive protein levels. May decrease potassium and hemoglobin levels.
● May increase erythrocyte sedimentation rate and WBC count.

CONTRAINDICATIONS & CAUTIONS
● Contraindicated in patients hypersensitive to drug.
● Use cautiously in patients with tuberculosis, hypertension, diabetes mellitus, osteoporosis, peptic ulcer disease, glaucoma, or cataracts; those with a family history of diabetes or glaucoma; and those with any other condition in which glucocorticoids may have unwanted effects.
● Glucocorticoids appear in breast milk, and infants may have adverse reactions. Use cautiously in breast-feeding women only if benefits outweigh risks.
⚠ *Overdose S&S:* Hypercorticism, adrenal suppression.

NURSING CONSIDERATIONS
- Reduced liver function affects elimination of this drug; systemic availability of drug may increase in patients with liver cirrhosis.
- Patients undergoing surgery or other stressful situations may need systemic glucocorticoid supplementation in addition to budesonide therapy.
- Carefully monitor patients transferred from systemic glucocorticoid therapy to budesonide for signs and symptoms of corticosteroid withdrawal. Watch for immunosuppression, especially in patients who haven't had diseases such as chickenpox or measles; these can be fatal in patients who are immunosuppressed or receiving glucocorticoids.
- Replacement of systemic glucocorticoids with this drug may unmask allergies, such as eczema and rhinitis, which were previously controlled by systemic drug.
- Long-term use of drug may cause hypercorticism and adrenal suppression.

PATIENT TEACHING
- Tell patient to swallow capsules whole and not to chew or break them.
- Advise patient to avoid grapefruit juice while taking drug.
- Tell patient to notify prescriber immediately if he is exposed to or develops chickenpox or measles.
- Tell patient to keep container tightly closed.

bumetanide
byoo-MET-a-nide

Therapeutic class: Diuretics
Pharmacologic class: Loop diuretics
Pregnancy risk category: C

AVAILABLE FORMS
Injection: 0.25 mg/mL
Tablets: 0.5 mg, 1 mg, 2 mg

INDICATIONS & DOSAGES
➤ **Edema caused by heart failure or hepatic or renal disease**
Adults: 0.5 to 2 mg P.O. once daily. If diuretic response isn't adequate, a second or third dose may be given at 4- to 5-hour intervals. Maximum dose is 10 mg daily. May be given parenterally if oral route isn't possible. Usual first dose is 0.5 to 1 mg given I.V. or I.M. If response isn't adequate, a second or third dose may be given at 2- to 3-hour intervals. Maximum, 10 mg daily.

ADMINISTRATION
P.O.
- Give drug with food to minimize GI upset.
- To prevent nocturia, give drug in morning. If second dose is needed, give in early afternoon.

I.V.
▼ For direct injection, give drug over 1 to 2 minutes using a 21G or 23G needle.
▼ For intermittent infusion, give diluted drug through an intermittent infusion device or piggyback into an I.V. line containing a free-flowing, compatible solution.
▼ **Incompatibilities:** Dobutamine, fenoldopam, midazolam.

I.M.
- Document injection site.

ACTION
Inhibits sodium and chloride reabsorption in the ascending loop of Henle.

Route	Onset	Peak	Duration
P.O.	30–60 min	1–2 hr	4–6 hr
I.V.	Within min	15–30 min	30–60 min
I.M.	40 min	Unknown	5–6 hr

Half-life: 1 to 1½ hours.

ADVERSE REACTIONS
CNS: dizziness, headache, vertigo.
CV: orthostatic hypotension.
GU: oliguria.
Metabolic: volume depletion and dehydration, hypokalemia, hypochloremic alkalosis, *hypomagnesemia,* asymptomatic hyperuricemia.
Skin: rash, pruritus.

INTERACTIONS
Drug-drug. *Aminoglycoside antibiotics:* May increase ototoxicity. Avoid using together if possible.
Antidiabetics: May decrease hypoglycemic effects. Monitor glucose level.
Antihypertensives: May increase hypotensive effects. Consider dosage adjustment.

Cardiac glycosides: May increase risk of digoxin toxicity from bumetanide-induced hypokalemia. Monitor potassium and digoxin levels.

Chlorothiazide, chlorthalidone, furosemide, hydrochlorothiazide, indapamide, metolazone: May cause excessive diuretic response, causing serious electrolyte abnormalities or dehydration. Adjust doses carefully, and monitor patient closely for signs and symptoms of excessive diuretic response.

Cisplatin: May increase risk of ototoxicity. Monitor patient closely.

Lithium: May decrease lithium clearance, increasing risk of lithium toxicity. Monitor lithium level.

Neuromuscular blockers: May prolong neuromuscular blockade. Monitor patient closely.

NSAIDs, probenecid: May inhibit diuretic response. Use together cautiously.

Other potassium-wasting drugs (such as amphotericin B, corticosteroids): May increase risk of hypokalemia. Use together cautiously.

Drug-herb. *Dandelion:* May interfere with drug activity. Discourage use together.

Licorice: May cause unexpected, rapid potassium loss. Discourage use together.

EFFECTS ON LAB TEST RESULTS
• May increase alkaline phosphatase, ALT, AST, bilirubin, cholesterol, creatinine, glucose, LDH, and urine urea levels. May decrease calcium, magnesium, potassium, sodium, and chloride levels.
• May decrease platelet count.

CONTRAINDICATIONS & CAUTIONS
• Contraindicated in patients hypersensitive to drug or sulfonamides (possible cross-sensitivity) and in patients with anuria, hepatic coma, or severe electrolyte depletion.
• Use cautiously in patients with hepatic cirrhosis and ascites, in elderly patients, and in those with decreased renal function.

⚠ *Overdose S&S:* Electrolyte depletion, weakness, dizziness, confusion, anorexia, lethargy, vomiting, cramps, dehydration, circulatory collapse, vascular thrombosis, and embolism.

NURSING CONSIDERATIONS
• Safest and most effective dosage schedule is alternate days or 3 or 4 consecutive days with 1 or 2 days off between cycles.
• Monitor fluid intake and output, weight, and electrolyte, BUN, creatinine, and carbon dioxide levels frequently.
• Watch for evidence of hypokalemia, such as muscle weakness and cramps. Instruct patient to report these symptoms.
• Consult prescriber and dietitian about a high-potassium diet. Foods rich in potassium include citrus fruits, tomatoes, bananas, dates, and apricots.
• Monitor glucose level in diabetic patients.
• Monitor uric acid level, especially in patients with history of gout.

Black Box Warning Monitor blood pressure and pulse rate during rapid diuresis. Profound water and electrolyte depletion may occur. ▉

• If oliguria or azotemia develops or increases, prescriber may stop drug.
• Drug can be safely used in patients allergic to furosemide; 1 mg of bumetanide equals about 40 mg of furosemide.

PATIENT TEACHING
• Instruct patient to take drug with food to minimize GI upset.
• Advise patient to take drug in morning to avoid need to urinate at night; if patient needs second dose, have him take it in early afternoon.
• Advise patient to avoid sudden posture changes and to rise slowly to avoid dizziness upon standing quickly.
• Instruct patient to notify prescriber about extreme thirst, muscle weakness, cramps, nausea, or dizziness.
• Instruct patient to weigh himself daily to monitor fluid status.

buprenorphine
byoo-pre-NOR-feen

Butrans

buprenorphine hydrochloride

Buprenex

Therapeutic class: Opioid analgesics
Pharmacologic class: Opioid agonist-antagonists–opioid partial agonists
Pregnancy risk category: C
Controlled substance schedule: III

AVAILABLE FORMS
Injection: 0.324 mg (equivalent to 0.3 mg base/mL)
Sublingual tablets: 2 mg, 8 mg (as base)
Transdermal patch: 5 mcg/hour, 10 mcg/hour, 20 mcg/hour

INDICATIONS & DOSAGES
➤ **Moderate to severe pain**
Adults and children age 13 and older:
0.3 mg I.M. or slow I.V. every 6 hours p.r.n., or around the clock; repeat dose (up to 0.3 mg), as needed, 30 to 60 minutes after first dose. May increase I.M. dosing to 0.6 mg/dose.
Children ages 2 to 12: 2 to 6 mcg/kg I.M. or I.V. every 4 to 6 hours.
Adjust-a-dose: In high-risk patients, such as debilitated or elderly patients, reduce dose by one-half.
➤ **Moderate to severe chronic pain in patients requiring continuous opioid analgesia for an extended period of time**
Adults (opioid-naive): 5 mcg/hour transdermal patch once every 7 days. To achieve adequate analgesia and minimize adverse effects, consider patient's tolerance, condition, and other medications and titrate dosage to maximum of 20 mcg/hour. Allow minimum of 72 hours between dosage increases.
Adults (non–opioid-naive): Buprenorphine may precipitate withdrawal in patients already on opioids. For conversion from other opioids to buprenorphine, taper patient's current around-the-clock opioids for up to

7 days to no more than morphine 30 mg or equivalent per day before beginning treatment with buprenorphine. Patients may use short-acting analgesics as needed until analgesic efficacy with buprenorphine is attained. For patients whose daily dose was less than morphine 30 mg orally or equivalent, initiate treatment with buprenorphine transdermal patch 5 mcg/hour. For patients whose daily dose was between 30 and 80 mg of morphine equivalents, initiate treatment with buprenorphine transdermal patch 10 mcg/hour. To achieve adequate analgesia with tolerable adverse effects, consider patient's tolerance, condition, and other medications and titrate dose to maximum of 20 mcg/hour transdermal patch once every 7 days. Allow minimum of 72 hours between dosage increases.
Adjust-a-dose: For patients with mild to moderate hepatic impairment, start with buprenorphine dosage of 5 mcg/hour. Thereafter, individually titrate dosage to level that provides adequate analgesia and tolerable adverse effects, under close supervision of prescriber.
➤ **Opioid dependence**
Adults: 8 mg S.L. on day 1 and 16 mg S.L. on day 2. Maintenance dose is 12 to 16 mg S.L. as a single daily dose.

ADMINISTRATION
I.V.
▼ When mixed in a 1:1 volume ratio, drug is compatible with atropine sulfate, diphenhydramine hydrochloride, droperidol, glycopyrrolate, haloperidol lactate, hydroxyzine hydrochloride, promethazine hydrochloride, scopolamine hydrochloride, D_5W, 5% dextrose in normal saline solution, sodium chloride solution, lactated Ringer solution, and normal saline solution injections.
▼ For direct injection, give slowly over at least 2 minutes into a vein or through tubing of a free-flowing, compatible I.V. solution.
▼ **Incompatibilities:** Diazepam, furosemide, lorazepam.
I.M.
● Give drug as deep I.M. injection.

S.L.

• Place all the tablets of the dose under the tongue until dissolved; if uncomfortable, patient should take at least two at the same time.

Transdermal

Black Box Warning Avoid exposing patch or surrounding area to direct external heat source or direct sunlight. Increased temperature may increase amount of drug released, which can result in overdose and death. ■

Black Box Warning Transdermal patch is indicated only for moderate to severe chronic pain that requires around-the-clock analgesia for an extended period of time. ■

• Each patch is intended to be worn for 7 days. If patch falls off during 7-day dosing interval, apply new patch to different site.

• Don't use if pouch seal is broken or patch is cut, damaged, or changed in any way. Apply patch to intact skin immediately after opening.

• Appropriate application sites are right or left upper outer arm, upper chest, upper back, or side of the chest only.

• Application site should be hairless; clip hair if needed but don't shave site. If needed, clean selected site with water only and allow to dry completely before applying patch.

• Edges of patch may be taped to the skin if needed.

• After removing patch, fold it in half, seal it in patch-disposal unit, and place it in trash.

• Wait minimum of 3 weeks before applying new patch to same application site.

ACTION

Unknown. Binds with opioid receptors in the CNS, altering perception of and emotional response to pain.

Route	Onset	Peak	Duration
I.V.	Immediate	2 min	6 hr
I.M.	15 min	1 hr	6 hr
S.L.	Unknown	Unknown	Unknown
Transdermal	17 hr	3–6 days	7 days

Half-life: 1 to 7 hours; transdermal, 26 hours.

ADVERSE REACTIONS

CNS: dizziness, sedation, vertigo, *increased intracranial pressure (ICP),* asthenia (tablets only), confusion, depression, dreaming, euphoria, fatigue, headache,

insomnia, nervousness, pain, paresthesia, psychosis, slurred speech, weakness.

CV: *bradycardia,* cyanosis, flushing, hypertension, hypotension, tachycardia.

EENT: blurred vision, conjunctivitis, diplopia, dry mouth (patch), miosis, rhinitis (tablets only), tinnitus, visual abnormalities.

GI: nausea, abdominal pain (tablets only), constipation, diarrhea (tablets only), vomiting.

GU: urine retention.

Respiratory: *respiratory depression,* dyspnea, hypoventilation.

Skin: application-site rash or erythema (patch), diaphoresis, injection-site reactions, pruritus, sweating.

Other: back pain (tablets only), chills, infection (tablets only), withdrawal syndrome.

INTERACTIONS

Drug-drug. *Benzodiazepines, CNS depressants, MAO inhibitors, opioids:* May cause additive effects. Use together cautiously.
Class IA or III antiarrhythmics: May increase risk of prolonged QT syndrome. Avoid use with transdermal patch.
CYP3A4 inducers (carbamazepine, phenobarbital, phenytoin, rifampin): May increase clearance of buprenorphine. Monitor patient for clinical effects of drug.
CYP3A4 inhibitors (erythromycin, indinavir, ketoconazole, ritonavir, saquinavir): May decrease clearance of buprenorphine. Monitor patient for increased adverse effects.
Skeletal muscle relaxants: May enhance neuromuscular blocking action and increase respiratory depression. Use together cautiously.

Drug-lifestyle. *Alcohol or illicit drug use:* May cause additive effects. Discourage use together.

EFFECTS ON LAB TEST RESULTS

None reported.

CONTRAINDICATIONS & CAUTIONS

• Contraindicated in patients hypersensitive to drug and during pregnancy or breast-feeding.

❸ *Alert:* Don't exceed dose of one 20-mcg/hour transdermal patch every 7 days due to risk of prolonging QTc interval.

• Use cautiously in elderly or debilitated patients; patients who are opioid dependent; in those undergoing biliary tract surgery and those with biliary tract disease or pancreatitis; and in those with head injury, intracranial lesions, and increased ICP; severe respiratory, liver, or kidney impairment; CNS depression or coma; those at risk for hypotension and circulatory shock; thyroid irregularities; adrenal insufficiency; and prostatic hypertrophy, urethral stricture, acute alcoholism, delirium tremens, or kyphoscoliosis.

⚠ Overdose S&S: Respiratory depression, pinpoint pupils, sedation, hypotension, death.

NURSING CONSIDERATIONS

Black Box Warning Buprenorphine has potential for abuse similar to other opioids and is a controlled substance. Patients at risk for opioid abuse include those with personal or family history of substance abuse or mental illness. Assess for risk or abuse before prescribing, and monitor patients regularly. ∎

Black Box Warning Accidental exposure to drug, especially in children, can cause a fatal overdose. ∎

• Taper dosage before discontinuing transdermal patch.

• Drug may worsen increased ICP and mask its signs and symptoms. Carefully monitor patient's pupillary reflexes and level of consciousness.

• Reassess patient's level of pain 15 and 30 minutes after parenteral administration.

• Buprenorphine 0.3 mg is equal to 10 mg of morphine and 75 mg of meperidine in analgesic potency. It has longer duration of action than morphine or meperidine.

☞ Alert: Naloxone won't completely reverse the respiratory depression caused by buprenorphine overdose; an overdose may require mechanical ventilation. Larger-than-usual doses of naloxone (more than 0.4 mg) and doxapram also may be indicated.

• Treat accidental skin exposure by removing exposed clothing and rinsing skin with water.

• Drug may cause constipation. Assess bowel function and need for stool softeners and stimulant laxatives.

☞ Alert: Drug's opioid antagonist properties may cause withdrawal syndrome in opioid-dependent patients.

• If dependence occurs, withdrawal symptoms may appear up to 14 days after drug is stopped.

• **Look alike–sound alike:** Don't confuse Buprenex with Bumex or bupropion.

PATIENT TEACHING

• Caution ambulatory patient about getting out of bed or walking.

• When drug is used after surgery, encourage patient to turn, cough, and breathe deeply to prevent breathing problems.

• Tell patient to place all the tablets of the dose under his tongue until dissolved; if this is uncomfortable, tell him to take at least two at the same time.

• Instruct patient in proper disposal of transdermal system.

• Teach patient proper patch application and advise him to read package instructions.

• Warn patient not to apply heat to patch application site or to cut patch.

• Tell patient and family to report adverse reactions to prescriber immediately.

• Warn patient not to take other long-acting opioids while using transdermal system.

---

buPROPion hydrobromide
byoo-PROE-pee-on

Aplenzin

buPROPion hydrochloride
Forfivo XL, Wellbutrin✦, Wellbutrin SR✦, Wellbutrin XL, Zyban✦

Therapeutic class: Antidepressants
Pharmacologic class: Aminoketones
Pregnancy risk category: B

AVAILABLE FORMS
bupropion hydrobromide
Tablets (extended-release): 174 mg, 348 mg, 522 mg
bupropion hydrochloride
Tablets (extended-release): 150 mg, 300 mg, 450 mg
Tablets (immediate-release): 75 mg, 100 mg
Tablets (sustained-release): 50 mg, 100 mg, 150 mg, 200 mg

INDICATIONS & DOSAGES

➤ **Major depressive disorder (Aplenzin only)**

Adults: Initially, 174 mg P.O. (equivalent to 150 mg/day bupropion HCl) given as a single daily dose in the morning. If the 174-mg initial dose is adequately tolerated, increase to the 348-mg/day target dose as early as day 4 of dosing. There should be an interval of at least 24 hours between successive doses. The full antidepressant effect may not be evident until after 4 weeks of treatment or longer. Consider increasing dosage to the maximum of 522 mg P.O. daily, given as a single dose, for patients in whom no clinical improvement is noted after several weeks of treatment at 348 mg/day. When switching patients from Wellbutrin, Wellbutrin SR, or Wellbutrin XL to Aplenzin, give the equivalent total daily dose when possible (522 mg bupropion HBr is equivalent to 450 mg bupropion HCl; 348 mg bupropion HBr is equivalent to 300 mg bupropion HCl; 174 mg bupropion HBr is equivalent to 150 mg bupropion HCl).

Adjust-a-dose: In patients with renal impairment or mild to moderate hepatic impairment, including hepatic cirrhosis, reduced frequency or dose should be considered. In patients with severe hepatic cirrhosis, don't exceed 174 mg every other day.

➤ **Seasonal affective disorder**

Adults: Start treatment in autumn before depressive symptoms appear. Wellbutrin XL: Initially, 150 mg extended-release P.O. once daily in the morning. After 1 week, increase to 300 mg once daily, if tolerated. Continue 300 mg daily during the autumn and winter and taper to 150 mg daily for 2 weeks before stopping the drug in the early spring. Aplenzin: 174 mg P.O. daily. May increase to 348 mg P.O. once daily after 7 days. Taper and discontinue drug in early spring.

➤ **Depression**

Adults: For immediate-release, initially, 100 mg P.O. b.i.d.; increase after 3 days to 100 mg P.O. t.i.d., if needed. If patient doesn't improve after several weeks of therapy, increase dosage to 150 mg t.i.d. No single dose should exceed 150 mg. Allow at least 6 hours between successive doses. Maximum dose is 450 mg daily. For sustained-release, initially, 150 mg P.O. every morning; increase to target dose of 150 mg P.O. b.i.d., as tolerated, as early as day 4 of dosing. Allow at least 8 hours between successive doses. Maximum dose is 400 mg daily. For extended-release, initially, 150 mg P.O. every morning; increase to target dosage of 300 mg P.O. daily, as tolerated, as early as day 4 of dosing. Allow at least 24 hours between successive doses. Maximum is 450 mg daily. Don't initiate treatment with Forfivo XL.

➤ **Aid to smoking-cessation treatment**

Adults: 150 mg Zyban P.O. daily for 3 days; increased to maximum of 300 mg daily in two divided doses at least 8 hours apart. Continue therapy for 7 to 12 weeks. Some patients may need continuous treatment.

Adjust-a-dose: In patients with mild to moderate hepatic cirrhosis or renal impairment, reduce frequency and dose. In patients with severe hepatic cirrhosis, don't exceed 75 mg immediate-release P.O. daily, 150 mg sustained-release P.O. every other day, or 150 mg extended-release P.O. every other day.

➤ **ADHD** ◆

Adults: 150 mg P.O. daily. May increase up to 450 mg P.O. daily.

Children and adolescents: Up to 3 mg/kg/day initially, titrated to maximum of 6 mg/kg/day or 300 mg/day. Single dose shouldn't exceed 150 mg. Usually given in two divided doses daily for children and three divided doses daily for adolescents.

ADMINISTRATION
P.O.

● Don't crush, split, or allow patients to chew tablets.

● When switching patients from immediate-release or sustained-release tablets to extended-release tablets, give the same total daily dose (when possible) as the once-daily dosage provided.

ACTION

Unknown. Drug doesn't inhibit MAO, but it weakly inhibits norepinephrine, dopamine, and serotonin reuptake. Noradrenergic or dopaminergic mechanisms, or both, may cause drug's effect.

Route	Onset	Peak	Duration
P.O. (extended-release)	Unknown	5 hr	Unknown
P.O. (immediate-release)	Unknown	2 hr	Unknown
P.O. (sustained-release)	Unknown	3 hr	Unknown

Half-life: 8 to 24 hours.

ADVERSE REACTIONS

CNS: abnormal dreams, insomnia, headache, sedation, tremor, agitation, dizziness, *seizures, suicidal behavior,* anxiety, confusion, delusions, euphoria, fever, hostility, impaired concentration, impaired sleep quality, akinesia, akathisia, fatigue, syncope, somnolence.
CV: tachycardia, *arrhythmias,* hypertension, hypotension, palpitations, chest pain.
EENT: blurred vision, rhinitis, auditory disturbances, epistaxis, pharyngitis, sinusitis, dry mouth.
GI: constipation, nausea, vomiting, anorexia, taste disturbance, dyspepsia, diarrhea, abdominal pain, flatulence.
GU: erectile dysfunction, menstrual complaints, urinary frequency, urine retention.
Metabolic: increased appetite, weight loss, weight gain.
Musculoskeletal: arthritis, myalgia, arthralgia, muscle spasm or twitch.
Respiratory: upper respiratory complaints, increase in coughing.
Skin: excessive sweating, pruritus, rash, cutaneous temperature disturbance, urticaria.
Other: chills, decreased libido, accidental injury, hot flashes.

INTERACTIONS

Drug-drug. *Amantadine, levodopa:* May increase risk of adverse reactions. If used together, give small first doses of bupropion and increase dosage gradually.
Antidepressants (desipramine, fluoxetine, imipramine, nortriptyline, sertraline), antipsychotics (haloperidol, risperidone, thioridazine), systemic corticosteroids, theophylline: May lower seizure threshold. Use cautiously together.

Beta blockers, class IC antiarrhythmics: May increase levels of these drugs and adverse reactions. Use a reduced dose if used with bupropion.
Carbamazepine, phenobarbital, phenytoin: May enhance metabolism of bupropion and decrease its effect. Monitor patient closely.
CYP2B6 substrates or inhibitors (cyclophosphamide, orphenadrine, thiotepa), efavirenz, fluvoxamine, nelfinavir, norfluoxetine, paroxetine, ritonavir, sertraline: May increase bupropion activity. Monitor patient for expected therapeutic effects and adverse effects.
Linezolid, methylene blue, SSRIs: May cause serotonin syndrome. Use extreme caution and monitor closely.
MAO inhibitors: May increase the risk of bupropion toxicity. Don't use drugs within 14 days of each other.
Nicotine replacement agents: May cause hypertension. Monitor blood pressure.
Drug-lifestyle. *Alcohol use:* May alter seizure threshold. Discourage use together.
Sun exposure: May increase risk of photosensitivity reactions. Advise patient to avoid excessive sunlight exposure.

EFFECTS ON LAB TEST RESULTS
● May increase LFT values.

CONTRAINDICATIONS & CAUTIONS
● Contraindicated in patients hypersensitive to drug, in those who have taken MAO inhibitors within previous 14 days, and in those with seizure disorders or history of bulimia or anorexia nervosa because of a higher risk of seizures.
◑ *Alert:* Concomitant use with SSRIs, linezolid, or methylene blue can cause serotonin syndrome (fever, mental status changes, muscle twitching, excessive sweating, shivering or shaking, diarrhea, loss of coordination). Use drug with SSRIs, linezolid, or methylene blue only for life-threatening or urgent conditions when the potential benefits outweigh the risks of toxicity.
● Contraindicated in patients abruptly stopping use of alcohol or sedatives (including benzodiazepines).
● Don't use with other drugs containing bupropion.

Reactions in bold italics are *life-threatening*. Interactions may have a *rapid onset* or a *delayed onset*.

Black Box Warning Bupropion hydrobromide (Aplenzin) isn't approved for smoking cessation treatment. ■

Black Box Warning Bupropion isn't approved for use in children. ■

• Use cautiously in patients with recent history of MI, unstable heart disease, renal or hepatic impairment, a history of seizures, head trauma, or other predisposition to seizures, and in those being treated with drugs that lower seizure threshold.

⚠ **Overdose S&S:** Seizures, ECG changes, hallucinations, loss of consciousness, sinus tachycardia, coma, fever, hypotension, muscle rigidity, rhabdomyolysis, respiratory failure, stupor.

NURSING CONSIDERATIONS

• Many patients experience a period of increased restlessness, including agitation, insomnia, and anxiety, especially at start of therapy.

🔊 **Alert:** To minimize the risk of seizures, don't exceed maximum recommended dose.

🔊 **Alert:** Patient with major depressive disorder may experience a worsening of depression and suicidal thoughts. Carefully monitor patient for worsening depression or suicidal thoughts, especially at the beginning of therapy and during dosage changes.

Black Box Warning Drug may increase the risk of suicidal thinking and behavior in children, adolescents, and young adults with major depressive disorder or other psychiatric disorder. ■

Black Box Warning Drug may cause hostility, agitation, and depressed mood. ■

🔊 **Alert:** If SSRIs, linezolid, or methylene blue must be given, bupropion must be stopped and the patient should be monitored for serotonin toxicity for 2 weeks or until 24 hours after the last dose of SSRIs, methylene blue, or linezolid, whichever comes first. Treatment with bupropion may be resumed 24 hours after last dose of SSRIs, methylene blue, or linezolid.

• Closely monitor patient with history of bipolar disorder. Antidepressants can cause manic episodes during the depressed phase of bipolar disorder. This may be less likely to occur with bupropion than with other antidepressants.

• Begin smoking-cessation treatment while patient is still smoking; about 1 week is needed to achieve steady-state drug levels.

• Stop smoking-cessation treatment if patient hasn't progressed toward abstinence by week 7. Treatment usually lasts up to 12 weeks. Patient can stop taking drug without tapering off.

Black Box Warning Zyban isn't indicated for treatment of depression. ■

• **Look alike–sound alike:** Don't confuse bupropion with buspirone or Wellbutrin with Wellcovorin. Don't confuse Zyban with Diovan. Don't confuse Wellbutrin SR with Wellbutrin XL.

PATIENT TEACHING

Black Box Warning Advise families and caregivers to closely observe patient for increased suicidal thinking and behavior and hostility, agitation, and depressed mood. ■

🔊 **Alert:** Explain that excessive use of alcohol, abrupt withdrawal from alcohol or other sedatives, and addiction to cocaine, opiates, or stimulants during therapy may increase risk of seizures. Seizure risk is also increased in those using OTC stimulants, in anorectics, and in diabetic patients using oral antidiabetics or insulin.

🔊 **Alert:** Teach patient to recognize and immediately report symptoms of serotonin toxicity (fever, mental status changes, muscle twitching, excessive sweating, shivering or shaking, diarrhea, loss of coordination).

• Tell patient not to chew, crush, or divide tablets.

• Advise patient to consult prescriber before taking other prescription or OTC drugs.

• Advise patient to avoid hazardous activities that require alertness and good psychomotor coordination until effects of drug are known.

🔊 **Alert:** Advise patient that Zyban and Wellbutrin contain the same active ingredient and shouldn't be used together.

• Tell patient that it may take 4 weeks to reach full antidepressant effect.

🔊 **Alert:** Advise patient to report mood swings or suicidal thoughts immediately.

• Inform patient that tablets may have an odor.

• Tell patient taking extended-release form that the empty shell may appear in stool.

busPIRone hydrochloride
byoo-SPYE-rone

Bustab†

Therapeutic class: Anxiolytics
Pharmacologic class:
Azaspirodecanedione derivatives
Pregnancy risk category: B

AVAILABLE FORMS
Tablets: 5 mg, 7.5 mg, 10 mg, 15 mg, 30 mg

INDICATIONS & DOSAGES
➤ **Anxiety disorders**
Adults: Initially, 7.5 mg P.O. b.i.d. Increase dosage by 5 mg daily at 2- to 3-day intervals. Usual maintenance dosage is 20 to 30 mg daily in divided doses. Don't exceed 60 mg daily.
➤ **Traumatic brain injury ♦**
Adults: 10 to 60 mg P.O. once daily for 3 or more months.

ADMINISTRATION
P.O.
● Don't give drug with grapefruit juice.
● Give drug at the same times each day, and always with or always without food.

ACTION
May inhibit neuronal firing and reduce serotonin turnover in cortical, amygdaloid, and septohippocampal tissue.

Route	Onset	Peak	Duration
P.O.	Unknown	40–90 min	Unknown

Half-life: 2 to 3 hours.

ADVERSE REACTIONS
CNS: dizziness, drowsiness, headache, nervousness, insomnia, light-headedness, fatigue, numbness, excitement, confusion, depression, anger, decreased concentration.
CV: tachycardia, nonspecific chest pain.
EENT: blurred vision.
GI: dry mouth, nausea, diarrhea, abdominal distress, constipation, vomiting.
Skin: rash, sweating or clamminess.

INTERACTIONS
Drug-drug. *Azole antifungals:* May inhibit first-pass metabolism of buspirone. Monitor patient closely for adverse effects; adjust dosage as needed.
CNS depressants: May increase CNS depression. Use together cautiously.
CYP3A4 inducers (such as carbamazepine, dexamethasone, phenobarbital, phenytoin, rifabutin, rifampin): May decrease buspirone level. Adjust dosage as needed.
Drugs metabolized by CYP3A4 (clarithromycin, diltiazem, erythromycin, fluvoxamine, itraconazole, ketoconazole, nefazodone, ritonavir, verapamil): May increase buspirone level. Monitor patient; decrease buspirone dosage and adjust carefully.
Linezolid, methylene blue: May cause serotonin syndrome. Use extreme caution and monitor closely.
MAO inhibitors: May elevate blood pressure. Avoid using together.
Drug-food. *Grapefruit juice:* May increase drug level, increasing adverse effects. Give with liquid other than grapefruit juice.
Drug-lifestyle. *Alcohol use:* May increase CNS depression. Discourage use together.

EFFECTS ON LAB TEST RESULTS
None reported.

CONTRAINDICATIONS & CAUTIONS
● Contraindicated in patients hypersensitive to drug and within 14 days of MAO inhibitor therapy.
🔔 **Alert:** Concomitant use with linezolid or methylene blue can cause serotonin syndrome (fever, mental status changes, muscle twitching, excessive sweating, shivering or shaking, diarrhea, loss of coordination). Use drug with linezolid or methylene blue only for life-threatening or urgent conditions when the potential benefits outweigh the risks of toxicity.
● Drug isn't recommended for patients with severe hepatic or renal impairment.
⚠ **Overdose S&S:** Nausea, vomiting, dizziness, drowsiness, miosis, gastric distress.

NURSING CONSIDERATIONS
● Monitor patient closely for adverse CNS reactions. Drug is less sedating than other

---

anxiolytics, but CNS effects may be unpredictable.

۞ Alert: Before starting therapy, don't stop a previous benzodiazepine regimen abruptly because a withdrawal reaction may occur.

۞ Alert: If linezolid or methylene blue must be given, buspirone must be stopped and the patient should be monitored for serotonin toxicity for 2 weeks or until 24 hours after the last dose of methylene blue or linezolid, whichever comes first. Treatment with buspirone may be resumed 24 hours after last dose of methylene blue or linezolid.

• Drug shows no potential for abuse and isn't classified as a controlled substance.

• **Look alike–sound alike:** Don't confuse buspirone with bupropion or risperidone.

PATIENT TEACHING

۞ Alert: Teach patient to recognize and immediately report symptoms of serotonin toxicity (fever, mental status changes, muscle twitching, excessive sweating, shivering or shaking, diarrhea, loss of coordination).

• Warn patient to avoid hazardous activities that require alertness and good coordination until effects of drug are known.

• Remind patient that drug effects may not be noticeable for several weeks.

• Warn patient not to abruptly stop a benzodiazepine because of risk of withdrawal symptoms.

• Tell patient to avoid use of alcohol during therapy.

• Advise patient to take consistently, that is, always with or always without food.

SAFETY ALERT!

busulfan
byoo-SUL-fan

Busulfex, Myleran

Therapeutic class: Antineoplastics
Pharmacologic class: Alkyl sulfonates
Pregnancy risk category: D

AVAILABLE FORMS
Injection: 6 mg/mL
Tablets: 2 mg

INDICATIONS & DOSAGES
➤ **Chronic myelocytic (granulocytic) leukemia (CML)**
Adults: 4 to 8 mg P.O. daily until WBC count falls to 15,000/mm³; stop drug until WBC count rises to 50,000/mm³, and then resume dosage as before. When remission is less than 3 months, may give maintenance therapy of 1 to 3 mg P.O. daily. Or, 0.8 mg/kg I.V. every 6 hours for 4 days (a total of 16 doses). Give cyclophosphamide 60 mg/kg I.V. over 1 hour daily for 2 days beginning 6 hours after the 16th dose of busulfan injection.
Children: 0.06 to 0.12 mg/kg daily or 1.8 to 4.6 mg/m² daily P.O. until WBC count falls to 15,000/mm³; stop drug until WBC count rises to 50,000/mm³ and then resume dosage as before.

ADMINISTRATION
P.O.
• Give drug on an empty stomach to minimize nausea and vomiting.
I.V.
▼ Give antiemetic before first dose of busulfan injection and then on a fixed schedule during therapy; give anticonvulsant to prevent seizures.
▼ Follow facility policy when preparing and handling drug. Label as a hazardous drug.
▼ Dilute drug in either D₅W or normal saline solution to at least 0.5 mg/mL.
▼ Use the 5-micron nylon filter to withdraw the calculated volume from the ampule. Then use a new needle to inject the drug into the I.V. bag or syringe.
▼ Invert several times to ensure mixing.
▼ Use a central venous access device.
▼ Flush access device with 5 mL of D₅W or normal saline solution before and after each infusion.
▼ Infuse over 2 hours through a central venous access device using a controlled-infusion device.
▼ Solutions are stable 8 hours at room temperature or 12 hours when diluted in normal saline solution and refrigerated. Infusions must be completed within these times.
▼ **Incompatibilities:** Don't mix or give with other I.V. solutions of unknown compatibility.

ACTION

Unknown. Thought to cross-link strands of cellular DNA and interfere with RNA transcription, causing an imbalance of growth that leads to cell death. Not specific to cell cycle.

Route	Onset	Peak	Duration
P.O.	1–2 wk	Unknown	Unknown
I.V.	Unknown	Unknown	Unknown

Half-life: About 2½ hours.

ADVERSE REACTIONS

CNS: fever, headache, asthenia, pain, insomnia, anxiety, dizziness, depression, delirium, agitation, *encephalopathy,* confusion, hallucination, lethargy, somnolence, *seizures.*

CV: edema, chest pain, tachycardia, hypertension, hypotension, *thrombosis,* vasodilation, *heart rhythm abnormalities,* cardiomegaly, *heart failure, pericardial effusion,* tachycardia.

EENT: rhinitis, epistaxis, pharyngitis, sinusitis, ear disorder, cataracts, corneal thinning, lens changes.

GI: nausea, stomatitis, vomiting, anorexia, diarrhea, abdominal pain and enlargement, dyspepsia, constipation, dry mouth, rectal disorder, *pancreatitis.*

GU: dysuria, oliguria, hematuria, hemorrhagic cystitis.

Hematologic: *granulocytopenia, thrombocytopenia, leukopenia,* anemia, *aplastic anemia.*

Hepatic: jaundice, hepatomegaly, hyperbilirubinemia, *hepatic veno-occlusive disease.*

Metabolic: *hypomagnesemia,* hyperglycemia, hypokalemia, hypocalcemia, hypervolemia, weight gain, hypophosphatemia, hyponatremia.

Musculoskeletal: back pain, myalgia, arthralgia.

Respiratory: lung disorder, cough, dyspnea, *irreversible pulmonary fibrosis, alveolar hemorrhage, asthma,* atelectasis, pleural effusion, hypoxia, hemoptysis.

Skin: inflammation at injection site, rash, pruritus, alopecia, exfoliative dermatitis, erythema nodosum, acne, skin discoloration, hyperpigmentation.

Other: Addison-like wasting syndrome, chills, allergic reaction, *infection,* hiccup.

INTERACTIONS

Drug-drug. *Acetaminophen, itraconazole:* May decrease busulfan clearance. Use together cautiously.

Anticoagulants, aspirin: May increase risk of bleeding. Avoid using together.

Cyclophosphamide: May increase risk of cardiac tamponade in patients with thalassemia. Monitor patient.

Metronidazole: May increase busulfan toxicity. Avoid using together.

Myelosuppressives: May increase myelosuppression. Monitor patient.

Other cytotoxic agents causing pulmonary injury: May cause additive pulmonary toxicity. Avoid using together.

Phenytoin: May decrease busulfan level. Monitor busulfan level.

Thioguanine: May cause hepatotoxicity, esophageal varices, or portal hypertension. Use together cautiously.

EFFECTS ON LAB TEST RESULTS

● May increase alkaline phosphatase, ALT, bilirubin, BUN, creatinine, and glucose levels. May decrease calcium, hemoglobin, magnesium, phosphorus, potassium, and sodium levels.

● May decrease WBC and platelet counts.

CONTRAINDICATIONS & CAUTIONS

● Contraindicated in patients with CML resistant to drug and in those with chronic lymphocytic leukemia, acute leukemia, or in the blastic crisis of CML.

● Use cautiously in patients recently given other myelosuppressives or radiation treatment and in those with depressed neutrophil or platelet count.

● Use cautiously in patients with history of head trauma or seizures and in those receiving other drugs that lower the seizure threshold because high-dose therapy has been linked to seizures.

⚠ *Overdose S&S:* GI toxicity with diarrhea, mucositis, nausea, vomiting, bone marrow depression, pancytopenia.

Reactions in bold italics are *life-threatening*. Interactions may have a *rapid onset* or a *delayed onset*.

NURSING CONSIDERATIONS

Black Box Warning Don't use busulfan unless a diagnosis of CML has been adequately established. ∎

Black Box Warning Reduce or discontinue the dosage if unusual depression of bone marrow function occurs. ∎

Black Box Warning Malignant tumors and acute leukemias have been reported in patients who have received busulfan therapy. ∎

• Therapeutic effects are commonly accompanied by toxicity.

• To prevent bleeding, avoid all I.M. injections when platelet count is less than 50,000/mm^3.

• Monitor patient response (increased appetite and sense of well-being, decreased total WBC count, reduced size of spleen), which usually begins in 1 to 2 weeks.

• Monitor for jaundice and liver function abnormalities in patients receiving high-dose busulfan.

• Anticipate possible blood transfusion during treatment because of cumulative anemia. Patients may receive injections of RBC colony-stimulating factor to promote RBC production and decrease the need for blood transfusions.

❸ Alert: Pulmonary fibrosis may occur as late as 8 months to 10 years after therapy. (Average length of therapy is 4 years.)

PATIENT TEACHING

• Advise patient to watch for signs of infection (fever, sore throat, fatigue) and bleeding (easy bruising, nosebleeds, bleeding gums, tarry stools). Tell patient to take temperature daily.

• Instruct patient to report signs and symptoms of toxicity so dosage can be adjusted. Persistent cough and progressive labored breathing with liquid in the lungs, suggestive of pneumonia, may be caused by drug toxicity.

• Advise patient to report sudden weakness, anorexia, melanoderma, nausea and vomiting, unusual fatigue, and weight loss.

• Instruct patient to avoid OTC products containing aspirin and NSAIDs.

• Inform patient that drug may cause skin darkening.

• Advise woman of childbearing age to avoid becoming pregnant during therapy.

Recommend that she consult prescriber before becoming pregnant.

• Advise patient not to breast-feed during therapy because of risk of toxicity to infant.

• Instruct patient to take drug on empty stomach to decrease nausea and vomiting.

• Because of risk of erectile dysfunction and sterility, advise men who want to father a child about sperm banking before therapy.

SAFETY ALERT!

butorphanol tartrate
byoo-TOR-fa-nole

Stadol

Therapeutic class: Opioid analgesics
Pharmacologic class: Opioid agonist-antagonists–opioid partial agonists
Pregnancy risk category: C
Controlled substance schedule: IV

AVAILABLE FORMS
Injection: 1 mg/mL, 2 mg/mL
Nasal spray: 10 mg/mL (1 mg/spray)

INDICATIONS & DOSAGES
➤ **Moderate to severe pain**
Adults: 1 to 4 mg I.M. every 3 to 4 hours p.r.n., or around the clock. Not to exceed 4 mg per dose. Or, 0.5 to 2 mg I.V. every 3 to 4 hours p.r.n., or around the clock. Or, 1 mg by nasal spray every 3 to 4 hours (1 spray in one nostril); repeat in 60 to 90 minutes if pain relief is inadequate. For severe pain, 2 mg (1 spray in each nostril) every 3 to 4 hours.

Adjust-a-dose: For patients with renal or hepatic impairment, increase dosage interval to 6 to 8 hours and give 50% of the normal dose. For elderly patients, give 1 mg I.M. or 0.5 mg I.V.; wait 6 hours before repeating dose. For nasal use, 1 mg (1 spray in one nostril). May give another 1 mg in 1.5 to 2 hours. Wait 6 hours before repeating sequence.

➤ **Labor for patients at full term; early labor (without signs of fetal distress)**
Adults: 1 or 2 mg I.V. or I.M.; repeat after 4 hours as needed. Don't give dose less than 4 hours before anticipated delivery.

➤ **Preoperative anesthesia or preanesthesia**
Adults: 2 mg I.M. 60 to 90 minutes before surgery.
➤ **Adjunct to balanced anesthesia**
Adults: 2 mg I.V. shortly before induction, or 0.5 to 1 mg I.V. in increments during anesthesia.
Elderly patients: One-half usual dose at twice the interval for I.V. use.

ADMINISTRATION

I.V.
▼ Compatible solutions include D₅W and normal saline solutions.
▼ Give by direct injection into a vein or into the tubing of a free-flowing I.V. solution.
▼ **Incompatibilities:** Dimenhydrinate, pentobarbital sodium.
I.M.
● Give drug I.M.; don't give subcutaneously.
Intranasal
● Watch for nasal congestion with nasal spray use.

ACTION
May bind with opioid receptors in the CNS, altering perception of and emotional response to pain.

Route	Onset	Peak	Duration
I.V.	1 min	4–5 min	2–4 hr
I.M.	10–30 min	30–60 min	3–4 hr
Nasal	15 min	1–2 hr	2½–5 hr

Half-life: About 2 to 9¼ hours.

ADVERSE REACTIONS
CNS: dizziness, insomnia, somnolence, anxiety, asthenia, confusion, euphoria, headache, lethargy, nervousness, paresthesia, tremor.
CV: flushing, palpitations, vasodilation.
EENT: nasal congestion, blurred vision, nasal irritation, pharyngitis, sinus congestion, sinusitis, rhinitis, tinnitus.
GI: nausea, unpleasant taste, vomiting, anorexia, constipation, dry mouth, stomach pain.
Respiratory: bronchitis, cough, dyspnea, upper respiratory tract infection.
Skin: clamminess, excessive diaphoresis, pruritus.
Other: sensation of heat.

INTERACTIONS
Drug-drug. *CNS depressants:* May cause additive effects. Use together cautiously.
Drug-lifestyle. *Alcohol use:* May cause additive effects. Discourage use together.

EFFECTS ON LAB TEST RESULTS
None reported.

CONTRAINDICATIONS & CAUTIONS
● Contraindicated in patients hypersensitive to drug or to preservative, benzethonium chloride, and in those with opioid addiction; may cause withdrawal syndrome.
● Use cautiously in patients with head injury, increased intracranial pressure, acute MI, ventricular dysfunction, coronary insufficiency, respiratory disease or depression, and renal or hepatic dysfunction.
● Use cautiously in patients who have recently received repeated doses of opioid analgesic.
⚠ *Overdose S&S:* Respiratory depression, CNS depression, CV insufficiency, coma, death.

NURSING CONSIDERATIONS
● Reassess patient's level of pain 15 and 30 minutes after administration.
● Respiratory depression apparently doesn't increase with larger dosage.
● Drug may cause constipation. Assess bowel function and need for stool softener and stimulant laxatives.
● Psychological and physical addiction may occur.
● Periodically monitor postoperative vital signs and bladder function. Because drug decreases both rate and depth of respirations, monitor arterial oxygen saturation to help assess respiratory depression.
● *Look alike–sound alike:* Don't confuse Stadol with sotalol.

PATIENT TEACHING
● Caution ambulatory patient about getting out of bed or walking. Warn outpatient to avoid driving and other hazardous activities that require mental alertness until it's clear how the drug affects the CNS.
● Teach patient how to take and store nasal spray.
● Instruct patient to avoid alcohol during therapy.

Reactions in bold italics are *life-threatening*. Interactions may have a *rapid onset* or a *delayed onset*.

calcitonin salmon
kal-si-TOE-nin

Fortical, Miacalcin

Therapeutic class: Antiosteoporotics
Pharmacologic class: Polypeptide hormones
Pregnancy risk category: C

AVAILABLE FORMS
Injection: 200 units/mL in 2-mL ampules
Nasal spray: 200 units/activation

INDICATIONS & DOSAGES
➤ **Paget disease of bone (osteitis defor-mans)**
Adults: Initially, 100 units daily I.M. or subcutaneously. Maintenance dosage is 50 units daily or every other day.
➤ **Hypercalcemia**
Adults: 4 units/kg every 12 hours I.M. or subcutaneously. If response is inade-quate after 1 or 2 days, increase dosage to 8 units/kg every 12 hours. If response re-mains unsatisfactory after 2 additional days, increase dosage to maximum of 8 units/kg every 6 hours.
➤ **Postmenopausal osteoporosis**
Adults: 200 units (one activation) daily intra-nasally, alternating nostrils daily. Or, 100 units I.M. or subcutaneously every other day. Patient should receive adequate vitamin D and calcium supplements (1.5 g calcium carbonate and 400 units of vitamin D) daily.

ADMINISTRATION
I.M.
● I.M. route is preferred if volume of dose exceeds 2 mL.
● Use freshly reconstituted solution within 2 hours.
● Give drug at bedtime, when possible, to minimize nausea and vomiting.
Intranasal
● Alternate nostrils daily.
● Give drug at bedtime, when possible, to minimize nausea and vomiting.
Subcutaneous
● Use freshly reconstituted solution within 2 hours.
● Give drug at bedtime, when possible, to minimize nausea and vomiting.
● Alternate injection sites.

ACTION
Decreases osteoclastic activity by inhibiting osteocytic osteolysis; decreases mineral release and matrix or collagen breakdown in bone.

Route	Onset	Peak	Duration
I.M., Subcut.	15 min	4 hr	8–24 hr
Intranasal	Rapid	30 min	1 hr

Half-life: 43 to 60 minutes.

ADVERSE REACTIONS
CNS: depression, headache, weakness, dizziness, paresthesia.
CV: chest pressure, facial flushing, edema of feet.
EENT: eye pain, nasal congestion, rhinitis, abnormal tearing, sinusitis, conjunctivitis.
GI: constipation, transient nausea, unusual taste, diarrhea, anorexia, vomiting, epigas-tric discomfort, abdominal pain.
GU: cystitis, increased urinary frequency, nocturia.
Musculoskeletal: arthrosis.
Respiratory: *bronchospasm,* upper respira-tory tract infection, shortness of breath.
Skin: rash, pruritus of ear lobes, inflamma-tion at injection site.
Other: hypersensitivity reactions, *ana-phylaxis,* chills, tender palms and soles, influenza-like symptoms.

INTERACTIONS
Drug-drug. *Bisphosphonates:* Prior use of bisphosphonates in patients with Paget disease may reduce the antiresorptive response to nasal spray. Monitor patient.

EFFECTS ON LAB TEST RESULTS
None reported.

CONTRAINDICATIONS & CAUTIONS
● Contraindicated in patients hypersensitive to drug.
⚠ *Overdose S&S:* Nausea, vomiting.

NURSING CONSIDERATIONS

• Skin test is usually done in patients with suspected drug sensitivity before therapy.

❸ Alert: Systemic allergic reactions are possible because hormone is protein. Keep epinephrine nearby.

❸ Alert: Observe patient for signs of hypocalcemic tetany during therapy (muscle twitching, tetanic spasms, and seizures when hypocalcemia is severe).

• Monitor calcium level closely. Watch for symptoms of hypercalcemia relapse: bone pain, renal calculi, polyuria, anorexia, nausea, vomiting, thirst, constipation, lethargy, bradycardia, muscle hypotonicity, pathologic fracture, psychosis, and coma.

• Periodic examinations of urine sediment are recommended.

• Monitor periodic alkaline phosphatase and 24-hour urine hydroxyproline levels to evaluate drug effect.

• In Paget disease, maximum reductions of alkaline phosphatase and urinary hydroxyproline excretion may take 6 to 24 months of continuous treatment.

• In patients with good first response to drug who have a relapse, expect to evaluate antibody response to the hormone protein.

• If symptoms have been relieved after 6 months, treatment may be stopped until symptoms or radiologic signs recur.

• Refrigerate drug at 36° to 46° F (2° to 8° C).

• **Look alike–sound alike:** Don't confuse calcitonin with calcifediol or calcitriol.

PATIENT TEACHING

• When drug is given for postmenopausal osteoporosis, remind patient to take adequate calcium and vitamin D supplements.

• Show home care patient and family member how to give drug. Tell them to do so at bedtime if only one dose is needed daily. If nasal spray is prescribed, tell patient to alternate nostrils daily.

• Advise patient to notify prescriber if significant nasal irritation or evidence of an allergic response occurs.

• Inform patient that facial flushing and warmth occur in 20% to 30% of patients within minutes of injection and usually last about 1 hour.

• Tell patient that nausea and vomiting may occur at the onset of therapy.

• Tell patient to inform prescriber promptly if signs and symptoms of hypercalcemia occur. Inform patient that, if drug loses its hypocalcemic activity, other drugs or increased dosages won't help.

calcitriol (1,25-dihydroxycholecalciferol)
kal-SIH-trye-ol

Calcijex, Rocaltrol, Vectical

Therapeutic class: Antihypocalcemics
Pharmacologic class: Vitamin D analogues
Pregnancy risk category: C

AVAILABLE FORMS
Capsules: 0.25 mcg, 0.5 mcg
Injection: 1 mcg/mL, 2 mcg/mL
Oral solution: 1 mcg/mL
Topical: 3 mcg/g

INDICATIONS & DOSAGES
➤ **Hypocalcemia in patients undergoing long-term dialysis**
Adults: Initially, 0.25 mcg P.O. daily. Increase by 0.25 mcg daily at 4- to 8-week intervals. Maintenance P.O. dosage is 0.25 mcg every other day up to 1 mcg daily. Or usual I.V. dosage is 1 to 2 mcg I.V. three times weekly. Increase dose by 0.5 to 1 mcg at 2- to 4-week intervals.
➤ **Hypoparathyroidism, pseudohypoparathyroidism**
Adults and children age 6 and older: Initially, 0.25 mcg P.O. daily in the morning. Dosage may be increased at 2- to 4-week intervals. Maintenance dosage is 0.25 to 2 mcg P.O. daily.
➤ **Hypoparathyroidism**
Children ages 1 to 5: Give 0.25 to 0.75 mcg P.O. daily.
➤ **To manage secondary hyperparathyroidism and resulting metabolic bone disease in predialysis patients (with CrCl of 15 to 55 mL/minute)**
Adults and children age 3 and older: Initially, 0.25 mcg P.O. daily. Dosage may be increased to 0.5 mcg/day if needed.

Children younger than age 3: Initially, 0.01 to 0.015 mcg/kg P.O. daily.
➤ **Mild to moderate plaque psoriasis**
Adults: Topically to affected area b.i.d. Maximum weekly dosage is 200 g.
➤ **Psoriasis** ◆
Children and adolescents: Topically to affected area b.i.d.

ADMINISTRATION
P.O.
● Give drug without regard for food.
● Don't give with magnesium-containing antacids.
I.V.
▼ For hypocalcemia in patient undergoing hemodialysis, give drug by rapid injection through catheter at end of hemodialysis session.
▼ **Incompatibilities:** None reported.
Topical
● Drug isn't for oral, ophthalmic, or intravaginal use.
● Gently rub into skin until no longer visible.

ACTION
Stimulates calcium absorption from the GI tract and promotes movement of calcium from bone to blood.

Route	Onset	Peak	Duration
P.O.	2–6 hr	3–6 hr	3–5 days
I.V.	Immediate	Unknown	3–5 days
Topical	Unknown	Unknown	Unknown

Half-life: 5 to 8 hours.

ADVERSE REACTIONS
CNS: headache, somnolence, weakness, irritability.
CV: hypertension, *arrhythmias.*
EENT: conjunctivitis, photophobia, rhinorrhea.
GI: nausea, vomiting, constipation, polydipsia, *pancreatitis,* metallic taste, dry mouth, anorexia.
GU: polyuria, nocturia, nephrocalcinosis, hypercalciuria.
Metabolic: weight loss.
Musculoskeletal: bone and muscle pain.
Skin: pruritus, skin discomfort at application area, psoriasis.
Other: hyperthermia, decreased libido.

INTERACTIONS
Drug-drug. *Cardiac glycosides:* May increase risk of arrhythmias. Use together cautiously.
Cholestyramine, colestipol, excessive use of mineral oil: May decrease absorption of oral vitamin D analogues. Avoid using together.
Corticosteroids: May counteract vitamin D analogue effects. Avoid using together.
Magnesium-containing antacids: May cause hypermagnesemia, especially in patients with chronic renal failure. Avoid using together.
Phenytoin, phenobarbital: May inhibit calcitriol synthesis. Dose may need to be increased.
Thiazides: May cause hypercalcemia. Use together cautiously.

EFFECTS ON LAB TEST RESULTS
● May increase AST, ALT, BUN, creatinine, cholesterol, urine albumin, and calcium levels.

CONTRAINDICATIONS & CAUTIONS
● Contraindicated in patients with hypercalcemia or vitamin D toxicity. Withhold all preparations containing vitamin D.
● Use cautiously in patients receiving cardiac glycosides and in those with sarcoidosis or hyperparathyroidism.
⚠ *Overdose S&S:* Hypercalcemia, hyperphosphatemia, weakness, headache, anorexia, nausea, vomiting, stomach cramps, dizziness.

NURSING CONSIDERATIONS
● Effective therapy is dependent on adequate calcium intake.
● Monitor calcium level; this level times the phosphate level shouldn't exceed 70. During dose adjustment, determine calcium level twice weekly. If hypercalcemia occurs, stop drug and notify prescriber but resume after calcium level returns to normal. Patient should receive adequate daily intake of calcium. Observe for hypocalcemia, bone pain, and weakness before and during therapy.
● Monitor phosphorus level, especially in hypoparathyroid patients and dialysis patients.
● Reduce dose as parathyroid hormone levels decrease in response to therapy.

• The symptoms of vitamin D intoxication include headache, somnolence, weakness, irritability, hypertension, arrhythmias, conjunctivitis, photophobia, rhinorrhea, nausea, vomiting, constipation, polydipsia, pancreatitis, metallic taste, dry mouth, anorexia, nephrocalcinosis, polyuria, nocturia, weight loss, bone and muscle pain, pruritus, hyperthermia, and decreased libido.

• Protect drug from heat and light.

• *Look alike–sound alike:* Don't confuse calcitriol with calcifediol or calcitonin.

PATIENT TEACHING
• Tell patient to immediately report early symptoms of vitamin D intoxication: weakness, nausea, vomiting, dry mouth, constipation, muscle or bone pain, or metallic taste.

• Instruct patient to adhere to diet and calcium supplementation and to avoid unapproved OTC drugs and antacids that contain magnesium.

• Warn patient to avoid excessive exposure of topically treated areas to either artificial or natural sunlight, including phototherapy.

☉ Alert: Tell patient that drug is the most potent form of vitamin D available and shouldn't be taken by anyone else.

---

calcium acetate
Eliphos, PhosLo Gelcaps, Phoslyra
calcium chloride

calcium citrate ◊
Cal-Citrate ◊, Citracal ◊, Citracal Liquitab ◊

calcium glubionate

calcium gluconate

calcium lactate ◊

calcium phosphate (tribasic)

Therapeutic class: Calcium supplements
Pharmacologic class: Calcium salts
Pregnancy risk category: NR; C (PhosLo)

AVAILABLE FORMS
calcium acetate
Contains 253 mg or 12.7 mEq of elemental calcium/g

Capsules: 667 mg
Gelcaps: 667 mg
Solution: 667 mg/5 mL
Tablets: 667 mg, 668 mg
calcium chloride
Contains 273 mg or 13.6 mEq of elemental calcium/g
Injection: 10% solution in 10-mL ampules, vials, and syringes
calcium citrate
Contains 211 mg or 10.6 mEq of elemental calcium/g
Capsules: 150 mg ◊
Granules for oral solution: 760 mg/3.5 g
Tablets: 200 mg ◊, 250 mg ◊, 950 mg ◊, 1,040 mg ◊
calcium glubionate
Contains 64 mg or 3.2 mEq elemental calcium/g
Syrup: 1.8 g/5 mL
calcium gluconate
Contains 90 mg or 4.5 mEq of elemental calcium/g
Capsules: 500 mg
Injection: 10% solution in 10-mL ampules and vials, 10-mL or 50-mL vials
Tablets: 50 mg, 500 mg ◊, 650 mg ◊
calcium lactate
Contains 130 mg or 6.5 mEq of elemental calcium/g
Capsules: 500 mg (96 mg elemental calcium)
Tablets: 100 mg, 325 mg, 648 mg, 750 mg
calcium phosphate (tribasic)
Contains 400 mg or 20 mEq of elemental calcium/g
Tablets: 600 mg ◊

INDICATIONS & DOSAGES
➤ **Hypocalcemic emergency**
Adults: 7 to 14 mEq calcium I.V. May give as a 10% calcium gluconate solution or 2% to 10% calcium chloride solution.
Children: 1 to 7 mEq calcium I.V.
Infants: Up to 1 mEq calcium I.V.
➤ **Hypocalcemic tetany**
Adults: 4.5 to 16 mEq calcium I.V. Repeat until tetany is controlled.
Children: 0.5 to 0.7 mEq/kg calcium I.V. t.i.d. to q.i.d. until tetany is controlled.
Neonates: 2.4 mEq/kg calcium I.V. daily in divided doses.

Reactions in bold italics are *life-threatening*. Interactions may have a *rapid onset* or a *delayed onset*.

➤ **Adjunctive treatment of magnesium intoxication**
Adults: Initially, 7 mEq I.V. Base subsequent doses on patient's response.
➤ **During exchange transfusions**
Adults: 1.35 mEq I.V. with each 100 mL citrated blood.
Neonates: 0.45 mEq I.V. after each 100 mL citrated blood.
➤ **Hyperphosphatemia**
Adults: 1,334 to 2,000 mg P.O. calcium acetate t.i.d. with meals. Most dialysis patients need 3 to 4 tablets with each meal.
➤ **Dietary supplement**
Adults: 500 mg to 2 g P.O. daily.
➤ **Hyperkalemia with secondary cardiac toxicity**
Adults: 2.25 to 14 mEq I.V. Repeat dose after 1 to 2 minutes, if needed.

ADMINISTRATION
P.O.
● Give drug with a full glass of water.
● Give 1 to 1½ hours after meals if GI upset occurs.
I.V.
▼ Calcium salts are not interchangeable; verify preparation before use.
▼ Give calcium chloride only by I.V. route. When adding to parenteral solutions that contain other additives (especially phosphorus or phosphate), watch for precipitate. Use an in-line filter.
▼ When giving calcium gluconate as injection, give only by I.V. route.
▼ Monitor ECG when giving calcium I.V. Stop drug and notify prescriber if patient complains of discomfort.
▼ Extravasation may cause severe necrosis and tissue sloughing. Calcium gluconate is less irritating to veins and tissues than calcium chloride.
Direct injection
▼ Don't use scalp veins in children.
▼ Warm solution to body temperature before giving it.
▼ For calcium chloride, give at 1 mL/minute (1.5 mEq/minute); for calcium gluconate, 2 mL/minute.
▼ Give slowly through a small needle into a large vein or through an I.V. line

containing a free-flowing, compatible solution.
▼ After injection, keep patient recumbent for 15 minutes.
Intermittent infusion
▼ Infuse diluted solution through an I.V. line containing a compatible solution.
▼ For calcium gluconate, don't exceed 200 mg/minute.
▼ **Incompatibilities:** Drug will precipitate if given with sodium bicarbonate or other alkaline drugs. Calcium chloride: amphotericin B, chlorpheniramine, dobutamine. Calcium gluconate: amphotericin B, dobutamine, fluconazole, indomethacin sodium trihydrate, methylprednisolone sodium succinate, prochlorperazine edisylate.

ACTION
Replaces calcium and maintains calcium level.

Route	Onset	Peak	Duration
P.O.	Unknown	Unknown	Unknown
I.V., I.M.	Immediate	Immediate	30 min–2 hr

Half-life: Unknown.

ADVERSE REACTIONS
CNS: tingling sensations, sense of oppression or heat waves with I.V. use, syncope with rapid I.V. use.
CV: *bradycardia, arrhythmias, cardiac arrest with rapid I.V. use,* mild drop in blood pressure, vasodilation.
GI: constipation, irritation, chalky taste, *hemorrhage,* nausea, vomiting, thirst, abdominal pain.
GU: polyuria, renal calculi.
Metabolic: hypercalcemia.
Skin: local reactions, including burning, necrosis, tissue sloughing, cellulitis, soft-tissue calcification with I.M. use.

INTERACTIONS
Drug-drug. *Atenolol, tetracyclines:* May decrease bioavailability of these drugs and calcium when oral preparations are taken together. Separate dosing times.
Cardiac glycosides: May increase digoxin toxicity. Give calcium cautiously, if at all, to digitalized patients.

Fosphenytoin, phenytoin: Use together may decrease absorption of both drugs. Avoid using together, or monitor levels carefully.
Iron supplements: May reduce iron absorption. Separate drug administration by 2 hours.
Sodium polystyrene sulfonate: May cause metabolic acidosis in patients with renal disease and a reduction of the resin's binding of potassium. Separate drugs by several hours.
Thiazide diuretics: May cause hypercalcemia. Avoid using together.
Verapamil: May reduce effects and toxicity of verapamil. Monitor patient closely.
Drug-food. *Foods containing oxalic acid (rhubarb, spinach), phytic acid (bran, whole-grain cereals), phosphorus (dairy products, milk):* May interfere with calcium absorption. Discourage use together.

EFFECTS ON LAB TEST RESULTS
• May increase calcium level.

CONTRAINDICATIONS & CAUTIONS
• Contraindicated in cancer patients with bone metastases and in those with ventricular fibrillation, hypercalcemia, hypophosphatemia, or renal calculi.
⚠ **Overdose S&S:** Hypercalcemia, confusion, delirium, stupor, coma.

NURSING CONSIDERATIONS
• Use all calcium products with extreme caution in digitalized patients and patients with sarcoidosis and renal or cardiac disease. Use calcium chloride cautiously in patients with cor pulmonale, respiratory acidosis, or respiratory failure.
🕭 **Alert:** Double-check that you are giving the correct form of calcium; resuscitation cart may contain both calcium gluconate and calcium chloride.
• Monitor calcium levels frequently. Maintain calcium level of 9 to 10.4 mg/dL. Don't allow level to exceed 12 mg/dL. Hypercalcemia may result after large doses in chronic renal failure. Report abnormalities.
• Signs and symptoms of severe hypercalcemia may include stupor, confusion, delirium, and coma. Signs and symptoms of mild hypercalcemia may include anorexia, nausea, and vomiting.

• **Look alike–sound alike:** Don't confuse calcium with calcitriol, calcium gluconate with calcium glubionate, or calcium chloride with calcium gluconate.

PATIENT TEACHING
• Tell patient to take oral calcium 1 to 1½ hours after meals if GI upset occurs.
• Tell patient to take oral calcium with a full glass of water.
• Tell patient to report anorexia, nausea, vomiting, constipation, abdominal pain, dry mouth, thirst, or polyuria.
• Warn patient that, in the meal before he takes calcium, he shouldn't have rhubarb, spinach, bran and whole-grain cereals, or dairy products; these foods may interfere with calcium absorption.
• Inform patient that some products may contain phenylalanine or tartrazine.

SAFETY ALERT!
✳ NEW DRUG

canagliflozin
KAN-a-gli-FLOE-zin

Invokana

Therapeutic class: Antidiabetics
Pharmacologic class: Sodium glucose cotransporter 2 inhibitors
Pregnancy risk category: C

AVAILABLE FORMS
Tablets: 100 mg, 300 mg

INDICATIONS & DOSAGES
➤ **Adjunct to diet and exercise to improve glycemic control in patients with type 2 diabetes**
Adults: 100 mg P.O. once daily before first meal of the day. May increase to 300 mg/day.
Adjust-a-dose: In patients tolerating 100 mg once daily who have an estimated GFR of 60 mL/minute/1.73 m^2 or greater and require additional glycemic control, may increase dosage to 300 mg once daily.
In those with moderate renal impairment (estimated GFR of 45 to <60 mL/minute/1.73 m^2), maximum dosage is 100 mg once daily. Don't initiate therapy

in patients with an estimated GFR of less than 45 mL/minute/1.73 m^2. Discontinue drug in patients with an estimated GFR persistently less than 45 mL/minute/1.73 m^2.

If patient is also taking UDP-glucurono-syltransferases (UGTs) inducers (for example, phenobarbital, phenytoin, rifampin, ritonavir), may increase canagliflozin dosage to 300 mg once daily if patient is currently tolerating canagliflozin 100 mg once daily, has an estimated GFR greater than 60 mL/minute/1.73 m^2, and requires additional glycemic control; if estimated GFR is 45 to less than 60 mL/minute/1.73 m^2, consider changing to another antihyperglycemic drug.

ADMINISTRATION
P.O.
- Give before first meal of the day.
- Store tablets at room temperature.

ACTION
Inhibits sodium glucose cotransporter 2, which reabsorbs glucose filtered by the kidneys, increasing amount of urinary glucose that is excreted.

Route	Onset	Peak	Duration
P.O.	Unknown	1–2 hr	Unknown

Half-life: 10.6 hours for 100-mg dose; 13.1 hours for 300-mg dose.

ADVERSE REACTIONS
CNS: fatigue, asthenia, syncope, postural dizziness.
CV: hypotension, orthostatic hypotension.
GI: thirst, constipation, nausea, abdominal pain, dehydration, *pancreatitis.*
GU: genital fungal infection, UTI, increased urination, vulvovaginal pruritus, renal impairment.
Hematologic: increased hemoglobin level.
Metabolic: *hypoglycemia, hyperkalemia,* hypercholesterolemia, hypermagnesemia, hyperphosphatemia.
Musculoskeletal: bone fracture.
Other: hypersensitivity reactions.

INTERACTIONS
Drug-drug. *ACE inhibitors (enalapril, lisinopril, moexipril, quinapril), ARBs (candesartan, losartan, olmesartan, valsartan),* *eplerenone, potassium-sparing diuretics (amiloride, spironolactone):* May increase risk of hyperkalemia. Monitor potassium level closely.
Antihypertensives: May increase hypotension. Monitor patient closely.
Digoxin: May increase digoxin level. Monitor digoxin level periodically.
Insulin and insulin secretagogues (glipizide, repaglinide): May increase risk of hypoglycemia. Consider lower dosage of insulin or insulin secretagogue.
Lomitapide: May increase lomitapide level. Limit maximum adult dosage of lomitapide to 30 mg daily.
Salicylates: May increase hypoglycemic effects. Monitor patient closely.
SSRIs (citalopram, fluoxetine, sertraline): May increase canagliflozin level. Monitor patient closely. Canagliflozin dosage may need adjustment if SSRI is discontinued.
UGT inducers (phenobarbital, phenytoin, rifampin, ritonavir): May decrease canagliflozin level. Adjust canagliflozin dosage based on estimated GFR.

EFFECTS ON LAB TEST RESULTS
- May increase serum creatinine, potassium, magnesium, phosphate, hemoglobin, LDL cholesterol, non-HDL cholesterol, and urine glucose levels.
- May decrease GFR and serum glucose level.

CONTRAINDICATIONS & CAUTIONS
- Contraindicated in patients hypersensitive to drug or its components, in those with type 1 diabetes, diabetic ketoacidosis, severe renal impairment (estimated GFR of <30 mL/minute/1.73 m^2), or ESRD, and in patients on dialysis.
- Drug isn't recommended for patients with severe hepatic disease.
- Drug increases serum creatinine level and decreases estimated GFR; patients with hypovolemia may be more susceptible to these changes. Renal function abnormalities can occur after drug initiation. More frequent renal function monitoring is recommended in patients with an estimated GFR of less than 60 mL/minute/1.73 m^2.

• Use cautiously in elderly patients and in those with volume depletion, impaired renal function, chronic low systolic blood pressure, or hypotension.
• Use in pregnant women only if potential benefit justifies potential risk to the fetus.
• It isn't known if drug appears in breast milk. Patient should discontinue breast-feeding or discontinue drug, taking into account the importance of drug to the mother.

NURSING CONSIDERATIONS
• Correct volume depletion before initiating drug. Observe for hypotension during therapy.
• Assess renal function at baseline and periodically throughout therapy.
• Monitor blood glucose level. Assess for signs and symptoms of hypoglycemia.
• Be aware that because of the drug's mechanism of action, urine test will be positive for glucose.
• Monitor electrolytes, such as potassium and magnesium. Correct levels as clinically indicated.
• Drug may increase lipid levels. Assess LDL cholesterol level periodically and treat as clinically indicated.
• Assess for genital mycotic (fungal) infections, especially in patients with a history of infection and in uncircumcised males. Treat appropriately.
• Monitor patient for hypersensitivity reaction (urticaria); reaction may occur hours to days after start of therapy. Discontinue drug and treat appropriately if hypersensitivity reaction occurs.

PATIENT TEACHING
• Advise patient to discontinue drug and immediately report hypersensitivity reaction (generalized urticarial rash).
• Warn female patient of possible risks to fetus and infant during pregnancy or breast-feeding. Instruct breast-feeding woman that she should discontinue drug or discontinue breast-feeding.
• Caution patient to avoid dehydration, which can cause hypotension. Instruct patient regarding adequate fluid intake and to report signs and symptoms of hypotension (postural dizziness, weakness, syncope).

• Instruct patient on general diabetes care, including importance of diet and exercise and monitoring blood glucose and glycosylated hemoglobin levels; signs and management of hypoglycemia and hyperglycemia; and assessing for diabetes complications.
• Advise patient to seek medical advice promptly during periods of stress (such as fever, trauma, infection, or surgery) because medication requirements may change.
• Instruct patient that if a dose is missed, to take it as soon as it's remembered unless it's almost time for the next dose, in which case patient should skip missed dose and take drug at next regularly scheduled time. Advise patient not to take two doses of drug at the same time.

candesartan cilexetil
kan-dah-SAR-tan

Atacand

Therapeutic class: Antihypertensives
Pharmacologic class: Angiotensin II receptor antagonists
Pregnancy risk category: D

AVAILABLE FORMS
Tablets: 4 mg, 8 mg, 16 mg, 32 mg

INDICATIONS & DOSAGES
Adjust-a-dose (for all indications): If patient takes a diuretic, consider a lower starting dose.
➤ **Hypertension (used alone or with other antihypertensives)**
Adults: Initially, 16 mg P.O. once daily when used alone; usual range is 8 to 32 mg P.O. daily as a single dose or in two divided doses.
➤ **Pediatric hypertension (used alone or with other antihypertensives)**
Children ages 6 to younger than 17: Initially for patients weighing more than 50 kg (110 lb), 8 to 16 mg P.O. once daily. May increase to 32 mg P.O. as single dose or divided doses as needed. Initially for patients weighing less than 50 kg, 4 to 8 mg P.O. once daily. May increase to 16 mg P.O. as single dose or divided doses as needed. *Children ages 1 to younger than 6:* Initially, 0.20 mg/kg P.O. once daily. Dosage range

is 0.05 to 0.4 mg/kg P.O. as single dose or divided doses.
➤ **Heart failure (New York Heart Association class II to IV)**
Adults: Initially, 4 mg P.O. once daily. Double the dose about every 2 weeks as tolerated to a target dose of 32 mg once daily.

ADMINISTRATION
P.O.
- Give drug without regard for food.
- Tablets may be made into suspension by pharmacist for patients unable to swallow pills.
- Suspension may be stored unopened at room temperature for 100 days.
- Shake suspension well before each use.
- Use suspension within 30 days of opening bottle.

ACTION
Inhibits vasoconstrictive action of angiotensin II by blocking angiotensin II receptor on the surface of vascular smooth muscle and other tissue cells.

Route	Onset	Peak	Duration
P.O.	Unknown	3–4 hr	24 hr

Half-life: 9 hours.

ADVERSE REACTIONS
CNS: dizziness, fatigue, headache.
CV: chest pain, peripheral edema.
EENT: pharyngitis, rhinitis, sinusitis.
GI: abdominal pain, diarrhea, nausea, vomiting.
GU: albuminuria.
Musculoskeletal: arthralgia, back pain.
Respiratory: coughing, bronchitis, upper respiratory tract infection.
Other: *angioedema.*

INTERACTIONS
Drug-drug. *Aliskiren:* May increase risk of renal impairment, hypotension, and hyperkalemia in diabetic patients and those with moderate to severe renal impairment (GFR <60 mL/minute). Concomitant use is contraindicated in diabetic patients. Avoid concomitant use in those with moderate to severe renal impairment.

Lithium: May increase lithium concentration. Monitor lithium levels closely.
NSAIDs (celecoxib, ibuprofen): May decrease antihypertensive effect of candesartan. Coadministration in patients who are elderly, volume-depleted (including those taking diuretics), or with decreased renal function may result in deteriorating renal function. Monitor blood pressure and renal function.
Potassium-sparing diuretics, potassium supplements: May cause hyperkalemia. Monitor patient closely.
Drug-herb. *Ma huang:* May decrease antihypertensive effects. Discourage use together.
Drug-food. *Salt substitutes containing potassium:* May cause hyperkalemia. Monitor patient closely.

EFFECTS ON LAB TEST RESULTS
- May increase potassium, BUN, and serum creatinine levels.

CONTRAINDICATIONS & CAUTIONS
- Contraindicated in patients hypersensitive to drug or its components, in children with GFR of less than 30 mL/min/1.73 m^2, and in children younger than age 1.
Black Box Warning Contraindicated in pregnant patients. ∎
- Use cautiously in patients whose renal function depends on the renin-angiotensin-aldosterone system (such as patients with heart failure) because of risk of oliguria and progressive azotemia with acute renal failure or death.
- Use cautiously in patients who are volume or salt depleted because they could develop symptoms of hypotension. Start therapy with a lower dosage range, and monitor blood pressure carefully.
⚠ Overdose S&S: Hypotension, dizziness, tachycardia; possible bradycardia from parasympathetic stimulation.

NURSING CONSIDERATIONS
Black Box Warning Drugs such as candesartan that act directly on the renin-angiotensin system can cause fetal and neonatal illness and death when given to pregnant women. If pregnancy is

detected, discontinue candesartan as soon as possible. ■

• If hypotension occurs after a dose of candesartan, place patient in the supine position and, if needed, give an I.V. infusion of normal saline solution.

• Most of drug's antihypertensive effect occurs within 2 weeks. Maximal effect may take 4 to 6 weeks. Diuretic may be added if blood pressure isn't controlled by drug alone.

• Carefully monitor elderly patients and those with renal disease for therapeutic response and adverse reactions.

PATIENT TEACHING

• Inform women of childbearing age of the consequences of exposure to drug during pregnancy. Prescriber should be notified immediately if pregnancy is suspected.

• Advise breast-feeding women of the risk of adverse effects on the infant and the need to stop either breast-feeding or drug.

• Instruct patient to store drug at room temperature and to keep container tightly sealed.

• Inform patient to report adverse reactions without delay.

• Tell patient that drug may be taken without regard to meals.

SAFETY ALERT!

capecitabine
kap-ah-SEAT-ah-been

Xeloda

Therapeutic class: Antineoplastics
Pharmacologic class: Pyrimidine analogues
Pregnancy risk category: D

AVAILABLE FORMS
Tablets: 150 mg, 500 mg

INDICATIONS & DOSAGES
Adjust-a-dose (for all indications): Round to nearest dose that gives a whole tablet; don't cut tablets in half.

➤ **With docetaxel or alone, metastatic breast cancer resistant to both paclitaxel and an anthracycline-containing** chemotherapy regimen or resistant to paclitaxel in patients for whom further anthracycline therapy isn't indicated; first-line treatment of metastatic colorectal cancer when fluoropyrimidine therapy alone is preferred; Duke stage C colon cancer after complete resection of primary tumor when fluoropyrimidine alone is preferred

Adults: 2,500 mg/m^2 daily P.O., in two divided doses, about 12 hours apart and after a meal, for 2 weeks, followed by a 1-week rest period; repeat every 3 weeks. Adjuvant treatment in patients with Duke C colon cancer is recommended for a total of eight cycles (24 weeks).

Adjust-a-dose: Follow National Cancer Institute of Canada (NCIC) common toxicity criteria when adjusting dosage. Toxicity criteria relate to degrees of severity of diarrhea, nausea, vomiting, stomatitis, and hand-foot syndrome. Refer to drug package insert for specific toxicity definitions. NCIC grade 1: Maintain dose level. NCIC grade 2: At first appearance, stop treatment until resolved to grade 0 to 1; then restart at 100% of starting dose for next cycle. At second appearance, stop treatment until resolved to grade 0 to 1 and use 75% of starting dose for next cycle. At third appearance, stop treatment until resolved to grade 0 to 1 and use 50% of starting dose for next cycle. At fourth appearance, stop treatment permanently. NCIC grade 3: At first appearance, stop treatment until resolved to grade 0 to 1 and use 75% of starting dose for next cycle. At second appearance, stop treatment until resolved to grade 0 to 1 and use 50% of starting dose for next cycle. At third appearance, stop treatment permanently. NCIC grade 4: At first appearance, stop treatment permanently or until resolved to grade 0 to 1, and use 50% of starting dose for next cycle. Reduce starting dose for patients with CrCl of 30 to 50 mL/minute to 75% of the starting dose (from 1,250 to 950 mg/m^3 P.O. b.i.d.).

ADMINISTRATION
P.O.
• Give drug whole with water within 30 minutes after breakfast and dinner.
• Don't cut or crush tablets.

• Use gloves and safety glasses to avoid exposure if tablets break.

ACTION

Converted to active 5-FU, which causes cellular injury by interfering with DNA synthesis to inhibit cell division and with RNA processing and protein synthesis.

Route	Onset	Peak	Duration
P.O.	Unknown	90–120 min	Unknown

Half-life: About 45 minutes.

ADVERSE REACTIONS

CNS: dizziness, fatigue, headache, insomnia, paresthesia, pyrexia, lethargy, peripheral neuropathy, asthenia.
CV: edema, chest pain, *venous thrombosis.*
EENT: eye irritation, epistaxis, increased lacrimation, rhinorrhea.
GI: diarrhea, nausea, vomiting, stomatitis, abdominal pain, constipation, anorexia, dyspepsia, taste perversion.
Hematologic: *neutropenia, thrombocytopenia,* anemia, *lymphopenia.*
Metabolic: dehydration.
Musculoskeletal: myalgia, limb pain, back pain.
Respiratory: dyspnea.
Skin: hand-foot syndrome, dermatitis, nail disorder, alopecia, rash.
Other: neutropenic fever.

INTERACTIONS

Drug-drug. *Antacids containing aluminum hydroxide and magnesium hydroxide:* May increase exposure to capecitabine and its metabolites. Monitor patient.
Leucovorin: May increase cytotoxic effects of 5-FU with enhanced toxicity. Monitor patient carefully.
Phenytoin: May increase toxicity or phenytoin effect. Monitor phenytoin level.
Black Box Warning *Warfarin:* May decrease clearance of warfarin and increase risk of bleeding. Monitor PT and INR. ∎

EFFECTS ON LAB TEST RESULTS

• May increase ALT and bilirubin levels. May decrease hemoglobin level. May increase or decrease calcium level.
• May decrease neutrophil, platelet, and WBC counts.

CONTRAINDICATIONS & CAUTIONS

• Contraindicated in patients hypersensitive to 5-FU, patients with known dihydropyrimidine dehydrogenase deficiency, and in those with severe renal impairment.
• Use cautiously in elderly patients and those with history of coronary artery disease, mild to moderate hepatic dysfunction from liver metastases, hyperbilirubinemia, and renal insufficiency. Use cautiously in patients also taking warfarin.
⚠ *Overdose S&S:* Nausea, vomiting, diarrhea, GI irritation and bleeding, bone marrow depression.

NURSING CONSIDERATIONS

• Patients older than age 80 may have a greater risk of adverse GI effects.
• Assess patient for severe diarrhea, and notify prescriber if it occurs. Give fluid and electrolyte replacement if patient becomes dehydrated. Drug may need to be immediately interrupted until diarrhea resolves or becomes less intense.
• Monitor patient for hand-foot syndrome (numbness, paresthesia, painless or painful swelling, erythema, desquamation, blistering, and severe pain of hands or feet), hyperbilirubinemia, and severe nausea. Drug therapy must be immediately adjusted. Hand-foot syndrome is staged from 1 to 4; drug may be stopped if severe or recurrent episodes occur.
• Hyperbilirubinemia may require stopping drug.
Black Box Warning Frequently monitor the INR and PT of patients also taking capecitabine and oral coumarin-derivative anticoagulant therapy; adjust anticoagulant dose accordingly. ∎
Black Box Warning Age older than 60 and a diagnosis of cancer independently predispose patients to an increased risk of coagulopathy. ∎
◑ *Alert:* Monitor patient carefully for toxicity, which may be managed by symptomatic treatment, dose interruptions, and dosage adjustments.
• *Look alike–sound alike:* Don't confuse Xeloda with Xenical.

PATIENT TEACHING

● Tell patient how to take drug. Drug is usually taken for 14 days, followed by 7-day rest period (no drug), as a 21-day cycle. Prescriber determines number of treatment cycles. Swallow tablets whole.

● *Alert:* Tell patient who also takes warfarin to report significant bleeding or bruising.

● Instruct patient to take drug with water within 30 minutes after breakfast and dinner.

● If a combination of tablets is prescribed, teach patient importance of correctly identifying the tablets to avoid possible dosing error.

● For missed doses, instruct patient not to take the missed dose and not to double the next one. Instead, he should continue with regular dosing schedule and check with prescriber.

● Instruct patient to inform prescriber if he's taking folic acid.

● Inform patient and caregiver about expected adverse effects of drug, especially nausea, vomiting, diarrhea, and hand-foot syndrome (pain, swelling, or redness of hands or feet). Tell him that patient-specific dosage adaptations during therapy are expected and needed.

● *Alert:* Instruct patient to stop taking drug and contact prescriber immediately if he develops diarrhea (more than four bowel movements daily or diarrhea at night), vomiting (two to five episodes in 24 hours), nausea, appetite loss or decrease in amount of food eaten each day, stomatitis (pain, redness, swelling, or sores in mouth), hand-foot syndrome, temperature of 100.5° F (38° C) or higher, or other evidence of infection.

● Tell patient that most adverse effects improve within 2 to 3 days after stopping drug. If patient doesn't improve, tell him to contact prescriber.

● Advise women of childbearing age to avoid becoming pregnant during therapy.

● Advise breast-feeding women to stop breast-feeding during therapy.

captopril
KAP-toe-pril

Capoten

Therapeutic class: Antihypertensives
Pharmacologic class: ACE inhibitors
Pregnancy risk category: C; D in 2nd and 3rd trimesters

AVAILABLE FORMS
Tablets: 12.5 mg, 25 mg, 50 mg, 100 mg

INDICATIONS & DOSAGES

➤ **Hypertension (alone or in combination with other antihypertensives)**
Adults: Initially, 25 mg P.O. b.i.d. or t.i.d. If dosage doesn't control blood pressure satisfactorily in 1 or 2 weeks, increase it to 50 mg b.i.d. or t.i.d. If that dosage doesn't control blood pressure satisfactorily after another 1 or 2 weeks, expect to add a diuretic. If patient needs further blood pressure reduction, dosage may be increased to 150 mg t.i.d. while continuing diuretic. Maximum daily dose is 450 mg.

➤ **Diabetic nephropathy**
Adults: 25 mg P.O. t.i.d.

➤ **Heart failure**
Adults: Initially, 25 mg P.O. t.i.d. Patients with normal or low blood pressure who have been vigorously treated with diuretics and who may be hyponatremic or hypovolemic may start with 6.25 or 12.5 mg P.O. t.i.d.; starting dosage may be adjusted over several days. Gradually increase dosage to 50 mg P.O. t.i.d.; once patient reaches this dosage, delay further dosage increases for at least 2 weeks. Maximum dosage is 450 mg daily.
Elderly patients: Initially, 6.25 mg P.O. b.i.d. Increase gradually as needed.

➤ **Left ventricular dysfunction after acute MI**
Adults: Start therapy as early as 3 days after MI with 6.25 mg P.O. for one dose, followed by 12.5 mg P.O. t.i.d. Increase over several days to 25 mg P.O. t.i.d.; then increase to 50 mg P.O. t.i.d. over several weeks.

ADMINISTRATION
P.O.
● Give 1 hour before meals to enhance drug absorption.

ACTION
Inhibits ACE, preventing conversion of angiotensin I to angiotensin II, a potent vasoconstrictor. Less angiotensin II decreases peripheral arterial resistance, decreasing aldosterone secretion, which reduces sodium and water retention and lowers blood pressure.

Route	Onset	Peak	Duration
P.O.	15–60 min	60–90 min	6–12 hr

Half-life: Less than 2 hours.

ADVERSE REACTIONS
CNS: dizziness, fainting, headache, malaise, fatigue, fever.
CV: tachycardia, hypotension, angina pectoris.
GI: abdominal pain, anorexia, constipation, diarrhea, dry mouth, dysgeusia, nausea, vomiting.
Hematologic: *leukopenia, agranulocytosis, thrombocytopenia, pancytopenia,* anemia.
Metabolic: hyperkalemia.
Respiratory: dry, persistent, nonproductive cough; dyspnea.
Skin: urticarial rash, maculopapular rash, pruritus, alopecia.
Other: *angioedema.*

INTERACTIONS
Drug-drug. *Aliskiren:* May increase risk of renal impairment, hypotension, and hyperkalemia in diabetic patients and those with moderate to severe renal impairment (GFR <60 mL/minute). Concomitant use is contraindicated in diabetic patients. Avoid concomitant use in those with moderate to severe renal impairment.
Antacids: May decrease captopril effect. Separate dosage times.
Diuretics, other antihypertensives: May cause excessive hypotension. May need to stop diuretic or reduce captopril dosage.
Insulin, oral antidiabetics: May cause hypoglycemia when captopril therapy is started. Monitor patient closely.

Lithium: May increase lithium level; symptoms of toxicity possible. Monitor lithium level and patient closely.
NSAIDs: May reduce antihypertensive effect. Monitor blood pressure.
Potassium-sparing diuretics, potassium supplements: May cause hyperkalemia. Avoid using together unless hypokalemia is confirmed.
Drug-herb. *Black catechu:* May cause additional hypotensive effect. Discourage use together.
Capsaicin: May worsen cough. Discourage use together.
Drug-food. *Salt substitutes containing potassium:* May cause hyperkalemia. Monitor patient closely.

EFFECTS ON LAB TEST RESULTS
● May increase alkaline phosphatase, bilirubin, BUN, serum creatinine, and potassium levels. May decrease sodium, glucose, and hemoglobin levels and hematocrit.
● May decrease granulocyte, platelet, RBC, and WBC counts.
● May cause false-positive urine acetone test results.

CONTRAINDICATIONS & CAUTIONS
● Contraindicated in patients hypersensitive to drug or other ACE inhibitors.
Black Box Warning Use during pregnancy can cause injury and death in the developing fetus. When pregnancy is detected, stop drug as soon as possible. ■
● Use cautiously in patients with impaired renal function or serious autoimmune disease, especially systemic lupus erythematosus, and in those who have been exposed to other drugs that affect WBC counts or immune response.
⚠ *Overdose S&S:* Hypotension.

NURSING CONSIDERATIONS
❂ *Alert:* Black patients who take ACE inhibitors as monotherapy for hypertension have a smaller reduction in blood pressure than nonblacks.
❂ *Alert:* Black patients taking ACE inhibitors have a higher incidence of angioedema than nonblacks.
● Monitor patient's blood pressure and pulse rate frequently.

❸ Alert: Elderly patients may be more sensitive to drug's hypotensive effects.

● Assess patient for signs of angioedema.

● Drug causes the most frequent occurrence of cough, compared with other ACE inhibitors.

● In patients with impaired renal function or collagen vascular disease, monitor WBC and differential counts before starting treatment, every 2 weeks for the first 3 months of therapy, and periodically thereafter.

● **Look alike–sound alike:** Don't confuse captopril with Capitrol or carvedilol.

PATIENT TEACHING

● Instruct patient to take drug 1 hour before meals; food in the GI tract may reduce absorption.

● Inform patient that light-headedness is possible, especially during first few days of therapy. Tell him to rise slowly to minimize this effect and to report occurrence to prescriber. If fainting occurs, he should stop drug and call prescriber immediately.

● Tell patient to use caution in hot weather and during exercise. Lack of fluids, vomiting, diarrhea, and excessive perspiration can lead to light-headedness and syncope.

● Advise patient to report signs and symptoms of infection, such as fever and sore throat.

● Tell women to notify prescriber if pregnancy occurs. Drug will need to be stopped.

● Urge patient to promptly report swelling of the face, lips, or mouth or difficulty breathing.

---

carbamazepine
kar-ba-MAZ-e-peen

Carbatrol, Epitol, Equetro, Mazepine†, Tegretol, Tegretol-XR, Teril

Therapeutic class: Anticonvulsants
Pharmacologic class: Iminostilbene derivatives
Pregnancy risk category: D

AVAILABLE FORMS
Capsules (extended-release): 100 mg, 200 mg, 300 mg

Oral suspension: 100 mg/5 mL
Tablets: 200 mg
Tablets (chewable): 100 mg
Tablets (extended-release): 100 mg, 200 mg, 400 mg

INDICATIONS & DOSAGES
➤ **Generalized tonic-clonic and complex partial seizures, mixed seizure patterns (except Carbatrol and Equetro)**
Adults and children older than age 12: Initially, 200 mg P.O. b.i.d. (conventional or extended-release tablets), or 100 mg suspension P.O. q.i.d. with meals. May be increased weekly by 200 mg P.O. daily in divided doses at 12-hour intervals for extended-release tablets or 6- to 8-hour intervals for conventional tablets or suspension, adjusted to minimum effective level. Maximum, 1,000 mg daily in children ages 12 to 15, and 1,200 mg daily in patients older than age 15. Usual maintenance dosage is 800 to 1,200 mg daily.
Children ages 6 to 12: Initially, 100 mg P.O. b.i.d. (conventional or extended-release tablets) or 50 mg suspension P.O. q.i.d. with meals, increased at weekly intervals by up to 100 mg P.O. in three to four divided doses daily (in two divided doses for extended-release form). Maximum, 1,000 mg daily. Usual maintenance dosage is 400 to 800 mg daily; or, 20 to 30 mg/kg in three or four divided doses.
Children younger than age 6: 10 to 20 mg/kg in two to three divided doses (conventional tablets) or four divided doses (suspension). Maximum dosage is 35 mg/kg in 24 hours.
➤ **Epilepsy (Carbatrol only)**
Adults and children older than age 12: 200 mg P.O. b.i.d. Increase at weekly intervals by adding up to 200 mg daily until optimal response is obtained. Dosage shouldn't exceed 1,000 mg daily in children ages 12 to 15 and 1,200 mg daily in patients older than age 15. Usual effective maintenance level is 800 to 1,200 mg daily.
➤ **Acute manic and mixed episodes associated with bipolar I disorder (Equetro only)**
Adults: Initially, 200 mg Equetro P.O. b.i.d. Increase by 200 mg daily to achieve

---

therapeutic response. Doses higher than 1,600 mg daily haven't been studied.

➤ **Trigeminal neuralgia (except Carbatrol and Equetro)**
Adults: Initially, 100 mg P.O. b.i.d. (conventional or extended-release tablets) or 50 mg suspension P.O. q.i.d. with meals, increased by 100 mg every 12 hours for tablets or 50 mg q.i.d. for suspension until pain is relieved. Maximum, 1,200 mg daily. Maintenance dosage is usually 200 to 400 mg P.O. b.i.d.

➤ **Trigeminal neuralgia (Carbatrol only)**
Adults: Initially, 200-mg capsule P.O. daily. Daily dosage may be increased by up to 200 mg/day every 12 hours, only as needed to achieve freedom from pain. Don't exceed 1,200 mg daily.

➤ **Borderline personality disorder ◆**
Adults: Initially, 400 mg P.O. daily in two divided doses (tablets or extended-release tablets or capsules) or four divided doses (oral suspension). May increase dosage in increments of 200 mg/day. Maximum dosage is 1,600 mg/day.

➤ **Alcohol withdrawal ◆**
Adults: 600 to 1,200 mg P.O. on day 1, tapered to 0 mg over 5 to 10 days.

ADMINISTRATION
P.O.
- Shake oral suspension well before measuring dose.
- Give tablets with meals.
- Contents of extended-release capsules may be sprinkled over applesauce if patient has difficulty swallowing capsules. Capsules and tablets shouldn't be crushed or chewed, unless labeled as chewable form.
- When giving by nasogastric tube, mix dose with an equal volume of water, normal saline solution, or D_5W. Flush tube with 100 mL of diluent after giving dose.
- Don't crush or split extended-release form or give broken or chipped tablets.
- Patients converting from immediate-release to extended-release form should receive the same total daily dosage.

ACTION
Thought to stabilize neuronal membranes and limit seizure activity by either increasing efflux or decreasing influx of sodium ions across cell membranes in the motor cortex during generation of nerve impulses.

Route	Onset	Peak	Duration
P.O.	Unknown	1½–12 hr	Unknown
P.O. (extended-release)	Unknown	4–8 hr	Unknown

Half-life: 25 to 65 hours with single dose; 8 to 29 hours with long-term use.

ADVERSE REACTIONS
CNS: ataxia, dizziness, drowsiness, somnolence, vertigo, *worsening of seizures,* confusion, fatigue, fever, headache, syncope, pain, depression including *suicidal ideation,* speech disorder.
CV: *arrhythmias, AV block, heart failure,* aggravation of coronary artery disease, hypertension, hypotension.
EENT: blurred vision, conjunctivitis, diplopia, dry pharynx, nystagmus.
GI: nausea, vomiting, abdominal pain, anorexia, diarrhea, dry mouth, dyspepsia, glossitis, stomatitis.
GU: albuminuria, glycosuria, erectile dysfunction, urinary frequency, urine retention.
Hematologic: *agranulocytosis, aplastic anemia, thrombocytopenia,* eosinophilia, leukocytosis.
Hepatic: *hepatitis.*
Metabolic: hyponatremia, SIADH.
Respiratory: pulmonary hypersensitivity.
Skin: *erythema multiforme, Stevens-Johnson syndrome,* excessive diaphoresis, rash, urticaria, pruritus.
Other: chills.

INTERACTIONS
Drug-drug. *Anticoagulants:* May reduce anticoagulant effect. Monitor PT when starting or stopping carbamazepine.
Atracurium, cisatracurium, pancuronium, rocuronium, vecuronium: May decrease the effects of nondepolarizing muscle relaxant, causing it to be less effective. May need to increase the dose of the nondepolarizing muscle relaxant.
Azole antifungals (itraconazole, ketoconazole): May increase carbamazepine level and decrease antifungal level. Monitor levels and effectiveness of drugs.

Cimetidine, danazol, diltiazem, fluoxetine, fluvoxamine, isoniazid, valproic acid, verapamil: May increase carbamazepine level. Use together cautiously.

Clarithromycin, erythromycin, troleandomycin: May inhibit metabolism of carbamazepine, increasing carbamazepine level and risk of toxicity. Avoid using together.

Doxycycline, felbamate, haloperidol, hormonal contraceptives, phenytoin, theophylline, tiagabine, topiramate, valproate: May decrease levels of these drugs. Watch for decreased effect.

Lamotrigine: May decrease lamotrigine level and increase carbamazepine level. Monitor patient for clinical effects and toxicity.

Lithium: May increase CNS toxicity of lithium. Avoid using together.

MAO inhibitors: May increase depressant and anticholinergic effects. Avoid using together. Discontinue MAO inhibitors at least 14 days before starting carbamazepine.

Nefazodone: May increase carbamazepine levels and toxicity while reducing nefazodone levels and therapeutic benefits. Use together is contraindicated.

Oral and other hormonal contraceptives: May cause breakthrough bleeding and reduced contraceptive effectiveness. Consider back-up method of birth control.

Phenobarbital, phenytoin, primidone: May decrease carbamazepine level. Watch for decreased effect.

SSRIs, TCAs: May increase carbamazepine level and decrease levels of antidepressant. Closely monitor patient and adjust dosage as needed.

Drug-food. *Grapefruit juice:* May increase carbamazepine level. Avoid use together.

Drug-herb. *Plantains (psyllium seed):* May inhibit GI absorption of drug. Discourage use together.

EFFECTS ON LAB TEST RESULTS

• May increase BUN level. May decrease sodium and hemoglobin levels and hematocrit.

• May increase LFT values and eosinophil and WBC counts. May decrease thyroid function test values and granulocyte and platelet counts.

• May cause false pregnancy test results.

CONTRAINDICATIONS & CAUTIONS

• Contraindicated in patients hypersensitive to this drug or TCAs and in those with a history of bone marrow suppression; also contraindicated in those who have taken an MAO inhibitor within 14 days.

• Use cautiously in patients with mixed seizure disorders because they may experience an increased risk of seizures. Also, use with caution in patients with hepatic dysfunction.

⚠ *Overdose S&S:* Conduction disorders, hypotension or hypertension, impairment of consciousness, irregular breathing, respiratory depression, tachycardia, shock, seizures, adiadochokinesia, ataxia, athetoid movements, ballism, dizziness, drowsiness, dysmetria, motor restlessness, muscular twitching, mydriasis, nystagmus, opisthotonos, psychomotor disturbances, tremor; hyperreflexia followed by anuria or oliguria, hyporeflexia, nausea and vomiting, urine retention.

NURSING CONSIDERATIONS

Black Box Warning Patients of Asian ancestry should get a genetic blood test to identify their risk for rare, but serious skin reactions (toxic epidermal necrolysis, Stevens-Johnson syndrome). Screen for HLA-B*1502 allele before starting treatment with carbamazepine. ∎

• Watch for worsening of seizures, especially in patients with mixed seizure disorders, including atypical absence seizures.

❂ *Alert:* Closely monitor all patients taking or starting antiepileptic drugs for changes in behavior indicating worsening of suicidal thoughts or behavior or depression. Symptoms such as anxiety, agitation, hostility, mania, and hypomania may be precursors to emerging suicidality.

• Obtain baseline determinations of urinalysis, BUN and iron levels, liver function, CBC, and platelet and reticulocyte counts. Monitor these values periodically thereafter.

Black Box Warning Aplastic anemia and agranulocytosis have been reported in association with carbamazepine therapy. Obtain complete pretreatment hematologic testing as a baseline. If patient in the course of treatment exhibits low or decreased WBC

Reactions in bold italics are *life-threatening*. Interactions may have a *rapid onset* or a *delayed onset*.

or platelet counts, monitor patient closely. Consider discontinuing drug if evidence of significant bone marrow depression develops. ■

• Never stop drug suddenly when treating seizures. Notify prescriber immediately if adverse reactions occur.

• Adverse reactions may be minimized by gradually increasing dosage.

• Therapeutic level is 4 to 12 mcg/mL. Monitor level and effects closely. Ask patient when last dose was taken to better evaluate drug level.

• When managing seizures, take appropriate precautions.

❸ Alert: Watch for signs of anorexia or subtle appetite changes, which may indicate excessive drug level.

• **Look alike–sound alike:** Don't confuse carbamazepine with oxcarbazepine. Don't confuse Tegretol or Tegretol-XR with Trental, Topamax, Toprol-XL, or Toradol. Don't confuse Carbatrol with carvedilol.

PATIENT TEACHING

• Instruct patient to take drug with food to minimize GI distress. Tell patient taking suspension form to shake container well before measuring dose.

• Tell patient not to crush or chew extended-release form and not to take broken or chipped tablets.

• Tell patient that Tegretol-XR tablet coating may appear in stool because it isn't absorbed.

• Advise patient to keep tablets in the original container and to keep the container tightly closed and away from moisture. Some formulations may harden when exposed to excessive moisture, so that less is available in the body, decreasing seizure control.

• Inform patient that when drug is used for trigeminal neuralgia, an attempt to decrease dosage or withdraw drug is usually made every 3 months.

• Advise patient to notify prescriber immediately if fever, sore throat, mouth ulcers, or easy bruising or bleeding occurs.

• Tell patient that drug may cause mild to moderate dizziness and drowsiness when first taken. Advise him to avoid hazardous activities until effects disappear, usually within 3 to 4 days.

• Advise patient that periodic eye examinations are recommended.

• Advise women of risks to fetus if pregnancy occurs while taking carbamazepine.

• Advise women that breast-feeding isn't recommended during therapy.

SAFETY ALERT!

carboplatin
KAR-bo-pla-tin

Therapeutic class: Antineoplastics
Pharmacologic class: Platinum-containing compounds
Pregnancy risk category: D

AVAILABLE FORMS

Aqueous solution for injection: 50 mg/5 mL, 150 mg/15 mL, 450 mg/45 mL, 600 mg/60 mL, 1 g/100 mL
Lyophilized powder for injection: 50-mg, 150-mg, 450-mg vials

INDICATIONS & DOSAGES

➤ **Advanced ovarian cancer**

Adults: 360 mg/m^2 I.V. on day 1 every 4 weeks. Or, 300 mg/m^2 on day 1 every 4 weeks for six cycles when used with other chemotherapy drugs. Or, use the Calvert formula to calculate initial dosage:

$$\text{Total dose (mg)} = (\text{target AUC}) \times (\text{GFR} + 25)$$

where target AUC (area under the curve) is usually 4 to 6 mg/mL and GFR is measured in mL/minute. Doses shouldn't be repeated until platelet count exceeds 100,000/mm^3 and neutrophil count exceeds 2,000/mm^3. Subsequent doses are based on blood counts: If platelet count is greater than 100,000/mm^3 and neutrophil count is greater than 2,000/mm^3, give 125% of dose. If platelet count is 50,000/mm^3 to 100,000/mm^3 and neutrophil count is 500/mm^3 to 2,000/mm^3, keep same dose. If platelet count is less than 50,000/mm^3 and neutrophil count is less than 500/mm^3, give 75% of dose.

Adjust-a-dose: If CrCl is 41 to 59 mL/minute, first dose is 250 mg/m^2. If CrCl is 16 to 40 mL/minute, first dose is

200 mg/m^2. Drug isn't recommended for patients with CrCl of 15 mL/minute or less.

ADMINISTRATION

I.V.

Black Box Warning Anaphylaxis may occur within minutes of administration. Keep epinephrine, corticosteroids, and antihistamines available when giving carboplatin. ∎

▼ Preparing and giving parenteral form of drug may be mutagenic, teratogenic, or carcinogenic. Follow facility policy to reduce risks.

▼ Don't use aluminum needles or I.V. administration sets because drug may precipitate or lose potency.

▼ For premixed aqueous solution of 10 mg/mL, dilute for infusion with normal saline solution or D$_5$W to a concentration as low as 0.5 mg/mL.

▼ For vials of lyophilized powder, reconstitute with sterile water for injection, D$_5$W, or normal saline solution. For 150-mg vial, use 15 mL solution to yield a concentration of 10 mg/mL.

▼ Give drug by continuous or intermittent infusion over at least 15 minutes.

▼ Store unopened vials at room temperature. Protect from light.

▼ Once reconstituted and diluted as directed, drug is stable at room temperature for 8 hours.

▼ Because drug contains no preservatives, discard after 8 hours.

▼ **Incompatibilities:** Amphotericin B cholesteryl sulfate complex, 5-FU, mesna, sodium bicarbonate.

ACTION

May cross-link strands of cellular DNA and interfere with RNA transcription, causing an imbalance of growth that leads to cell death. Not specific to cell cycle.

Route	Onset	Peak	Duration
I.V.	Unknown	Unknown	Unknown

Half-life: 5 hours.

ADVERSE REACTIONS

CNS: dizziness, confusion, *stroke,* peripheral neuropathy, *central neurotoxicity,* pain, asthenia.

CV: *heart failure, embolism.*
EENT: ototoxicity.
GI: abdominal pain, constipation, diarrhea, nausea, vomiting, mucositis, change in taste, stomatitis.
GU: renal toxicity.
Hematologic: *thrombocytopenia, leukopenia, neutropenia,* anemia, *bone marrow suppression, bleeding.*
Skin: alopecia.
Other: hypersensitivity reactions.

INTERACTIONS

Drug-drug. *Bone marrow suppressants, including radiation therapy:* May increase hematologic toxicity. Monitor CBC with differential closely.
Nephrotoxic drugs, especially aminoglycosides and amphotericin B: May enhance nephrotoxicity of carboplatin. Use together cautiously.
Phenytoin: May decrease phenytoin level. Monitor serum level and patient for decreased effectiveness.

EFFECTS ON LAB TEST RESULTS

● May increase alkaline phosphatase, AST, BUN, and creatinine levels. May decrease electrolyte and hemoglobin levels and hematocrit.
● May decrease neutrophil, platelet, RBC, and WBC counts.

CONTRAINDICATIONS & CAUTIONS

● Contraindicated in patients with severe bone marrow suppression or bleeding or with history of hypersensitivity to cisplatin, platinum-containing compounds, or mannitol.
⚠ *Overdose S&S:* Bone marrow suppression, hepatotoxicity.

NURSING CONSIDERATIONS

Black Box Warning Carboplatin should be administered under the supervision of a physician experienced in the use of chemotherapeutic agents. ∎
● Determine electrolyte, creatinine, and BUN levels; CBC; platelet count; and CrCl before first infusion and before each course of treatment.
☻ *Alert:* When using the Calvert formula, the total dose is calculated in mg, not mg/m^2.

• Monitor CBC and platelet count frequently during therapy and, when indicated, until recovery. Lowest WBC and platelet counts usually occur by day 21. Levels usually return to baseline by day 28. Don't repeat unless platelet count exceeds 100,000/mm³.

Black Box Warning Bone marrow suppression is dose related and may be severe, resulting in infection or bleeding. ∎

Black Box Warning Vomiting is another frequent drug-related side effect. ∎

• Bone marrow suppression may be more severe in patients with CrCl below 60 mL/minute; adjust dosage.

⟳ Alert: Carefully check ordered dose against laboratory test results. Only one increase in dosage is recommended. Subsequent doses shouldn't exceed 125% of starting dose.

• Therapeutic effects are commonly accompanied by toxicity.

• Drug has less nephrotoxicity and neurotoxicity than cisplatin, but it causes more severe myelosuppression.

• To prevent bleeding, avoid all I.M. injections when platelet count is below 50,000/mm³.

• Monitor vital signs during infusion.

• Give antiemetic to reduce nausea and vomiting.

Black Box Warning Anemia may be cumulative and may require transfusion support. ∎

• Patients older than age 65 are at greater risk for neurotoxicity.

• **Look alike–sound alike:** Don't confuse carboplatin with cisplatin.

PATIENT TEACHING

• Advise patient of most common adverse reactions: nausea, vomiting, bone marrow suppression, anemia, and reduction in blood platelets.

• Advise patient to watch for signs of infection (fever, sore throat, fatigue) and bleeding (easy bruising, nosebleeds, bleeding gums, tarry stools). Tell patient to take temperature daily.

• Instruct patient to avoid OTC products containing aspirin and NSAIDs.

• Advise women to stop breast-feeding during therapy because of risk of toxicity to infant.

• Because of risk of sterility and menstruation cessation, counsel both men and women of childbearing age before starting therapy. Also recommend that women consult prescriber before becoming pregnant.

carboprost tromethamine
KAR-boe-prost

Hemabate

Therapeutic class: Oxytocics
Pharmacologic class: Prostaglandins
Pregnancy risk category: C

AVAILABLE FORMS
Injection: 250 mcg/mL

INDICATIONS & DOSAGES
➤ **To terminate pregnancy between weeks 13 and 20 of gestation**
Adults: Initially, 250 mcg deep I.M.; optionally, a 100-mcg I.M. test dose may be given. Give subsequent doses of 250 mcg at intervals of 1½ to 3½ hours, depending on uterine response. Dosage may be increased in increments to 500 mcg if contractility is inadequate after several 250-mcg doses. Total dose shouldn't exceed 12 mg or continuous administration for more than 2 days.

➤ **Postpartum hemorrhage from uterine atony not managed by conventional methods**
Adults: 250 mcg by deep I.M. injection. Repeat doses every 15 to 90 minutes as needed. Maximum total dose is 2 mg.

ADMINISTRATION
I.M.
⟳ Alert: Only trained personnel in a hospital setting should give drug, with strict adherence to recommended dosages.

• Give deep in the muscle using a tuberculin syringe.

• Store drug in refrigerator.

ACTION
Produces strong, prompt contractions of uterine smooth muscle, possibly mediated by calcium and cAMP.

Route	Onset	Peak	Duration
I.M.	Unknown	15–60 min	24 hr

Half-life: Unknown.

ADVERSE REACTIONS
CNS: fever, headache, anxiety, paresthesia, syncope, weakness.
CV: *arrhythmias,* chest pain, flushing.
EENT: blurred vision, eye pain.
GI: vomiting, diarrhea, nausea.
GU: *uterine rupture,* endometritis, uterine or vaginal pain.
Musculoskeletal: backache, leg cramps.
Respiratory: coughing, wheezing.
Skin: rash, diaphoresis.
Other: breast tenderness, chills, hot flashes.

INTERACTIONS
Drug-drug. *Other oxytocics:* May increase action. Avoid using together.

EFFECTS ON LAB TEST RESULTS
None reported.

CONTRAINDICATIONS & CAUTIONS
• Contraindicated in patients hypersensitive to drug and in those with acute pelvic inflammatory disease or active cardiac, pulmonary, renal, or hepatic disease.
• Use cautiously in patients with history of asthma, hypotension, hypertension, anemia, jaundice, or diabetes; and those with seizure disorders, previous uterine surgery, or CV, adrenal, renal, or hepatic disease.

NURSING CONSIDERATIONS
• Unlike other prostaglandin abortifacients, drug is given by I.M. injection. Injectable form avoids risk of expelling vaginal suppositories if patient has profuse vaginal bleeding.
• Pretreating and giving with antiemetics and antidiarrheals decreases the risk of common GI effects.

PATIENT TEACHING
• Explain use and administration of drug to patient and family.
• Instruct patient to report adverse reactions promptly.

carisoprodol
kar-eye-soe-PROE-dol

Soma♦

Therapeutic class: Skeletal muscle relaxants
Pharmacologic class: Carbamate derivatives
Pregnancy risk category: C
Controlled substance schedule: IV

AVAILABLE FORMS
Tablets: 250 mg, 350 mg

INDICATIONS & DOSAGES
➤ **Adjunctive treatment for acute, painful musculoskeletal conditions**
Adults: 250 to 350 mg P.O. t.i.d. and at bedtime for a maximum of 2 to 3 weeks.

ADMINISTRATION
P.O.
• Give drug with food or milk if GI upset occurs.

ACTION
May modify central perception of pain without modifying pain reflexes. Muscle relaxant effects may be related to sedative properties.

Route	Onset	Peak	Duration
P.O.	½ hr	1½–2 hr	4–6 hr

Half-life: 2 hours for carisoprodol, 10 hours for active metabolite.

ADVERSE REACTIONS
CNS: drowsiness, dizziness, vertigo, ataxia, tremor, agitation, irritability, headache, depressive reactions, fever, insomnia, syncope.
Respiratory: *asthmatic episodes.*
Skin: *erythema multiforme,* pruritus, rash.
Other: *angioedema, anaphylaxis.*

INTERACTIONS
Drug-drug. *CNS depressants:* May increase CNS depression. Avoid using together.
CYP2C19 inducers (such as rifampin): May increase active metabolite (meprobamate) exposure and decrease available carisoprodol. Use cautiously together.

Reactions in bold italics are *life-threatening*. Interactions may have a *rapid onset* or a *delayed onset*.

CYP2C19 inhibitors (such as fluvoxamine, omeprazole): May decrease metabolism of carisoprodol to meprobamate, increasing exposure to carisoprodol. Use cautiously together.

Meprobamate: May increase meprobamate level. Avoid use together.

Drug-herb. *St. John's wort:* May increase active metabolite (meprobamate) exposure and decrease available carisoprodol. Use cautiously together.

Drug-lifestyle. *Alcohol use:* May increase CNS depression. Discourage use together.

EFFECTS ON LAB TEST RESULTS
• May increase eosinophil count.

CONTRAINDICATIONS & CAUTIONS
• Contraindicated in patients hypersensitive to related compounds (such as meprobamate) and in those with intermittent porphyria.

❸ Alert: Drug has been classified as a Schedule IV controlled substance; cases of dependence, withdrawal, and abuse have occurred with prolonged use.

• Use cautiously in patients with impaired hepatic or renal function.

• Safety and effectiveness in adults older than age 65 and children younger than age 16 haven't been established.

⚠ Overdose S&S: Stupor, coma, seizures, shock, respiratory depression, drowsiness, dizziness, headache, diplopia, nystagmus, delirium, dystonia, muscular incoordination.

NURSING CONSIDERATIONS
❸ Alert: Watch for idiosyncratic reactions after first to fourth doses (weakness, ataxia, visual and speech difficulties, fever, skin eruptions, and mental changes) and for severe reactions, including bronchospasm, hypotension, and anaphylactic shock. After unusual reactions, withhold dose and notify prescriber immediately.

• Record amount of relief to help prescriber determine whether dosage can be reduced.

• Don't stop drug abruptly, which may cause mild withdrawal effects, such as insomnia, headache, nausea, or abdominal cramps.

• Drug may be habit forming.

PATIENT TEACHING
• Warn patient to avoid activities that require alertness until CNS effects of drug are known. Drowsiness is transient.

• Advise patient to avoid combining drug with alcohol or other CNS depressants.

• Tell patient to ask prescriber before using OTC cold or hay fever remedies.

• Instruct patient to follow prescriber's orders regarding rest and physical therapy.

• Advise patient to avoid sudden changes in posture if dizziness occurs.

• Tell patient to take drug with food or milk if GI upset occurs.

SAFETY ALERT!

carmustine (BCNU)
kar-MUS-teen

BiCNU, Gliadel Wafer

Therapeutic class: Antineoplastics
Pharmacologic class: Nitrosoureas
Pregnancy risk category: D

AVAILABLE FORMS
Injection: 100-mg vial (lyophilized), with a 3-mL vial of absolute alcohol supplied as a diluent
Wafer: 7.7 mg, for intracavitary use

INDICATIONS & DOSAGES
➤ **Brain tumor, Hodgkin lymphoma, malignant lymphoma, multiple myeloma**
Adults: 150 to 200 mg/m^2 I.V. by slow infusion every 6 weeks; may be divided into daily injections of 75 to 100 mg/m^2 on 2 successive days; repeat dose every 6 weeks if platelet count is greater than 100,000/mm^3 and WBC count is greater than 4,000/mm^3.

Adjust-a-dose: Dosage is reduced by 30% when WBC nadir is 2,000 to 2,999/mm^3 and platelet nadir is 25,000 to 74,999/mm^3. Dosage is reduced by 50% when WBC nadir is less than 2,000/mm^3 and platelet nadir is less than 25,000/mm^3.

➤ **Adjunct to surgery to prolong survival in patients with recurrent glioblastoma multiforme for whom surgical resection is indicated; adjunct to surgery and**

radiation in patients with newly diagnosed high-grade malignant glioma
Adults: 8 wafers placed in the resection cavity if size and shape of cavity allow. If 8 wafers can't be accommodated, use maximum number of wafers allowed.

ADMINISTRATION

I.V.

▼ Preparing and giving parenteral form of drug may be mutagenic, teratogenic, or carcinogenic. Follow facility policy to reduce risks. Wear gloves when handling any form of drug.

▼ Prepare drug only in glass containers. Solution is unstable in plastic I.V. bags.

▼ If powder liquefies or appears oily, discard because decomposition has occurred.

▼ To reconstitute, dissolve 100 mg of drug in 3 mL of absolute alcohol provided by manufacturer.

▼ Dilute solution with 27 mL of sterile water for injection. Resulting solution contains 3.3 mg of carmustine/mL in 10% alcohol.

▼ For infusion, dilute in D_5W.

▼ Don't use polyvinyl chloride I.V. tubing. May use polyethylene I.V. tubing.

▼ Don't mix with other drugs during administration.

▼ Give at least 250 mL over 1 to 2 hours.

▼ To reduce pain on infusion, dilute further or slow infusion rate.

▼ Solution may be stored in refrigerator for 24 hours or at room temperature for 8 hours. It may decompose at temperatures above 80° F (27° C). Protect from light.

▼ **Incompatibilities:** Sodium bicarbonate.

Intracavitary

● Unopened foil pouches of wafer may be kept at room temperature for a maximum of 6 hours.

● Wafers broken in half may be used; however, discard wafers broken into more than two pieces.

ACTION

Inhibits enzymatic reactions involved with DNA synthesis, cross-links strands of cellular DNA, and interferes with RNA transcription, causing an imbalance of growth that leads to cell death. Not specific to cell cycle.

Route	Onset	Peak	Duration
I.V., intra-cavitary	Unknown	Unknown	Unknown

Half-life: 15 to 30 minutes.

ADVERSE REACTIONS

(I.V. and intracavitary wafer)
CNS: ataxia, *brain edema, seizures.*
EENT: visual disturbances.
GI: nausea, vomiting, anorexia, diarrhea, dysphagia, *GI hemorrhage.*
GU: *nephrotoxicity,* renal impairment.
Hematologic: *cumulative bone marrow suppression, leukopenia, thrombocytopenia, acute leukemia or bone marrow dysplasia,* anemia, *hemorrhage.*
Hepatic: *hepatotoxicity.*
Metabolic: hyperglycemia, *hypokalemia,* hyponatremia.
Respiratory: *pulmonary fibrosis.*
Other: intense pain at infusion site from venous spasm.

(Intracavitary wafer only)
CNS: headache, hemiplegia, confusion, aphasia, depression, somnolence, speech disorder, amnesia, *intracranial hypertension,* personality disorder, anxiety, facial paralysis, neuropathy, hypoesthesia, abnormal thinking, abnormal gait, hallucinations, insomnia, incoordination, hypokinesia, pain.
CV: deep vein thrombophlebitis, *hemorrhage,* chest pain.
GI: constipation, abdominal pain.
GU: UTI, urinary incontinence.
Musculoskeletal: back pain, myasthenia.
Respiratory: *pulmonary embolus,* dyspnea, pneumonia.
Skin: rash, facial edema, abscess.
Other: fever, allergic reaction, accidental injury, abnormal healing.

INTERACTIONS

Drug-drug. *Cimetidine:* May increase carmustine's bone marrow toxicity. Avoid using together.
Digoxin, phenytoin: May decrease levels of these drugs. Monitor patient.
Live-virus vaccines: May increase risk of infection in immunocompromised patients. Don't use together.

Reactions in bold italics are *life-threatening*. Interactions may have a *rapid onset* or a *delayed onset*.

Myelosuppressives: May increase myelosuppression. Monitor patient.

EFFECTS ON LAB TEST RESULTS
• May increase alkaline phosphatase, AST, bilirubin, hemoglobin, and urine urea levels.
• May decrease platelet and WBC counts.

CONTRAINDICATIONS & CAUTIONS
• Contraindicated in patients hypersensitive to drug.
• Drug may increase risk of secondary malignancies.

NURSING CONSIDERATIONS
Black Box Warning Carmustine for injection should be administered under the supervision of a physician experienced in the use of cancer chemotherapeutic agents. ∎
Black Box Warning Bone marrow suppression, notably thrombocytopenia and leukopenia, is the most common and severe of the toxic effects. ∎
Black Box Warning Pulmonary toxicity appears to be dose related. Patients receiving greater than 1,400 mg/m^2 cumulative dose are at higher risk. Pulmonary toxicity can occur years after treatment and can result in death, particularly in patients treated in childhood. ∎
• Obtain pulmonary function tests before and during therapy.
Black Box Warning Bone marrow suppression is delayed with carmustine. Blood counts should be monitored weekly for at least 6 weeks after a dose and drug shouldn't be given more often than every 6 weeks. ∎
• Give antiemetic before drug to reduce nausea.
• If drug touches skin, wash off thoroughly. Avoid contact with skin because drug will stain skin brown.
• Perform liver, renal, and pulmonary function tests periodically.
• Monitor CBC with differential. The ANC may be used to better calculate the patient's immunosuppressive state.
• Monitor uric acid level. To prevent hyperuricemia with resulting uric acid nephropathy, allopurinol may be used with adequate hydration.
• Therapeutic levels are commonly toxic.

• Acute leukemia or bone marrow dysplasia may occur after long-term use.
• To prevent bleeding, avoid using I.M. when platelet count is less than 50,000/mm^3.
• Anticipate blood transfusions during treatment because of cumulative anemia.
• Monitor patient for secondary malignancies.

PATIENT TEACHING
• Advise patient about common adverse reactions to drug.
• Tell patient to watch for signs and symptoms of infection (fever, sore throat, fatigue) and bleeding (easy bruising, nosebleeds, bleeding gums, tarry stools). Tell him to take temperature daily.
• Instruct patient to avoid OTC products containing aspirin and NSAIDs unless prescribed by health care provider.
• Advise women to stop breast-feeding during therapy because of possible risk of toxicity to infant.
• Caution woman of childbearing age to avoid becoming pregnant during therapy. Recommend that she consult prescriber before becoming pregnant.

carteolol hydrochloride
KAR-tee-oh-lol

Ocupress

Therapeutic class: Antiglaucoma drugs
Pharmacologic class: Nonselective beta blockers
Pregnancy risk category: C

AVAILABLE FORMS
Ophthalmic solution: 1%

INDICATIONS & DOSAGES
➤ **Chronic open-angle glaucoma, intraocular hypertension**
Adults: One drop into conjunctival sac of each affected eye b.i.d.

ADMINISTRATION
Ophthalmic
• Don't touch tip of dropper to eye or surrounding tissue.

• Apply light finger pressure on lacrimal sac for 1 minute after instilling to minimize systemic absorption.
• If more than one ophthalmic drug is being used, give at least 5 minutes apart.

ACTION
Exact mechanism unknown. Reduces intraocular pressure by decreasing aqueous humor production.

Route	Onset	Peak	Duration
Ophthalmic	Unknown	2 hr	12 hr

Half-life: Unknown.

ADVERSE REACTIONS
CNS: asthenia, dizziness, headache, insomnia.
CV: *arrhythmias, bradycardia,* hypotension, palpitations.
EENT: burning, conjunctival hyperemia, edema, ocular tearing, transient eye irritation, abnormal corneal staining, blepharoconjunctivitis, blurred and cloudy vision, corneal sensitivity, decreased night vision, photophobia, ptosis, sinusitis.
GI: constipation, diarrhea, nausea, taste perversion, vomiting.
Respiratory: *bronchospasm,* dyspnea.

INTERACTIONS
Drug-drug. *Catecholamine-depleting drugs such as reserpine, oral beta blockers:* May cause additive effects and development of hypotension or bradycardia. Monitor patient closely; monitor vital signs.
Insulin: May mask symptoms of hypoglycemia as a result of beta blockade (such as tachycardia). Use together cautiously in patients with diabetes.
Drug-lifestyle. *Sun exposure:* May cause photophobia. Advise patient to wear sunglasses.

EFFECTS ON LAB TEST RESULTS
None reported.

CONTRAINDICATIONS & CAUTIONS
• Contraindicated in patients hypersensitive to drug or its components and in those with bronchial asthma, severe COPD, sinus bradycardia, second- or third-degree AV

block, overt cardiac failure, or cardiogenic shock.
• Use cautiously in patients hypersensitive to other beta blockers; in those with non-allergic bronchospastic disease, diabetes mellitus, hyperthyroidism, or decreased pulmonary function; and in breast-feeding women.
⚠ *Overdose S&S:* Bradycardia, bronchospasm, heart failure, hypotension.

NURSING CONSIDERATIONS
• Monitor vital signs.
⚠ *Alert:* Stop drug at first sign of cardiac failure, and notify prescriber.

PATIENT TEACHING
• If patient is using more than one topical ophthalmic drug, tell him to apply them at least 5 minutes apart.
• Teach patient how to instill drops. Advise him to wash hands before and after instillation, and warn him not to touch tip of dropper to eye or surrounding tissue.
• Advise patient to apply light finger pressure on lacrimal sac for 1 minute after drug instillation to minimize systemic absorption.
• Tell patient to remove contact lenses before instilling drug.
• Instruct patient to keep bottle tightly closed when not in use and to protect it from light.
• Tell patient that drug is a beta blocker and, although given topically, may be absorbed systemically, causing adverse effects. Advise patient to monitor heart rate and blood pressure closely, to report slow heart rate to prescriber and, if signs or symptoms of serious adverse reactions or hypersensitivity occur, to stop drug and notify prescriber immediately.
• Stress importance of compliance with recommended therapy.
• Advise patient to ease sun sensitivity by wearing sunglasses.

carvedilol
kar-VAH-da-lol

Coreg

carvedilol phosphate
Coreg CR

Therapeutic class: Antihypertensives
Pharmacologic class: Alpha-nonselective beta blockers
Pregnancy risk category: C

AVAILABLE FORMS
Capsules (extended-release): 10 mg, 20 mg, 40 mg, 80 mg
Tablets: 3.125 mg, 6.25 mg, 12.5 mg, 25 mg

INDICATIONS & DOSAGES
Adjust-a-dose (for all indications): In patient with pulse rate below 55 beats/minute, reduce dosage.

➤ **Hypertension**
Adults: Dosage highly individualized. For immediate-release tablets, initially, 6.25 mg P.O. b.i.d. Measure standing blood pressure 1 hour after first dose. If tolerated, continue dosage for 7 to 14 days. May increase to 12.5 mg P.O. b.i.d. for 7 to 14 days, following same blood pressure monitoring protocol as before. Maximum dose is 25 mg P.O. b.i.d. as tolerated. May be switched to extended-release capsule after controlled on immediate-release tablets. Or, for extended-release capsule, initially 20 mg P.O. once daily. Measure standing blood pressure 1 hour after dose. May increase every 7 to 14 days to maximum of 80 mg P.O. once daily.

➤ **Left ventricular dysfunction after MI**
Adults: Dosage individualized. Start therapy after patient is hemodynamically stable and fluid retention has been minimized. For immediate-release tablets, initially, 6.25 mg P.O. b.i.d. Increase after 3 to 10 days to 12.5 mg b.i.d., then again to a target dose of 25 mg b.i.d. Or start with 3.25 mg b.i.d., or adjust dosage more slowly if indicated. May be switched to extended-release capsule after controlled on immediate-release tablets. Or, 10 to 20 mg extended-release capsules P.O. once daily. May increase after 3 to 10 days to 40 mg P.O. once daily, then again to target dose of 80 mg P.O. once daily.

➤ **Mild to severe heart failure**
Adults: Dosage highly individualized. For immediate-release tablets, initially, 3.125 mg P.O. b.i.d. for 2 weeks; if tolerated, may increase to 6.25 mg P.O. b.i.d. Dosage may be doubled every 2 weeks, as tolerated. Maximum dose for patients who weigh less than 85 kg (187 lb) is 25 mg P.O. b.i.d.; for those weighing more than 85 kg, dose is 50 mg P.O. b.i.d. May be switched to extended-release capsule after controlled on immediate-release tablets. Or, 10-mg extended-release capsule P.O. once daily for 2 weeks. May increase to 20, 40, and 80 mg over successive intervals of at least 2 weeks.

➤ **Chronic, stable angina ◆**
Adults: 12.5 to 50 mg P.O. b.i.d. for 2 to 12 weeks. May be switched to extended-release capsule after controlled on immediate-release tablets.

➤ **Idiopathic cardiomyopathy ◆**
Adults: Initially, 2.5 mg P.O. once daily. May increase dosage as tolerated up to 75 mg/day.

ADMINISTRATION
P.O.
● Give drug with food.
● Capsules may be opened, mixed in cool applesauce, and taken immediately; don't store.
● Give capsules in the morning.
● Extended-release equivalent of 3.125 mg immediate-release b.i.d. is 10 mg, 6.25 mg immediate-release b.i.d. is 20 mg, 12.5 mg immediate-release b.i.d. is 40 mg, and 25 mg immediate-release b.i.d. is 80 mg. Dosage may be further titrated based on clinical response.
● Administer extended-release form and drugs that contain alcohol 2 hours apart.

ACTION
Nonselective beta blocker with alpha-blocking activity.

Route	Onset	Peak	Duration
P.O.	Rapid	1–2 hr	7–10 hr
P.O. (extended-release)	30 min	5 hr	Unknown

Half-life: Immediate-release: 7 to 10 hours; extended-release: unknown.

ADVERSE REACTIONS

CNS: asthenia, dizziness, fatigue, *stroke,* pain, headache, malaise, fever, hypesthesia, vertigo, somnolence, depression, insomnia, syncope, paresthesia.

CV: hypotension, orthostatic hypotension, *AV block, bradycardia,* edema, syncope, angina pectoris, peripheral edema, hypovolemia, fluid overload, hypertension, palpitations, chest pain.

EENT: abnormal vision, blurred vision.

GI: diarrhea, vomiting, nausea, melena, periodontitis, abdominal pain, dyspepsia.

GU: erectile dysfunction, abnormal renal function, albuminuria, hematuria, UTI.

Hematologic: *thrombocytopenia,* purpura.

Metabolic: hyperglycemia, weight gain, *hyperkalemia, hypoglycemia,* weight loss, hypercholesterolemia, hyperuricemia, hyponatremia, glycosuria, diabetes mellitus, gout.

Musculoskeletal: arthralgia, muscle cramps.

Respiratory: *lung edema,* cough, rales.

Other: hypersensitivity reactions.

INTERACTIONS

Drug-drug. *Amiodarone:* May increase risk of bradycardia, AV block, and myocardial depression. Monitor patient's ECG and vital signs.

Catecholamine-depleting drugs such as MAO inhibitors, reserpine: May cause bradycardia or severe hypotension. Monitor patient closely.

Cimetidine: May increase bioavailability of carvedilol. Monitor vital signs closely.

Clonidine: May increase blood pressure- and heart rate-lowering effects. Monitor vital signs closely.

Cyclosporine: May increase cyclosporine level. Monitor cyclosporine level.

CYP4502D6 inhibitors, such as fluoxetine, paroxetine, propafenone, quinidine: May increase level of carvedilol. Monitor patient for hypotension and dizziness.

Digoxin: May increase digoxin level by about 15% when given together. Monitor digoxin level.

Diltiazem, verapamil: May cause isolated conduction disturbances. Monitor patient's heart rhythm and blood pressure.

Insulin, oral antidiabetics: May enhance hypoglycemic properties. Monitor glucose level.

NSAIDs, salicylates: May decrease antihypertensive effects. Monitor blood pressure.

Rifampin: May reduce carvedilol level by 70%. Monitor vital signs closely.

Drug-herb. *Ma huang:* May decrease antihypertensive effects. Discourage use together.

EFFECTS ON LAB TEST RESULTS

● May increase alkaline phosphatase, ALT, AST, BUN, cholesterol, creatinine, GGT, nonprotein nitrogen, potassium, triglyceride, sodium, and uric acid levels. May increase or decrease glucose level.

● May decrease PT and platelet count.

CONTRAINDICATIONS & CAUTIONS

● Contraindicated in patients hypersensitive to drug and in those with New York Heart Association class IV decompensated cardiac failure requiring I.V. inotropic therapy.

● Contraindicated in those with bronchial asthma or related bronchospastic conditions, second- or third-degree AV block, sick sinus syndrome (unless a permanent pacemaker is in place), cardiogenic shock, severe bradycardia, or symptomatic hepatic impairment.

● Use cautiously in hypertensive patients with left-sided heart failure, perioperative patients who receive anesthetics that depress myocardial function (such as cyclopropane and trichloroethylene), and diabetic patients receiving insulin or oral antidiabetics, and in those subject to spontaneous hypoglycemia.

● Use cautiously in patients with thyroid disease (may mask hyperthyroidism; withdrawal may precipitate thyroid storm or exacerbation of hyperthyroidism), pheochromocytoma, Prinzmetal or variant angina, bronchospastic disease (in those who can't tolerate other antihypertensives), or peripheral vascular disease (may precipitate or aggravate symptoms of arterial insufficiency).

● Use cautiously in breast-feeding women.

● Safety and effectiveness in children younger than age 18 haven't been established.

Reactions in bold italics are *life-threatening*. Interactions may have a *rapid onset* or a *delayed onset*.

⚠ *Overdose S&S:* Hypotension, bradycardia, cardiac insufficiency, cardiogenic shock, cardiac arrest, respiratory problems, bronchospasm, vomiting, lapses of consciousness, generalized seizures.

NURSING CONSIDERATIONS

🕀 *Alert:* Patients who have a history of severe anaphylactic reaction to several allergens may be more reactive to repeated challenge (accidental, diagnostic, or therapeutic). They may be unresponsive to dosages of epinephrine typically used to treat allergic reactions.

• Mild hepatocellular injury may occur during therapy. At first sign of hepatic dysfunction, perform tests for hepatic injury or jaundice; if present, stop drug.

• If drug must be stopped, do so gradually over 1 to 2 weeks, if possible.

• Monitor patient with heart failure for worsened condition, renal dysfunction, or fluid retention; diuretics may need to be increased.

• Monitor diabetic patient closely; drug may mask signs of hypoglycemia, or hyperglycemia may be worsened.

• Observe patient for dizziness or lightheadedness for 1 hour after giving each new dose.

• Monitor elderly patients carefully; drug levels are about 50% higher in elderly patients than in younger patients.

• *Look alike–sound alike:* Don't confuse carvedilol with carteolol or captopril.

PATIENT TEACHING

• Tell patient not to interrupt or stop drug without medical approval.

• Inform patient that improvement of heart failure symptoms might take several weeks of drug therapy.

• Advise patient with heart failure to call prescriber if weight gain or shortness of breath occurs.

• Inform patient that he may experience low blood pressure when standing. If dizziness or fainting occurs (rare), advise him to sit or lie down and to notify prescriber if symptoms persist.

• Caution patient against performing hazardous tasks during start of therapy.

• Advise diabetic patient to promptly report changes in glucose level.

• Inform patient who wears contact lenses that his eyes may feel dry.

• Tell patient to take drug with food. Extended-release capsule may be opened and contents mixed with cool applesauce and taken immediately; don't store.

• Advise patient that capsules shouldn't be crushed, chewed, or contents divided.

caspofungin acetate
KAS-po-fun-gin

Cancidas

Therapeutic class: Antifungals
Pharmacologic class: Echinocandins
Pregnancy risk category: C

AVAILABLE FORMS
Lyophilized powder for injection: 50-mg, 70-mg single-use vials

INDICATIONS & DOSAGES
Adjust-a-dose (for all indications): For adults receiving rifampin, give 70 mg I.V. daily. Adults receiving nevirapine, efavirenz, carbamazepine, dexamethasone, or phenytoin may also require 70 mg I.V. once daily. For patients with Child-Pugh score of 7 to 9, after initial 70-mg loading dose (when indicated), give 35 mg/day. Dosage adjustment in patients with Child-Pugh score of more than 9 is unknown.

➤ **Invasive aspergillosis in patients who are refractory to or intolerant of other therapies (amphotericin B, lipid forms of amphotericin B, or itraconazole); candidemia and *Candida*-caused intra-abdominal abscesses, peritonitis, and pleural space infections**

Adults: Single 70-mg I.V. loading dose on day 1, followed by 50 mg/day I.V. over about 1 hour. Base treatment duration on severity of patient's underlying disease, recovery from immunosuppression, and clinical response.

Children age 3 months to 17 years: Single 70-mg/m² I.V. loading dose on day 1, followed by 50 mg/m² daily thereafter. May increase daily maintenance dose to

70 mg/m^2. Maximum loading dose and daily maintenance dose shouldn't exceed 70 mg.

➤ **Empirical treatment of presumed fungal infections in febrile, neutropenic patients**

Adults: Single 70-mg I.V. loading dose on day 1, followed by 50 mg/day I.V. over 1 hour thereafter. Continue empirical therapy until neutropenia resolves. If fungal infection is confirmed, treat for a minimum of 14 days and continue therapy for at least 7 days after neutropenia and symptoms resolve. May increase daily dose to 70 mg if the 50-mg dose is well tolerated but clinical response is suboptimal.

Children age 3 months to 17 years: Single 70-mg/m^2 I.V. loading dose on day 1, followed by 50 mg/m^2 daily thereafter. May increase daily maintenance dose to 70 mg/m^2. Maximum loading dose and daily maintenance dose shouldn't exceed 70 mg.

➤ **Esophageal candidiasis**

Adults: 50 mg I.V. daily over 1 hour for 7 to 14 days after symptoms resolve.

Children age 3 months to 17 years: Single 70-mg/m^2 I.V. loading dose on day 1, followed by 50 mg/m^2 daily thereafter. May increase daily maintenance dose to 70 mg/m^2. Maximum loading dose and daily maintenance dose shouldn't exceed 70 mg.

ADMINISTRATION

I.V.

▼ Let refrigerated vial warm to room temperature.

▼ For patients on fluid restriction, dilute the 35-mg and 50-mg doses in 100 mL normal saline solution. For other patients, dilute 35-mg, 50-mg, and 70-mg doses in 250 mL normal saline solution.

▼ Give drug by slow infusion over about 1 hour.

▼ Monitor site carefully for phlebitis.

▼ Use reconstituted vials within 1 hour or discard.

▼ The final product for infusion (solution in I.V. bag or bottle) can be stored at room temperature for 24 hours or at 36° to 46° F (2° to 8° C) for 48 hours.

▼ **Incompatibilities:** Don't mix or infuse with other drugs or dextrose solutions.

ACTION

Inhibits synthesis of 1,3-β-D-glucan, an essential component of the cell wall, in susceptible *Aspergillus* and *Candida* species. Drug is extensively distributed and has a prolonged half-life.

Route	Onset	Peak	Duration
I.V.	Unknown	Unknown	Unknown

Half-life: 9 to 11 hours.

ADVERSE REACTIONS

CNS: paresthesia, fever, headache.

CV: tachycardia, phlebitis, infused vein complications, hypotension.

GI: anorexia, nausea, vomiting, diarrhea, abdominal pain.

GU: proteinuria, hematuria.

Hematologic: anemia, eosinophilia.

Metabolic: hypokalemia.

Musculoskeletal: pain, myalgia.

Respiratory: dyspnea, crackles, cough, pneumonia, tachypnea.

Skin: histamine-mediated symptoms, including rash, facial swelling, pruritus, sensation of warmth.

Other: chills, sweating, mucosal inflammation.

INTERACTIONS

Drug-drug. *Cyclosporine:* May increase caspofungin level. May increase risk of elevated ALT level; avoid using together unless benefit outweighs risk.

Inducers of drug clearance or mixed inducer-inhibitors (carbamazepine, dexamethasone, efavirenz, nelfinavir, nevirapine, phenytoin, rifampin): May reduce caspofungin level. May need to adjust dosage upwards to 70 mg in patients who are clinically unresponsive.

Tacrolimus: May reduce tacrolimus level. Monitor tacrolimus level; expect to adjust dosage.

EFFECTS ON LAB TEST RESULTS

● May increase glucose, alkaline phosphatase, and liver enzyme levels. May decrease albumin, calcium, hemoglobin, potassium, magnesium, and protein levels.

● May increase eosinophil count.

Reactions in bold italics are *life-threatening*. Interactions may have a *rapid onset* or a *delayed onset*.

CONTRAINDICATIONS & CAUTIONS
• Contraindicated in patients hypersensitive to drug or its components.
• Safety and effectiveness in neonates and infants younger than 3 months aren't known.
• It's unknown if drug appears in breast milk. Use cautiously in breast-feeding women.

NURSING CONSIDERATIONS
• Safety information is limited, but drug is well tolerated for therapy lasting longer than 2 weeks.
• Observe patients for histamine-mediated reactions, including rash, facial swelling, pruritus, and a sensation of warmth.

PATIENT TEACHING
• Instruct patient to report signs and symptoms of phlebitis.
• Instruct patient to immediately report any signs of a hypersensitivity reaction.

cefadroxil
sef-a-DROX-ill

Therapeutic class: Antibiotics
Pharmacologic class: First-generation cephalosporins
Pregnancy risk category: B

AVAILABLE FORMS
Capsules: 500 mg
Oral suspension: 250 mg/5 mL, 500 mg/5 mL
Tablets: 1 g

INDICATIONS & DOSAGES
➤ **UTIs caused by** *Escherichia coli,* **Proteus mirabilis, and** *Klebsiella* **species; skin and soft-tissue infections caused by staphylococci and streptococci; pharyngitis or tonsillitis caused by group A beta-hemolytic streptococci**
Adults: 1 to 2 g P.O. daily, depending on infection being treated. Usually given once daily or in two divided doses.
Children: 30 mg/kg P.O. daily in two divided doses every 12 hours.
Adjust-a-dose: In patients with renal impairment, give first dose of 1 g. Reduce additional doses based on CrCl. If clearance is 25 to 50 mL/minute, give 500 mg

P.O. every 12 hours. If CrCl is 10 to 25 mL/minute, give 500 mg P.O. every 24 hours; if CrCl is less than 10 mL/minute, give 500 mg P.O. every 36 hours.

ADMINISTRATION
P.O.
• Before administration, ask patient if he's allergic to penicillins or cephalosporins.
• Obtain specimen for culture and sensitivity tests before giving first dose. Begin therapy while awaiting results.
• Give drug with food or milk to lessen GI discomfort.

ACTION
Inhibits cell-wall synthesis, promoting osmotic instability; usually bactericidal.

Route	Onset	Peak	Duration
P.O.	Unknown	1–2 hr	Unknown

Half-life: About 1 to 2 hours.

ADVERSE REACTIONS
CNS: *seizures,* fever.
GI: *pseudomembranous colitis,* glossitis, abdominal cramps.
GU: genital pruritus, candidiasis, vaginitis, renal dysfunction.
Hematologic: *transient neutropenia, leukopenia, agranulocytosis, thrombocytopenia,* anemia, eosinophilia
Skin: maculopapular and erythematous rashes, urticaria.
Other: *anaphylaxis, angioedema,* hypersensitivity reactions.

INTERACTIONS
Drug-drug. *Aminoglycosides:* May increase risk of nephrotoxicity. Avoid using together.
Live-virus vaccines: May decrease vaccine effectiveness. Don't give together.
Probenecid: May inhibit excretion and increase cefadroxil level. Use together cautiously.

EFFECTS ON LAB TEST RESULTS
• May increase alkaline phosphatase, ALT, AST, bilirubin, GGT, and LDH levels. May decrease hemoglobin level.
• May increase eosinophil count. May decrease granulocyte, neutrophil, platelet, and WBC counts.

• May falsely increase serum or urine creatinine level in tests using Jaffe reaction. May cause false-positive results of Coombs test and urine glucose tests that use cupric sulfate, such as Benedict reagent and Clinitest.

CONTRAINDICATIONS & CAUTIONS
• Contraindicated in patients hypersensitive to drug or other cephalosporins.
• Use cautiously in patients with a history of sensitivity to penicillin or GI diseases (colitis) and in breast-feeding women.
• Use cautiously in patients with impaired renal function; adjust dosage as needed.
۞ Alert: Seizures have occurred, particularly in patients with renal impairment when the dosage wasn't reduced. If seizures occur, discontinue drug and treat if clinically indicated.
۞ Alert: Drug can cause pseudomembranous colitis ranging from mild to life-threatening. Monitor patient for diarrhea and treat appropriately.

NURSING CONSIDERATIONS
• If CrCl is less than 50 mL/minute, lengthen dosage interval so drug doesn't accumulate. Monitor renal function in patients with renal dysfunction.
• If large doses are given, therapy is prolonged, or patient is high risk, monitor patient for superinfection.
• **Look alike–sound alike:** Don't confuse drug with other cephalosporins that sound alike.

PATIENT TEACHING
• Instruct patient to take drug with food or milk to lessen GI discomfort.
• Tell patient to take entire amount of drug exactly as prescribed, even after he feels better.
• Advise patient to notify prescriber if rash develops or if signs and symptoms of superinfection appear, such as recurring fever, chills, and malaise.

cefazolin sodium
sef-AH-zoe-lin

Ancef, Kefzol

Therapeutic class: Antibiotics
Pharmacologic class: First-generation cephalosporins
Pregnancy risk category: B

AVAILABLE FORMS
Infusion: 1 g/50-mL bag, 2 g/50-mL bag
Injection (parenteral): 500 mg, 1 g, 2 g, 10 g, 20 g

INDICATIONS & DOSAGES
Adjust-a-dose (for all indications): For adults with CrCl of 35 to 54 mL/minute, give full dose every 8 hours; if CrCl is 11 to 34 mL/minute, give 50% of usual dose every 12 hours; if CrCl is below 10 mL/minute, give 50% of usual dose every 18 to 24 hours.
➤ **Perioperative prevention in contaminated surgery**
Adults: 1 g I.M. or I.V. 30 to 60 minutes before surgery; then 0.5 to 1 g I.M. or I.V. every 6 to 8 hours for 24 hours. In operations lasting longer than 2 hours, give another 0.5- to 1-g dose I.M. or I.V. intraoperatively. Continue treatment for 3 to 5 days if life-threatening infection is likely.
➤ **Infections of respiratory, biliary, and GU tracts; skin, soft-tissue, bone, and joint infections; septicemia; endocarditis caused by *Escherichia coli, Enterobacteriaceae*, gonococci, *Haemophilus influenzae, Klebsiella* species, *Proteus mirabilis, Staphylococcus aureus, Streptococcus pneumoniae*, and group A beta-hemolytic streptococci**
Adults: 250 to 500 mg I.M. or I.V. every 8 hours for mild infections or 500 mg to 1.5 g I.M. or I.V. every 6 to 8 hours for moderate to severe or life-threatening infections. Maximum 12 g/day in life-threatening situations.
Children older than age 1 month: 25 to 50 mg/kg/day I.M. or I.V. in three or four divided doses. In severe infections, dose may be increased to 100 mg/kg/day.

Reactions in bold italics are *life-threatening*. Interactions may have a *rapid onset* or a *delayed onset*.

Adjust-a-dose: For children with CrCl of 40 to 70 mL/minute, give 60% of normal daily dose divided every 12 hours; if CrCl is 20 to 40 mL/minute, give 25% of usual daily dose divided every 12 hours; if CrCl is 5 to 20 mL/minute, give 10% of usual dose every 24 hours.

➤ **Catheter-related bloodstream infections caused by methicillin-susceptible *S. aureus* or methicillin-susceptible, coagulase-negative *Staphylococcus* species ◆**

Adults: 2 g I.V. every 8 hours.

Adjust-a-dose: For dialysis patients, give 20 mg/kg (actual body weight), rounded to the nearest 500-mg increment, after dialysis.

ADMINISTRATION

I.V.

▼ Before giving first dose, obtain specimen for culture and sensitivity tests. Begin therapy while awaiting results.

▼ Before giving drug, ask patient if he's allergic to penicillins or cephalosporins.

▼ Give commercially available frozen solutions in D_5W only by intermittent or continuous I.V. infusion.

▼ Reconstitute drug with sterile water, bacteriostatic water, or normal saline solution as follows: Add 2 mL to 500-mg vial or 2.5 mL to 1-g vial, yielding 225 mg/mL or 330 mg/mL, respectively.

▼ Shake well until dissolved.

▼ For direct injection, further dilute with 5 mL of sterile water for injection.

▼ Inject into a large vein or into the tubing of a free-flowing I.V. solution over 3 to 5 minutes.

▼ For intermittent infusion, add reconstituted drug to 50 to 100 mL of compatible solution or use premixed solution.

▼ If I.V. therapy lasts longer than 3 days, alternate injection sites. Use of small I.V. needles in larger available veins may be preferable.

▼ Reconstituted drug is stable 24 hours at room temperature or 10 days refrigerated.

▼ **Incompatibilities:** Aminoglycosides, amiodarone, amobarbital, ascorbic acid injection, bleomycin, calcium gluconate, cimetidine, colistimethate, hydrocortisone, idarubicin, lidocaine, norepinephrine,

oxytetracycline, pentobarbital sodium, polymyxin B, ranitidine, tetracycline, theophylline, vitamin B complex with C.

I.M.

● Before giving first dose, obtain specimen for culture and sensitivity tests. Begin therapy while awaiting results.

● After reconstitution, inject drug I.M. without further dilution. This drug isn't as painful as other cephalosporins. Give injection deep into a large muscle.

ACTION

Inhibits cell-wall synthesis, promoting osmotic instability; usually bactericidal.

Route	Onset	Peak	Duration
I.V.	Immediate	Immediate	Unknown
I.M.	Unknown	1–2 hr	Unknown

Half-life: About 1 to 2 hours.

ADVERSE REACTIONS

CV: phlebitis, thrombophlebitis with I.V. injection.

GI: diarrhea, *pseudomembranous colitis,* anorexia, glossitis, dyspepsia, abdominal cramps, anal pruritus, oral candidiasis.

GU: genital pruritus, candidiasis, vaginitis.

Hematologic: *neutropenia, leukopenia, thrombocytopenia,* eosinophilia.

Skin: maculopapular and erythematous rashes, urticaria, pruritus, pain, induration, sterile abscesses, tissue sloughing at injection site, *Stevens-Johnson syndrome.*

Other: *anaphylaxis,* hypersensitivity reactions, drug fever.

INTERACTIONS

Drug-drug. *Aminoglycosides:* May increase risk of nephrotoxicity. Avoid using together.

Anticoagulants: May increase anticoagulant effects. Monitor PT and INR.

Live-virus vaccines: May decrease effectiveness of live-virus vaccines. Concurrent use isn't recommended.

Probenecid: May inhibit excretion and increase cefazolin level. Use together cautiously.

EFFECTS ON LAB TEST RESULTS

● May increase alkaline phosphatase, ALT, AST, bilirubin, GGT, and LDH levels.

• May increase eosinophil count. May decrease neutrophil, platelet, and WBC counts.

• May falsely increase serum or urine creatinine level in tests using Jaffe reaction. May cause false-positive results of Coombs test and urine glucose tests that use cupric sulfate, such as Benedict reagent and Clinitest.

CONTRAINDICATIONS & CAUTIONS

• Contraindicated in patients hypersensitive to drug or other cephalosporins.

• Use cautiously in patients hypersensitive to penicillin because of the possibility of cross-sensitivity with other beta-lactam antibiotics.

• Use cautiously in breast-feeding women and in patients with a history of colitis or renal insufficiency.

⚠ *Overdose S&S:* Pain, inflammation, and phlebitis at injection site; dizziness, paresthesia, headache, seizures; elevated creatinine, BUN, liver enzymes, and bilirubin levels; positive Coombs test; thrombocytosis, thrombocytopenia, eosinophilia, leukopenia; prolonged PT.

NURSING CONSIDERATIONS

• If CrCl falls below 55 mL/minute, adjust dosage.

• If large doses are given, therapy is prolonged, or patient is at high risk, monitor patient for signs and symptoms of superinfection.

• *Look alike–sound alike:* Don't confuse drug with other cephalosporins that sound alike.

PATIENT TEACHING

• Instruct patient to report adverse reactions promptly.

• Tell patient to report discomfort at I.V. injection site.

• Advise patient to notify prescriber if a rash develops or if signs and symptoms of superinfection, such as recurring fever, chills, and malaise, appear.

cefdinir
sef-DIN-er

Therapeutic class: Antibiotics
Pharmacologic class: Third-generation cephalosporins
Pregnancy risk category: B

AVAILABLE FORMS
Capsules: 300 mg
Suspension: 125 mg/5 mL, 250 mg/5 mL

INDICATIONS & DOSAGES
Adjust-a-dose (for all indications): If CrCl is less than 30 mL/minute, reduce dosage to 300 mg P.O. once daily for adults and 7 mg/kg (up to 300 mg) P.O. once daily for children. In patients receiving long-term hemodialysis, give 300 mg or 7 mg/kg P.O. at end of each dialysis session and then every other day.

➤ **Mild to moderate infections caused by susceptible strains of microorganisms in community-acquired pneumonia, acute worsening of chronic bronchitis, acute maxillary sinusitis, acute bacterial otitis media, and uncomplicated skin and skin-structure infections**
Adults and children age 13 and older: 300 mg P.O. every 12 hours or 600 mg P.O. every 24 hours for 10 days. Give every 12 hours for pneumonia and skin infections.
Children ages 6 months to 12 years: 7 mg/kg P.O. every 12 hours or 14 mg/kg P.O. every 24 hours for 10 days, up to maximum dose of 600 mg daily. Give every 12 hours for skin infections.

➤ **Pharyngitis, tonsillitis**
Adults and children age 13 and older: 300 mg P.O. every 12 hours for 5 to 10 days or 600 mg P.O. every 24 hours for 10 days.
Children ages 6 months to 12 years: 7 mg/ kg P.O. every 12 hours for 5 to 10 days; or 14 mg/kg P.O. every 24 hours for 10 days.

ADMINISTRATION
P.O.
• Before administration, ask patient if he's allergic to penicillins or cephalosporins.
• Give antacids and iron supplements 2 hours before or after a dose of cefdinir.
• Give drug without regard for meals.

Reactions in bold italics are *life-threatening*. Interactions may have a *rapid onset* or a *delayed onset*.

ACTION

Inhibits cell-wall synthesis, promoting osmotic instability; usually bactericidal. Some microorganisms resistant to penicillins and cephalosporins are susceptible to cefdinir. Active against a broad range of gram-positive and gram-negative aerobic microorganisms.

Route	Onset	Peak	Duration
P.O.	Unknown	2–4 hr	Unknown

Half-life: 1¾ hours.

ADVERSE REACTIONS

CNS: headache.
GI: diarrhea, *pseudomembranous colitis,* abdominal pain, nausea.
GU: vaginitis, increased urine proteins.
Hematologic: increased WBC and RBC counts.
Other: hypersensitivity reactions, *anaphylaxis.*

INTERACTIONS

Drug-drug. *Aminoglycosides:* May increase risk of nephrotoxicity. Avoid using together.
Antacids containing aluminum and magnesium, iron supplements, multivitamins containing iron: May decrease rate of absorption and bioavailability of cefdinir. Give such preparations 2 hours before or after cefdinir.
Live-virus vaccines: May decrease effectiveness of live-virus vaccines. Concurrent use isn't recommended.
Probenecid: May inhibit renal excretion of cefdinir. Monitor patient for adverse reactions.

EFFECTS ON LAB TEST RESULTS

● May increase alkaline phosphatase, GGT, and LDH levels. May decrease bicarbonate levels.
● May increase WBC, RBC, eosinophil, lymphocyte, and platelet counts.
● May falsely increase serum or urine creatinine level in tests using Jaffe reaction. May cause false-positive results of Coombs test and urine glucose tests that use cupric sulfate, such as Benedict reagent and Clinitest.

CONTRAINDICATIONS & CAUTIONS

● Contraindicated in patients hypersensitive to drug or other cephalosporins.
● Use cautiously in patients hypersensitive to penicillin because of the possibility of cross-sensitivity with other beta-lactam antibiotics.
● Use cautiously in patients with history of colitis or renal insufficiency.

NURSING CONSIDERATIONS

● Prolonged drug treatment may result in emergence and overgrowth of resistant organisms. Monitor patient for signs and symptoms of superinfection.
● Pseudomembranous colitis has been reported with cefdinir and should be considered in patients with diarrhea after antibiotic therapy and in those with history of colitis.
● *Look alike–sound alike:* Don't confuse drug with other cephalosporins that sound alike.

PATIENT TEACHING

● Instruct patient to take antacids and iron supplements 2 hours before or after a dose of cefdinir.
● Inform diabetic patient that each teaspoon of suspension contains 2.86 g of sucrose.
● Tell patient that drug may be taken without regard to meals.
● Tell patient to take drug as prescribed, even after he feels better.
● Advise patient to report severe diarrhea or diarrhea with abdominal pain.
● Tell patient to report adverse reactions or signs and symptoms of superinfection promptly.

cefepime hydrochloride
SEF-ah-peem

Maxipime

Therapeutic class: Antibiotics
Pharmacologic class: Fourth-generation cephalosporins
Pregnancy risk category: B

AVAILABLE FORMS

Injection: 500-mg vial, 1-g/100-mL piggyback bottle, 1-g ADD-Vantage vial,

1-g vial, 2-g/100-mL piggyback bottle, 2-g ADD-Vantage vial, 2-g vial

INDICATIONS & DOSAGES
Adjust-a-dose (for all indications): Adjust adult dosage based on CrCl, as shown in the table. For patients receiving hemodialysis, about 68% of drug is removed after a 3-hour dialysis session. Cefepime dosage for patients receiving hemodialysis is 1 g on day 1, followed by 500 mg every 24 hours for treatment of all infections except febrile neutropenia. For patients with febrile neutropenia, give 1 g every 24 hours. Give cefepime after hemodialysis and at the same time each day. For patients receiving continuous ambulatory peritoneal dialysis, give normal dose every 48 hours. Because pediatric and adult cefepime pharmacokinetics are similar, change the pediatric dosing regimen proportional to the adult regimen.

➤ **Mild to moderate UTI caused by** *Escherichia coli, Klebsiella pneumoniae,* **or** *Proteus mirabilis,* **including concurrent bacteremia with these microorganisms**
Adults and children age 16 and older: 0.5 to 1 g I.M. or I.V. over 30 minutes every 12 hours for 7 to 10 days. Use I.M. only for *E. coli* infection when I.M. route is considered more appropriate route of administration.

➤ **Severe UTI, including pyelonephritis, caused by** *E. coli* **or** *K. pneumoniae*
Adults and children age 16 and older: 2 g I.V. over 30 minutes every 12 hours for 10 days.

➤ **Moderate to severe pneumonia caused by** *Streptococcus pneumoniae, Pseudomonas aeruginosa, K. pneumoniae,* **or** *Enterobacter* **species**
Adults and children age 16 and older: 1 to 2 g I.V. over 30 minutes every 12 hours for 10 days.

➤ **Moderate to severe skin infection, uncomplicated skin infection, and skin-structure infection caused by** *Streptococcus pyogenes* **or methicillin-susceptible strains of** *Staphylococcus aureus*
Adults and children age 16 and older: 2 g I.V. over 30 minutes every 12 hours for 10 days.

➤ **Complicated intra-abdominal infection caused by** *E. coli,* **viridans group streptococci,** *P. aeruginosa, K. pneumoniae, Enterobacter* **species, or** *Bacteroides fragilis*
Adults and children age 16 and older: 2 g I.V. over 30 minutes every 12 hours for 7 to 10 days. Give with metronidazole.

➤ **Empirical therapy for febrile neutropenia**
Adults and children age 16 and older: 2 g I.V. every 8 hours for 7 days or until neutropenia resolves.

➤ **Uncomplicated and complicated UTI (including pyelonephritis), uncomplicated skin and skin-structure infection, pneumonia, empirical therapy for febrile neutropenic children**
Children ages 2 months to 16 years weighing up to 40 kg (88 lb): 50 mg/kg/dose I.V. over 30 minutes every 12 hours for 10 days. For febrile neutropenia, give 50 mg/kg every 8 hours for 7 days or until neutropenia resolves. For UTI, treat for 7 to 10 days. Don't exceed 2 g/dose.

➤ **Catheter-related bloodstream infections ◆**
Adults: 2 g I.V. every 8 hours for 7 to 10 days. *Infants age 2 weeks and older and children weighing up to 40 kg (88 lb):* 50 mg/kg I.V. every 12 hours for 7 to 10 days. Maximum dose is 2 g.
Infants age 2 weeks and younger: 30 mg/kg I.V. every 12 hours for 7 to 10 days.

Adult dosage adjustments for renal impairment (cefepime hydrochloride)				
	If normal dosage would be			
CrCl (mL/min)	500 mg every 12 hr	1 g every 12 hr	2 g every 12 hr	2 g every 8 hr
30–60	500 mg every 24 hr	1 g every 24 hr	2 g every 24 hr	2 g every 12 hr
11–29	500 mg every 24 hr	500 mg every 24 hr	1 g every 24 hr	2 g every 24 hr
<11	250 mg every 24 hr	250 mg every 24 hr	500 mg every 24 hr	1 g every 24 hr

Reactions in bold italics are *life-threatening*. Interactions may have a *rapid onset* or a *delayed onset*.

ADMINISTRATION

I.V.

▼ Before giving drug, ask patient if he's allergic to penicillins or cephalosporins.

▼ Obtain specimen for culture and sensitivity tests before giving. Begin therapy while awaiting results.

▼ Follow manufacturer's guidelines closely when reconstituting drug. They vary with concentration of drug ordered and how drug is packaged (piggyback vial, ADD-Vantage vial, or regular vial).

▼ The type of diluent varies with the product used. Use only solutions recommended by the manufacturer.

▼ Give intermittent I.V. infusion with a Y-type administration and compatible solutions.

▼ Stop the main I.V. fluid while infusing.

▼ Infuse over about 30 minutes.

▼ **Incompatibilities:** Aminophylline, amphotericin B, amphotericin B cholesteryl sulfate complex, ciprofloxacin, gentamicin, metronidazole, tobramycin, vancomycin.

I.M.

● Before giving drug, ask patient if he's allergic to penicillins or cephalosporins.

● Obtain specimen for culture and sensitivity tests before giving. Begin therapy while awaiting results.

● Reconstitute drug using sterile water for injection, normal saline solution for injection, D_5W injection, 0.5% or 1% lidocaine hydrochloride, or bacteriostatic water for injection with parabens or benzyl alcohol. Follow manufacturer's guidelines for quantity of diluent to use.

● Inspect solution for particulate matter before use. The powder and its solutions tend to darken, depending on storage conditions. If stored as recommended, potency isn't adversely affected.

● Pain may occur at injection site.

ACTION

Inhibits bacterial cell-wall synthesis, promotes osmotic instability, and destroys bacteria.

Route	Onset	Peak	Duration
I.V., I.M.	30 min	1–2 hr	Unknown

Half-life: Adults: 2 to 2½ hours. Children: 1½ to 2 hours.

ADVERSE REACTIONS

CNS: fever, headache.

CV: phlebitis.

GI: diarrhea, nausea, vomiting.

Skin: rash, pruritus.

Other: *anaphylaxis,* pain, inflammation, hypersensitivity reactions.

INTERACTIONS

Drug-drug. *Aminoglycosides:* May increase risk of nephrotoxicity. Monitor renal function closely.

Live-virus vaccines: May decrease effectiveness of live-virus vaccines. Concurrent use isn't recommended.

Potent diuretics: May increase risk of nephrotoxicity. Monitor renal function closely.

Probenecid: May inhibit renal excretion of cefepime. Monitor patient for adverse reactions.

EFFECTS ON LAB TEST RESULTS

● May increase ALT and AST levels. May decrease phosphorus level.

● May increase eosinophil count. May alter PT and PTT.

● May falsely increase serum or urine creatinine level in tests using Jaffe reaction. May cause false-positive results of Coombs test and urine glucose tests that use cupric sulfate, such as Benedict reagent and Clinitest.

CONTRAINDICATIONS & CAUTIONS

● Contraindicated in patients hypersensitive to drug, cephalosporins, beta-lactam antibiotics, or penicillins.

● *Alert:* Drug may increase risk of nonconvulsive status epilepticus (altered mental status, confusion, decreased responsiveness), especially in patients with renal impairment. To decrease risk, follow dosage adjustment guidelines for patients with CrCl of 60 mL/minute or less. Discontinue drug in patients with seizures associated with drug.

● Use cautiously in patients hypersensitive to penicillin because of possibility of cross-sensitivity with other beta-lactam antibiotics.

● Use cautiously in breast-feeding women and in patients with history of colitis or renal insufficiency.

⚠ **Overdose S&S:** Encephalopathy, myoclonus, seizures, neuromuscular excitability.

NURSING CONSIDERATIONS

• Monitor patient for superinfection. Drug may cause overgrowth of nonsusceptible bacteria or fungi.

• Drug may reduce PT activity. Patients at risk include those with renal or hepatic impairment or poor nutrition and those receiving prolonged therapy. Monitor PT and INR in these patients. Give vitamin K, as indicated.

• **Look alike–sound alike:** Don't confuse drug with other cephalosporins that sound alike.

PATIENT TEACHING

• Warn patient receiving drug I.M. that pain may occur at injection site.

• Advise patient to notify prescriber if a rash develops or if signs and symptoms of superinfection appear, such as recurring fever, chills, and malaise.

• Instruct patient to report adverse reactions promptly.

---

cefotaxime sodium
sef-oh-TAKS-eem

Claforan

Therapeutic class: Antibiotics
Pharmacologic class: Third-generation cephalosporins
Pregnancy risk category: B

AVAILABLE FORMS
Infusion: 1-g, 2-g premixed package
Injection: 500-mg, 1-g, 2-g, 10-g vials

INDICATIONS & DOSAGES
Adjust-a-dose (for all indications): For patients with CrCl less than 20 mL/minute/1.73 m^2, give half of usual dose at regular time interval. For patients receiving hemodialysis, give 0.5 to 2 g supplement after dialysis. For patients receiving continuous ambulatory peritoneal dialysis, give 0.5 to 1 g every 24 hours.

➤ **Perioperative prophylaxis in contaminated surgery**

Adults: 1 g I.M. or I.V. 30 to 90 minutes before surgery. In patients undergoing bowel surgery, provide preoperative mechanical bowel cleansing and give a nonabsorbable anti-infective, such as neomycin. In patients undergoing cesarean delivery, give 1 g I.M. or I.V. as soon as the umbilical cord is clamped; then 1 g I.M. or I.V. 6 and 12 hours later.

➤ **Uncomplicated gonorrhea caused by penicillinase-producing strains or non–penicillinase-producing strains of *Neisseria gonorrhoeae***
Adults and adolescents: 500 mg I.M. as a single dose.

➤ **Rectal gonorrhea**
Men: 1 g I.M. as a single dose.
Women: 500 mg I.M. as a single dose.

➤ **Serious infection of the lower respiratory and urinary tract, CNS, skin, bone, and joints; gynecologic and intra-abdominal infection; bacteremia; septicemia caused by susceptible microorganisms, such as streptococci (including *Streptococcus pneumoniae* and *S. pyogenes, Staphylococcus aureus* [penicillinase- and non–penicillinase-producing], and *S. epidermidis*), *Escherichia coli, Klebsiella, Haemophilus influenzae, Serratia marcescens,* and species of *Pseudomonas* (including *P. aeruginosa*), *Enterobacter, Proteus,* and *Peptostreptococcus***
Adults and children weighing 50 kg (110 lb) or more: 1 to 2 g I.V. or I.M. every 6 to 8 hours. Up to 12 g daily can be given for life-threatening infections.
Children ages 1 month to 12 years weighing less than 50 kg (110 lb): 50 to 180 mg/kg/day I.M. or I.V. in four to six divided doses.
Neonates ages 1 to 4 weeks: 50 mg/kg I.V. every 8 hours.
Neonates to age 1 week: 50 mg/kg I.V. every 12 hours.

➤ **Disseminated gonococcal infection ◆**
Adults: 1 g I.V. every 8 hours for 24 to 48 hours after symptom improvement.

➤ **Disseminated gonococcal infection and gonococcal scalp abscesses ◆**
Neonates: 25 mg/kg I.V. or I.M. every 12 hours for 7 days or for 10 to 14 days with documented meningitis.

➤ **Lyme neuroborreliosis** ◆
Adults: 2 g I.V. every 8 hours for 14 days.
Children: 150 to 200 mg/kg/day in three to four divided doses (maximum, 6 g/day) for 14 days.

ADMINISTRATION
I.V.
▼ Before giving drug, ask patient if he's allergic to penicillins or cephalosporins.
▼ Obtain specimen for culture and sensitivity tests before giving. Begin therapy while awaiting results.
▼ For direct injection, reconstitute drug in 500-mg, 1-g, or 2-g vials with 10 mL of sterile water for injection. Solutions containing 1 g/14 mL are isotonic.
▼ Inject drug over 3 to 5 minutes into a large vein or into the tubing of a free-flowing I.V. solution.
▼ For infusion, reconstitute drug in infusion vials with 50 to 100 mL of D_5W or normal saline solution.
▼ Interrupt flow of primary I.V. solution, and infuse this drug over 20 to 30 minutes.
▼ **Incompatibilities:** Allopurinol, aminoglycosides, aminophylline, azithromycin, doxapram, filgrastim, fluconazole, hetastarch, pentamidine isethionate, sodium bicarbonate injection, vancomycin.

I.M.
● Before giving drug, ask patient if he's allergic to penicillins or cephalosporins.
● Obtain specimen for culture and sensitivity tests before giving. Begin therapy while awaiting results.
● Reconstitute 500-mg vial with 2 mL, 1-g vial with 3 mL, and 2-g vial with 5 mL sterile water for injection.
● For doses of 2 g, divide the dose and give at different sites.
● Inject deep into a large muscle, such as the gluteus maximus or the side of the thigh.

ACTION
Inhibits cell-wall synthesis, promoting osmotic instability; usually bactericidal.

Route	Onset	Peak	Duration
I.V.	Immediate	Immediate	Unknown
I.M.	Unknown	30 min	Unknown

Half-life: 1 to 2 hours.

ADVERSE REACTIONS
CNS: fever, headache.
CV: phlebitis, thrombophlebitis.
GI: diarrhea, *pseudomembranous colitis,* nausea, vomiting.
Hematologic: *agranulocytosis, thrombocytopenia, transient neutropenia,* eosinophilia, hemolytic anemia.
Skin: maculopapular and erythematous rashes, urticaria, pain, induration, sterile abscesses, temperature elevation, tissue sloughing at I.M. injection site.
Other: *anaphylaxis,* hypersensitivity reactions, serum sickness.

INTERACTIONS
Drug-drug. *Aminoglycosides:* May increase risk of nephrotoxicity. Monitor patient's renal function tests.
Live-virus vaccines: May decrease effectiveness of live-virus vaccines. Concurrent use isn't recommended.
Probenecid: May inhibit excretion and increase cefotaxime. Use together cautiously.

EFFECTS ON LAB TEST RESULTS
● May increase alkaline phosphatase, ALT, AST, bilirubin, GGT, and LDH levels. May decrease hemoglobin level.
● May increase eosinophil count. May decrease granulocyte, neutrophil, and platelet counts.
● May cause positive Coombs test results.

CONTRAINDICATIONS & CAUTIONS
● Contraindicated in patients hypersensitive to drug or other cephalosporins.
● Use cautiously in patients hypersensitive to penicillin because of possibility of cross-sensitivity with other beta-lactam antibiotics.
● Use cautiously in breast-feeding women and in patients with history of colitis or renal insufficiency.
⚠ **Overdose S&S:** Elevated BUN and creatinine levels.

NURSING CONSIDERATIONS
● If large doses are given, therapy is prolonged, or patient is at high risk, monitor patient for superinfection.
● **Look alike–sound alike:** Don't confuse drug with other cephalosporins that sound alike.

PATIENT TEACHING
● Tell patient to report adverse reactions and signs and symptoms of superinfection promptly.
● Instruct patient to report discomfort at I.V. insertion site.

cefoxitin sodium
se-FOX-i-tin

Therapeutic class: Antibiotics
Pharmacologic class: Second-generation cephalosporins
Pregnancy risk category: B

AVAILABLE FORMS
Infusion: 1 g, 2 g in 50-mL or 100-mL container
Injection: 1 g, 2 g, 10 g

INDICATIONS & DOSAGES
Adjust-a-dose (for all indications): For adults with renal insufficiency, give loading dose of 1 to 2 g. For adults with CrCl of 30 to 50 mL/minute, give 1 to 2 g every 8 to 12 hours; if CrCl is 10 to 29 mL/minute, 1 to 2 g every 12 to 24 hours; if CrCl is 5 to 9 mL/minute, 0.5 to 1 g every 12 to 24 hours; and if CrCl is less than 5 mL/minute, 0.5 to 1 g every 24 to 48 hours. For patients receiving hemodialysis, give a loading dose of 1 to 2 g after each hemodialysis session; then give the maintenance dose based on creatinine level. For patients receiving continuous ambulatory peritoneal dialysis, give 1 g every 24 hours.
➤ **Serious infection of the respiratory and GU tracts; skin, soft-tissue, bone, or joint infection; bloodstream or intra-abdominal infection caused by susceptible organisms (such as** *Escherichia coli* **and other coliform bacteria, penicillinase- and non–penicillinase-producing** *Staphylococcus aureus,* *S. epidermidis,* **streptococci,** *Klebsiella, Haemophilus influenzae,* **and** *Bacteroides,* **including** *B. fragilis***)**
Adults: 1 to 2 g I.V. every 6 to 8 hours for uncomplicated infections. Up to 12 g daily may be used in life-threatening infections.
Children older than age 3 months: 80 to 160 mg/kg daily I.V., given in four to six equally divided doses. Maximum daily dose is 12 g.
➤ **Perioperative prophylaxis**
Adults: 2 g I.V. 30 to 60 minutes before surgery; then 2 g I.V. every 6 hours for up to 24 hours. For patients undergoing cesarean section, give 2 g I.V. as soon as the umbilical cord is clamped; may give additional 2-g doses 4 and 8 hours after initial dose.
Children age 3 months and older: 30 to 40 mg/kg I.V. 30 to 60 minutes before surgery; then 30 to 40 mg/kg every 6 hours for up to 24 hours.

ADMINISTRATION
I.V.
▼ Before giving drug, ask patient if he's allergic to penicillins or cephalosporins.
▼ Obtain specimen for culture and sensitivity tests before giving. Begin therapy while awaiting results.
▼ Reconstitute 1 g with at least 10 mL of sterile water for injection and 2 g with 10 to 20 mL of sterile water for injection. Solutions of D_5W and normal saline solution for injection also may be used.
▼ After reconstitution, drug may be stored for 24 hours (6 hours for non–ADD-Vantage vials) at room temperature or 1 week under refrigeration.
▼ For direct injection, give drug over 3 to 5 minutes into a large vein or into the tubing of a free-flowing I.V. solution.
▼ For intermittent infusion, add reconstituted drug to 50 or 100 mL of D_5W or normal saline solution for injection.
▼ Interrupt flow of primary solution during infusion.
▼ Assess site often to detect evidence of thrombophlebitis.
▼ **Incompatibilities:** Aminoglycosides, filgrastim, hetastarch, pentamidine isethionate, ranitidine.

ACTION
Inhibits cell-wall synthesis, promoting osmotic instability; usually bactericidal.

Route	Onset	Peak	Duration
I.V.	Immediate	Immediate	Unknown

Half-life: About ½ to 1 hours.

ADVERSE REACTIONS
CNS: fever.
CV: phlebitis, thrombophlebitis, hypotension.
GI: diarrhea, *pseudomembranous colitis,* nausea, vomiting.
GU: *acute renal failure.*
Hematologic: *thrombocytopenia, transient neutropenia,* eosinophilia, hemolytic anemia, anemia.
Respiratory: dyspnea.
Skin: maculopapular and erythematous rashes, urticaria, pain, induration, sterile abscesses, tissue sloughing at injection site, exfoliative dermatitis.
Other: *anaphylaxis,* hypersensitivity reactions, serum sickness.

INTERACTIONS
Drug-drug. *Aminoglycosides:* May increase risk of nephrotoxicity. Monitor patient's renal function tests.
Live-virus vaccines: May decrease effectiveness of live-virus vaccines. Concurrent use isn't recommended.
Probenecid: May inhibit excretion and increase cefoxitin level. Probenecid may be used for this effect.
Warfarin: May increase anticoagulation. Monitor PT and adjust warfarin dosage as needed.

EFFECTS ON LAB TEST RESULTS
• May increase alkaline phosphatase, ALT, AST, bilirubin, and LDH levels. May decrease hemoglobin level.
• May increase eosinophil count. May decrease neutrophil and platelet counts.
• May prolong PT.
• May falsely increase serum or urine creatinine level in tests using Jaffe reaction. May cause false-positive results of Coombs test and urine glucose tests that use cupric sulfate, such as Benedict reagent and Clinitest.

CONTRAINDICATIONS & CAUTIONS
• Contraindicated in patients hypersensitive to drug or other cephalosporins.
• Use cautiously in patients hypersensitive to penicillin because of possibility of cross-sensitivity with other beta-lactam antibiotics.

• Use cautiously in breast-feeding women and in patients with history of colitis or renal insufficiency.
• Drug can cause overgrowth of nonsusceptible organisms. Monitor patient for superinfection and treat appropriately.

NURSING CONSIDERATIONS
❸ Alert: The premixed frozen product is for I.V. use only.
• If large doses are given, therapy is prolonged, or patient is at high risk, monitor patient for signs and symptoms of superinfection.
• *Look alike–sound alike:* Don't confuse drug with other cephalosporins that sound alike.

PATIENT TEACHING
• Tell patient to report adverse reactions and signs and symptoms of superinfection promptly.
• Instruct patient to report discomfort at I.V. site.
• Advise patient to notify prescriber about loose stools or diarrhea.

cefpodoxime proxetil
SEF-pod-OX-eem

Therapeutic class: Antibiotics
Pharmacologic class: Third-generation cephalosporins
Pregnancy risk category: B

AVAILABLE FORMS
Oral suspension: 50 mg/5 mL or 100 mg/5 mL in 50-, 75-, or 100-mL bottles
Tablets (film-coated): 100 mg, 200 mg

INDICATIONS & DOSAGES
Adjust-a-dose (for all indications): For patients with CrCl less than 30 mL/minute, increase dosage interval to every 24 hours. Give to dialysis patients three times weekly after dialysis.
➤ **Acute community-acquired pneumonia caused by strains of** *Haemophilus influenzae* **or** *Streptococcus pneumoniae*
Adults and children age 12 and older: 200 mg P.O. every 12 hours for 14 days.
➤ **Acute bacterial worsening of chronic bronchitis caused by** *S. pneumoniae* **or**

H. influenzae (strains that don't produce beta-lactamase only), or *Moraxella catarrhalis*
Adults and children age 12 and older:
200 mg P.O. every 12 hours for 10 days.
➤ **Uncomplicated gonorrhea in men and women; rectal gonococcal infections in women**
Adults and children age 12 and older:
200 mg P.O. as a single dose.
➤ **Uncomplicated skin and skin-structure infections caused by** *Staphylococcus aureus* or *Streptococcus pyogenes*
Adults and children age 12 and older:
400 mg P.O. every 12 hours for 7 to 14 days.
➤ **Acute otitis media caused by** *S. pneumoniae* (penicillin-susceptible strains only), *S. pyogenes, H. influenzae,* or *M. catarrhalis*
Children ages 2 months to 12 years:
5 mg/kg P.O. every 12 hours for 5 days. Don't exceed 200 mg per dose.
➤ **Pharyngitis or tonsillitis caused by** *S. pyogenes*
Adults: 100 mg P.O. every 12 hours for 5 to 10 days.
Children ages 2 months to 12 years:
5 mg/kg P.O. every 12 hours for 5 to 10 days. Don't exceed 100 mg per dose.
➤ **Uncomplicated UTIs caused by** *Escherichia coli, Klebsiella pneumoniae, Proteus mirabilis,* or *Staphylococcus saprophyticus*
Adults: 100 mg P.O. every 12 hours for 7 days.
➤ **Mild to moderate acute maxillary sinusitis caused by** *H. influenzae, S. pneumoniae,* or *M. catarrhalis*
Adults and adolescents age 12 and older:
200 mg P.O. every 12 hours for 10 days.
Children ages 2 months to 12 years:
5 mg/kg P.O. every 12 hours for 10 days; maximum is 200 mg/dose.

ADMINISTRATION
P.O.
● Before administration, ask patient if he's allergic to penicillins or cephalosporins.
● Obtain specimen for culture and sensitivity tests before giving. Begin therapy while awaiting results.

● Give drug with food to enhance absorption. May give oral suspension without regard to food. Shake suspension well before using.
● Store suspension in the refrigerator (36° to 46° F [2° to 8° C]). Discard unused portion after 14 days.

ACTION
Inhibits cell-wall synthesis, promoting osmotic instability; usually bactericidal.

Route	Onset	Peak	Duration
P.O.	Unknown	2–3 hr	Unknown

Half-life: 2 to 3 hours.

ADVERSE REACTIONS
CNS: headache.
GI: diarrhea, *pseudomembranous colitis,* nausea, vomiting, abdominal pain.
GU: vaginal fungal infections.
Skin: rash.
Other: *anaphylaxis,* hypersensitivity reactions.

INTERACTIONS
Drug-drug. *Aminoglycosides:* May increase risk of nephrotoxicity. Monitor renal function tests closely.
Antacids, H$_2$-receptor antagonists: May decrease absorption of cefpodoxime. Avoid using together.
Live-virus vaccines: May decrease effectiveness of live-virus vaccines. Concurrent use isn't recommended.
Probenecid: May decrease excretion of cefpodoxime. Monitor patient for toxicity.
Warfarin: May prolong PT and INR. Monitor levels closely and adjust warfarin dosage.

EFFECTS ON LAB TEST RESULTS
● May falsely increase serum or urine creatinine level in tests using Jaffe reaction.
● May decrease WBC, absolute neutrophil, platelet, and lymphocyte counts.
● May cause false-positive results of Coombs test and urine glucose tests that use cupric sulfate, such as Benedict reagent and Clinitest.

Reactions in bold italics are *life-threatening*. Interactions may have a *rapid onset* or a *delayed onset*.

CONTRAINDICATIONS & CAUTIONS
• Contraindicated in patients hypersensitive to drug or other cephalosporins.
⊙ **Alert:** Drug can cause pseudomembranous colitis ranging from mild to life-threatening. Monitor patient for diarrhea and treat appropriately.
• Use cautiously in patients with a history of penicillin hypersensitivity because of risk of cross-sensitivity.
• Use cautiously in patients receiving nephrotoxic drugs because other cephalosporins have been shown to have nephrotoxic potential.
• Use cautiously in breast-feeding women because drug appears in breast milk.

NURSING CONSIDERATIONS
• Monitor renal function and compare with baseline.
• Monitor patient for superinfection. Drug may cause overgrowth of nonsusceptible bacteria or fungi.
• *Look alike–sound alike:* Don't confuse drug with other cephalosporins that sound alike.

PATIENT TEACHING
• Tell patient to take drug as prescribed, even after he feels better.
• Instruct patient to take drug with food. If patient is using suspension, tell him to shake container before measuring dose and to keep container refrigerated.
• Tell patient to call prescriber if rash or signs and symptoms of superinfection occur.
• Instruct patient to notify prescriber about loose stools or diarrhea.

cefprozil
sef-PRO-zil

Therapeutic class: Antibiotics
Pharmacologic class: Second-generation cephalosporins
Pregnancy risk category: B

AVAILABLE FORMS
Oral suspension: 125 mg/5 mL, 250 mg/5 mL
Tablets: 250 mg, 500 mg

INDICATIONS & DOSAGES
Adjust-a-dose (for all indications): If CrCl is less than 30 mL/minute, give 50% of standard dose at standard intervals. If patient is receiving dialysis, give dose after hemodialysis is completed; drug is removed by hemodialysis.
➤ **Pharyngitis or tonsillitis caused by** *Streptococcus pyogenes*
Adults and children age 13 and older: 500 mg P.O. daily for at least 10 days.
Children ages 2 to 12: 7.5 mg/kg P.O. every 12 hours for 10 days. Don't exceed adult dose.
➤ **Otitis media caused by** *Streptococcus pneumoniae, Haemophilus influenzae,* **and** *Moraxella catarrhalis*
Infants and children ages 6 months to 12 years: 15 mg/kg P.O. every 12 hours for 10 days.
➤ **Secondary bacterial infections of acute bronchitis and acute bacterial worsening of chronic bronchitis caused by** *S. pneumoniae, H. influenzae,* **and** *M. catarrhalis*
Adults and children age 13 and older: 500 mg P.O. every 12 hours for 10 days.
➤ **Uncomplicated skin and skin-structure infections caused by** *Staphylococcus aureus* **and** *S. pyogenes*
Adults and children age 13 and older: 250 or 500 mg P.O. every 12 hours or 500 mg daily for 10 days.
Children ages 2 to 12: 20 mg/kg P.O. every 24 hours. Don't exceed adult dose.
➤ **Acute sinusitis caused by** *S. pneumoniae, H. influenzae* **(beta-lactamase–positive and –negative strains), and** *M. catarrhalis* **(including strains that produce beta-lactamase)**
Adults and children age 13 and older: 250 mg P.O. every 12 hours for 10 days; for moderate to severe infection, 500 mg P.O. every 12 hours for 10 days.
Children ages 6 months to 12 years: 7.5 mg/kg P.O. every 12 hours for 10 days; for moderate to severe infections, 15 mg/kg P.O. every 12 hours for 10 days.

ADMINISTRATION
P.O.
• Obtain specimen for culture and sensitivity tests before giving first dose. Start therapy while awaiting results.

• Before giving, ask patient if he's allergic to penicillins or cephalosporins.
• Shake suspension well before using.

ACTION
Inhibits cell-wall synthesis, promoting osmotic instability; usually bactericidal.

Route	Onset	Peak	Duration
P.O.	Unknown	1½ hr	Unknown

Half-life: 1¼ hours in patients with normal renal function; 2 hours in patients with impaired hepatic function; and 5¼ to 6 hours in patients with ESRD.

ADVERSE REACTIONS
CNS: dizziness.
GI: diarrhea, nausea, vomiting, abdominal pain.
GU: genital pruritus, vaginitis.
Hematologic: eosinophilia.
Skin: diaper rash.
Other: *anaphylaxis,* superinfection, hypersensitivity reactions, serum sickness.

INTERACTIONS
Drug-drug. *Aminoglycosides:* May increase risk of nephrotoxicity. Monitor renal function tests closely.
Live-virus vaccines: May decrease effectiveness of live-virus vaccines. Concurrent use isn't recommended.
Probenecid: May inhibit excretion and increase cefprozil level. Use together cautiously.

EFFECTS ON LAB TEST RESULTS
• May increase alkaline phosphatase, ALT, AST, bilirubin, BUN, creatinine, and LDH levels.
• May increase eosinophil count. May decrease platelet and WBC counts.
• May prolong PT and PTT.
• May falsely increase serum or urine creatinine level in tests using Jaffe reaction. May cause false-positive results of Coombs test and urine glucose tests that use cupric sulfate, such as Benedict reagent and Clinitest.

CONTRAINDICATIONS & CAUTIONS
• Contraindicated in patients hypersensitive to drug or other cephalosporins.

• Use cautiously in patients hypersensitive to penicillin because of possibility of cross-sensitivity with other beta-lactam antibiotics.
• Use cautiously in breast-feeding women and in patients with history of colitis and renal insufficiency.

NURSING CONSIDERATIONS
• Monitor renal function and LFT results.
• Monitor patient for superinfection. May cause overgrowth of nonsusceptible bacteria or fungi.
• ● *Look alike–sound alike:* Don't confuse drug with other cephalosporins that sound alike.

PATIENT TEACHING
• Advise patient to take drug as prescribed, even after he feels better.
• Tell patient to shake suspension well before measuring dose.
• Inform patient or parent that oral suspension is bubble gum–flavored to improve palatability and promote compliance in children. Tell him to refrigerate reconstituted suspension and to discard unused drug after 14 days.
• Instruct patient to notify prescriber if rash or signs and symptoms of superinfection occur.

ceftaroline fosamil
sef-TAR-oh-leen

Teflaro

Therapeutic class: Antibiotics
Pharmacologic class: Fifth-generation cephalosporins
Pregnancy risk category: B

AVAILABLE FORMS
Injection: 400-mg, 600-mg single-use vials

INDICATIONS & DOSAGES
➤ **Acute bacterial skin and skin-structure infections caused by susceptible isolates of *Staphylococcus aureus, Streptococcus pyogenes, Streptococcus agalactiae, Escherichia coli, Klebsiella pneumoniae, Klebsiella oxytoca;* community-acquired bacterial pneumonia (CABP) caused by susceptible isolates of *Streptococcus***

C

pneumoniae, S. aureus, Haemophilus influenzae, K. pneumoniae, K. oxytoca, and *E. coli*
Adults: 600 mg I.V. over 1 hour every 12 hours. For skin and skin-structure infections, continue treatment for 5 to 14 days; for CABP, continue treatment for 5 to 7 days.
Adjust-a-dose: For patients with CrCl of 31 to 50 mL/minute, give 400 mg I.V. every 12 hours. If CrCl is 15 to 30 mL/minute, give 300 mg I.V. every 12 hours. For patients with ESRD, including those on hemodialysis, give 200 mg I.V. every 12 hours. Administer after dialysis treatment.

ADMINISTRATION

I.V.
▼ Obtain specimen for culture before administration.
▼ Before administration, ask patient if he's allergic to penicillins or cephalosporins.
▼ Reconstitute drug with 20 mL sterile water for injection. Mix gently.
▼ Inspect solution for particulate matter. Color of solution ranges from clear to light to dark yellow.
▼ Further dilute in 50 to 250 mL I.V. fluid for infusion using normal saline injection, 5% dextrose injection, 2.5% dextrose in half normal saline injection, or lactated Ringer injection.
▼ Final solution of ceftaroline is stable for 6 hours at room temperature or for 24 hours if refrigerated at 36° to 46° F (2° to 8° C).
▼ **Incompatibilities:** Other drugs, I.V. solutions not listed above.

ACTION

Bactericidal by binding penicillin-binding proteins.

Route	Onset	Peak	Duration
I.V.	Unknown	1 hr	Unknown

Half-life: 1.6 to 2.7 hours.

ADVERSE REACTIONS

CNS: dizziness, *seizures,* pyrexia.
CV: *bradycardia,* palpitations, phlebitis.
GI: diarrhea, nausea, constipation, vomiting, abdominal pain, *colitis.*
GU: *renal failure.*
Hematologic: anemia, eosinophilia, *neutropenia, thrombocytopenia.*
Hepatic: hepatitis.
Metabolic: *hypokalemia, hyperkalemia,* hyperglycemia.
Skin: rash, urticaria.
Other: hypersensitivity, *anaphylaxis.*

INTERACTIONS

Live-virus vaccines: May decrease effectiveness of live-virus vaccines. Concurrent use isn't recommended.

EFFECTS ON LAB TEST RESULTS

● May increase serum glucose and transaminase levels.
● May decrease eosinophil, neutrophil, platelet, and RBC counts.
● May increase or decrease potassium level.
● May cause seroconversion of direct Coombs test from negative to positive.

CONTRAINDICATIONS & CAUTIONS

● Contraindicated in patients hypersensitive to drug or other cephalosporins, penicillins, or carbapenem drugs.
● Use cautiously in patients with history of beta-lactam allergy, renal failure, or drug-resistant infections.
● May cause *Clostridium difficile*–associated diarrhea, which can range from mild to severe and may be fatal.
● Use cautiously in pregnant and breast-feeding women.
● Safety and effectiveness in children haven't been established.

NURSING CONSIDERATIONS

● Prescribing drug without proven or strongly suspected bacterial infection is unlikely to provide benefit and increases the risk of drug resistance.
● Obtain a list of patient's known allergies before beginning treatment.
● Monitor patient for signs of *C. difficile* diarrhea (frequent watery or bloody diarrhea).
● Monitor patient for signs and symptoms of anemia during and after therapy. A diagnostic workup, including direct Coombs test for drug-induced hemolytic anemia, should be considered.

• Monitor renal function periodically during therapy, especially in elderly patients and in those with decreased renal function.

• *Look alike–sound alike:* Don't confuse ceftaroline with other cephalosporins that sound alike (such as ceftazidime and ceftriaxone).

PATIENT TEACHING

• Instruct patient to tell his health care provider if he's allergic to penicillin or cephalosporins before beginning treatment.

• Caution patient to immediately report itching, hives, throat swelling, or shortness of breath.

• Tell patient that blood tests may be required to assess his tolerance to treatment.

• Warn patient that diarrhea may occur and to immediately report watery or bloody diarrhea.

• Advise female patient to tell prescriber if she's pregnant or breast-feeding.

ceftazidime
sef-TAZ-i-deem

Fortaz, Tazicef

Therapeutic class: Antibiotics
Pharmacologic class: Third-generation cephalosporins
Pregnancy risk category: B

AVAILABLE FORMS
Infusion: 1 g, 2 g in 50-mL and 100-mL vials (premixed)
Injection (with sodium carbonate): 500 mg, 1 g, 2 g, 6 g

INDICATIONS & DOSAGES
Adjust-a-dose (for all indications): If CrCl is 31 to 50 mL/minute, give 1 g every 12 hours; if CrCl is 16 to 30 mL/minute, give 1 g every 24 hours; if CrCl is 6 to 15 mL/minute, give 500 mg every 24 hours; if CrCl is less than 5 mL/minute, give 500 mg every 48 hours. Ceftazidime is removed by hemodialysis; give a loading dose of 1 g, followed by 1 g after each hemodialysis period. If patient is receiving continuous ambulatory peritoneal dialysis, give a loading dose of 1 g, followed

by 500 mg every 24 hours. Or, add 250 mg per 2 L of dialysis fluid.

➤ **Serious UTI and lower respiratory tract infection; skin, gynecologic, intra-abdominal, bone and joint, and CNS infection; bacteremia; and septicemia caused by susceptible microorganisms, such as streptococci (including *Streptococcus pneumoniae* and *S. pyogenes*), penicillinase- and non–penicillinase-producing *Staphylococcus aureus, Escherichia coli, Klebsiella, Proteus, Enterobacter, Haemophilus influenzae, Pseudomonas,* and some strains of *Bacteroides***

Adults and children age 12 and older: 1 to 2 g I.V. or I.M. every 8 to 12 hours; up to 6 g daily in life-threatening infections.

Children ages 1 month to 12 years: 30 to 50 mg/kg I.V. every 8 hours. Maximum dose is 6 g/day. Use sodium carbonate formulation.

Neonates up to age 4 weeks: 30 mg/kg I.V. every 12 hours. Use sodium carbonate formulation.

➤ **Uncomplicated UTI**
Adults: 250 mg I.V. or I.M. every 12 hours.

➤ **Complicated UTI**
Adults and children age 12 and older: 500 mg to 1 g I.V. or I.M. every 8 to 12 hours.

➤ **Uncomplicated pneumonia**
Adults and children age 12 and older: 500 mg to 1 g I.V. or I.M. every 8 hours.

➤ **Lung infections caused by *Pseudomonas* in patients with cystic fibrosis with healthy renal function**
Adults and children age 12 and older: 30 to 50 mg/kg I.V. every 8 hours. Maximum dose is 6 g/day.

➤ **Catheter-related bloodstream infections ◆**
Infants and children younger than age 12: 100 to 150 mg/kg/day I.V. every 8 hours in divided doses for 7 to 14 days. Maximum dose is 6 g/day.
Neonates: 100 to 150 mg/kg/day I.V. every 8 to 12 hours in divided doses for 7 to 14 days. Maximum dose is 6 g/day.

Reactions in bold italics are *life-threatening*. Interactions may have a *rapid onset* or a *delayed onset*.

C

ADMINISTRATION

I.V.

▼ Before administration, ask patient if he's allergic to penicillins or cephalosporins.

▼ Obtain specimen for culture and sensitivity tests before giving. Begin therapy while awaiting results.

▼ Each brand of drug includes specific instructions for reconstitution. Read and follow them carefully.

▼ To reconstitute solution that contains sodium carbonate, add 5 mL sterile water for injection to a 500-mg vial, or add 10 mL to a 1-g or 2-g vial. Shake well to dissolve drug. Because carbon dioxide is released during dissolution, positive pressure will develop in vial.

▼ Infuse drug over 15 to 30 minutes.

▼ **Incompatibilities:** Aminoglycosides, aminophylline, amiodarone, amphotericin B cholesteryl sulfate complex, azithromycin, clarithromycin, fluconazole, idarubicin, midazolam, pentamidine isethionate, ranitidine hydrochloride, sargramostim, sodium bicarbonate solutions, vancomycin.

I.M.

● Before administration, ask patient if he's allergic to penicillins or cephalosporins.

● Obtain specimen for culture and sensitivity tests before giving. Begin therapy while awaiting results.

● Inject deep into a large muscle, such as the gluteus maximus or the side of the thigh.

ACTION

Inhibits cell-wall synthesis, promoting osmotic instability; usually bactericidal.

Route	Onset	Peak	Duration
I.V.	Immediate	Immediate	Unknown
I.M.	Unknown	1 hr	Unknown

Half-life: 1½ to 2 hours.

ADVERSE REACTIONS

CNS: *seizures.*
CV: phlebitis, thrombophlebitis.
GI: *pseudomembranous colitis,* nausea, vomiting, diarrhea, abdominal cramps.
Hematologic: *agranulocytosis, leukopenia, thrombocytopenia,* eosinophilia, thrombocytosis, hemolytic anemia.

Skin: maculopapular and erythematous rashes, urticaria, pain, induration, sterile abscesses, tissue sloughing at injection site.
Other: *anaphylaxis,* hypersensitivity reactions, serum sickness.

INTERACTIONS

Drug-drug. *Aminoglycosides:* May cause additive or synergistic effect against some strains of *Pseudomonas aeruginosa* and *Enterobacteriaceae;* may increase risk of nephrotoxicity. Monitor patient for effects and monitor renal function.
Chloramphenicol: May cause antagonistic effect. Avoid using together.
Live-virus vaccines: May decrease effectiveness of live-virus vaccines. Concurrent use isn't recommended.
Warfarin: May increase anticoagulation effect. Monitor PT and INR closely.

EFFECTS ON LAB TEST RESULTS

● May increase alkaline phosphatase, ALT, AST, bilirubin, and LDH levels. May decrease hemoglobin level.
● May increase eosinophil count. May decrease granulocyte and WBC counts. May increase or decrease platelet count.
● May increase PTT, PT, and INR.
● May falsely increase serum or urine creatinine level in tests using Jaffe reaction. May cause false-positive results of Coombs test and urine glucose tests that use cupric sulfate, such as Benedict reagent and Clinitest.

CONTRAINDICATIONS & CAUTIONS

● Contraindicated in patients hypersensitive to drug or other cephalosporins.
● Use cautiously in patients hypersensitive to penicillin because of possibility of cross-sensitivity with other beta-lactam antibiotics.
● Use cautiously in breast-feeding women and in patients with history of colitis or renal insufficiency.
⚠ Overdose S&S: Seizures, encephalopathy, asterixis, neuromuscular excitability, coma (in patients with renal failure).

NURSING CONSIDERATIONS

● If large doses are given, therapy is prolonged, or patient is at high risk, monitor

patient for signs and symptoms of superinfection.
● *Look alike–sound alike:* Don't confuse drug with other cephalosporins that sound alike.

PATIENT TEACHING
● Tell patient to report adverse reactions or signs and symptoms of superinfection promptly.
● Instruct patient to report discomfort at I.V. insertion site.
● Advise patient to notify prescriber about loose stools or diarrhea.

ceftriaxone sodium
sef-try-AX-ohn

Rocephin

Therapeutic class: Antibiotics
Pharmacologic class: Third-generation cephalosporins
Pregnancy risk category: B

AVAILABLE FORMS
Infusion: 1 g, 2 g, 1 g/50 mL, 2 g/50 mL premixed
Injection: 250 mg, 500 mg, 1 g, 2 g

INDICATIONS & DOSAGES
➤ **Uncomplicated gonococcal vulvovaginitis**
Adults: 250 mg I.M. as a single dose, plus azithromycin 1 g P.O. as a single dose or doxycycline 100 mg P.O. b.i.d. for 7 days.
➤ **UTI; lower respiratory tract, gynecologic, bone or joint, intra-abdominal, skin, or skin-structure infection; septicemia**
Adults and children older than age 12: 1 to 2 g I.M. or I.V. daily or in equally divided doses every 12 hours. Total daily dose shouldn't exceed 4 g. Treat for 4 to 14 days. Complicated infections may require longer treatment.
Children age 12 and younger: 50 to 75 mg/kg I.M. or I.V., not to exceed 2 g/day, given in divided doses every 12 hours or given once daily.

➤ **Meningitis**
Adults: 1 to 2 g I.M. or I.V. once daily or in two equally divided doses daily for 4 to 14 days.
Children: Initially, 100 mg/kg I.M. or I.V.; then 100 mg/kg/day as a single dose or in divided doses every 12 hours for 7 to 14 days. Maximum dose is 4 g/day.
➤ **Perioperative prophylaxis**
Adults: 1 g I.V. as a single dose 30 minutes to 2 hours before surgery.
➤ **Acute bacterial otitis media**
Adults: 1 to 2 g I.M. or I.V. once daily or in two equally divided doses daily for 4 to 14 days.
Children: 50 mg/kg I.M. as a single dose. Don't exceed 1 g.
➤ **Lyme disease ◆**
Adults: 2 g I.V. daily for 14 days.
Children: 50 to 75 mg/kg/day I.V. for 14 days.
➤ **Epididymitis ◆**
Adults: 250 mg I.M. in a single dose plus doxycycline 100 mg P.O. b.i.d. for 10 days.
➤ **Chancroid ◆**
Adults: 250 mg I.M. as a single dose.
➤ **Disseminated gonococcal infection ◆**
Adults: 1 g I.V. or I.M. once daily. Continue for 24 to 48 hours after symptomatic improvement, then switch to oral antibiotic therapy with cefixime 400 mg P.O. b.i.d. to complete a total of 1 week of antimicrobial therapy.
➤ **Gonococcal meningitis and endocarditis ◆**
Adults: 1 to 2 g I.V. every 12 hours. Continue therapy for 10 to 14 days for meningitis; continue for a minimum of 4 weeks for endocarditis.
➤ **Infective endocarditis in patients with native valves and infections with highly penicillin-susceptible viridans-group streptococci or *Streptococcus bovis* ◆**
Adults: 2 g I.V. or I.M. once daily for 4 weeks as monotherapy. In combination with gentamicin, duration of therapy is 2 weeks. The 2-week regimen isn't intended for patients with cardiac or extracardiac abscess or for those with CrCl of less than 20 mL/minute, impaired eighth cranial nerve function, or infection with *Abiotrophia, Granulicatella,* or *Gemella* species.
Children and adolescents: 100 mg/kg/day I.V. or I.M. once daily for 4 weeks as

monotherapy. In combination with gentamicin, duration of therapy is 2 weeks. The 2-week regimen isn't intended for patients with cardiac or extracardiac abscess or for those with CrCl of less than 20 mL/minute, impaired eighth cranial nerve function, or infection with *Abiotrophia, Granulicatella,* or *Gemella* species.

➤ **Infective endocarditis in patients with native valves and infections with penicillin-resistant viridans-group streptococci or *S. bovis* relatively resistant to penicillins ◆**

Adults: 2 g I.V. or I.M. once daily for 4 weeks with gentamicin.

Children and adolescents: 100 mg/kg/day I.V. or I.M. once daily for 4 weeks with gentamicin.

➤ **Infective endocarditis in patients with prosthetic valves and infection with viridans-group streptococci or *S. bovis* ◆**

Adults: For patients with penicillin-susceptible strain (minimum inhibitory concentration [MIC] 0.12 mcg/mL or less), give 2 g I.V. or I.M. once daily for 6 weeks as monotherapy or in combination with gentamicin. For patients with penicillin relatively or fully resistant strain (MIC more than 0.12 mcg/mL), give 2 g I.V. or I.M. once daily for 6 weeks with gentamicin.

Children and adolescents: For patients with penicillin-susceptible strain (MIC 0.12 mcg/mL or less), give 100 mg/kg/day I.V. or I.M. once daily for 6 weeks as monotherapy or in combination with gentamicin.

➤ **Infective endocarditis in patients with *Enterococcus faecalis* infections resistant to penicillin, aminoglycosides, and vancomycin ◆**

Adults: 4 g I.V. or I.M. daily in two equally divided doses for at least 8 weeks in combination with ampicillin.

Children and adolescents: 100 mg/kg/day I.V. or I.M. in two equally divided doses for at least 8 weeks in combination with ampicillin.

➤ **Infective endocarditis in patients with *Haemophilus parainfluenzae, Haemophilus aphrophilus, Haemophilus paraphrophilus, Haemophilus influenzae, Actinobacillus actinomycetemcomitans, Cardiobacterium hominis, Eikenella**

corrodens, Kingella kingae, and *Kingella denitrificans* (HACEK) infections ◆**

Adults: 2 g I.V. or I.M. once daily for 4 weeks. Cefotaxime or another third- or fourth-generation cephalosporin may be substituted.

Children and adolescents: 100 mg/kg/day I.V. or I.M. once daily for 4 weeks. Cefotaxime or another third- or fourth-generation cephalosporin may be substituted.

➤ **Infective endocarditis in patients with suspected *Bartonella* infection with a negative culture ◆**

Adults: 2 g I.V. or I.M. once daily for 6 weeks in combination with gentamicin. Doxycycline may also be added to therapy. Patients with *Bartonella* endocarditis should be treated in consultation with an infectious diseases specialist.

Children and adolescents: 100 mg/kg/day I.V. or I.M. once daily for 6 weeks in combination with gentamicin. Doxycycline may also be added to therapy. Patients with *Bartonella* endocarditis should be treated in consultation with an infectious diseases specialist.

➤ **Mild to moderately severe pelvic inflammatory disease ◆**

Adults: 250 mg I.M. as a single dose with doxycycline 100 mg P.O. b.i.d. for 14 days, with or without metronidazole 500 mg P.O. b.i.d. for 14 days.

➤ **Proctitis, proctocolitis, enteritis ◆**

Adults: Single 250-mg I.M. dose in conjunction with doxycycline 100 mg P.O. b.i.d. for 7 days.

➤ **Acute otitis media ◆**

Children: 50 mg/kg/day I.V. or I.M. for 3 consecutive days in patients unresponsive to initial antibiotic therapy and in penicillin-allergic patients with a temperature of 102° F (39° C) or higher or severe otalgia.

Neonates age 7 days and older weighing more than 2 kg (4.4 lb): 50 to 75 mg/kg I.V. or I.M. every 24 hours.

Neonates age 7 days and older weighing 1.2 to 2 kg (2.6 to 4.4 lb): 50 mg/kg I.V. or I.M. every 24 hours.

Neonates age 0 to younger than 7 days weighing at least 1.2 kg (2.6 lb): 50 mg/kg I.V. or I.M. every 24 hours.

Neonates age 0 to 28 days weighing less than 1.2 kg (2.6 lb): 50 mg/kg I.V. or I.M. every 24 hours.

ADMINISTRATION

I.V.

▼ Before giving drug, ask patient if he's allergic to penicillins or cephalosporins.

▼ Obtain specimen for culture and sensitivity tests before giving first dose. Begin therapy while awaiting results.

▼ Reconstitute drug with sterile water for injection, normal saline solution for injection, D_5W, or a combination of normal saline solution and dextrose injection and other compatible solutions.

▼ Add 2.4 mL of diluent to the 250-mg vial, 4.8 mL to the 500-mg vial, 9.6 mL to the 1-g vial, and 19.2 mL to the 2-g vial. All reconstituted solutions average 100 mg/mL. For intermittent infusion, dilute further to achieve desired concentration, and give over 30 minutes.

▼ Diluted I.V. preparation is stable for 48 hours at room temperature or 10 days if refrigerated.

❸ Alert: Don't mix or coadminister ceftriaxone with calcium-containing I.V. solutions, including parenteral nutrition. This includes the use of different infusion lines at different sites. Don't administer within 48 hours of each other in any patient.

▼ **Incompatibilities:** Aminoglycosides, aminophylline, amphotericin B cholesteryl sulfate complex, azithromycin, calcium, clindamycin phosphate, filgrastim, fluconazole, gentamicin, labetalol, linezolid, metronidazole, pentamidine isethionate, theophylline, vancomycin, vinorelbine tartrate.

I.M.

● Before giving drug, ask patient if he's allergic to penicillins or cephalosporins.

● Obtain specimen for culture and sensitivity tests before giving first dose. Begin therapy while awaiting results.

● Inject deep into a large muscle, such as the gluteus maximus or the lateral aspect of the thigh.

ACTION

Inhibits cell-wall synthesis, promoting osmotic instability; usually bactericidal.

Route	Onset	Peak	Duration
I.V.	Immediate	Immediate	Unknown
I.M.	Unknown	1½–4 hr	Unknown

Half-life: 5½ to 11 hours.

ADVERSE REACTIONS

GI: *pseudomembranous colitis,* diarrhea.
Hematologic: eosinophilia, thrombocytosis, *leukopenia.*
Skin: pain, induration, tenderness at injection site, rash.
Other: hypersensitivity reactions, serum sickness, *anaphylaxis.*

INTERACTIONS

Drug-drug. *Aminoglycosides:* May increase nephrotoxicity and cause synergistic effect against some strains of *Pseudomonas aeruginosa* and *Enterobacteriaceae* species. Monitor patient.
Live-virus vaccines: May decrease effectiveness of live-virus vaccines. Concurrent use isn't recommended.
Probenecid: High doses (1 or 2 g daily) may enhance hepatic clearance of ceftriaxone and shorten its half-life. Avoid using together.
Warfarin: May increase anticoagulation effect. Monitor PT and INR closely.

EFFECTS ON LAB TEST RESULTS

● May increase alkaline phosphatase, ALT, AST, bilirubin, BUN, and LDH levels.
● May increase eosinophil and platelet counts. May decrease WBC count.
● May increase PTT, PT, and INR.
● May falsely increase serum or urine creatinine level in tests using Jaffe reaction. May cause false-positive results of Coombs test and urine glucose tests that use cupric sulfate, such as Benedict reagent and Clinitest.

CONTRAINDICATIONS & CAUTIONS

● Contraindicated in patients hypersensitive to drug or other cephalosporins.
● Use cautiously in patients hypersensitive to penicillin because of possibility of cross-sensitivity with other beta-lactam antibiotics.
● Use cautiously in breast-feeding women and in patients with history of colitis and renal insufficiency.

Reactions in bold italics are *life-threatening*. Interactions may have a *rapid onset* or a *delayed onset*.

NURSING CONSIDERATIONS
• If large doses are given, therapy is prolonged, or patient is at high risk, monitor patient for signs and symptoms of superinfection.
• Monitor PT and INR in patients with impaired vitamin K synthesis or low vitamin K stores. Vitamin K therapy may be needed.
• Drug is commonly used in home antibiotic programs for outpatient treatment of serious infections, such as osteomyelitis and community-acquired pneumonia.
• *Look alike–sound alike:* Don't confuse drug with other cephalosporins that sound alike.

PATIENT TEACHING
• Tell patient to report adverse reactions promptly.
• Instruct patient to report discomfort at I.V. insertion site.
• Teach patient and family receiving home care how to prepare and give drug.
• If home care patient is diabetic and is testing his urine for glucose, tell him drug may affect results of cupric sulfate tests; he should use an enzymatic test instead.
• Tell patient to notify prescriber about loose stools or diarrhea.

cefuroxime axetil
se-fyoor-OX-eem

Ceftin

cefuroxime sodium
Zinacef

Therapeutic class: Antibiotics
Pharmacologic class: Second-generation cephalosporins
Pregnancy risk category: B

AVAILABLE FORMS
cefuroxime axetil
Suspension: 125 mg/5 mL, 250 mg/5 mL
Tablets: 125 mg, 250 mg, 500 mg
cefuroxime sodium
Infusion: 750-mg, 1.5-g vials, infusion packs, and ADD-Vantage vials
Injection: 750 mg, 1.5 g

INDICATIONS & DOSAGES
Adjust-a-dose (for all indications): For injectable form in adults with CrCl of 10 to 20 mL/minute, give 750 mg I.V. or I.M. every 12 hours; if CrCl is less than 10 mL/minute, give 750 mg I.V. or I.M. every 24 hours. Give patients on hemodialysis an additional dose after hemodialysis.
➤ **Serious lower respiratory tract infection, UTI, skin or skin-structure infections, bone or joint infection, septicemia, meningitis, and gonorrhea**
Adults and children age 13 and older: 750 mg to 1.5 g cefuroxime sodium I.V. or I.M. every 8 hours for 5 to 10 days. For life-threatening infections and infections caused by less susceptible organisms, 1.5 g I.V. or I.M. every 6 hours; for bacterial meningitis, up to 3 g I.V. every 8 hours.
Children ages 3 months to 12 years: 50 to 100 mg/kg/day cefuroxime sodium I.V. or I.M. in equally divided doses every 6 to 8 hours. Use higher dosage of 100 mg/kg/day, not to exceed maximum adult dosage, for more severe or serious infections. For bacterial meningitis, 200 to 240 mg/kg/day cefuroxime sodium I.V. in divided doses every 6 to 8 hours.
➤ **Perioperative prophylaxis**
Adults: 1.5 g I.V. 30 to 60 minutes before surgery; in lengthy operations, 750 mg I.V. or I.M. every 8 hours. For open heart surgery, 1.5 g I.V. at induction of anesthesia and then every 12 hours for a total dose of 6 g.
➤ **Bacterial exacerbations of chronic bronchitis or secondary bacterial infection of acute bronchitis**
Adults and children age 13 and older: 250 or 500 mg P.O. b.i.d. for 10 days (chronic bronchitis) or 5 to 10 days (acute bronchitis).
➤ **Acute bacterial maxillary sinusitis**
Adults and children age 13 and older: 250 mg P.O. b.i.d. for 10 days.
Children ages 3 months to 12 years: 250 mg P.O. b.i.d. for 10 days. For children who can't swallow tablets whole, 30 mg/kg/day oral suspension in two divided doses for 10 days. Maximum daily dose for suspension is 1,000 mg.

➤ **Pharyngitis and tonsillitis**
Adults and children age 13 and older:
250 mg P.O. b.i.d. for 10 days.
Children ages 3 months to 12 years:
125 mg P.O. b.i.d. for 10 days. For children who can't swallow tablets whole, give 20 mg/kg daily of oral suspension in two divided doses for 10 days. Maximum daily dose for suspension is 500 mg.

➤ **Otitis media**
Children ages 3 months to 12 years:
250 mg P.O. b.i.d. for 10 days. For children who can't swallow tablets whole, give 30 mg/kg/day of oral suspension divided b.i.d. for 10 days. Maximum daily dose for suspension is 1,000 mg.

➤ **Uncomplicated skin and skin-structure infection**
Adults and children age 13 and older:
250 or 500 mg P.O. b.i.d. for 10 days.

➤ **Uncomplicated UTI**
Adults: 250 mg P.O. b.i.d. for 7 to 10 days.

➤ **Uncomplicated gonorrhea**
Adults: 1,000 mg P.O. as a single dose. Or, 1.5 g I.M. with 1 g probenecid P.O. for one dose.

➤ **Early Lyme disease**
Adults and children age 13 and older:
500 mg P.O. b.i.d. for 20 days.

➤ **Impetigo**
Children ages 3 months to 12 years:
30 mg/kg/day of oral suspension in two divided doses for 10 days. Maximum daily dose, 1,000 mg.

ADMINISTRATION
P.O.
● Before giving drug, ask patient if he's allergic to penicillins or cephalosporins.
● Obtain specimen for culture and sensitivity tests before giving first dose. Therapy may begin while awaiting results.
● Shake suspension well before each use.
● Give tablets without regard for meals; give oral suspension with food.
● Crush tablets, if absolutely necessary, for patients who can't swallow tablets. Tablets may be dissolved in small amounts of apple, orange, or grape juice or chocolate milk. However, the drug has a bitter taste that is difficult to mask, even with food.
● Store suspension at room temperature or under refrigeration. Discard after 10 days.

I.V.
▼ Before giving drug, ask patient if he's allergic to penicillins or cephalosporins.
▼ Obtain specimen for culture and sensitivity tests before giving first dose. Therapy may begin while awaiting results.
▼ Reconstitute each 750-mg vial with 8 mL and each 1.5-g vial with 16 mL of sterile water for injection.
▼ Withdraw entire contents of vial for a dose.
▼ For direct injection, inject over 3 to 5 minutes into a large vein or into the tubing of a free-flowing I.V. solution.
▼ For intermittent infusion, add reconstituted drug to 100 mL D_5W, normal saline solution for injection, or other compatible I.V. solution.
▼ Infuse over 15 to 60 minutes.
▼ **Incompatibilities:** Aminoglycosides, azithromycin, ciprofloxacin, cisatracurium, clarithromycin, cyclophosphamide, doxapram, filgrastim, fluconazole, gentamicin, midazolam, ranitidine, sodium bicarbonate injection, vancomycin, vinorelbine tartrate.

I.M.
● Before giving drug, ask patient if he's allergic to penicillins or cephalosporins.
● Obtain specimen for culture and sensitivity tests before giving first dose. Therapy may begin while awaiting results.
● Reconstitute 750-mg vial with 3 mL sterile water for injection.
● Inject deep into a large muscle, such as the gluteus maximus or the side of the thigh.

ACTION
Inhibits cell-wall synthesis, promoting osmotic instability; usually bactericidal.

Route	Onset	Peak	Duration
P.O.	Unknown	15–60 min	Unknown
I.V.	Immediate	Immediate	Unknown
I.M.	Unknown	2 hr	Unknown

Half-life: 1 to 2 hours.

ADVERSE REACTIONS
CV: phlebitis, thrombophlebitis.
GI: diarrhea, *pseudomembranous colitis,* nausea, anorexia, vomiting.

C

Hematologic: hemolytic anemia, ***thrombocytopenia, transient neutropenia,*** eosinophilia.
Skin: maculopapular and erythematous rashes, urticaria, pain, induration, sterile abscesses, temperature elevation, tissue sloughing at I.M. injection site.
Other: ***anaphylaxis,*** hypersensitivity reactions, serum sickness.

INTERACTIONS
Drug-drug. *Aminoglycosides:* May cause synergistic activity against some organisms; may increase nephrotoxicity. Monitor patient's renal function closely.
Live-virus vaccines: May decrease effectiveness of live-virus vaccines. Concurrent use isn't recommended.
Loop diuretics: May increase risk of adverse renal reactions. Monitor renal function test results closely.
Probenecid: May inhibit excretion and increase cefuroxime level. Probenecid may be used for this effect.
Warfarin: May increase anticoagulation effects. Monitor PT and INR closely.

EFFECTS ON LAB TEST RESULTS
• May increase alkaline phosphatase, ALT, AST, bilirubin, and LDH levels. May decrease hemoglobin level and hematocrit.
• May increase PT and INR and eosinophil count. May decrease neutrophil and platelet counts.
• May falsely increase serum or urine creatinine level in tests using Jaffe reaction. May cause false-positive results of Coombs test and urine glucose tests that use cupric sulfate, such as Benedict reagent and Clinitest.

CONTRAINDICATIONS & CAUTIONS
• Contraindicated in patients hypersensitive to drug or other cephalosporins.
• Use cautiously in patients hypersensitive to penicillin because of possibility of cross-sensitivity with other beta-lactam antibiotics.
• Use cautiously in breast-feeding women and in patients with history of colitis or renal insufficiency.
🕄 **Alert:** Drug may cause pseudomembranous colitis ranging from mild to life-

threatening. Monitor patient for diarrhea and treat appropriately.
• Some cephalosporins have been associated with seizures in patients with renal impairment when the dosage wasn't reduced. If drug-associated seizures occur, discontinue drug and treat with anticonvulsant therapy if indicated.

NURSING CONSIDERATIONS
🕄 **Alert:** Tablets and suspension aren't bioequivalent and can't be substituted milligram-for-milligram.
• Monitor patient for signs and symptoms of superinfection.
• **Look alike–sound alike:** Don't confuse drug with other cephalosporins that sound alike.

PATIENT TEACHING
• Tell patient to take drug as prescribed, even after he feels better.
• If patient has difficulty swallowing tablets, show him how to dissolve or crush tablets, but warn him that the bitter taste is hard to mask, even with food.
• Tell parent to shake suspension well before measuring dose. Suspension may be stored at room temperature or refrigerated, but must be discarded after 10 days.
• Instruct caregiver to give oral suspension with food.
• Instruct patient to notify prescriber about rash, loose stools, diarrhea, or evidence of superinfection.
• Advise patient receiving drug I.V. to report discomfort at I.V. insertion site.

celecoxib
sell-ah-COCKS-ib

Celebrex⌀

Therapeutic class: NSAIDs
Pharmacologic class: Cyclooxygenase-2 inhibitors
Pregnancy risk category: C; D in 3rd trimester

AVAILABLE FORMS
Capsules: 50 mg, 100 mg, 200 mg, 400 mg

INDICATIONS & DOSAGES
Adjust-a-dose (for all indications): For elderly patients and those weighing less than 50 kg (110 lb), start at lowest dosage. For patients with Child-Pugh class B hepatic impairment, reduce dosage by about 50%. For patients who are poor metabolizers of CYP2C9, start treatment at half the lowest recommended dose.

➤ **To relieve signs and symptoms of osteoarthritis**
Adults: 200 mg P.O. daily as a single dose or in two equally divided doses.

➤ **To relieve signs and symptoms of rheumatoid arthritis**
Adults: 100 to 200 mg P.O. b.i.d.

➤ **To relieve signs and symptoms of ankylosing spondylitis**
Adults: 200 mg P.O. once daily or in two divided doses. If no response after 6 weeks, may increase dose to 400 mg daily. If no response after 6 more weeks, consider other treatment.

➤ **To relieve signs and symptoms of juvenile rheumatoid arthritis**
Children age 2 and older weighing 10 to 25 kg (22 to 55 lb): 50 mg P.O. b.i.d.
Children age 2 and older weighing more than 25 kg: 100 mg P.O. b.i.d.

➤ **Acute pain and primary dysmenorrhea**
Adults: 400 mg P.O., initially, followed by another 200-mg dose if needed. On subsequent days, 200 mg P.O. b.i.d. as needed.

ADMINISTRATION
P.O.
● May give dosages up to 200 mg b.i.d. without regard to food.
● For patients who have difficulty swallowing capsules, capsule contents can be added to applesauce. Carefully empty entire contents of capsule onto a level teaspoon of cool or room-temperature applesauce and give immediately with water.

ACTION
Thought to inhibit prostaglandin synthesis, impeding cyclooxygenase-2, to produce anti-inflammatory, analgesic, and antipyretic effects.

Route	Onset	Peak	Duration
P.O.	Unknown	3 hr	Unknown

Half-life: 11 hours.

ADVERSE REACTIONS
CNS: headache, dizziness, insomnia.
CV: hypertension, peripheral edema.
EENT: pharyngitis, rhinitis, sinusitis.
GI: abdominal pain, diarrhea, dyspepsia, flatulence, GI reflux, nausea.
Metabolic: hyperchloremia.
Musculoskeletal: back pain.
Respiratory: dyspnea, upper respiratory tract infection.
Skin: *erythema multiforme, exfoliative dermatitis, Stevens-Johnson syndrome, toxic epidermal necrolysis,* rash.
Other: accidental injury.

INTERACTIONS
Drug-drug. *ACE inhibitors, angiotensin II antagonists:* May decrease antihypertensive effects. Monitor patient's blood pressure.
Antacids containing aluminum or magnesium: May decrease celecoxib level. Separate doses.
Antiplatelets (clopidogrel, prasugrel): May increase bleeding risk. Use cautiously.
Aspirin: May increase risk of ulcers; low aspirin dosages can be used safely to reduce the risk of CV events. Monitor patient for signs and symptoms of GI bleeding.
Corticosteroids, SSRIs: May increase risk of GI bleeding. Use together cautiously.
CYP2C9 inhibitors (amiodarone, metronidazole, ritonavir, zafirlukast): May affect celecoxib metabolism. Use together cautiously.
Fluconazole, voriconazole: May increase celecoxib level. Reduce dosage of celecoxib to minimal effective dose.
Furosemide, thiazides: May reduce sodium excretion caused by diuretics, leading to sodium retention. Monitor patient for swelling and increased blood pressure.
Lithium: May increase lithium level. Monitor lithium level closely during treatment.
Warfarin: May increase PT and bleeding complications. Monitor PT and INR, and check for signs and symptoms of bleeding.
Drug-herb. *Dong quai, feverfew, garlic, ginger, horse chestnut, red clover:* May

---

Reactions in bold italics are *life-threatening*. Interactions may have a *rapid onset* or a *delayed onset*.

increase risk of bleeding. Discourage use together.

White willow: Herb and drug contain similar components. Discourage use together.

Drug-lifestyle. *Long-term alcohol use, smoking:* May cause GI irritation or bleeding. Check for signs and symptoms of bleeding.

EFFECTS ON LAB TEST RESULTS
• May increase ALT, AST, BUN, creatinine, and chloride levels.
• May decrease phosphate level.

CONTRAINDICATIONS & CAUTIONS
Black Box Warning Contraindicated for the treatment of perioperative pain after CABG. ∎
• Contraindicated in patients hypersensitive to drug, sulfonamides, aspirin, or other NSAIDs.
• Contraindicated in those with severe hepatic impairment.
• Avoid use in the third trimester of pregnancy and with any dose of a nonaspirin NSAID.
• Use cautiously in patients with history of ulcers or GI bleeding, advanced renal disease, dehydration, anemia, symptomatic liver disease, hypertension, edema, heart failure, or asthma, and in poor CYP2C9 metabolizers.
• Use cautiously in elderly or debilitated patients.
⚠ *Overdose S&S:* Lethargy, drowsiness, nausea, vomiting, epigastric pain, GI bleeding, hypertension, acute renal failure, respiratory depression, coma, anaphylaxis.

NURSING CONSIDERATIONS
⊕ *Alert:* Patients allergic to or with a history of anaphylactic reactions to sulfonamides, aspirin, or other NSAIDs may be allergic to this drug.
Black Box Warning NSAIDs cause an increased risk of serious GI adverse events, including bleeding, ulceration, and perforation of the stomach or intestines, which can be fatal. Elderly patients are at greater risk. ∎
• Patient with history of ulcers or GI bleeding is at higher risk for GI bleeding while taking NSAIDs such as celecoxib. Other

risk factors for GI bleeding include treatment with corticosteroids or anticoagulants, longer duration of NSAID treatment, smoking, alcoholism, older age, and poor overall health.
• Although drug may be used with low aspirin dosages, the combination may increase risk of GI bleeding.
• Watch for signs and symptoms of overt and occult bleeding.
Black Box Warning NSAIDs may increase the risk of serious thrombotic events, MI, or stroke. The risk may be greater with longer use or in patients with CV disease or risk factors for CV disease. ∎
• Drug can cause fluid retention; monitor patient with hypertension, edema, or heart failure.
• Assess patient for CV risk factors before therapy.
• Drug may be hepatotoxic; watch for signs and symptoms of liver toxicity.
• Before starting drug therapy, rehydrate dehydrated patient.
• Monitor patient's renal function; renal insufficiency is possible in patients with preexisting renal disease. Long-term administration may cause renal papillary necrosis and other renal injury.
• *Look alike–sound alike:* Don't confuse Celebrex with Cerebyx or Celexa.

PATIENT TEACHING
• Tell patient to report history of allergic reactions to sulfonamides, aspirin, or other NSAIDs before therapy.
• Instruct patient to promptly report signs of GI bleeding, such as blood in vomit, urine, or stool; or black, tarry stools.
⊕ *Alert:* Advise patient to immediately report rash, unexplained weight gain, or swelling.
• Tell woman to notify prescriber if she becomes pregnant or is planning to become pregnant during drug therapy.
• Instruct patient to take drug with food if stomach upset occurs.
• Tell patient who has trouble swallowing capsule whole that contents of capsule may be taken with applesauce.
• Tell patient that drug may harm the liver. Advise patient to stop therapy and notify prescriber immediately if he experiences signs and symptoms of hepatic toxicity,

including nausea, fatigue, lethargy, itching, yellowing of skin or eyes, right upper quadrant tenderness, and flulike syndrome.
• Inform patient that it may take several days before he feels consistent pain relief.
• Advise patient that using OTC NSAIDs with celecoxib may increase the risk of GI toxicity.

cephalexin
sef-a-LEX-in

Apo-Cephalex†, Keflex, Novo-Lexin†

Therapeutic class: Antibiotics
Pharmacologic class: First-generation cephalosporins
Pregnancy risk category: B

AVAILABLE FORMS
Capsules: 250 mg, 500 mg, 750 mg
Oral suspension: 125 mg/5 mL, 250 mg/5 mL
Tablets: 250 mg, 500 mg

INDICATIONS & DOSAGES
➤ **Respiratory tract, GI tract, GU tract, skin, soft-tissue, bone, and joint infections and otitis media caused by** *Escherichia coli* **and other coliform bacteria, group A beta-hemolytic streptococci,** *Klebsiella* **species,** *Proteus mirabilis,* *Streptococcus pneumoniae,* **and staphylococci**
Adults: 250 mg to 1 g P.O. every 6 hours or 500 mg every 12 hours. Maximum 4 g daily.
Children: 25 to 50 mg/kg/day P.O. in two to four equally divided doses. For otitis media and severe infections, dose can be doubled. Don't exceed recommended adult dosage.
Adjust-a-dose: For patients with impaired renal function, safe dosage may be lower than that usually recommended.

ADMINISTRATION
P.O.
• Before giving, ask patient if he's allergic to penicillins or cephalosporins.
• Obtain specimen for culture and sensitivity tests before giving. Begin therapy while awaiting results.

• To prepare oral suspension, add required amount of water to powder in two portions. Shake well after each addition. After mixing, store in refrigerator. Mixture will remain stable for 14 days. Keep tightly closed and shake well before using.
• Give drug with food or milk to lessen GI discomfort.

ACTION
Inhibits cell-wall synthesis, promoting osmotic instability; usually bactericidal.

Route	Onset	Peak	Duration
P.O.	Unknown	1 hr	Unknown

Half-life: 30 minutes to 1 hour.

ADVERSE REACTIONS
CNS: dizziness, headache, fatigue, agitation, confusion, hallucinations.
GI: anorexia, diarrhea, *pseudomembranous colitis,* gastritis, glossitis, dyspepsia, abdominal pain, anal pruritus, tenesmus, oral candidiasis.
GU: genital pruritus, candidiasis, vaginitis, interstitial nephritis.
Hematologic: *neutropenia, thrombocytopenia,* eosinophilia, anemia.
Musculoskeletal: arthritis, arthralgia, joint pain.
Skin: maculopapular and erythematous rashes, urticaria.
Other: *anaphylaxis,* hypersensitivity reactions, serum sickness.

INTERACTIONS
Drug-drug. *Aminoglycosides:* May increase risk of nephrotoxicity. Avoid using together.
Live-virus vaccines: May decrease effectiveness of live-virus vaccines. Concurrent use isn't recommended.
Metformin: May increase metformin level. Monitor blood glucose level closely.
Probenecid: May increase cephalosporin level. Use probenecid for this effect.

EFFECTS ON LAB TEST RESULTS
• May increase alkaline phosphatase, ALT, AST, bilirubin, and LDH levels. May decrease hemoglobin level.
• May increase eosinophil count. May decrease neutrophil and platelet counts.

• May falsely increase serum or urine creatinine level in tests using Jaffe reaction. May cause false-positive results of Coombs test and urine glucose tests that use cupric sulfate, such as Benedict reagent and Clinitest.

CONTRAINDICATIONS & CAUTIONS
• Contraindicated in patients hypersensitive to cephalosporins.
• Use cautiously in patients hypersensitive to penicillin because of possibility of cross-sensitivity with other beta-lactam antibiotics.
• Use cautiously in breast-feeding women and in patients with history of colitis or renal insufficiency.
🕄 *Alert:* Drug can cause pseudomembranous colitis ranging from mild to life-threatening. Monitor patient for diarrhea and treat appropriately.
⚠ *Overdose S&S:* Nausea, vomiting, epigastric distress, diarrhea, hematuria.

NURSING CONSIDERATIONS
• If large doses are given or if therapy is prolonged, monitor patient for superinfection, especially if patient is high risk.
• Treat group A beta-hemolytic streptococcal infections for a minimum of 10 days.
• *Look alike–sound alike:* Don't confuse Keflex with Keppra. Don't confuse drug with other cephalosporins that sound alike.

PATIENT TEACHING
• Tell patient to take drug exactly as prescribed, even if feeling better.
• Instruct patient to take drug with food or milk to lessen GI discomfort. If patient is taking suspension form, instruct him to shake container well before measuring dose and to store in refrigerator.
• Tell patient to notify prescriber if rash or signs and symptoms of superinfection develop.

certolizumab pegol
SERT-oh-LIZ-u-mahb PEGH-ol

Cimzia

Therapeutic class: Immune response modifiers
Pharmacologic class: TNF blockers
Pregnancy risk category: B

AVAILABLE FORMS
Lyophilized powder for injection: 200 mg
Prefilled syringe: 200 mg/mL

INDICATIONS & DOSAGES
➤ **Crohn disease when response to conventional therapy is inadequate**
Adults: Initially and at weeks 2 and 4, 400 mg subcutaneously (given as two injections of 200 mg each), followed by a maintenance dose of 400 mg subcutaneously every 4 weeks, if adequate response.
➤ **Rheumatoid arthritis**
Adults: Initially and at weeks 2 and 4, 400 mg subcutaneously (given as two injections of 200 mg each), followed by maintenance dose of 200 mg every other week or 400 mg every 4 weeks.
✴ *NEW INDICATION:* **Psoriatic arthritis; active ankylosing spondylitis**
Adults: 400 mg subcutaneously (given as two injections of 200 mg each) initially; repeat dose at week 2 and then again at week 4. Maintenance dosage is 200 mg subcutaneously every other week, or 400 mg subcutaneously every 4 weeks.

ADMINISTRATION
Subcutaneous
• Bring drug to room temperature before reconstituting.
• Each 400-mg dose requires two vials. Reconstitute each vial with 1 mL of sterile water for injection, using a 20G needle. Gently swirl the vial without shaking. May take up to 30 minutes to fully reconstitute. Inspect vial for particulate matter and discoloration, and discard if present.
• Draw up each vial in its own syringe, switching each 20G needle to a 23G needle. Inject prepared or prefilled syringes into separate sites in the abdomen or thigh.

● Reconstituted drug is stable for 2 hours at room temperature or for up to 24 hours if refrigerated.

● Give at room temperature.

ACTION

Selectively neutralizes TNFα, a proinflammatory cytokine responsible for stimulating the production of inflammatory mediators.

Route	Onset	Peak	Duration
Subcut.	Unknown	54–171 hr	Unknown

Half-life: 14 days.

ADVERSE REACTIONS

CNS: anxiety, bipolar disorder, *suicide attempt.*
CV: angina pectoris, *arrhythmias, heart failure,* hypertensive heart disease, *MI,* pericardial effusion and pericarditis, vasculitis.
EENT: optic neuritis, retinal hemorrhage, uveitis.
GI: abdominal pain.
GU: UTI.
Hematologic: anemia, *leukopenia,* lymphadenopathy, *pancytopenia,* thrombophilia.
Hepatic: elevated liver enzymes, *hepatitis.*
Musculoskeletal: arthralgia, extremity pain.
Respiratory: upper respiratory tract infection.
Skin: alopecia, dermatitis, peripheral edema, erythema nodosum, urticaria, injection-site pain and erythema.
Other: *tuberculosis and opportunistic infection, Stevens-Johnson syndrome, toxic epidermal necrolysis, erythema multiforme.*

INTERACTIONS

Drug-drug. *Abatacept, anakinra, natalizumab, rituximab:* May increase risk of serious infection and neutropenia. Avoid using together.
Live-virus vaccines: May cause infection. Avoid using together.

EFFECTS ON LAB TEST RESULTS

● May falsely elevate PTT.

CONTRAINDICATIONS & CAUTIONS

● Use cautiously in patients with known hypersensitivity to other TNF blockers and those with underlying conditions that may increase the risk of infections.

Black Box Warning Patients treated with certolizumab are at increased risk for serious infections that may lead to hospitalization or death. Most patients who developed these infections were taking concomitant immunosuppressants, such as methotrexate or corticosteroids. ■

Black Box Warning Prophylactic antifungal therapy should be considered for patients at risk for invasive fungal infections who develop severe systemic illness. ■

● Use cautiously in those with a history of recurrent infections or concomitant immunosuppressive therapy, or in those who have resided in regions where tuberculosis and histoplasmosis are endemic. Avoid use in patients with active infections.

● Use cautiously in patients with a history of CNS demyelinating disorder, hematologic disorders, or heart failure.

● Use during pregnancy only when benefits to mother outweigh the risks to fetus.

● It isn't known whether drug appears in breast milk. Advise stopping breast-feeding during therapy.

Black Box Warning Certolizumab isn't indicated for use in children because of the risk of lymphoma and other malignancies reported with the use of TNF blockers. ■

● Use cautiously in elderly patients because of increased risk for infection.

NURSING CONSIDERATIONS

Black Box Warning Monitor patient for signs and symptoms of tuberculosis, invasive fungal infection, and other opportunistic infections during and after treatment. Discontinue treatment if serious infection develops. Fatal infections have occurred. ■

● Before initiating therapy, evaluate patient for tuberculosis risk factors and test for latent tuberculosis infection.

● Before therapy, consider antituberculosis therapy in patients with past history of latent or active tuberculosis when adequate treatment can't be confirmed.

Reactions in bold italics are *life-threatening.* Interactions may have a *rapid onset* or a *delayed onset.*

• Before therapy, evaluate patients at risk for hepatitis B virus (HBV) infection and test for previous HBV infection.

PATIENT TEACHING

Black Box Warning Teach patient to seek prompt medical attention if persistent fever, cough, shortness of breath, or fatigue develops. ▪

• Advise patient to seek immediate medical attention for signs and symptoms of infection or for unusual bruising or bleeding.

• Instruct patient to seek immediate medical attention if any symptoms of severe allergic reaction develop.

• Tell patient to report signs and symptoms of heart failure.

• Show patient how to self-administer prefilled syringes and how to properly dispose of needles and syringes.

---

cetirizine hydrochloride
se-TEER-i-zeen

All Day Allergy ◊, Zyrtec ◊

Therapeutic class: Antihistamines
Pharmacologic class: Piperazine derivatives
Pregnancy risk category: B

AVAILABLE FORMS

Capsules: 10 mg ◊
Syrup: 5 mg/5 mL ◊
Tablets: 5 mg ◊, 10 mg ◊
Tablets (chewable): 5 mg ◊, 10 mg ◊

INDICATIONS & DOSAGES

Adjust-a-dose (for all indications): For adults and children age 6 and older receiving hemodialysis, those with hepatic impairment, those with CrCl less than 31 mL/minute, and patients age 65 and older, give 5 mg P.O. daily. Don't use in children younger than age 6 with renal or hepatic impairment.

➤ **Seasonal allergic rhinitis**
Adults and children age 6 and older: 5 to 10 mg P.O. once daily.
Children ages 2 to 5: 2.5 mg P.O. once daily. Maximum daily dose is 5 mg.

➤ **Perennial allergic rhinitis, chronic urticaria**
Adults and children age 6 and older: 5 to 10 mg P.O. once daily.
Children ages 6 months to 5 years: 2.5 mg P.O. once daily; in children ages 1 to 5, increase to maximum of 5 mg daily. Children ages 12 to 23 months should receive the 5-mg dose as two divided doses.

ADMINISTRATION
P.O.
• Give drug without regard for food.

ACTION
A long-acting, nonsedating antihistamine that selectively inhibits peripheral H_1 receptors.

Route	Onset	Peak	Duration
P.O.	Rapid	60 min	24 hr

Half-life: About 8 hours.

ADVERSE REACTIONS
CNS: somnolence, fatigue, dizziness, headache.
EENT: pharyngitis.
GI: dry mouth, nausea, vomiting, abdominal distress.

INTERACTIONS
Drug-drug. *CNS depressants:* May cause additive effect. Monitor patient closely for excessive sedation or other adverse effects.
Theophylline: May decrease cetirizine clearance. Monitor patient closely.
Drug-lifestyle. *Alcohol use:* May cause additive effects. Discourage use together.

EFFECTS ON LAB TEST RESULTS
• May prevent, reduce, or mask positive result in diagnostic skin test.

CONTRAINDICATIONS & CAUTIONS
• Contraindicated in patients hypersensitive to drug or to hydroxyzine and in breast-feeding women.
• Use cautiously in patients with renal or hepatic impairment.
⚠ *Overdose S&S:* Somnolence; initial restlessness and irritability, then drowsiness.

NURSING CONSIDERATIONS
- Stop drug 4 days before diagnostic skin testing because antihistamines can prevent, reduce, or mask positive skin test response.
- *Look alike–sound alike:* Don't confuse cetirizine with sertraline. Don't confuse Zyrtec with Lipitor, Zocor, Zyprexa, or Zantac.

PATIENT TEACHING
- Warn patient not to perform hazardous activities until CNS effects of drug are known. Somnolence is a common adverse reaction.
- Advise patient not to use alcohol or other CNS depressants while taking drug.
- Inform patient that sugarless gum, hard candy, or ice chips may relieve dry mouth.

SAFETY ALERT!

cetuximab
seh-TUX-eh-mab

Erbitux

Therapeutic class: Antineoplastics
Pharmacologic class: Monoclonal antibodies
Pregnancy risk category: C

AVAILABLE FORMS
Injection: 2 mg/mL

INDICATIONS & DOSAGES
Adjust-a-dose (for all indications): If patient develops a grade 1 or 2 National Cancer Institute Common Toxicity Criteria (NCI-CTC) infusion reaction or a nonserious grade 3 NCI-CTC infusion reaction, permanently reduce infusion rate by 50%. If patient develops a serious infusion reaction requiring medical intervention or hospitalization, stop drug immediately and permanently. If patient develops a severe acneiform rash, follow these guidelines:
- After first occurrence, delay infusion 1 to 2 weeks. If patient improves, continue at 250 mg/m^2. If patient doesn't improve, stop drug.
- After second occurrence, delay infusion 1 to 2 weeks. If patient improves, reduce dose to 200 mg/m^2. If patient doesn't improve, stop drug.
- After third occurrence, delay infusion 1 to 2 weeks. If patient improves, reduce dose to 150 mg/m^2. If patient doesn't improve, stop drug.
- After fourth occurrence, stop drug.

➤ **Squamous cell carcinoma of the head and neck**
Adults: A loading dose of 400 mg/m^2 I.V. over 2 hours (maximum rate, 10 mg/minute) followed by weekly maintenance dose of 250 mg/m^2 I.V. over 1 hour. If used with radiation therapy, begin drug 1 week before radiation course or on day of initiation of platinum-based therapy with 5-FU. Complete administration 1 hour before radiation or platinum-based therapy with 5-FU. Continue for the duration (6 or 7 weeks) of radiation therapy or until disease progression or unacceptable toxicity occurs. If used as monotherapy for recurrent or metastatic disease after failure of platinum-based therapy, continue until disease progresses or unacceptable toxicity occurs.
➤ **K-Ras mutation-negative (wild type), epidermal growth factor receptor–expressing, metastatic colorectal cancer as determined by FDA-approved tests in combination with FOLFIRI (irinotecan, 5-FU, leucovorin) chemotherapy regimen for first-line treatment, or in combination with irinotecan in patients refractory to irinotecan-based chemotherapy, or as a single agent in patients who have failed oxaliplatin- and irinotecan-based chemotherapy or who are intolerant to irinotecan**
Adults: Loading dose, 400 mg/m^2 I.V. over 2 hours (maximum, 10 mg/minute). Complete drug administration 1 hour before initiating FOLFIRI regimen. Maintenance dosage, 250 mg/m^2 I.V. weekly over 1 hour (maximum, 10 mg/minute) until disease progression or unacceptable toxicity occurs.

ADMINISTRATION
I.V.
▼ Premedicate with an H$_1$-antagonist such as diphenhydramine 50 mg I.V. 30 to 60 minutes before first dose. Premedication before subsequent doses should be based on clinical judgment and severity of prior infusion reactions.

Reactions in bold italics are *life-threatening*. Interactions may have a *rapid onset* or a *delayed onset*.

▼ Solution should be clear and colorless and may contain a small amount of particulates.

▼ Don't shake or dilute.

▼ Drug can be given by infusion pump or syringe pump, piggybacked into the patient's infusion line. Don't give drug by I.V. push or bolus.

▼ Give drug through a low–protein-binding 0.22-micrometer in-line filter.

▼ Flush line with normal saline solution at the end of the infusion.

▼ Store vials at 36° to 46° F (2° to 8° C). Don't freeze.

▼ Solution in infusion container is stable up to 12 hours at 36° to 46° F (2° to 8° C) and up to 8 hours at 68° to 77° F (20° to 25° C).

▼ **Incompatibilities:** Don't dilute with other solutions.

ACTION

An epidermal growth factor receptor (EGFR) antagonist that binds to the EGFR on normal and tumor cells, inhibiting epidermal growth factor from binding, which interrupts cell growth, induces cell death, and decreases growth factor production.

Route	Onset	Peak	Duration
I.V.	Unknown	Unknown	Unknown

Half-life: 4.6 days.

ADVERSE REACTIONS

CNS: asthenia, depression, fever, headache, insomnia, pain.
CV: edema, *cardiopulmonary arrest.*
EENT: conjunctivitis.
GI: abdominal pain, anorexia, constipation, diarrhea, dyspepsia, dysphagia, mucositis, nausea, stomatitis, vomiting, xerostomia.
GU: *acute renal failure.*
Hematologic: anemia, *leukopenia.*
Metabolic: dehydration, *hypomagnesemia,* weight loss.
Musculoskeletal: back pain.
Respiratory: cough, dyspnea, *pulmonary embolus.*
Skin: alopecia, maculopapular rash, nail disorder, pruritus, radiation dermatitis, acneiform rash.
Other: *anaphylactoid reaction,* chills, infection, infusion reaction, *sepsis.*

INTERACTIONS

Drug-drug. *Live-virus vaccines:* May decrease immune response. Avoid using together.
Drug-lifestyle. *Sun exposure:* May worsen skin reactions. Advise patient to avoid excessive sun exposure.

EFFECTS ON LAB TEST RESULTS

● May decrease magnesium, calcium, and potassium levels.

CONTRAINDICATIONS & CAUTIONS

● Use cautiously in patients hypersensitive to drug, its components, or murine proteins. If used with radiation, use cautiously in patients with a history of coronary artery disease, arrhythmias, and heart failure.
● Determine *K-Ras* mutation and epidermal growth factor receptor–expression status using FDA-approved tests before initiating treatment for colorectal cancer. Drug isn't indicated for treatment of *K-Ras* mutation–positive colorectal cancer.
● Drug is a potential teratogen. Follow safe handling procedures when preparing or administering.

NURSING CONSIDERATIONS

Black Box Warning Severe infusion reactions, including acute airway obstruction, urticaria, and hypotension, may occur, usually with the first infusion. If a severe infusion reaction occurs, stop drug immediately and give symptomatic treatment. ∎

● Keep epinephrine, corticosteroids, I.V. antihistamines, bronchodilators, and oxygen available for severe infusion reactions.
● Manage mild to moderate infusion reactions by decreasing infusion rate and premedicating with an antihistamine for subsequent infusions.
● Monitor patient for infusion reactions for 1 hour after infusion ends.
● Assess patient for acute onset or worsening of pulmonary symptoms. If interstitial lung disease is confirmed, stop drug.
● Monitor patient for skin toxicity, which starts most often during first 2 weeks of therapy. Treat with topical and oral antibiotics.
● Periodically monitor serum electrolyte levels during and for at least 8 weeks after therapy ends.

Black Box Warning In patients also receiving radiation therapy or platinum-based therapy with 5-FU, closely monitor electrolytes, especially magnesium, potassium, and calcium, during and after therapy. Cardiopulmonary arrest or sudden death has occurred. ■

● It's unknown if drug appears in breast milk. Women shouldn't breast-feed until 60 days after last dose.

PATIENT TEACHING
● Tell patient to promptly report adverse reactions.
● Inform patient that skin reactions may occur, typically during the first 2 weeks of treatment.
● Advise patient to avoid prolonged or unprotected sun exposure during and 2 months after treatment.

SAFETY ALERT!

chlordiazepoxide hydrochloride
klor-dye-az-e-POX-ide

Librium

Therapeutic class: Anxiolytics
Pharmacologic class: Benzodiazepines
Pregnancy risk category: D
Controlled substance schedule: IV

AVAILABLE FORMS
Capsules: 5 mg, 10 mg, 25 mg

INDICATIONS & DOSAGES
Adjust-a-dose (for all indications): In elderly or debilitated patients give 5 mg P.O. b.i.d. to q.i.d. Use the smallest effective dose to prevent oversedation or ataxia.
➤ **Mild to moderate anxiety**
Adults: 5 to 10 mg P.O. t.i.d. or q.i.d.
Children older than age 6: 5 mg P.O. b.i.d. to q.i.d. Maximum, 10 mg P.O. b.i.d. or t.i.d.
➤ **Severe anxiety**
Adults: 20 to 25 mg P.O. t.i.d. or q.i.d.
➤ **Withdrawal symptoms of acute alcoholism**
Adults: 50 to 100 mg P.O. Repeat as needed, up to 300 mg daily.

➤ **Preoperative apprehension and anxiety**
Adults: 5 to 10 mg P.O. t.i.d. or q.i.d. on day before surgery.

ADMINISTRATION
P.O.
● **Alert:** 5-mg and 25-mg capsules may look similar in color through the packaging. Verify contents and read label carefully.

ACTION
A benzodiazepine that may potentiate the effects of GABA, depress the CNS, and suppress the spread of seizure activity.

Route	Onset	Peak	Duration
P.O.	Unknown	½–4 hr	Unknown

Half-life: 24 to 48 hours.

ADVERSE REACTIONS
CNS: drowsiness, lethargy, ataxia, confusion, extrapyramidal reactions, minor changes in EEG patterns.
CV: edema.
GI: nausea, constipation.
GU: menstrual irregularities.
Hematologic: *agranulocytosis.*
Hepatic: jaundice.
Skin: swelling and pain at injection site, skin eruptions.
Other: altered libido.

INTERACTIONS
Drug-drug. *Cimetidine:* May decrease chlordiazepoxide clearance and increase risk of adverse reactions. Monitor patient carefully.
CNS depressants: May increase CNS depression. Use together cautiously.
Digoxin: May increase digoxin level and risk of toxicity. Monitor patient and digoxin level closely.
Disulfiram: May decrease clearance and increase half-life of chlordiazepoxide. Monitor patient for enhanced effects. Consider dosage adjustment.
Fluconazole, itraconazole, ketoconazole, miconazole: May increase and prolong chlordiazepoxide levels, CNS depression, and psychomotor impairment. Avoid using together.

Reactions in bold italics are *life-threatening*. Interactions may have a *rapid onset* or a *delayed onset*.

Levodopa: May decrease control of parkinsonian symptoms in patients with Parkinson disease. Use together cautiously.

Drug-herb. *Kava:* May increase sedation. Discourage use together.

Drug-lifestyle. *Alcohol use:* May cause additive CNS effects. Discourage use together.

Smoking: May decrease effectiveness of drug. Monitor patient closely.

EFFECTS ON LAB TEST RESULTS
• May increase LFT values. May decrease granulocyte count.

• May cause a false-positive pregnancy test result. May alter urinary 17-ketosteroid (Zimmerman reaction), urine alkaloid (Frings thin-layer chromatography method), and urinary glucose determinations (with Chemstrip uG and Diastix).

CONTRAINDICATIONS & CAUTIONS
• Contraindicated in patients hypersensitive to drug and in pregnant women, especially in first trimester.

• Use cautiously in elderly patients and in patients with mental depression, history of substance abuse, porphyria, or hepatic or renal disease.

⚠ **Overdose S&S:** Somnolence, confusion, coma, diminished reflexes.

NURSING CONSIDERATIONS
• In patients receiving repeated or prolonged therapy, monitor hepatic, renal, and hematopoietic function periodically.

• Watch for paradoxical reaction in psychiatric patients and hyperactive, aggressive children.

• **Alert:** Use of this drug may lead to abuse and addiction. Don't withdraw drug abruptly after long-term use because withdrawal symptoms may occur.

• **Look alike–sound alike:** Don't confuse chlordiazepoxide with chlorpromazine. Don't confuse Librium with Librax.

PATIENT TEACHING
• Warn patient to avoid hazardous activities that require alertness and coordination until effects of drug are known.

• Tell patient to avoid use of alcohol while taking drug.

• Notify patient that smoking may decrease drug's effectiveness.

• Warn patient that drug may cause psychological and physical dependence. Tell patient not to increase dose or abruptly stop the drug because withdrawal symptoms may occur.

• Warn women to avoid use during pregnancy.

chloroquine phosphate
KLO-ro-kwin

Aralen

Therapeutic class: Antimalarials
Pharmacologic class: Aminoquinolines
Pregnancy risk category: C

AVAILABLE FORMS
Tablets: 250 mg (equivalent to 150 mg base), 500 mg (equivalent to 300 mg base)

INDICATIONS & DOSAGES
Black Box Warning Prescribers should be completely familiar with this drug before prescribing. ∎

➤ **Acute malarial attacks caused by** *Plasmodium vivax, P. malariae, P. ovale,* **and susceptible strains of** *P. falciparum*
Adults: Initially, 600 mg base P.O.; then 300 mg base at 6, 24, and 48 hours.
Children: Initially, 10 mg/kg base P.O.; then 5 mg/kg base at 6, 24, and 48 hours. Don't exceed adult dose.

➤ **To prevent malaria**
Adults: 300 mg base P.O. once weekly on the same day each week, for 1 to 2 weeks before entering a malaria-endemic area and continued for 8 weeks after leaving the area. If treatment begins after exposure, give 600 mg base P.O. initially, in two divided doses 6 hours apart, followed by the usual dosing regimen.
Children: 5 mg/kg base P.O. once weekly on the same day each week, for 1 to 2 weeks before entering a malaria-endemic area and continued for 4 to 8 weeks after leaving the area. Don't exceed 300 mg base. If treatment begins after exposure, give 10 mg/kg base P.O. initially, in two divided doses 6 hours apart, followed by the usual dosing regimen.

➤ **Extraintestinal amebiasis**
Adults: 600 mg base P.O. once daily for
2 days; then 300 mg base daily for 2 to
3 weeks. Treatment is usually combined
with an intestinal amebicide.

ADMINISTRATION
P.O.
🟊 *Alert:* Drug dosage may be discussed in "mg"
or "mg base"; be aware of the difference.
● To improve compliance when drug is used
for prevention, advise patient to take drug
immediately before or after a meal on the
same day each week.

ACTION
May bind to and alter the properties of DNA
in susceptible parasites.

Route	Onset	Peak	Duration
P.O.	Unknown	1–3 hr	Unknown

Half-life: 1 to 2 months.

ADVERSE REACTIONS
CNS: *seizures,* mild and transient headache,
psychic stimulation, neuropathy.
CV: hypotension, ECG changes.
EENT: blurred vision, difficulty in focusing, reversible corneal changes; typically
irreversible, sometimes progressive or delayed retinal changes such as narrowing
of arterioles, macular lesions, pallor of
optic disk, optic atrophy, patchy retinal pigmentation, typically leading to blindness;
ototoxicity, nerve deafness, vertigo, tinnitus.
GI: anorexia, abdominal cramps, diarrhea,
nausea, vomiting.
Hematologic: *agranulocytosis, aplastic
anemia, thrombocytopenia,* hemolytic
anemia.
Skin: pruritus, lichen planus eruptions,
skin and mucosal pigmentary changes,
pleomorphic skin eruptions.

INTERACTIONS
Drug-drug. *Aluminum salts (kaolin), magnesium:* May decrease GI absorption. Separate dose times.
Cimetidine: May decrease hepatic metabolism
of chloroquine. Monitor patient for toxicity.
Drug-lifestyle. *Sun exposure:* May worsen
drug-induced dermatoses. Advise patient to
avoid excessive sun exposure.

EFFECTS ON LAB TEST RESULTS
● May decrease hemoglobin level.
● May decrease granulocyte and platelet
counts.

CONTRAINDICATIONS & CAUTIONS
● Contraindicated in patients hypersensitive
to drug and in those with retinal or visual
field changes or porphyria.
● Use cautiously in patients with severe
GI, neurologic, or blood disorders; hepatic
disease or alcoholism; or G6PD deficiency
or psoriasis.
⚠ *Overdose S&S:* Headache, drowsiness,
visual disturbances, nausea, vomiting, CV
collapse, seizures, sudden and early respiratory and cardiac arrest; atrial standstill,
nodal rhythm, prolonged intraventricular
conduction time, progressive bradycardia
leading to ventricular fibrillation or arrest.

NURSING CONSIDERATIONS
● Ensure that baseline and periodic ophthalmic examinations are performed. Check
periodically for ocular muscle weakness
after long-term use.
● Make sure patient is tested with an audiometer before, during, and after therapy,
especially if therapy is long-term.
● Monitor CBC and LFTs periodically
during long-term therapy. If a severe blood
disorder—not caused by the disease—
develops, drug may need to be stopped.
🟊 *Alert:* Monitor patient for overdose, which
can quickly lead to toxic symptoms. Children are extremely susceptible to toxicity;
avoid long-term treatment.

PATIENT TEACHING
● To improve compliance when using drug
for prevention, advise patient to take drug
immediately before or after a meal on the
same day each week.
● Instruct patient to avoid excessive sun
exposure to prevent worsening of drug-
induced dermatoses.
● Tell patient to report adverse reactions
promptly, especially blurred vision, increased sensitivity to light, tinnitus, hearing
loss, or muscle weakness.
● Instruct patient to keep drug out of reach
of children. Overdose may be fatal.

Reactions in bold italics are *life-threatening*. Interactions may have a *rapid onset* or a *delayed onset*.

chlorpheniramine maleate
klor-fen-IR-a-meen

Allergy Time ◇, ChlorTabs ◇,
Chlor-Trimeton ◇, Chlor-Trimeton
Allergy 12 Hour ◇, Diabetic Tussin
Allergy ◇

Therapeutic class: Antihistamines
Pharmacologic class: Alkylamines
Pregnancy risk category: C

AVAILABLE FORMS
Syrup ◇*:* 2 mg/5 mL*
Tablets ◇*:* 4 mg
Tablets (extended-release) ◇*:* 8 mg, 12 mg

INDICATIONS & DOSAGES
➤ **Allergic rhinitis**
Adults and children age 12 and older:
4 mg P.O. every 4 to 6 hours, not to exceed
24 mg daily. Or, 8 to 12 mg extended-release
P.O. every 8 to 12 hours, not to exceed
24 mg daily. Or, 16 mg extended-release
P.O. once daily.
Children ages 6 to 12: 2 mg P.O. every 4 to
6 hours, not to exceed 12 mg daily.
Children ages 2 to 6: 1 mg P.O. every 4 to
6 hours, not to exceed 6 mg daily.

ADMINISTRATION
P.O.
• May be given without regard for food.
• Give extended-release tablets whole and
not crushed or divided.
• Measure and give syrup using dosing
syringe, dosing spoon, or dosing cup.

ACTION
Competes with histamine for H_1-receptor
sites on effector cells. Drug prevents, but
doesn't reverse, histamine-mediated responses.

Route	Onset	Peak	Duration
P.O.	15–60 min	2–6 hr	24 hr

Half-life: Adults with normal renal and hepatic
function, 12 to 43 hours; children with normal
renal and hepatic function, 9½ to 13 hours; chronic
renal failure on hemodialysis, 11½ to 13¾ days.

ADVERSE REACTIONS
CNS: drowsiness, stimulation, sedation,
excitability in children.
CV: hypotension, palpitations, weak pulse.
GI: dry mouth, epigastric distress.
GU: urine retention.
Respiratory: thick bronchial secretions.
Skin: rash, urticaria, pallor.

INTERACTIONS
Drug-drug. *CNS depressants:* May increase
sedation. Use together cautiously.
MAO inhibitors: May increase anticholiner-
gic effects. Avoid using together.
Drug-lifestyle. *Alcohol use:* May increase
CNS depression. Discourage use together.

EFFECTS ON LAB TEST RESULTS
• May prevent, reduce, or mask positive
result in diagnostic skin test.

CONTRAINDICATIONS & CAUTIONS
• Contraindicated in patients having acute
asthmatic attacks and in those with angle-
closure glaucoma, symptomatic prostatic
hyperplasia, pyloroduodenal obstruction, or
bladder neck obstruction.
• Contraindicated in breast-feeding women
and in patients taking MAO inhibitors.
• Use cautiously in elderly patients and in
those with increased intraocular pressure,
hyperthyroidism, hypertension, bronchial
asthma, urine retention, prostatic hyperplasia, stenosing peptic ulcerations, and CV,
liver, or renal disease.
⚠ **Overdose S&S:** CNS depression or stimulation, tinnitus, blurred vision, dizziness,
ataxia, hypotension, dry mouth, fixed dilated
pupils, flushing, hypothermia, GI symptoms.

NURSING CONSIDERATIONS
• Stop drug 4 days before diagnostic skin
testing because antihistamines can prevent,
reduce, or mask positive skin test response.

PATIENT TEACHING
• Warn patient to avoid alcohol and haz-
ardous activities that require alertness until
CNS effects of drug are known.
• Inform patient that sugarless gum, hard
candy, or ice chips may relieve dry mouth.

• Instruct patient to notify prescriber if tolerance develops because a different antihistamine may need to be prescribed.
• Advise patient that extended-release tablets should be swallowed whole and not crushed, chewed, or divided.
• Advise patient or caregiver to measure and give oral syrup by dosing syringe, dosing spoon, or dosing cup for accuracy.

chlorproMAZINE hydrochloride
klor-PROE-ma-zeen

Therapeutic class: Antipsychotics
Pharmacologic class: Phenothiazines
Pregnancy risk category: Undetermined

AVAILABLE FORMS
Injection: 25 mg/mL
Tablets: 10 mg, 25 mg, 50 mg, 100 mg, 200 mg

INDICATIONS & DOSAGES
➤ **Psychosis, mania**
Adults and children older than age 12: For hospitalized patients with acute disease, 25 mg I.M.; may give an additional 25 to 50 mg I.M. in 1 hour if needed. Increase over several days to 400 mg every 4 to 6 hours. Switch to oral therapy as soon as possible. Or, 25 mg P.O. t.i.d. initially; then gradually increase to 400 mg daily in divided doses. For outpatients, 30 to 75 mg daily in two to four divided doses. Increase dosage by 20 to 50 mg twice weekly until symptoms are controlled.
➤ **Nausea and vomiting**
Adults and children older than age 12: 10 to 25 mg P.O. every 4 to 6 hours, p.r.n. Or, 25 mg I.M. initially. If no hypotension occurs, 25 to 50 mg I.M. every 3 to 4 hours may be given, p.r.n., until vomiting stops.
Children ages 6 months to 12 years: 0.55 mg/kg P.O. every 4 to 6 hours or I.M. every 6 to 8 hours. Maximum I.M. dose in children younger than age 5 or weighing less than 23 kg (50 lb) is 40 mg. Maximum I.M. dose in children ages 5 to 12 or weighing 23 to 45 kg (50 to 100 lb) is 75 mg.

➤ **Acute intermittent porphyria, intractable hiccups**
Adults and children older than age 12: 25 to 50 mg P.O. t.i.d. or q.i.d. If hiccups persist for 2 to 3 days, 25 to 50 mg I.M. If hiccups still persist, 25 to 50 mg diluted in 500 to 1,000 mL of normal saline solution and infused slowly with patient in supine position.
➤ **Tetanus**
Adults and children older than age 12: 25 to 50 mg I.V. or I.M. t.i.d. or q.i.d.
Children ages 6 months to 12 years: 0.55 mg/kg I.M. or I.V. every 6 to 8 hours. Maximum parenteral dosage in children weighing less than 23 kg (50 lb) is 40 mg daily; for children weighing 23 to 45 kg (50 to 100 lb), 75 mg, except in severe cases. If giving I.V., dilute to 1 mg/mL with normal saline solution and give at a rate of 0.5 mg/minute.
➤ **Behavioral disorders; hyperactivity**
Children ages 6 months to 12 years: For outpatients: 0.55 mg/kg P.O. every 4 to 6 hours or I.M. every 6 to 8 hours, as needed. For hospitalized patients, start with low oral doses and increase gradually. In severe behavioral disorders, 50 to 100 mg P.O. daily or, in older children, 200 mg/day or more P.O. may be necessary. There is little evidence that improvement in severely disturbed mentally retarded patients is enhanced by doses beyond 500 mg/day. In hospitalized patients age 5 or younger or weighing less than 23 kg (50 lb), don't exceed 40 mg/day I.M. In children ages 5 to 12 weighing 23 to 45 kg (50 to 100 lb), don't exceed 75 mg/day I.M., except in unmanageable cases.
➤ **Surgery**
Adults and children older than age 12: Preoperatively, 25 to 50 mg P.O. 2 to 3 hours before surgery or 12.5 to 25 mg I.M. 1 to 2 hours before surgery; during surgery, 12.5 mg I.M., repeated in 30 minutes, if needed, or fractional 2-mg doses I.V. at 2-minute intervals to maximum dose of 25 mg.
Children ages 6 months to 12 years: Preoperatively, 0.55 mg/kg P.O. 2 to 3 hours before surgery or I.M. 1 to 2 hours before surgery. During surgery, 0.25 mg/kg I.M., repeated in 30 minutes if needed, or

---

Reactions in bold italics are ***life-threatening***. Interactions may have a ***rapid onset*** or a ***delayed onset***.

fractional 1-mg doses I.V. at 2-minute intervals to maximum of 0.25 mg/kg. May repeat fractional I.V. regimen in 30 minutes if needed.

Elderly patients: Lower dosages are sufficient; dosage increments should be more gradual than in adults.

ADMINISTRATION
P.O.
• Give drug without regard to food.
I.V.
▼ Wear gloves when preparing solutions and avoid contact with skin and clothing. Parenteral forms can cause contact dermatitis.
▼ Drug is compatible with most common I.V. solutions, including D_5W, Ringer injection, lactated Ringer injection, and normal saline solution for injection.
▼ For direct injection, dilute with normal saline solution for injection and give into a large vein or through the tubing of a free-flowing I.V. solution.
▼ Don't exceed 1 mg/minute for adults or 0.5 mg/minute for children.
▼ For intermittent infusion, dilute with 50 or 100 mL of a compatible solution.
▼ Infuse over 30 minutes.
▼ **Incompatibilities:** Aminophylline, amphotericin B, ampicillin, chloramphenicol sodium succinate, chlorothiazide, cimetidine, dimenhydrinate, furosemide, heparin sodium, linezolid, melphalan, methohexital, paclitaxel, penicillin, pentobarbital, phenobarbital, solutions with a pH of 4 to 5, thiopental.
I.M.
• Wear gloves when preparing solutions and avoid contact with skin and clothing. Parenteral forms can cause contact dermatitis.
• Slight yellowing of injection is common and doesn't affect potency. Discard markedly discolored solutions.
• Monitor blood pressure before and after I.M. administration; keep patient supine for 1 hour afterward and have him get up slowly.
• Give deep I.M. only in upper outer quadrant of buttocks. Consider giving injection by Z-track method. Massage slowly afterward to prevent sterile abscess. Injection stings. Rotate injection sites.

ACTION
A piperidine phenothiazine that may block postsynaptic dopamine receptors in the brain.

Route	Onset	Peak	Duration
P.O.	30–60 min	Unknown	4–6 hr
I.V., I.M.	Unknown	Unknown	Unknown

Half-life: 20 to 24 hours.

ADVERSE REACTIONS
CNS: extrapyramidal reactions, sedation, tardive dyskinesia, pseudoparkinsonism, *neuroleptic malignant syndrome, seizures,* dizziness, drowsiness.
CV: orthostatic hypotension, tachycardia, quinidine-like ECG effects.
EENT: ocular changes, blurred vision, nasal congestion.
GI: dry mouth, constipation, nausea.
GU: urine retention, menstrual irregularities, inhibited ejaculation, priapism.
Hematologic: *leukopenia, agranulocytosis, aplastic anemia, thrombocytopenia,* eosinophilia, hemolytic anemia.
Hepatic: jaundice.
Skin: mild photosensitivity reactions, pain at I.M. injection site, allergic reactions, sterile abscess, skin pigmentation changes.
Other: gynecomastia, lactation, galactorrhea.

INTERACTIONS
Drug-drug. *Antacids:* May inhibit absorption of oral phenothiazines. Separate antacid and phenothiazine doses by at least 2 hours.
Anticholinergics such as TCAs, antiparkinsonians: May increase anticholinergic activity, aggravating parkinsonian symptoms. Use together cautiously.
Anticonvulsants: May lower seizure threshold. Monitor patient closely.
Barbiturates, lithium: May decrease phenothiazine effect. Monitor patient.
Centrally acting antihypertensives: May decrease antihypertensive effect. Monitor blood pressure.
CNS depressants: May increase CNS depression. Use together cautiously.
Drugs that prolong QT interval (such as antiarrhythmics, fluoroquinolones, tacrolimus, ziprasidone): May have additive effects. Monitor ECG and patient closely.

Electroconvulsive therapy, insulin: May cause severe reactions. Monitor patient closely.

Lithium: May increase neurologic effects. Monitor patient closely.

Meperidine: May cause excessive sedation and hypotension. Don't use together.

Propranolol: May increase levels of both propranolol and chlorpromazine. Monitor patient closely.

Warfarin: May decrease effect of oral anticoagulants. Monitor PT and INR.

Drug-herb. *St. John's wort:* May cause photosensitivity reactions. Advise patient to avoid excessive sunlight exposure.

Drug-lifestyle. *Alcohol use:* May increase CNS depression, particularly psychomotor skills. Strongly discourage alcohol use.

Sun exposure: May increase risk of photosensitivity reactions. Advise patient to avoid excessive sunlight exposure.

EFFECTS ON LAB TEST RESULTS

● May decrease hemoglobin level and hematocrit.

● May increase LFT values and eosinophil count. May decrease granulocyte, platelet, and WBC counts.

● May cause false-positive results for phenylketonuria, urinary porphyrin, urobilinogen, amylase, and 5-hydroxyindoleacetic acid tests and for urine pregnancy tests that use human chorionic gonadotropin.

CONTRAINDICATIONS & CAUTIONS

● Contraindicated in patients hypersensitive to drug; in those with CNS depression, bone marrow suppression, or subcortical damage; and in those in coma.

● Use cautiously in elderly or debilitated patients and in patients with hepatic or renal disease, severe CV disease (may suddenly decrease blood pressure), respiratory disorders, hypocalcemia, glaucoma, or prostatic hyperplasia. Also use cautiously in those exposed to extreme heat or cold (including antipyretic therapy) or organophosphate insecticides.

● Use cautiously in acutely ill or dehydrated children.

⚠ *Overdose S&S:* CNS depression, somnolence, coma, hypotension, extrapyramidal symptoms, agitation, restlessness, seizures, fever, dry mouth, ileus, ECG changes, cardiac arrhythmias.

NURSING CONSIDERATIONS

● Obtain baseline blood pressure measurements before therapy, and monitor regularly. Watch for orthostatic hypotension, especially with parenteral administration.

● Monitor patient for tardive dyskinesia, which may occur after prolonged use. It may not appear until months or years later and may disappear spontaneously or persist for life, despite stopping drug.

● After abrupt withdrawal of long-term therapy, gastritis, nausea, vomiting, dizziness, or tremor may occur.

⚠ *Alert:* Watch for evidence of neuroleptic malignant syndrome (extrapyramidal effects, hyperthermia, autonomic disturbance), which is rare but life-threatening. It may not be related to length of drug use or type of neuroleptic; more than 60% of affected patients are men.

● If jaundice, symptoms of blood dyscrasia (fever, sore throat, infection, cellulitis, weakness), or persistent extrapyramidal reactions (longer than a few hours) develop, or if such reactions occur in children or pregnant women, withhold dose and notify prescriber.

● Don't withdraw drug abruptly unless required by severe adverse reactions.

Black Box Warning Elderly patients with dementia-related psychosis treated with atypical or conventional antipsychotics are at increased risk for death. Antipsychotics aren't approved for the treatment of dementia-related psychosis. ▮

● *Look alike–sound alike:* Don't confuse chlorpromazine with chlordiazepoxide, clomipramine, or chlorpropamide, a hypoglycemic.

PATIENT TEACHING

● Warn patient to avoid activities that require alertness and good coordination until effects of drug are known. Drowsiness and dizziness usually subside after first few weeks.

● Tell patient to avoid alcohol while taking drug.

Reactions in bold italics are *life-threatening*. Interactions may have a *rapid onset* or a *delayed onset*.

- Have patient report signs of urine retention or constipation.
- Tell patient to use sunblock and to wear protective clothing to avoid oversensitivity to the sun. This drug is more likely to cause sun sensitivity than other drugs in its class.
- Tell patient to relieve dry mouth with sugarless gum or hard candy.
- Advise patient receiving drug by any method other than by mouth to remain lying down for 1 hour afterward and to rise slowly.

cholestyramine
koe-LESS-tir-a-meen

Prevalite

Therapeutic class: Antilipemics
Pharmacologic class: Bile acid sequestrants
Pregnancy risk category: C

AVAILABLE FORMS
Powder: 378-g cans, 9-g single-dose packets; each scoop of powder or single-dose packet contains 4 g of cholestyramine resin

INDICATIONS & DOSAGES
➤ **Primary hyperlipidemia or pruritus caused by partial bile obstruction, adjunct for reduction of increased cholesterol level in patients with primary hypercholesterolemia**
Adults: 4 g P.O. once daily or b.i.d. Maintenance dose is 8 to 16 g daily divided into two doses. Maximum daily dose is 24 g.
Children: 240 mg/kg P.O. daily in two to three divided doses, not to exceed 8 g/day.
➤ **Diarrhea ♦**
Adults: Up to 4 g P.O. q.i.d. for 2 weeks.

ADMINISTRATION
P.O.
- Mix thoroughly with 60 to 180 mL of water or other noncarbonated beverage.
- Give drug with a meal.
- Give other drugs 1 hour before or at least 4 hours after cholestyramine to avoid impeding absorption.

ACTION
Binds bile acids in the intestinal tract, impeding their absorption and causing their elimination in feces. In response to this bile acid depletion, LDL cholesterol levels decrease as the liver uses LDL cholesterol to replenish reduced bile acid stores.

Route	Onset	Peak	Duration
P.O.	Unknown	Unknown	2–4 wk

Half-life: Unknown.

ADVERSE REACTIONS
CNS: dizziness, headache, vertigo, anxiety, fatigue, insomnia, syncope, tinnitus.
GI: abdominal discomfort, constipation, fecal impaction, nausea, anorexia, diarrhea, flatulence, *GI bleeding,* hemorrhoids, steatorrhea, vomiting.
GU: dysuria, hematuria.
Hematologic: anemia, bleeding tendencies, ecchymoses.
Metabolic: hyperchloremic acidosis.
Musculoskeletal: backache, muscle and joint pains, osteoporosis.
Skin: rash; irritation of skin, tongue, and perianal area.
Other: vitamin A, D, E, and K deficiencies from decreased absorption.

INTERACTIONS
Drug-drug. *Acetaminophen, beta blockers, cardiac glycosides, corticosteroids, estrogens, fat-soluble vitamins (A, D, E, and K), iron preparations, niacin, penicillin G, phenobarbital, progestins, tetracycline, thiazide diuretics, thyroid hormones, warfarin and other coumarin derivatives:* May decrease absorption of these drugs. Give other drugs 1 hour before or 4 to 6 hours after cholestyramine.

EFFECTS ON LAB TEST RESULTS
- May increase alkaline phosphatase and triglyceride levels. May decrease hemoglobin level and hematocrit.
- May increase PT.
- May cause abnormal results in cholecystography that uses iopanoic acid because iopanoic acid is also bound by cholestyramine.

CONTRAINDICATIONS & CAUTIONS

• Contraindicated in patients hypersensitive to bile-acid sequestering resins and in those with complete biliary obstruction.

• Use cautiously in patients predisposed to constipation and in those with conditions aggravated by constipation, such as severe, symptomatic coronary artery disease.

⚠ *Overdose S&S:* GI tract obstruction.

NURSING CONSIDERATIONS

• Monitor cholesterol and triglyceride levels regularly during therapy.

• Monitor levels of cardiac glycosides in patients receiving cardiac glycosides and cholestyramine together. If cholestyramine therapy is stopped, adjust dosage of cardiac glycosides, if necessary, to avoid toxicity.

• Monitor bowel habits. Encourage a diet high in fiber and fluids. If severe constipation develops, decrease dosage, add a stool softener, or stop drug.

• Watch for hyperchloremic acidosis with long-term use or very high doses.

• Long-term use may lead to deficiencies of vitamins A, D, E, and K and folic acid.

• For patients with phenylketonuria, light form contains 28.1 mg of phenylalanine per 6.4-g dose.

PATIENT TEACHING

◑ *Alert:* Tell patient never to take drug in its dry form because it may irritate the esophagus or cause severe constipation.

• Tell patient to prepare drug in a large glass containing water, milk, or juice (especially pulpy fruit juice). Tell him to sprinkle powder on the surface of the beverage, let the mixture stand for a few minutes, and then stir thoroughly. Discourage mixing with carbonated beverages because of excessive foaming. After drinking preparation, patient should swirl a small additional amount of liquid in the same glass and then drink again to make sure he has taken the entire dose.

• Tell patient to avoid sipping or holding the suspension in the mouth because drug may damage tooth surfaces. Advise patient to maintain good oral hygiene.

• Advise patient to take at mealtime, if possible.

• Advise patient to take all other drugs at least 1 hour before or 4 to 6 hours after cholestyramine to avoid blocking their absorption.

• Teach patient about proper dietary management of fats. When appropriate, recommend weight control, exercise, and smoking cessation programs.

• Tell patient that drug may deplete body stores of vitamins A, D, E, and K and folic acid. Patient should discuss need for supplements with prescriber.

ciclesonide (inhalation)
si-CLEH-son-ide

Alvesco

Therapeutic class: Corticosteroids
Pharmacologic class: Corticosteroids
Pregnancy risk category: C

AVAILABLE FORMS
Oral inhalation aerosol: 80 mcg, 160 mcg

INDICATIONS & DOSAGES
➤ **Preventative during asthma maintenance**

Adults and children age 12 and older who were previously taking bronchodilators alone: Initially, inhaled dose of 80 mcg b.i.d. to maximum of 160 mcg b.i.d.

Adults and children age 12 and older who were previously taking inhaled corticosteroids: Initially, 80 mcg b.i.d. to maximum of 320 mcg b.i.d.

Adults and children age 12 and older who were previously taking oral corticosteroids: 320 mcg b.i.d.

ADMINISTRATION
Inhalational

• Patient should rinse mouth after inhalation.

ACTION
May decrease inflammation by inhibiting macrophages, eosinophils, and mediators such as leukotrienes involved in the asthmatic response.

Route	Onset	Peak	Duration
Inhalation	Unknown	1 hr	Unknown

Half-life of drug and its active metabolite: Less than an hour and 6 to 7 hours, respectively.

Reactions in bold italics are *life-threatening*. Interactions may have a *rapid onset* or a *delayed onset*.

ADVERSE REACTIONS
CNS: headache, back pain.
EENT: nasopharyngitis, sinusitis, pharyngolaryngeal pain, upper respiratory tract infection, nasal congestion.
Musculoskeletal: arthralgia, pain in the extremities or back.

INTERACTIONS
Drug-drug. *Delavirdine:* May increase serum ciclesonide level. Use together cautiously.
Ketoconazole, other inhibitors of CYP450: May increase ciclesonide level and adverse effects. Use together cautiously; adjust ciclesonide dosage as needed.
Protease inhibitors (such as ritonavir): May increase serum level and effects of ciclesonide. Use lowest effective ciclesonide dosage and monitor patient closely for Cushing syndrome.

EFFECTS ON LAB TEST RESULTS
None reported.

CONTRAINDICATIONS & CAUTIONS
• Contraindicated as primary treatment of status asthmaticus or other acute asthmatic episodes, and in patients hypersensitive to drug or its components.
• Use cautiously, if at all, in patients with active or quiescent respiratory tuberculosis infection; untreated systemic fungal, bacterial, viral, or parasitic infections; or ocular herpes simplex.
• Use cautiously in pregnant and breast-feeding women.
⚠ *Overdose S&S:* Hypercorticism.

NURSING CONSIDERATIONS
🔆 *Alert:* Don't use for acute bronchospasm or acute asthma.
• Assess patient for bone loss during long-term use.
• Watch for evidence of localized mouth infections, glaucoma, cataracts, and immunosuppression.
• Closely monitor children for growth suppression.
• Use drug only if benefits to mother justify risks to fetus. If a woman takes a corticosteroid during pregnancy, monitor neonate for hypoadrenalism.

• After asthma stability has been achieved, titrate to lowest effective dosage to minimize systemic effects.

PATIENT TEACHING
• Inform patient that drug isn't indicated for the relief of acute bronchospasm.
• Instruct patient to rinse his mouth with water and spit out after inhalation.
• Advise patient to use drug at regular intervals, as directed.
• Inform patient that therapeutic results may take several weeks.
• Warn patient to avoid exposure to chickenpox, measles, or other infections, and if exposed to consult prescriber immediately.
• Instruct patient to contact prescriber if symptoms don't improve after 4 weeks of treatment or if condition worsens.
• Advise parents of child receiving long-term therapy that child should have periodic growth measurements.

ciclesonide (intranasal)
si-CLEH-son-ide

Omnaris, Zetonna

Therapeutic class: Corticosteroids
Pharmacologic class: Nonhalogenated glucocorticoids
Pregnancy risk category: C

AVAILABLE FORMS
Nasal aerosol solution: 37 mcg/metered spray
Nasal spray: 50 mcg/metered spray

INDICATIONS & DOSAGES
➤ **Symptoms of perennial allergic rhinitis**
Adults and children age 12 and older:
2 sprays Omnaris in each nostril once daily (200 mcg/day). Or, 1 actuation Zetonna per nostril once daily.
➤ **Symptoms of seasonal allergic rhinitis**
Adults and children age 12 and older:
1 actuation Zetonna per nostril once daily.
Adults and children age 6 and older:
2 sprays Omnaris in each nostril once daily (200 mcg/day).

ADMINISTRATION
Intranasal
• Before first use of Omnaris, gently shake container, then prime by spraying eight times. If not used for 4 consecutive days, gently shake and reprime with 1 spray or until a fine mist appears.
• Before first use of Zetonna, prime by actuating three times. If not used for 10 consecutive days, prime by actuating three times.

ACTION
Hydrolyzed by the nasal mucosa to a biologically active metabolite with anti-inflammatory properties.

Route	Onset	Peak	Duration
Intranasal	1–2 days	1–5 wk	Unknown

Half-life: Unknown.

ADVERSE REACTIONS
CNS: headache.
EENT: epistaxis, nasopharyngitis, ear pain, nasal discomfort.
Metabolic: growth retardation.

INTERACTIONS
Drug-drug. *Delavirdine:* May increase serum ciclesonide level. Use with caution.
Ketoconazole, other CYP450 inhibitors: May increase ciclesonide level and adverse effects. Use together cautiously.
Protease inhibitors (ritonavir): May increase serum level and effects of ciclesonide. Use lowest effective ciclesonide dosage and monitor patient closely for Cushing syndrome.

EFFECTS ON LAB TEST RESULTS
None reported.

CONTRAINDICATIONS & CAUTIONS
• Contraindicated in patients hypersensitive to the drug or its components.
• Contraindicated in patients who have had recent nasal septal ulcers, nasal surgery, or nasal trauma until healing has occurred.
• Use cautiously in patients who have changed from systemic to inhaled corticosteroids; renal insufficiency, steroid withdrawal (pain, lassitude, depression), or acute worsening of symptoms may occur.

• Use cautiously in immunosuppressed patients or in those with wounds; corticosteroids suppress the immune system.
• Use cautiously in children; may cause a decline in growth rate.
• Use cautiously in breast-feeding women.
⚠ *Overdose S&S:* Hyperadrenocorticism.

NURSING CONSIDERATIONS
• Monitor infants born to mothers using drug during pregnancy for hypoadrenalism.
• Monitor patients who are switched from systemic to inhaled corticosteroids for worsening of symptoms and other side effects of withdrawal.
• Monitor children for decline in growth rate; potential to regain growth after drug is stopped hasn't been studied.
• Monitor patient for nasal side effects.

PATIENT TEACHING
• Teach patient how to use the spray properly. Refer patient to package insert.
• Instruct patient to contact his prescriber if he has no relief from symptoms after 1 week.
• Advise patient to use drug around the same time every day, as directed.
• Warn patient to avoid exposure to people with infections, such as chickenpox or measles; corticosteroids have immunosuppressant effects.
• Tell patient to discard the Omnaris bottle after 120 actuations following initial priming or 4 months after removal from foil pouch, whichever occurs first.
• Tell patient to replace Zetonna nasal aerosol when indicator shows zero.

cidofovir
sye-DOE-fo-veer

Vistide

Therapeutic class: Antivirals
Pharmacologic class: Nucleosides–nucleotides
Pregnancy risk category: C

AVAILABLE FORMS
Injection: 75 mg/mL in 5-mL vial

INDICATIONS & DOSAGES

Black Box Warning Cidofovir is indicated only for the treatment of CMV retinitis in patients with AIDS. ■

➤ **CMV retinitis in patients with AIDS**
Adults: Initially, 5 mg/kg I.V. infused over 1 hour once weekly for 2 consecutive weeks; then maintenance dose of 5 mg/kg I.V. infused over 1 hour once every 2 weeks. Give probenecid and prehydration with normal saline solution I.V. simultaneously to reduce risk of nephrotoxicity.

Adjust-a-dose: For patients with creatinine level of 0.3 to 0.4 mg/dL above baseline, reduce dosage to 3 mg/kg at same rate and frequency. If creatinine level reaches 0.5 mg/dL or more above baseline, or patient develops 3+ or higher proteinuria, stop drug.

ADMINISTRATION

I.V.

Black Box Warning Drug has mutagenic effects; prepare it in a class II laminar flow biological safety cabinet and wear surgical gloves and a closed-front surgical gown with knit cuffs. ■

▼ If drug contacts skin, wash and flush thoroughly with water.

▼ Place excess drug and all materials used to prepare and give it in a leak-proof, puncture-proof container.

▼ Let drug reach room temperature before use.

▼ Using a syringe, withdraw prescribed dose and add to an I.V. bag containing 100 mL of normal saline solution.

▼ Infuse over 1 hour using an infusion pump.

▼ Because of the risk of nephrotoxicity, don't exceed recommended dosages or frequency or rate of infusion.

▼ Discard any partially used vials.

▼ Give within 24 hours of preparing. Admixture may be refrigerated at 36° to 46° F (2° to 8° C) for up to 24 hours.

🔃 *Alert:* Due to increased risk of nephrotoxicity, give 1 L normal saline solution I.V. over 1- to 2-hour period, immediately before giving drug. Also give probenecid with each cidofovir infusion.

▼ Compatibility of admixture with Ringer, lactated Ringer, and bacteriostatic solutions hasn't been evaluated.

▼ **Incompatibilities:** Other drugs or supplements.

ACTION

Suppresses CMV replication by selective inhibition of viral DNA synthesis.

Route	Onset	Peak	Duration
I.V.	Unknown	Unknown	Unknown

Half-life: Unknown.

ADVERSE REACTIONS

CNS: asthenia, fever, headache, *seizures,* abnormal gait, amnesia, anxiety, confusion, depression, dizziness, hallucinations, insomnia, neuropathy, paresthesia, somnolence, malaise.

CV: hypotension, orthostatic hypotension, pallor, syncope, tachycardia, vasodilation.

EENT: ocular hypotony, abnormal vision, amblyopia, conjunctivitis, eye disorders, iritis, pharyngitis, retinal detachment, rhinitis, sinusitis, uveitis.

GI: abdominal pain, anorexia, diarrhea, nausea, vomiting, aphthous stomatitis, colitis, constipation, dry mouth, dyspepsia, dysphagia, flatulence, gastritis, melena, mouth ulcers, oral candidiasis, rectal disorders, stomatitis, taste perversion, tongue discoloration.

GU: proteinuria, *nephrotoxicity,* glycosuria, hematuria, urinary incontinence, UTI.

Hematologic: anemia, *neutropenia, thrombocytopenia.*

Hepatic: hepatomegaly.

Metabolic: fluid imbalance, hyperglycemia, hyperlipidemia, hypocalcemia, hypokalemia, weight loss.

Musculoskeletal: arthralgia, myalgia, myasthenia; pain in back, chest, or neck.

Respiratory: dyspnea, asthma, bronchitis, coughing, hiccups, increased sputum, lung disorders, pneumonia.

Skin: alopecia, rash, acne, dry skin, pruritus, skin discoloration, sweating, urticaria.

Other: chills, infections, *sarcoma, sepsis,* allergic reactions, facial edema, herpes simplex.

INTERACTIONS

Drug-drug. Black Box Warning *Nephrotoxic drugs (such as aminoglycosides, amphotericin B, foscarnet, I.V. pentamidine):* May increase nephrotoxicity. Avoid using together. ∎

Zidovudine: Stop zidovudine or reduce dosage by 50% on the days cidofovir is given; probenecid reduces metabolic clearance of zidovudine.

EFFECTS ON LAB TEST RESULTS

● May increase alkaline phosphatase, ALT, AST, BUN, creatinine, glucose, cholesterol, LDH, and urine protein levels. May decrease bicarbonate, calcium, potassium, and hemoglobin levels.

● May decrease neutrophil and platelet counts.

CONTRAINDICATIONS & CAUTIONS

● Contraindicated in patients hypersensitive to drug, probenecid, and other sulfa drugs. Black Box Warning Renal failure has occurred with as few as one or two doses of cidofovir. Monitor renal function within 48 hours before each dose and modify dosage as needed. Contraindicated in patients receiving other drugs with nephrotoxic potential (stop such drugs at least 7 days before starting cidofovir therapy) and in those with creatinine level exceeding 1.5 mg/dL, CrCl of 55 mL/minute or less, or urine protein level of 100 mg/dL or more (equivalent to 2+ proteinuria or more). ∎

● Use within 1 month of placement of a ganciclovir ocular implant may cause profound hypotony.

● Direct intraocular injection is contraindicated and is associated with iritis, ocular hypotony, and permanent vision impairment.

● Safety and effectiveness in children haven't been established.

● Use cautiously in patients with renal impairment. Monitor renal function tests and patient's fluid balance.

NURSING CONSIDERATIONS

Black Box Warning Safety and effectiveness of drug haven't been established for treating other CMV infections, congenital or neonatal CMV disease, or CMV disease in patients not infected with HIV. ∎

Black Box Warning Due to increased risk of nephrotoxicity and bone marrow suppression, monitor creatinine and urine protein levels and WBC counts with differential before each dose. ∎

● Drug may cause Fanconi syndrome and decreased bicarbonate level with renal tubular damage. Monitor patient closely.

● Drug may cause granulocytopenia.

PATIENT TEACHING

● Inform patient that drug doesn't cure CMV retinitis and that regular ophthalmologic examinations are needed.

● Alert patient taking zidovudine that he'll need to obtain dosage guidelines on days cidofovir is given.

● Tell patient that close monitoring of kidney function will be needed and that abnormalities may require a change in therapy.

● Stress importance of completing a full course of probenecid with each cidofovir dose. Tell patient to take probenecid after a meal to decrease nausea.

● Patients with AIDS should use effective contraception, especially during and for 1 month after treatment.

● Advise men to practice barrier contraception during and for 3 months after treatment.

cilostazol
sill-AHS-tah-zoll

Pletal

Therapeutic class: Antiplatelet drugs
Pharmacologic class: cAMP phosphodiesterase inhibitors
Pregnancy risk category: C

AVAILABLE FORMS
Tablets: 50 mg, 100 mg

INDICATIONS & DOSAGES

➤ **To reduce symptoms of intermittent claudication**

Adults: 100 mg P.O. b.i.d., at least 30 minutes before or 2 hours after breakfast and dinner.

Adjust-a-dose: Decrease dose to 50 mg P.O. b.i.d. when giving with drugs that may interact to cause an increase in cilostazol level.

ADMINISTRATION

P.O.

• Give drug at least 30 minutes before or 2 hours after breakfast and dinner.

• Don't give with grapefruit juice.

ACTION

Thought to inhibit the enzyme phosphodiesterase III, thus inhibiting platelet aggregation and causing vasodilation.

Route	Onset	Peak	Duration
P.O.	Unknown	2–4 hr	Unknown

Half-life: 11 to 13 hours.

ADVERSE REACTIONS

CNS: dizziness, headache, vertigo.
CV: palpitations, peripheral edema, tachycardia.
EENT: pharyngitis, rhinitis.
GI: abnormal stools, diarrhea, abdominal pain, dyspepsia, flatulence, nausea.
Hematologic: bleeding.
Musculoskeletal: back pain, myalgia.
Respiratory: increased cough.
Other: infection.

INTERACTIONS

Drug-drug. *Diltiazem:* May increase cilostazol level. Reduce cilostazol dosage to 50 mg b.i.d.
Erythromycin, other macrolides: May increase level of cilostazol and its metabolites. Reduce cilostazol dosage to 50 mg b.i.d.
Omeprazole: May increase level of cilostazol metabolite. Reduce cilostazol dosage to 50 mg b.i.d.
Strong inhibitors of CYP3A4 (such as fluconazole, fluoxetine, fluvoxamine, itraconazole, ketoconazole, miconazole, nefazodone, sertraline): May increase level of cilostazol and its metabolites. Reduce cilostazol dosage to 50 mg b.i.d.
Drug-food. *Grapefruit juice:* May increase drug level. Discourage use together.
Drug-herb. *Ginkgo biloba:* May prolong bleeding time. Discourage use together.
Drug-lifestyle. *Smoking:* May decrease drug exposure. Discourage smoking.

EFFECTS ON LAB TEST RESULTS

• May reduce triglyceride levels. May increase HDL level.

CONTRAINDICATIONS & CAUTIONS

• Contraindicated in patients hypersensitive to drug or its components.

Black Box Warning Contraindicated in patients with heart failure of any severity. ∎

• Contraindicated in patients with hemostatic disorders or active bleeding, such as bleeding peptic ulcer and intracranial bleeding.

• Use cautiously in patients with severe underlying heart disease; also use cautiously with other drugs having antiplatelet activity.

• Use cautiously in patients with severe renal impairment (CrCl <25 mL/minute) and in those with moderate to severe hepatic impairment.

⚠ *Overdose S&S:* Severe headache, diarrhea, hypotension, tachycardia, cardiac arrhythmias.

NURSING CONSIDERATIONS

• Beneficial effects may not be seen for up to 12 weeks after therapy starts.

Black Box Warning Cilostazol and similar drugs that inhibit the enzyme phosphodiesterase decrease the likelihood of survival in patients with class III and IV heart failure. ∎

☉ *Alert:* CV risk is unknown in patients who use drug on long-term basis and in those with severe underlying heart disease.

• Dosage can be reduced or stopped without such rebound effects as platelet hyperaggregation.

• If aspirin is added to drug therapy, monitor patient for aspirin-related adverse reactions.

PATIENT TEACHING

• Instruct patient to take drug on an empty stomach, at least 30 minutes before or 2 hours after breakfast and dinner.

• Tell patient that beneficial effect of drug on cramping pain isn't likely to be noticed for 2 to 4 weeks and that it may take as long as 12 weeks.

• Advise patient to avoid drinking grapefruit juice during drug therapy.

• Inform patient that CV risk is unknown in patients who use drug on a long-term basis and in those with severe underlying heart disease.

● Tell patient that drug may cause dizziness. Caution patient not to drive or perform other activities that require alertness until response to drug is known.

cimetidine
sye-MET-i-deen

Tagamet, Tagamet HB ◊

cimetidine hydrochloride
Tagamet

Therapeutic class: Antiulcer drugs
Pharmacologic class: H₂ receptor
antagonists
Pregnancy risk category: B

AVAILABLE FORMS
Injection: 300 mg/2 mL
Oral liquid: 300 mg/5 mL*
Tablets: 200 mg ◊, 300 mg, 400 mg, 800 mg

INDICATIONS & DOSAGES
Adjust-a-dose (for all indications): In patients with renal impairment, decrease dosage to 300 mg P.O. or I.V. every 12 hours, increasing frequency to every 8 hours with caution. A renally impaired patient who also has liver dysfunction may require even further dosage reduction. Schedule dose at the end of hemodialysis.
➤ **Short-term treatment of duodenal ulcer; maintenance therapy**
Adults and children age 16 and older:
800 mg P.O. at bedtime. Or, 400 mg P.O. b.i.d. or 300 mg q.i.d. (with meals and at bedtime). Or, 200 mg t.i.d. with a 400-mg bedtime dose. Treatment lasts 4 to 6 weeks unless endoscopy shows healing. For maintenance therapy, 400 mg at bedtime. For parenteral therapy, 300 mg diluted to 20 mL total volume with normal saline solution or other compatible I.V. solution by I.V. push over at least 5 minutes every 6 to 8 hours; or 300 mg diluted in 50 mL D₅W or other compatible I.V. solution by I.V. infusion over 15 to 20 minutes every 6 to 8 hours; or 300 mg I.M. every 6 to 8 hours (no dilution needed). To increase dosage, give 300-mg

doses more frequently to maximum of 2,400 mg daily, as needed. Or, 900 mg/day (37.5 mg/hour) I.V. diluted in 100 to 1,000 mL of compatible solution by continuous I.V. infusion.
➤ **Active benign gastric ulceration**
Adults: 800 mg P.O. at bedtime or 300 mg P.O. q.i.d. (with meals and at bedtime) for up to 8 weeks.
➤ **Pathologic hypersecretory conditions, such as Zollinger-Ellison syndrome, systemic mastocytosis, and multiple endocrine adenomas**
Adults and children age 16 and older:
300 mg P.O. q.i.d. with meals and at bedtime, adjusted to patient needs. Maximum oral amount, 2,400 mg daily.

For parenteral therapy, 300 mg diluted in 20 mL normal saline solution or other compatible I.V. solution by I.V. push over at least 5 minutes every 6 to 8 hours; or 300 mg diluted in 50 mL D₅W or other compatible I.V. solution by I.V. infusion over 15 to 20 minutes every 6 to 8 hours. Increase parenteral dosage by giving 300-mg doses more frequently to maximum of 2,400 mg daily, as needed.
➤ **GERD with erosive esophagitis**
Adults: 800 mg P.O. b.i.d. or 400 mg q.i.d. before meals and at bedtime for up to 12 weeks.
➤ **Heartburn**
Adults and children age 12 and older:
200 mg Tagamet HB P.O. with water as symptoms occur, or as directed, up to b.i.d. For prevention, 200 mg right before or up to 30 minutes before eating food or drinking beverages that cause heartburn. Maximum, 400 mg daily. Drug shouldn't be taken daily for longer than 2 weeks.

ADMINISTRATION
P.O.
● Give dose at end of hemodialysis.
I.V.
▼ Dilute I.V. solutions with normal saline solution, D₅W, dextrose 10% in water (and combinations of these), lactated Ringer solution, or 5% sodium bicarbonate injection.
▼ For direct injection, give over 5 minutes. Rapid I.V. injection may result in arrhythmias and hypotension.

Reactions in bold italics are *life-threatening*. Interactions may have a *rapid onset* or a *delayed onset*.

▼ For intermittent infusion, give drug over at least 30 minutes to minimize risk of adverse cardiac effects.

▼ For continuous infusion, if giving a total volume of 250 mL over 24 hours or less, use an infusion pump.

▼ **Incompatibilities:** Allopurinol, amphotericin B, barbiturates, cefazolin, cefepime, chlorpromazine, combination atropine sulfate and pentobarbital sodium, indomethacin sodium trihydrate, pentobarbital sodium, secobarbital, warfarin. Don't dilute with sterile water for injection.

I.M.

● I.M. injection may be given undiluted.

● Give dose at end of hemodialysis.

ACTION

Competitively inhibits action of histamine on the H_2 receptor sites of parietal cells, decreasing gastric acid secretion.

Route	Onset	Peak	Duration
P.O.	¼–3 hr	45–90 min	4–5 hr
I.V.	¼–3 hr	Immediate	4–5 hr
I.M.	¼–3 hr	Unknown	4–5 hr

Half-life: 2 hours.

ADVERSE REACTIONS

CNS: confusion, dizziness, hallucinations, headache, peripheral neuropathy, somnolence.

GI: mild and transient diarrhea.

GU: erectile dysfunction.

Musculoskeletal: arthralgia, muscle pain.

Other: mild gynecomastia if used longer than 1 month, hypersensitivity reactions.

INTERACTIONS

Drug-drug. *Antacids:* May interfere with cimetidine absorption. Separate doses by at least 1 hour, if possible.

Carmustine: May enhance the bone marrow suppressant effects of carmustine. Avoid use together.

Digoxin, fluconazole, indomethacin, iron salts, ketoconazole, tetracycline: May decrease drug absorption. Separate doses by at least 2 hours.

Fosphenytoin, phenytoin, some benzodiazepines, theophylline, warfarin: May inhibit hepatic microsomal enzyme metabolism of these drugs. Monitor drug level.

I.V. lidocaine: May decrease clearance of lidocaine, increasing the risk of toxicity. Consider using a different H_2 antagonist, if possible. Monitor lidocaine level closely.

Metoprolol, propranolol, timolol: May increase the effects of beta blocker. Consider another H_2 antagonist or decrease the dose of beta blocker.

Procainamide: May increase procainamide level. Avoid this combination, if possible. Monitor procainamide level closely and adjust the dose as necessary.

Drug-herb. *Pennyroyal:* May change rate at which herb's toxic metabolites form. Monitor patient.

Yerba maté: May decrease clearance of herb's methylxanthines and cause toxicity. Discourage use together.

Drug-lifestyle. *Alcohol use:* May increase blood alcohol level. Discourage use together.

Smoking: May decrease drug's ability to inhibit nocturnal gastric secretion. Urge patient to quit smoking.

EFFECTS ON LAB TEST RESULTS

● May increase ALT, AST, and creatinine levels.

● May antagonize pentagastrin's effect during gastric acid secretion tests. May cause false-negative results in skin tests using allergen extracts. May impair interpretation of Hemoccult and Gastroccult test results on gastric content aspirate because of FD&C blue dye number 2 used in tablets.

CONTRAINDICATIONS & CAUTIONS

● Contraindicated in patients hypersensitive to drug.

● Use cautiously in elderly or debilitated patients because they may be more susceptible to drug-induced confusion.

⚠ **Overdose S&S:** Mental deterioration, unresponsiveness, death.

NURSING CONSIDERATIONS

● Assess patient for abdominal pain. Note blood in emesis, stool, or gastric aspirate.

● Identify tablet strength when obtaining a drug history.

● Schedule dose at end of hemodialysis treatment because hemodialysis reduces drug levels.

• Wait at least 15 minutes after giving tablet before drawing sample for Hemoccult or Gastroccult test, and follow test manufacturer's instructions closely.

• Treatment of gastric ulcer isn't as effective as treatment of duodenal ulcer.

• *Look alike–sound alike:* Don't confuse cimetidine with simethicone.

PATIENT TEACHING

• Remind patient taking drug once daily to take it at bedtime and to take multiple daily doses with meals.

• Instruct patient taking Tagamet HB not to exceed recommended dosage and not to take daily for longer than 14 days.

• Warn patient receiving drug I.M. that injection may be painful.

• Urge patient to avoid cigarette smoking because it may increase gastric acid secretion and worsen disease.

• Advise patient to report abdominal pain, blood in stools or emesis, black tarry stools, and coffee-ground emesis.

• Tell patient to check with prescriber or pharmacist before taking other drugs.

cinacalcet hydrochloride
sin-ah-KAL-set

Sensipar

Therapeutic class: Hyperparathyroidism drugs
Pharmacologic class: Calcimimetics
Pregnancy risk category: C

AVAILABLE FORMS
Tablets: 30 mg, 60 mg, 90 mg

INDICATIONS & DOSAGES
➤ **Primary hyperparathyroidism**
Adults: Initially, 30 mg P.O. b.i.d. Titrate every 2 to 4 weeks through sequential doses of 30 mg b.i.d., 60 mg b.i.d., 90 mg b.i.d., and 90 mg t.i.d. or q.i.d. to normalize calcium levels.
➤ **Secondary hyperparathyroidism in patients with chronic kidney disease undergoing dialysis**
Adults: Initially, 30 mg P.O. once daily; adjust no more than every 2 to 4 weeks

through sequential doses of 60 mg, 90 mg, 120 mg, and 180 mg P.O. once daily to reach target range of 150 to 300 picograms (pg)/mL for intact parathyroid hormone (PTH).
➤ **Hypercalcemia in patients with parathyroid carcinoma**
Adults: Initially, 30 mg P.O. b.i.d.; adjust every 2 to 4 weeks through sequential doses of 30 mg, 60 mg, and 90 mg P.O. b.i.d., and 90 mg P.O. t.i.d. or q.i.d. daily if needed to normalize calcium level.

ADMINISTRATION
P.O.
• Don't break or crush tablets; give them whole, with food or shortly after a meal.

ACTION
Increases sensitivity of calcium-sensing receptor to extracellular calcium, letting calcium be absorbed despite decreased PTH.

Route	Onset	Peak	Duration
P.O.	Unknown	2–6 hr	Unknown

Half-life: Terminal half-life, 30 to 40 hours.

ADVERSE REACTIONS
CNS: dizziness, asthenia, *seizures,* depression, fatigue, headache, paresthesia.
CV: chest pain, hypertension.
GI: diarrhea, nausea, vomiting, anorexia, constipation.
Hematologic: anemia.
Metabolic: hypocalcemia, dehydration, hypercalcemia.
Musculoskeletal: myalgia, arthralgia, fracture, limb pain.
Respiratory: upper respiratory tract infection.
Other: access infection.

INTERACTIONS
Drug-drug. *Amitriptyline:* Amitriptyline and nortriptyline exposure increases by 20% in patients who are CYP2D6 extensive metabolizers. Avoid using together, if possible.
Drugs metabolized mainly by CYP2D6 with a narrow therapeutic index (such as flecainide, thioridazine, most TCAs, vinblastine): May strongly inhibit CYP2D6, decreasing metabolism and increasing

C

levels of these drugs. Adjust dosage of other drugs, as needed.

Drugs that strongly inhibit CYP3A4 (such as erythromycin, itraconazole, ketoconazole): May increase cinacalcet level. Use together cautiously, monitoring PTH and calcium level closely and adjusting cinacalcet dosage, as needed.

EFFECTS ON LAB TEST RESULTS
• May decrease calcium, phosphorus, and testosterone levels.

CONTRAINDICATIONS & CAUTIONS
• Contraindicated in patients hypersensitive to drug or its components and in patients with calcium level less than 8.4 mg/dL.
• Use cautiously in patients with history of seizures and in those with moderate to severe hepatic impairment.
⚠ *Overdose S&S:* Hypocalcemia.

NURSING CONSIDERATIONS
◑ *Alert:* Monitor calcium level closely, especially if patient has a history of seizures, because decreased calcium level lowers seizure threshold.
• Patients with moderate to severe hepatic impairment may need dosage adjustment based on PTH and calcium level. Monitor these patients closely.
• Give drug alone or with vitamin D sterols, phosphate binders, or both.
• Measure calcium level within 1 week after starting therapy or adjusting dosage. After maintenance dose is established, measure calcium level monthly for patients with chronic kidney disease receiving dialysis and every 2 months for those with parathyroid carcinoma.
• Watch carefully for evidence of hypocalcemia: paresthesias, myalgias, cramping, tetany, and seizures.
• If calcium level is 7.5 to 8.4 mg/dL or patient develops symptoms of hypocalcemia, give calcium-containing phosphate binders, vitamin D sterols, or both, to raise calcium level. If calcium level is below 7.5 mg/dL or hypocalcemia symptoms persist and the vitamin D dose can't be increased, withhold drug until calcium level reaches 8.0 mg/dL, hypocalcemia symptoms resolve, or both. Resume therapy with the next lowest dose.

• Measure intact PTH level 1 to 4 weeks after therapy starts or dosage changes. After the maintenance dose is established, monitor PTH level every 1 to 3 months. Levels in patients with chronic kidney disease receiving dialysis should be 150 to 300 pg/mL.
• Adynamic bone disease may develop if intact PTH levels are suppressed below 100 pg/mL. If this occurs, notify prescriber. The dosage of cinacalcet or vitamin D sterols may need to be reduced or stopped.
◑ *Alert:* Don't use drug in patients with chronic kidney disease who aren't receiving dialysis because they have an increased risk of hypocalcemia.

PATIENT TEACHING
• Tell patient not to divide tablets but to take them whole, with food or shortly after a meal.
• Advise patient to report to prescriber adverse reactions and signs of hypocalcemia, which include paresthesias, muscle weakness, muscle cramping, and muscle spasm.

ciprofloxacin
si-proe-FLOX-a-sin

Cipro◈, Cipro I.V., Cipro XR

Therapeutic class: Antibiotics
Pharmacologic class: Fluoroquinolones
Pregnancy risk category: C

AVAILABLE FORMS
Infusion (premixed): 200 mg in 100 mL D_5W, 400 mg in 200 mL D_5W
Injection: 200 mg, 400 mg
Suspension (oral): 250 mg/5 mL (5%), 500 mg/5 mL (10%)
Tablets (extended-release, film-coated): 500 mg, 1,000 mg
Tablets (film-coated): 100 mg, 250 mg, 500 mg, 750 mg

INDICATIONS & DOSAGES
Adjust-a-dose (for all indications): For patients with a CrCl of 30 to 50 mL/minute, give 250 to 500 mg P.O. every 12 hours or the usual I.V. dose; if CrCl is 5 to 29 mL/minute, give 250 to 500 mg P.O.

every 18 hours or 200 to 400 mg I.V. every 18 to 24 hours. If patient is receiving hemodialysis, give 250 to 500 mg P.O. every 24 hours after dialysis.

➤ **Complicated intra-abdominal infection**
Adults: 500 mg P.O. or 400 mg I.V. every 12 hours for 7 to 14 days. Give with metronidazole.

➤ **Severe or complicated bone or joint infection, severe respiratory tract infection, severe skin or skin-structure infection**
Adults: 750 mg P.O. every 12 hours or 400 mg I.V. every 8 hours.

➤ **Severe or complicated UTI; mild to moderate bone or joint infection; mild to moderate respiratory infection; mild to moderate skin or skin-structure infection; infectious diarrhea; typhoid fever**
Adults: 500 mg P.O. or 400 mg I.V. every 12 hours. Or, 1,000 mg extended-release tablets P.O. every 24 hours.

➤ **Complicated UTI or pyelonephritis**
Adults: 500 mg P.O. every 12 hours for 7 to 14 days. Or 1,000 mg extended-release tablets P.O. every 24 hours for 7 to 14 days.
Children ages 1 to 17: 6 to 10 mg/kg I.V. every 8 hours for 10 to 21 days. Maximum I.V. dose, 400 mg. Or, 10 to 20 mg/kg P.O. every 12 hours. Maximum P.O. dose, 750 mg. Don't exceed maximum dose, even in patients who weigh more than 51 kg (112 lb).
Adjust-a-dose: If CrCl is less than 30 mL/minute, reduce the dosage of extended-release form from 1,000 to 500 mg daily. Administer extended-release form after hemodialysis or peritoneal dialysis is completed.

➤ **Nosocomial pneumonia**
Adults: 400 mg I.V. every 8 hours for 10 to 14 days.

➤ **Mild to moderate UTI**
Adults: 250 mg P.O. or 200 mg I.V. every 12 hours for 7 to 14 days.

➤ **Uncomplicated UTI**
Adults: 500 mg extended-release tablet P.O. once daily for 3 days.

➤ **Chronic bacterial prostatitis**
Adults: 500 mg P.O. every 12 hours or 400 mg I.V. every 12 hours for 28 days.

➤ **Mild to moderate acute sinusitis**
Adults: 500 mg P.O. or 400 mg I.V. every 12 hours for 10 days.

➤ **Empirical therapy in febrile neutropenic patients**
Adults: 400 mg I.V. every 8 hours used with piperacillin 50 mg/kg I.V. every 4 hours (not to exceed 24 g/day of piperacillin).

➤ **Inhalation anthrax (postexposure)**
Adults: 400 mg I.V. every 12 hours initially until susceptibility test results are known; then 500 mg P.O. b.i.d. Give drug with one or two additional antimicrobials. Switch to oral therapy when appropriate. Treat for 60 days (I.V. and P.O. combined).
Children: 10 mg/kg I.V. every 12 hours; then 15 mg/kg P.O. every 12 hours. Don't exceed 800 mg/day I.V. or 1,000 mg/day P.O. Give drug with one or two additional antimicrobials. Switch to oral therapy when appropriate. Treat for 60 days (I.V. and P.O. combined).

➤ **Anthrax prophylaxis** ◆
Adults with zoonotic cutaneous anthrax without head or neck involvement: 500 mg P.O. b.i.d. for 7 to 10 days.
Adults with inhalational, GI, or oropharyngeal/cutaneous anthrax with systemic, edematous, or head or neck involvement: 400 mg I.V. every 12 hours; switch to 500 mg P.O. b.i.d. for a total of 60 days.
Children with inhalational/systemic/cutaneous anthrax: 10 to 15 mg/kg I.V. every 12 hours (maximum, 800 mg/day). Convert to 10 to 15 mg/kg P.O. every 12 hours (maximum, 1 g/day) when clinically indicated. Duration of therapy is 60 days.

➤ **Plague** ◆
Adults: 400 mg I.V. b.i.d. Treat for 7 days after last known or suspected exposure or until exposure has been excluded. Continue treatment for 10 to 14 days.
Children: 10 to 15 mg/kg I.V. b.i.d. Treat for 7 days after last known or suspected exposure or until exposure has been excluded. Continue treatment for 10 to 14 days.

➤ **Traveler's diarrhea** ◆
Adults: 500 mg P.O. b.i.d. for 3 days.

➤ **Tularemia** ◆
Adults: 400 mg I.V. b.i.d. for 10 days.
Children: 15 mg/kg I.V. b.i.d. (maximum, 1 g/day) for 10 days.

➤ **Infective endocarditis from** *Haemophilus parainfluenzae, Haemophilus aphrophilus, Haemophilus*

C

paraphrophilus, Haemophilus influenzae, Actinobacillus actinomycetemcomitans, Cardiobacterium hominis, Eikenella corrodens, Kingella kingae, and *Kingella denitrificans* (HACEK) infections ♦
Adults: 800 mg I.V. daily or 1,000 mg P.O. daily in two divided doses for 4 weeks in native valve infections and for 6 weeks for infections of prosthetic valves or other cardiac prosthetic materials. Fluoroquinolone therapy is recommended only for patients unable to tolerate cephalosporin and ampicillin therapy; levofloxacin, gatifloxacin, or moxifloxacin may be substituted.
Children and adolescents: 20 to 30 mg/kg/day I.V. or P.O. in two divided doses for 4 weeks in native valve infections and for 6 weeks for infections of prosthetic valves or other cardiac prosthetic materials. Fluoroquinolone therapy is recommended only for patients unable to tolerate cephalosporin and ampicillin therapy; levofloxacin, gatifloxacin, or moxifloxacin may be substituted. Fluoroquinolones aren't generally recommended for patients younger than age 18.
➤ **Infective endocarditis (culture-negative), including *Bartonella* infection, in patients with native valve** ♦
Adults: 800 mg I.V. daily or 1,000 mg P.O. daily in two divided doses for 4 to 6 weeks in combination with vancomycin and gentamicin.
Children and adolescents: 20 to 30 mg/kg/day I.V. or P.O. in two divided doses for 4 to 6 weeks in combination with vancomycin and gentamicin.
➤ **Surgical prophylaxis** ♦
Adults: 400 mg I.V. infused over 60 minutes and repeated every 4 to 10 hours. Or, 500 mg P.O. every 12 hours or a one-time dose of 1,500 mg.
➤ **Chancroid** ♦
Adults: 500 mg P.O. b.i.d. for 3 days.
➤ **Granuloma inguinale (donovanosis)** ♦
Adults: 750 mg P.O. b.i.d. for at least 3 weeks. Treatment should continue until all lesions have completely healed.
➤ **Infection prophylaxis in cancer-related neutropenia** ♦
Adults: 500 mg P.O. b.i.d. initiated at time of stem cell infusion, first day of cytotoxic therapy, or day after last dose of cytotoxic

therapy. Discontinue ciprofloxacin when recovery from neutropenia occurs or empirical antibiotic therapy for fever is initiated.

ADMINISTRATION
P.O.
● Cipro XR and immediate-release oral forms aren't interchangeable.
● Obtain specimen for culture and sensitivity tests before giving first dose. Begin therapy while awaiting results.
● To avoid decreasing the effects of ciprofloxacin, separate dosage of certain drugs by up to 6 hours. Food doesn't affect absorption but may delay peak levels.
● Caffeine should be avoided during therapy with this drug because of potential for increased caffeine effects.
● Give drug with plenty of fluids to reduce risk of urine crystals.
● Don't crush or split the extended-release tablets.
I.V.
▼ Obtain specimen for culture and sensitivity tests before giving first dose. Begin therapy while awaiting results.
▼ Dilute drug to 1 to 2 mg/mL using D_5W or normal saline solution for injection.
▼ If giving drug through a Y-type set, stop the other I.V. solution while infusing.
▼ Infuse over 1 hour into a large vein to minimize discomfort and vein irritation.
▼ **Incompatibilities:** Aminophylline, ampicillin–sulbactam, azithromycin, cefepime, clindamycin phosphate, dexamethasone sodium phosphate, furosemide, heparin sodium, methylprednisolone sodium succinate, phenytoin sodium.

ACTION
Inhibits bacterial DNA synthesis, mainly by blocking DNA gyrase; bactericidal.

Route	Onset	Peak	Duration
P.O.	Unknown	30–120 min	Unknown
P.O. (extended-release)	Unknown	1–4 hr	Unknown
I.V.	Unknown	Immediate	Unknown

Half-life: 4 hours; Cipro XR, 6 hours in adults with normal renal function.

ADVERSE REACTIONS
CNS: *seizures,* confusion, headache, restlessness.

GI: *pseudomembranous colitis,* diarrhea, nausea, vomiting.
GU: crystalluria, interstitial nephritis.
Hematologic: *leukopenia, neutropenia, thrombocytopenia,* eosinophilia.
Musculoskeletal: tendon rupture.
Skin: rash, *Stevens-Johnson syndrome, toxic epidermal necrolysis.*
Other: hypersensitivity reactions.

INTERACTIONS
Drug-drug. *Aluminum hydroxide, aluminum-magnesium hydroxide, calcium carbonate, didanosine (chewable tablets, buffered tablets, or pediatric powder for oral solution), magnesium hydroxide, products containing zinc:* May decrease ciprofloxacin absorption and effects. Give ciprofloxacin 2 hours before or 6 hours after these drugs.
Cyclosporine: May increase risk for cyclosporine toxicity. Monitor cyclosporine level.
Iron salts: May decrease absorption of ciprofloxacin, reducing anti-infective response. Give at least 2 hours apart.
NSAIDs: May increase risk of CNS stimulation. Monitor patient closely.
Probenecid: May elevate level of ciprofloxacin. Monitor patient for toxicity.
Black Box Warning *Steroids:* May increase risk of tendinitis and tendon rupture. ∎
Sucralfate: May decrease ciprofloxacin absorption, reducing anti-infective response. If use together can't be avoided, give at least 6 hours apart.
Theophylline: May increase theophylline level and prolong theophylline half-life. Monitor level of theophylline and watch for adverse effects.
Tizanidine: Increases tizanidine levels, causing low blood pressure, somnolence, dizziness, and slowed psychomotor skills. Avoid using together.
Warfarin: May increase anticoagulant effects. Monitor PT and INR closely.
Drug-herb. *Dong quai, St. John's wort:* May cause photosensitivity. Advise patient to avoid excessive sunlight exposure.
Yerba maté: May decrease clearance of herb's methylxanthines and cause toxicity. Discourage use together.
Drug-food. *Caffeine:* May increase effect of caffeine. Monitor patient closely.

Dairy products, other foods: May delay peak drug levels. Advise patient to take drug on an empty stomach.
Orange juice fortified with calcium: May decrease GI absorption of drug, reducing its effects. Discourage use together.
Drug-lifestyle. *Sun exposure:* May cause photosensitivity reactions. Advise patient to avoid excessive sunlight exposure.

EFFECTS ON LAB TEST RESULTS
● May increase alkaline phosphatase, ALT, AST, bilirubin, BUN, creatinine, LDH, and GGT levels.
● May increase eosinophil count. May decrease WBC, neutrophil, and platelet counts.

CONTRAINDICATIONS & CAUTIONS
● Contraindicated in patients sensitive to fluoroquinolones.
● Use cautiously in patients with CNS disorders, such as severe cerebral arteriosclerosis or seizure disorders, and in those at risk for seizures. Drug may cause CNS stimulation.
Black Box Warning Drug is associated with increased risk of tendinitis and tendon rupture, especially in patients older than age 60 and those with heart, kidney, or lung transplants. ∎
Black Box Warning Drug may exacerbate muscle weakness in patients with myasthenia gravis. Avoid use of fluoroquinolones in patients with a known history of myasthenia gravis. ∎
☉ Alert: Oral or parenteral fluoroquinolones may increase the risk of peripheral neuropathy of the arms or legs. Symptoms can occur anytime during treatment and can last for months to years or be permanent. Stop drug immediately if patient develops symptoms and switch to a non-fluoroquinolone antibacterial drug unless the benefits of continued treatment outweigh the risks.

NURSING CONSIDERATIONS
● Monitor patient's intake and output and observe patient for signs of crystalluria.
Black Box Warning Tendon rupture may occur in patients receiving quinolones. If pain or inflammation occurs or if patient ruptures a tendon, stop drug. ∎

Reactions in bold italics are *life-threatening*. Interactions may have a *rapid onset* or a *delayed onset*.

❸ Alert: Monitor patient for symptoms of peripheral neuropathy (pain, burning, tingling, numbness, weakness, or a change in sensation to light touch, pain or temperature, or sense of body position) and report them immediately to the practitioner.

• Long-term therapy may result in overgrowth of organisms resistant to drug.

• Cutaneous anthrax patients with signs of systemic involvement, extensive edema, or lesions on the head or neck need I.V. therapy and a multidrug approach.

• Additional antimicrobials for anthrax multidrug regimens can include rifampin, vancomycin, penicillin, ampicillin, chloramphenicol, imipenem, clindamycin, and clarithromycin.

• Steroids may be used as adjunctive therapy for anthrax patients with severe edema and for meningitis.

• Follow current Centers for Disease Control and Prevention recommendations for anthrax.

• Pregnant women and immunocompromised patients should receive the usual doses and regimens for anthrax.

PATIENT TEACHING

• Tell patient to take drug as prescribed, even after he feels better.

• Advise patient to drink plenty of fluids to reduce risk of urine crystals.

• Advise patient not to crush, split, or chew the extended-release tablets.

❸ Alert: Warn patient to contact practitioner immediately if symptoms of peripheral neuropathy occur.

• Warn patient to avoid hazardous tasks that require alertness, such as driving, until effects of drug are known.

• Instruct patient to avoid caffeine while taking drug because of potential for increased caffeine effects.

• Advise patient that hypersensitivity reactions may occur even after first dose. If a rash or other allergic reaction occurs, tell him to stop drug immediately and notify prescriber.

• Tell patient that tendon rupture can occur with drug and to notify prescriber if he experiences pain or inflammation.

• Tell patient to avoid excessive sunlight or artificial ultraviolet light during therapy.

• Because drug appears in breast milk, advise women to stop breast-feeding during treatment or to consider treatment with another drug.

ciprofloxacin hydrochloride
si-proe-FLOX-a-sin

Ciloxan

Therapeutic class: Antibiotics
Pharmacologic class: Fluoroquinolones
Pregnancy risk category: C

AVAILABLE FORMS
Ophthalmic ointment: 0.3% (base)
Ophthalmic solution: 0.3% (base)

INDICATIONS & DOSAGES
➤ **Corneal ulcers caused by *Pseudomonas aeruginosa*, *Staphylococcus aureus*, *Staphylococcus epidermidis*, *Streptococcus pneumoniae*, and possibly *Serratia marcescens* and *Streptococcus viridans***
Adults and children older than age 1: Give 2 drops in affected eye every 15 minutes for first 6 hours; then 2 drops every 30 minutes for remainder of first day. On the second day, 2 drops hourly. On days 3 to 14, 2 drops every 4 hours. Treatment may be continued after day 14 if reepithelialization hasn't occurred.
➤ **Bacterial conjunctivitis caused by *Haemophilus influenzae*, *S. aureus*, *S. epidermidis*, and possibly *S. pneumoniae***
Adults and children older than age 1: Give 1 or 2 drops into conjunctival sac of affected eye every 2 hours while awake for first 2 days. Then, 1 or 2 drops every 4 hours while awake for next 5 days.
Adults and children older than age 2: ½-inch ribbon into the conjunctival sac t.i.d. for the first 2 days, then ½-inch ribbon b.i.d. for the next 5 days.

ADMINISTRATION
Ophthalmic

• Apply light finger pressure on lacrimal sac for 1 minute after drops are instilled.

ACTION

Inhibits bacterial DNA gyrase, an enzyme needed for bacterial replication.

Route	Onset	Peak	Duration
Ophthalmic	Unknown	Unknown	Unknown

Half-life: 3 to 5 hours.

ADVERSE REACTIONS

EENT: local burning or discomfort, white crystalline precipitate in superficial portion of corneal defect in patients with corneal ulcers, allergic reactions, conjunctival hyperemia, foreign body sensation, itching.
GI: bad or bitter taste in mouth.

INTERACTIONS

None significant.

EFFECTS ON LAB TEST RESULTS

None reported.

CONTRAINDICATIONS & CAUTIONS

• Contraindicated in patients hypersensitive to drug or other fluoroquinolones.
• It's unknown if drug appears in breast milk after application to eye; however, drug given systemically appears in breast milk. Use cautiously in breast-feeding women.

NURSING CONSIDERATIONS

☣ Alert: Stop drug at first sign of hypersensitivity, such as rash, and notify prescriber. Serious hypersensitivity reactions, including anaphylaxis, may occur in patients receiving systemic drug.
• A topical overdose may be flushed from eyes with warm tap water.
• If corneal epithelium is still compromised after 14 days of treatment, continue therapy.
• Institute appropriate therapy if superinfection occurs. Prolonged use may result in overgrowth of nonsusceptible organisms, including fungi.
• **Look alike–sound alike:** Don't confuse Ciloxan with Cytoxan.

PATIENT TEACHING

• Tell patient to clean eye area of excessive discharge before instilling.
• Teach patient how to instill drops or apply ointment. Advise him to wash hands before and after using drug and not to touch tip of dropper to eye or surrounding tissues.
• Instruct patient to apply light finger pressure on lacrimal sac for 1 minute after drops are instilled.
• Advise patient that drug may cause temporary blurring of vision or stinging after administration. If these symptoms become pronounced or worsen, contact prescriber.
• Tell patient to avoid wearing contacts while treating bacterial conjunctivitis. If approved by prescriber, tell patient to wait at least 15 minutes after instilling drops before inserting contact lenses.
• Tell patient not to share drug, washcloths, or towels with family members and to notify prescriber if anyone develops same signs or symptoms.
• Stress importance of compliance with recommended therapy.

SAFETY ALERT!

cisatracurium besylate
sis-ah-trah-KYOO-ee-hum

Nimbex

Therapeutic class: Skeletal muscle relaxants
Pharmacologic class: Nondepolarizing neuromuscular blockers
Pregnancy risk category: B

AVAILABLE FORMS

Injection: 2 mg/mL, 10 mg/mL*

INDICATIONS & DOSAGES

➤ **Adjunct to general anesthesia to facilitate endotracheal intubation and relax skeletal muscles during surgery**
Adults: First dose of 0.15 mg/kg I.V.; then maintenance dosages of 0.03 mg/kg I.V. every 40 to 50 minutes p.r.n. Or, first dose of 0.2 mg/kg I.V.; then maintenance dosages of 0.03 mg/kg I.V. every 50 to 60 minutes p.r.n. Or, as a continuous infusion in operating room, after initial bolus dose, give a maintenance infusion at 3 mcg/kg/minute and reduce to 1 to 2 mcg/kg/minute as needed.
Children ages 2 to 12: 0.1 to 0.15 mg/kg I.V. over 5 to 10 seconds. After first dose, give a maintenance infusion of 3 mcg/kg/minute,

then reduce to 1 to 2 mcg/kg/minute as needed.

Children ages 1 to 23 months: 0.15 mg/kg over 5 to 10 seconds. No information is available for continuous infusion.

Adjust-a-dose: During coronary artery bypass surgery with induced hypothermia, reduce infusion rate by 50%.

➤ **To maintain neuromuscular blockade during mechanical ventilation in intensive care unit (ICU)**

Adults: Principles for infusion in operating room apply to use in ICU. After first dose, give 3 mcg/kg/minute by I.V. infusion. Range, 0.5 to 10.2 mcg/kg/minute.

Adjust-a-dose: In patients with neuromuscular disease, such as myasthenia gravis or Eaton-Lambert syndrome, don't exceed 0.02 mg/kg. Patients with burns may need increased amount.

ADMINISTRATION

I.V.

▼ Drug is colorless to slightly yellow or green-yellow. Inspect vials for particulates and discoloration before use. Don't use unclear solutions or those with visible particulates.

▼ The 20-mL vial is intended for use only in the ICU.

▼ Use only under direct supervision of medical staff skilled in using neuromuscular blockers and maintaining airway patency. Don't give drug unless resources for intubation, mechanical ventilation, and oxygen therapy are within reach.

▼ Keep refrigerated; don't freeze. Use drug within 21 days after removing from refrigeration.

▼ Use drug within 24 hours when diluted to a concentration of 0.1 mg/mL in D_5W, normal saline solution, or 5% dextrose and normal saline solution.

▼ **Incompatibilities:** Acyclovir, alkaline solutions with pH higher than 8.5, aminophylline, amphotericin B, amphotericin B cholesteryl sulfate complex, ampicillin, ampicillin sodium–sulbactam sodium, cefazolin, cefotaxime, cefoxitin, ceftazidime, ceftizoxime, cefuroxime, diazepam, furosemide, ganciclovir, heparin sodium, ketorolac, lactated Ringer injection, methylprednisolone sodium

succinate, piperacillin, piperacillin sodium–tazobactam sodium, propofol, sodium bicarbonate, sodium nitroprusside, thiopental sodium, ticarcillin disodium–clavulanate potassium, sulfamethoxazole-trimethoprim.

ACTION

Binds to cholinergic receptors on the motor end plate, antagonizing acetylcholine and blocking neuromuscular transmission.

Route	Onset	Peak	Duration
I.V.	1–2 min	2–5 min	25–44 min

Half-life: 22 to 29 minutes; about 3 hours for laudanosine.

ADVERSE REACTIONS

CV: ***bradycardia,*** hypotension, flushing.
Respiratory: ***bronchospasm, prolonged apnea.***
Skin: rash.

INTERACTIONS

Drug-drug. *Aminoglycosides, bacitracin, clindamycin, colistimethate sodium, colistin, lithium, local anesthetics, magnesium salts, polymyxins, procainamide, quinidine, quinine, tetracyclines:* May enhance neuromuscular blocking action of cisatracurium. Use together cautiously.

Carbamazepine, phenytoin: May decrease the effects of cisatracurium. May need to increase cisatracurium dose.

Enflurane or isoflurane given with nitrous oxide or oxygen: May prolong cisatracurium duration of action. Patient may need less frequent maintenance doses, lower maintenance doses, or reduced infusion rate of cisatracurium. Effects are dependent on duration of volatile agent administration.

Succinylcholine: May shorten time to onset of maximal neuromuscular block. Monitor patient.

EFFECTS ON LAB TEST RESULTS

None reported.

CONTRAINDICATIONS & CAUTIONS

• Contraindicated in patients who are hypersensitive to drug, to other bisbenzylisoquinolinium drugs, or to benzyl alcohol (found in 10 mg/mL vial).

• Use cautiously in pregnant or breast-feeding women.

⚠ *Overdose S&S:* Prolonged neuromuscular blockade.

NURSING CONSIDERATIONS

• Drug isn't recommended for rapid-sequence endotracheal intubation because of its intermediate onset.

• Dosage requirements vary widely among patients.

❸ *Alert:* Drug has no known effect on consciousness, pain threshold, or cerebration. To avoid patient distress, don't induce neuromuscular block before unconsciousness.

❸ *Alert:* Never give by I.M. injection.

• Monitor neuromuscular function with nerve stimulator during drug administration. If stimulation doesn't elicit a response, stop infusion until response returns.

• To avoid inaccurate dosing, perform neuromuscular monitoring on a nonparetic arm or leg in patients with hemiparesis or paraparesis.

• Monitor acid-base balance and electrolyte levels. Abnormalities may potentiate or antagonize the action of cisatracurium.

• Monitor patient for malignant hyperthermia.

• Give analgesics, if indicated. Patient can feel pain but can't indicate its presence.

❸ *Alert:* Careful dosage calculation is essential. Always verify dosage with another health care professional.

PATIENT TEACHING

• Explain purpose of drug.

• Assure patient that monitoring will be continuous.

• Explain all procedures and events because patient can still hear.

SAFETY ALERT!

cisplatin (CDDP)
SIS-pla-tin

Therapeutic class: Antineoplastics
Pharmacologic class: Platinum-containing compounds
Pregnancy risk category: D

AVAILABLE FORMS
Injection: 1 mg/mL

INDICATIONS & DOSAGES

Adjust-a-dose (for all indications): If CrCl is 10 to 50 mL/minute, give 75% of normal dose; if CrCl is less than 10 mL/minute, give 50% of normal dose but consider avoiding use. For hemodialysis patients, give 50% of usual dose; give after dialysis on dialysis days. For peritoneal dialysis patients, give 50% of usual dose. For patients receiving continuous renal replacement therapy, give 75% of usual dose.

➤ **Adjunctive therapy in metastatic testicular cancer**
Adults: 20 mg/m² I.V. daily for 5 days. Repeat every 3 weeks for three cycles.

➤ **Adjunctive therapy in metastatic ovarian cancer**
Adults: 100 mg/m² I.V.; repeat every 4 weeks. Or, 75 to 100 mg/m² I.V. once every 4 weeks with cyclophosphamide.

➤ **Advanced bladder cancer**
Adults: 50 to 70 mg/m² I.V. every 3 to 4 weeks. Give 50 mg/m² every 4 weeks in patients who have received other antineoplastics or radiation therapy.

ADMINISTRATION
I.V.

▼ Preparing and giving parenteral form of drug may be mutagenic, teratogenic, or carcinogenic. Follow facility policy to reduce risks.

▼ Hydrate patient with normal saline solution for 8 to 12 hours before giving drug. Maintain urine output of at least 100 mL/hour for 4 consecutive hours before therapy and for 24 hours after therapy.

Black Box Warning Anaphylactic-type reactions may occur within minutes of administration. Have emergency equipment available. ∎

▼ Infusions are most stable in solutions containing chloride (such as normal or half-normal saline solution and 0.22% sodium chloride). Don't use D₅W alone.

▼ Further dilute with dextrose 5% in 0.3% sodium chloride injection or dextrose 5% in half-normal saline solution for injection with 37.5 g mannitol added.

▼ Administer over 6 to 8 hours.

▼ Solutions are stable for 20 hours at room temperature. Don't refrigerate.

Reactions in bold italics are *life-threatening*. Interactions may have a *rapid onset* or a *delayed onset*.

▼ **Incompatibilities:** Aluminum administration sets, amifostine, amphotericin B cholesteryl sulfate complex, cefepime, D_5W, etoposide–mannitol–potassium chloride, 5-FU, mesna, 0.1% sodium chloride solution, paclitaxel, piperacillin sodium–tazobactam sodium, sodium bicarbonate, sodium bisulfate, sodium thiosulfate, solutions with a chloride content less than 2%, thiotepa.

ACTION
May cross-link strands of cellular DNA and interfere with RNA transcription, causing an imbalance of growth that leads to cell death. Not specific to cell cycle.

Route	Onset	Peak	Duration
I.V.	Unknown	Unknown	Several days

Half-life: Initial phase, 25 to 79 minutes; terminal phase, 58 to 78 hours.

ADVERSE REACTIONS
CNS: peripheral neuritis, *seizures.*
EENT: tinnitus, hearing loss.
GI: anorexia, diarrhea, loss of taste, nausea, vomiting.
GU: *prolonged renal toxicity with repeated courses of therapy.*
Hematologic: *myelosuppression, leukopenia, thrombocytopenia,* anemia.
Metabolic: *hypomagnesemia, hypokalemia, hypocalcemia.*
Other: *anaphylactoid reaction.*

INTERACTIONS
Drug-drug. *Aminoglycosides:* May increase nephrotoxicity. Carefully monitor renal function study results.
Aminoglycosides, bumetanide, ethacrynic acid, furosemide, torsemide: May increase ototoxicity. Avoid using together, if possible.
Aspirin, NSAIDs: May increase risk of bleeding. Avoid using together.
Fosphenytoin, phenytoin: May decrease phenytoin and fosphenytoin levels. Monitor levels.
Myelosuppressives: May increase myelosuppression. Monitor patient.

EFFECTS ON LAB TEST RESULTS
● May increase uric acid level. May decrease calcium, hemoglobin, magnesium, phosphate, potassium, and sodium levels.
● May decrease platelet and WBC counts.

CONTRAINDICATIONS & CAUTIONS
● Contraindicated in patients hypersensitive to drug or other platinum-containing compounds and in those with preexisting severe renal disease, hearing impairment, or myelosuppression.
● Use cautiously in patients previously treated with radiation or cytotoxic drugs and in those with peripheral neuropathies; also use cautiously with other ototoxic and nephrotoxic drugs.
⚠ *Overdose S&S:* Renal failure, liver failure, deafness, ocular toxicity, significant myelosuppression, intractable nausea and vomiting, neuritis, death.

NURSING CONSIDERATIONS
Black Box Warning Drug should be administered under the supervision of a physician experienced in the use of cancer chemotherapeutic agents. ∎
Black Box Warning Be careful to avoid overdose. Doses greater than 100 mg/m^2 per cycle every 3 to 4 weeks are rare. Confirm that dose is total dose per cycle, not daily dose. ∎
� *Alert:* Cisplatin is considered a vesicant if more than 20 mL is administered or if it's given at a concentration of 0.5 mg/mL or more. Stop infusion immediately if extravasation occurs and prepare for the provider to infiltrate the area with sodium thiosulfate and institute other treatments.
● Monitor CBC, electrolyte levels (especially potassium and magnesium), platelet count, and renal function studies before initial and subsequent doses.
Black Box Warning Ototoxicity, which may be more pronounced in children, is manifested by tinnitus or loss of high-frequency hearing and, occasionally, deafness. ∎
● To detect hearing loss, obtain audiometry tests before initial and subsequent doses.
● Prehydration and mannitol diuresis may significantly reduce renal toxicity and ototoxicity.

• Therapeutic effects are frequently accompanied by toxicity.

• Patients may experience vomiting 3 to 5 days after treatment, requiring prolonged antiemetic treatment. Monitor intake and output. Continue I.V. hydration until patient can tolerate adequate oral intake.

Black Box Warning Renal toxicity is cumulative; don't give next dose until renal function returns to normal. ∎

• Don't repeat dose unless platelet count exceeds 100,000/mm^3, WBC count exceeds 4,000/mm^3, creatinine level is below 1.5 mg/dL, BUN level is below 25 mg/dL, and auditory acuity is within normal limits.

• To prevent bleeding, avoid all I.M. injections when platelet count is less than 50,000/mm^3.

• Anticipate need for blood transfusions during treatment because of cumulative anemia.

Black Box Warning Immediately give epinephrine, corticosteroids, or antihistamines for anaphylactoid reactions. ∎

• Safety of drug in children hasn't been established.

• **Look alike–sound alike:** Don't confuse cisplatin with carboplatin; they aren't interchangeable.

PATIENT TEACHING

• Advise patient to watch for signs and symptoms of infection (fever, sore throat, fatigue) and bleeding (easy bruising, nosebleeds, bleeding gums, tarry stools). Tell patient to take temperature daily.

• Tell patient to immediately report ringing in the ears or numbness in hands or feet.

• Instruct patient to avoid OTC products containing aspirin.

• Advise women to stop breast-feeding during therapy because of risk of toxicity to infant.

• Advise women of childbearing age to consult prescriber before becoming pregnant.

citalopram hydrobromide
si-TAL-oh-pram

Celexa✧

Therapeutic class: Antidepressants
Pharmacologic class: SSRIs
Pregnancy risk category: C

AVAILABLE FORMS
Solution: 10 mg/5 mL
Tablets: 10 mg, 20 mg, 40 mg

INDICATIONS & DOSAGES
Adjust-a-dose (for all indications): For patients with hepatic impairment and for those who are CYP2C19 poor metabolizers, are taking cimetidine or another CYP2C19 inhibitor, or are older than age 60, the maximum dosage is 20 mg/day.

➤ **Depression**
Adults: Initially, 20 mg P.O. once daily, increasing to 40 mg daily after no less than 1 week. Maximum recommended dose is 40 mg daily.
Elderly patients: 20 mg P.O. daily.

➤ **Premenstrual disorders** ♦
Adults: Intermittent dosing consists of initiating treatment on the estimated day of ovulation. Give 5 mg P.O. Each day increase dose by 5 mg to a maximum dose of 30 mg P.O. daily until first day of menstruation. On first day of menstruation, reduce dose to 20 mg P.O. daily. On second day, reduce dose to 10 mg P.O. daily. No drug is given from menstruation day 3 until estimated ovulation begins.

➤ **Obsessive-compulsive disorder** ♦
Adults: Initially, 20 mg P.O. daily, titrated to a target dose of 40 mg P.O. daily. Maximum dosage is 40 mg/day. Significant improvement is generally seen 4 to 6 weeks after the start of therapy.

ADMINISTRATION
P.O.
• Give drug without regard for food.

ACTION
Probably linked to potentiation of serotonergic activity in the CNS resulting from inhibition of neuronal reuptake of serotonin.

Route	Onset	Peak	Duration
P.O.	Unknown	4 hr	Unknown

Half-life: 35 hours.

ADVERSE REACTIONS

CNS: somnolence, insomnia, *suicide attempt,* anxiety, agitation, dizziness, paresthesia, migraine, impaired concentration, amnesia, depression, apathy, tremor, confusion, fatigue, fever.
CV: tachycardia, orthostatic hypotension, hypotension.
EENT: rhinitis, sinusitis, abnormal accommodation.
GI: dry mouth, nausea, diarrhea, anorexia, dyspepsia, vomiting, abdominal pain, taste perversion, increased saliva, flatulence, increased appetite.
GU: dysmenorrhea, amenorrhea, ejaculation disorder, erectile dysfunction, anorgasmia, polyuria.
Metabolic: decreased or increased weight.
Musculoskeletal: arthralgia, myalgia.
Respiratory: upper respiratory tract infection, coughing.
Skin: rash, pruritus.
Other: increased sweating, yawning, decreased libido.

INTERACTIONS

Drug-drug. *Amphetamines, buspirone, dextromethorphan, dihydroergotamine, meperidine, other SSRIs or SSNRIs (duloxetine, venlafaxine), TCAs,* **tramadol,** *trazodone, tryptophan:* May increase the risk of serotonin syndrome. Avoid other drugs that increase the availability of serotonin in the CNS; monitor patient closely if used together.
Antiarrhythmics (Class IA [procainamide, quinidine], Class III [amiodarone, sotalol]), antibiotics (gatifloxacin, moxifloxacin), antipsychotics (chlorpromazine, thioridazine), drugs that prolong QTc interval (levomethadyl acetate, methadone, pentamidine): May cause QTc prolongation and increase risk of torsades de pointes. Use together isn't recommended.
Carbamazepine: May increase citalopram clearance. Monitor patient for effects.

CNS drugs: May cause additive effects. Use together cautiously.
Drugs that affect coagulation (such as aspirin, NSAIDs): May increase bleeding risk. Monitor patient closely.
Drugs that inhibit CYP3A4 and CYP2C19: May cause decreased clearance of citalopram. Monitor patient for increased adverse effects.
Imipramine, other TCAs: May increase level of imipramine metabolite desipramine by about 50%. Use together cautiously.
Linezolid, methylene blue: May cause serotonin syndrome. Use with extreme caution and monitor closely.
Lithium: May enhance serotonergic effect of citalopram. Use together cautiously, and monitor lithium level.
MAO inhibitors (phenelzine, selegiline, tranylcypromine): May cause serotonin syndrome or signs and symptoms resembling neuroleptic malignant syndrome. Avoid using within 14 days of MAO inhibitor therapy.
Sumatriptan: May cause weakness, hyperreflexia, and incoordination. Monitor patient closely.
Drug-herb. *St. John's wort:* May increase the risk of serotonin syndrome. Discourage use together.
Drug-lifestyle. *Alcohol use:* May increase CNS effects. Discourage use together.

EFFECTS ON LAB TEST RESULTS
None reported.

CONTRAINDICATIONS & CAUTIONS
• Contraindicated in patients hypersensitive to drug or its inactive components, within 14 days of MAO inhibitor therapy, and in patients taking pimozide.
❸ **Alert:** Drug isn't recommended for patients with congenital long QT syndrome, bradycardia, hypokalemia, hypomagnesemia, recent acute MI, or uncompensated heart failure. Use with extreme caution.
❸ **Alert:** High doses can prolong the QT interval and cause torsades de pointes, a potentially fatal heart rhythm. Maximum dose is 40 mg/day.

❸ Alert: Discontinue drug in patients with persistent QTc interval measurement longer than 500 ms.

❸ Alert: Concomitant use with linezolid or methylene blue can cause serotonin syndrome (fever, mental status changes, muscle twitching, excessive sweating, shivering or shaking, diarrhea, loss of coordination). Use with linezolid or methylene blue only for life-threatening or urgent conditions when the potential benefits outweigh the risks of toxicity.

• Use cautiously in patients with history of mania, seizures, suicidal thoughts, or hepatic or renal impairment.

• Use in third trimester of pregnancy may be linked to neonatal complications at birth. Consider the risk versus benefit of treatment during this time.

• Drug appears in breast milk. Consider benefits to the mother versus risks to the infant when deciding whether to continue drug or allowing patient to breast-feed.

Black Box Warning Drug isn't approved for use in children. ∎

⚠ Overdose S&S: Dizziness, sweating, nausea, vomiting, tremor, somnolence, sinus tachycardia, amnesia, confusion, coma, seizures, hyperventilation, cyanosis, rhabdomyolysis, ECG changes.

NURSING CONSIDERATIONS

• Correct electrolyte disturbances before starting drug; monitor patients at high risk for electrolyte disturbances periodically during therapy.

• Although drug hasn't been shown to impair psychomotor performance, any psychoactive drug has the potential to impair judgment, thinking, or motor skills.

• The possibility of a suicide attempt is inherent in depression and may persist until significant remission occurs. Closely supervise high-risk patients at start of drug therapy. Reduce risk of overdose by limiting amount of drug available per refill.

Black Box Warning Drug may increase the risk of suicidal thinking and behavior in children, adolescents, and young adults with major depressive disorder or other psychiatric disorders. ∎

• At least 14 days should elapse between MAO inhibitor therapy and citalopram therapy.

❸ Alert: Combining triptans with an SSRI or an SSNRI may cause serotonin syndrome or neuroleptic malignant syndrome–like reactions. Signs and symptoms of serotonin syndrome may include restlessness, hallucinations, loss of coordination, fast heartbeat, rapid changes in blood pressure, increased body temperature, overactive reflexes, nausea, vomiting, and diarrhea. Serotonin syndrome may be more likely to occur when starting or increasing the dose of the triptan, SSRI, or SNRI.

❸ Alert: If linezolid or methylene blue must be given, stop drug and monitor the patient for serotonin toxicity for 2 weeks, or until 24 hours after the last dose of methylene blue or linezolid, whichever comes first. Treatment may be resumed 24 hours after last dose of methylene blue or linezolid.

• **Look alike–sound alike:** Don't confuse Celexa with Zyprexa, Celebrex, or Cerebyx.

PATIENT TEACHING

Black Box Warning Advise families and caregivers to closely observe patient for increased suicidal thinking and behavior. ∎

❸ Alert: Teach patient to recognize and immediately report symptoms of serotonin toxicity (fever, mental status changes, muscle twitching, excessive sweating, shivering or shaking, diarrhea, loss of coordination).

• Caution patient against use of MAO inhibitors while taking citalopram.

• Inform patient that, although improvement may take 1 to 4 weeks, he should continue therapy as prescribed.

• Advise patient not to stop drug abruptly.

• Tell patient that drug may be taken in the morning or evening without regard to meals. If drowsiness occurs, he should take drug in evening.

• Instruct patient to exercise caution when driving or operating hazardous machinery; drug may impair judgment, thinking, and motor skills.

• Advise patient to consult prescriber before taking other prescription or OTC drugs.

• Advise women of childbearing age to consult prescriber before breast-feeding.

C

- Warn patient to avoid alcohol during drug therapy.
- Instruct women of childbearing age to use contraceptives during drug therapy and to notify prescriber immediately if pregnancy is suspected.

clarithromycin
klar-ITH-ro-my-sin

Biaxin◆, Biaxin XL◆

Therapeutic class: Antibiotics
Pharmacologic class: Macrolides
Pregnancy risk category: C

AVAILABLE FORMS
Suspension: 125 mg/5 mL, 250 mg/5 mL
Tablets (extended-release): 500 mg
Tablets (film-coated): 250 mg, 500 mg

INDICATIONS & DOSAGES
Adjust-a-dose (for all indications): In patients with CrCl of less than 30 mL/minute, reduce dosage by 50% or double frequency interval. For concomitant use with atazanavir or ritonavir in patients with CrCl of 30 to 60 mL/minute, reduce dosage by 50%; if CrCl is less than 30 mL/minute, reduce dosage by 75%.
➤ **Pharyngitis or tonsillitis caused by** *Streptococcus pyogenes*
Adults: 250 mg P.O. every 12 hours for 10 days.
Children: 15 mg/kg/day P.O. divided every 12 hours for 10 days.
➤ **Acute maxillary sinusitis caused by** *Streptococcus pneumoniae, Haemophilus influenzae,* **or** *Moraxella catarrhalis*
Adults: 500 mg P.O. every 12 hours for 14 days. Or, if using extended-release form, give two 500-mg tablets P.O. daily for 14 days.
Children: 15 mg/kg/day P.O. divided every 12 hours for 10 days.
➤ **Acute worsening of chronic bronchitis caused by** *M. catarrhalis, S. pneumoniae;* **community-acquired pneumonia caused by** *H. influenzae, S. pneumoniae, Mycoplasma pneumoniae,* **or** *Chlamydia pneumoniae*

Adults: 250 mg P.O. every 12 hours for 7 days (*H. influenzae*) or 7 to 14 days (other bacteria).
➤ **Acute worsening of chronic bronchitis caused by** *H. influenzae* **or** *Haemophilus parainfluenzae*
Adults: 500 mg P.O. every 12 hours for 7 days (*H. parainfluenzae*) or 7 to 14 days (*H. influenzae*).
➤ **Acute worsening of chronic bronchitis caused by** *M. catarrhalis, S. pneumoniae, H. parainfluenzae,* **or** *H. influenzae*
Adults: Two 500-mg extended-release tablets P.O. daily for 7 days.
➤ **Mild to moderate community-acquired pneumonia caused by** *H. influenzae, H. parainfluenzae, M. catarrhalis, S. pneumoniae, C. pneumoniae,* **or** *M. pneumoniae*
Adults: 250 mg P.O. b.i.d. for 7 to 14 days. Or, two 500-mg extended-release tablets P.O. daily for 7 days.
➤ **Community-acquired pneumonia caused by** *S. pneumoniae, C. pneumoniae,* **and** *M. pneumoniae*
Children: 15 mg/kg/day P.O. divided every 12 hours for 10 days.
➤ **Uncomplicated skin and skin-structure infections caused by** *Staphylococcus aureus* **or** *S. pyogenes*
Adults: 250 mg P.O. every 12 hours for 7 to 14 days.
Children: 15 mg/kg/day P.O. divided every 12 hours for 10 days.
➤ **Acute otitis media**
Children: 15 mg/kg/day P.O. divided every 12 hours for 10 days.
➤ **To prevent and treat disseminated infection caused by** *Mycobacterium avium* **complex**
Adults: 500 mg P.O. b.i.d.
Children age 20 months and older: 7.5 mg/kg P.O. b.i.d., up to 500 mg b.i.d.
➤ *Helicobacter pylori,* **to reduce risk of duodenal ulcer recurrence**
Adults: 500 mg clarithromycin with 30 mg lansoprazole and 1 g amoxicillin, all given P.O. every 12 hours for 10 to 14 days. Or, 500 mg clarithromycin with 20 mg omeprazole and 1 g amoxicillin, all given P.O. every 12 hours for 10 days. Or, two-drug regimen with 500 mg clarithromycin P.O. every 8 hours and 40 mg omeprazole P.O. once

daily for 14 days. Continue omeprazole for 14 additional days.

ADMINISTRATION
P.O.
- Obtain specimen for culture and sensitivity tests before giving. Begin therapy while awaiting results.
- Give drug with or without food.
- Don't refrigerate the suspension form; discard unused portion after 14 days.

ACTION
Binds to the 50S subunit of bacterial ribosomes, blocking protein synthesis; bacteriostatic or bactericidal, depending on concentration.

Route	Onset	Peak	Duration
P.O.	Unknown	2–4 hr	Unknown
P.O. (extended)	Unknown	5–6 hr	Unknown

Half-life: 5 to 7 hours.

ADVERSE REACTIONS
CNS: headache.
GI: *pseudomembranous colitis,* abdominal pain or discomfort, diarrhea, nausea, taste perversion, vomiting (in children).
Hematologic: coagulation abnormalities.
Skin: rash (in children).

INTERACTIONS
Drug-drug. *Alprazolam, midazolam, triazolam:* May decrease clearance of these drugs, causing adverse reactions. Use together cautiously.
Carbamazepine, phenytoin: May inhibit metabolism of these drugs, increasing serum levels and risk of toxicity. Avoid using together.
Cyclosporine: May increase cyclosporine levels. Monitor cyclosporine level.
Digoxin: May increase digoxin level. Monitor patient for digoxin toxicity.
Dihydroergotamine, ergotamine: May cause acute ergot toxicity. Avoid using together.
Fluconazole: May increase clarithromycin level. Monitor patient closely.
HMG-CoA reductase inhibitors: May increase levels of these drugs; may rarely cause rhabdomyolysis. Use together cautiously.

Other drugs that prolong the QTc interval (amiodarone, antipsychotics, disopyramide, fluoroquinolones, procainamide, quinidine, sotalol, TCAs): May have additive effects. Monitor ECG for QTc interval prolongation. Avoid using together if possible.
Pimozide: May cause torsades de pointes. Use together is contraindicated.
Rifamycin: May decrease therapeutic effects of clarithromycin while increasing adverse effects of rifamycin. Monitor patient.
Ritonavir: May increase level of clarithromycin. May need to reduce clarithromycin dosage in renally impaired patients.
Sildenafil: May prolong absorption of sildenafil. May need to reduce sildenafil dosage.
Theophylline: May increase theophylline level. Monitor drug level.
Warfarin: May increase PT and INR. Monitor PT and INR carefully.
Zidovudine: May alter zidovudine level. Monitor patient closely.
Drug-food. *Grapefruit juice:* May inhibit metabolism, increasing adverse effects. Don't take with grapefruit juice.

EFFECTS ON LAB TEST RESULTS
- May increase BUN level.
- May increase PT and INR.

CONTRAINDICATIONS & CAUTIONS
- Contraindicated in patients hypersensitive to clarithromycin, erythromycin, or other macrolides and in those receiving pimozide or other drugs that prolong QT interval or cause cardiac arrhythmias.
- Use cautiously in patients with hepatic or renal impairment.
- Safety and effectiveness in children younger than age 6 months haven't been established.
- Use during pregnancy only if potential benefit justifies potential risk to fetus.

NURSING CONSIDERATIONS
- **Alert:** The safety and effectiveness of the extended-release form haven't been established for treating other infections for which the original form has been approved.
- Monitor patient for superinfection. Drug may cause overgrowth of nonsusceptible bacteria or fungi.

• Giving clarithromycin with a drug metabolized by CYP3A may increase drug levels and prolong therapeutic and adverse effects.

PATIENT TEACHING
• Tell patient to take drug as prescribed, even after he feels better.
• Advise patient to report persistent adverse reactions.
• Inform patient that drug may be taken with or without food.
• Tell patient not to refrigerate the suspension form, but to discard unused portion after 14 days.

clevidipine butyrate
cle-VIH-deh-peen

Cleviprex

Therapeutic class: Antihypertensives
Pharmacologic class: Dihydropyridine calcium channel blockers
Pregnancy risk category: C

AVAILABLE FORMS
Injection: 0.5 mg/mL in 50- and 100-mL single-use vials

INDICATIONS & DOSAGES
➤ **To lower blood pressure when oral therapy isn't feasible or desirable**
Adults: Begin infusion at 1 to 2 mg/hour and titrate by doubling the dose every 90 seconds. When blood pressure approaches goal, titrate every 5 to 10 minutes at less than double the dose. Maximum dose is 1,000 mL (average of 21 mg/hour) per 24-hour period. Drug isn't recommended for use beyond 72 hours.

ADMINISTRATION
I.V.
▼ Store vials in cartons in refrigerator because drug is photosensitive. May store at controlled room temperature (77°F [25°C]) for up to 2 months.
▼ Maintain aseptic technique when handling solution. Drug can support growth of microorganisms; don't use if solution might be contaminated.
▼ Invert vial several times to mix emulsion before use.

▼ Inspect solution and discard if particulate matter or discoloration is present before use. Don't dilute.
▼ Use a continuous infusion pump to regulate flow.
▼ Discard unused portion within 12 hours.
▼ **Incompatibilities:** Don't administer drug in same I.V. line with other medications.

ACTION
Inhibits calcium ion influx across cardiac and smooth-muscle cells, decreasing contractility and oxygen demand. Dilates coronary arteries and arterioles, decreasing systemic vascular resistance.

Route	Onset	Peak	Duration
I.V.	2–4 min	Unknown	5–15 min

Half-life: 15 minutes; metabolite, 9 hours.

ADVERSE REACTIONS
CNS: headache.
CV: atrial fibrillation.
GI: nausea, vomiting.
GU: *acute renal failure.*

INTERACTIONS
None reported.

EFFECTS ON LAB TEST RESULTS
• May increase bilirubin, AST, and ALT levels.

CONTRAINDICATIONS & CAUTIONS
• Contraindicated in patients hypersensitive to soy beans, soy products, eggs, or egg products.
• Contraindicated in those with defective lipid metabolism or severe aortic stenosis.
• Use cautiously in patients with heart failure.
• Use during pregnancy only if the potential benefit justifies the potential risk to the fetus. It's not known if drug appears in breast milk. Advise patient to stop breast-feeding during therapy.
• Safety and effectiveness in children younger than age 18 haven't been established
⚠ *Overdose S&S:* Hypotension, reflex tachycardia.

NURSING CONSIDERATIONS

• Monitor blood pressure and heart rate continuously, especially when starting drug and during dosage adjustments.

• Drug may exacerbate heart failure; monitor patient closely.

• Titrate dose slowly; rapid titration may cause hypotension and reflex tachycardia. If either occurs, decrease clevidipine dosage.

• Monitor patient who received prolonged infusion for rebound hypertension for at least 8 hours after infusion is stopped if no other antihypertensive is prescribed.

• Because drug contains lipids, restrict lipid intake in those with lipid metabolism disorders.

• Drug isn't a beta-adrenergic blocker; if given with beta-adrenergic blocker, gradually reduce beta-adrenergic blocker dosage to avoid withdrawal symptoms.

• Discard unopened vials that have been stored at room temperature for longer than 2 months.

PATIENT TEACHING

• Tell patient to report adverse reactions promptly.

• Advise patient to seek medical attention immediately if signs and symptoms of hypertensive emergency occur (visual changes, neurologic symptoms, heart failure).

clindamycin hydrochloride
klin-da-MYE-sin

Cleocin Hydrochloride, Dalacin C†

clindamycin palmitate hydrochloride
Cleocin Pediatric, Dalacin C Flavored Granules†

clindamycin phosphate (injection)
Cleocin Phosphate, Dalacin C Phosphate Sterile Solution†

Therapeutic class: Antibiotics
Pharmacologic class: Lincomycin derivatives
Pregnancy risk category: B

AVAILABLE FORMS
clindamycin hydrochloride
Capsules: 75 mg, 150 mg, 300 mg
clindamycin palmitate hydrochloride
Granules for oral solution: 75 mg/5 mL
clindamycin phosphate (injection)
Injectable infusion (in D₅W): 300 mg (50 mL), 600 mg (50 mL), 900 mg (50 mL)
Injection: 150-mg base/mL, 300-mg base/2 mL, 600-mg base/4 mL, 900-mg base/6 mL

INDICATIONS & DOSAGES
➤ **Infections caused by sensitive staphylococci, streptococci, pneumococci, *Bacteroides, Fusobacterium, Clostridium perfringens,* and other sensitive aerobic and anaerobic organisms**
Adults: 150 to 450 mg P.O. every 6 hours; or 300 to 600 mg I.M. or I.V. every 6, 8, or 12 hours. In more severe infections, dosage may be increased to 1,200 to 2,700 mg/day I.M. or I.V. in two, three, or four divided doses. In life-threatening infections, dosages as high as 4,800 mg daily can be given.
Children ages 1 month to 16 years: 20 to 40 mg/kg/day I.M. or I.V. in three or four equal doses. In beta-hemolytic streptococcal infections, treatment should continue for at least 10 days.

C

Neonates younger than age 1 month: 15 to 20 mg/kg/day I.M. or I.V. in three or four equal doses.

➤ **Pelvic inflammatory disease ♦**
Adults and adolescents: 900 mg I.V. every 8 hours, with gentamicin. Continue until 24 hours after symptoms improve; then switch to oral clindamycin 450 mg q.i.d. for total of 10 to 14 days or doxycycline 100 mg P.O. every 12 hours for total of 10 to 14 days.

➤ **Acute otitis media in infants and children with penicillin allergies if infection is known or presumed to be caused by penicillin-resistant *Streptococcus pneumoniae* ♦**
Children age 6 and older with mild to moderate disease: 30 to 40 mg/kg/day P.O. divided into three doses daily for 5 to 7 days.
Children younger than age 6 and those with severe disease: 30 to 40 mg/kg/day P.O. divided into three doses daily for 10 days.

ADMINISTRATION

P.O.
● Obtain specimen for culture and sensitivity tests before giving first dose. Begin therapy while awaiting results.
● Give capsule form with a full glass of water to prevent esophageal irritation.
● Don't refrigerate reconstituted oral solution because it will thicken. Drug is stable for 2 weeks at room temperature.

I.V.
▼ Obtain specimen for culture and sensitivity tests before giving first dose. Begin therapy while awaiting results.
▼ Never give undiluted as a bolus.
▼ For infusion, dilute each 300 mg in 50 mL solution and give over 10 to 60 minutes at no more than 30 mg/minute.
▼ Check site daily for phlebitis and irritation.
▼ Drug may contain benzyl alcohol. Benzyl alcohol has been associated with a fatal gasping syndrome in premature infants.
▼ **Incompatibilities:** Allopurinol, aminophylline, ampicillin, azithromycin, barbiturates, calcium gluconate, cefazolin, ceftriaxone, ciprofloxacin hydrochloride, doxapram, filgrastim, fluconazole, gen-

tamicin sulfate, idarubicin, magnesium sulfate, phenytoin sodium, ranitidine, rubber closures such as those on I.V. tubing, tobramycin sulfate.

I.M.
● Obtain specimen for culture and sensitivity tests before giving first dose. Begin therapy while awaiting results.
● Inject deep into muscle. Rotate sites. Don't exceed 600 mg per injection.

ACTION

Inhibits bacterial protein synthesis by binding to the 50S subunit of the ribosome.

Route	Onset	Peak	Duration
P.O.	Unknown	45–60 min	Unknown
I.V.	Immediate	Immediate	Unknown
I.M.	Unknown	3 hr	Unknown

Half-life: 2½ to 3 hours.

ADVERSE REACTIONS

CV: thrombophlebitis.
GI: nausea, *pseudomembranous colitis,* abdominal pain, diarrhea, vomiting.
Hematologic: *thrombocytopenia, transient leukopenia,* eosinophilia.
Hepatic: jaundice.
Skin: maculopapular rash, urticaria.
Other: *anaphylaxis.*

INTERACTIONS

Drug-drug. *Erythromycin:* May block access of clindamycin to its site of action. Avoid using together.
Kaolin: May decrease absorption of oral clindamycin. Separate dosage times.
Neuromuscular blockers: May increase neuromuscular blockade. Monitor patient closely.
Paclitaxel: May increase paclitaxel effects. Observe patient for toxicity.
Drug-food. *Diet foods with sodium cyclamate:* May decrease drug level. Discourage patient from eating these foods.

EFFECTS ON LAB TEST RESULTS

● May increase alkaline phosphatase, AST, and bilirubin levels.
● May increase eosinophil count. May decrease platelet and WBC counts.

CONTRAINDICATIONS & CAUTIONS
• Contraindicated in patients hypersensitive to drug or lincomycin.
• Clindamycin use may result in overgrowth of nonsusceptible organisms, particularly yeasts. Monitor patient for sign of superinfection.
• Use cautiously in neonates and patients with renal or hepatic disease, asthma, history of GI disease, or significant allergies.
Black Box Warning Clindamycin therapy has been associated with severe, possibly fatal, colitis; its use should be reserved for serious infections. ∎

NURSING CONSIDERATIONS
• I.M. injection may raise CK level in response to muscle irritation.
• Monitor renal, hepatic, and hematopoietic functions during prolonged therapy.
• Observe patient for signs and symptoms of superinfection.
❸ Alert: Don't give opioid antidiarrheals to treat drug-induced diarrhea; they may prolong and worsen this condition.
Black Box Warning Diarrhea, colitis, and pseudomembranous colitis have developed up to several weeks after cessation of drug therapy. ∎
• Drug doesn't penetrate blood-brain barrier.

PATIENT TEACHING
• Advise patient to take capsule form with a full glass of water to prevent esophageal irritation.
• Warn patient that I.M. injection may be painful.
• Tell patient to report discomfort at I.V. insertion site.
• Instruct patient to notify prescriber of adverse reactions (especially diarrhea). Warn him not to treat diarrhea himself because drug may cause life-threatening colitis.

clindamycin phosphate (topical)
klin-da-MYE-sin

Cleocin, Cleocin T, Clinda-Derm, Clindagel, Clindamax, Clindasol†, Clinda-T†, Clindesse, Clindets, Dalacin†, Evoclin

Therapeutic class: Antibiotics
Pharmacologic class: Lincomycin derivatives
Pregnancy risk category: B

AVAILABLE FORMS
Foam: 1%
Gel: 1%
Lotion: 1%
Pledget: 1%*
Topical cream: 1%, 2%
Topical solution: 1%*
Vaginal cream: 2%
Vaginal suppositories: 100 mg

INDICATIONS & DOSAGES
➤ **Inflammatory acne vulgaris**
Adults and children age 12 and older:
Apply to skin b.i.d., morning and evening, or once daily if using Clindagel or Evoclin.
➤ **Bacterial vaginosis**
Adults: 1 applicatorful vaginally at bedtime for 3 to 7 days in nonpregnant women or 7 days in pregnant women, or 1 suppository vaginally at bedtime for 3 days, or 1 applicatorful of Clindesse vaginally as a single dose.

ADMINISTRATION
Topical
• Wash area with warm water and soap, rinse, pat dry, and wait 30 minutes after washing or shaving to apply.
• Avoid excessive washing of affected area.
• Apply to entire area, but avoid contact with eyes, nose, mouth, and other mucous membranes.
• Tell patient to remove pledgets from foil just before use.
• Advise patient to use pledgets only once and then discard. Also, more than 1 pledget may be used per application.

C

Vaginal

● Make sure patient knows how to use applicators that come with drug.

ACTION

Bacteriostatic or bactericidal based on drug level and susceptibility of organism; suppresses growth of susceptible organisms in sebaceous glands by blocking protein synthesis.

Route	Onset	Peak	Duration
Topical, vaginal	Unknown	Unknown	Unknown

Half-life: 1½ to 2½ hours for topical and vaginal cream; 11 hours for vaginal suppositories.

ADVERSE REACTIONS

CNS: headache.
EENT: pharyngitis.
GI: abdominal pain, bloody diarrhea, colitis including *pseudomembranous colitis,* constipation, diarrhea, GI upset.
GU: *Candida albicans* overgrowth, cervicitis, vaginitis, vulvar irritation, UTI, vaginal discharge, vaginal moniliasis.
Skin: dryness, redness, burning, contact dermatitis, irritation, rash, pruritus, swelling.

INTERACTIONS

Drug-drug. *Erythromycin:* May antagonize clindamycin's effect. Separate doses.
Isotretinoin: May cause cumulative dryness, resulting in excessive skin irritation. Use together cautiously.
Neuromuscular blockers: May increase action of neuromuscular blocker. Use together cautiously.
Drug-lifestyle. *Abrasive or medicated soaps or cleansers, acne products, or other preparations containing peeling drugs (benzoyl peroxide, resorcinol, salicylic acid, sulfur, tretinoin), alcohol-containing products (aftershave, cosmetics, perfumed toiletries, shaving creams or lotions), astringent soaps or cosmetics, medicated cosmetics or cover-ups:* May cause cumulative dryness, resulting in excessive skin irritation. Urge caution.

EFFECTS ON LAB TEST RESULTS

● May increase liver enzyme levels.

CONTRAINDICATIONS & CAUTIONS

● Contraindicated in patients hypersensitive to clindamycin or lincomycin and in those with history of ulcerative colitis, regional enteritis, or antibiotic-related colitis.
⚠ *Overdose S&S:* Systemic effects.

NURSING CONSIDERATIONS

● For treating acne, drug may be used with tretinoin or benzoyl peroxide, as well as systemic antibiotics.
● Drug can cause excessive dryness.
● Topical solution and pledgets contain alcohol base, which may irritate eyes.
● Monitor elderly patients for systemic effects.

PATIENT TEACHING

● Tell patient to wash area with warm water and soap, rinse, pat dry, and wait 30 minutes after washing or shaving to apply.
● Warn patient to avoid excessive washing of area. Tell patient to cover entire affected area but to avoid contact with eyes, nose, mouth, and other mucous membranes.
● Instruct patient to use other prescribed acne medicines at a different time.
● Tell patient to use only as prescribed.
● Instruct patient to dab, not roll, applicator-tipped bottle. If tip becomes dry, patient should invert bottle and depress tip several times to moisten.
● Warn patient not to smoke while applying topical solution.
● For vaginal treatment, instruct patient how to use vaginal applicators.
● Advise patient that the vaginal form contains mineral oil, which can weaken latex or rubber products, such as condoms and diaphragms, and that she should use another form of birth control during and within 3 days of therapy.
● Advise patient to avoid sexual intercourse during vaginal treatment.
● Advise patient to avoid use of tampons or douches during vaginal treatment.
● Instruct patient to notify prescriber immediately if abdominal pain or diarrhea occurs. Inform patient that an antidiarrheal may worsen condition and should only be used as directed by prescriber.
● Tell patient to remove pledgets from foil before use.

- Advise patient to use pledgets only once and then discard. Also, more than 1 pledget may be used per application.
- Advise patient to complete entire course of therapy.

clobazam
KLOE-ba-zam

Onfi

Therapeutic class: Anticonvulsants
Pharmacologic class: Benzodiazepines
Pregnancy risk category: C
Controlled substance schedule: IV

AVAILABLE FORMS
Oral suspension: 2.5 mg/mL
Tablets: 5 mg, 10 mg, 20 mg

INDICATIONS & DOSAGES
➤ **Adjunctive treatment of seizures associated with Lennox-Gastaut syndrome**
Adults and children age 2 and older weighing more than 30 kg (66 lb): Initially, 5 mg P.O. b.i.d. for 6 days. On day 7, increase to 10 mg P.O. b.i.d.; on day 14, titrate to 20 mg P.O. b.i.d. as tolerated.
Adults and children age 2 and older weighing 30 kg or less: Initially, 5 mg P.O. once daily for 6 days. On day 7, increase to 5 mg P.O. b.i.d.; on day 14, titrate to 10 mg P.O. b.i.d. as tolerated.
Adjust-a-dose: For elderly patients, those with mild to moderate hepatic impairment (Child-Pugh score 5 to 9), and those who are poor CYP2C19 metabolizers, initially 5 mg P.O. daily. Then titrate according to weight but at half the recommended dose. If necessary, may start an additional titration to the maximum dosage (20 or 40 mg/day depending on weight) on day 21. There are no dosage recommendations for patients with severe hepatic or renal impairment.

ADMINISTRATION
P.O.
- May give tablets whole or crushed and mixed in applesauce.
- May give with or without food.

- Shake oral suspension well before every dose and use only oral dosing syringe supplied with product.
- To discontinue drug, taper gradually by 5 to 10 mg/day on a weekly basis.

ACTION
Thought to involve potentiating GABA neurotransmission, which results from binding at the benzodiazepine site of the GABA$_A$ receptor.

Route	Onset	Peak	Duration
P.O.	Rapid	½–4 hr	Unknown

Half-life: 36 to 42 hours.

ADVERSE REACTIONS
CNS: somnolence, lethargy, pyrexia, irritability, fatigue, sedation, ataxia, psychomotor hyperactivity, insomnia, aggression.
EENT: drooling.
GI: vomiting, constipation, dysphagia.
GU: UTI.
Metabolic: increased or decreased appetite.
Musculoskeletal: dysarthria.
Respiratory: upper respiratory tract infection, pneumonia, cough, bronchitis.

INTERACTIONS
Drug-drug. *CNS depressants (opioids, TCAs):* May increase sedation. Avoid use together.
Drugs metabolized by CYP2C19 inhibitors (fluconazole, fluvoxamine, ketoconazole, omeprazole, ticlopidine): May increase levels of clobazam or its metabolite. Decrease clobazam dosage if needed.
Drugs metabolized by CYP2D6 inhibitors (dextromethorphan): May increase levels of drugs metabolized by CYP2D6 inhibitors. Decreased dosages of these drugs may be needed.
Hormonal contraceptives: May diminish contraceptive effectiveness. Patient should use nonhormonal contraceptives as needed.
Drug-lifestyle. *Alcohol use:* May increase clobazam level by up to 50% and increase CNS depression. Discourage alcohol use.

EFFECTS ON LAB TEST RESULTS
None reported.

Reactions in bold italics are *life-threatening*. Interactions may have a *rapid onset* or a *delayed onset*.

CONTRAINDICATIONS & CAUTIONS

• Contraindicated in patients hypersensitive to drug.
• Withdraw clobazam gradually to minimize risk of precipitating seizures, seizure exacerbation, status epilepticus, or withdrawal signs and symptoms (seizures, psychosis, hallucinations, behavioral disorder, tremor, anxiety).
• Use cautiously in patients with history of dependence.
• Drug may increase risk of suicidal thoughts or behavior.
• Neonatal flaccidity, respiratory and feeding difficulties, hypothermia, and withdrawal signs and symptoms have occurred in infants born to women who received benzodiazepines, including clobazam, late in pregnancy. Use during pregnancy only if benefit to the mother outweighs risks to the fetus.
• Drug appears in breast milk, but the full effects of exposure are unknown. Fetal sedation is possible. Discuss risks with patient.
⚠ Overdose S&S: Drowsiness, confusion, lethargy, respiratory depression, hypotension, ataxia, coma.

NURSING CONSIDERATIONS

• Monitor patients for signs and symptoms of abuse or physical dependence.
• Monitor patients for depression, suicidal thoughts or behavior, or other mood changes.
• Monitor patients for somnolence. This can occur at all dosage ranges, is usually seen within the first month, then may subside with continued therapy.
• Monitor patients for dependence. Dependence may occur at the recommended dosage range over only a few weeks. Risk increases with increasing dosage and duration of treatment. Risk is increased in those with a history of alcohol or drug abuse.
• Advise pregnant patients to enroll in the North American Antiepileptic Drug Pregnancy Registry by calling 1-888-233-2334 or going online at www.aedpregnancyregistry.org/.
• Use oral suspension within 90 days of first opening; discard any remaining product.

PATIENT TEACHING

• Advise patient and caregivers to notify health care providers before taking or giving clobazam with other CNS depressants (other benzodiazepines, opioids, TCAs, sedating antihistamines, alcohol).
• Inform patient to use caution if operating heavy machinery, including cars, when taking drug until its effects are known.
• Caution patient and caregivers not to stop drug or change dosage without first discussing with prescriber.
• Advise women using hormonal contraceptives to use nonhormonal methods during therapy and to continue these methods for 28 days after stopping drug.
• Caution patient and caregivers that drug may increase risk of suicidal thoughts. Tell them to report signs and symptoms of depression or changes in mood or behavior.
• Instruct female patient to inform health care provider if she is pregnant, plans to become pregnant, or plans to breast-feed during therapy.
• Instruct patient or caregiver to discard any remaining oral suspension within 90 days of first opening the bottle.
• Teach patient or caregiver how to use the dosing syringe for the oral suspension.

clobetasol propionate
kloe-BAY-ta-sol

Clobex, Cormax, Embeline, Embeline E, Olux, Olux-E, Temovate, Temovate E

Therapeutic class: Corticosteroids
Pharmacologic class: Corticosteroids
Pregnancy risk category: C

AVAILABLE FORMS

Cream: 0.05%
Foam: 0.05%*
Gel: 0.05%
Lotion: 0.05%
Ointment: 0.05%
Scalp application: 0.05%*
Shampoo: 0.05%*
Solution: 0.05%*
Spray: 0.05%*

INDICATIONS & DOSAGES
➤ **Short-term topical treatment for moderate to severe plaque-type psoriasis of nonscalp regions, excluding the face and intertriginous areas**
Adults: Apply thin layer of lotion or cream to affected skin areas b.i.d., morning and evening, for up to 14 days. Or, apply spray directly onto affected skin areas b.i.d. and rub in gently and completely. For localized lesions (less than 10% of body surface area) that haven't improved sufficiently, continue treatment for up to 2 more weeks. Total dose shouldn't exceed 50 g (50 mL) weekly.

➤ **Inflammation and pruritus from corticosteroid-responsive dermatoses; short-term topical treatment of mild to moderate plaque-type psoriasis of nonscalp regions, excluding the face and intertriginous areas**
Adults and children age 12 and older: Apply thin layer to affected skin areas b.i.d., morning and evening, for maximum of 14 days. Total dose shouldn't exceed 50 g (50 mL) per week.

➤ **Inflammation and pruritus of moderate to severe corticosteroid-responsive dermatoses of the scalp**
Adults: Apply foam or solution to the affected scalp area b.i.d., morning and evening. Massage into affected scalp area gently and completely. Don't use more than 1½ capfuls of foam at each application. Limit treatment to 14 days, with no more than 50 g (50 mL) weekly.

➤ **Moderate to severe scalp psoriasis**
Adults: Apply Clobex shampoo to affected areas of dry scalp in thin film once daily. Leave in place for 15 minutes before lathering and rinsing. Limit treatment to 4 consecutive weeks. Maximum dose is 50 g (50 mL) per week.

ADMINISTRATION
Topical
● Gently wash skin before applying. To prevent skin damage, rub medication in gently and completely. When treating hairy sites, part hair and apply directly to lesions.
● To dispense foam, hold the can upside down and depress the actuator.

● Avoid applying near eyes or mucous membranes or in ear canal.
⊖ *Alert:* Don't use occlusive dressings or bandages. Don't cover or wrap treated areas unless directed by prescriber.

ACTION
Unclear. Diffuses across cell membranes to form complexes with receptors, showing anti-inflammatory, antipruritic, vasoconstrictive, and antiproliferative activity. Considered a very-high-potency to high-potency drug, according to vasoconstrictive properties.

Route	Onset	Peak	Duration
Topical	Unknown	Unknown	Unknown

Half-life: Unknown.

ADVERSE REACTIONS
GU: glycosuria.
Metabolic: hyperglycemia.
Skin: burning, pruritus, irritation, dryness, erythema, folliculitis, perioral dermatitis, allergic contact dermatitis, hypopigmentation, hypertrichosis, acneiform eruptions, skin atrophy, telangiectasia.
Other: *hypothalamic-pituitary-adrenal (HPA) axis suppression,* Cushing syndrome, finger numbness.

INTERACTIONS
None significant.

EFFECTS ON LAB TEST RESULTS
● May increase glucose level.

CONTRAINDICATIONS & CAUTIONS
● Contraindicated in patients hypersensitive to corticosteroids and in those with primary scalp infections.
● Don't use as monotherapy for primary bacterial infections (impetigo, paronychia, erysipelas, cellulitis, angular cheilitis, erythrasma), rosacea, perioral dermatitis, or acne.
● Don't use very-high-potency or high-potency agents on the face, groin, or axilla areas.
● Drug isn't for ophthalmic use.
● Use cautiously in children and in pregnant or breast-feeding women.
⚠ *Overdose S&S:* Systemic effects.

NURSING CONSIDERATIONS

• If antifungal or antibiotic combined with corticosteroid fails to provide prompt improvement, stop corticosteroid until infection is controlled.

• Stop drug and notify prescriber if skin infection, striae, or atrophy occurs.

• HPA axis suppression occurs at doses as low as 2 g daily.

PATIENT TEACHING

• Teach patient how to apply drug and to avoid contact with eyes.

• Tell patient to wash hands after application.

• Tell patient to stop drug and report signs of systemic absorption, skin irritation or ulceration, hypersensitivity, or infection.

• Warn patient to use drug for no longer than 14 consecutive days.

• Tell patient using the foam to invert can and dispense a small amount of Olux foam (up to a golfball-size dollop) into the cap of the can, onto a saucer or other cool surface, or directly on the lesion, taking care to avoid contact with the eyes. Dispensing directly onto hands isn't recommended because the foam will melt immediately on contact with warm skin. Tell him to move hair away from affected area of scalp so that foam can be applied to each affected area.

• Tell patient using foam that contents are flammable and under pressure, so he should avoid smoking during and immediately after application and keep can away from flames. Also tell him not to puncture or incinerate container.

clomiPHENE citrate
KLOE-mi-feen

Clomid, Serophene

Therapeutic class: Ovulation stimulants
Pharmacologic class: Chlorotrianisene derivatives
Pregnancy risk category: X

AVAILABLE FORMS
Tablets: 50 mg

INDICATIONS & DOSAGES
➤ **To induce ovulation**

Women: 50 mg P.O. daily for 5 days, starting on day 5 of menstrual cycle (first day of menstrual flow is day 1) if bleeding occurs, or at any time if patient hasn't had recent uterine bleeding. If ovulation doesn't occur, may increase dose to 100 mg P.O. daily for 5 days as soon as 30 days after previous course. Repeat until conception occurs or until three courses of therapy are completed.

ADMINISTRATION
P.O.

• Protect drug from heat, light, and excessive humidity.

• Give drug without regard for food.

ACTION

Appears to stimulate release of follicle-stimulating hormone, luteinizing hormone, and pituitary gonadotropins, resulting in maturation of the ovarian follicle, ovulation, and development of the corpus luteum.

Route	Onset	Peak	Duration
P.O.	Unknown	Unknown	Unknown

Half-life: 5 days.

ADVERSE REACTIONS

CNS: headache.
EENT: blurred vision, diplopia, scotoma, photophobia.
GI: nausea, vomiting, bloating, distention.
GU: ovarian enlargement, urinary frequency and polyuria, abnormal uterine bleeding, ovarian cyst that regresses spontaneously when drug is stopped.
Metabolic: weight gain.
Skin: reversible alopecia, urticaria, rash, dermatitis.
Other: hot flashes, breast discomfort.

INTERACTIONS
None significant.

EFFECTS ON LAB TEST RESULTS
None reported.

CONTRAINDICATIONS & CAUTIONS

• Contraindicated in pregnant women and in those with undiagnosed abnormal genital bleeding, ovarian cyst not related to polycystic ovary syndrome, hepatic disease or dysfunction, uncontrolled thyroid or adrenal dysfunction, or organic intracranial lesion (such as a pituitary tumor).

⚠ **Overdose S&S:** Nausea; vomiting; vasomotor flushes; visual blurring, spots, or flashes; scotomata; ovarian enlargement with pelvic or abdominal pain.

NURSING CONSIDERATIONS
• Monitor patient closely because of potentially serious adverse reactions.
• Long-term cyclic therapy isn't recommended.
• **Look alike–sound alike:** Don't confuse clomiphene with clomipramine or clonidine. Don't confuse Serophene with Sarafem.

PATIENT TEACHING
• Tell patient about the risk of multiple births, which increases with higher doses.
• Teach patient to take and chart basal body temperature to ascertain if ovulation has occurred.
• Reinforce importance of compliance with drug regimen.
• Reassure patient that ovulation typically occurs after first course of therapy. If pregnancy doesn't occur, therapy may be repeated twice.
• Advise patient to stop drug and contact prescriber immediately if pregnancy is suspected because drug may have teratogenic effect.
🌙 **Alert:** Advise patient to stop drug and contact prescriber immediately if abdominal symptoms or pain occur; these symptoms may indicate ovarian enlargement or ovarian cyst. Also, tell patient to immediately notify prescriber if signs and symptoms of impending visual toxicity occur, such as blurred vision, double vision, vision defect in one part of the eye (scotoma), or sensitivity to the sun.
• Warn patient to avoid hazardous activities, such as driving or operating machinery, until CNS effects are known. Drug may cause dizziness and visual disturbances.

clomiPRAMINE hydrochloride
kloe-MI-pra-meen

Anafranil

Therapeutic class: Antidepressants
Pharmacologic class: Tricyclic antidepressants
Pregnancy risk category: C

AVAILABLE FORMS
Capsules: 25 mg, 50 mg, 75 mg

INDICATIONS & DOSAGES
➤ **Obsessive-compulsive disorder**
Adults: Initially, 25 mg P.O. daily with meals, gradually increased to 100 mg daily in divided doses during first 2 weeks. Thereafter, increase to maximum dose of 250 mg daily in divided doses with meals, as needed. After adjustment, give total daily dose at bedtime.
Children age 10 and older and adolescents: Initially, 25 mg P.O. daily with meals, gradually increased over first 2 weeks to daily maximum of 3 mg/kg or 100 mg P.O. in divided doses, whichever is smaller. Maximum daily dose is 3 mg/kg or 200 mg, whichever is smaller; give at bedtime after adjustment. Reassess and adjust dosage periodically.
➤ **Panic disorder** ◆
Adults: Initially, 10 mg P.O. daily and increased to a maximum dosage of 150 mg P.O. daily.

ADMINISTRATION
P.O.
• Give drug without regard for food.

ACTION
Unknown. Inhibits reuptake of serotonin and norepinephrine at the presynaptic neuron.

Route	Onset	Peak	Duration
P.O.	Unknown	2–6 hr	Unknown

Half-life: Parent compound, 32 hours; active metabolite, 69 hours.

Reactions in bold italics are *life-threatening*. Interactions may have a *rapid onset* or a *delayed onset*.

ADVERSE REACTIONS
CNS: somnolence, tremor, dizziness, headache, insomnia, nervousness, myoclonus, fatigue, *seizures,* EEG changes.
CV: orthostatic hypotension, palpitations, tachycardia.
EENT: pharyngitis, rhinitis, visual changes.
GI: dry mouth, constipation, nausea, dyspepsia, increased appetite, anorexia, abdominal pain, diarrhea.
GU: urinary hesitancy, UTI, dysmenorrhea, ejaculation failure, erectile dysfunction.
Hematologic: purpura.
Metabolic: weight gain.
Musculoskeletal: myalgia.
Respiratory: bronchospasm, coughing, dyspnea.
Skin: diaphoresis, rash, pruritus, dry skin.
Other: altered libido.

INTERACTIONS
Drug-drug. *Antiarrhythmics, chlorpromazine, dolasetron, droperidol, mefloquine, mesoridazine, moxifloxacin, pentamidine, pimozide, tacrolimus, thioridazine, ziprasidone:* May prolong QT interval. Monitor patient closely.
Barbiturates: May decrease TCA level. Watch for decreased antidepressant effect.
Cimetidine, **fluoxetine, fluvoxamine, paroxetine, sertraline:** May increase TCA level. Monitor drug level and patient for signs of toxicity.
Clonidine: May cause life-threatening hypertension. Avoid using together.
CNS depressants: May enhance CNS depression. Avoid using together.
CYP2D6 inhibitors (phenothiazines, SSRIs): May increase clomipramine plasma concentrations. Monitor patient and adjust dosage as needed.
Epinephrine, norepinephrine: May increase hypertensive effect. Use together cautiously.
Haloperidol, methylphenidate: May increase plasma concentrations of these drugs. Monitor patient.
Linezolid, methylene blue: May cause serotonin syndrome. Use with extreme caution and monitor closely.
MAO inhibitors: May cause hyperpyretic crisis, seizures, coma, or death. Avoid using within 14 days of MAO inhibitor therapy.

Quinolones: May increase the risk of life-threatening arrhythmias. Avoid using together.
Drug-herb. *Evening primrose oil:* May cause additive or synergistic effect, resulting in lower seizure threshold and increasing the risk of seizure. Discourage use together.
St. John's wort, SAM-e, yohimbe: May cause serotonin syndrome. Discourage use together.
Drug-lifestyle. *Alcohol use:* May enhance CNS depression. Discourage use together.
Sun exposure: May increase risk of photosensitivity reactions. Advise patient to avoid excessive sunlight exposure.

EFFECTS ON LAB TEST RESULTS
None reported.

CONTRAINDICATIONS & CAUTIONS
• Contraindicated in patients hypersensitive to drug or other TCAs, in those who have taken MAO inhibitors within previous 14 days, in those receiving linezolid or methylene blue I.V., and in patients in acute recovery period after MI.
• Use cautiously in patients with history of seizure disorders or with brain damage of varying cause; in patients receiving other seizure threshold–lowering drugs; in patients at risk for suicide; in patients with history of urine retention or angle-closure glaucoma, increased intraocular pressure, CV disease, impaired hepatic or renal function, or hyperthyroidism; in patients with tumors of the adrenal medulla; in patients receiving thyroid drug or electroconvulsive therapy; and in those undergoing elective surgery.
Black Box Warning Clomipramine isn't approved for use in children except for those with obsessive-compulsive disorder. ■
⚠ **Overdose S&S:** Cardiac arrhythmias, severe hypotension, seizures, CNS depression, coma, ECG changes, drowsiness, stupor, ataxia, restlessness, agitation, delirium, severe perspiration, hyperactive reflexes, muscle rigidity, athetoid and choreiform movements, tachycardia, congestive heart failure, cardiac arrest, respiratory depression, cyanosis, shock, vomiting, hyperpyrexia, mydriasis, oliguria or anuria.

NURSING CONSIDERATIONS

• Monitor mood and watch for suicidal tendencies. Allow patient to have only the minimum amount of drug.

Black Box Warning Drug may increase risk of suicidal thinking and behavior in children, adolescents, and young adults ages 18 to 24 during the first 2 months of treatment, especially in those with major depressive disorder or other psychiatric disorder. ∎

☼ Alert: If linezolid or methylene blue must be given, stop drug and monitor the patient for serotonin toxicity for 2 weeks, or until 24 hours after the last dose of methylene blue or linezolid, whichever comes first. Treatment may be resumed 24 hours after last dose of methylene blue or linezolid.

• Don't withdraw drug abruptly.

• Because patients may suffer hypertensive episodes during surgery, stop drug gradually several days before surgery.

• Relieve dry mouth with sugarless candy or gum. Saliva substitutes may be needed.

• **Look alike–sound alike:** Don't confuse clomipramine with chlorpromazine or clomiphene. Don't confuse Anafranil with enalapril, nafarelin, or alfentanil.

PATIENT TEACHING

• Warn patient to avoid hazardous activities requiring alertness and good coordination, especially during adjustment. Daytime sedation and dizziness may occur.

• Tell patient to avoid alcohol during drug therapy.

☼ Alert: Teach patient to recognize and immediately report symptoms of serotonin toxicity (fever, mental status changes, muscle twitching, excessive sweating, shivering or shaking, diarrhea, loss of coordination).

• Warn patient not to stop drug suddenly.

• Advise patient to use sunblock, wear protective clothing, and avoid prolonged exposure to strong sunlight to prevent oversensitivity to the sun.

Black Box Warning Advise family members and caregivers to closely observe patient for increased suicidal thinking and behavior. ∎

SAFETY ALERT!

clonazepam
kloe-NAZ-e-pam

Klonopin✎

Therapeutic class: Anticonvulsants
Pharmacologic class: Benzodiazepines
Pregnancy risk category: D
Controlled substance schedule: IV

AVAILABLE FORMS

Tablets: 0.5 mg, 1 mg, 2 mg
Tablets (orally disintegrating): 0.125 mg, 0.25 mg, 0.5 mg, 1 mg, 2 mg

INDICATIONS & DOSAGES

➤ **Lennox-Gastaut syndrome, atypical absence seizures, akinetic and myoclonic seizures**

Adults and children older than age 10 or weighing more than 30 kg (66 lb): Initially, no more than 1.5 mg P.O. daily in three divided doses. May be increased by 0.5 to 1 mg every 3 days until seizures are controlled. If given in unequal doses, give largest dose at bedtime. Maximum recommended daily dose is 20 mg.

Children age 10 and younger or weighing 30 kg (66 lb) or less: Initially, 0.01 to 0.03 mg/kg P.O. daily (not to exceed 0.05 mg/kg daily) in two or three divided doses. Increase by 0.25 to 0.5 mg every third day to maximum maintenance dose of 0.1 to 0.2 mg/kg P.O. daily divided into three equal doses, as needed.

➤ **Panic disorder**

Adults: Initially, 0.25 mg P.O. b.i.d.; increase to target dose of 1 mg daily after 3 days. Some patients may benefit from dosages up to maximum of 4 mg daily. To achieve 4 mg daily, increase dosage in increments of 0.125 to 0.25 mg b.i.d. every 3 days, as tolerated, until panic disorder is controlled. Taper drug with decrease of 0.125 mg b.i.d. every 3 days until drug is stopped.

➤ **Bipolar disorder (manic or mixed episodes) ◆**

Adults: 2 to 16 mg/day P.O. for up to 4 years as monotherapy or adjunctive therapy.

Reactions in bold italics are *life-threatening*. Interactions may have a *rapid onset* or a *delayed onset*.

> **Tic disorders** ♦
Adults and children: 0.5 to 12 mg P.O. after
dosage titration for up to 48 weeks.

ADMINISTRATION
P.O.
● Peel back the foil of the orally disinte-
grating tablet (ODT) pouch carefully. Don't
push ODT through foil.
● Give ODT to patient with or without water.

ACTION
Unknown. Probably acts by facilitating the
effects of the inhibitory neurotransmitter
GABA.

Route	Onset	Peak	Duration
P.O.	Unknown	1–2 hr	Unknown

Half-life: 18 to 50 hours.

ADVERSE REACTIONS
CNS: amnesia, aphonia, choreiform movements, coma, confusion, depression,
dysarthria, dysdiadochokinesis, "glassy-
eyed" appearance, hallucinations, headache,
hemiparesis, hypotonia, hysteria, increased
libido, insomnia, psychosis, slurred speech,
tremor, vertigo, paradoxical reactions (aggressive behavior, agitation, anxiety, excitability, hostility, irritability, nervousness,
nightmares and vivid dreams, sleep disturbances), fever, ataxia, abnormal coordination, somnolence, dizziness, nervousness,
reduced intellectual ability.
CV: palpitations.
EENT: abnormal eye movements, diplopia,
nystagmus, blurred vision, pharyngitis,
rhinitis, sinusitis.
GI: anorexia, coated tongue, constipation,
diarrhea, dry mouth, encopresis, gastritis,
increased or decreased appetite, nausea, sore
gums, abdominal pain.
GU: dysuria, enuresis, nocturia, urine retention, colpitis, dysmenorrhea, delayed
ejaculation, erectile dysfunction, urinary
frequency, UTI.
Hematologic: anemia, eosinophilia,
leukopenia, thrombocytopenia.
Hepatic: hepatomegaly, transient elevations of serum transaminases and alkaline
phosphatase.
Metabolic: dehydration, weight loss or
gain.

Musculoskeletal: muscle weakness, muscle
pains.
Respiratory: chest congestion, hypersecretion in upper respiratory tract passages,
respiratory depression, rhinorrhea, shortness of breath, bronchitis, upper respiratory
tract infection, cough.
Skin: hair loss, hirsutism, rash.
Other: ankle and facial edema, general
deterioration, lymphadenopathy, allergic
reaction, influenza.

INTERACTIONS
Drug-drug. *Carbamazepine, phenobarbital, phenytoin:* May lower clonazepam
levels. Monitor patient closely.
Cimetidine: May increase effects of clonazepam. Adjust clonazepam dosage as
needed.
Clozapine: May cause delirium, sedation,
sialorrhea, ataxia, severe orthostatic hypotension, and respiratory depression.
Don't start drugs simultaneously. Adding
clonazepam to an established clozapine
regimen may carry less risk than adding
clozapine to clonazepam. Monitor patient
carefully, especially during the first 48 hours
of coadministration.
CNS depressants: May increase CNS
depression. Avoid using together.
Digoxin: May increase digoxin level and
toxicity. Monitor digoxin level.
Disulfiram: May increase toxic effects of
clonazepam. Reduce clonazepam dosage as
needed.
*Fluconazole, itraconazole, ketoconazole,
miconazole:* May increase and prolong drug
levels, CNS depression, and psychomotor
impairment. Avoid using together.
Methadone: May increase potential for fatal
respiratory depression. Use cautiously.
Omeprazole: May increase effects and toxicities of clonazepam. Adjust clonazepam
dosage as needed or discontinue one or both
drugs.
Protease inhibitors (nelfinavir, ritonavir):
May cause severe respiratory depression.
Monitor patient carefully.
Theophylline: May decrease clonazepam
effects. Monitor patient closely.
Valproic acid: May increase clonazepam
toxicity and increase seizure risk and

teratogenic effects of both drugs in first trimester. Use cautiously.

Drug-herb. *St. John's wort:* May increase hepatic metabolism, resulting in decreased drug effects. Adjust clonazepam dosage as needed.

Drug-lifestyle. *Alcohol use:* May cause additive CNS effects. Discourage use together. *Smoking:* May increase clearance of clonazepam. Monitor patient for decreased drug effects.

EFFECTS ON LAB TEST RESULTS
● May increase LFT values and eosinophil count. May decrease platelet and WBC counts.

CONTRAINDICATIONS & CAUTIONS
● Contraindicated in patients hypersensitive to benzodiazepines and in those with significant hepatic disease or acute angle-closure glaucoma.
● Use cautiously in patients with mixed-type seizures because drug may cause generalized tonic-clonic seizures.
● Use cautiously in children and in patients with chronic respiratory disease, open-angle glaucoma, or a history of drug or alcohol addiction.
● Use cautiously in elderly patients. Drug may accumulate due to potential decrease in hepatic and renal function.
⚠ Overdose S&S: Somnolence, confusion, coma, diminished reflexes.

NURSING CONSIDERATIONS
⊙ Alert: Closely monitor all patients for changes in behavior that may indicate worsening of suicidal thoughts or behavior or depression.
● Don't stop drug abruptly because this may worsen seizures. Call prescriber at once if adverse reactions develop.
● Assess elderly patient's response closely. Elderly patients are more sensitive to drug's CNS effects.
● Monitor patient for oversedation.
● Monitor CBC and LFTs.
● Withdrawal symptoms are similar to those of barbiturates.
● To reduce inconvenience of somnolence when drug is used for panic disorder, giving one dose at bedtime may be desirable.

● *Look alike–sound alike:* Don't confuse clonazepam with clonidine, clozapine, or lorazepam. Don't confuse Klonopin with clonidine.

PATIENT TEACHING
● Advise patient to avoid driving and other hazardous activities that require mental alertness until drug's CNS effects are known.
● Instruct parent to monitor child's school performance because drug may interfere with attentiveness.
● Warn patient and parents not to stop drug abruptly because seizures may occur.
● Advise patient that drug isn't for use during pregnancy or breast-feeding.
● Tell patient to open pouch of ODTs and peel back the foil. He shouldn't push the tablet *through* the foil.
● Tell patient to use dry hands when removing the ODT.
● Tell patient that ODTs can be taken with or without water.

clonidine
KLOE-ni-deen

clonidine hydrochloride
Catapres, Catapres-TTS, Dixarit†, Duraclon, Kapvay

Therapeutic class: Antihypertensives
Pharmacologic class: Centrally acting alpha agonists
Pregnancy risk category: C

AVAILABLE FORMS
Injection for epidural use: 100 mcg/mL
Injection for epidural use, concentrate: 500 mcg/mL
Tablets: 0.025 mg†, 0.1 mg, 0.2 mg, 0.3 mg
Tablets (extended-release): 0.1 mg, 0.2 mg
Transdermal: 0.1 mg/24 hours, 0.2 mg/24 hours, 0.3 mg/24 hours

INDICATIONS & DOSAGES
➤ **Essential and renal hypertension**
Adults and children age 12 and older:
Initially, 0.1 mg P.O. b.i.d.; then increased by 0.1 mg daily on a weekly basis. Usual range is 0.2 to 0.6 mg daily in divided doses;

infrequently, dosages as high as 2.4 mg daily are used.

Or, apply transdermal patch once every 7 days, starting with 0.1-mg system and adjusted with another 0.1-mg or larger system after 1 or 2 weeks if desired blood pressure reduction isn't achieved.

➤ **Severe cancer pain that is unresponsive to epidural or spinal opiate analgesia or other more conventional methods of analgesia**
Adults: Initially, 30 mcg/hour by continuous epidural infusion. Experience with rates greater than 40 mcg/hour is limited.
Children: Initially, 0.5 mcg/kg/hour by epidural infusion. Dosage should be cautiously adjusted, based on response.

➤ **ADHD as monotherapy or as adjunctive therapy to stimulant medications**
Children ages 6 to 17: Initially, 0.1 mg extended-release tablet (Kapvay) P.O. at bedtime. Adjust by 0.1 mg/day at weekly intervals to desired response. With first dosage increase, give tablets b.i.d., with equal or higher dose given at bedtime. Maximum dose is 0.4 mg/day.

➤ **Pheochromocytoma diagnosis** ◆
Adults: 0.3 mg P.O. for a single dose.

➤ **Growth hormone stimulation test** ◆
Adults: 200 mcg or 0.15 mg/m^2 P.O. as a single dose.

➤ **Vasomotor symptoms of menopause** ◆
Adults: 0.05 to 0.4 mg P.O. b.i.d. or 0.1-mg/ 24-hour patch applied once every 7 days.

➤ **Ulcerative colitis** ◆
Adults: 0.3 mg P.O. t.i.d. for 6 weeks.

➤ **Opiate dependence** ◆
Adults: Initially, 0.005 or 0.006 mg/kg test dose, followed by 0.017 mg/kg P.O. daily in three or four divided doses for 10 days. Or, initially, 0.1 mg P.O. t.i.d, with dosage adjusted by 0.1 to 0.2 mg daily. Dosage range is 0.3 to 1.2 mg P.O. daily. Stop drug gradually. Follow protocols.

➤ **Symptom suppression during methadone withdrawal** ◆
Adults: 0.2 mg P.O. t.i.d or q.i.d. for 2 to 3 weeks. Primary dose and dosage titration should be individualized.

➤ **Smoking cessation** ◆
Adults: Initially, 0.1 mg P.O. b.i.d., beginning on or shortly before the day of smoking cessation. Increase dosage every 7 days

by 0.1 mg daily, if needed. Or, 0.2-mg/ 24-hour transdermal patch applied every 7 days. Therapy should begin on or shortly before the day of smoking cessation. Increase dosage by 0.1 mg/24 hours at weekly intervals, if needed.

➤ **ADHD (immediate-release tablets)** ◆
Children: 0.05 mg P.O. daily. May increase by 0.05 mg every 3 to 7 days to maximum dosage of 0.3 to 0.4 mg daily.

➤ **Postanesthetic shivering** ◆
Adults: 2 to 3 mcg/kg or 150 mcg I.V. as a single dose at anesthesia induction, end of surgery, or when laryngeal reflexes and spontaneous breathing return.

ADMINISTRATION
P.O.
● Don't crush, break, or allow patient to chew extended-release tablets.
● Immediate-release and extended-release forms can't be substituted on a milligram-per-milligram basis.
● Give last dose immediately before bedtime.
● Reduce dosage gradually over 2 to 4 days before discontinuing. Decrease dosage of extended-release form by no more than 0.1 mg every 3 to 7 days.
Transdermal
● Apply patch to nonhairy area of intact skin on upper arm or torso.
Epidural
Black Box Warning The injection form concentrate containing 500 mcg/mL must be diluted in normal saline injection before use to yield 100 mcg/mL. ∎

ACTION
Unknown. Thought to stimulate alpha$_2$ receptors and inhibit the central vasomotor centers, decreasing sympathetic outflow to the heart, kidneys, and peripheral vasculature, and lowering peripheral vascular resistance, blood pressure, and heart rate.

Route	Onset	Peak	Duration
P.O.	30–60 min	2–4 hr	12–24 hr
Transdermal	2–3 days	2–3 days	7–8 days
Epidural	Unknown	30–60 min	Unknown

Half-life: 6 to 20 hours.

ADVERSE REACTIONS

CNS: drowsiness, dizziness, sedation, weakness, fatigue, malaise, agitation, depression.
CV: *bradycardia, severe rebound hypertension,* orthostatic hypotension.
GI: constipation, dry mouth, nausea, vomiting, anorexia.
GU: urine retention, erectile dysfunction.
Metabolic: weight gain.
Skin: pruritus, dermatitis with transdermal patch, rash.
Other: loss of libido.

INTERACTIONS

Drug-drug. *Amitriptyline, amoxapine, clomipramine, desipramine, doxepin, imipramine, nortriptyline, protriptyline, trimipramine:* May cause loss of blood pressure control with life-threatening elevations in blood pressure. Avoid using together.
Beta blockers: May cause life-threatening hypertension. Closely monitor blood pressure.
CNS depressants: May increase CNS depression. Use together cautiously.
Digoxin, verapamil: May cause AV block and severe hypotension. Monitor BP and ECG.
Diuretics, other antihypertensives: May increase hypotensive effect. Monitor patient closely.
Levodopa: May reduce effectiveness of levodopa. Monitor patient.
MAO inhibitors, prazosin: May decrease antihypertensive effect. Use together cautiously.
Propranolol, other beta blockers: May cause paradoxical hypertensive response. Monitor patient carefully.
Drug-herb. *Capsicum:* May reduce antihypertensive effectiveness. Discourage use together.
Ma huang: May decrease antihypertensive effects. Discourage use together.

EFFECTS ON LAB TEST RESULTS

● May decrease urinary excretion of vanillylmandelic acid and catecholamines. May cause a weakly positive Coombs test result.

CONTRAINDICATIONS & CAUTIONS

● Contraindicated in patients hypersensitive to drug.
● Transdermal form is contraindicated in patients hypersensitive to any component of the adhesive layer of transdermal system.
● Epidural form is contraindicated in patients receiving anticoagulant therapy, in those with bleeding diathesis, in those with an injection-site infection, and in those who are hemodynamically unstable or have severe CV disease.
● Use cautiously in patients with severe coronary insufficiency, conduction disturbances, recent MI, cerebrovascular disease, chronic renal failure, or impaired liver function.

⚠ *Overdose S&S:* Early hypertension, then hypotension; bradycardia; respiratory and CNS depression; hypothermia; drowsiness; decreased or absent reflexes; weakness; irritability; miosis. With large overdoses: Reversible cardiac conduction defects or arrhythmias, apnea, coma, seizures.

NURSING CONSIDERATIONS

● Drug may be given to lower blood pressure rapidly in some hypertensive emergencies.
● Monitor blood pressure and pulse rate frequently. Dosage is usually adjusted to patient's blood pressure and tolerance.
● Elderly patients may be more sensitive than younger ones to drug's hypotensive effects.
● Observe patient for tolerance to drug's therapeutic effects, which may require increased dosage.
● Noticeable antihypertensive effects of transdermal clonidine may take 2 to 3 days. Oral antihypertensive therapy may have to be continued in the interim.
◆ *Alert:* Remove transdermal patch before defibrillation to prevent arcing.
● Stop drug gradually by reducing dosage over 2 to 4 days to avoid rapid rise in blood pressure, agitation, headache, and tremor. When stopping therapy in patients receiving both clonidine and a beta blocker, gradually withdraw the beta blocker several days before gradually stopping clonidine to minimize adverse reactions.
● Don't stop drug before surgery.

Reactions in bold italics are *life-threatening*. Interactions may have a *rapid onset* or a *delayed onset.*

C

• When drug is given epidurally, carefully monitor infusion pump, and inspect catheter tubing for obstruction or dislodgment.

Black Box Warning Epidural clonidine isn't recommended for obstetric, postpartum, or perioperative pain management due to the risk of hemodynamic instability. ∎

• *Look alike–sound alike:* Don't confuse clonidine with clonazepam, clozapine, Klonopin, quinidine, or clomiphene. Don't confuse Catapres with Cetapred or Combipres.

PATIENT TEACHING

• Instruct patient to take drug exactly as prescribed.

• Advise patient that stopping drug abruptly may cause severe rebound high blood pressure. Tell him dosage must be reduced gradually over 2 to 4 days, as instructed by prescriber.

• Tell patient to take the last dose immediately before bedtime.

• Reassure patient that the transdermal patch usually remains attached despite showering and other routine daily activities. Instruct him on the use of the adhesive overlay to provide additional skin adherence, if needed. Also tell him to place patch at a different site each week.

• Caution patient that drug may cause drowsiness but that this adverse effect usually diminishes over 4 to 6 weeks.

• Inform patient that dizziness upon standing can be minimized by rising slowly from a sitting or lying position and avoiding sudden position changes.

• Advise patient that, if he is scheduled for an MRI, he should alert the facility that he is wearing a transdermal patch.

clopidogrel bisulfate
cloe-PID-oh-grel

Plavix✒

Therapeutic class: Antiplatelet drugs
Pharmacologic class: Platelet aggregation inhibitors
Pregnancy risk category: B

AVAILABLE FORMS
Tablets: 75 mg, 300 mg

INDICATIONS & DOSAGES

➤ **To reduce thrombotic events in patients with atherosclerosis documented by recent stroke, MI, or peripheral arterial disease**
Adults: 75 mg P.O. daily.

➤ **To reduce thrombotic events in patients with acute coronary syndrome (unstable angina and non–Q-wave MI), including those receiving drugs and those undergoing percutaneous coronary intervention (with or without stent) or CABG**
Adults: Initially, a single 300-mg P.O. loading dose; then 75 mg P.O. once daily. Start and continue aspirin (75 to 325 mg once daily) with clopidogrel.

➤ **ST-segment elevation acute MI**
Adults: 75 mg P.O. once daily, with aspirin, with or without thrombolytics. A 300-mg loading dose is optional.

➤ **Loading-dose regimen in patients undergoing coronary stent placement ♦**
Adults: 150 to 600 mg P.O., followed by 75 or 150 mg P.O. daily.

ADMINISTRATION
P.O.
• Give drug without regard to meals.

ACTION
Inhibits the binding of adenosine diphosphate (ADP) to its platelet receptor, impeding ADP-mediated activation and subsequent platelet aggregation, and irreversibly modifies the platelet ADP receptor.

Route	Onset	Peak	Duration
P.O.	2 hr	Unknown	5 days

Half-life: 8 hours.

ADVERSE REACTIONS
CNS: confusion, *fatal intracranial bleeding,* hallucinations.
CV: hypotension.
EENT: epistaxis, rhinitis, taste disorder.
GI: *hemorrhage,* abdominal pain, constipation, diarrhea, dyspepsia, gastritis, ulcers.
GU: UTI, hematuria.
Hematologic: purpura.
Musculoskeletal: arthralgia, myalgia, arthritis.
Respiratory: *bronchospasm,* interstitial pneumonitis, respiratory tract bleeding.

Skin: rash, pruritus, bruising, eczema, erythema multiforme, urticaria, *Stevens-Johnson syndrome, toxic epidermal necrolysis.*
Other: flulike syndrome, *angioedema, anaphylaxis,* serum sickness.

INTERACTIONS

Drug-drug. *Aspirin, NSAIDs:* May increase risk of GI bleeding. Monitor patient.
Bupropion: May elevate bupropion plasma concentration. Closely monitor patient and adjust bupropion dosage as needed when clopidogrel is started or stopped.
Macrolides: May inhibit antiplatelet effect. Adjust clopidogrel dosage as needed. Consider using azithromycin if a macrolide is necessary.
Rifamycins: May increase antiplatelet effect. Carefully monitor platelet function when starting, stopping, or changing rifamycin dosage. Adjust clopidogrel dosage as needed.
Salicylates: May increase the risk of serious bleeding in patients with TIA or ischemic stroke. Avoid use together.
Strong or moderate CYP2C19 inhibitors (cimetidine, etravirine, felbamate, fluconazole, fluoxetine, fluvoxamine, ketoconazole, proton pump inhibitors, ticlopidine, voriconazole): May decrease effects of clopidogrel. Avoid use together. If proton pump inhibitor must be used, consider pantoprazole.
Warfarin: May increase risk of bleeding. Use together cautiously.
Drug-herb. *Red clover:* May increase risk of bleeding. Discourage use together.

EFFECTS ON LAB TEST RESULTS

• May decrease platelet count.

CONTRAINDICATIONS & CAUTIONS

• Contraindicated in patients hypersensitive to drug or its components and in those with pathologic bleeding (such as peptic ulcer or intracranial hemorrhage).
• Use cautiously in patients at risk for increased bleeding from trauma, surgery, or other pathologic conditions and in those with renal or hepatic impairment.
⚠ **Overdose S&S:** Prolonged bleeding time, bleeding complications.

NURSING CONSIDERATIONS

Black Box Warning Drug effectiveness depends on the drug's activation to an active metabolite by the cytochrome P450 system, principally CYP2C19. Patients who are poor metabolizers exhibit higher CV event rates after acute coronary syndrome or percutaneous coronary intervention than patients with normal CYP2C19 function. Tests are available to assess a patient's CYP2C19 genotype. Consider alternative treatment for patients identified as poor metabolizers. ■
• Platelet aggregation won't return to normal for at least 5 days after drug has been stopped.
◐ *Alert:* Drug may cause fatal thrombotic thrombocytopenic purpura (thrombocytopenia, hemolytic anemia, neurologic findings, renal dysfunction, and fever) that requires urgent treatment, including plasmapheresis.
• *Look alike–sound alike:* Don't confuse Plavix with Paxil.

PATIENT TEACHING

• Advise patient that it may take longer than usual to stop bleeding. Tell him to refrain from activities in which trauma and bleeding may occur, and encourage him to wear a seat belt when in a car.
• Instruct patient to notify prescriber if unusual bleeding or bruising occurs.
• Tell patient to inform all health care providers, including dentists, before undergoing procedures or starting new drug therapy, that he is taking drug.
• Inform patient that drug may be taken without regard to meals.

Reactions in bold italics are *life-threatening*. Interactions may have a *rapid onset* or a *delayed onset*.

C

clotrimazole
kloe-TRIM-a-zole

Canesten†, Clotrimaderm†, Cruex ◇,
Gyne-Lotrimin ◇, Lotrimin AF ◇,
Mycelex, Mycelex-7 ◇,
Trivagizole 3 ◇

Therapeutic class: Antifungals
Pharmacologic class: Imidazole
derivatives
Pregnancy risk category: B; C (for
lozenges)

AVAILABLE FORMS
Combination pack: Vaginal tablets 100 mg
and vulvar cream 1% ◇, vaginal tablets
200 mg and vulvar cream 1% ◇
Topical cream: 1%
Topical lotion: 1%
Topical solution: 1%
Troches (lozenges): 10 mg
Vaginal cream: 1% ◇, 2% ◇, 10%† ◇
Vaginal suppositories: 100 mg ◇, 200 mg ◇
Vaginal tablets: 100 mg ◇, 200 mg† ◇,
500 mg† ◇

INDICATIONS & DOSAGES
➤ **Superficial fungal infections (tinea
corporis, tinea cruris, tinea pedis, tinea
versicolor, candidiasis)**
Adults and children age 2 and older: Apply
thin film and massage into affected and
surrounding area, morning and evening, for
2 to 4 weeks. If improvement doesn't occur
after 4 weeks, reevaluate patient.
➤ **Vulvovaginal candidiasis**
Adults and children age 12 and older: One
100-mg vaginal suppository inserted daily
at bedtime for 7 consecutive days. Or, one
200-mg vaginal suppository at bedtime for
3 days. Or, 1 applicatorful of vaginal cream
daily at bedtime for 3 days (2%) or 7 days
(1%).
➤ **Oropharyngeal candidiasis**
Adults and children age 3 and older:
Dissolve lozenge in mouth over 15 to
30 minutes five times daily for 14 consecutive days.
➤ **To prevent oropharyngeal candidiasis in patients immunocompromised
by chemotherapy, radiotherapy, or cor-**

ticosteroid therapy in the treatment of
leukemia, solid tumors, or renal transplantation
Adults: Dissolve lozenge in mouth over
15 to 30 minutes t.i.d. for duration of
chemotherapy or until corticosteroid is
reduced to maintenance levels.

ADMINISTRATION
P.O.
● Lozenges should dissolve in mouth and
not be chewed, for full benefit.
Topical
● Clean and dry area before applying drug.
● Don't use occlusive wrappings or dress-
ings.
Vaginal
● Insert suppository high into vagina.
● Applicators for cream and some supposi-
tories are disposable. If not disposable, wash
with soap and warm water immediately after
use. Rinse thoroughly and dry.

ACTION
Fungistatic or fungicidal, depending on
level. Alters fungal cell-wall permeability
and produces osmotic instability.

Route	Onset	Peak	Duration
P.O.	Unknown	Unknown	3 hr
Topical, vaginal	Unknown	Unknown	Unknown

Half-life: Unknown.

ADVERSE REACTIONS
GI: lower abdominal cramps, nausea and
vomiting with lozenges.
GU: mild vaginal burning or irritation,
urinary frequency.
Skin: erythema, blistering, burning, edema,
general irritation, peeling, pruritus, skin
fissures, stinging, urticaria.

INTERACTIONS
None significant.

EFFECTS ON LAB TEST RESULTS
● May increase liver enzyme levels.

CONTRAINDICATIONS & CAUTIONS
● Contraindicated in patients hypersensitive
to drug.
● Contraindicated for ophthalmic use.

NURSING CONSIDERATIONS
• Consult prescriber before using topical preparations in children younger than age 2. Don't use troches in children younger than age 3; don't use vaginal preparations in children younger than age 12.
• Watch for irritation or sensitivity; stop if irritation occurs, and notify prescriber.
• Improvement usually occurs within 1 week; if no improvement is seen within 4 weeks, review diagnosis.

PATIENT TEACHING
• Reassure patient that hypopigmentation from tinea versicolor will resolve gradually.
• Warn patient not to use occlusive wrappings or dressings.
• Warn patient to avoid contact with eyes.
• Caution patient that frequent or persistent yeast infections may suggest a more serious medical problem.
• Tell patient to refrain from sexual intercourse during vaginal treatment.
• Warn patient that topical preparation may stain clothing.
• Tell patient that using a sanitary napkin protects clothing when using vaginal preparation.
• Stress need to continue use of vaginal preparations, as prescribed, even if menstruation begins.
• Tell patient with athlete's foot to change shoes and cotton socks daily and to dry between the toes after bathing.
• Tell patient to allow lozenges to dissolve in mouth and not to chew, for full benefit.
• Stress need to continue treatment for full course and to notify prescriber if no improvement occurs after 4 weeks.

SAFETY ALERT!

clozapine
KLOE-za-peen

Clozaril⬥, FazaClo, Versacloz

Therapeutic class: Antipsychotics
Pharmacologic class: Dibenzapine derivatives
Pregnancy risk category: B

AVAILABLE FORMS
Oral suspension: 50 mg/mL
Tablets: 12.5 mg, 25 mg, 50 mg, 100 mg, 200 mg
Tablets (orally disintegrating): 12.5 mg, 25 mg, 100 mg, 150 mg, 200 mg

INDICATIONS & DOSAGES
➤ **Schizophrenia in severely ill patients unresponsive to other therapies; to reduce risk of recurrent suicidal behavior in schizophrenia or schizoaffective disorders**
Adults: Initially, 12.5 mg P.O. once daily or b.i.d. Adjust dose upward by 25 to 50 mg daily (if tolerated) to 300 to 450 mg daily by end of 2 weeks. Individual dosage is based on clinical response, patient tolerance, and adverse reactions. Subsequent dosage shouldn't be increased more than once or twice weekly and shouldn't exceed 50- to 100-mg increments. Many patients respond to dosages of 200 to 600 mg daily, but some may need as much as 900 mg daily. Don't exceed 900 mg daily.

ADMINISTRATION
P.O.
• Peel the foil from the orally disintegrating tablet (ODT) blister and gently remove the tablet immediately before giving.
• Give ODT with or without water.
• Shake bottle for 10 seconds before withdrawing suspension using provided oral syringe and syringe adaptor.

ACTION
Unknown. Binds selectively to dopaminergic receptors in the CNS and may interfere with adrenergic, cholinergic, histaminergic, and serotonergic receptors.

Reactions in bold italics are *life-threatening*. Interactions may have a *rapid onset* or a ***delayed onset***.

Route	Onset	Peak	Duration
P.O.	Unknown	2½ hr	4–12 hr

Half-life: Proportional to dose; may range from 8 to 12 hours.

ADVERSE REACTIONS

CNS: drowsiness, sedation, dizziness, vertigo, headache, *seizures,* syncope, tremor, disturbed sleep or nightmares, restlessness, hypokinesia or akinesia, agitation, rigidity, akathisia, confusion, fatigue, insomnia, hyperkinesia, weakness, lethargy, ataxia, slurred speech, depression, myoclonus, anxiety, fever.
CV: tachycardia, *cardiomyopathy, myocarditis, pulmonary embolism, cardiac arrest,* hypotension, hypertension, chest pain, ECG changes, orthostatic hypotension.
EENT: visual disturbances.
GI: constipation, excessive salivation, dry mouth, nausea, vomiting, heartburn, diarrhea.
GU: urinary frequency or urgency, urine retention, incontinence, abnormal ejaculation.
Hematologic: *leukopenia, agranulocytosis, granulocytopenia,* eosinophilia.
Metabolic: hyperglycemia, weight gain, hypercholesterolemia, hypertriglyceridemia.
Musculoskeletal: muscle pain or spasm, muscle weakness.
Respiratory: *respiratory arrest.*
Skin: rash, diaphoresis.

INTERACTIONS

Drug-drug. *Anticholinergics:* May potentiate anticholinergic effects of clozapine. Use together cautiously.
Antihypertensives: May potentiate hypotensive effects. Monitor blood pressure.
Black Box Warning *Benzodiazepines, other psychotropic drugs:* May increase risk of sedation and CV and respiratory arrest. Use together cautiously. ∎
Bone marrow suppressants: May increase bone marrow toxicity. Avoid using together.
Citalopram, *fluoroquinolones,* **fluoxetine, fluvoxamine,** *paroxetine,* **sertraline:** May increase clozapine levels and toxicity. Adjust clozapine dose as needed.
CYP1A2 inducers (tobacco smoking): May decrease clozapine (oral suspension) effectiveness. Increase clozapine dosage as necessary.

CYP2D6 or CYP3A4 inhibitors (bupropion, cimetidine, duloxetine, erythromycin, escitalopram, fluoxetine, paroxetine, quinidine, sertraline, terbinafine); moderate or weak CYP1A2 inhibitors (caffeine, oral contraceptives): Monitor patient for adverse reactions. Reduce clozapine oral suspension dosage if necessary.
Digoxin, other highly protein-bound drugs, warfarin: May increase levels of these drugs. Monitor patient closely for adverse reactions.
Phenytoin: May decrease clozapine level and cause breakthrough psychosis. Monitor patient for psychosis and adjust clozapine dosage.
Psychoactive drugs: May cause additive effects. Use together cautiously.
Ritonavir: May increase clozapine levels and toxicity. Avoid using together.
Strong CYP3A4 inducers (carbamazepine, phenytoin, rifampin): May decrease clozapine effectiveness. Use together isn't recommended. If coadministration is necessary, consider increasing clozapine dosage.
Strong CYP1A2 inhibitors (ciprofloxacin, fluvoxamine): May increase clozapine level. Reduce clozapine (oral suspension) dosage to one-third during coadministration.
Drug-herb. *St. John's wort:* May decrease drug level. Discourage use together.
Drug-lifestyle. *Alcohol use:* May increase CNS depression. Discourage use together.
Smoking: May decrease drug level. Urge patient to quit smoking. Monitor patient for effectiveness and adjust dosage.

EFFECTS ON LAB TEST RESULTS

● May increase glucose, cholesterol, and triglyceride levels.
● May increase eosinophil count. May decrease granulocyte and WBC counts.

CONTRAINDICATIONS & CAUTIONS

◑ *Alert:* Neonates exposed to antipsychotics during the third trimester of pregnancy are at risk for developing extrapyramidal signs and symptoms (repetitive muscle movements of the face and body) and withdrawal symptoms (agitation, abnormally increased or decreased muscle tone, tremors, sleepiness, severe difficulty breathing, and difficulty feeding) following delivery. Use in pregnancy only if the potential benefit to the mother justifies the risk to the fetus.

• Contraindicated in patients with uncontrolled epilepsy, history of clozapine-induced agranulocytosis, WBC count below 3,500/mm³, severe CNS depression or coma, paralytic ileus, and myelosuppressive disorders.

• Contraindicated in patients taking other drugs that suppress bone marrow function.

• Use cautiously in patients with prostatic hyperplasia or angle-closure glaucoma because drug has potent anticholinergic effects.

⚠ *Overdose S&S:* Altered state of consciousness, drowsiness, delirium, coma, tachycardia, hypotension, respiratory depression or failure, hypersalivation, aspiration pneumonia, cardiac arrhythmias, seizures.

NURSING CONSIDERATIONS

• ODTs contain phenylalanine.

Black Box Warning Drug carries significant risk of agranulocytosis. If possible, give patient at least two trials of standard antipsychotic before starting clozapine. Obtain baseline WBC and differential counts before clozapine therapy. Baseline WBC count must be at least 3,500/mm³ and baseline ANC at least 2,000/mm³. Monitor WBC and ANC values weekly for at least 4 weeks after stopping drug, regardless of how often you were monitoring when therapy stopped. ∎

• During the first 6 months of therapy, monitor patient weekly and dispense no more than a 1-week supply of drug. If acceptable WBC and ANC values (WBC 3,500/mm³ or higher and ANC 2,000/mm³ or higher) are maintained during the first 6 months of continuous therapy, reduce monitoring to every other week. After 6 months of every-other-week monitoring without interruption by leukopenia, reduce frequency of monitoring WBC and ANC to monthly.

• If WBC count drops below 3,500/mm³ after therapy begins or if it drops substantially from baseline, monitor patient closely for signs and symptoms of infection. If WBC count is 3,000 to 3,500/mm³ and granulocyte count is above 1,500/mm³, perform WBC and differential count twice weekly. If WBC count drops to 2,000/mm³

to 3,000/mm³ or granulocyte count drops to 1,000 to 1,500/mm³, interrupt therapy and notify prescriber. Monitor WBC and differential daily until WBC exceeds 3,000/mm³ and ANC exceeds 1,500/mm³, and monitor patient for signs and symptoms of infection. Continue monitoring WBC and differential counts twice weekly until WBC count exceeds 3,500/mm³ and ANC exceeds 2,000/mm³. Then, restart therapy with weekly monitoring for 1 year before returning to the usual monitoring schedule of every 2 weeks for 6 months and then every 4 weeks.

• If WBC count drops below 2,000/mm³ and granulocyte count drops below 1,000/mm³, patient may need protective isolation. Bone marrow aspiration may be needed to assess bone marrow function. Future clozapine therapy is contraindicated in these patients.

Black Box Warning Drug increases the risk of fatal myocarditis, especially during, but not limited to, the first month of therapy. In patients in whom myocarditis is suspected (unexplained fatigue, dyspnea, tachypnea, chest pain, tachycardia, fever, palpitations, and other signs or symptoms of heart failure or ECG abnormalities, such as ST-T wave abnormalities or arrhythmias), stop therapy immediately and don't restart. ∎

🕓 *Alert:* Drug may cause hyperglycemia. Monitor patients with diabetes regularly. In patients with risk factors for diabetes, obtain fasting blood glucose test results at baseline and periodically.

🕓 *Alert:* Monitor patient for metabolic syndrome, including significant weight gain and increased body mass index, hypertension, hyperglycemia, hypercholesterolemia, and hypertriglyceridemia.

• Monitor patient for signs and symptoms of cardiomyopathy.

Black Box Warning Orthostatic hypotension, with or without syncope, can occur. Rarely, collapse can be profound and be accompanied by respiratory or cardiac arrest. Orthostatic hypotension is more likely to occur during initial titration with rapid dose escalation. In patients who have had even a brief interval off clozapine (2 or more days since the last dose), start treatment with 12.5 mg once daily or b.i.d. ∎

Black Box Warning Seizures may occur, especially in patients receiving high doses. ■
- Some patients experience transient fever with temperature higher than 100.4° F (38° C), especially in the first 3 weeks of therapy. Monitor these patients closely.

Black Box Warning Drug isn't indicated for use in elderly patients with dementia-related psychoses because of an increased risk for death from CV disease or infection. ■

- After abrupt withdrawal of long-term therapy, abrupt recurrence of psychosis is possible.
- If therapy must be stopped, withdraw drug gradually over 1 or 2 weeks. If changes in patient's medical condition (including development of leukopenia) require that drug be stopped immediately, monitor patient closely for recurrence of psychosis.
- If therapy is reinstated in patients withdrawn from drug, follow usual guidelines for dosage increase. Reexposure of patient to drug may increase severity and risk of adverse reactions. If therapy was stopped because WBC counts were below 2,000/mm^3 or granulocyte counts were below 1,000/mm^3, don't restart.
- **Look alike–sound alike:** Don't confuse clozapine with clonidine, clofazimine, clonazepam, or Klonopin. Don't confuse Clozaril with Colazal.

PATIENT TEACHING
- Tell patient about need for weekly blood tests to check for blood-cell deficiency. Advise him to report flulike symptoms, fever, sore throat, lethargy, malaise, or other signs of infection.
- Warn patient to avoid hazardous activities that require alertness and good coordination while taking drug.
- Tell patient to check with prescriber before taking alcohol or OTC drugs.
- Advise patient that smoking may decrease drug effectiveness.
- Tell patient to rise slowly to avoid dizziness.
- Tell patient to keep ODTs in the blister package until he is ready to take them.
- Inform patient that ice chips or sugarless candy or gum may help relieve dry mouth.

SAFETY ALERT!

codeine phosphate
koe-DEEN

codeine sulfate

Therapeutic class: Opioid analgesics
Pharmacologic class: Opioids
Pregnancy risk category: C
Controlled substance schedule: II

AVAILABLE FORMS
codeine phosphate
Injection: 15 mg/mL, 30 mg/mL, 60 mg/mL†
Syrup: 5 mg/mL†
Tablets: 15 mg†, 30 mg†
codeine sulfate
Oral solution: 30 mg/5 mL
Tablets: 15 mg, 30 mg, 60 mg

INDICATIONS & DOSAGES
➤ **Mild to moderate pain**
Adults: 15 to 60 mg P.O. or 15 to 60 mg (phosphate) subcutaneously, I.M., or I.V. every 4 to 6 hours p.r.n.
Children older than age 1: 0.5 mg/kg P.O., subcutaneously, or I.M. every 4 to 6 hours p.r.n. Don't give I.V. in children.

ADMINISTRATION
P.O.
- Give drug with milk or meals to avoid GI upset.

I.V.
▼ Don't give discolored solution.
▼ Give drug by direct injection into a large vein. Give very slowly.
▼ **Incompatibilities:** Aminophylline, ammonium chloride, amobarbital, bromides, chlorothiazide, heparin, iodides, pentobarbital, phenobarbital, phenytoin, salts of heavy metals, sodium bicarbonate, sodium iodide, thiopental.

I.M.
- Document injection site.
Subcutaneous
- Assess injection site for local irritation, pain, and induration.

ACTION
May bind with opioid receptors in the CNS, altering perception of and emotional

response to pain. Also suppresses the cough reflex by direct action on the cough center in the medulla.

Route	Onset	Peak	Duration
P.O.	30–45 min	1–2 hr	4–6 hr
I.V.	Immediate	Immediate	4–6 hr
I.M.	10–30 min	30–60 min	4–6 hr
Subcut.	10–30 min	Unknown	4–6 hr

Half-life: 2½ to 4 hours.

ADVERSE REACTIONS

CNS: clouded sensorium, sedation, dizziness, euphoria, light-headedness, physical dependence.
CV: *bradycardia,* flushing, hypotension.
GI: constipation, dry mouth, ileus, nausea, vomiting.
GU: urine retention.
Respiratory: *respiratory depression.*
Skin: diaphoresis, pruritus.

INTERACTIONS

Drug-drug. *CNS depressants, general anesthetics, hypnotics, MAO inhibitors, other opioid analgesics, sedatives, TCAs, tranquilizers:* May cause additive effects. Use together cautiously; monitor patient response.
Drug-lifestyle. *Alcohol use:* May cause additive effects. Discourage use together.

EFFECTS ON LAB TEST RESULTS

• May increase amylase and lipase levels.

CONTRAINDICATIONS & CAUTIONS

• Contraindicated in patients hypersensitive to drug.
• I.V. use contraindicated in children.
Black Box Warning Children who receive codeine for pain relief following a tonsillectomy and/or adenoidectomy have an increased risk of death. Codeine is contraindicated for pain management after these surgeries. ∎
❸ Alert: For managing pain (not associated with tonsillectomy and/or adenoidectomy), codeine should be used in children only if the benefits outweigh the risks.
• Use cautiously in elderly or debilitated patients and in those with head injury, increased intracranial pressure, increased CSF pressure, hepatic or renal disease, hypothy-roidism, Addison disease, acute alcoholism, seizures, severe CNS depression, bronchial asthma, COPD, respiratory depression, and shock.
• Don't administer drug during labor when delivery of a premature infant is anticipated.
❸ Alert: Breast-feeding women may put their infants at increased risk for morphine overdose if the mother is an ultra-rapid codeine metabolizer.
⚠ Overdose S&S: CNS depression, respiratory depression, apnea, flaccid skeletal muscles, bradycardia, hypotension, circulatory collapse, death.

NURSING CONSIDERATIONS

• Reassess patient's level of pain at least 15 and 30 minutes after use.
• Codeine and aspirin or acetaminophen are commonly prescribed together to provide enhanced pain relief.
• For full analgesic effect, give drug before patient has intense pain.
• Drug is an antitussive and shouldn't be used when cough is a valuable diagnostic sign or is beneficial (as after thoracic surgery).
• Monitor cough type and frequency.
• Monitor respiratory and circulatory status.
• Opioids may cause constipation. Assess bowel function and need for stool softeners and stimulant laxatives.
• Codeine may delay gastric emptying, increase biliary tract pressure from contraction of the sphincter of Oddi, and interfere with hepatobiliary imaging studies.
• **Look alike–sound alike:** Don't confuse codeine with Cardene, Lodine, or Cordran.

PATIENT TEACHING

❸ Alert: Caution parents and caregivers to observe children for signs of toxicity (unusual sleepiness, confusion, or difficult or noisy breathing). If signs occur, stop drug and seek medical attention immediately.
• Advise patient that GI distress caused by taking drug P.O. can be eased by taking drug with milk or meals.
• Instruct patient to ask for or to take drug before pain is intense.
• Caution ambulatory patient about getting out of bed or walking. Warn outpatient to avoid driving and other hazardous activities

---

Reactions in bold italics are *life-threatening*. Interactions may have a *rapid onset* or a *delayed onset*.

that require mental alertness until drug's effects on the CNS are known.
• Advise patient to avoid alcohol during therapy.
• Warn breast-feeding woman to watch for increased sleepiness, difficulty breast-feeding or breathing, or limpness of infant. Tell her to immediately seek medical attention if this occurs.

SAFETY ALERT!

codeine phosphate–acetaminophen
koe-DEEN/a-seet-a-MIN-a-fen

Capital and Codeine,
Tylenol with Codeine #3🖉,
Tylenol with Codeine #4

Therapeutic class: Analgesics
Pharmacologic class: Opioids–para aminophenol derivatives
Pregnancy risk category: C
Controlled substance schedule: III (tablets); V (liquid)

AVAILABLE FORMS
Oral solution or suspension: 12 mg codeine and 120 mg acetaminophen/5 mL*
Tablets: 15 mg codeine and 300 mg acetaminophen, 30 mg codeine and 300 mg acetaminophen, 60 mg codeine and 300 mg acetaminophen

INDICATIONS & DOSAGES
Adjust-a-dose (for all indications): Consider decreased dosage in patients with renal impairment, elderly patients, and patients overly sensitive to effects of opioids. For patients with hepatic impairment, maximum total daily acetaminophen dose is 2,000 mg.
➤ **Mild to moderately severe pain**
Adults and children older than age 12: Codeine 15 to 60 mg and acetaminophen 300 to 1,000 mg P.O. every 4 hours as needed for pain; adjust dosage based on pain severity and patient response. Maximum total daily dosage: acetaminophen 4,000 mg and codeine 360 mg.
Children ages 7 to 12: Codeine 0.5 to 1 mg/kg/dose every 4 to 6 hours; acetaminophen 10 to 15 mg/kg/dose every 4 hours as needed.

Children ages 3 up to 7: 5 mL oral solution or suspension P.O. t.i.d. or q.i.d. as needed.
➤ **Analgesic-antipyretic therapy in presence of aspirin allergy, hemostatic disturbances, bleeding diatheses, upper GI disease, and gouty arthritis**
Adults and children older than age 12: Codeine 15 to 60 mg and acetaminophen 300 to 1,000 mg P.O. every 4 hours as needed (varies according to product). Maximum total daily dosage is codeine, 360 mg and acetaminophen, 4,000 mg.
Children ages 7 to 12: 10 mL oral solution P.O. t.i.d. or q.i.d as needed.
Children ages 3 up to 7: 5 mL oral solution P.O. t.i.d. or q.i.d. as needed.

ADMINISTRATION
P.O.
• Store tablets at room temperature.
• Give with milk or meals to avoid GI upset.

ACTION
Codeine may bind with opioid receptors in the CNS, altering perception and emotional response to pain. Acetaminophen is thought to produce analgesia by inhibiting prostaglandin and other substances that sensitize pain receptors.

Route	Onset	Peak	Duration
P.O. (codeine)	30–45 min	1–2 hr	4–6 hr
P.O. (acetaminophen)	Rapid	½–2 hr	3–4 hr

Half-life: Codeine, 2.9 hours; acetaminophen, 1.25 to 3 hours.

ADVERSE REACTIONS
CNS: drowsiness, light-headedness, dizziness, sedation, euphoria, dysphoria.
GI: nausea, vomiting, constipation, abdominal pain.
Hematologic: *thrombocytopenia, agranulocytosis.*
Respiratory: shortness of breath.
Skin: pruritus, rash.
Other: allergic reactions.

INTERACTIONS
Drug-drug. *Antipsychotics, general anesthetics, opioid analgesics, sedative-hypnotics, tranquilizers, other CNS depressants:* May increase CNS depression. Use together cautiously.

Cimetidine: May enhance effects of codeine, increasing toxicity. Monitor patient carefully.

Drug-lifestyle. *Alcohol use:* May increase CNS depression. Discourage use together.

EFFECTS ON LAB TEST RESULTS
● May increase serum amylase level.
● May cause false-positive results for urinary 5-hydroxyindoleacetic acid.

CONTRAINDICATIONS & CAUTIONS
● Contraindicated in patients hypersensitive to codeine or acetaminophen.
Black Box Warning Children who receive codeine for pain relief following a tonsillectomy and/or adenoidectomy have an increased risk of death. Codeine is contraindicated for pain management after these surgeries. ■
◆ *Alert:* For managing pain (not associated with tonsillectomy and/or adenoidectomy), codeine should be used in children only if the benefits outweigh the risks.
● Use cautiously in patients with head injury, intracranial lesions, increased intracranial pressure, or acute abdominal conditions.
Black Box Warning Acetaminophen has been associated with acute liver failure, usually at doses greater than 4,000 mg/day and often when more than one acetaminophen-containing product is used. Liver failure may result in liver transplant or death. ■
◆ *Alert:* May cause serious, potentially fatal skin reactions, including Stevens-Johnson syndrome, toxic epidermal necrolysis, and acute generalized exanthematous pustulosis. Reaction may occur with first or subsequent use when acetaminophen is used as monotherapy or when it is one component of combination drug therapy. Monitor for reddening of the skin, rash, blisters, and detachment of the upper surface of the skin. Stop drug immediately if skin reaction is suspected.
● Use cautiously in patients with asthma or sulfite sensitivity because allergy-type reactions, anaphylaxis, and asthmatic episodes may occur.
● Use cautiously in elderly or debilitated patients; in those with severe renal or hepatic impairment, hypothyroidism, urethral

stricture, Addison disease, or prostatic hypertrophy; in patients identified as ultra-rapid metabolizers of codeine; and in those with identified polymorphism of CYP2D6 genotype.
● Use in pregnant women only if benefit justifies risk; dependence in newborns may occur. Use in breast-feeding women only if benefit justifies risk; both components appear in breast milk.
⚠ *Overdose S&S:* Extreme sleepiness, confusion, shallow breathing. Codeine: Pinpoint pupils, respiratory depression, loss of consciousness, seizures. Acetaminophen: Hepatic necrosis, nausea, vomiting, diaphoresis, malaise, renal tubular necrosis, hypoglycemia, coma, coagulation defects.

NURSING CONSIDERATIONS
● Prescribe lowest effective dosage for shortest period of time and inform patients of risks and signs and symptoms of acetaminophen and codeine toxicity.
● Carefully monitor patients identified as ultra-rapid metabolizers of codeine and those with identified polymorphism of CYP2D6 genotype. Overdose signs and symptoms and exaggerated adverse effects may occur at normal doses in these patients.
● Monitor serial liver or renal function tests in patients with severe hepatic or renal disease.

PATIENT TEACHING
◆ *Alert:* Caution parents and caregivers to observe children for signs of toxicity (unusual sleepiness, confusion, or difficult or noisy breathing). If signs occur, stop drug and seek medical attention immediately.
◆ *Alert:* Warn patient to stop drug and seek medical attention immediately if skin rash or reaction occurs while using acetaminophen.
● Inform patient with severe hepatic or renal disease that serial liver or renal function tests will be needed.
● Caution patient not to drive a car or operate heavy machinery while taking this drug.
● Discourage alcohol use during therapy.
● Warn patient that codeine may be habit-forming and to take only as long as it's prescribed and in the amounts prescribed.

Reactions in bold italics are *life-threatening*. Interactions may have a *rapid onset* or a *delayed onset*.

• Advise breast-feeding women who are ultra-rapid metabolizers to consult prescriber immediately, call 911, or go to the nearest emergency department if the infant shows signs and symptoms of codeine toxicity (sleepiness, difficulty breast-feeding, breathing difficulties, limpness).

colchicine
KOL-chih-seen

Colcrys♪

Therapeutic class: Antigout drugs
Pharmacologic class: Colchicum autumnale alkaloids
Pregnancy risk category: C

AVAILABLE FORMS
Tablets: 0.6 mg

INDICATIONS & DOSAGES
➤ **Prevention of gout flares**
Adults: 0.6 mg P.O. once daily or b.i.d. Maximum daily dose is 1.2 mg.
Adjust-a-dose: For patients with CrCl of less than 30 mL/minute, give 0.3 mg/day.
➤ **Gout flares**
Adults: 1.2 mg P.O. at first sign of a flare, followed by 0.6 mg 1 hour later; maximum dosage is 1.8 mg over a 1-hour period.
Adjust-a-dose: For patients with CrCl of 10 to 50 mL/minute, give 50% to 100% of usual daily dose; for CrCl of less than 10 mL/minute or for patients on peritoneal dialysis, give 25% of usual dose. For patients with hepatic impairment or CrCl of less than 30 mL/minute and on maintenance colchicine for gout prophylaxis, treatment of flares isn't recommended.
➤ **Familial Mediterranean fever (FMF)**
Adults: 1.2 to 2.4 mg P.O. daily; may increase by 0.3 mg/day to maximum daily dosage given once daily or in two divided doses.
Adolescents older than age 12: 1.2 to 2.4 mg P.O. once daily or in two divided doses.
Children ages 6 to 12: 0.9 to 1.8 mg P.O. once daily or in two divided doses.
Children ages 4 to 6: 0.3 to 1.8 mg P.O. once daily or in two divided doses.
Adjust-a-dose: For patients with CrCl of less than 30 mL/minute, initially 0.3 mg/day, carefully increasing dosage as needed.

➤ **Acute pericarditis** ♦
Adults: Initial loading dose of 1 to 2 mg P.O. daily, followed by maintenance dose of 0.5 to 1 mg P.O. daily for at least 3 months.
➤ **Recurrent pericarditis** ♦
Adults: Initial loading dose of 1 to 3 mg P.O. daily, followed by maintenance dose of 0.5 to 2 mg P.O. daily for at least 6 months.
➤ **Behçet syndrome** ♦
Adults: 1 to 2 mg P.O. daily in divided doses (0.5 or 0.6 mg t.i.d.) as primary or adjunctive therapy.

ADMINISTRATION
P.O.
• Give drug with or without food.

ACTION
Exact mechanism of action is not fully known; thought to involve a reduction in lactic acid produced by leukocytes, reducing uric acid deposits and phagocytosis, thereby decreasing the inflammatory process.

Route	Onset	Peak	Duration
P.O.	Unknown	2 hr	Unknown

Half-life: 27 to 31 hours.

ADVERSE REACTIONS
CNS: fatigue, headache.
EENT: pharyngolaryngeal pain.
GI: diarrhea, nausea, vomiting.
Hematologic: *aplastic anemia, granulocytopenia, leukopenia, pancytopenia, thrombocytopenia.*
Other: gout.

INTERACTIONS
Drug-drug. *Acidifying agents:* May inhibit action of colchicine. Avoid use together.
Alkalinizing agents: May increase action of colchicine. Avoid use together.
CNS depressants, sympathomimetics (such as phenylephrine): May increase sensitivity to these drugs. Monitor patient closely and adjust dosage as needed.
Digoxin, HMG-CoA reductase inhibitors (such as atorvastatin, simvastatin): May increase risk of myopathy or rhabdomyolysis. Avoid use together. If coadministration can't be avoided, monitor patient carefully. Discontinue colchicine if signs or symptoms occur.

†Canada   ◇OTC   ♦Off-label use   ♪Photoguide   *Liquid contains alcohol.

Moderate CYP3A4 inhibitors (such as amprenavir, aprepitant, diltiazem, erythromycin, fluconazole, fosamprenavir, verapamil), P-glycoprotein inhibitors (such as cyclosporine, ranolazine), strong CYP3A4 inhibitors (such as atazanavir, clarithromycin, indinavir, itraconazole, ketoconazole, nefazodone, nelfinavir, ritonavir, saquinavir, telithromycin): May increase colchicine level, increasing the risk of toxic effects. Reduce colchicine dose, if alternative treatment isn't available.

Drug-food. *Grapefruit juice:* May increase drug level. Discourage use together.

EFFECTS ON LAB TEST RESULTS
• May increase AST, ALT, and CK levels.
• May decrease hemoglobin and hematocrit levels.
• May decrease leukocyte, granulocyte, and platelet counts.
• May cause false-positive results when urine is tested for RBCs or hemoglobin.

CONTRAINDICATIONS & CAUTIONS
• Contraindicated in patients with renal or hepatic impairment who are taking P-glycoprotein inhibitors or strong CYP3A4 inhibitors.
• Use only during pregnancy if benefit to patient outweighs risk to fetus.
• Drug appears in breast milk; patient shouldn't breast-feed while taking drug.
⚠ **Overdose S&S:** Abdominal pain, nausea, vomiting, diarrhea, hypovolemia, multiorgan failure, death.

NURSING CONSIDERATIONS
• Safety and effectiveness of repeat treatment for gout flares haven't been established.
🕐 **Alert:** Colcrys is the only FDA-approved single-ingredient colchicine product.
• Drug isn't an analgesic and shouldn't be used to treat pain from other causes.
• Obtain baseline laboratory studies, including CBC, before starting therapy and periodically thereafter; watch for myelosuppression, leukopenia, granulocytopenia, thrombocytopenia, pancytopenia, and aplastic anemia.

• Monitor patient who has used drug for a prolonged period for neuromuscular toxicity and rhabdomyolysis.
• When used for gout prophylaxis, colchicine must be given with allopurinol or a uricosuric drug (such as probenecid) to decrease serum uric acid level. However, colchicine should be started before the other agent because a sudden change in uric acid level may cause a gout attack.
• *Look alike–sound alike:* Don't confuse colchicine with Cortrosyn.

PATIENT TEACHING
• Tell patient that drug can be taken without regard to food.
• Advise female patient not to breast-feed and to use an alternative method for feeding the baby.
• Advise patient to report muscle pain or weakness, tingling or numbness in fingers or toes, unusual bleeding or bruising, increased infections, weakness, tiredness, severe diarrhea or vomiting, or cyanosis.

colesevelam hydrochloride
koe-leh-SEVE-eh-lam

Welchol♦

Therapeutic class: Antilipemics
Pharmacologic class: Bile acid sequestrants
Pregnancy risk category: B

AVAILABLE FORMS
Oral suspension: 1.875-g, 3.75-g packets
Tablets: 625 mg

INDICATIONS & DOSAGES
➤ **Adjunct to diet and exercise, either alone or with an HMG-CoA reductase inhibitor, to reduce elevated LDL cholesterol in patients with primary hypercholesterolemia (Fredrickson type IIa)**
Adults: 3 tablets (1,875 mg) P.O. b.i.d. or 6 tablets (3,750 mg) once daily. Or, one 1.875-g packet P.O. b.i.d. or one 3.75-g packet P.O. once daily.
Children ages 10 to 17: One 1.875-g packet P.O. b.i.d. with meals or one 3.75-g packet P.O. once daily with a meal.

➤ **Adjunct to diet and exercise to improve glycemic control in type 2 diabetes mellitus**
Adults: 3 tablets (1,875 mg) P.O. b.i.d. or 6 tablets (3,750 mg) P.O. once daily. Or, one 1.875-g packet P.O. b.i.d. or one 3.75-g packet P.O. once daily.

ADMINISTRATION
P.O.
• Give drug with a meal and plenty of fluids.
• Store tablets at room temperature and protect them from moisture.
• Empty entire contents of one packet into glass and add 4 to 8 ounces of water, fruit juice, or diet soft drink. Stir well and give immediately.

ACTION
Binds bile acids in the intestinal tract, impeding their absorption and causing their elimination in feces. In response to this bile acid depletion, LDL cholesterol levels decrease as the liver uses LDL cholesterol to replenish reduced bile acid stores.

Route	Onset	Peak	Duration
P.O.	Unknown	2 wk	Unknown

Half-life: Unknown.

ADVERSE REACTIONS
CNS: headache, asthenia, pain.
EENT: pharyngitis, rhinitis, sinusitis.
GI: constipation, flatulence, abdominal pain, diarrhea, dyspepsia, nausea.
Musculoskeletal: back pain, myalgia.
Respiratory: increased cough.
Other: infection, accidental injury, flulike syndrome.

INTERACTIONS
Glyburide: May decrease glyburide level. Administer glyburide at least 4 hours before colesevelam dose.
Hormonal contraceptives containing ethinyl estradiol and norethindrone: May decrease levels of these contraceptives. Administer hormonal contraceptive at least 4 hours before colesevelam dose.
Phenytoin: May decrease phenytoin level and increase seizure activity. Administer phenytoin 4 hours before colesevelam dose and monitor phenytoin level.

Thyroid hormones: Coadministration may increase thyroid-stimulating hormone level. Administer thyroid hormone replacement 4 hours before colesevelam dose.
Warfarin: May decrease INR. Monitor INR and patient closely.

EFFECTS ON LAB TEST RESULTS
• May increase triglyceride levels.

CONTRAINDICATIONS & CAUTIONS
• Contraindicated in patients hypersensitive to drug or any of its components, in patients with triglyceride levels greater than 500 mg/dL, and in patients with bowel obstruction.
• Contraindicated for glycemic control in patients with type 1 diabetes and for the treatment of diabetic ketoacidosis.
• Use cautiously in patients susceptible to vitamin K or fat-soluble vitamin deficiencies and in patients with swallowing disorders, severe GI motility disorders, or major GI tract surgery.
• Use cautiously in patients with triglyceride levels greater than 300 mg/dL.
⚠ Overdose S&S: Severe local GI reactions, especially constipation.

NURSING CONSIDERATIONS
• Before starting drug, assess patient for underlying causes of hypercholesterolemia, such as poorly controlled diabetes, hypothyroidism, nephrotic syndrome, dysproteinemias, obstructive liver disease, other drug therapy, and alcoholism.
• Monitor patient's bowel habits. If severe constipation develops, decrease dosage, add a stool softener, or stop drug.
• Monitor the effects of patient's other drugs to identify drug interactions.
• Monitor INR and total and LDL cholesterol and triglyceride levels periodically during therapy.
• Use only when clearly needed in breast-feeding women because it's not known if drug appears in breast milk.

PATIENT TEACHING
• Instruct patient to take drug with a meal and plenty of fluids.
• Teach patient to monitor bowel habits. Encourage a diet high in fiber and fluids.

Instruct patient to notify prescriber promptly if severe constipation develops.

● Encourage patient to follow prescribed diet, exercise, and monitoring of cholesterol and triglyceride levels.

● Tell patient to notify prescriber if she's pregnant or breast-feeding.

conivaptan hydrochloride
kah-nih-VAP-tan

Vaprisol

Therapeutic class: Vasopressin antagonists
Pharmacologic class: Arginine vasopressin receptor antagonists
Pregnancy risk category: C

AVAILABLE FORMS
Injection (premixed): 0.2 mg/mL in 100 mL D_5W

INDICATIONS & DOSAGES
➤ **Euvolemic hyponatremia (as from SIADH, hypothyroidism, adrenal insufficiency, pulmonary disorders) and hypervolemic hyponatremia in hospitalized patients**
Adults: Loading dose of 20 mg I.V. over 30 minutes; then 20 mg I.V. by continuous infusion over 24 hours for 1 to 3 days. If sodium level isn't rising at desired rate, increase to 40 mg/day by continuous infusion. Don't give for more than 4 days after loading dose.
Adjust-a-dose: If sodium level rises more than 12 mEq/L in 24 hours, stop infusion. If hyponatremia persists or recurs and the patient has had no adverse neurologic effects from the rapid rise in sodium level, restart infusion at a reduced dose. If patient develops hypotension or hypovolemia, stop infusion. Monitor vital signs and volume status often. If hyponatremia persists once the patient is no longer hypotensive and volume returns to normal, restart infusion at a reduced dose. In patients with hepatic impairment (Child-Pugh class A to C) or with CrCl of 30 to 60 mL/minute, give a loading dose of 10 mg followed by a continuous infusion of 10 mg over 24 hours for

2 to 4 days. If serum sodium level isn't rising at desired rate, drug may be titrated upward to 20 mg over 24 hours. Don't use if CrCl is less than 30 mL/minute.

ADMINISTRATION
I.V.
▼ Give via a large vein, and change infusion site every 24 hours.
▼ Protect premixed solution from light until ready to use.
▼ **Incompatibilities:** Lactated Ringer solution, normal saline solution. Don't mix or infuse with other I.V. drugs.

ACTION
Increases free water eliminated by kidneys, inhibiting inappropriate or excessive arginine vasopressin (antidiuretic hormone) secretion. Typically, this causes increased net fluid loss, increased urine output, and decreased urine osmolality.

Route	Onset	Peak	Duration
I.V.	Unknown	2–4 hr	12 hr

Half-life: 5 hours.

ADVERSE REACTIONS
CNS: headache, confusion, fever, insomnia.
CV: atrial fibrillation, hypertension, hypotension, orthostatic hypotension.
EENT: pharyngolaryngeal pain.
GI: constipation, diarrhea, dry mouth, nausea, oral candidiasis, vomiting.
GU: frequency, hematuria, polyuria, UTI.
Hematologic: anemia.
Metabolic: *hypoglycemia,* hypokalemia, dehydration, hyperglycemia, *hypomagnesemia,* hyponatremia.
Respiratory: pneumonia.
Skin: erythema.
Other: infusion-site reactions, thirst.

INTERACTIONS
Drug-drug. *Amlodipine:* May increase amlodipine level and half-life. Monitor blood pressure.
Digoxin: May increase digoxin level. Monitor patient, and adjust digoxin dose, as needed.
Midazolam: May increase midazolam level. Monitor patient for respiratory depression and hypotension.

Reactions in bold italics are *life-threatening*. Interactions may have a *rapid onset* or a *delayed onset*.

Potent CYP3A4 inhibitors (clarithromycin, indinavir, itraconazole, ketoconazole, ritonavir): May seriously increase levels and toxic effects. Use together is contraindicated.
Simvastatin: May increase simvastatin level. Monitor patient for signs of rhabdomyolysis, including muscle pain, weakness, and tenderness.

EFFECTS ON LAB TEST RESULTS
• May decrease potassium, magnesium, sodium, and hemoglobin levels and hematocrit. May increase or decrease blood glucose level.

CONTRAINDICATIONS & CAUTIONS
• Contraindicated in patients with hypovolemic hyponatremia; patients hypersensitive to drug or its components, corn, or corn products; and those taking potent CYP3A4 inhibitors, such as clarithromycin, indinavir, itraconazole, ketoconazole, or ritonavir.
• Use cautiously in hyponatremic patients with underlying heart failure and patients with hepatic or renal impairment.
⚠ **Overdose S&S:** Hypotension, thirst.

NURSING CONSIDERATIONS
• Monitor sodium level and neurologic status regularly during therapy.
❸ **Alert:** Rapid correction of sodium level may cause osmotic demyelination syndrome. Monitor patient's sodium level and volume status.
• Drug may cause significant infusion-site reactions, even with proper dilution and administration. Rotate infusion site every 24 hours to reduce risk of reaction.

PATIENT TEACHING
• Inform patient that he may experience low blood pressure when standing. If he feels dizzy or faint, advise him to sit or lie down.
• Advise patient to promptly report signs and symptoms of hypoglycemia, such as feeling shaky, nervous, tired, sweaty, cold, hungry, confused, irritable, or impatient.
• Emphasize the importance of reporting an unusually fast heartbeat or weakness.
• Tell patient that analgesics and moist heating pads can be used to treat pain and inflammation at the infusion site.

• Inform patient that the infusion will be given for a maximum of 4 days after the loading dose.

SAFETY ALERT!

crizotinib
kriz-OH-ti-nib

Xalkori

Therapeutic class: Antineoplastics
Pharmacologic class: Tyrosine kinase inhibitors
Pregnancy risk category: D

AVAILABLE FORMS
Capsules: 200 mg, 250 mg

INDICATIONS & DOSAGES
➤ **Locally advanced or metastatic non–small-cell lung cancer (NSCLC) that is anaplastic lymphoma kinase (ALK)–positive as detected by an FDA-approved test**
Adults: 250 mg P.O. b.i.d.
Adjust-a-dose: For patients with grade 3 hematologic toxicity, withhold drug until recovery to grade 2 or lower; then resume at same dosing schedule. For patients with grade 4 hematologic toxicity, withhold drug until recovery to grade 2 or lower; then reduce dosage to 200 mg P.O. b.i.d. If recurrence occurs, withhold drug until recovery to grade 2 or lower; then resume at 250 mg P.O. once daily. Permanently discontinue drug for patients with grade 4 recurrence. For patients with grade 3 QTc-interval prolongation, withhold drug until recovery to grade 1 or lower; then resume at 200 mg b.i.d. If grade 3 QTc-interval prolongation recurs, withhold drug until recovery to grade 1 or lower; then resume at 250 mg once daily. If grade 3 QTc-interval prolongation recurs or patient develops grade 4 QTc-interval prolongation, permanently discontinue drug. For patients with grade 3 or 4 ALT or AST elevation with grade 1 or lower total bilirubin, withhold drug until recovery to grade 1 or lower or to baseline; then resume at 200 mg P.O. b.i.d. For patients with grade 2, 3, or 4 ALT or AST elevation with concurrent grade 2, 3, or 4 total bilirubin elevation (in the absence

of cholestasis or hemolysis), permanently discontinue drug.

ADMINISTRATION

P.O.

• Drug may only be prescribed to patients diagnosed by FDA-approved test to detect ALK-positive NSCLC.

• Give capsules whole; don't crush, open, or dissolve them.

• Don't touch or handle crushed or broken capsules.

• May give drug with or without food.

ACTION

Inhibits tyrosine kinase receptors, including ALK and other growth factors, decreasing tumor-cell proliferation.

Route	Onset	Peak	Duration
P.O.	Unknown	4–6 hr	Unknown

Half-life: 42 hours.

ADVERSE REACTIONS

CNS: dizziness, neuropathy, headache, insomnia, fatigue, fever.
CV: chest pain, edema, bradycardia.
EENT: visual disorders.
GI: nausea, diarrhea, vomiting, constipation, esophageal disorder, abdominal pain, stomatitis, decreased appetite, dysgeusia.
Musculoskeletal: arthralgia, back pain.
Respiratory: cough, pneumonia, dyspnea, *pulmonary embolism,* upper respiratory tract infection, *pneumonitis.*
Skin: rash.

INTERACTIONS

Drug-drug. *CYP3A substrates (alfentanil, cyclosporine, dihydroergotamine, ergotamine, fentanyl, pimozide, quinidine, sirolimus, tacrolimus):* May increase levels of these drugs. Avoid use together.
Moderate CYP3A inhibitors (aprepitant, diltiazem, erythromycin, fluconazole, verapamil): May increase crizotinib level. Use together cautiously.
P-glycoprotein substrates (daunorubicin, saquinavir, vinca alkaloids): May increase levels of these drugs. Avoid use together.
Strong CYP3A inducers (carbamazepine, phenobarbital, phenytoin, rifabutin,

rifampin): May decrease crizotinib level. Avoid use together.
Strong CYP3A inhibitors (atazanavir, clarithromycin, indinavir, itraconazole, ketoconazole, nefazodone, nelfinavir, ritonavir, saquinavir, telithromycin, troleandomycin, voriconazole): May increase crizotinib level. Avoid use together.
Drug-herb. *St. John's wort:* May decrease crizotinib level. Avoid use together.
Drug-food. *Grapefruit, grapefruit juice:* May increase crizotinib level. Avoid use together.

EFFECTS ON LAB TEST RESULTS

• May increase ALT and AST levels.
• May decrease neutrophil, platelet, and lymphocyte counts.

CONTRAINDICATIONS & CAUTIONS

• Contraindicated in patients hypersensitive to drug or its components.
• Contraindicated in pregnant and breast-feeding women.
• Use cautiously in patients with hepatic disease, congestive heart failure, bradyarrhythmias, or electrolyte abnormalities; in patients at risk for pneumonitis; and in patients taking medications that prolong QTc interval.
• Use cautiously in patients with hepatic impairment, severe renal impairment (CrCl of less than 30 mL/minute), or ESRD.
• Use cautiously in Asian patients; drug levels at standard doses may be higher in this population.

NURSING CONSIDERATIONS

• Monitor patient for signs and symptoms of long QTc interval (such as dizziness or syncope).
• Monitor ECG in patients with congestive heart failure, bradyarrhythmias, or electrolyte abnormalities and in patients taking medications that prolong QTc interval.
• Monitor electrolyte levels; correct levels as needed.
• Monitor patient for pulmonary signs and symptoms; discontinue drug if treatment-related pneumonitis occurs.
• Monitor LFTs and CBC at least monthly or as clinically indicated.

C

PATIENT TEACHING
• Warn patient to swallow capsules whole and to avoid touching crushed or broken tablets.
• Advise patient to avoid grapefruit and grapefruit juice while taking drug.
• Instruct patient in the use of standard antiemetics, antidiarrheals, and laxatives to treat most frequent GI adverse effects.
• Tell patient to report visual disturbances, such as flashes of light, blurred vision, light sensitivity, or floaters.
• Teach patient that if he misses a dose, to take missed dose as soon as he remembers unless it's less than 6 hours until next dose; in that case, patient shouldn't take missed dose. Instruct patient to never take two doses at the same time to make up for a missed dose.
• Caution patient not to change dosage or stop drug without discussing with health care provider.
• Advise patient of potential risk to fetus. Women and partners should use adequate contraceptive methods during therapy and for at least 90 days after therapy ends.

✱ NEW DRUG

crofelemer
kro-FEL-e-mer

Fulyzaq

Therapeutic class: Antidiarrheals
Pharmacologic class: Antidiarrheals
Pregnancy risk category: C

AVAILABLE FORMS
Tablets (delayed-release): 125 mg

INDICATIONS & DOSAGES
➤ **Noninfectious diarrhea in patients with HIV/AIDS on antiretroviral therapy**
Adults: 125 mg P.O. b.i.d.

ADMINISTRATION
P.O.
• May give without regard to food.
• Don't crush, split, or allow patient to chew tablet. Patient must swallow tablet whole.
• Store at room temperature.

ACTION
Blocks the chloride ion secretion and accompanying high-volume water loss in diarrhea, normalizing the flow of chloride and water in the GI tract.

Route	Onset	Peak	Duration
P.O.	Unknown	Unknown	Unknown

Half-life: Unknown.

ADVERSE REACTIONS
CNS: anxiety, depression, dizziness.
EENT: seasonal allergies, sinusitis, nasopharyngitis.
GI: constipation, flatulence, nausea, abdominal distention, abdominal pain, dry mouth, dyspepsia, gastroenteritis, hemorrhoids, giardiasis.
GU: UTI, nephrolithiasis, frequent urination.
Hematologic: decreased WBC count.
Musculoskeletal: back pain, arthralgia, extremity pain, musculoskeletal pain.
Respiratory: upper respiratory tract infection, bronchitis, cough.
Skin: acne, dermatitis.
Other: herpes zoster, procedural pain.

INTERACTIONS
None reported.

EFFECTS ON LAB TEST RESULTS
• May increase bilirubin, ALT, and AST levels.
• May decrease WBC count.

CONTRAINDICATIONS & CAUTIONS
• Contraindicated in patients hypersensitive to drug or its components, in those with infectious diarrhea, and in breast-feeding women.
• Use cautiously in pregnant women and only if clearly needed.

NURSING CONSIDERATIONS
• Rule out the possibility of infectious diarrhea before initiation of therapy.
• If infectious diarrhea occurs during treatment, discontinue drug.

PATIENT TEACHING
• Instruct patient not to crush or chew tablets but to swallow them whole.

• Caution patient to report pregnancy to health care provider.

cyclobenzaprine hydrochloride
sye-kloe-BEN-za-preen

Amrix

Therapeutic class: Skeletal muscle relaxants
Pharmacologic class: Tricyclic antidepressant derivatives
Pregnancy risk category: B

AVAILABLE FORMS
Capsules (extended-release): 15 mg, 30 mg
Tablets: 5 mg, 7.5 mg, 10 mg

INDICATIONS & DOSAGES
➤ **Adjunct to rest and physical therapy to relieve muscle spasm from acute, painful musculoskeletal conditions**
Adults and children age 15 and older: 5 mg P.O. t.i.d. Based on response, dose may be increased to 10 mg t.i.d. Don't exceed 30 mg/day. Or, 15 to 30 mg extended-release capsule P.O. once daily (adults only). Use for longer than 2 or 3 weeks isn't recommended.
Adjust-a-dose: In elderly patients and in those with mild hepatic impairment, start with 5-mg conventional tablets and adjust slowly upward. Drug isn't recommended in patients with moderate to severe hepatic impairment. Don't use extended-release capsules in children, elderly patients, or those with impaired hepatic function.

ADMINISTRATION
P.O.
• Don't split the generic 10-mg tablets because of the high risk of inconsistent doses.
• Give extended-release capsules whole; don't crush or break.

ACTION
Unknown. Relieves skeletal muscle spasm of local origin without disrupting muscle function.

Route	Onset	Peak	Duration
P.O.	1 hr	4 hr	12–24 hr
P.O. (extended-release)	1.5 hr	7–8 hr	Unknown

Half-life: 1 to 3 days; 32 hours for extended-release capsules.

ADVERSE REACTIONS
CNS: dizziness, drowsiness, *seizures,* headache, tremor, insomnia, fatigue, asthenia, nervousness, confusion, paresthesia, depression, attention disturbances, dysarthria, ataxia, syncope.
CV: *arrhythmias,* palpitations, hypotension, tachycardia.
EENT: visual disturbances, blurred vision.
GI: dry mouth, dyspepsia, abnormal taste, constipation, nausea.
Skin: rash, pruritus, acne.

INTERACTIONS
Drug-drug. *CNS depressants:* May increase CNS depression. Avoid using together.
Guanethidine: May block guanethidine's antihypertensive effect. Monitor patient's blood pressure.
MAO inhibitors: May cause hyperpyretic crisis, seizures, and death when MAO inhibitors are used with TCAs; may also occur with cyclobenzaprine. Avoid using within 2 weeks of MAO inhibitor therapy.
Naproxen: May increase drowsiness. Make patient aware of this interaction.
Tramadol: May increase risk of seizures. Use together cautiously.
Drug-lifestyle. *Alcohol use:* May increase CNS depression. Discourage use together.

EFFECTS ON LAB TEST RESULTS
None reported.

CONTRAINDICATIONS & CAUTIONS
• Contraindicated in patients hypersensitive to drug; in those with hyperthyroidism, heart block, arrhythmias, conduction disturbances, or heart failure; in those who have received MAO inhibitors within 14 days; and in those in the acute recovery phase of an MI.
• Use cautiously in elderly or debilitated patients and in those with a history of urine

---

Reactions in bold italics are *life-threatening*. Interactions may have a *rapid onset* or a *delayed onset*.

retention, acute angle-closure glaucoma, or increased intraocular pressure.
• Safety and effectiveness in children younger than age 15 haven't been established.
⚠ *Overdose S&S:* Drowsiness, tachycardia, tremor, agitation, coma, ataxia, hypertension, slurred speech, confusion, dizziness, nausea, vomiting, hallucinations, cardiac arrest, chest pain, cardiac arrhythmias, ECG changes (changes in QRS axis or width).

NURSING CONSIDERATIONS
• Drug may cause toxic reactions similar to those caused by TCAs. Observe same precautions as when giving TCAs.
• Monitor patient for nausea, headache, and malaise, which may occur if drug is stopped abruptly after long-term use.
🔵 *Alert:* Notify prescriber immediately of signs and symptoms of overdose, including cardiac toxicity.

PATIENT TEACHING
• Advise patient to report urinary hesitancy or urine retention. If constipation is a problem, suggest that patient increase fluid intake and use a stool softener.
• Warn patient to avoid activities that require alertness until CNS effects of drug are known.
• Warn patient not to combine with alcohol or other CNS depressants, including OTC cold or allergy remedies.
• Instruct patient not to split the generic 10-mg tablets because of the high risk of inconsistent doses.
• Advise patient that using drug for longer than 2 to 3 weeks isn't recommended.

SAFETY ALERT!

cyclophosphamide
sye-kloe-FOSS-fa-mide

Cytoxan (Lyophilized), Procytox†

Therapeutic class: Antineoplastics
Pharmacologic class: Nitrogen mustards
Pregnancy risk category: D

AVAILABLE FORMS
Injection: 200-mg†, 500-mg, 1-g, 2-g vials
Tablets: 25 mg, 50 mg

INDICATIONS & DOSAGES
Adjust-a-dose (for all indications): Consider dosage reduction to 75% of usual dosage in patients with severe renal failure (CrCl of 0 to 10 mL/minute). Adjust dosage for patients with hepatic dysfunction as follows: If bilirubin level is 3.1 to 5 mg/dL or AST level is greater than 180 units/L, give 75% of dose. Don't give if bilirubin level is greater than 5 mg/dL.
➤ **Breast or ovarian cancer, Hodgkin lymphoma, chronic lymphocytic leukemia, chronic myelocytic leukemia, acute lymphoblastic leukemia, acute myelocytic and monocytic leukemia, neuroblastoma, retinoblastoma, malignant lymphoma, multiple myeloma, mycosis fungoides, sarcoma**
Adults and children: Initially for induction, 40 to 50 mg/kg I.V. in divided doses over 2 to 5 days. Or, 10 to 15 mg/kg I.V. every 7 to 10 days, 3 to 5 mg/kg I.V. twice weekly, or 1 to 5 mg/kg P.O. daily, based on patient tolerance.
Adjust subsequent doses according to evidence of antitumor activity or leukopenia.
➤ **Minimal-change nephrotic syndrome**
Children: 2.5 to 3 mg/kg P.O. daily for 60 to 90 days.

ADMINISTRATION
P.O.
• Don't give drug at bedtime; infrequent urination during the night may increase possibility of cystitis.
I.V.
▼ Preparing and giving parenteral form of drug may be mutagenic, teratogenic, or carcinogenic. Follow facility policy to reduce risks.
▼ Reconstitute powder using sterile water for injection or bacteriostatic water for injection containing only parabens.
▼ Add 25 mL to 500-mg vial, 50 mL to 1-g vial, or 100 mL to 2-g vial to produce a solution containing 20 mg/mL. Shake vigorously to dissolve. If powder doesn't dissolve completely, let vial stand for a few minutes.
▼ Check reconstituted solution for small particles. Filter solution, if needed.
▼ Give by direct I.V. injection or infusion.

▼ For infusion, further dilute with D₅W, dextrose 5% in normal saline solution for injection, dextrose 5% in Ringer injection, lactated Ringer injection, sodium lactate injection, or half-normal saline solution for injection.

▼ Reconstituted solution is stable 6 days if refrigerated or 24 hours at room temperature. Use stored solutions cautiously because drug contains no preservatives.

▼ **Incompatibilities:** Amphotericin B cholesteryl sulfate complex.

ACTION

Cross-links strands of cellular DNA and interferes with RNA transcription, causing an imbalance of growth that leads to cell death. Not specific to cell cycle.

Route	Onset	Peak	Duration
P.O.	Unknown	Unknown	Unknown
I.V.	Unknown	2–3 hr	Unknown

Half-life: 3 to 12 hours.

ADVERSE REACTIONS

CV: *cardiotoxicity with very high doses and with doxorubicin.*
GI: nausea and vomiting, anorexia, stomatitis.
GU: *hemorrhagic cystitis,* impaired fertility.
Hematologic: *leukopenia, thrombocytopenia,* anemia.
Hepatic: *hepatotoxicity.*
Metabolic: hyperuricemia, SIADH.
Respiratory: *pulmonary fibrosis with high doses.*
Skin: alopecia.
Other: *secondary malignant disease, anaphylaxis,* hypersensitivity reactions.

INTERACTIONS

Drug-drug. *Allopurinol, myelosuppressants:* May increase myelosuppression. Monitor patient for toxicity.
Anticoagulants: May increase anticoagulant effect. Monitor patient for bleeding.
Aspirin, NSAIDs: May increase risk of bleeding. Avoid using together.
Azole antifungals (itraconazole): May increase exposure to cyclophosphamide and its metabolites. Closely monitor patient for cyclophosphamide adverse reactions.

Barbiturates: May enhance cyclophosphamide toxicity. Monitor patient closely.
Carbamazepine: May increase cyclophosphamide level. Monitor patient carefully and adjust cyclophosphamide dosage as needed.
Cardiotoxic drugs: May increase adverse cardiac effects. Monitor patient for toxicity.
Chloramphenicol, corticosteroids: May reduce activity of cyclophosphamide. Use together cautiously.
Ciprofloxacin: May decrease antimicrobial effect. Monitor patient for effect.
Digoxin: May decrease digoxin level. Monitor level closely.
Live-virus vaccines: May increase vaccine-induced adverse reactions. Don't give together.
Pentostatin: May cause respiratory distress, hypotension, hypothermia, and death. Avoid use together if possible.
Phenytoin: May increase risk of cyclophosphamide toxicity. If coadministration can't be avoided, monitor patient carefully and consider reducing initial dose of cyclophosphamide.
Quinolones: May decrease the antimicrobial effects of quinolones. Monitor patient.
Succinylcholine: May prolong neuromuscular blockade. Avoid using together.
Thiazide diuretics: May prolong antineoplastic-induced leukopenia. Monitor patient closely.
TNF blockers: May increase the incidence of noncutaneous solid malignancies. Use together isn't recommended.

EFFECTS ON LAB TEST RESULTS

● May increase uric acid level. May decrease hemoglobin and pseudocholinesterase levels.
● May decrease platelet, RBC, and WBC counts.
● May suppress positive reaction to *Candida,* mumps, *Trichophyton,* and tuberculin skin test results. May cause a false-positive Papanicolaou test result.

CONTRAINDICATIONS & CAUTIONS

● Contraindicated in patients hypersensitive to drug and in those with severe bone marrow suppression.
● Use cautiously in patients with leukopenia, thrombocytopenia, malignant cell

---

Reactions in bold italics are *life-threatening*. Interactions may have a *rapid onset* or a *delayed onset*.

infiltration of bone marrow, or hepatic or renal disease and in those who have recently undergone radiation therapy or chemotherapy.

⚠ **Overdose S&S:** Infection, myelosuppression, cardiotoxicity.

NURSING CONSIDERATIONS

• If cystitis occurs, stop drug and notify prescriber. Cystitis can occur months after therapy ends. Mesna may be given to reduce frequency and severity of bladder toxicity. Test urine for blood.

• Adequately hydrate patients before and after dose to decrease risk of cystitis.

• Use caution to ensure correct dose to decrease risk of cardiac toxicity.

• Monitor CBC and renal and liver function test results.

• Monitor patient closely for leukopenia (nadir between days 8 and 15, recovery in 17 to 28 days).

• Monitor uric acid level. To prevent hyperuricemia with resulting uric acid nephropathy, allopurinol may be used with adequate hydration.

• To prevent bleeding, avoid all I.M. injections when platelet count is less than 50,000/mm^3.

• Anticipate blood transfusions because of cumulative anemia.

• Therapeutic effects are often accompanied by toxicity.

• In boys, using drug for nephrotic syndrome for more than 60 days increases the incidence of oligospermia and azoospermia. Use for more than 90 days increases the risk of sterility.

• Drug may be used to treat nononcologic disorders, such as lupus, nephritis, and rheumatoid arthritis.

PATIENT TEACHING

• Warn patient that hair loss is likely to occur but is reversible.

• Advise patient to watch for signs and symptoms of infection (fever, sore throat, fatigue) and bleeding (easy bruising, nosebleeds, bleeding gums, tarry stools). Tell patient to take temperature daily.

• Instruct patient to avoid OTC products that contain aspirin.

• To minimize risk of hemorrhagic cystitis, encourage patient to urinate every 1 to

2 hours while awake and to drink at least 3 L of fluid daily.

• If patient is taking tablets, tell him not to take it at bedtime because infrequent urination increases risk of cystitis.

• Advise both men and women to practice contraception during therapy and for 4 months afterward; drug may cause birth defects.

• Advise women to stop breast-feeding during therapy because of risk of toxicity to infant.

• Drug can cause irreversible sterility in both men and women. Before therapy, counsel patients who are considering parenthood. Also recommend that women consult prescriber before becoming pregnant.

cycloSPORINE
sye-kloe-SPOR-een

Sandimmune

cycloSPORINE (modified)
Gengraf, Neoral

Therapeutic class: Immunosuppressants
Pharmacologic class: Immunosuppressants
Pregnancy risk category: C

AVAILABLE FORMS
Capsules for microemulsion (modified) *:
25 mg, 50 mg, 100 mg
Capsules (nonmodified): 25 mg, 50 mg, 100 mg
Injection: 50 mg/mL
Oral solution (modified and nonmodified): 100 mg/mL*

INDICATIONS & DOSAGES
➤ **To prevent organ rejection in renal, hepatic, or cardiac transplantation**
Adults and children: 15 mg/kg P.O. 4 to 12 hours before transplantation and continue daily for 1 to 2 weeks postoperatively. Then reduce dosage by 5% each week to maintenance level of 5 to 10 mg/kg daily. Or, 5 to 6 mg/kg I.V. concentrate 4 to 12 hours before transplantation as a slow I.V. infusion over 2 to 6 hours. Postoperatively, repeat dose daily until patient can tolerate P.O. forms.

For conversion from Sandimmune to Gengraf or Neoral, use same daily dose as previously used for Sandimmune. Monitor blood levels every 4 to 7 days after conversion, and monitor blood pressure and creatinine level every 2 weeks during the first 2 months.

➤ **Severe, active rheumatoid arthritis (RA) that hasn't adequately responded to methotrexate**

Adults: 2.5 mg/kg Gengraf or Neoral daily P.O., taken as two divided doses. Dosage may be increased by 0.5 to 0.75 mg/kg daily after 8 weeks and again after 12 weeks to a maximum of 4 mg/kg daily. If no response is seen after 16 weeks, stop therapy.

Adjust-a-dose: If hypertension, serum creatinine elevations (30% above the patient's pretreatment level), or clinically significant laboratory abnormalities occur, decrease dosage by 25% to 50% to control adverse reactions. If dosage reduction doesn't control abnormalities, or if the adverse reaction or abnormality is severe, discontinue drug.

➤ **Psoriasis**

Adults: 1.25 mg/kg Gengraf or Neoral daily P.O. b.i.d. for at least 4 weeks. Increase dosage by 0.5 mg/kg daily once every 2 weeks as needed to a maximum of 4 mg/kg daily.

Adjust-a-dose: If clinically significant laboratory abnormalities occur, decrease dosage by 25% to 50% to control adverse reactions. If the serum creatinine level is 25% or more above the patient's pretreatment level, serum creatinine measurement should be repeated within 2 weeks. If the serum creatinine level remains at 25% or more above baseline, reduce dosage by 25% to 50%. If at any time the serum creatinine level increases by 50% or more above pretreatment level, reduce dosage by 25% to 50%. If reversibility (within 25% of baseline) of the serum creatinine level isn't achievable after two dosage modifications, discontinue drug.

If the patient with no history of hypertension before initiation of therapy develops hypertension, reduce dosage by 25% to 50%. If the patient continues to be hypertensive despite multiple dosage reductions, discontinue drug. For patients with previously treated hypertension, adjust their antihypertensive medication. Discontinue

cyclosporine if a change in hypertension management isn't effective or tolerable.

ADMINISTRATION

P.O.

● Give Neoral or Gengraf on an empty stomach.

● Measure oral solution doses carefully in an oral syringe. Don't rinse dosing syringe with water. If syringe is cleaned, it must be completely dry before reuse.

● To improve the taste of Sandimmune oral solution, mix it with milk, chocolate milk, or orange juice. Gengraf or Neoral oral solution may be mixed with orange or apple juice (not grapefruit juice); it's less palatable when mixed with milk.

● Use a glass container to mix, and have patient drink at once.

I.V.

▼ This form is usually reserved for patients who can't tolerate oral drugs.

▼ Immediately before use, dilute each milliliter of concentrate in 20 to 100 mL of D₅W or normal saline solution for injection. Give at one-third the oral dose.

▼ Infuse over 2 to 6 hours.

▼ Protect diluted drug from light.

▼ **Incompatibilities:** Amphotericin B cholesteryl sulfate complex, magnesium sulfate.

ACTION

May inhibit proliferation and function of T lymphocytes and inhibit production and release of lymphokines.

Route	Onset	Peak	Duration
P.O.	Unknown	90 min–3 hr	Unknown
I.V.	Unknown	Unknown	Unknown

Half-life: Initial phase, about 1 hour; terminal phase, 8½ to 27 hours.

ADVERSE REACTIONS

CNS: tremor, headache, confusion, paresthesia, *seizures.*

CV: hypertension, flushing.

EENT: gum hyperplasia, sinusitis.

GI: nausea, vomiting, diarrhea, abdominal discomfort.

GU: *nephrotoxicity.*

Hematologic: anemia, *leukopenia, thrombocytopenia.*

Reactions in bold italics are *life-threatening*. Interactions may have a *rapid onset* or a *delayed onset*.

Hepatic: *hepatotoxicity.*
Metabolic: hyperglycemia.
Skin: hirsutism, acne.
Other: infections, *anaphylaxis.*

INTERACTIONS

Drug-drug. *Acyclovir, aminoglycosides, amphotericin B, cimetidine, diclofenac, gentamicin, ketoconazole, melphalan, NSAIDs, ranitidine, sulfamethoxazole–trimethoprim, tacrolimus, tobramycin, vancomycin:* May increase risk of nephrotoxicity. Avoid using together.

Allopurinol, **azole antifungals,** *bromocriptine,* **caspofungin,** *cimetidine, clarithromycin, danazol, diltiazem, erythromycin, imipenem–cilastatin, methylprednisolone, metoclopramide,* **micafungin,** *nicardipine, prednisolone, verapamil:* May increase cyclosporine level. Monitor patient for increased toxicity.

Azathioprine, corticosteroids, cyclophosphamide, verapamil: May increase immunosuppression. Monitor patient closely.

Carbamazepine, isoniazid, nafcillin, octreotide, **orlistat,** *phenobarbital,* **phenytoin,** *rifabutin,* **rifampin,** *ticlopidine:* May decrease immunosuppressant effect from low cyclosporine level. Cyclosporine dosage may need to be increased.

Digoxin, HMG-CoA reductase inhibitors (such as lovastatin), prednisolone: May decrease clearance of these drugs. Use together cautiously.

Mycophenolate mofetil: May decrease mycophenolate level. Monitor patient closely when cyclosporine is added to or removed from therapy.

Potassium-sparing diuretics: May induce hyperkalemia. Monitor patient closely.

Sirolimus: May increase sirolimus level. Take sirolimus at least 4 hours after cyclosporine dose. If separating doses isn't possible, monitor patient for increased adverse effects.

Vaccines: May decrease immune response. Delay routine immunization.

Drug-herb. *Astragalus, echinacea, licorice:* May interfere with drug's effect. Discourage use together.

St. John's wort: May reduce drug level, resulting in transplant failure. Discourage use together.

Drug-food. *Alfalfa sprouts:* May interfere with drug's effect. Discourage use together.

Grapefruit and grapefruit juice: May increase drug level and cause toxicity. Advise patient to avoid use together.

Drug-lifestyle. *Sun exposure:* May increase risk of sensitivity to sunlight. Advise patient to avoid excessive sun exposure.

EFFECTS ON LAB TEST RESULTS

● May increase ALT, AST, bilirubin, BUN, creatinine, glucose, and LDL levels. May decrease hemoglobin and magnesium levels.
● May decrease platelet and WBC counts.

CONTRAINDICATIONS & CAUTIONS

● Contraindicated in patients hypersensitive to drug or polyoxyethylated castor oil (found in injectable form).
● Contraindicated in patients with RA or psoriasis with abnormal renal function, uncontrolled hypertension, or malignancies (Neoral or Gengraf).

NURSING CONSIDERATIONS

Black Box Warning Only experienced physicians should prescribe this drug. ▮

Black Box Warning Psoriasis patients previously treated with psoralen and ultraviolet A light, methotrexate or other immunosuppressive agents, ultraviolet B light, coal tar, or radiation therapy are at an increased risk for skin malignancies when taking Neoral or Gengraf. ▮

● Drug can cause hepatotoxicity.

Black Box Warning Neoral and Gengraf may increase the susceptibility to infection and the development of neoplasia. ▮

◔ **Alert:** Drugs causing immunosuppression increase the risk of opportunistic infections, including activation of latent viral infections such as BK virus–associated neuropathy, which may lead to serious outcomes, including kidney graft loss.

● Monitor elderly patient for renal impairment and hypertension.

Black Box Warning Monitor Sandimmune level at regular intervals. Absorption of oral solution can be erratic during long-term administration. ▮

Black Box Warning Neoral and Gengraf have greater bioavailability than Sandimmune. A lower dose of Neoral or Gengraf may be needed to provide blood level similar to that achieved with Sandimmune. Monitor blood level when switching patients between these two brands. ∎

Black Box Warning Gengraf is bioequivalent to and interchangeable with Neoral capsules, but neither is interchangeable with Sandimmune. ∎

Black Box Warning Always give with corticosteroids; however, don't give Sandimmune with other immunosuppressants. ∎

Black Box Warning Drug can cause systemic hypertension and nephrotoxicity. ∎

• Use Neoral or Gengraf to treat RA or psoriasis.

• *Look alike–sound alike:* Don't confuse cyclosporine with cyclophosphamide or cycloserine. Don't confuse Sandimmune with Sandostatin.

RA

• Before starting treatment, measure blood pressure at least twice and obtain two creatinine levels to estimate baseline.

• Evaluate blood pressure and creatinine level every 2 weeks during first 3 months and then monthly if patient is stable.

• Monitor blood pressure and creatinine level after an increase in NSAID dosage or introduction of a new NSAID. Monitor CBC and LFTs monthly if patient also receives methotrexate.

Psoriasis

• Measure blood pressure at least twice to determine a baseline. Monitor blood pressure after dosage changes.

• Evaluate patient for occult infection and tumors initially and throughout treatment.

• Obtain baseline creatinine level (on two occasions), CBC, and BUN, magnesium, uric acid, potassium, and lipid levels.

• Evaluate blood pressure, CBC, and uric acid, potassium, lipid, magnesium, creatinine, and BUN levels every 2 weeks during first 3 months and then monthly thereafter if patient is stable.

• Monitor creatinine level after increasing NSAID dose or starting a new NSAID.

• Improvement in psoriasis takes 12 to 16 weeks of therapy.

PATIENT TEACHING

• Encourage patient to take drug at same time each day and to be consistent with relation to meals.

• Teach patient how to measure dosage and mask taste of oral solution. Tell him not to take drug with grapefruit juice.

• Instruct patient to fill glass with water after dose and drink it to make sure he consumes all of drug.

• Advise patient to take drug with meals if nausea occurs.

• Advise patient to take Neoral or Gengraf on an empty stomach.

• Tell patient being treated for psoriasis that improvement may not occur until after 12 to 16 weeks of therapy.

• Stress that drug shouldn't be stopped without prescriber's approval.

• Explain to patient the importance of frequent laboratory monitoring while receiving therapy.

• Tell patient to avoid people with infections because drug lowers resistance to infection.

• Advise patient to perform careful oral care and to see a dentist regularly because drug can cause gum disease.

• Advise women to use barrier contraception, not hormonal contraceptives, during therapy. Advise patient of the potential risk during pregnancy and the increased risk of tumors, high blood pressure, and renal problems.

• Warn patient to wear protection in the sun and to avoid excessive sun exposure.

SAFETY ALERT!

cytarabine (ara-C, cytosine arabinoside)
sye-TARE-a-been

Cytosar†, Cytosar-U, DepoCyt

Therapeutic class: Antineoplastics
Pharmacologic class: Pyrimidine analogues
Pregnancy risk category: D

AVAILABLE FORMS
Injection: 20 mg/mL, 100 mg/mL
Liposomal intrathecal injection: 10 mg/mL
Powder for injection: 100-mg, 500-mg, 1-g, 2-g vials

INDICATIONS & DOSAGES

Adjust-a-dose (for all indications): For conventional form, consider dosage reduction in patients with poor renal function.

➤ **Acute nonlymphocytic leukemia**
Adults and children: 100 mg/m^2 I.V. daily by continuous I.V. infusion or 100 mg/m^2 I.V. every 12 hours by rapid I.V. injection or I.V. infusion on days 1 to 7 in a course of therapy or daily until remission is attained.

➤ **Acute lymphocytic leukemia**
Consult literature for current recommendations.

➤ **Meningeal leukemia**
Adults and children: Varies from 5 to 75 mg/m^2 intrathecally. Frequency varies from once daily for 4 days to once every 4 days. The most frequently used dose is 30 mg/m^2 every 4 days until CSF is normal; then one additional dose.

➤ **Lymphomatous meningitis (liposomal)**
Adults: For induction, give 50 mg liposomal injection intrathecally every 14 days for two doses (weeks 1 and 3); then, for consolidation therapy, give 50 mg liposomal injection intrathecally every 14 days for three doses (weeks 5, 7, and 9) followed by one additional dose at week 13. Maintenance dose, 50 mg liposomal injection intrathecally every 28 days for four doses (weeks 17, 21, 25, and 29).

Adjust-a-dose: For patients with neurotoxicity, reduce dose to 25 mg. If neurotoxicity persists, stop therapy.

ADMINISTRATION

I.V.

▼ Preparing and giving parenteral drug may be mutagenic, teratogenic, or carcinogenic. Follow facility policy to reduce risks.

▼ To reduce nausea, give antiemetic before drug. Nausea and vomiting are more likely with large doses given by I.V. push. Dizziness may occur with rapid infusion.

▼ Except for neonates or intrathecal use, reconstitute drug using the provided diluent, which is bacteriostatic water for injection containing benzyl alcohol.

▼ Reconstitute 100-mg vial with 5 mL of diluent, 500-mg or 1 g vials with 10 mL of diluent or 2 g vial with 20 mL of diluent.

▼ Discard cloudy reconstituted solution.

▼ For I.V. infusion, further dilute using normal saline solution for injection or D$_5$W.

▼ Reconstituted solution is stable for 48 hours.

▼ **Incompatibilities:** Allopurinol sodium, amphotericin B cholesteryl sulfate complex, 5-FU, ganciclovir sodium, heparin sodium, hydrocortisone sodium succinate, insulin, methylprednisolone sodium succinate, nafcillin, oxacillin, penicillin.

Intrathecal

Black Box Warning Give liposomal form with dexamethasone to help decrease the symptoms of chemical arachnoiditis, which may be life-threatening. ∎

● For intrathecal administration, use preservative-free normal saline solution. Use immediately after reconstitution. Discard unused drug.

● Withdraw intrathecal cytarabine liposomal injection from the vial immediately before administration. It is a single-use vial, doesn't contain any preservative, and should be used within 4 hours of withdrawal from the vial. Discard unused portions of each vial properly.

● Don't use in-line filters when giving intrathecal cytarabine liposomal injection.

● After drug administration by lumbar puncture, instruct patient to lie flat for 1 hour.

● Patients should be observed by the physician for immediate toxic reactions.

● Refrigerate liposomal form at 36° to 46° F (2° to 8° C).

ACTION

Inhibits DNA synthesis.

Route	Onset	Peak	Duration
I.V., in-trathecal	Unknown	Unknown	Unknown

Half-life: Initial, 8 minutes; terminal, 1 to 3 hours; in CSF, 2 hours.

ADVERSE REACTIONS

CNS: *neurotoxicity,* malaise, dizziness, headache, cerebellar syndrome, fever.
CV: thrombophlebitis, edema.
EENT: conjunctivitis.
GI: nausea, vomiting, diarrhea, anorexia, anal ulceration, abdominal pain, oral ulcers in 5 to 10 days, projectile vomiting, *bowel necrosis with high doses given by rapid I.V.*

GU: urine retention, renal dysfunction.
Hematologic: *leukopenia,* anemia, reticulocytopenia, *thrombocytopenia,* megaloblastosis.
Hepatic: *hepatotoxicity,* jaundice.
Metabolic: hyperuricemia.
Musculoskeletal: myalgia, bone pain.
Respiratory: *pulmonary edema,* shortness of breath, pulmonary hypersensitivity.
Skin: rash, pruritus, alopecia, freckling.
Other: flulike syndrome, infection, *anaphylaxis.*

INTERACTIONS
Drug-drug. *Digoxin, except oral liquid:* May decrease oral digoxin absorption. Monitor digoxin level closely.
Flucytosine: May decrease flucytosine activity. Avoid using together.
Gentamicin: May decrease activity against *Klebsiella pneumoniae.* Avoid using together.

EFFECTS ON LAB TEST RESULTS
• May increase bilirubin, phosphorus, potassium, and uric acid levels. May decrease hemoglobin level.
• May increase megaloblast count. May decrease platelet, RBC, reticulocyte, and WBC counts.

CONTRAINDICATIONS & CAUTIONS
• Contraindicated in patients hypersensitive to drug and active meningeal infection (liposomal cytarabine).
• Use cautiously in patients with hepatic or renal impairment, gout, or myelosuppression.
⚠ **Overdose S&S:** Irreversible CNS toxicity, death (conventional form); severe chemical arachnoiditis (liposomal form).

NURSING CONSIDERATIONS
Black Box Warning Cytarabine should be administered by physicians experienced in cancer chemotherapy. For induction therapy, patients should be treated in a facility with laboratory and supportive resources sufficient to monitor drug tolerance and protect and maintain a patient compromised by drug toxicity. The physician must judge possible benefit to the patient against known toxic effects of cytarabine. ∎

• Drug is an irritant. If extravasation occurs, stop the infusion immediately and follow facility policy for monitoring and treatment.
• Monitor fluid intake and output carefully. Maintain high fluid intake and give allopurinol to avoid urate nephropathy in leukemia-induction therapy. Monitor uric acid level.
• Monitor hepatic and renal function studies and CBC.
• Therapy may be modified or stopped if granulocyte count is below 1,000/mm^3 or platelet count is below 50,000/mm^3.
• Corticosteroid eye drops help prevent drug-induced conjunctivitis.
• Provide diligent mouth care to help minimize stomatitis.
🛈 **Alert:** Assess patient receiving high doses for neurotoxicity, which may first appear as nystagmus but can progress to ataxia and cerebellar dysfunction.
• To prevent bleeding, avoid all I.M. injections when platelet count is below 50,000/mm^3.
• Anticipate blood transfusions because of cumulative anemia. Patient may receive RBC colony-stimulating factors to promote RBC production and decrease need for blood transfusions.
Black Box Warning Monitor patient for toxic effects, including bone marrow suppression, nausea, vomiting, diarrhea, oral ulceration, and hepatic dysfunction. ∎
• In leukopenia, initial WBC count nadir occurs 7 to 9 days after drug is stopped. A second, more severe nadir occurs 15 to 24 days after drug is stopped. In thrombocytopenia, platelet count nadir occurs on days 12 to 15.
🛈 **Alert:** A cytarabine syndrome has been described and is characterized by fever, myalgia, bone pain, occasionally chest pain, maculopapular rash, conjunctivitis, and malaise. It usually occurs 6 to 12 hours after drug administration. Corticosteroids have been shown to be beneficial in the treatment or prevention of this syndrome.
• **Look alike–sound alike:** Don't confuse conventional cytarabine with liposomal cytarabine.

Reactions in bold italics are *life-threatening*. Interactions may have a *rapid onset* or a *delayed onset*.

PATIENT TEACHING
• Instruct patient to watch for signs and symptoms of infection (fever, sore throat, fatigue) and bleeding (easy bruising, nosebleeds, bleeding gums, tarry stools). Tell patient to take temperature daily.
• Advise patient to report visual changes, blurred vision, or eye pain to prescriber.
• Advise breast-feeding women to stop breast-feeding during therapy because of risk of toxicity to infant.
• Caution women of childbearing age to consult prescriber before becoming pregnant because drug may harm fetus.

SAFETY ALERT!

dabigatran etexilate mesylate
da-bye-GAT-ran

Pradaxa◆

Therapeutic class: Anticoagulants
Pharmacologic class: Direct thrombin inhibitors
Pregnancy risk category: C

AVAILABLE FORMS
Capsules: 75 mg, 150 mg

INDICATIONS & DOSAGES
➤ **To reduce the risk of stroke and systemic embolism in patients with nonvalvular atrial fibrillation**
Adults: 150 mg P.O. b.i.d. When converting from warfarin to dabigatran, stop warfarin and start dabigatran when INR is below 2. When converting from dabigatran to warfarin and CrCl is more than 50 mL/minute, start warfarin 3 days before stopping dabigatran; if CrCl is 31 to 50 mL/minute, start warfarin 2 days before stopping dabigatran; if CrCl is 15 to 30 mL/minute, start warfarin 1 day before stopping dabigatran. When converting from parenteral anticoagulants to dabigatran, start dabigatran 0 to 2 hours before the next scheduled dose of the parenteral anticoagulant, or at the time of discontinuing a continuously administered parenteral drug (such as unfractionated heparin). When converting from dabigatran to parenteral anticoagulation and CrCl is 30 mL/minute or more, wait 12 hours or,

if CrCl is less than 30 mL/minute, wait 24 hours after the last dose of dabigatran before beginning parenteral treatment.
Adjust-a-dose: For patients with CrCl of 15 to 30 mL/minute, give 75 mg P.O. b.i.d. Don't use in patients with CrCl of less than 15 mL/minute.

ADMINISTRATION
P.O.
• Give without regard to food.
• Don't crush capsule, empty its contents, or allow patient to chew capsule. Capsule must be swallowed whole.
• Temporarily discontinue drug before invasive or surgical procedures. Restart drug promptly after procedure.
Black Box Warning Discontinuing drug increases risk of thrombotic events. If drug must be discontinued for a reason other than pathologic bleeding, consider coverage with another anticoagulant. ■

ACTION
Inhibits thrombin formation, preventing the development of a thrombus.

Route	Onset	Peak	Duration
P.O.	Unknown	1–2 hr	Unknown

Half-life: 12 to 17 hours.

ADVERSE REACTIONS
GI: dyspepsia, abdominal pain, abdominal discomfort, gastritis-like symptoms, GERD, esophagitis, erosive gastritis, *gastric hemorrhage, hemorrhagic erosive gastritis,* GI ulcer, diarrhea, nausea, *GI bleeding.*
Hematologic: *life-threatening bleeding,* major bleeding, any bleeding.

INTERACTIONS
Drug-drug. *Antiplatelets, aspirin, fibrinolytic therapy, heparin, long-term use of dronedarone, ketoconazole:* May increase effectiveness of dabigatran. Consider reducing dabigatran dosage to 75 mg b.i.d. when giving concomitantly to patients with moderate renal impairment (CrCl of 30 to 50 mL/minute).
NSAIDs: May increase risk of bleeding. Avoid use together.
Rifampin: May reduce dabigatran level. Avoid use together.

Drug-herb. *St. John's wort:* May decrease dabigatran pharmacologic effects and plasma concentration. Avoid concurrent use.

EFFECTS ON LAB TEST RESULTS
• May increase activated partial thromboplastin time (aPTT), ecarin clotting time (ECT), and thrombin time.

CONTRAINDICATIONS & CAUTIONS
• Contraindicated in patients hypersensitive to drug and in those with active pathologic bleeding.
• Contraindicated in patients with mechanical prosthetic valves. Use in patients with atrial fibrillation in the setting of other forms of valvular heart disease, including the presence of a bioprosthetic heart valve, isn't recommended.
• Use cautiously in patients with history of bleeding and in pregnant women. Give drug only if benefit to mother outweighs risk to fetus. It isn't known if drug appears in breast milk.
• Because of risk of clot formation and stroke, avoid lapses in therapy when possible. Restart therapy as soon as possible.
Black Box Warning Discontinuing drug increases risk of thrombotic events. If drug must be discontinued for a reason other than pathologic bleeding, consider coverage with another anticoagulant. ∎
⚠ *Overdose S&S:* Hemorrhagic complications.

NURSING CONSIDERATIONS
• Monitor patient for signs of bleeding. If bleeding occurs, stop drug, investigate cause, and provide supportive measures. There is no antidote for dabigatran.
• Monitor ECT or aPPT to assess treatment effectiveness.
• Discontinue dabigatran 1 to 2 days before invasive or surgical procedures in patients with CrCl of 50 mL/minute or more and 3 to 5 days in patients with CrCl of less than 50 mL/minute. Consider longer times for patients undergoing major surgery, spinal puncture, or placement of a spinal or epidural catheter or port, in whom complete hemostasis may be required.

PATIENT TEACHING
• Tell patient that drug may be taken without regard to food.
• Advise patient to take dabigatran at approximately the same times each day. A missed dose may be skipped only if it can't be taken at least 6 hours before the next scheduled dose.
• Teach patient to swallow the capsule whole and not to open, crush, or chew it.
• Caution patient to take drug as prescribed and not to stop or change dosage without first consulting health care provider.
• Advise patient to tell all of his health care providers that he's taking this drug.
• Counsel patient to tell his health care provider if he's taking other medications, including OTC medications, vitamins, and herbal preparations.
• Warn patient he may bruise more easily and bleed longer while taking this drug.
• Instruct patient to report bleeding when brushing teeth or shaving; blood in vomit, urine, or stool; heavier menstrual bleeding; or nosebleeds.
• Tell patient he will need to have regular blood tests to monitor drug's effects.
• Instruct patient to inform his health care provider of scheduled invasive procedures, including dental work. Drug may need to be stopped temporarily.
• Advise patient to keep drug in the original bottle to protect from moisture, to remove only one capsule from the opened bottle at the time of use, to tightly close bottle immediately after removing drug, and not to put drug in pill boxes or pill organizers.

SAFETY ALERT!

dacarbazine (DTIC)
da-KAR-ba-zeen

DTIC-Dome

Therapeutic class: Antineoplastics
Pharmacologic class: Triazenes
Pregnancy risk category: C

AVAILABLE FORMS
Injection: 100 mg, 200 mg

INDICATIONS & DOSAGES
➤ **Metastatic malignant melanoma**
Adults: 2 to 4.5 mg/kg I.V. daily for 10 days; repeat every 4 weeks as tolerated. Or, 250 mg/m² I.V. daily for 5 days; repeat every 3 weeks.
➤ **Hodgkin lymphoma**
Adults: 150 mg/m² I.V. daily (with other drugs) for 5 days; repeat every 4 weeks. Or, 375 mg/m² on first day of combination regimen; repeat every 15 days.

ADMINISTRATION
I.V.
▼ Preparing and giving parenteral drug may be mutagenic, teratogenic, or carcinogenic. Follow facility policy to reduce risks.
▼ Reconstitute drug using sterile water for injection. Add 9.9 mL to 100-mg vial or 19.7 mL to 200-mg vial to yield a concentration of 10 mg/mL.
▼ For infusion, dilute with up to 250 mL of normal saline solution or D₅W.
▼ Infuse over at least 15 to 30 minutes.
▼ To decrease pain at insertion site, dilute drug further or decrease infusion rate.
▼ Watch for irritation and infiltration during infusion; extravasation can cause severe pain, tissue damage, and necrosis. If solution infiltrates, stop immediately, apply ice to area for 24 to 48 hours, and notify prescriber.
▼ Reconstituted solutions in the vial are stable 8 hours at room temperature and with normal lighting conditions, or up to 3 days if refrigerated.
▼ Solution should be colorless to clear yellow. If solution turns pink, it has decomposed. Discard it.
▼ Diluted solutions are stable 8 hours at room temperature and with normal lighting, or up to 24 hours if refrigerated.
▼ **Incompatibilities:** Allopurinol sodium, cefepime, hydrocortisone sodium succinate, piperacillin–tazobactam.

ACTION
May cross-link strands of cellular DNA and interfere with RNA and protein synthesis. Not specific to cell cycle.

Route	Onset	Peak	Duration
I.V.	Unknown	Unknown	Unknown

Half-life: Initial phase, 19 minutes; terminal phase, 5 hours.

ADVERSE REACTIONS
GI: anorexia, severe nausea and vomiting, stomatitis.
Hematologic: *leukopenia, thrombocytopenia.*
Skin: alopecia.
Other: *anaphylaxis,* severe pain with infiltration or a too-concentrated solution, tissue damage.

INTERACTIONS
Drug-lifestyle. *Sun exposure:* May cause photosensitivity reaction, especially during first 2 days of therapy. Advise patient to avoid excessive sunlight exposure.

EFFECTS ON LAB TEST RESULTS
• May increase BUN and liver enzyme levels.
• May decrease platelet, RBC, and WBC counts.

CONTRAINDICATIONS & CAUTIONS
• Contraindicated in patients hypersensitive to drug.
Black Box Warning Use cautiously because drug may be carcinogenic and teratogenic. ■
• Use cautiously in patients with impaired bone marrow function and those with severe renal or hepatic dysfunction.

NURSING CONSIDERATIONS
Black Box Warning Dacarbazine should be administered under the supervision of a physician experienced in the use of cancer chemotherapeutic agents. ■
Black Box Warning The physician must carefully weigh the possibility of therapeutic benefit against the risk of toxicity for each patient. ■
• Give antiemetics before giving this drug. Nausea and vomiting may subside after several doses.
• To prevent bleeding, avoid all I.M. injections when platelet count is below 50,000/mm³.

Black Box Warning Hematopoietic depression is the most common toxicity. ∎
• Anticipate need for blood transfusions to combat anemia.
• Therapeutic effects commonly occur with toxicity. Monitor CBC and platelet count.
Black Box Warning Hepatic necrosis may occur. Monitor LFTs. ∎
• For Hodgkin lymphoma, drug is usually given with bleomycin, vinblastine, and doxorubicin.
• *Look alike–sound alike:* Don't confuse dacarbazine with procarbazine.

PATIENT TEACHING
• Tell patient to watch for evidence of infection (fever, sore throat, fatigue) and bleeding (easy bruising, nosebleeds, bleeding gums, tarry stools). Tell him to take temperature daily.
• Tell patient to avoid people with upper respiratory tract infections.
• Instruct patient to avoid OTC products that contain aspirin or NSAIDs.
• Advise patient to avoid sunlight and sunlamps for first 2 days after treatment.
• Reassure patient that fever, malaise, and muscle pain, beginning 7 days after treatment ends and possibly lasting 7 to 21 days, may be treated with mild fever reducers such as acetaminophen.
• Tell patient that restricting food intake for 4 to 6 hours before dose may help to decrease adverse GI effects.
• Reassure patient that hair loss is reversible.
• Advise women to avoid pregnancy and breast-feeding during therapy.

dalfampridine
dal-FAM-prih-deen

Ampyra

Therapeutic class: MS drugs
Pharmacologic class: Potassium channel blockers
Pregnancy risk category: C

AVAILABLE FORMS
Tablets (extended-release): 10 mg

INDICATIONS & DOSAGES
➤ **To improve walking in patients with MS**
Adults: 10 mg P.O. every 12 hours.

ADMINISTRATION
P.O.
• May give with or without food approximately 12 hours apart.
• Give tablets whole; don't divide, crush, dissolve, or allow patient to chew tablets.

ACTION
Thought to increase conduction of action potentials in demyelinated axons by inhibiting potassium channels.

Route	Onset	Peak	Duration
P.O.	Rapid	3–4 hr	Unknown

Half-life: About 6 hours.

ADVERSE REACTIONS
CNS: asthenia, balance disorder, dizziness, headache, insomnia, MS relapse, paresthesia, *seizures.*
EENT: nasopharyngitis, pharyngolaryngeal pain.
GI: constipation, dyspepsia, nausea.
GU: UTI.
Musculoskeletal: back pain.

INTERACTIONS
None known.

EFFECTS ON LAB TEST RESULTS
None known.

CONTRAINDICATIONS & CAUTIONS
❸ *Alert:* Contraindicated in patients with history of hypersensitivity to Ampyra or 4-aminopyridine. Drug can cause anaphylaxis and severe allergic reactions.
• Contraindicated in patients with moderate or severe renal impairment and in those with history of seizures.
❸ *Alert:* Use cautiously in those with mild renal impairment (CrCl of 51 to 80 mL/minute) and in patients over age 50, who may have age-related decreased renal function.
• Use during pregnancy only if benefit outweighs risk to fetus.

Reactions in bold italics are *life-threatening*. Interactions may have a *rapid onset* or a *delayed onset*.

• It isn't known if drug appears in breast milk. Because of risk of adverse effects, patient should stop breast-feeding or stop drug.

⚠ **Overdose S&S:** Seizures, confusion, tremors, diaphoresis, amnesia.

NURSING CONSIDERATIONS
• Monitor patient for seizures.

🜂 **Alert:** The risk of seizures increases with higher doses. Maximum dosage is 10 mg b.i.d.

• Monitor renal function before and during therapy.

• Monitor patient's walking for improvement.

PATIENT TEACHING
• Tell patient to take drug without regard to food.

• Instruct patient to take tablets whole and not to divide, crush, dissolve, or chew them.

• Advise patient to stop drug and seek medical attention if seizures occur.

• Instruct patient not to take more than two tablets in 24 hours.

SAFETY ALERT!

dalteparin sodium
DAHL-tep-ah-rin

Fragmin

Therapeutic class: Anticoagulants
Pharmacologic class: Low–molecular-weight heparins
Pregnancy risk category: B

AVAILABLE FORMS
Injection: 2,500 antifactor Xa international units/0.2 mL syringe, 5,000 antifactor Xa international units/0.2 mL syringe, 7,500 antifactor Xa international units/0.3 mL syringe, 10,000 antifactor Xa international units/0.4 mL syringe, 10,000 antifactor Xa international units/1 mL syringe, 12,500 antifactor Xa international units/0.5 mL syringe, 15,000 antifactor Xa international units/0.6 mL syringe, 18,000 antifactor Xa international units/0.72 mL syringe, 95,000 antifactor Xa international units/3.8 mL vial, 95,000 antifactor Xa international units/9.5 mL vial

INDICATIONS & DOSAGES
Adjust-a-dose (for all indications): For patients with CrCl of 30 mL/minute or less, monitor anti-Xa levels to determine appropriate dose. Target anti-Xa range is 0.5 to 1.5 international units/mL. Draw anti-Xa 4 to 6 hours after dose and only after the patient has received three to four doses.

➤ **To prevent DVT in patients undergoing abdominal surgery who are at moderate to high risk for thromboembolic complications**
Adults: 2,500 international units subcutaneously daily, starting 1 to 2 hours before surgery and repeated once daily for 5 to 10 days postoperatively. Or, for patients at high risk, give 5,000 international units subcutaneously the evening before surgery, then once daily postoperatively for 5 to 10 days. Or, in patients with malignancy, give 2,500 international units subcutaneously 1 to 2 hours before surgery followed by 2,500 international units subcutaneously 12 hours later, then 5,000 international units subcutaneously once daily for 5 to 10 days postoperatively.

➤ **To prevent DVT in patients undergoing hip replacement surgery**
Adults: 2,500 international units subcutaneously within 2 hours before surgery and second dose of 2,500 international units subcutaneously in the evening after surgery (at least 6 hours after first dose). Starting on first postoperative day, give 5,000 international units subcutaneously once daily for 5 to 10 days. Or, give 5,000 international units subcutaneously on the evening before surgery; then 5,000 international units subcutaneously once daily starting on the evening of surgery for 5 to 10 days postoperatively.

➤ **Unstable angina; non-Q-wave MI**
Adults: 120 international units/kg subcutaneously every 12 hours with aspirin (75 to 165 mg daily) P.O., unless contraindicated. Maximum dose, 10,000 international units. Treatment usually lasts 5 to 8 days.

➤ **To prevent DVT in patients at risk for thromboembolic complications because**

---

of severely restricted mobility during acute illness
Adults: 5,000 international units subcutaneously once daily for 12 to 14 days.
➤ **Symptomatic venous thromboembolism in cancer patients**
Adults: Initially, 200 international units/kg (maximum, 18,000 international units) subcutaneously daily for 30 days; then 150 international units/kg (maximum, 18,000 international units) subcutaneously daily months 2 through 6.
Adjust-a-dose: In patients with platelet count 50,000 to 100,000/mm³, reduce dose by 2,500 international units until platelet count exceeds 100,000/mm³. In patients with platelet count less than 50,000/mm³, stop drug until platelet count exceeds 50,000/mm³.

ADMINISTRATION
Subcutaneous
● Before giving injection, obtain complete list of all prescribed and OTC medications and supplements, including herbs.
● Have patient sit or lie supine when giving drug.
● Injection sites include a U-shaped area around the navel, upper outer side of thigh, and upper outer quadrangle of buttock. Rotate sites daily.
● When area around the navel or thigh is used, use thumb and forefinger to lift up a fold of skin while giving injection.
● Give subcutaneous injection deeply, inserting the entire length of needle at a 45- to 90-degree angle.

ACTION
Enhances inhibition of factor Xa and thrombin by antithrombin.

Route	Onset	Peak	Duration
Subcut.	Unknown	4 hr	Unknown

Half-life: 3 to 5 hours.

ADVERSE REACTIONS
CNS: fever.
GU: hematuria.
Hematologic: *thrombocytopenia, hemorrhage,* ecchymoses, bleeding complications.
Skin: pruritus, rash, hematoma at injection site, injection-site pain.
Other: *anaphylaxis.*

INTERACTIONS
Drug-drug. *Antiplatelet drugs (aspirin, NSAIDs, clopidogrel, dipyridamole, ticlodipine), oral anticoagulants, SSRIs (fluoxetine), thrombolytics:* May increase risk of bleeding. Use together cautiously.
Drug-herb. *Angelica (dong quai), boldo, bromelains, capsicum, chamomile, dandelion, danshen, devil's claw, fenugreek, feverfew, garlic, ginger, ginkgo, ginseng, horse chestnut, licorice, meadowsweet, onion, passion flower, red clover, willow:* May increase risk of bleeding. Discourage use together.

EFFECTS ON LAB TEST RESULTS
● May increase ALT and AST levels.
● May decrease platelet count.

CONTRAINDICATIONS & CAUTIONS
● Contraindicated in patients hypersensitive to drug, heparin, or pork products; in those with active major bleeding; and in those with thrombocytopenia and antiplatelet antibodies in presence of drug.
● Contraindicated in patients with unstable angina or non-Q-wave MI who are undergoing regional anesthesia because of an increased risk of bleeding associated with the dose of dalteparin recommended for these indications.
● Use with caution in patients with history of heparin-induced thrombocytopenia and in patients at increased risk for hemorrhage, such as those with severe uncontrolled hypertension, bacterial endocarditis, congenital or acquired bleeding disorders, active ulceration, angiodysplastic GI disease, or hemorrhagic stroke; also use with caution shortly after brain, spinal, or ophthalmic surgery. Monitor vital signs.
● Use with caution in patients with bleeding diathesis, thrombocytopenia, platelet defects, severe hepatic or renal insufficiency, hypertensive or diabetic retinopathy, or recent GI bleeding.
⚠ *Overdose S&S:* Hemorrhagic complications.

NURSING CONSIDERATIONS

Black Box Warning Patients who have received epidural or spinal anesthesia or spinal puncture are at increased risk for developing an epidural or spinal hematoma, which may result in long-term or permanent paralysis. Monitor these patients closely for neurologic impairment and treat urgently. ∎

• DVT is a risk factor in patients who are candidates for therapy, including those older than age 40, those who are obese, those undergoing surgery under general anesthesia lasting longer than 30 minutes, and those who have additional risk factors (such as malignancy or history of DVT or pulmonary embolism).

• Never give drug I.M.

• Don't mix with other injections or infusions unless specific compatibility data support such mixing.

• Multidose vial shouldn't be used in pregnant women because of benzyl alcohol content. Benzyl alcohol has been associated with fatal "gasping syndrome" in premature neonates.

۞ Alert: Drug isn't interchangeable (unit for unit) with unfractionated heparin or other low–molecular-weight heparin.

• Periodic, routine CBC and fecal occult blood tests are recommended during therapy. Patients don't need regular monitoring of PT or activated PTT.

• Monitor patient closely for thrombocytopenia.

• Stop drug if a thromboembolic event occurs despite dalteparin prophylaxis.

• Obtain a complete list of patient's prescription and OTC drugs and supplements, including herbs.

PATIENT TEACHING

• Instruct patient and family to watch for and report signs of bleeding (bruising and blood in stools).

• Tell patient to avoid OTC drugs containing aspirin or other salicylates unless ordered by prescriber.

• Advise patient to consult with prescriber before initiating any herbal therapy; many herbs have anticoagulant, antiplatelet, and fibrinolytic properties.

• Tell patient to use a soft toothbrush and electric razor during treatment.

dantrolene sodium
DAN-troe-leen

Dantrium, Dantrium Intravenous

Therapeutic class: Skeletal muscle relaxants
Pharmacologic class: Hydantoin derivatives
Pregnancy risk category: C

AVAILABLE FORMS
Capsules: 25 mg, 50 mg, 100 mg
Injection: 20 mg/vial

INDICATIONS & DOSAGES

➤ **Spasticity and sequelae from severe chronic disorders, such as MS, cerebral palsy, spinal cord injury, and stroke**
Adults: 25 mg P.O. daily. Increase by 25-mg increments, up to 100 mg t.i.d. to q.i.d. Maintain each dosage level for 7 days to determine response. Maximum, 400 mg daily.
Children age 5 and older: Initially, 0.5 mg/ kg P.O. daily for 7 days; then 0.5 mg/kg t.i.d. for 7 days, 1 mg/kg t.i.d. for 7 days, and finally, 2 mg/kg t.i.d. for 7 days. May increase up to 3 mg/kg b.i.d. to q.i.d. if necessary. Maximum, 100 mg q.i.d.

➤ **To manage malignant hyperthermic crisis**
Adults and children: Initially, 1 mg/kg I.V. push. Repeat, as needed, up to cumulative dose of 10 mg/kg.

➤ **To prevent or attenuate malignant hyperthermic crisis in susceptible patients who need surgery**
Adults and children: 4 to 8 mg/kg P.O. daily in three or four divided doses for 1 or 2 days before procedure. Give final dose 3 or 4 hours before procedure. Or, 2.5 mg/kg I.V. about 1.25 hours before anesthesia; infuse over 1 hour.

➤ **To prevent recurrence of malignant hyperthermic crisis**
Adults: 4 to 8 mg/kg P.O. daily in four divided doses for up to 3 days after hyperthermic crisis.

ADMINISTRATION
P.O.
• Give drug with food or milk.
• Prepare oral suspension for single dose by dissolving capsule contents in juice or other liquid. For multiple doses, use acid vehicle and refrigerate. Use within several days.
I.V.
▼ Reconstitute drug by adding 60 mL of sterile water for injection and shaking vial until clear. Don't use a diluent that contains a bacteriostatic drug.
▼ Protect solution from light, and use within 6 hours.
▼ **Incompatibilities:** D₅W, normal saline solution, other I.V. drugs mixed in a syringe.

ACTION
Acts directly on skeletal muscle to decrease excitation and contraction coupling and reduce muscle strength by interfering with intracellular calcium movement.

Route	Onset	Peak	Duration
P.O.	Unknown	5 hr	Unknown
I.V.	Unknown	Unknown	3 hr after infusion

Half-life: P.O., 9 hours; I.V., 4 to 8 hours.

ADVERSE REACTIONS
CNS: drowsiness, dizziness, malaise, fatigue, *seizures,* headache, light-headedness, confusion, nervousness, insomnia, fever, depression.
CV: tachycardia, blood pressure changes, phlebitis, thrombophlebitis, heart failure.
EENT: excessive lacrimation, speech disturbance, diplopia, visual disturbances.
GI: anorexia, constipation, cramping, dysphagia, metallic taste, severe diarrhea, *GI bleeding,* vomiting.
GU: urinary frequency, hematuria, incontinence, nocturia, dysuria, crystalluria, difficult erection, urine retention.
Hematologic: *leukopenia, thrombocytopenia, lymphocytic lymphoma,* anemia.
Hepatic: *hepatitis.*
Musculoskeletal: muscle weakness, myalgia, back pain.
Respiratory: pleural effusion with pericarditis, *pulmonary edema.*

Skin: eczematous eruption, pruritus, urticaria, abnormal hair growth, diaphoresis, photosensitivity.
Other: chills.

INTERACTIONS
Drug-drug. *Clofibrate, warfarin:* May decrease protein binding of dantrolene. Use together cautiously.
CNS depressants: May increase CNS depression. Avoid using together.
Estrogens: May increase risk of hepatotoxicity. Use together cautiously.
I.V. verapamil and other calcium channel blockers: May cause hyperkalemia, ventricular fibrillation, and myocardial depression. Stop verapamil before giving I.V. dantrolene.
Vecuronium: May increase neuromuscular blockade effect. Use together cautiously.
Drug-lifestyle. *Alcohol use:* May increase CNS depression. Discourage use together.
Sun exposure: May cause photosensitivity reactions. Advise patient to avoid excessive sunlight exposure.

EFFECTS ON LAB TEST RESULTS
• May increase ALT, AST, alkaline phosphatase, LDH, bilirubin, and BUN levels.

CONTRAINDICATIONS & CAUTIONS
• Contraindicated for spasms in rheumatic disorders and when spasticity is used to maintain motor function.
• Contraindicated in breast-feeding patients and patients with upper motor neuron disorders or active hepatic disease.
Black Box Warning Risk of hepatic injury is increased in women, patients older than age 35, and patients with hepatic disease (such as cirrhosis or hepatitis) or severely impaired cardiac or pulmonary function. ▋
⚠ *Overdose S&S:* Muscle weakness, altered level of consciousness, vomiting, diarrhea, crystalluria.

NURSING CONSIDERATIONS
• Start therapy as soon as malignant hyperthermia reaction is recognized.
Black Box Warning Liver damage may occur with short- or long-term use. Use the lowest possible effective dose for each

---

Reactions in bold italics are *life-threatening*. Interactions may have a *rapid onset* or a *delayed onset*.

patient. If benefits don't occur within 45 days, stop therapy. ■
Black Box Warning Obtain LFT results at start of therapy. Monitor hepatic function, including AST and ALT, frequently. ■
۞ Alert: Watch for fever, jaundice, severe diarrhea, weakness, and sensitivity reactions, including skin eruptions. Withhold dose and notify prescriber.
• **Look alike–sound alike:** Don't confuse Dantrium with Daraprim.

PATIENT TEACHING
• Instruct patient to take drug with meals or milk.
• Tell patient to eat carefully to avoid choking. Some patients may have trouble swallowing during therapy.
• Warn patient to avoid driving and other hazardous activities until CNS effects of drug are known.
• Advise patient to avoid combining drug with alcohol or other CNS depressants.
• Advise patient to notify prescriber if skin or eyes turn yellow, skin itches, or fever develops.
• Tell patient to avoid photosensitivity reactions by using sunblock and wearing protective clothing, to report abdominal discomfort or GI problems immediately, and to follow prescriber's orders regarding rest and physical therapy.

daptomycin
dap-toe-MYE-sin

Cubicin

Therapeutic class: Antibiotics
Pharmacologic class: Cyclic lipopeptides
Pregnancy risk category: B

AVAILABLE FORMS
Powder for injection: 500-mg vial

INDICATIONS & DOSAGES
➤ **Bacteremia caused by** *Staphylococcus aureus* **(including right-sided endocarditis caused by methicillin-susceptible and methicillin-resistant strains)**
Adults: 6 mg/kg I.V. infusion over 30 minutes or I.V. injection over 2 minutes every 24 hours for at least 2 to 6 weeks based on patient response.
Adjust-a-dose: For bacteremic patients with CrCl of less than 30 mL/minute, give 6 mg/kg I.V. every 48 hours. When possible, give drug after hemodialysis.
➤ **Complicated skin or skin-structure infection (SSSI) caused by susceptible strains of** *S. aureus* **(including methicillin-resistant strains),** *Streptococcus pyogenes,* *Streptococcus agalactiae, Streptococcus dysgalactiae,* **and** *Enterococcus faecalis* **(vancomycin-susceptible strains only)**
Adults: 4 mg/kg I.V. infusion over 30 minutes or I.V. injection over 2 minutes every 24 hours for 7 to 14 days.
Adjust-a-dose: In patients with SSSI and CrCl of less than 30 mL/minute, including those receiving hemodialysis or continuous ambulatory peritoneal dialysis, give 4 mg/kg I.V. every 48 hours.
➤ **Device-related osteoarticular infections (MRSA)** ◆
Adults and children: 6 mg/kg I.V. once daily.

ADMINISTRATION
I.V.
▼ Obtain specimen for culture and sensitivity tests before giving first dose. Begin therapy while awaiting results.
▼ Reconstitute 500-mg vial with 10 mL of normal saline solution.
▼ Further dilute with normal saline solution for I.V. infusion and infuse over 30 minutes.
▼ For I.V. injection over 2 minutes, give at a concentration of 50 mg/mL.
▼ Refrigerate vials at 36° to 46° F (2° to 8° C).
▼ Vials are for single use; discard excess.
▼ Reconstituted and diluted solutions are stable 12 hours at room temperature or 48 hours at 36° to 46° F (2° to 8° C).
▼ **Incompatibilities:** Dextrose-containing solutions and other I.V. drugs. If an I.V. line is used for several drugs, flush the line with normal saline solution or lactated Ringer injection between drugs.

ACTION
Binds to and depolarizes bacterial membranes to inhibit protein, DNA, and RNA synthesis, thus causing bacterial cell death.

Route	Onset	Peak	Duration
I.V.	Rapid	<1 hr	Unknown

Half-life: About 8 hours.

ADVERSE REACTIONS

CNS: anxiety, confusion, dizziness, fever, headache, insomnia.
CV: *cardiac failure,* chest pain, edema, hypertension, hypotension.
EENT: sore throat.
GI: *pseudomembranous colitis,* abdominal pain, constipation, decreased appetite, diarrhea, nausea, vomiting.
GU: *renal failure,* UTI.
Hematologic: anemia.
Metabolic: *hypoglycemia,* hyperglycemia, hypokalemia.
Musculoskeletal: limb and back pain, myopathy.
Respiratory: cough, dyspnea.
Skin: cellulitis, injection-site reactions, pruritus, rash.
Other: fungal infections.

INTERACTIONS

Drug-drug. *HMG-CoA reductase inhibitors:* May increase risk of myopathy. Consider stopping these drugs while giving daptomycin.
Tobramycin: May affect levels of both drugs. Use together cautiously.
Warfarin: May alter anticoagulant activity. Monitor PT and INR for the first several days of daptomycin therapy.

EFFECTS ON LAB TEST RESULTS

● May increase alkaline phosphatase and CK levels. May decrease potassium and hemoglobin levels and hematocrit. May increase or decrease glucose level.
● May increase LFT values.
● May cause false elevation of INR and false prolongation of PT.

CONTRAINDICATIONS & CAUTIONS

● Contraindicated in patients hypersensitive to drug.
● Use cautiously in patients with renal insufficiency and those who are older than age 65, pregnant, or breast-feeding.
● Safety and effectiveness haven't been established in patients younger than age 18.

NURSING CONSIDERATIONS

● Monitor CBC and renal and liver function tests periodically.
⚠ *Alert:* Because drug may increase the risk of myopathy, monitor CK level weekly. If CK level rises, monitor it more often. In patients with myopathy and CK elevation over 1,000 units/L or more than 10 times the upper limit of normal, stop drug. Consider stopping all other drugs linked with myopathy (such as HMG-CoA reductase inhibitors) during therapy.
● Monitor patient for superinfection because drug may cause overgrowth of non-susceptible organisms.
⚠ *Alert:* Drug may cause eosinophilic pneumonia, a rare type of pneumonia in which eosinophil-type WBCs fill the lungs, causing fever, cough, shortness of breath, and difficulty breathing. Monitor patient closely.
● Watch for evidence of *Clostridium difficile*–associated diarrhea and treat accordingly.
● Monitor patient for muscle pain or weakness, particularly of the distal extremities.
● *Look alike–sound alike:* Don't confuse daptomycin with dactinomycin.

PATIENT TEACHING

● Advise patient to immediately report muscle weakness and infusion-site irritation.
● Tell patient to report severe diarrhea, rash, and infection.
● Inform patient about possible adverse reactions.

SAFETY ALERT!

darbepoetin alfa
dar-bah-poe-E-tin

Aranesp

Therapeutic class: Colony stimulating factors
Pharmacologic class: Recombinant human erythropoietins
Pregnancy risk category: C

AVAILABLE FORMS

Injection (with albumin or polysorbate solution): 25 mcg/mL, 40 mcg/mL, 60 mcg/mL, 100 mcg/mL, 150 mcg/

0.75 mL, 200 mcg/mL, 300 mcg/mL
in single-dose vials
Prefilled syringe or autoinjector (with al-bumin or polysorbate solution): 25 mcg/
0.42 mL, 40 mcg/0.4 mL, 60 mcg/0.3 mL,
100 mcg/0.5 mL, 150 mcg/0.3 mL,
200 mcg/0.4 mL, 300 mcg/0.6 mL,
500 mcg/mL

INDICATIONS & DOSAGES
➤ **Anemia from chronic renal failure**
Adults: 0.45 mcg/kg I.V. or subcutaneously
once weekly. The I.V. route is preferred for
patients on dialysis. Or give an initial dose
of 0.75 mcg/kg I.V. or subcutaneously once
every 2 weeks. For patients not on dialysis,
give 0.45 mcg/kg I.V. or subcutaneously at
4-week intervals. Give the lowest effective
dose to gradually increase hemoglobin
to a level at which blood transfusion isn't
necessary. Don't increase dose more often
than once a month. In adults and children
older than age 1 who are on dialysis and
converting from epoetin alfa, base starting
dose on the previous epoetin alfa dose (see
table on next page). Don't use as initial
treatment of anemia in children with chronic
renal failure.

Previous epoetin alfa dose (units/wk)	Darbepoetin alfa dose (mcg/wk): Adults	Darbepoetin alfa dose (mcg/wk): Children
<1,500	6.25	Unknown
1,500–2,499	6.25	6.25
2,500–4,999	12.5	10
5,000–10,999	25	20
11,000–17,999	40	40
18,000–33,999	60	60
34,000–89,999	100	100
≥90,000	200	200

Give darbepoetin alfa less often than epoetin alfa. If patient was receiving epoetin
alfa two to three times weekly, give darbepoetin alfa once weekly. If patient was
receiving epoetin alfa once weekly, give
darbepoetin alfa once every 2 weeks.
Adjust-a-dose: For patients with chronic
renal disease who aren't on dialysis, if the
hemoglobin level exceeds 10 g/dL, reduce
dosage or interrupt therapy; use the lowest
dosage sufficient to reduce the need for

RBC transfusions. For patients with chronic
renal disease who are on dialysis, if the
hemoglobin level approaches or exceeds
11 g/dL, reduce dosage or interrupt therapy.
➤ **Anemia from chemotherapy in pa-tients with nonmyeloid malignancies**
Adults: 2.25 mcg/kg subcutaneously once
weekly or 500 mcg subcutaneously once
every 3 weeks.
Adjust-a-dose: For either dosing schedule,
adjust dose to maintain a target hemoglobin
below 12 g/dL. Give the lowest effective
dose to gradually increase hemoglobin to a
level at which blood transfusion isn't necessary. If hemoglobin exceeds 12 g/dL, hold
drug until hemoglobin drops to 11 g/dL,
then resume at 40% of previous dose. If
hemoglobin increases more than 1 g/dL in a
2-week period, or when hemoglobin exceeds
11 g/dL, reduce dose by 40%. For patients
receiving the drug on a once-a-week schedule, if hemoglobin level increases less than 1
g/dL after 6 weeks of therapy, increase dose
up to 4.5 mcg/kg.
  If after 8 weeks of therapy there is no response as measured by hemoglobin levels or
if transfusions are still required, discontinue
drug. Discontinue drug after completion of
chemotherapy course.

ADMINISTRATION
I.V.
🛈 *Alert:* The needle cover of the pre-
filled syringe contains dry natural rubber
(a derivative of latex). Assess patient for a
history of latex allergy.
▼ Don't shake. Shaking can denature drug.
▼ If drug contains particles or is discol-
ored, don't use.
▼ Give undiluted by I.V. injection.
▼ Single-dose vials contain no preserva-
tives; don't pool unused portions.
▼ Store drug in refrigerator; don't freeze.
Protect drug from light.
▼ **Incompatibilities:** Other I.V. drugs or
solutions.
Subcutaneous
🛈 *Alert:* The needle cover of the prefilled sy-
ringe contains dry natural rubber (a deriva-
tive of latex). Assess patient for a history of
latex allergy.
● Don't give subcutaneously in patients with
chronic renal failure on dialysis.

• Don't shake. Shaking can denature drug.
• Store drug in refrigerator; don't freeze. Protect drug from light.

ACTION

Mimics effects of erythropoietin. Functions as a growth factor and as a differentiating factor, enhancing RBC production.

Route	Onset	Peak	Duration
I.V.	Unknown	Unknown	Unknown
Subcut.	Slow	48 hr	Unknown

Half-life: 21 hours (I.V.); 74 hours (subcutaneous).

ADVERSE REACTIONS

CNS: *seizures,* dizziness, fatigue, fever, headache, asthenia, transient ischemic attack.
CV: *cardiac arrest, cardiac arrhythmia,* edema, hypertension, hypotension, peripheral edema, *acute MI, heart failure, stroke, thrombosis,* angina, chest pain, vascular access thrombosis.
GI: abdominal pain, constipation, diarrhea, nausea, vomiting, *GI hemorrhage.*
Metabolic: dehydration.
Musculoskeletal: arthralgia, limb pain, myalgia, back pain.
Respiratory: cough, dyspnea, upper respiratory tract infection, *pulmonary embolism,* bronchitis, pneumonia.
Skin: pruritus, rash.
Other: infection, *bacteremia, hemorrhage at access site, peritonitis, sepsis,* abscess, access infection, fluid overload, flulike symptoms, injection-site pain.

INTERACTIONS

None reported.

EFFECTS ON LAB TEST RESULTS

None reported.

CONTRAINDICATIONS & CAUTIONS

• Contraindicated in patients hypersensitive to drug or its components and in those with uncontrolled hypertension.
• Safety and effectiveness haven't been established in patients with underlying hematologic disease, such as hemolytic anemia, sickle cell anemia, thalassemia, or porphyria. Use with caution.
⚠ *Overdose S&S:* CV and thrombotic reactions, polycythemia.

NURSING CONSIDERATIONS

Black Box Warning Erythropoiesis-stimulating agents increase risk of death, MI, stroke, venous thromboembolism, thrombosis of vascular access, and tumor progression or recurrence. ■

Black Box Warning Patients with chronic renal disease have an increased risk of death and serious CV events, including stroke, when erythropoiesis-stimulating agents are used to increase hemoglobin level to greater than 11 g/dL. Therapy should be individualized for each patient and the lowest possible dose sufficient to reduce the need for RBC transfusions should be used. ■

Black Box Warning In patients with non–small-cell lung cancer and breast, head and neck, lymphoid, and cervical cancers, there is a risk of tumor growth and short-ened survival when hemoglobin levels of 12 g/dL are achieved. Target dosage to achieve hemoglobin level of less than 12 g/dL. Use the lowest dosage needed to avoid RBC transfusions. Use only for treatment of anemia due to concomitant myelosuppressive chemotherapy and discontinue drug after chemotherapy course. ■

Black Box Warning Health care providers and hospitals must enroll in and comply with the ESA APPRISE Oncology Program to prescribe or dispense darbepoetin alfa to patients with cancer. ■

• When initiating therapy or adjusting dosage, monitor hemoglobin levels at least weekly until stable; then, at least monthly.
• Hemoglobin level may not increase until 2 to 6 weeks after starting therapy.
• If patient has a minimal response or lack of response at recommended dose, check for deficiencies in folic acid, iron, or vitamin B_{12}. Other contributing factors include infection, malignancy, and occult blood loss.
☻ *Alert:* If patient develops a sudden loss of response with severe anemia and low reticulocyte count, withhold drug and test patient for antierythropoietin antibodies. If antibodies are present, stop treatment. Don't switch to another erythropoietic protein because a cross-reaction is possible.
• Control blood pressure and monitor it carefully.

Reactions in bold italics are *life-threatening*. Interactions may have a *rapid onset* or a *delayed onset*.

● Monitor renal function and electrolytes in predialysis patients.
● Patients who are marginally dialyzed may need adjustments in dialysis prescriptions.
● Serious allergic reactions, including skin rash and urticaria, may occur. If an anaphylactic reaction occurs, stop the drug and give appropriate therapy.

PATIENT TEACHING
● Instruct patients on proper administration and use and disposal of needles.
● Advise patient of possible side effects and allergic reactions.
● Inform patient of the need for frequent monitoring of blood pressure and hemoglobin level; stress compliance with his treatment for high blood pressure.
● Instruct patient how to take drug correctly at home, including how to store drug and dispose of supplies properly.

darifenacin hydrobromide
da-ree-FEN-ah-sin

Enablex✏

Therapeutic class: Antispasmodics
Pharmacologic class: Anticholinergics
Pregnancy risk category: C

AVAILABLE FORMS
Tablets (extended-release): 7.5 mg, 15 mg

INDICATIONS & DOSAGES
➤ **Urge incontinence, urgency, and frequency from an overactive bladder**
Adults: Initially, 7.5 mg P.O. once daily. After 2 weeks, may increase to 15 mg P.O. once daily if needed.
Adjust-a-dose: If patient has hepatic impairment (Child-Pugh class B) or takes a potent CYP3A4 inhibitor, such as clarithromycin, itraconazole, ketoconazole, nefazodone, nelfinavir, or ritonavir, don't exceed 7.5 mg P.O. once daily. Drug isn't recommended for use in patients with severe hepatic impairment (Child-Pugh class C).

ADMINISTRATION
P.O.
● Don't crush tablet; patient should swallow whole.
● Give drug without regard for food.

ACTION
Relaxes smooth muscle of bladder by antagonizing muscarinic receptors, relieving symptoms of overactive bladder.

Route	Onset	Peak	Duration
P.O.	Unknown	7 hr	Unknown

Half-life: 13 to 19 hours.

ADVERSE REACTIONS
CNS: asthenia, dizziness, pain, headache.
CV: hypertension, peripheral edema.
EENT: abnormal vision, dry eyes, pharyngitis, rhinitis, sinusitis.
GI: dry mouth, constipation, abdominal pain, diarrhea, dyspepsia, nausea, vomiting.
GU: urinary tract disorder, UTI, vaginitis, urine retention.
Metabolic: weight gain.
Musculoskeletal: arthralgia, back pain.
Respiratory: bronchitis.
Skin: dry skin, pruritus, rash.
Other: accidental injury, flulike syndrome.

INTERACTIONS
Drug-drug. *Anticholinergics:* May increase anticholinergic effects, such as dry mouth, blurred vision, and constipation. Monitor patient closely.
Digoxin: May increase digoxin level. Monitor digoxin level.
Drugs metabolized by CYP2D6 (such as flecainide, TCAs, thioridazine): May increase levels of these drugs. Use together cautiously.
Midazolam: May increase midazolam level. Monitor patient carefully.
Potent CYP3A4 inhibitors (such as clarithromycin, itraconazole, ketoconazole, nefazodone, nelfinavir, ritonavir): May increase darifenacin level. Maintain dosage no higher than 7.5 mg P.O. daily.
Drug-lifestyle. *Hot weather:* May cause heat prostration from decreased sweating. Urge caution.

EFFECTS ON LAB TEST RESULTS
None reported.

CONTRAINDICATIONS & CAUTIONS
• Contraindicated in patients hypersensitive to drug or its ingredients.
• Contraindicated in patients who have or who are at risk for urine retention, gastric retention, or uncontrolled angle-closure glaucoma.
• Avoid use in patients with severe hepatic impairment (Child-Pugh class C).
• Use cautiously in patients with bladder outflow or GI obstruction, ulcerative colitis, myasthenia gravis, severe constipation, controlled angle-closure glaucoma, decreased GI motility, or Child-Pugh class B hepatic impairment.
⚠ **Overdose S&S:** Severe antimuscarinic effects (mydriasis, decreased secretions, ileus, urine retention, tachycardia, altered mental status).

NURSING CONSIDERATIONS
• Assess bladder function, and monitor drug effects.
• If patient has bladder outlet obstruction, watch for urine retention.
• Assess patient for decreased gastric motility and constipation.
• Use during pregnancy only if maternal benefit outweighs fetal risk.
• It's unknown if drug appears in breast milk.

PATIENT TEACHING
• Tell patient to swallow tablet whole with plenty of liquid; caution against crushing or chewing tablet.
• Inform patient that drug may be taken with or without food.
• Tell patient to use caution, especially when performing hazardous tasks, until drug effects are known.
• Tell patient to report blurred vision, constipation, and urine retention.
• Discourage use of other drugs that may cause dry mouth, constipation, urine retention, or blurred vision.
• Tell patient that drug decreases sweating, and advise cautious use in hot environments and during strenuous activity.

darunavir ethanolate
duh-ROO-nah-veer

Prezista

Therapeutic class: Antiretrovirals
Pharmacologic class: Protease inhibitors
Pregnancy risk category: C

AVAILABLE FORMS
Oral suspension: 100 mg/mL
Tablets: 75 mg, 150 mg, 400 mg, 600 mg, 800 mg

INDICATIONS & DOSAGES
➤ **HIV infection, with ritonavir and other antiretrovirals**
Adults who are treatment-experienced with at least one darunavir resistance–associated substitution or when genotypic testing isn't feasible (testing is recommended): 600 mg P.O. b.i.d., given with 100 mg ritonavir P.O. b.i.d. and food.
Adults who are treatment-naive with no darunavir resistance–associated substitutions: 800 mg P.O. once daily, given with ritonavir 100 mg P.O. once daily and food.
Children ages 3 to younger than 18 who are treatment-naive or treatment-experienced with no darunavir resistance–associated substitutions: Don't exceed recommended dosage for treatment-experienced adults. For those weighing 40 kg (88 lb) or more, give 800 mg P.O. once daily with ritonavir 100 mg once daily and food; for those weighing 30 to less than 40 kg (66 to less than 88 lb), give 675 mg (may round dose to 680 mg for oral suspension) P.O. once daily with ritonavir 100 mg once daily and food; for those weighing 15 to less than 30 kg (33 to less than 66 lb), give 600 mg P.O. once daily with ritonavir 100 mg once daily and food; for those weighing 14 to less than 15 kg (31 to less than 33 lb), give 490 mg (may round dose to 500 mg for oral suspension) P.O. once daily with ritonavir 96 mg once daily and food; for those weighing 13 to less than 14 kg (29 to less than 31 lb), give 455 mg (may round dose to 460 mg for oral suspension) P.O. once daily with ritonavir 80 mg once daily and food; for those weighing 12 to less than 13 kg (26 to

less than 29 lb), give 420 mg P.O. once daily with ritonavir 80 mg once daily and food; for those weighing 11 to less than 12 kg (24 to less than 26 lb), give 385 mg (may round dose to 400 mg for oral suspension) P.O. once daily with ritonavir 64 mg once daily and food; for those weighing 10 to less than 11 kg (22 to less than 24 lb), give 350 mg (may round dose to 360 mg for oral suspension) P.O. once daily with ritonavir 64 mg once daily and food.

Children ages 3 to younger than 18 who are treatment-experienced with at least one darunavir resistance–associated substitution: Don't exceed recommended dosage for treatment-experienced adults. For those weighing 40 kg (88 lb) or more, give 600 mg P.O. b.i.d. with ritonavir 100 mg b.i.d. and food; for those weighing 30 to less than 40 kg (66 to less than 88 lb), give 450 mg (may round dose to 460 mg for oral suspension) P.O. b.i.d. with ritonavir 60 mg b.i.d. and food; for those weighing 15 to less than 30 kg (33 to less than 66 lb), give 375 mg (may round dose to 380 mg for oral suspension) P.O. b.i.d. with ritonavir 48 mg b.i.d. and food; for those weighing 14 to less than 15 kg (31 to less than 33 lb), give 280 mg P.O. b.i.d. with ritonavir 48 mg b.i.d. and food; for those weighing 13 to less than 14 kg (29 to less than 31 lb), give 260 mg P.O. b.i.d. with ritonavir 40 mg b.i.d. and food; for those weighing 12 to less than 13 kg (26 to less than 29 lb), give 240 mg P.O. b.i.d. with ritonavir 40 mg b.i.d. and food; for those weighing 11 to less than 12 kg (24 to less than 26 lb), give 220 mg P.O. b.i.d. with ritonavir 32 mg b.i.d. and food; for those weighing 10 to less than 11 kg (22 to less than 24 lb), give 200 mg P.O. b.i.d. with ritonavir 32 mg b.i.d. and food.

ADMINISTRATION
P.O.
- Always give with ritonavir and food.
- Shake oral suspension well before using.
- Use provided oral dosing syringe to administer oral suspension.

ACTION
Binds to the protease-active site and inhibits enzyme activity. This prevents mature viral particles from forming.

Route	Onset	Peak	Duration
P.O.	Unknown	2½–4 hr	Unknown

Half-life: About 15 hours when combined with ritonavir.

ADVERSE REACTIONS
CNS: headache, asthenia, fatigue.
GI: diarrhea, nausea, abdominal distention, abdominal pain, anorexia, constipation, dry mouth, dyspepsia, flatulence, vomiting.
Hematologic: *leukopenia, neutropenia, thrombocytopenia.*
Hepatic: *hepatotoxicity.*
Metabolic: diabetes mellitus, hypercholesterolemia, hyperlipidemia, hypernatremia, hyperuricemia, hyponatremia, obesity.
Musculoskeletal: myalgia.
Skin: *erythema multiforme, Stevens-Johnson syndrome,* rash.
Other: immune reconstitution syndrome.

INTERACTIONS
Drug-drug. *Amiodarone, bepridil, cyclosporine, felodipine, fluticasone, lidocaine, nicardipine, nifedipine, quinidine, rifabutin, sildenafil, sirolimus, tacrolimus, tadalafil, trazodone, vardenafil:* May increase levels of these drugs, increasing the risk of adverse reactions. Use caution, and monitor patient carefully.
Clarithromycin: May increase clarithromycin level. Reduce clarithromycin dose in patients with renal impairment.
CYP3A inducers (carbamazepine, dexamethasone, phenobarbital, phenytoin, rifabutin, rifampin), efavirenz, lopinavir, saquinavir: May increase darunavir clearance and decrease darunavir level. Avoid using together.
Ergot derivatives, midazolam, pimozide, terfenadine, triazolam: May cause life-threatening reactions. Use together is contraindicated.
Ethinyl estradiol, norethindrone: May decrease estrogen level. Recommend alternative or additional contraception.
HMG-CoA reductase inhibitors (atorvastatin, lovastatin, pravastatin, rosuvastatin,

D

simvastatin): May increase risk of serious reactions, including myopathy and rhabdomyolysis. Start with lowest possible dose of atorvastatin, pravastatin, or rosuvastatin with careful monitoring, or consider using fluvastatin. Coadministration with lovastatin and simvastatin is contraindicated.

Itraconazole, ketoconazole: May increase levels of these drugs and darunavir. Don't exceed 200 mg of itraconazole or ketoconazole daily.

Methadone: May decrease methadone level. Monitor patient for opioid abstinence syndrome, and consider increasing methadone dosage.

Rifabutin: May decrease darunavir level. If used together, give rifabutin as 150 mg every other day.

SSRIs (paroxetine, sertraline): May decrease levels of these drugs. Adjust dosage carefully based on antidepressant response.

Trazodone: May increase trazodone level and risk of toxicity. Decrease trazodone dosage.

Warfarin: May decrease warfarin level. Monitor patient carefully.

Drug-herb. *St. John's wort:* May decrease drug level significantly. Discourage use together.

Drug-food. *Food:* Increases drug absorption, which is needed for adequate therapeutic effect. Advise patient to take with food.

EFFECTS ON LAB TEST RESULTS
● May increase AST, ALT, GGT, alkaline phosphatase, bilirubin, pancreatic amylase, pancreatic lipase, cholesterol, triglyceride, and uric acid levels. May decrease albumin, bicarbonate, and calcium levels. May increase or decrease sodium and glucose levels.
● May decrease WBC, neutrophil, lymphocyte, and platelet counts.

CONTRAINDICATIONS & CAUTIONS
● Contraindicated in patients hypersensitive to any component of drug and patient taking drugs metabolized by CYP3A (alfuzosin, dihydroergotamine, ergonovine, ergotamine, lovastatin, methylergonovine, midazolam, pimozide, rifampin, sildenafil, simvastatin, triazolam).

● Use cautiously in patients with hepatic or renal impairment, diabetes mellitus, hemophilia, known sulfonamide allergy, or a history of opportunistic infections.
● Use in patients with severe hepatic impairment isn't recommended.

NURSING CONSIDERATIONS
۞ Alert: Because of an increased risk of hepatotoxicity, especially in patients with prior hepatic dysfunction, check LFTs before beginning treatment and periodically thereafter. Discontinue treatment in patients with elevated liver enzyme levels and signs and symptoms of liver dysfunction.
● During initial phase of treatment, patients responding to antiretroviral therapy may develop an inflammatory response to indolent or residual opportunistic infections (CMV, *Mycobacterium avium* complex, *Pneumocystis jiroveci* pneumonia, tuberculosis), which may necessitate further evaluation and treatment. Autoimmune disorders (such as Graves disease, polymyositis, and Guillain-Barré syndrome) have also been reported in the setting of immune reconstitution; however, time to onset is more variable, and can occur many months after initiation of antiretroviral treatment.
● Make sure patient isn't taking any drugs that are incompatible with darunavir.
● If patient has diabetes, monitor glucose level.
● Risks and benefits of drug in treatment-naive patients aren't known.
● Refer to ritonavir prescribing information for contraindications and adverse effects because of required coadministration with darunavir.

PATIENT TEACHING
● Explain that many drugs interact with darunavir; advise patient to report all drugs he takes, including OTC products.
۞ Alert: Instruct patient to take darunavir and ritonavir at the same time every day, with food.
● Tell patient that drug doesn't cure HIV infection or AIDS and doesn't reduce the risk of passing HIV to others.
● Explain that opportunistic infections and other complications of HIV infection may still develop.

Reactions in bold italics are **life-threatening**. Interactions may have a *rapid onset* or a **delayed onset**.

• For b.i.d. dosing, if patient misses a dose by more than 6 hours, tell him to wait and take the next dose at the regularly scheduled time. If he remembers within 6 hours, tell him to take the missed dose immediately.
• For once-daily dosing, if patient misses a dose by more than 12 hours, tell him to wait and take the next dose at the regularly scheduled time. If he remembers within 12 hours, tell him to take the missed dose immediately.
• Tell patient to never double a dose if a dose is skipped.

SAFETY ALERT!

dasatinib
duh-SAH-tin-nib

Sprycel

Therapeutic class: Antineoplastics
Pharmacologic class: Protein–tyrosine kinase inhibitors
Pregnancy risk category: D

AVAILABLE FORMS
Tablets: 20 mg, 50 mg, 70 mg, 80 mg, 100 mg, 140 mg

INDICATIONS & DOSAGES
Adjust-a-dose (for all indications): If patient has hematologic toxicity, such as neutropenia or thrombocytopenia, consider reducing dose or interrupting or stopping therapy. If patient has severe, nonhematologic toxicity, hold dose until condition resolves; then resume at previous or reduced dose as appropriate.
➤ **Accelerated, myeloid, or lymphoid blast-phase chronic myeloid leukemia (CML) with resistance or intolerance to earlier treatment, including imatinib; Philadelphia chromosome–positive acute lymphoblastic leukemia with resistance or intolerance to prior therapy**
Adults: 140 mg P.O. once daily. If patient tolerates this dose but fails to respond to treatment, increase to 180 mg P.O. once daily. Continue until disease progresses or intolerable adverse effects occur.
Adjust-a-dose: If ANC is less than 0.5 × 10^9/L or platelet count is less than 10 ×

10^9/L, take the following steps: (1) Check if cytopenia is related to leukemia (marrow aspirate or biopsy). (2) If cytopenia is unrelated to leukemia, stop dasatinib until ANC is 1 × 10^9/L or more and platelet count is 20 × 10^9/L or more; resume at the original starting dose. (3) If cytopenia recurs, repeat step 1 and resume dasatinib at a reduced dosage of 100 mg once daily (second episode) or 80 mg once daily (third episode). (4) If cytopenia is related to leukemia, consider dosage escalation to 180 mg once daily.
➤ **Newly diagnosed Philadelphia chromosome-positive chronic-phase CML or chronic-phase CML resistant or intolerant to previous therapy, including imatinib**
Adults: 100 mg P.O. daily. May increase to 140 mg daily.
Adjust-a-dose: If ANC is less than 0.5 × 10^9/L or platelet count is less than 50 × 10^9/L, take the following steps: (1) Stop dasatinib until ANC is 1 × 10^9/L or more and platelet count is 50 × 10^9/L or more. (2) Resume treatment with dasatinib at the original starting dose if recovery occurs in 7 days or less. (3) If platelet count is less than 25 × 10^9/L or there is a recurrence of ANC of less than 0.5 × 10^9/L for more than 7 days, repeat step 1 and resume dasatinib at a reduced dosage of 80 mg once daily (second episode). (4) For the third episode, further reduce dosage to 50 mg once daily (for newly diagnosed patients) or discontinue dasatinib (for patients resistant to or intolerant of prior therapy, including imatinib).

ADMINISTRATION
P.O.
• Give drug without regard for food.
⚠ *Alert:* Don't crush or cut tablets. If tablet is crushed or broken, wear chemotherapy gloves to dispose of it. Pregnant women shouldn't handle broken tablets.

ACTION
Reduces leukemic cell growth by inhibiting a tyrosine kinase enzyme. As a result, bone marrow can resume production of normal RBCs, WBCs, and platelets.

Route	Onset	Peak	Duration
P.O.	Unknown	½–6 hr	Unknown

Half-life: 3 to 5 hours.

ADVERSE REACTIONS

CNS: asthenia, chills, dizziness, fatigue, headache, neuropathy, ***bleeding,*** pyrexia, ***seizures,*** anxiety, confusion, depression, insomnia, somnolence, syncope, tremor, vertigo, affect lability.

CV: ***arrhythmias,*** chest pain, edema, ***cardiac dysfunction, heart failure,*** hypertension, hypotension, pericardial effusion, cardiomegaly, flushing, palpitations, ***MI.***

EENT: mucositis, stomatitis, conjunctivitis, dry eyes, dysgeusia, tinnitus.

GI: abdominal distention and pain, anorexia, constipation, diarrhea, nausea, vomiting, ***bleeding,*** anal fissure, colitis, dyspepsia, dysphagia, gastritis.

GU: ***renal failure,*** urinary frequency.

Hematologic: anemia, ***febrile neutropenia, pancytopenia, thrombocytopenia.***

Metabolic: weight loss or gain, hyperuricemia, appetite changes.

Musculoskeletal: arthralgia, myalgia, pain, inflammation, muscle stiffness, weakness.

Respiratory: cough, dyspnea, upper respiratory tract infection, pleural effusion, pneumonia, asthma, ***pulmonary edema, pulmonary hypertension,*** lung infiltrates, pneumonitis.

Skin: pruritus, rash, acne, alopecia, dry skin, nail or pigment disorders, sweating, dermatitis, photosensitivity reactions, urticaria.

Other: infection, ***tumor lysis syndrome,*** ascites, gynecomastia, herpes infection, fluid retention.

INTERACTIONS

Drug-drug. *Antacids:* May decrease dasatinib absorption. Give antacid 2 hours before or 2 hours after dasatinib.

CYP3A4 inducers (carbamazepine, dexamethasone, phenobarbital, phenytoin, rifampin): May decrease dasatinib level. Avoid using together, or increase dasatinib dose in 20-mg increments.

CYP3A4 inhibitors (atazanavir, clarithromycin, erythromycin, indinavir, itraconazole, ketoconazole, nefazodone, nelfin-avir, ritonavir, saquinavir, telithromycin): May increase dasatinib level and toxicity. Avoid using together; if unavoidable, monitor patient closely and consider decreasing dasatinib dose to 20 to 40 mg daily.

CYP3A4 substrates (cyclosporine, ergot alkaloids, fentanyl, pimozide, quinidine, sirolimus, tacrolimus): May alter levels of these drugs. Use cautiously together, and monitor patient.

H₂-blockers, proton pump inhibitors: May decrease dasatinib level because of gastric acid suppression. Avoid using together. Consider antacids as an alternative.

Simvastatin: May increase simvastatin level. Monitor patient.

Drug-herb. *St. John's wort:* May decrease drug level. Discourage use together.

Drug-food. *Grapefruit juice:* May increase dasatinib level. Avoid use together.

EFFECTS ON LAB TEST RESULTS

● May increase uric acid, bilirubin, creatinine, AST, ALT, CK, and troponin levels. May decrease phosphate and calcium levels.

● May decrease RBC, platelet, and neutrophil counts.

CONTRAINDICATIONS & CAUTIONS

⊗ *Alert:* May increase risk of pulmonary arterial hypertension (PAH). Assess for cardiopulmonary disease before starting and periodically during treatment. Discontinue drug if PAH is confirmed.

● Use cautiously in patients receiving antiarrhythmics, antiplatelets, or anticoagulants; patients receiving cumulative high-dose anthracycline therapy; patients with a prolonged QT interval or risk of prolonged QT interval (those with hypokalemia, hypomagnesemia, or current use of drugs that prolong the QT interval); patients with liver impairment; and patients who are lactose intolerant.

⚠ *Overdose S&S:* Severe myelosuppression, bleeding.

NURSING CONSIDERATIONS

● Monitor CBC weekly for the first 2 months of treatment, then monthly thereafter, or as indicated.

Reactions in bold italics are *life-threatening*. Interactions may have a *rapid onset* or a *delayed onset*.

• Correct electrolyte imbalances, especially of potassium and magnesium, before treatment.
• Monitor for fluid retention and heart failure.
• Drug contains lactose.
• Drug may cause fetal harm. Don't use in pregnant women. If used, mother should be warned of potential harm.
• Drug affects older and younger adults similarly, although older adults may be more sensitive to drug's effects.
• It's unknown if drug appears in breast milk; mothers shouldn't breast-feed during treatment.

PATIENT TEACHING
• Tell patient to take the tablets at about the same time every day.
• Caution patient not to crush or cut the tablets.
• Warn women of childbearing age to use reliable contraception during treatment. Men who take drug should use condoms to avoid impregnating their partners.
• Tell patient to report weight gain, swelling, and shortness of breath.
• Advise patient to notify prescriber immediately about easy or unusual bruising.
• Tell patient to avoid grapefruit juice.

SAFETY ALERT!

DAUNOrubicin citrate liposomal
daw-nah-ROO-buh-sin

DaunoXome

Therapeutic class: Antineoplastics
Pharmacologic class: Anthracycline glycoside antibiotics
Pregnancy risk category: D

AVAILABLE FORMS
Injection: 2 mg/mL (equivalent to 50 mg daunorubicin base)

INDICATIONS & DOSAGES
➤ **First-line cytotoxic therapy for advanced HIV-related Kaposi sarcoma**
Adults: 40 mg/m^2 I.V. over 60 minutes once every 2 weeks. Repeat blood counts before

each dose; withhold drug if absolute granulocyte count is less than 750 cells/mm^3. Continue treatment until progressive disease becomes evident or until other complications of HIV infection preclude continuation of therapy.

Adjust-a-dose: For patients with impaired hepatic and renal function, if bilirubin level is 1.2 to 3 mg/dL, give three-fourths normal dose; if bilirubin or creatinine level exceeds 3 mg/dL, give one-half normal dose.

ADMINISTRATION
I.V.
▼ Preparing and giving drug may be mutagenic, teratogenic, or carcinogenic. Follow facility policy to reduce risks.
▼ To dilute, withdraw calculated volume of drug from vial and transfer into an equal amount of D$_5$W. Recommended concentration after dilution is 1 mg/mL.
▼ Use immediately after dilution.
▼ Don't use an in-line filter.
▼ Give over 60 minutes.
Black Box Warning Back pain, flushing, and chest tightness may develop during first 5 minutes of infusion. These symptoms subside after infusion stops and usually don't recur when drug is infused more slowly. ∎
▼ Monitor I.V. site closely; watch for irritation and infiltration, which can cause tissue damage and necrosis. If it occurs, stop infusion, apply ice, and notify prescriber.
▼ If needed, drug may be refrigerated at 36° to 46° F (2° to 8° C) for up to 6 hours.
▼ **Incompatibilities:** Bacteriostatic agents, other I.V. drugs, saline and other solutions.

ACTION
Maximizes selectivity of daunorubicin for solid tumors in situ. After penetrating tumor, drug is released over time to exert antineoplastic activity by inhibiting DNA synthesis and DNA-dependent RNA synthesis.

Route	Onset	Peak	Duration
I.V.	Unknown	Unknown	Unknown

Half-life: 4½ hours.

ADVERSE REACTIONS

CNS: headache, neuropathy, depression, dizziness, insomnia, amnesia, anxiety, ataxia, confusion, *seizures,* hallucination, tremor, hypertonia, *meningitis,* fatigue, malaise, emotional lability, abnormal gait, hyperkinesia, somnolence, abnormal thinking, fever.

CV: chest pain, hypertension, palpitations, *arrhythmias, pericardial effusion, cardiac arrest,* angina pectoris, *pulmonary hypertension,* flushing, edema, tachycardia, *MI, heart failure.*

EENT: rhinitis, stomatitis, sinusitis, abnormal vision, conjunctivitis, tinnitus, eye pain, deafness, earache.

GI: taste disturbances, dry mouth, gingival bleeding, nausea, diarrhea, abdominal pain, vomiting, anorexia, constipation, *GI hemorrhage,* gastritis, dysphagia, stomatitis, increased appetite, melena, hemorrhoids, tenesmus.

GU: dysuria, nocturia, polyuria.

Hematologic: *neutropenia, thrombocytopenia.*

Hepatic: hepatomegaly.

Metabolic: dehydration.

Musculoskeletal: rigors, back pain, arthralgia, myalgia.

Respiratory: cough, dyspnea, hemoptysis, hiccups, pulmonary infiltration, increased sputum.

Skin: alopecia, pruritus, increased sweating, dry skin, seborrhea, folliculitis, injection-site inflammation.

Other: splenomegaly, lymphadenopathy, tooth caries, *allergic reactions,* flulike symptoms.

INTERACTIONS
None significant.

EFFECTS ON LAB TEST RESULTS
● May decrease neutrophil and platelet counts.

CONTRAINDICATIONS & CAUTIONS
● Contraindicated in patients who have experienced severe hypersensitivity reaction to drug or its components.
● Use cautiously in patients with myelosuppression, cardiac disease, previous radiotherapy encompassing the heart, previous anthracycline use (doxorubicin cumulative dose is 300 mg/m^2 or above), or hepatic or renal dysfunction.

⚠ *Overdose S&S:* Increased severity of observed dose-limiting toxicities of therapeutic doses, myelosuppression (especially granulocytopenia), fatigue, nausea, vomiting.

NURSING CONSIDERATIONS
● Drug can cause extravasation. Take proper precautions during administration.
● Drug causes less nausea, vomiting, alopecia, neutropenia, thrombocytopenia, and potentially less cardiotoxicity than conventional daunorubicin.

Black Box Warning Give only under supervision of prescriber specializing in chemotherapy. ∎

Black Box Warning Monitor cardiac function regularly. Assess patient before giving each dose because of risk of cardiac toxicity and heart failure. Cardiac monitoring is especially advised in patients who have received prior anthracyclines, have preexisting cardiac disease, or have had prior radiotherapy encompassing the heart. ∎

● Determine LVEF at total cumulative doses of 320 mg/m^2 and every 160 mg/m^2 thereafter. Total cumulative doses generally shouldn't exceed 550 mg/m^2.

Black Box Warning Provide careful hematologic monitoring because severe myelosuppression may occur. ∎

● Monitor patient closely for signs and symptoms of opportunistic infection, especially because patients with HIV infection are immunocompromised.

Black Box Warning Reduce dosage in patients with impaired hepatic function. ∎

● *Look alike–sound alike:* Don't confuse daunorubicin citrate liposomal with daunorubicin hydrochloride or doxorubicin hydrochloride.

PATIENT TEACHING
● Inform patient that hair loss may occur but that it's usually reversible.
● Instruct patient to call prescriber if sore throat, fever, or other signs or symptoms of infection occur. Tell patient to avoid exposure to people with infections.

Reactions in bold italics are *life-threatening*. Interactions may have a *rapid onset* or a *delayed onset*.

• Advise women to report suspected or confirmed pregnancy during therapy.
• Tell patient to report back pain, flushing, or chest tightness during infusion.

SAFETY ALERT!

DAUNOrubicin hydrochloride
daw-nah-ROO-buh-sin

Cerubidine

Therapeutic class: Antineoplastics
Pharmacologic class: Anthracycline glycoside antibiotics
Pregnancy risk category: D

AVAILABLE FORMS
Injection: 5 mg/mL
Powder for injection: 20-mg vials

INDICATIONS & DOSAGES
Adjust-a-dose (for all indications): For patients with impaired hepatic and renal function, reduce dosage as follows: If bilirubin level is 1.2 to 3 mg/dL, give three-fourths normal dose; if bilirubin or creatinine level exceeds 3 mg/dL, give one-half normal dose. Dosages vary. Check treatment protocol with prescriber.

➤ **To induce remission in acute non-lymphocytic (myelogenous, monocytic, erythroid) leukemia**
Adults age 60 and older: In combination, 30 mg/m^2 per day I.V. on days 1, 2, and 3 of first course and on days 1 and 2 of subsequent courses with cytarabine infusions. Maximum lifetime cumulative dose is 500 mg/m^2; in patients who received mediastinal radiation, maximum lifetime cumulative dose is 400 mg/m^2.
Adults younger than age 60: In combination, 45 mg/m^2 per day I.V. on days 1, 2, and 3 of first course and on days 1 and 2 of subsequent courses with cytarabine infusions. Maximum lifetime cumulative dose is 500 mg/m^2; in patients who received mediastinal radiation, maximum lifetime cumulative dose is 400 mg/m^2.

➤ **To induce remission in acute lymphocytic leukemia (with combination therapy)**

Adults: 45 mg/m^2 per day I.V. on days 1, 2, and 3 of first course. Maximum lifetime cumulative dose is 550 mg/m^2; in patients who received mediastinal radiation, maximum lifetime cumulative dose is 400 mg/m^2.
Children age 2 and older: 25 mg/m^2 I.V. on day 1 every week for up to 6 weeks, if needed. Maximum lifetime cumulative dose is 300 mg/m^2.
Children younger than age 2 or with body surface area less than 0.5 m^2: 1 mg/kg/dose for 1 to 3 days (dose based on body weight, not surface area). Administration frequency is specific to each combination chemotherapy regimen. Maximum lifetime cumulative dose is 10 mg/kg.

ADMINISTRATION
I.V.
▼ Preparing and giving parenteral drug may be mutagenic, teratogenic, or carcinogenic. Follow facility policy to reduce risks.
▼ Reconstitute with 4 mL sterile water for injection to yield 5 mg/mL.
▼ Withdraw desired dose into syringe containing 10 to 15 mL of normal saline solution for injection.
▼ Inject as a slow I.V. push over 2 to 3 minutes into tubing of a free-flowing I.V. solution of D$_5$W or normal saline solution for injection.
Black Box Warning Give drug into a rapidly infusing I.V. infusion. Do not give I.M. or subcutaneously. Severe local tissue necrosis will result from extravasation. ∎
▼ If extravasation occurs, stop infusion immediately, apply ice to area for 24 to 48 hours, and notify prescriber. Because drug is a vesicant, extravasation could cause severe tissue necrosis.
▼ Use vial contents or discard remainder within 6 hours of initial needle puncture if opened within an ISO Class 5 biological safety cabinet, or within 1 hour of initial needle puncture if opened outside of such an environment.
▼ Reconstituted solution is stable 24 hours at room temperature, 48 hours if refrigerated.
▼ **Incompatibilities:** Other I.V. drugs. If mixed with dexamethasone or heparin, drug may precipitate; don't mix together.

ACTION
May interfere with DNA-dependent RNA synthesis by intercalation.

Route	Onset	Peak	Duration
I.V.	Unknown	Unknown	Unknown

Half-life: Initial, 45 minutes; terminal, 18½ hours.

ADVERSE REACTIONS
CNS: fever.
CV: *irreversible cardiomyopathy,* ECG changes.
GI: nausea, vomiting, diarrhea, abdominal pain, mucositis.
Hematologic: *bone marrow suppression.*
Metabolic: hyperuricemia.
Skin: reversible alopecia, severe cellulitis and tissue sloughing with drug extravasation, rash, darkening or redness of previously irradiated areas, contact dermatitis, urticaria.

INTERACTIONS
Drug-drug. *Doxorubicin:* May cause additive cardiotoxicity. Monitor patient for toxicity.
Hepatotoxic drugs: May increase risk of additive hepatotoxicity. Monitor hepatic function closely.
Myelosuppressives: May increase risk of myelosuppression. Monitor patient closely.

EFFECTS ON LAB TEST RESULTS
• May increase alkaline phosphatase, AST, bilirubin, and uric acid levels. May decrease hemoglobin level and hematocrit.
• May decrease platelet and WBC counts.

CONTRAINDICATIONS & CAUTIONS
• Contraindicated in patients hypersensitive to the drug.
• Use cautiously in patients with myelosuppression or impaired cardiac, renal, or hepatic function.

NURSING CONSIDERATIONS
Black Box Warning Only physicians experienced in leukemia chemotherapy should administer drug. The physician and institution must be capable of responding rapidly and completely to severe hemorrhage or overwhelming infection. Adequate laboratory and supportive resources must be available. ∎
• Take preventive measures (including adequate hydration) before starting treatment. Hyperuricemia may result from rapid lysis of leukemic cells. Allopurinol may be ordered.
Black Box Warning Myocardial toxicity may occur when total cumulative dosage exceeds 400 to 550 mg/m^2 in adults, 300 mg/m^2 in children older than 2 years, or 10 mg/kg in children younger than 2 years. This may occur during therapy and for several months to years after therapy. ∎
• Perform cardiac function studies, including ECG and LVEF, before treatment and then periodically throughout therapy.
❸ *Alert:* Cumulative adult dosage is limited to 400 to 550 mg/m^2 (450 mg/m^2 when patient is also receiving or has received cyclophosphamide or radiation therapy to cardiac area).
Black Box Warning Reduce dosage in patients with renal or hepatic impairment. ∎
• Monitor CBC and LFTs; monitor ECG every month during therapy.
❸ *Alert:* If signs of heart failure, cardiomyopathy, or arrhythmia develop, stop drug immediately and notify prescriber.
• Watch for nausea and vomiting, which may last 24 to 48 hours.
Black Box Warning Severe myelosuppression occurs when used in therapeutic doses; this may lead to infection or hemorrhage. ∎
• Blood transfusions may be needed to combat anemia.
• Lowest blood counts occur 10 to 14 days after dose.
• *Look alike–sound alike:* Reddish color of drug is similar to that of doxorubicin; don't confuse the two. Don't confuse daunorubicin hydrochloride with daunorubicin citrate liposomal or doxorubicin.

PATIENT TEACHING
• Advise patient to report any pain or burning at site of injection during or after administration.
• Advise patient to watch for signs and symptoms of infection (fever, sore throat, fatigue) and bleeding (easy bruising,

---

Reactions in bold italics are *life-threatening*. Interactions may have a *rapid onset* or a *delayed onset*.

nosebleeds, bleeding gums, tarry stools) and to take temperature daily.
• Inform patient that red urine for 1 to 2 days is normal and doesn't indicate the presence of blood in urine.
• Advise patient that hair loss may occur but that it's usually reversible.
• Caution woman of childbearing age to avoid becoming pregnant during therapy. Recommend that she consult prescriber before becoming pregnant.

deferasirox
deh-fah-RASS-ih-rocks

Exjade

Therapeutic class: Chelating agents
Pharmacologic class: Heavy metal antagonists
Pregnancy risk category: C

AVAILABLE FORMS
Tablets for oral suspension: 125 mg, 250 mg, 500 mg

INDICATIONS & DOSAGES
Adjust-a-dose (for all indications): Contraindicated in patients with serum creatinine level greater than two times the age-appropriate upper limit of normal (ULN) or CrCl less than 40 mL/minute. Discontinue drug if necessary. Start elderly patients at the low end of the dosing range. Avoid use in patients with severe (Child-Pugh class C) hepatic impairment. Reduce starting dose by 50% in patients with moderate (Child-Pugh class B) hepatic impairment. Closely monitor all patients with mild (Child-Pugh class A) or moderate hepatic impairment for effectiveness and adverse reactions.
➤ **Chronic iron overload caused by blood transfusions (transfusional hemosiderosis)**
Adults and children age 2 and older: Initially, 20 mg/kg P.O. daily on an empty stomach 30 minutes before eating. Monitor serum ferritin level monthly and adjust dose every 3 to 6 months by 5 or 10 mg/kg based on ferritin trends. Don't exceed 40 mg/kg daily. Consider stopping therapy if serum ferritin level drops below 500 mcg/L.

Adjust-a-dose: For adults with serum creatinine level of more than 33% above average baseline seen at two consecutive visits that isn't attributable to other causes, decrease daily dosage by 10 mg/kg. For children age 15 and younger with serum creatinine level of more than 33% above normal limits at two consecutive visits, decrease dosage by 10 mg/kg.
✳ **NEW INDICATION: Chronic iron overload in patients with non-transfusion-dependent thalassemia syndromes and with a liver iron (Fe) concentration (LIC) of at least 5 mg Fe per gram of dry weight (dw) and a serum ferritin level greater than 300 mcg/L**
Adults and children age 10 and older: Initially 10 mg/kg P.O. once daily. Calculate dose to the nearest whole tablet. If baseline LIC is greater than 15 mg Fe/g dw, may increase to 20 mg/kg/day after 4 weeks. Interrupt treatment when serum ferritin level is less than 300 mcg/L and obtain LIC to determine if LIC is less than 3 mg Fe/g dw. If LIC remains greater than 7 mg Fe/g dw after 6 months of therapy, increase dosage to maximum of 20 mg/kg/day. If LIC is 3 to 7 mg Fe/g dw after 6 months, continue treatment at maximum of 10 mg/kg/day. If LIC is less than 3 mg Fe/g dw, stop treatment.
Adjust-a-dose: For adults and adolescents age 16 and older: If serum creatinine level increases by 33% or more above the average baseline measurement, repeat serum creatinine within 1 week and, if still elevated by 33% or more, interrupt therapy if dose is 5 mg/kg, or reduce by 50% if dose is 10 or 20 mg/kg. For children ages 10 to 15: Reduce dose by 5 mg/kg if serum creatinine level increases to greater than 33% above the average baseline measurement and greater than the age-appropriate ULN.

ADMINISTRATION
P.O.
• Give drug to patient at same time each day, about 30 minutes before he eats.
• Dissolve tablets in water, orange juice, or apple juice. If dose is less than 1 g, dissolve in 3½ ounces (100 mL) of liquid. If dose is more than 1 g, dissolve in 7 ounces (200 mL) of liquid.

● Make sure that patient doesn't chew or swallow tablets whole.

ACTION
Binds with high affinity to iron, allowing mainly fecal excretion.

Route	Onset	Peak	Duration
P.O.	Unknown	1½–4 hr	Unknown

Half-life: 8 to 16 hours.

ADVERSE REACTIONS
CNS: fever.
GI: abdominal pain, diarrhea, nausea, vomiting.
GU: *acute renal failure.*
Hematologic: *agranulocytosis, neutropenia, thrombocytopenia.*
Hepatic: *liver toxicity.*
Skin: rash, urticaria, leukocytoclastic vasculitis.
Other: influenza, hypersensitivity reactions (including *anaphylaxis* and *angioedema*).

INTERACTIONS
Drug-drug. *Aluminum-containing antacids:* May decrease iron chelation. Avoid using together.
Anticoagulants: May increase risk of hemorrhage. Monitor patient closely.
Bile acid sequestrants (such as cholestyramine, colesevelam, colestipol): Decrease deferasirox level. If drugs must be used together, consider increasing initial dose of deferasirox by 50%, and monitor serum ferritin level and clinical response for further dosage modification.
Bisphosphonates, NSAIDs, prednisone: May increase risk of GI irritation and ulcers. Use together cautiously.
Cholestyramine, potent UGT (UDP-glucuronosyltransferase) inducers (phenobarbital, phenytoin, rifampin, ritonavir): May decrease deferasirox level. If drugs must be used together, consider increasing initial deferasirox dosage by 50%. Monitor serum ferritin level and clinical response before further dosage adjustment.
Cyclosporine: May decrease effectiveness of cyclosporine. Monitor drug levels and patient for decreased immunosuppression. Adjust cyclosporine dosage as needed.

Hormonal contraceptives: May decrease efficacy of contraceptive. Recommend use of a nonhormonal form of contraception.
Midazolam: May decrease levels of both drugs. Use together cautiously. Monitor patient for effectiveness and adjust midazolam dosage as needed.
Other iron chelators: May increase risk of toxic effects. Avoid using together.
Paclitaxel: May increase paclitaxel level and risk of toxicity. Use together cautiously. Adjust dosage as needed.
Repaglinide: May increase effects of repaglinide. Monitor blood glucose level and adjust repaglinide dosage as needed.
Simvastatin: May decrease simvastatin level. Monitor patient response and adjust simvastatin dosage as needed.
Drug-food. *Any food:* May decrease drug effects. Give to patient on an empty stomach at least 30 minutes before eating.

EFFECTS ON LAB TEST RESULTS
● May increase transaminase and creatinine levels.

CONTRAINDICATIONS & CAUTIONS
● Contraindicated in patients hypersensitive to deferasirox or any component of the drug.
Black Box Warning Drug may cause hepatic or renal impairment, including failure, or GI hemorrhage, which may be fatal. Risk is higher in elderly patients and in those with high risk of myelodysplastic syndrome (MDS), underlying renal or hepatic impairment, or low platelet count. ∎
● Contraindicated in patients with CrCl of less than 40 mL/minute or serum creatinine level greater than age-appropriate 2 times ULN, in those with poor performance status and high risk of MDS or advanced malignancies, and in patients with platelet count of less than 50,000/mm^3.
● Use cautiously in breast-feeding women and patients with renal impairment, hepatic impairment, hearing loss, or vision disturbances.
⚠ *Overdose S&S:* Hepatitis, nausea, diarrhea.

NURSING CONSIDERATIONS
Black Box Warning Monitor renal and liver function tests closely. Monitor serum creatinine level or CrCl before initiation

---

Reactions in bold italics are *life-threatening*. Interactions may have a *rapid onset* or a *delayed onset*.

of therapy and monthly thereafter; in patients with underlying renal impairment or risk factors for renal impairment, monitor serum creatinine level or CrCl weekly for first month, then monthly. Monitor serum transaminase and bilirubin levels before initiation of therapy, every 2 weeks during first month, and monthly thereafter. ■
Black Box Warning Avoid using deferasirox in patients with severe (Child-Pugh class C) hepatic impairment and reduce dosage in patients with moderate (Child-Pugh class B) hepatic impairment. ■

• Before starting therapy, obtain baseline serum ferritin and iron levels.

• Deferasirox therapy should only be considered when a patient with a non-transfusion-dependent thalassemia syndrome has an LIC of at least 5 mg Fe/g dw and a serum ferritin level greater than 300 mcg/L.

• Periodically evaluate patient for proteinuria.

• Test patient's hearing and visual acuity before starting drug and yearly thereafter.

• Monitor patient for rash. If mild or moderate, treatment may continue. If severe, drug may be stopped or dose reduced. Patient also may need corticosteroids.

• Maintain adequate hydration for patients experiencing nausea and vomiting.

PATIENT TEACHING
• Tell patient to take drug at about the same time each day, on an empty stomach, 30 minutes before eating.

• Caution patient not to chew or swallow tablets.

• Instruct patient to dissolve tablets in water, orange juice, or apple juice; drink the mixture; swirl a small amount of the same liquid in the glass to pick up any remaining drug; and swallow that as well.

• Tell patient not to take aluminum-containing antacids at the same time as the drug.

• Inform patient of the need for regular blood tests to evaluate the effectiveness of therapy and detect possible side effects.

• Tell patient to report changes in hearing or vision, rash, abdominal pain, yellowing of skin or eyes, pale stools, or dark urine.

• Urge patient to avoid driving or operating hazardous equipment if he becomes dizzy.

SAFETY ALERT!

degarelix acetate
day-gah-REL-ix

Firmagon

D

Therapeutic class: Antineoplastics
Pharmacologic class: Gonadotropin-releasing hormone receptor antagonists
Pregnancy risk category: X

AVAILABLE FORMS
Injection: 80-mg, 120-mg vial

INDICATIONS & DOSAGES
➤ **Advanced prostate cancer**
Adult men: Initially, 240 mg subcutaneously, administered as two 120-mg injections. Maintenance dose is 80 mg subcutaneously every 28 days starting 28 days after first dose.

ADMINISTRATION
Subcutaneous
• To minimize exposure, always wear gloves when working with degarelix.

• Give drug within 1 hour of reconstitution.

• For 120-mg initial dose, draw up 3 mL sterile water for injection with a reconstitution needle (21G/2″). For 80-mg maintenance dose, draw up 4.2 mL sterile water for injection.

• Inject sterile water for injection slowly into degarelix 80-mg or 120-mg vial. To keep product and syringe sterile, don't remove syringe and needle.

• Keeping vial in an upright position, swirl it very gently until liquid looks clear and has no undissolved powder or particles. If powder adheres to vial over the liquid surface, vial can be tilted slightly to dissolve powder. Avoid shaking, to prevent foam formation. A ring of small air bubbles on surface of liquid is acceptable. The reconstitution procedure may take up to 15 minutes.

• Tilt vial slightly and keep needle in lowest part of vial. Withdraw 3 mL of degarelix 120 mg or 4.2 mL of degarelix 80 mg without turning vial upside down.

• Exchange reconstitution needle with administration needle for deep subcutaneous injection (27G/1¼″). Remove any air bubbles.

• Inject 3 mL degarelix 120 mg or 4.2 mL degarelix 80 mg subcutaneously immediately after reconstitution. Grasp skin of abdomen, and elevate subcutaneous tissue. Insert needle deeply at angle of not less than 45 degrees. Gently pull back plunger to check if blood is aspirated. If blood appears in syringe, reconstituted product can no longer be used. Discontinue procedure and discard syringe and needle. Reconstitute new dose.

• Repeat reconstitution procedure for second 120-mg initial dose. Choose different injection site and inject 3 mL.

ACTION

Reversibly binds to the pituitary GnRH receptors, reducing the release of gonadotropins, and consequently testosterone.

Route	Onset	Peak	Duration
Subcut.	Unknown	2 days	53 days

Half-life: About 53 days.

ADVERSE REACTIONS

CNS: asthenia, dizziness, fatigue, fever, headache, insomnia, nausea.
CV: hypertension, hot flashes.
GI: constipation, diarrhea.
GU: erectile dysfunction, UTI, testicular atrophy.
Metabolic: weight gain, increased GGT.
Musculoskeletal: arthralgia, back pain, decrease in bone density.
Skin: injection-site reactions (including pain, erythema, swelling, induration, and nodule formation), night sweats, hyperhidrosis.
Other: chills, gynecomastia.

INTERACTIONS

Drug-drug. *Class IA, Class III antiarrhythmics (such as amiodarone, procainamide, quinidine, sotalol):* May prolong QT interval. Avoid use together.

EFFECTS ON LAB TEST RESULTS

• May increase prostate-specific antigen (PSA), AST, ALT, and GGT levels.

CONTRAINDICATIONS & CAUTIONS

• Contraindicated in patients hypersensitive to drug or its components.
• Use cautiously in patients with congenital long QT syndrome, electrolyte abnormalities, or heart failure and in those taking Class IA or Class III antiarrhythmics.
• Use cautiously in patients with CrCl of less than 50 mL/minute or severe hepatic impairment.

NURSING CONSIDERATIONS

• Monitor QT interval in patients with congenital long QT syndrome, electrolyte abnormalities, or heart failure, and in those taking Class IA or Class III antiarrhythmics.
• Monitor PSA level; if level is elevated, monitor testosterone level.
• Monitor bone density tests periodically.
• Monitor LFT values.

PATIENT TEACHING

• Teach injection technique and methods of record-keeping to patient or family if they will be giving drug.
• Emphasize to patient the importance of notifying health care provider of heart problems, such as heart failure, irregular heart rhythm, or salt imbalance, before taking drug.
• Advise patient to inform all health care providers that he's taking drug.

delavirdine mesylate
dell-ah-VUR-den

Rescriptor

Therapeutic class: Antiretrovirals
Pharmacologic class: Nonnucleoside reverse transcriptase inhibitors
Pregnancy risk category: C

AVAILABLE FORMS
Tablets: 100 mg, 200 mg

INDICATIONS & DOSAGES
➤ **HIV-1 infection**
Adults and adolescents age 16 and older: 400 mg P.O. t.i.d. with other appropriate antiretrovirals.

Resistant virus emerges rapidly when delavirdine is administered as monotherapy.

Reactions in bold italics are *life-threatening*. Interactions may have a *rapid onset* or a *delayed onset.*

Always administer with appropriate antiretroviral therapy.

ADMINISTRATION
P.O.
● Patient may take drug with or without food.
● For patient with achlorhydria (absence of gastric acid in the stomach), drug should be taken with an acidic beverage, such as orange juice or cranberry juice.
● Patient should separate doses of delavirdine and antacid by at least 1 hour.
● Drug may be dispersed in water before ingestion. Add four 100-mg tablets to at least 3 ounces (90 mL) of water, allow to stand for a few minutes, and stir until a uniform dispersion occurs. Tell patient to drink dispersion promptly, rinse glass, and swallow the rinse to ensure that entire dose is consumed. Don't try to disperse 200-mg tablets because they don't disperse well; take 200-mg tablets intact.

ACTION
A nonnucleoside reverse transcriptase inhibitor of HIV-1 that binds directly to reverse transcriptase and blocks RNA- and DNA-dependent DNA polymerase activities.

Route	Onset	Peak	Duration
P.O.	Unknown	1 hr	Unknown

Half-life: 5¼ hours.

ADVERSE REACTIONS
CNS: asthenia, fatigue, headache, depression, fever, insomnia, pain.
EENT: pharyngitis, sinusitis.
GI: nausea, abdominal cramps, diarrhea, distention or pain, vomiting.
GU: epididymitis, hematuria, hemospermia, erectile dysfunction, metrorrhagia, nocturia, polyuria, proteinuria, renal calculi, renal pain, vaginal candidiasis.
Respiratory: bronchitis, cough, upper respiratory tract infection.
Skin: rash.
Other: flulike syndrome.

INTERACTIONS
Drug-drug. *Amphetamines, nonsedating antihistamines, benzodiazepines, calcium channel blockers, clarithromycin, dapsone, ergot alkaloid preparations, indinavir,*

rifabutin, sedative-hypnotics, warfarin: May increase or prolong therapeutic and adverse effects of these drugs. Avoid using together or, if use together is unavoidable, reduce doses of indinavir and clarithromycin.
Antacids: May reduce absorption of delavirdine. Separate doses by at least 1 hour.
Antiarrhythmics (amiodarone, bepridil, flecainide, lidocaine systemic, quinidine, propafenone): May increase risk of arrhythmias. Use cautiously and monitor drug levels if possible.
Carbamazepine, phenobarbital, phenytoin: May decrease delavirdine level. Use together cautiously.
Didanosine: May decrease absorption of both drugs by 20%. Separate doses by at least 1 hour.
Fluoxetine, ketoconazole: May cause a 50% increase in delavirdine bioavailability. Monitor patient and reduce dose of clarithromycin.
H₂-receptor antagonists: May increase gastric pH and reduce absorption of delavirdine. Long-term use together isn't recommended.
HMG-CoA reductase inhibitors, such as atorvastatin, lovastatin, simvastatin: May increase levels of these drugs, which increases risk of myopathy, including rhabdomyolysis. Avoid using together.
Rifabutin, rifampin: May decrease delavirdine level. May increase rifabutin level by 100%. Avoid using together.
Saquinavir: May increase bioavailability of saquinavir fivefold. Monitor AST and ALT levels frequently when used together.
Sildenafil: May increase sildenafil level and may increase sildenafil adverse events, including hypotension, visual changes, and priapism. Tell patient not to exceed 25 mg of sildenafil in 48 hours.
Drug-herb. *St. John's wort:* May decrease drug level. Discourage use together.

EFFECTS ON LAB TEST RESULTS
● May increase alkaline phosphatase, ALT, amylase, AST, CK, creatinine, GGT, and lipase levels. May decrease glucose and hemoglobin levels and hematocrit.
● May increase eosinophil count, PT, and PTT. May decrease granulocyte, neutrophil, platelet, RBC, and WBC counts.

CONTRAINDICATIONS & CAUTIONS
• Contraindicated in patients hypersensitive to drug or its components.
• Use cautiously in elderly patients and in patients with impaired hepatic function.

NURSING CONSIDERATIONS
• Because drug's effects in patients with hepatic or renal impairment haven't been studied, monitor renal and liver function test results carefully.
• Drug-induced diffuse, maculopapular, erythematous, pruritic rash occurs most commonly on upper body and arms of patients with lower CD4 cell counts, usually within first 3 weeks of treatment. Dosage adjustment doesn't seem to affect rash. Treat symptoms with diphenhydramine, hydroxyzine, or topical corticosteroids.
• Drug doesn't reduce risk of transmission of HIV-1.
• Monitor patient's fluid balance and weight.

PATIENT TEACHING
• Tell patient to stop drug and call prescriber if severe rash or such symptoms as fever, fatigue, headache, nausea, abdominal pain, or cough occur.
• Inform patient that drug doesn't cure HIV-1 infection and that he may continue to acquire illnesses, including opportunistic infections related to HIV-1 infection. Therapy hasn't been shown to reduce the risk or frequency of such illnesses. Drug hasn't been shown to reduce transmission of HIV.
• Advise patient to remain under medical supervision when taking drug because the long-term effects aren't known.
• Tell patient to take drug as prescribed and not to alter doses without prescriber's approval. If a dose is missed, tell patient to take the next dose as soon as possible; he shouldn't double the next dose.
• Inform patient that drug may be dispersed in water before ingestion. Add four 100-mg tablets to at least 3 ounces (90 mL) of water, allow to stand for a few minutes, and stir until a uniform dispersion occurs. Tell patient to drink dispersion promptly, rinse glass, and swallow the rinse to ensure that entire dose is consumed.

• Instruct patient to take 200-mg tablets whole; 200-mg tablets don't disperse well in water.
• Tell patient that drug may be taken with or without food.
• Tell patient with achlorhydria to take drug with an acidic beverage, such as orange or cranberry juice.
• Instruct patient to take drug and antacids at least 1 hour apart.
• Advise patient to report use of other prescription or nonprescription drugs, including herbal remedies.
• Advise patient taking sildenafil about an increased risk of sildenafil-related adverse events, including low blood pressure, visual changes, and painful penile erection. Tell him to promptly report any symptoms to his prescriber. Tell patient not to exceed 25 mg of sildenafil in 48 hours.

denosumab
deh-KNOW-sue-mab

Prolia, Xgeva

Therapeutic class: Antiosteoporotics–antiresorptives
Pharmacologic class: Monoclonal antibodies
Pregnancy risk category: X (Prolia), D (Xgeva)

AVAILABLE FORMS
Injection: 60-mg/mL prefilled syringe; 60-mg/mL, 70-mg/mL single-use vial

INDICATIONS & DOSAGES
➤ **Osteoporosis in men and post-menopausal women at risk for fracture (Prolia only)**
Adults: 60 mg subcutaneously every 6 months. All patients should receive 1,000 mg of calcium daily and at least 400 international units of vitamin D daily.
➤ **Bone metastases from solid tumors (Xgeva only)**
Adults: 120 mg subcutaneously every 4 weeks with calcium and vitamin D as necessary to prevent or treat hypocalcemia.
➤ **Increase bone mass in men at high risk for fracture who are receiving androgen**

Reactions in bold italics are *life-threatening*. Interactions may have a *rapid onset* or a *delayed onset*.

deprivation therapy for nonmetastatic prostate cancer and in women who are receiving adjuvant aromatase inhibitor therapy for breast cancer (Prolia only)

Adults: 60 mg subcutaneously in the upper arm, upper thigh, or abdomen once every 6 months. All patients should receive calcium 1,000 mg daily and at least 400 international units of vitamin D daily.

✳ *NEW INDICATION:* Giant cell tumor of bone (Xgeva only)

Adults: 120 mg subcutaneously every 4 weeks with additional 120-mg doses on days 8 and 15 of first month of therapy. Administer calcium and vitamin D as necessary to prevent or treat hypocalcemia.

ADMINISTRATION
Subcutaneous

• Don't use if solution is discolored or cloudy or contains many particles or foreign particulate matter.

• Before administration, drug may be removed from refrigerator and brought to room temperature (up to 77° F [25° C]) by letting stand in original container. This generally takes 15 to 30 minutes. Don't warm drug in any other way. Avoid vigorous shaking of drug.

• Use 27G needle to withdraw drug from single-use vial and inject entire contents of vial. Don't reenter vial.

• Administer via subcutaneous injection in upper arm, upper thigh, or abdomen.

ACTION

Inhibits osteoclast activity, thereby decreasing bone resorption and increasing bone mass and strength.

Route	Onset	Peak	Duration
Subcut.	Unknown	10 days	4–5 mo

Half-life: About 25 days.

ADVERSE REACTIONS

CNS: asthenia, insomnia, sciatica, vertigo.
CV: angina, atrial fibrillation, peripheral edema.
EENT: pharyngitis.
GI: flatulence, GERD, upper abdominal pain.
GU: cystitis.
Hematologic: anemia.

Metabolic: hypercholesterolemia, *hypocalcemia.*
Musculoskeletal: back pain, bone pain, extremity pain, musculoskeletal pain, myalgia, spinal osteoarthritis.
Respiratory: pneumonia, upper respiratory tract infection.
Skin: pruritus, rash.
Other: herpes zoster.

INTERACTIONS
None reported.

EFFECTS ON LAB TEST RESULTS
• May increase cholesterol level. May decrease calcium level.

CONTRAINDICATIONS & CAUTIONS

• Contraindicated in patients with hypocalcemia.

• Xgeva isn't for use in prevention of skeletal-related events due to multiple myeloma.

• Use cautiously in patients with history of hypoparathyroidism, thyroid surgery, parathyroid surgery, malabsorption syndromes, excision of small intestine, or severe renal impairment.

• Use cautiously in patients taking immunosuppressants and in those with an impaired immune system.

• Prolia and Xgeva are contraindicated in pregnant women. It isn't known if drug appears in breast milk. Because of risk of adverse effects, a decision should be made to discontinue either drug or breast-feeding.

NURSING CONSIDERATIONS

• Make sure patient has adequate intake of calcium and vitamin D.

• Monitor calcium, vitamin D, magnesium, and phosphorus levels before and during therapy.

• Drug may cause osteonecrosis of the jaw, which can occur spontaneously and is commonly associated with tooth extraction, local infection with delayed healing, or both.

• Consider stopping drug if severe skin reactions occur.

❸ *Alert:* Needle cap on single-use syringe contains latex; keep away from those with latex allergy.

⊙ Alert: Prolia and Xgeva contain the same active ingredient, denosumab. Patients receiving Prolia should not receive Xgeva.

PATIENT TEACHING

● Caution patient to read medication guide that comes with prescription before starting treatment and at every prescription refill.

● Warn patient to immediately report signs and symptoms of low calcium (spasms, twitching or muscle cramps, and numbness or tingling of fingers or toes or around mouth); emphasize the importance of maintaining normal calcium levels.

● Advise patient to have a dental exam before treatment and to follow good oral hygiene practices during therapy.

● Instruct patient that, before dental procedures, she should tell dentist that she is taking drug, and to inform dentist or prescriber if persistent pain or slow healing of mouth or jaw occurs after dental surgery.

● Tell patient to report jaw pain, swelling, or numbness; loose teeth; or dramatic gum loss.

● Advise patient to seek prompt medical care if signs and symptoms of severe infection occur, including cellulitis or skin reactions (such as dermatitis, rash, or eczema).

● Instruct patient with severe renal impairment about signs and symptoms of hypocalcemia and the importance of maintaining normal calcium levels.

● Tell patient to take calcium and vitamin D supplement, as directed by prescriber.

● Caution women who may become pregnant to use highly effective contraception during therapy and for at least 5 months after last dose of denosumab.

● Advise patient who becomes pregnant while taking Prolia to stop taking drug and contact her health care provider. Tell patient who becomes pregnant while taking Xgeva to consider the risks and benefits and to contact her health care provider. Advise pregnant women taking either Prolia or Xgeva to enroll in Amgen's Pregnancy Surveillance Program at 1-800-772-6436.

● Advise male patient taking denosumab who has a pregnant partner that denosumab may be present in seminal fluid and fetal exposure to the drug may occur during unprotected sexual intercourse.

desipramine hydrochloride
dess-IP-ra-meen

Norpramin

Therapeutic class: Antidepressants
Pharmacologic class: Tricyclic antidepressants
Pregnancy risk category: NR

AVAILABLE FORMS
Tablets: 10 mg, 25 mg, 50 mg, 75 mg, 100 mg, 150 mg

INDICATIONS & DOSAGES
➤ **Depression**
Adults: 100 to 200 mg P.O. daily in divided doses; increase to maximum of 300 mg daily. Or, give entire dose at bedtime.
Adolescents and elderly patients: 25 to 100 mg P.O. daily in divided doses; increase gradually to maximum of 150 mg daily, if needed.
➤ **Postherpetic neuralgia ◆**
Adults: Mean dose, 94 to 167 mg P.O. daily for at least 6 weeks.
➤ **Bulimia nervosa ◆**
Adults: 25 mg P.O. t.i.d. titrated to 200 to 300 mg/day depending on response and adverse effects.
➤ **Irritable bowel syndrome ◆**
Adults: 10 to 50 mg P.O. daily as maintenance dose. Initiate at low dose and titrate up based on response to therapy.

ADMINISTRATION
P.O.
● Give drug without regard for food.

ACTION
Unknown. Increases the amount of norepinephrine, serotonin, or both in the CNS by blocking their reuptake by the presynaptic neurons.

Route	Onset	Peak	Duration
P.O.	Unknown	4–6 hr	Unknown

Half-life: Unknown.

ADVERSE REACTIONS
CNS: drowsiness, dizziness, *seizures,* excitation, tremor, weakness, confusion, anxiety, restlessness, agitation, headache,

---

Reactions in bold italics are *life-threatening*. Interactions may have a *rapid onset* or a *delayed onset*.

nervousness, EEG changes, extrapyramidal reactions.
CV: tachycardia, orthostatic hypotension, ECG changes, hypertension.
EENT: blurred vision, tinnitus, mydriasis.
GI: dry mouth, constipation, nausea, vomiting, anorexia, paralytic ileus.
GU: urine retention.
Metabolic: *hypoglycemia,* hyperglycemia.
Skin: rash, urticaria, photosensitivity reactions, diaphoresis, alopecia.
Other: *sudden death in children,* hypersensitivity reactions.

INTERACTIONS
Drug-drug. *Barbiturates, CNS depressants:* May enhance CNS depression. Avoid using together.
Cimetidine, **fluoxetine, fluvoxamine, paroxetine, sertraline:** May increase desipramine level. Monitor drug levels and patient for signs of toxicity.
Clonidine: May cause life-threatening blood pressure elevations. Avoid using together.
Epinephrine, norepinephrine: May increase hypertensive effect. Use together cautiously.
Linezolid, methylene blue: May cause serotonin syndrome. Use with extreme caution and monitor closely.
MAO inhibitors: May cause severe excitation, hyperpyrexia, or seizures, usually with high doses. Avoid using within 14 days of MAO inhibitor therapy.
Quinolones: May increase the risk of life-threatening arrhythmias. Avoid using together.
Drug-herb. *Evening primrose oil:* May cause additive or synergistic effect, resulting in lower seizure threshold and increasing the risk of seizure. Discourage use together.
St. John's wort, *SAM-e, yohimbe:* May cause serotonin syndrome. Discourage use together.
Drug-lifestyle. *Alcohol use:* May enhance CNS depression. Discourage use together.
Smoking: May lower drug level. Monitor patient for lack of effect.
Sun exposure: May increase risk of photosensitivity reactions. Advise patient to avoid excessive sunlight exposure.

EFFECTS ON LAB TEST RESULTS
● May increase or decrease glucose level.
● May increase LFT values.

CONTRAINDICATIONS & CAUTIONS
● Contraindicated in patients hypersensitive to drug and in those who have taken MAO inhibitors within previous 14 days.
⊛ **Alert:** Concomitant use with linezolid or methylene blue can cause serotonin syndrome (fever, mental status changes, muscle twitching, excessive sweating, shivering or shaking, diarrhea, loss of coordination). Use with linezolid or methylene blue only for life-threatening or urgent conditions when the potential benefits outweigh the risks of toxicity.
● Contraindicated during acute recovery phase after MI.
Black Box Warning Desipramine isn't approved for use in children. ■
● Use with extreme caution in patients with CV disease; in those with a family history of sudden death, cardiac arrhythmias, or cardiac conduction disturbances; in those with history of urine retention, glaucoma, seizure disorders, or thyroid disease; and in those taking thyroid drug.
⊛ **Alert:** Treatment of patients who require as much as 300 mg desipramine should be initiated in hospitals where access to skilled health care providers and frequent ECGs is available. High doses may cause prolongation of the QRS or QT interval.
⚠ *Overdose S&S:* Cardiac arrhythmias, severe hypotension, seizures, CNS depression, coma, ECG changes, confusion, disturbed concentration, transient visual hallucinations, dilated pupils, agitation, hyperactive reflexes, stupor, drowsiness, muscle rigidity, vomiting, hypothermia, hyperpyrexia.

NURSING CONSIDERATIONS
⊛ **Alert:** Drug has been shown to lower the seizure threshold. Seizures precede cardiac arrhythmias and death in some patients.
● Monitor patient for nausea, headache, and malaise after abrupt withdrawal of long-term therapy; these symptoms don't indicate addiction.
● Don't withdraw drug abruptly.

• Because patients may suffer hypertensive episodes during surgery, stop drug gradually several days before surgery.

❸ Alert: If linezolid or methylene blue must be given, stop drug and monitor the patient for serotonin toxicity for 2 weeks or until 24 hours after the last dose of methylene blue or linezolid, whichever comes first. Treatment may be resumed 24 hours after last dose of methylene blue or linezolid.

• If signs or symptoms of psychosis occur or increase, notify prescriber. Record mood changes. Monitor patient for suicidal tendencies.

Black Box Warning Drug may increase risk of suicidal thinking and behavior in children, adolescents, and young adults ages 18 to 24, especially during the first few months of treatment, especially in those with major depressive disorder or other psychiatric disorder. ∎

• Recommend sugarless hard candy or gum to relieve dry mouth. Saliva substitutes may be needed.

❸ Alert: Norpramin may contain tartrazine.

• **Look alike–sound alike:** Don't confuse desipramine with disopyramide or imipramine.

PATIENT TEACHING

Black Box Warning Advise families and caregivers to observe patient closely for increased suicidal thinking and behavior. ∎

• Advise patient to take full dose at bedtime to avoid daytime sedation; if insomnia occurs, tell him to take drug in the morning.

• Warn patient to avoid hazardous activities that require alertness and good coordination until effects of drug are known. Drowsiness and dizziness usually subside after a few weeks.

❸ Alert: Teach patient to recognize and immediately report symptoms of serotonin toxicity (fever, mental status changes, muscle twitching, excessive sweating, shivering or shaking, diarrhea, loss of coordination).

• Advise patient to call prescriber if fever and sore throat occur. Blood counts may need to be obtained.

• Tell patient to avoid alcohol during therapy because it may antagonize effects of drug.

• Tell patient to consult prescriber before taking other prescription or OTC drugs.

• Warn patient not to stop drug suddenly.

• To prevent sensitivity to the sun, advise patient to use sunblock, wear protective clothing, and avoid prolonged exposure to strong sunlight.

SAFETY ALERT!

desirudin
deh-SIHR-uh-din

Iprivask

Therapeutic class: Anticoagulants
Pharmacologic class: Thrombin inhibitors
Pregnancy risk category: C

AVAILABLE FORMS
Injection: 15 mg desirudin lyophilized powder and 0.6 mL mannitol (3%) diluent

INDICATIONS & DOSAGES
➤ **To prevent deep vein thrombosis in patients undergoing hip replacement surgery**
Adults: 15 mg subcutaneously every 12 hours for 9 to 12 days. Give first injection 5 to 15 minutes before surgery, after induction of regional block anesthesia, if used.
Adjust-a-dose: If CrCl is 31 to 60 mL/minute, give 5 mg subcutaneously every 12 hours. If CrCl is less than 31 mL/minute, give 1.7 mg subcutaneously every 12 hours. Check activated PTT (aPTT) and creatinine daily. If aPTT exceeds two times control, stop therapy until it's within two times control; then resume at a reduced dose.

ADMINISTRATION
Subcutaneous
• Reconstitute each 15-mg vial with 0.5 mL of provided diluent (mannitol 3%).
• Shake vial gently until powder is dissolved. Once reconstituted, each 0.5 mL contains 15.75 mg of desirudin.
• Inspect vial. If solution contains visible particles, don't use it.
• Use reconstituted solution immediately or store it at room temperature for up to 24 hours protected from light.

Reactions in bold italics are *life-threatening*. Interactions may have a *rapid onset* or a *delayed onset*.

• Use a syringe with a ½″ 26G or 27G needle to withdraw all the reconstituted solution.

• With the patient lying down, inject entire contents of syringe by deep subcutaneous injection. Insert entire length of needle into a skinfold held between thumb and forefinger.

• Rotate sites between the right and left thigh or right and left anterolateral and posterolateral abdominal walls.

• **Incompatibilities:** Don't mix with any other drugs.

ACTION

Selectively inhibits free and clot-bound thrombin, which prolongs plasma clotting time.

Route	Onset	Peak	Duration
Subcut.	30 min	60–180 min	Unknown

Half-life: 2 to 3 hours.

ADVERSE REACTIONS

CNS: cerebrovascular disorder, dizziness, fever.
CV: *thrombosis,* deep thrombophlebitis, hypotension.
EENT: epistaxis.
GI: *hematemesis,* nausea, vomiting.
GU: hematuria.
Hematologic: *hemorrhage,* anemia.
Other: *anaphylaxis,* impaired healing, injection-site mass, leg edema, leg pain, wound seeping.

INTERACTIONS

Drug-drug. *Abciximab, aspirin, clopidogrel, dipyridamole, glycoprotein IIb/IIIa antagonists, ketorolac, salicylates, sulfinpyrazone, ticlopidine:* May increase the risk of bleeding. Use together cautiously.
Anticoagulants, dextran 40, glucocorticoids, thrombolytics: May increase the risk of bleeding. Avoid using together.
Drug-herb. *Alfalfa, angelica (dong quai), anise, boldo, bromelains, capsicum, chamomile, dandelion, danshen, devil's claw, fenugreek, feverfew, garlic, ginger, ginkgo, ginseng, horse chestnut, licorice, meadowsweet, onion, passion flower, red clover, willow:* May increase the risk of bleeding. Discourage use together.

EFFECTS ON LAB TEST RESULTS

• May decrease hemoglobin level and hematocrit.

CONTRAINDICATIONS & CAUTIONS

• Contraindicated in patients hypersensitive to natural or recombinant hirudins and in patients with active bleeding or irreversible coagulation disorders.

• Use cautiously in patients with a CrCl less than 60 mL/minute; patients undergoing spinal or epidural anesthesia; patients with hepatic insufficiency or injury; patients with GI or pulmonary bleeding within 3 months; patients with severe uncontrolled hypertension, bacterial endocarditis, or a hemostatic disorder; and patients with an increased risk of bleeding, such as those with recent major surgery, organ biopsy, puncture of a noncompressible vessel (within 1 month), intracranial or intraocular bleeding, or hemorrhagic or ischemic stroke.

⚠ Overdose S&S: Hemorrhagic complications, excessively high aPTT values.

NURSING CONSIDERATIONS

• Don't give this drug I.M.

⊙ Alert: If the patient has either an unexplained decline in hematocrit or blood pressure or other unexplained symptoms, consider the possibility of hemorrhage.

• Monitor coagulation tests, hemoglobin level, hematocrit, and renal function throughout therapy.

• Watch venipuncture sites for bleeding, hematoma, or inflammation.

Black Box Warning Patients who receive epidural or spinal anesthesia or spinal puncture are at increased risk of an epidural or spinal hematoma, which may result in long-term or permanent paralysis. Monitor these patients closely for neurologic impairment. ∎

PATIENT TEACHING

• Advise patient that this drug can cause bleeding. Stress the need to report unusual bruising or bleeding (nosebleeds, blood in urine, tarry stools) immediately.

• Caution patient not to take any other drugs that increase the risk of bleeding, such as aspirin or NSAIDs, while receiving desirudin.

• Advise patient to consult with prescriber before starting any herbal therapy; many herbs have anticoagulant, antiplatelet, or fibrinolytic properties.

• Advise against activities that risk injury.

• Tell patient to use a soft toothbrush and electric razor during therapy.

desloratadine
dess-lor-AT-a-deen

Clarinex✔, Clarinex RediTabs

Therapeutic class: Antihistamines
Pharmacologic class: Piperidines
Pregnancy risk category: C

AVAILABLE FORMS
Syrup: 0.5 mg/mL
Tablets: 5 mg
Tablets (orally disintegrating): 2.5 mg, 5 mg

INDICATIONS & DOSAGES
➤ **Seasonal allergic rhinitis (patients age 2 and older); perennial allergic rhinitis and chronic idiopathic urticaria (patients age 6 months and older)**
Adults and children age 12 and older: 5 mg P.O. tablets or syrup once daily.
Children ages 6 to 11: 2.5 mg orally disintegrating tablet (ODT) or syrup P.O. once daily.
Children ages 12 months to 5 years: 1.25 mg P.O. once daily.
Infants ages 6 to 11 months: 1 mg P.O. once daily.
Adjust-a-dose: In adults with hepatic or renal impairment, start dosage at 5 mg P.O. every other day.

ADMINISTRATION
P.O.
• Give drug without regard for meals.
• Place ODTs on tongue immediately after opening blister pack.
• Give ODTs with or without water.

ACTION
Long-acting tricyclic antihistamine with selective H_1-receptor antagonist activity. It inhibits histamine release from human mast cells in vitro.

Route	Onset	Peak	Duration
P.O.	<1 hr	3 hr	Up to 24 hr
P.O. (orally disintegrating)	<1 hr	2½–4 hr	Up to 24 hr

Half-life: 27 hours.

ADVERSE REACTIONS
CNS: headache, somnolence, fatigue, dizziness.
EENT: pharyngitis, dry throat.
GI: nausea, dry mouth, dyspepsia.
GU: dysmenorrhea.
Musculoskeletal: myalgia.

INTERACTIONS
None reported.

EFFECTS ON LAB TEST RESULTS
• May prevent, reduce, or mask positive result in diagnostic skin test.

CONTRAINDICATIONS & CAUTIONS
• Contraindicated in breast-feeding women and in patients hypersensitive to drug, to any of its components, or to loratadine.
• Use cautiously in elderly patients because of the greater likelihood of decreased hepatic, renal, or cardiac function and concomitant disease or other drug therapy.
⚠ *Overdose S&S:* Somnolence, increased QTc interval.

NURSING CONSIDERATIONS
• Stop drug 4 days before diagnostic skin testing because antihistamines can prevent, reduce, or mask positive skin test response.

PATIENT TEACHING
• Advise patient not to exceed recommended dosage. Higher doses don't increase effectiveness and may cause somnolence.
• Tell patient that drug can be taken without regard to meals.
• Instruct patient to remove ODTs from blister pack and place on tongue immediately to dissolve.

Reactions in bold italics are *life-threatening*. Interactions may have a *rapid onset* or a *delayed onset*.

- ODTs may be taken with or without water.
- Tell patient to report adverse effects.

desmopressin acetate
des-moe-PRESS-in

DDAVP, Minirin, Stimate

Therapeutic class: Hemostatics
Pharmacologic class: Posterior pituitary hormones
Pregnancy risk category: B

AVAILABLE FORMS
Injection: 4 mcg/mL
Metered nasal spray: 10 mcg/spray, 150 mg/spray
Nasal solution: 0.1 mg/mL, 1.5 mg/mL
Tablets: 0.1 mg, 0.2 mg

INDICATIONS & DOSAGES
➤ **Nonnephrogenic diabetes insipidus, temporary polyuria, and polydipsia related to pituitary trauma**
Intranasal, I.V., or subcutaneous
Adults and children older than age 12: 0.1 to 0.4 mL (10 to 40 mcg) intranasally daily in one to three doses. Most adults need 0.2 mL (20 mcg) daily in two divided doses. Or, give 0.5 to 1 mL (2 to 4 mcg) I.V. or subcutaneously daily, usually in two divided doses.
P.O.
Adults and children older than age 4: Initially, 0.05 mg (half of the 0.1-mg tablet) P.O. b.i.d.; adjust dosage to patient response. If patient previously received the drug intranasally, begin oral therapy 12 hours after last intranasal dose. Maximum dose is 1.2 mg/day for patients with diabetes insipidus.
Intranasal
Children ages 3 months to 12 years: 0.05 to 0.3 mL (5 to 30 mcg) intranasally daily in one or two doses.
➤ **Hemophilia A and von Willebrand disease**
Adults and children: 0.3 mcg/kg diluted in normal saline solution and infused I.V. over 15 to 30 minutes. Repeat dose, if needed, as indicated by laboratory response and patient's condition. If used preoperatively,

give 30 minutes prior to the scheduled procedure. Or, 300 mcg (one spray in each nostril) of solution containing 1.5 mcg/mL. Dose of 150 mcg (one spray of solution containing 1.5 mg/mL into a single nostril) may be adequate for patients weighing less than 50 kg (110 lb). Give drug 2 hours before surgery.
➤ **Primary nocturnal enuresis**
Adults and children age 6 and older: Initially, 0.2 mg P.O. at bedtime, and adjust dose up to 0.6 mg to achieve desired response.

ADMINISTRATION
P.O.
- Discontinue in patient with acute illness that may result in fluid or electrolyte imbalance.
- Store at controlled room temperature.
I.V.
▼ Don't give injection to patients with hemophilia A with factor VIII of up to 5% or with severe von Willebrand disease.
▼ For adults and children weighing more than 10 kg (22 lb), dilute with 50 mL sterile physiologic saline solution. For children weighing 10 kg or less, 10 mL of diluent is recommended.
▼ Inspect drug for particulates and discoloration before infusing.
▼ Monitor blood pressure and pulse during infusion.
▼ The comparable antidiuretic dose of the injection is about one-tenth of the intranasal dose.
▼ **Incompatibilities:** None reported.
Intranasal
- Ensure nasal passages are intact, clean, and free of obstruction before giving intranasally.
- Nasal spray pump delivers only doses of 10 mcg DDAVP or 150 mcg Stimate. If doses other than those are required, use the nasal tube delivery system or injection.
Subcutaneous
- Teach patient to rotate injection sites to prevent tissue damage.

ACTION
Increases the permeability of renal tubular epithelium to adenosine monophosphate and water, enabling the epithelium to

promote reabsorption of water and produce a concentrated urine. Also increases factor VIII activity by releasing endogenous factor VIII from plasma storage sites.

Route	Onset	Peak	Duration
P.O.	1 hr	1–1½ hr	8–12 hr
I.V.	15–30 min	1½–2 hr	4–12 hr
Intranasal	1 hr	1–5 hr	8–12 hr
Subcut.	Unknown	Unknown	Unknown

Half-life: Oral, 1.5 to 2.5 hours; I.V. and intranasal, 7.8 minutes (initial phase) and 75.5 minutes (terminal phase).

ADVERSE REACTIONS

CNS: headache, *seizures.*
CV: flushing, slight rise in blood pressure.
EENT: rhinitis, epistaxis, sore throat.
GI: nausea, abdominal cramps.
GU: vulvar pain.
Metabolic: hyponatremia.
Respiratory: cough.
Skin: local erythema, swelling, or burning after injection.

INTERACTIONS

Drug-drug. *Carbamazepine, chlorpropamide:* May increase ADH; may increase desmopressin effect. Avoid using together.
Clofibrate: May enhance and prolong effects of desmopressin. Monitor patient closely.
Demeclocycline, epinephrine, heparin, lithium: May increase risk of adverse effects. Monitor patient closely.
Pressor agents: May enhance pressor effects with large doses of desmopressin. Monitor patient closely.
Drug-lifestyle. *Alcohol use:* May increase risk of adverse effects. Discourage use together.

EFFECTS ON LAB TEST RESULTS

● May decrease sodium level.

CONTRAINDICATIONS & CAUTIONS

● Contraindicated in patients hypersensitive to drug and in those with type IIB von Willebrand disease, moderate to severe renal impairment, or hyponatremia.
● Use cautiously in patients with coronary artery insufficiency, hypertensive CV disease, and conditions linked to fluid and electrolyte imbalances, such as cystic fibrosis, because these patients are susceptible to hyponatremia.
● Use cautiously in patients at risk for water intoxication with hyponatremia.
● Use cautiously in breast-feeding women; it's unknown if drug appears in breast milk.
⚠ Overdose S&S: Confusion, drowsiness, continuing headache, problems passing urine, rapid weight gain due to fluid retention.

NURSING CONSIDERATIONS

● Morning and evening doses are adjusted separately for adequate diurnal rhythm of water turnover.
● Intranasal use can cause changes in the nasal mucosa, resulting in erratic, unreliable absorption. Report worsening condition to prescriber, who may recommend injectable DDAVP.
● Restrict fluid intake to reduce risk of water intoxication and sodium depletion, especially in children or elderly patients.
◆ Alert: Overdose may cause oxytocic or vasopressor activity. Withhold drug and notify prescriber. If fluid retention is excessive, give furosemide.
● **Look alike–sound alike:** Don't confuse desmopressin with vasopressin.

PATIENT TEACHING

● Some patients may have trouble measuring and inhaling drug into nostrils. Teach patient and caregivers correct administration method.
● Instruct patient to clear nasal passages before giving drug.
● Instruct patient to press down four times to prime pump. Tell him to discard the bottle after 25 (150 mcg/spray) or 50 doses (10 mcg/spray), depending on the strength, because the amount left may be less than desired dose.
● Advise patient to report nasal congestion, allergic rhinitis, or upper respiratory tract infection to prescriber; dosage adjustment may be needed.
● Teach patient using subcutaneous drug to rotate injection sites to prevent tissue damage.
● Warn patient to drink only enough water to satisfy thirst.

Reactions in bold italics are *life-threatening*. Interactions may have a *rapid onset* or a *delayed onset*.

- Inform patient with hemophilia A or von Willebrand disease that taking desmopressin may prevent hazards of using blood products.
- Advise patient to carry medical identification indicating use of drug.

desoximetasone
dess-OX-ee-MET-ah-sone

Topicort

Therapeutic class: Corticosteroids
Pharmacologic class: Corticosteroids
Pregnancy risk category: C

AVAILABLE FORMS
Cream: 0.05%, 0.25%
Gel: 0.05%*
Ointment: 0.05%, 0.25%
Spray: 0.25%

INDICATIONS & DOSAGES
➤ **Inflammation from corticosteroid-responsive dermatoses**
Adults and children: Clean area; apply a thin film and rub in gently b.i.d. Don't use ointment on children younger than age 10.
✱ *NEW INDICATION:* **Plaque psoriasis (spray only)**
Adults: Apply a thin film to affected areas and rub in gently b.i.d. Treatment beyond 4 weeks isn't recommended.

ADMINISTRATION
Topical
- Gently wash skin before applying. To prevent skin damage, rub in gently, leaving thin coat. When treating hairy sites, part hair and apply directly to lesions.
- Avoid applying near eyes, mucous membranes, or in ear canal.
- **Alert:** Don't bandage, cover, or wrap the treated skin area unless ordered.
- Stop drug and notify prescriber if skin infection, striae, or atrophy occur.
- Continue drug for a few days after lesions clear.
- Avoid using spray on face, axilla, or groin or if atrophy is present.

ACTION
Unclear. Diffuses across cell membranes to form complexes with receptors, showing anti-inflammatory, antipruritic, vasoconstrictive, and antiproliferative activity.

Route	Onset	Peak	Duration
Topical	Unknown	Unknown	Unknown

Half-life: Unknown.

ADVERSE REACTIONS
GU: glycosuria.
Metabolic: hyperglycemia.
Skin: burning, pruritus, irritation, dryness, erythema, folliculitis, hypertrichosis, acneiform eruptions, perioral dermatitis, hypopigmentation, allergic contact dermatitis, maceration, secondary infection, atrophy, striae, miliaria with occlusive dressings.
Other: *hypothalamic-pituitary-adrenal (HPA) axis suppression,* Cushing syndrome.

INTERACTIONS
None significant.

EFFECTS ON LAB TEST RESULTS
- May increase glucose level.

CONTRAINDICATIONS & CAUTIONS
- Contraindicated in patients hypersensitive to drug or its components.
- Don't use as monotherapy in primary bacterial infections (impetigo, paronychia, erysipelas, cellulitis, angular cheilitis), treatment of rosacea, perioral dermatitis, or acne.
- Don't use very-high-potency or high-potency agents on the face, groin, or axillae.
- Drug isn't for ophthalmic use.
- Use cautiously in children and pregnant or breast-feeding women. Spray isn't recommended for use in children.
⚠ Overdose S&S: Systemic effects.

NURSING CONSIDERATIONS
- If fever develops and occlusive dressing is in place, notify prescriber and remove occlusive dressing.
- If antifungal or antibiotic combined with corticosteroid fails to provide prompt improvement, stop corticosteroid until infection is controlled.

• Systemic absorption is likely with use of occlusive dressings, prolonged treatment, or extensive body surface treatment. Watch for symptoms of HPA axis suppression, Cushing syndrome, hyperglycemia, and glycosuria.

• Avoid using plastic pants or tight-fitting diapers on treated areas in young children. Children may absorb larger amounts of drug and be more susceptible to systemic toxicity.

• Gel contains alcohol and may cause burning or irritation in open lesions.

• **Look alike–sound alike:** Don't confuse desoximetasone with dexamethasone.

PATIENT TEACHING
• Teach patient how to apply drug.
• Tell patient this drug is for external use only and to avoid contact with the eyes.
• If an occlusive dressing is ordered, advise patient to leave it in place for no longer than 12 hours each day and not to use the dressing on infected or weeping lesions.
• Tell patient to stop drug and report signs of systemic absorption, skin irritation or ulceration, hypersensitivity, or infection.

desvenlafaxine succinate
des-ven-lah-FAX-in

Pristiq

Therapeutic class: Antidepressants
Pharmacologic class: SSNRIs
Pregnancy risk category: C

AVAILABLE FORMS
Tablets (extended-release): 50 mg, 100 mg

INDICATIONS & DOSAGES
➤ **Major depressive disorder**
Adults: 50 mg P.O. once daily.
Adjust-a-dose: For patients with CrCl less than 30 mL/minute, give 50 mg P.O. every other day. Don't give supplemental doses after dialysis. For patients with hepatic impairment, maximum dosage is 100 mg/day.

ADMINISTRATION
P.O.
• Administer at approximately the same time each day with or without food.

• Patient must swallow tablets whole with fluid and not divide, crush, chew, or dissolve them.

ACTION
Thought to stimulate receptors, increasing the release of serotonin and norepinephrine.

Route	Onset	Peak	Duration
P.O.	Unknown	7½ hr	Unknown

Half-life: About 11 hours.

ADVERSE REACTIONS
CNS: abnormal dreams, anxiety, asthenia, chills, dizziness, fatigue, jittery feeling, headache, insomnia, irritability, paresthesia, somnolence, tremor.
CV: hot flashes, hypertension, palpitations, tachycardia.
EENT: blurred vision, mydriasis, tinnitus.
GI: constipation, diarrhea, dry mouth, dysgeusia, *GI bleeding,* nausea, vomiting.
GU: proteinuria.
Metabolic: decreased appetite, weight loss.
Skin: hyperhidrosis, rash.
Other: sexual dysfunction, yawning.

INTERACTIONS
Drug-drug. *Aspirin, NSAIDs, warfarin, other drugs that affect coagulation:* May increase risk of bleeding. Use together cautiously.
CNS drugs: Drug may cause additive effect. Avoid using together.
CYP3A4 inhibitors (ketoconazole): May increase desvenlafaxine levels. Use together cautiously.
Desipramine, other drugs metabolized by CYP2D6: May increase levels of these drugs. Use together cautiously.
Linezolid, methylene blue: May cause serotonin syndrome. Use with extreme caution and monitor closely.
MAO inhibitors: May cause serotonin syndrome or signs and symptoms resembling neuroleptic malignant syndrome. Avoid using within 7 days of MAO inhibitor therapy.
Midazolam, other drugs metabolized by CYP3A4: May decrease levels of these drugs. Use together cautiously.
SSNRIs, SSRIs: May increase risk of serotonin syndrome. Monitor patient closely if used together.

Reactions in bold italics are *life-threatening*. Interactions may have a *rapid onset* or a *delayed onset*.

Venlafaxine: Drug is a major active metabolite of venlafaxine. Avoid using together.
Drug-lifestyle. *Alcohol use:* May enhance CNS depression. Discourage use together.

EFFECTS ON LAB TEST RESULTS
● May increase total cholesterol, LDL, triglyceride, and sodium levels.

CONTRAINDICATIONS & CAUTIONS
● Contraindicated in patients hypersensitive to drug or within 14 days of MAO inhibitor therapy.
◆ **Alert:** Concomitant use with linezolid or methylene blue can cause serotonin syndrome (fever, mental status changes, muscle twitching, excessive sweating, shivering or shaking, diarrhea, loss of coordination). Use with linezolid or methylene blue only for life-threatening or urgent conditions when the potential benefits outweigh the risks of toxicity.
● Use cautiously in elderly patients and in patients with renal impairment, diseases or conditions that could affect hemodynamic responses or metabolism, and in those with a history of mania or seizures. Use only in pregnant or breast-feeding women when the benefits outweigh the possible risks to the fetus.
Black Box Warning Desvenlafaxine isn't approved for use in children. ■
⚠ **Overdose S&S:** Headache, vomiting, agitation, dizziness, nausea, constipation, diarrhea, dry mouth, paresthesia, tachycardia, change in level of consciousness, mydriasis, seizures, ECG changes.

NURSING CONSIDERATIONS
Black Box Warning Closely monitor patient being treated for depression for signs and symptoms of clinical worsening and suicidal ideation, especially at the beginning of therapy and with dosage adjustments. Symptoms may include agitation, insomnia, anxiety, aggressiveness, or panic attacks. ■
◆ **Alert:** If linezolid or methylene blue must be given, stop drug and monitor the patient for serotonin toxicity for 7 days, or until 24 hours after the last dose of methylene blue or linezolid, whichever comes first. Treatment may be resumed 24 hours after last dose of methylene blue or linezolid.

● Carefully monitor blood pressure. Drug may cause dose-related increases in blood pressure.
● Monitor intraocular pressure in patients at risk for angle-closure glaucoma.
● Record mood changes. Monitor patient for suicidal tendencies and allow patient only a minimum supply of the drug.
● Monitor patient for signs and symptoms of bleeding.
● Monitor lipid and sodium levels before and during therapy.
◆ **Alert:** Don't stop drug abruptly. Withdrawal or discontinuation syndrome may occur if drug is stopped abruptly. Signs and symptoms of withdrawal syndrome include dizziness, nausea, headache, irritability, insomnia, diarrhea, anxiety, fatigue, abnormal dreams, and hyperhidrosis. Taper drug slowly.
● Monitor respiratory status. Drug may cause interstitial lung disease or eosinophilic pneumonia. If patient develops dyspnea, cough, or chest discomfort, discontinue drug.

PATIENT TEACHING
● Advise a woman of childbearing age to contact prescriber if she becomes pregnant, intends to become pregnant during therapy, or is breast-feeding.
Black Box Warning Warn family members to closely monitor patient for signs and symptoms of worsening condition or suicidal ideation. ■
◆ **Alert:** Teach patient to recognize and immediately report symptoms of serotonin toxicity (fever, mental status changes, muscle twitching, excessive sweating, shivering or shaking, diarrhea, loss of coordination).
● Tell patient to avoid alcohol and to consult prescriber before taking other prescription or OTC drugs.
● Warn patient to avoid hazardous activities that require alertness and good coordination until effects of drug are known.
● If medication is to be stopped, tell patient to stop drug gradually by tapering the dosage as instructed by prescriber and not to abruptly stop taking drug.
● Tell patient not to divide, crush, chew, or dissolve tablets.

D

dexamethasone (ophthalmic)
dex-a-METH-a-sone

Maxidex, Ozurdex

Therapeutic class: Anti-inflammatory drugs (ophthalmic)
Pharmacologic class: Corticosteroids
Pregnancy risk category: C

AVAILABLE FORMS
Intraocular implant: 0.7 mg
Ophthalmic suspension: 0.1%

INDICATIONS & DOSAGES
➤ **Uveitis; iridocyclitis; inflammatory conditions of eyelids, conjunctiva, cornea, and anterior segment of globe; corneal injury from chemical or thermal burns or penetration of foreign bodies; allergic conjunctivitis; suppression of graft rejection after keratoplasty; acne rosacea**
Adults and children: Initially, 1 or 2 drops of solution into conjunctival sac every 1 to 2 hours. Decrease to 1 drop every 4 hours when favorable response is noted. As condition improves, taper to 1 drop t.i.d. or q.i.d. to control symptoms, then to b.i.d., then once daily. Treatment may extend from a few days to several weeks. Or, give 1 or 2 drops of suspension in the conjunctival sac. In severe disease, drops may be used hourly, being tapered to discontinuation as inflammation subsides. In mild disease, drops may be used up to six times daily.
➤ **Macular edema; posterior-segment uveitis**
Adults: 1 implant (0.7 mg) injected intravitreally into each affected eye.

ADMINISTRATION
Ophthalmic
• Shake suspension well before use.
• Apply light finger pressure on lacrimal sac for 1 minute after instillation.
• Implant should be injected under controlled aseptic conditions, with adequate anesthesia and administration of a broad-spectrum microbicide.

ACTION
Suppresses edema, fibrin deposition, capillary dilation, leukocyte migration, capillary proliferation, and collagen deposition.

Route	Onset	Peak	Duration
Ophthalmic	Unknown	Unknown	Unknown

Half-life: Unknown.

ADVERSE REACTIONS
EENT: burning, stinging, or red eyes; cataracts, corneal ulceration, defects in visual acuity and visual field, discharge, discomfort, dry eyes, foreign body sensation, glaucoma worsening, increased intraocular pressure (IOP), increased susceptibility to viral or fungal corneal infection, interference with corneal wound healing, mild blurred vision, optic nerve damage with excessive or long-term use, ocular pain, photophobia, thinning of cornea.
Other: adrenal suppression with excessive or long-term use, systemic effects.

INTERACTIONS
None significant.

EFFECTS ON LAB TEST RESULTS
None reported.

CONTRAINDICATIONS & CAUTIONS
• Contraindicated in patients hypersensitive to drug or its ingredients. Drug contains sulfite.
• Contraindicated in those with ocular tuberculosis or acute superficial herpes simplex (dendritic keratitis), vaccinia, varicella, or other fungal or viral diseases of cornea and conjunctiva; in patients with acute, purulent, untreated infections of eye; and in those who have had uncomplicated removal of superficial corneal foreign body. Ocular implant is also contraindicated in patients with advanced glaucoma.
• Use cautiously in patients with corneal abrasions that may be infected (especially with herpes).
• Use cautiously in patients with glaucoma (any form) because IOP may increase. Dosage of glaucoma drugs may need to be increased to compensate.
• Safe use in pregnant and breast-feeding women hasn't been established.

NURSING CONSIDERATIONS
- Drug isn't for long-term use.
- Watch for corneal ulceration, which may require stopping drug.
- Corneal viral and fungal infections may be worsened by corticosteroid application.
- After injection of implant, monitor patient for elevated IOP and endophthalmitis.
- **Look alike–sound alike:** Don't confuse dexamethasone with desoximetasone. Don't confuse Maxidex with Maxzide.

PATIENT TEACHING
- Tell patient to shake suspension well before use.
- Teach patient how to instill drops. Advise him to wash hands before and after applying solution, and warn him not to touch tip of dropper to eye or surrounding tissue.
- Tell patient to apply light finger pressure on lacrimal sac for 1 minute after instillation.
- Advise patient that he may use eye pad with ointment.
- Warn patient not to use leftover drug for new eye inflammation; doing so may cause serious problems.
- **❸ Alert:** Warn patient to call prescriber immediately and to stop drug if visual acuity changes or visual field diminishes.
- Tell patient not to share drug, washcloths, or towels with family members and to notify prescriber if anyone develops same signs or symptoms.
- Stress importance of compliance with recommended therapy.
- Tell patient who wears contact lenses to check with prescriber before using lenses again.

D

dexamethasone (oral; injection)
dex-a-METH-a-sone

Dexamethasone Intensol*, Dexpak

dexamethasone sodium phosphate (injection)

Therapeutic class: Corticosteroids
Pharmacologic class: Glucocorticoids
Pregnancy risk category: C

AVAILABLE FORMS
dexamethasone
Elixir: 0.5 mg/5 mL*
Oral concentrate: 1 mg/mL
Oral solution: 0.5 mg/5 mL, 0.5 mg/0.5 mL*
Tablets: 0.5 mg, 0.75 mg, 1 mg, 1.5 mg, 2 mg, 4 mg, 6 mg
dexamethasone sodium phosphate
Injection: 4 mg/mL, 10 mg/mL

INDICATIONS & DOSAGES
➤ **Cerebral edema**
Adults: Initially, 10 mg phosphate I.V.; then 4 mg I.M. every 6 hours until symptoms subside (usually 2 to 4 days); then taper over 5 to 7 days. Oral therapy (1 to 3 mg t.i.d.) should replace I.M. dosing as soon as possible.
➤ **Palliative management of recurrent or inoperable brain tumors**
Adults: 2 mg I.M. or I.V. b.i.d. to t.i.d. for maintenance therapy.
➤ **Inflammatory conditions, neoplasias**
Adults: 0.75 to 9 mg/day P.O. or 0.5 to 9 mg/day phosphate I.M., depending on size and location of affected area.
➤ **Acute, self-limited allergic disorders; acute exacerbations of chronic allergic disorders**
Adults: On day one, give 4 or 8 mg I.M. (using 4 mg/mL preparation). On days two and three, give four 0.75-mg tablets P.O. in two divided doses. On day four, give two 0.75-mg tablets P.O. in two divided doses. On days five and six, give one 0.75-mg tablet P.O. A follow-up visit should take place on day eight.
➤ **Shock**
Adults: 20 mg phosphate as single first dose; then 3 mg/kg/24 hours via continuous I.V.

infusion. Or, 1 to 6 mg/kg phosphate I.V. as single dose. Or, 40 mg phosphate I.V. every 2 to 6 hours, as needed, continued only until patient is stabilized (usually not longer than 48 to 72 hours).

➤ **Dexamethasone suppression test for Cushing syndrome**
Adults: Determine baseline 24-hour urine levels of 17-hydroxycorticosteroids; then, give 0.5 mg P.O. every 6 hours for 48 hours. Repeat 24-hour urine collection to determine 17-hydroxycorticosteroid excretion during second 24 hours of dexamethasone administration. Or, 1 mg P.O. as single dose at 11:00 p.m. with determination of plasma cortisol at 8 a.m. the next morning.

➤ **Adrenocortical insufficiency**
Children: 0.02 to 0.3 mg/kg or 0.6 to 9 mg/m^2 P.O. daily, in three or four divided doses.

➤ **Tuberculous meningitis**
Adults: 8 to 12 mg phosphate I.M. daily; taper over 6 to 8 weeks.

➤ **Acute exacerbation of MS**
Adults: 30 mg P.O. daily for 1 week, followed by 4 to 12 mg every other day for 1 month.

➤ **Adjunctive therapy for short-term administration in synovitis of osteoarthritis, rheumatoid arthritis, bursitis, acute gouty arthritis, epicondylitis, acute non-specific tenosynovitis, posttraumatic osteoarthritis; lesions (keloids; localized, hypertrophic, infiltrated, inflammatory lesions of lichen planus, psoriatic plaques, granuloma annulare, or lichen simplex chronicus; discoid lupus erythematosus; necrobiosis lipoidica diabeticorum; alopecia areata; cystic tumors of an aponeurosis or tendon [ganglia])**
Adults: 0.2 to 6 mg intra-articular or intralesional injection ranging from one single injection to injection every 3 to 5 days to once every 2 to 3 weeks. Dosage and frequency of injection vary depending on condition and site of injection.

ADMINISTRATION
P.O.
● Give oral dose with food when possible. Patient may need measures to prevent GI irritation.

I.V.
▼ For direct injection, inject undiluted over at least 1 minute.
▼ For intermittent or continuous infusion, dilute solution according to manufacturer's instructions and give over prescribed duration.
▼ During continuous infusion, change solution every 24 hours.
▼ **Incompatibilities:** Ciprofloxacin, daunorubicin, diphenhydramine, doxapram, doxorubicin, glycopyrrolate, idarubicin, midazolam, vancomycin.

I.M.
● Give I.M. injection deep into gluteal muscle. Rotate injection sites to prevent muscle atrophy. Avoid subcutaneous injection because atrophy and sterile abscesses may occur.

Intra-articular, intralesional
● Frequent intra-articular injection may damage joint tissues.

ACTION
Unclear. Decreases inflammation, mainly by stabilizing leukocyte lysosomal membranes; suppresses immune response; stimulates bone marrow; and influences protein, fat, and carbohydrate metabolism.

Route	Onset	Peak	Duration
P.O.	1–2 hr	1–2 hr	2½ days
I.V.	1 hr	1 hr	Variable
I.M.	1 hr	1 hr	6 days
Intra-articular, intralesional	Unknown	Unknown	Unknown

Half-life: About 1 to 2 days.

ADVERSE REACTIONS
CNS: euphoria, insomnia, psychotic behavior, *pseudotumor cerebri,* vertigo, headache, paresthesia, *seizures,* depression.
CV: *heart failure,* hypertension, edema, *arrhythmias,* thrombophlebitis, *thromboembolism.*
EENT: cataracts, glaucoma.
GI: peptic ulceration, GI irritation, increased appetite, *pancreatitis,* nausea, vomiting.
GU: menstrual irregularities, increased urine glucose and calcium levels.

Reactions in bold italics are *life-threatening*. Interactions may have a *rapid onset* or a *delayed onset*.

Metabolic: hypokalemia, hyperglycemia, carbohydrate intolerance, hypercholesterolemia, hypocalcemia, sodium retention.
Musculoskeletal: growth suppression in children, muscle weakness, osteoporosis, tendon rupture, myopathy.
Skin: hirsutism, delayed wound healing, acne, various skin eruptions, atrophy at I.M. injection site.
Other: cushingoid state, susceptibility to infections, acute adrenal insufficiency after increased stress or abrupt withdrawal after long-term therapy, *angioedema.*
After abrupt withdrawal: rebound inflammation, fatigue, weakness, arthralgia, fever, dizziness, lethargy, fainting, orthostatic hypotension, dyspnea, anorexia, *hypoglycemia. After prolonged use, sudden withdrawal may be fatal.*

INTERACTIONS
Drug-drug. *Aminoglutethimide:* May cause loss of dexamethasone-induced adrenal suppression. Use together cautiously.
Antidiabetics, including insulin: May decrease response. May need dosage adjustment.
Aspirin, indomethacin, other NSAIDs: May increase risk of GI distress and bleeding. Use together cautiously.
Barbiturates, carbamazepine, phenytoin, rifampin: May decrease corticosteroid effect. Increase corticosteroid dosage.
Cardiac glycosides: May increase risk of arrhythmia resulting from hypokalemia. May need dosage adjustment.
Cyclosporine: May increase toxicity. Monitor patient closely.
Ephedrine: May cause decreased half-life and increased clearance of dexamethasone. Monitor patient.
Oral anticoagulants: May alter dosage requirements. Monitor PT and INR closely.
Potassium-depleting drugs such as thiazide diuretics: May enhance potassium-wasting effects of dexamethasone. Monitor potassium level.
Salicylates: May decrease salicylate level. Monitor patient for lack of salicylate effectiveness.
Skin-test antigens: May decrease response. Postpone skin testing until therapy is completed.

Toxoids, vaccines: May decrease antibody response and may increase risk of neurologic complications. Avoid using together.
Drug-lifestyle. *Alcohol use:* May increase risk of gastric irritation and GI ulceration. Discourage use together.

EFFECTS ON LAB TEST RESULTS
• May increase cholesterol and glucose levels. May decrease calcium, potassium, T_3, and T_4 levels.
• May decrease ^{131}I uptake and protein-bound iodine levels in thyroid function tests.
• May cause false-negative results in nitroblue tetrazolium test for systemic bacterial infections. May alter reactions to skin tests.

CONTRAINDICATIONS & CAUTIONS
• Contraindicated in patients hypersensitive to drug or its ingredients, in those with systemic fungal infections, and in those receiving immunosuppressive doses together with live-virus vaccines. I.M. administration is contraindicated in patients with idiopathic thrombocytopenic purpura.
• Use with caution in patient with recent MI.
• Use cautiously in patients with GI ulcer, renal disease, hypertension, osteoporosis, diabetes mellitus, hypothyroidism, cirrhosis, diverticulitis, nonspecific ulcerative colitis, recent intestinal anastomoses, thromboembolic disorders, seizures, myasthenia gravis, heart failure, tuberculosis, active hepatitis, ocular herpes simplex, emotional instability, or psychotic tendencies and in women who are breast-feeding.
• Because some forms contain sulfite preservatives, also use cautiously in patients sensitive to sulfites.

NURSING CONSIDERATIONS
• Most adverse reactions to corticosteroids are dose- or duration-dependent.
• For better results and less toxicity, give once-daily dose in morning.
• Always adjust to lowest effective dose.
• Monitor patient's weight, blood pressure, and electrolyte levels.
• Monitor patient for cushingoid effects, including moon face, buffalo hump, central obesity, thinning hair, hypertension, and increased susceptibility to infection.

• Watch for depression or psychotic episodes, especially in high-dose therapy.
• Diabetic patient may need increased insulin; monitor glucose levels.
• Drug may mask or worsen infections, including latent amebiasis.
• Elderly patients may be more susceptible to osteoporosis with long-term use.
• Inspect patient's skin for petechiae.
• Gradually reduce dosage after long-term therapy.
• *Look alike–sound alike:* Don't confuse dexamethasone with desoximetasone.

PATIENT TEACHING
• Tell patient not to stop drug abruptly or without prescriber's consent.
• Instruct patient to take drug with food or milk.
• Teach patient signs and symptoms of early adrenal insufficiency: fatigue, muscle weakness, joint pain, fever, anorexia, nausea, shortness of breath, dizziness, and fainting.
• Instruct patient to carry medical identification indicating his need for supplemental systemic glucocorticoids during stress, especially when dosage is decreased. This card should contain prescriber's name, drug name, and dosage of drug.
• Warn patient on long-term therapy about cushingoid effects (moon face, buffalo hump) and the need to notify prescriber about sudden weight gain or swelling.
• Warn patient about easy bruising.
• Advise patient receiving long-term therapy to consider exercise or physical therapy. Tell him to ask prescriber about vitamin D or calcium supplement.
• Instruct patient receiving long-term therapy to have periodic eye examinations.
• Advise patient to avoid exposure to infections (such as measles and chickenpox) and to notify prescriber if such exposure occurs.
• Tell patient to avoid alcohol.

dexlansoprazole
decks-lan-SOH-prah-zole

Dexilant⊘

Therapeutic class: Antiulcer drugs
Pharmacologic class: Proton pump inhibitors
Pregnancy risk category: B

AVAILABLE FORMS
Capsules: 30 mg, 60 mg

INDICATIONS & DOSAGES
Adjust-a-dose (for all indications): For patients with moderate hepatic impairment (Child-Pugh class B), maximum dose is 30 mg P.O. daily.
➤ **Erosive esophagitis**
Adults: Initially, 60 mg P.O. once daily for up to 8 weeks; maintenance dose is 30 mg P.O. once daily for up to 6 months.
➤ **Symptomatic nonerosive GERD**
Adults: 30 mg P.O. once daily for 4 weeks.

ADMINISTRATION
P.O.
• Give drug with or without food.
• Capsules should be swallowed whole. Or, they can be opened and the intact granules sprinkled on 1 tablespoon of applesauce and swallowed immediately.

ACTION
Inhibits proton pump activity by binding to hydrogen–potassium adenosine triphosphatase, located at the secretory surface of the gastric parietal cells, to suppress gastric acid secretion.

Route	Onset	Peak	Duration
P.O.	Unknown	4 hr	Unknown

Half-life: 1 to 2 hours.

ADVERSE REACTIONS
GI: abdominal discomfort, abdominal tenderness, diarrhea, flatulence, nausea, vomiting.
Respiratory: upper respiratory tract infection.

Reactions in bold italics are *life-threatening*. Interactions may have a *rapid onset* or a *delayed onset*.

INTERACTIONS

Drug-drug. *Atazanavir:* May decrease atazanavir level. Don't use together.

Azole antifungals (itraconazole, ketoconazole): May decrease antifungal level. Avoid concomitant use if possible. If concomitant use is necessary, have patient take antifungal with an acidic beverage (cola) to increase absorption.

Clopidogrel: May reduce clopidogrel's plasma concentration and clinical effect. Avoid use together.

Drugs with pH-dependent absorption (ampicillin, digoxin, ketoconazole, iron): May decrease absorption of these drugs. Use together cautiously.

Fluvoxamine: May increase dexlansoprazole level. Monitor patient for dexlansoprazole-related adverse reactions.

Warfarin: May increase INR and the risk of bleeding. Monitor patient closely.

EFFECTS ON LAB TEST RESULTS

● May increase alkaline phosphatase, ALT, and AST levels. May increase creatinine, gastrin, protein, glucose, and potassium levels.

● May increase or decrease bilirubin level. May decrease magnesium level.

● May decrease platelet count.

CONTRAINDICATIONS & CAUTIONS

● Contraindicated in patients hypersensitive to drug or its components.

⚠ **Alert:** There may be an increased risk of hip, wrist, and spine fractures associated with proton pump inhibitors.

● Use cautiously in patients with suspected gastric malignancy. Response to treatment doesn't eliminate the possibility of malignancy.

● Use in pregnant women only if benefit to the mother outweighs risk to the fetus. It isn't known if drug appears in breast milk; use cautiously in breast-feeding women.

● Safety and effectiveness in children haven't been established.

NURSING CONSIDERATIONS

● Monitor patient periodically for improvement in the signs and symptoms of GERD and erosive esophagitis to assess success of therapy.

● Monitor LFT results and glucose and electrolyte levels periodically during therapy.

● Monitor patient for bleeding during therapy.

⚠ **Alert:** Prolonged use of proton pump inhibitors may cause low magnesium levels. Monitor magnesium levels before starting treatment and periodically thereafter.

⚠ **Alert:** Monitor patient for symptoms of low magnesium, such as abnormal heart rate or rhythm, palpitations, muscle spasms, tremor, or seizures. In children, abnormal heart rates may present as fatigue, upset stomach, dizziness, and light-headedness. Magnesium supplementation or drug discontinuation may be required.

⚠ **Alert:** Drug may cause *Clostridium difficile*–associated diarrhea (CDAD). Evaluate for CDAD in patients who develop diarrhea that doesn't improve.

PATIENT TEACHING

● Tell patient to report hypersensitivity reactions immediately.

● Urge patient to swallow capsule whole and not to crush, split, or chew it. Capsule may also be opened and its contents sprinkled on applesauce if desired.

● Advise patient that drug can be taken without regard to meals.

● Advise female patient to notify prescriber if she is pregnant, plans to become pregnant, or is breast-feeding.

● Tell patient to report persistent diarrhea.

● Teach patient to recognize and report symptoms of low magnesium levels.

dexmethylphenidate hydrochloride

decks-meth-ill-FEN-i-date

Focalin, Focalin XR⬥

Therapeutic class: CNS stimulants
Pharmacologic class: Methylphenidate derivatives
Pregnancy risk category: C
Controlled substance schedule: II

AVAILABLE FORMS

Capsules (extended-release): 5 mg, 10 mg, 15 mg, 20 mg, 25 mg, 30 mg, 35 mg, 40 mg
Tablets: 2.5 mg, 5 mg, 10 mg

INDICATIONS & DOSAGES
➤ **ADHD**
Immediate-release tablets
Adults and children age 6 and older:
For patients who aren't now taking
methylphenidate, initially, 2.5 mg P.O. b.i.d.,
given at least 4 hours apart. Increase weekly
by 2.5 to 5 mg daily, up to a maximum of
20 mg daily in divided doses.

For patients who are now taking
methylphenidate, initially give half the
current methylphenidate dosage, up to a
maximum of 20 mg P.O. daily in divided
doses.
Extended-release capsules
Adults: For patients who aren't now taking
dexmethylphenidate or methylphenidate,
or who are on stimulants other than methylphenidate, give 10 mg P.O. once daily in the
morning. May adjust in weekly increments
of 10 mg to a maximum dose of 20 mg daily.

For patients who are now taking
methylphenidate, initially give half the total
daily dose of methylphenidate. Patients who
are now taking the immediate-release form
of dexmethylphenidate may be switched
to the same daily dose of extended-release
form. Maximum daily dose is 20 mg.
Children age 6 and older: For patients who
aren't now taking dexmethylphenidate or
methylphenidate, or who are on stimulants
other than methylphenidate, give 2.5 mg
P.O. b.i.d. May adjust in weekly increments
of 5 mg to a maximum daily dose of 20 mg.

For patients who are now taking
methylphenidate, initially give half the total
daily dose of methylphenidate. Patients who
are now taking the immediate-release form
of dexmethylphenidate may be switched
to the same daily dose of extended-release
form. Maximum daily dose is 30 mg.

ADMINISTRATION
P.O.
● Capsules may be swallowed whole or the
contents sprinkled on a small amount of
applesauce and eaten immediately.
● Don't crush or divide the capsule or its
contents.

ACTION
Blocks presynaptic reuptake of norepinephrine and dopamine and increases their
release, increasing concentration in the
synapse.

Route	Onset	Peak	Duration
P.O. (immediate-release)	Unknown	1–1½ hr	Unknown
P.O. (extended-release)	Unknown	1–4 hr; 4½–7 hr	Unknown

Half-life: 2 to 3 hours.

ADVERSE REACTIONS
CNS: headache, anxiety, feeling jittery,
nervousness, insomnia, fever, dizziness.
CV: tachycardia.
GI: anorexia, abdominal pain, nausea,
dyspepsia, dry mouth.
Musculoskeletal: twitching (motor or vocal
tics).
Other: hypersensitivity reactions.

INTERACTIONS
Drug-drug. *Antacids, acid suppressants:*
May alter the release of extended-release
form. Avoid using together.
*Anticoagulants, phenobarbital, phenytoin,
primidone, TCAs:* May inhibit metabolism
of these drugs. May need to decrease dosage
of these drugs; monitor drug levels.
Antihypertensives: May decrease effectiveness of these drugs. Use together cautiously;
monitor blood pressure.
*Clonidine, other centrally acting alpha
agonists:* May cause serious adverse effects.
Use together cautiously.
MAO inhibitors: May increase risk of hypertensive crisis. Using together within
14 days of MAO inhibitor therapy is
contraindicated.

EFFECTS ON LAB TEST RESULTS
None reported.

CONTRAINDICATIONS & CAUTIONS
● Contraindicated in patients hypersensitive
to methylphenidate or other components.
● Contraindicated in patients with severe
anxiety, tension, or agitation; glaucoma;
motor tics; a family history or diagnosis of
Tourette syndrome; or within 14 days of
MAO inhibitor therapy.
۞ Alert: Contraindicated in patients with
serious heart problems and in patients intolerant of increased blood pressure or heart
rate.

Reactions in bold italics are *life-threatening*. Interactions may have a *rapid onset* or a *delayed onset*.

Black Box Warning Use cautiously in patients with a history of substance abuse, including alcoholism. Chronic abuse can lead to marked tolerance and psychological dependence. Psychotic episodes can occur. Withdraw patient carefully from abusive use because severe depression can occur. ■

• Use cautiously in patients with a psychiatric illness, bipolar disorder, depression, or family history of suicide, and in patients with seizures, hypertension, hyperthyroidism, heart failure, or recent MI.

• Use in pregnant women only if the benefits outweigh the risks; drug may delay skeletal ossification, suppress weight gain, and impair organ development in the fetus.

• Use cautiously in breast-feeding women. It's unknown if drug appears in breast milk.

▲ Overdose S&S: Agitation, cardiac arrhythmias, confusion, seizures, delirium, dryness of mucous membranes, euphoria, flushing, hallucinations, headache, hyperpyrexia, hyperreflexia, hypertension, muscle twitching, mydriasis, palpitations, sweating, tachycardia, tremors, vomiting.

NURSING CONSIDERATIONS

• Diagnosis of ADHD must be based on complete history and evaluation of the patient by psychological and educational experts.

• Obtain a detailed patient history, including a family history for mental disorders, family suicide, ventricular arrhythmias, or sudden death.

• Refer patient for psychological, educational, and social support.

• Periodically reevaluate the long-term usefulness of the drug.

• Monitor CBC and differential and platelet counts during prolonged therapy.

• Don't use for severe depression or normal fatigue states.

• Stop treatment or reduce dosage if symptoms worsen or adverse reactions occur.

• Long-term stimulant use may temporarily suppress growth. Monitor children for growth and weight gain. If growth slows or weight gain is lower than expected, stop drug.

❸ Alert: Periodically monitor patient for changes in heart rate or blood pressure.

• Monitor patient for signs of drug dependence or abuse.

• If seizures occur, stop drug.

• **Look alike–sound alike:** Don't confuse dexmethylphenidate with methadone.

PATIENT TEACHING

• Stress the importance of taking the correct dose of drug at the same time every day. Report accidental overdose immediately.

❸ Alert: Warn patient that the misuse of amphetamines can have serious effects, including sudden death.

• Advise patients unable to swallow capsules to empty the contents of the capsule onto a spoonful of applesauce and eat immediately.

❸ Alert: Tell patient not to cut, crush, or chew the contents of the extended-release beaded capsule.

• Advise parents to monitor child for medication abuse or sharing. Also inform parents to watch for increased aggression or hostility and to report worsening behavior.

❸ Alert: Instruct patient to immediately report chest pain, shortness of breath, or fainting.

• Advise parents to monitor child's height and weight and to tell the prescriber if they suspect growth is slowing.

• Caution patient to expect blurred vision or difficulty with accommodation and to exercise caution while performing activities that require a clear visual field. Advise patient to report blurred vision to the prescriber.

dextroamphetamine sulfate
dex-troe-am-FET-a-meen

Dexedrine*

Therapeutic class: CNS stimulants
Pharmacologic class: Amphetamines
Pregnancy risk category: C
Controlled substance schedule: II

AVAILABLE FORMS
Capsules (extended-release): 5 mg, 10 mg, 15 mg
Oral solution: 5 mg/5 mL
Tablets: 5 mg, 10 mg

INDICATIONS & DOSAGES
➤ **Narcolepsy**
Adults: 5 to 60 mg P.O. daily in divided doses.
Children age 12 and older: 10 mg P.O. daily. Increase by 10 mg at weekly intervals, as needed. Give first dose on awakening; give additional doses (one or two) at intervals of 4 to 6 hours.
Children ages 6 to 12: 5 mg P.O. daily. Increase by 5 mg at weekly intervals as needed.
➤ **ADHD**
Adults and children age 6 and older: 5 mg P.O. once daily or b.i.d. Increase by 5 mg at weekly intervals, as needed. It's rarely necessary to exceed 40 mg/day.
Children ages 3 to 5: 2.5 mg P.O. daily. Increase by 2.5 mg at weekly intervals as needed.

ADMINISTRATION
P.O.
● Avoid late-evening doses, particularly with extended-release capsules, due to resulting insomnia.
● Certain formulations may contain tartrazine.

ACTION
Unknown. Probably promotes nerve impulse transmission by releasing stored dopamine and norepinephrine from nerve terminals in the brain. Main sites of activity appear to be the cerebral cortex and the reticular activating system.

Route	Onset	Peak	Duration
P.O.	30–60 min	2 hr	4 hr
P.O. (extended-release)	60 min	2 hr	8 hr

Half-life: 10 to 12 hours.

ADVERSE REACTIONS
CNS: insomnia, nervousness, restlessness, tremor, dizziness, headache, chills, overstimulation, dysphoria, euphoria.
CV: tachycardia, palpitations, *arrhythmias,* hypertension.
GI: dry mouth, taste perversion, diarrhea, constipation, anorexia, other GI disturbances.
GU: erectile dysfunction.

Metabolic: weight loss.
Skin: urticaria.
Other: increased libido.

INTERACTIONS
Drug-drug. *Acetazolamide, alkalizing drugs, antacids, sodium bicarbonate:* May increase renal reabsorption. Monitor patient for enhanced amphetamine effects.
Acidifying drugs, ammonium chloride, ascorbic acid: May decrease level and increase renal clearance of dextroamphetamine. Monitor patient for decreased amphetamine effects.
Adrenergic blockers: May inhibit adrenergic blocking effects. Avoid using together.
Chlorpromazine: May inhibit central stimulant effects of amphetamines. May use to treat amphetamine poisoning.
Insulin, oral antidiabetics: May decrease antidiabetic requirements. Monitor glucose level.
MAO inhibitors: May cause severe hypertension or hypertensive crisis. Avoid using within 14 days of MAO inhibitor therapy.
Meperidine: May potentiate analgesic effect. Use together cautiously.
Methenamine: May increase urinary excretion of amphetamines and reduce effectiveness. Monitor drug effects.
Norepinephrine: May enhance adrenergic effect of norepinephrine. Monitor patient.
Phenobarbital, phenytoin: May delay absorption of these drugs. Monitor patient closely.
Drug-food. *Caffeine:* May increase amphetamine and related amine effects. Urge caution.
Fruit juice: May decrease effectiveness of oral solution. Avoid giving together.

EFFECTS ON LAB TEST RESULTS
● May increase corticosteroid level.

CONTRAINDICATIONS & CAUTIONS
● Contraindicated in patients hypersensitive to or with idiosyncratic reactions to sympathomimetic amines and in those with hyperthyroidism, moderate to severe hypertension, symptomatic CV disease, glaucoma, advanced arteriosclerosis, or history of drug abuse.

Reactions in bold italics are *life-threatening*. Interactions may have a *rapid onset* or a *delayed onset*.

❸ Alert: Contraindicated in patients with serious heart problems and in patients intolerant of increased blood pressure or heart rate.

• Use cautiously in agitated patients and patients with motor tics, phonic tics, or Tourette syndrome. Also use cautiously in patients whose underlying condition may be worsened by an increase in blood pressure or heart rate (preexisting hypertension, heart failure, recent MI); patients with a psychiatric illness, bipolar disorder, depression, or family history of suicide; and those with a seizure disorder.

• Don't use in children or adolescents with structural cardiac abnormalities or other serious heart problems.

⚠ Overdose S&S: Assaultiveness, confusion, hallucinations, hyperreflexia, rapid respiration, restlessness, rhabdomyolysis, tremor, hyperpyrexia, panic states, fatigue, depression, arrhythmias, hypertension, hypotension, circulatory collapse, nausea, vomiting, diarrhea, abdominal cramps, seizures, coma.

NURSING CONSIDERATIONS

• Obtain a detailed patient history, including a family history for mental disorders, family suicide, ventricular arrhythmias, or sudden death.

• Monitor patients beginning treatment for ADHD for aggressive behavior or hostility.

• Drug shouldn't be used to prevent fatigue.

Black Box Warning Drug has a high abuse potential and may cause dependence. Monitor patient closely. ∎

❸ Alert: Periodically monitor patient for changes in heart rate or blood pressure.

• Monitor for growth retardation in children.

• **Look alike–sound alike:** Don't confuse Dexedrine with dextran or Excedrin.

PATIENT TEACHING

Black Box Warning Warn patient that the misuse of amphetamines can cause serious CV adverse events, including sudden death. ∎

❸ Alert: Instruct patient to immediately report chest pain, shortness of breath, or fainting.

• Warn patient to avoid activities that require alertness, a clear visual field, or good coordination until CNS effects of drug are known.

• Tell patient he may get tired as drug effects wear off.

• Ask patient to report signs and symptoms of excessive stimulation.

• Inform parents that children may show increased aggression or hostility and to report worsening of behavior.

• Advise patient to consume caffeine-containing products cautiously.

• Tell patient not to drink fruit juice at same time as oral solution.

• Warn patient with a seizure disorder that drug may decrease seizure threshold. Instruct him to notify prescriber if seizures occur.

dextromethorphan hydrobromide

dex-troe-meth-OR-fan

Balminil DM† ◇, Buckley's Cough Mixture, Creomulsion ◇, Creo-Terpin ◇*, Delsym ◇, ElixSure Cough ◇, Hold DM ◇, Koffex DM† ◇, Little Colds Cough Formula ◇, PediaCare ◇, Robitussin ◇, Robitussin Pediatric ◇, Scot-Tussin ◇, Simply Cough ◇, St. Joseph Cough Suppressant ◇, Sucrets Cough ◇, Triaminic ◇*, Trocal ◇, Vicks Formula 44 ◇

Therapeutic class: Antitussives
Pharmacologic class: Levorphanol derivatives
Pregnancy risk category: C

AVAILABLE FORMS

Freezer pops (oral): 7.5 mg/25 mL ◇
Gelcaps: 15 mg ◇, 30 mg ◇
Liquid (extended-release): 30 mg/5 mL ◇
Lozenges: 5 mg ◇, 7.5 mg ◇, 10 mg ◇
Solution: 3.5 mg/5 mL, 5 mg/5 mL ◇*, 7.5 mg/5 mL ◇, 10 mg/5 mL ◇*, 12.5 mg/ 5 mL ◇, 15 mg/5 mL ◇*, 15 mg/15 mL ◇*
Strips (orally disintegrating): 7.5 mg ◇*, 15 mg ◇*

INDICATIONS & DOSAGES
➤ **Nonproductive cough**
Adults and children age 12 and older: 10 to 20 mg P.O. every 4 hours, or 30 mg every 6 to 8 hours. Or, 60 mg extended-release liquid b.i.d. Maximum, 120 mg daily. Or, give lozenges, 5 to 15 mg, every 1 to 4 hours, up to 120 mg/day.
Children ages 6 to 11: 5 to 10 mg P.O. every 4 hours, or 15 mg every 6 to 8 hours. Or, 30 mg extended-release liquid b.i.d. Maximum, 60 mg daily. Or, give lozenges, 5 to 10 mg, every 1 to 4 hours, up to 60 mg/day, or two freezer pops every 6 to 8 hours. Don't exceed four doses in 24 hours.
Children ages 2 to 5: 2.5 to 5 mg P.O. every 4 hours, or 7.5 mg every 6 to 8 hours. Or, 15 mg extended-release liquid b.i.d. Maximum, 30 mg daily. Or, 1 freezer pop every 6 to 8 hours. Don't exceed four doses in 24 hours.

ADMINISTRATION
P.O.
● Store at controlled room temperature (59° to 86° F [15° to 30° C]), except for freezer pops.
● Allow orally disintegrating strips to dissolve on the tongue.

ACTION
Suppresses the cough reflex by direct action on the cough center in the medulla.

Route	Onset	Peak	Duration
P.O.	<30 min	Unknown	3–6 hr
P.O. (extended-release)	Unknown	Unknown	Unknown

Half-life: About 11 hours.

ADVERSE REACTIONS
CNS: drowsiness, dizziness.
GI: nausea, vomiting, stomach pain.

INTERACTIONS
Drug-drug. *MAO inhibitors:* May cause risk of hypotension, coma, hyperpyrexia, and death. Avoid using together.
Quinidine: May increase the risk of dextromethorphan adverse effects. Consider decreasing dextromethorphan dose if needed.

Drug-herb. *Parsley:* May promote or produce serotonin syndrome. Discourage use together.

EFFECTS ON LAB TEST RESULTS
None reported.

CONTRAINDICATIONS & CAUTIONS
● Contraindicated in patients currently taking MAO inhibitors or within 2 weeks of stopping MAO inhibitors.
● Use cautiously in atopic children, sedated or debilitated patients, and patients confined to the supine position.
● Use cautiously in patients sensitive to aspirin or tartrazine dyes.
❸ **Alert:** Use of OTC cough products is not recommended for neonates and children younger than age 2.
⚠ **Overdose S&S:** Altered sensory perception, ataxia, dysphoria, slurred speech; seizures, respiratory depression (in children).

NURSING CONSIDERATIONS
● Don't use dextromethorphan when cough is a valuable diagnostic sign or is beneficial (such as after thoracic surgery).
● Dextromethorphan 15 to 30 mg is equivalent to codeine 8 to 15 mg as an antitussive.
● Drug produces no analgesia or addiction and little or no CNS depression.
● Use drug with chest percussion and vibration.
● Monitor cough type and frequency.

PATIENT TEACHING
● Instruct patient to take drug exactly as prescribed and not to exceed recommended doses.
● Tell patient to report adverse reactions.
● Tell patient to contact health care provider if cough lasts longer than 1 week, recurs frequently, or is accompanied by high fever, rash, or severe headache.

---

diazepam
dye-AZ-e-pam

Diastat*, Diastat Acudial,
Diazemuls†, Diazepam Intensol*,
Novo-Dipam†, Valium✔

Therapeutic class: Anxiolytics
Pharmacologic class: Benzodiazepines
Pregnancy risk category: D
Controlled substance schedule: IV

AVAILABLE FORMS
Injection: 5 mg/mL
Oral solution: 5 mg/5 mL, 5 mg/mL*
Rectal gel twin packs:* 2.5 mg (pediatric);
10 mg, 20 mg (adult)
Tablets: 2 mg, 5 mg, 10 mg

INDICATIONS & DOSAGES
Adjust-a-dose (for all indications): For elderly
or debilitated patients, give 2 to 2.5 mg P.O.
daily or b.i.d. initially; increase gradually
as needed and tolerated. Or, when using
injection, use lower doses (2 to 5 mg) and
increase dosage more gradually.
➤ **Anxiety**
Adults: Depending on severity, 2 to 10 mg
P.O. b.i.d. to q.i.d. Or, 2 to 10 mg I.M. or I.V.
every 3 to 4 hours, p.r.n.
Children age 6 months and older: 1 to
2.5 mg P.O. t.i.d. or q.i.d., increased gradually, as needed and tolerated.
Elderly patients: Initially, 2 to 2.5 mg P.O.
once daily or b.i.d.; increase gradually.
➤ **Acute alcohol withdrawal**
Adults: 10 mg P.O. t.i.d. or q.i.d. first
24 hours; reduce to 5 mg P.O. t.i.d. or q.i.d.,
p.r.n. Or, initially, 10 mg I.V. or I.M. Then,
5 to 10 mg I.V. or I.M. every 3 to 4 hours,
p.r.n.
➤ **Before endoscopic procedures**
Adults: Adjust I.V. dose to desired sedative
response (up to 20 mg). Or, 5 to 10 mg I.M.
30 minutes before procedure.
➤ **Muscle spasm**
Adults: 2 to 10 mg P.O. b.i.d. to q.i.d. as
an adjunct. Or, 5 to 10 mg I.V. or I.M. initially; then 5 to 10 mg I.V. or I.M. every 3 to
4 hours, p.r.n.
Children age 5 and older: 5 to 10 mg I.V. or
I.M. every 3 to 4 hours, p.r.n.

Children ages 1 month to 5 years: 1 to 2 mg
I.V. or I.M. slowly; repeat every 3 to 4 hours,
p.r.n.
➤ **Preoperative sedation**
Adults: 10 mg I.M. or I.V. before surgery.
➤ **Cardioversion**
Adults: 5 to 15 mg I.V. within 5 to 10 min-
utes before procedure.
➤ **Adjunct treatment for seizure disorders**
Adults: 2 to 10 mg P.O. b.i.d. to q.i.d.
Children age 6 months and older: 1 to
2.5 mg P.O. t.i.d. or q.i.d. initially; increase
as needed and as tolerated.
➤ **Status epilepticus, severe recurrent
seizures**
Adults: 5 to 10 mg I.V. or I.M. initially. Use
I.M. route only if I.V. access is unavailable.
Repeat every 10 to 15 minutes, p.r.n., up to
maximum dose of 30 mg. Repeat every 2 to
4 hours, if needed.
Children age 5 and older: 1 mg I.V. every
2 to 5 minutes up to maximum of 10 mg.
Repeat every 2 to 4 hours, p.r.n.
Children ages 1 month to 5 years: 0.2 to
0.5 mg I.V. slowly every 2 to 5 minutes up
to maximum of 5 mg. Repeat every 2 to
4 hours, p.r.n.
➤ **Patients on stable regimens of
antiepileptic drugs who need diazepam
intermittently to control bouts of increased seizure activity**
Adults and children age 12 and older:
0.2 mg/kg P.R., rounding up to the nearest
available dose form. A second dose may be
given 4 to 12 hours later.
Children ages 6 to 11: 0.3 mg/kg P.R.,
rounding up to the nearest available dose
form. A second dose may be given 4 to
12 hours later.
Children ages 2 to 5: 0.5 mg/kg P.R., rounding up to the nearest available dose form.
A second dose may be given 4 to 12 hours
later.
➤ **Tetanus**
Adults: Initially, 5 to 10 mg I.V. or I.M. then
5 to 10 mg in 3 to 4 hours, p.r.n. Larger
doses may be required.
Children age 5 and older: 5 to 10 mg I.M. or
I.V. repeated every 3 to 4 hours, p.r.n.
*Children ages 1 month to younger than
5 years:* 1 to 2 mg I.M. or I.V. slowly
repeated every 3 to 4 hours, p.r.n.

ADMINISTRATION
P.O.
● When using oral solution, dilute dose just before giving with liquid or semisolid food, such as water, juices, soda or sodalike beverages, applesauce, or pudding.

I.V.
▼ Keep emergency resuscitation equipment and oxygen at bedside.
▼ Avoid infusion sets or containers made from polyvinyl chloride.
▼ If possible, inject directly into a large vein. If not, inject slowly through infusion tubing as near to the insertion site as possible. Give at no more than 5 mg/minute. Watch closely for phlebitis at injection site.
▼ Monitor respirations every 5 to 15 minutes and before each dose.
▼ Don't store parenteral solution in plastic syringes.
▼ **Incompatibilities:** All other I.V. drugs, most I.V. solutions.

I.M.
● Use the I.M. route if I.V. administration is impossible.

Rectal
● Use Diastat rectal gel to treat no more than five episodes per month and no more than one episode every 5 days because tolerance may develop.
◑ *Alert:* Only caregivers who can distinguish the distinct cluster of seizures or events from the patient's ordinary seizure activity, who have been instructed and can give the treatment competently, who understand which seizures may be treated with Diastat, and who can monitor the clinical response and recognize when immediate professional medical evaluation is needed should give Diastat rectal gel.

ACTION
A benzodiazepine that probably potentiates the effects of GABA, depresses the CNS, and suppresses the spread of seizure activity.

Route	Onset	Peak	Duration
P.O.	30 min	2 hr	20–80 hr
I.V.	1–5 min	1–5 min	15–60 min
I.M.	Unknown	2 hr	Unknown
P.R.	Unknown	90 min	Unknown

Half-life: About 1 to 12 days.

ADVERSE REACTIONS
CNS: drowsiness, dysarthria, slurred speech, tremor, transient amnesia, fatigue, ataxia, headache, insomnia, paradoxical anxiety, hallucinations, minor changes in EEG patterns, pain.
CV: *CV collapse, bradycardia,* hypotension.
EENT: diplopia, blurred vision, nystagmus.
GI: nausea, constipation, diarrhea with rectal form.
GU: incontinence, urine retention.
Hematologic: *neutropenia.*
Hepatic: jaundice.
Respiratory: *respiratory depression, apnea.*
Skin: rash, phlebitis at injection site.
Other: altered libido, physical or psychological dependence.

INTERACTIONS
Drug-drug. *Cimetidine, disulfiram, fluoxetine, fluvoxamine, hormonal contraceptives, isoniazid, metoprolol, propoxyphene, propranolol, valproic acid:* May decrease clearance of diazepam and increase risk of adverse effects. Monitor patient for excessive sedation and impaired psychomotor function.
CNS depressants: May increase CNS depression. Use together cautiously.
Digoxin: May increase digoxin level and risk of toxicity. Monitor patient and digoxin level closely.
Diltiazem: May increase CNS depression and prolong effects of diazepam. Reduce dose of diazepam.
Fluconazole, itraconazole, ketoconazole, miconazole: May increase and prolong diazepam level, CNS depression, and psychomotor impairment. Avoid using together.
Levodopa: May decrease levodopa effectiveness. Monitor patient.
Phenobarbital: May increase effects of both drugs. Use together cautiously.
Valproate: May increase CNS depression. Monitor patient closely.
Drug-herb. *Kava:* May increase sedation. Discourage use together.
Drug-lifestyle. *Alcohol use:* May cause additive CNS effects. Discourage use together.
Smoking: May decrease effectiveness of drug. Monitor patient closely.

Reactions in bold italics are *life-threatening*. Interactions may have a *rapid onset* or a *delayed onset*.

EFFECTS ON LAB TEST RESULTS
• May increase LFT values.
• May decrease neutrophil count.

CONTRAINDICATIONS & CAUTIONS
• Contraindicated in patients hypersensitive to drug or soy protein; in patients experiencing shock, coma, or acute alcohol intoxication (parenteral form); in pregnant women, especially in first trimester; and in infants younger than age 6 months (oral form).
• Diazepam is contraindicated in patients with acute angle-closure glaucoma.
• Use cautiously in patients with liver or renal impairment, depression, history of substance abuse, or chronic open-angle glaucoma. Use cautiously in elderly and debilitated patients.
⚠ **Overdose S&S:** Somnolence, confusion, coma, diminished reflexes.

NURSING CONSIDERATIONS
• Monitor periodic hepatic, renal, and hematopoietic function studies in patients receiving repeated or prolonged therapy.
• Monitor elderly patients for dizziness, ataxia, and mental status changes. Patients are at an increased risk for falls.
⟩ **Alert:** Use of drug may lead to abuse and addiction. Don't withdraw drug abruptly after long-term use; withdrawal symptoms may occur.
• **Look alike–sound alike:** Don't confuse diazepam with diazoxide or Ditropan. Don't confuse Valium with Valcyte.

PATIENT TEACHING
• Warn patient to avoid activities that require alertness and good coordination until effects of drug are known.
• Tell patient to avoid alcohol while taking drug.
• Notify patient that smoking may decrease drug's effectiveness.
• Warn patient not to abruptly stop drug because withdrawal symptoms may occur.
• Warn women to avoid use during pregnancy.
• Instruct patient's caregiver on the proper use of Diastat rectal gel.

diclofenac epolamine (topical)
dye-KLOE-fen-ak

Flector

diclofenac sodium (topical)
Pennsaid, Solaraze, Voltaren

Therapeutic class: NSAIDs
Pharmacologic class: NSAIDs
Pregnancy risk category: B (topical gel); C (topical patch); C (topical prior to 30 weeks' gestation; D starting at 30 weeks' gestation)

AVAILABLE FORMS
Topical gel: 1%, 3%
Topical patch: 1.3%
Topical solution: 1.5%

INDICATIONS & DOSAGES
➤ **Actinic keratosis (Solaraze only)**
Adults: Apply gently to lesion b.i.d. for 60 to 90 days.
➤ **Osteoarthritis (Voltaren only)**
Adults: Apply 4 g of gel to affected foot, knee, or ankle q.i.d. Maximum dose of 16 g to any single joint of the lower extremities. Or apply 2 g of gel to affected hand, elbow, or wrist q.i.d. Maximum dose of 8 g to any single joint of the upper extremities. Total dose shouldn't exceed 32 g daily for all affected joints.
➤ **Acute pain due to minor strains, sprains, and contusions**
Adults: Apply 1 patch to most painful area b.i.d.
➤ **Osteoarthritis of the knee**
Adults: Count 10 drops of topical solution onto hand or directly onto knee. Apply to each side, front and back, spreading evenly, using a total of 40 drops q.i.d.

ADMINISTRATION
Topical
• Apply to clean, dry skin.
• Don't apply to open wounds or broken skin.
• Avoid contact with eyes.

• Use enough gel to cover the lesion; for example, use 0.5 g of gel on a 5 × 5-cm lesion.

• Don't apply Flector patch to nonintact or damaged skin, including from exudative dermatitis, eczema, infected lesions, burns, or wounds.

• Patient shouldn't wear patch while bathing or showering.

• Measure gel using supplied dosing cards in package.

• Wear gloves to gently massage Voltaren into skin of entire joint.

• Wash hands after applying.

ACTION
Unknown. May produce anti-inflammatory and analgesic effects by ability to inhibit prostaglandin synthesis.

Route	Onset	Peak	Duration
Topical	Unknown	4–12 hr	Unknown
Transdermal	Unknown	10–20 hr	Unknown

Half-life: 1 to 3 hours; 12 hours for patch.

ADVERSE REACTIONS
CNS: paresthesia, headache, pain, asthenia, migraine, hypokinesia.
CV: chest pain, hypertension.
EENT: sinusitis, pharyngitis, rhinitis, conjunctivitis, eye pain.
GI: diarrhea, dyspepsia, abdominal pain.
GU: hematuria, renal impairment.
Hepatic: liver impairment.
Metabolic: hypercholesterolemia, hyperglycemia.
Musculoskeletal: arthralgia, arthrosis, back pain, myalgia, neck pain.
Respiratory: *asthma,* dyspnea, pneumonia.
Skin: reaction at application site, contact dermatitis, dry skin, exfoliation, localized pain, pruritus, rash, localized edema, acne, alopecia, photosensitivity reactions, skin ulcer.
Other: *anaphylaxis,* flulike syndrome, infection, allergic reaction.

INTERACTIONS
Drug-drug. *Oral NSAIDs:* May increase drug effects. Minimize use together.
Drug-lifestyle. *Sun exposure:* May increase risk of photosensitivity reactions. Advise patient to avoid excessive sun exposure.

EFFECTS ON LAB TEST RESULTS
• May increase ALT, AST, cholesterol, creatinine, glucose, and transaminase levels.

CONTRAINDICATIONS & CAUTIONS
• Contraindicated in patients hypersensitive to diclofenac, benzyl alcohol, polyethylene glycol monomethyl ether 350, or hyaluronic acid.
Black Box Warning Contraindicated for perioperative pain for CABG surgery. ▪
• Avoid use during late pregnancy.
• Use cautiously in patients with the aspirin triad; these patients are usually asthmatics who develop rhinitis, with or without nasal polyps, after taking aspirin or other NSAIDs.
• Use cautiously in patients with active GI bleeding or ulceration and in those with severe renal or hepatic impairment.
• Use cautiously in breast-feeding women; it's unknown if drug appears in breast milk. Patient should either stop breast-feeding or stop treatment, taking into account importance of drug to mother.

NURSING CONSIDERATIONS
Black Box Warning NSAIDs may increase the risk of serious CV thrombotic events. The risk may increase with duration of use. Patients with CV disease or risk factors for CV disease may be at greater risk. ▪
Black Box Warning NSAIDs increase the risk of serious GI adverse reactions, including bleeding, ulceration, and perforation of the stomach or intestines, which can be fatal. These reactions can occur at any time and without warning. Elderly patients are at greater risk. ▪
• Evaluate patient with signs or symptoms of liver dysfunction or with abnormal LFT results for development of more severe hepatic reaction while taking drug.
• If clinical signs or symptoms of liver disease develop, or if systemic manifestation (eosinophilia, rash) occurs, discontinue drug.
• Safety and effectiveness of sunscreens, cosmetics, or other topical medications used with drug are unknown.
• Complete healing or optimal therapeutic effect may not be seen until 30 days after therapy is complete.

Reactions in bold italics are *life-threatening*. Interactions may have a *rapid onset* or a ***delayed onset***.

- Reevaluate lesions that don't respond to therapy.
- Because of the risk of premature closure of the ductus arteriosus, avoid drug in late pregnancy.

PATIENT TEACHING
- Inform patient about risk of skin reactions (rash, itchiness, pain, irritation) at the application site. Urge patient to seek medical attention if adverse reactions persist or worsen.
- Encourage patient to minimize sun exposure during therapy. Explain that sunscreen may be helpful but that the safety of using sunscreen with drug is unknown.
- Advise patient needing an MRI to inform the facility that he's wearing a transdermal patch.
- Tell patient using Solaraze that complete healing or optimal therapeutic effect may not occur for up to 30 days after stopping therapy.
- Caution patient not to apply gel to open wounds or broken skin.
- Instruct patient to avoid contact with eyes.
- Instruct patient not to apply other topical drugs or cosmetics to affected area while using drug, unless directed.
- Advise patient to use only on intact skin unless otherwise directed.
- Inform patient that if Flector patch begins to peel off, the edges may be taped down. Instruct patient not to wear Flector patch during bathing or showering. Bathing should take place in between scheduled patch removal and application.
- Tell patient to wash his hands after applying gel unless the hands are the treated area and to wait at least 1 hour after application before washing hands.
- Instruct patient not to cover area with clothing for at least 10 minutes after applying gel and to wait at least 1 hour before showering or bathing.
- Tell women to notify prescriber if pregnant or breast-feeding.

diclofenac potassium (oral)
Apo-Diclo Rapide†, Cambia, Cataflam, Voltaren Rapide†, Zipsor

diclofenac sodium (oral)
Apo-Diclo†, Nu-Diclo†, Voltaren-XR, Voltaren SR†

Therapeutic class: NSAIDs
Pharmacologic class: NSAIDs
Pregnancy risk category: C; D in 3rd trimester

AVAILABLE FORMS
diclofenac potassium
Capsules: 25 mg*
Powder for solution: 50 mg/packet
Tablets: 50 mg
diclofenac sodium
Tablets (delayed-release): 25 mg, 50 mg, 75 mg
Tablets (extended-release): 100 mg

INDICATIONS & DOSAGES
➤ **Ankylosing spondylitis**
Adults: 25 mg delayed-release diclofenac sodium P.O. q.i.d.; may add another 25-mg dose at bedtime.
➤ **Osteoarthritis**
Adults: 50 mg P.O. b.i.d. or t.i.d., or 75 mg P.O. b.i.d. diclofenac potassium or delayed-release diclofenac sodium only. Or, 100 mg P.O. daily extended-release diclofenac sodium only.
➤ **Rheumatoid arthritis**
Adults: 50 mg P.O. t.i.d. or q.i.d., or 75 mg P.O. b.i.d. diclofenac potassium or delayed-release diclofenac sodium only. Or, 100 mg P.O. daily or b.i.d. extended-release diclofenac sodium only.
➤ **Analgesia, primary dysmenorrhea**
Adults: 50 mg diclofenac potassium P.O. t.i.d. For some patients, the first dose on the first day may be 100 mg, followed by 50 mg for the second and third doses; maximum dose for first day is 200 mg. Don't exceed 150 mg daily after the first day.
➤ **Migraine**
Adults: 50 mg (1 packet) P.O. as a single dose.

ADMINISTRATION

P.O.

- Give drug with milk, meals, or antacids.
- Don't crush or break enteric-coated tablets.
- Mix powder in water only. Use no other liquid.
- Mix solution well and have patient drink immediately.
- Powder may be less effective if taken with food.

ACTION

May inhibit prostaglandin synthesis, to produce anti-inflammatory, analgesic, and antipyretic effects.

Route	Onset	Peak	Duration
P.O. (delayed-release)	30 min	2–3 hr	8 hr
P.O. (extended-release)	Unknown	5–6 hr	Unknown
P.O.	10 min	1 hr	8 hr

Half-life: 1 to 2 hours.

ADVERSE REACTIONS

CNS: *aseptic meningitis,* anxiety, depression, dizziness, drowsiness, headache, insomnia, irritability.
CV: *heart failure,* edema, fluid retention, hypertension.
EENT: *laryngeal edema,* blurred vision, epistaxis, eye pain, night blindness, reversible hearing loss, swelling of the lips and tongue, tinnitus.
GI: abdominal distention, abdominal pain or cramps, *bleeding,* constipation, diarrhea, flatulence, indigestion, melena, nausea, peptic ulceration, taste disorder, bloody diarrhea, appetite change, colitis.
GU: nephrotic syndrome, *acute renal failure,* fluid retention, interstitial nephritis, oliguria, papillary necrosis, proteinuria.
Hepatic: jaundice, *hepatitis, hepatotoxicity.*
Metabolic: *hypoglycemia,* hyperglycemia.
Musculoskeletal: back, leg, or joint pain.
Respiratory: *asthma.*
Skin: *Stevens-Johnson syndrome,* allergic purpura, alopecia, bullous eruption, dermatitis, eczema, photosensitivity reactions, pruritus, rash, urticaria.
Other: *anaphylactoid reactions, anaphylaxis, angioedema.*

INTERACTIONS

Drug-drug. *Anticoagulants, including warfarin:* May cause bleeding. Monitor patient closely.
Aspirin: May decrease effectiveness of diclofenac and increase GI toxicity. Avoid using together.
Beta blockers: May decrease antihypertensive effects. Monitor patient closely.
Cyclosporine, digoxin, lithium, methotrexate: May reduce renal clearance of these drugs and increase risk of toxicity. Monitor patient closely.
Diuretics: May decrease effectiveness of diuretics. Avoid using together.
Insulin, oral antidiabetics: May alter requirements for antidiabetics. Monitor patient closely.
Potassium-sparing diuretics: May enhance retention and increase level of potassium. Monitor potassium level.
Drug-herb. *Dong quai, feverfew, garlic, ginger, horse chestnut, red clover:* May cause bleeding based on the known effects or components. Discourage use together.
White willow: Herb and drug contain similar components. Discourage use together.
Drug-lifestyle. *Sun exposure:* May cause photosensitivity reactions. Advise patient to avoid excessive sunlight exposure.

EFFECTS ON LAB TEST RESULTS

- May increase ALT, AST, bilirubin, BUN, and creatinine levels.
- May increase or decrease glucose level.

CONTRAINDICATIONS & CAUTIONS

Black Box Warning Contraindicated for the treatment of perioperative pain after CABG surgery. ■

- Contraindicated in patients hypersensitive to drug and in those with hepatic porphyria or history of asthma, urticaria, or other allergic reactions after taking aspirin or other NSAIDs. Zipsor is contraindicated in patients hypersensitive to bovine protein.
- Avoid use during late pregnancy or while breast-feeding.
- Use cautiously in patients with history of peptic ulcer disease, hepatic dysfunction, cardiac disease, hypertension, fluid retention, or impaired renal function.

Reactions in bold italics are *life-threatening*. Interactions may have a *rapid onset* or a *delayed onset*.

⚠ Overdose S&S: Drowsiness, confusion, hypotonia, loss of consciousness, vomiting, aspiration, pneumonitis, increased intracranial pressure.

NURSING CONSIDERATIONS

• Because NSAIDs impair the synthesis of renal prostaglandins, they can decrease renal blood flow and lead to reversible renal impairment, especially in patients with renal or heart failure or liver dysfunction, in elderly patients, and in those taking diuretics. Monitor these patients closely.

• LFT values may increase during therapy. Monitor transaminase, especially ALT, levels periodically in patients undergoing long-term therapy. Make first transaminase measurement no later than 8 weeks after therapy begins.

Black Box Warning NSAIDs cause an increased risk of serious GI adverse events, including bleeding, ulceration, and perforation of the stomach or intestines, which can be fatal. Elderly patients are at greater risk. ■

Black Box Warning NSAIDs may increase the risk of serious thrombotic events, MI, or stroke, which can be fatal. The risk may be greater with longer use or in patients with CV disease or risk factors for CV disease. ■

☰ Alert: Different formulations of oral diclofenac are not bioequivalent even if the milligram strength is the same.

• Because of their antipyretic and anti-inflammatory actions, NSAIDs may mask the signs and symptoms of infection.

• **Look alike–sound alike:** Don't confuse diclofenac with Diflucan.

PATIENT TEACHING

• Tell patient to take tablets or capsules with milk, meals, or antacids to minimize GI distress.

• Instruct patient not to crush, break, or chew enteric-coated tablets.

• Tell patient to mix powder form of drug well in water only and to drink immediately.

• Advise patient not to take this drug with any other diclofenac-containing products (such as Arthrotec).

• Teach patient signs and symptoms of GI bleeding, including blood in vomit, urine, or stool; coffee-ground vomit; and black,

tarry stool. Tell him to notify prescriber immediately if any of these occurs.

• Teach patient the signs and symptoms of damage to the liver, including nausea, fatigue, lethargy, itching, yellowed skin or eyes, right upper quadrant tenderness, and flulike symptoms. Tell patient to contact prescriber immediately if these symptoms occur.

• Advise patient to avoid drinking alcohol or taking aspirin during drug therapy.

• Tell patient to wear sunscreen or protective clothing because drug may cause sensitivity to sunlight.

• Warn patient to avoid hazardous activities that require alertness until it is known whether the drug causes CNS symptoms.

• Tell pregnant women to avoid use of drug during last trimester.

• Advise patient that use of OTC NSAIDs and diclofenac may increase the risk of GI toxicity.

---

dicyclomine hydrochloride
dye-SYE-kloe-meen

Bentyl, Bentylol†, Formulex†, Protylol†

Therapeutic class: Antispasmodics
Pharmacologic class: Anticholinergics–antimuscarinics
Pregnancy risk category: B

AVAILABLE FORMS
Capsules: 10 mg
Injection: 10 mg/mL
Syrup: 10 mg/5 mL
Tablets: 10 mg†, 20 mg

INDICATIONS & DOSAGES
➤ **Irritable bowel syndrome, other functional GI disorders**
Adults: Initially, 20 mg P.O. q.i.d., increased to 40 mg q.i.d. Or, 20 mg I.M. q.i.d. Don't use I.M. form for longer than 1 to 2 days.

ADMINISTRATION

P.O.
● Give drug 30 to 60 minutes before meals and at bedtime. Bedtime dose can be larger; give at least 2 hours after last meal of day.
● Store in light-resistant container.

I.M.
◐ *Alert:* Don't give subcutaneously or I.V.
● Aspirate syringe before injecting to avoid I.V. injection; thrombosis may occur if drug is inadvertently injected I.V.
◐ *Alert:* The dicyclomine labeling may be misleading. Injection concentration is 10 mg/mL. Carefully calculate appropriate amount of solution for administering correct dose.

ACTION

Inhibits action of acetylcholine on post-ganglionic, parasympathetic muscarinic receptors, decreasing GI motility. Drug possesses local anesthetic properties that may be partly responsible for spasmolysis.

Route	Onset	Peak	Duration
P.O., I.M.	Unknown	1–1½ hr	Unknown

Half-life: Initial, about 2 hours; secondary, 9 to 10 hours.

ADVERSE REACTIONS

CNS: asthenia, headache, dizziness, fever, insomnia, light-headedness, drowsiness, nervousness, confusion; excitement (in elderly patients), somnolence.
CV: palpitations, tachycardia.
EENT: blurred vision, increased intraocular pressure, mydriasis, photophobia.
GI: constipation, dry mouth, thirst, vomiting, nausea, abdominal distention, heartburn, paralytic ileus.
GU: urinary hesitancy, urine retention, erectile dysfunction.
Skin: urticaria, decreased sweating or inability to sweat, local irritation.
Other: allergic reactions, heat prostration.

INTERACTIONS

Drug-drug. *Amantadine, antihistamines, antiparkinsonians, disopyramide, glutethimide, meperidine, phenothiazines, procainamide, quinidine, TCAs:* May have additive adverse effects. Avoid using together.

Antacids: May interfere with dicyclomine absorption. Give dicyclomine at least 1 hour before antacid.
Drug-lifestyle. *Alcohol use:* May cause additive sedative effects. Avoid use together.

EFFECTS ON LAB TEST RESULTS

None reported.

CONTRAINDICATIONS & CAUTIONS

● Contraindicated in patients hypersensitive to anticholinergics and in those with obstructive uropathy, obstructive disease of the GI tract, reflux esophagitis, severe ulcerative colitis, toxic megacolon, myasthenia gravis, unstable CV status in acute hemorrhage, tachycardia secondary to cardiac insufficiency or thyrotoxicosis, or glaucoma.
● Contraindicated in breast-feeding patients and in children younger than age 6 months.
● Use cautiously in patients with autonomic neuropathy, hyperthyroidism, coronary artery disease, arrhythmias, heart failure, hypertension, hiatal hernia, hepatic or renal disease, prostatic hyperplasia, known or suspected GI infection, and ulcerative colitis.
● Use cautiously in patients in hot or humid environments; drug can cause heatstroke.
⚠ *Overdose S&S:* Headache; nausea; vomiting; blurred vision; dilated pupils; hot, dry skin; dry mouth; dysphagia; CNS stimulation; muscle weakness; paralysis.

NURSING CONSIDERATIONS

● Adjust dosage based on patient's needs and response. Dosages up to 40 mg P.O. q.i.d. have been used in adults, but safety and effectiveness for longer than 2 weeks haven't been established.
● Dicyclomine may have atropine-like adverse reactions.
◐ *Alert:* Overdose may cause curare-like effects, such as respiratory paralysis. Keep emergency equipment available.
● Monitor patient's vital signs and urine output carefully.
● *Look alike–sound alike:* Don't confuse dicyclomine with dyclonine or doxycycline. Don't confuse Bentyl with Aventyl or Benadryl.

Reactions in bold italics are *life-threatening*. Interactions may have a *rapid onset* or a *delayed onset*.

PATIENT TEACHING

• Tell patient when to take drug, and stress importance of doing so on time and at evenly spaced intervals.

• Advise patient to avoid driving and other hazardous activities if drowsiness, dizziness, or blurred vision occurs; to drink plenty of fluids to help prevent constipation; and to report rash or other skin eruption.

• Warn patient that heat prostration may occur during therapy when environmental temperatures are high. If symptoms (fever, decreased sweating) occur, instruct patient to stop drug and contact his physician.

---

didanosine (ddl, dideoxyinosine)
dye-DAN-oh-seen

Videx, Videx EC

Therapeutic class: Antiretrovirals
Pharmacologic class: Nucleoside–nucleotide reverse transcriptase inhibitors
Pregnancy risk category: B

AVAILABLE FORMS
Capsules (delayed-release): 125 mg, 200 mg, 250 mg, 400 mg
Powder for oral solution (pediatric): 2 g/4-ounce glass bottle, 4 g/8-ounce glass bottle

INDICATIONS & DOSAGES
➤ **HIV infection**
Adults weighing 60 kg (132 lb) or more: 400-mg capsule P.O. daily. Or, 200 mg b.i.d. (preferred dosing) or 400 mg of the pediatric powder for oral solution P.O. once daily.
Adults weighing 25 to less than 60 kg (55 to less than 132 lb): 250-mg capsule P.O. daily. Or, 125 mg b.i.d. (preferred dosing) or 250 mg of the pediatric powder for oral solution P.O. once daily.
Adults weighing 20 to less than 25 kg (44 to less than 55 lb): 200-mg capsule P.O. daily. Or, 125 mg b.i.d. (preferred dosing) or 250 mg of the pediatric powder for oral solution P.O. once daily.
Children older than age 8 months: 120 mg/m^2 of the pediatric powder for oral solution P.O. b.i.d. Or, for children weighing 60 kg or more, 400-mg capsule P.O. daily; for children weighing 25 to less than 60 kg, 250-mg capsule P.O. daily; for children weighing 20 to less than 25 kg, 200-mg capsule P.O. daily.
Children ages 2 weeks to 8 months: 100 mg/m^2 of the pediatric powder for oral solution P.O. b.i.d.
Adjust-a-dose: For dialysis patients weighing 60 kg (132 lb) or more, 100 mg of the pediatric powder for oral solution once daily. For dialysis patients weighing less than 60 kg, 75 mg of the pediatric powder for oral solution once daily. For dialysis patients weighing 60 kg or more, 125 mg of Videx EC once daily. Don't use in dialysis patients who weigh less than 60 kg. If CrCl is less than 10 mL/minute, don't give a supplemental dose after hemodialysis for either drug.

In adults weighing 60 kg or more with CrCl of 30 to 59 mL/minute, 200-mg capsule once daily; or 200 mg once daily or 100 mg b.i.d. of the pediatric powder for oral solution. If CrCl is 10 to 29 mL/minute, 125-mg capsule or 150 mg of the pediatric powder for oral solution once daily. If CrCl is less than 10 mL/minute, give 125-mg capsule or 100 mg of the pediatric powder for oral solution once daily.

In adults weighing less than 60 kg with a CrCl of 30 to 59 mL/minute, 125-mg capsule once daily; or 150 mg once daily or 75 mg b.i.d. of the pediatric powder for oral solution. If CrCl is 10 to 29 mL/minute, 125-mg capsule or 100 mg of the pediatric powder for oral solution once daily. For CrCl less than 10 mL/minute, 75 mg of the pediatric powder for oral solution once daily; capsule not indicated for these patients.

For adult patients taking tenofovir who weigh 60 kg or more with a CrCl of 60 mL/minute or more, reduce Videx dose to 250 mg once daily. Avoid concomitant therapy in patients with CrCl less than 60 mL/minute. For adult patients taking tenofovir who weigh less than 60 kg with a CrCl of 60 mL/minute or more, reduce Videx dose to 200 mg once daily. Avoid concomitant therapy in patients with CrCl less than 60 mL/minute.

ADMINISTRATION
P.O.
● Give drug on an empty stomach, at least 30 minutes before or 2 hours after eating; giving drug with meals can decrease absorption by 50%.

◑ **Alert:** The pediatric powder for oral solution must be prepared by a pharmacist before dispensing. It must be constituted with purified USP water and then diluted with an antacid (Mylanta Maximum Strength) to a final concentration of 10 mg/mL. The admixture is stable for 30 days at 36° to 46° F (2° to 8° C). Shake the solution well before measuring dose.

ACTION
Inhibits the enzyme HIV-RNA–dependent DNA polymerase (reverse transcriptase) and terminates DNA chain growth.

Route	Onset	Peak	Duration
P.O.	Unknown	15–90 min	Unknown
P.O., E.C.	Unknown	2 hr	Unknown

Half-life: 48 minutes.

ADVERSE REACTIONS
CNS: dizziness, fever, headache, peripheral neuropathy, *seizures,* abnormal thinking, asthenia, pain.
EENT: optic neuritis, retinal changes.
GI: abdominal pain, diarrhea, nausea, vomiting, *pancreatitis,* anorexia, dry mouth.
Hematologic: *leukopenia, thrombocytopenia,* anemia.
Hepatic: *hepatic failure.*
Metabolic: hyperuricemia.
Musculoskeletal: myopathy.
Skin: alopecia, pruritus, rash.
Other: chills, *sarcoma,* allergic reactions, infection.

INTERACTIONS
Drug-drug. *Allopurinol:* Increases didanosine level. Don't administer together.
Amprenavir, delavirdine, indinavir, nelfinavir, ritonavir, saquinavir: May alter pharmacokinetics of didanosine or these drugs. Separate dosage times.
Antacids containing magnesium or aluminum hydroxides: May enhance adverse effects of the antacid component (including diarrhea or constipation) when given with

didanosine tablets or pediatric suspension. Avoid using together.
Dapsone, drugs that require gastric acid for adequate absorption, ketoconazole: May decrease absorption from buffering action. Give these drugs 2 hours before didanosine.
Fluoroquinolones, tetracyclines: May decrease absorption from buffering products in didanosine tablets or antacids in pediatric suspension. Separate dosage times by at least 2 hours.
Itraconazole: May decrease itraconazole level. Avoid using together.
Ribavirin: Increases risk of fatal hepatic failure, peripheral neuropathy, pancreatitis, and systematic hyperlactemia/lactic acidosis. Don't use together.
Black Box Warning *Stavudine, other antiretrovirals:* Fatal lactic acidosis has been reported in pregnant women. Use only if potential benefits clearly outweigh potential risks. ■
Sulfamethoxazole–trimethoprim, pentamidine, other drugs linked to pancreatitis: May increase risk of pancreatic toxicity. Use together cautiously; consider temporarily stopping didanosine during administration of these drugs.
Tenofovir: May increase didanosine levels and risk of life-threatening adverse effects, including lactic acidosis and pancreatitis. Adjust didanosine dosage.
Drug-herb. *St. John's wort:* May decrease drug level, decreasing therapeutic effects. Discourage use together.
Drug-food. *Any food:* May decrease rate of absorption. Advise patient to take drug on an empty stomach at least 30 minutes before a meal.

EFFECTS ON LAB TEST RESULTS
● May increase alkaline phosphatase, ALT, AST, bilirubin, and uric acid levels. May decrease hemoglobin level.
● May decrease granulocyte, platelet, and WBC counts.

CONTRAINDICATIONS & CAUTIONS
● Contraindicated in patients hypersensitive to drug or its components.
◑ **Alert:** Administration with allopurinol or ribavirin is contraindicated.

Black Box Warning Contraindicated in patients with confirmed pancreatitis. ∎

Black Box Warning Use cautiously in patients with history of pancreatitis; deaths have occurred. ∎

Black Box Warning Lactic acidosis and severe hepatomegaly with steatosis, including fatal cases, have been reported. ∎

• Use cautiously in patients with peripheral neuropathy, renal or hepatic impairment, or hyperuricemia. Monitor liver and renal function tests.

⚠ Overdose S&S: Pancreatitis, peripheral neuropathy, diarrhea, hyperuricemia, hepatic dysfunction.

NURSING CONSIDERATIONS

• Patients with advanced HIV disease or history of peripheral neuropathy may develop numbness, tingling, or pain in the hands and feet.

• Drug dosage may need to be reduced, or drug may need to be stopped.

• Patients may tolerate a reduced dose of Videx after symptoms of peripheral neuropathy resolve; if symptoms recur, consider permanently stopping drug.

• Because of a high rate of early virologic failure and emergence of resistance, using tenofovir with didanosine and lamivudine isn't recommended as a new treatment regimen for therapy-naive or therapy-experienced patients with HIV infection. Patients on this regimen should be considered for treatment modification.

• **Look alike–sound alike:** Don't confuse drug with other antiretrovirals that use abbreviations for identification.

PATIENT TEACHING

• Instruct patient to take drug on an empty stomach, 30 minutes before or 2 hours after eating.

• Inform patient that drug doesn't cure HIV infection, that opportunistic infections and other complications of HIV infection may continue to occur, and that transmission of HIV to others through sexual contact or blood contamination is still possible.

• Tell patient to report symptoms of inflammation of the pancreas, such as abdominal pain, nausea, vomiting, diarrhea, or symptoms of peripheral neuropathy.

difluprednate
die-FLU-pred-nate

Durezol

Therapeutic class: Anti-inflammatory drugs (ophthalmic)
Pharmacologic class: Corticosteroids
Pregnancy risk category: C

AVAILABLE FORMS
Ophthalmic emulsion: 0.05%

INDICATIONS & DOSAGES
➤ **Inflammation and pain associated with ocular surgery**
Adults: One drop into the conjunctival sac of the affected eye q.i.d. beginning 24 hours after surgery for 2 weeks, then decrease to b.i.d. for 1 week, and then taper according to response.
➤ **Endogenous anterior uveitis**
Adults: One drop into the conjunctival sac of the affected eye q.i.d. for 14 days, then taper as clinically indicated.

ADMINISTRATION
Ophthalmic
• Shake well before each use.
• Don't touch tip of dropper to any surface, including eye.

ACTION
May inhibit the release of arachidonic acid, a precursor of inflammatory mediators, such as prostaglandins and leukotrienes.

Route	Onset	Peak	Duration
Ophthalmic	Rapid	Unknown	Unknown

Half-life: Unknown.

ADVERSE REACTIONS
EENT: anterior chamber cells, anterior chamber flare, blepharitis, ciliary and conjunctival hyperemia, conjunctival edema, corneal edema, eye inflammation, eye pain, iritis, photophobia, posterior capsule

opacification, punctate keratitis, reduced visual acuity.

INTERACTIONS
None reported.

EFFECTS ON LAB TEST RESULTS
None reported.

CONTRAINDICATIONS & CAUTIONS
• Contraindicated in patients with ocular tuberculosis, epithelial herpes simplex keratitis (dendritic keratitis), vaccinia, varicella, or other fungal or viral diseases of ocular structures.
• Use cautiously in patients with glaucoma (any form) because intraocular pressure (IOP) may increase.
• Use cautiously in patients with a history of herpes simplex; drug may prolong or worsen the condition.

NURSING CONSIDERATIONS
• Drug isn't intended for long-term use; if used for 10 days or more, monitor IOP. Watch for ocular bacterial, fungal, or viral infections.
• Drug may delay healing after cataract surgery; examine with slit-lamp biomicroscopy and, if appropriate, fluorescein staining if used for more than 28 days.
• Safe use in pregnant women hasn't been established.
• Appearance of drug in breast milk isn't known. Use cautiously in breast-feeding women.
• Safety and effectiveness haven't been established in children.

PATIENT TEACHING
• Teach patient how to instill drops. Advise him to wash his hands before and after applying the drug, and warn him not to touch tip of dropper to eye or surrounding tissue.
• Advise patient to contact prescriber if pain develops or redness, itching, or inflammation worsens.
• Tell patient who wears contact lenses to check with prescriber before using lenses again.
• Advise patient to store drug at room temperature in protective carton away from light, and to keep unused vials in foil pouch.

SAFETY ALERT!

digoxin
di-JOX-in

Apo-Digoxin†, Lanoxin*, Lanoxin Pediatric, Toloxin†

Therapeutic class: Inotropes
Pharmacologic class: Cardiac glycosides
Pregnancy risk category: C

AVAILABLE FORMS
Elixir∗: 0.05 mg/mL (pediatric)
Injection∗: 0.05 mg/mL†, 0.1 mg/mL (pediatric), 0.25 mg/mL
Tablets: 0.0625 mg†, 0.125 mg, 0.25 mg

INDICATIONS & DOSAGES
Adjust-a-dose (for all indications): If CrCl is 10 to 50 mL/minute, give 25% to 75% of the normal dose or usual dose every 36 hours. If CrCl is less than 10 mL/minute or the patient is on hemodialysis, give 10% to 25% of the normal dose or usual dose every 48 hours.
➤ **Heart failure, rapid digitalization**
Tablets
Adults: For rapid digitalization, give a single initial dose of 500 to 750 mcg (0.5 to 0.75 mg) of digoxin tablets P.O. (usually produces a detectable effect in ½ to 2 hours, which becomes maximal in 2 to 6 hours). Give additional doses of 125 to 375 mcg (0.125 to 0.375 mg) cautiously at 6- to 8-hour intervals until clinical evidence of an adequate effect is noted. The usual dosage (tablets) required by a 70-kg (154-lb) patient to achieve 8- to 12-mcg/kg (0.008- to 0.012-mg/kg) peak body stores is 750 to 1,250 mcg (0.75 to 1.25 mg).
Elixir
In pediatric patients, if a loading dose is needed, it can be administered with roughly half the total given as the first dose. Additional fractions of this planned total dose may be given at 4- to 8-hour intervals, with careful assessment of clinical response before each additional dose. If the patient's clinical response necessitates a change from the calculated loading dose of digoxin, base the calculation of the maintenance dose

on the amount actually given as the loading dose.

Children older than age 10: Loading dose is 10 to 15 mcg/kg P.O. in divided doses, followed by maintenance dose of 3 to 4.5 mcg/kg P.O. once daily.

Children ages 5 to 10: Loading dose is 20 to 35 mcg/kg P.O. in divided doses, followed by maintenance dose of 2.8 to 5.6 mcg/kg P.O. b.i.d.

Children ages 2 to 5: Loading dose is 30 to 45 mcg/kg P.O. in divided doses, followed by maintenance dose of 4.7 to 6.6 mcg/kg P.O. b.i.d.

Infants ages 1 to 24 months: Loading dose is 35 to 60 mcg/kg P.O. in divided doses, followed by maintenance dose of 5.6 to 9.4 mcg/kg P.O. b.i.d.

Full-term infants: Loading dose is 25 to 35 mcg/kg P.O. in divided doses, followed by maintenance dose of 3.8 to 5.6 mcg/kg P.O. b.i.d.

Preterm infants: Loading dose is 20 to 30 mcg/kg P.O. in divided doses, followed by maintenance dose of 2.3 to 3.9 mcg/kg P.O. b.i.d.

I.V.

Adults: Initially, 400 to 600 mcg (0.4 to 0.6 mg) I.V., followed by 100 to 300 mcg (0.1 to 0.3 mg) I.V. every 6 to 8 hours as needed and tolerated. The usual amount of digoxin injection required by a 70-kg (154 lb) patient to achieve 8- to 12-mcg/kg (0.008- to 0.012-mg/kg) peak body stores is 600 to 1,000 mcg (0.6 to 1 mg).

For children, administer the loading dose in several portions, with roughly half of the total given as the first dose. Give additional fractions of this planned total dose at 4- to 8-hour intervals, with careful assessment of clinical response before each additional dose. If the patient's clinical response necessitates a change from the calculated loading dose of digoxin, base the calculation of the maintenance dose on the amount actually given.

Children older than age 10: Digitalizing dose is 8 to 12 mcg/kg I.V. in divided doses, followed by a daily I.V. maintenance dose that is 25% to 35% of the I.V. digitalizing dose.

Children ages 5 to 10: Digitalizing dose is 15 to 30 mcg/kg I.V. in divided doses, fol-

lowed by a total daily I.V. maintenance dose that is 25% to 35% of the I.V. digitalizing dose. Give maintenance dose in divided doses.

Children ages 2 to 5: Digitalizing dose is 25 to 35 mcg/kg I.V. in divided doses, followed by a total daily I.V. maintenance dose that is 25% to 35% of the I.V. digitalizing dose. Give maintenance dose in divided doses.

Infants ages 1 to 24 months: Digitalizing dose is 30 to 50 mcg/kg I.V. in divided doses, followed by a total daily I.V. maintenance dose that is 25% to 35% of the I.V. digitalizing dose. Give maintenance dose in divided doses.

Full-term infants: Digitalizing dose is 20 to 30 mcg/kg I.V. in divided doses, followed by a total daily I.V. maintenance dose that is 25% to 35% of the I.V. digitalizing dose. Give maintenance dose in divided doses.

Preterm infants: Digitalizing dose is 15 to 25 mcg/kg I.V. in divided doses, followed by a total daily I.V. maintenance dose that is 20% to 30% of the I.V. digitalizing dose. Give maintenance dose in divided doses.

➤ **Heart failure, gradual digitalization**
Tablets

Adults: For gradual digitalization, therapy is generally initiated at a dosage of 250 mcg (0.25 mg) P.O. once daily in patients younger than age 70 with good renal function, 125 mcg (0.125 mg) once daily in patients older than age 70 or with impaired renal function, and 62.5 mcg (0.0625 mg) once daily in patients with marked renal impairment. May increase dosages every 2 weeks according to clinical response. Maintenance dosages range from 125 to 500 mcg (0.125 to 0.5 mg) once daily.

Children age 10 and older: 3 to 5 mcg/kg P.O. daily.

Children ages 5 to 10: 7 to 10 mcg/kg P.O. daily in divided doses.

Children ages 2 to 5: 10 to 15 mcg/kg P.O. daily in divided doses.

Elixir

More gradual attainment of digoxin levels can also be accomplished by beginning an appropriate maintenance dosage. In general, divided daily dosing is recommended for infants and children younger than age 10. In newborns, renal clearance of digoxin is diminished and suitable dosage adjustments must be observed, especially in preterm infants. Beyond the immediate newborn period, children generally require proportionally larger doses than adults on the basis of body weight or surface area. Children older than age 10 require adult dosages in proportion to their body weight.

Children older than age 10: 3 to 4.5 mcg/kg P.O. once daily.

Children ages 5 to 10: 2.8 to 5.6 mcg/kg P.O. b.i.d.

Children ages 2 to 5: 4.7 to 6.6 mcg/kg P.O. b.i.d.

Infants ages 1 to 24 months: 5.6 to 9.4 mcg/kg P.O. b.i.d.

Full-term infants: 3.8 to 5.6 mcg/kg P.O. b.i.d.

Preterm infants: 2.3 to 3.9 mcg/kg P.O. b.i.d.
I.V.

Adults: Initially, 250 mcg (0.25 mg) I.V. once daily in patients younger than age 70 with good renal function, 125 mcg (0.125 mg) I.V. once daily in patients older than age 70 or with impaired renal function, and 62.5 mcg (0.0625 mg) I.V. once daily in patients with marked renal impairment. Increase dosages every 2 weeks according to clinical response. The digoxin dose has been generally titrated according to the patient's age, lean body weight, and renal function.

Children older than age 10: Give a total daily I.V. maintenance dose that is 25% to 35% of the 8- to 12-mcg/kg I.V. digitalizing dose.

Children ages 5 to 10: Give a total daily I.V. maintenance dose (in divided doses) that is 25% to 35% of the 15- to 30-mcg/kg I.V. digitalizing dose.

Children ages 2 to 5: Give a total daily I.V. maintenance dose (in divided doses) that is 25% to 35% of the 25- to 35-mcg/kg I.V. digitalizing dose.

Infants ages 1 to 24 months: Give a total daily I.V. maintenance dose (in divided doses) that is 25% to 35% of the 30- to 50-mcg/kg I.V. digitalizing dose.

Full-term infants: Give a total daily I.V. maintenance dose (in divided doses) that is 25% to 35% of the 20- to 30-mcg/kg I.V. digitalizing dose.

Preterm infants: Give a total daily I.V. maintenance dose (in divided doses) that is 20%

to 30% of the 15- to 25-mcg/kg I.V. digitalizing dose.

➤ **Atrial fibrillation**
P.O., I.V.

Adults: Peak digoxin body stores larger than the 8 to 12 mcg/kg (0.008 to 0.012 mg/kg) required for most patients with heart failure and healthy sinus rhythm have been used for control of ventricular rate in patients with atrial fibrillation. Titrate digoxin dosages used for the treatment of chronic atrial fibrillation to the minimum dosage that achieves the desired ventricular rate control without causing undesirable adverse effects.

ADMINISTRATION
P.O.

● Before giving loading dose, obtain baseline data (heart rate and rhythm, blood pressure, and electrolytes) and ask patient about use of cardiac glycosides within the previous 2 to 3 weeks.

● Before giving drug, take apical-radial pulse for 1 minute. Record and notify prescriber of significant changes (sudden increase or decrease in pulse rate, pulse deficit, irregular beats and, particularly, regularization of a previously irregular rhythm). If these occur, check blood pressure and obtain a 12-lead ECG.

I.V.

▼ Before giving loading dose, obtain baseline data (heart rate and rhythm, blood pressure, and electrolytes) and ask patient about use of cardiac glycosides within the previous 2 to 3 weeks.

▼ Before giving drug, take apical-radial pulse for 1 minute. Record and notify prescriber of significant changes (sudden increase or decrease in pulse rate, pulse deficit, irregular beats and, particularly, regularization of a previously irregular rhythm). If these occur, check blood pressure and obtain a 12-lead ECG.

▼ Dilute fourfold with D_5W, normal saline solution, or sterile water for injection to reduce the chance of precipitation.

▼ Infuse drug slowly over at least 5 minutes.

▼ Protect solution from light.

▼ **Incompatibilities:** Amiodarone, amphotericin B cholesteryl sulfate complex, dobutamine, doxapram, fluconazole, fos-carnet, propofol, remifentanil. Mixing with other drugs isn't recommended.

ACTION
Inhibits sodium-potassium–activated adeno-sine triphosphatase, promoting movement of calcium from extracellular to intracellular cytoplasm and strengthening myocardial contraction. Also acts on CNS to enhance vagal tone, slowing conduction through the SA and AV nodes.

Route	Onset	Peak	Duration
P.O.	30–120 min	2–6 hr	3–4 days
I.V.	5–30 min	1–4 hr	3–4 days

Half-life: 30 to 40 hours.

ADVERSE REACTIONS
CNS: agitation, fatigue, generalized mus-cle weakness, hallucinations, dizziness, headache, malaise, paresthesia, stupor, vertigo.
CV: *arrhythmias, heart block.*
EENT: blurred vision, diplopia, light flashes, photophobia, yellow-green halos around visual images.
GI: anorexia, nausea, diarrhea, vomiting.

INTERACTIONS
Drug-drug. *Amiloride:* May decrease digoxin effect and increase renal clearance of digoxin. Monitor patient for altered digoxin effect.
Amiodarone, *diltiazem, indomethacin, nifedipine,* **quinidine, verapamil:** May in-crease digoxin level. Monitor patient for toxicity.
Amphotericin B, carbenicillin, cortico-steroids, **diuretics (such as chlorthalidone, loop diuretics, metolazone, thiazides),** *ticarcillin:* May cause hypokalemia, predis-posing patient to digitalis toxicity. Monitor potassium level.
Antacids, kaolin-pectin: May decrease absorption of oral digoxin. Separate doses as much as possible.
Antibiotics (azole antifungals, macrolides, telithromycin, tetracyclines), propafenone, ritonavir: May increase risk of toxicity. Monitor patient for toxicity.

Anticholinergics: May increase digoxin absorption of oral digoxin tablets. Monitor drug level and observe for toxicity.
Beta blockers, calcium channel blockers: May have additive effects on AV node con-duction, causing advanced or complete heart block. Use cautiously.
Cholestyramine, colestipol, metoclo-pramide: May decrease absorption of oral digoxin. Monitor patient for decreased digoxin level and effect. Give digoxin 1½ hours before or 2 hours after other drugs.
Parenteral calcium, thiazides: May cause hypercalcemia and hypomagnesemia, predisposing patient to digitalis toxicity. Monitor calcium and magnesium levels.
Drug-herb. *Betel palm, foxglove, fumitory, goldenseal, hawthorn, lily of the valley, motherwort, rue, shepherd's purse:* May increase cardiac effects. Discourage use together.
Gossypol, horsetail, licorice, oleander, Siberian ginseng, squill: May increase toxicity. Monitor patient closely.
Plantain, St. John's wort: May decrease effectiveness of drug. Discourage use together.

EFFECTS ON LAB TEST RESULTS
● May prolong PR interval or depress ST segment.

CONTRAINDICATIONS & CAUTIONS
● Contraindicated in patients hypersensitive to drug and in those with digitalis-induced toxicity, ventricular fibrillation, or ven-tricular tachycardia unless caused by heart failure.
● Don't use in patients with Wolff-Parkinson-White syndrome unless the conduction accessory pathway has been pharmacologically or surgically disabled.
● Use with extreme caution in elderly pa-tients and in those with acute MI, incom-plete AV block, sinus bradycardia, PVCs, chronic constrictive pericarditis, hyper-trophic cardiomyopathy, renal insufficiency, severe pulmonary disease, or hypothy-roidism.
⚠ Overdose S&S: Ventricular tachycardia, ventricular fibrillation, bradycardia, heart block, cardiac arrest, hyperkalemia.

†Canada   ◇OTC   ◆Off-label use   ✔Photoguide   *Liquid contains alcohol.

NURSING CONSIDERATIONS

• Drug-induced arrhythmias may increase the severity of heart failure and hypotension.

• In children, cardiac arrhythmias, including sinus bradycardia, are usually early signs of toxicity.

• Patients with hypothyroidism are extremely sensitive to cardiac glycosides and may need lower doses.

• Loading dose is usually divided over the first 24 hours with about half the loading dose given in the first dose.

• Toxic effects on the heart may be life-threatening and require immediate attention.

• Monitor digoxin level. Therapeutic level ranges from 0.8 to 2 nanograms/mL. Obtain blood for digoxin level at least 6 to 8 hours after last oral dose, preferably just before next scheduled dose.

❸ *Alert:* Excessively slow pulse rate (60 beats/minute or less) may be a sign of digitalis toxicity. Withhold drug and notify prescriber.

• Monitor potassium level carefully. Take corrective action before hypokalemia occurs. Hyperkalemia may result from digoxin toxicity.

• Reduce drug dose for 1 or 2 days before elective cardioversion. Adjust dosage after cardioversion.

• *Look alike–sound alike:* Don't confuse digoxin with doxepin.

PATIENT TEACHING

• Teach patient and a responsible family member about drug action, dosage regimen, how to take pulse, reportable signs, and follow-up care.

• Tell patient to report pulse less than 60 beats/minute or more than 110 beats/minute, or skipped beats or other rhythm changes.

• Instruct patient to report adverse reactions promptly. Nausea, vomiting, diarrhea, appetite loss, and visual disturbances may be indicators of toxicity.

• Encourage patient to eat a consistent amount of potassium-rich foods.

• Tell patient not to substitute one brand for another.

• Advise patient to avoid the use of herbal drugs or to consult his prescriber before taking one.

diltiazem hydrochloride
dil-TYE-a-zem

Apo-Diltiaz†, Cardizem✲, Cardizem CD✲, Cardizem LA✲, Cartia XT, Dilacor XR, Dilt-CD, Diltzac, Taztia XT, Tiazac, Tiazac XC†

Therapeutic class: Antihypertensives
Pharmacologic class: Calcium channel blockers
Pregnancy risk category: C

AVAILABLE FORMS
Capsules (extended-release): 60 mg, 90 mg, 120 mg, 180 mg, 240 mg, 300 mg, 360 mg, 420 mg
Injection: 5 mg/mL in 5-, 10-, 25-mL vials
Powder for injection: 100 mg
Tablets: 30 mg, 60 mg, 90 mg, 120 mg
Tablets (extended-release): 120 mg, 180 mg, 240 mg, 300 mg, 360 mg, 420 mg

INDICATIONS & DOSAGES
➤ **To manage Prinzmetal or variant angina or chronic stable angina pectoris**
Adults: 30 mg P.O. q.i.d. before meals and at bedtime. Increase dose gradually to maximum of 360 mg/day divided into three or four doses, as indicated. Or, give 120- or 180-mg extended-release capsule or 180-mg extended-release tablet P.O. once daily. Adjust over a 7- to 14-day period as needed and tolerated up to a maximum dose of 360 mg/day (Cardizem LA), 480 mg/day (Cardizem CD, Cartia XT, Dilacor XR), or 540 mg/day (Tiazac).
➤ **Hypertension, alone or as combination therapy**
Adults: Initially 180 to 240 mg P.O. once daily as monotherapy or 120 to 480 mg extended-release capsule P.O. once daily. Adjust dosage based on patient response to a maximum dose of 480 mg/day. Or, 120 to 540 mg extended-release tablet P.O. once daily. Dosage can be adjusted about every 2 weeks to a maximum of 540 mg daily.
➤ **Atrial fibrillation or flutter; paroxysmal supraventricular tachycardia**
Adults: 0.25 mg/kg I.V. as a bolus injection over 2 minutes. Repeat after 15 minutes if response isn't adequate with a dose of 0.35 mg/kg I.V. over 2 minutes. Follow

bolus with continuous I.V. infusion at 5 to 15 mg/hour (for up to 24 hours).
➤ **Idiopathic muscle cramps** ◆
Adults: 30 mg P.O. once daily.

ADMINISTRATION
P.O.
• Don't crush or allow patient to chew extended-release tablets; they should be swallowed whole.
• Tiazac extended-release capsules can be opened and the contents sprinkled onto a spoonful of applesauce. The applesauce must be eaten immediately and without chewing, followed by a glass of cool water.
I.V.
▼ For direct injection, you need not dilute the 5 mg/mL injection.
▼ For continuous infusion, add 25 mL of drug to 100 mL solution, 50 mL of drug to 250 mL solution, or 50 mL of drug to 500 mL solution of 5 mg/mL injection to yield 1 mg/mL, 0.83 mg/mL, or 0.45 mg/mL, respectively. Compatible solutions include normal saline solution, D$_5$W, or 5% dextrose and half-normal saline solution.
▼ For direct injection or continuous infusion; give slowly while monitoring ECG and blood pressure continuously.
▼ Don't infuse for longer than 24 hours.
▼ **Incompatibilities:** Acetazolamide, acyclovir, aminophylline, ampicillin, ampicillin sodium–sulbactam sodium, cefoperazone, diazepam, furosemide, heparin, hydrocortisone, insulin, methylprednisolone, nafcillin, phenytoin, rifampin, sodium bicarbonate, thiopental.

ACTION
A calcium channel blocker that inhibits calcium ion influx across cardiac and smooth-muscle cells, decreasing myocardial contractility and oxygen demand. Drug also dilates coronary arteries and arterioles.

Route	Onset	Peak	Duration
P.O.	30–60 min	2–3 hr	6–8 hr
P.O. (extended-release capsule)	2–3 hr	10–14 hr	12–24 hr
P.O. (Cardizem LA)	3–4 hr	11–18 hr	6–9 hr
I.V.	<3 min	2–7 min	1–10 hr

Half-life: 3 to 9 hours.

ADVERSE REACTIONS
CNS: headache, dizziness, asthenia, somnolence.
CV: edema, *arrhythmias, AV block, bradycardia, heart failure,* flushing, hypotension, conduction abnormalities, abnormal ECG.
GI: nausea, constipation, abdominal discomfort.
Hepatic: *acute hepatic injury.*
Skin: rash.

INTERACTIONS
Drug-drug. *Anesthetics:* May increase effects of anesthetics. Monitor patient.
Atazanavir, cimetidine: May inhibit diltiazem metabolism, increasing additive AV node conduction slowing. Monitor patient for toxicity.
Buspirone, quinidine, sirolimus, tacrolimus: May increase level of these drugs. Monitor drug levels and patient for toxicity.
Carbamazepine: May increase level of carbamazepine. Monitor carbamazepine level, and watch for signs and symptoms of toxicity.
Cyclosporine: May increase cyclosporine level. Monitor cyclosporine level with each dosage change.
Diazepam, midazolam, triazolam: May increase CNS depression and prolonged effects of these drugs. Use lower dose of these benzodiazepines.
Digoxin: May increase digoxin level. Monitor patient for digoxin toxicity.
Furosemide: May form a precipitate when mixed with diltiazem injection. Give through separate I.V. lines.
HMG-CoA reductase inhibitors (lovastatin, simvastatin): May increase risk of myopathy, rhabdomyolysis, and kidney failure. Use lower starting and maintenance doses of both agents.
Lithium: May reduce lithium levels, causing loss of mania control, and neurotoxic and psychotic symptoms. Monitor patient for signs of neurotoxicity.
Propranolol, other beta blockers: May precipitate heart failure or prolong conduction time. Use together cautiously.
Rifampin: May lower diltiazem levels significantly. Avoid use together.

Theophylline: May enhance action of theophylline, causing intoxication. Monitor theophylline levels.

EFFECTS ON LAB TEST RESULTS
None reported.

CONTRAINDICATIONS & CAUTIONS
• Contraindicated in patients hypersensitive to drug and in those with sick sinus syndrome or second- or third-degree AV block in the absence of an artificial pacemaker, cardiogenic shock, ventricular tachycardia, systolic blood pressure below 90 mm Hg, acute MI, or pulmonary congestion (documented by X-ray).
• Contraindicated in I.V. form for patients who have atrial fibrillation or flutter with an accessory bypass tract, as in Wolff-Parkinson-White syndrome or short PR interval syndrome.
• Use cautiously in elderly patients and in those with heart failure or impaired hepatic or renal function.
⚠ *Overdose S&S:* Bradycardia, hypotension, heart block, cardiac failure.

NURSING CONSIDERATIONS
• Patients controlled on drug alone or with other drugs may be switched to Cardizem LA tablets once a day at the nearest equivalent total daily dose.
• Monitor blood pressure and heart rate when starting therapy and during dosage adjustments.
• Maximal antihypertensive effect may not be seen for 14 days.
• If systolic blood pressure is below 90 mm Hg or heart rate is below 60 beats/minute, withhold dose and notify prescriber.
• *Look alike–sound alike:* Don't confuse Dilacor XR with Pilocar. Don't confuse Tiazac with Ziac.

PATIENT TEACHING
• Instruct patient to take drug as prescribed, even when he feels better.
• Advise patient to avoid hazardous activities during start of therapy.
• If nitrate therapy is prescribed during dosage adjustment, stress patient compliance. Tell patient that S.L. nitroglycerin may be taken with drug, as needed, when angina symptoms are acute.
⏲ *Alert:* Tell patient to swallow extended-release tablets whole, and not to crush or chew them.
• If patient is taking Tiazac extended-release capsules, inform him that these capsules can be opened and the contents sprinkled onto a spoonful of applesauce. He must eat the applesauce immediately and without chewing, and then drink a glass of cool water.

dimenhyDRINATE
dye-men-HYE-dri-nate

Dinate† ◇, Dramamine ◇, Gravol† ◇, Nauseatol† ◇, Travel Tabs† ◇

Therapeutic class: Antivertigo drugs
Pharmacologic class: Anticholinergics
Pregnancy risk category: B

AVAILABLE FORMS
Injection: 50 mg/mL
Tablets: 50 mg ◇
Tablets (chewable): 25 mg, 50 mg ◇

INDICATIONS & DOSAGES
➤ **To prevent and treat motion sickness**
Adults and children age 12 and older: 50 to 100 mg P.O. every 4 to 6 hours; 50 mg I.M., as needed; or 50 mg I.V. diluted in 10 mL normal saline solution for injection, injected over 2 minutes. Maximum, 400 mg daily. For prevention, use drug 30 minutes before motion exposure.
Children ages 6 to 11: 25 to 50 mg P.O. every 6 to 8 hours, not to exceed 150 mg in 24 hours. Or, 1.25 mg/kg or 37.5 mg/m^2 I.M. or P.O. q.i.d.
Children ages 2 to 5: 12.5 to 25 mg P.O. every 6 to 8 hours, not to exceed 75 mg in 24 hours. Or, 1.25 mg/kg or 37.5 mg/m^2 I.M. or P.O. q.i.d. Maximum, 300 mg daily.

ADMINISTRATION
P.O.
• May be given without regard for food.
• Give at least 30 minutes before activity or travel.

I.V.

▼ Dilute each milliliter (50 mg) of drug with 10 mL sterile water for injection, D$_5$W, or normal saline solution for injection.

▼ Give by direct injection over at least 2 minutes.

▼ Don't give if drug has particulate matter or discoloration.

▼ **Incompatibilities:** Aminophylline, ammonium chloride, amobarbital, butorphanol, chlorpromazine, glycopyrrolate, heparin, hydrocortisone sodium succinate, hydroxyzine hydrochloride, midazolam, pentobarbital sodium, phenobarbital sodium, phenytoin, prochlorperazine edisylate, promethazine hydrochloride, thiopental.

I.M.

● Inspect drug for particulate matter or discoloration; don't give if present.

ACTION

May affect neural pathways originating in the labyrinth to inhibit nausea and vomiting.

Route	Onset	Peak	Duration
P.O.	15–30 min	Unknown	3–6 hr
I.V.	Immediate	Unknown	3–6 hr
I.M.	20–30 min	Unknown	3–6 hr

Half-life: Unknown.

ADVERSE REACTIONS

CNS: drowsiness, confusion, dizziness, excitation, headache, insomnia, lassitude, nervousness, tingling and weakness of hands, vertigo.

CV: hypotension, palpitations, tachycardia.

EENT: blurred vision, diplopia, dry respiratory passages, nasal congestion.

GI: anorexia, constipation, diarrhea, dry mouth, epigastric distress, nausea, vomiting.

GU: urine retention.

Respiratory: thickened bronchial secretions, wheezing.

Skin: photosensitivity reactions, rash, urticaria.

Other: *anaphylaxis,* tightness of chest.

INTERACTIONS

Drug-drug. *CNS depressants:* May cause additive CNS depression. Avoid using together.

Ototoxic drugs: Dimenhydrinate may mask symptoms of ototoxicity. Use together cautiously.

TCAs, other anticholinergics: May increase anticholinergic activity. Monitor patient.

Drug-lifestyle. *Alcohol use:* May cause additive CNS depression. Discourage use together.

EFFECTS ON LAB TEST RESULTS

● May prevent, reduce, or mask diagnostic skin test response. May alter xanthine (caffeine, aminophylline) test results.

CONTRAINDICATIONS & CAUTIONS

● Contraindicated in patients hypersensitive to drug or its components.

● Use cautiously in elderly patients, patients receiving ototoxic drugs, and patients with seizures, acute angle-closure glaucoma, or enlarged prostate gland.

⚠ *Overdose S&S:* Drowsiness, seizures, coma, respiratory depression.

NURSING CONSIDERATIONS

● Elderly patients may be more susceptible to adverse CNS effects.

● Undiluted solution irritates veins and may cause sclerosis.

● Stop drug 4 days before diagnostic skin tests to prevent falsifying test response.

● Dramamine may contain tartrazine.

🖐 *Alert:* Drug may mask symptoms of ototoxicity, brain tumor, or intestinal obstruction.

● *Look alike–sound alike:* Don't confuse dimenhydrinate with diphenhydramine.

PATIENT TEACHING

● Advise patient to avoid activities that require alertness until CNS effects of drug are known.

● Instruct patient to report adverse reactions promptly.

✳ NEW DRUG

dimethyl fumarate
dye-METH-il

Tecfidera

Therapeutic class: Immunomodulators
Pharmacologic class: Nuclear factor–like
2 pathway activators
Pregnancy risk category: C

AVAILABLE FORMS
Capsules (delayed-release): 120 mg,
240 mg

INDICATIONS & DOSAGES
➤ **Relapsing multiple sclerosis**
Adults: Initially, 120 mg P.O. b.i.d. for
7 days; then increase to maintenance dosage
of 240 mg b.i.d.

ADMINISTRATION
P.O.
- Make sure patient swallows capsules
whole and intact. Don't allow patient to
chew capsules, and don't crush or open
capsule and sprinkle on food.
- Give without regard to meals.
- Store capsules in their original container
to prevent exposure to light; once bottle
has been opened, discard medication after
90 days. Store at room temperature.

ACTION
Unknown. The drug and its metabolite,
monomethyl fumarate, have been shown
to activate the nuclear factor–like 2 pathway, which reduces oxidative stress that
contributes to myelin damage.

Route	Onset	Peak	Duration
P.O.	Unknown	2–2½ hr	Unknown

Half-life: 1 hour.

ADVERSE REACTIONS
CV: flushing.
GI: abdominal pain, diarrhea, nausea,
vomiting, dyspepsia.
GU: albuminuria.
Hematologic: *lymphopenia.*
Skin: pruritus, rash, erythema.

INTERACTIONS
None reported.

EFFECTS ON LAB TEST RESULTS
- May increase AST and ALT levels.
- May decrease lymphocyte count.

CONTRAINDICATIONS & CAUTIONS
- Contraindicated in patients hypersensitive
to drug or its components.
- Use cautiously in patients with lymphopenia and in those with increased risk of ac-
quiring serious infections.
- Use cautiously in pregnant women and
only if benefit outweighs possible risk to
fetus.
- It isn't known if drug appears in breast
milk. Use cautiously in breast-feeding
women.

NURSING CONSIDERATIONS
- Obtain baseline CBC within 6 months
before the start of therapy to determine if
patient has preexisting low lymphocyte
count.
- Monitor CBC annually, and as clinically
appropriate.
- Transient increase in eosinophil count
may occur during the first 2 months of
therapy.
- If patient has a serious infection, consider
withholding treatment until the infection is
resolved.
- If patient experiences flushing during
therapy, giving drug with food may decrease
severity.

PATIENT TEACHING
- Instruct patients to swallow capsule whole
and intact.
- Reassure patient that GI side effects usually decrease after the first month of therapy.
- Inform patient that flushing may occur
after starting the medication and that taking
it with food may help.
- Advise patient that a blood test may be
needed before starting this medication and
then yearly to check for a low lymphocyte
count.
- Instruct female patient that if she is pregnant or plans to become pregnant during
therapy to inform her prescriber.

• Advise female patient who is pregnant to enroll in the pregnancy registry by calling 1-800-456-2255.

diphenhydrAMINE hydrochloride
dye-fen-HYE-drah-meen

Aler-Cap ◇, Aler-Dryl ◇, Aler-Tab ◇, Altaryl Children's Allergy† ◇, Anti-Hist ◇, Banophen ◇, Benadryl ◇, Ben-Tann ◇, Children's Pedia Care Nighttime Cough† ◇, Compoz Nighttime SleepAid ◇, Diphenhist ◇, Dormin ◇, 40 Winks ◇, Genahist ◇, Geri-Dryl ◇, Nytol ◇, PediaCare Childrens Allergy ◇, Q-Dryl ◇, Quenalin ◇, Scot-Tussin Allergy Relief ◇, Siladryl ◇*, Silphen ◇, Simply Allergy ◇, Simply Sleep ◇, Sominex ◇, Tetra-Formula Nighttime Sleep ◇, TGT Allergy Melts Childrens ◇, TH Allergy Relief ◇, TH Childrens Allergy ◇, TH Rest Simply ◇, TH Sleep Aid ◇, TheraFlu Multi-Symptom ◇, Total Allergy ◇, Triaminic MultiSymptom ◇*, Unisom SleepMelts ◇, Wal-Dryl Allergy Release Childrens ◇, ZzzQuil ◇

Therapeutic class: Antihistamines
Pharmacologic class: Ethanolamines
Pregnancy risk category: B

AVAILABLE FORMS
Capsules: 25 mg ◇, 50 mg ◇
Elixir: 12.5 mg/5 mL ◇*
Injection: 50 mg/mL
Strips (orally disintegrating): 12.5 mg ◇*, 25 mg ◇*
Syrup: 12.5 mg/5 mL ◇*
Tablets: 25 mg ◇, 50 mg ◇
Tablets (chewable): 12.5 mg ◇, 25 mg
Tablets (orally disintegrating): 12.5 mg ◇

INDICATIONS & DOSAGES
➤ **Rhinitis, allergy symptoms, motion sickness, Parkinson disease**
Adults and children age 12 and older: 25 to 50 mg P.O. every 4 to 6 hours. Maximum, 300 mg P.O. daily. Or, 10 to 50 mg I.V. or deep I.M. Maximum I.V. or I.M. dosage, 400 mg daily.

Children ages 6 to 11: 12.5 to 25 mg P.O. every 4 to 6 hours. Maximum dose is 150 mg daily. Or, 5 mg/kg deep I.M. or I.V. divided into four doses. Maximum dose is 300 mg daily.
Children younger than age 6 and weighing more than 9 kg (approximately 20 lb) (prescription products only): 5 mg/kg P.O. daily or 150 mg/m² P.O. daily; maximum, 300 mg daily. Or, 5 mg/kg daily deep I.M. or I.V. divided into four doses. Maximum dose is 300 mg daily. Don't use in neonates and premature infants.
➤ **Nighttime sleep aid**
Adults: 50 mg P.O. at bedtime.
➤ **Nonproductive cough**
Adults and children age 12 and older: 25 mg (syrup) P.O. every 4 hours. Don't exceed 150 mg daily. Or, 25 to 50 mg (liquid) every 4 hours. Don't exceed 300 mg daily.
Children ages 6 to 11: 12.5 mg (syrup) P.O. every 4 hours. Don't exceed 75 mg daily. Or, 12.5 to 25 mg (liquid) P.O. every 4 hours. Don't exceed 150 mg daily.

ADMINISTRATION
P.O.
• Give drug with food or milk to reduce GI distress.
I.V.
▼ Don't exceed 25 mg/minute.
▼ **Incompatibilities:** Allopurinol, amobarbital, amphotericin B, cefepime, dexamethasone, foscarnet, haloperidol lactate, pentobarbital, phenobarbital, phenytoin, thiopental.
I.M.
• Give I.M. injection deep into large muscle.
• Alternate injection sites to prevent irritation.

ACTION
Competes with histamine for H_1-receptor sites. Prevents, but doesn't reverse, histamine-mediated responses, particularly those of the bronchial tubes, GI tract, uterus, and blood vessels.

Route	Onset	Peak	Duration
P.O.	15 min	1–4 hr	6–8 hr
I.V.	Immediate	1–4 hr	6–8 hr
I.M.	Unknown	1–4 hr	6–8 hr

Half-life: About 2½ to 9½ hours.

ADVERSE REACTIONS

CNS: drowsiness, sedation, sleepiness, dizziness, incoordination, *seizures,* confusion, insomnia, headache, vertigo, fatigue, restlessness, tremor, nervousness.
CV: palpitations, hypotension, tachycardia.
EENT: diplopia, blurred vision, nasal congestion, tinnitus.
GI: dry mouth, nausea, epigastric distress, vomiting, diarrhea, constipation, anorexia.
GU: dysuria, urine retention, urinary frequency.
Hematologic: *thrombocytopenia, agranulocytosis,* hemolytic anemia.
Respiratory: thickening of bronchial secretions.
Skin: urticaria, photosensitivity, rash.
Other: *anaphylactic shock.*

INTERACTIONS

Drug-drug. *CNS depressants:* May increase sedation. Use together cautiously.
MAO inhibitors: May increase anticholinergic effects. Avoid using together.
Other products that contain diphenhydramine (including topical therapy): May increase risk of adverse reactions. Avoid using together.
Drug-lifestyle. *Alcohol use:* May increase CNS depression. Discourage use together.
Sun exposure: May cause photosensitivity reactions. Advise patient to avoid extensive sunlight exposure.

EFFECTS ON LAB TEST RESULTS

• May decrease hemoglobin level and hematocrit.
• May decrease granulocyte and platelet counts.
• May prevent, reduce, or mask positive result in diagnostic skin test.

CONTRAINDICATIONS & CAUTIONS

• Contraindicated in patients hypersensitive to drug; newborns; premature neonates; breast-feeding women; patients with angle-closure glaucoma, stenosing peptic ulcer, symptomatic prostatic hyperplasia, bladder neck obstruction, or pyloroduodenal obstruction; and those having an acute asthmatic attack.
• Avoid use in patients taking MAO inhibitors.

• Use with caution in patients with prostatic hyperplasia, asthma, COPD, increased intraocular pressure, hyperthyroidism, CV disease, and hypertension.
• Children younger than age 12 should use drug only as directed by prescriber.
⚠ *Overdose S&S:* Dry mouth, fixed or dilated pupils, flushing, GI symptoms.

NURSING CONSIDERATIONS

• Stop drug 4 days before diagnostic skin testing.
• Injection form is for I.V. or I.M. administration only.
• Dizziness, excessive sedation, syncope, toxicity, paradoxical stimulation, and hypotension are more likely to occur in elderly patients.
• *Look alike–sound alike:* Don't confuse diphenhydramine with dimenhydrinate. Don't confuse Benadryl with Bentyl or benazepril.

PATIENT TEACHING

• Warn patient not to take this drug with any other products that contain diphenhydramine (including topical therapy) because of increased adverse reactions.
• Instruct patient to take drug 30 minutes before travel to prevent motion sickness.
• Tell patient to take diphenhydramine with food or milk to reduce GI distress.
• Warn patient to avoid alcohol and hazardous activities that require alertness until CNS effects of drug are known.
• Inform patient that sugarless gum, hard candy, or ice chips may relieve dry mouth.
• Tell patient to notify prescriber if tolerance develops because a different antihistamine may need to be prescribed.
• Drug is in many OTC sleep and cold products. Advise patient to consult prescriber before using these products.
• Warn patient of possible photosensitivity reactions. Advise use of a sunblock.

Reactions in bold italics are *life-threatening*. Interactions may have a *rapid onset* or a *delayed onset*.

diphenoxylate hydrochloride–atropine sulfate
dye-fen-OKS-ul-ate and A-troe-peen

Lomotil*, Lonox

Therapeutic class: Antidiarrheals
Pharmacologic class: Opioids
Pregnancy risk category: C
Controlled substance schedule: V

AVAILABLE FORMS
Liquid: 2.5 mg/5 mL (with atropine sulfate 0.025 mg/5 mL)*
Tablets: 2.5 mg (with atropine sulfate 0.025 mg)

INDICATIONS & DOSAGES
➤ **Acute, nonspecific diarrhea**
Adults and children older than age 12:
Initially, 5 mg P.O. q.i.d.; then adjust as needed. Maximum dosage 20 mg/day.
Children ages 2 to 12: 0.3 to 0.4 mg/kg liquid form P.O. daily in four divided doses. For maintenance, reduce dose when initial control of symptoms is achieved. Dosage may be reduced by as much as 75%. Maximum dosage 20 mg/day.

ADMINISTRATION
P.O.
● Give drug without regard for food.

ACTION
Probably increases smooth muscle tone in GI tract, inhibits motility and propulsion, and diminishes secretions.

Route	Onset	Peak	Duration
P.O.	45–60 min	3 hr	3–4 hr

Half-life: Diphenoxylate, 2½ hours; its major metabolite, diphenoxylic acid, 4½ hours; atropine, 2½ hours.

ADVERSE REACTIONS
CNS: dizziness, sedation, confusion, depression, drowsiness, euphoria, headache, lethargy, malaise, numbness in limbs, restlessness.
CV: tachycardia.
EENT: blurred vision.

GI: dry mouth, *pancreatitis,* paralytic ileus, abdominal discomfort or distention, anorexia, fluid retention in bowel or megacolon, nausea, swollen gums, vomiting.
GU: urine retention.
Respiratory: *respiratory depression.*
Skin: dry skin, pruritus, rash.
Other: *anaphylaxis, angioedema,* possible physical dependence with long-term use.

INTERACTIONS
Drug-drug. *Barbiturates, CNS depressants, opioids, tranquilizers:* May enhance CNS depression. Monitor patient closely.
MAO inhibitors: May cause hypertensive crisis. Avoid using together.
Drug-lifestyle. *Alcohol use:* May enhance CNS depression. Discourage use together.

EFFECTS ON LAB TEST RESULTS
None reported.

CONTRAINDICATIONS & CAUTIONS
● Contraindicated in children younger than age 2 and in patients hypersensitive to diphenoxylate or atropine, in those with obstructive jaundice, and in those with acute diarrhea resulting from poison, organisms that penetrate intestinal mucosa, or antibiotic-induced pseudomembranous enterocolitis.
● Use cautiously in children age 2 and older; in patients with hepatic disease, opioid dependence, or acute ulcerative colitis; and in pregnant women.
⚠ *Overdose S&S:* Dry skin and mucous membranes, mydriasis, restlessness, flushing, hyperthermia, tachycardia, lethargy, coma, hypotonic reflexes, nystagmus, respiratory depression.

NURSING CONSIDERATIONS
☞ *Alert:* Monitor fluid and electrolyte balance. Correct fluid and electrolyte disturbances before starting drug. Dehydration, especially in young children, may increase risk of delayed toxicity. Fluid retention in bowel or megacolon may occur with drug use and may mask depletion of extracellular fluid and electrolytes, especially in young children treated for acute gastroenteritis.
● Stop therapy immediately and notify prescriber if abdominal distention or other

signs or symptoms of toxic megacolon develop.
• Don't use for antibiotic-induced diarrhea.
• Drug is unlikely to be effective if no response occurs within 48 hours.
• Risk of physical dependence increases with high dosage and long-term use. Atropine sulfate helps discourage abuse.
• Monitor for signs of overdose, which may initially include restlessness, flushing, hyperthermia, and tachycardia, followed by lethargy, coma, pinpoint pupils, hypotonicity, and respiratory depression.
• *Look alike–sound alike:* Don't confuse Lomotil with Lamictal.

PATIENT TEACHING
• Tell patient not to exceed recommended dosage.
• Warn patient not to use drug to treat acute diarrhea for longer than 2 days and to seek medical attention if diarrhea continues.
• Advise patient to avoid hazardous activities, such as driving, until CNS effects of drug are known.

dipyridamole
dye-peer-IH-duh-mohl

Persantine

Therapeutic class: Antiplatelet drugs
Pharmacologic class: Pyrimidine analogues
Pregnancy risk category: B

AVAILABLE FORMS
Injection: 5 mg/mL in 2- and 10-mL vials
Tablets: 25 mg, 50 mg, 75 mg

INDICATIONS & DOSAGES
➤ **To inhibit platelet adhesion in prosthetic heart valves (given together with warfarin)**
Adults and children older than age 12: 75 to 100 mg P.O. q.i.d.
➤ **Alternative to exercise in evaluation of coronary artery disease during thallium myocardial perfusion scintigraphy**
Adults: 0.57 mg/kg as an I.V. infusion at a constant rate over 4 minutes (0.142 mg/kg/minute).

ADMINISTRATION
P.O.
• If GI distress develops, give drug 1 hour before meals or with meals.
I.V.
▼ For use as a diagnostic drug, dilute in half-normal or normal saline solution or D_5W in at least a 1:2 ratio for a total volume of 20 to 50 mL.
▼ Inject thallium-201 within 5 minutes after completing the 4-minute dipyridamole infusion.
▼ Don't mix in same syringe or infusion container with other drugs.
▼ **Incompatibilities:** Other drugs.

ACTION
May involve drug's ability to increase adenosine, which is a coronary vasodilator and platelet aggregation inhibitor.

Route	Onset	Peak	Duration
P.O.	Unknown	75 min	Unknown
I.V.	Unknown	2 min	Unknown

Half-life: 1 to 12 hours; alpha half-life of oral form, 40 minutes; beta half-life of oral form, 10 hours.

ADVERSE REACTIONS
CNS: dizziness, headache.
CV: angina pectoris, chest pain, *ECG abnormalities,* flushing.
GI: nausea, abdominal distress, diarrhea, vomiting.
Skin: rash, pruritus.

INTERACTIONS
Drug-drug. *Adenosine:* May increase levels and cardiac effects of adenosine. Adjust adenosine dose as needed.
Cholinesterase inhibitors: May counteract anticholinesterase effects and aggravate myasthenia gravis. Monitor patient.
Heparin: May increase risk of bleeding. Monitor patient closely.
Theophylline, other xanthine derivatives: May prevent coronary vasodilation by I.V. dipyridamole, causing a false-negative thallium-imaging result. Avoid using together.

EFFECTS ON LAB TEST RESULTS
• May increase liver enzyme levels.

CONTRAINDICATIONS & CAUTIONS
• Contraindicated in patients hypersensitive to drug.
• Use cautiously in patients with hypotension and those with severe coronary artery disease.
⚠ *Overdose S&S:* Hypotension, warm feeling, flushes, sweating, restlessness, weakness, dizziness, tachycardia.

NURSING CONSIDERATIONS
• Observe for adverse reactions, especially with large doses. Monitor blood pressure.
• Observe for signs and symptoms of bleeding; note prolonged bleeding time (especially with large doses or long-term therapy).
• The value of drug as part of an antithrombotic regimen is controversial; its use may not provide significantly better results than aspirin alone.
• Dipyridamole injection may contain tartrazine, which may cause allergic reactions in some patients.
• *Look alike–sound alike:* Don't confuse dipyridamole with disopyramide. Don't confuse Persantine with Periactin or bosentan.

PATIENT TEACHING
• Instruct patient to take drug exactly as prescribed.
• Tell patient to report adverse reactions promptly.
• Tell patient receiving drug I.V. to report discomfort at insertion site.

---

disulfiram
dye-SUL-fi-ram

Antabuse

Therapeutic class: Alcohol deterrents
Pharmacologic class: Aldehyde dehydrogenase inhibitors
Pregnancy risk category: C

AVAILABLE FORMS
Tablets: 250 mg, 500 mg

INDICATIONS & DOSAGES
➤ **Adjunct to management of alcohol abstinence**
Adults: 250 to 500 mg P.O. as single dose in morning for 1 to 2 weeks or in evening if drowsiness occurs. Maintenance dosage is 125 to 500 mg P.O. daily (average 250 mg) until permanent self-control is established. Treatment may continue for months or years.

ADMINISTRATION
P.O.
❸ *Alert:* Never give until patient has abstained from alcohol for at least 12 hours. He should clearly understand consequences of drug and give permission for its use. Use drug only in patients who are cooperative, well motivated, and receiving supportive psychiatric therapy.

ACTION
Blocks oxidation of alcohol at the acetaldehyde stage. Excess acetaldehyde produces a highly unpleasant reaction in the presence of even small amounts of alcohol.

Route	Onset	Peak	Duration
P.O.	1–2 hr	Unknown	14 days

Half-life: Unknown.

ADVERSE REACTIONS
CNS: drowsiness, headache, fatigue, delirium, depression, neuritis, peripheral neuritis, polyneuritis, restlessness, psychotic reactions.
EENT: optic neuritis.
GI: metallic or garlicky aftertaste.
GU: erectile dysfunction.
Skin: acneiform or allergic dermatitis, occasional eruptions.
Other: *disulfiram reaction precipitated by alcohol use.*

INTERACTIONS
Drug-drug. *Barbiturates:* May prolong duration of barbiturate effect. Closely monitor patient.
CNS depressants: May increase CNS depression. Use together cautiously.
Coumarin anticoagulants: May increase anticoagulant effect. Adjust dosage of anticoagulant.

Isoniazid: May cause ataxia or marked change in behavior. Avoid using together.

Metronidazole: May cause psychotic reaction. Avoid using together.

Midazolam: May increase midazolam level. Use together cautiously.

Paraldehyde: May cause toxic level of acetaldehyde. Avoid using together.

Phenytoin: May increase toxic effect of phenytoin. Monitor phenytoin level closely, and adjust dose as necessary.

TCAs, especially amitriptyline: May cause transient delirium. Closely monitor patient.

Drug-herb. *Herbal preparations containing alcohol:* May cause disulfiram reaction. Warn patient against using together. Alcohol reaction may occur as long as 2 weeks after single drug dose.

Drug-food. *Caffeine:* May increase elimination half-life of caffeine. Tell patient to watch for effects.

Drug-lifestyle. *Alcohol use:* May cause disulfiram reaction, including flushing, tachycardia, bronchospasm, sweating, nausea and vomiting, or death. Warn patient not to use products containing alcohol, including back rub preparations, cough syrups, liniments, and shaving lotion, or to drink alcoholic beverages.

EFFECTS ON LAB TEST RESULTS
• May increase cholesterol level.

CONTRAINDICATIONS & CAUTIONS
• Contraindicated in patients hypersensitive to drug or other thiram derivatives used in pesticides and rubber vulcanization; in those with psychoses, myocardial disease, or coronary occlusion; in those receiving metronidazole, paraldehyde, alcohol, or alcohol-containing products; and in those experiencing alcohol intoxication or who have ingested alcohol in preceding 12 hours.

• Don't give drug during pregnancy.

• Use with caution in patients also receiving phenytoin therapy and in those with diabetes mellitus, hypothyroidism, seizure disorder, cerebral damage, nephritis, or hepatic cirrhosis or insufficiency.

NURSING CONSIDERATIONS
Black Box Warning Never give drug to a patient who is in a state of alcohol intoxication or without the patient's full knowledge. ▪

• Perform complete physical examination and laboratory studies, including CBC, SMA-12, and transaminase level, before therapy and repeat regularly.

• Disulfiram reaction may result from alcohol use, with flushing, throbbing headache, dyspnea, nausea, copious vomiting, diaphoresis, thirst, chest pain, palpitations, hyperventilation, hypotension, syncope, anxiety, weakness, blurred vision, confusion, and arthropathy.

❸ *Alert:* A severe disulfiram reaction can cause respiratory depression, CV collapse, arrhythmias, MI, acute heart failure, seizures, unconsciousness, and death.

• Mild reactions may occur in sensitive patient with blood alcohol levels of 5 to 10 mg/dL; symptoms are fully developed at 50 mg/dL; unconsciousness typically occurs at 125 to 150 mg/dL level. Reaction may last from 30 minutes to several hours or as long as alcohol remains in blood.

• The longer the patient remains on the drug, the more sensitive he becomes to alcohol.

• *Look alike–sound alike:* Don't confuse Antabuse with Anturane.

PATIENT TEACHING
Black Box Warning Caution patient's family that drug should never be given to patient without his knowledge; severe reaction or death could result if patient drinks alcohol. ▪

• Reassure patient that drug-induced adverse reactions (unrelated to alcohol use), such as drowsiness, fatigue, impotence, headache, peripheral neuritis, and metallic or garlic taste, subside after about 2 weeks of therapy.

• Advise patient not to drink alcoholic beverages or use products containing alcohol, including topical preparations and mouthwash.

• Have patient verify content of OTC products with pharmacist before use.

• Advise patient to carry a medical identification card stating that he's taking disulfiram.

SAFETY ALERT!

DOBUTamine hydrochloride
DOE-byoo-ta-meen

Therapeutic class: Inotropes
Pharmacologic class: Adrenergics–
beta$_1$ agonists
Pregnancy risk category: B

AVAILABLE FORMS
Dobutamine in 5% dextrose: 0.5 mg/mL
(250 mg); 1 mg/mL (250 or 500 mg);
2 mg/mL (500 mg); 4 mg/mL (1,000 mg)
Injection: 12.5 mg/mL in 20-mL and 40-mL
vials (parenteral)

INDICATIONS & DOSAGES
➤ **Increased cardiac output in short-term
treatment of cardiac decompensation
caused by depressed contractility, such as
during refractory heart failure; adjunctive therapy in cardiac surgery**
Adults and children: 0.5 to 1 mcg/kg/minute
I.V. infusion, titrating to optimum dosage
of 2 to 20 mcg/kg/minute. Usual effective
range to increase cardiac output is 2.5 to
10 mcg/kg/minute. Rarely, rates up to
40 mcg/kg/minute may be needed.

ADMINISTRATION
I.V.
▼ Before starting therapy, give a plasma
volume expander to correct hypovolemia
and a cardiac glycoside.
▼ Dilute concentrate before injecting.
Compatible solutions include D$_5$W, D$_{10}$W,
half-normal or normal saline solution
for injection, lactated Ringer injection,
Isolyte-M with D$_5$W, Normosol-M in
D$_5$W, and 20% Osmitrol.
▼ Diluting one vial (250 mg) with
1,000 mL of solution yields 250 mcg/mL.
Diluting with 500 mL yields 500 mcg/mL.
Diluting with 250 mL yields 1,000
mcg/mL.
▼ Oxidation may slightly discolor admixture. This doesn't indicate a significant loss
of potency, provided drug is used within
24 hours of reconstitution.
▼ Give through a central venous catheter
or large peripheral vein using an infusion
pump.

▼ Titrate rate according to patient's condition.
▼ Infusions lasting up to 72 hours produce no more adverse effects than shorter
infusions.
▼ Watch for irritation and infiltration;
extravasation can cause tissue damage and
necrosis. Change I.V. sites regularly to
avoid phlebitis.
▼ Solution remains stable for 24 hours.
Don't freeze.
▼ **Incompatibilities:** Acyclovir, alkaline solutions, alteplase, aminophylline,
bretylium, bumetanide, calcium chloride, calcium gluconate, cefazolin, cefepime, diazepam, digoxin, ethacrynate,
furosemide, heparin, hydrocortisone
sodium succinate, indomethacin, insulin,
magnesium sulfate, midazolam, penicillin,
phenytoin, phytonadione, piperacillin–
tazobactam, potassium chloride, sodium
bicarbonate, thiopental, verapamil, warfarin. Don't give through same line with
other drugs.

ACTION
Stimulates heart's beta$_1$ receptors to increase myocardial contractility and stroke
volume. At therapeutic dosages, drug increases cardiac output by decreasing peripheral vascular resistance, reducing ventricular
filling pressure, and facilitating AV node
conduction.

Route	Onset	Peak	Duration
I.V.	1–2 min	10 min	<5 min after infusion

Half-life: 2 minutes.

ADVERSE REACTIONS
CNS: headache.
CV: hypertension, increased heart rate,
angina, PVCs, phlebitis, nonspecific chest
pain, palpitations, ventricular ectopy, hypotension.
GI: nausea, vomiting.
Respiratory: *asthma attack,* shortness of
breath.
Other: *anaphylaxis,* hypersensitivity
reactions.

INTERACTIONS
Drug-drug. *Beta blockers:* May antagonize
dobutamine effects. Avoid using together.

Bretylium: May increase risk of arrhythmias. Monitor ECG.

General anesthetics: May have greater risk of ventricular arrhythmias. Monitor ECG closely.

Guanethidine, oxytocic drugs: May increase pressor response, causing severe hypertension. Monitor blood pressure closely.

TCAs: May potentiate pressor response and cause arrhythmias. Use together cautiously.

Drug-herb. *Rue:* May increase inotropic potential. Discourage use together.

EFFECTS ON LAB TEST RESULTS
• May decrease potassium level.
• May decrease platelet count.

CONTRAINDICATIONS & CAUTIONS
• Contraindicated in patients hypersensitive to drug or its components and in those with idiopathic hypertrophic subaortic stenosis.
• Use cautiously in patients with history of hypertension because drug may increase pressor response.
• Use cautiously after acute MI.
• Use cautiously in patients with history of sulfite sensitivity.
⚠ *Overdose S&S:* Anorexia, nausea, vomiting, tremor, anxiety, palpitations, headache, shortness of breath, anginal and nonspecific chest pain, hypertension, tachyarrhythmias, myocardial ischemia, ventricular fibrillation, hypotension.

NURSING CONSIDERATIONS
🖖 *Alert:* Because drug increases AV node conduction, patients with atrial fibrillation may develop a rapid ventricular rate.
• Continuously monitor ECG, blood pressure, pulmonary artery wedge pressure, cardiac output, and urine output.
• Monitor electrolyte levels. Drug may lower potassium level.
• *Look alike–sound alike:* Don't confuse dobutamine with dopamine.

PATIENT TEACHING
• Tell patient to report adverse reactions promptly, especially labored breathing and drug-induced headache.
• Instruct patient to report discomfort at I.V. insertion site.

SAFETY ALERT!

docetaxel
dohs-eh-TAX-ell

Docefrez, Taxotere

Therapeutic class: Antineoplastics
Pharmacologic class: Taxoids
Pregnancy risk category: D

AVAILABLE FORMS
Injection: 20 mg, 80 mg, 160 mg in single-dose vials

INDICATIONS & DOSAGES
➤ **Locally advanced or metastatic breast cancer after failure of previous chemotherapy**
Adults: 60 to 100 mg/m^2 I.V. over 1 hour every 3 weeks.
Adjust-a-dose: In patients receiving 100 mg/m^2 who experience febrile neutropenia, neutrophil count of less than 500/mm^3 for longer than 1 week, severe or cumulative cutaneous reactions, or severe peripheral neuropathy, reduce subsequent dose by 25%, to 75 mg/m^2. In patients who continue to experience reactions with decreased dose, either decrease it further to 55 mg/m^2 or stop drug.
➤ **Adjuvant postsurgery treatment of operable, node-positive breast cancer (excluding Docefrez)**
Adults: 75 mg/m^2 I.V. as a 1-hour infusion given 1 hour after doxorubicin 50 mg/m^2 and cyclophosphamide 500 mg/m^2 every 3 weeks for six cycles.
Adjust-a-dose: Patients who experience febrile neutropenia should receive granulocyte colony-stimulating factor (G-CSF) in all subsequent cycles. If febrile neutropenia doesn't resolve, continue G-CSF and reduce docetaxel dose to 60 mg/m^2. For patients who experience severe or cumulative cutaneous reactions or moderate neurosensory signs and symptoms, reduce dose to 60 mg/m^2. If these reactions persist at the reduced dosage, stop treatment.
➤ **Locally advanced or metastatic non–small-cell lung cancer (NSCLC) after failure of previous cisplatin-based chemotherapy**

Reactions in bold italics are *life-threatening*. Interactions may have a *rapid onset* or a *delayed onset*.

Adults: 75 mg/m² I.V. over 1 hour every 3 weeks.

Adjust-a-dose: In patients who experience febrile neutropenia, neutrophil count of less than 500/mm³ for longer than 1 week, severe or cumulative cutaneous reactions, or other grade 3 or 4 nonhematologic toxicities, withhold drug until toxicity resolves; then restart at 55 mg/m². In patients in whom grade 3 peripheral neuropathy or above develops, stop drug.

➤ **With cisplatin, unresectable, locally advanced, or metastatic NSCLC not previously treated with chemotherapy (excluding Docefrez)**
Adults: 75 mg/m² docetaxel I.V. over 1 hour, immediately followed by cisplatin 75 mg/m² I.V. over 30 to 60 minutes every 3 weeks.

Adjust-a-dose: In patients whose lowest platelet count during the previous course of therapy was less than 25,000/mm³, and those with febrile neutropenia or serious nonhematologic toxicities, decrease docetaxel dosage to 65 mg/m². For patients who require a further dosage reduction, a dosage of 50 mg/m² is recommended. For cisplatin dosage adjustments, see manufacturers' prescribing information.

➤ **Androgen-independent metastatic prostate cancer, with prednisone**
Adults: 75 mg/m² I.V., as a 1-hour infusion every 3 weeks, given with 5 mg prednisone P.O. b.i.d. continuously. Premedicate with dexamethasone 8 mg P.O. at 12 hours, 3 hours, and 1 hour before docetaxel infusion.

Adjust-a-dose: In patients who experience febrile neutropenia, neutrophil count less than 500/mm³ for more than 1 week, severe or cumulative cutaneous reactions, or moderate neurosensory signs or symptoms, reduce subsequent dose to 60 mg/m². In patients who continue to experience reactions with the decreased dose, stop treatment.

➤ **Advanced gastric adenocarcinoma, in combination with cisplatin and 5-FU (excluding Docefrez)**
Adults: Premedicate with antiemetics and hydration per cisplatin recommendations. Give 75 mg/m² docetaxel I.V. over 1 hour, followed by cisplatin 75 mg/m² I.V. over 1 to 3 hours both on day 1 only, then, 5-FU

750 mg/m² I.V. daily as a 24-hour continuous infusion for 5 days beginning at the end of cisplatin infusion. Repeat cycle every 3 weeks.

Adjust-a-dose: Patients who experience febrile neutropenia should receive G-CSF in subsequent cycles. If episode recurs, reduce dose to 60 mg/m². If subsequent episodes of complicated neutropenia occur, reduce dose to 45 mg/m². In patients who experience grade 4 thrombocytopenia, reduce dosage to 60 mg/m². Don't retreat until neutrophil count is greater than 1,500/mm³ and platelet count is greater than 100,000/mm³. Stop treatment if toxicity persists.

For patients who experience diarrhea, adjust dosage as follows: for first episode of grade 3 diarrhea, reduce 5-FU dose by 20%; for second episode, reduce docetaxel dose by 20%; for first episode of grade 4 diarrhea, reduce docetaxel and 5-FU doses by 20%; for second episode, stop drug.

For patients who experience stomatitis, adjust dosage as follows: for first episode of grade 3 stomatitis, reduce 5-FU dose by 20%; for second episode, stop 5-FU in subsequent cycles; for third episode, reduce docetaxel dose by 20%. For first episode of grade 4 stomatitis, stop 5-FU in subsequent cycles; for second episode, reduce docetaxel dose by 20%.

For patients who experience liver dysfunction, reduce docetaxel dose by 20%. If AST or ALT is greater than 5 times upper limit of normal (ULN) or alkaline phosphatase is greater than 5 times ULN, stop treatment.

➤ **Induction treatment of inoperable locally advanced squamous cell cancer of the head and neck (SCCHN), with cisplatin and 5-FU (excluding Docefrez)**
Adults: 75 mg/m² I.V. infusion over 1 hour, followed by cisplatin 75 mg/m² I.V. infusion over 1 hour, on day 1, followed by 5-FU 750 mg/m² daily as a continuous I.V. infusion for 5 days. Repeat this regimen every 3 weeks for four cycles. After chemotherapy, patients should receive radiotherapy. Premedicate with antiemetics and appropriate hydration before and after giving cisplatin.

Adjust-a-dose: Use the same dosage adjustment schedule as for advanced gastric adenocarcinoma.

---

†Canada   ◇OTC   ◆ Off-label use   ✐ Photoguide   *Liquid contains alcohol.

➤ **Induction treatment for locally advanced SCCHN with cisplatin and 5-FU before chemoradiotherapy (excluding Docefrez)**

Adults: 75 mg/m² I.V. infusion over 1 hour, followed by cisplatin 100 mg/m² I.V. infusion over 30 minutes to 3 hours on day 1, followed by 5-FU 1,000 mg/m² daily as a continuous I.V. infusion from day 1 to day 4. Repeat this regimen every 3 weeks for three cycles. After chemotherapy, patients should receive chemoradiotherapy. Premedicate with antiemetics and oral corticosteroids.

Adjust-a-dose: Use the same dosage adjustment schedule as for advanced gastric adenocarcinoma.

ADMINISTRATION

I.V.

▼ Wear gloves to prepare and give drug. If solution contacts skin, wash immediately and thoroughly with soap and water. If solution contacts mucous membranes, flush thoroughly with water.

▼ Dilute using supplied diluent. Let drug and diluent stand at room temperature for 5 minutes before mixing. After adding all the diluent to drug vial, gently rotate vial for about 45 seconds. Let solution stand for a few minutes so foam dissipates. All foam need not dissipate before preparing infusion solution.

▼ Prepare infusion solution by withdrawing needed amount of premixed solution from vial and injecting it into 250 mL normal saline solution or D₅W to yield 0.3 to 0.74 mg/mL. Doses of more than 200 mg need a larger volume to stay below 0.74 mg/mL of drug. Mix infusion thoroughly by manual rotation.

▼ Prepare and store infusion solution in bottles (glass or polypropylene) or plastic bags, and give through polyethylene-lined administration sets.

▼ Contact between undiluted concentrate and polyvinyl chloride equipment or devices isn't recommended.

▼ If solution isn't clear or if it contains precipitate, discard.

▼ The first dilution is stable for 8 hours. Use infusion solution within 4 hours.

▼ Infuse over 1 hour.

▼ Store unopened vials between 36° and 77° F (2° and 2.5°C).

▼ Mark all waste materials with CHEMOTHERAPY HAZARD labels.

▼ **Incompatibilities:** None reported.

ACTION

Promotes formation and stabilization of nonfunctional microtubules. This prevents mitosis and leads to cell death.

Route	Onset	Peak	Duration
I.V.	Rapid	Unknown	Unknown

Half-life: Alpha phase, 4 minutes; beta phase, 36 minutes; terminal phase, 11 hours.

ADVERSE REACTIONS

CNS: asthenia, paresthesia, peripheral neuropathy.

CV: fluid retention, peripheral edema, *arrhythmias,* chest tightness, flushing, hypotension.

EENT: altered hearing, tearing.

GI: anorexia, diarrhea, dysphagia, esophagitis, nausea, stomatitis, vomiting.

Hematologic: *febrile neutropenia, leukopenia, myelosuppression, neutropenia, thrombocytopenia,* anemia.

Hepatic: *hepatotoxicity.*

Musculoskeletal: myalgia, arthralgia, back pain.

Respiratory: dyspnea, *pulmonary edema.*

Skin: alopecia, desquamation, skin eruptions, nail pigmentation alterations, nail pain, rash, reaction at injection site.

Other: infection, chills, drug fever, hypersensitivity reactions.

INTERACTIONS

Drug-drug. *Compounds that induce, inhibit, or are metabolized by CYP3A4, such as cyclosporine, erythromycin, ketoconazole, troleandomycin:* May modify metabolism of docetaxel. Use together cautiously.

Ketoconazole or other CYP3A4 inhibitors: May increase docetaxel level and toxicity, including neutropenia. Monitor patient closely.

Reactions in bold italics are *life-threatening*. Interactions may have a *rapid onset* or a *delayed onset*.

EFFECTS ON LAB TEST RESULTS
• May increase alkaline phosphatase, ALT, AST, and bilirubin levels. May decrease hemoglobin level.
• May decrease platelet and WBC counts.

CONTRAINDICATIONS & CAUTIONS
• Contraindicated in patients severely hypersensitive to drug or to other forms containing polysorbate 80 and in those with neutrophil count below 1,500/mm³.

Black Box Warning Treatment-related mortality increases in patients with abnormal liver function, those receiving higher doses, and patients with NSCLC and a history of prior treatment with platinum-based chemotherapy who receive docetaxel as a single agent at a dose of 100 mg/m². ■

Black Box Warning Patients with severe hepatic impairment shouldn't receive this drug. Don't give drug to patients with bilirubin levels exceeding the ULN, or those with ALT or AST levels above 1½ times ULN and alkaline phosphatase levels above 2½ times ULN. ■

• Safety and effectiveness in children haven't been established.

⚠ **Overdose S&S:** Severe neutropenia, mild asthenia, cutaneous reactions, mild paresthesia, bone marrow suppression, peripheral neurotoxicity, mucositis.

NURSING CONSIDERATIONS
Black Box Warning Drug should be administered only under the supervision of a physician experienced with antineoplastics. ■

• Give oral corticosteroid such as dexamethasone 16 mg P.O. (8 mg b.i.d.) daily for 3 days, starting 1 day before docetaxel administration, to reduce risk or severity of fluid retention and hypersensitivity reactions.

Black Box Warning Don't give drug to patients with baseline neutrophil count less than 1,500/mm³. ■

• Bone marrow toxicity is the most frequent and dose-limiting toxicity. Frequent blood count monitoring is needed during therapy.

Black Box Warning Monitor patient closely for hypersensitivity reactions, especially during first and second infusions. Severe

and even fatal reactions have occurred in patients who have received recommended 3-day dexamethasone premedication. ■

Black Box Warning Fluid retention is dose related and may be severe. Monitor patient closely. ■

🔴 **Alert:** When indicated, cisplatin dose should follow dose of docetaxel.

• **Look alike–sound alike:** Don't confuse docetaxel with paclitaxel. Don't confuse Taxotere with Taxol.

PATIENT TEACHING
• Caution women of childbearing age to avoid pregnancy or breast-feeding during therapy.
• Remind patient that he will need premedication with dexamethasone.
• Advise patient to report any pain or burning at injection site during or after administration.
• Warn patient that hair loss occurs in almost 80% of patients and reverses when treatment stops.
• Tell patient to promptly report sore throat, fever, or unusual bruising or bleeding, as well as signs and symptoms of fluid retention, such as swelling or shortness of breath.

dofetilide
doe-FE-ti-lyed

Tikosyn

Therapeutic class: Antiarrhythmics
Pharmacologic class: Antiarrhythmics
Pregnancy risk category: C

AVAILABLE FORMS
Capsules: 125 mcg, 250 mcg, 500 mcg

INDICATIONS & DOSAGES
➤ **To maintain normal sinus rhythm in patients with symptomatic atrial fibrillation or atrial flutter lasting longer than 1 week who have been converted to normal sinus rhythm; to convert atrial fibrillation and atrial flutter to normal sinus rhythm**
Adults: Individualized dosage based on CrCl and baseline QTc interval (or QT interval

if heart rate is below 60 beats/minute), determined before first dose; usually 500 mcg P.O. b.i.d. for patients with CrCl greater than 60 mL/minute.

Adjust-a-dose: If CrCl is 40 to 60 mL/minute, starting dose is 250 mcg P.O. b.i.d.; if CrCl is 20 to 39 mL/minute, starting dose is 125 mcg P.O. b.i.d. Don't use drug at all if CrCl is less than 20 mL/minute.

Determine QTc interval 2 to 3 hours after first dose. If QTc interval has increased by more than 15% above baseline or if it's more than 500 msec (550 msec in patients with ventricular conduction abnormalities), adjust dosage as follows: If starting dose based on CrCl was 500 mcg P.O. b.i.d., give 250 mcg P.O. b.i.d. If starting dose based on CrCl was 250 mcg b.i.d., give 125 mcg b.i.d. If starting dose based on CrCl was 125 mcg b.i.d., give 125 mcg once a day.

Determine QTc interval 2 to 3 hours after each subsequent dose while patient is in hospital. If at any time after second dose the QTc interval exceeds 500 msec (550 msec in patients with ventricular conduction abnormalities), stop drug.

ADMINISTRATION
P.O.
● Give drug without regard for food or antacid administration.
● Don't give drug with grapefruit juice.

ACTION
Prolongs repolarization without affecting conduction velocity. Drug doesn't affect sodium channels, alpha-adrenergic receptors, or beta-adrenergic receptors.

Route	Onset	Peak	Duration
P.O.	Unknown	2–3 hr	Unknown

Half-life: 10 hours.

ADVERSE REACTIONS
CNS: headache, *stroke,* dizziness, insomnia, anxiety, migraine, cerebral ischemia, asthenia, paresthesia, syncope.
CV: chest pain, *ventricular fibrillation, ventricular tachycardia, torsades de pointes, AV block, heart block, bradycardia, cardiac arrest, MI,* bundle-branch block, angina, atrial fibrillation, hypertension, palpitations, edema.

GI: nausea, diarrhea, abdominal pain.
GU: UTI.
Hepatic: liver damage.
Musculoskeletal: back pain, arthralgia, facial paralysis.
Respiratory: respiratory tract infection, dyspnea, increased cough.
Skin: rash, sweating.
Other: *angioedema,* flu syndrome, peripheral edema.

INTERACTIONS
Drug-drug. *Antiarrhythmics (classes I and III):* May increase dofetilide level. Withhold other antiarrhythmics for at least three plasma half-lives before giving dofetilide.
*CYP3A4 inhibitors (amiodarone, **azole antifungals,** cannabinoids, diltiazem, **macrolides,** nefazodone, norfloxacin, protease inhibitors, quinine, SSRIs, zafirlukast):* May decrease metabolism and increase dofetilide level. Use together cautiously.
Drugs secreted by renal tubular cationic transport (amiloride, metformin, triamterene): May increase dofetilide level. Use together cautiously; monitor patient for adverse effects.
Drugs that prolong QT interval: May increase risk of QT interval prolongation. Avoid using together.
Inhibitors of renal cationic secretion (cimetidine, ketoconazole, megestrol, prochlorperazine, sulfamethoxazole–trimethoprim), trimethoprim, verapamil: May increase dofetilide level. Use together is contraindicated.
Potassium-depleting diuretics: May increase risk of hypokalemia or hypomagnesemia. Monitor potassium and magnesium levels.
Thiazide diuretics: May cause hypokalemia and arrhythmias. Use together is contraindicated.
Drug-food. *Grapefruit juice:* May decrease hepatic metabolism and increase drug level. Discourage use together.

EFFECTS ON LAB TEST RESULTS
None reported.

CONTRAINDICATIONS & CAUTIONS
● Contraindicated in patients hypersensitive to drug, in those with congenital or acquired

long QT interval syndromes or with base-line QTc interval greater than 440 msec (500 msec in patients with ventricular conduction abnormalities), and in those with CrCl less than 20 mL/minute.

• Contraindicated for use with thiazide diuretics, verapamil, and cation transport system inhibitors (cimetidine, ketoconazole, megestrol, prochlorperazine, sulfamethoxazole–trimethoprim, trimethoprim).

• Use cautiously in patients with severe hepatic impairment.

⚠ *Overdose S&S:* Prolonged QT interval, ventricular fibrillation, torsades de pointes, cardiac arrest.

NURSING CONSIDERATIONS

Black Box Warning When dofetilide is initiated or reinitiated, patients should be hospitalized for a minimum of 3 days in a facility that can provide calculations of CrCl, continuous ECG monitoring, and cardiac resuscitation. Dofetilide is available only to hospitals and prescribers who have received appropriate dofetilide dosing and treatment initiation education. ∎

• Don't discharge patient within 12 hours of conversion to normal sinus rhythm.

• Monitor patient for prolonged diarrhea, sweating, and vomiting. Report these signs to prescriber because electrolyte imbalance may increase potential for arrhythmia development.

• Monitor renal function and QTc interval every 3 months.

• Use of potassium-depleting diuretics may cause hypokalemia and hypomagnesemia, increasing the risk of torsades de pointes. Give dofetilide after potassium level reaches and stays in normal range.

• If patient doesn't convert to normal sinus rhythm within 24 hours of starting dofetilide, consider electrical conversion.

• Before starting dofetilide, stop previous antiarrhythmics while carefully monitoring patient for a minimum of three plasma half-lives. Don't give drug after amiodarone therapy until amiodarone level falls below 0.3 mcg/mL or until amiodarone has been stopped for at least 3 months.

• If dofetilide must be stopped to allow dosing with interacting drugs, allow at least 2 days before starting other drug therapy.

PATIENT TEACHING

• Tell patient to report any change in OTC or prescription drug use, or supplement or herb use.

• Inform patient that drug can be taken without regard to meals or antacid administration.

• Tell patient to immediately report excessive or prolonged diarrhea, sweating, vomiting, or loss of appetite or thirst.

• Advise patient not to take drug with grapefruit juice.

• Advise patient to use antacids, such as Zantac 75 mg, Pepcid, Prilosec, Axid, or Prevacid, instead of Tagamet HB if needed for ulcers or heartburn.

• Instruct patient to tell prescriber if she becomes pregnant.

• Advise patient not to breast-feed while taking dofetilide because drug appears in breast milk.

• If a dose is missed, tell patient not to double a dose but to skip that dose and take the next regularly scheduled dose.

dolasetron mesylate
doe-LAZ-e-tron

Anzemet

Therapeutic class: Antiemetics
Pharmacologic class: Selective serotonin receptor antagonists
Pregnancy risk category: B

AVAILABLE FORMS
Injection: 12.5 mg/0.625 mL, 20 mg/mL
Tablets: 50 mg, 100 mg

INDICATIONS & DOSAGES
➤ **To prevent nausea and vomiting from cancer chemotherapy (P.O. only)**
Adults: 100 mg P.O. given as a single dose 1 hour before chemotherapy.
Children ages 2 to 16: 1.8 mg/kg P.O. given 1 hour before chemotherapy. Injectable formulation can be mixed with apple or

apple-grape juice and given P.O. Maximum dose is 100 mg.

➤ **To prevent postoperative nausea and vomiting**
Adults: 100 mg P.O. given within 2 hours before surgery. Or, 12.5 mg as a single I.V. dose about 15 minutes before cessation of anesthesia or as soon as nausea or vomiting presents.
Children ages 2 to 16: 1.2 mg/kg P.O. given within 2 hours before surgery, to maximum of 100 mg. Or, 0.35 mg/kg, up to 12.5 mg given as a single I.V. dose about 15 minutes before stopping anesthesia or as soon as nausea or vomiting starts. I.V. form can be mixed with apple juice and given P.O.

➤ **Postoperative nausea and vomiting**
Adults: 12.5 mg as a single I.V. dose as soon as nausea or vomiting occurs.
Children ages 2 to 16: 0.35 mg/kg, to maximum dosage of 12.5 mg, given as a single I.V. dose as soon as nausea or vomiting occurs.

ADMINISTRATION
P.O.
● Mix injection for oral use in apple or apple-grape juice immediately before giving.
● Injection for oral use is stable in juice for 2 hours at room temperature.

I.V.
▼ Drug can be injected as rapidly as 100 mg over 30 seconds or diluted in 50 mL of compatible solution and infused over 15 minutes.
▼ **Incompatibilities:** Other I.V. drugs.

ACTION
Blocks the action of serotonin and prevents serotonin from stimulating the vomiting reflex.

Route	Onset	Peak	Duration
P.O.	Rapid	1 hr	8 hr
I.V.	Rapid	36 min	7 hr

Half-life: 8 hours.

ADVERSE REACTIONS
CNS: headache, dizziness, drowsiness, fatigue, fever.
CV: *arrhythmias,* ECG changes, edema, hypertension, hypotension, tachycardia.

GI: diarrhea, abdominal pain, anorexia, constipation, dyspepsia.
GU: hematuria, polyuria, urine retention.
Skin: pruritus, rash.
Other: chills, pain at injection site.

INTERACTIONS
Drug-drug. *Drugs that prolong ECG intervals, such as antiarrhythmics:* May increase risk of arrhythmia. Monitor patient closely.
Drugs that inhibit CYP enzymes, such as cimetidine: May increase level of hydrodolasetron, an active metabolite of dolasetron. Monitor patient for adverse effects.
Drugs that induce CYP enzymes, such as rifampin: May decrease level of hydrodolasetron, an active metabolite of dolasetron. Monitor patient for decreased effectiveness of antiemetic.

EFFECTS ON LAB TEST RESULTS
● May increase ALT and AST levels.
● May increase PTT.

CONTRAINDICATIONS & CAUTIONS
● Contraindicated in patients hypersensitive to drug and in those with congenital long-QT syndrome.
❸ *Alert:* Give with caution in patients who have or may develop prolonged cardiac conduction intervals, such as those with electrolyte abnormalities, history of arrhythmia, and history of cumulative high-dose anthracycline therapy.
❸ *Alert:* Don't use the injection form in children and adults for the prevention of nausea and vomiting associated with cancer chemotherapy because of the increased risk of developing abnormal and sometimes fatal arrhythmias, including torsades de pointes. The tablet form, however, may be used for this indication.
● Drug isn't recommended for use in children younger than age 2. Use cautiously in breast-feeding women.
⚠ *Overdose S&S:* Hypotension; dizziness; prolonged PR, QRS, and QTc intervals.

NURSING CONSIDERATIONS
● Correct hypovolemia and hypomagnesemia before giving drug, and closely monitor electrolyte levels.

Reactions in bold italics are *life-threatening*. Interactions may have a *rapid onset* or a *delayed onset*.

• Use ECG monitoring in elderly patients and in patients with heart failure, underlying heart disease, bradycardia, or renal impairment.
• Monitor patient for CV complications, such as heart block and tachyarrhythmias.
• **Look alike–sound alike:** Don't confuse Anzemet with Aldomet or Avandamet.

PATIENT TEACHING
• Tell patient about possible adverse effects.
• Instruct patient to mix injection in juice for oral use immediately before giving.
• Tell patient to report nausea or vomiting.
• Tell patient to report a racing heartbeat, shortness of breath, dizziness, or fainting.

donepezil hydrochloride
doe-NEP-ah-zill

Aricept⬦, Aricept ODT

Therapeutic class: Anti-Alzheimer drugs
Pharmacologic class: Acetyl-cholinesterase inhibitors
Pregnancy risk category: C

AVAILABLE FORMS
Tablets: 5 mg, 10 mg, 23 mg
Tablets (orally disintegrating): 5 mg, 10 mg

INDICATIONS & DOSAGES
➤ **Mild to moderate Alzheimer dementia**
Adults: 5 or 10 mg P.O. once daily.
➤ **Moderate to severe Alzheimer disease**
Adults: Initially, 5 mg P.O. once daily for 4 to 6 weeks; dose may then be increased to 10 mg P.O. once daily. The dose may be increased to 23 mg P.O. once daily after patients have been taking 10 mg daily for 3 months.
➤ **Traumatic brain injury** ◆
Adults: 5 to 10 mg P.O. daily through subacute or long-term periods of recovery if response is adequate.
➤ **Lewy body dementia** ◆
Adults: 5 mg P.O. once daily. May be increased to 10 mg P.O. daily after 4 weeks. May start therapy at 2.5 mg daily in patients sensitive to adverse effects or frail patients.

ADMINISTRATION
P.O.
• Allow orally disintegrating tablet (ODT) to dissolve on tongue; then follow with water.
• Give drug at bedtime, without regard for food.
• Don't split or crush tablets.

ACTION
Thought to increase acetylcholine level by inhibiting cholinesterase enzyme, which causes acetylcholine hydrolysis.

Route	Onset	Peak	Duration
P.O.	Unknown	3–4 hr	Unknown

Half-life: 70 hours.

ADVERSE REACTIONS
CNS: headache, insomnia, *seizures,* dizziness, fatigue, depression, somnolence, syncope, pain.
CV: chest pain, hypertension, atrial fibrillation, hypotension, *bradycardia, heart block.*
EENT: cataract, blurred vision, eye irritation, sore throat.
GI: nausea, diarrhea, vomiting, anorexia, fecal incontinence, *GI bleeding,* weight loss.
GU: urinary frequency.
Metabolic: weight loss, dehydration.
Musculoskeletal: muscle cramps, arthritis, bone fracture.
Respiratory: dyspnea, bronchitis.
Skin: pruritus, urticaria, diaphoresis, ecchymoses.
Other: toothache, influenza, increased libido.

INTERACTIONS
Drug-drug. *Anticholinergics:* May decrease donepezil effects. Avoid using together.
Anticholinesterases, cholinomimetics: May have synergistic effect. Monitor patient closely.
Bethanechol, succinylcholine: May have additive effects. Monitor patient closely.
Carbamazepine, dexamethasone, phenobarbital, phenytoin, rifampin: May increase rate of donepezil elimination. Monitor patient.

NSAIDs: May increase gastric acid secretions. Monitor for active or occult GI bleeding.

EFFECTS ON LAB TEST RESULTS
• May increase CK level.

CONTRAINDICATIONS & CAUTIONS
• Contraindicated in patients hypersensitive to drug or piperidine derivatives and in breast-feeding women.
• Use cautiously in pregnant women and in patients who take NSAIDs or have CV disease, asthma, obstructive pulmonary disease, urinary outflow impairment, or history of ulcer disease.
⚠ ***Overdose S&S:*** Severe nausea, vomiting, salivation, sweating, bradycardia, hypotension, respiratory depression, collapse, seizures, increasing muscle weakness.

NURSING CONSIDERATIONS
• Monitor patient for evidence of active or occult GI bleeding.
• Monitor patient for bradycardia because of potential for vagotonic effects.
• ***Look alike–sound alike:*** Don't confuse Aricept with Ascriptin.

PATIENT TEACHING
• Stress that drug doesn't alter underlying degenerative disease but can temporarily stabilize or relieve symptoms. Effectiveness depends on taking drug at regular intervals.
• Tell caregiver to give drug just before patient's bedtime.
• Tell patient and caregiver not to break or crush tablets.
• ODTs may be taken with or without food. Have patient allow tablet to dissolve on his tongue, then swallow with a sip of water.
• Advise patient and caregiver to report immediately significant adverse effects or changes in overall health status and to inform health care team that patient is taking drug before he receives anesthesia.
• Tell patient to avoid OTC cold or sleep remedies because of risk of increased anticholinergic effects.

SAFETY ALERT!

DOPamine hydrochloride
DOE-pa-meen

Therapeutic class: Vasopressors
Pharmacologic class: Adrenergics
Pregnancy risk category: C

AVAILABLE FORMS
Injection: 40 mg/mL, 80 mg/mL, 160 mg/mL parenteral concentrate for injection for I.V. infusion; 0.8 mg/mL (200 or 400 mg) in D_5W; 1.6 mg/mL (400 or 800 mg) in D_5W; 3.2 mg/mL (800 mg) in D_5W parenteral injection for I.V. infusion

INDICATIONS & DOSAGES
➤ **To treat shock and correct hemodynamic imbalances; to improve perfusion to vital organs; to increase cardiac output; to correct hypotension**
Adults and children: Initially, 2 to 5 mcg/kg/ minute by I.V. infusion. Titrate dosage to desired hemodynamic or renal response. Increase by 1 to 4 mcg/kg/minute at 10- to 30-minute intervals. In seriously ill patients, start with 5 mcg/kg/minute and increase gradually in increments of 5 to 10 mcg/kg/minute to a rate of 20 to 50 mcg/kg/minute, as needed.
Adjust-a-dose: In patients with occlusive vascular disease, initial dose is 1 mcg/kg/minute or less. Initial dopamine dosages shouldn't exceed one-tenth of the usual dosage in patients who have received MAO inhibitors within the prior 2 to 3 weeks.

ADMINISTRATION
I.V.
▼ Dilute with D_5W, normal saline solution, D_5W in normal saline or 0.45% saline, lactated Ringer, or D_5W in lactated Ringer. Mix just before use.
▼ Use a central line or large vein, as in the antecubital fossa, to minimize risk of extravasation.
▼ Use a continuous infusion pump to regulate flow rate. Avoid inadvertent administration of a bolus of the drug.

Reactions in bold italics are *life-threatening*. Interactions may have a *rapid onset* or a *delayed onset*.

Black Box Warning Watch infusion site carefully for extravasation; if it occurs, stop infusion immediately and call prescriber. To prevent sloughing and necrosis in ischemic areas, you may need to infiltrate area with 5 to 10 mg phentolamine in 10 to 15 mL normal saline solution as soon as possible. ∎

▼ Because solution will deteriorate rapidly, discard after 24 hours or earlier if it's discolored.

▼ **Incompatibilities:** Acyclovir sodium, additives with dopamine and dextrose solution, alteplase, amphotericin B, cefepime, furosemide, gentamicin, indomethacin sodium trihydrate, iron salts, insulin, oxidizing agents, penicillin G potassium, sodium bicarbonate or other alkaline solutions, thiopental. Don't mix other drugs in I.V. container with dopamine.

ACTION

Stimulates dopaminergic and alpha and beta receptors of the sympathetic nervous system, resulting in a positive inotropic effect and increased cardiac output. Action is dose-related; large doses cause mainly alpha stimulation.

Route	Onset	Peak	Duration
I.V.	5 min	Unknown	<10 min after infusion

Half-life: 2 minutes.

ADVERSE REACTIONS

CNS: headache, anxiety.
CV: hypotension, *ventricular arrhythmias (high doses),* ectopic beats, tachycardia, angina, palpitations, vasoconstriction.
GI: nausea, vomiting.
Metabolic: azotemia, hyperglycemia.
Respiratory: *asthmatic episodes,* dyspnea.
Skin: necrosis and tissue sloughing with extravasation, piloerection.
Other: *anaphylactic reactions.*

INTERACTIONS

Drug-drug. *Alpha and beta blockers:* May antagonize dopamine effects. Monitor patient closely.
Diuretics (furosemide): May potentiate diuresis. Use together cautiously and monitor fluid volume closely.

Ergot alkaloids: May cause extremely high blood pressure. Avoid using together.
Inhaled anesthetics: May increase risk of arrhythmias or hypertension. Monitor patient closely.
MAO inhibitors (phenelzine, tranylcypromine): May cause fever, hypertensive crisis, or severe headache. Avoid using together; if patient received an MAO inhibitor in the past 2 to 3 weeks, initial dopamine dose is less than or equal to 10% of the usual dose.
Oxytocics: May cause severe, persistent hypertension. Use together cautiously.
Phenytoin: May cause severe hypotension, bradycardia, and cardiac arrest. Monitor patient carefully.
TCAs: May decrease pressor response. Monitor patient closely.

EFFECTS ON LAB TEST RESULTS

● May increase catecholamine, glucose, and urine urea levels.

CONTRAINDICATIONS & CAUTIONS

● Contraindicated in patients with uncorrected tachyarrhythmias, pheochromocytoma, or ventricular fibrillation.
● Use cautiously in patients with occlusive vascular disease, cold injuries, diabetic endarteritis, and arterial embolism; in pregnant or breast-feeding women; in those with a history of sulfite sensitivity; and in those taking MAO inhibitors.
⚠ *Overdose S&S:* Excessive blood pressure elevation.

NURSING CONSIDERATIONS

● Most patients receive less than 20 mcg/kg/minute. Doses of 0.5 to 2 mcg/kg/minute mainly stimulate dopamine receptors and dilate the renal vasculature. Doses of 2 to 10 mcg/kg/minute stimulate beta receptors for a positive inotropic effect. Higher doses also stimulate alpha receptors, constricting blood vessels and increasing blood pressure.
● Drug isn't a substitute for blood or fluid volume deficit. If deficit exists, replace fluid before giving vasopressors.
● During infusion, frequently monitor ECG, blood pressure, cardiac output, central venous pressure, pulmonary artery wedge pressure, pulse rate, urine output, and color and temperature of limbs.

• If diastolic pressure rises disproportionately with a significant decrease in pulse pressure, decrease infusion rate, and watch carefully for further evidence of predominant vasoconstrictor activity, unless such an effect is desired.

• Observe patient closely for adverse reactions; dosage may need to be adjusted or drug stopped.

• Check urine output often. If urine flow decreases without hypotension, notify prescriber because dosage may need to be reduced.

⊙ *Alert:* After drug is stopped, watch closely for sudden drop in blood pressure. Taper dosage slowly to evaluate stability of blood pressure.

• Acidosis decreases effectiveness of drug.

• *Look alike–sound alike:* Don't confuse dopamine with dobutamine.

PATIENT TEACHING
• Tell patient to report adverse reactions promptly.

• Instruct patient to report discomfort at I.V. insertion site.

doripenem
dor-eh-PEN-em

Doribax

Therapeutic class: Antibiotics
Pharmacologic class: Carbapenems
Pregnancy risk category: B

AVAILABLE FORMS
Injection: 250-mg, 500-mg vial

INDICATIONS & DOSAGES
Adjust-a-dose (for all indications): In patients with CrCl of 30 to 50 mL/minute, give 250 mg I.V. every 8 hours; with CrCl of more than 10 to less than 30 mL/minute, give 250 mg I.V. every 12 hours.

➤ **Complicated intra-abdominal infections caused by** *Escherichia coli, Klebsiella pneumoniae, Pseudomonas aeruginosa, Bacteroides caccae, B. fragilis, B. thetaiotaomicron, B. uniformis, B. vulgatas, Streptococcus intermedius,*

S. constellatus, **or** *Peptostreptococcus micros*
Adults: 500 mg I.V. every 8 hours for 5 to 14 days.

➤ **Complicated urinary tract infections, including pyelonephritis caused by** *E. coli, K. pneumoniae, Proteus mirabilis, Pseudomonas aeruginosa,* **or** *Acinetobacter baumannii*
Adults: 500 mg I.V. every 8 hours for 10 days. May be given for 14 days to patient with concurrent bacteremia.

➤ **Catheter-related bloodstream infections ♦**
Adults: 500 mg I.V. every 8 hours for 7 to 14 days.

➤ **Community-acquired pneumonia ♦**
Adults: 500 mg I.V. every 8 hours for at least 5 days.

ADMINISTRATION
I.V.
▼ Assess for history of allergies to beta-lactams (carbapenems, penicillins, cephalosporins).

▼ Obtain specimen for culture and sensitivity tests before beginning treatment.

▼ Dilute drug in single-use vials with 10 mL sterile water for injection or normal saline for injection; shake gently to form a concentration of 25 mg/mL when using 250-mg vial or 50 mg/mL when using 500-mg vial.

▼ Add reconstituted 250-mg suspension to 50 or 100 mL normal saline or D₅W. Add reconstituted 500-mg suspension to 100 mL normal saline or D₅W for a final concentration of 4.5 mg/mL.

▼ Inspect solution for particulate matter and discoloration. Solution should be clear to slightly yellow.

▼ Solution prepared with normal saline solution may be stored at room temperature for 8 hours; D₅W, for 4 hours. If refrigerated, solution may be stored for 24 hours.

▼ Give only by infusion over 1 hour.

▼ **Incompatibilities:** Other I.V. drugs.

ACTION
Inhibits bacterial cell-wall biosynthesis by inactivating multiple penicillin-binding proteins, causing cell death.

Reactions in bold italics are *life-threatening*. Interactions may have a *rapid onset* or a *delayed onset*.

Route	Onset	Peak	Duration
I.V.	Rapid	1¼ hr	Unknown

Half-life: 1 hour.

ADVERSE REACTIONS
CNS: headache, *seizures.*
GI: *pseudomembranous colitis,* diarrhea, nausea.
GU: renal insufficiency, *renal failure.*
Hematologic: anemia.
Respiratory: interstitial pneumonia.
Skin: phlebitis, pruritus, rash, *Stevens-Johnson syndrome, toxic epidermal necrolysis.*
Other: *anaphylaxis,* infection.

INTERACTIONS
Drug-drug. *Probenecid:* May increase drug level. Avoid using together.
Valproic acid: May decrease valproic acid level, causing seizures. Monitor valproic acid levels. May need to switch to another antibacterial or anticonvulsant if levels can't be maintained.

EFFECTS ON LAB TEST RESULTS
• May increase ALT, AST, transaminase, and other hepatic enzyme levels.
• May decrease RBC count.

CONTRAINDICATIONS & CAUTIONS
• Contraindicated in patients hypersensitive to drug, its components, or other beta-lactams.
• Use caution in those with moderate to severe renal impairment, especially elderly patients.
• Patients with preexisting CNS disorders (such as stroke or history of seizures) and those taking doses greater than 500 mg every 8 hours are at increased risk for seizures.

NURSING CONSIDERATIONS
• Monitor patient closely for pseudomembranous colitis, which can occur up to 2 months after drug administration.
• Monitor renal function.
❸ Alert: If allergic reaction occurs, stop drug, use supportive measures, and contact the prescriber.
• To report suspected adverse reactions, contact the FDA at 1-800-FDA-1088 or fda.gov/medwatch.

• Safety and effectiveness haven't been established in pregnant or pediatric patients. It's unknown whether drug is excreted in breast milk.

PATIENT TEACHING
• Tell patient to report any serious adverse effects such as dyspnea, skin reaction, pain at injection site, or diarrhea.
❸ Alert: Severe and life-threatening diarrhea can occur up to 2 months after drug is given; tell patient to report immediately.
• Advise woman to tell prescriber if she's pregnant or breast-feeding.
• Advise patient with preexisting CNS disorder or history of stroke or seizures, or who is taking doses greater than 500 mg every 8 hours of increased risk of seizures.

dorzolamide hydrochloride
dor-ZOLE-ah-mide

Trusopt

Therapeutic class: Antiglaucoma drugs
Pharmacologic class: Carbonic anhydrase inhibitors–sulfonamides
Pregnancy risk category: C

AVAILABLE FORMS
Ophthalmic solution: 2%

INDICATIONS & DOSAGES
➤ **Increased intraocular pressure (IOP) in patients with ocular hypertension or open-angle glaucoma**
Adults and children: One drop into conjunctival sac of each affected eye t.i.d.

ADMINISTRATION
Ophthalmic
• Don't touch tip of dropper to eye or surrounding tissue.
• Apply light finger pressure on lacrimal sac for 1 minute after instilling to minimize systemic absorption.
• If more than one ophthalmic drug is being used, give at least 10 minutes apart.

ACTION
Decreases aqueous humor secretion, presumably by slowing the formation of

bicarbonate ions. This reduces sodium and fluid transport, reducing IOP.

Route	Onset	Peak	Duration
Ophthalmic	1–2 hr	2–3 hr	8 hr

Half-life: 4 months.

ADVERSE REACTIONS
CNS: asthenia, fatigue, headache.
EENT: blurred vision; dryness; lacrimation; ocular allergic reaction; ocular burning, stinging, and discomfort; photophobia; superficial punctate keratitis; iridocyclitis.
GI: bitter taste, nausea.
GU: urolithiasis.
Skin: rash.

INTERACTIONS
Drug-drug. *Oral carbonic anhydrase inhibitors, salicylates:* May cause additive effects. Avoid using together.

EFFECTS ON LAB TEST RESULTS
None reported.

CONTRAINDICATIONS & CAUTIONS
• Contraindicated in patients hypersensitive to drug or its components.
• Use cautiously in patients hypersensitive to sulfonamides and in those with hepatic or renal impairment.
⚠ *Overdose S&S:* Electrolyte imbalance, acidosis, CNS effects.

NURSING CONSIDERATIONS
• Normal IOP is 10 to 21 mm Hg.
• Monitor patient who is hypersensitive to sulfonamides carefully. Drug may cause reactions similar to those seen with oral sulfonamides.

PATIENT TEACHING
• Teach patient how to instill drops. Advise him to wash hands before and after instillation, and warn him not to touch tip of dropper to eye or surrounding tissue.
• Tell patient that drug is a sulfonamide and, although it's given topically, it can be absorbed systemically. Advise patient to apply light finger pressure on lacrimal sac for 1 minute after drug instillation to minimize systemic absorption.

• Tell patient to stop drug and notify prescriber immediately if signs or symptoms of serious adverse reactions or hypersensitivity occur, including eye inflammation and eyelid reactions.
• Tell patient not to wear soft contact lenses during therapy.
• Stress importance of compliance with recommended therapy.

doxazosin mesylate
dox-AY-zo-sin

Cardura♦, Cardura XL

Therapeutic class: Antihypertensives
Pharmacologic class: Alpha blockers
Pregnancy risk category: C

AVAILABLE FORMS
Tablets: 1 mg, 2 mg, 4 mg, 8 mg
Tablets (extended-release): 4 mg, 8 mg

INDICATIONS & DOSAGES
➤ **Essential hypertension**
Adults: Initially, 1 mg P.O. daily; determine effect on standing and supine blood pressure at 2 to 6 hours and 24 hours after dose. May increase at 2-week intervals to 2 mg and, thereafter, 4 mg and 8 mg once daily, if needed. Maximum daily dose is 16 mg, but doses over 4 mg daily increase the risk of adverse reactions. Don't use extended-release formulation to treat hypertension.
➤ **BPH**
Adults: Initially, 1 mg P.O. once daily in the morning or evening; may increase at 1- or 2-week intervals to 2 mg and, thereafter, 4 mg and 8 mg once daily, if needed. Or, one 4-mg extended-release tablet once daily with breakfast. May increase to 8 mg at 3- to 4-week intervals.
➤ **Pediatric hypertension ♦**
Children: Initially, 1 mg P.O. daily. May increase, as needed, at 2-week intervals to maximum dosage of 4 mg/day.
➤ **Ureteral stones ♦**
Adults: 4 mg P.O. daily as adjunctive therapy for up to 1 month or until expulsion.

ADMINISTRATION
P.O.
● Patient should swallow extended-release tablets whole and not chew, divide, cut, or crush them.
● Give extended-release tablet with breakfast.
● Don't give evening dose the night before switching to extended-release tablets from immediate-release formula.

ACTION
An alpha blocker that acts on the peripheral vasculature to reduce peripheral vascular resistance and produce vasodilation. Drug also decreases smooth muscle tone in the prostate and bladder neck.

Route	Onset	Peak	Duration
P.O.	1–2 hr	2–3 hr	24 hr

Half-life: 19 to 22 hours.

ADVERSE REACTIONS
CNS: dizziness, asthenia, headache, vertigo, somnolence, drowsiness, pain.
CV: orthostatic hypotension, *arrhythmias*, hypotension, edema, palpitations, tachycardia.
EENT: rhinitis, pharyngitis, abnormal vision, dry mouth.
GI: nausea, vomiting, diarrhea, constipation.
GU: erectile dysfunction.
Hematologic: *leukopenia, neutropenia.*
Musculoskeletal: arthralgia, myalgia, back pain.
Respiratory: dyspnea.
Skin: rash, pruritus.

INTERACTIONS
Drug-drug. *Antihypertensives, diuretics:* May increase hypotensive effects. Adjust dosages as necessary.
Midodrine: May decrease the effectiveness of midodrine. Monitor patient for therapeutic effect.
PDE5 inhibitors (sildenafil, tadalafil, vardenafil): May cause additive hypotensive effects and symptomatic hypotension. Initiate PDE5 therapy at lowest possible dosage.
Drug-herb. *Butcher's broom:* May decrease effect of doxazosin. Discourage use together.

Ma huang: May decrease antihypertensive effects. Discourage use together.

EFFECTS ON LAB TEST RESULTS
● May decrease WBC and neutrophil counts.

CONTRAINDICATIONS & CAUTIONS
● Contraindicated in patients hypersensitive to drug and quinazoline derivatives (including prazosin and terazosin).
● Use cautiously in patients with impaired hepatic function.
⚠ *Overdose S&S:* Hypotension.

NURSING CONSIDERATIONS
● Monitor blood pressure closely.
● If syncope occurs, place patient in a recumbent position and treat supportively. A transient hypotensive response isn't considered a contraindication to continued therapy.
● Initial extended-release dose is 4 mg. If patient stops medication briefly, he should resume at 4-mg dose and titrate back to 8 mg if appropriate.
● Wait 3 to 4 weeks before increasing extended-release dose.
● *Look alike–sound alike:* Don't confuse doxazosin with doxapram, doxorubicin, or doxepin. Don't confuse Cardura with Coumadin, K-Dur, Cardene, or Cordarone.

PATIENT TEACHING
● Instruct patient to take drug exactly as prescribed.
● *Alert:* Advise patient that he is susceptible to a first-dose effect (marked low blood pressure on standing up with dizziness or fainting). This is most common after first dose but also can occur during dosage adjustment or interruption of therapy.
● Advise patient to consult prescriber if dizziness or palpitations are bothersome.
● Advise patient to rise slowly from sitting or lying position.
● Advise patient to avoid driving and other hazardous activities until drug's effects are known.

doxepin hydrochloride
DOKS-eh-pin

Silenor

Therapeutic class: Antidepressants
Pharmacologic class: Tricyclic antidepressants
Pregnancy risk category: C

AVAILABLE FORMS
Capsules: 10 mg, 25 mg, 50 mg, 75 mg, 100 mg, 150 mg
Oral concentrate: 10 mg/mL
Tablets: 3 mg, 6 mg

INDICATIONS & DOSAGES
➤ **Depression; anxiety**
Adults: Initially, 75 mg P.O. daily. Usual dosage range is 75 to 150 mg daily to maximum of 300 mg daily in divided doses. Mild symptoms may require only 25 to 50 mg/day. Or, entire maintenance dose may be given once daily. Maximum dosage is 300 mg/day.
➤ **Insomnia**
Adults: 6 mg P.O. once daily within 30 minutes of bedtime.
Adjust-a-dose: For elderly patients, give 3 mg P.O. once daily within 30 minutes of bedtime. Daily dose may be increased to 6 mg if indicated.
➤ **Migraine prevention** ◆
Adults: 75 to 150 mg P.O. daily. Dose up to 300 mg daily may be needed.

ADMINISTRATION
P.O.
● Dilute oral concentrate with 4 ounces (120 mL) of water, milk, or juice (orange, grapefruit, tomato, prune, or pineapple, but not grape); don't mix preparation with carbonated beverages.
● Give at bedtime, if possible, because it may cause drowsiness and dizziness.
● Don't give Silenor within 3 hours of a meal.

ACTION
Unknown. Increases amount of norepinephrine, serotonin, or both in the CNS by blocking their reuptake by the presynaptic neurons.

Route	Onset	Peak	Duration
P.O.	Unknown	2 hr	Unknown

Half-life: 6 to 8 hours.

ADVERSE REACTIONS
CNS: drowsiness, dizziness, *seizures,* confusion, numbness, hallucinations, paresthesia, ataxia, weakness, headache, extrapyramidal reactions.
CV: orthostatic hypotension, tachycardia, ECG changes.
EENT: blurred vision, tinnitus.
GI: dry mouth, constipation, nausea, vomiting, anorexia.
GU: urine retention.
Metabolic: *hypoglycemia,* hyperglycemia.
Skin: diaphoresis, rash, urticaria, photosensitivity reactions.
Other: hypersensitivity reactions.

INTERACTIONS
Drug-drug. *Barbiturates, CNS depressants:* May enhance CNS depression. Avoid using together.
Cimetidine, **fluoxetine, fluvoxamine, paroxetine, sertraline:** May increase doxepin level. Monitor drug levels and patient for signs of toxicity.
Clonidine: May cause life-threatening hypertension. Avoid using together.
Epinephrine, norepinephrine: May increase hypertensive effect. Use together cautiously.
Linezolid, methylene blue: May cause serotonin syndrome. Use with extreme caution and monitor closely.
MAO inhibitors: May cause severe excitation, hyperpyrexia, or seizures. Avoid using within 14 days of MAO inhibitor therapy.
Quinolones: May increase the risk of life-threatening arrhythmias. Avoid using together.
Drug-herb. *Evening primrose oil:* May cause additive or synergistic effect, resulting in lower seizure threshold and increasing the risk of seizure. Discourage use together.
St. John's wort, SAM-e, yohimbe: May cause serotonin syndrome. Discourage use together.
Drug-lifestyle. *Alcohol use:* May enhance CNS depression. Discourage use together.

D

Sun exposure: May increase risk of photosensitivity reactions. Advise patient to avoid excessive sunlight exposure.

EFFECTS ON LAB TEST RESULTS
• May increase or decrease glucose level.
• May increase LFT values.

CONTRAINDICATIONS & CAUTIONS
• Contraindicated in patients hypersensitive to drug and in those with glaucoma or tendency toward urine retention; also contraindicated in those who have received an MAO inhibitor within past 14 days and during acute recovery phase of an MI.
Black Box Warning Doxepin isn't approved for use in pediatric patients. Clinicians considering the use of doxepin in a child, adolescent, or young adult must balance risk with clinical need. ■
۞ Alert: Concomitant use with linezolid or methylene blue can cause serotonin syndrome (fever, mental status changes, muscle twitching, excessive sweating, shivering or shaking, diarrhea, loss of coordination). Use with linezolid or methylene blue only for life-threatening or urgent conditions when the potential benefits outweigh the risks of toxicity.
⚠ Overdose S&S: Cardiac arrhythmias, severe hypotension, seizures, CNS depression, coma, confusion, disturbed concentration, transient visual hallucinations, dilated pupils, agitation, hyperactive reflexes, stupor, drowsiness, muscle rigidity, vomiting, hypothermia, hyperpyrexia.

NURSING CONSIDERATIONS
• Don't withdraw drug abruptly.
• Monitor patient for nausea, headache, and malaise after abrupt withdrawal of long-term therapy; these symptoms don't indicate addiction.
۞ Alert: Because hypertensive episodes may occur during surgery in patients receiving drug, stop it gradually several days before surgery.
۞ Alert: If linezolid or methylene blue must be given, stop drug and monitor the patient for serotonin toxicity for 2 weeks, or until 24 hours after the last dose of methylene blue or linezolid, whichever comes first.

Treatment may be resumed 24 hours after last dose of methylene blue or linezolid.
• If signs or symptoms of psychosis occur or increase, expect prescriber to reduce dosage. Record mood changes. Monitor patient for suicidal tendencies, and allow only a minimum supply of drug.
Black Box Warning Drug may increase risk of suicidal thinking and behavior in children, adolescents, and young adults ages 18 to 24, especially during the first few months of treatment, especially in those with major depressive disorder or other psychiatric disorder. ■
• Drug has strong anticholinergic effects and is one of the most sedating tricyclic antidepressants. Adverse anticholinergic effects can occur rapidly.
• Recommend use of sugarless hard candy or gum to relieve dry mouth.
• **Look alike–sound alike:** Don't confuse doxepin with doxazosin, digoxin, doxapram, or Doxidan.

PATIENT TEACHING
۞ Alert: Teach patient to recognize and immediately report symptoms of serotonin toxicity (fever, mental status changes, muscle twitching, excessive sweating, shivering or shaking, diarrhea, loss of coordination).
• Tell patient to dilute oral concentrate with 4 ounces (120 mL) of water, milk, or juice (orange, grapefruit, tomato, prune, or pineapple, but not grape); preparation shouldn't be mixed with carbonated beverages.
Black Box Warning Advise families and caregivers to closely observe patient for increased suicidal thinking and behavior. ■
• Tell patient to take full dose at bedtime whenever he can, but warn him of possible morning dizziness on standing up quickly.
• Tell patient that, to minimize the potential for next-day effect, he should not take Silenor within 3 hours of a meal.
• Advise patient to consult prescriber before taking other prescription or OTC drugs.
• Warn patient to avoid hazardous activities that require alertness and good psychomotor coordination until effects of drug are known. Drowsiness and dizziness usually subside after a few weeks.

• Tell patient to avoid alcohol during drug therapy.

• Tell patient that maximal effect may not be evident for 2 to 3 weeks.

• Warn patient not to stop drug suddenly.

• To prevent sensitivity to the sun, advise patient to use sunblock, wear protective clothing, and avoid prolonged exposure to strong sunlight.

SAFETY ALERT!

DOXOrubicin hydrochloride
dox-oh-ROO-bi-sin

Therapeutic class: Antineoplastics
Pharmacologic class: Anthracycline glycoside antibiotics
Pregnancy risk category: D

AVAILABLE FORMS
Injection (preservative-free): 2 mg/mL
Powder for injection: 10 mg, 20 mg, 50 mg

INDICATIONS & DOSAGES
➤ **Bladder, breast, lung, ovarian, stomach, and thyroid cancers; non-Hodgkin lymphoma; Hodgkin lymphoma; acute lymphoblastic and myeloblastic leukemia; Wilms tumor; neuroblastoma; lymphoma; soft-tissue and bone sarcomas**
Adults and children: 60 to 75 mg/m^2 I.V. as single dose every 3 weeks; or when used in combination with other chemotherapy drugs, 40 to 60 mg/m^2 I.V. every 21 to 28 days.

Adjust-a-dose: Reduce dosage for patients with myelosuppression or impaired liver function. Elderly patients may need reduced dosages. Patients older than age 70 should receive no more than 300 mg/m^2 as a maximum lifetime cumulative dose. Be prepared to decrease dosage if bilirubin level rises: Give 50% of dose when bilirubin level is 1.2 to 3 mg/100 mL; 25% when it's 3.1 to 5 mg/100 mL. For patients with CrCl of less than 10 mL/minute, consider reducing dosage to 75% of usual dose.

ADMINISTRATION
I.V.
Black Box Warning Never give drug I.M. or subcutaneously. ∎

▼ Preparing and giving parenteral drug may be mutagenic, teratogenic, or carcinogenic. Follow facility policy to reduce risks.

▼ Reconstitute with preservative-free normal saline solution for injection to yield 2 mg/mL; add 5 mL to 10-mg vial, 10 mL to 20-mg vial, or 25 mL to 50-mg vial. Shake vial to dissolve drug.

▼ Don't place I.V. catheter over joints or in limbs with poor venous or lymphatic drainage.

▼ Give by direct injection over at least 3 minutes into the tubing of a free-flowing I.V. solution containing D$_5$W or normal saline solution for injection.

▼ If vein streaking occurs, slow administration rate. If welts appear, stop drug and notify prescriber.

▼ Some protocols give doxorubicin as a prolonged infusion, which requires central venous access.

Black Box Warning If extravasation occurs, stop infusion immediately and notify prescriber. Monitor area closely because extravasation may be progressive. Apply ice to the site for 15 minutes four times daily for 3 days. Drug is a strong vesicant and may cause tissue necrosis; two treatments for extravasation include topical dimethyl sulfoxide and dexrazoxane I.V. Early consultation with a plastic surgeon may be advisable. ∎

▼ Refrigerated, reconstituted solution is stable 15 days; at room temperature, it's stable 7 days.

▼ **Incompatibilities:** Allopurinol, aluminum, aminophylline, bacteriostatic diluents, cefepime, dexamethasone sodium phosphate, diazepam, 5-FU, furosemide, ganciclovir, heparin sodium, hydrocortisone sodium succinate, piperacillin–tazobactam.

ACTION
May interfere with DNA-dependent RNA synthesis by intercalation.

Route	Onset	Peak	Duration
I.V.	Unknown	Unknown	Unknown

Half-life: Initial, 30 minutes; terminal, 16½ hours.

Reactions in bold italics are *life-threatening*. Interactions may have a *rapid onset* or a *delayed onset*.

ADVERSE REACTIONS

CV: cardiac depression, *arrhythmias, acute left ventricular failure, irreversible cardiomyopathy.*

GI: nausea, vomiting, diarrhea, stomatitis, esophagitis, anorexia.

GU: transient red urine.

Hematologic: *leukopenia, thrombocytopenia, myelosuppression.*

Metabolic: hyperuricemia.

Skin: severe cellulitis and tissue sloughing with drug extravasation, urticaria, facial flushing, complete alopecia within 3 to 4 weeks, hyperpigmentation of nail beds and dermal creases, radiation recall effect.

Other: chills, *anaphylaxis, secondary malignancy (acute myelogenous leukemia [AML], myelodysplastic syndrome).*

INTERACTIONS

Drug-drug. *Aminophylline, cephalothin, dexamethasone, 5-FU, heparin, hydrocortisone:* May form a precipitate. Don't mix together.

Calcium channel blockers: May increase cardiotoxic effects. Monitor patient's ECG closely.

Cyclosporine: May increase doxorubicin concentration. Monitor patient for toxicity.

Digoxin: May decrease digoxin level. Monitor digoxin level closely.

Fosphenytoin, phenytoin: May decrease level of phenytoin or fosphenytoin. Monitor drug level.

Paclitaxel: May decrease doxorubicin clearance. Monitor patient for toxicity.

Phenobarbital: May increase doxorubicin clearance. Monitor patient closely.

Progesterone: May enhance neutropenia and thrombocytopenia. Monitor patient and laboratory values closely.

Streptozocin: May increase and prolong doxorubicin level. Doxorubicin dosage may have to be adjusted.

EFFECTS ON LAB TEST RESULTS

- May increase uric acid level.
- May decrease platelet and WBC counts.

CONTRAINDICATIONS & CAUTIONS

- Contraindicated in patients with a history of sensitivity reactions to drug or its components.
- Contraindicated in patients with marked myelosuppression induced by previous treatment with other antitumor drugs or radiotherapy and in those who have received a lifetime cumulative dose of 550 mg/m^2 of doxorubicin or daunorubicin.

NURSING CONSIDERATIONS

Black Box Warning Drug should be administered under the supervision of a physician experienced with cancer chemotherapeutic agents. ∎

- Perform cardiac function studies, including ECG and LVEF, before treatment and then periodically throughout therapy.
- Take preventive measures, including adequate hydration of the patient, before starting treatment. Rapid lysis of leukemic cells may cause hyperuricemia. Allopurinol may be ordered.
- Premedicate with antiemetic to reduce nausea.
- If skin or mucosal contact occurs, immediately wash with soap and water.

Black Box Warning Reduce dosage in patients with hepatic impairment. ∎

Black Box Warning Severe myelosuppression may occur. ∎

Black Box Warning Risk of secondary AML or myelodysplastic syndrome increases with doxorubicin use, especially when given with DNA-damaging antineoplastics or radiotherapy, when patients have been heavily pretreated with cytotoxic drugs, when doses have been escalated, or when patients age 50 and older had an existing increased risk of secondary AML or myelodysplastic syndrome. Pediatric patients are also at risk for developing secondary AML. ∎

- Monitor CBC with differential and LFTs; monitor ECG monthly during therapy. If WBC count falls below 2,000/mm^3 or granulocyte count falls below 1,000/mm^3, follow institutional policy for infection control in immunocompromised patients.
- Monitor ECG for changes, such as sinus tachycardia, T-wave flattening, ST-segment depression, and voltage reduction.
- Leukopenia may occur during days 10 to 15, with recovery by day 21.

• If tachycardia develops, stop drug or slow rate of infusion, and notify prescriber.

Black Box Warning Myocardial toxicity may occur during therapy or months to years after termination of therapy. Pediatric patients are at increased risk for developing delayed cardiotoxicity. ∎

❸ *Alert:* If signs of heart failure develop, stop drug and notify prescriber. Heart failure can often be prevented by limiting cumulative dose to 550 mg/m^2 (400 mg/m^2 when patient is also receiving or has received cyclophosphamide or radiation therapy to cardiac area).

❸ *Alert:* Reddish color of drug is similar to that of daunorubicin; don't confuse the two drugs.

• Esophagitis is common in patients who also have received radiation therapy.

❸ *Alert:* If patient has previously received radiation therapy, he's susceptible to radiation recall effect.

• *Look alike–sound alike:* Don't confuse doxorubicin with doxorubicin liposomal, daunorubicin, or idarubicin.

PATIENT TEACHING

• Advise patient to report any pain or burning at site of injection during or after administration.

• Advise patient to watch for signs and symptoms of infection (fever, sore throat, fatigue) and bleeding (easy bruising, nosebleeds, bleeding gums, tarry stools) and to take temperature daily.

• Advise patient that orange to red urine for 1 to 2 days is normal and doesn't indicate presence of blood.

• Inform patient that hair loss may occur but that it's usually reversible. Hair may regrow 2 to 5 months after drug is stopped.

SAFETY ALERT!

DOXOrubicin hydrochloride liposomal
dox-oh-ROO-bi-sin

Doxil

Therapeutic class: Antineoplastics
Pharmacologic class: Anthracycline glycoside antibiotics
Pregnancy risk category: D

AVAILABLE FORMS
Injection: 20 mg/10 mL, 50 mg/25 mL

INDICATIONS & DOSAGES
Adjust-a-dose (for all indications): For patients with impaired hepatic function, reduce dosage as follows: If bilirubin level is 1.2 to 3 mg/dL, give half normal dose; if bilirubin level is more than 3 mg/dL, give one-fourth normal dose. Dose modifications may be needed for stomatitis, myelosuppression, and hand-foot syndrome, based on toxicity grade. Refer to manufacturer's directions.

Don't exceed lifetime maximum cumulative dose of 550 mg/m^2 (400 mg/m^2 for adults having received mediastinal radiation or other cardiotoxic drugs and 300 mg/m^2 for patients older than age 70 with or without mediastinal radiation).

➤ **Metastatic ovarian carcinoma refractory to both paclitaxel- and platinum-based chemotherapy regimens**
Women: 50 mg/m^2 I.V. initially at 1 mg/minute once every 4 weeks for minimum of four courses. Continue as long as condition doesn't progress, patient shows no evidence of cardiotoxicity, and patient continues to tolerate treatment. If no infusion-related adverse reactions develop, increase infusion rate to complete administration over 1 hour.

➤ **AIDS-related Kaposi sarcoma refractory to previous combination chemotherapy and in patients intolerant of such therapy**
Adults: 20 mg/m^2 I.V. over 60 minutes once every 3 weeks. Initial rate should be 1 mg/minute to minimize infusion-related reactions. Continue as long as patient responds satisfactorily and tolerates treatment.

Reactions in bold italics are *life-threatening*. Interactions may have a *rapid onset* or a *delayed onset*.

➤ **Multiple myeloma**
Adults: 30 mg/m² I.V. on day 4 following bortezomib, which is given at 1.3 mg/m² bolus on days 1, 4, 8, and 11, every 3 weeks. Initial rate of first dose of doxorubicin hydrochloride liposomal should be 1 mg/minute to minimize infusion-related reactions. If no infusion-related adverse reactions occur, increase infusion rate to complete administration over 1 hour. Treatment may continue for up to eight cycles, until disease progression or occurrence of unacceptable toxicity.

ADMINISTRATION

I.V.
▼ Don't give I.M. or subcutaneously.
▼ Follow procedures for proper handling and disposal of antineoplastics.
▼ Dilute appropriate dose (maximum, 90 mg) in 250 mL D₅W using aseptic technique.
Black Box Warning Carefully check label on I.V. bag before giving drug. Accidentally substituting doxorubicin hydrochloride liposomal for conventional doxorubicin hydrochloride may cause severe adverse reactions. The two products can't be substituted on a milligram-per-milligram basis. ▋
▼ Don't use an in-line filter.
▼ Infuse over 60 minutes. Monitor patient carefully during infusion.
Black Box Warning Serious, sometimes fatal, allergic infusion reactions can occur. Make sure emergency equipment and medications are available. Acute infusion-related reactions include flushing, shortness of breath, facial swelling, headache, chills, back pain, tightness in chest or throat, and hypotension. They may resolve when infusion rate is slowed, or over several hours to a day when infusion is stopped. ▋
▼ If extravasation occurs, stop infusion immediately. Apply ice at the site for about 30 minutes to help alleviate local reaction. Restart infusion in another vein.
▼ Refrigerate diluted solution at 36° to 46° F (2° to 8° C) and give within 24 hours.
▼ **Incompatibilities:** Other I.V. drugs.

ACTION

Consists of doxorubicin hydrochloride encapsulated in liposomes. Action may involve drug's ability to bind DNA and inhibit nucleic acid synthesis.

Route	Onset	Peak	Duration
I.V.	Unknown	Unknown	Unknown

Half-life: 5 hours in first phase; 55 hours in second phase with doses of 10 to 20 mg/m².

ADVERSE REACTIONS

CNS: asthenia, paresthesia, headache, somnolence, dizziness, depression, insomnia, anxiety, malaise, emotional lability, fatigue, fever.
CV: chest pain, hypotension, tachycardia, peripheral edema, *cardiomyopathy, heart failure, arrhythmias,* pericardial effusion.
EENT: pharyngitis, rhinitis, conjunctivitis, retinitis, optic neuritis.
GI: nausea, vomiting, constipation, anorexia, diarrhea, abdominal pain, dyspepsia, oral candidiasis, enlarged abdomen, esophagitis, dysphagia, stomatitis, taste perversion, glossitis.
Hematologic: *leukopenia, neutropenia, thrombocytopenia,* anemia.
Hepatic: hyperbilirubinemia.
Metabolic: dehydration, weight loss, hypocalcemia, hyperglycemia.
Musculoskeletal: myalgia, back pain.
Respiratory: dyspnea, increased cough, pneumonia.
Skin: rash, alopecia, dry skin, pruritus, skin discoloration, skin disorder, exfoliative dermatitis, sweating, palmar-plantar erythrodysesthesia.
Other: allergic reaction, chills, herpes zoster, infection, infusion-related reactions.

INTERACTIONS

None reported. However, drug may interact with drugs that interact with conventional form of doxorubicin hydrochloride.

EFFECTS ON LAB TEST RESULTS

● May increase bilirubin and glucose levels. May decrease calcium and hemoglobin levels.
● May increase PT and INR. May decrease neutrophil, platelet, and WBC counts.

D

CONTRAINDICATIONS & CAUTIONS

• Contraindicated in patients hypersensitive to conventional formulation of doxorubicin hydrochloride or any component in the liposomal form.

• Contraindicated in patients with marked myelosuppression and those who have received a lifetime cumulative dose of 550 mg/m^2 (400 mg/m^2 in patients who have received radiotherapy to the mediastinal area or therapy with other cardiotoxic drugs such as cyclophosphamide and 300 mg/m^2 in patients older than age 70 with or without mediastinal radiation).

• Use cautiously in patients who have received other anthracyclines.

⚠ **Overdose S&S:** Leukopenia, mucositis, thrombocytopenia.

NURSING CONSIDERATIONS

• Consider previous or current therapy with related compounds such as daunorubicin when calculating total dose of drug to be given. Heart failure and cardiomyopathy may occur after stopping therapy.

Black Box Warning Cumulative dose over 550 mg/m^2 increases risk of cardiotoxicity. Cardiotoxicity may occur at lower cumulative doses in patients with prior mediastinal irradiation and in patients receiving concurrent cyclophosphamide therapy. The lifetime maximum cumulative dose for these patients is 400 mg/m^2. The lifetime maximum cumulative dose for patients older than age 70 with or without mediastinal radiation is 300 mg/m^2. ∎

• Give drug to patient with history of CV disease only when benefit outweighs risk to patient.

🔆 **Alert:** Monitor patient for signs and symptoms of palmar-plantar erythrodysesthesia, hematologic toxicity, or stomatitis. These adverse reactions may be managed with dosage delays and adjustments.

Black Box Warning Evaluate patient's hepatic function before therapy, and reduce dosage accordingly. ∎

• Drug may increase toxicity of other antineoplastics.

• Closely monitor cardiac function by endomyocardial biopsy, echocardiography, or gated radionuclide scans. If results indicate possible cardiac injury, the benefit of continued therapy must be weighed against the risk of myocardial injury.

Black Box Warning Severe myelosuppression may occur. ∎

• Monitor CBC, including platelets, before each dose and frequently throughout therapy. Leukopenia is usually transient. Persistent severe myelosuppression may result in superinfection or hemorrhage. Patient may need granulocyte colony-stimulating factor (or granulocyte-macrophage colony-stimulating factor) to support blood counts.

• **Look alike–sound alike:** Don't confuse doxorubicin with daunorubicin. Don't confuse Doxil with Paxil.

PATIENT TEACHING

• Tell patient to notify prescriber if he experiences signs and symptoms of hand-foot syndrome (such as tingling or burning, redness, flaking, bothersome swelling, small blisters, or small sores on palms of hands or soles of feet).

• To reduce the risk of hand-foot syndrome, advise the patient to follow these guidelines at least 1 day before and for 3 to 5 days after treatment:

– Avoid direct sunlight and use sunblock SPF 15 or higher on all exposed skin.

– Wear loose clothing and comfortable, well-ventilated, low-heeled shoes.

– Avoid contact with hot water and take cool, short showers or baths.

– Don't put pressure on your skin. (Avoid kneeling, leaning on your elbows, wearing tight jewelry or undergarments, and chopping hard foods.)

• Advise patient to report signs and symptoms of mouth inflammation (such as painful redness, swelling, or sores in mouth).

• Warn patient to avoid exposure to people with infections. Tell patient to report temperature of 100.5° F (38° C) or higher.

• Tell patient to report nausea, vomiting, tiredness, weakness, rash, or mild hair loss.

• Advise women of childbearing age to avoid pregnancy during therapy.

D

doxycycline
dox-i-SYE-kleen

Oracea

doxycycline calcium
Vibramycin

doxycycline hyclate
Atridox, Doryx, Doxy 100, Doxy 200,
Morgidox, Periostat, Vibramycin,
Vibra-Tabs

doxycycline monohydrate
Monodox, Vibramycin

Therapeutic class: Antibiotics
Pharmacologic class: Tetracyclines
Pregnancy risk category: D

AVAILABLE FORMS
doxycycline
Capsules: 40 mg, 50 mg, 75 mg, 100 mg,
150 mg
Injection: 100 mg/vial
Oral suspension: 25 mg/5 mL
Tablets: 50 mg, 75 mg, 100 mg, 150 mg
doxycycline calcium
Syrup: 50 mg/5 mL
doxycycline hyclate
Capsules: 50 mg, 100 mg
Capsules (coated pellets): 100 mg
Injection: 100 mg, 200 mg
Tablets: 20 mg, 100 mg
Tablets (delayed-release): 50 mg, 75 mg,
100 mg, 150 mg, 200 mg
doxycycline monohydrate
Capsules: 50 mg, 75 mg, 100 mg
Oral suspension: 25 mg/5 mL
Tablets: 50 mg, 75 mg, 100 mg, 150 mg

INDICATIONS & DOSAGES
➤ **Infections caused by susceptible gram-positive and gram-negative organisms (including *Haemophilus ducreyi, Yersinia pestis,* and *Campylobacter fetus*), *Rickettsiae* species, *Mycoplasma pneumoniae, Chlamydia trachomatis,* and *Borrelia burgdorferi* (Lyme disease); psittacosis; granuloma inguinale**

Adults and children older than age 8 weighing at least 45 kg (99 lb): 100 mg P.O. every 12 hours on first day; then 100 mg P.O. daily as a single dose or in two divided doses. Or, 200 mg I.V. on first day in one or two infusions; then 100 to 200 mg I.V. daily. Daily doses of 200 mg I.V. can be given as a single dose or in two divided doses.
Children older than age 8 weighing less than 45 kg: 4.4 mg/kg P.O. or I.V. daily, in divided doses every 12 hours on first day; then 2.2 to 4.4 mg/kg daily given as a single dose or in two divided doses.

Give I.V. infusion slowly (minimum 1 hour). Infusion must be completed within 12 hours (within 6 hours in lactated Ringer solution or dextrose 5% in lactated Ringer solution).
➤ **Gonorrhea in patients allergic to penicillin**
Adults: 100 mg P.O. b.i.d. for 7 days. For epididymitis, use for 10 days and give a single dose of ceftriaxone 250 mg I.M.
➤ **Syphilis in patients allergic to penicillin (except Doryx, Monodox)**
Adults: 100 mg P.O. b.i.d. for 14 days (early). If more than 1-year duration, 100 mg P.O. daily for 4 weeks.
➤ **Primary or secondary syphilis in patients allergic to penicillin (Doryx, Monodox only)**
Adults: 300 mg P.O. daily in divided doses for at least 10 days.
➤ **Uncomplicated urethral, endocervical, or rectal infections caused by *C. trachomatis* or *Ureaplasma urealyticum***
Adults: 100 mg P.O. b.i.d. for at least 7 days. For epididymitis, use for 10 days and give a single dose of ceftriaxone 250 mg I.M. if caused by *C. trachomatis.* In those with lymphogranuloma venereum, treat for at least 21 days.
➤ **To prevent malaria**
Adults: 100 mg P.O. daily beginning 1 to 2 days before travel to endemic area and continued for 4 weeks after travel.
Children older than age 8: Give 2 mg/kg P.O. once daily beginning 1 to 2 days before travel to endemic area and continued for 4 weeks after travel. Don't exceed daily dose of 100 mg.

➤ **Adjunct to other antibiotics for inhalation, GI, and oropharyngeal anthrax**
Adults: 100 mg every 12 hours I.V. initially until susceptibility test results are known. Switch to 100 mg P.O. b.i.d. when appropriate. Treat for 60 days total.
Children older than age 8 weighing more than 45 kg (99 lb): 100 mg every 12 hours I.V.; then switch to 100 mg P.O. b.i.d. when appropriate. Treat for 60 days total.
Children older than age 8 weighing 45 kg or less: 2.2 mg/kg every 12 hours I.V.; then switch to 2.2 mg/kg (up to 100 mg) P.O. b.i.d. when appropriate. Treat for 60 days total.
Children age 8 and younger: 2.2 mg/kg every 12 hours I.V.; then switch to 2.2 mg/kg (up to 100 mg) P.O. b.i.d. when appropriate. Treat for 60 days total.

➤ **Cutaneous anthrax**
Adults: 100 mg P.O. every 12 hours for 60 days.
Children older than age 8 weighing more than 45 kg (99 lb): 100 mg P.O. every 12 hours for 60 days.
Children older than age 8 weighing 45 kg or less: 2.2 mg/kg (up to 100 mg) every 12 hours P.O. for 60 days.
Children age 8 and younger: 2.2 mg/kg (up to 100 mg) P.O. every 12 hours for 60 days.

➤ **Adjunct to scaling and root planing to improve attachment and reduce pocket depth in periodontitis**
Adults: 20 mg P.O. Periostat b.i.d., more than 1 hour before or 2 hours after the morning and evening meals and after scaling and root planing. Effective for 9 months.

➤ **Inflammatory lesions of rosacea**
Adults: 40 mg Oracea P.O. once daily in the morning, 1 hour before or 2 hours after a meal. Give with a full glass of water. Reevaluate treatment after 16 weeks.

➤ **Cervicitis** ◆
Adults: 100 mg P.O. b.i.d. for 7 days.

➤ **Device-related osteoarticular methicillin-resistant *Staphylococcus aureus* (MRSA) infection** ◆
Adults: 100 mg P.O. every 12 hours.

➤ **Epididymitis** ◆
Adults: 100 mg P.O. b.i.d. for 10 days. Give in conjunction with a single dose of I.M. ceftriaxone 250 mg.

➤ **Infective endocarditis (suspected *Bartonella* infection with a negative culture)** ◆
Adults: 200 mg P.O. every 24 hours in two equally divided doses for 6 weeks in combination with gentamicin and ceftriaxone.
Children: 2 to 4 mg/kg P.O. every 24 hours in two equally divided doses for 6 weeks in combination with gentamicin and ceftriaxone.

➤ **Infective endocarditis (documented *Bartonella* infection with a positive culture)** ◆
Adults: 200 mg P.O. every 24 hours in two equally divided doses for 6 weeks in combination with gentamicin or rifampin.
Children: 2 to 4 mg/kg P.O. every 24 hours in two equally divided doses for 6 weeks in combination with gentamicin or rifampin.

➤ **Early Lyme disease (erythema migrans)** ◆
Adults: 100 mg P.O. b.i.d. for 14 days (range, 10 to 21 days).
Children age 8 and older: 2 mg/kg b.i.d., up to a maximum dose of 100 mg.

➤ **Lyme disease with early neurologic manifestations (without meningitis)** ◆
Adults: 100 to 200 mg P.O. b.i.d. for 10 to 28 days.
Children age 8 and older: 2 to 4 mg/kg b.i.d., up to a maximum dose of 100 to 200 mg.

➤ **Lyme disease with meningitis or radiculopathy (if intolerant of beta-lactam antibiotics)** ◆
Adults: 100 to 200 mg b.i.d. P.O. or I.V. for 14 days.
Children age 8 and older: 2 to 4 mg/kg b.i.d., up to a maximum dose of 100 to 200 mg.

➤ **Late Lyme disease arthritis (without neurologic manifestations)** ◆
Adults: 100 mg P.O. b.i.d. for 28 days.
Children age 8 and older: 2 mg/kg b.i.d., up to a maximum dose of 100 mg.

➤ **Pelvic inflammatory disease** ◆
Adults and adolescents: 100 mg P.O. b.i.d. for 14 days in conjunction with a single dose of ceftriaxone, cefoxitin, or another third-generation parenteral cephalosporin (such as ceftizoxime or cefotaxime). Metronidazole 500 mg P.O. b.i.d. may be added to the regimen if concerns of anaerobic infection exist.

Reactions in bold italics are *life-threatening*. Interactions may have a *rapid onset* or a *delayed onset*.

➤ Proctitis, proctocolitis, enteritis ◆
Adults: 100 mg P.O. b.i.d for 7 days. Give with a one-time I.M. dose of ceftriaxone 125 mg. Patients diagnosed with lymphogranuloma venereum should receive 21 days of doxycycline therapy.

ADMINISTRATION
P.O.
● Obtain specimen for culture and sensitivity tests before giving. Begin therapy while awaiting results.
⊕ Alert: Check expiration date. Outdated or deteriorated tetracyclines may cause reversible nephrotoxicity (Fanconi syndrome).
● Give drug with food or milk if stomach upset occurs.
● Increase fluid intake and don't administer tablets or capsules within 1 hour of bedtime because of possible esophageal irritation or ulceration.
● Give Oracea with a full glass of water.
● Tablets may be crushed and mixed with low-fat or chocolate milk, chocolate pudding, or apple juice mixed equally with sugar. Store mixtures in refrigerator (except apple juice mixture, which can be stored at room temperature) and discard after 24 hours.

I.V.
▼ Obtain specimen for culture and sensitivity tests before giving. Begin therapy while awaiting results.
▼ Reconstitute powder for injection with sterile water for injection. Use 10 mL in 100-mg vial and 20 mL in 200-mg vial. Further dilute solution to a concentration of 0.1 mg/mL to 1 mg/mL; don't infuse solution that contains more than 1 mg/mL.
▼ Don't expose drug to light or heat. Protect it from sunlight during infusion.
▼ Infusion time varies with dose but usually ranges from 1 to 4 hours. Infusion must be completed within 12 hours.
▼ Monitor infusion site for evidence of thrombophlebitis.
▼ Reconstituted injectable solution is stable 72 hours if refrigerated and protected from light.
▼ **Incompatibilities:** Allopurinol; drugs that are unstable in acidic solutions, such as barbiturates; erythromycin lactobionate; heparin; meropenem; nafcillin; penicillin G potassium; piperacillin–tazobactam; riboflavin; sulfonamides.

ACTION
May exert bacteriostatic effect by binding to the 30S and possibly 50S ribosomal subunits of microorganisms and inhibiting protein synthesis. May also alter the cytoplasmic membrane of susceptible microorganisms.

Route	Onset	Peak	Duration
P.O.	Unknown	1½–4 hr	Unknown
P.O. (delayed-release)	Unknown	2–4 hr	Unknown
I.V.	Immediate	Unknown	Unknown

Half-life: About 1 day after multiple dosing.

ADVERSE REACTIONS
CNS: *intracranial hypertension.*
CV: pericarditis, thrombophlebitis.
GI: diarrhea, epigastric distress, nausea, anorexia, glossitis, dysphagia, vomiting, oral candidiasis, enterocolitis, anogenital inflammation.
Hematologic: *neutropenia, thrombocytopenia,* eosinophilia, hemolytic anemia.
Musculoskeletal: bone growth retardation in children younger than age 8.
Skin: maculopapular and erythematous rashes, photosensitivity reactions, increased pigmentation, urticaria.
Other: *anaphylaxis,* hypersensitivity reactions, superinfection, permanent discoloration of teeth, enamel defects.

INTERACTIONS
Drug-drug. *Antacids and laxatives containing aluminum, magnesium, or calcium, antidiarrheals:* May decrease antibiotic absorption. Give antibiotic 1 hour before or 2 hours after these drugs.
Carbamazepine, phenobarbital, rifamycins: May decrease antibiotic effect. Avoid using together.
Ferrous sulfate and other iron products, zinc: May decrease antibiotic absorption. Give drug 2 hours before or 3 hours after iron.
Hormonal contraceptives: May decrease contraceptive effectiveness and increase risk

of breakthrough bleeding. Advise use of a nonhormonal contraceptive.

Isotretinoin: May increase risk of pseudotumor cerebri. Avoid using together.

Methoxyflurane: May cause nephrotoxicity with tetracyclines. Avoid using together.

Oral anticoagulants: May increase anticoagulant effect. Monitor PT and INR, and adjust dosage.

Penicillins: May interfere with bactericidal action of penicillins. Avoid using together.

Drug-lifestyle. *Alcohol use:* May decrease drug's effect. Discourage use together.

Sun exposure: May cause photosensitivity reactions. Advise patient to avoid excessive sunlight exposure.

EFFECTS ON LAB TEST RESULTS
● May increase BUN and liver enzyme levels. May decrease hemoglobin level.
● May increase eosinophil count. May decrease platelet, neutrophil, and WBC counts.
● May falsely elevate fluorometric tests for urine catecholamines. May cause false-negative results in urine glucose tests using glucose oxidase reagent (Diastix or Chemstrip uG). Parenteral form may cause false-positive Clinitest results.

CONTRAINDICATIONS & CAUTIONS
● Contraindicated in patients hypersensitive to drug or other tetracyclines.
● Use cautiously in patients with impaired renal or hepatic function.
● In a fetus in the last half of gestation or a child younger than age 8, drug may cause permanently discolored teeth, enamel defects, and bone growth retardation.
⚠ *Overdose S&S:* Dizziness, nausea, vomiting.

NURSING CONSIDERATIONS
● If patient receives large doses or prolonged therapy or if patient is at high risk, watch for signs and symptoms of superinfection. If superinfection occurs, drug should be discontinued and appropriate therapy instituted.
● Cutaneous anthrax with signs of systemic involvement, extensive edema, or lesions on the head or neck requires I.V. therapy and a multidrug approach.

● Ciprofloxacin and doxycycline are first-line therapies for anthrax. If anthrax patient also has meningitis, ciprofloxacin is preferred because of better distribution to the CNS.
● In pregnant women and immunocompromised patients, use the usual dosage schedule for anthrax. In pregnant women, adverse effects on fetal teeth and bones are dose-limited, so drug may be used for 7 to 14 days before the third trimester.
● Check patient's tongue for signs of fungal infection. Emphasize good oral hygiene.
● Photosensitivity reactions may occur within a few minutes to several hours after exposure and may last after therapy ends.
● ***Look alike–sound alike:*** Don't confuse doxycycline with doxylamine or dicyclomine. Don't confuse Oracea with Orencia.

PATIENT TEACHING
● Tell patient to take entire amount of drug exactly as prescribed, even after he feels better.
● Instruct patient to report adverse reactions promptly. If drug is being given I.V., tell him to report discomfort at I.V. site.
● Advise patient to take oral form of drug with food or milk if stomach upset occurs.
● Advise patient to increase fluid intake and not to take oral tablets or capsules within 1 hour of bedtime because of possible esophageal irritation or ulceration.
● Advise parent giving drug to a child that tablets may be crushed and mixed with low-fat or chocolate milk, chocolate pudding, or apple juice mixed equally with sugar. Tell parent to store mixtures in refrigerator (except apple juice mixture, which can be stored at room temperature) and to discard after 24 hours.
● Warn patient to avoid direct sunlight and ultraviolet light, wear protective clothing, and use sunscreen.
● Tell patient to report signs and symptoms of superinfection to prescriber.
● Tell patient taking Oracea to take drug with a full glass of water.

doxylamine succinate–pyridoxine hydrochloride
docks-ILL-ah-meen–peer-reh-DOCK-seen

Diclegis

Therapeutic class: Antiemetics
Pharmacologic class: Antihistamines–B₆ vitamin analogs
Pregnancy risk category: A

AVAILABLE FORMS
Tablets (delayed-release): doxylamine succinate 10 mg and pyridoxine hydrochloride 10 mg

INDICATIONS & DOSAGES
➤ **Nausea and vomiting of pregnancy in women who don't respond to conservative management**
Adults: Initially, doxylamine 20 mg and pyridoxine 20 mg at bedtime on day 1. If that dosage adequately controls symptoms the next day, continue. If symptoms persist into the afternoon of day 2, patients should take doxylamine 20 mg and pyridoxine 20 mg at bedtime that night, then take doxylamine 10 mg and pyridoxine 10 mg in the morning and doxylamine 20 mg and pyridoxine 20 mg at bedtime on day 3. If that dosage adequately controls symptoms on day 4, patients should continue taking doxylamine 10 mg and pyridoxine 10 mg in the morning and doxylamine 20 mg and pyridoxine 20 mg at bedtime. Otherwise, they should take doxylamine 10 mg and pyridoxine 10 mg in the morning, doxylamine 10 mg and pyridoxine 10 mg midafternoon, and doxylamine 20 mg and pyridoxine 20 mg at bedtime on day 4.

ADMINISTRATION
P.O.
• Give tablets whole on an empty stomach with a glass of water. Don't crush, split, or allow patient to chew tablets.
• Patient should take tablets daily and not p.r.n.
• Store bottle at room temperature. Keep bottle tightly closed and protect from moisture. Don't remove desiccant canister from bottle.

ACTION
Unknown. The combination of antihistamine and vitamin B₆ may cause anticholinergic effects, decreasing nausea.

Route	Onset	Peak	Duration
P.O. (doxylamine)	Unknown	7½ hr	Unknown
P.O. (pyridoxine)	Unknown	5½ hr	Unknown

Half-life: Doxylamine, 12½ hours; pyridoxine, ½ hour.

ADVERSE REACTIONS
CNS: somnolence.

INTERACTIONS
Drug-drug. *CNS depressants (hypnotic sedatives and tranquilizers):* May have additive effects. Don't use together.
MAO inhibitors (selegiline, tranylcypromine): May prolong and intensify CNS anticholinergic effects. Use together is contraindicated.
Other ethanolamine derivative antihistamines (diphenhydramine): May have additive effects. Avoid use together.
Drug-lifestyle. *Alcohol use:* May have additive effects. Discourage use together.

EFFECTS ON LAB TEST RESULTS
• None reported.

CONTRAINDICATIONS & CAUTIONS
• Contraindicated in women hypersensitive to drug or its components.
• Contraindicated in breast-feeding women. Drug appears in breast milk.
• Use cautiously in patients with asthma, increased intraocular pressure, angle-closure glaucoma, stenosing peptic ulcer, or pyloroduodenal obstruction or urinary bladder neck obstruction because of anticholinergic effects.
⚠ *Overdose S&S:* Restlessness, dry mouth, dilated pupils, sleepiness, vertigo, mental confusion, tachycardia, seizures, rhabdomyolysis, acute renal failure, death.

NURSING CONSIDERATIONS
• Reassess for continued need for drug as the pregnancy progresses.

- Drug hasn't been studied in women with hyperemesis gravidarum.
- Monitor patient for anticholinergic effects (dry mouth, tachycardia, urine retention, constipation, ataxia).
- Monitor patient for somnolence, increased falls, and other CNS depressant effects.

PATIENT TEACHING
- Warn patient about side effects, including somnolence, increased falls, and other CNS depressant effects.
- Advise patient to avoid alcohol and sedating medications, including antihistamine cough and cold products, opioids, and sleep aids, while taking this drug because of increased risk of additive effects.
- Caution patient to avoid driving and operating heavy equipment or other activities that require complete mental alertness.

dronabinol (delta-9-tetrahydrocannabinol)
droe-NAB-i-nol

Marinol

Therapeutic class: Antiemetics
Pharmacologic class: Cannabinoids
Pregnancy risk category: C
Controlled substance schedule: III

AVAILABLE FORMS
Capsules: 2.5 mg, 5 mg, 10 mg

INDICATIONS & DOSAGES
➤ **Nausea and vomiting from cancer chemotherapy**
Adults: 5 mg/m^2 P.O. 1 to 3 hours before chemotherapy session. Then, same dose every 2 to 4 hours after chemotherapy, for total of four to six doses daily. If needed, increase dosage in 2.5-mg/m^2 increments to maximum of 15 mg/m^2 per dose.
➤ **Anorexia and weight loss in patients with AIDS**
Adults: 2.5 mg P.O. b.i.d. before lunch and dinner. If patient can't tolerate it, decrease to 2.5 mg P.O. given as a single dose daily in evening or at bedtime. May gradually increase to maximum of 20 mg daily given in divided doses.

ADMINISTRATION
P.O.
- Give 1 to 3 hours before chemotherapy.
- Store in cool environment, but protect from freezing.

ACTION
Unknown. A derivative of marijuana.

Route	Onset	Peak	Duration
P.O.	30–60 min	2–4 hr	4–6 hr

Half-life: 1 to 1½ days.

ADVERSE REACTIONS
CNS: ataxia, dizziness, drowsiness, euphoria, paranoia, amnesia, asthenia, confusion, depersonalization, hallucinations, muddled thinking, somnolence.
CV: orthostatic hypotension, palpitations, tachycardia, vasodilation.
EENT: visual disturbances.
GI: abdominal pain, dry mouth, nausea, vomiting, diarrhea.

INTERACTIONS
Drug-drug. *CNS depressants, psychomimetic substances, sedatives:* May cause additive CNS depression. Avoid using together.
Drug-lifestyle. *Alcohol use:* May cause additive CNS depression. Discourage use together.

EFFECTS ON LAB TEST RESULTS
None reported.

CONTRAINDICATIONS & CAUTIONS
- Contraindicated in patients hypersensitive to sesame oil or cannabinoids.
- Use cautiously in the elderly, in pregnant or breast-feeding women, and in those with heart disease, psychiatric illness, or history of drug abuse.
- ⚠ *Overdose S&S:* Mild—drowsiness, euphoria, heightened sensory awareness, altered time perception, reddened conjunctiva, dry mouth, tachycardia; moderate—memory impairment, depersonalization, mood alteration, urine retention, decreased bowel motility; severe—decreased motor coordination, lethargy, slurred speech, orthostatic hypotension.

Reactions in bold italics are *life-threatening*. Interactions may have a *rapid onset* or a *delayed onset*.

NURSING CONSIDERATIONS

● Expect drug to be prescribed only for patients who haven't responded satisfactorily to other antiemetics.

◑ **Alert:** Drug is the principal active substance in *Cannabis sativa* (marijuana), which can produce both physiologic and psychological dependence and has a high risk of abuse.

● Monitor patient for hypotension, hypertension, syncope, and tachycardia.

● Monitor patient for worsening signs and symptoms of psychiatric illness.

● CNS effects are intensified at higher dosages.

● Drug effects may persist for days after treatment ends.

● **Look alike–sound alike:** Don't confuse dronabinol with droperidol.

PATIENT TEACHING

● Tell patient that drug may induce unusual changes in mood or other adverse behavioral effects.

● Advise patient against performing activities that require alertness until CNS effects of drug are known.

● Warn caregivers to supervise patient during and immediately after treatment.

● Advise patient to take drug 1 to 3 hours before chemotherapy.

---

dronedarone
dro-neh-DAR-rone

Multaq

Therapeutic class: Antiarrhythmics
Pharmacologic class: Benzofuran derivatives
Pregnancy risk category: X

AVAILABLE FORMS
Tablets: 400 mg

INDICATIONS & DOSAGES
➤ **To reduce risk of hospitalization in patients with recent episode of paroxysmal or persistent atrial fibrillation or flutter who have CV risk factors, such as age older than 70, diabetes, hypertension, stroke, left atrial diameter greater than 50 mm, or LVEF less than 40%, who are** in normal sinus rhythm or who will be cardioverted

Adults: 400 mg P.O. b.i.d.

ADMINISTRATION
P.O.
● Give drug with morning and evening meals.
● Don't give grapefruit juice to patient taking this drug.

ACTION

Unknown. Exhibits properties of all four Vaughan-Williams antiarrhythmic classes; it's unclear which of these is important in producing drug's clinical effects.

Route	Onset	Peak	Duration
P.O.	Unknown	3–6 hr	Unknown

Half-life: 13 to 19 hours.

ADVERSE REACTIONS
CNS: asthenia.
CV: *bradycardia, heart failure, QT interval prolongation.*
GI: abdominal pain, diarrhea, dyspepsia, nausea, vomiting.
Skin: allergic dermatitis, dermatitis, eczema, pruritus, rash.

INTERACTIONS
Drug-drug. *Beta blockers:* May cause bradycardia. Initially, give low dose of beta blocker and increase dosage only after monitoring ECG for tolerance.
Calcium channel blockers: May cause additive effects. Reduce initial dosage of calcium channel blocker; increase dosage only after monitoring ECG for tolerance.
CYP2C9 substrates (losartan, warfarin): May increase metabolite levels. Monitor patient closely; monitor INR in patient taking warfarin.
CYP3A inducers (carbamazepine, phenobarbital, phenytoin, rifampin): May decrease dronedarone level. Use together is contraindicated.
CYP3A inhibitors (clarithromycin, erythromycin, itraconazole, ketoconazole, ritonavir, voriconazole): May increase dronedarone level. Use together is contraindicated.

CYP3A substrates (sirolimus, tacrolimus): May increase levels of these drugs. Monitor drug levels.

Digoxin: May increase digoxin level and electrophysiologic effects of dronedarone. Avoid use together; if necessary to use together, decrease digoxin dosage by 50%.

Drugs that prolong QT interval (class I and III antiarrhythmics, macrolide antibiotics, phenothiazines, tricyclic antidepressants): May further increase QT interval, leading to torsades de pointes. Use together is contraindicated.

Statins: May increase statin level. Use together cautiously.

Drug-herb. *St John's wort:* May decrease drug level. Discourage use together.

Drug-lifestyle. *Grapefruit juice:* May increase drug level. Discourage use together.

EFFECTS ON LAB TEST RESULTS

● May increase serum creatinine level.

● May decrease potassium and magnesium levels (in patients taking potassium-depleting diuretics).

CONTRAINDICATIONS & CAUTIONS

Black Box Warning Contraindicated in patients with New York Heart Association class IV heart failure or class II to III heart failure with recent decompensation requiring hospitalization or referral to a heart failure clinic. ∎

Black Box Warning Contraindicated in patients with atrial fibrillation who won't or can't be restored to normal sinus rhythm. Drug doubles risk of death, stroke, and hospitalization for heart failure in patients with permanent atrial fibrillation. ∎

● Contraindicated in second- or third-degree AV block or sick sinus syndrome (unless a functioning pacemaker is in place), bradycardia (less than 50 beats/minute), severe hepatic impairment, QTc interval of 500 ms or greater, or PR interval greater than 280 ms.

● Contraindicated with concomitant use of CYP3A inhibitors and drugs or herbal preparations that prolong QT interval.

۞ Alert: Drug may increase risk of severe hepatic injury or failure.

● Use cautiously in patients with new or worsening heart failure.

● Use in pregnant women is contraindicated. Women of childbearing age should use effective birth control during therapy.

● It isn't known if drug appears in breast milk. Women should stop breast-feeding before using this drug.

⚠ Overdose S&S: QTc interval prolongation.

NURSING CONSIDERATIONS

● Potassium-depleting diuretics may cause hypokalemia and hypomagnesemia, increasing the risk of torsades de pointes. Initiate dronedarone therapy after potassium and magnesium levels reach and stay within normal range.

● Monitor CV status, ECG, and QTc interval routinely.

● Monitor renal function and electrolyte levels regularly.

● Monitor hepatic serum enzyme levels, especially during the first 6 months of therapy. Discontinue drug if hepatic injury is suspected.

PATIENT TEACHING

● Instruct patient to take drug with morning and evening meals.

● Warn patient to avoid grapefruit juice.

● Advise patient to report weight gain, dyspnea, fatigue, and peripheral edema, which may indicate worsening heart failure.

● Tell patient to report changes in OTC or prescription drug use, or in supplement or herb use.

● If patient misses a dose, tell patient not to double the dose but to skip that dose and take the next regularly scheduled dose.

● Instruct patient to report slowed heartbeat, diarrhea, nausea, vomiting, abdominal pain, indigestion, fatigue, or rash.

● Advise women of childbearing age to use an effective method of birth control while taking drug and to notify prescriber if becoming pregnant or thinking of becoming pregnant.

● Advise women not to breast-feed while taking dronedarone because drug may appear in breast milk.

drospirenone–ethinyl estradiol

droh-SPYE-re-none and ETH-i-nill
es-tra-DYE-ole

Yasmin, YAZ

Therapeutic class: Contraceptives
Pharmacologic class: Estrogen–
progestin combinations
Pregnancy risk category: X

AVAILABLE FORMS
Tablets: 3 mg drospirenone and 0.03 mg
ethinyl estradiol as 21 yellow tablets and
7 white (inert) tablets (Yasmin); 3 mg
drospirenone and 0.02 mg ethinyl estradiol as 24 light pink active tablets and
4 white (inert) tablets (YAZ)

INDICATIONS & DOSAGES
➤ Contraception
Women: 1 yellow Yasmin tablet P.O. daily
for 21 days beginning on day 1 of menstrual
cycle or first Sunday after onset of menstruation. Then 1 white inert tablet P.O. daily
on days 22 through 28. Or 1 light pink YAZ
tablet P.O. daily for 24 days beginning on
day 1 of menstrual cycle or first Sunday
after onset of menstruation. Then 1 white
inert tablet P.O. daily on days 25 through 28.
Begin next and all subsequent 28-day regimens on same day of week that first regimen
began, following same schedule. Restart
yellow or light pink tablets on next day after
last white tablet.
➤ Premenstrual dysphoric disorder
Women: 1 light pink YAZ tablet P.O. daily
for 24 days beginning on day 1 of menstrual
cycle or first Sunday after menstruation
begins. Then 1 white inert tablet P.O. daily
on days 25 through 28. Begin next and all
subsequent 28-day regimens on same day
of week that first regimen began, following
same schedule. Restart light pink tablets on
next day after last white tablet.
➤ Acne
Women: Follow guidelines of use for timing
and initiation of dosing with YAZ. The
28-day dosing regimen consists of 1 active
tablet P.O. for 24 consecutive days followed
by 1 inert tablet P.O. daily for 4 days. After

28 tablets are taken, new course is started
next day.

ADMINISTRATION
P.O.
● Give pill at same time each day.

ACTION
Reduces chance of conception by inhibiting
ovulation, inhibiting sperm progression, and
reducing chance of implantation.

Route	Onset	Peak	Duration
P.O.	Unknown	1–3 hr	Unknown

Half-life: drospirenone, 30 hours; ethinyl estradiol,
24 hours.

ADVERSE REACTIONS
CNS: *cerebral hemorrhage, cerebral
thrombosis,* asthenia, depression, dizziness,
emotional lability, headache, migraine,
nervousness.
CV: *arterial thromboembolism, mesenteric
thrombosis, MI, pulmonary embolism,*
hypertension, thrombophlebitis, fluid retention, edema.
EENT: cataracts, steepening of corneal
curvature, intolerance to contact lenses,
pharyngitis, retinal thrombosis, sinusitis.
GI: abdominal pain, abdominal cramping,
bloating, changes in appetite, colitis, diarrhea, gastroenteritis, nausea, vomiting,
gallbladder disease.
GU: amenorrhea, breakthrough bleeding,
change in cervical erosion and secretion,
change in menstrual flow, cystitis, cystitis-
like syndrome, dysmenorrhea, impaired
renal function, leukorrhea, menstrual disorder, premenstrual syndrome, spotting,
temporary infertility after discontinuing
treatment, UTI, vaginal candidiasis,
vaginitis.
Hepatic: *Budd-Chiari syndrome, hepatic
adenomas,* cholestatic jaundice, benign
liver tumors.
Metabolic: reduced glucose tolerance,
porphyria, weight change, *hyperkalemia.*
Musculoskeletal: back pain.
Respiratory: bronchitis, upper respiratory
tract infection.
Skin: *erythema multiforme,* acne, erythema
nodosum, hemorrhagic eruption, hirsutism,
loss of scalp hair, melasma, pruritus, rash.

Other: changes in libido, breast tenderness, *hemolytic-uremic syndrome.*

INTERACTIONS
Drug-drug. *ACE inhibitors, aldosterone antagonists, angiotensin II receptor antagonists, NSAIDs, potassium-sparing diuretics:* May increase risk of hyperkalemia. Monitor potassium level.
Acetaminophen: May increase level of contraceptive and decrease effectiveness of acetaminophen. Monitor patient for adverse effects. Adjust acetaminophen dose as needed.
Antibiotics, griseofulvin, penicillins, tetracycline: May decrease contraceptive effect. Advise patient to use additional method of birth control while taking the antibiotic.
Ascorbic acid, atorvastatin: May increase level of contraceptive. Monitor patient for adverse effects.
Carbamazepine, modafinil, oxcarbazepine, phenobarbital, phenytoin, protease inhibitors: May increase metabolism of ethinyl estradiol and decrease contraceptive effectiveness. Advise patient to use another method of birth control.
Clofibrate, morphine, salicylic acid, temazepam: May decrease levels and increase clearance of these drugs. Monitor patient for effectiveness.
Cyclosporine, prednisolone, theophylline: May increase levels of these drugs. Monitor patient for adverse effects and toxicity.
Phenylbutazone, rifampin: May decrease contraceptive effectiveness and increase menstrual irregularities. Advise patient to use another method of birth control.
Troleandomycin: May increase risk of intrahepatic cholestasis and decrease contraceptive effect. Advise patient to use an alternative method of birth control.
Drug-herb. *St. John's wort:* May decrease contraceptive effectiveness and increase breakthrough bleeding. Discourage use together, or advise use of additional method of birth control.
Drug-lifestyle. *Smoking:* May increase risk of CV adverse effects. Advise patient to avoid smoking.

EFFECTS ON LAB TEST RESULTS
● May increase potassium, corticoid, prothrombin, thyroid-binding globulin, total circulating sex steroid, total thyroid hormone, triglyceride, amylase, GGT, transferrin, prolactin, renin activity, vitamin A, and factor VII, VIII, IX, and X levels, as well as iron-binding capacity. May decrease antithrombin III level, folate, albumin, zinc, and vitamin B_{12}.
● May increase norepinephrine-induced platelet aggregation. May decrease glucose tolerance and free T_3 resin uptake.

CONTRAINDICATIONS & CAUTIONS
● Contraindicated in women with hepatic dysfunction, tumor, or disease; renal or adrenal insufficiency; thrombophlebitis, thromboembolic disorders, or history of deep vein thrombosis or thromboembolic disorders; cerebrovascular or coronary artery disease; headaches with focal neurologic symptoms; known or suspected breast cancer, endometrial cancer, or other estrogen-dependent neoplasia; abnormal genital bleeding; or cholestatic jaundice of pregnancy or jaundice with other hormonal contraceptive use.
● Contraindicated in women who are or may be pregnant and in women age 65 or older.
● Use cautiously in patients with CV risk factors such as hypertension, hyperlipidemias, obesity, and diabetes.
● Use cautiously in patients with conditions aggravated by fluid retention.
⚠ *Overdose S&S:* Nausea, withdrawal uterine bleeding.

NURSING CONSIDERATIONS
⚠ *Alert:* The use of contraceptives causes increased risk of MI, thromboembolism, stroke, hepatic neoplasia, gallbladder disease, and hypertension. Risk increases in patients with hypertension, diabetes, hyperlipidemia, and obesity.
▐ Black Box Warning ▐ Smoking increases the risk of serious CV adverse effects. The risk increases with age (especially age older than 35 years) and in patients who smoke 15 or more cigarettes daily. ■
● The relationship between the use of hormonal contraceptives and breast and

cervical cancers is unclear. Encourage women to schedule a complete gynecologic examination at least yearly and to perform breast self-examinations monthly.

• In patients scheduled to have elective surgery that may increase the risk of thromboembolism, stop contraceptive use from at least 4 weeks before until 2 weeks after surgery. Also stop use during and after prolonged immobilization.

• Because of increased risk of thromboembolism in the postpartum period, don't start contraceptive earlier than 4 to 6 weeks after delivery.

• Stop use and evaluate patient if loss of vision, proptosis, diplopia, papilledema, or retinal vascular lesions occur. Recommend that contact lens wearers be evaluated by an ophthalmologist if visual changes or lens intolerance occurs.

• If patient misses two consecutive periods, she should obtain a negative pregnancy test result before continuing use of contraceptive.

• Immediately stop use if pregnancy is confirmed.

• Closely monitor patient with diabetes. Glucose intolerance may occur.

• Closely monitor patient with hypertension or a history of depression. Stop drug if these events occur.

• In patient at high risk for hyperkalemia and patient taking medications that may increase potassium, check potassium level during the first treatment cycle.

• Stop drug and evaluate patient if persistent, severe headaches occur or if migraines occur or are worsened.

• Evaluate patient for malignancy or pregnancy if she experiences breakthrough bleeding or spotting.

• Closely monitor patient with hyperlipidemias.

• Stop use if jaundice occurs.

• **Look alike–sound alike:** Don't confuse YAZ with Yasmin.

PATIENT TEACHING

• Advise patient to use additional method of birth control during the first 7 days of the first cycle of hormonal contraceptive.

• Inform patient that pills don't protect against sexually transmitted diseases such as HIV.

• Advise patient of the dangers of smoking while taking hormonal contraceptives. Suggest smokers choose a different form of birth control.

• Tell patient to schedule gynecologic examinations yearly and perform breast self-examination monthly.

• Inform patient that spotting, light bleeding, or stomach upset may occur during the first one to three packs of pills. Tell her to continue taking the pills and to notify her health care provider if these symptoms persist.

• Tell patient to take the pill at the same time each day.

• Tell patient to immediately report sharp chest pain, coughing of blood or sudden shortness of breath, calf pain, crushing chest pain or chest heaviness, sudden severe headache or vomiting, dizziness or fainting, visual or speech disturbances, weakness or numbness in an arm or leg, vision loss, breast lumps, severe stomach pain or tenderness, difficulty sleeping, lack of energy, fatigue, or change in mood; jaundice with fever, fatigue, loss of appetite, dark urine, or light-colored bowel movements.

• Tell patient to notify health care provider if she wears contact lenses and notices a change in vision or has trouble wearing the lenses.

• Tell patient that the risk of pregnancy increases with each active yellow or light pink tablet she forgets to take. Inform patient what to do if she misses pills.

• Tell patient to use an additional method of birth control and to notify health care provider if she isn't sure what to do about missed pills.

• Small amounts of hormonal contraceptives appear in breast milk. Quality and quantity of breast milk may be decreased. Yellow skin and eyes (jaundice) and breast enlargement may occur in breast-fed neonates. Advise breast-feeding women to use alternative method of birth control until infant is completely weaned.

duloxetine hydrochloride
do-LOCKS-ah-teen

Cymbalta◆

Therapeutic class: Antidepressants
Pharmacologic class: SSNRIs
Pregnancy risk category: C

AVAILABLE FORMS
Capsules (delayed-release): 20 mg, 30 mg,
60 mg

INDICATIONS & DOSAGES
Adjust-a-dose (for all indications): Duloxetine
isn't recommended for patients with ESRD,
severe renal dysfunction, or hepatic dysfunction. Consider a lower starting dose and
gradual dosage increase for those with renal
impairment.
➤ **Major depressive disorder**
Adults: Initially, 20 mg P.O. b.i.d.; then,
60 mg P.O. once daily or divided in two
equal doses. May also start at 30 mg/day
for 1 week to allow patients to adjust to
medication. Maximum, 60 mg daily.
➤ **Generalized anxiety disorder**
Adults: 60 mg P.O. daily. Or, 30 mg P.O.
daily for 1 week; then increase to 60 mg P.O.
daily. May increase in increments of 30 mg
daily to 120 mg P.O. once daily.
➤ **Fibromyalgia**
Adults: Initially, 30 mg P.O. once daily for
1 week; increase to 60 mg P.O. once daily
after a week. Some patients may respond
to the starting dose. Maximum dose is
60 mg/day. Base continued treatment on
individual patient response.
➤ **Neuropathic pain related to diabetic**
peripheral neuropathy
Adults: 60 mg P.O. once daily.
➤ **Chronic musculoskeletal pain**
Adults: Initially, 30 mg P.O. once daily for
1 week; then increase to 60 mg P.O. once
daily.
➤ **Stress urinary incontinence ◆**
Adults: 80 mg P.O. once daily or in two
divided doses (range, 20 to 120 mg) for
12 weeks.

ADMINISTRATION
P.O.
● Give drug whole; don't crush or open
capsule.

ACTION
May inhibit serotonin and norepinephrine
reuptake in the CNS.

Route	Onset	Peak	Duration
P.O.	Unknown	6 hr	Unknown

Half-life: 12 hours.

ADVERSE REACTIONS
CNS: dizziness, fatigue, headache, insomnia, somnolence, *suicidal thoughts,* fever,
hypoesthesia, irritability, lethargy, nervousness, nightmares, restlessness, sleep
disorder, anxiety, asthenia, tremor.
CV: hot flashes, hypertension, increased
heart rate.
EENT: blurred vision, nasopharyngitis,
pharyngolaryngeal pain.
GI: constipation, diarrhea, dry mouth,
nausea, dyspepsia, gastritis, vomiting.
GU: abnormal orgasm, abnormally increased frequency of urinating, delayed or
dysfunctional ejaculation, dysuria, erectile
dysfunction, urinary hesitation.
Metabolic: decreased appetite, *hypo-*
glycemia, increased appetite, weight gain or
loss, hyponatremia.
Musculoskeletal: muscle cramps, myalgia.
Respiratory: cough.
Skin: increased sweating, night sweats,
pruritus, rash.
Other: decreased libido, rigors.

INTERACTIONS
Drug-drug. *Anticoagulants (such as as-*
pirin, NSAIDs, warfarin): May increase
bleeding risk. Monitor patient closely.
Class IC antiarrhythmics (flecainide,
propafenone), phenothiazines: May increase levels of these drugs. Use together
cautiously.
CNS drugs: May increase adverse effects.
Use together cautiously.
CYP1A2 inhibitors (cimetidine, fluvox-
amine, certain quinolones): May increase
duloxetine level. Avoid using together.

Reactions in bold italics are *life-threatening*. Interactions may have a *rapid onset* or a *delayed onset*.

CYP2D6 inhibitors (fluoxetine, paroxetine, quinidine): May increase duloxetine level. Use together cautiously.

Drugs that reduce gastric acidity: May cause premature breakdown of duloxetine's protective coating and early release of the drug. Monitor patient for effects.

Linezolid, methylene blue: May cause serotonin syndrome. Use with extreme caution and monitor closely.

Lithium, SSNRIs, SSRIs, tramadol: May increase risk of serotonin syndrome. Avoid use together.

MAO inhibitors (phenelzine, rasagiline, selegiline): May cause hyperthermia, rigidity, myoclonus, autonomic instability, rapid fluctuations of vital signs, agitation, delirium, and coma. Avoid use within 2 weeks after MAO inhibitor therapy; wait at least 5 days after stopping duloxetine before starting MAO inhibitor.

TCAs (amitriptyline, imipramine, nortriptyline): May increase levels of these drugs. Reduce TCA dose, and monitor drug levels closely.

Thioridazine: May prolong the QT interval and increase risk of serious ventricular arrhythmias and sudden death. Avoid using together.

Triptans: May cause serotonin syndrome (restlessness, hallucinations, loss of coordination, fast heartbeat, rapid changes in blood pressure, increased body temperature, hyperreflexia, nausea, vomiting, and diarrhea) or neuroleptic malignant syndrome. Use cautiously and with increased monitoring, especially when starting or increasing dosages.

Drug-herb. *St. John's wort:* May increase sedative-hypnotic effects and risk of serotonin syndrome. Discourage use together.

Drug-lifestyle. *Alcohol use:* May increase risk of liver damage. Discourage use together.

EFFECTS ON LAB TEST RESULTS
• May increase alkaline phosphatase, ALT, AST, bilirubin, and CK levels.

CONTRAINDICATIONS & CAUTIONS
• Contraindicated in patients hypersensitive to drug or its ingredients, patients taking MAO inhibitors, patients with uncontrolled angle-closure glaucoma, and patients with a CrCl less than 30 mL/minute. Drug isn't recommended for patients with hepatic dysfunction or ESRD.

Black Box Warning Duloxetine isn't approved for use in children. ∎

⟁ Alert: Concomitant use with linezolid or methylene blue can cause serotonin syndrome (fever, mental status changes, muscle twitching, excessive sweating, shivering or shaking, diarrhea, loss of coordination). Use with linezolid or methylene blue only for life-threatening or urgent conditions when the potential benefits outweigh the risks of toxicity.

• Use cautiously in patients with a history of mania or seizures, patients who drink substantial amounts of alcohol, patients with hypertension, patients with controlled angle-closure glaucoma, and those with conditions that slow gastric emptying.

⚠ Overdose S&S: Coma, hypotension, hypertension, seizures, serotonin syndrome, somnolence, syncope, tachycardia, vomiting.

NURSING CONSIDERATIONS
Black Box Warning Drug may increase risk of suicidal thinking and behavior in children, adolescents, and young adults ages 18 to 24, especially during the first few months of treatment, especially in those with major depressive disorder or other psychiatric disorder. ∎

• Monitor patient for worsening of depression or suicidal behavior, especially when therapy starts or dosage changes.

⟁ Alert: If linezolid or methylene blue must be given, stop drug and monitor the patient for serotonin toxicity for 2 weeks, or until 24 hours after the last dose of methylene blue or linezolid, whichever comes first. Treatment may be resumed 24 hours after last dose of methylene blue or linezolid.

• Treatment of overdose is symptomatic. Don't induce emesis; gastric lavage or activated charcoal may be performed soon after ingestion or if patient is still symptomatic. Because drug undergoes extensive distribution, forced diuresis, dialysis, hemoperfusion, and exchange transfusion aren't useful. Contact a poison control center for information.

• If taken with TCAs, duloxetine metabolism will be prolonged, and patient will need extended monitoring.

• Periodically reassess patient to determine the need for continued therapy.

• Decrease dosage gradually, and watch for symptoms that may arise when drug is stopped, such as dizziness, nausea, headache, paresthesia, vomiting, irritability, and nightmares.

• If intolerable symptoms arise when decreasing or stopping drug, restart at previous dose and decrease even more gradually.

• Monitor blood pressure periodically during treatment.

• Use during the third trimester of pregnancy may cause neonatal complications, including respiratory distress, cyanosis, apnea, seizures, vomiting, hypoglycemia, and hyperreflexia, which may require prolonged hospitalization, respiratory support, and tube feeding. Consider potential benefit of drug to the mother versus risks to the fetus.

• Older patients may be more sensitive to drug effects than younger adults.

◑ *Alert:* Combining triptans with an SSRI or an SSNRI may cause serotonin syndrome or neuroleptic malignant syndrome–like reactions. Signs and symptoms of serotonin syndrome may include restlessness, hallucinations, loss of coordination, fast heartbeat, rapid changes in blood pressure, increased body temperature, overactive reflexes, nausea, vomiting, and diarrhea. Serotonin syndrome may be more likely to occur when starting or increasing the dose of triptan, SSRI, or SSNRI.

• *Look alike–sound alike:* Don't confuse duloxetine with fluoxetine or paroxetine. Don't confuse Cymbalta with Symbyax.

PATIENT TEACHING
Black Box Warning Warn families or caregivers to report signs of worsening depression (such as agitation, irritability, insomnia, hostility, impulsivity) and signs of suicidal behavior to prescriber immediately. ∎

◑ *Alert:* Teach patient to recognize and immediately report symptoms of serotonin toxicity (fever, mental status changes, muscle twitching, excessive sweating, shivering or shaking, diarrhea, loss of coordination).

• Tell patient to consult his prescriber or pharmacist if he plans to take other prescription or OTC drugs or an herbal or other dietary supplement.

• Instruct patient to swallow capsules whole and not to chew, crush, or open them because they have an enteric coating.

• Urge patient to avoid activities that are hazardous or require mental alertness until he knows how the drug affects him.

• Warn against drinking alcohol during therapy.

• If patient takes drug for depression, explain that it may take 1 to 4 weeks to notice an effect.

dutasteride
doo-TAS-teh-ride

Avodart✐

Therapeutic class: BPH drugs
Pharmacologic class: 5-alpha-reductase enzyme inhibitors
Pregnancy risk category: X

AVAILABLE FORMS
Capsules: 0.5 mg

INDICATIONS & DOSAGES
➤ **To treat and improve the symptoms of BPH, reduce the risk of acute urine retention, and reduce the need for BPH-related surgery**
Men: 0.5 mg P.O. once daily as monotherapy. May be given with tamsulosin 0.4 mg P.O. once daily as combination therapy.

ADMINISTRATION
P.O.
• Don't crush or break capsules.
• Give drug without regard for food.
◑ *Alert:* Drug is considered a teratogen. Follow safe-handling procedures when preparing, administering, or dispensing drug.

ACTION
Inhibits conversion of testosterone to dihydrotestosterone, the androgen primarily responsible for the initial development and

subsequent enlargement of the prostate gland.

Route	Onset	Peak	Duration
P.O.	Unknown	2–3 hr	Unknown

Half-life: About 5 weeks.

ADVERSE REACTIONS
GU: erectile dysfunction, decreased libido, ejaculation disorder.
Other: gynecomastia.

INTERACTIONS
Drug-drug. *CYP3A4 inhibitors (such as cimetidine, ciprofloxacin, diltiazem, ketoconazole, ritonavir, verapamil):* May increase dutasteride level. Use together cautiously.

EFFECTS ON LAB TEST RESULTS
• May lower prostate-specific antigen (PSA) level.

CONTRAINDICATIONS & CAUTIONS
• Contraindicated in women and children and in patients hypersensitive to dutasteride or its ingredients or to other 5-alpha-reductase inhibitors.
◑ Alert: 5-Alpha-reductase inhibitors may increase the risk of high-grade prostate cancer. Before start of therapy, patients should be evaluated to rule out other urologic conditions, including prostate cancer, that might mimic BPH. Any increase in PSA level in patient receiving dutasteride should be considered significant, and the patient should be evaluated for prostate cancer.
• Use cautiously in patients with hepatic disease and in those taking long-term potent CYP450 inhibitors.

NURSING CONSIDERATIONS
• Because drug may be absorbed through the skin, women who are or may become pregnant shouldn't handle the drug.
• If contact is made with leaking capsules, wash the contact area immediately with soap and water.
• Carefully monitor patients with a large residual urine volume or severely diminished urine flow, or both, for obstructive uropathy.
• Patients should wait at least 6 months after their last dose before donating blood.

• Establish a new baseline PSA level in men treated for 3 to 6 months and use it to assess potentially cancer-related changes in PSA level.
• To interpret PSA values in men treated for 6 months or more, double the PSA value for comparison with normal values in untreated men.
• Evaluate patients for prostate cancer prior to initiating therapy and periodically thereafter.

PATIENT TEACHING
• Tell patient to swallow the capsule whole.
• Inform patient that ejaculate volume may decrease but that sexual function should remain normal.
• Teach women who are pregnant or may become pregnant not to handle drug. A male fetus exposed to drug by the mother's swallowing or absorbing the drug through her skin may be born with abnormal sex organs.
◑ Alert: Tell patient not to donate blood for at least 6 months after final dose to prevent drug administration to a pregnant female transfusion recipient.
• Tell patient he'll need periodic blood tests to monitor therapeutic effects.

ecallantide
ee-KAL-lan-tide

Kalbitor

Therapeutic class: Protein inhibitors
Pharmacologic class: Human plasma kallikrein inhibitors
Pregnancy risk category: C

AVAILABLE FORMS
Injection: 10-mg/mL vials

INDICATIONS & DOSAGES
➤ **Acute attacks of hereditary angioedema**
Adults and adolescents age 16 and older: 30 mg subcutaneously given as three 10-mg injections; give additional 30-mg dose within 24 hours if attack persists.

ADMINISTRATION
Subcutaneous

Black Box Warning Drug should be administered only by health care provider with medical support available to treat anaphylaxis. ■

• Visually inspect each vial for particulate matter and discoloration before administration. If there is particulate matter or discoloration, don't use vial.

• Using aseptic technique, withdraw 1 mL (10 mg) of ecallantide from vial using large-bore needle. Then change needle on syringe to one suitable for subcutaneous injection (27G).

• Inject subcutaneously into skin of abdomen, thigh, or upper arm.

• Site for each injection may be in same or in different anatomic location (abdomen, thigh, or upper arm); there is no need for site rotation. Separate injection sites by at least 2 inches (5 cm) and avoid anatomic site of attack.

ACTION
Inhibits kallikrein within the inflammatory pathways, preventing excess bradykinin production.

Route	Onset	Peak	Duration
Subcut.	Unknown	2–3 hr	Unknown

Half-life: About 2 hours.

ADVERSE REACTIONS
CNS: fatigue, fever, headache.
EENT: nasopharyngitis.
GI: abdominal pain, diarrhea, nausea, vomiting.
Respiratory: upper respiratory tract infection.
Skin: injection-site reactions, pruritus, rash, urticaria.
Other: *anaphylaxis.*

INTERACTIONS
None reported.

EFFECTS ON LAB TEST RESULTS
None reported.

CONTRAINDICATIONS & CAUTIONS
Black Box Warning Contraindicated in patients hypersensitive to drug or its components. ■

Black Box Warning Anaphylaxis has occurred after administration (usually within first hour after dosing). Monitor patient closely. ■

• Use during pregnancy only if clearly needed.

• It isn't known if drug appears in breast milk. Use cautiously in breast-feeding women.

• Use cautiously in elderly patients because they may be at increased risk for adverse reactions.

NURSING CONSIDERATIONS
Black Box Warning Be aware that signs and symptoms of hypersensitivity reactions and acute hereditary angioedema may be very similar. Anaphylaxis has occurred after administration (usually within first hour after dosing). Monitor patient closely. ■

• Monitor patient closely for signs and symptoms of hypersensitivity reactions (including chest discomfort, flushing, pharyngeal edema, pruritus, rhinorrhea, sneezing, nasal congestion, throat irritation, urticaria, wheezing, and hypotension), especially within first hour after dosing.

PATIENT TEACHING
• Advise patient to immediately report wheezing, cough, chest tightness, trouble breathing, dizziness, fainting, throat tightness, itchiness, hives, and swelling of tongue or throat.

• Inform patient that drug must be given by health care provider in health care setting, in case serious allergic reaction occurs.

efavirenz
eff-ah-VYE-renz

Sustiva

Therapeutic class: Antiretrovirals
Pharmacologic class: NNRTIs
Pregnancy risk category: D

AVAILABLE FORMS
Capsules: 50 mg, 200 mg
Tablets: 600 mg

Reactions in bold italics are *life-threatening*. Interactions may have a *rapid onset* or a *delayed onset*.

INDICATIONS & DOSAGES
➤ **HIV-1 infection, with a protease inhibitor with or without nucleoside analogue reverse transcriptase inhibitors**
Adults and children age 3 months and older weighing 40 kg (88 lb) or more: 600 mg (three 200-mg capsules or one 600-mg tablet) P.O. once daily on an empty stomach, preferably at bedtime.
Children age 3 months and older weighing 32.5 to less than 40 kg (72 to less than 88 lb): 400 mg P.O. once daily on an empty stomach, preferably at bedtime.
Children age 3 months and older weighing 25 to less than 32.5 kg (55 to less than 72 lb): 350 mg P.O. once daily on an empty stomach, preferably at bedtime.
Children age 3 months and older weighing 20 to less than 25 kg (44 to less than 55 lb): 300 mg P.O. once daily on an empty stomach, preferably at bedtime.
Children age 3 months and older weighing 15 to less than 20 kg (33 to less than 44 lb): 250 mg P.O. once daily on an empty stomach, preferably at bedtime.
Children age 3 months and older weighing 7.5 to less than 15 kg (16.5 to less than 33 lb): 200 mg P.O. once daily on an empty stomach, preferably at bedtime.
Children age 3 months and older weighing 5 to less than 7.5 kg (11 to less than 16.5 lb): 150 mg P.O. once daily on an empty stomach, preferably at bedtime.
Children age 3 months and older weighing 3.5 to less than 5 kg (7.7 to less than 11 lb): 100 mg P.O. once daily on an empty stomach, preferably at bedtime.
Adjust-a-dose: For adults also taking voriconazole, increase voriconazole maintenance dose to 400 mg every 12 hours and decrease efavirenz capsules to 300 mg once daily. For adults and children weighing 50 kg (110 lb) or more who are also taking rifampin, recommended efavirenz dosage is 800 mg once daily.

ADMINISTRATION
P.O.
● Give drug at bedtime to decrease CNS adverse effects.
● Don't break tablets.
● Give on an empty stomach.

● For patients who can't swallow capsules or tablets, capsule contents may be given with a small amount (5 to 10 mL) of food. For patients who can tolerate solid foods, mix with soft food, such as applesauce, grape jelly, or yogurt.
● For young infants, dose can be gently mixed into 10 mL of reconstituted room-temperature infant formula in a medicine cup. Draw up dose mixture into a 10-mL dosing syringe to administer; then add an additional 10 mL to mixing cup and stir to disperse any remaining residue. Administer to infant.
● Give efavirenz food or formula mixture within 30 minutes of mixing. Patient shouldn't consume any additional food for 2 hours after administration.

ACTION
Inhibits the transcription of HIV-1 RNA to DNA, a critical step in the viral replication process, suppressing viral replication.

Route	Onset	Peak	Duration
P.O.	Unknown	3–5 hr	Unknown

Half-life: 40 to 76 hours.

ADVERSE REACTIONS
CNS: dizziness, abnormal dreams or thinking, agitation, amnesia, confusion, depersonalization, depression, euphoria, fever, fatigue, hallucinations, headache, hypoesthesia, impaired concentration, insomnia, nervousness, somnolence.
GI: diarrhea, nausea, abdominal pain, anorexia, dyspepsia, vomiting.
Skin: rash, *erythema multiforme, Stevens-Johnson syndrome, toxic epidermal necrolysis,* increased sweating, pruritus.

INTERACTIONS
Drug-drug. *Amprenavir, clarithromycin, indinavir, lopinavir:* May decrease levels of these drugs. Consider alternative therapy or dosage adjustment.
Atorvastatin, calcium channel blockers, itraconazole, pravastatin, rifampin, simvastatin: May decrease levels of these drugs. Dosage adjustments may be necessary.
Axitinib, bortezomib, bosutinib, cabazitaxel: May decrease pharmacologic effects of these drugs. Avoid concurrent use.

Bepridil, ergot derivatives, midazolam, pimozide, triazolam: May inhibit metabolism of these drugs and cause serious or life-threatening adverse events (such as arrhythmias, prolonged sedation, or respiratory depression). Avoid using together.

Bupropion: May decrease plasma concentrations and clinical effects of bupropion. Guide bupropion dosage by clinical response.

Drugs that induce the CYP450 enzyme system (such as phenobarbital, phenytoin, rifampin): May result in lower drug levels of efavirenz. Avoid using together.

Estrogens, ritonavir: May increase drug levels. Monitor patient.

Hormonal contraceptives: May increase ethinyl estradiol level. Advise use of a reliable method of barrier contraception in addition to use of hormonal contraceptives.

Nevirapine: May decrease clinical effectiveness and increase risk of adverse reactions. Avoid using together.

Psychoactive drugs: May cause additive CNS effects. Avoid using together.

Rifabutin: May decrease rifabutin level. Increase daily rifabutin dosage by 50%. Consider doubling rifabutin dosage when rifabutin is given two or three times per week.

Ritonavir: May increase levels of both drugs. Monitor patient and liver function closely.

Saquinavir: May decrease saquinavir level and efavirenz exposure to the body. Don't use with saquinavir as sole protease inhibitor.

Voriconazole (in standard doses): Decreases voriconazole levels significantly, while efavirenz levels significantly increase. Avoid using together unless doses of each are adjusted.

Warfarin: May increase or decrease level and effects of warfarin. Monitor INR.

Drug-herb. *St. John's wort:* May decrease response and lead to possible resistance to efavirenz or all drugs in the class. Don't use together.

Drug-food. *High-fat meals:* May increase absorption of drug. Instruct patient to maintain a proper low-fat diet.

Drug-lifestyle. *Alcohol use:* May enhance CNS effects. Discourage use together.

EFFECTS ON LAB TEST RESULTS
● May increase ALT, AST, and cholesterol levels.
● May cause false-positive urine cannabinoid test results.

CONTRAINDICATIONS & CAUTIONS
● Contraindicated in patients hypersensitive to drug or its components, in those with moderate or severe hepatic impairment, and in those taking bepridil, midazolam, pimozide, triazolam, ergot derivatives, or St. John's wort.
● Use cautiously in patients with mild hepatic impairment and in those receiving hepatotoxic drugs. Monitor LFTs in patients with history of hepatitis B or C and in those taking ritonavir.
⚠ **Overdose S&S:** Increased nervous system symptoms, involuntary muscle contractions.

NURSING CONSIDERATIONS
● Monitor cholesterol level.
⚠ **Alert:** Drug shouldn't be used as monotherapy or added on as a single drug to a regimen failing because of viral resistance.
● Using drug with ritonavir may increase liver enzyme levels and adverse effects (such as dizziness, nausea, paresthesia).
● Pregnancy must be ruled out before starting therapy in women of childbearing age.
● Children may be more prone to adverse reactions, especially diarrhea, nausea, vomiting, and rash.

PATIENT TEACHING
● Instruct patient to take drug with water, preferably at bedtime and on an empty stomach. Tell patient not to break tablets.
● Inform patient about need for scheduled blood tests to monitor liver function and cholesterol level.
● Tell patient to use a barrier contraceptive with a hormonal contraceptive and to notify prescriber immediately if pregnancy is suspected; drug is a known risk to the fetus.
● Inform patient that drug doesn't cure HIV infection, that opportunistic infections and other complications of HIV infection may continue to occur, and that transmission of HIV to others through sexual contact or blood contamination is still possible.

Reactions in bold italics are *life-threatening*. Interactions may have a *rapid onset* or a *delayed onset*.

E

- Instruct patient to take drug at the same time daily and always with other antiretrovirals.
- Tell patient to take drug exactly as prescribed and not to stop it without medical approval. Also instruct patient to report adverse reactions.
- Inform patient that rash is the most common adverse effect. Tell patient to report rash immediately because it may be serious in rare cases.
- Advise patient to report use of other drugs, including OTC drugs and herbal supplements.
- Advise patient that dizziness, difficulty sleeping or concentrating, drowsiness, or unusual dreams may occur during the first few days of therapy. Reassure him that these symptoms typically resolve after 2 to 4 weeks and may be less problematic if drug is taken at bedtime.
- Tell patient to avoid alcohol, driving, or operating machinery until the drug's effects are known.

eletriptan hydrobromide
ell-ah-TRIP-tan

Relpax◆

Therapeutic class: Antimigraine drugs
Pharmacologic class: Serotonin 5-HT₁ receptor agonists
Pregnancy risk category: C

AVAILABLE FORMS
Tablets: 20 mg, 40 mg

INDICATIONS & DOSAGES
➤ **Acute migraine with or without aura**
Adults: 20 to 40 mg P.O. at first migraine symptom. If headache recurs, dose may be repeated at least 2 hours later to a maximum of 80 mg daily.

ADMINISTRATION
P.O.
- Give drug without regard for food.
- Give drug whole; don't crush or break tablet.
- Give drug with a full glass of water.

ACTION
Binds to 5-HT₁ receptors and may constrict intracranial blood vessels and inhibit proinflammatory neuropeptide release.

Route	Onset	Peak	Duration
P.O.	½ hr	1½–2 hr	Unknown

Half-life: About 4 hours.

ADVERSE REACTIONS
CNS: asthenia, dizziness, headache, hypertonia, hypesthesia, pain, paresthesia, somnolence, vertigo.
CV: chest tightness, pain, and pressure; flushing, palpitations.
EENT: pharyngitis.
GI: abdominal pain, discomfort, or cramps; dry mouth, dyspepsia, dysphagia, nausea.
Musculoskeletal: back pain.
Skin: increased sweating.
Other: chills.

INTERACTIONS
Drug-drug. *CYP3A4 inhibitors (such as clarithromycin, itraconazole, ketoconazole, nefazodone, nelfinavir, ritonavir, troleandomycin):* May decrease eletriptan metabolism. Avoid use within 72 hours of these drugs.
Ergotamine-containing or ergot-type drugs (such as dihydroergotamine or methysergide), other triptans: May prolong vasospastic reactions. Avoid use within 24 hours of these drugs.
SSRIs: May increase the risk of serotonin syndrome (weakness, hyperreflexia, and incoordination). If used together, observe patient closely.

EFFECTS ON LAB TEST RESULTS
None known.

CONTRAINDICATIONS & CAUTIONS
- Contraindicated in patients hypersensitive to drug or its components and in those with severe hepatic impairment; ischemic heart disease, such as angina pectoris, a history of MI, or silent ischemia; coronary artery vasospasm, including Prinzmetal variant angina; and other significant CV conditions.
- Contraindicated in patients with cerebrovascular syndromes, such as stroke or transient ischemic attack; peripheral

vascular disease, including ischemic bowel disease; uncontrolled hypertension; or hemiplegic or basilar migraine.
- Contraindicated within 24 hours of another 5-HT$_1$ agonist, drugs containing ergotamine, or ergot-type drug.
- Contraindicated in patients with risk factors for coronary artery disease (CAD), such as hypertension, hypercholesterolemia, smoking, obesity, diabetes, strong family history of CAD, postmenopausal women, or men older than age 40, unless patient is free from cardiac disease. Monitor patient closely after first dose.
- Safety of treating more than three migraine headaches in 30 days hasn't been established.

⚠ **Overdose S&S:** Hypertension, more serious CV reactions.

NURSING CONSIDERATIONS
- Drug isn't intended for migraine prevention.
- ☻ **Alert:** Combining a triptan with an SSRI or an SSNRI may cause serotonin syndrome. Signs and symptoms may include restlessness, hallucinations, loss of coordination, fast heartbeat, rapid changes in blood pressure, increased body temperature, hyperreflexia, nausea, vomiting, and diarrhea. Serotonin syndrome may be more likely to occur when starting or increasing the dose of a triptan, SSRI, or SSNRI.
- Use drug only when patient has a clear diagnosis of migraine. If the first use produces no response, reconsider the migraine diagnosis.
- ☻ **Alert:** Serious cardiac events, including acute MI, arrhythmias, and death, occur rarely within a few hours after use of 5-HT$_1$ agonists.
- Ophthalmologic effects may occur with long-term use.
- Older patients may develop higher blood pressure than younger patients after taking drug.

PATIENT TEACHING
- Instruct patient to take dose at the first sign of a migraine headache. If the headache comes back after the first dose, he may take a second dose after 2 hours. Caution patient not to take more than 80 mg in 24 hours.

- Warn patient to avoid driving and operating machinery if he feels dizzy or fatigued after taking the drug.
- Tell patient to immediately report pain, tightness, heaviness, or pressure in the chest, throat, neck, or jaw.
- Tell patient to swallow tablet whole and not to split, crush, or chew.
- Instruct patient to take each dose with a full glass of water.

elvitegravir–cobicistat–emtricitabine–tenofovir disoproxil fumarate
el-vye-TEG-gra-veer–koe-BIK-i-stat–em-tra-SYE-tah-ben–te-NOE-fo-veer

Stribild

Therapeutic class: Antiretrovirals
Pharmacologic class: Antivirals–cytochrome P450 inhibitors–nucleoside and nucleotide reverse transcriptase inhibitors
Pregnancy risk category: B

AVAILABLE FORMS
Tablets: 150 mg elvitegravir, 150 mg cobicistat, 200 mg emtricitabine, and 300 mg tenofovir disoproxil fumarate

INDICATIONS & DOSAGES
➤ **HIV-1 infection in treatment-naive patients**
Adults: 1 tablet P.O. once daily.
Adjust-a-dose: Discontinue drug in patients with estimated CrCl of less than 50 ml/minute.

ADMINISTRATION
P.O.
- Give with food.
- Drug is used as a complete treatment; don't give with other antiretrovirals.

ACTION
Combination of agents with differing mechanisms of action (integrase strand transfer inhibition, pharmacokinetic enhancement, nucleoside and nucleotide analogue HIV-1 reverse transcriptase inhibition) working

together via differing mechanisms to inhibit HIV replication.

Route	Onset	Peak	Duration
P.O. (elvitegravir)	Unknown	4 hr	Unknown
P.O. (cobicistat, emtricitabine)	Unknown	3 hr	Unknown
P.O. (tenofovir)	Unknown	2 hr	Unknown

Half-life: Elvitegravir, 13 hours; cobicistat, 3½ hours; emtricitabine and tenofovir, unknown.

ADVERSE REACTIONS

CNS: headache, dizziness, insomnia, abnormal dreams, fatigue, somnolence.
GI: diarrhea, nausea, flatulence.
GU: proteinuria, hematuria.
Skin: rash.

INTERACTIONS

Drug-drug. *Acyclovir, cidofovir, ganciclovir, valacyclovir, valganciclovir:* May increase concentrations of these drugs, emtricitabine, and tenofovir due to competition for renal excretion. Use together carefully.

Additional antiretrovirals: May increase risk of drug interactions and altered pharmacokinetics of drug components. Use together is contraindicated.

Alfuzosin: May increase alfuzosin level and risk of severe hypotension. Use together is contraindicated.

Antacids: May decrease elvitegravir concentration. Separate administration times by 2 hours.

Antiarrhythmics, digoxin: May increase levels of these drugs. Use together cautiously and monitor drug levels if possible.

Antidepressants (SSRIs, TCAs, trazodone): May increase levels of these drugs. Use together cautiously and titrate antidepressant according to response.

Antifungals (itraconazole, ketoconazole, voriconazole): May increase levels of these drugs, elvitegravir, and cobicistat. Use together cautiously. Don't exceed 200 mg/day of ketoconazole or itraconazole.

Beta blockers (metoprolol, timolol): May increase beta blocker concentration. Monitor patient carefully and decrease beta blocker dosage as necessary.

Bosentan: May increase bosentan level. Give bosentan dose based on manufacturer's instructions and adjust according to patient tolerance.

Calcium channel blockers (amlodipine, diltiazem, felodipine, nicardipine, nifedipine, verapamil): May increase level of calcium channel blocker. Use together cautiously and monitor patient closely.

Carbamazepine, oxcarbazepine, phenobarbital, phenytoin: May significantly decrease elvitegravir and cobicistat levels; may increase carbamazepine level. Use together isn't recommended. Consider alternative anticonvulsants.

Clarithromycin, telithromycin: May increase level of clarithromycin, telithromycin, and cobicistat. Use together cautiously. Decrease clarithromycin dosage by 50% if CrCl is between 50 and 60 mL/minute.

Clonazepam, ethosuximide: May increase levels of these drugs. Use together cautiously.

Colchicine: May increase colchicine concentration. Adjust dosage according to manufacturer's instructions. Use together is contraindicated in patients with renal or hepatic impairment.

CYP2D6, CYP3 A, P-glycoprotein substrates: May alter plasma concentrations of the four drug components (elvitegravir, cobicistat, emtricitabine, or tenofovir). Use together cautiously.

Dexamethasone: May significantly decrease cobicistat and elvitegravir levels. Monitor patient carefully for loss of therapeutic effect (elvitegravir, cobicistat) and development of resistance.

Ergot derivatives (dihydroergotamine, ergotamine): May increase levels of these drugs. Use together is contraindicated.

Fluticasone: May increase fluticasone level. Choose an alternative corticosteroid.

HMG-CoA reductase inhibitors (atorvastatin, lovastatin, simvastatin): May increase statin drug level and risk of myopathy. Start statin at lowest dosage and titrate carefully.

Hormonal contraceptives: May alter levels of these drugs. Consider nonhormonal forms of birth control.

Immunosuppressants (cyclosporine, sirolimus, tacrolimus): May increase immunosuppressant level. Use together cautiously.

Midazolam: May increase midazolam level. Use with oral midazolam is contraindicated. Use parenteral form cautiously and monitor patient closely.

Neuroleptics (perphenazine, risperidone, thioridazine): May increase neuroleptic level. Decrease neuroleptic dosage as needed.

PDE5 inhibitors (sildenafil, tadalafil, vardenafil): May increase effects of PDE5 inhibitors. Adjust dosage according to manufacturer's instructions. Use with sildenafil for pulmonary arterial hypertension is contraindicated.

Pimozide: May increase risk of cardiac adverse effects. Use together is contraindicated.

Rifabutin, rifapentine: May decrease cobicistat and elvitegravir levels. Avoid use together.

Rifampin: May increase elvitegravir and cobicistat concentrations. Use together is contraindicated.

Salmeterol: May increase risk of CV effects of salmeterol, including QT-interval prolongation, palpitations, and tachycardia. Avoid use together.

Sedative/hypnotics (buspirone, clorazepate, diazepam, estazolam, flurazepam, triazolam, zolpidem): May increase concentrations of sedative/hypnotics. Use cautiously together and monitor patient carefully.

Warfarin: May increase warfarin concentration. Monitor INR carefully.

Drug-herb. *St. John's wort:* May reduce concentrations of drug components and decrease therapeutic effect. Discourage use together.

EFFECTS ON LAB TEST RESULTS
- May increase AST, amylase, CK, total cholesterol, HDL, LDL, and triglyceride levels.
- May increase urine RBC count.

CONTRAINDICATIONS & CAUTIONS
- Contraindicated in patients hypersensitive to drugs or their components and in those with CrCl of less than 70 mL/minute or severe hepatic impairment (Child-Pugh class C).
- Contraindicated in breast-feeding women because of risk of HIV transmission and

potential for serious adverse effects in infant.
- Use cautiously in new-onset or worsening renal impairment and in Fanconi syndrome.
- Use cautiously in patients with a history of pathologic fracture or other risk factors for osteoporosis or bone loss.

Black Box Warning Drug isn't approved for the treatment of chronic hepatitis B virus (HBV) infection; safety and efficacy of drug haven't been established in patients coinfected with HBV and HIV-1. Severe acute exacerbations of hepatitis B have been reported in patients who are coinfected with HBV and HIV-1 and have discontinued emtricitabine (Emtriva) or tenofovir (Viread), which are components of this drug. Monitor hepatic function closely with both clinical and laboratory follow-up for at least several months in patients who are coinfected with HIV-1 and HBV and discontinue this drug. If appropriate, initiation of anti–hepatitis B therapy may be warranted. ■
- Use in pregnancy only if benefit outweighs risk to fetus. Register pregnant patients in the Antiretroviral Pregnancy Registry at 800-258-4263.

NURSING CONSIDERATIONS
Black Box Warning Lactic acidosis and severe hepatomegaly with steatosis, including fatal cases, have been reported with the use of nucleoside analogues, including tenofovir disoproxil fumarate, a component of Stribild, in combination with other antiretrovirals. ■
- Suspend treatment in patients who develop signs and symptoms suggestive of lactic acidosis or pronounced hepatotoxicity (including nausea, vomiting, unusual or unexpected stomach discomfort, and weakness).
- Test for HBV before starting therapy; severe acute exacerbations of hepatitis B have been reported in patients coinfected with HBV and HIV-1.
- Avoid concurrent or recent use of a nephrotoxic agent because renal impairment is possible.
- Assess CrCl, urine glucose, and urine protein before initiating and periodically during treatment.

• Monitor serum phosphorus level in patients at risk for renal impairment.
• Closely monitor patients with a confirmed increase in serum creatinine of greater than 0.4 mg/dL from baseline for renal safety.
• Consider assessing bone mineral density (BMD) in patients with a history of pathologic bone fracture or other risk factors for osteoporosis or bone loss because of risk of drug-related decreased BMD.
• Redistribution or accumulation of body fat may occur in patients receiving antiretrovirals. The cause and long-term health effects of these conditions aren't known.
• Monitor patients for infection and development of immune reconstitution syndrome (inflammatory response to indolent or residual opportunistic infections, such as *Mycobacterium avium* infection, cytomegalovirus, *Pneumocystis jiroveci* pneumonia, or tuberculosis), which may necessitate further evaluation and treatment.
• Autoimmune disorders (such as Graves disease, polymyositis, and Guillain-Barré syndrome) have also been reported in the setting of immune reconstitution; however, the time to onset is more variable, and the disorder can occur many months after initiation of treatment.

PATIENT TEACHING
• Caution patient to remain under the care of a health care provider and comply with routine monitoring to decrease risk of adverse events.
• Inform patient that this drug isn't a cure for HIV-1 infection; patient must stay on continuous HIV therapy to control HIV-1 infection and decrease HIV-related illnesses.
• Instruct patient to avoid behaviors that can spread HIV-1 infection to others (such as sharing needles or other injection equipment; sharing personal items that may have blood or body fluids on them, such as toothbrushes and razor blades; or having sex without the protection of a latex or polyurethane condom).
• Warn female patient not to breast-feed because HIV-1 can be passed to the infant in breast milk.
• Teach patient to take drug on a regular dosing schedule with food and not to miss doses.

• Advise patient to immediately report nausea, vomiting, unusual or unexpected stomach discomfort, and weakness.
• Instruct patient not to change dose or stop drug without first consulting health care provider.
• Inform patient that redistribution or accumulation of body fat may occur.
• Caution patient to report signs and symptoms of infection.
• Teach patient to report yellowing of skin or sclera, dark urine, light-colored stools, loss of appetite, or nausea.

emtricitabine
em-tra-SYE-tah-ben

Emtriva

Therapeutic class: Antiretrovirals
Pharmacologic class: Nucleotide–nucleotide reverse transcriptase inhibitors
Pregnancy risk category: B

AVAILABLE FORMS
Capsules: 200 mg
Oral solution: 10 mg/mL

INDICATIONS & DOSAGES
➤ HIV-1 infection, with other antiretrovirals
Adults: One 200-mg capsule or 240 mg (24 mL) oral solution P.O. once daily.
Children ages 3 months to 17 years: For children weighing more than 33 kg (73 lb) who can swallow intact capsules, give one 200-mg capsule P.O. once daily. Otherwise, give 6 mg/kg, up to a maximum dose of 240 mg (24 mL) oral solution once daily.
Children younger than age 3 months: 3 mg/kg oral solution P.O. once daily.
Adjust-a-dose: In adults with CrCl of 30 to 49 mL/minute, give one 200-mg capsule every 48 hours or 120 mg oral solution every 24 hours; if CrCl is 15 to 29 mL/minute, give one 200-mg capsule every 72 hours or 80 mg oral solution every 24 hours; if CrCl is less than 15 mL/minute or patient is receiving dialysis, give one 200-mg capsule every 96 hours or 60 mg oral solution every 24 hours. Give dose after dialysis session. In children with renal

insufficiency, consider a dose reduction or increased dosing interval.

Black Box Warning Emtricitabine isn't indicated for the treatment of chronic hepatitis B virus (HBV) infection; safety and effectiveness of drug haven't been established in patients coinfected with HBV and HIV. ∎

ADMINISTRATION
P.O.
● Give drug with or without food.
● Refrigerate oral solution; if stored at room temperature, use within 3 months.

ACTION
Inhibits replication of HIV by blocking viral DNA synthesis and inhibits reverse transcriptase by acting as an alternative for the enzyme's substrate, deoxycytidine triphosphate.

Route	Onset	Peak	Duration
P.O.	Unknown	1–2 hr	Unknown

Half-life: About 10 hours.

ADVERSE REACTIONS
CNS: abnormal dreams, asthenia, dizziness, headache, insomnia, depression, fatigue, neuritis, paresthesia, peripheral neuropathy.
EENT: rhinitis.
GI: abdominal pain, diarrhea, nausea, dyspepsia, vomiting.
Hepatic: *hepatotoxicity.*
Musculoskeletal: arthralgia, myalgia.
Respiratory: increased cough.
Skin: allergic skin reaction, discoloration, maculopapular rash, pruritus, urticarial and purpuric lesions, vesiculobullous rash.

INTERACTIONS
None reported.

EFFECTS ON LAB TEST RESULTS
● May increase ALT, amylase, AST, bilirubin, CK, lipase, glucose, and triglyceride levels.
● May decrease neutrophil count.

CONTRAINDICATIONS & CAUTIONS
● Contraindicated in patients hypersensitive to drug or its ingredients.

● In elderly patients, use cautiously because of the potential for other diseases and drug therapies and for decreased hepatic, renal, or cardiac function.
● Use cautiously in patients with impaired renal function.

Black Box Warning Lactic acidosis and severe hepatomegaly, including fatal cases, have been reported. ∎

NURSING CONSIDERATIONS
● Test all patients for HBV before starting drug.

Black Box Warning Hepatitis B may worsen after emtricitabine therapy stops. Patients with both HIV and HBV need close clinical and laboratory follow-up for several months or longer after stopping drug. ∎
● Like other antiretrovirals, emtricitabine may cause changes or increases in body fat, including central obesity, buffalo hump, peripheral wasting, facial wasting, breast enlargement, and a cushingoid appearance.
● Use drug only if clearly needed in pregnant women.

PATIENT TEACHING
● Remind patient that anti-HIV medicine must be taken for life.
● Inform patient that drug doesn't cure HIV infection, that opportunistic infections and other complications of HIV infection may continue to occur, and that transmission of HIV to others through sexual contact or blood contamination is still possible.
● Explain possible adverse reactions, including lactic acidosis, hepatotoxicity, and changes or increases in body fat.
● Tell woman to notify prescriber immediately if she is or could be pregnant.
● Inform patient the drug may be taken with or without food.
● Tell patient to refrigerate oral solution but if stored at room temperature, to use within 3 months.

---

enalaprilat
eh-NAH-leh-prel-at

enalapril maleate
Vasotec*⬦*

Therapeutic class: Antihypertensives
Pharmacologic class: ACE inhibitors
Pregnancy risk category: C; D in 2nd and
3rd trimesters

AVAILABLE FORMS
enalaprilat
Injection: 1.25 mg/mL
enalapril maleate
Tablets: 2.5 mg, 5 mg, 10 mg, 20 mg

INDICATIONS & DOSAGES
➤ **Hypertension**
Adults: In patients not taking diuretics,
initially, 5 mg P.O. once daily; then adjusted
based on response. Usual dosage range is
10 to 40 mg daily as a single dose or two
divided doses. Or, 1.25 mg I.V. infusion over
5 minutes every 6 hours.
Children ages 1 month to 16 years:
0.08 mg/kg (up to 5 mg) P.O. once daily;
dosage should be adjusted as needed up to
0.58 mg/kg (maximum 40 mg). Don't use if
CrCl is less than 30 mL/minute.
Adjust-a-dose: If patient is taking diuretics
or CrCl is 30 mL/minute or less, initially,
2.5 mg P.O. once daily. Or, 0.625 mg I.V.
over 5 minutes, and repeat in 1 hour, if
needed; then 1.25 mg I.V. every 6 hours.
➤ **To convert from I.V. therapy to oral
therapy in patients receiving diuretics**
Adults: Initially, 2.5 mg P.O. once daily; if
patient was receiving 0.625 mg I.V. every
6 hours, then 2.5 mg P.O. once daily. Adjust
dosage based on response.
➤ **To convert from oral therapy to I.V.
therapy**
Adults: 1.25 mg I.V. over 5 minutes every
6 hours.
➤ **To convert from I.V. therapy to oral
therapy**
Adults: 5 mg P.O. once daily.
Adjust-a-dose: For patients with CrCl of
30 mL/minute or less, give 2.5 mg P.O. once
daily.

➤ **To manage symptomatic heart failure**
Adults: Initially, 2.5 mg P.O. daily or b.i.d.,
increased gradually over several weeks.
Maintenance is 5 to 20 mg daily in two
divided doses. Maximum daily dose is
40 mg in two divided doses.
➤ **Asymptomatic left ventricular
dysfunction**
Adults: Initially, 2.5 mg P.O. b.i.d. Increase
as tolerated to target daily dose of 20 mg
P.O. in divided doses.

ADMINISTRATION
P.O.
● Give drug without regard for food.
● Request oral suspension for patient who
has difficulty swallowing.
I.V.
▼ Visually inspect solution for particulate
matter and discoloration before administration.
▼ Compatible solutions include D_5W,
normal saline solution for injection,
dextrose 5% in lactated Ringer injection,
dextrose 5% in normal saline solution for
injection, and Isolyte E.
▼ Inject drug slowly over at least 5 minutes, or dilute in 50 mL of a compatible
solution and infuse over 15 minutes.
▼ **Incompatibilities:** Amphotericin B,
cefepime hydrochloride, phenytoin sodium.

ACTION
May inhibit ACE, preventing conversion of
angiotensin I to angiotensin II, a potent
vasoconstrictor. Less angiotensin II
decreases peripheral arterial resistance,
decreasing aldosterone secretion, reducing
sodium and water retention, and lowering
blood pressure.

Route	Onset	Peak	Duration
P.O.	1 hr	4–6 hr	24 hr
I.V.	15 min	1–4 hr	6 hr

Half-life: 11 hours.

ADVERSE REACTIONS
CNS: asthenia, headache, dizziness,
fatigue, vertigo, syncope.
CV: hypotension, chest pain, angina
pectoris.
GI: diarrhea, nausea, abdominal pain,
vomiting.

GU: decreased renal function (in patients with bilateral renal artery stenosis or heart failure).
Hematologic: bone marrow depression.
Respiratory: dry, persistent, tickling, nonproductive cough; dyspnea.
Skin: rash.
Other: *angioedema.*

INTERACTIONS

Drug-drug. *Aldosterone blockers (eplerenone), aliskiren, angiotensin II receptor antagonists (candesartan, telmisartan), trimethoprim:* May increase risk of hyperkalemia. Monitor potassium level and clinical response.
Azathioprine: May increase risk of anemia or leukopenia. Monitor hematologic study results if used together.
Diuretics: May excessively reduce blood pressure. Use together cautiously.
Insulin, oral antidiabetics: May cause hypoglycemia, especially at start of enalapril therapy. Monitor patient closely.
Lithium: May cause lithium toxicity. Monitor lithium level.
NSAIDs: May reduce antihypertensive effect. Monitor blood pressure.
Potassium-sparing diuretics, potassium supplements: May cause hyperkalemia. Avoid using together unless hypokalemia is confirmed.
Drug-herb. *Capsaicin:* May cause cough. Discourage use together.
Ma huang: May decrease antihypertensive effects. Discourage use together.
Drug-food. *Salt substitutes containing potassium:* May cause hyperkalemia. Monitor patient closely.

EFFECTS ON LAB TEST RESULTS

● May increase bilirubin, BUN, creatinine, and potassium levels. May decrease sodium and hemoglobin levels and hematocrit.
● May increase LFT values.

CONTRAINDICATIONS & CAUTIONS

● Contraindicated in patients hypersensitive to drug and in those with a history of angioedema related to previous treatment with an ACE inhibitor.
Black Box Warning Use during pregnancy can cause injury and death to the developing fetus. When pregnancy is detected, stop drug as soon as possible. ■
● Use cautiously in renally impaired patients or those with aortic stenosis or hypertrophic cardiomyopathy.
⚠ Overdose S&S: Hypotension.

NURSING CONSIDERATIONS

● Closely monitor blood pressure response to drug.
● Monitor CBC with differential counts before and during therapy.
● Diabetic patients, those with impaired renal function or heart failure, and those receiving drugs that can increase potassium level may develop hyperkalemia. Monitor potassium intake and potassium level.
● Black patients who take ACE inhibitors as monotherapy for hypertension have a smaller reduction in blood pressure than non-Black patients. Black patients taking ACE inhibitors have a higher incidence of angioedema than non-Blacks.
● **Look alike–sound alike:** Don't confuse enalapril with Anafranil or Eldepryl.
● **Look alike–sound alike:** Similar packaging and labeling of enalaprilat injection and pancuronium, a neuromuscular-blocking drug, could result in a fatal medication error. Check all labels carefully.

PATIENT TEACHING

● Instruct patient to report breathing difficulty or swelling of face, eyes, lips, or tongue. Swelling of the face and throat (including swelling of the larynx) may occur, especially after first dose.
● Advise patient to report signs of infection, such as fever and sore throat.
● Inform patient that light-headedness can occur, especially during first few days of therapy. Tell him to rise slowly to minimize this effect and to notify prescriber if symptoms develop. If he faints, he should stop taking drug and call prescriber immediately.
● Tell patient to use caution in hot weather and during exercise. Inadequate fluid intake, vomiting, diarrhea, and excessive perspiration can lead to light-headedness and fainting.
● Advise patient to avoid salt substitutes; these products may contain potassium,

---

Reactions in bold italics are *life-threatening*. Interactions may have a *rapid onset* or a *delayed onset*.

which can cause high potassium levels in patients taking this drug.

• Tell women of childbearing age to notify prescriber if pregnancy occurs. Drug will need to be stopped.

enfuvirtide
en-foo-VEER-tide

Fuzeon

Therapeutic class: Antiretrovirals
Pharmacologic class: Fusion inhibitors
Pregnancy risk category: B

AVAILABLE FORMS
Powder for injection: 108-mg single-use vials (90 mg/mL after reconstitution)

INDICATIONS & DOSAGES
➤ **To help control HIV-1 infection, with other antiretrovirals, in patients who have continued HIV-1 replication despite antiretroviral therapy**
Adults: 90 mg subcutaneously b.i.d., injected into the upper arm, anterior thigh, or abdomen.
Children ages 6 to 16: 2 mg/kg subcutaneously b.i.d.; maximum 90 mg per dose.

ADMINISTRATION
Subcutaneous
• Reconstitute vial with 1.1 mL sterile water for injection. Tap vial for 10 seconds and then gently roll to prevent foaming. Let drug stand for up to 45 minutes to ensure reconstitution. Or, gently roll vial between hands until product is completely dissolved. Then draw up correct dose and inject drug.
• If you won't be using drug immediately after reconstitution, refrigerate in original vial and use within 24 hours. Don't inject drug until it's at room temperature.
• Vial is for single use; discard unused portion.
• Rotate injection sites. Don't inject into the same site for two consecutive doses, and don't inject into moles, scar tissue, bruises, or the navel, where large nerves course close to the skin.

• Store unreconstituted vials at room temperature.

ACTION
Interferes with entry of HIV-1 into cells by inhibiting fusion of HIV-1 to cell membranes.

Route	Onset	Peak	Duration
Subcut.	Unknown	4–8 hr	Unknown

Half-life: 4 hours.

ADVERSE REACTIONS
CNS: fatigue, insomnia, anxiety, asthenia, depression, peripheral neuropathy.
EENT: conjunctivitis, sinusitis, taste disturbance.
GI: diarrhea, nausea, *pancreatitis,* abdominal pain, constipation, dry mouth.
Metabolic: anorexia, weight decrease.
Musculoskeletal: myalgia.
Respiratory: *bacterial pneumonia,* cough.
Skin: injection-site reactions, pruritus, skin papilloma.
Other: herpes simplex, influenza, influenza-like illness, lymphadenopathy.

INTERACTIONS
None reported.

EFFECTS ON LAB TEST RESULTS
• May increase ALT, amylase, AST, CK, GGT, lipase, and triglyceride levels. May decrease hemoglobin level.
• May decrease eosinophil count.

CONTRAINDICATIONS & CAUTIONS
• Contraindicated in patients hypersensitive to drug and in those not infected with HIV.
• Use in pregnant women only if clearly needed. Pregnant women can be registered in the Antiretroviral Pregnancy Registry by calling 1-800-258-4263.
• Safety and effectiveness haven't been established in children younger than age 6.

NURSING CONSIDERATIONS
• Injection-site reactions (pain, discomfort, induration, erythema, pruritus, nodules, cysts, ecchymosis) are common and may require analgesics or rest.
🟢 *Alert:* Monitor patient closely for evidence of bacterial pneumonia. Patients at

E

high risk include those with a low initial CD4 count or high initial viral load, those who use I.V. drugs or smoke, and those with history of lung disease.

• Hypersensitivity may occur with the first dose or later doses. If symptoms occur, stop drug.

PATIENT TEACHING

• Teach patient how to prepare and give drug and how to safely dispose of used needles and syringes.

• Tell patient to rotate injection sites and to watch for cellulitis or local infection.

• Urge patient to immediately report evidence of pneumonia, such as cough with fever, rapid breathing, or shortness of breath.

• Tell patient to stop taking drug and seek medical attention if evidence of hypersensitivity develops, such as rash, fever, nausea, vomiting, chills, rigors, and hypotension.

• Teach patient that drug doesn't cure HIV infection and that it must be taken with other antiretrovirals.

• Tell patient to inform prescriber if she's pregnant, plans to become pregnant, or is breast-feeding while taking this drug. Because HIV could be transmitted to the infant, HIV-infected mothers shouldn't breast-feed.

• Tell patient that drug may affect his ability to drive or operate machinery.

• Tell patient that information on self-administration is available by calling 1-877-4FUZEON or at www.fuzeon.com.

SAFETY ALERT!

enoxaparin sodium
en-OCKS-a-par-in

Lovenox

Therapeutic class: Anticoagulants
Pharmacologic class: Low–molecular-weight heparins
Pregnancy risk category: B

AVAILABLE FORMS
Syringes (graduated prefilled): 60 mg/0.6 mL, 80 mg/0.8 mL, 100 mg/mL, 120 mg/0.8 mL, 150 mg/mL

Syringes (prefilled): 30 mg/0.3 mL, 40 mg/0.4 mL
Vial * *(multidose):* 300 mg/3 mL (contains 15 mg/mL of benzyl alcohol)

INDICATIONS & DOSAGES
➤ **To prevent PE and DVT after hip or knee replacement surgery**
Adults: 30 mg subcutaneously every 12 hours for 7 to 10 days. Treatment for up to 14 days has been well tolerated. Give initial dose between 12 and 24 hours postoperatively, as long as hemostasis has been established. Continue treatment during postoperative period until risk of DVT has diminished. Hip replacement patients may receive 40 mg subcutaneously given 12 hours preoperatively. After initial phase of therapy, hip replacement patients should continue with 40 mg subcutaneously daily for 3 weeks.
Adjust-a-dose: In patients with CrCl of less than 30 mL/minute, give 30 mg subcutaneously once daily.
➤ **To prevent PE and DVT after abdominal surgery**
Adults: 40 mg subcutaneously daily with initial dose 2 hours before surgery. Give subsequent dose, as long as hemostasis has been established, 24 hours after initial preoperative dose and continue once daily for 7 to 10 days. Treatment for up to 12 days has been well tolerated. Continue treatment during postoperative period until risk of DVT has diminished.
Adjust-a-dose: In patients with CrCl of less than 30 mL/minute, give 30 mg subcutaneously once daily.
➤ **To prevent PE and DVT in patients with acute illness who are at increased risk because of decreased mobility**
Adults: 40 mg subcutaneously once daily for 6 to 11 days. Treatment for up to 14 days has been well tolerated.
Adjust-a-dose: In patients with CrCl of less than 30 mL/minute, give 30 mg subcutaneously once daily.
➤ **To prevent ischemic complications of unstable angina and non–Q-wave MI with oral aspirin therapy**
Adults: 1 mg/kg subcutaneously every 12 hours until clinical stabilization (minimum 2 days) with aspirin 100 to 325 mg

---

P.O. once daily. Usual duration of treatment is 2 to 8 days.

Adjust-a-dose: In patients with CrCl of less than 30 mL/minute, give 1 mg/kg subcutaneously once daily.

➤ **Acute ST-segment elevation MI**
Adults younger than age 75: 30 mg single I.V. bolus plus 1 mg/kg subcutaneously followed by 1 mg/kg subcutaneously every 12 hours (maximum of 100 mg for the first two doses only) with aspirin 75 to 325 mg P.O. once daily. When given with a thrombolytic, give enoxaparin from 15 minutes before to 30 minutes after the start of fibrinolytic therapy. For patients undergoing percutaneous coronary intervention (PCI), if the last subcutaneous dose was given less than 8 hours before balloon inflation, no additional dose is needed. If the last dose was given more than 8 hours before balloon inflation, give 0.3 mg/kg I.V. bolus.
Adults age 75 and older: Don't use an initial I.V. bolus. Give 0.75 mg/kg subcutaneously every 12 hours (maximum 75 mg for the first two doses only).

Adjust-a-dose: In adults younger than age 75 with severe renal impairment (CrCl of less than 30 mL/minute), 30 mg single I.V. bolus plus 1 mg/kg subcutaneously followed by 1 mg/kg subcutaneously once daily. In adults age 75 and older with severe renal impairment, 1 mg/kg subcutaneously once daily with no initial bolus. Give with aspirin.

➤ **Inpatient treatment of acute DVT with and without PE when given with warfarin sodium**
Adults: 1 mg/kg subcutaneously every 12 hours. Or, 1.5 mg/kg subcutaneously once daily (at same time daily) for 5 to 7 days until therapeutic oral anticoagulant effect (INR 2 to 3) is achieved. Warfarin sodium therapy is usually started within 72 hours of enoxaparin injection.

Adjust-a-dose: In patients with CrCl of less than 30 mL/minute, give 1 mg/kg subcutaneously once daily.

➤ **Outpatient treatment of acute DVT without PE when given with warfarin sodium**
Adults: 1 mg/kg subcutaneously every 12 hours for 5 to 7 days until therapeutic

oral anticoagulant effect (INR 2 to 3) is achieved. Warfarin sodium therapy usually is started within 72 hours of enoxaparin injection.

Adjust-a-dose: In patients with CrCl of less than 30 mL/minute, give 1 mg/kg subcutaneously once daily.

ADMINISTRATION
I.V.
▼ If using multidose vial, use a tuberculin syringe to withdraw appropriate volume of drug.
▼ Flush I.V. access with sufficient amount of saline or dextrose solution before and after I.V. bolus administration.
▼ **Incompatibilities:** Don't mix with other I.V. drugs.
Subcutaneous
● With patient lying down, give by deep subcutaneous injection, alternating doses between left and right anterolateral and posterolateral abdominal walls.
● Don't massage after subcutaneous injection. Watch for signs of bleeding at site. Rotate sites and keep record.

ACTION
Accelerates formation of antithrombin III–thrombin complex and deactivates thrombin, preventing conversion of fibrinogen to fibrin. Drug has a higher antifactor-Xa-to-antifactor-IIa activity ratio than heparin.

Route	Onset	Peak	Duration
Subcut.	Unknown	4 hr	Unknown

Half-life: 4½ hours after a single dose; 7 hours after repeated dosing.

ADVERSE REACTIONS
CNS: confusion, fever, pain.
CV: edema, peripheral edema.
GI: nausea, diarrhea.
Hematologic: *thrombocytopenia, hemorrhage,* ecchymoses, bleeding complications, hypochromic anemia.
Respiratory: dyspnea.
Skin: irritation, pain, hematoma, and erythema at injection site; rash; urticaria.
Other: *angioedema, anaphylaxis.*

INTERACTIONS

Drug-drug. *Anticoagulants, antiplatelet drugs, NSAIDs:* May increase risk of bleeding. Use together cautiously. Monitor PT and INR.

SSRIs: May increase risk of severe bleeding. Monitor PT, INR, and patient. Adjust therapy as needed.

Drug-herb. *Angelica (dong quai), boldo, bromelains, capsicum, chamomile, dandelion, danshen, devil's claw, fenugreek, feverfew, garlic, ginger, ginkgo, ginseng, horse chestnut, licorice, meadowsweet, onion, passion flower, red clover, willow:* May increase risk of bleeding. Discourage use together.

EFFECTS ON LAB TEST RESULTS
- May increase ALT and AST levels. May decrease hemoglobin level.
- May decrease platelet count.

CONTRAINDICATIONS & CAUTIONS
- Contraindicated in patients hypersensitive to drug, heparin, or pork products; in those with active major bleeding; and in those with thrombocytopenia and antiplatelet antibodies in presence of drug.
- Use cautiously in patients with history of heparin-induced thrombocytopenia, aneurysms, cerebrovascular hemorrhage, spinal or epidural punctures (as with anesthesia), uncontrolled hypertension, or threatened abortion.
- Use cautiously in elderly patients and in those with conditions that place them at increased risk for hemorrhage, such as bacterial endocarditis, congenital or acquired bleeding disorders, ulcer disease, angiodysplastic GI disease, hemorrhagic stroke, or recent spinal, eye, or brain surgery.
- Use cautiously in patients with prosthetic heart valves, with regional or lumbar block anesthesia, blood dyscrasias, recent childbirth, pericarditis or pericardial effusion, renal insufficiency, or severe CNS trauma.
- **⚠ Overdose S&S:** Hemorrhagic complications.

NURSING CONSIDERATIONS
- It's important to achieve hemostasis at the puncture site after PCI. The vascular access sheath for instrumentation should remain in place for 6 hours after a dose if manual compression method is used; give next dose no sooner than 6 to 8 hours after sheath removal. Monitor vital signs and site for hematoma and bleeding.
- Monitor pregnant women closely. Warn pregnant women and women of childbearing age about the potential risk of therapy to her and the fetus.
- Multidose vial shouldn't be used in pregnant women because of benzyl alcohol content.
- Monitor anti-Xa levels in pregnant women with mechanical heart valves and in patients with significant renal impairment.
- **Black Box Warning** Patients who receive epidural or spinal anesthesia or spinal puncture during therapy are at increased risk for developing an epidural or spinal hematoma, which may result in long-term or permanent paralysis. Monitor these patients closely for neurologic impairment, as urgent treatment is necessary. ■
- Draw blood to establish baseline coagulation parameters before therapy.
- Never give drug I.M.
- **◑ Alert:** Don't try to expel the air bubble from the 30- or 40-mg prefilled syringes. This may lead to loss of drug and an incorrect dose.
- Avoid I.M. injections of other drugs to prevent or minimize hematoma.
- Monitor platelet counts regularly. Patients with normal coagulation won't need close monitoring of PT or PTT.
- Regularly inspect patient for bleeding gums, bruises on arms or legs, petechiae, nosebleeds, melena, tarry stools, hematuria, and hematemesis.
- To treat severe overdose, give protamine sulfate (a heparin antagonist) by slow I.V. infusion at concentration of 1% to equal dose of drug injected.
- **◑ Alert:** Drug isn't interchangeable with heparin or other low–molecular-weight heparins.

PATIENT TEACHING
- Instruct patient and family to watch for signs of bleeding or abnormal bruising and to notify prescriber immediately if any occur.

Reactions in bold italics are *life-threatening*. Interactions may have a *rapid onset* or a *delayed onset*.

• Tell patient to avoid OTC drugs containing aspirin or other salicylates unless ordered by prescriber.
• Advise patient to consult with prescriber before initiating any herbal therapy; many herbs have anticoagulant, antiplatelet, or fibrinolytic properties.

entacapone
en-tah-KAP-own

Comtan

Therapeutic class: Antiparkinsonians
Pharmacologic class: Catechol-O-methyltransferase inhibitors
Pregnancy risk category: C

AVAILABLE FORMS
Tablets: 200 mg

INDICATIONS & DOSAGES
➤ **Adjunct to levodopa–carbidopa for treatment of idiopathic Parkinson disease in patients with signs and symptoms of end-of-dose wearing-off**
Adults: 200 mg P.O. with each dose of levodopa–carbidopa, up to eight times daily. Maximum, 1,600 mg daily. May need to reduce daily levodopa dose or extend the interval between doses to optimize patient's response.

ADMINISTRATION
P.O.
• Give drug with immediate- or sustained-release levodopa–carbidopa.
• Give drug without regard for food.

ACTION
A reversible catechol-O-methyltransferase (COMT) inhibitor given with levodopa–carbidopa. The combination is thought to cause higher levels of levodopa and optimal control of parkinsonian symptoms.

Route	Onset	Peak	Duration
P.O.	1 hr	1 hr	6 hr

Half-life: About ½ to ¾ hour for first phase and about 2½ hours for second phase.

ADVERSE REACTIONS
CNS: dyskinesia, hyperkinesia, hypokinesia, dizziness, anxiety, somnolence, agitation, fatigue, asthenia, hallucinations.
GI: nausea, diarrhea, abdominal pain, constipation, vomiting, dry mouth, dyspepsia, flatulence, gastritis, taste perversion.
GU: urine discoloration.
Hematologic: purpura.
Musculoskeletal: back pain.
Respiratory: dyspnea.
Skin: sweating.
Other: bacterial infection.

INTERACTIONS
Drug-drug. *Ampicillin, chloramphenicol, cholestyramine, erythromycin, probenecid, rifampin:* May block biliary excretion, resulting in higher levels of entacapone. Use together cautiously.
CNS depressants: May cause additive effect. Use together cautiously.
Drugs metabolized by COMT (dobutamine, dopamine, epinephrine, isoetharine, isoproterenol, norepinephrine): May cause higher levels of these drugs, resulting in increased heart rate, changes in blood pressure, or arrhythmias. Use together cautiously.
Nonselective MAO inhibitors (such as phenelzine, tranylcypromine): May inhibit normal catecholamine metabolism. Avoid using together.
Drug-lifestyle. *Alcohol use:* May cause additive CNS effects. Discourage use together.

EFFECTS ON LAB TEST RESULTS
None reported.

CONTRAINDICATIONS & CAUTIONS
• Contraindicated in patients hypersensitive to drug.
• Use cautiously in patients with hepatic impairment, biliary obstruction, or orthostatic hypotension.
⚠ Overdose S&S: Abdominal pain, loose stools.

NURSING CONSIDERATIONS
• Use drug only with levodopa–carbidopa; no antiparkinsonian effects occur when drug is given as monotherapy.
• Levodopa–carbidopa dosage requirements are usually lower when drug is given with

entacapone; lower levodopa–carbidopa dose or increase dosing interval to avoid adverse effects.

- Drug may cause or worsen dyskinesia, even if levodopa dose is lowered.
- Hallucinations may occur or worsen during therapy with this drug.
- Monitor blood pressure closely, and watch for orthostatic hypotension.
- Diarrhea most often begins within 4 to 12 weeks of starting therapy but may begin as early as 1 week or as late as many months after starting treatment.
- Drug may discolor urine.
- Rarely, rhabdomyolysis has occurred with drug use.

❶ **Alert:** Rapid withdrawal or abrupt reduction in dose could lead to signs and symptoms of Parkinson disease; it may also lead to hyperpyrexia and confusion, a group of symptoms resembling neuroleptic malignant syndrome. Stop drug gradually, and monitor patient closely. Adjust other dopaminergic treatments, as needed.

PATIENT TEACHING

- Instruct patient not to crush or break tablet and to take it at same time as levodopa–carbidopa.
- Warn patient to avoid hazardous activities until CNS effects of drug are known.
- Advise patient to avoid alcohol during treatment.
- Instruct patient to use caution when standing after a prolonged period of sitting or lying down because dizziness may occur. This effect is more common during initial therapy.
- Warn patient that hallucinations, increased difficulty with voluntary movements, nausea, and diarrhea could occur.
- Inform patient that drug may turn urine brownish orange.
- Advise patient to notify prescriber about planned, suspected, or known pregnancy, and to notify prescriber if she's breast-feeding.

entecavir
en-TEK-ah-veer

Baraclude

Therapeutic class: Antivirals
Pharmacologic class: Nucleosides–nucleotides
Pregnancy risk category: C

AVAILABLE FORMS
Oral solution: 0.05 mg/mL
Tablets: 0.5 mg, 1 mg

INDICATIONS & DOSAGES
➤ **Chronic hepatitis B virus (HBV) infection in patients with active viral replication and either persistently increased aminotransferase levels or histologically active disease**
Adults and adolescents age 16 and older who have had no previous nucleoside treatment: 0.5 mg P.O. once daily at least 2 hours before or after a meal.
Adjust-a-dose: If CrCl is 30 to 49 mL/minute, give 0.25 mg P.O. once daily or 0.5 mg P.O. every 48 hours. If CrCl is 10 to less than 30 mL/minute, give 0.15 mg P.O. once daily or 0.5 mg P.O. every 72 hours. If CrCl is less than 10 mL/minute or patient is undergoing hemodialysis or continuous ambulatory peritoneal dialysis, give 0.05 mg P.O. once daily or 0.5 mg P.O. every 7 days.
Adults and adolescents age 16 and older who have a history of viremia and are taking lamivudine or have resistance mutations, or patients with decompensated liver disease: 1 mg P.O. once daily at least 2 hours before or after a meal.
Adjust-a-dose: If CrCl is 30 to 49 mL/minute, give 0.5 mg P.O. once daily or 1 mg P.O. every 48 hours. If CrCl is 10 to less than 30 mL/minute, give 0.3 mg P.O. once daily or 1 mg P.O. every 72 hours. If CrCl is less than 10 mL/minute or patient is undergoing hemodialysis or continuous ambulatory peritoneal dialysis, give 0.1 mg P.O. once daily or 1 mg P.O. every 7 days.

Reactions in bold italics are *life-threatening*. Interactions may have a *rapid onset* or a *delayed onset*.

ADMINISTRATION

P.O.
● Drug should be taken on an empty stomach at least 2 hours before or after a meal to increase absorption.

ACTION

Inhibits HBV polymerase and reduces viral DNA levels.

Route	Onset	Peak	Duration
P.O.	Unknown	½–1½ hr	Unknown

Half-life: About 5 or 6 days.

ADVERSE REACTIONS

CNS: dizziness, fatigue, headache.
GI: diarrhea, dyspepsia, nausea.
GU: glycosuria, hematuria.
Hepatic: hepatomegaly.
Metabolic: *lactic acidosis.*

INTERACTIONS

Drug-drug. *Cyclosporine, tacrolimus:* May further decrease renal function. Monitor renal function carefully.
Drugs that reduce renal function or compete for active tubular secretion: May increase level of either drug. Monitor renal function, and watch for adverse effects.
Drug-food. *All foods:* Delays absorption and decreases drug level. Give drug at least 2 hours before or after a meal.

EFFECTS ON LAB TEST RESULTS

● May increase ALT, amylase, AST, blood glucose, creatinine, lipase, and total bilirubin levels.
● May decrease platelet count.

CONTRAINDICATIONS & CAUTIONS

● Contraindicated in patients hypersensitive to drug or its components.
Black Box Warning Don't use in patients coinfected with HIV and HBV who aren't also receiving highly active antiretroviral therapy. ■
● Use cautiously in patients with renal impairment and in patients who have had a liver transplant.

NURSING CONSIDERATIONS

Black Box Warning Drug may cause life-threatening lactic acidosis and severe hepatomegaly with steatosis. ■
Black Box Warning HBV infection may worsen severely after therapy stops. Monitor hepatic function for several months in patients who stop therapy. If appropriate, start therapy for HBV infection. ■
● Use cautiously in pregnant women only if maternal benefit outweighs fetal risk. For monitoring of fetal outcome data, call the Antiretroviral Pregnancy Registry at 1-800-258-4263.
● It's unknown if drug appears in breast milk. Avoid use in breast-feeding women.
● In elderly patients, adjust dosage for age-related decrease in renal function.

PATIENT TEACHING

● Tell patient to take drug on an empty stomach at least 2 hours before or after a meal.
● Caution against mixing or diluting oral solution with any other substance. Teach proper use of dosing spoon.
● Tell patient to report to prescriber any new adverse effects from this drug and any new drugs he's taking.
● Explain that drug doesn't reduce the risk of HBV transmission to others.
● Teach patient the signs and symptoms of lactic acidosis, such as muscle pain, weakness, dyspnea, GI distress, cold hands and feet, dizziness, or fast or irregular heartbeat.
● Teach patient the signs and symptoms of hepatotoxicity, such as jaundice, dark urine, light-colored stool, loss of appetite, nausea, and stomach pain.
● Warn patient not to stop drug abruptly.

epinastine hydrochloride

ep-ih-NAS-teen

Elestat

Therapeutic class: Antihistamines
Pharmacologic class: H_1-receptor antagonists–mast cell stabilizers
Pregnancy risk category: C

AVAILABLE FORMS

Ophthalmic solution: 0.05%

INDICATIONS & DOSAGES
➤ **To prevent pruritus from allergic conjunctivitis**
Adults and children age 3 and older: Instill 1 drop into each eye b.i.d. Continue treatment as long as allergen is present, even if symptoms resolve.

ADMINISTRATION
Ophthalmic
● Drug is for ophthalmic use only. Don't inject or give orally.
● Keep bottle tightly closed when not in use.
● Don't touch tip of dropper to any surface.

ACTION
Inhibits release of mediators from cells involved in hypersensitivity reactions, temporarily preventing pruritus.

Route	Onset	Peak	Duration
Ophthalmic	Immediate	Unknown	8 hr

Half-life: About 12 hours.

ADVERSE REACTIONS
CNS: headache.
EENT: cold symptoms, burning eyes, hyperemia, increased lymph nodes near eyes, pharyngitis, pruritus, rhinitis, sinusitis.
Respiratory: increased cough, upper respiratory tract infection.

INTERACTIONS
None reported.

EFFECTS ON LAB TEST RESULTS
None reported.

CONTRAINDICATIONS & CAUTIONS
● Contraindicated in patients hypersensitive to drug or its components.
● Contraindicated for irritation related to contact lenses.
● Use cautiously in pregnant or breast-feeding women.
● Safety and effectiveness haven't been established in children younger than age 3.

NURSING CONSIDERATIONS
● Monitor patient for signs and symptoms of infection.

● Soft contact lenses may absorb the preservative benzalkonium.

PATIENT TEACHING
● Teach patient proper instillation technique. Instruct him not to touch any surface, eyelid, or surrounding areas with tip of dropper.
● Caution patient not to use drops to treat contact lens–related eye irritation and not to wear contact lenses if eyes are red.
● Tell patient to remove contact lenses before instillation and to wait at least 10 minutes after instilling drug before reinserting lenses.
● Warn patient that soft contact lenses may absorb the preservative benzalkonium.
● Advise patient to report adverse reactions to drug.
● Tell patient to keep bottle tightly closed when not in use.

SAFETY ALERT!

epinephrine (adrenaline)
ep-i-NEF-rin

epinephrine hydrochloride

Adrenaclick, Adrenalin Chloride, Asthmanefrin, Auvi-Q ◊, EpiPen, EpiPen Jr, microNefrin ◊, S2 ◊

Therapeutic class: Vasopressors
Pharmacologic class: Adrenergics
Pregnancy risk category: C

AVAILABLE FORMS
Injection: 0.1 mg/mL (1:10,000), 1 mg/mL (1:1,000) parenteral
Injection device: 0.15 mg/0.15 mL, 0.3 mg/0.3 mL
Nasal solution: 2.25%
Nebulizer solution: 2.25% ◊

INDICATIONS & DOSAGES
➤ **Anaphylaxis**
Adults: 0.3 to 0.5 mg Adrenalin I.M. or subcutaneously, repeated every 5 to 10 minutes as needed. Or, 0.2 to 1 mg of generic 1:1,000 solution I.M. or subcutaneously. Repeat every 10 to 15 minutes as needed. Or, 0.1 to 0.25 mg of 1:10,000 solution

E

I.V. slowly over 5 to 10 minutes. May repeat every 5 to 15 minutes as needed, or follow with a continuous I.V. infusion, starting at 1 mcg/minute and increasing to 4 mcg/minute, as needed. Or, 0.3 mg I.M. or subcutaneously with autoinjector into outer aspect of thigh, through clothing if necessary. Repeat as needed.

Children weighing 30 kg (66 lb) or more: 0.3 to 0.5 mg Adrenalin I.M. or subcutaneously, repeated every 5 to 10 minutes as needed.

Children weighing less than 30 kg (66 lb): 0.1 mg/kg Adrenalin I.M. or subcutaneously, repeated every 5 to 10 minutes as needed.

Children: 0.01 mg/kg (10 mcg) of generic 1:1,000 solution subcutaneously. Repeat every 15 minutes for two doses, then every 4 hours as needed. Maximum single dose shouldn't exceed 0.5 mg. Or, 0.3 mg of 1:10,000 solution I.V. Repeat every 15 minutes for three or four doses p.r.n. Or, 0.15 mg by autoinjector if patient weighs 15 to 29 kg (33 to 64 lb) or 0.3 mg by autoinjector if patient weighs 30 kg (66 lb) or more, I.M. or subcutaneously, into outer aspect of thigh, through clothing if necessary. Repeat p.r.n.

➤ **Asthma (not Adrenalin)**
Adults: 0.2 to 1 mg of 1:1,000 solution subcutaneously. Start with small dose and increase if needed. Or, 0.1 to 0.25 mg of 1:10,000 solution given slowly I.V.

Children: 0.01 mg/kg (or 0.3 mg/m^2) of 1:1,000 solution subcutaneously to a maximum of 0.5 mg, repeated every 4 hours as needed.

Infants: 0.05 mg solution subcutaneously. May be repeated at 20- to 30-minute intervals.

Neonates: 0.01 mg/kg of 1:1,000 solution subcutaneously.

Adults and children age 4 and older: One inhalation, repeated once if needed after at least 1 minute; don't give subsequent doses for at least 3 hours. Or, 1 to 3 deep inhalations using a hand-bulb nebulizer containing 1% (1:100) solution of epinephrine repeated every 3 hours, as needed.

➤ **Cardiac stimulation (not Adrenalin)**
Adults: 0.1 mg/mL of 1:10,000 solution I.V. May follow with 0.3 mg of 1:1,000 solution subcutaneously. Or, 0.1 to 1 mg of 1:10,000

solution I.V., repeated every 5 minutes, if needed.

Children: 0.005 to 0.01 mg/kg of 1:10,000 solution I.V., repeated every 5 minutes, if needed.

➤ **Induction and maintenance of mydriasis during intraocular surgery (Adrenalin only)**
Adults and children: Dilute 1 mL of epinephrine 1:1,000 (1 mg/mL) in 100 to 1,000 mL of an ophthalmic irrigation fluid to create a concentration of 1:100,000 to 1:1,000,000. Irrigate eye as needed for surgical procedure. Or, dilute to 1:1,000,000 to 1:4,000,000 (10 to 2.5 mcg/mL) for injection intracamerally as a bolus dose.

➤ **Nasal decongestant**
Adults and children age 6 and older: Apply locally as drops or spray with a sterile swab, as required.

ADMINISTRATION
I.V.
▼ Keep solution in light-resistant container, and don't remove before use.
▼ Just before use, mix with D$_5$W, normal saline solution for injection, lactated Ringer injection, or combinations of dextrose in saline solution.
▼ Monitor blood pressure, heart rate, and ECG when therapy starts and frequently thereafter.
▼ Discard solution if it's discolored or contains precipitate or after 24 hours.
▼ Don't give autoinjectors I.V.
▼ **Incompatibilities:** Aminophylline; ampicillin sodium; furosemide; hyaluronidase; Ionosol D-CM, PSL, and T solutions with D$_5$W; mephentermine; thiopental sodium. Compatible with most other I.V. solutions. Rapidly destroyed by alkalies or oxidizing drugs, including halogens, nitrates, nitrites, permanganates, sodium bicarbonate, and salts of easily reducible metals, such as iron, copper, and zinc. Don't mix with alkaline solutions.
I.M.
● Avoid I.M. use of parenteral suspension into buttocks. Gas gangrene may occur because drug reduces oxygen tension of the tissues, encouraging growth of contaminating organisms.

• Massage site after I.M. injection to counteract vasoconstriction. Repeated local injection can cause necrosis at injection site.
• Don't give if solution is discolored or contains precipitate.
• Don't give autoinjectors I.V.

Subcutaneous
• Don't refrigerate; protect from light.
• Don't give if solution is discolored or contains precipitate.
• Don't give autoinjectors I.V.
• Preferred route. Don't inject too deeply and enter muscle.

Inhalational
• Teach patient to perform oral inhalation correctly. See "Patient teaching" for complete instructions.
• Epinephrine 1:100 will turn from pink to brown if exposed to air, light, heat, alkalies, and some metals. Don't use solution that's discolored or has a precipitate.

Intranasal
• Dilute to prescribed strength according to manufacturer's instructions.
• Don't use solution if it's pinkish or darker than slightly yellow, or if it contains precipitate.
• Apply locally as spray or drops, or with a sterile swab.
• Protect from light and freezing; store between 59° and 77° F (15° and 25° C).

Intraocular
• Must dilute before administration.

ACTION
Relaxes bronchial smooth muscle by stimulating beta$_2$ receptors and alpha and beta receptors in the sympathetic nervous system.

Route	Onset	Peak	Duration
I.V.	Immediate	5 min	Short
I.M.	Variable	Unknown	1–4 hr
Subcut.	5–15 min	30 min	1–4 hr
Inhalation	1–5 min	Unknown	1–3 hr
Intranasal	Unknown	Unknown	Unknown
Intraocular	Unknown	Unknown	Unknown

Half-life: Unknown.

ADVERSE REACTIONS
CNS: drowsiness, headache, nervousness, tremor, *cerebral hemorrhage, stroke,* vertigo, pain, disorientation, agitation, fear, dizziness, weakness, *subarachnoid hemorrhage.*
CV: palpitations, *ventricular fibrillation, shock,* widened pulse pressure, hypertension, tachycardia, anginal pain, altered ECG (including a decreased T-wave amplitude).
GI: nausea, vomiting.
Respiratory: dyspnea.
Skin: urticaria, hemorrhage at injection site, pallor.
Other: tissue necrosis, sweating.

INTERACTIONS
Drug-drug. *Alpha blockers:* May cause hypotension from unopposed beta-adrenergic effects. Avoid using together.
Antihistamines, thyroid hormones: When given with sympathomimetics, may cause severe adverse cardiac effects. Avoid using together.
Cardiac glycosides, general anesthetics (halogenated hydrocarbons): May increase risk of ventricular arrhythmias. Monitor ECG closely.
Carteolol, nadolol, penbutolol, pindolol, propranolol, timolol: May cause hypertension followed by bradycardia. Stop beta blocker 3 days before starting epinephrine.
Doxapram, methylphenidate: May enhance CNS stimulation or pressor effects. Monitor patient closely.
Ergot alkaloids: May decrease vasoconstrictor activity. Monitor patient closely.
Guanadrel, guanethidine: May enhance pressor effects of epinephrine. Monitor patient closely.
Levodopa: May enhance risk of arrhythmias. Monitor ECG closely.
MAO inhibitors: May increase risk of hypertensive crisis. Monitor blood pressure closely.
TCAs: May potentiate the pressor response and cause arrhythmias. Use together cautiously.

EFFECTS ON LAB TEST RESULTS
• May increase BUN, glucose, and lactic acid levels.

CONTRAINDICATIONS & CAUTIONS
• Contraindicated in patients with angle-closure glaucoma, shock (other than anaphylactic shock), organic brain damage,

---

Reactions in bold italics are *life-threatening*. Interactions may have a *rapid onset* or a *delayed onset*.

heart failure, cardiac dilation, arrhythmias, coronary insufficiency, or cerebral arteriosclerosis.
• Contraindicated in patients receiving general anesthesia with halogenated hydrocarbons or cyclopropane and in patients in labor (may delay second stage).
• Commercial products containing sulfites contraindicated in patients with sulfite allergies, except when epinephrine is being used to treat serious allergic reactions or other emergency situations.
• Contraindicated for use in fingers, toes, ears, nose, or genitalia when used with local anesthetic.
• Use cautiously in patients with long-standing bronchial asthma or emphysema who have developed degenerative heart disease.
• Use cautiously in elderly patients and in those with hyperthyroidism, CV disease, hypertension, psychoneurosis, and diabetes.
⚠ **Overdose S&S:** Precordial distress, vomiting, headache, dyspnea, hypertension, peripheral vascular constriction, pulmonary edema, cerebral hemorrhage, arrhythmias, extreme pallor and coldness of the skin, metabolic acidosis, kidney failure.

NURSING CONSIDERATIONS
• In patients with Parkinson disease, drug increases rigidity and tremor.
• Drug interferes with tests for urinary catecholamines.
• Note that 1 mg equals 1 mL of 1:1,000 solution or 10 mL of 1:10,000 solution.
• Epinephrine is drug of choice in emergency treatment of acute anaphylactic reactions.
• Observe patient closely for adverse reactions. Notify prescriber if adverse reactions develop; adjusting dosage or stopping drug may be necessary.
• If blood pressure increases sharply, give rapid-acting vasodilators, such as nitrates and alpha blockers, to counteract the marked pressor effect of large doses.
• Drug is rapidly destroyed by oxidizing products, such as iodine, chromates, nitrites, oxygen, and salts of easily reducible metals (such as iron).

• When treating patient with reactions caused by other drugs given I.M. or subcutaneously, inject this drug into the site where the other drug was given to minimize further absorption.
• **Look alike–sound alike:** Don't confuse epinephrine with ephedrine or norepinephrine.

PATIENT TEACHING
• Teach patient to perform oral inhalation correctly. Give the following instructions for using a metered-dose inhaler:
– Shake canister.
– Clear nasal passages and throat.
– Breathe out, expelling as much air from lungs as possible.
– Place mouthpiece well into mouth, and inhale deeply as you release dose from inhaler. Or, hold inhaler about 1 inch (two fingerwidths) from open mouth, and inhale while releasing dose.
– Hold breath for several seconds, remove mouthpiece, and exhale slowly.
• If more than one inhalation is prescribed, advise patient to wait at least 2 minutes before repeating procedure.
• Tell patient that use of a spacer device may improve drug delivery to lungs.
• If patient is also using a corticosteroid inhaler, instruct him to use the bronchodilator first and then to wait about 5 minutes before using the corticosteroid. This lets the bronchodilator open the air passages for maximal effectiveness.
• Instruct patient to remove canister and wash inhaler with warm, soapy water at least once weekly.
• If patient has acute hypersensitivity reactions (such as to bee stings), you may need to teach him to self-inject drug.
• Instruct patient in autoinjector use.
• Tell patient to give autoinjector in outer thigh and not into the buttock.
• Caution patient or caregiver to only give two sequential doses unless under direct medical supervision. Patient should seek immediate medical care for acute hypersensitivity reactions.

SAFETY ALERT!

epirubicin hydrochloride
ep-uh-ROO-bi-sin

Ellence

Therapeutic class: Antineoplastics
Pharmacologic class: Anthracycline glycoside antibiotics
Pregnancy risk category: D

AVAILABLE FORMS
Injection: 2 mg/mL
Powder for injection: 50 mg, 200 mg

INDICATIONS & DOSAGES
➤ **Adjuvant therapy in patients with evidence of axillary node tumor involvement after resection of primary breast cancer**
Adults: 100 to 120 mg/m^2 I.V. infusion over 3 to 20 minutes, depending on dosage and infusion volume, through a free-flowing I.V. solution on day 1 of each cycle, or divided equally in two doses on days 1 and 8 of each cycle; cycle repeated every 3 to 4 weeks for six cycles; used with regimens containing cyclophosphamide and fluorouracil.

Dosage modification after first cycle is based on toxicity. For patients with platelet count nadir below 50,000/mm^3, ANC below 250/mm^3, neutropenic fever, or grade 3 or 4 nonhematologic toxicity, reduce day 1 dose in subsequent cycles to 75% of day 1 dose given in current cycle. Delay day 1 therapy in subsequent cycles until platelet count is at least 100,000/mm^3, ANC is at least 1,500/mm^3, and nonhematologic toxicities recover to grade 1.

For patients receiving divided doses (days 1 and 8), day 8 dose should be 75% of day 1 dose if platelet count is 75,000 to 100,000/mm^3 and ANC is 1,000 to 1,499/mm^3. If day 8 platelet count is below 75,000/mm^3, ANC is below 1,000/mm^3, or grade 3 or 4 nonhematologic toxicity has occurred, omit day 8 dose.
Adjust-a-dose: For patients with bone marrow dysfunction (heavily pretreated patients, patients with bone marrow depression, or those with neoplastic bone marrow infiltration), start at lower doses of 75 to 90 mg/m^2.

Black Box Warning For patients with hepatic dysfunction, if bilirubin is 1.2 to 3 mg/dL or AST is 2 to 4 times upper limit of normal (ULN), give half recommended starting dose. If bilirubin level is above 3 mg/dL or AST is more than 4 times ULN, give one-fourth recommended starting dose. ∎

For patients with severe renal dysfunction (creatinine level over 5 mg/dL), consider lower doses.

ADMINISTRATION
I.V.
▼ Wear protective clothing (goggles, gown, disposable gloves) when handling drug, which is a vesicant.
Black Box Warning Never give drug I.M. or subcutaneously; severe tissue necrosis may result. Always give I.V. through free-flowing normal saline solution or D$_5$W over 3 to 20 minutes depending on dosage and volume of infusion solution. ∎
Black Box Warning Avoid veins over joints or in limbs with compromised venous or lymphatic drainage. ∎
▼ Avoid repeated injection into the same vein.
▼ Facial flushing and erythematous streaking along vein may indicate overly rapid delivery.
Black Box Warning If burning or stinging occurs, stop infusion immediately and restart in another vein. ∎
▼ After vial has been penetrated, discard unused solution after 24 hours.
▼ **Incompatibilities:** Fluorouracil, heparin, ifosfamide with mesna, any alkaline pH solutions, other I.V. drugs.

ACTION
May form a complex with DNA by getting between nucleotide base pairs, inhibiting DNA, RNA, and protein synthesis; DNA cleavage occurs, resulting in cytocidal activity. Drug may also interfere with replication and transcription of DNA and may generate cytotoxic free radicals.

Route	Onset	Peak	Duration
I.V.	Unknown	Unknown	Unknown

Half-life: 31 to 35 hours.

Reactions in bold italics are *life-threatening*. Interactions may have a *rapid onset* or a *delayed onset*.

ADVERSE REACTIONS
CNS: lethargy, fever.
CV: *cardiomyopathy, heart failure.*
EENT: conjunctivitis, keratitis.
GI: nausea, vomiting, diarrhea, anorexia, mucositis.
GU: amenorrhea, red urine.
Hematologic: *leukopenia, neutropenia, febrile neutropenia,* anemia, *thrombocytopenia.*
Skin: alopecia, rash, pruritus, skin changes, local toxicity.
Other: infection, hot flashes.

INTERACTIONS
Drug-drug. *Calcium channel blockers, other cardioactive compounds:* May increase risk of heart failure. Monitor cardiac function closely.
Cimetidine: May increase epirubicin level by 50%. Avoid using together.
Cytotoxic drugs: May cause additive toxicities (especially hematologic and GI). Monitor patient closely.
Live-virus vaccines: May increase risk of vaccine-induced adverse reactions. Avoid concomitant use.

EFFECTS ON LAB TEST RESULTS
● May decrease hemoglobin level.
● May decrease neutrophil, platelet, and WBC counts.

CONTRAINDICATIONS & CAUTIONS
● Contraindicated in patients hypersensitive to drug, other anthracyclines, or anthracenediones, and in patients with baseline neutrophil counts below 1,500/mm^3, severe myocardial insufficiency, recent MI, serious arrhythmias, or severe hepatic dysfunction.
● Contraindicated in patients who have had previous treatment with anthracyclines to the maximum total cumulative doses.
● Use cautiously in patients with active or dormant cardiac disease, previous or current radiotherapy to mediastinal and pericardial areas, or previous therapy with other anthracyclines or anthracenediones.
● Use cautiously in patients receiving other cardiotoxic drugs.
⚠ *Overdose S&S:* Bone marrow aplasia, grade 4 mucositis, GI bleeding, hyperther-

mia, multiple organ failure, lactic acidosis, increased LDH level, anuria, death.

NURSING CONSIDERATIONS
Black Box Warning Give drug under supervision of prescriber experienced in cancer chemotherapy. ∎
● Don't handle drug if you are pregnant.
● For patients taking 120 mg/m^2, give prophylactic sulfamethoxazole–trimethoprim or fluoroquinolones.
● Give antiemetic before drug to reduce nausea and vomiting.
● Before therapy, obtain total bilirubin, AST, and creatinine levels; CBC including ANC; and LVEF.
● Monitor LVEF regularly during therapy. Stop drug at first sign of impaired cardiac function. Early signs of cardiac toxicity include sinus tachycardia, ECG abnormalities, tachyarrhythmias, bradycardia, AV block, and bundle-branch block.
Black Box Warning Cardiac toxicity may occur during therapy or months to years after treatment ends; indications include reduced LVEF and signs and symptoms of heart failure (tachycardia, dyspnea, pulmonary edema, dependent edema, hepatomegaly, ascites, pleural effusion, and gallop rhythm). Delayed cardiac toxicity depends on cumulative dose of epirubicin. Don't exceed cumulative dose of 900 mg/m^2. ∎
Black Box Warning Severe myelosuppression may occur. ∎
● Obtain total and differential WBC, CBC, platelet count, and LFTs before and during each cycle of therapy.
● WBC nadir is usually reached 10 to 14 days after drug administration, and returns to normal by day 21.
● Monitor uric acid, potassium, calcium, phosphate, and creatinine levels immediately after initial chemotherapy administration in patients susceptible to tumor lysis syndrome. Hydration, urine alkalinization, and prophylaxis with allopurinol may prevent hyperuricemia and minimize potential complications of tumor lysis syndrome.
● Drug may enhance the effects of radiation therapy or cause an inflammatory cell

reaction at irradiation site. Monitor patient closely.

Black Box Warning Secondary acute myeloid leukemia has been reported in patients with breast cancer treated with anthracyclines, including epirubicin. ∎

PATIENT TEACHING
• Advise patient to report any pain or burning at injection site during or after administration.
• Advise patient to report nausea, vomiting, mouth inflammation, dehydration, fever, evidence of infection, or symptoms of heart failure (rapid heart beat, labored breathing, swelling).
• Tell patient that urine will be reddish pink for 1 to 2 days after treatment.
• Inform patient of risk of heart damage and treatment-related leukemia with use of drug.
• Advise men to use effective contraception during treatment.
• Advise women that irreversible, premature menopause may occur.
• Tell patient that hair usually regrows within 2 to 3 months after therapy stops.

eplerenone
ep-LER-eh-nown

Inspra

Therapeutic class: Antihypertensives
Pharmacologic class: Selective aldosterone receptor antagonists
Pregnancy risk category: B

AVAILABLE FORMS
Tablets: 25 mg, 50 mg

INDICATIONS & DOSAGES
➤ **Hypertension**
Adults: 50 mg P.O. once daily. If response is inadequate after 4 weeks, increase dosage to 50 mg P.O. b.i.d. Maximum daily dose, 100 mg.
Adjust-a-dose: In patients taking weak CYP3A4 inhibitors (erythromycin, fluconazole, saquinavir, verapamil), reduce eplerenone starting dose to 25 mg P.O. once daily.

➤ **Heart failure after an MI**
Adults: Initially, 25 mg P.O. once daily. Increase within 4 weeks, as tolerated and according to potassium level, to 50 mg P.O. once daily.
Adjust-a-dose: If potassium level is less than 5 mEq/L, increase dosage from 25 mg every other day to 25 mg daily; or increase dosage from 25 mg daily to 50 mg daily. If potassium level is 5 to 5.4 mEq/L, don't adjust dosage. If potassium level is 5.5 to 5.9 mEq/L, decrease dosage from 50 mg daily to 25 mg daily; or decrease dosage from 25 mg daily to 25 mg every other day; or if dosage was 25 mg every other day, withhold drug. If potassium level is greater than 6 mEq/L, withhold drug. May restart drug at 25 mg every other day when potassium level is less than 5.5 mEq/L.

ADMINISTRATION
P.O.
• Give drug without regard for meals.
• Don't give with grapefruit juice.

ACTION
Binds to mineralocorticoid receptors and blocks aldosterone, which increases blood pressure through induction of sodium reabsorption and possibly other mechanisms.

Route	Onset	Peak	Duration
P.O.	Unknown	90 min	Unknown

Half-life: 4 to 6 hours.

ADVERSE REACTIONS
CNS: dizziness, fatigue.
GI: diarrhea, abdominal pain.
GU: albuminuria, abnormal vaginal bleeding.
Metabolic: *hyperkalemia.*
Respiratory: cough.
Other: flulike syndrome, gynecomastia.

INTERACTIONS
Drug-drug. *ACE inhibitors, angiotensin II receptor antagonists:* May increase risk of hyperkalemia. Use together cautiously.
Azole antifungals (itraconazole, ketoconazole), macrolides (clarithromycin), nefazodone, protease inhibitors (nelfinavir, ritonavir): Inhibits the CYP3A4 metabolism of eplerenone. Use together is contraindicated.

Lithium: May increase risk of lithium toxicity. Monitor lithium level.

NSAIDs: May reduce the antihypertensive effect and cause severe hyperkalemia in patients with impaired renal function. Monitor blood pressure and potassium level.

Potassium supplements, potassium-sparing diuretics (amiloride, spironolactone, triamterene): May increase risk of hyperkalemia and sometimes-fatal arrhythmias. Use together is contraindicated.

Weak CYP3A4 inhibitors (erythromycin, fluconazole, saquinavir, verapamil): May increase eplerenone level. Reduce eplerenone starting dose to 25 mg P.O. once daily.

Drug-herb. *St. John's wort:* May decrease eplerenone level over time. Discourage use together.

Drug-food. *Grapefruit juice:* May increase eplerenone level by about 25%.

EFFECTS ON LAB TEST RESULTS
● May increase ALT, BUN, cholesterol, creatinine, GGT, potassium, triglyceride, and uric acid levels. May decrease sodium level.

CONTRAINDICATIONS & CAUTIONS
● When used for hypertension, contraindicated in patients with type 2 diabetes with microalbuminuria, creatinine level greater than 2 mg/dL in men or greater than 1.8 mg/dL in women, or CrCl less than 50 mL/minute and in patients taking potassium supplements or potassium-sparing diuretics (amiloride, spironolactone, or triamterene).
● Contraindicated in patients with potassium level greater than 5.5 mEq/mL or CrCl of 30 mL/minute or less and in patients taking strong CYP3A4 inhibitors, such as ketoconazole, clarithromycin, ritonavir, nelfinavir, nefazodone, and itraconazole.
● Use cautiously in patient with mild to moderate hepatic impairment.
● Use in pregnant women only if the potential benefits justify the potential risk to the fetus. Use cautiously in breast-feeding women; it's unknown if drug appears in breast milk.
⚠ Overdose S&S: Hypotension, hyperkalemia.

NURSING CONSIDERATIONS
● Drug may be used alone or with other antihypertensives.
● Full therapeutic effect of the drug occurs in 4 weeks.
● In patients with heart failure, measure potassium level at baseline, within the first week, at 1 month after starting therapy, and periodically thereafter.
● Monitor patient for signs and symptoms of hyperkalemia.
● **Look alike–sound alike:** Don't confuse Inspra with Spiriva.

PATIENT TEACHING
● Inform patient that drug may be taken with or without food.
● Advise patient to avoid potassium supplements and salt substitutes during treatment.
● Tell patient to report adverse reactions.

SAFETY ALERT!

epoetin alfa (erythropoietin)
e-poe-E-tin

Epogen, Eprex†, Procrit

Therapeutic class: Colony stimulating factors
Pharmacologic class: Recombinant human erythropoietins
Pregnancy risk category: C

AVAILABLE FORMS
Injection: 2,000 units/mL, 3,000 units/mL, 4,000 units/mL, 10,000 units/mL, 20,000 units/mL, 40,000 units/mL

INDICATIONS & DOSAGES
➤ **Anemia caused by chronic renal disease**
Adults: Dosage is individualized. For patients on hemodialysis, start treatment only if hemoglobin level is less than 10 g/dL. For patients not on hemodialysis, start treatment only if hemoglobin level is less than 10 g/dL and the decline of hemoglobin level indicates that patient will require an RBC transfusion and reducing the risk of alloimmunization and other RBC transfusion–related risks is a treatment goal. Starting dose is 50 to

100 units/kg subcutaneously or I.V. three times weekly. I.V. route is preferred for patients receiving hemodialysis. Maintenance dosage is highly individualized. Give the lowest effective dose to gradually increase hemoglobin to a level where blood transfusion isn't necessary.

Children age 1 month and older who are on dialysis: Initially, 50 units/kg I.V. or subcutaneously three times weekly. I.V. route is preferred for patients receiving hemodialysis. Maintenance dosage is highly individualized to keep hemoglobin level within target range. Give the lowest effective dose to gradually increase hemoglobin to a level at which blood transfusion isn't necessary.

Adjust-a-dose: Don't increase dosage more frequently than every 4 weeks. Reduce dosage by 25% when target hemoglobin level approaches 12 g/dL or if it rises more than 1 g/dL in any 2-week period. If hemoglobin level continues to increase, hold dose until hemoglobin level begins to decrease; then restart at 25% below previous dose. Increase dosage by 25% if hemoglobin level is less than 10 g/dL and hasn't increased by 1 g/dL after 4 weeks or hemoglobin level falls below 10 g/dL. For patients on dialysis, if hemoglobin level approaches or exceeds 10 g/dL, reduce dosage or interrupt therapy. For patients not on dialysis, if hemoglobin level exceeds 10 g/dL, reduce dosage or interrupt therapy.

➤ **Anemia from zidovudine therapy (4,200 mg/week or less) in HIV-infected patients**

Adults: Initially, 100 units/kg I.V. or subcutaneously three times weekly for 8 weeks or until target hemoglobin level is reached. If response isn't satisfactory after 8 weeks, increase dosage by 50 to 100 units/kg I.V. or subcutaneously three times weekly. Evaluate response every 4 to 8 weeks thereafter; further increase dosage in increments of 50 to 100 units/kg three times weekly, up to maximum of 300 units/kg I.V. or subcutaneously three times weekly. Give the lowest effective dose to gradually increase hemoglobin to a level where blood transfusion isn't necessary. Withhold drug if hemoglobin level exceeds 12 g/dL. Restart drug at 25% below the previous dosage

if hemoglobin level declines to less than 11 g/dL.

➤ **Anemia from chemotherapy**

Adults: Start therapy if hemoglobin level is less than 10 g/dL and a minimum of 2 additional months of chemotherapy is planned. Initially, 150 units/kg subcutaneously three times weekly. If response isn't satisfactory after 4 weeks, increase dosage up to 300 units/kg subcutaneously three times weekly. Give the lowest effective dose to gradually increase hemoglobin to a level at which blood transfusion isn't necessary. Discontinue drug after 8 weeks if no response, as measured by hemoglobin level or if tranfusions are still required.

Children ages 5 to 18: 600 units/kg I.V. once weekly. If hemoglobin level hasn't increased by at least 1 g/dL (in the absence of RBC transfusion) and remains below 10 g/dL, increase dosage to 900 units/kg I.V. (maximum, 60,000 units). Discontinue drug after 8 weeks if no response, as measured by hemoglobin level or if transfusions are still required.

Adjust-a-dose: Withhold drug if hemoglobin level exceeds level needed to avoid an RBC transfusion. Restart drug at dosage 25% below previous dosage when hemoglobin level approaches a level at which an RBC transfusion may be required. Reduce dosage by 25% if hemoglobin level increases more than 1 g/dL in a 2-week period or reaches a level needed to avoid an RBC transfusion.

➤ **To reduce need for allogenic blood transfusion in anemic patients scheduled to have elective, noncardiac, nonvascular surgery**

Adults: 300 units/kg subcutaneously daily for 10 days before surgery, on day of surgery, and for 4 days after surgery. Or, 600 units/kg subcutaneously in once-weekly doses (21, 14, and 7 days before surgery), plus a fourth dose on day of surgery.

ADMINISTRATION

I.V.

▼ Store solution in refrigerator and protect from light.

▼ Don't shake.

▼ Give by direct injection without dilution.

▼ If patient is having dialysis, drug may be given into venous return line after

---

dialysis session. To keep drug from adhering to tubing, inject drug with blood still in the line. Then flush with normal saline solution.

▼ Single-dose vials contain no preservatives. Discard unused portion.

🕄 *Alert:* Multidose vials contain benzyl alcohol, which has been associated with sometimes fatal neurologic and other complications in premature infants.

▼ **Incompatibilities:** Other I.V. drugs.

Subcutaneous

• Store solution in refrigerator and protect from light.

• Don't shake.

• Don't use if solution is discolored or has particulate matter.

• Give in upper arm, abdomen, mid-thigh, or outer buttocks.

• Single-use vial without preservative may be admixed in a syringe with bacteriostatic normal saline solution for injection with benzyl alcohol 0.9% (bacteriostatic saline) at a 1:1 ratio to provide local anesthetic.

• Rotate injection sites and document.

ACTION

Mimics effects of erythropoietin. Functions as a growth factor and as a differentiating factor, enhancing RBC production.

Route	Onset	Peak	Duration
I.V.	Immediate	Immediate	Unknown
Subcut.	Unknown	5–24 hr	Unknown

Half-life: 4 to 13 hours.

ADVERSE REACTIONS

CNS: asthenia, dizziness, fatigue, headache, paresthesia, pyrexia, *seizures.*
CV: edema, hypertension, increased clotting of arteriovenous grafts.
EENT: pharyngitis.
GI: abdominal pain and constipation (in children), diarrhea, nausea, vomiting.
Metabolic: hyperglycemia, *hypokalemia,* hyperphosphatemia, hyperuricemia.
Musculoskeletal: arthralgia, myalgia, bone pain, muscle spasm.
Respiratory: cough, shortness of breath, upper respiratory tract infection.
Skin: injection-site reactions, rash, urticaria.

INTERACTIONS

None significant.

EFFECTS ON LAB TEST RESULTS

• May increase BUN, creatinine, phosphate, potassium, and uric acid levels.

CONTRAINDICATIONS & CAUTIONS

• Contraindicated in patients hypersensitive to products derived from mammal cells or albumin (human), in those with uncontrolled hypertension, and in patients receiving myelosuppressive chemotherapy when the anticipated outcome is cure.

• Use cautiously in breast-feeding women.

⚠ *Overdose S&S:* Severe hypertension.

NURSING CONSIDERATIONS

Black Box Warning Patients with chronic renal disease have an increased risk of death and serious CV adverse events, including stroke, when erythropoiesis-stimulating agents are used to increase hemoglobin level to more than 11 g/dL. Individualize therapy and use the lowest dosage needed to reduce the need for RBC transfusion. ∎

• Before starting therapy, evaluate patient's iron status. Patient should receive adequate iron supplementation beginning no later than when epoetin alfa treatment starts and continuing throughout therapy. Patient also may need vitamin B_{12} and folic acid.

• Monitor blood pressure before therapy. Most patients with chronic renal failure have hypertension. Blood pressure may increase, especially when hematocrit increases in the early part of therapy.

Black Box Warning In patients with non-small-cell lung cancer and breast, head and neck, lymphoid, and cervical cancers, there is a risk of tumor growth and shortened survival when hemoglobin levels of 12 g/dL are achieved. Use the lowest dosage needed to avoid RBC transfusions. Use only for treatment of anemia due to concomitant myelosuppressive chemotherapy and discontinue drug following chemotherapy course. ∎

• Institute diet restrictions or drug therapy to control blood pressure.

• Monitor hemoglobin level twice weekly until it stabilizes in the target range and maintenance dose is established, then continue to monitor at regular intervals. Resume twice-weekly testing after any dosage adjustments.

• When used in HIV-infected adults, dosage recommendations are for those with endogenous erythropoietin levels of 500 units/L or less and cumulative zidovudine doses of 4.2 g/week or less.

• Monitor blood counts; elevated hematocrit may cause excessive clotting. For patients with chronic renal disease, monitor hemoglobin levels weekly until stable and then at least monthly.

• Patient may need additional heparin to prevent clotting during dialysis treatments. **Black Box Warning** Due to increased risk of DVT, consider prophylaxis. ▌

❸ *Alert:* Evaluate patient who experiences a lack or loss of effect for pure red cell aplasia.

• *Look alike–sound alike:* Don't confuse Epogen with Neupogen.

PATIENT TEACHING

• Inform patient that pain or discomfort in limbs (long bones) and pelvis, feelings of cold, and sweating may occur after injection (usually within 2 hours). Symptoms may last for 12 hours and then disappear.

• Advise patient to avoid driving or operating heavy machinery at start of therapy. There may be a relationship between too-rapid increase in hematocrit and seizures.

• Tell patient to monitor blood pressure at home and to adhere to dietary restrictions.

• Advise women that they may resume menstruating after therapy and to consider the need for contraception.

---

eprosartan mesylate
ep-row-SAR-tan

Teveten

Therapeutic class: Antihypertensives
Pharmacologic class: Angiotensin II receptor antagonists
Pregnancy risk category: C; D in 2nd and 3rd trimesters

AVAILABLE FORMS
Tablets: 400 mg, 600 mg

INDICATIONS & DOSAGES
➤ **Hypertension (alone or with other antihypertensives)**
Adults: Initially, 600 mg P.O. daily. Dosage ranges from 400 to 800 mg daily, given as single daily dose or two divided doses.

ADMINISTRATION
P.O.
• Give drug without regard for meals.

ACTION
An angiotensin II receptor antagonist that reduces blood pressure by blocking the vasoconstrictor and aldosterone-secreting effects of angiotensin II. Drug selectively blocks the binding of angiotensin II to its receptor sites found in many tissues, such as vascular smooth muscle and the adrenal gland.

Route	Onset	Peak	Duration
P.O.	1–2 hr	1–3 hr	24 hr

Half-life: 20 hours after multiple oral doses.

ADVERSE REACTIONS
CNS: depression, fatigue, headache, dizziness.
CV: chest pain, dependent edema.
EENT: pharyngitis, rhinitis, sinusitis.
GI: abdominal pain, dyspepsia, diarrhea.
GU: UTI.
Hematologic: *neutropenia.*
Musculoskeletal: arthralgia, myalgia.
Respiratory: cough, upper respiratory tract infection, bronchitis.
Other: injury, viral infection.

INTERACTIONS
Drug-drug. *ACE inhibitors:* May increase risk of renal impairment and hyperkalemia. Use with caution, and closely monitor renal function and potassium level.
Direct renin inhibitors (aliskiren): May cause renal impairment, hypotension, and hyperkalemia. Use together in patients with diabetes is contraindicated. Avoid using together in patients with renal impairment and GFR of less than 60 mL/minute.
Lithium: May increase lithium concentration, leading to toxicity. Adjust lithium dosage as needed.

Reactions in bold italics are *life-threatening*. Interactions may have a *rapid onset* or a *delayed onset*.

NSAIDs: May decrease antihypertensive effects. Monitor blood pressure. Also may result in renal function deterioration, including possible acute renal failure, in volume-depleted elderly patients and those with compromised renal function.

Potassium preparations: May decrease renal excretion of potassium, increasing risk of hyperkalemia and possibly resulting in cardiac arrhythmias or cardiac arrest. Adjust potassium-preparation dosage as needed.

Potassium-sparing diuretics, trimethoprim: May increase risk of hyperkalemia. Adjust eprosartan dosage as needed.

Drug-herb. *Ma huang:* May decrease antihypertensive effects. Discourage use together.

EFFECTS ON LAB TEST RESULTS
• May increase BUN and triglyceride levels.

CONTRAINDICATIONS & CAUTIONS
• Contraindicated in patients hypersensitive to eprosartan or its components.
• Use cautiously in patients with renal artery stenosis; in patients with an activated renin-angiotensin system, such as volume- or salt-depleted patients; and in patients whose renal function may depend on the renin-angiotensin-aldosterone system, such as those with severe heart failure.
• Safety and effectiveness in children haven't been established.

Black Box Warning Use during pregnancy can cause injury and death to the developing fetus. When pregnancy is detected, stop drug as soon as possible. ∎

NURSING CONSIDERATIONS
• Correct hypovolemia and hyponatremia before starting therapy to reduce risk of symptomatic hypotension.
• Monitor blood pressure closely for 2 hours at start of treatment. If hypotension occurs, place patient in a supine position and, if needed, give an I.V. infusion of normal saline solution.
• A transient episode of hypotension isn't a contraindication to continued treatment. Drug may be restarted once patient's blood pressure has stabilized.
• Drug may be used alone or with other antihypertensives, such as diuretics and calcium channel blockers. Maximal blood pressure response may take 2 or 3 weeks.
• Monitor patient for facial or lip swelling because angioedema has occurred with other angiotensin II receptor antagonists.
• Closely observe infants exposed to eprosartan in utero for hypotension, oliguria, and hyperkalemia.

PATIENT TEACHING
• Advise women of childbearing age to use a reliable form of contraception and to notify prescriber immediately if pregnancy is suspected. Treatment may need to be stopped under medical supervision.
• Advise patient to report facial or lip swelling and signs and symptoms of infection, such as fever and sore throat.
• Tell patient to notify prescriber before taking OTC medication to treat a dry cough.
• Inform patient that drug may be taken without regard to meals.
• Advise breast-feeding women to stop either therapy or breast-feeding because of potential for adverse reactions in infant.

SAFETY ALERT!

eptifibatide
ep-tiff-IB-ah-tide

Integrilin

Therapeutic class: Antiplatelet drugs
Pharmacologic class: Glycoprotein IIb/IIIa inhibitors
Pregnancy risk category: B

AVAILABLE FORMS
Injection: 10-mL (2 mg/mL), 100-mL (0.75 mg/mL) vials

INDICATIONS & DOSAGES
➤ **Acute coronary syndrome (unstable angina or non–ST-segment elevation MI) in patients receiving drug therapy and in those undergoing a percutaneous coronary intervention (PCI)**
Adults: 180 mcg/kg I.V. bolus as soon as possible after diagnosis, followed by a continuous I.V. infusion at a rate of 2 mcg/kg/minute until hospital discharge or start of CABG surgery, for up to 72 hours.

If patient is having a PCI, continue infusion until hospital discharge or for 18 to 24 hours after the procedure, whichever comes first, for up to 96 hours.

Adjust-a-dose: If CrCl is less than 50 mL/minute, give 180 mcg/kg I.V. bolus as soon as possible after diagnosis, followed by a continuous I.V. infusion at 1 mcg/kg/minute.

➤ **PCI**

Adults: 180 mcg/kg I.V. bolus given just before the procedure, immediately followed by an infusion of 2 mcg/kg/minute and a second I.V. bolus of 180 mcg/kg given 10 minutes after the first bolus. Continue infusion until hospital discharge or for 18 to 24 hours, whichever comes first; the minimum duration of infusion is 12 hours.

Adjust-a-dose: If CrCl is less than 50 mL/minute, give 180 mcg/kg I.V. bolus just before the procedure, immediately followed by a continuous I.V. infusion at 1 mcg/kg/minute and a second bolus of 180 mcg/kg given 10 minutes after the first bolus.

ADMINISTRATION

I.V.

▼ Inspect solution for particles before use; if they appear, drug may not be sterile. Discard it.

▼ Protect drug from light before giving.

▼ Drug may be given in same line with normal saline solution, D_5W, alteplase, atropine, dobutamine, heparin, lidocaine, meperidine, metoprolol, midazolam, morphine, nitroglycerin, or verapamil. Main infusion may also contain up to 60 mEq/L of potassium chloride.

▼ For I.V. push, withdraw bolus dose from 10-mL vial into a syringe and give over 1 or 2 minutes.

▼ For infusion, give undiluted drug directly from 100-mL vial using an infusion pump.

▼ If patient needs thrombolytics, stop infusion.

▼ Refrigerate vials at 36° to 46° F (2° to 8° C). Store vials at room temperature for no longer than 2 months; afterward, discard them.

▼ **Incompatibilities:** Furosemide.

ACTION

Reversibly binds to the glycoprotein IIb/IIIa (GPIIb/IIIa) receptor on human platelets and inhibits platelet aggregation.

Route	Onset	Peak	Duration
I.V.	Immediate	Immediate	4–6 hr

Half-life: 2½ hours.

ADVERSE REACTIONS

CV: hypotension.

GU: hematuria.

Hematologic: *thrombocytopenia, major bleeding,* minor bleeding.

Other: bleeding at femoral artery access site.

INTERACTIONS

Drug-drug. *Clopidogrel, dipyridamole, NSAIDs, oral anticoagulants (warfarin), thrombolytics, ticlopidine:* May increase risk of bleeding. Monitor patient closely for signs of bleeding.

Other inhibitors of GPIIb/IIIa: May cause serious bleeding. Avoid using together.

EFFECTS ON LAB TEST RESULTS

● May decrease platelet count.

CONTRAINDICATIONS & CAUTIONS

● Contraindicated in patients hypersensitive to drug or its ingredients and in those with history of bleeding diathesis or evidence of active abnormal bleeding within previous 30 days; severe hypertension (systolic blood pressure higher than 200 mm Hg or diastolic blood pressure higher than 110 mm Hg) not adequately controlled with antihypertensives; major surgery within previous 6 weeks; history of stroke within 30 days or history of hemorrhagic stroke; current or planned use of another parenteral GPIIb/IIIa inhibitor; or platelet count less than 100,000/mm³.

● Contraindicated in patients with creatinine level of 4 mg/dL or higher and in patients dependent on renal dialysis.

● Use cautiously in patients at increased risk for bleeding, in those with platelet count less than 150,000/mm³, in those with hemorrhagic retinopathy, and in those weighing more than 143 kg (315 lb).

NURSING CONSIDERATIONS

• Drug is intended for use with heparin and aspirin.

• At least 4 hours before hospital discharge, stop this drug and heparin and achieve sheath hemostasis by standard compressive techniques.

• Remove sheath during infusion only after heparin has been stopped and its effects largely reversed.

• If patient is to have a CABG, stop infusion before surgery.

• Minimize use of arterial and venous punctures, I.M. injections, urinary catheters, and nasotracheal and nasogastric tubes.

• When obtaining I.V. access, avoid use of noncompressible sites (such as subclavian or jugular veins).

• Monitor patient for bleeding.

⊙ Alert: If patient's platelet count is less than 100,000/mm^3, stop this drug and heparin.

• Perform baseline laboratory tests before start of drug therapy; also determine hemoglobin level, hematocrit, PT, INR, activated PTT, platelet count, and creatinine level.

PATIENT TEACHING

• Advise patient to inform health care provider of all drugs and supplements he takes.

• Explain that drug is a blood thinner used to prevent chest pain and heart attack.

• Explain that benefits of drug far outweigh risk of serious bleeding.

• Tell patient to report to prescriber chest discomfort or other adverse effects immediately.

• Tell patient to report unusual bleeding, bruising, or blood in stools.

SAFETY ALERT!

eribulin mesylate
er-ih-BYOO-lin

Halaven

Therapeutic class: Antineoplastics
Pharmacologic class: Microtubule inhibitors
Pregnancy risk category: D

AVAILABLE FORMS
Injection: 1 mg/2-mL vial

INDICATIONS & DOSAGES

➤ **To treat metastatic breast cancer in patients who have received at least two chemotherapeutic regimens for the treatment of metastatic disease, and whose treatments have included an anthracycline and a taxane in either the adjuvant or metastatic setting**

Adults: 1.4 mg/m^2 I.V. over 2 to 5 minutes on days 1 and 8 of a 21-day cycle.

Adjust-a-dose: In mild hepatic impairment (Child-Pugh class A) and in patients with moderate renal impairment (CrCl of 30 to 50 mL/minute), give 1.1 mg/m^2 I.V. over 2 to 5 minutes on days 1 and 8 of a 21-day cycle. In moderate hepatic impairment (Child-Pugh class B), give 0.7 mg/m^2 I.V. over 2 to 5 minutes on days 1 and 8 of a 21-day cycle. If toxicities occur, refer to package insert for dosage adjustments.

ADMINISTRATION
I.V.

▼ Draw up required amount from vial and administer undiluted, or dilute in 100 mL normal saline solution.

▼ May store undiluted drug in a syringe or diluted solutions for 4 hours at room temperature or 24 hours if refrigerated.

▼ Discard unused portion of vial.

▼ **Incompatibilities:** Dextrose, other I.V. drugs.

ACTION
Causes cell death by inhibiting cell division.

Route	Onset	Peak	Duration
I.V.	Unknown	Unknown	Unknown

Half-life: About 40 hours.

ADVERSE REACTIONS
CNS: peripheral neuropathy, headache, asthenia, fatigue, pyrexia.
CV: *QT-interval prolongation,* peripheral edema.
EENT: increased lacrimation, mucosal inflammation.
GI: anorexia, dysgeusia, dyspepsia, abdominal pain, stomatitis, dry mouth, constipation, diarrhea, nausea, vomiting.
GU: UTI.

Hematologic: *neutropenia,* anemia.
Metabolic: weight loss, *hypokalemia.*
Musculoskeletal: muscle spasms, muscle weakness, arthralgia, myalgia, back pain, bone pain, pain in extremity.
Respiratory: upper respiratory tract infection, cough, dyspnea.
Skin: rash, alopecia.

INTERACTIONS
Drug-drug. *Class IA and III antiarrhythmics, other drugs known to prolong QT interval:* May further prolong QT interval. Use together cautiously and monitor patient carefully.
Disulfiram: May produce acute and severe alcohol intolerance. Avoid concurrent use and all ethanol-containing products during disulfiram therapy.
Live-virus vaccines: May increase risk of live-virus vaccine–induced adverse reactions. Concurrent use isn't recommended.

EFFECTS ON LAB TEST RESULTS
● May increase ALT and bilirubin levels. May decrease potassium level.
● May decrease hemoglobin level and neutrophil and platelet counts.

CONTRAINDICATIONS & CAUTIONS
● Contraindicated in patients hypersensitive to drug or its components.
● Avoid use in patients with existing congenital long QT syndrome.
● Use cautiously in patients with liver or renal insufficiency and in those at risk for neutropenia or peripheral motor or sensory neuropathy.
● Use cautiously in patients with congestive heart failure, bradyarrhythmias, or electrolyte imbalance and in those taking drugs known to prolong QT interval or with a history of prolonged QT interval.
● Use during pregnancy only if benefits outweigh risk and patient is aware of potential hazard to fetus.
● Safety and effectiveness in children haven't been established.
⚠ *Overdose S&S:* Neutropenia, hypersensitivity reaction.

NURSING CONSIDERATIONS
● Assess patient for peripheral neuropathy.
● Monitor patient for hypokalemia and hypomagnesemia before and periodically during therapy.
● Monitor patient for signs and symptoms of infection.
● Monitor blood counts and obtain CBC before each dose.
● Monitor liver and kidney function tests during therapy.
● Monitor ECG for changes, especially QT-interval prolongation.
● Consider prophylactic antiemetics for nausea and vomiting.

PATIENT TEACHING
● Tell patient to report a temperature of 100.5° F (38° C) or greater and other signs or symptoms of infection, such as chills, cough, or burning or pain on urination.
● Advise patient that drug may cause nerve damage and to contact prescriber if burning, tingling, or radiating pain occurs in any extremity.
● Caution patient to immediately report irregular heartbeat.
● Warn patient to avoid pregnancy and to use effective contraception during treatment.
● Tell patient to consult prescriber before breast-feeding.

SAFETY ALERT!

erlotinib
ur-LOE-tih-nib

Tarceva

Therapeutic class: Antineoplastics
Pharmacologic class: Epidermal growth factor receptor inhibitors
Pregnancy risk category: D

AVAILABLE FORMS
Tablets: 25 mg, 100 mg, 150 mg

INDICATIONS & DOSAGES
Adjust-a-dose (for all indications): In patients with severe skin reactions or severe diarrhea refractory to loperamide, reduce dose in 50-mg decrements or stop therapy.

In patients with severe hepatic impairment (AST greater than 3 times upper limit of normal [ULN]), reduce initial dose to 75 mg/day and gradually increase as tolerated. Interrupt therapy or discontinue drug if total bilirubin level doubles or transaminase levels triple when pretreatment levels are outside normal range. Interrupt therapy or discontinue drug if total bilirubin level is more than 3 times ULN or transaminase levels are 5 times ULN when pretreatment levels are within normal range.

➤ **With gemcitabine, first-line treatment of locally advanced, unresectable, or metastatic pancreatic cancer**
Adults: 100 mg P.O. once daily taken at least 1 hour before or 2 hours after meals. Continue until disease progresses or intolerable toxicity occurs.

➤ **Maintenance therapy for locally advanced or metastatic non–small-cell lung cancer (NSCLC) in patients whose disease hasn't progressed after four cycles of platinum-based, first-line chemotherapy; locally advanced or metastatic NSCLC after failure of at least one chemotherapy regimen**
Adults: 150 mg P.O. once daily at least 1 hour before or 2 hours after meals. Continue until disease progresses or intolerable toxicity occurs.

✹ *NEW INDICATION:* **Metastatic NSCLC in patients with tumors with epidermal growth factor receptor (EGFR) exon 19 deletions or exon 21 (L858R) substitution mutations as detected by an FDA-approved test**
Adults: 150 mg P.O. once daily at least 1 hour before or 2 hours after a meal. Continue until disease progresses or intolerable toxicity occurs.

ADMINISTRATION
P.O.
● Give drug 1 hour before or 2 hours after a meal.

ACTION
Probably inhibits tyrosine kinase activity in EGFRs, which are expressed on the surface of normal and cancer cells. Is particularly selective for human EGFR 1.

Route	Onset	Peak	Duration
P.O.	Unknown	4 hr	Unknown

Half-life: About 36 hours.

ADVERSE REACTIONS
CNS: fatigue, syncope, ***stroke,*** anxiety, depression, dizziness, headache, insomnia, neuropathies, pyrexia.
CV: arrhythmias, edema, ***MI, DVT.***
EENT: conjunctivitis, keratoconjunctivitis sicca.
GI: abdominal pain, anorexia, diarrhea, nausea, stomatitis, vomiting, constipation, dyspepsia, flatulence, ***pancreatitis.***
GU: renal insufficiency.
Hematologic: hemolytic anemia.
Metabolic: decreased weight.
Musculoskeletal: bone pain, myalgia.
Respiratory: cough, dyspnea, ***pulmonary toxicity.***
Skin: acne, dry skin, pruritus, rash, alopecia, paronychia.
Other: infection, rigors.

INTERACTIONS
Drug-drug. *Antacids, H$_2$-receptor antagonists, proton pump inhibitors:* May reduce bioavailability of drug. Separate doses by several hours.
Anticoagulants, such as warfarin: May increase risk of bleeding. Monitor PT and INR.
Ciprofloxacin: May increase erlotinib plasma concentration. Consider reducing erlotinib dosage if severe adverse reactions occur.
CYP3A4 inducers, such as carbamazepine, phenobarbital, phenytoin, rifabutin, rifampin: May increase erlotinib metabolism. Increase erlotinib dosage, as needed.
Strong CYP3A4 inhibitors, such as atazanavir, clarithromycin, indinavir, itraconazole, ketoconazole, nefazodone, nelfinavir, ritonavir, saquinavir, telithromycin, troleandomycin, voriconazole: May decrease erlotinib metabolism. Use together cautiously, and consider reducing erlotinib dosage.
Drug-food. *Any food:* May increase bioavailability of drug. Give drug 1 hour before or 2 hours after meals.

Grapefruit or grapefruit juice: May increase drug level. Avoid use together.

Drug-herb. *St. John's wort:* May increase drug metabolism. Drug dosage may need to be increased. Discourage use together.

Drug-lifestyle. *Cigarette smoking:* May decrease drug level. Encourage smoking cessation.

EFFECTS ON LAB TEST RESULTS
- May increase ALT, AST, and bilirubin levels.
- May increase INR and PT.

CONTRAINDICATIONS & CAUTIONS
- Use cautiously in patients with pulmonary disease or liver impairment. Also use cautiously in patients who have received or are receiving chemotherapy because it may worsen adverse pulmonary effects.
- Use cautiously in patients receiving other antiangiogenic agents, corticosteroids, NSAIDs, or taxane-based chemotherapy, and in those with a history of peptic ulcer disease because of increased risk of GI perforation.
- Interrupt therapy or discontinue drug in patients with acute or worsening ocular disorders and in those with dehydration at risk for renal failure.

⚠ *Overdose S&S:* Severe adverse reactions (such as diarrhea, ALT or AST elevation, rash).

NURSING CONSIDERATIONS
- Monitor renal function tests and LFTs periodically during therapy.
- ➍ *Alert:* GI perforation with fatalities has been reported. Permanently discontinue drug if GI perforation occurs.
- ➍ *Alert:* Rarely, serious interstitial lung disease may occur. If patient develops dyspnea, cough, and fever, notify prescriber. Therapy may need to be interrupted or stopped.
- Monitor patient for severe diarrhea, and give loperamide if needed.
- Monitor patient for eye ulcers, bullous blistering, and exfoliative skin conditions.
- Women shouldn't breast-feed while taking this drug.
- Drug has been used off label to treat squamous cell head and neck cancer.

PATIENT TEACHING
- ➍ *Alert:* Tell patient to immediately report new or worsened cough, shortness of breath, eye irritation, or severe or persistent diarrhea, nausea, anorexia, or vomiting.
- Instruct patient to take drug 1 hour before or 2 hours after food.
- Advise women to avoid pregnancy while taking this drug and for 2 weeks after treatment ends. Drug can harm fetus.
- Explain the likelihood of serious interactions with other drugs and herbal supplements and the need to tell prescriber about any change in drugs and supplements taken.
- Counsel patient about smoking cessation, as smoking may decrease drug level and effectiveness.

ertapenem sodium
er-tah-PEN-em

Invanz

Therapeutic class: Antibiotics
Pharmacologic class: Carbapenems
Pregnancy risk category: B

AVAILABLE FORMS
Injection: 1 g

INDICATIONS & DOSAGES
Adjust-a-dose (for all indications): In adult patients with CrCl of 30 mL/minute or less, give 500 mg/day. In hemodialysis patients receiving daily 500-mg dose less than 6 hours before hemodialysis, give supplementary 150-mg dose afterward. In hemodialysis patients receiving dose 6 hours or more before hemodialysis, no supplementary dose is needed.

➤ **Complicated intra-abdominal infection caused by** *Escherichia coli, Clostridium clostridioforme, Eubacterium lentum, Peptostreptococcus* **species,** *Bacteroides fragilis, B. distasonis, B. ovatus, B. thetaiotaomicron,* **or** *B. uniformis*
Adults and children age 13 and older: 1 g I.V. or I.M. once daily for 5 to 14 days.
Infants and children ages 3 months to 13 years: 15 mg/kg I.V. or I.M. every 12 hours for 5 to 14 days. Don't exceed 1 g daily.

E

➤ Complicated skin or skin-structure infection, including diabetic foot infections without osteomyelitis caused by *Staphylococcus aureus* (methicillin-susceptible strains), *Streptococcus agalactiae*, *Streptococcus pyogenes*, *E. coli*, *Klebsiella pneumoniae*, *Proteus mirabilis*, *B. fragilis*, *Peptostreptococcus* species, *Porphyromonas asaccharolytica*, or *Prevotella bivia*

Adults and children age 13 and older: 1 g I.V. or I.M. once daily for 7 to 14 days. Diabetic foot infections may need up to 28 days of treatment.

Infants and children ages 3 months to 13 years: 15 mg/kg I.V. or I.M. every 12 hours for 7 to 14 days. Don't exceed 1 g daily.

➤ Community-acquired pneumonia from *S. pneumoniae* (penicillin-susceptible strains), *Haemophilus influenzae* (beta-lactamase–negative strains), or *Moraxella catarrhalis;* complicated UTI, including pyelonephritis caused by *E. coli* or *K. pneumoniae*

Adults and children age 13 and older: 1 g I.V. or I.M. once daily for 10 to 14 days. If patient improves after at least 3 days of treatment, use appropriate oral therapy to complete the full course of therapy.

Infants and children ages 3 months to 13 years: 15 mg/kg I.V. or I.M. every 12 hours for 10 to 14 days. Don't exceed 1 g daily. If patient improves after at least 3 days of treatment, use appropriate oral therapy to complete the full course of therapy.

➤ Acute pelvic infection, including postpartum endomyometritis, septic abortion, and postsurgical gynecologic infections caused by *S. agalactiae, E. coli, B. fragilis, P. asaccharolytica, Peptostreptococcus* species, or *P. bivia*

Adults and children age 13 and older: 1 g I.V. or I.M. once daily for 3 to 10 days.

Infants and children ages 3 months to 13 years: 15 mg/kg I.V. or I.M. every 12 hours for 3 to 10 days. Don't exceed 1 g daily.

➤ Prevention of surgical site infection after elective colorectal surgery

Adults: 1 g I.V. 1 hour before surgical incision.

➤ Catheter-related bloodstream infections caused by gram-negative bacilli that are extended-spectrum beta-lactamase–positive, *Enterobacter* species, *Serratia marcescens*, and *Ochrobactrum anthropi* ◆

Adults: 1 g I.V. over 30 minutes once daily for up to 14 days.

➤ Hospital-acquired pneumonia, ventilator-associated pneumonia, and health care–associated pneumonia (as both empirical therapy in patients without known risk factors for multidrug-resistant pathogens and infections caused by extended-spectrum, beta-lactamase–producing gram-negative bacteria) ◆

Adults: 1 g I.V. daily over 30 minutes for 7 to 14 days.

ADMINISTRATION

I.V.

▼ Obtain specimens for culture and sensitivity testing before giving. Begin therapy while awaiting results.

▼ Before giving first dose, check for previous hypersensitivity to penicillin, cephalosporin, beta-lactam, or local amide-type anesthetics.

▼ Reconstitute 1-g vial with 10 mL of sterile water for injection, normal saline solution for injection, or bacteriostatic water for injection.

▼ Shake well to dissolve, and then immediately transfer contents to 50 mL of normal saline solution.

▼ Infuse over 30 minutes.

▼ Complete the infusion within 6 hours of reconstitution or refrigerate for up to 24 hours. Infuse within 4 hours once removed from refrigeration. Don't freeze.

▼ **Incompatibilities:** Diluents containing dextrose (alpha-D-glucose), other I.V. drugs.

I.M.

● Obtain specimens for culture and sensitivity testing before giving. Begin therapy while awaiting results.

● Before giving first dose, check for previous hypersensitivity to penicillin, cephalosporin, beta-lactam, or local amide-type anesthetics.

● Reconstitute 1-g vial with 3.2 mL of 1% lidocaine hydrochloride injection (without epinephrine). Shake vial thoroughly to form solution. Immediately withdraw the contents of the vial and give by deep I.M. injection into a large muscle, such as the gluteal muscles or lateral part of the thigh. Use the reconstituted I.M. solution within 1 hour after preparation. Don't give reconstituted solution I.V.

ACTION

Inhibits cell-wall synthesis through penicillin-binding proteins.

Route	Onset	Peak	Duration
I.V.	Immediate	30 min	24 hr
I.M.	Unknown	2 hr	24 hr

Half-life: 4 hours.

ADVERSE REACTIONS

CNS: altered mental status, anxiety, asthenia, dizziness, fatigue, fever, headache, insomnia.
CV: chest pain, edema, hypertension, hypotension, infused vein complication, phlebitis, swelling, tachycardia, thrombophlebitis.
EENT: pharyngitis.
GI: diarrhea, abdominal pain, acid regurgitation, constipation, dyspepsia, nausea, oral candidiasis, vomiting.
GU: renal dysfunction, vaginitis.
Hematologic: *leukopenia, neutropenia, thrombocytopenia,* anemia, coagulation abnormalities, eosinophilia, *thrombocytosis.*
Hepatic: jaundice.
Metabolic: *hyperkalemia, hypokalemia,* hyperglycemia.
Musculoskeletal: leg pain.
Respiratory: cough, dyspnea, rales, *respiratory distress,* rhonchi.
Skin: erythema, extravasation, infusion-site pain and redness, pruritus, rash.
Other: hypersensitivity reactions.

INTERACTIONS

Drug-drug. *Probenecid:* May reduce renal clearance and may increase half-life. Don't give together with probenecid to extend half-life.
Valproic acid: May decrease valproic acid levels, leading to loss of seizure control. Monitor valproic acid levels, and observe patient for signs of seizure activity.

EFFECTS ON LAB TEST RESULTS

● May increase albumin, ALT, alkaline phosphatase, AST, bilirubin, creatinine, glucose, and potassium levels. May decrease hemoglobin level and hematocrit.
● May increase eosinophil count, PT, and urine RBC or urine WBC counts. May decrease segmented neutrophil and serum WBC counts. May increase or decrease platelet count.

CONTRAINDICATIONS & CAUTIONS

● Contraindicated in patients hypersensitive to any component of the drug or to other drugs in the same class and in patients who have had anaphylactic reactions to beta-lactams. I.M. use is contraindicated in patients hypersensitive to local anesthetics of the amide type (because of drug's diluent, lidocaine hydrochloride).
● Use cautiously in patients with CNS disorders, compromised renal function, or both, as seizures may occur in these patients.
⚠ *Overdose S&S:* Nausea, diarrhea, dizziness.

NURSING CONSIDERATIONS

● If patient has diarrhea during therapy, notify prescriber and collect stool specimen for culture to rule out pseudomembranous colitis.
● Vomiting occurs more frequently in children than adults. Monitor children closely for signs and symptoms of dehydration and electrolyte imbalance.
● If allergic reaction occurs, stop drug immediately.
● Anaphylactic reactions require immediate emergency treatment with epinephrine, oxygen, I.V. steroids, and airway management.
● Anticonvulsants may continue in patients with seizure disorders. If focal tremors, myoclonus, or seizures occur, notify prescriber. Drug may need to be decreased or stopped.
● Monitor renal, hepatic, and hematopoietic function during prolonged therapy.
● Methicillin-resistant staphylococci and *Enterococcus* species are resistant to drug.
● *Look alike–sound alike:* Don't confuse Invanz with Avinza.

PATIENT TEACHING
● Tell patient about adverse reactions.
● Tell patient to alert nurse if discomfort occurs at injection site.
● Tell patient that diarrhea is common and to report diarrhea as soon as possible.

erythromycin (ophthalmic)
er-ith-roe-MYE-sin

Therapeutic class: Antibiotics
Pharmacologic class: Macrolides
Pregnancy risk category: B

AVAILABLE FORMS
Ophthalmic ointment: 0.5%

INDICATIONS & DOSAGES
➤ **Acute and chronic conjunctivitis, other eye infections**
Adults and children: Apply a ribbon of ointment about 1 cm long directly to infected eye up to six times daily, depending on severity of infection.
➤ **To prevent ophthalmia neonatorum caused by *Neisseria gonorrhoeae* or *Chlamydia trachomatis***
Neonates: Apply a ribbon of ointment about 1 cm long in lower conjunctival sac of each eye shortly after birth.

ADMINISTRATION
Ophthalmic
● Don't use for infection unless causative organism has been identified.
● To prevent ophthalmia neonatorum, apply ointment no later than 1 hour after birth. Use drug in neonates born either vaginally or by cesarean birth. Gently massage eyelids for 1 minute to spread ointment. Use new tube for each neonate.

ACTION
Inhibits protein synthesis; usually bacteriostatic, but may be bactericidal in high concentrations or against highly susceptible organisms.

Route	Onset	Peak	Duration
Ophthalmic	Unknown	Unknown	Unknown

Half-life: Unknown.

ADVERSE REACTIONS
EENT: minor ocular irritations, redness.
Other: hypersensitivity reactions.

INTERACTIONS
None significant.

EFFECTS ON LAB TEST RESULTS
● May interfere with fluorometric determinations of urine catecholamines.

CONTRAINDICATIONS & CAUTIONS
● Contraindicated in patients hypersensitive to drug.
● Use cautiously in breast-feeding women.

NURSING CONSIDERATIONS
● For infants born to mothers with clinically apparent gonorrhea, give I.V. or I.M. injections of aqueous crystalline penicillin G; a single dose of 50,000 units for term infants or 20,000 units for infants of low birth height.
● Store drug at room temperature in tightly closed, light-resistant container.

PATIENT TEACHING
● Tell patient to clean eye area of excessive discharge before application.
● Teach patient how to apply drug. Advise him to wash hands before and after applying ointment, and warn him not to touch tip of applicator to eye or surrounding tissue.
● Tell patient that vision may be blurred for a few minutes after applying ointment. Instruct patient to keep eyes closed for 1 to 2 minutes after applying drug.
● Advise patient to watch for and report signs and symptoms of sensitivity (itching lids, redness, swelling, or constant burning).
● Tell patient not to share drug, washcloths, or towels with family members and to notify prescriber if anyone develops same signs or symptoms.
● Stress importance of compliance with recommended therapy.

erythromycin (topical)
er-ith-roe-MYE-sin

Akne-mycin, Ery-Sol†, Erythra-Derm, Erythro-Statin

Therapeutic class: Antiacne drugs
Pharmacologic class: Macrolides
Pregnancy risk category: C (topical solution); B (other topical preparations)

AVAILABLE FORMS
Ointment: 2%
Pledgets: 2%
Topical gel: 2%
Topical solution: 2%*

INDICATIONS & DOSAGES
➤ **Inflammatory acne vulgaris**
Adults and children: Apply to affected areas b.i.d., morning and evening. If no improvement in 6 to 8 weeks, discontinue drug; prescriber should reevaluate treatment.

ADMINISTRATION
Topical
● Wash, rinse, and pat dry affected areas before application.
● Use pledget once, and then discard.
● Wash hands after each application.

ACTION
Usually bacteriostatic, but may be bactericidal in high concentrations or against highly susceptible organisms. Disrupts protein synthesis in susceptible bacteria.

Route	Onset	Peak	Duration
Topical	Unknown	Unknown	Unknown

Half-life: Unknown.

ADVERSE REACTIONS
Skin: burning, dryness, pruritus, erythema, irritation, oily skin, peeling, sensitivity reactions.

INTERACTIONS
Drug-drug. *Clindamycin:* May antagonize clindamycin's effect. Avoid using together.
Isotretinoin: May cause cumulative dryness, resulting in excessive skin irritation. Use together cautiously.

Drug-lifestyle. *Abrasive or medicated soaps or cleansers, acne products, or other preparations containing peeling drugs (benzoyl peroxide, resorcinol, salicylic acid, sulfur, tretinoin), alcohol-containing products (aftershave, cosmetics, perfumed toiletries, shaving creams or lotions), astringent soaps or cosmetics, medicated cosmetics or cover-ups:* May cause cumulative dryness, resulting in excessive skin irritation. Urge caution.

EFFECTS ON LAB TEST RESULTS
● May interfere with fluorometric determinations of urine catecholamines.

CONTRAINDICATIONS & CAUTIONS
● Contraindicated in patients hypersensitive to drug or its components.
● Safety and effectiveness in children haven't been established.

NURSING CONSIDERATIONS
● Prolonged use may be needed when treating acne vulgaris, which may result in overgrowth of nonsusceptible organisms.
۞ Alert: Pseudomembranous colitis has been reported with nearly all antibacterial agents. Consider this diagnosis in patients who present with diarrhea.

PATIENT TEACHING
● Advise patient to wash, rinse, and dry face thoroughly before each use.
● Advise patient to avoid use near eyes, nose, mouth, or other mucous membranes.
● Tell patient to wash hands after each application.
● Tell patient to stop using drug and notify prescriber if no improvement occurs or if condition worsens in 3 to 12 weeks.
● Advise patient not to share towels or washcloths.
● Instruct patient to use each pledget once, then discard.
● Caution patient to keep drug away from heat and open flame.

erythromycin base
er-ith-roe-MYE-sin

Apo-Erythro Base†, Apo-Erythro
E-C†, Erybid†, Eryc✐, Ery-Tab✐,
Erythromycin Delayed-Release,
Erythromycin Filmtabs, PCE

erythromycin ethylsuccinate
Apo-Erythro-ES†, E.E.S. Granules,
EryPed

erythromycin lactobionate
Erythrocin

erythromycin stearate
Apo-Erythro-S†, Erythrocin
Stearate

Therapeutic class: Antibiotics
Pharmacologic class: Macrolides
Pregnancy risk category: B

AVAILABLE FORMS
erythromycin base
Capsules (delayed-release): 250 mg
Tablets (enteric-coated): 250 mg, 333 mg,
500 mg
Tablets (filmtabs): 250 mg, 500 mg
erythromycin ethylsuccinate
Oral suspension: 200 mg/5 mL,
400 mg/5 mL
Powder for oral suspension: 200 mg/5 mL,
400 mg/5 mL
Tablets: 400 mg
erythromycin lactobionate
Injection: 500-mg, 1-g vials
erythromycin stearate
Tablets (film-coated): 250 mg

INDICATIONS & DOSAGES
➤ **Acute pelvic inflammatory disease
caused by *Neisseria gonorrhoeae***
Adults: 500 mg I.V. every 6 hours for 3 days;
then 500 mg P.O. every 12 hours or 333 mg
P.O. every 8 hours for 7 days.
➤ **Intestinal amebiasis caused by *Entamoeba histolytica***
Adults: 500 mg P.O. every 12 hours, 333 mg
P.O. every 8 hours, or 250 mg P.O. every
6 hours for 10 to 14 days.

Children: 30 to 50 mg/kg P.O. daily, in
divided doses, for 10 to 14 days.
➤ **To prevent rheumatic fever recurrence
in patients allergic to penicillin and sulfonamides**
Adults: 250 mg base or stearate P.O. b.i.d.,
or 400 mg ethylsuccinate P.O. b.i.d.
➤ **Mild to moderately severe respiratory
tract, skin, or soft-tissue infection from
sensitive group A beta-hemolytic streptococci, *Streptococcus pneumoniae, Mycoplasma pneumoniae, Corynebacterium
diphtheriae,* or *Bordetella pertussis; Listeria monocytogenes* infection**
Adults: 250 mg P.O. every 6 hours, 333 mg
P.O. every 8 hours, or 500 mg P.O. every
12 hours. Maximum dose is 4 g daily. Or
15 to 20 mg/kg I.V. daily, as continuous infusion or in divided doses every 6 hours for
10 days (3 weeks for *Mycoplasma* species
infection). Maximum dosage is 4 g/day.
Children: 30 to 50 mg/kg P.O. daily, in
divided doses every 6 hours; or 15 to
20 mg/kg I.V. daily, in divided doses
every 4 to 6 hours for 10 days (3 weeks
for *Mycoplasma* species infection).
➤ **Nongonococcal urethritis caused by
*Ureaplasma urealyticum***
Adults: 500 mg P.O. every 6 hours or 666 mg
P.O. every 8 hours for at least 7 days.
➤ **Legionnaires disease**
Adults: 1 to 4 g P.O. daily in divided doses
for 10 to 14 days alone or with rifampin. I.V.
route may be used initially in severe cases.
➤ **Uncomplicated urethral, endocervical,
or rectal infection caused by *Chlamydia
trachomatis,* when tetracyclines are contraindicated**
Adults: 500 mg base P.O. q.i.d. for at least
7 days, or 666 mg P.O. every 8 hours for
at least 7 days, or 250 mg P.O. q.i.d. for
14 days if patient can't tolerate higher doses.
➤ **Urogenital *C. trachomatis* infection
during pregnancy**
Adults: 500 mg base or stearate P.O. q.i.d.
for at least 7 days or 250 mg base or stearate
or 400 mg ethylsuccinate P.O. q.i.d. for at
least 14 days.
➤ **Conjunctivitis of the newborn caused
by *C. trachomatis***
Neonates: 50 mg/kg/day P.O. in divided
doses for at least 2 weeks.

E

➤ **Pneumonia in infants caused by**
C. trachomatis
Infants: 50 mg/kg/day base or stearate P.O. in four divided doses for 21 days, or 15 to 20 mg/kg/day lactobionate I.V. as a continuous infusion or in four divided doses.

➤ **Pertussis**
Adults: 40 to 50 mg/kg/day P.O. in divided doses for 5 to 14 days.

➤ **Preoperative prophylaxis for elective colorectal surgery**
Adults: Two 500-mg tablets, three 333-mg tablets, or four 250-mg tablets P.O. at 1 p.m., 2 p.m., and 11 p.m. on preoperative day 1 before 8 a.m. surgery.

➤ **Primary syphilis**
Adults: 30 to 40 g base or stearate P.O. or 48 to 64 g ethylsuccinate P.O. in divided doses for 10 to 15 days.

➤ **Chancroid caused by** *Haemophilus*
ducreyi ◆
Adults: 500 mg base P.O. t.i.d. for 7 days.

➤ **Granuloma inguinale** ◆
Adults: 500 mg q.i.d. for at least 3 weeks; continue treatment until all lesions have completely heated.

➤ **Acne vulgaris** ◆
Adults and children: 333 mg P.O. t.i.d. for 4 weeks, followed by 333 mg P.O. once daily for 8 weeks.

ADMINISTRATION
P.O.
● Obtain specimen for culture and sensitivity tests before giving. Begin therapy while awaiting results.
● When giving suspension, note the concentration.
● Give drug with full glass of water 2 hours before or 2 hours after meals for best absorption.
● Give drug with food if GI upset occurs. Don't give drug with fruit juice. Make sure patient doesn't swallow chewable tablets whole.
● Coated tablets or encapsulated pellets cause less GI upset, so they may be better tolerated by patients who have trouble tolerating drug.
I.V.
▼ Obtain specimen for culture and sensitivity tests before giving. Begin therapy while awaiting results.

▼ Reconstitute drug according to manufacturer's directions.
▼ Dilute each 250 mg in at least 100 mL of normal saline solution.
▼ Infuse over 1 hour.
▼ **Incompatibilities:** Ascorbic acid injection, colistimethate, dextrose 2.5% in half-strength lactated Ringer solution, dextrose 5% in lactated Ringer solution, dextrose 5% in normal saline solution, dextrose 5% in Normosol-M, dextrose 10% in water, D_5W, furosemide, heparin sodium, linezolid, metoclopramide, Normosol-R, Ringer injection, vitamin B complex with C.

ACTION
Inhibits bacterial protein synthesis by binding to the 50S subunit of the ribosome. Bacteriostatic or bactericidal, depending on concentration.

Route	Onset	Peak	Duration
P.O.	Unknown	1½ hr	Unknown
I.V.	Immediate	1½ hr	Unknown

Half-life: 1½ hours.

ADVERSE REACTIONS
CNS: fever.
CV: vein irritation or thrombophlebitis after I.V. injection, *ventricular arrhythmias.*
GI: *pseudomembranous colitis,* abdominal pain and cramping, diarrhea, nausea, vomiting.
Hepatic: hepatic dysfunction.
Skin: eczema, rash, urticaria.
Other: *anaphylaxis,* overgrowth of nonsusceptible bacteria or fungi.

INTERACTIONS
Drug-drug. *Azole antifungals (ketoconazole):* May increase erythromycin concentrations, leading to increased risk of adverse reactions, including sudden death from cardiac causes. Avoid use together.
Carbamazepine: May inhibit metabolism of carbamazepine, increasing blood level and risk of toxicity. Avoid using together.
Clindamycin, lincomycin: May be antagonistic. Avoid using together.
Clopidogrel: May inhibit antiplatelet effect of clopidogrel. Monitor platelet function

---

Reactions in bold italics are *life-threatening*. Interactions may have a *rapid onset* or a *delayed onset*.

when starting or stopping erythromycin.
Adjust clopidogrel dosage as needed.
Colchicine: May increase colchicine level
and risk of colchicine-related adverse reactions. Use cautiously and monitor patient for
colchicine-related toxicity.
Cyclosporine: May increase cyclosporine
level. Monitor drug level.
Digoxin: May increase digoxin level. Monitor patient for digoxin toxicity.
Disopyramide: May increase disopyramide
level, which may cause arrhythmias and
prolonged QT intervals. Monitor ECG.
Ergot alkaloids: May cause acute ergot
toxicity with severe peripheral vasospasm
and dysesthesias. Monitor carefully.
Fluoroquinolones, *other drugs that prolong
the QTc interval (amiodarone, antipsychotics,
procainamide, quinidine, sotalol, TCAs):*
May have additive effects. Monitor ECG
for QTc interval prolongation. Avoid using
together, if possible.
*HMG-CoA reductase inhibitors (lovastatin,
simvastatin):* May increase concentrations
of HMG-CoA reductase inhibitors; rhabdomyolysis has occurred rarely. Monitor CK
and serum transaminase levels.
Midazolam, triazolam: May increase effects
of these drugs. Monitor patient closely.
Oral anticoagulants: May increase anticoagulant effect. Monitor PT and INR closely.
Rifamycins (rifabutin, rifampin, rifapentine):
May decrease therapeutic effects of erythromycin while increasing adverse effects
of rifamycin. Monitor patient.
*Strong CYP3A inhibitors (such as diltiazem,
verapamil, troleandomycin):* May increase
the risk of sudden death from cardiac
causes. Don't use together.
Theophylline: May decrease erythromycin
level and increase theophylline toxicity. Use
together cautiously.
Drug-herb. *Pill-bearing spurge:* May
inhibit CYP3A enzymes, affecting drug
metabolism. Urge caution.
Drug-food. *Any food:* Can delay absorption;
don't give within 2 hours of a meal.
Grapefruit juice: May inhibit drug's
metabolism; caution patient to avoid grapefruit juice during therapy.

EFFECTS ON LAB TEST RESULTS

● May increase alkaline phosphatase, ALT,
AST, and bilirubin levels.
● May interfere with fluorometric determination of urine catecholamines and with
colorimetric assays.

CONTRAINDICATIONS & CAUTIONS

● Contraindicated in those hypersensitive to
drug or other macrolides.
● Use erythromycin salts cautiously in
patients with impaired hepatic function.
● May cause infantile hypertrophic pyloric
stenosis (HPS) requiring surgery. Benefit of
therapy needs to be weighed against risk of
developing HPS.
● Prolonged or repeated use may result in
superinfection. If superinfection occurs,
discontinue drug.
● Drug appears in breast milk. Use cautiously in breast-feeding women.
● Don't use drug to treat neurosyphilis.

NURSING CONSIDERATIONS

● Monitor patient for superinfection. Drug
may cause overgrowth of nonsusceptible
bacteria or fungi.
● Monitor hepatic function. Drug may cause
hepatotoxicity.
● Elderly patients may be more at risk for
developing drug-induced hearing loss.
Monitor patient for new hearing loss.

PATIENT TEACHING

● Tell patient to take drug as prescribed,
even after he feels better.
● Instruct patient to take oral form of drug
with full glass of water 2 hours before or
2 hours after meals for best absorption.
● Drug may be taken with food if GI upset
occurs. Tell patient not to take drug with
fruit juice or to swallow the chewable tablets
whole.
● Instruct patient to report adverse reactions, especially nausea, abdominal pain,
vomiting, and fever.
● Instruct parents or caregivers to report
vomiting or irritability immediately.

E

escitalopram oxalate
ess-si-TAL-oh-pram

Lexapro◆

Therapeutic class: Antidepressants
Pharmacologic class: SSRIs
Pregnancy risk category: C

AVAILABLE FORMS
Oral solution: 5 mg/5 mL
Tablets: 5 mg, 10 mg, 20 mg

INDICATIONS & DOSAGES
Adjust-a-dose (for all indications): For elderly patients and those with hepatic impairment, 10 mg P.O. daily, initially and as maintenance dosages. In pregnant patients, consider tapering dosage in the third trimester.
➤ **Treatment and maintenance therapy for patients with major depressive disorder**
Adults and adolescents: Initially, 10 mg P.O. once daily, increasing to 20 mg if needed after at least 1 week.
➤ **Generalized anxiety disorder**
Adults: Initially, 10 mg P.O. once daily, increasing to 20 mg if needed after at least 1 week.
➤ **Posttraumatic stress disorder (PTSD)** ◆
Adults: 10 mg P.O. once daily. Increase to 20 mg once daily after 4 weeks. Consider tapering, over 2 weeks to 1 month, after 6 to 12 months in patients with acute PTSD, after 12 to 24 months in patients with chronic PTSD who have had an excellent response to therapy, and after at least 24 months in patients with chronic PTSD and residual symptoms.

ADMINISTRATION
P.O.
• Give drug without regard for food.

ACTION
Action may be linked to increase of serotonergic activity in the CNS from inhibition of neuronal reuptake of serotonin. Drug is closely related to citalopram, which may be the active component.

Route	Onset	Peak	Duration
P.O.	Unknown	5 hr	Unknown

Half-life: 27 to 32 hours.

ADVERSE REACTIONS
CNS: ***suicidal behavior,*** fever, insomnia, dizziness, somnolence, paresthesia, lightheadedness, migraine, tremor, vertigo, abnormal dreams, irritability, impaired concentration, fatigue, lethargy.
CV: palpitations, hypertension, flushing, chest pain.
EENT: rhinitis, sinusitis, blurred vision, tinnitus, earache.
GI: nausea, diarrhea, constipation, indigestion, abdominal pain, vomiting, increased or decreased appetite, dry mouth, flatulence, heartburn, cramps, gastroesophageal reflux.
GU: ejaculation disorder, erectile dysfunction, anorgasmia, menstrual cramps, UTI, urinary frequency.
Metabolic: weight gain or loss, hyponatremia.
Musculoskeletal: arthralgia, myalgia, muscle cramps, pain in arms or legs.
Respiratory: bronchitis, cough.
Skin: rash, increased sweating.
Other: decreased libido, yawning, flulike symptoms.

INTERACTIONS
Drug-drug. *Antiparkinsonians (such as rasagiline, selegiline):* May cause serotonin syndrome. Avoid use together.
Aspirin, NSAIDs, other drugs known to affect coagulation: May increase the risk of bleeding. Use together cautiously.
Beta blockers: May cause bradycardia and increase risk of CNS toxicity. Monitor patient closely.
Boceprevir, telaprevir: May decrease escitalopram concentration. Monitor clinical response and adjust escitalopram dosage as needed.
Buspirone, methylphenidate: May increase risk of serotonin syndrome. Monitor patient closely.
Carbamazepine: May increase escitalopram clearance. Monitor patient for expected antidepressant effect and adjust dose as needed.

Reactions in bold italics are *life-threatening*. Interactions may have a *rapid onset* or a *delayed onset*.

Cimetidine: May increase escitalopram level. Monitor patient for increased adverse reactions to escitalopram.

Citalopram: May cause additive effects. Using together is contraindicated.

CNS drugs: May cause additive effects. Use together cautiously.

Desipramine, other drugs metabolized by CYP2D6: May increase levels of these drugs. Use together cautiously.

Linezolid, methylene blue: May cause serotonin syndrome. Use extreme caution and monitor closely.

Lithium: May enhance serotonergic effect of escitalopram. Use together cautiously, and monitor lithium level.

MAO inhibitors: May cause fatal serotonin syndrome or signs and symptoms resembling neuroleptic malignant syndrome. Avoid using within 14 days of MAO inhibitor therapy.

Triptans: May increase serotonergic effects, leading to weakness, hyperreflexia, incoordination, rapid changes in blood pressure, nausea, and diarrhea. Use together cautiously, especially at the start of therapy or at dosage increases.

Tramadol: May cause serotonin syndrome. Monitor patient closely.

Drug-herb. *St. John's wort:* May cause serotonin syndrome. Use with caution.

Drug-lifestyle. *Alcohol use:* May increase CNS effects. Discourage use together.

EFFECTS ON LAB TEST RESULTS
None reported.

CONTRAINDICATIONS & CAUTIONS
• Contraindicated in patients taking pimozide, MAO inhibitors, or within 14 days of MAO inhibitor therapy and in those hypersensitive to escitalopram, citalopram, or any of its inactive ingredients.

Black Box Warning Escitalopram isn't approved for use in children age 11 and younger. ■

☉ Alert: Concomitant use with methylene blue or linezolid can cause serotonin syndrome (fever, mental status changes, muscle twitching, sweating, shivering, shaking, diarrhea, loss of coordination). Use drug with methylene blue or linezolid only for life-threatening or urgent conditions when the potential benefits outweigh the risks of toxicity.

☉ Alert: If linezolid or methylene blue must be given, the serotonergic drug must be stopped and the patient should be monitored for serotonin toxicity for 2 weeks or until 24 hours after the last dose of methylene blue or linezolid, whichever comes first. Treatment with serotonergic drugs may be resumed 24 hours after the last dose of methylene blue or linezolid.

• Use cautiously in patients with a history of mania, seizure disorders, suicidal thoughts, or renal or hepatic impairment.

• Use cautiously in patients with diseases that produce altered metabolism or hemodynamic responses.

• Use with caution in elderly patients because they may have greater sensitivity to drug.

• Use in third trimester of pregnancy may cause complications at birth. Consider the risk versus benefit of treatment during this time.

• Drug appears in breast milk. Patient should either stop breast-feeding or stop taking drug.

⚠ Overdose S&S: Seizures, coma, dizziness, ECG changes, hypotension, insomnia, nausea, sinus tachycardia, somnolence, vomiting, acute renal failure.

NURSING CONSIDERATIONS
Black Box Warning Drug may increase risk of suicidal thinking and behavior in children, adolescents, and young adults ages 18 to 24, especially during the first few months of treatment, especially in those with major depressive disorder or other psychiatric disorder. ■

• Closely monitor patients at high risk of suicide.

• Evaluate patient for history of drug abuse, and observe for signs of misuse or abuse.

• Periodically reassess patient to determine need for maintenance treatment and appropriate dosing.

☉ Alert: Combining triptans with an SSRI or an SSNRI may cause serotonin syndrome or neuroleptic malignant syndrome–like reactions. Serotonin syndrome may be more likely to occur when starting or increasing the dose of triptan, SSRI, or SSNRI.

E

● **Look alike–sound alike:** Don't confuse
escitalopram with estazolam.

PATIENT TEACHING
● Inform patient that symptoms should
improve gradually over several weeks, rather
than immediately.
● Tell patient that although improvement
may occur within 1 to 4 weeks, he should
continue drug as prescribed.
Black Box Warning Caution patient and
patient's family to report signs of worsening
depression (such as agitation, irritability, insomnia, hostility, impulsivity) and
signs of suicidal behavior to prescriber
immediately. ■
❸ Alert: Teach patient to recognize and immediately report symptoms of serotonin
toxicity (fever, mental status changes, muscle twitching, excessive sweating, shivering
or shaking, diarrhea, loss of coordination).
● Tell patient to use caution while driving
or operating hazardous machinery because
of drug's potential to impair judgment,
thinking, and motor skills.
● Advise patient to consult health care
provider before taking other prescription or
OTC drugs.
● Tell patient that drug may be taken in the
morning or evening without regard to meals.
● Encourage patient to avoid alcohol while
taking drug.
● Tell women to notify health care provider
if pregnant or breast-feeding.

SAFETY ALERT!

esmolol hydrochloride
ESS-moe-lol

Brevibloc

Therapeutic class: Antiarrhythmics
Pharmacologic class: Selective beta
blockers
Pregnancy risk category: C

AVAILABLE FORMS
Injection: 10 mg/mL
Premixed bags in sodium chloride:
10 mg/mL in 100-mL bags; 20 mg/mL in
100-mL bags

INDICATIONS & DOSAGES
➤ **Supraventricular tachycardia; non-
compensatory sinus tachycardias**
Adults: 500 mcg/kg/minute as loading
dose by I.V. infusion over 1 minute;
then 4-minute maintenance infusion of
50 mcg/kg/minute. If adequate response
doesn't occur within 5 minutes, may repeat loading dose and follow with maintenance infusion of 100 mcg/kg/minute for
4 minutes. May repeat loading dose and
increase maintenance infusion by increments of 50 mcg/kg/minute. Maximum
maintenance infusion for tachycardia is
200 mcg/kg/minute.
➤ **Intraoperative and postoperative
tachycardia or hypertension**
Adults: For immediate control: 1 mg/kg
as a bolus dose over 30 seconds, followed
by 150 mcg/kg/minute I.V. infusion, if
needed. Maximum dose for tachycardia
is 200 mcg/kg/minute; maximum dose
for hypertension is 300 mcg/kg/minute.
For gradual control (stepwise dosing):
Loading dose is 500 mcg/kg over
1 minute, then 50 mcg/kg/minute for
4 minutes. Optional loading dose if needed,
then 100 mcg/kg/minute for 4 minutes.
Optional loading dose if needed, then
150 mcg/kg/minute for 4 minutes. If necessary, may increase to 200 mcg/kg/minute.
Maximum doses are 200 mcg/kg/minute
for tachycardia and 300 mcg/kg/minute for
hypertension.
➤ **Hypertensive emergency ♦**
Children ages 1 to 17: 100 to 500 mcg/kg/
minute by I.V. infusion.
➤ **Cardiac risk reduction during surgery ♦**
Adults: Start therapy at standard doses well
before planned procedure, titrated by heart
rate. Drug is usually continued for 7 to
30 days postoperatively.

ADMINISTRATION
I.V.
▼ Don't dilute 10-mg/mL single-dose,
ready-to-use vials.
▼ Give with an infusion-control device
rather than by I.V. push.
▼ If concentration exceeds 10 mg/mL, give
drug through a central line.
▼ Don't use for longer than 48 hours.
Watch infusion site carefully for signs of

Reactions in bold italics are *life-threatening*. Interactions may have a *rapid onset* or a *delayed onset*.

extravasation; if they occur, stop infusion immediately and call prescriber.

▼ **Incompatibilities:** Amphotericin B cholesteryl sulfate complex, diazepam, furosemide, procainamide, sodium bicarbonate 5%, thiopental sodium, warfarin sodium.

ACTION

A class II antiarrhythmic and ultra–short-acting selective beta blocker that decreases heart rate, contractility, and blood pressure.

Route	Onset	Peak	Duration
I.V.	Immediate	30 min	30 min after infusion

Half-life: About 9 minutes.

ADVERSE REACTIONS

CNS: dizziness, somnolence, headache, agitation, confusion.
CV: hypotension, peripheral ischemia.
GI: nausea, vomiting.
Skin: inflammation or induration at infusion site.

INTERACTIONS

Drug-drug. *Antidiabetic agents:* May increase blood glucose–lowering effect of antidiabetic agent. Closely monitor blood glucose concentration.
Calcium channel blockers (diltiazem, nicardipine, nifedipine, verapamil), flecainide: May potentiate pharmacologic effects of both drugs. I.V. administration in close proximity is contraindicated. Monitor cardiac function closely and adjust therapy as needed.
Clonidine: May cause life-threatening blood pressure increases. Closely monitor blood pressure. Discontinue either agent gradually, preferably esmolol first.
Digoxin: May increase digoxin level by 10% to 20%. Monitor digoxin level.
Lidocaine: May increase lidocaine concentration. Monitor patient closely and adjust dosage as needed.
MAO inhibitors: May worsen bradycardia or hypertension. Discontinue esmolol or reduce esmolol dosage if needed.
Morphine: May increase esmolol level. Adjust esmolol dosage carefully.

NSAIDs: May impair antihypertensive effect of esmolol. Monitor blood pressure and adjust esmolol dosage as needed.
Prazosin: May increase risk of orthostatic hypertension. Help patient to stand slowly until effects are known.
Reserpine, other catecholamine-depleting drugs: May increase bradycardia and hypertension. Adjust esmolol dosage carefully.
Salicylates (aspirin): May impair antihypertensive effect of esmolol. Monitor patient and consider alternative therapy as needed.
Succinylcholine: May prolong neuromuscular blockade. Monitor patient closely.
Vasoconstrictive and positive inotropic agents (dopamine, epinephrine, norepinephrine): May increase risk of reduced cardiac contractility in presence of high systemic vascular resistance. Don't use together.
Verapamil: May increase effects of both drugs. Monitor cardiac function closely and decrease dosages as necessary.

EFFECTS ON LAB TEST RESULTS
None reported.

CONTRAINDICATIONS & CAUTIONS
• Contraindicated in patients with sinus bradycardia, second- or third-degree heart block, cardiogenic shock, or overt heart failure.
• Use cautiously in patients with renal impairment, diabetes, or bronchospasm.
⚠ *Overdose S&S:* Bradycardia, hypotension, loss of consciousness, cardiac arrest, pulseless electrical activity.

NURSING CONSIDERATIONS
• Dosage for postoperative treatment of tachycardia and hypertension is same as for supraventricular tachycardia.
✿ *Alert:* Monitor ECG and blood pressure continuously during infusion. Nearly half of patients will develop hypotension. Diaphoresis and dizziness may accompany hypotension. Monitor patient closely, especially if he had low blood pressure before treatment.
• Hypotension can usually be reversed within 30 minutes by decreasing the dose or, if needed, by stopping the infusion. Notify prescriber if this becomes necessary.

• If a local reaction develops at the infusion site, change to another site. Avoid using butterfly needles.
• When patient's heart rate becomes stable, replace drug with an alternative antiarrhythmic, such as propranolol, digoxin, or verapamil. Reduce infusion rate by half 30 minutes after the first dose of the new drug. Monitor patient response and, if heart rate is controlled for 1 hour after administration of the second dose of the replacement drug, stop esmolol infusion.

PATIENT TEACHING
• Instruct patient to report adverse reactions promptly.
• Tell patient to report discomfort at I.V. site.

esomeprazole magnesium
ess-oh-ME-pray-zol

Nexium◆

esomeprazole sodium
Nexium I.V.

esomeprazole strontium

Therapeutic class: Antiulcer drugs
Pharmacologic class: Proton pump inhibitors
Pregnancy risk category: B (esomeprazole magnesium, esomeprazole sodium); C (esomeprazole strontium)

AVAILABLE FORMS
esomeprazole magnesium
Capsules (delayed-release): 20 mg, 40 mg
Powder for suspension (delayed-release): 2.5 mg, 5 mg, 10 mg, 20 mg, 40 mg
esomeprazole sodium
Powder for injection: 20-mg, 40-mg single-use vials
esomeprazole strontium
Capsules (delayed-release): 24.65 mg, 49.3 mg

INDICATIONS & DOSAGES
Adjust-a-dose (for all indications): For patients with severe hepatic failure, maximum daily dose is 20 mg.

➤ **GERD; to heal erosive esophagitis**
Adults: 20 or 40 mg P.O. daily for 4 to 8 weeks. Maintenance dose for healing erosive esophagitis is 20 mg P.O. for up to 6 months.
Children ages 1 to 11 weighing less than 20 kg (44 lb): 10 mg P.O. once daily for up to 8 weeks.
Children ages 1 to 11 weighing 20 kg or more: 10 or 20 mg P.O. once daily for up to 8 weeks.
➤ **Symptomatic GERD**
Adults: 20 mg P.O. daily for 4 weeks. If symptoms are unresolved, may continue treatment for 4 more weeks. Or, 24.65 mg or 49.3 mg (delayed-release) P.O. once daily for 4 to 8 weeks.
Children and adolescents ages 12 to 17: 20 mg P.O. once daily for up to 4 weeks.
Children ages 1 to 11: 10 mg P.O. once daily for up to 8 weeks.
➤ **Short-term therapy (up to 10 days) of GERD in patients with a history of erosive esophagitis who are unable to take drug orally**
Adult: Reconstitute 20 or 40 mg with 5 mL of D₅W, normal saline solution, or lactated Ringer injection and give by I.V. bolus over 3 minutes. Or, further dilute to a total volume of 50 mL and give I.V. over 10 to 30 minutes. Switch patient to oral therapy as soon as he can tolerate it.
Children ages 1 to 17 weighing 55 kg (121 lb) or more: 20 mg I.V. infusion once daily over 10 to 30 minutes.
Children ages 1 to 17 weighing less than 55 kg: 10 mg I.V. infusion once daily over 10 to 30 minutes.
Children ages 1 month to younger than 1 year: 0.5 mg/kg I.V. infusion once daily over 10 to 30 minutes.
➤ **Erosive esophagitis due to acid-mediated GERD only**
Infants ages 1 to 11 months weighing more than 7.5 to 12 kg (17 to 26 lb): 10 mg P.O. once daily for up to 6 weeks.
Infants ages 1 to 11 months weighing more than 5 to 7.5 kg (11 to 17 lb): 5 mg P.O. once daily for up to 6 weeks.
Infants ages 1 to 11 months weighing 3 to 5 kg (7 to 11 lb): 2.5 mg P.O. once daily for up to 6 weeks.

Reactions in bold italics are *life-threatening*. Interactions may have a *rapid onset* or a ***delayed onset***.

E

➤ **To reduce the risk of gastric ulcers in patients receiving continuous NSAID therapy**

Adults: 20 or 40 mg P.O. once daily for up to 6 months. Or, 24.65 or 49.3 mg (delayed-release) P.O. once daily for up to 6 months.

➤ **Long-term treatment of pathologic hypersecretory conditions, including Zollinger-Ellison syndrome**

Adults: 40 mg P.O. b.i.d. Adjust dosage based on patient response. Or, 49.3 mg (delayed-release) P.O. b.i.d.

➤ **To eliminate *Helicobacter pylori***

Adults: 40 mg esomeprazole magnesium or 49.3 mg (delayed-release) P.O. daily, 1,000 mg amoxicillin P.O. b.i.d., and 500 mg clarithromycin P.O. b.i.d., given together for 10 days to reduce duodenal ulcer recurrence.

ADMINISTRATION
P.O.

● Give drug at least 1 hour before meals. If patient has difficulty swallowing the capsule, contents of the capsule can be emptied and mixed with 1 tablespoon of applesauce and swallowed (without chewing the enteric-coated pellets).

● If giving capsule via nasogastric (NG) tube, open capsule and empty the granules into a 60-mL syringe. Mix with 50 mL of water. Replace the plunger and shake vigorously for 15 seconds. Flush NG tube with additional water after use. Don't give if pellets have dissolved or disintegrated.

● For oral suspension, mix contents of a 2.5- or 5-mg packet with 5 mL of water; mix contents of a 10-, 20-, or 40-mg packet with 15 mL of water. Then let it sit for 2 to 3 minutes to thicken. Stir the suspension and drink within 30 minutes.

● To give oral suspension via NG tube, add 5 mL of water to a syringe, then add contents of 2.5- or 5-mg packet; or add 15 mL of water to a syringe, then add contents of 10-, 20-, or 40-mg packet. Shake syringe and leave for 2 to 3 minutes to thicken. Shake syringe again and inject through NG or gastric tube within 30 minutes.

I.V.

▼ Flush I.V. line with D$_5$W, normal saline solution, or lactated Ringer injection before and after administration.

▼ Use reconstituted solution within 12 hours.

▼ Use admixture diluted with D$_5$W within 6 hours.

▼ If diluted with normal saline solution or lactated Ringer injection, use within 12 hours.

▼ Store reconstituted solution and admixture at room temperature.

▼ **Incompatibilities:** Other I.V. drugs.

ACTION

Reduces gastric acid secretion and decreases gastric acidity.

Route	Onset	Peak	Duration
P.O.	Unknown	1½ hr	13–17 hr
I.V.	Unknown	Unknown	Unknown

Half-life: 1 to 1½ hours.

ADVERSE REACTIONS

CNS: headache, dizziness.
GI: abdominal pain, constipation, diarrhea, dry mouth, flatulence, nausea, vomiting.
Skin: pruritus.

INTERACTIONS

Drug-drug. *Azole antifungals (such as itraconazole, ketoconazole):* May decrease bioavailability of antifungal. Avoid use together.

Azole antifungals (such as voriconazole): May significantly increase esomeprazole level. Adjust dosage in patients receiving higher doses.

Calcium salts (calcium carbonate): May interfere with GI absorption of calcium salts. Closely monitor clinical response to calcium; larger dosages of calcium may be needed.

Cilostazol: May increase concentrations of cilostazol and its active metabolite. Consider a cilostazol dose reduction when esomeprazole is given concurrently.

Clopidogrel: May decrease antiplatelet activity. Use esomeprazole magnesium or esomeprazole sodium cautiously with clopidogrel. Avoid concomitant use with esomeprazole strontium.

Clozapine: May increase clozapine plasma concentration and risk of toxicity. Closely monitor clinical status and laboratory values.

Diazepam: May decrease clearance of diazepam. Monitor patient for diazepam toxicity.

Digoxin: May increase serum digoxin level. Monitor digoxin concentration and clinical response. If an interaction is suspected, adjust digoxin dosage as needed.

Drugs metabolized by CYP2C19: May alter clearance of esomeprazole, especially in elderly patients or patients with hepatic insufficiency. Monitor patient for toxicity.

Fluvoxamine: May increase risk of adverse reactions. Use cautiously.

Iron salts (ferrous sulfate): May interfere with absorption of iron salts. Temporary cessation of esomeprazole may be required to achieve appropriate clinical response to oral iron. If stopping esomeprazole isn't an option, parenteral iron may be a suitable alternative.

Macrolide antibiotics (clarithromycin): May increase esomeprazole level. Monitor patient for toxicity.

Methotrexate: May increase methotrexate concentration and risk of toxicity. Monitor patient closely.

Mycophenolate: May decrease mycophenolate plasma concentration and pharmacologic effects. Monitor clinical response and adjust mycophenolate dosage as needed.

Protease inhibitors (atazanavir, nelfinavir, saquinavir): May reduce plasma levels of atazanavir or nelfinavir. Use together isn't recommended. May increase saquinavir levels. Monitor carefully and reduce dosage if needed.

Rifampin: May decrease esomeprazole levels. Avoid using together.

Rilpivirine: May cause loss of virologic response or resistance. Use together is contraindicated.

Tacrolimus: May increase pharmacologic effects of tacrolimus and risk of adverse reactions. Closely monitor tacrolimus trough concentration when starting or stopping esomeprazole. Adjust tacrolimus dosage as needed.

Warfarin: May prolong PT and INR, causing abnormal bleeding. Monitor the patient and his PT and INR.

Drug-herb. *St. John's wort:* May decrease esomeprazole level. Avoid use together.

Drug-food. *Any food:* May reduce drug level. Advise patient to take drug 1 hour before food.

EFFECTS ON LAB TEST RESULTS

• May decrease magnesium level.

CONTRAINDICATIONS & CAUTIONS

• Contraindicated in patients hypersensitive to drug or components of esomeprazole or omeprazole (a drug similar to this one).

• In patients with severe liver impairment the maximum dose of delayed-release formulation is 24.65 mg daily.

❸ Alert: There may be an increased risk of hip, wrist, and spine fractures associated with proton pump inhibitors.

• Use esomeprazole magnesium and esomeprazole sodium cautiously in patients with hepatic insufficiency and in pregnant or breast-feeding women. It's unknown if this drug appears in breast milk, but omeprazole does. Patients taking esomeprazole strontium shouldn't breast-feed.

• Use cautiously in patients receiving continuous NSAID therapy who are at increased risk for gastric ulcers (those age 60 and older and those with a history of gastric ulcers).

⚠ Overdose S&S: Blurred vision, confusion, tremor, ataxia, intermittent clonic seizures, diaphoresis, drowsiness, flushing, headache, nausea, tachycardia.

NURSING CONSIDERATIONS

• Antacids can be used while taking drug, unless otherwise directed by prescriber.

• Monitor patient for rash or signs and symptoms of hypersensitivity. Monitor GI symptoms for improvement or worsening. Monitor LFTs, especially in patients with preexisting hepatic disease.

❸ Alert: Prolonged use may cause low magnesium levels that require magnesium supplementation and possibly discontinuation of drug. Monitor magnesium level

---

before treatment and periodically during treatment. Monitor patient for signs and symptoms of low magnesium level, such as abnormal heart rate or rhythm, palpitations, muscle spasms, tremor, and seizures. In children, abnormal heart rate may present as fatigue, upset stomach, dizziness, and light-headedness.

❸ **Alert:** May increase risk of *Clostridium difficile*–associated diarrhea (CDAD). Evaluate for CDAD in patients who develop diarrhea that doesn't improve.

• Long-term therapy may cause atrophic gastritis.

• **Look alike–sound alike:** Don't confuse Nexium with Nexavar.

PATIENT TEACHING
• Instruct patient to take drug exactly as prescribed.

• Tell patient to take drug at least 1 hour before a meal.

• Advise patient that antacids can be used while taking drug unless otherwise directed by prescriber.

• Warn patient not to chew or crush drug pellets because this inactivates the drug.

• If patient has difficulty swallowing capsule, tell him to mix contents of capsule with 1 tablespoon of soft applesauce and swallow immediately.

• Advise patient to store capsules at room temperature in a tight container.

• Tell patient to inform prescriber of worsening signs and symptoms, pain, or diarrhea that doesn't improve.

• Instruct patient to alert prescriber if rash or other signs and symptoms of allergy occur.

• Warn patient to immediately report symptoms of low magnesium level.

---

esterified estrogens
ESS-tehr-eh-fide ESS-troe-jenz

Menest, Neo-Estrone†

Therapeutic class: Estrogens
Pharmacologic class: Estrogens
Pregnancy risk category: X

E

AVAILABLE FORMS
Tablets (film-coated): 0.3 mg, 0.625 mg, 1.25 mg, 2.5 mg

INDICATIONS & DOSAGES
➤ **Inoperable progressing prostate cancer**
Men: 1.25 to 2.5 mg P.O. t.i.d.
➤ **Palliative treatment for metastatic breast cancer**
Men and postmenopausal women: 10 mg P.O. t.i.d. for 3 or more months.
➤ **Hypogonadism**
Women: 2.5 to 7.5 mg P.O. daily in divided doses in cycles of 20 days on, 10 days off.
➤ **Castration, primary ovarian failure**
Women: 1.25 mg P.O. daily in cycles of 3 weeks on, 1 week off. Adjust for symptoms. Can be given continuously.
➤ **Vasomotor menopausal symptoms**
Women: 1.25 mg P.O. daily in cycles of 3 weeks on, 1 week off. Dosage may be increased to 2.5 to 3.75 mg P.O. daily, if needed.
➤ **Moderate to severe menopausal vulvar and vaginal atrophy**
Women: 0.3 to 1.25 mg or more P.O. daily in cycles of 3 weeks on, 1 week off.

ADMINISTRATION
P.O.
• Use lowest effective dose needed for specific indication.

ACTION
Mimics the actions of endogenous estrogens; increases synthesis of DNA, RNA, and protein in responsive tissues; reduces release of follicle-stimulating and luteinizing hormones from pituitary gland.

Route	Onset	Peak	Duration
P.O.	Unknown	Unknown	Unknown

Half-life: Unknown.

ADVERSE REACTIONS

CNS: headache, dizziness, chorea, depression, *stroke, seizures.*
CV: thrombophlebitis, *thromboembolism,* hypertension, edema, *PE, MI.*
EENT: worsening myopia or astigmatism, intolerance of contact lenses.
GI: nausea, vomiting, abdominal cramps, bloating, anorexia, increased appetite, *pancreatitis,* increased risk of gallbladder disease.
GU: breakthrough bleeding, altered menstrual flow, dysmenorrhea, amenorrhea, *increased risk of endometrial cancer,* cervical erosion, altered cervical secretions, enlargement of uterine fibromas, vaginal candidiasis, testicular atrophy, impotence.
Hepatic: cholestatic jaundice, *hepatic adenoma.*
Metabolic: hypercalcemia, weight changes, hypertriglyceridemia.
Skin: melasma, rash, hirsutism or hair loss, erythema nodosum, *erythema multiforme,* dermatitis.
Other: breast tenderness, enlargement, or secretion; gynecomastia; *increased risk of breast cancer.*

INTERACTIONS

Drug-drug. *Carbamazepine, fosphenytoin, phenobarbital, phenytoin, rifampin:* May decrease effectiveness of estrogen therapy. Monitor patient closely.
Clarithromycin, erythromycin, itraconazole, ketoconazole, ritonavir: May increase estrogen plasma levels and side effects. Monitor patient.
Corticosteroids: May increase corticosteroid effects. Monitor patient closely.
Cyclosporine: May increase risk of toxicity. Use together with caution, and monitor cyclosporine level frequently.
Dantrolene, hepatotoxic drugs: May increase risk of hepatotoxicity. Monitor liver function closely.
Oral anticoagulants: May decrease anticoagulant effects. Adjust dosage if needed. Monitor PT and INR.

Tamoxifen: May interfere with tamoxifen effectiveness. Avoid using together.
Drug-herb. *St. John's wort:* May decrease effects of drug. Discourage use together.
Drug-food. *Caffeine:* May increase caffeine level. Urge caution.
Grapefruit, grapefruit juice: May increase risk of adverse effects. Discourage use together.
Drug-lifestyle. *Smoking:* May increase risk of CV effects. If smoking continues, may need another form of therapy.

EFFECTS ON LAB TEST RESULTS

● May increase calcium, thyroid-binding globulin, serum triglyceride, serum phospholipid, and clotting factor VII, VIII, IX, and X levels.
● May increase norepinephrine-induced platelet aggregation and PT.
● May reduce metyrapone test results and cause impaired glucose tolerance.

CONTRAINDICATIONS & CAUTIONS

● Contraindicated in pregnant women, in patients hypersensitive to drug, and in patients with breast cancer (except metastatic disease), estrogen-dependent neoplasia, active thrombophlebitis, thromboembolic disorders, undiagnosed abnormal genital bleeding, or history of thromboembolic disease.
● Use cautiously in patients with history of hypertension, mental depression, cardiac or renal dysfunction, liver impairment, gallbladder disease, bone disease, migraine, seizures, or diabetes.
⚠ *Overdose S&S:* Nausea, withdrawal bleeding in females.

NURSING CONSIDERATIONS

◑ *Alert:* Drug is considered a high-risk medication for elderly patients.
● When used for vasomotor symptoms in menstruating women, cyclic administration is started on day 5 of bleeding.
● When given cyclically for short-term use, administration should be cyclic and attempts to discontinue or taper the medication should be made at 3- to 6-month intervals.
● Make sure patient has thorough physical examination before starting estrogen

---

therapy. Patients receiving long-term therapy should have annual examinations. Periodically monitor body weight, blood pressure, lipid levels, and hepatic function.

• Notify pathologist about patient's estrogen therapy when sending specimens to laboratory for evaluation.

❸ Alert: Because of risk of thromboembolism, stop therapy at least 1 month before procedures that cause prolonged immobilization or increased risk of thromboembolism, such as knee or hip surgery.

Black Box Warning Estrogens have been reported to increase the risk of endometrial carcinoma. ■

Black Box Warning Estrogens should not be used during pregnancy. ■

• Glucose tolerance may be impaired. Monitor glucose level closely in patients with diabetes.

PATIENT TEACHING

• Tell patient to read package insert describing estrogen's adverse effects; also, give patient verbal explanation.

• Emphasize importance of regular physical examinations. Postmenopausal women who use estrogen replacement for longer than 5 years to treat menopausal symptoms may be at increased risk for endometrial cancer. This risk is reduced by using cyclic rather than continuous therapy and the lowest possible estrogen dosage. Adding progestins to the regimen decreases risk of endometrial hyperplasia, but it's unknown whether progestins affect risk of endometrial cancer.

❸ Alert: Warn patient to immediately report abdominal pain; pain, numbness, or stiffness in legs or buttocks; pressure or pain in chest or shortness of breath; severe headaches; visual disturbances, such as blind spots, flashing lights, or blurriness; vaginal bleeding or discharge; breast lumps; swelling of hands or feet; yellow skin or sclera; dark urine; or light-colored stools.

• Tell diabetic patient to report elevated glucose level so that antidiabetic dosage can be adjusted.

• Explain to woman receiving cyclic therapy for postmenopausal symptoms that she may experience withdrawal bleeding during week off drug. Tell her to report unusual vaginal bleeding.

• Teach woman to perform routine breast self-examination.

• Advise woman of childbearing age to consult prescriber before taking drug and to advise prescriber immediately if she becomes pregnant.

• Teach patient methods to decrease risk of blood clots.

• Encourage patient to stop smoking or reduce number of cigarettes smoked because of the risk of CV complications.

estradiol (oestradiol)
ess-tra-DYE-ole

Alora, Climara, Estrace Vaginal Cream, Estraderm, Estring Vaginal Ring, Evamist, Menostar, Minivelle, Vivelle, Vivelle-Dot

estradiol acetate
Femring, Femtrace

estradiol cypionate
Depo-Estradiol

estradiol gel
Divigel, Elestrin, EstroGel

estradiol hemihydrate
Estrasorb, Vagifem

estradiol valerate (oestradiol valerate)
Delestrogen

Therapeutic class: Estrogens
Pharmacologic class: Estrogens
Pregnancy risk category: X

AVAILABLE FORMS
estradiol
Spray, topical solution: 1.53 mg/spray
Tablets (micronized): 0.5 mg, 1 mg, 2 mg
Transdermal: 0.014 mg/24 hours, 0.025 mg/24 hours, 0.0375 mg/24 hours, 0.05 mg/24 hours, 0.06 mg/24 hours, 0.075 mg/24 hours, 0.1 mg/24 hours
Vaginal cream (in nonliquefying base): 0.1 mg/g
Vaginal ring (extended-release): 0.0075 mg/24 hours

estradiol acetate
Tablets: 0.45 mg, 0.9 mg, 1.8 mg
Vaginal ring: 0.05 mg/24 hours; 0.1 mg/24 hours
estradiol cypionate
Injection (in oil): 5 mg/mL
estradiol gel
Transdermal gel: 0.06% (1.25 g/metered dose), 0.06% (0.87 g/activation), 0.1% (in 0.25-, 0.5-, and 1-g single-dose packets)
estradiol hemihydrate
Topical emulsion: 0.25%
Vaginal tablets: 10 mcg
estradiol valerate
Injection (in oil): 10 mg/mL, 20 mg/mL, 40 mg/mL

INDICATIONS & DOSAGES
➤ **Vasomotor menopausal symptoms, female hypogonadism, female castration, primary ovarian failure**
Women: 1 to 2 mg P.O. estradiol daily. Or, for vasomotor symptoms, 1 to 5 mg cypionate I.M. once every 3 to 4 weeks; for female hypogonadism, 1.5 to 2 mg cypionate I.M. once every month.
Transdermal patch
Women: Apply patch according to manufacturer's instructions. Alora, Estraderm, Vivelle, and Vivelle-Dot are applied twice weekly. Climara and Menostar are applied once a week. Apply to clean, dry area of the trunk. Adjust dose, if necessary, after the first 2 or 3 weeks of therapy; then every 3 to 6 months as needed. Rotate application sites weekly with an interval of at least 1 week between particular sites used. Adjust dosage as needed.
➤ **Postmenopausal urogenital symptoms**
Women: One ring inserted into the upper third of the vagina. Ring is kept in place for 3 months.
➤ **Vulvar and vaginal atrophy**
Women: 0.05 mg/24 hours Estraderm applied twice weekly in a cyclic regimen. Or, 0.05 mg/24 hours Climara applied weekly in a cyclic regimen. Or, 2 to 4 g vaginal applications of cream daily for 1 to 2 weeks. When vaginal mucosa is restored, maintenance dose is 1 g one to three times weekly in a cyclic regimen. If using Vagifem for atrophic vaginitis, give 1 tablet vaginally once daily for 2 weeks. Maintenance

dose is 1 tablet inserted vaginally twice weekly. Or, 10 to 20 mg valerate I.M. every 4 weeks as needed. Or, 1 to 5 mg cypionate I.M. once every 3 to 4 weeks. Or, 0.05 to 0.1 mg daily by vaginal ring. Replace vaginal ring every 3 months.
➤ **Moderate to severe vasomotor symptoms, as well as vulvar and vaginal atrophy associated with menopause**
Women: 1.25 g EstroGel applied once daily to skin in a thin layer from wrist to shoulder of one upper extremity.
➤ **Palliative treatment of advanced, inoperable breast cancer**
Men and postmenopausal women: 10 mg P.O. estradiol t.i.d. for 3 months.
➤ **Palliative treatment of advanced, inoperable prostate cancer**
Men: 30 mg valerate I.M. every 1 to 2 weeks, or 1 to 2 mg estradiol P.O. t.i.d.
➤ **To prevent postmenopausal osteoporosis**
Women: Place a 6.5-cm^2 (0.025 mg/24 hours) Climara patch once weekly on clean, dry skin of lower abdomen or upper quadrant of buttock. Or, place a 3.25-cm^2 (0.014 mg/24 hours) Menostar patch once weekly to clean, dry area of the lower abdomen. Or, place a 0.5 mg/24 hours Estraderm patch twice weekly in a cyclic regimen in women with an intact uterus. In women with a hysterectomy, apply one Estraderm patch twice weekly in a continuous regimen. For each system, press firmly in place for about 10 seconds; ensure complete contact, especially around edges. Or, 0.025-mg/24 hours Vivelle, Vivelle-Dot, or Alora system applied to a clean, dry area of the trunk twice weekly. Or, 0.5 mg P.O. daily for 23 days, followed by 5 days without drug.
➤ **Moderate to severe vasomotor symptoms from menopause**
Women: Apply contents of two 1.74-g foil pouches (total 3.48 g) of Estrasorb daily. Or, Divigel 0.1% at dose of 0.25, 0.5, or 1 g/day. Start with Divigel 0.25 g daily and adjust dose based on individual patient response. Or, 1 pump per day of Elestrin applied to the upper arm. Or, Evamist 1 spray per day initially; may adjust dose based on clinical response. Or, 0.05 to 0.1 mg daily by vaginal ring. Replace vaginal ring every 3 months.

Reactions in bold italics are *life-threatening*. Interactions may have a *rapid onset* or a *delayed onset*.

ADMINISTRATION

P.O.
• Give without regard for food. If stomach upset occurs, give with food.
• Don't give drug with grapefruit juice.
• Store at controlled room temperature.

I.M.
• To give I.M. injection, make sure drug is well dispersed by rolling vial between palms. Inject deep into large muscle. Rotate injection sites to prevent muscle atrophy. Never give drug I.V.

Transdermal
• Open each pouch of Estrasorb individually and use contents of one pouch for each leg. Rub emulsion into thigh and calf for 3 minutes until thoroughly absorbed; rub emulsion remaining on hands onto the buttocks. Allow areas to dry before covering with clothing. Wash hands with soap and water to remove excess drug.
• Apply Elestrin once daily to the upper arm.
• Apply EstroGel over the entire area of one arm.
• Apply Evamist each morning to adjacent, nonoverlapping areas on the inner surface of the forearm, starting near the elbow. Allow to dry for 2 minutes and do not wash the site for 30 minutes.
• Apply Divigel once daily on skin of either right or left upper thigh. Application surface area should be about 5 by 7 inches (about the size of two palm prints). Apply entire contents of a unit-dose packet each day. To avoid potential skin irritation, apply Divigel to right or left upper thigh on alternating days. Don't apply Divigel on face, breasts, or irritated skin, or in or around the vagina. After application, allow gel to dry before dressing. Don't wash application site within 1 hour after applying Divigel. Avoid contact of gel with eyes. Wash hands after application.
• Apply transdermal patch to clean, dry, hairless, intact skin on abdomen or buttock. Don't apply to breasts, waistline, or other areas where clothing can loosen patch. When applying, ensure thorough contact between patch and skin, especially around edges, and hold in place for about 10 seconds. Apply patch immediately after opening and removing protective cover. Rotate application sites.

Vaginal
• Using the applicator, insert Vagifem as far into vagina as it can comfortably go, without using force.
• Remove vaginal ring from its pouch. Squeeze sides together and insert ring into vagina where comfortable.

ACTION

Increases synthesis of DNA, RNA, and protein in responsive tissues; reduces release of follicle-stimulating and luteinizing hormones from the pituitary gland.

Route	Onset	Peak	Duration
P.O., I.M., vaginal	Unknown	Unknown	Unknown
Transdermal (Estrasorb)	Immediate	Unknown	Unknown
Transdermal gel (EstroGel)	Immediate	1 hr	24–36 hr

Half-life: Alora transdermal patch, 1.75 ± 2.87 hours; Vivelle transdermal patch, 4.4 ± 2.3 hours; Vivelle-Dot transdermal patch, 5.9 to 7.7 hours; other forms, unknown.

ADVERSE REACTIONS

CNS: *stroke,* headache, dizziness, chorea, depression, *seizures,* insomnia (Vagifem).
CV: thrombophlebitis, *thromboembolism,* hypertension, edema, *PE, MI.*
EENT: worsening myopia or astigmatism, intolerance of contact lenses, sinusitis (Vagifem).
GI: nausea, vomiting, abdominal cramps, bloating, increased appetite, *pancreatitis,* anorexia, gallbladder disease, dyspepsia (Vagifem).
GU: breakthrough bleeding, altered menstrual flow, dysmenorrhea, amenorrhea, *increased risk of endometrial cancer,* cervical erosion, abnormal Pap smear, altered cervical secretions, enlargement of uterine fibromas, vaginal candidiasis in women, testicular atrophy, erectile dysfunction, genital pruritus, hematuria, vaginal discomfort, vaginitis (Vagifem).
Hepatic: cholestatic jaundice, *hepatic adenoma.*
Metabolic: weight changes, hypothyroidism, hypercalcemia (in patients with breast cancer and bone metastases).
Respiratory: upper respiratory tract infection, allergy, bronchitis (Vagifem).

Skin: melasma, urticaria, erythema nodosum, dermatitis, hair loss, pruritus.
Other: gynecomastia; *increased risk of breast cancer;* hot flashes; pain (Vagifem); breast tenderness, enlargement, or secretion; flulike syndrome.

INTERACTIONS

Drug-drug. *Carbamazepine, fosphenytoin, phenobarbital, phenytoin, rifampin:* May decrease effectiveness of estrogen therapy. Monitor patient closely.
Clarithromycin, erythromycin, itraconazole, ketoconazole, ritonavir: May increase estrogen plasma levels and side effects. Monitor patient.
Corticosteroids: May enhance effects of corticosteroids. Monitor patient closely.
Cyclosporine: May increase risk of toxicity. Use together with caution, and monitor cyclosporine level frequently.
Dantrolene, other hepatotoxic drugs: May increase risk of hepatotoxicity. Monitor liver function closely.
Oral anticoagulants: May decrease anticoagulant effect. Dosage adjustments may be needed. Monitor PT and INR.
Tamoxifen: May interfere with tamoxifen effectiveness. Avoid using together.
Thyroid hormones: May change thyroid hormone concentrations. May increase thyroid hormone requirements.
Drug-herb. *Black cohosh:* May increase drug's adverse effects. Discourage use together.
Saw palmetto: May negate drug's effects. Discourage use together.
St. John's wort: May decrease effects of drug. Discourage use together.
Drug-food. *Caffeine:* May increase caffeine level. Advise patient to avoid or minimize use of caffeine.
Grapefruit juice: May elevate drug level. Tell patient to take drug with liquid other than grapefruit juice.
Drug-lifestyle. *Smoking:* May increase risk of adverse CV effects. If smoking continues, may need another therapy.
Sunscreen use: May increase absorption of Estrasorb. Tell patient to separate application times.

EFFECTS ON LAB TEST RESULTS
● May increase clotting factor VII, VIII, IX, and X; total T_4; thyroid-binding globulin; LFT results; and triglyceride levels.
● May increase norepinephrine-induced platelet aggregation and PT.
● May decrease metyrapone test results.

CONTRAINDICATIONS & CAUTIONS
● Contraindicated in pregnant patients and patients with thrombophlebitis or thromboembolic disorders, estrogen-dependent neoplasia, breast or reproductive organ cancer (except for palliative treatment), undiagnosed abnormal genital bleeding, or history of thrombophlebitis or thromboembolic disorders linked to previous estrogen use (except for palliative treatment of breast and prostate cancer).
● Contraindicated in patients with liver dysfunction or disease.
● Use cautiously in patients with cerebrovascular or coronary artery disease, asthma, bone disease, migraine, seizures, or cardiac or renal dysfunction.
● Use cautiously in women who have a strong family history (grandmother, mother, sister) of breast cancer, breast nodules, fibrocystic breasts, or abnormal mammogram findings.
۞ Alert: Postmenopausal women ages 50 to 79 who are taking estrogen and progestin have an increased risk of MI, stroke, invasive breast cancer, PE, and thrombosis. Postmenopausal women age 65 or older also have an increased risk of dementia.
⚠ Overdose S&S: Nausea, vomiting, withdrawal uterine bleeding.

NURSING CONSIDERATIONS
● Ensure that patient has physical examination before starting therapy. Patients receiving long-term therapy should have yearly examinations. Monitor lipid levels, blood pressure, body weight, and hepatic function.
● Ask patient about allergies, especially to foods and plants. Estradiol is available as an aqueous solution or as a solution in peanut oil; estradiol cypionate, as a solution in cottonseed oil; estradiol valerate, as a solution in castor oil or sesame oil.

Reactions in bold italics are *life-threatening*. Interactions may have a *rapid onset* or a *delayed onset*.

Black Box Warning Estrogen increases the risk of endometrial cancer. Use adequate diagnostic measures, including endometrial sampling when indicated, to rule out malignancy in all cases of undiagnosed persistent or recurring abnormal vaginal bleeding. ∎

Black Box Warning Do not use estrogens with or without progestins to prevent CV disease or dementia. ∎

• When estrogen is prescribed for a postmenopausal woman with a uterus, also initiate a progestin to reduce the risk of endometrial cancer.

❸ *Alert:* EstroGel contains alcohol. Avoid fire, flame, or smoking until area dries in 2 to 5 minutes.

• In women also taking oral estrogen, treatment with the Estraderm transdermal patch can begin 1 week after withdrawal of oral therapy, or sooner if menopausal symptoms appear before the end of the week.

• Transdermal systems may be used continually rather than cyclically. Other alternative regimens are 1 to 5 mg cypionate I.M. every 3 to 4 weeks and 10 to 20 mg valerate I.M. every 4 weeks, as needed.

• Instruct patients using Vagifem who have severely atrophic vaginal mucosa to be careful when inserting the applicator. After gynecologic surgery, tell patient to use any vaginal applicator cautiously and only if clearly indicated.

• The prescriber should assess the patient's need to continue estradiol therapy. Make attempts to stop or taper at 3- to 6-month intervals.

• Because of risk of thromboembolism, stop therapy at least 1 month before high-risk procedures or those that cause prolonged immobilization, such as knee or hip surgery.

• Glucose tolerance may be impaired. Monitor glucose level closely in patients with diabetes.

• Notify pathologist about estrogen therapy when sending specimens to laboratory for evaluation.

PATIENT TEACHING

• Tell patient to read package insert describing estrogen's adverse effects and give verbal explanation.

❸ *Alert:* Advise patient not to allow contact between children and Evamist application site. Accidental exposure may cause premature puberty in children. If contact occurs, immediately wash child's skin with soap and water.

• Emphasize importance of regular physical examinations. Postmenopausal women who use estrogen replacement for longer than 5 years may be at increased risk for endometrial cancer. Risk is reduced by using cyclic rather than continuous therapy and the lowest possible dosages of estrogen. Adding progestins to the regimen decreases risk of endometrial hyperplasia; however, it isn't known whether progestins affect risk of endometrial cancer. No increased risk of breast cancer has been reported.

• Teach woman how to use cream. She should wash vaginal area with soap and water before applying and insert cream high into the vagina (about two-thirds the length of the applicator). She should take drug at bedtime, or lie flat for 30 minutes after instillation to minimize drug loss.

• Tell patient using topical emulsion not to apply it with sunscreen.

• Tell patient to use transdermal system correctly, to rotate sites, to avoid breasts and waistline, and to reapply patch if it falls off.

• Teach patient using transdermal gel (EstroGel) to apply in a thin layer on one arm and allow to dry before smoking, getting near flames, dressing, or touching the arm. Recommend bathing before application to maintain full dosage.

• Tell patient that estradiol gel should never be applied directly to the breast.

• Tell patient to insert Vagifem by the applicator as far into vagina as it can comfortably go, without using force.

❸ *Alert:* Warn patient to immediately report abdominal pain, pressure or pain in chest, shortness of breath, severe headaches, visual disturbances, vaginal bleeding or discharge, breast lumps, swelling of hands or feet, yellow skin or sclera, dark urine, light-colored stools, and pain, numbness, or stiffness in legs or buttocks.

• Explain to patient receiving cyclic therapy for postmenopausal symptoms that withdrawal bleeding may occur during week off drug. Tell her to report unusual vaginal bleeding.

• Tell diabetic patient to report elevated glucose level so that antidiabetic dosage can be adjusted.

• Teach woman how to perform routine breast self-examination.

• Teach patient methods to decrease risk of blood clots.

• Advise woman not to become pregnant during estrogen therapy.

• Advise woman of childbearing age to consult prescriber before taking drug and to advise prescriber immediately if she becomes pregnant.

• Encourage patient to stop or reduce smoking because of the risk of CV complications.

• Advise patient not to allow pets to lick or touch Evamist application site. If signs of illness occur, patient should contact pet's veterinarian.

estradiol–norethindrone acetate transdermal system
ess-tra-DYE-ole–nor-ETH-in-drone

CombiPatch

Therapeutic class: Estrogens
Pharmacologic class: Estrogen–progestin combinations
Pregnancy risk category: X

AVAILABLE FORMS
Transdermal: 9-cm^2 system releasing 0.05 mg estradiol and 0.14 mg norethindrone acetate daily; 16-cm^2 system releasing 0.05 mg estradiol and 0.25 mg norethindrone acetate daily

INDICATIONS & DOSAGES
➤ **Moderate to severe vasomotor symptoms from menopause; vulval and vaginal atrophy; hypoestrogenemia from hypogonadism, castration, or primary ovarian failure in women with intact uterus**
Continuous combined regimen
Women: Wear 9-cm^2 patch system continuously on lower abdomen. Replace system

twice weekly during 28-day cycle. May increase to 16-cm^2 patch.
Continuous sequential regimen
Women: For use in sequential regimen with an estradiol transdermal system (such as Alora, Estraderm, Vivelle), wear 0.05-mg estradiol transdermal patch for first 14 days of 28-day cycle; replace system twice weekly. Wear 9-cm^2 patch system on lower abdomen for rest of 28-day cycle; replace system twice weekly. May increase to 16-cm^2 patch system as needed.

ADMINISTRATION
Transdermal
• Apply patch system to a smooth (fold-free), clean, dry, nonirritated area of skin on lower abdomen, avoiding the waistline. Rotate application sites, with an interval of at least 1 week between applications to same site.

• Don't apply patch on or near breasts.

• Avoid applying to areas that may get prolonged sun exposure.

• Reapply patch, if needed, to another area of lower abdomen. If patch fails to adhere, replace with a new one.

ACTION
A matrix transdermal system in which estradiol and norethindrone are released continuously. Estrogen replacement therapy can reduce menopausal symptoms and release of follicle-stimulating and luteinizing hormones in postmenopausal women.

Route	Onset	Peak	Duration
Transdermal	12–24 hr	Unknown	3–4 days

Half-life: 2 to 23 hours (estradiol); 6 to 8 hours (norethindrone).

ADVERSE REACTIONS
CNS: asthenia, *stroke,* depression, insomnia, nervousness, dizziness, headache, pain.
CV: *thromboembolism,* thrombophlebitis, hypertension, edema, *PE, MI.*
EENT: pharyngitis, rhinitis, sinusitis, retinal vascular thrombosis, intolerance to contact lenses.
GI: abdominal pain, diarrhea, dyspepsia, changes in appetite, flatulence, nausea, constipation, gallbladder disease.

Reactions in bold italics are *life-threatening*. Interactions may have a *rapid onset* or a *delayed onset*.

GU: dysmenorrhea, leukorrhea, menstrual disorder, suspicious Papanicolaou smears, vaginitis, menorrhagia, *vaginal hemorrhage.*
Hepatic: cholestatic jaundice.
Metabolic: weight changes, hypercalcemia, hypertriglyceridemia.
Musculoskeletal: arthralgia, back pain.
Respiratory: respiratory disorder, bronchitis.
Skin: application-site reactions, acne, melasma, chloasma.
Other: accidental injury, flulike syndrome, breast pain, tooth disorder, peripheral edema, breast enlargement, infection, changes in libido.

INTERACTIONS
Drug-drug. *Carbamazepine, fosphenytoin, phenobarbital, phenytoin, rifampin:* May decrease estrogen therapy effectiveness. Monitor patient closely.
Clarithromycin, erythromycin, itraconazole, ketoconazole, ritonavir: May increase estrogen plasma levels and side effects. Monitor patient.
Corticosteroids: May enhance effects of corticosteroids. Monitor patient closely.
Cyclosporine: May increase risk of toxicity. Use together with caution; monitor cyclosporine level frequently.
Dantrolene, hepatotoxic drugs: May increase risk of hepatotoxicity. Monitor liver function closely.
Oral anticoagulants: May decrease effect of anticoagulant. May need to adjust dose. Monitor PT and INR.
Tamoxifen: May interfere with tamoxifen effectiveness. Avoid using together.
Drug-herb. *Black cohosh:* May increase adverse effects of drug. Discourage use together.
Saw palmetto: May cause antiestrogenic effects. Discourage use together.
St. John's wort: May decrease effects of drug. Discourage use together.
Drug-food. *Caffeine:* May increase caffeine level. Advise patient to avoid or minimize use of caffeine.
Grapefruit juice: May elevate estrogen level. Advise patient to take with liquid other than grapefruit juice.

Drug-lifestyle. *Smoking:* May increase risk of adverse CV effects. If smoking continues, may need alternative therapy.

EFFECTS ON LAB TEST RESULTS
• May increase T_3 and T_4, HDL, and triglyceride levels. May decrease LDL levels.
• May increase fibrinogen activity and platelet count. May decrease T_3 resin uptake. May alter activated PTT, INR, and platelet aggregation times.
• May reduce metyrapone test values. May alter glucose tolerance test results.

CONTRAINDICATIONS & CAUTIONS
• Contraindicated in women hypersensitive to estrogen, progestin, or any component of the patch; in pregnant patients; and in patients with known or suspected breast cancer, known or suspected estrogen-dependent neoplasia, undiagnosed abnormal genital bleeding, active thrombophlebitis, thromboembolic disorders, or stroke.
• Use cautiously in breast-feeding women and in patients with impaired liver function, asthma, epilepsy, migraine, or cardiac or renal dysfunction.
⚠ *Overdose S&S:* Nausea, withdrawal bleeding.

NURSING CONSIDERATIONS
Black Box Warning Do not use estrogens, with or without progestins, to prevent CV disease or dementia. ▮
Black Box Warning Postmenopausal women treated for 5 years have an increased risk of MI, stroke, invasive breast cancer, PE, and DVT. ▮
• Women not receiving continuous estrogen or combined estrogen–progestin therapy may start therapy at any time.
• Women receiving continuous hormone replacement therapy should complete the current cycle before starting therapy. Women commonly have withdrawal bleeding at completion of cycle; first day of withdrawal bleeding is an appropriate time to start therapy.
• Store patches in refrigerator before dispensing. Patient may then store patches at room temperature for up to 6 months, or the expiration date, whichever comes first.

• Reevaluate therapy at 3- to 6-month intervals.
• A combined estrogen–progestin regimen is indicated for a woman with an intact uterus. Progestins taken with estrogen significantly reduce, but don't eliminate, risk of endometrial cancer linked to use of estrogen alone.
• Because of risk of thromboembolism, stop therapy at least 4 to 6 weeks before surgery associated with an increased risk of thromboembolism, or during periods of prolonged immobilization.
• Blood pressure increases have been linked to estrogen use. Monitor patient's blood pressure regularly.
• Treatment of postmenopausal symptoms usually starts during menopausal stage when vasomotor symptoms occur.
• Monitor glucose level closely in patients with diabetes.
• **Alert:** Don't interchange CombiPatch with other estrogen patches. Verify therapy before application.

PATIENT TEACHING

• Teach woman how to apply patch properly. She should wear only one patch at any time during therapy. Tell her to apply patch immediately after opening protective cover.
• Tell patient that an oil-based cream or lotion may help remove adhesive from the skin after patch has been removed and the area allowed to dry for 15 minutes.
• Advise woman not to use patch if she's pregnant or plans to become pregnant.
• Urge woman of childbearing age to consult prescriber before applying patch and to advise prescriber immediately if she becomes pregnant.
• Instruct patient that the continuous combined regimen may lead to irregular bleeding, particularly in the first 6 months, but that it usually decreases with time and often stops completely.
• Tell patient that, for the continuous sequential regimen, monthly withdrawal bleeding is common.
• Advise patient to alert prescriber and remove patch at first sign of clotting disorders (thrombophlebitis, cerebrovascular disorders, and PE).

• Instruct patient to stop using patch and call prescriber about any loss of vision, sudden onset of protrusion of the eyeball (proptosis), double vision, or migraine.
• Encourage patient to stop or reduce smoking because of the risk of CV complications.
• Tell patient to perform monthly breast self-examinations and to have annual gynecologic and breast examinations by a health care provider.
• Advise patient not to store patches where extreme temperatures can occur.
• Tell patient undergoing an MRI to alert facility that she's using a transdermal patch.

estradiol valerate–estradiol valerate with dienogest
ess-tra-DYE-ole VAL-er-ate–dye-EN-oh-jest

Natazia

Therapeutic class: Estrogens
Pharmacologic class: Estrogen–progestin combinations
Pregnancy risk category: X

AVAILABLE FORMS
Tablets: 28-day blister pack containing two 3-mg estradiol valerate, five 2-mg estradiol valerate with 2-mg dienogest, seventeen 2-mg estradiol valerate with 3-mg dienogest, two 1-mg estradiol valerate, and two inert tablets

INDICATIONS & DOSAGES
➤ **Contraception**
Women: 1 tablet P.O. daily beginning on first day of menstrual cycle as directed on blister pack at same time each day. When changing from another combination hormonal contraceptive, begin on first day of withdrawal bleeding. When changing from combination hormonal vaginal ring or transdermal patch, begin on day vaginal ring or transdermal patch is removed. When changing from progestin-only contraceptive, begin next day. When changing from implant contraceptive or intrauterine system, begin day of implant or intrauterine system removal. When changing from injection contraceptive, begin day next injection is due.

Reactions in bold italics are *life-threatening*. Interactions may have a *rapid onset* or a *delayed onset*.

ADMINISTRATION

P.O.

● Give at same time each day; don't delay by more than 12 hours.

● Tablets must be given in order indicated on blister pack.

ACTION

Prevents pregnancy by suppressing ovulation. May also cause changes in endometrium and cervical mucus, inhibiting sperm penetration and reducing likelihood of implantation.

Route	Onset	Peak	Duration
P.O.	Unknown	3 hr (estradiol); 1½ hr (dienogest)	Unknown

Half-life: 14 hours (estradiol); 11 hours (dienogest).

ADVERSE REACTIONS

CNS: depression, headache.

CV: *MI, DVT,* hypertension.

GI: nausea, vomiting.

GU: amenorrhea, irregular uterine bleeding, metrorrhagia, oligomenorrhea, *uterine leiomyoma, ruptured ovarian cyst.*

Metabolic: weight gain, hyperglycemia.

Skin: acne.

Other: breast pain, tenderness, or discomfort.

INTERACTIONS

Drug-drug. *Antibiotics:* May reduce contraceptive effectiveness. Advise use of back-up contraception during therapy.

HIV protease inhibitors: May either increase or decrease estrogen and progesterone levels. Use together cautiously and monitor patient for effectiveness of hormone treatment.

Lamotrigine: May decrease lamotrigine serum level, reducing seizure control. Adjust lamotrigine dosage as necessary.

Strong CYP3A4 inducers (such as barbiturates, carbamazepine, phenytoin, rifampin): May reduce contraceptive effectiveness or increase breakthrough bleeding. An alternative method of birth control should be used.

Strong and moderate inhibitors of CYP3A4 (such as cimetidine, erythromycin, ketoconazole, SSRIs, verapamil): May increase levels of hormones. Avoid use together. If drugs must be used together, monitor patient for adverse effects.

Thyroid hormone: May increase serum concentration of thyroid-binding globulin, leading to decreased effectiveness of thyroid replacement therapy. Monitor patient; thyroid hormone dosage may need adjustment.

Drug-herb. *St John's wort:* May reduce contraceptive effectiveness or increase breakthrough bleeding. Recommend alternative method of birth control.

Drug-food. *Grapefruit juice:* May increase levels of hormones. Avoid use together.

Drug-lifestyle. **Black Box Warning** *Smoking:* Increases risk of medical problems, such as stroke, emboli, or heart disease. Recommend smoking cessation. ∎

EFFECTS ON LAB TEST RESULTS

● May increase thyroid-binding globulin, glucose, cholesterol, and lipid levels.

● May increase coagulation factors.

CONTRAINDICATIONS & CAUTIONS

● Contraindicated in pregnant patients and in those with benign or malignant liver tumors; liver disease; breast cancer or history of breast cancer; undiagnosed abnormal genital bleeding; headaches with focal neurologic symptoms or migraine headaches with or without aura if older than age 35; diabetes with vascular disease; uncontrolled hypertension; hypertension with vascular disease; inherited or acquired hypercoagulopathies; thrombogenic valvular or thrombogenic rhythm disease of heart, such as endocarditis or atrial fibrillation; coronary artery disease; cerebrovascular disease; DVT; or current or past PE.

Black Box Warning Contraindicated in women who smoke and who are older than age 35. ∎

● Use cautiously in women with CV disease risk factors, history of cholestasis, history of well-controlled hypertension, prediabetes or well-controlled diabetes, history of hyperlipidemia, new-onset headaches, history of bleeding irregularities, history of emotional disorders, angioedema, or chloasma.

● Safety and effectiveness in women with BMI greater than 30 kg/m^2 haven't been evaluated.

• Drug hasn't been studied in post-menopausal women and isn't indicated in this population.

• When possible, breast-feeding women should use other forms of contraception while breast-feeding because estrogen may reduce milk production and a small amount of drug is present in breast milk.

• Safety and effectiveness in women of reproductive age have been established. Use of this product before menarche isn't indicated.

⚠ **Overdose S&S:** Nausea, withdrawal bleeding.

NURSING CONSIDERATIONS

• Start drug no earlier than 4 weeks after delivery in women who aren't breast-feeding. Risk of postpartum venous thrombotic event (VTE) decreases and ovulation risk increases after third postpartum week.

• Ensure that oral contraceptives aren't given to pregnant women. Evaluate reported amenorrhea.

• Monitor blood pressure; elevations are possible in nonhypertensive women.

• Monitor coagulation factors as appropriate.

• Monitor glucose and cholesterol levels regularly, especially in women who are prediabetic and in those with history of elevated lipid levels.

• Monitor women for headache. New-onset headaches may require discontinuing oral contraceptives.

• Carefully monitor women with history of depression for recurrence or exacerbation.

• Stop drug if arterial or deep VTE occurs. Highest risk of VTE is during first year of contraceptive use. If feasible, stop tablets at least 4 weeks before and for 2 weeks after major surgery.

• Oral contraceptives are associated with increased risk of thrombotic and hemorrhagic strokes, especially in women older than age 35, in those with hypertension, and in smokers. Stop drug if unexplained vision loss, proptosis, diplopia, papilledema, or retinal vascular changes occur. Evaluate retinal vein thrombosis immediately.

• Risk of drug causing breast cancer or cervical or endometrial cancer is controversial and uncertain. As a precaution, women

should have regular Papanicolaou tests, breast examinations, and mammograms.

• Discontinue drug if jaundice develops. Women who take oral contraceptives are at slightly higher risk for developing liver tumors and gallstones. Monitor patient for skin color changes and pain in right upper quadrant.

PATIENT TEACHING

• Teach patient to take tablet once daily and not to skip doses or delay taking tablet by more than 12 hours. Advise patient that tablets should be taken in the order marked on each pack.

• Instruct patient to read package insert for information on missed tablets or to contact her pharmacist or prescriber and that back-up contraception must be used.

• Tell patient starting drug for first time to begin taking tablets on day 1 of her period and to use back-up contraceptive method for first 9 days.

• Instruct patient that spotting or light bleeding is normal at first.

• Advise patient that she may feel nauseous, especially during first few months, but that this symptom usually disappears and she shouldn't stop taking tablets. Tell patient to report to prescriber if nausea doesn't resolve.

• Warn patient to start drug no earlier than 4 weeks after giving birth.

• Advise patient to notify prescriber if she is pregnant before taking drug.

• Tell patient that breast-feeding while taking tablets isn't recommended because milk production may be reduced and small amounts of drug appear in breast milk.

• Inform patient taking tablets that blood tests may be needed to check blood glucose and cholesterol levels, as well as how her blood is clotting, and that her blood pressure may also be checked.

• Tell patient to inform prescriber of all prescription, over-the-counter, and herbal supplements she is taking.

• Advise patient, if appropriate, to quit smoking before taking drug.

Black Box Warning Advise patient who smokes that she is at increased risk for serious CV events from combination oral contraceptive use. Risk increases with age,

---

Reactions in bold italics are *life-threatening*. Interactions may have a *rapid onset* or a *delayed onset*.

especially after age 35, and with number of cigarettes smoked. ■

• Inform patient that contraceptive use doesn't protect against HIV infection or other sexually transmitted diseases.

• Tell patient that a missed period may occur but that pregnancy should be ruled out if she misses two or more consecutive menstrual cycles.

• Warn patient to call prescriber immediately if she experiences persistent leg pain; sudden shortness of breath; sudden blindness (partial or complete); severe chest pain; sudden, severe headache; weakness or numbness in an arm or leg; trouble speaking; or yellowing of skin or eyes.

• Advise patient with tendency to chloasma to avoid sun exposure and ultraviolet radiation.

• Advise patient to stop smoking while taking oral contraceptive because of increased risk of stroke and other thromboembolic events.

estrogens (conjugated) (estrogenic substances, conjugated; oestrogens, conjugated)
ESS-troe-jenz

Cenestin, C F S.†, Enjuvia, Premarin🖉

Therapeutic class: Estrogens
Pharmacologic class: Estrogens
Pregnancy risk category: X

AVAILABLE FORMS
Injection: 25 mg/5 mL*
Tablets: 0.3 mg, 0.45 mg, 0.625 mg, 0.9 mg, 1.25 mg
Vaginal cream: 0.625 mg/g

INDICATIONS & DOSAGES
➤ **Abnormal uterine bleeding (hormonal imbalance)**
Adults: 25 mg I.V. (preferred) or I.M. Repeat dose in 6 to 12 hours, if necessary.
➤ **Vulvar or vaginal atrophy**
Adults: 0.5 to 2 g cream intravaginally once daily in cycles of 3 weeks on, 1 week off.

➤ **Castration and primary ovarian failure**
Adults: Initially, 1.25 mg Premarin P.O. daily in cycles of 3 weeks on, 1 week off. Adjust dose as needed.
➤ **Female hypogonadism**
Adults: 0.3 to 0.625 mg Premarin P.O. daily, given cyclically 3 weeks on, 1 week off.
➤ **Moderate to severe vasomotor symptoms with or without moderate to severe symptoms of vulvar and vaginal atrophy associated with menopause**
Adults: Initially, 0.3 mg Premarin or Enjuvia P.O. daily. Premarin may also be given cyclically 25 days on, 5 days off. Adjust dosage based on patient response.
➤ **Moderate to severe vasomotor symptoms from menopause**
Adults: 0.45 mg Cenestin P.O. daily. Adjust dose based on patient response.
➤ **Moderate to severe symptoms of vulvar and vaginal atrophy from menopause**
Adults: 0.3 mg Cenestin P.O. daily.
➤ **To prevent osteoporosis**
Adults: 0.3 mg Premarin P.O. daily, or cyclically 25 days on, 5 days off. Adjust dose based on response of bone mineral density testing.
➤ **Palliative treatment of inoperable prostatic cancer**
Adults: 1.25 to 2.5 mg Premarin P.O. t.i.d.
➤ **Palliative treatment of breast cancer**
Adults: 10 mg Premarin P.O. t.i.d. for at least 3 months.

ADMINISTRATION
P.O.
• Give drug at same time each day.
I.V.
▼ Refrigerate before reconstituting.
▼ Reconstitute only with diluent provided. Agitate gently after adding diluent.
▼ Drug is compatible with normal saline, dextrose, or invert sugar solutions.
▼ Use reconstituted solution within a few hours, if possible. Reconstituted solution is stable under refrigeration for 60 days. Don't use if solution darkens or precipitates.
▼ Give direct injection slowly to avoid flushing reaction.
▼ **Incompatibilities:** Acidic solutions, ascorbic acid, protein hydrolysate.

E

I.M.
● Reconstitute only with diluent provided. Agitate gently after adding diluent.
● Inject deep into large muscle. Rotate injection sites to prevent muscle atrophy.
Vaginal
● Wash the vaginal area with soap and water, insert about two-thirds the length of the applicator into the vagina, and release drug. Give drug at bedtime or when the patient will lie flat for 30 minutes after use to minimize drug loss.

ACTION

Increases synthesis of DNA, RNA, and protein in responsive tissues. Also reduces release of follicle-stimulating and luteinizing hormones from the pituitary gland.

Route	Onset	Peak	Duration
P.O., I.V., I.M., vaginal	Unknown	Unknown	Unknown

Half-life: Unknown.

ADVERSE REACTIONS

CNS: headache, dizziness, chorea, depression, *stroke, seizures.*
CV: flushing with rapid I.V. administration, thrombophlebitis, *thromboembolism,* hypertension, edema, *PE, MI.*
EENT: worsening myopia or astigmatism, intolerance of contact lenses.
GI: nausea, vomiting, abdominal cramps, bloating, anorexia, increased appetite, *pancreatitis,* gallbladder disease.
GU: breakthrough bleeding, altered menstrual flow, dysmenorrhea, amenorrhea, *increased risk of endometrial cancer,* cervical erosion, altered cervical secretions, enlargement of uterine fibromas, vaginal candidiasis, testicular atrophy, impotence.
Hepatic: cholestatic jaundice, *hepatic adenoma.*
Metabolic: weight changes, hypercalcemia, hypertriglyceridemia.
Skin: melasma, chloasma, urticaria, hirsutism or hair loss, erythema nodosum, dermatitis.
Other: breast tenderness, enlargement, or secretion; gynecomastia; *increased risk of breast cancer;* changes in libido.

INTERACTIONS

Drug-drug. *Carbamazepine, fosphenytoin, phenobarbital, phenytoin, rifampin:* May decrease effectiveness of estrogen therapy. Monitor patient closely.
Corticosteroids: May enhance corticosteroid effects. Monitor patient closely.
Cyclosporine: May increase risk of toxicity. Use together with caution, and monitor cyclosporine level frequently.
Dantrolene, other hepatotoxic drugs: May increase risk of hepatotoxicity. Monitor liver function closely.
Itraconazole, ketoconazole, macrolide antibiotics, ritonavir: May increase estrogen plasma levels and side effects. Monitor patient.
Oral anticoagulants: May decrease anticoagulant effects. May need to adjust dosage. Monitor PT and INR.
Tamoxifen: May interfere with tamoxifen effectiveness. Avoid using together.
Thyroid hormones: May increase serum thyroxine-binding globulin levels, which may increase thyroid hormone requirements.
Drug-herb. *Black cohosh:* May increase adverse effects of drug. Discourage use together.
Red clover: May interfere with hormonal therapies. Discourage use together.
Saw palmetto: May have antiestrogenic effects. Discourage use together.
St. John's wort: May decrease effects of drug. Discourage use together.
Drug-food. *Caffeine:* May increase caffeine level. Advise caution.
Grapefruit juice: May increase concentration of estrogen. Avoid using together.
Drug-lifestyle. *Smoking:* May increase risk of adverse CV effects. If smoking continues, recommend nonhormonal contraception.

EFFECTS ON LAB TEST RESULTS

● May increase clotting factor VII, VIII, IX, and X; total T_4; phospholipid; thyroid-binding globulin; and triglyceride levels.
● May increase norepinephrine-induced platelet aggregation and PT.
● May cause a false-positive metyrapone test result.

Reactions in bold italics are *life-threatening*. Interactions may have a *rapid onset* or a *delayed onset*.

CONTRAINDICATIONS & CAUTIONS

Black Box Warning Contraindicated in pregnant patients. ∎

• Contraindicated in patients with thrombophlebitis, thromboembolic disorders, estrogen-dependent neoplasia, breast or reproductive cancer (except for palliative treatment), or undiagnosed abnormal genital bleeding.

• Use cautiously in patients with cerebrovascular or coronary artery disease, asthma, bone disease, migraine, seizures, or cardiac, hepatic, or renal dysfunction.

• Use cautiously in women who have a strong family history (mother, grandmother, sister) of breast or genital tract cancer, breast nodules, fibrocystic breasts, or abnormal mammogram findings.

⚠ Overdose S&S: Nausea, vomiting, breast tenderness, abdominal pain, drowsiness or fatigue, withdrawal uterine bleeding.

NURSING CONSIDERATIONS

• Make sure patient has thorough physical examination before starting therapy; patients receiving long-term therapy should have yearly examinations. Periodically monitor lipid levels, blood pressure, body weight, and hepatic function.

• Rapid treatment of dysfunctional uterine bleeding or reduction of surgical bleeding usually requires delivery by I.V. or I.M. route.

Black Box Warning Don't use to prevent CV disease. In postmenopausal women receiving therapy for more than 5 years, drug may increase risks of MI, stroke, invasive breast cancer, PE, and DVT. Use the lowest effective doses for the shortest time, considering the benefits and risks. ∎

Black Box Warning In postmenopausal women receiving therapy for more than 5 years, drug may increase risk of endometrial cancer. Cyclic therapy and the lowest possible dose reduces risk. Adding progestins decreases risk of endometrial hyperplasia, but it's unknown whether they affect risk of endometrial cancer. ∎

Black Box Warning In postmenopausal women age 65 or older receiving 4 years of treatment with conjugated estrogens plus medroxyprogesterone acetate, drug may increase the risk of dementia. ∎

• When used solely for the treatment of vulval and vaginal atrophy, consider topical products.

• Notify pathologist about estrogen therapy when sending specimens to laboratory for evaluation.

• Because of thromboembolism risk, stop therapy at least 1 month before procedures that prolong immobilization or raise the risk of thromboembolism, such as knee or hip surgery.

• Glucose tolerance may be impaired. Monitor glucose level closely in patients with diabetes.

• Reevaluate need for therapy at 3- to 6-month intervals.

• Look alike–sound alike: Don't confuse Premarin with Primaxin, Provera, or Remeron.

PATIENT TEACHING

• Tell patient to read package insert describing estrogen's adverse effects and to explain them back to you.

• Emphasize importance of regular physical examinations.

• Teach woman how to use vaginal cream. Tell patient to wash the vaginal area with soap and water, insert about two-thirds the length of the applicator into the vagina, and release drug. Tell her to use drug at bedtime or to lie flat for 30 minutes after use to minimize drug loss.

• Explain to patient that cyclic therapy for postmenopausal symptoms may cause withdrawal bleeding during week off drug. Tell her to report unusual vaginal bleeding.

✸ Alert: Warn patient to immediately report abdominal pain; pain, numbness, or stiffness in legs or buttocks; pressure or pain in chest; shortness of breath; severe headaches; visual disturbances, such as blind spots, flashing lights, or blurriness; vaginal bleeding or discharge; breast lumps; swelling of hands or feet; yellow skin or sclera; dark urine; and light-colored stools.

• Tell diabetic patient to report elevated glucose level so that antidiabetic dosage can be adjusted.

• Teach woman how to perform routine breast self-examination.

• Advise woman not to become pregnant during estrogen therapy.

● Advise woman of childbearing age to consult prescriber before taking drug and to advise prescriber immediately if she becomes pregnant.

● Encourage patient to stop smoking or reduce number of cigarettes smoked because of the risk of CV complications.

● Tell patient using drug for osteoporosis prevention to ensure adequate intake of calcium and vitamin D.

● Inform patient that vaginal cream has been reported to weaken latex condoms and to use an alternative method of birth control.

---

estropipate (piperazine estrone sulfate)
ess-troe-PIH-pate

Ogen .625, Ogen 1.25, Ogen 2.5, Ogen 5, Ortho-Est

Therapeutic class: Estrogens
Pharmacologic class: Estrogens
Pregnancy risk category: X

AVAILABLE FORMS
Tablets: 0.75 mg, 1.5 mg, 3 mg, 6 mg

INDICATIONS & DOSAGES
➤ **Vulval and vaginal atrophy**
Women: 0.75 to 6 mg P.O. daily, 3 weeks on and 1 week off.
➤ **Primary ovarian failure, female castration, female hypogonadism**
Women: 1.5 to 9 mg P.O. daily for first 3 weeks; then a rest period of 8 to 10 days. If bleeding doesn't occur by end of rest period, cycle is repeated.
➤ **Moderate to severe vasomotor menopausal symptoms**
Women: 0.75 to 6 mg P.O. daily in cyclic method, 3 weeks on and 1 week off. Can be given continuously.
➤ **To prevent osteoporosis**
Women: 0.75 mg P.O. daily for 25 consecutive days of a 31-day cycle, followed by 6 days without drug. Repeat regimen as indicated.

ADMINISTRATION
P.O.
● Give drug with meals to minimize GI upset.

ACTION
Increases synthesis of DNA, RNA, and proteins in responsive tissues; reduces follicle-stimulating and luteinizing hormones.

Route	Onset	Peak	Duration
P.O.	Unknown	Unknown	Unknown

Half-life: Unknown.

ADVERSE REACTIONS
CNS: depression, headache, dizziness, migraine, *seizures, stroke.*
CV: edema, thrombophlebitis, hypertension, *PE, MI, thromboembolism.*
EENT: steepening of corneal curvature, intolerance to contact lenses.
GI: nausea, vomiting, gallbladder disease, abdominal cramps, bloating.
GU: increased size of uterine fibromas, *endometrial cancer,* vaginal candidiasis, cystitis-like syndrome, dysmenorrhea, amenorrhea, breakthrough bleeding, condition resembling premenstrual syndrome.
Hepatic: cholestatic jaundice, *hepatic adenoma.*
Metabolic: weight changes, hypercalcemia, hypertriglyceridemia.
Skin: hemorrhagic eruption, erythema nodosum, *erythema multiforme,* hirsutism or hair loss, melasma.
Other: breast engorgement or enlargement, *breast cancer,* breast tenderness, changes in libido.

INTERACTIONS
Drug-drug. *Carbamazepine, fosphenytoin, phenobarbital, phenytoin, rifampin:* May decrease estrogen effect. Monitor patient closely.
Clarithromycin, erythromycin, itraconazole, ketoconazole, ritonavir: May increase estrogen plasma levels and side effects. Monitor patient.
Corticosteroids: May enhance corticosteroid effect. Monitor patient closely.
Cyclosporine: May increase risk of toxicity. Use together with caution; frequently monitor cyclosporine level.

Dantrolene, other hepatotoxic drugs: May increase risk of hepatotoxicity. Monitor liver function closely.

Oral anticoagulants: May decrease anticoagulant effect. Dosage adjustments may be needed. Monitor PT and INR.

Tamoxifen: May interfere with tamoxifen effect. Avoid using together.

Drug-herb. *Black cohosh:* May increase adverse effects of estrogen. Discourage use together.

Red clover: May interfere with hormonal therapies. Discourage use together.

Saw palmetto: May have antiestrogenic effect. Discourage use together.

St. John's wort: May decrease estrogen effect. Discourage use together.

Drug-food. *Caffeine:* May increase caffeine level. Advise caution.

Drug-lifestyle. *Smoking:* May increase risk of adverse CV effects. If smoking continues, may need alternative therapy.

EFFECTS ON LAB TEST RESULTS
● May increase clotting factor VII, VIII, IX, and X; total T_4; phospholipid; thyroid-binding globulin; and triglyceride levels.
● May increase norepinephrine-induced platelet aggregation and PT.
● May reduce metyrapone test results.

CONTRAINDICATIONS & CAUTIONS
Black Box Warning Contraindicated during pregnancy or during the immediate postpartum period. ∎
● Contraindicated in patients with active thrombophlebitis; thromboembolic disorders; estrogen-dependent neoplasia; undiagnosed genital bleeding; and breast, reproductive organ, or genital cancer.
● Use cautiously in patients with cerebrovascular or coronary artery disease; asthma; mental depression; bone disease; migraine; seizures; or cardiac, hepatic, or renal dysfunction.
● Use cautiously in women who have a family history (mother, grandmother, sister) of breast or genital tract cancer, breast nodules, fibrocystic breasts, or abnormal mammogram findings.
⚠ **Overdose S&S:** Nausea, vomiting, withdrawal uterine bleeding.

NURSING CONSIDERATIONS
● Make sure patient has thorough physical examination before starting estrogen therapy. Patients receiving long-term therapy should have examinations yearly. Periodically monitor lipid levels, blood pressure, body weight, and hepatic function.

Black Box Warning Estrogens and progestins shouldn't be used to prevent CV disease. The Women's Health Initiative study reported increased risks of MI, stroke, invasive breast cancer, PE, and DVT in postmenopausal women during 5 years of combination therapy. Because of these risks, estrogens and progestins should be prescribed at the lowest effective doses and for the shortest duration consistent with treatment goals and risks for the individual woman. ∎

Black Box Warning Estrogens may increase the risk of endometrial cancer in postmenopausal women. ∎

● When used to treat hypogonadism, duration of therapy needed to produce withdrawal bleeding depends on patient's endometrial response to drug. If satisfactory withdrawal bleeding doesn't occur, an oral progestin is added to the regimen. Explain to patient that, despite return of withdrawal bleeding, pregnancy can't occur because she doesn't ovulate.
● Because of risk of thromboembolism, stop therapy at least 1 month before procedures that prolong immobilization or raise the risk of thromboembolism, such as knee or hip surgery.
● Glucose tolerance may be impaired. Monitor glucose level closely in patients with diabetes.

PATIENT TEACHING
● Tell patient to read package insert describing estrogen's adverse effects; also, explain effects verbally.
● Tell diabetic patient to report elevated glucose level to prescriber.
● Stress importance of regular physical examinations. Postmenopausal women who use estrogen replacement for longer than 5 years may have increased risk of endometrial cancer. Using cyclic therapy and lowest possible estrogen dosage reduces risk. Adding progestins to regimen

E

decreases risk of endometrial hyperplasia; however, it isn't known whether progestins affect risk of endometrial cancer.

⚠ Alert: Warn patient to immediately report abdominal pain; pain, stiffness, or numbness in legs or buttocks; pressure or pain in chest; shortness of breath; severe headaches; visual disturbances, such as blind spots or flashing lights; vaginal bleeding or discharge; breast lumps; swelling of hands or feet; yellow skin or sclera; dark urine; and light-colored stools.

• Teach woman how to perform routine breast self-examination.

• Advise woman not to become pregnant while on estrogen therapy.

• Encourage patient to stop or reduce smoking because of the risk of CV complications.

• Advise woman of childbearing age to consult prescriber before taking drug and to tell prescriber immediately if she becomes pregnant.

• Teach patient at risk for osteoporosis about the importance of adequate calcium and vitamin D intake.

SAFETY ALERT!

eszopiclone
ess-ZOP-ah-klone

Lunesta✒

Therapeutic class: Hypnotics
Pharmacologic class: Pyrrolopyrazine derivatives
Pregnancy risk category: C
Controlled substance schedule: IV

AVAILABLE FORMS
Tablets: 1 mg, 2 mg, 3 mg

INDICATIONS & DOSAGES
➤ **Insomnia**
Adults: 2 mg P.O. immediately before bedtime. Increase to 3 mg as needed.
Elderly patients having trouble falling asleep: 1 mg P.O. immediately before bedtime. Increase to 2 mg as needed.
Elderly patients having trouble staying asleep: 2 mg P.O. immediately before bedtime.

Adjust-a-dose: In patients with severe hepatic impairment, start with 1 mg P.O. In patients who also take a potent CYP3A4 inhibitor, start with 1 mg and increase to 2 mg as needed.

ADMINISTRATION
P.O.
• Avoid giving drug after a high-fat meal.
• Give drug immediately before bedtime because drug may cause dizziness or lightheadedness.
• Patient must swallow tablet whole.

ACTION
Probably interacts with GABA receptors at binding sites close or connected to benzodiazepine receptors.

Route	Onset	Peak	Duration
P.O.	Rapid	1 hr	Unknown

Half-life: 6 hours.

ADVERSE REACTIONS
CNS: abnormal dreams, anxiety, complex sleep-related behavior, confusion, decreased libido, depression, dizziness, hallucinations, headache, nervousness, pain, somnolence, neuralgia.
EENT: unpleasant taste.
GI: diarrhea, dry mouth, dyspepsia, nausea, vomiting.
GU: dysmenorrhea, UTI.
Respiratory: respiratory tract infection.
Skin: pruritus, rash.
Other: *anaphylaxis, angioedema,* accidental injury, gynecomastia, viral infection.

INTERACTIONS
Drug-drug. *CNS depressants:* May have additive CNS effects. Adjust dosage of either drug as needed.
CYP3A4 inhibitors (clarithromycin, itraconazole, ketoconazole, nefazodone, nelfinavir, ritonavir, troleandomycin): May decrease eszopiclone elimination, increasing the risk of toxicity. Use together cautiously.
Olanzapine: May impair cognitive function or memory. Use together cautiously.
Rifampin: May decrease eszopiclone activity. Don't use together.
Drug-food. *High-fat meals:* May decrease drug absorption and effects. Discourage

---

Reactions in bold italics are *life-threatening*. Interactions may have a *rapid onset* or a *delayed onset*.

high-fat meals with or just before taking drug.

Drug-lifestyle. *Alcohol use:* May decrease psychomotor ability. Discourage use together.

EFFECTS ON LAB TEST RESULTS
None reported.

CONTRAINDICATIONS & CAUTIONS
• Use cautiously in elderly and debilitated patients, and in patients with diseases or conditions that could affect metabolism or hemodynamic responses. Also use cautiously in patients with compromised respiratory function, severe hepatic impairment, or signs and symptoms of depression.

⚠ *Overdose S&S:* CNS depression.

NURSING CONSIDERATIONS
⊘ *Alert:* Anaphylaxis and angioedema may occur as early as the first dose; monitor the patient closely.
• Evaluate patient for physical and psychiatric disorders before treatment.
• Use the lowest effective dose.
⊘ *Alert:* Give drug immediately before patient goes to bed or after patient has gone to bed and has trouble falling asleep.
• Use only for short periods (for example, 7 to 10 days). If patient still has trouble sleeping, check for other psychological disorders.
• Risk of abuse and dependence increases with the dose and duration of treatment and the concurrent use of other psychoactive drugs.
• Monitor patient for changes in behavior, such as decreased inhibition, aggression, and agitation, and including those that suggest depression or suicidal thinking. Amnesia and other neuropsychiatric symptoms may occur unpredictably.

PATIENT TEACHING
⊘ *Alert:* Warn patient that drug may cause allergic reactions, facial swelling, and complex sleep-related behaviors, such as driving, eating, and making phone calls while asleep. Advise patient to report these adverse effects.

• Urge patient to take drug immediately before going to bed because drug may cause dizziness or light-headedness.
• Caution patient not to take drug unless he can't get a full night's sleep.
• Advise patient to avoid taking drug after a high-fat meal.
• Tell patient to avoid activities that require mental alertness until the drug's effects are known.
• Tell patient to swallow tablet whole.
• Advise patient to avoid alcohol while taking drug.
• Urge patient to immediately report changes in behavior and thinking.
• Warn patient not to stop drug abruptly or change dose without consulting the prescriber.
• Inform patient that tolerance or dependence may develop if drug is taken for a prolonged period.

etanercept
ee-tan-ER-sept

Enbrel

Therapeutic class: Antiarthritics
Pharmacologic class: TNF blockers
Pregnancy risk category: B

AVAILABLE FORMS
Injection: 25-mg multiuse vial
Prefilled syringe: 25 mg/0.5 mL, 50 mg/mL

INDICATIONS & DOSAGES
➤ **To reduce signs and symptoms of moderately to severely active polyarticular-course juvenile rheumatoid arthritis (RA) in patients whose response to one or more disease-modifying antirheumatic drugs has been inadequate**
Children ages 2 to 17: For children weighing 63 kg (138 lb) or more, 50 mg subcutaneously weekly using the prefilled syringe. For children weighing less than 63 kg, 0.8 mg/kg subcutaneously weekly as two injections, either on the same day or 3 or 4 days apart using the multiuse vial. Maximum dosage is 50 mg/week. Glucocorticoids, NSAIDs, or analgesics may be continued during treatment. Use

with methotrexate hasn't been studied in pediatric patients.

➤ **RA, psoriatic arthritis, ankylosing spondylitis**

Adults: 50 mg subcutaneously once weekly using the 50-mg/mL single-use prefilled syringe. Methotrexate, glucocorticoids, salicylates, NSAIDs, or analgesics may be continued during treatment.

➤ **Chronic moderate to severe plaque psoriasis in patients who are candidates for systemic therapy or phototherapy**

Adults: 50 mg subcutaneously twice weekly, 3 to 4 days apart, for 3 months. Then, reduce dose to 50 mg subcutaneously once weekly. Give dose using 50-mg/mL single-use prefilled syringes.

ADMINISTRATION
Subcutaneous

● Give 50-mg dose as one subcutaneous injection using a 50-mg/mL single-use pre-filled syringe or as two 25-mg subcutaneous injections using multiuse vial. Give the two 25-mg injections on the same day or 3 to 4 days apart.

● Store prefilled syringe at 36° to 46° F (2° to 8° C), but let it reach room temperature (15 to 30 minutes) before use.

● Reconstitute multiple-use vial aseptically with 1 mL of supplied sterile bacteriostatic water for injection (0.9% benzyl alcohol). Use a 25G needle rather than the supplied vial adapter if the vial will be used for multiple doses. Don't filter reconstituted solution when preparing or giving drug. Inject diluent slowly into vial. Refrigerate in vial for up to 14 days at 36° to 46° F (2° to 8° C).

● Minimize foaming by gently swirling during dissolution rather than shaking. Dissolution takes less than 10 minutes.

● Don't use solution if it's discolored or cloudy, or if it contains particulate matter.

● Separate injection sites by at least 1 inch (2.5 cm), rotate regularly, and never use areas where skin is tender, bruised, red, or hard. Use sites on the thigh, abdomen, and upper arm.

❸ Alert: Needle covers of diluent syringe and prefilled syringe contain latex and shouldn't be handled by persons sensitive to latex.

● **Incompatibilities:** Don't add other drugs or diluents to solution.

ACTION
Binds specifically to TNF and blocks its action with cell-surface TNF receptors, reducing inflammatory and immune responses found in RA.

Route	Onset	Peak	Duration
Subcut.	Unknown	72 hr	Unknown

Half-life: About 5 days.

ADVERSE REACTIONS
CNS: headache, asthenia, dizziness.
CV: peripheral edema.
EENT: rhinitis, pharyngitis, sinusitis, mouth ulcers.
GI: abdominal pain, dyspepsia, nausea, vomiting, diarrhea.
Respiratory: upper respiratory tract infections, cough, respiratory disorder.
Skin: injection-site reaction, rash, alopecia, urticaria, pruritus.
Other: infections, *malignancies.*

INTERACTIONS
Drug-drug. *Anakinra:* Increased rate of serious infection when used together. Use together cautiously.
Cyclophosphamide: May increase risk of solid malignancies. Concurrent use not recommended.
Sulfasalazine: May cause decreased neutrophil count. Monitor patient carefully.
Live-virus vaccines: Etanercept may affect normal immune response. Postpone live-virus vaccine until therapy stops.

EFFECTS ON LAB TEST RESULTS
None reported.

CONTRAINDICATIONS & CAUTIONS
● Contraindicated in patients hypersensitive to drug or its components, in those with sepsis, and in those receiving a live-virus vaccine.

● Drug isn't indicated for use in children younger than age 2.

● Use cautiously in patients with underlying diseases that predispose them to infection, such as diabetes, heart failure, or history of active or chronic infections. Also use cautiously in RA patients with preexisting or recent onset of demyelinating disorders, including MS, myelitis, and optic neuritis.

Reactions in bold italics are *life-threatening*. Interactions may have a *rapid onset* or a *delayed onset.*

NURSING CONSIDERATIONS
• Methotrexate, glucocorticoids, salicylates, NSAIDs, or analgesics may be continued during treatment in adults.

Black Box Warning Patients treated with anti-TNF therapies are at increased risk for developing serious, sometimes fatal, infections. Most patients who developed serious infections were also receiving immunosuppressants, such as methotrexate or corticosteroids. If serious infection occurs, stop therapy and notify prescriber. ■

Black Box Warning Infections, including bacterial sepsis and tuberculosis, have been reported. Evaluate patient's risk factors and test for latent tuberculosis. Begin treatment for latent tuberculosis before therapy with etanercept. ■

◑ Alert: Don't give live-virus vaccines during therapy.

• If possible, bring patients with juvenile RA up to date with all immunizations before starting treatment.

Black Box Warning Histoplasmosis, coccidioidomycosis, blastomycosis, and other opportunistic infections may develop with use of this drug. Consider empirical antifungal therapy in patients at risk for invasive fungal infections who develop severe systemic illness. ■

Black Box Warning Lymphoma and other malignancies, sometimes fatal, have been reported in children and adolescents. ■

PATIENT TEACHING
• If patient will be self-administering drug, advise him about mixing and injection techniques, including rotation of injection sites.
• Instruct patient to use puncture-resistant container for disposal of needles and syringes.
• Tell patient that injection-site reactions generally occur within first month of therapy and decrease thereafter.
• Inform patient of importance of avoiding live-virus vaccine administration during therapy.
• Stress importance of alerting other health care providers of etanercept use.
• Instruct patient to promptly report signs and symptoms of infection, including persistent fever, cough, shortness of breath, or fatigue, to prescriber.

• Advise women to stop breast-feeding during therapy.

---

ethacrynate sodium
eth-uh-KRIH-nayt

Edecrin Sodium

ethacrynic acid
Edecrin

Therapeutic class: Diuretics
Pharmacologic class: Loop diuretics
Pregnancy risk category: B

AVAILABLE FORMS
ethacrynate sodium
Injection: 50 mg/vial
ethacrynic acid
Tablets: 25 mg

INDICATIONS & DOSAGES
➤ **Acute pulmonary edema**
Adults: 50 mg or 0.5 to 1 mg/kg I.V. Usually only one dose is needed, although a second dose may be needed.
➤ **Edema**
Adults: 50 to 200 mg P.O. daily. May increase to 200 mg b.i.d. for desired effect.
Children age 13 months and older: First dose is 25 mg P.O., increased cautiously by 25 mg daily until desired effect is achieved.
Adjust-a-dose: If added to an existing diuretic regimen, first dose is 25 mg and dosage adjustments are made in 25-mg increments.

ADMINISTRATION
P.O.
• Give drug in morning to prevent nocturia.
I.V.
▼ Add 50 mL of D_5W or normal saline solution to vial.
▼ Don't use cloudy or opalescent solution.
▼ Give over several minutes through tubing of running infusion.
▼ If more than one I.V. dose is needed, use a new injection site to avoid thrombophlebitis.
▼ Discard unused solution after 24 hours.
▼ **Incompatibilities:** Hydralazine, Normosol-M, procainamide, ranitidine,

reserpine, solutions or drugs with pH below 5, tolazoline, triflupromazine, whole blood and its derivatives.

ACTION

Potent loop diuretic; inhibits sodium and chloride reabsorption at the proximal and distal tubules and the ascending loop of Henle.

Route	Onset	Peak	Duration
P.O.	30 min	2 hr	6–8 hr
I.V.	5 min	15–30 min	2 hr

Half-life: 1 hour.

ADVERSE REACTIONS

CNS: malaise, confusion, fatigue, apprehension, vertigo, headache, fever.
CV: orthostatic hypotension.
EENT: transient or permanent deafness with over-rapid I.V. injection, blurred vision, tinnitus, hearing loss.
GI: cramping, diarrhea, anorexia, nausea, vomiting, *GI bleeding, pancreatitis.*
GU: oliguria, hematuria, nocturia, polyuria, frequent urination.
Hematologic: *agranulocytosis, neutropenia, thrombocytopenia,* azotemia.
Metabolic: asymptomatic hyperuricemia; hypokalemia; hypochloremic alkalosis; fluid and electrolyte imbalances, including dilutional hyponatremia, hypocalcemia, and hypomagnesemia; hyperglycemia and impaired glucose tolerance; volume depletion and dehydration.
Skin: rash.
Other: chills.

INTERACTIONS

Drug-drug. *Aminoglycoside antibiotics:* May increase ototoxic adverse reactions of both drugs. Use together cautiously.
Antidiabetics: May decrease hypoglycemic effects. Monitor glucose level.
Antihypertensives: May increase risk of hypotension. Use together cautiously.
Cardiac glycosides: May increase risk of digoxin toxicity from ethacrynate-induced hypokalemia. Monitor potassium and digoxin levels.
Chlorothiazide, chlorthalidone, hydrochlorothiazide, indapamide, metolazone: May cause excessive diuretic response, causing serious electrolyte abnormalities or dehydration. Adjust doses carefully, and monitor patient closely for signs and symptoms of excessive diuretic response.
Cisplatin: May increase risk of ototoxicity. Avoid using together.
Lithium: May decrease lithium clearance, increasing risk of lithium toxicity. Monitor lithium level.
Neuromuscular blockers: May enhance neuromuscular blockade. Monitor patient closely.
NSAIDs: May decrease diuretic effect. Use together cautiously.
Other potassium-wasting drugs (amphotericin B, corticosteroids): May increase risk of hypocalcemia. Use together cautiously.
Probenecid: May decrease diuretic effect. Avoid using together.
Warfarin: May increase anticoagulant effect. Use together cautiously.
Drug-herb. *Dandelion:* May interfere with diuretic activity. Discourage use together.
Licorice: May cause unexpected rapid potassium loss. Discourage use together.

EFFECTS ON LAB TEST RESULTS

● May increase glucose and uric acid levels. May decrease calcium, magnesium, potassium, and sodium levels.
● May decrease granulocyte, neutrophil, and platelet counts.

CONTRAINDICATIONS & CAUTIONS

● Contraindicated in infants, patients hypersensitive to drug, and patients with anuria.
🖐 **Alert:** Drug is potent diuretic and can cause severe diuresis with water and electrolyte depletion. Monitor patient closely.
● Use cautiously in patients with electrolyte abnormalities or hepatic impairment.
⚠ **Overdose S&S:** Dehydration, electrolyte depletion.

NURSING CONSIDERATIONS

● Monitor fluid intake and output, weight, blood pressure, and electrolyte levels.
● Watch for signs of hypokalemia, such as muscle weakness and cramps.
● Monitor glucose level in diabetic patients.
● Consult prescriber and dietitian about providing a high-potassium diet. Foods rich

---

in potassium include citrus fruits, tomatoes, bananas, dates, and apricots. Potassium chloride and sodium supplements may be needed.
• Dosage may be on an alternate-day schedule, or more prolonged periods of diuretic therapy may be interspersed with rest periods. Intermittent dosage schedule allows time to correct electrolyte imbalance and may provide a more efficient diuretic response.
• Drug may increase risk of gastric hemorrhage caused by steroid treatment.
• Monitor elderly patients, who are especially susceptible to excessive diuresis.
• Monitor uric acid level, especially in patients with history of gout.
ⓘ Alert: If patient develops severe diarrhea, stop drug. Patient shouldn't receive drug again after diarrhea has resolved.

PATIENT TEACHING
• Instruct patient to take drug with food to minimize GI upset.
• Advise patient to take drug in morning to avoid need to urinate at night; if patient needs second dose, have him take it in early afternoon.
• Advise patient to avoid sudden posture changes and to rise slowly to avoid dizziness upon standing quickly.
• Tell patient to notify prescriber about muscle weakness, cramps, nausea, diarrhea, or dizziness.
• Caution patient not to perform hazardous activities if drug causes drowsiness.
• Advise diabetic patient to closely monitor glucose level.

ethambutol hydrochloride
e-THAM-byoo-tole

Etibi†, Myambutol

Therapeutic class: Antituberculotics
Pharmacologic class: Synthetic antituberculotics
Pregnancy risk category: C

AVAILABLE FORMS
Tablets: 100 mg, 400 mg

INDICATIONS & DOSAGES
➤ **Adjunctive treatment for pulmonary tuberculosis**
Adults and children age 13 and older: In patients who haven't received prior antitubercular therapy, 15 mg/kg P.O. daily as a single dose once every 24 hours, combined with other antituberculotics. For retreatment, 25 mg/kg P.O. every 24 hours as a single dose for 60 days (or until bacteriologic smears and cultures become negative) with at least one other antituberculotic; after 60 days, decrease to 15 mg/kg/day as a single dose every 24 hours.
Adjust-a-dose: Reduce dosage in patients with impaired renal function.

ADMINISTRATION
P.O.
• Always give drug with other antituberculotics to prevent development of resistant organisms.
• Giving drug with food doesn't significantly alter absorption.
• Administer on a once-every-24-hour basis only.

ACTION
May inhibit synthesis of one or more metabolites of susceptible bacteria, changing cell metabolism during cell division; bacteriostatic.

Route	Onset	Peak	Duration
P.O.	Unknown	2–4 hr	Unknown

Half-life: About 3½ hours.

ADVERSE REACTIONS
CNS: dizziness, fever, hallucinations, headache, malaise, mental confusion, peripheral neuritis.
EENT: optic neuritis, irreversible blindness.
GI: abdominal pain, anorexia, GI upset, nausea, vomiting.
Hematologic: *thrombocytopenia, leukopenia, neutropenia.*
Metabolic: hyperuricemia.
Musculoskeletal: joint pain.
Skin: *toxic epidermal necrolysis,* dermatitis, pruritus.
Other: *anaphylactoid reactions,* precipitation of acute gout.

INTERACTIONS
Drug-drug. *Aluminum salts:* May delay and reduce absorption of ethambutol. Separate doses by several hours.

EFFECTS ON LAB TEST RESULTS
• May increase ALT, AST, bilirubin, and uric acid levels. May decrease glucose level.
• May decrease platelet count.

CONTRAINDICATIONS & CAUTIONS
• Contraindicated in children younger than age 13, patients hypersensitive to drug, and patients with optic neuritis.
• Use cautiously in patients with impaired renal function, cataracts, recurrent eye inflammation, gout, or diabetic retinopathy.

NURSING CONSIDERATIONS
• Perform visual acuity and color discrimination tests before and during therapy.
• Ensure that any changes in vision don't result from an underlying condition.
• Obtain AST and ALT levels before therapy, and monitor these levels every 3 to 4 weeks.
• In patients with impaired renal function, base dosage on drug level.
• Monitor uric acid level; observe patient for signs and symptoms of gout.

PATIENT TEACHING
• Reassure patient that visual disturbances usually disappear several weeks to months after drug is stopped. Inflammation of the optic nerve is related to dosage and duration of treatment.
• Inform patient that drug is given with other antituberculotics.
• Stress importance of compliance with drug therapy.
• Advise patient to report adverse reactions to prescriber.

ethinyl estradiol–desogestrel
ETH-i-nill–DAY-so-jest-rul

Monophasic
Desogen, Emoquette, Ortho-Cept

Biphasic
Kariva, Mircette, Viorele

Triphasic
Cyclessa, Velivet

ethinyl estradiol–ethynodiol diacetate
Monophasic
Kelnor 1/35, Zovia 1/35E-28, Zovia 1/50E-28

ethinyl estradiol–levonorgestrel
Monophasic
Altavera, Aviane-28, Falmina, Introvale, Lessina-28, Levora 0.15/30-28, Lybrel, Marlissa, Nordette-28, Orsythia, Portia-28, Quasense, Seasonale

Biphasic
Lo Seasonique, Seasonique

Triphasic
Enpresse-28, Levonest, Myzilra, Trivora-28

ethinyl estradiol–norethindrone
Monophasic
Alyacen 1/35, Alyacen 777, Aranelle, Balziva-28, Brevicon 28-Day, Briellyn, Cyclafem 1/35, Dasetta 1/35, Modicon-28, Norethin 1/35E, Norinyl 1+35, Nortrel 0.5/35, Nortrel 1/35, Ortho-Novum 1/35-28, Ovcon-35, Ovcon-50, Philith, Wera

Triphasic
Alyacen 7/7/7, Aranelle, Cyclafem 7/7/7, Dasetta 7/7/7, Nortrel 7/7/7, Ortho-Novum 7/7/7-28, Tri-Norinyl 28-day

ethinyl estradiol–norethindrone acetate
Monophasic
Junel 1/20, Junel 1.5/30, Junel Fe 1/20, Junel Fe 1.5/30, Loestrin 21 1.5/30, Loestrin 21 1/20, Microgestin 1.5/30, Microgestin 1/20

ethinyl estradiol–norgestimate
Monophasic
Mono-Linyah, Ortho-Cyclen-28, Previfem, Sprintec

Triphasic
Ortho Tri-Cyclen, Ortho Tri-Cyclen Lo, Tri-Linyah, Tri-Lo-Sprintec, Tri-Previfem, Tri-Sprintec

ethinyl estradiol–norgestrel
Monophasic
Cryselle, Elinest, Lo/Ovral-28, Low-Ogestrel, Ogestrel 0.5/50-28

ethinyl estradiol–norethindrone acetate–ferrous fumarate
Monophasic
Femcon Fe, Gildess Fe 1/20, Gildess Fe 1.5/30, Loestrin 24 Fe, Loestrin Fe 1/20, Loestrin Fe 1.5/30, Lo Loestrin Fe, Microgestin Fe 1/20, Microgestin Fe 1.5/30

Triphasic
Estrostep Fe, Tri-Legest Fe

mestranol–norethindrone
Monophasic
Norinyl 1+50

Therapeutic class: Contraceptives
Pharmacologic class: Estrogen–progestin combinations
Pregnancy risk category: X

AVAILABLE FORMS
Monophasic hormonal contraceptives
ethinyl estradiol–desogestrel
Tablets: ethinyl estradiol 30 mcg and desogestrel 0.15 mg (Desogen, Emoquette, Ortho-Cept)

ethinyl estradiol–ethynodiol diacetate
Tablets: ethinyl estradiol 35 mcg and ethynodiol diacetate 1 mg (Kelnor 1/35, Zovia 1/35E-28); ethinyl estradiol 50 mcg and ethynodiol diacetate 1 mg (Zovia 1/50E-28)
ethinyl estradiol–levonorgestrel
Tablets: ethinyl estradiol 20 mcg and levonorgestrel 0.1 mg (Aviane-28, Falmina, Lessina-28, Orsythia); ethinyl estradiol 20 mcg and levonorgestrel 0.9 mg (Lybrel); ethinyl estradiol 30 mcg and levonorgestrel 0.15 mg (Altavera, Introvale, Levora 0.15/30-28, Marlissa, Nordette-28, Portia-28, Quasense, Seasonale); ethinyl estradiol 30 mcg and 0.15 mg levonorgestrel (84 tablets), and 10 mcg ethinyl estradiol (7 tablets) (Seasonale)
ethinyl estradiol–norethindrone
Tablets: ethinyl estradiol 35 mcg and norethindrone 0.4 mg (Balziva-28, Briellyn, Ovcon-35, Philith); ethinyl estradiol 35 mcg and norethindrone 0.5 mg (Brevicon 28-Day, Modicon-28, Nortrel 0.5/35-28, Wera); ethinyl estradiol 35 mcg and norethindrone 0.75 mg (Alyacen 777); ethinyl estradiol 35 mcg and norethindrone 1 mg (Alyacen 1/35, Alyacen 777, Cyclafem 1/35, Dasetta 1/35, Norethin 1/35E, Norinyl 1 + 35, Nortrel 1/35, Ortho-Novum 1/35-28); ethinyl estradiol 50 mcg and norethindrone 1 mg (Ovcon-50)
ethinyl estradiol–norethindrone acetate
Tablets: ethinyl estradiol 20 mcg and norethindrone acetate 1 mg (Junel 1/20, Loestrin 21 1/20, Microgestin 1/20); ethinyl estradiol 30 mcg and norethindrone acetate 1.5 mg (Junel 1.5/30, Loestrin 21 1.5/30, Microgestin 1.5/30)
ethinyl estradiol–norgestimate
Tablets: ethinyl estradiol 35 mcg and norgestimate 0.25 mg (Mono-Linyah, Ortho-Cyclen-28, Previfem, Sprintec)
ethinyl estradiol–norgestrel
Tablets: ethinyl estradiol 30 mcg and norgestrel 0.3 mg (Cryselle, Elinest, Lo/Ovral-28, Low-Ogestrel); ethinyl estradiol 50 mcg and norgestrel 0.5 mg (Ogestrel 0.5/50-28)
ethinyl estradiol–norethindrone acetate–ferrous fumarate
Chewable tablets: norethindrone 0.4 mg/ethinyl estradiol 35 mcg; inactive tablets contain ferrous fumarate 75 mg

Tablets: ethinyl estradiol 10 mcg, norethindrone acetate 1 mg, and ferrous fumarate 75 mg (Lo Loestrin Fe); ethinyl estradiol 20 mcg, norethindrone acetate 1 mg, and ferrous fumarate 75 mg (Gildess Fe 1/20, Loestrin Fe 1/20, Loestrin 24 Fe, Microgestin Fe 1/20); ethinyl estradiol 30 mcg, norethindrone acetate 1.5 mg, and ferrous fumarate 75 mg (Gildess Fe 1.5/30, Loestrin Fe 1.5/30, Microgestin Fe 1.5/30)

mestranol–norethindrone
Tablets: mestranol 50 mcg and norethindrone 1 mg (Norinyl 1 + 50)

Biphasic hormonal contraceptives
ethinyl estradiol–desogestrel
Tablets: ethinyl estradiol 20 mcg and desogestrel 0.15 mg (21 days), then inert tablets (2 days), then ethinyl estradiol 10 mcg (5 days) (Kariva, Mircette, Viorele)

ethinyl estradiol–levonorgestrel
Tablets: ethinyl estradiol 0.02 mg and levonorgestrel 0.1 mg (84 days), then ethinyl estradiol 0.01 mg (7 days) (Lo Seasonique); ethinyl estradiol 30 mcg and levonorgestrel 0.15 mg (84 days), then ethinyl estradiol 10 mcg (7 days) (Seasonique)

Triphasic hormonal contraceptives
ethinyl estradiol–desogestrel
Tablets: 0.1 mg desogestrel and 25 mcg ethinyl estradiol (7 tablets); 0.125 mg desogestrel and 25 mcg ethinyl estradiol (7 tablets); 0.15 mg desogestrel and 25 mcg ethinyl estradiol (7 tablets) (Cyclessa, Velivet)

ethinyl estradiol–levonorgestrel
Tablets: ethinyl estradiol 30 mcg and levonorgestrel 0.05 mg (6 days); ethinyl estradiol 40 mcg and levonorgestrel 0.075 mg (5 days); ethinyl estradiol 30 mcg and levonorgestrel 0.125 mg (10 days) (Enpresse-28, Levonest, Myzilra, Trivora-28)

ethinyl estradiol–norethindrone
Tablets: ethinyl estradiol 30 mcg and norethindrone 0.5 mg (7 days); ethinyl estradiol 35 mcg and norethindrone 1 mg (9 days); ethinyl estradiol 35 mcg and norethindrone 0.5 mg (5 days) (Aranelle, Tri-Norinyl 28-day); ethinyl estradiol 35 mcg and norethindrone 0.5 mg (7 days); ethinyl estradiol 35 mcg and norethindrone 0.75 mg (7 days); ethinyl estradiol 35 mcg and norethindrone 1 mg (7 days)

(Alyacen 7/7/7, Cyclafem 7/7/7, Dasetta 7/7/7, Nortrel 7/7/7, Ortho-Novum 7/7/7-28)

ethinyl estradiol–norethindrone acetate
Tablets: ethinyl estradiol 20 mcg and norethindrone acetate 1 mg (5 days); ethinyl estradiol 30 mcg and norethindrone acetate 1 mg (7 days); ethinyl estradiol 35 mcg and norethindrone acetate 1 mg (9 days) (Tri-Legest 21)

ethinyl estradiol–norgestimate
Tablets: ethinyl estradiol 25 mcg and norgestimate 0.18 mg (7 days); ethinyl estradiol 25 mcg and norgestimate 0.215 mg (7 days); ethinyl estradiol 25 mcg and norgestimate 0.25 mg (7 days) (Ortho Tri-Cyclen Lo, Tri-Lo Sprintec); ethinyl estradiol 35 mcg and norgestimate 0.18 mg (7 days); ethinyl estradiol 35 mcg and norgestimate 0.215 mg (7 days); ethinyl estradiol 35 mcg and norgestimate 0.25 mg (7 days) (Ortho Tri-Cyclen, Tri-Linyah, Tri-Previfem, Tri-Sprintec)

ethinyl estradiol–norethindrone acetate–ferrous fumarate
Tablets: ethinyl estradiol 20 mcg and norethindrone acetate 1 mg (5 days); ethinyl estradiol 30 mcg and norethindrone acetate 1 mg (7 days); ethinyl estradiol 35 mcg and norethindrone acetate 1 mg (9 days); 75-mg ferrous fumarate tablets (7 days) (Estrostep Fe, Tri-Legest Fe)

INDICATIONS & DOSAGES

➤ **Contraception**
Monophasic hormonal contraceptives
Women: 1 tablet P.O. daily beginning on first day of menstrual cycle or first Sunday after menstrual cycle begins. With 20- and 21-tablet package, new cycle begins 7 days after last tablet taken. With 28-tablet package, dosage is 1 tablet daily without interruption; extra tablets taken on days 22 to 28 are placebos or contain iron. Or, for Seasonale, 1 pink tablet P.O. daily beginning on first Sunday after menstrual cycle begins, for 84 consecutive days, followed by 7 days of white (inert) tablets. Or, for Lybrel, 1 tablet P.O. daily beginning on the first day of menstrual cycle. When changing from 21-day or 28-day combination oral contraceptive, begin on first day of

withdrawal bleeding, at the latest 7 days after last active tablet. When changing from progestin-only pill, begin the next day. When changing from implant contraceptive, begin the day of implant removal. When changing from injection contraceptive, begin the day when next injection is due.

Biphasic hormonal contraceptives
Women: 1 color tablet P.O. daily for 10 days; then next color tablet for 11 days. With 21-tablet packages, new cycle begins 7 days after last tablet taken. With 28-tablet packages, dosage is 1 tablet daily without interruption. Or, for Seasonique, 1 light blue-green tablet P.O. once daily for 84 consecutive days followed by 1 yellow tablet for 7 consecutive days; then repeat cycle.

Triphasic hormonal contraceptives
Women: 1 tablet P.O. daily in the sequence specified by the brand. With 21-tablet packages, new dosing cycle begins 7 days after last tablet taken. With 28-tablet packages, dosage is 1 tablet daily without interruption.

➤ **Moderate acne vulgaris in women age 15 and older who have no known contraindications to hormonal contraceptive therapy, who want oral contraception for at least 6 months, who have reached menarche, and who are unresponsive to topical antiacne drugs**
Women age 15 and older: 1 tablet Ortho Tri-Cyclen or Estrostep P.O. daily (21 tablets contain active ingredients and 7 are inert).

ADMINISTRATION
P.O.
• Give drug at the same time each day; give at night to reduce nausea and headaches.
• Chewable tablet may be swallowed whole or chewed and followed with a full glass of liquid.

ACTION
Inhibit ovulation and may prevent transport of the ovum (if ovulation should occur) through the fallopian tubes.

Estrogen suppresses follicle-stimulating hormone, blocking follicular development and ovulation.

Progestin suppresses luteinizing hormone so that ovulation can't occur even if the follicle develops; it also thickens cervical mucus, interfering with sperm migration, and prevents implantation of the fertilized ovum.

Route	Onset	Peak	Duration
P.O.	Unknown	2 hr (ethinyl estradiol), 0.5–4 hr (varies by progestin)	Unknown

Half-life: 6 to 20 hours (ethinyl estradiol); 5 to 45 hours (varies by progestin).

ADVERSE REACTIONS
CNS: headache, dizziness, depression, lethargy, migraine, *stroke, cerebral hemorrhage.*
CV: *thromboembolism,* hypertension, edema, *PE, MI.*
EENT: worsening myopia or astigmatism, intolerance of contact lenses, exophthalmos, diplopia.
GI: nausea, vomiting, abdominal cramps, bloating, anorexia, changes in appetite, gallbladder disease, *pancreatitis.*
GU: breakthrough bleeding, spotting, granulomatous colitis, dysmenorrhea, amenorrhea, cervical erosion or abnormal secretions, enlargement of uterine fibromas, vaginal candidiasis.
Hepatic: cholestatic jaundice, *liver tumors,* gallbladder disease.
Metabolic: weight change, additive insulin resistance in diabetics.
Skin: rash, acne, *erythema multiforme,* melasma, hirsutism.
Other: breast tenderness, enlargement, or secretion; *anaphylaxis; hemolytic-uremic syndrome.*

INTERACTIONS
Drug-drug. *Anti-infectives (chloramphenicol, fluconazole, griseofulvin, neomycin, nitrofurantoin, penicillins, sulfonamides, tetracyclines):* May decrease contraceptive effect. Advise patient to use another method of contraception.
Atorvastatin: May increase norethindrone and ethinyl estradiol levels. Monitor patient for adverse effects.
Benzodiazepines: May decrease or increase benzodiazepine levels. Adjust dosage, if necessary.
Beta blockers: May increase beta blocker level. Dosage adjustment may be necessary.

Carbamazepine, fosphenytoin, phenobarbital, phenytoin, rifampin: May decrease estrogen effect. Use together cautiously.

Corticosteroids: May enhance corticosteroid effect. Monitor patient closely.

Insulin, sulfonylureas: Glucose intolerance may decrease antidiabetic effects. Monitor these effects.

NNRTIs, protease inhibitors: May decrease hormonal contraceptive effect. Avoid using together, if possible.

Oral anticoagulants: May decrease anticoagulant effect. Dosage adjustments may be needed. Monitor PT and INR.

Tamoxifen: May inhibit tamoxifen effect. Avoid using together.

Drug-herb. *Black cohosh:* May increase adverse effects of estrogen. Discourage use together.

Red clover: May interfere with drug. Discourage use together.

Saw palmetto: May have antiestrogenic effect. Discourage use together.

St. John's wort: May decrease drug effect because of increased hepatic metabolism. Discourage use together, or advise patient to use an additional method of contraception.

Drug-food. *Caffeine:* May increase caffeine level. Urge caution.

Grapefruit juice: May increase estrogen level. Advise patient to take with liquid other than grapefruit juice.

Drug-lifestyle. *Smoking:* May increase risk of adverse CV effects. If smoking continues, may need alternative therapy.

EFFECTS ON LAB TEST RESULTS

• May increase clotting factors II, VII, VIII, IX, and X; fibrinogen; phospholipid; plasminogen; thyroid-binding globulin; total T_4; and triglyceride levels.

• May increase norepinephrine-induced platelet aggregation and PT.

• May reduce metyrapone test results. May cause false-positive result in nitroblue tetrazolium test.

CONTRAINDICATIONS & CAUTIONS

• Contraindicated in patients with thromboembolic disorders, cerebrovascular or coronary artery disease, diplopia or ocular lesions arising from ophthalmic vascular disease, classic migraine, MI, known or

suspected breast cancer, known or suspected estrogen-dependent neoplasia, benign or malignant liver tumors, active liver disease or history of cholestatic jaundice with pregnancy or previous use of hormonal contraceptives, and undiagnosed abnormal vaginal bleeding.

• Contraindicated in women who are or may be pregnant or breast-feeding.

• Use cautiously in patients with hyperlipidemia, hypertension, migraines, seizure disorders, asthma, bleeding irregularities, gallbladder disease, ocular disease, diabetes, emotional disorders, and cardiac, renal, or hepatic insufficiency.

⚠ *Overdose S&S:* Nausea, withdrawal uterine bleeding.

NURSING CONSIDERATIONS

Black Box Warning Cigarette smoking increases the risk of serious CV side effects from oral contraceptives. This risk increases with age and with heavy smoking (at least 15 cigarettes daily) and is quite marked in women older than age 35. Women who use oral contraceptives should not smoke. ■

• Triphasic hormonal contraceptives may cause fewer adverse reactions, such as breakthrough bleeding and spotting.

• The Centers for Disease Control and Prevention reports that use of hormonal contraceptives may decrease risk of ovarian and endometrial cancers and doesn't seem to increase risk of breast cancer. However, the FDA reports that some studies suggest that hormonal contraceptives may be linked to an increase in cervical cancer.

• Monitor lipid levels, blood pressure, body weight, and hepatic function.

❸ *Alert:* Many hormonal contraceptives share similar names. Make sure to check the hormone strength for verification.

• Estrogens and progestins may alter glucose tolerance, thus changing dosage requirements for antidiabetics. Monitor glucose level.

• Stop hormonal contraceptives for a few weeks before adrenal function tests.

• Stop hormonal contraceptive and notify prescriber if patient develops granulomatous colitis.

• Stop drug at least 1 week before surgery to decrease risk of thromboembolism. Tell

---

patient to use an alternative method of birth control.

• Women who are nonlactating mothers or those who have had second-trimester abortion must wait 28 days before starting oral contraception.

• In case of first-trimester abortion, patient may start Lybrel immediately without additional contraceptive method.

PATIENT TEACHING

• Tell patient to take tablets at same time each day; nighttime doses may reduce nausea and headaches.

• Advise patient to use additional method of birth control, such as condom or diaphragm with spermicide, for first week of first cycle.

• Tell patient that missing doses in midcycle greatly increases likelihood of pregnancy.

• Tell patient that missing a dose may cause spotting or light bleeding.

• Tell patient that hormonal contraceptives don't protect against HIV or other sexually transmitted diseases.

• Tell patient using Seasonale that there will be four planned menses per year, but spotting or bleeding between menses may occur.

• If 1 pill is missed, tell patient to take it as soon as possible (2 pills if remembered on the next day) and then to continue regular schedule. Advise an additional method of contraception for remainder of cycle. If 2 consecutive pills are missed, tell patient to take 2 pills a day for next 2 days and then resume regular schedule. Advise an additional method of contraception for the next 7 days or preferably for the remainder of cycle. If 2 consecutive pills are missed in the 3rd or 4th week or if patient misses 3 consecutive pills, tell patient to contact prescriber for instructions.

• Warn patient of common adverse effects, such as headache, nausea, dizziness, breast tenderness, spotting, and breakthrough bleeding, which usually diminish after 3 to 6 months.

• Instruct patient to weigh herself at least twice a week and to report any sudden weight gain or swelling to prescriber.

• Warn patient to avoid exposure to ultraviolet light or prolonged exposure to sunlight.

⚠ **Alert:** Warn patient to immediately report abdominal pain; numbness, stiffness, or pain in legs or buttocks; pressure or pain in chest; shortness of breath; severe headache; visual disturbances, such as blind spots, blurriness, or flashing lights; undiagnosed vaginal bleeding or discharge; two consecutive missed menstrual periods; lumps in the breast; swelling of hands or feet; or severe pain in the abdomen (tumor rupture in liver).

• Advise patient of increased risks created by simultaneous use of cigarettes and hormonal contraceptives.

• If one menstrual period is missed and tablets have been taken on schedule, tell patient to continue taking them. If two consecutive menstrual periods are missed, tell patient to stop drug and have pregnancy test. Progestins may cause birth defects if taken early in pregnancy.

• Tell patient to chew chewable tablet and follow with a full glass of liquid or swallow whole.

• Advise patient not to take same drug for longer than 12 months without consulting prescriber. Stress importance of Papanicolaou tests and annual gynecologic examinations.

• Advise patient to check with prescriber about how soon pregnancy may be attempted after hormonal therapy is stopped. Many prescribers recommend that women not become pregnant within 2 months after stopping drug.

• Warn patient of possible delay in achieving pregnancy when drug is stopped.

• Teach women how to perform routine breast self-examination.

• Teach patient methods to decrease risk of thromboembolism.

• Advise patient taking hormonal contraceptives to use additional form of birth control during concurrent treatment with certain antibiotics.

• Advise patient that hormonal contraceptives may change the fit of contact lenses.

etodolac
ee-toe-DOE-lak

Therapeutic class: NSAIDs
Pharmacologic class: NSAIDs
Pregnancy risk category: C

AVAILABLE FORMS
Capsules: 200 mg, 300 mg
Tablets: 400 mg, 500 mg
Tablets (extended-release): 400 mg, 500 mg, 600 mg

INDICATIONS & DOSAGES
➤ **Acute pain**
Adults: 200 to 400 mg P.O. every 6 to 8 hours p.r.n., not to exceed 1,000 mg daily.
➤ **Short- and long-term management of osteoarthritis and rheumatoid arthritis**
Adults: 600 to 1,000 mg P.O. daily, divided into two or three doses. Maximum daily dose is 1,200 mg. For extended-release tablets, 400 to 1,000 mg P.O. daily. Maximum daily dose is 1,200 mg.
➤ **Juvenile rheumatoid arthritis (extended-release tablets)**
Children ages 6 to 16 weighing 20 to 30 kg (44 to 66 lb): 400 mg P.O. once daily.
Children ages 6 to 16 weighing 31 to 45 kg (68 to 99 lb): 600 mg P.O. once daily.
Children ages 6 to 16 weighing 46 to 60 kg (101 to 132 lb): 400 mg P.O. b.i.d.
Children ages 6 to 16 weighing 61 kg (134 lb) or more: 500 mg P.O. b.i.d.

ADMINISTRATION
P.O.
● Give drug with milk or meals to minimize GI discomfort.

ACTION
Unknown. Produces anti-inflammatory, analgesic, and antipyretic effects, possibly by inhibiting prostaglandin synthesis.

Route	Onset	Peak	Duration
P.O.	30 min	1–2 hr	4–12 hr
P.O. (extended-release)	Unknown	3–12 hr	6–12 hr

Half-life: 7¼ hours.

ADVERSE REACTIONS
CNS: asthenia, malaise, dizziness, depression, drowsiness, nervousness, insomnia, syncope, fever.
CV: hypertension, *heart failure,* flushing, palpitations, edema, fluid retention.
EENT: blurred vision, tinnitus, photophobia.
GI: dyspepsia, flatulence, abdominal pain, diarrhea, nausea, constipation, gastritis, melena, vomiting, anorexia, *peptic ulceration with or without GI bleeding or perforation,* ulcerative stomatitis, thirst, dry mouth.
GU: dysuria, urinary frequency, *renal failure.*
Hematologic: anemia, *leukopenia,* hemolytic anemia.
Hepatic: *hepatitis.*
Metabolic: weight gain.
Respiratory: *asthma.*
Skin: pruritus, rash, cutaneous vasculitis, *Stevens-Johnson syndrome.*
Other: chills.

INTERACTIONS
Drug-drug. *Antacids:* May decrease etodolac's peak level. Watch for decreased effect of etodolac.
Aspirin: May decrease protein-binding of etodolac without altering its clearance. May increase GI toxicity. Avoid using together.
Beta blockers, diuretics: May blunt effects of these drugs. Monitor patient closely.
Cyclosporine: May increase risk of nephrotoxicity. Avoid using together.
Digoxin, lithium, methotrexate: May impair elimination of these drugs, increasing risk of toxicity. Monitor drug levels.
Phenytoin: May increase phenytoin level. Monitor patient for toxicity.
Warfarin: May decrease the protein binding of warfarin but doesn't change its clearance. Although no dosage adjustment is needed, monitor INR closely and watch for bleeding.
Drug-herb. *Dong quai, feverfew, garlic, ginger, horse chestnut, red clover:* May increase risk of bleeding. Discourage use together.
White willow: Herb and drug contain similar components. Discourage use together.
Drug-lifestyle. *Alcohol use:* May increase risk of adverse effects. Discourage use together.

Reactions in bold italics are *life-threatening*. Interactions may have a *rapid onset* or a *delayed onset*.

Sun exposure: May cause photosensitivity reactions. Advise patient to avoid excessive sunlight exposure.

EFFECTS ON LAB TEST RESULTS
• May increase BUN and creatinine. May decrease uric acid and hemoglobin levels and hematocrit.
• May decrease WBC count.
• May cause a false-positive test result for urine bilirubin, possibly from phenolic metabolites and ketone bodies.

CONTRAINDICATIONS & CAUTIONS
Black Box Warning Contraindicated for the treatment of perioperative pain after CABG surgery. ∎
• Contraindicated in patients hypersensitive to drug and in those with history of aspirin- or NSAID-induced asthma, rhinitis, urticaria, or other allergic reactions.
• Use cautiously in elderly patients and in patients with history of renal or hepatic impairment, preexisting asthma, or GI bleeding, ulceration, and perforation.
⚠ Overdose S&S: Lethargy, drowsiness, nausea, vomiting, epigastric pain, GI bleeding, coma, hypertension, acute renal failure, respiratory depression, anaphylaxis.

NURSING CONSIDERATIONS
• Because NSAIDs impair the synthesis of renal prostaglandins, they can decrease renal blood flow and lead to reversible renal impairment, especially in patients with renal or heart failure or liver dysfunction, in elderly patients, and in those taking diuretics. Monitor these patients closely.
Black Box Warning NSAIDs cause an increased risk of serious GI adverse events, including bleeding, ulceration, and perforation of the stomach or intestines, which can be fatal. Elderly patients are at greater risk. ∎
Black Box Warning NSAIDs may increase the risk of serious thrombotic events, MI, or stroke, which can be fatal. The risk may be greater with longer use or in patients with CV disease or risk factors for CV disease. ∎

PATIENT TEACHING
• Tell patient to take drug with milk or meals to minimize GI discomfort.

• Teach patient signs and symptoms of GI bleeding, including blood in vomit, urine, or stool; coffee-ground vomit; and black, tarry stool. Tell him to notify prescriber immediately if any of these occurs.
• Advise patient to avoid consuming alcohol or aspirin while taking drug.
• Warn patient to avoid hazardous activities that require alertness until harmful CNS effects of drug are known.
• Teach patient signs and symptoms of liver damage, including nausea, fatigue, lethargy, itching, yellowed skin or eyes, right upper quadrant tenderness, and flulike symptoms. Tell him to contact prescriber immediately if any of these symptoms occurs.
• Advise patient to use a sunblock, wear protective clothing, and avoid prolonged exposure to sunlight because of possible sensitivity to sunlight.
• Tell pregnant women to avoid use of drug during third trimester.
• Advise patient that use of OTC NSAIDs and etodolac may increase the risk of GI toxicity.

etonogestrel–ethinyl estradiol vaginal ring
e-toe-noe-JES-trel and ETH-i-nill

NuvaRing

Therapeutic class: Contraceptives
Pharmacologic class: Estrogen–progestin combinations
Pregnancy risk category: X

AVAILABLE FORMS
Vaginal ring: Delivers 0.12 mg etonogestrel and 0.015 mg ethinyl estradiol daily

INDICATIONS & DOSAGES
➤ **Contraception**
Women: Insert one ring into the vagina and leave in place for 3 weeks. Insert new ring 1 week after the previous ring is removed.

ADMINISTRATION
Vaginal
• In women who did not use hormonal contraception during the previous month, therapy should be initiated on the first day

of the menstrual cycle. A woman using a combination oral contraceptive may switch to NuvaRing on any day, but at the latest on the day following the usual hormone-free interval.

• Leave ring in place continuously for a full 3 weeks to maintain effect. It's then removed for 1 week. During this time, withdrawal bleeding occurs (usually starting 2 or 3 days after removal). Insert a new ring 1 week after removal of the previous one, regardless of whether patient is still menstruating.

ACTION

Suppresses gonadotropins, which inhibits ovulation, increases the viscosity of cervical mucus (decreasing the ability of sperm to enter the uterus), and alters the endometrial lining (reducing potential for implantation).

Route	Onset	Peak	Duration
Vaginal	Immediate	200 hr (etonogestrel), 60 hr (ethinyl estradiol)	Unknown

Half-life: etonogestrel, 29 hours; ethinyl estradiol, 45 hours.

ADVERSE REACTIONS

CNS: headache, emotional lability, *cerebral thrombosis, cerebral hemorrhage.*
CV: hypertension, *thromboembolic events, MI.*
EENT: sinusitis, changes in corneal curvature, intolerance to contact lenses.
GI: nausea.
GU: vaginitis, leukorrhea, device-related events (for example, foreign body sensation, coital difficulties, device expulsion), vaginal discomfort, breakthrough bleeding.
Hematologic: *coagulation abnormalities.*
Hepatic: *hepatic adenomas,* benign liver tumors, cholestatic jaundice.
Metabolic: weight gain.
Respiratory: upper respiratory tract infection.
Skin: melasma.

INTERACTIONS

Drug-drug. *Acetaminophen:* May decrease acetaminophen level and increase ethinyl estradiol level. Monitor patient for effects.
Ampicillin, barbiturates, carbamazepine, felbamate, griseofulvin, oxcarbazepine, *phenylbutazone, phenytoin, rifampin, tetracyclines, topiramate:* May decrease contraceptive effect and increase risk of pregnancy, breakthrough bleeding, or both. Tell patient to use an additional form of contraception while taking these drugs.
Ascorbic acid, atorvastatin, itraconazole: May increase ethinyl estradiol level. Monitor patient for adverse effects.
Clofibrate, morphine, salicylic acid, temazepam: May increase clearance of these drugs. Monitor patient for effectiveness.
Cyclosporine, prednisolone, theophylline: May increase levels of these drugs. Monitor levels if appropriate and adjust dosage.
HIV protease inhibitors: May affect contraceptive effect. Refer to the specific protease inhibitor drug literature. May need to use a backup method of contraception.
Miconazole (oil-based vaginal capsule): May increase serum concentrations of etonogestrel and ethinyl estradiol. Monitor patient for adverse effects.
Drug-herb. *St. John's wort:* May reduce drug effectiveness and increase the risk of breakthrough bleeding and pregnancy. Discourage use together.
Drug-lifestyle. *Smoking:* May increase risk of serious CV adverse effects, especially in those older than age 35 who smoke 15 or more cigarettes daily. Urge patient to avoid smoking.

EFFECTS ON LAB TEST RESULTS

• May increase clotting factors VII, VIII, IX, and X; prothrombin; thyroid-binding globulin (leading to increased circulating total thyroid hormone levels); sex hormone–binding globulin (and other binding proteins); and triglyceride levels. May decrease antithrombin III and folate levels.

• May increase norepinephrine-induced platelet aggregation. May decrease T_3 resin uptake.

CONTRAINDICATIONS & CAUTIONS

• Contraindicated in patients hypersensitive to any component of drug, patients who are or may be pregnant, patients older than age 35 who smoke 15 or more cigarettes daily, and patients with thrombophlebitis, thromboembolic disorder, history of deep vein thrombophlebitis, cerebrovascular or coronary artery disease (current or previous), valvular heart disease with complications, severe hypertension, diabetes with vascular complications, headache with focal neurologic symptoms, major surgery with prolonged immobilization, known or suspected cancer of the endometrium or breast, estrogen-dependent neoplasia, abnormal undiagnosed genital bleeding, jaundice related to pregnancy or previous use of hormonal contraceptive, active liver disease, or benign or malignant hepatic tumors.

• Use cautiously in patients with hypertension, hyperlipidemias, obesity, or diabetes.

• Use cautiously in patients with conditions that could be aggravated by fluid retention, and in patients with a history of depression.

NURSING CONSIDERATIONS

◑ Alert: Drug may increase the risk of MI, thromboembolism, stroke, hepatic neoplasia, and gallbladder disease.

Black Box Warning Cigarette smoking increases the risk of serious adverse cardiac effects. The risk increases with age and in patients who smoke 15 or more cigarettes daily. ■

• Stop drug at least 4 weeks before and for 2 weeks after procedures that may increase the risk of thromboembolism, and during and after prolonged immobilization.

• Stop drug and notify prescriber if patient develops unexplained partial or complete loss of vision, proptosis, diplopia, papilledema, retinal vascular lesions, migraines, depression, or jaundice.

• Monitor blood pressure closely if patient has hypertension or renal disease.

• Rule out pregnancy if woman hasn't adhered to the prescribed regimen and a period is missed, if prescribed regimen has been adhered to and two periods are missed, or if the patient has retained the ring for longer than 4 weeks.

PATIENT TEACHING

• Stress importance of having regular annual physical examinations to check for adverse effects or developing contraindications.

• Tell patient that drug doesn't protect against HIV and other sexually transmitted diseases.

• Advise patient not to smoke while using contraceptive.

• Tell patient to use backup method of contraception until ring has been used continuously for 7 days. Tell patient not to use diaphragm if backup method is needed.

• Tell patient who wears contact lenses to contact an ophthalmologist if vision or lens tolerance changes.

• Advise patient to follow manufacturer's instructions for use if switching from different form of hormonal contraceptive.

• Tell patient to insert ring into vagina (using fingers) and keep it in place continuously for 3 weeks to maintain effect, saving foil package for later disposal. Explain that it is then removed for 1 full week and that, during this time, withdrawal bleeding occurs (usually starting 2 or 3 days after removal). Tell patient to insert new ring 1 week after removing previous one, regardless of menstrual bleeding. Tell patient to reseal ring in the package after removing it from vagina.

• Advise patient that, if the ring is removed or expelled (such as while removing a tampon, straining, or moving bowels), it should be washed with cool to lukewarm (not hot) water and reinserted immediately. Stress that contraceptive effect may be compromised if the ring stays out for longer than 3 hours and that she should use a backup method of contraception until the newly reinserted ring has been used continuously for 7 days.

• Tell patient that there's no danger of the vaginal ring being pushed too far up in the vagina or getting lost.

etoposide (VP-16-213)
e-toe-POE-side

etoposide phosphate
Etopophos

Therapeutic class: Antineoplastics
Pharmacologic class: Podophyllotoxin derivatives
Pregnancy risk category: D

AVAILABLE FORMS
etoposide
Capsules: 50 mg
Injection: 20 mg/mL in 5-, 12.5-, and 25-mL vials
etoposide phosphate
Injection: 119.3-mg vials equivalent to 100 mg etoposide

INDICATIONS & DOSAGES
Adjust-a-dose (for all indications): For patients with CrCl of 15 to 50 mL/minute, reduce dose by 25%. For patients with CrCl of less than 10 mL/minute and patients receiving hemodialysis or peritoneal dialysis, reduce dose by 50%. For patients receiving continuous renal replacement therapy, reduce dose by 25%. For patients with hepatic impairment, if bilirubin level is 1.5 to 3 mg/dL and AST level is 60 to 180 units/L, give 50% of usual dose. If bilirubin level is 3 to 5 mg/dL and AST level is greater than 180 units/L, give 25% of usual dose. Withhold drug if bilirubin level is greater than 5 mg/dL.

➤ **Refractory testicular cancer in combination with other chemotherapeutic agents**
Adults: 50 to 100 mg/m² daily I.V. on 5 consecutive days every 3 to 4 weeks. Or, 100 mg/m² daily I.V. on days 1, 3, and 5 every 3 to 4 weeks for three or four courses of therapy.

➤ **Small-cell carcinoma of the lung in combination with other chemotherapeutic agents**
Adults: 35 mg/m² daily I.V. for 4 days. Or, 50 mg/m² daily I.V. for 5 days. Repeat cycles every 3 to 4 weeks. P.O. dose is two times I.V. dose, rounded to nearest 50 mg.

ADMINISTRATION
P.O.
● Give drug without regard for food.
● Don't give drug with grapefruit juice.
I.V.
▼ Preparing and giving parenteral drug may be mutagenic, teratogenic, or carcinogenic. Follow facility policy to reduce risks.
▼ For etoposide infusion, dilute to 0.2 or 0.4 mg/mL in either D_5W or normal saline solution. Higher concentrations may crystallize.
▼ Give etoposide by slow infusion over at least 30 minutes to prevent severe hypotension.
▼ For etoposide phosphate, give without further dilution or dilute to as low as 0.1 mg/mL in either D_5W or normal saline solution.
▼ Give etoposide phosphate over 5 to 210 minutes.
▼ Check blood pressure every 15 minutes during infusion. Hypotension may occur if infusion is too rapid. If systolic pressure falls below 90 mm Hg, stop infusion and notify prescriber.
▼ Etoposide diluted to 0.2 mg/mL is stable 96 hours at room temperature in plastic or glass, unprotected from light; at 0.4 mg/mL, it's stable 24 hours under same conditions. Diluted etoposide phosphate solution is stable for same times at room temperature or 24 hours refrigerated.
▼ **Incompatibilities:** Cefepime hydrochloride, filgrastim, gallium nitrate, idarubicin.

ACTION
Inhibits topoisomerase II enzyme, causing inability to repair DNA strand breaks, which leads to cell death. Cell-cycle specific to G_2 portion of cell cycle.

Route	Onset	Peak	Duration
P.O., I.V.	Unknown	Unknown	Unknown

Half-life: Initial phase, ½ to 2 hours; terminal phase, 5¼ hours.

ADVERSE REACTIONS
CNS: peripheral neuropathy.
CV: hypotension.
GI: anorexia, diarrhea, nausea, vomiting, abdominal pain, stomatitis, mucositis.

Reactions in bold italics are *life-threatening*. Interactions may have a *rapid onset* or a *delayed onset*.

Hematologic: *leukopenia, neutropenia, thrombocytopenia,* anemia, *myelosuppression.*
Hepatic: *hepatotoxicity.*
Skin: reversible alopecia, rash.
Other: *anaphylaxis,* hypersensitivity reactions.

INTERACTIONS
Drug-drug. *Cyclosporine:* May increase etoposide level and toxicity. Monitor CBC and adjust etoposide dose.
Live-virus vaccines: May increase risk of live-virus vaccine–induced adverse reactions. Concurrent use isn't recommended.
Phosphatase inhibitors: May decrease etoposide effectiveness. Monitor drug effects.
Warfarin: May further prolong PT. Monitor PT and INR closely.
Drug-food. *Grapefruit juice:* May reduce etoposide concentrations. Avoid using together.

EFFECTS ON LAB TEST RESULTS
• May decrease hemoglobin level.
• May decrease neutrophil, platelet, RBC, and WBC counts.

CONTRAINDICATIONS & CAUTIONS
• Contraindicated in patients hypersensitive to drug.
• Use cautiously in patients who have had cytotoxic or radiation therapy and in those with hepatic impairment.

NURSING CONSIDERATIONS
Black Box Warning Give drug under the supervision of a physician experienced in the use of cancer chemotherapy. ∎
• Obtain baseline blood pressure before starting therapy.
• Anticipate need for antiemetics.
• Have diphenhydramine, hydrocortisone, epinephrine, and emergency equipment available to establish an airway in case anaphylaxis occurs.
• Store capsules in refrigerator.
Black Box Warning Monitor CBC. Watch for evidence of bone marrow suppression. ∎
• Observe patient's mouth for signs of ulceration.

• To prevent bleeding, avoid all I.M. injections when platelet count is below 50,000/mm³.
• Etoposide phosphate dose is expressed as etoposide equivalents; 119.3 mg of etoposide phosphate is equivalent to 100 mg of etoposide.

PATIENT TEACHING
• Tell patient to watch for signs and symptoms of infection (fever, sore throat, fatigue) and bleeding (easy bruising, nosebleeds, bleeding gums, tarry stools). Tell patient to take temperature daily.
• Inform patient of need for frequent blood pressure readings during I.V. administration.
• Caution women of childbearing age to avoid pregnancy and breast-feeding during therapy.

etravirine
eh-trah-VIGH-reen

Intelence

Therapeutic class: Antiretrovirals
Pharmacologic class: Antivirals
Pregnancy risk category: B

AVAILABLE FORMS
Tablets: 25 mg, 100 mg, 200 mg

INDICATIONS & DOSAGES
➤ **HIV-1 in patients who have had previous treatment and have replication of HIV-1 strains resistant to an NNRTI and other antiretrovirals**
Adults: 200 mg P.O. b.i.d. after meals. Given with other antiretrovirals.
Children age 6 and older weighing 30 kg (66 lb) or more: 200 mg P.O. b.i.d.
Children age 6 and older weighing 25 kg (55 lb) to less than 30 kg: 150 mg P.O. b.i.d.
Children age 6 and older weighing 20 kg (44 lb) to less than 25 kg: 125 mg P.O. b.i.d.
Children age 6 and older weighing 16 kg (35 lb) to less than 20 kg: 100 mg P.O. b.i.d.

ADMINISTRATION
P.O.
• Give drug after meals.
• If patient can't swallow tablets, disperse tablets in a glass of water. Stir the dispersion

well and have the patient drink immediately. Rinse the glass with water several times and have patient swallow each rinse completely.

ACTION

Binds to reverse transcriptase, an enzyme that replicates HIV.

Route	Onset	Peak	Duration
P.O.	Unknown	2.5–4 hours	Unknown

Half-life: About 41 hours.

ADVERSE REACTIONS

CNS: abnormal dreams, amnesia, anxiety, confusion, disorientation, fatigue, headache, hypoesthesia, insomnia, paresthesia, peripheral neuropathy, *seizures,* sluggishness, syncope, tremors.
CV: angina, *atrial fibrillation,* hypertension, *MI.*
EENT: blurred vision, vertigo.
GI: abdominal distension, abdominal pain, anorexia, constipation, diarrhea, dry mouth, flatulence, gastritis, GERD, hematemesis, nausea, *pancreatitis,* retching, stomatitis, vomiting.
GU: *renal failure.*
Hepatic: *hepatitis,* hepatomegaly, increased liver enzyme levels.
Hematologic: anemia, hemolytic anemia.
Metabolic: *diabetes,* dyslipidemia.
Respiratory: *bronchospasm,* dyspnea.
Skin: rash.
Other: facial wasting, fat redistribution or accumulation, gynecomastia, hypersensitivity, immune reconstitution syndrome.

INTERACTIONS

Drug-drug. *Amiodarone, bepridil, disopyramide, flecainide, lidocaine, mexiletine, propafenone, quinidine:* May decrease levels of these drugs. Use caution, and monitor patient closely.
Amprenavir and ritonavir: May increase amprenavir level. Avoid use together.
Atazanavir and ritonavir: May decrease atazanavir level and increase etravirine level. Avoid use together.
Atorvastatin, lovastatin, simvastatin: May decrease levels of these drugs. Adjust dosage, if needed.
Clarithromycin: May decrease clarithromycin level and increase etravirine

level. Consider using azithromycin for treating *Mycobacterium avium* complex.
CYP3A4 inhibitors (such as itraconazole, ketoconazole): May decrease levels of these drugs. Adjust dosage, if needed.
CYP450 inducers (such as carbamazepine, phenobarbital, phenytoin): May decrease etravirine level. Avoid use together.
Delavirdine: May increase etravirine level. Avoid use together.
Dexamethasone: May decrease etravirine level. Avoid use together.
Diazepam: May increase diazepam level. Reduce diazepam dose, as needed.
Efavirenz, nevirapine: May decrease etravirine level. Avoid use together.
Fluconazole, posaconazole: May increase etravirine level. Use together cautiously.
Fluvastatin: May increase fluvastatin level. Adjust dosage, if needed.
Immunosuppressants (such as cyclosporine, sirolimus, tacrolimus): May decrease levels of these drugs. Use together cautiously, and monitor patient closely.
Lopinavir–ritonavir: May increase etravirine level. Use together cautiously.
Methadone: May cause withdrawal symptoms. Monitor patient, and consider increasing methadone dosage.
PDE5 inhibitors (sildenafil, tadalafil, vardenafil): May decrease effectiveness of these drugs. Adjust dosage, as needed.
Protease inhibitors (such as atazanavir, fosamprenavir, indinavir, nelfinavir): May alter protease inhibitor level if given without ritonavir. Avoid use together unless given with low-dose ritonavir.
Rifabutin: May decrease etravirine and rifabutin levels. If etravirine isn't given with a protease inhibitor and ritonavir, give rifabutin 300 mg daily. If etravirine is given with darunavir and ritonavir or with raquinavir and ritonavir, avoid rifabutin.
Rifampin, rifapentine: May decrease etravirine level. Avoid use together.
Ritonavir: May decrease etravirine level. Avoid use together.
Ritonavir and tipranavir: May decrease etravirine level. Avoid use together.
Warfarin: May increase warfarin level. Monitor INR closely, and adjust warfarin dosage if needed.

Reactions in bold italics are *life-threatening*. Interactions may have a *rapid onset* or a *delayed onset*.

Drug-herb. *St. John's wort:* May decrease etravirine level. Avoid use together.

EFFECTS ON LAB TEST RESULTS
● May increase amylase, lipase, creatinine, total cholesterol, LDL, triglyceride, AST, ALT, and glucose levels. May decrease hemoglobin level.
● May decrease RBC, neutrophil, and platelet counts.

CONTRAINDICATIONS & CAUTIONS
● Contraindicated in patients hypersensitive to etravirine or its components.
● Use cautiously in elderly patients and patients with hepatic impairment or hepatitis B or C.
● For children, don't exceed adult dosage or give to children younger than age 6.
● Pregnant women should take etravirine only if potential benefits to mother outweigh risks to fetus.
● Pregnant women who take etravirine should be enrolled in the Antiretroviral Pregnancy Registry, which monitors maternal-fetal outcomes, by calling 1-800-258-4263.

NURSING CONSIDERATIONS
۞ Alert: Etravirine may interact with many drugs. Review patient's complete drug regimen.
● If patient can't swallow the tablet whole, dissolve it in water and have patient drink it immediately. To make sure patient receives entire dose, refill the glass several times and have patient drink.
۞ Alert: Monitor patient closely for skin reactions. Fatalities have occurred due to toxic epidermal necrolysis and hypersensitivity reactions that may be accompanied by hepatic failure. Discontinue drug if severe skin or hypersensitivity reactions develop.
● Monitor patient for signs of fat redistribution, including central obesity, buffalo hump, peripheral wasting, breast enlargement, and cushingoid appearance.
● Notify prescriber if signs, symptoms, or laboratory abnormalities suggest pancreatitis. Monitor amylase and lipase levels.
● Monitor patient's CBC, platelet count, and renal and liver function studies. Report abnormalities.

PATIENT TEACHING
● Advise patient to take etravirine after a meal.
● Warn patient to tell prescriber about any other prescription drugs, OTC drugs, and herbal supplements he takes.
● Advise patient to report adverse effects to prescriber.
● Inform patient that drug doesn't cure HIV infection, that opportunistic infections and other complications of HIV infection may still occur, and that HIV may still be transmitted to others through sexual contact or blood contamination.
● Advise patient to take drug as prescribed and not to alter dose or stop drug without medical approval.
● If patient misses a dose, tell him to take it as soon as possible and then return to his normal schedule. Advise patient not to double the dose.
● Tell patient that routine blood tests will be needed to assess how he is tolerating drug therapy.

SAFETY ALERT!

everolimus
eh-ver-OH-lih-mus

Afinitor, Afinitor Disperz, Zortress

Therapeutic class: Antineoplastics
Pharmacologic class: Kinase inhibitors
Pregnancy risk category: D

AVAILABLE FORMS
Tablets (Afinitor): 2.5 mg, 5 mg, 7.5 mg, 10 mg
Tablets (Afinitor Disperz): 2 mg, 3 mg, 5 mg
Tablets (Zortress): 0.25 mg, 0.5 mg, 0.75 mg

INDICATIONS & DOSAGES
➤ **Advanced renal cell carcinoma after treatment with sunitinib or sorafenib fails (Afinitor)**
Adults: 10 mg P.O. once daily.
Adjust-a-dose: For severe or intolerable adverse effects, reduce dosage to 5 mg P.O. daily or interrupt therapy. For mild hepatic impairment (Child-Pugh class A), reduce dosage to 7.5 mg P.O. daily; may decrease to 5 mg if not well tolerated. For moderate hepatic impairment (Child-Pugh class B),

reduce dosage to 5 mg P.O. daily; may decrease to 2.5 mg if not well tolerated. For severe hepatic impairment (Child-Pugh class C), reduce dosage to 2.5 mg P.O. daily and use only if benefit outweighs risk; don't exceed 2.5 mg. If concomitant use of drugs that are moderate inhibitors of CYP3A4 or P-glycoprotein (P-gp) are required, decrease dosage to 2.5 mg P.O. daily; if tolerated, may increase to 5 mg daily. If concomitant use of drugs that are strong inducers of CYP3A4 can't be avoided, increase dosage in 5-mg increments to a maximum dosage of 20 mg P.O. daily.

✸ *NEW INDICATION:* **Prevention of organ rejection in liver transplantation (Zortress only)**
Adults: 1 mg P.O. b.i.d. starting at least 30 days after transplant in combination with reduced-dose tacrolimus and corticosteroids. Adjust dosage based on trough concentrations obtained 4 to 5 days after previous dosing change to a target therapeutic range of 3 to 8 ng/mL.
Adjust-a-dose: In patients with mild hepatic impairment, reduce initial dose by one-third. In patients with moderate to severe hepatic impairment, reduce initial dose by one-half.

➤ **Prevention of kidney transplant rejection in patients at low to moderate immunologic risk (Zortress only)**
Adults: Initially, 0.75 mg P.O. b.i.d. in combination with basiliximab induction and a reduced dose of cyclosporine and corticosteroids as soon as possible after transplantation. Dosage adjustments may be made at 4- to 5-day intervals based on patient response and clinical situation.
Adjust-a-dose: In patients with moderate hepatic impairment, give half the recommended initial daily dose and monitor blood concentrations.

➤ **Subependymal giant cell astrocytoma with tuberous sclerosis in patients who aren't surgical candidates (Afinitor or Afinitor Disperz)**
Adults and children age 1 and older: Initially, 4.5 mg/m^2 P.O. once daily. Adjust dosage in 2-week intervals to trough concentration of 5 to 15 ng/mL. Don't combine the two dosage forms (Afinitor tablets and Afinitor Disperz tablets) to achieve the desired dose. Use one dosage form or the other.

Adjust-a-dose: The recommended starting dose for patients with severe hepatic impairment (Child-Pugh class C) or requiring moderate CYP3A4 or P-gp inhibitors is 2.5 mg/m^2, once daily. The recommended starting dose for patients requiring a concomitant strong CYP3A4 inducer is 9 mg/m^2 once daily. Assess trough concentrations approximately 2 weeks after initiation of treatment, a change in dose, a change in coadministration of CYP3A4 or P-gp inducers or inhibitors, a change in hepatic function, or a change in dosage form between Afinitor tablets and Afinitor Disperz. For severe or intolerable adverse reactions, reduce dose by approximately 50%. If dose reduction falls below lowest available strength, give every other day.

➤ **Progressive pancreatic neuroendocrine tumors (unresectable, locally advanced, or metastatic) (Afinitor)**
Adults: 10 mg P.O. daily.
Adjust-a-dose: For severe or intolerable adverse effects, reduce dosage to 5 mg P.O. daily or interrupt therapy. For mild hepatic impairment (Child-Pugh class A), reduce dosage to 7.5 mg P.O. daily; may decrease to 5 mg if not well tolerated. For moderate hepatic impairment (Child-Pugh class B), reduce dosage to 5 mg P.O. daily; may decrease to 2.5 mg if not well tolerated. For severe hepatic impairment (Child-Pugh class C), reduce dosage to 2.5 mg P.O. daily and use only if benefit outweighs risk; don't exceed 2.5 mg. If concomitant use of drugs that are moderate inhibitors of CYP3A4 or P-gp is required, reduce dosage to 2.5 mg P.O. daily; if tolerated, may increase to 5 mg daily. If concomitant use of drugs that are strong inducers of CYP3A4 can't be avoided, increase dosage in 5-mg increments to a maximum of 20 mg P.O. daily.

➤ **Renal angiomyolipoma with tuberous sclerosis complex (Afinitor); advanced hormone-receptor positive, *HER2*-negative breast cancer in postmenopausal women in combination with exemestane for recurrence or progression after treatment with letrozole or anastrozole (Afinitor)**
Adults: 10 mg P.O. daily.
Adjust-a-dose: For severe or intolerable adverse effects, reduce dosage to 5 mg P.O.

daily or interrupt therapy. For mild hepatic failure (Child Pugh class A), reduce dosage to 7.5 mg P.O. daily; may decrease to 5 mg if not well tolerated. For moderate hepatic failure (Child Pugh class B), reduce dosage to 5 mg P.O. daily; may decrease to 2.5 mg if not well tolerated. For severe hepatic impairment (Child Pugh class C), reduce dosage to 2.5 mg P.O. daily and use only if benefit outweighs risk; don't exceed 2.5 mg. If concomitant use of drugs that are moderate inhibitors of CYP3A4 or P-gp are needed, decrease dosage to 2.5 mg P.O. daily; if tolerated, may increase to 5 mg daily. If concomitant use of drugs that are strong inducers of CYP3A4 can't be avoided, increase dosage in 5-mg increments to a maximum of 20 mg P.O. daily.

ADMINISTRATION
P.O. (Afinitor, Zortress)
● Give drug at same time each day, consistently with or consistently without food.
● Have patient swallow tablets whole with a glass of water. Tablets shouldn't be chewed or crushed.
● Patient should avoid grapefruit or grapefruit juice while taking drug.
P.O. (Afinitor Disperz)
● Give Afinitor Disperz (everolimus tablets for oral suspension) as a suspension only.
● Give drug orally once daily at the same time every day, either consistently with food or consistently without food.
● Administer suspension immediately after preparation. Discard suspension if not administered within 60 minutes after preparation. Prepare suspension in water only.
● To administer drug using an oral syringe, place the prescribed dose into a 10-mL syringe. Do not exceed a total of 10 mg per syringe. If higher doses are required, prepare an additional syringe. Do not break or crush tablets. Draw approximately 5 mL of water and 4 mL of air into the syringe. Place the filled syringe into a container (tip up) for 3 minutes, until the tablets are in suspension. Gently invert the syringe 5 times immediately prior to administration. After administration of the prepared suspension, draw approximately 5 mL of water and 4 mL of air into the same syringe, and swirl the contents to suspend remaining particles. Administer the entire contents of the syringe.
● To administer using a small drinking glass, place the prescribed dose into a small drinking glass (maximum size 100 mL) containing approximately 25 mL of water. Do not exceed a total of 10 mg per glass. If higher doses are required, prepare an additional glass. Do not break or crush tablets. Allow 3 minutes for suspension to occur. Stir the contents gently with a spoon, immediately prior to drinking. After administration of the prepared suspension, add 25 mL of water and stir with the same spoon to re-suspend remaining particles. Administer the entire contents of the glass.

ACTION
Binds to an intracellular protein, thereby inhibiting mammalian target rapamycin (mTOR), a kinase. Inhibiting mTOR reduces cancer cell proliferation, angiogenesis, and glucose uptake.

Route	Onset	Peak	Duration
P.O.	Unknown	1–2 hr	Unknown

Half-life: 30 hours.

ADVERSE REACTIONS
CNS: asthenia, dizziness, dysgeusia, headache, insomnia, paresthesia, fever, fatigue.
CV: chest pain, *heart failure,* hypertension, tachycardia.
EENT: conjunctivitis, eyelid edema, epistaxis, mucosal inflammation, nasopharyngitis, pharyngolaryngeal pain, rhinorrhea, sinusitis.
GI: abdominal pain, anorexia, diarrhea, dry mouth, dysphagia, hemorrhoids, nausea, stomatitis, vomiting.
GU: renal failure, UTI.
Hematologic: *hemorrhage.*
Metabolic: exacerbation of diabetes mellitus, weight loss.
Musculoskeletal: extremity pain, jaw pain.
Respiratory: bronchitis, cough, dyspnea, pleural effusion, pneumonia, *pneumonitis.*
Skin: acneiform dermatitis, dry skin, erythema, hand-foot syndrome, nail disorder, pruritus, onychoclasis, rash, skin lesion.
Other: chills, peripheral edema.

INTERACTIONS
Drug-drug. Black Box Warning *Cyclosporine:* Increased nephrotoxicity can occur with standard cyclosporine dosing in combination with everolimus. Decrease cyclosporine dosage and monitor serum cyclosporine and everolimus levels. ■
Strong CYP3A4 inducers (carbamazepine, dexamethasone, phenobarbital, phenytoin, rifabutin, rifampin): May decrease everolimus level. Avoid using together; if drugs must be used together, increase everolimus dosage at 5 mg-increments up to 20 mg daily.
Strong or moderate CYP3A4 inhibitors (amprenavir, aprepitant, atazanavir, clarithromycin, delavirdine, diltiazem, erythromycin, fluconazole, fosamprenavir, indinavir, itraconazole, ketoconazole, nefazodone, nelfinavir, ritonavir, saquinavir, telithromycin, verapamil, voriconazole) and P-gp inhibitors (amiodarone, atorvastatin, spironolactone): May increase everolimus level. Avoid using together.
Drug-herb. *St. John's wort:* May alter drug level. Discourage use together.
Drug-food. *Grapefruit, grapefruit juice:* May increase drug level. Don't use together.

EFFECTS ON LAB TEST RESULTS
● May increase creatinine, cholesterol, triglyceride, and glucose levels.
● May decrease hemoglobin level and lymphocyte, neutrophil, and platelet counts.

CONTRAINDICATIONS & CAUTIONS
Black Box Warning Use of Zortress has been shown to increase mortality in a heart transplant clinical trial. Use in heart transplant patients isn't recommended. ■
● Contraindicated in patients hypersensitive to drug, its components, other rapamycin derivatives, or sirolimus (Zortress only).
● Avoid use in patients with severe hepatic impairment or severe infection.
● Avoid use in pregnant women because of potential hazards to fetus.
● It isn't known if drug appears in breast milk. Women shouldn't breast-feed while taking drug.

NURSING CONSIDERATIONS
Black Box Warning Zortress should only be prescribed by providers experienced in immunosuppressive therapy and management of transplant patients. ■
● Don't crush tablets. Avoid direct contact with skin or mucous membranes. If contact occurs, wash area thoroughly.
Black Box Warning Zortress increases risk of infection and malignancies, such as lymphoma and skin cancer, due to immunosuppression. ■
● *Alert:* Drug may cause immunosuppression, predisposing patients to bacterial, fungal, viral, or protozoal infections, including reactivation of hepatitis B virus. Infections may be severe or even fatal. Complete treatment of preexisting invasive fungal infections before starting therapy. Consider holding or stopping everolimus if infection occurs. Discontinue drug if invasive systemic fungal infection is diagnosed, and treat infection appropriately.
● Monitor patient for signs of infection (fever, chills, sore throat, fatigue).
Black Box Warning There is an increased risk of arterial and venous renal thrombosis leading to graft loss in patients taking Zortress, usually in first 30 days after transplant. ■
● Monitor renal function studies and CBC before and during therapy.
● Avoid mouthwash containing alcohol or peroxide in patients who develop mouth ulcers, stomatitis, or oral mucositis.
● Monitor respiratory status for signs and symptoms of noninfectious pneumonitis (hypoxia, pleural effusion, cough, dyspnea). For severe cases, discontinue therapy and administer corticosteroids.

PATIENT TEACHING
● Advise women of childbearing age to use an effective method of contraception during therapy and for 8 weeks after therapy ends.
● Tell patient to swallow the Afinitor or Zortress tablets whole with a full glass of water.
● Teach patient to take the drug at the same time each day, consistently with or consistently without food.
● Instruct caregiver how to prepare and administer Afinitor Disperz for oral suspension.
● Instruct patient that if he misses a dose of Afinitor, he may still take it up to 6 hours

after he would normally take it. If more than 6 hours have elapsed, tell patient to skip the dose for that day and take it at the usual time the next day.

• Advise patient to notify health care provider if he experiences mouth ulcers, fever, shortness of breath, cough, rash, headache, loss of appetite, nausea, vomiting, diarrhea, swelling of the extremities or face, weakness, tiredness, or nosebleeds.

• Tell patient not to receive live-virus vaccines and to avoid close contact with anyone who has received a live-virus vaccine.

SAFETY ALERT!

exenatide
eks-EHN-uh-tyde

Bydureon, Byetta

Therapeutic class: Antidiabetics
Pharmacologic class: Incretin mimetics
Pregnancy risk category: C

AVAILABLE FORMS
Injection: 5 mcg/dose in 1.2-mL prefilled pen (60 doses); 10 mcg/dose in 2.4-mL prefilled pen (60 doses)
Injection (extended-release): 2 mg/dose in single-use vial

INDICATIONS & DOSAGES
➤ **Adjunct to diet and exercise to improve glycemic control in patients with type 2 diabetes**
Adults: 5 mcg subcutaneously b.i.d. within 60 minutes before morning and evening meals. If needed, increase to 10 mcg b.i.d. after 1 month. Or, 2 mg (extended-release) subcutaneously every 7 days.
Adjust-a-dose: Use caution when escalating doses of Byetta (injection) from 5 to 10 mcg in patients with moderate renal impairment (CrCl of 50 to 80 mL/minute). Bydureon and Byetta aren't recommended for patients with ESRD or severe renal impairment (CrCl of less than 30 mL/minute).

ADMINISTRATION
Subcutaneous
Bydureon
• Give Bydureon at any time during the day and without regard to meals.

• To administer: Attach vial connector to vial.
— Connect prefilled diluent syringe to vial.
— Push on syringe's plunger to inject diluent into vial. Continue to push on plunger while shaking vial to thoroughly mix powder and diluent. Solution will be cloudy.
— Invert vial and withdraw solution to the black-dashed dose line on syringe.
— Remove vial connector and attach needle.
— Give immediately as a subcutaneous injection in the thigh, abdomen, or back of upper arm.
• Store in refrigerator at 36° to 46° F (2° to 8° C). May store at room temperature (68° to 77° F [20° to 25° C]) for up to 4 weeks. Don't freeze.
Byetta
• Drug comes in two strengths; check cartridge carefully before use.
• Give as a subcutaneous injection in the thigh, abdomen, or upper arm.
• Before first use, store drug in refrigerator at 36° to 46° F (2° to 8° C). After first use, drug can be kept at room temperature up to 77° F (25° C). Don't freeze, and don't use drug if it has been frozen. Protect drug from light. Discard pen 30 days after first use, even if some drug remains.

ACTION
Reduces fasting and postprandial glucose levels in type 2 diabetes by stimulating insulin production in response to elevated glucose levels, inhibiting glucagon release after meals, and slowing gastric emptying.

Route	Onset	Peak	Duration
Subcut.	Unknown	2 hr	Unknown
Subcut. (extended-release)	Unknown	2 wk, 6–7 wk	10 wk

Half-life: 2½ hours, extended-release unknown.

ADVERSE REACTIONS
CNS: dizziness, headache, jittery feeling, weakness.
GI: anorexia, constipation, diarrhea, dyspepsia, nausea, *pancreatitis,* vomiting, reflux.
Metabolic: *hypoglycemia.*
Skin: excessive sweating, pruritis, urticaria, rash.
Other: hypersensitivity reactions, injection-site reaction, *angioedema, anaphylaxis.*

INTERACTIONS
Drug-drug. *Acetaminophen:* May decrease acetaminophen concentration. Give acetaminophen at least 1 hour before or 4 hours after exenatide injection.
Digoxin, lisinopril, lovastatin: May decrease concentrations of these drugs. Monitor patient.
Drugs that are rapidly absorbed: May slow gastric emptying and reduce absorption of some oral drugs. Separate administration by 1 hour.
Oral drugs that need to maintain a threshold concentration to maintain effectiveness (antibiotics, hormonal contraceptives): May reduce rate and extent of absorption of these drugs. Give these drugs at least 1 hour before giving exenatide.
Other hypoglycemic agents (insulin, meglitinides [repaglinide]): May increase risk of hypoglycemia. Closely monitor blood glucose concentrations when exenatide is started or stopped, and reinforce patient instructions for hypoglycemia management, especially in patients receiving insulin.
Sulfonylureas: May increase the risk of hypoglycemia. Reduce sulfonylurea dose as needed, and monitor patient closely.
Warfarin: May increase INR and increase bleeding risk when administered together. Monitor INR frequently, especially when starting drug or changing dosage.

EFFECTS ON LAB TEST RESULTS
● May increase INR.

CONTRAINDICATIONS & CAUTIONS
Black Box Warning Extended-release form (Bydureon) is contraindicated in patients with personal or family history of medullary thyroid carcinoma and in patients with multiple endocrine neoplasia syndrome type 2. ■
● Contraindicated in patients hypersensitive to drug or its components.
● Don't use in patients with type 1 diabetes or diabetic ketoacidosis.
● Don't use in patients with ESRD, CrCl less than 30 mL/minute, or severe GI disease (including gastroparesis).
● Use cautiously in pregnant or breast-feeding women, and in patients with renal transplant.
⚠ **Overdose S&S:** Severe nausea, severe vomiting, hypoglycemia.

NURSING CONSIDERATIONS
● Assess GI and renal function before and during treatment.
❸ **Alert:** Drug-related nausea, vomiting, and diarrhea resulting in dehydration have led to increased serum creatinine levels and acute renal failure.
● Monitor glucose level regularly and glycosylated hemoglobin level periodically.
❸ **Alert:** Stop drug if pancreatitis is suspected. Initiate appropriate treatment and monitor patient carefully. Drug shouldn't be readministered.
● **Look alike–sound alike:** Don't confuse exenatide with ezetimibe.

PATIENT TEACHING
Black Box Warning Explain to patient taking Bydureon the risk and signs and symptoms of thyroid tumors. ■
● Explain the risks of drug.
● Review proper use and storage of medication, particularly the one-time setup for each new pen or reconstitution procedure for powder.
● Inform patient that prefilled pen doesn't include a needle; the prescriber will indicate which needle length and gauge is appropriate.
● Instruct patient to inject Byetta in the thigh, abdomen, or upper arm within 60 minutes before morning and evening meals. Caution against injecting drug after a meal.
● Instruct patient to inject Bydureon in the thigh, abdomen, or back of upper arm immediately after mixing with diluent.
● Advise patient that drug may decrease appetite, food intake, and body weight, and that these changes don't warrant a change in dosage.
● Advise patient to seek immediate medical care if unexplained, persistent, severe abdominal pain, with or without vomiting, occurs.
● Review steps for managing hypoglycemia, especially if patient takes a sulfonylurea or insulin.
● Inform patient of potential risk of worsening renal function and signs and symptoms of renal dysfunction.
● Tell patient changing from Byetta to Bydureon that transient blood glucose

---

Reactions in bold italics are *life-threatening*. Interactions may have a *rapid onset* or a *delayed onset*.

elevations are possible during the first 2 weeks of therapy.

• Stress importance of proper storage (refrigerated), infection prevention, and timing of exenatide dose in relation to other oral drugs.

• Tell patient that if a dose of Byetta is missed to resume treatment as prescribed with the next scheduled dose.

• Tell patient that if a dose of Bydureon is missed to administer it as soon as noticed, provided the next regularly scheduled dose is due at least 3 days later, and then to resume once-every-7-days dosing schedule. If a dose is missed and the next regularly scheduled dose is due in 1 to 2 days, tell patient not to administer the missed dose and instead to resume therapy with next regularly scheduled dose.

ezetimibe
ee-ZET-ah-mibe

Zetia🖋

Therapeutic class: Antilipemics
Pharmacologic class: Selective cholesterol absorption inhibitors
Pregnancy risk category: C

AVAILABLE FORMS
Tablets: 10 mg

INDICATIONS & DOSAGES
➤ **Adjunct to diet and exercise to reduce total cholesterol, LDL-C, and apolipoprotein B (apo B) levels in patients with primary hypercholesterolemia, alone or combined with HMG-CoA reductase inhibitors (statins) or bile acid sequestrants; adjunct to other lipid-lowering drugs (combined with atorvastatin or simvastatin) in patients with homozygous familial hypercholesterolemia; adjunct to diet in patients with homozygous sitosterolemia to reduce sitosterol and campesterol levels; adjunct to fenofibrate and diet to reduce total cholesterol, LDL-C, apo B, and non–HDL-C levels in patients with mixed hyperlipidemia**
Adults and children age 10 and older: 10 mg P.O. daily.

ADMINISTRATION
P.O.
• Give drug without regard for meals.
• May give dose at same time as an HMG-CoA reductase inhibitor or fenofibrate.
• Give at least 2 hours before or at least 4 hours after administration of a bile acid sequestrant.

ACTION
Inhibits absorption of cholesterol by the small intestine, unlike other drugs used for cholesterol reduction; causes reduced hepatic cholesterol stores and increased cholesterol clearance from the blood.

Route	Onset	Peak	Duration
P.O.	Unknown	4–12 hr	Unknown

Half-life: 22 hours.

ADVERSE REACTIONS
CNS: dizziness, fatigue, headache.
EENT: nasopharyngitis, sinusitis.
GI: abdominal pain, diarrhea.
Musculoskeletal: arthralgia, back pain, pain in extremity, myalgia.
Respiratory: upper respiratory tract infection.
Other: viral infection.

INTERACTIONS
Drug-drug. *Bile acid sequestrant (cholestyramine):* May decrease ezetimibe level. Give ezetimibe at least 2 hours before or 4 hours after cholestyramine.
Cyclosporine, fenofibrate: May increase ezetimibe level. Monitor patient for adverse reactions.
Fibrates: May increase excretion of cholesterol into the gallbladder bile. Avoid using together.

EFFECTS ON LAB TEST RESULTS
• May increase LFT values.

CONTRAINDICATIONS & CAUTIONS
• Contraindicated in patients allergic to any component of the drug.
• Contraindicated with HMG-CoA reductase inhibitor in pregnant or breast-feeding women and in patients with active hepatic disease or unexplained increased transaminase level.
• Use cautiously in elderly patients.

NURSING CONSIDERATIONS
● Before starting treatment, assess patient for underlying causes of dyslipidemia.
● Obtain baseline triglyceride and total cholesterol, LDL-C, and HDL-C levels.
● Using drug with an HMG-CoA reductase inhibitor significantly decreases total cholesterol and LDL-C, apo B, and triglyceride levels and (except with pravastatin) increases HDL-C level more than use of an HMG-CoA reductase inhibitor alone. Check LFT values when therapy starts and thereafter according to the HMG-CoA reductase inhibitor manufacturer's recommendations.
● Patient should maintain a cholesterol-lowering diet during treatment.
● Monitor patient for muscle pain, weakness, or tenderness.

PATIENT TEACHING
● Emphasize importance of following a cholesterol-lowering diet during drug therapy.
● Tell patient he may take drug without regard for meals.
● Advise patient to notify prescriber of unexplained muscle pain, weakness, or tenderness.
● Urge patient to tell prescriber about any herbal or dietary supplements he's taking.
● Advise patient to visit prescriber for routine follow-ups and blood tests.
● Tell woman to notify prescriber if she becomes pregnant.

ezogabine
e-ZOG-a-been

Potiga

Therapeutic class: Anticonvulsants
Pharmacologic class: Potassium channel activators
Pregnancy risk category: C
Controlled substance schedule: V

AVAILABLE FORMS
Tablets: 50 mg, 200 mg, 300 mg, 400 mg

INDICATIONS & DOSAGES
➤ **Adjunctive treatment of partial-onset seizures**
Adults: 100 mg P.O. t.i.d. Increase at weekly intervals by no more than 50 mg t.i.d. Maximum dosage is 400 mg P.O. t.i.d.
Adjust-a-dose: For patients older than age 65 and those with hepatic impairment (Child-Pugh score between 7 and 9), initially give 50 mg P.O. t.i.d.; may increase dosage at weekly intervals by no more than 50 mg P.O. t.i.d. to a maximum of 250 mg P.O. t.i.d. For patients with CrCl of less than 50 mL/minute, ESRD, or severe hepatic impairment (Child-Pugh score greater than 9), initially give 50 mg P.O. t.i.d. May increase dosage at weekly intervals by no more than 50 mg P.O. t.i.d. to a maximum of 200 mg P.O. t.i.d.

ADMINISTRATION
P.O.
● May give with or without food.
● Patient should swallow tablets whole, and shouldn't crush, chew, or dissolve them.

ACTION
Unknown. Thought to activate potassium channels, which stabilize the resting membrane potential and reduce brain excitability.

Route	Onset	Peak	Duration
P.O.	Rapid	½–2 hr	Unknown

Half-life: 7 to 11 hours.

ADVERSE REACTIONS
CNS: fatigue, dizziness, somnolence, tremor, abnormal coordination, confusion, aphasia, dysarthria, vertigo, asthenia, impaired memory, paresthesia, amnesia, anxiety, disorientation, psychosis, hallucinations, *suicidal thoughts or behaviors,* worsening depression, withdrawal seizures, disturbance in attention, gait, or balance.
CV: *QT-interval prolongation.*
EENT: diplopia, blurred vision.
GI: nausea, constipation, dyspepsia, dysphagia.
GU: dysuria, urinary hesitation, urine retention, hematuria, chromaturia.
Metabolic: weight gain.
Other: influenza.

Reactions in bold italics are *life-threatening*. Interactions may have a *rapid onset* or a *delayed onset*.

INTERACTIONS

Drug-drug. *Carbamazepine, phenytoin:* May decrease ezogabine level. Consider increasing ezogabine dosage.

Digoxin: May inhibit renal clearance of digoxin, increasing digoxin level. Monitor digoxin level closely.

Drug-lifestyle. *Alcohol use:* May increase ezogabine level and risk of adverse effects. Use together cautiously, if at all.

EFFECTS ON LAB TEST RESULTS

● May cause falsely elevated serum and urine bilirubin levels.

CONTRAINDICATIONS & CAUTIONS

● Contraindicated in patients hypersensitive to drug and in breast-feeding women.

● Use cautiously in patients with increased risk of urine retention, such as those with BPH, those unable to communicate symptoms, and those who use medications such as anticholinergics that affect voiding.

● Use cautiously in patients with prolonged QT interval, congestive heart failure, ventricular hypertrophy, hypokalemia, or hypomagnesemia, and in those who are taking other drugs known to prolong QT interval.

● Use cautiously in patients with hepatic or renal insufficiency.

● Use in pregnant women only if benefits to the mother outweigh potential risk to the fetus. Encourage patients to enroll in the North American Antiepileptic Drug Pregnancy Registry by calling 1-888-233-2334 or going online to www.aedpregnancyregistry.org.

⚠ Overdose S&S: Agitation, aggressive behavior, irritability, cardiac arrhythmia.

NURSING CONSIDERATIONS

● Avoid stopping drug abruptly. Gradually reduce dosage over at least 3 weeks, unless safety concerns require abrupt withdrawal. May cause blue skin discoloration.

Black Box Warning May cause pigment changes in the retina. Obtain eye examination at baseline and periodically (every 6 months) during therapy. Discontinue drug if skin discoloration or ophthalmic changes occur, unless no other treatment options are available and the benefits of treatment outweigh the potential risk of vision loss. ∎

● Monitor patient for urine retention, weak urine stream, or pain on urination.

● Monitor patient for confusion, psychosis, hallucinations, dizziness, and somnolence.

● Monitor QT interval in patients with known prolonged QT interval, congestive heart failure, ventricular hypertrophy, hypokalemia, or hypomagnesemia, or when patient is taking other drugs known to prolong the QT interval.

● Monitor patient for warning signs and symptoms of suicidal thoughts or behaviors, such as worsening depression or unusual changes in mood or behavior.

PATIENT TEACHING

Black Box Warning Warn patient to contact health care provider immediately if changes in vision occur. ∎

● Tell patient to report discoloration of the skin, including lips and nail beds.

● Warn patient not to stop drug without first consulting health care provider, because seizures may worsen. Patient should contact prescriber if more than one dose is missed.

● Advise patient to report signs and symptoms of urine retention (bloating, bladder discomfort), weakening of urine stream, or painful urination.

● Warn patient not to drive, operate machinery, or perform other dangerous activities until the effects of ezogabine are known.

⟲ Alert: Inform patient, caregivers, and family about the risk of confusion, psychosis, hallucinations, and suicidal thoughts and behavior. Caution them to immediately report changes in behavior to prescriber.

● Caution patient that drug can lead to abuse or dependence. Discuss careful follow-up with prescriber and protecting drug from theft; discourage patient from giving drug to anyone else.

● Instruct female patient to report pregnancy or plans to become pregnant to her provider. Caution patient not to breast-feed while taking this drug.

famciclovir
fam-SYE-kloe-vir

Famvir⚬

Therapeutic class: Antivirals
Pharmacologic class: Nucleosides–nucleotides
Pregnancy risk category: B

AVAILABLE FORMS
Tablets: 125 mg, 250 mg, 500 mg

INDICATIONS & DOSAGES
➤ **Acute herpes zoster infection (shingles)**
Adults: 500 mg P.O. every 8 hours for 7 days.
Adjust-a-dose: For patients with CrCl of 40 to 59 mL/minute, give 500 mg P.O. every 12 hours; if CrCl is 20 to 39 mL/minute, give 500 mg P.O. every 24 hours; if CrCl is less than 20 mL/minute, give 250 mg P.O. every 24 hours. For hemodialysis patients, give 250 mg P.O. after each hemodialysis session.
➤ **Recurrent genital herpes**
Adults: 1,000 mg P.O. b.i.d. for a single day. Begin therapy at the first sign or symptom.
Adjust-a-dose: For patients with CrCl of 40 to 59 mL/minute, give 500 mg every 12 hours for 1 day; for CrCl of 20 to 39 mL/minute, give 500 mg P.O. as a single dose; if CrCl is less than 20 mL/minute, give 250 mg as a single dose. For hemodialysis patient, give 250 mg single dose following dialysis session.
➤ **Suppression of recurrent genital herpes**
Adults: 250 mg P.O. b.i.d. for up to 1 year.
Adjust-a-dose: For patients with CrCl of 20 to 39 mL/minute, give 125 mg P.O. every 12 hours; if CrCl is less than 20 mL/minute, give 125 mg P.O. every 24 hours. For hemodialysis patients, give 125 mg P.O. after each hemodialysis session.
➤ **Recurrent mucocutaneous herpes simplex infections in HIV-infected patients**
Adults: 500 mg P.O. b.i.d. for 7 days.
Adjust-a-dose: For patients with CrCl of 20 to 39 mL/minute, give 500 mg P.O. every 24 hours; if CrCl is less than 20 mL/minute, give 250 mg P.O. every 24 hours. For hemodialysis patients, give 250 mg P.O. after each hemodialysis session.
➤ **Recurrent herpes labialis (cold sores)**
Adults: 1,500 mg P.O. for one dose. Give at the first sign or symptom of cold sore.
Adjust-a-dose: For patients with CrCl of 40 to 59 mL/minute, give 750 mg as a single dose; for CrCl of 20 to 39 mL/minute, give 500 mg P.O. as a single dose; if CrCl is less than 20 mL/minute, give 250 mg as a single dose. For hemodialysis patient, give 250 mg single dose following dialysis session.

ADMINISTRATION
P.O.
● Give drug without regard for meals.

ACTION
A guanosine nucleoside that is converted to penciclovir, which enters viral cells and inhibits DNA polymerase and viral DNA synthesis.

Route	Onset	Peak	Duration
P.O.	Unknown	1 hr	Unknown

Half-life: 2 to 3 hours.

ADVERSE REACTIONS
CNS: headache, fatigue, dizziness, paresthesia, somnolence.
GI: nausea, abdominal pain, diarrhea, vomiting.
GU: dysmenorrhea.
Skin: pruritus.
Other: zoster-related signs, symptoms, and complications.

INTERACTIONS
Drug-drug. *Probenecid:* May increase level of penciclovir, the active metabolite of famciclovir. Monitor patient for increased adverse reactions.
Zoster vaccine (live, attenuated): May diminish effect of zoster vaccine. When possible, discontinue famciclovir for at least 24 hours before and 14 days after receiving zoster vaccine.

EFFECTS ON LAB TEST RESULTS
● None reported.

CONTRAINDICATIONS & CAUTIONS
• Contraindicated in patients hypersensitive to drug.
• Use cautiously in patients with renal or hepatic impairment.

NURSING CONSIDERATIONS
• In patients with renal or hepatic impairment, adjust dosage as needed.
• Monitor renal and liver function tests.

PATIENT TEACHING
• Inform patient that drug doesn't cure genital herpes but can decrease the length and severity of symptoms.
• Teach patient how to avoid spreading infection to others.
• Urge patient to recognize the early signs and symptoms of herpes infection, such as tingling, itching, and pain, and to report them. Therapy is more effective if started within 48 hours of rash onset.

---

famotidine
fa-MOE-ti-deen

Pepcid✐, Pepcid AC ◇

Therapeutic class: Antiulcer drugs
Pharmacologic class: H_2-receptor antagonists
Pregnancy risk category: B

AVAILABLE FORMS
Gelcaps: 10 mg ◇
Injection: 10 mg/mL
Powder for oral suspension: 40 mg/5 mL after reconstitution
Premixed injection: 20 mg/50 mL in normal saline solution
Tablets: 10 mg ◇, 20 mg ◇, 40 mg
Tablets (chewable): 10 mg ◇, 20 mg ◇

INDICATIONS & DOSAGES
Adjust-a-dose (for all indications): For patients with CrCl below 50 mL/minute, give half the dose, or increase dosing interval to every 36 to 48 hours.
➤ **Short-term treatment for duodenal ulcer**
Adults: For acute therapy, 40 mg P.O. once daily at bedtime or 20 mg P.O. b.i.d. Healing

usually occurs within 4 weeks. For maintenance therapy, 20 mg P.O. once daily at bedtime.
➤ **Short-term treatment for benign gastric ulcer**
Adults: 40 mg P.O. daily at bedtime or 20 mg P.O. b.i.d. for 8 weeks.
Children ages 1 to 16: 0.5 mg/kg/day P.O. at bedtime or in two divided doses, up to 40 mg daily.
➤ **Pathologic hypersecretory conditions (such as Zollinger-Ellison syndrome)**
Adults: 20 mg P.O. every 6 hours, up to 160 mg every 6 hours.
➤ **Hospitalized patients who can't take oral drug or who have intractable ulcers or hypersecretory conditions**
Adults: 20 mg I.V. every 12 hours.
➤ **GERD**
Adults: 20 mg P.O. b.i.d. for up to 6 weeks. For esophagitis caused by GERD, 20 to 40 mg b.i.d. for up to 12 weeks.
Children ages 1 to 16: 1 mg/kg/day P.O. in two divided doses up to 40 mg b.i.d.
Children ages 3 months to younger than 1 year: 0.5 mg/kg/dose oral suspension b.i.d. for up to 8 weeks.
Children younger than age 3 months: 0.5 mg/kg/dose oral suspension once daily for up to 8 weeks.
➤ **To prevent or treat heartburn**
Adults: 10 mg Pepcid AC P.O. 1 hour before meals to prevent symptoms, or 10 mg Pepcid AC P.O. with water when symptoms occur. Maximum daily dose is 20 mg. Drug shouldn't be taken daily for longer than 2 weeks.
➤ **Stress ulcer prevention in certain populations (such as general intensive-care patients and head and thermal injury patients) ◆**
Adults: 20 mg P.O. b.i.d. via nasogastric (NG) tube. Or, 20 mg I.V. b.i.d. or 1.7 mg/hour by continuous I.V. infusion.
Adjust-a-dose: For patients with CrCl of less than 30 mL/minute, give 20 mg P.O. once daily via NG tube. Or, 20 mg I.V. b.i.d. or 0.85 mg/hour by continuous I.V. infusion.

ADMINISTRATION
P.O.
• Reconstitute and shake oral suspension before use.

• Store reconstituted oral suspension below 86° F (30° C). Discard after 30 days.

I.V.

▼ Compatible solutions include sterile water for injection, normal saline solution for injection, D_5W or dextrose 10% in water for injection, 5% sodium bicarbonate injection, and lactated Ringer injection. Drug also can be added to total parenteral nutrition solutions.

▼ For direct injection, dilute 2 mL (20 mg) with compatible solution to a total volume of either 5 or 10 mL.

▼ Inject over at least 2 minutes.

▼ For intermittent infusion, dilute 20 mg (2 mL) in 100-mL compatible solution. The premixed 50-mL solution doesn't need further dilution.

▼ Infuse over 15 to 30 minutes.

▼ After dilution, solution is stable 48 hours at 36° to 46° F (2° to 8° C).

▼ **Incompatibilities:** Amphotericin B cholesteryl sulfate complex, azithromycin, cefepime, piperacillin–tazobactam.

ACTION

Competitively inhibits action of histamine on the H_2-receptor sites of parietal cells, decreasing gastric acid secretion.

Route	Onset	Peak	Duration
P.O.	1 hr	1–3 hr	12 hr
I.V.	1 hr	1–4 hr	12 hr

Half-life: 2½ to 3½ hours.

ADVERSE REACTIONS

CNS: headache, dizziness.
GI: constipation, diarrhea.

INTERACTIONS

None significant.

EFFECTS ON LAB TEST RESULTS

• May increase BUN, creatinine, and liver enzyme levels.

• May cause false-negative results in skin tests using allergen extracts. May antagonize pentagastrin in gastric acid secretion tests.

CONTRAINDICATIONS & CAUTIONS

• Contraindicated in patients hypersensitive to drug.

NURSING CONSIDERATIONS

• Assess patient for abdominal pain.

• Look for blood in emesis, stool, or gastric aspirate.

PATIENT TEACHING

• Instruct patient in proper use of OTC product, if appropriate.

• Warn patient with phenylketonuria that Pepcid AC chewable tablets contain phenylalanine.

• Tell patient to take prescription drug with a snack, if desired.

• Advise patient to limit use of prescription drug to no longer than 8 weeks, unless ordered by prescriber, and OTC drug to no longer than 2 weeks.

• With prescriber's knowledge, let patient take antacids together, especially at beginning of therapy when pain is severe.

• Urge patient to avoid cigarette smoking because it may increase gastric acid secretion and worsen disease.

• Advise patient to report abdominal pain, blood in stools or vomit, black tarry stools, or coffee-ground emesis.

febuxostat

feh-BUCKS-oh-stat

Uloric

Therapeutic class: Antigout drugs
Pharmacologic class: Xanthine oxidase inhibitors
Pregnancy risk category: C

AVAILABLE FORMS

Tablets: 40 mg, 80 mg

INDICATIONS & DOSAGES

➤ **Hyperuricemia associated with gout**
Adults: 40 mg P.O. daily. May increase dosage to 80 mg after 2 weeks if uric acid level remains above 6 mg/dL.

ADMINISTRATION

P.O.

• Give drug without regard to food or antacid use.

ACTION

Reduces uric acid production by inhibiting xanthine oxidase.

Route	Onset	Peak	Duration
P.O.	Rapid	1–1½ hr	Unknown

Half-life: 5 to 8 hours.

ADVERSE REACTIONS

CNS: dizziness.
GI: nausea.
Hepatic: liver function abnormalities.
Musculoskeletal: arthralgia.
Skin: rash.

INTERACTIONS

Drug-drug. *Azathioprine, didanosine, mercaptopurine:* May increase levels of these drugs, leading to toxicity. Use together is contraindicated.
Theophylline: May increase theophylline level. Use cautiously together.

EFFECTS ON LAB TEST RESULTS

• May increase alkaline phosphatase, AST, and ALT levels.

CONTRAINDICATIONS & CAUTIONS

• Contraindicated in patients hypersensitive to drug or its components and in those taking azathioprine, mercaptopurine, or didanosine.
• Use cautiously in patients with severe hepatic impairment (Child-Pugh class C) or renal impairment (CrCl of less than 30 mL/minute).
• Use during pregnancy only if benefit to the mother outweighs risk to the fetus. It isn't known if drug appears in breast milk; use cautiously in breast-feeding women.
• Safety and effectiveness in children haven't been established.

NURSING CONSIDERATIONS

• Acute gouty flares may occur during first 6 weeks of therapy; colchicine or another anti-inflammatory may be added prophylactically and drug should be continued.
• Monitor hepatic function at 2 months and 4 months after starting therapy and periodically thereafter.
• Monitor uric acid level.

• Patient taking drug may be at risk for thromboembolic events, such as MI and stroke. Monitor patient closely.

PATIENT TEACHING

• Warn patient about the risk of gout flares and the importance of taking an NSAID or colchicine during the first 6 weeks of treatment.
• Instruct women of childbearing age to notify prescriber if pregnant or breast-feeding or planning a pregnancy during therapy.
• Inform patient that drug may increase the risk of MI or stroke. Advise him to report rash, chest pain, dyspnea, or neurologic symptoms of a stroke.

felodipine
fell-OH-di-peen

Plendil, Renedil†

Therapeutic class: Antihypertensives
Pharmacologic class: Calcium channel blockers
Pregnancy risk category: C

AVAILABLE FORMS

Tablets (extended-release): 2.5 mg, 5 mg, 10 mg

INDICATIONS & DOSAGES

➤ **Hypertension**
Adults: Initially, 5 mg P.O. daily. Adjust dosage based on patient response, usually at intervals of not less than 2 weeks. Usual dosage is 2.5 to 10 mg daily; maximum dosage is 10 mg daily.
Elderly patients: 2.5 mg P.O. daily; adjust dosage as for adults. Maximum dosage is 10 mg daily.
Adjust-a-dose: For patients with impaired hepatic function, 2.5 mg P.O. daily; adjust dosage as for adults. Maximum daily dose is 10 mg.

ADMINISTRATION

P.O.
• Give drug whole; don't crush or cut tablets.

- Give drug without food or with a light meal.
- Don't give drug with grapefruit juice.

ACTION

Unknown. A dihydropyridine-derivative calcium channel blocker that prevents entry of calcium ions into vascular smooth muscle and cardiac cells; shows some selectivity for smooth muscle compared with cardiac muscle.

Route	Onset	Peak	Duration
P.O.	2–5 hr	2½–5 hr	24 hr

Half-life: 11 to 16 hours.

ADVERSE REACTIONS

CNS: headache, dizziness, paresthesia, asthenia.
CV: peripheral edema, chest pain, palpitations, flushing.
EENT: rhinorrhea, pharyngitis.
GI: abdominal pain, nausea, constipation, diarrhea, dyspepsia.
Musculoskeletal: muscle cramps, back pain.
Respiratory: upper respiratory tract infection, cough, sneezing.
Skin: rash.

INTERACTIONS

Drug-drug. *Anticonvulsants:* May decrease felodipine level. Avoid using together.
CYP3A4 inhibitors (such as azole antifungals, cimetidine, erythromycin): May decrease clearance of felodipine. Reduce doses of felodipine; monitor patient for toxicity.
Metoprolol: May alter pharmacokinetics of metoprolol. Monitor patient for adverse reactions.
NSAIDs: May decrease antihypertensive effects. Monitor blood pressure.
Tacrolimus: May increase tacrolimus level. Monitor patient closely.
Theophylline: May slightly decrease theophylline level. Monitor patient response closely.
Drug-herb. *Ma huang:* May decrease antihypertensive effects. Discourage use together.

Drug-food. *Grapefruit, lime:* May increase drug level and adverse effects. Discourage use together.

EFFECTS ON LAB TEST RESULTS

None reported.

CONTRAINDICATIONS & CAUTIONS

- Contraindicated in patients hypersensitive to drug.
- Use cautiously in patients with heart failure, particularly those receiving beta blockers, and in patients with impaired hepatic function.
⚠ *Overdose S&S:* Peripheral vasodilation, hypotension, bradycardia.

NURSING CONSIDERATIONS

- Monitor blood pressure for response.
- Monitor patient for peripheral edema, which appears to be both dose- and age-related. It's more common in patients taking higher doses, especially those older than age 60.

PATIENT TEACHING

- Tell patient to swallow tablets whole and not to crush or chew them.
- Tell patient to take drug without food or with a light meal.
- Advise patient not to take drug with grapefruit juice.
- Advise patient to continue taking drug even when he feels better, to watch his diet, and to check with prescriber or pharmacist before taking other drugs, including OTC drugs, nutritional supplements, or herbal remedies.
- Advise patient to observe good oral hygiene and to see a dentist regularly; use of drug may cause mild gum problems.

Reactions in bold italics are *life-threatening*. Interactions may have a *rapid onset* or a *delayed onset*.

fenofibrate
fee-no-FYE-brate

Antara, Fenoglide, Lipofen, TriCor✐, Triglide

fenofibric acid
Trilipix

Therapeutic class: Antilipemics
Pharmacologic class: Fibric acid derivatives
Pregnancy risk category: C

AVAILABLE FORMS
fenofibrate
Capsules: 50 mg, 150 mg
Capsules (micronized): 43 mg, 67 mg, 130 mg, 134 mg, 200 mg
Tablets: 40 mg, 48 mg, 50 mg, 54 mg, 107 mg, 120 mg, 145 mg, 160 mg
fenofibric acid
Capsules (delayed-release): 45 mg, 135 mg
Tablets: 35 mg, 105 mg

INDICATIONS & DOSAGES
Adjust-a-dose (for all indications): If CrCl is less than 50 mL/minute or in elderly patients, initially 43 mg daily for Antara, 50 mg daily for Lipofen, 48 mg daily for TriCor, 50 mg daily for Triglide, 40 mg/day for Fenoglide, or 45 mg once daily for Trilipix. Increase only after evaluating effects on renal function and triglyceride level at this dose.

➤ **Hypertriglyceridemia (Fredrickson types IV and V hyperlipidemia) in patients who don't respond adequately to diet alone**
Adults: For Antara, initial dose is 43 to 130 mg P.O. daily, with maximum dose of 130 mg daily. For Lipofen, initial dose is 50 to 150 mg daily, with maximum dose of 150 mg daily. For TriCor, initial dose is 48 to 145 mg daily, with maximum dose of 145 mg daily. For Triglide, initial dose is 50 to 160 mg daily, with maximum dose of 160 mg daily. For Fenoglide, initial dose is 40 to 120 mg/day. For Trilipix, initial dose is 45 to 135 mg once daily, with maximum dose of 135 mg once daily. For all forms, adjust dose based on patient response and repeat lipid determinations every 4 to 8 weeks.

➤ **Primary hypercholesterolemia or mixed dyslipidemia (Fredrickson types IIa and IIb) in patients who don't respond adequately to diet alone**
Adults: For Antara, initial dose is 130 mg P.O. daily. For Lipofen, initial dose is 150 mg daily. For TriCor, initial dose is 145 mg daily. For Triglide, initial dose is 160 mg daily. For Fenoglide, initial dose is 120 mg/day. For Trilipix, initial dose is 135 mg once daily. May reduce dose if lipid levels fall significantly below the target range.

➤ **Mixed dyslipidemia in combination with HMG-CoA reductase inhibitors (Trilipix)**
Adults: 135 mg P.O. once daily with a statin. May give daily dose at the same time as the statin, following the dosing recommendations for each medication. Avoid administering with maximum dose of a statin unless the benefits are expected to outweigh the risks.

➤ **Hyperuricemia ♦**
Adults: 200 mg/day (micronized formulation) P.O. for up to 12 months or 100 mg t.i.d. for 6 weeks.

ADMINISTRATION
P.O.
• Give Lipofen capsules with food to enhance absorption; give other preparations without regard for food.

ACTION
May lower triglyceride levels by inhibiting triglyceride synthesis with less very–low-density lipoproteins released into circulation. Drug may also stimulate breakdown of triglyceride-rich protein.

Route	Onset	Peak	Duration
P.O.	Unknown	6–8 hr	Unknown

Half-life: 20 hours.

ADVERSE REACTIONS
CNS: dizziness, headache, asthenia, fatigue, insomnia, localized pain, paresthesia.
CV: *arrhythmias.*
EENT: blurred vision, conjunctivitis, earache, eye discomfort, eye floaters, rhinitis, sinusitis.

GI: abdominal pain, constipation, diarrhea, dyspepsia, eructation, flatulence, increased appetite, nausea, vomiting.
GU: polyuria, vaginitis.
Musculoskeletal: arthralgia.
Respiratory: cough.
Skin: pruritus, rash.
Other: infection, decreased libido, flulike syndrome, hypersensitivity reactions.

INTERACTIONS

Drug-drug. *Bile acid sequestrants:* May bind and inhibit absorption of fenofibrate. Give drug 1 hour before or 4 to 6 hours after bile acid sequestrants.
Coumarin-type anticoagulants: May potentiate anticoagulant effect, prolonging PT and INR. Monitor PT and INR closely. May need to reduce anticoagulant dosage.
Cyclosporine, immunosuppressants, nephrotoxic drugs: May induce renal dysfunction that may affect fenofibrate elimination. Use together cautiously.
HMG-CoA reductase inhibitors: May increase risk of adverse musculoskeletal effects. Avoid using together, unless potential benefit outweighs risk.
Drug-food. *Any food:* May increase capsule absorption. Advise patient to take capsule with meals.
Drug-lifestyle. *Alcohol use:* May increase triglyceride levels. Discourage use together.

EFFECTS ON LAB TEST RESULTS

● May increase ALT, AST, BUN, CK, and creatinine levels. May decrease uric acid and hemoglobin levels and hematocrit.
● May decrease WBC count.

CONTRAINDICATIONS & CAUTIONS

● Contraindicated in patients hypersensitive to drug and in those with gallbladder disease, hepatic dysfunction, primary biliary cirrhosis, severe renal dysfunction, or unexplained persistent liver function abnormalities.
● Use cautiously in patients with a history of pancreatitis.
● Select Trilipix dosage cautiously for elderly patients and those with renal impairment because of the increased risk of adverse reactions.

NURSING CONSIDERATIONS

● Obtain baseline lipid levels and LFT results before therapy, and monitor liver function periodically during therapy. Stop drug if enzyme levels persist above 3 times normal.
◑ *Alert:* Watch for signs and symptoms of pancreatitis, myositis, rhabdomyolysis, cholelithiasis, and renal failure. Monitor patient for muscle pain, tenderness, or weakness, especially with malaise or fever.
● If an adequate response isn't obtained after 2 months of treatment with maximum daily dose, stop therapy.
● Drug lowers uric acid level by increasing uric acid excretion in patients with or without hyperuricemia.
● Beta blockers, estrogens, and thiazide diuretics may increase triglyceride levels; evaluate need for continued use of these drugs.
● Hemoglobin level, hematocrit, and WBC count may decrease when therapy starts but will stabilize with long-term administration.

PATIENT TEACHING

● Inform patient that drug therapy doesn't reduce need for following a triglyceride-lowering diet.
● Advise patient to promptly report unexplained muscle weakness, pain, or tenderness, especially with malaise or fever.
● Tell patient to take capsules with meals for best drug absorption.
● Advise patient to continue weight control measures, including diet and exercise, and to limit alcohol before therapy.
● Instruct patient who is also taking a bile acid sequestrant to take fenofibrate 1 hour before or 4 to 6 hours after the bile acid sequestrant.
● Advise patient about risk of tumor growth.
● Tell breast-feeding women to either stop breast-feeding or stop taking drug.

---

fentanyl citrate
FEN-ta-nil

Sublimaze

fentanyl nasal spray
Lazanda

fentanyl sublingual spray
SUBSYS

fentanyl transdermal system
Duragesic-12, Duragesic-25,
Duragesic-50, Duragesic-75,
Duragesic-100

fentanyl transmucosal
Abstral, Actiq, Fentora, Onsolis

Therapeutic class: Opioid analgesics
Pharmacologic class: Opioid agonists
Pregnancy risk category: C
Controlled substance schedule: II

F

AVAILABLE FORMS
Injection: 50 mcg/mL
Nasal spray: 100 mcg, 400 mcg
Transdermal system: Patches that release
12.5 mcg, 25 mcg, 50 mcg, 75 mcg, or
100 mcg of drug per hour
Transmucosal (buccal soluble film):
200 mcg, 400 mcg, 600 mcg, 800 mcg,
1,200 mcg
Transmucosal (buccal tablet): 100 mcg,
200 mcg, 400 mcg, 600 mcg, 800 mcg
Transmucosal (lozenge): 200 mcg, 400 mcg,
600 mcg, 800 mcg, 1,200 mcg, 1,600 mcg
Transmucosal (sublingual spray): 100 mcg,
200 mcg, 400 mcg, 600 mcg, 800 mcg
Transmucosal (sublingual tablet): 100 mcg,
200 mcg, 300 mcg, 400 mcg, 600 mcg,
800 mcg

INDICATIONS & DOSAGES
➤ **Adjunct to general anesthetic**
Adults: For low-dose therapy, 2 mcg/kg I.V.
For moderate-dose therapy, 2 to 20 mcg/kg
I.V.; then 25 to 100 mcg I.V. or I.M. p.r.n.
For high-dose therapy, 20 to 50 mcg/kg I.V.;
then 25 mcg to one-half initial loading dose
I.V. p.r.n.

➤ **Adjunct to regional anesthesia**
Adults: 50 to 100 mcg I.M. or slowly I.V.
over 1 to 2 minutes p.r.n.
➤ **To induce and maintain anesthesia**
Children ages 2 to 12: 2 to 3 mcg/kg I.V.
➤ **Postoperative pain, restlessness,
tachypnea, and emergence delirium**
Adults: 50 to 100 mcg I.M. every 1 to
2 hours p.r.n.
➤ **Preoperative medication**
Adults: 50 to 100 mcg I.M. 30 to 60 minutes
before surgery.
➤ **To manage persistent, moderate to
severe chronic pain in opioid-tolerant
patients who require around-the-clock
opioid analgesics for an extended time**
Adults and children age 2 and older: When
converting to transdermal system, base the
first dose on the daily dose, potency, and
characteristics of the current opioid therapy;
the reliability of the relative potency estimates used to calculate the needed dose; the
degree of opioid tolerance; and the patient's
condition. Each patch may be worn for
72 hours, although some adult patients may
need a patch to be applied every 48 hours
during the first dosage period. May increase
dose 3 days after the first dose, then every
6 days thereafter.
Adjust-a-dose: For elderly, cachectic, or
debilitated patients, start transdermal
system doses at no higher than 25 mcg/hr
unless these patients are already tolerating around-the-clock opioid at a dose and
potency comparable to fentanyl 25 mcg/hr
transdermal system.
➤ **To manage breakthrough cancer pain
in patients already receiving and tolerating an opioid**
Adults: 200 mcg Actiq initially; may give
second dose 15 minutes after completing
the first (30 minutes after first lozenge is
placed in mouth). Maximum dose is
2 lozenges per breakthrough episode. If
several episodes of breakthrough pain
requiring 2 lozenges occur, dose may be
increased to the next available strength.
After a successful dosage has been reached,
patient should limit use to no more than 4
lozenges daily.

Or, initially 100 mcg buccal tablet between the upper cheek and gum. May repeat
same dose once per breakthrough episode

after at least 30 minutes. Adjust in 100-mcg increments. Doses above 400 mcg can be increased by 200 mcg. Generally, dosage should be increased when patient requires more than one dose per breakthrough episode. Once a successful maintenance dose has been established, reevaluate if patient experiences more than four breakthrough episodes per day.

Or, initially 100 mcg sublingual tablet. If adequate analgesia is obtained within 30 minutes, continue to treat subsequent episodes with this dose. If adequate analgesia isn't obtained, may give a second sublingual tablet after 30 minutes. Use no more than two doses per episode of breakthrough pain; it's essential to wait at least 2 hours before treating another episode. Dosage escalation may be performed in a stepwise manner over consecutive breakthrough episodes until adequate analgesia with tolerable adverse effects is achieved. Limit drug consumption to treat four or fewer breakthrough pain episodes per day once a successful dose is found.

Or, initially 100 mcg nasal spray. Titrate as needed to an effective dosage (from 100, to 200, to 400 mcg, up to maximum of 800 mcg) that gives adequate analgesia with tolerable adverse effects. Dose is a single spray into one nostril or single spray into each nostril per episode. Don't give more than two doses per 24 hours. Wait at least 2 hours before treating another episode. During an episode, if analgesia isn't achieved within 30 minutes, patient may use a rescue medication as directed by the health care provider.

Or, initially 100 mcg sublingual spray. If pain isn't relieved after 30 minutes during each breakthrough pain episode treated, one additional dose of the same strength may be given for that episode. May use a maximum of two doses for any breakthrough pain episode, and 4 hours must elapse before treating another episode of breakthrough pain with a higher dose. Titrate dosage level as needed to an effective dosage (from 100 to 200, to 400, to 600, to 800, to 1,200, to 1,600 mcg) that gives adequate analgesia with tolerable adverse effects using a single dose per breakthrough cancer pain episode. When drug has been titrated to an effective

dosage, patients should generally use only one dose of the appropriate strength per breakthrough pain episode.

Or, initially 200 mcg transmucosal buccal film. Use drug only once per breakthrough cancer pain episode. If adequate pain relief isn't achieved after initial dose, titrate using multiples of 200-mcg film in each subsequent episode, separated by at least 2 hours, until adequate analgesia with tolerable adverse effects is achieved. Multiple 200-mcg films shouldn't be placed on top of each other, but may be placed on both sides of the mouth. Don't use more than four 200-mcg films (800 mcg) simultaneously. If pain isn't relieved after titrating to 800 mcg and adverse effects are tolerable, treat next episode using one 1,200-mcg film. Maximum dosage is 1,200 mcg. During an episode, if analgesia isn't achieved within 30 minutes, patient may use a rescue medication as directed by the health care provider.

➤ **Switching from Actiq to Fentora to manage breakthrough cancer pain in opioid-tolerant patients**
Adults: If current Actiq dose is 200 to 400 mcg, start with 100 mcg Fentora; if current Actiq dose is 600 to 800 mcg, use 200 mcg Fentora; if current Actiq dose is 1,200 to 1,600 mcg, use 400 mcg Fentora. Actiq and Fentora aren't bioequivalent.
Adjust-a-dose: For patients with renal or hepatic impairment, use lowest possible dose.

ADMINISTRATION
I.V.
▼ Only those trained to give I.V. anesthetics and manage adverse effects should give this form.
▼ Keep opioid antagonist (naloxone) and resuscitation equipment available.
▼ I.V. form often used with droperidol to produce neuroleptanalgesia.
▼ Inject slowly over 1 to 2 minutes.
▼ **Incompatibilities:** Azithromycin, fluorouracil, lidocaine, methohexital, pentobarbital sodium, phenytoin, thiopental.
I.M.
● Document administration site.

Intranasal

• Prime the device by spraying into the pouch (4 sprays in total).

• Insert the nozzle about ½ inch (1 cm) into the nose and point toward the bridge of the nose, tilting the bottle slightly.

• Press down firmly until a click is heard and the number in the counting window advances by one.

Transdermal

• Dosage equivalent charts are available to calculate the fentanyl transdermal dose based on the daily morphine intake; for example, for every 90 mg of oral morphine or 15 mg of I.M. morphine per 24 hours, 25 mcg/hour of transdermal fentanyl is needed.

• Clip hair at application site but don't use a razor, which may irritate skin. Wash area with clear water, if needed, but not with soaps, oils, lotions, alcohol, or other substances that may irritate skin or prevent adhesion. Dry area completely before application.

• Remove transdermal system from package just before applying, hold in place for 30 seconds, and be sure edges of patch stick to skin.

• Don't cut or otherwise alter transdermal patch before applying.

• Place transdermal patch on the upper back for a child or patient who's cognitively impaired to reduce the chance the patch will be removed and placed in the mouth.

Black Box Warning Heat from fever or heating pads, electric blankets, heat lamps, hot tubs, or water beds may increase transdermal delivery and cause toxicity. ∎

Transmucosal

• Remove foil just before giving.

• For Actiq: Place lozenge between patient's cheek and gum and allow to dissolve over about 15 to 20 minutes; it must not be bitten, sucked, or chewed. Lozenge may be moved from one side to the other using the stick. Discard stick in the trash after use or, if any drug matrix remains on the stick, place under hot running tap water until dissolved. Or, place in child-resistant container provided and discard as for schedule II drugs.

• For buccal tablet: Place tablet between patient's cheek and gum and leave there

until disintegrated, usually 14 to 25 minutes. Tablet shouldn't be sucked, chewed, or swallowed; this results in lower plasma concentrations. After 30 minutes, if remnants from tablet remain, they may be swallowed with a glass of water.

• For sublingual tablet: Place on the floor of the mouth directly under the tongue. Patient should let tablet completely dissolve and shouldn't chew, suck, or swallow it. Water may be used to moisten buccal mucosa before administration.

• For sublingual spray: Open blister package with scissors immediately before use. Carefully spray contents of unit into the mouth under the tongue. Advise patients and caregivers to properly dispose of used unit-dose systems immediately after use.

• For buccal film: Have patient use tongue to wet the inside of the cheek or rinse the mouth with water to wet the area before use. Open package immediately before use; don't cut or tear film before use. Place entire film near the tip of a dry finger with the pink side facing up, and hold in place. Place the pink side of the film against the inside of the cheek. Press and hold film in place for 5 seconds; it should then stay in place on its own. Patient shouldn't manipulate it with the tongue or finger after placement. Film will dissolve within 15 to 30 minutes after application. Patient may consume liquids after 5 minutes; however, patient should avoid eating food until the film has dissolved.

ACTION

Unknown. Binds with opioid receptors in the CNS, altering perception of and emotional response to pain.

Route	Onset	Peak	Duration
I.V.	1–2 min	3–5 min	30–60 min
I.M.	7–15 min	20–30 min	1–2 hr
Intranasal	15–21 min	25–35 min	Unknown
Transdermal	12–24 hr	1–3 days	Variable
Transmucosal	5–15 min	20–30 min	Unknown

Half-life: 3½ hours after parenteral use; 15 to 24.9 hours after intranasal use; 5 to 15 hours after transmucosal use; 18 hours after transdermal use.

ADVERSE REACTIONS
CNS: asthenia, clouded sensorium, confusion, euphoria, sedation, somnolence, *seizures,* anxiety, depression, dizziness, hallucinations, headache, nervousness.
CV: *arrhythmias,* chest pain, hypertension, hypotension, *DVT, PE.*
EENT: pharyngitis, dry eyes, swelling, strabismus, ptosis, epistaxis, nasal discomfort, rhinorrhea, nasal congestion, postnasal drip, rhinitis (intranasal).
GI: constipation, abdominal pain, anorexia, diarrhea, dyspepsia, dry mouth, ileus, nausea, vomiting.
GU: urine retention.
Musculoskeletal: skeletal muscle rigidity (dose-related).
Respiratory: *apnea, hypoventilation, respiratory depression,* dyspnea, cough, upper respiratory tract infection, bronchitis.
Skin: diaphoresis, pruritus, erythema at application site (transdermal).
Other: physical dependence.

INTERACTIONS
Drug-drug. *Amiodarone:* May cause hypotension, bradycardia, and decreased cardiac output. Monitor patient closely.
CNS depressants, general anesthetics, hypnotics, MAO inhibitors, other opioid analgesics, sedatives, TCAs: May cause additive effects. Use together cautiously. Reduce dosages of these drugs and reduce fentanyl dose by one-fourth to one-third.
CYP3A4 inducers (carbamazepine, phenytoin, rifampin): May decrease analgesic effects. Monitor patient for adequate pain relief.
Black Box Warning *CYP3A4 inhibitors (such as cyclosporine, itraconazole, ketoconazole):* May increase fentanyl level and cause fatal respiratory depression. Carefully monitor patient and adjust fentanyl dosage as needed. ∎
Diazepam: May cause CV depression when given with high doses of fentanyl. Monitor patient closely.
Droperidol: May cause hypotension and decrease pulmonary arterial pressure. Use together cautiously.
Protease inhibitors: May increase fentanyl levels and adverse effects. Monitor patient closely for respiratory depression.

Drug-lifestyle. *Alcohol use:* May cause additive effects. Discourage use together.

EFFECTS ON LAB TEST RESULTS
• May increase amylase and lipase levels.

CONTRAINDICATIONS & CAUTIONS
• Contraindicated in patients intolerant to drug.
Black Box Warning Transdermal form contraindicated in patients hypersensitive to adhesives, those who are opioid-naive, those who need postoperative pain management, and those with acute, mild, or intermittent pain that can be managed with nonopioids. Don't use in patients with increased intracranial pressure, head injury, impaired consciousness, or coma. ∎
Black Box Warning Transmucosal forms contraindicated in those who need acute or postoperative pain management. ∎
Black Box Warning Nasal spray is contraindicated in opioid-nontolerant patients and in those who need acute or postoperative pain management. ∎
• Fentora contraindicated in patients with mucositis more severe than grade 1.
• Use with caution in patients with brain tumors, COPD, decreased respiratory reserve, potentially compromised respirations, hepatic or renal disease, or cardiac bradyarrhythmias.
• Use with caution in elderly or debilitated patients.
⚠ **Overdose S&S:** CNS depression, respiratory depression, apnea, flaccid skeletal muscles, bradycardia, hypotension, circulatory collapse.

NURSING CONSIDERATIONS
Black Box Warning Respiratory depression or death can occur even when transdermal drug has been used as recommended and not misused or abused. Drug should only be prescribed by health care providers knowledgeable in the use of potent opioids for management of long-term pain. Drug is contraindicated for use in conditions in which the risk of life-threatening respiratory depression is significantly increased. ∎
• For better analgesic effect, give drug before patient has intense pain.

Reactions in bold italics are *life-threatening*. Interactions may have a *rapid onset* or a *delayed onset*.

◑ *Alert:* High doses can produce muscle rigidity, which can be reversed with neuromuscular blockers; however, patient must be artificially ventilated.

• Monitor circulatory and respiratory status and urinary function carefully. Drug may cause respiratory depression, hypotension, urine retention, nausea, vomiting, ileus, or altered level of consciousness, no matter how it's given.

• Periodically monitor postoperative vital signs and bladder function. Because drug decreases both rate and depth of respirations, monitoring of arterial oxygen saturation (SaO_2) may help assess respiratory depression. Immediately report respiratory rate below 12 breaths/minute, decreased respiratory volume, or decreased SaO_2.

• Drug may cause constipation. Assess bowel function and need for stool softeners and stimulant laxatives.

Black Box Warning Fentanyl is an opioid agonist and schedule II controlled substance with potential for abuse. Be alert for signs of misuse, abuse, or diversion. ∎

Transdermal form

Black Box Warning Transdermal drug levels peak between 24 and 72 hours after initial application and dose increases. Monitor patients for life-threatening hypoventilation, especially during these times. ∎

• Fentanyl patches should be used only in patients age 2 or older who are opioid-tolerant, who have chronic moderate to severe pain poorly controlled by other drugs, and who need a total daily opioid dose at least equivalent to the 25-mcg/hour fentanyl patch.

• When converting a patient from another opioid, determine the initial fentanyl dosage with great care; overestimating the dosage could be dangerous or fatal.

• Identify all daily drugs, particularly CYP3A4 inhibitors, which may increase fentanyl levels.

• Monitor patients closely, and provide immediate care for evidence of overdose, such as slow or shallow breathing, a slow heartbeat, severe sleepiness, cold and clammy skin, trouble walking and talking, and feeling faint, dizzy, or confused.

• Give patients detailed instructions for using fentanyl patches correctly and safely.

• Make dosage adjustments gradually in patient using the transdermal system. Reaching steady-state level of a new dosage may take up to 6 days; delay dosage adjustment until after at least two applications.

• Monitor patient who develops adverse reactions to the transdermal system for at least 12 hours after removal. Drug level drops gradually; it may take as long as 17 hours to decline by 50%.

• Most patients experience good control of pain for 3 days while wearing the transdermal system, but a few may need a new application after 48 hours.

• Because the drug level rises for the first 24 hours after application, analgesic effect can't be evaluated on the first day. Make sure patient has adequate supplemental analgesic to prevent breakthrough pain.

• When reducing opioid therapy or switching to a different analgesic, withdraw the transdermal system gradually. Because the drug level drops gradually after removal, give half the equianalgesic dose of the new analgesic 12 to 18 hours after removal.

◑ *Alert:* Transdermal patches must be stored, used, and disposed of properly to prevent poisonings or other harm, especially to children and pets. A patch that has been worn for 3 days may still contain enough fentanyl to cause harm, or even kill a child or pet. Patches should only be handled by patient or patient's caregivers.

Intranasal and transmucosal forms

Black Box Warning Intranasal and transmucosal forms are used only to manage breakthrough cancer pain in patients who are already receiving and tolerating opioids. ∎

Black Box Warning Intranasal and transmucosal forms aren't bioequivalent and can't be substituted on a microgram-per-microgram basis. ∎

• ***Look alike–sound alike:*** Don't confuse fentanyl with alfentanil.

PATIENT TEACHING

• When drug is used for pain control, instruct patient to request drug before pain becomes intense.

• When drug is used after surgery, encourage patient to turn, cough, and breathe deeply to prevent lung problems.

● Instruct patient to avoid hazardous activities until CNS effects subside.

● Tell home care patient to avoid drinking alcohol or taking other CNS-type drugs because additive effects can occur.

● Advise patient not to stop drug abruptly.

● Teach patient about proper application of transdermal patch. Tell patient to clip hair at application site but not to use a razor, which may irritate skin. Wash area with clear water, if needed, but not with soaps, oils, lotions, alcohol, or other substances that may irritate skin or prevent adhesion. Dry area completely before application.

● Tell patient to remove transdermal system from package just before applying, hold in place for 30 seconds, and be sure the edges of patch stick to skin.

❸ Alert: Teach patient not to alter the transdermal patch (such as by cutting it) before applying.

● Advise parent or caregiver to place transdermal patch on the upper back for a child or a patient who's cognitively impaired, to reduce the chance the patch will be removed and placed in the mouth.

● Teach patient to dispose of the transdermal patch by folding it so the adhesive side adheres to itself and then flushing it down the toilet.

● Tell patient that, if another patch is needed after 48 to 72 hours, he should apply it to a different skin site.

● Tell patient that pain relief with the patch may not occur for several hours after the patch is applied. Oral, immediate-release opioids may be needed for initial pain relief.

Black Box Warning Inform patient that heat from fever or environment, such as from heating pads, electric blankets, heat lamps, hot tubs, or water beds, may increase transdermal delivery and cause toxicity requiring dosage adjustment. Instruct patient to notify prescriber if fever occurs or if he'll be spending time in a hot climate. ∎

● Instruct patient that, if he requires an MRI, to inform the facility that he is wearing a transdermal patch.

● Teach patient proper administration of transmucosal forms.

● Teach patient proper administration of the nasal spray. Tell him that a fine mist is not always felt and to rely on the audible click and advancement of the dose counter.

Black Box Warning Warn patient and patient's family that the amount of drug in transmucosal and intranasal forms can be fatal to a child. Advise patient to keep medicine well secured and out of children's reach. ∎

ferrous fumarate
FAIR-us

Euro-Fer† ◊, Femiron ◊, Feostat ◊, Ferrate† ◊, Ferretts ◊, Ferrocite ◊, Hemocyte ◊, Iron ◊, Neo-Fer† ◊, Nephro-Fer ◊, Palafer† ◊

Therapeutic class: Iron supplements
Pharmacologic class: Hematinics
Pregnancy risk category: A

AVAILABLE FORMS
Each 100 mg of ferrous fumarate provides 33 mg of elemental iron.
Tablets: 90 mg ◊, 150 mg ◊, 200 mg ◊, 300 mg† ◊, 324 mg ◊, 325 mg ◊, 350 mg ◊
Tablets (chewable): 100 mg ◊
Tablets (extended-release): 18 mg ◊

INDICATIONS & DOSAGES
➤ **Iron deficiency**
Adults: One or two tablets P.O. daily between meals or as directed by prescriber. Or, 100-mg chewable tablet P.O. once daily to q.i.d. For extended-release tablets, give one tablet P.O. daily.

➤ **As a supplement during pregnancy**
Women: 30 mg elemental iron P.O. daily.

ADMINISTRATION
P.O.
● Between-meal doses are preferable. Drug can be given with some foods, although absorption may be decreased.
● Give tablets with juice (preferably orange juice) or water but not with milk or antacids.
● Don't crush tablets.

Reactions in bold italics are *life-threatening*. Interactions may have a *rapid onset* or a *delayed onset*.

ACTION
Provides elemental iron, an essential component in the formation of hemoglobin.

Route	Onset	Peak	Duration
P.O.	4 days	7–10 days	2–4 mo

Half-life: Unknown.

ADVERSE REACTIONS
GI: nausea, vomiting, constipation, diarrhea, black stools, GI irritation.

INTERACTIONS
Drug-drug. *Antacids, cholestyramine resin, H_2 antagonists, proton pump inhibitors:* May decrease iron absorption. Separate doses by at least 2 hours.
Chloramphenicol: May delay response to iron therapy. Monitor patient.
Fluoroquinolones, penicillamine, tetracyclines: May decrease GI absorption of these drugs, possibly causing decreased levels or effect. Separate doses by 2 to 4 hours.
Levodopa, methyldopa: May decrease absorption and effectiveness of levodopa and methyldopa. Watch for decreased effect of these drugs.
L-thyroxine: May decrease L-thyroxine absorption. Separate doses by at least 2 hours. Monitor thyroid function.
Mycophenolate mofetil: May decrease absorption of mycophenolate. Avoid simultaneous administration.
Vitamin C: May increase iron absorption. Use together for therapeutic effect.
Drug-herb. *Black cohosh, chamomile, feverfew, gossypol, hawthorn, nettle, plantain, St. John's wort:* May decrease iron absorption. Discourage use together.
Oregano: May decrease iron absorption. Tell patient to separate ingestion of herb from ingestion of food containing iron or iron supplement by at least 2 hours.
Drug-food. *Cereals, cheese, coffee, eggs, milk, tea, whole-grain breads, yogurt:* May decrease iron absorption. Discourage use together.

EFFECTS ON LAB TEST RESULTS
● May yield false-positive guaiac test results. May decrease uptake of technetium-99m and interfere with skeletal imaging.

CONTRAINDICATIONS & CAUTIONS
● Contraindicated in patients with primary hemochromatosis or hemosiderosis, hemolytic anemia (unless patient also has iron deficiency anemia), peptic ulcer disease, regional enteritis, or ulcerative colitis.
● Contraindicated in those receiving repeated blood transfusions.
● Use cautiously on long-term basis.
⚠ *Overdose S&S:* Lethargy, nausea, vomiting, abdominal pain, tarry stools, weak rapid pulse, hypotension, diminished tissue perfusion, metabolic acidosis, fever, leukocytosis, hyperglycemia, dyspnea, coma, diffuse vascular congestion, pulmonary edema, shock, seizures, anuria, death.

NURSING CONSIDERATIONS
● GI upset may be related to dose.
● Enteric-coated products reduce GI upset but also reduce amount of iron absorbed.
● Check for constipation; record color and amount of stools.
☽ *Alert:* Oral iron may turn stools black. Although this unabsorbed iron is harmless, it could mask presence of melena.
● Monitor hemoglobin level, hematocrit, and reticulocyte count during therapy.
● Combination products such as Ferro-Sequels contain stool softeners, which help prevent constipation—a common adverse reaction.

PATIENT TEACHING
Black Box Warning Inform parents that as few as five or six tablets of a high-potency form can cause fatal poisoning in children. Tell parents to keep all iron-containing products out of the reach of children and to immediately call prescriber or poison control center if an accidental overdose occurs. ▪
● Tell patient to take tablets with juice (preferably orange juice) or water but not with milk or antacids.
● Tell patient to take suspension with straw and place drops at back of throat to avoid staining teeth.
● Caution patient not to crush tablets.
● Advise patient not to substitute one iron salt for another; the amount of elemental iron may vary.

● Advise patient to report constipation and change in stool color or consistency.

ferrous gluconate
FAIR-us

Fergon ◊, Novo-ferrogluc† ◊

Therapeutic class: Iron supplements
Pharmacologic class: Hematinics
Pregnancy risk category: A

AVAILABLE FORMS
Each 100 mg of ferrous gluconate provides 11.6 mg of elemental iron.
Tablets: 225 mg ◊, 240 mg ◊, 324 mg ◊, 325 mg ◊

INDICATIONS & DOSAGES
➤ **Iron deficiency**
Adults: 100 to 200 mg P.O. elemental iron daily in three divided doses.
Adolescent boys up to age 18: 120 mg/day P.O.
➤ **As a supplement during pregnancy**
Adults: 15 to 30 mg elemental iron P.O. daily during last two trimesters.

ADMINISTRATION
P.O.
● Between-meal doses are preferable. Drug can be given with some foods, although absorption may be decreased.
● Give tablets with juice (preferably orange juice) or water but not with milk or antacids.

ACTION
Provides elemental iron, an essential component in the formation of hemoglobin.

Route	Onset	Peak	Duration
P.O.	4 days	7–10 days	2–4 mo

Half-life: Unknown.

ADVERSE REACTIONS
GI: nausea, vomiting, constipation, diarrhea, black stools, GI irritation.

INTERACTIONS
Drug-drug. *Antacids, cholestyramine resin, H_2 antagonists, proton pump inhibitors:* May decrease iron absorption. Separate doses by at least 2 hours.

Chloramphenicol: Delays response to iron therapy. Monitor patient.
Fluoroquinolones, penicillamine, tetracyclines: May decrease GI absorption of these drugs, possibly causing decreased level or effect. Separate doses by 2 to 4 hours.
Levodopa, methyldopa: May decrease levodopa and methyldopa absorption and effect. Watch for decreased effect of these drugs.
L-thyroxine: May decrease L-thyroxine absorption. Separate doses by at least 2 hours. Monitor thyroid function.
Mycophenolate mofetil: May decrease absorption of mycophenolate. Avoid simultaneous administration.
Vitamin C: May increase iron absorption. Use together for therapeutic effect.
Drug-herb. *Black cohosh, chamomile, feverfew, gossypol, hawthorn, nettle, plantain, St. John's wort:* May decrease iron absorption. Discourage use together.
Oregano: May decrease iron absorption. Tell patient to separate ingestion of herb from ingestion of food containing iron or iron supplement by at least 2 hours.
Drug-food. *Cereals, cheese, coffee, eggs, milk, tea, whole-grain breads, yogurt:* May decrease iron absorption. Discourage using together.

EFFECTS ON LAB TEST RESULTS
● May yield false-positive guaiac test results. May decrease uptake of technetium-99m and interfere with skeletal imaging.

CONTRAINDICATIONS & CAUTIONS
● Contraindicated in patients with peptic ulceration, regional enteritis, ulcerative colitis, hemosiderosis, primary hemochromatosis, or hemolytic anemia (unless patient also has iron deficiency anemia) and in those receiving repeated blood transfusions.
● Use cautiously on long-term basis.
⚠ *Overdose S&S:* Lethargy, nausea, vomiting, abdominal pain, tarry stools, weak rapid pulse, hypotension, diminished tissue perfusion, metabolic acidosis, fever, leukocytosis, hyperglycemia, dyspnea, coma, diffuse vascular congestion, pulmonary edema, shock, seizures, anuria, death.

NURSING CONSIDERATIONS

Black Box Warning Accidental overdose of iron-containing products is a leading cause of fatal poisoning in children younger than age 6. Keep out of reach of children. In case of accidental overdose, seek emergency treatment. ∎

- GI upset may be related to dose.
- Enteric-coated products reduce GI upset but also reduce amount of iron absorbed.
- Check for constipation; record color and amount of stools.
- **❸ Alert:** Oral iron may turn stools black. Although this unabsorbed iron is harmless, it could mask melena.
- Monitor hemoglobin level, hematocrit, and reticulocyte count during therapy.

PATIENT TEACHING

- Tell patient to take tablets with juice (preferably orange juice) or water, but not with milk or antacids.
- Caution patient not to substitute one iron salt for another because the amounts of elemental iron vary.
- Advise patient to report constipation and change in stool color or consistency.

ferrous sulfate
FAIR-us

Foocol ◊*, Fer Gen Sol ◊*, Fer-In-Sol ◊*, FeroSul ◊

ferrous sulfate (dried)
Feosol ◊, Feratab ◊, Novo-ferrosulfate† ◊, Slow FE ◊, Slow Release Iron ◊

Therapeutic class: Iron supplements
Pharmacologic class: Hematinics
Pregnancy risk category: A

AVAILABLE FORMS

Each 100 mg of ferrous sulfate provides 20 mg of elemental iron or 30 mg of elemental iron in ferrous sulfate dried products.
Caplets (extended-release) ◊: 160 mg (dried)
Capsules: 190 mg (dried)
Drops ◊: 125 mg/mL
Elixir ◊: 220 mg/5 mL ◊*
Liquid ◊: 150 mg/5 mL†, 300 mg/5 mL
Tablets ◊: 195 mg, 200 mg (dried), 300 mg (dried), 325 mg
Tablets (slow-release) ◊: 142 mg, 160 mg (dried)

INDICATIONS & DOSAGES
➤ **Iron deficiency**
Adults: One 325-mg tablet P.O. b.i.d. to t.i.d. Or, 5 mL (300 mg) P.O. t.i.d. between meals.
Children age 12 and older: 5 mL (300 mg) P.O. t.i.d. between meals beginning with 5 mL the first day, 10 mL the second day, until the recommended dosage is reached.
Children age 4 and younger: 0.6 mL (75 mg ferrous sulfate) P.O. daily or as prescribed.

ADMINISTRATION
P.O.
- Between-meal doses are preferable. Drug can be given with some foods, although absorption may be decreased.
- Give tablets with juice (preferably orange juice) or water, but not with milk or antacids.
- Don't crush extended-release form.

ACTION
Provides elemental iron, an essential component in the formation of hemoglobin.

Route	Onset	Peak	Duration
P.O.	4 days	7–10 days	2–4 mo

Half-life: Unknown.

ADVERSE REACTIONS
GI: nausea, constipation, black stools, diarrhea, GI discomfort.
Other: temporarily stained teeth from liquid forms.

INTERACTIONS
Drug-drug. *Antacids, cholestyramine resin, H_2 antagonists, proton pump inhibitors:* May decrease iron absorption. Separate doses if possible.
Chloramphenicol: May delay response to iron therapy. Monitor patient.
Fluoroquinolones: May decrease GI absorption of fluoroquinolones. Avoid use together.

F

Levodopa, methyldopa: May decrease absorption and effect of levodopa and methyldopa. Watch for decreased effect of these drugs.

L-thyroxine: May decrease L-thyroxine absorption. Separate doses by at least 2 hours. Monitor thyroid function.

Mycophenolate mofetil: May decrease absorption of mycophenolate. Avoid simultaneous administration.

Penicillamine: May decrease absorption and effect of penicillamine. Separate doses by 2 hours.

Tetracyclines: May decrease absorption of both drugs. Separate doses by at least 2 hours.

Vitamin C: May increase iron absorption. Use together for therapeutic effect.

Drug-herb. *Black cohosh, chamomile, feverfew, gossypol, hawthorn, nettle, plantain, St. John's wort:* May decrease iron absorption. Discourage use together.

Oregano: May decrease iron absorption. Tell patient to separate ingestion of herb from ingestion of food containing iron or iron supplement by at least 2 hours.

Drug-food. *Cereals, cheese, coffee, eggs, milk, tea, whole-grain breads, yogurt:* May decrease iron absorption. Discourage use together.

EFFECTS ON LAB TEST RESULTS
● May yield false-positive guaiac test results. May decrease uptake of technetium-99m and interfere with skeletal imaging.

CONTRAINDICATIONS & CAUTIONS
● Contraindicated in patients with hemosiderosis, primary hemochromatosis, hemolytic anemia (unless patient also has iron deficiency anemia), peptic ulceration, ulcerative colitis, or regional enteritis and in those receiving repeated blood transfusions.
● Use cautiously on long-term basis.
⚠ *Overdose S&S:* Abdominal pain, coma, diminished tissue perfusion, dyspnea, fever, hyperglycemia, hypotension, lethargy, leukocytosis, metabolic acidosis, nausea, tarry stools, vomiting, weak rapid pulse, anuria, seizures, pulmonary edema, shock, diffuse vascular congestion, death.

NURSING CONSIDERATIONS
Black Box Warning Accidental overdose is a leading cause of fatal poisoning in children younger than age 6. Keep out of reach of children. In case of accidental overdose, seek immediate emergency treatment. ■
● GI upset may be related to dose.
● Enteric-coated products reduce GI upset but also reduce amount of iron absorbed.
◑ *Alert:* Oral iron may turn stools black. Although this unabsorbed iron is harmless, it could mask melena.
● Monitor hemoglobin level, hematocrit, and reticulocyte count during therapy.
● *Look alike–sound alike:* Don't confuse different iron salts; elemental content may vary.

PATIENT TEACHING
● Tell patient to take tablets with juice (preferably orange juice) or water, but not with milk or antacids.
● Instruct patient not to crush or chew extended-release form.
● Caution patient not to substitute one iron salt for another because amounts of elemental iron vary.
● Advise patient to report constipation and change in stool color or consistency.

fesoterodine fumarate
fezz-oh-TER-ah-deen

Toviaz

Therapeutic class: Antispasmodics
Pharmacologic class: Muscarinic receptor antagonists
Pregnancy risk category: C

AVAILABLE FORMS
Tablets (extended-release): 4 mg, 8 mg

INDICATIONS & DOSAGES
➤ **Urge incontinence, urinary urgency, and urinary frequency from overactive bladder**
Adults: 4 mg P.O. once daily; increase to 8 mg if needed.
Adjust-a-dose: Don't exceed 4 mg in patients with severe renal insufficiency and in those taking CYP3A4 inhibitors.

ADMINISTRATION
P.O.
● Give drug with or without food.
● Don't divide or crush tablets. Give with liquid and have patient swallow whole.

ACTION
Antagonizes muscarinic (M3) receptors, increasing bladder capacity and decreasing unstable detrusor contractions.

Route	Onset	Peak	Duration
P.O.	Unknown	5 hr	Unknown

Half-life: 7 hours.

ADVERSE REACTIONS
CNS: insomnia.
CV: peripheral edema.
EENT: dry eyes.
GI: dry mouth, constipation, dyspepsia, nausea, abdominal pain.
GU: UTI, dysuria, urine retention.
Musculoskeletal: back pain.
Respiratory: upper respiratory tract infection, dry throat, cough.
Skin: rash.

INTERACTIONS
Drug-drug. *Anticholinergics, antimuscarinics:* May increase risk of anticholinergic effects (such as constipation, blurred vision, urine retention). Use together cautiously.
Potassium preparations: May slow GI motility, arresting or delaying transport of solid dosage forms of potassium. Use together is contraindicated.
Strong CYP3A4 inhibitors (such as clarithromycin, itraconazole, ketoconazole): May increase fesoterodine concentrations. Avoid use together.
Drug-lifestyle. *Alcohol use:* May cause additive CNS depression. Discourage use together.

EFFECTS ON LAB TEST RESULTS
● May increase ALT and GGT levels.

CONTRAINDICATIONS & CAUTIONS
● Contraindicated in patients with hypersensitivity to drug or its components and in those with urine retention, gastric retention, or uncontrolled angle-closure glaucoma.

● Avoid use in patients with severe hepatic impairment.
● Use cautiously in patients with bladder outlet obstruction, decreased GI motility, myasthenia gravis, or controlled angle-closure glaucoma.
● Use in pregnant women only if benefit to the mother outweighs risk to the fetus. It isn't known if drug appears in breast milk. Women shouldn't breast-feed while taking drug.
⚠ Overdose S&S: Confusion, blurred vision, tachycardia, constipation, dry mouth, light-headedness, difficulty starting and continuing urination, urinary incontinence.

NURSING CONSIDERATIONS
● Give drug without regard to food.
● Monitor patient for urinary symptoms and adverse reactions.

PATIENT TEACHING
● Warn patient to avoid hot environments because drug may decrease sweating, causing severe heat illness.
● Advise patient to avoid driving, operating machinery, and other dangerous activities until drug's effects are known.
● Tell patient to avoid alcohol as it may cause drowsiness.
● Tell patient to report stomach or intestinal problems, constipation, difficulty emptying the bladder, weak urine stream, glaucoma, kidney or liver problems, or myasthenia gravis.
● Instruct woman of childbearing age to consult prescriber if she's pregnant, trying to become pregnant, or is breast-feeding.
● Tell patient to take drug with water and to swallow tablet whole. Tell him not to chew, crush, or divide tablet.

---

fexofenadine hydrochloride
fecks-oh-FEN-a-deen

Allegra Allergy ◇, Allegra Allergy
Children's ◇, Allegra ODT, EQL
Aller-Ease ◇, GNP Allergy Relief ◇,
KLS Aller-Fex ◇

Therapeutic class: Antihistamines
Pharmacologic class: Piperidines
Pregnancy risk category: C

AVAILABLE FORMS
Oral suspension: 30 mg/5 mL ◇
Tablets: 30 mg ◇, 60 mg ◇, 180 mg ◇
Tablets (orally disintegrating): 30 mg

INDICATIONS & DOSAGES
Adjust-a-dose (for all indications): For patients with impaired renal function or a
need for dialysis, give adults and children
age 12 and older 60 mg P.O. daily, children
ages 2 to 11, 30 mg daily, and children ages
6 months to 2 years, 15 mg daily.
➤ **Seasonal allergic rhinitis**
Adults and children age 12 and older:
60 mg P.O. b.i.d. or 180 mg P.O. once daily.
Children ages 2 to 11: 30 mg P.O. b.i.d.
either as a tablet or 5 mL oral suspension.
➤ **Chronic idiopathic urticaria**
Adults and children age 12 and older:
60 mg P.O. b.i.d. or 180 mg P.O. once daily.
Children ages 2 to 11: 30 mg P.O. b.i.d.
either as a tablet or 5 mL oral suspension.
*Children ages 6 months to younger than
2 years:* 15 mg (2.5 mL) P.O. b.i.d.

ADMINISTRATION
P.O.
• Don't give aluminum- or magnesium-
containing antacid within 2 hours of this
drug.
• Give orally disintegrating tablets (ODTs)
to patient with an empty stomach. Allow
ODT to disintegrate on the patient's tongue;
it may be swallowed with or without
water.
• Don't remove ODT from blister package
until time of administration.

ACTION
A long-acting nonsedating antihistamine
that selectively inhibits peripheral H_1 receptors.

Route	Onset	Peak	Duration
P.O.	Rapid	3 hr	14 hr

Half-life: 14½ hours.

ADVERSE REACTIONS
CNS: fatigue, drowsiness, fever, headache.
EENT: otitis media.
GI: nausea, dyspepsia, vomiting.
GU: dysmenorrhea.
Musculoskeletal: back pain.
Respiratory: cough, rhinorrhea, upper
respiratory tract infection.
Other: viral infection.

INTERACTIONS
Drug-drug. *Aluminum or magnesium
antacids:* May decrease fexofenadine level.
Separate dosage times.
Erythromycin, ketoconazole: May increase
fexofenadine level. Monitor patient for side
effects.
Rifampin: May decrease pharmacologic
effects of fexofenadine. Monitor patient
carefully.
Drug-food. *Apple juice, grapefruit juice,
orange juice:* May decrease drug effects.
Patients should take drug with liquid other
than these juices.
Drug-lifestyle. *Alcohol use:* May increase
CNS depression. Discourage use together.

EFFECTS ON LAB TEST RESULTS
• May prevent, reduce, or mask positive
result in diagnostic skin test.

CONTRAINDICATIONS & CAUTIONS
• Contraindicated in patients hypersensitive
to drug or its components.
• Use cautiously in patients with impaired
renal function.
⚠ *Overdose S&S:* Dizziness, drowsiness, dry
mouth.

NURSING CONSIDERATIONS
• Stop drug 4 days before patient undergoes diagnostic skin tests because drug can
prevent, reduce, or mask positive skin test
response.

Reactions in bold italics are *life-threatening*. Interactions may have a *rapid onset* or a *delayed onset*.

• It's unknown if drug appears in breast milk; use caution when using drug in breast-feeding women.

PATIENT TEACHING
• Instruct patient or parent not to exceed prescribed dosage and to use drug only when needed.
• Warn patient to avoid alcohol and hazardous activities that require alertness until CNS effects of drug are known. Explain that drug may cause drowsiness.
• Tell patient not to take antacids within 2 hours of this drug.
• Advise patient with dry mouth to try sugarless gum, hard candy, or ice chips.
• Tell parents to keep the oral suspension in a cool, dry place, tightly closed, and to shake well before using.
• Instruct patient to let ODT disintegrate on the tongue and then swallow with or without water.
• Tell patient ODT should be taken on an empty stomach.
• Tell patient to keep ODT in original blister package until time of use.

fidaxomicin
fye-DAX-oh-MYE sin

Dificid

Therapeutic class: Antibiotics
Pharmacologic class: Macrolides
Pregnancy risk category: B

AVAILABLE FORMS
Tablets: 200 mg

INDICATIONS & DOSAGES
➤ *Clostridium difficile*–associated diarrhea
Adults: 200 mg P.O. b.i.d. for 10 days.

ADMINISTRATION
P.O.
• May give without regard for food.
• Store at room temperature.

ACTION
Acts on *C. difficile* locally in the GI tract by inhibiting RNA synthesis through RNA polymerases.

Route	Onset	Peak	Duration
P.O.	<1 hr	1–5 hr	Unknown

Half-life: About 12 hours.

ADVERSE REACTIONS
GI: nausea, vomiting, abdominal pain or discomfort, *GI bleeding,* dyspepsia, flatulence, intestinal obstruction.
Hematologic: anemia, *neutropenia.*
Metabolic: hyperglycemia, *metabolic acidosis.*
Skin: drug eruption, rash, pruritus.

INTERACTIONS
None reported.

EFFECTS ON LAB TEST RESULTS
• May increase alkaline phosphatase, hepatic enzyme, and blood glucose levels.
• May decrease serum bicarbonate level and platelet count.

CONTRAINDICATIONS & CAUTIONS
• Drug isn't an effective treatment for systemic *Clostridium* infections. Don't prescribe fidaxomicin unless a *C. difficile* infection has been proven or is strongly suspected because this may lead to the development of drug-resistant bacteria.
• Drug's effects in pregnant women are unknown; use cautiously in these patients. Use cautiously in breast-feeding women; it isn't known if drug appears in breast milk.

NURSING CONSIDERATIONS
• Obtain specimen for culture before start of treatment. Monitor patient's response to treatment.
• Monitor glucose level, especially in diabetic patients.
• Monitor patient for abdominal pain or bleeding.

PATIENT TEACHING
• Inform patient that drug can be taken with or without food.
• Advise patient that drug is used to treat *C. difficile*–associated diarrhea only and shouldn't be used to treat other infections.
• Counsel patient to take the drug exactly as directed. Missing or skipping doses, or not completing the full course of therapy, may

lead to reinfection, continued infection, or bacterial resistance.

filgrastim (G-CSF; granulocyte colony-stimulating factor)
fill-GRASS-tim

Neupogen

Therapeutic class: Colony stimulating factors
Pharmacologic class: Hematopoietics
Pregnancy risk category: C

AVAILABLE FORMS
Injection: 300 mcg/0.5 mL, 300 mcg/mL, 480 mcg/0.8 mL, 480 mcg/1.6 mL

INDICATIONS & DOSAGES
➤ **To decrease risk of infection in patients with nonmyeloid malignant disease receiving myelosuppressive antineoplastics**
Adults and children: 5 mcg/kg daily I.V. (as continuous or intermittent infusion), subcutaneous infusion, or subcutaneously as a single dose given no sooner than 24 hours after cytotoxic chemotherapy. Doses may be increased in increments of 5 mcg/kg for each chemotherapy cycle, depending on duration and severity of the nadir of ANC. Administer daily for up to 2 weeks.
➤ **To decrease risk of infection in patients with nonmyeloid malignant disease receiving myelosuppressive antineoplastics followed by bone marrow transplantation**
Adults and children: 10 mcg/kg daily I.V. infusion of 4 or 24 hours or as continuous 24-hour subcutaneous infusion at least 24 hours after cytotoxic chemotherapy and bone marrow infusion. Adjust subsequent dosages based on neutrophil response.
Adjust-a-dose: For patients with ANC above 1,000/mm^3 for 3 consecutive days, reduce dosage to 5 mcg/kg daily; if ANC remains above 1,000/mm^3 for 3 more consecutive days, stop drug. If ANC decreases to below 1,000/mm^3, resume therapy at 5 mcg/kg daily.

➤ **Congenital neutropenia**
Adults: 6 mcg/kg subcutaneously b.i.d. Adjust dosage based on patient response.
Adjust-a-dose: For patients with an ANC persistently above 10,000/mm^3, reduce dosage, as directed.
➤ **Idiopathic or cyclic neutropenia**
Adults: 5 mcg/kg subcutaneously daily. Adjust dosage based on patient response.
➤ **Peripheral blood progenitor cell collection and therapy in cancer patients**
Adults: 10 mcg/kg subcutaneously (as bolus or continuous infusion) daily. Give 4 days before leukapheresis and continue until last leukapheresis.
Adjust-a-dose: Patients with WBC count over 100,000/mm^3 may need dosage adjustment.
➤ **To reduce time to neutrophil recovery and fever duration after induction or consolidation chemotherapy treatment of adults with acute myeloid leukemia**
Adults: 5 mcg/kg/day subcutaneously beginning 24 hours after last dose of chemotherapy until neutrophil recovery (ANC 1,000/mm^3 for 3 consecutive days or 10,000/mm^3 for 1 day) or for a maximum of 35 days.
➤ **Neutropenic fever ◆**
Adults: 5 mcg/kg subcutaneously daily 24 to 72 hours after administration of myelotoxic chemotherapeutic agents. Continue until ANC is at least 2 to 3×10^9/L.

ADMINISTRATION
I.V.
▼ Dilute in 50 to 100 mL of D$_5$W. Dilution to less than 5 mcg/mL isn't recommended.
▼ Don't dilute with normal saline solution.
▼ If drug yield is 5 to 15 mcg/mL, add albumin at 2 mg/mL (0.2%) to minimize binding of drug to plastic containers or tubing.
▼ Give by intermittent infusion over 15 to 60 minutes or by continuous infusion over 24 hours.
▼ **Incompatibilities:** Amphotericin B, cefepime, cefonicid, cefotaxime, cefoxitin, ceftizoxime, ceftriaxone, cefuroxime, clindamycin, dactinomycin, etoposide, fluorouracil, furosemide, heparin sodium, mannitol, methylprednisolone sodium succinate, metronidazole, mitomycin,

---

Reactions in bold italics are *life-threatening*. Interactions may have a *rapid onset* or a *delayed onset*.

piperacillin, prochlorperazine edisylate, sodium solutions, thiotepa.

Subcutaneous
• Rotate administration sites and record.

ACTION

Binds cell receptors to stimulate proliferation, differentiation, commitment, and end-cell function of neutrophils.

Route	Onset	Peak	Duration
I.V.	5–60 min	24 hr	1–7 days
Subcut.	5–60 min	2–8 hr	1–7 days

Half-life: 3½ hours.

ADVERSE REACTIONS

CNS: fever, headache, weakness, fatigue.
CV: *MI, arrhythmias,* chest pain, hypotension.
EENT: sore throat.
GI: nausea, vomiting, diarrhea, mucositis, stomatitis, constipation.
Hematologic: *thrombocytopenia,* leukocytosis, *neutropenic fever.*
Metabolic: hyperuricemia.
Musculoskeletal: bone pain.
Respiratory: dyspnea, cough.
Skin: alopecia, rash, cutaneous vasculitis.
Other: hypersensitivity reactions.

INTERACTIONS

Drug-drug. *Chemotherapeutic drugs:* Rapidly dividing myeloid cells may be sensitive to cytotoxic drugs. Don't use within 24 hours before or after a dose of one of these drugs.
Lithium: May potentiate release of neutrophils, causing a greater increase in WBC count than expected. Use together cautiously.

EFFECTS ON LAB TEST RESULTS

• May increase alkaline phosphatase, creatinine, LDH, and uric acid levels.
• May increase WBC count. May decrease platelet count.

CONTRAINDICATIONS & CAUTIONS

• Contraindicated in patients hypersensitive to drug or its components or to proteins derived from *Escherichia coli.*
• Use cautiously in breast-feeding women.
⚠ *Overdose S&S:* Excessive leukocytosis.

NURSING CONSIDERATIONS

• Obtain baseline CBC and platelet count before therapy.
• Once a dose is withdrawn, don't reuse vial. Discard unused portion. Vials are for single-dose use and contain no preservatives.
• Obtain CBC and platelet count two to three times weekly during therapy. Patients who receive drug also may receive high doses of chemotherapy, which may increase risk of toxicities.
• A transiently increased neutrophil count is common 1 or 2 days after therapy starts. Give daily for up to 2 weeks or until ANC has returned to 10,000/mm^3 after the expected chemotherapy-induced neutrophil nadir.
• *Look alike–sound alike:* Don't confuse Neupogen with Epogen or Neumega.

PATIENT TEACHING

• If patient will give drug, teach him how to do so and how to dispose of used needles, syringes, drug containers, and unused medicine.
🛑 *Alert:* Rarely, splenic rupture may occur. Advise patient to immediately report left upper abdominal or shoulder tip pain.
• Instruct patient to report persistent or serious adverse reactions promptly.

finasteride
fin-AS-teh-ride

Propecia, Proscar⚘

Therapeutic class: BPH drugs
Pharmacologic class: 5-alpha-reductase enzyme inhibitors
Pregnancy risk category: X

AVAILABLE FORMS
Tablets: 1 mg, 5 mg

INDICATIONS & DOSAGES
➤ **To improve symptoms of BPH and reduce risk of acute urine retention and need for surgery, including transurethral resection of prostate and prostatectomy (Proscar)**
Men: 5 mg P.O. daily.

➤ **With doxazosin, to reduce risk of BPH symptom progression (Proscar)**
Men: 5 mg P.O. daily.
➤ **Male pattern hair loss (androgenetic alopecia) in men only (Propecia)**
Men: 1 mg P.O. daily.
➤ **Women with hirsutism related to polycystic ovary syndrome ♦**
Adults: 2.5 to 5 mg P.O. daily.
➤ **Chronic pelvic pain syndrome ♦**
Adults: 5 mg P.O. once daily.

ADMINISTRATION
P.O.
● Give drug without regard for food.
⊕ *Alert:* Drug is a potential teratogen. Follow safe handling procedures when preparing, administering, or dispensing drug.

ACTION
Inhibits conversion of testosterone to dihydrotestosterone (DHT), the androgen primarily responsible for the initial development and subsequent enlargement of the prostate gland. In male pattern baldness, the scalp contains miniaturized hair follicles and increased DHT level; drug decreases scalp DHT level in such cases.

Route	Onset	Peak	Duration
P.O.	Unknown	1–2 hr	24 hr

Half-life: 6 hours; 8 hours in elderly patients.

ADVERSE REACTIONS
CNS: dizziness, asthenia, headache.
CV: hypotension, orthostatic hypotension.
GU: erectile dysfunction, decreased volume of ejaculate, decreased libido.
Other: gynecomastia.

INTERACTIONS
Drug-herb. *St. John's wort:* May decrease finasteride level. Avoid use together.

EFFECTS ON LAB TEST RESULTS
● May decrease prostate-specific antigen (PSA) level.

CONTRAINDICATIONS & CAUTIONS
● Contraindicated in patients hypersensitive to drug or to other 5-alpha-reductase inhibitors, such as dutasteride. Drug is also contraindicated in pregnancy.

⊕ *Alert:* Drug may increase the risk of high-grade prostate cancer. Before starting drug, patient should be evaluated to rule out other urologic conditions, including prostate cancer, that might mimic BPH. An increase in PSA level during therapy should be considered significant and the patient should be evaluated for prostate cancer.
● Use cautiously in patients with liver dysfunction.

NURSING CONSIDERATIONS
● Before therapy, evaluate patient for conditions that mimic BPH, including hypotonic bladder, prostate cancer, infection, or stricture.
● Carefully monitor patients who have a large residual urine volume or severely diminished urine flow.
● Sustained increase in PSA level could indicate noncompliance with therapy.
● A minimum of 6 months of therapy may be needed for treatment of BPH.

PATIENT TEACHING
● Tell patient that drug may be taken with or without meals.
● Warn woman who is or may become pregnant not to handle crushed tablets because of risk of adverse effects on male fetus.
● Inform patient that signs of improvement may require at least 3 months of daily use when drug is used to treat hair loss or at least 6 months when taken for BPH.
● Reassure patient that drug may decrease volume of ejaculate without impairing normal sexual function.
● Instruct patient to report breast changes, such as lumps, pain, or nipple discharge.

---

fingolimod
fin-GOL-ih-mod

Gilenya

Therapeutic class: Immunosuppressants
Pharmacologic class: Sphingosine 1-phosphate receptor modulators
Pregnancy risk category: C

AVAILABLE FORMS
Capsules: 0.5 mg

INDICATIONS & DOSAGES
➤ **To reduce frequency of clinical exacerbations and to delay accumulation of physical disability in relapsing forms of MS**
Adults: 0.5 mg P.O. once daily.

ADMINISTRATION
P.O.
● May give drug without regard for food.
● Monitor patient for signs and symptoms of bradycardia for 6 hours after first dose.

ACTION
Unclear. May reduce migration of lymphocytes into CNS.

Route	Onset	Peak	Duration
P.O.	Unknown	12–16 hr	Unknown

Half-life: 6 to 9 days.

ADVERSE REACTIONS
CNS: asthenia, depression, dizziness, paresthesia, headache, migraine.
CV: *bradycardia,* hypertension.
EENT: sinusitis, blurred vision, eye pain.
GI: gastroenteritis, diarrhea.
Hematologic: *lymphopenia, leukopenia.*
Hepatitis: *hepatotoxicity.*
Metabolic: hypertriglyceridemia, weight loss.
Musculoskeletal: back pain.
Respiratory: bronchitis, cough, dyspnea.
Skin: tinea infections, alopecia, eczema, pruritus.
Other: influenza, herpes viral infections.

INTERACTIONS
Drug-drug. *Antineoplastics, immunomodulators, immunosuppressants:* May increase risk of immunosuppression. Use cautiously together.
◑ *Alert:Beta blockers, heart rate–lowering calcium channel blockers (diltiazem, verapamil), digoxin:* May increase risk of severe bradycardia or heart block. If possible, switch patient to cardiac drug that doesn't cause bradycardia before starting fingolimod. If change isn't possible, monitor patient with continuous ECG overnight after first dose to determine effects.
Class IA or III antiarrhythmics (amiodarone, procainamide, quinidine, sotalol): May increase risk of bradycardia or torsades de pointes. Contraindicated together.
Ketoconazole: May increase fingolimod level and risk of adverse effects. Use cautiously and monitor patient closely.
Live attenuated virus vaccines: May decrease vaccination effects or increase infection risk. Don't use together or give vaccine within 60 days of prior fingolimod use.

EFFECTS ON LAB TEST RESULTS
● May increase ALT, AST, GGT, and triglyceride levels.
● May decrease lymphocyte and neutrophil counts.

CONTRAINDICATIONS & CAUTIONS
● Contraindicated in patients hypersensitive to drug and in those with active acute or chronic infection.
◑ *Alert:* Contraindicated in patients with MI, unstable angina, stroke, transient ischemic attack, decompensated heart failure requiring hospitalization, or Class III/IV heart failure within the past 6 months; in those with history or presence of Mobitz Type II second- or third-degree AV block or sick sinus syndrome unless the patient has a functioning pacemaker; and in those with baseline QTc interval of 500 ms or greater.
◑ *Alert:* Use cautiously after cardiac evaluation in patients with ischemic heart disease, history of MI, congestive heart failure, history of cardiac arrest, cerebrovascular disease, history of symptomatic bradycardia, recurrent syncope, severe untreated sleep apnea, AV block, or SA heart block. Monitor patient with continuous ECG overnight in medical facility after first dose.
● Use cautiously in patients with history of bradycardia, syncope, sick sinus syndrome, ischemic heart disease, or heart failure and in patients taking class IA or III antiarrhythmics, beta blockers, or calcium channel blockers.
● Use cautiously in patients with history of infection, macular edema, decreased pulmonary function test results, or liver disease, and in women of childbearing age.
● Use in pregnant women only if benefit justifies risk. Pregnant women should enroll in the Gilenya Pregnancy Registry at 1-877-598-7237.

F

• It isn't known if drug appears in breast milk. Because of potential for serious adverse effects in breast-feeding infant, give drug only if potential benefit to mother outweighs potential risk to infant.

• Use cautiously in patients older than age 65 who have concomitant disease or are taking other drugs.

• Safety and effectiveness in children haven't been established.

⚠ **Overdose S&S:** Chest tightness or discomfort.

NURSING CONSIDERATIONS

⚠ **Alert:** Monitor hourly heart rate and blood pressure for at least 6 hours after first dose in all patients. Obtain ECG before first dose and at the end of the observation period. Monitor blood pressure routinely during treatment.

⚠ **Alert:** Monitor high-risk patients and those who may not tolerate bradycardia with continuous ECG overnight. High-risk patients include those who develop severe bradycardia after receiving the first dose, those with preexisting conditions who may not tolerate bradycardia, those receiving other drugs that slow the heart rate or AV conduction, those with QT-interval prolongation before taking fingolimod or prolonged QT interval that occurs during monitoring period, those receiving other drugs that prolong QT interval, and those at risk for QT-interval prolongation due to hypokalemia, hypomagnesemia, or congenital long-QT syndrome.

⚠ **Alert:** If CV symptoms occur (heart rate less than 45 beats/minute or at it lowest value 6 hours after dose, or new-onset second-degree or higher AV block 6 hours after dose), continue monitoring until symptoms resolve.

⚠ **Alert:** Repeat first-dose monitoring guidelines after second dose in patients who required pharmacologic intervention for symptomatic bradycardia after first dose.

• Obtain baseline ECG if one wasn't done within 6 months before start of therapy, especially in patients receiving antiarrhythmics, beta blockers, or calcium channel blockers and in those with cardiac risk factors or slow or irregular heart rates on physical examination.

• Test for varicella antibodies before treatment initiation, especially if patient has no history of chickenpox or immunization; consider vaccination against varicella zoster 1 month before start of fingolimod therapy.

• Obtain baseline ophthalmic examination and monitor patient for macular edema at 3 to 4 months after treatment initiation and if patient complains of visual disturbances. Although macular edema is a rare adverse reaction, patients with uveitis and diabetes are at increased risk.

• Monitor patient for signs and symptoms of infection during treatment and for 2 months after discontinuation of therapy. Obtain baseline CBC with differential within 6 months of beginning therapy. Consider suspending treatment if patient has active infection.

• Monitor patient for hepatic impairment (unexplained nausea, vomiting, abdominal pain, fatigue, anorexia, jaundice, dark urine). Obtain LFTs at baseline and as needed during therapy. Most enzyme elevations occur within 3 to 4 months of treatment initiation.

• Monitor patient for respiratory changes. Obtain spirometry and diffusion lung capacity tests if clinically indicated.

• Restart therapy as at initiation if patient discontinues treatment for more than 2 weeks.

PATIENT TEACHING

⚠ **Alert:** Teach patient to immediately contact the health care provider if signs and symptoms of a slowing heart rate, such as dizziness, tiredness, irregular heartbeat, or palpitations, occur.

• Instruct patient to report visual disturbances, trouble breathing, changes in heart rate (low heart rate, dizziness, fatigue, chest pain) or rhythm (palpitations), or infection (pain, fever, malaise).

• Tell patient to immediately report unexplained nausea, vomiting, abdominal pain, fatigue, anorexia, jaundice, or dark urine.

• Advise patient to notify prescriber of any medication changes.

• Warn woman of childbearing potential about possible risk to fetus; advise her to use effective contraception during treatment and for 2 months after treatment ends.

Reactions in bold italics are *life-threatening*. Interactions may have a *rapid onset* or a *delayed onset*.

• Advise women to notify prescriber immediately if they are or plan to become pregnant.

flecainide acetate
FLEH-kay-nighd

Tambocor

Therapeutic class: Antiarrhythmics
Pharmacologic class: Benzamide derivatives
Pregnancy risk category: C

AVAILABLE FORMS
Tablets: 50 mg, 100 mg, 150 mg

INDICATIONS & DOSAGES
➤ **Prevention of paroxysmal supraventricular tachycardia, including AV nodal reentrant tachycardia and AV reentrant tachycardia or paroxysmal atrial fibrillation or flutter in patients without structural heart disease; life-threatening ventricular arrhythmias such as sustained ventricular tachycardia**
Adults: For paroxysmal supraventricular tachycardia or paroxysmal atrial fibrillation or flutter, 50 mg P.O. every 12 hours. Increase in increments of 50 mg b.i.d. every 4 days. Maximum dose is 300 mg/day. For life-threatening ventricular arrhythmias, 100 mg P.O. every 12 hours. Increase in increments of 50 mg b.i.d. every 4 days until desired effect occurs. Maximum dose for most patients is 400 mg/day.
Adjust-a-dose: If CrCl is 35 mL/minute or less, first dose is 100 mg P.O. once daily or 50 mg P.O. b.i.d.

ADMINISTRATION
P.O.
• Give drug without regard for food.

ACTION
A class IC antiarrhythmic that decreases excitability, conduction velocity, and automaticity by slowing atrial, AV node, His-Purkinje system, and intraventricular conduction; prolongs refractory periods in these tissues.

Route	Onset	Peak	Duration
P.O.	Unknown	2–3 hr	Unknown

Half-life: 12 to 27 hours.

ADVERSE REACTIONS
CNS: dizziness, headache, lightheadedness, syncope, fatigue, fever, tremor, anxiety, insomnia, depression, malaise, paresthesia, ataxia, vertigo, asthenia.
CV: *new or worsened arrhythmias, heart failure, cardiac arrest,* chest pain, palpitations, edema, flushing.
EENT: blurred vision and other visual disturbances, eye pain, eye irritation.
GI: nausea, constipation, abdominal pain, dyspepsia, vomiting, diarrhea, anorexia.
Respiratory: dyspnea.
Skin: rash.

INTERACTIONS
Drug-drug. *Amiodarone, cimetidine, CYP2D6 inhibitors (clozapine, quinidine):* May increase level of flecainide. Watch for toxicity. In the presence of amiodarone, reduce usual flecainide dose by 50% and monitor the patient for adverse effects.
Digoxin: May increase digoxin level by 15% to 25%. Monitor digoxin level.
Disopyramide, verapamil: May increase negative inotropic properties. Avoid using together.
Propranolol, other beta blockers: May increase flecainide and propranolol levels by 20% to 30%. Watch for propranolol and flecainide toxicity.
Ritonavir: May significantly increase flecainide levels and toxicity. Use together is contraindicated.
Urine-acidifying and urine-alkalinizing drugs: May cause extremes of urine pH, which may alter flecainide excretion. Monitor patient for flecainide toxicity or decreased effectiveness.
Drug-lifestyle. *Smoking:* May decrease flecainide level. Monitor patient closely.

EFFECTS ON LAB TEST RESULTS
None reported.

F

CONTRAINDICATIONS & CAUTIONS

• Contraindicated in patients hypersensitive to drug and in those with second- or third-degree AV block or right bundle-branch block with a left hemiblock (in the absence of an artificial pacemaker), recent MI, or cardiogenic shock, and in patients taking ritonavir.

Black Box Warning Patients who received flecainide for atrial fibrillation or flutter were at increased risk for ventricular tachycardia and ventricular fibrillation. Its use for these conditions isn't recommended. ∎

• Use cautiously in patients with heart failure, cardiomyopathy, severe renal disease, prolonged QT interval, sick sinus syndrome, or blood dyscrasia.

• In patients with hepatic disease, use drug only if potential benefits outweigh risk, and use frequent and early drug-level monitoring to guide dosage.

• When transferring patient from another antiarrhythmic to flecainide, allow two to four plasma half-lives to elapse for the drug being discontinued before starting flecainide at the usual dosage. Consider hospitalizing patients in whom withdrawal of a previous antiarrhythmic produced life-threatening arrhythmias.

NURSING CONSIDERATIONS

Black Box Warning When used to prevent ventricular arrhythmias, reserve drug for patients with documented life-threatening arrhythmias. For patients with sustained ventricular tachycardia, initiate therapy in the hospital and monitor rhythm. ∎

Black Box Warning Patients treated with flecainide for atrial flutter have a 1:1 AV conduction due to slowing of the atrial rate. A paradoxical increase in the ventricular rate may occur. Concomitant negative chronotropic therapy with digoxin or beta blockers may lower the risk of this complication. ∎

• Check that pacing threshold was determined 1 week before and after starting therapy in a patient with a pacemaker; flecainide can alter endocardial pacing thresholds.

• Correct hypokalemia or hyperkalemia before giving flecainide because these electrolyte disturbances may alter drug's effect.

• Monitor ECG rhythm for proarrhythmic effects.

• Most patients can be adequately maintained on an every-12-hours dosing schedule, but some need to receive flecainide every 8 hours.

• Monitor flecainide level, especially if patient has renal or heart failure. Therapeutic flecainide levels range from 0.2 to 1 mcg/mL. Risk of adverse effects increases when trough blood level exceeds 1 mcg/mL.

PATIENT TEACHING

• Stress importance of taking drug exactly as prescribed.

• Instruct patient to report adverse reactions promptly and to limit fluid and sodium intake to minimize fluid retention.

fluconazole
floo-KON-a-zole

Diflucan✦

Therapeutic class: Antifungals
Pharmacologic class: Bis-triazole derivatives
Pregnancy risk category: D; C for vaginal candidiasis

AVAILABLE FORMS
Injection: 100 mg/50 mL, 200 mg/100 mL, 400 mg/200 mL
Powder for oral suspension: 10 mg/mL, 40 mg/mL, 50 mg/5 mL, 200 mg/5 mL
Tablets: 50 mg, 100 mg, 150 mg, 200 mg

INDICATIONS & DOSAGES
Adjust-a-dose (for all indications): (Applies to all indications except vulvovaginal candidiasis.) If CrCl is less than 50 mL/minute and patient isn't receiving dialysis, reduce dosage by 50%. Patients receiving regular hemodialysis treatment should receive usual dose after each dialysis session.

➤ **Oropharyngeal candidiasis**
Adults: 200 mg P.O. or I.V. on first day, then 100 mg once daily for at least 2 weeks.
Children: 6 mg/kg P.O. or I.V. on first day, then 3 mg/kg daily for 2 weeks.

➤ **Esophageal candidiasis**
Adults: 200 mg P.O. or I.V. on first day, then 100 mg once daily. Up to 400 mg daily has

---

been used, depending on patient's condition and tolerance of treatment. Patients should receive drug for at least 3 weeks and for 2 weeks after symptoms resolve.

Children: 6 mg/kg P.O. or I.V. on first day, then 3 mg/kg daily for at least 3 weeks and for at least 2 weeks after symptoms resolve. Maximum daily dose 12 mg/kg.

➤ **Vulvovaginal candidiasis**
Adults: 150 mg P.O. for one dose only.

➤ **Systemic candidiasis**
Adults: 400 mg P.O. or I.V. on first day, then 200 mg once daily for at least 4 weeks and for 2 weeks after symptoms resolve. Doses up to 400 mg/day may be used.
Children: 6 to 12 mg/kg/day P.O. or I.V.

➤ **Cryptococcal meningitis**
Adults: 400 mg P.O. or I.V. on first day, then 200 mg once daily for 10 to 12 weeks after CSF culture result is negative. Doses up to 400 mg/day may be used.
Children: 12 mg/kg/day P.O. or I.V. on first day, then 6 mg/kg/day for 10 to 12 weeks after CSF culture result is negative.

➤ **To prevent candidiasis in bone marrow transplant and cancer patients**
Adults: 400 mg P.O. or I.V. once daily. Start treatment several days before anticipated agranulocytosis, and continue for 7 days after neutrophil count exceeds 1,000/mm^3.

➤ **To suppress relapse of cryptococcal meningitis in patients with AIDS**
Adults: 200 mg P.O. or I.V. daily.
Children: 6 mg/kg/day P.O. or I.V. once daily.

ADMINISTRATION

P.O.
• Give drug without regard for food.
• Add 24 mL of distilled or purified water to the bottle and shake oral suspension well before giving.

I.V.
▼ To ensure product sterility, don't remove protective wrap from I.V. bag until just before use.
▼ The plastic container may show some opacity from moisture absorbed during sterilization. This doesn't affect drug and diminishes over time.
▼ To prevent air embolism, don't connect in series with other infusions.

▼ Use an infusion pump.
▼ Give by continuous infusion at no more than 200 mg/hour.
▼ **Incompatibilities:** Amphotericin B, amphotericin B cholesteryl sulfate complex, ampicillin sodium, calcium gluconate, cefotaxime sodium, ceftazidime, ceftriaxone, cefuroxime sodium, chloramphenicol sodium succinate, clindamycin phosphate, diazepam, digoxin, erythromycin lactobionate, furosemide, haloperidol lactate, hydroxyzine hydrochloride, imipenem–cilastatin sodium, pentamidine, piperacillin sodium, ticarcillin disodium, sulfamethoxazole–trimethoprim. Don't add other drugs to I.V. bag.

ACTION

Inhibits fungal CYP450 (responsible for fungal sterol synthesis); weakens fungal cell walls.

Route	Onset	Peak	Duration
P.O.	Unknown	1–2 hr	30 hr
I.V.	Immediate	Immediate	Unknown

Half-life: 20 to 50 hours.

ADVERSE REACTIONS

CNS: headache, dizziness.
GI: nausea, vomiting, abdominal pain, diarrhea, dyspepsia, taste perversion.
Hematologic: *leukopenia, thrombocytopenia.*
Skin: rash.
Other: *anaphylaxis.*

INTERACTIONS

Drug-drug. *Alprazolam, chlordiazepoxide, clonazepam, clorazepate, diazepam, estazolam, flurazepam, midazolam, quazepam, triazolam:* May increase and prolong levels of these drugs, CNS depression, and psychomotor impairment. Avoid using together.
Cimetidine: May decrease fluconazole level. Monitor patient's response to fluconazole.
Cyclosporine, phenytoin, theophylline: May increase levels of these drugs. Monitor cyclosporine, phenytoin, and theophylline levels.
Erythromycin: May cause prolonged QT interval and sudden death. Don't use together.

HMG-CoA reductase inhibitors (atorvastatin, fluvastatin, lovastatin, pravastatin, simvastatin): May increase levels and adverse effects of these drugs. Avoid using together or reduce dosage of HMG-CoA reductase inhibitor.

Isoniazid, oral sulfonylureas, phenytoin, rifampin, valproic acid: May increase hepatic transaminase level. Monitor LFT results closely.

Oral sulfonylureas (such as glipizide, glyburide): May increase levels of these drugs. Monitor patient for enhanced hypoglycemic effect.

Proton pump inhibitors: May decrease fluconazole effect. Give fluconazole 2 hours or more before proton pump inhibitors.

Rifampin: May enhance fluconazole metabolism. Monitor patient for lack of response to fluconazole.

Tacrolimus: May increase tacrolimus level and nephrotoxicity. Monitor patient carefully.

Warfarin: May increase risk of bleeding. Monitor PT and INR.

Zidovudine: May increase zidovudine activity. Monitor patient closely.

Zolpidem: May increase therapeutic effects of zolpidem. Monitor patient closely. A decrease in dosage may be needed.

EFFECTS ON LAB TEST RESULTS
• May increase alkaline phosphatase, ALT, AST, bilirubin, and GGT levels.
• May decrease platelet and WBC counts.

CONTRAINDICATIONS & CAUTIONS
❸ Alert: Long-term treatment with high doses (400 to 800 mg/day) during the first trimester of pregnancy may be associated with fetal birth defects.
• Contraindicated in patients hypersensitive to drug and in breast-feeding patients.
• Use cautiously in patients hypersensitive to other antifungal azole compounds.
• Oral suspension contains sucrose and shouldn't be used in patients with hereditary fructose, glucose, or galactose malabsorption or sucrase-isomaltase deficiency.
⚠ Overdose S&S: Hallucinations, paranoid behavior.

NURSING CONSIDERATIONS
❸ Alert: Serious hepatotoxicity has occurred in patients with underlying medical conditions.
• If patient develops mild rash, monitor him closely. Stop drug if lesions progress.
• Likelihood of adverse reactions may be greater in HIV-infected patients.

PATIENT TEACHING
• Tell patient to take drug as directed, even after he feels better.
• Instruct patient to report adverse reactions promptly.

SAFETY ALERT!

fludarabine phosphate
floo-DAR-a-been

Therapeutic class: Antineoplastics
Pharmacologic class: Purine antagonists
Pregnancy risk category: D

AVAILABLE FORMS
Liquid for injection: 50 mg/2 mL
Powder for injection: 50 mg

INDICATIONS & DOSAGES
➤ B-cell chronic lymphocytic leukemia in patients with no or inadequate response to at least one standard alkylating drug regimen
Adults: 25 mg/m² I.V. daily over 30 minutes for 5 consecutive days. Repeat cycle every 28 days. The optimal duration of treatment hasn't been established.
Adjust-a-dose: In patients with CrCl of 50 to 79 mL/minute, starting dose is 20 mg/m². In patients with CrCl of 30 to 49 mL/minute, starting dose is 15 mg/m². If CrCl is less than 30 mL/minute, don't give drug.

ADMINISTRATION
I.V.
▼ Preparing and giving parenteral drug may be mutagenic, teratogenic, or carcinogenic. Follow facility policy to reduce risks.
▼ To prepare, add 2 mL of sterile water for injection to the vial. If using powder for injection, dissolution should occur within 15 seconds.

▼ Each milliliter contains 25 mg of drug.
▼ Dilute further in 100 or 125 mL of D₅W or normal saline solution for injection.
▼ Use within 8 hours of reconstitution.
▼ Store drug in refrigerator at 36° to 46° F (2° to 8° C).
▼ **Incompatibilities:** Acyclovir sodium, amphotericin B, chlorpromazine, daunorubicin, ganciclovir, hydroxyzine hydrochloride, prochlorperazine edisylate.

ACTION
Unknown. After conversion to its active metabolite, drug interferes with DNA synthesis by inhibiting DNA polymerase alpha, ribonucleotide reductase, and DNA primase.

Route	Onset	Peak	Duration
I.V.	Unknown	Unknown	Unknown

Half-life: About 20 hours.

ADVERSE REACTIONS
CNS: fatigue, malaise, weakness, paresthesia, peripheral neuropathy, *stroke,* headache, sleep disorder, depression, cerebellar syndrome, *transient ischemic attack,* agitation, confusion, fever, *coma,* pain.
CV: edema, angina, phlebitis, *arrhythmias, heart failure, MI,* supraventricular tachycardia, *DVT, aneurysm, hemorrhage.*
EENT: visual disturbances, hearing loss, delayed blindness, sinusitis, pharyngitis, epistaxis.
GI: nausea, vomiting, diarrhea, constipation, anorexia, stomatitis, *GI bleeding,* esophagitis, mucositis.
GU: dysuria, UTI, urinary hesitancy, proteinuria, hematuria, *renal failure.*
Hematologic: hemolytic anemia, *myelosuppression.*
Hepatic: *liver failure,* cholelithiasis.
Metabolic: hypocalcemia, hyperkalemia, hyperglycemia, dehydration, hyperuricemia, hyperphosphatemia.
Musculoskeletal: myalgia.
Respiratory: cough, pneumonia, dyspnea, upper respiratory tract infection, allergic pneumonitis, hemoptysis, hypoxia, bronchitis.
Skin: rash, pruritus, alopecia, seborrhea, diaphoresis.

Other: chills, *tumor lysis syndrome, infection, anaphylaxis.*

INTERACTIONS
Drug-drug. *Cytarabine:* May decrease metabolism of subsequently given fludarabine and inhibition of fludarabine activity. Monitor patient closely.
Myelosuppressives: May increase toxicity. Avoid using together, if possible.
Black Box Warning *Pentostatin:* May increase risk of pulmonary toxicity, which can be fatal. Avoid using together. ∎

EFFECTS ON LAB TEST RESULTS
● May increase glucose, phosphate, potassium, and uric acid levels.
● May decrease calcium and hemoglobin levels. May decrease platelet, RBC, and WBC counts.

CONTRAINDICATIONS & CAUTIONS
● Contraindicated in patients hypersensitive to drug or its components.
● Use cautiously in patients with renal insufficiency.
⚠ *Overdose S&S:* Delayed blindness, coma, thrombocytopenia, neutropenia, death.

NURSING CONSIDERATIONS
Black Box Warning Administer under the supervision of a physician experienced in the use of antineoplastic therapy. ∎
Black Box Warning Higher than recommended doses are associated with severe neurologic toxicity, including blindness, coma, and death. ∎
⊙ *Alert:* Monitor patient closely and expect modified dosage based on toxicity. Most toxic effects are dose dependent. Advanced age, renal insufficiency, and bone marrow impairment may predispose patients to increased or excessive toxicity.
Black Box Warning Careful hematologic monitoring is needed, especially of neutrophil and platelet counts. Bone marrow suppression can be severe. ∎
Black Box Warning Monitor patient for development of hemolysis. ∎
● To prevent bleeding, avoid all I.M. injections when platelet count is below 50,000/mm³.

• Give blood transfusions because of cumulative anemia. Patients should be given irradiated blood only, to minimize transfusion-associated graft-versus-host disease.

• Hyperuricemia, hypocalcemia, hyperkalemia, and renal failure may result from rapid lysis of tumor cells. Take preventive measures against tumor lysis syndrome, such as I.V. hydration, alkalinization of urine, and treatment with allopurinol as appropriate.

• Avoid vaccination with live-virus vaccines during and after treatment.

• **Look alike–sound alike:** Don't confuse fludarabine with floxuridine, fluorouracil, or flucytosine.

PATIENT TEACHING

• Instruct patient to watch for signs and symptoms of infection (fever, sore throat, fatigue) and bleeding (easy bruising, nosebleeds, bleeding gums, tarry stools). Tell patient to take temperature daily.

• Advise women to consult prescriber before becoming pregnant.

• Caution women to stop breast-feeding during therapy because of risk of toxicity to infant.

flunisolide (inhalation)
floo-NISS-oh-lide

AeroSpan HFA

Therapeutic class: Corticosteroids
Pharmacologic class: Corticosteroids
Pregnancy risk category: C

AVAILABLE FORMS

Oral inhalant in a hydrofluoroalkane (HFA) inhaler: 80 mcg/metered dose (AeroSpan HFA)

INDICATIONS & DOSAGES

➤ **Chronic asthma**

Adults and children age 12 and older: 2 inhalations (160 mcg) with AeroSpan HFA inhaler b.i.d. Don't exceed 320 mcg b.i.d.

Children ages 6 to 11: 1 inhalation (80 mcg) with AeroSpan HFA inhaler b.i.d. Don't exceed 160 mcg b.i.d.

Children ages 6 to 15: 2 inhalations with AeroSpan HFA inhaler b.i.d. for a total daily dose of 1 mg.

ADMINISTRATION

Inhalational

• For best results, the canister should be at room temperature before use.

• Allow 1 minute between doses.

ACTION

A corticosteroid that may decrease inflammation of asthma by inhibiting macrophages, T cells, eosinophils, and mediators such as leukotrienes while reducing the number of mast cells within the airway.

Route	Onset	Peak	Duration
Inhalation	1–4 wk	Unknown	Unknown

Half-life: About 1¾ hours.

ADVERSE REACTIONS

CNS: headache, dizziness, insomnia, migraine.

CV: chest pain, edema.

EENT: conjunctivitis, ear pain, laryngitis, voice alteration, taste perversion, epistaxis, rhinitis, pharyngitis, sinusitis.

GI: dyspepsia, vomiting, diarrhea, gastroenteritis, nausea, oral moniliasis, abdominal pain.

GU: UTI, dysmenorrhea, vaginitis.

Musculoskeletal: neck pain, myalgia.

Respiratory: cough, bronchitis.

Skin: *erythema multiforme.*

Other: infection, allergic reaction.

INTERACTIONS

Drug-drug. *Aldesleukin:* May diminish antineoplastic effect of aldesleukin. Avoid using together.

Amphotericin B: May enhance hypokalemic effect of amphotericin B. Monitor patient.

Antidiabetic agents: May diminish hypoglycemic effect of antidiabetic agent. Monitor patient.

Bacille Calmette-Guérin (BCG) vaccine: May diminish therapeutic effect of BCG vaccine. Avoid using together.

Vaccines (inactivated): Therapeutic effect of vaccines may be diminished. Monitor therapy.

Reactions in bold italics are *life-threatening*. Interactions may have a *rapid onset* or a *delayed onset*.

Conivaptan, dasatinib: May increase serum concentration of CYP3A4 substrates. Avoid using together.
Corticorelin: May diminish therapeutic effect of corticorelin. Monitor therapy.
Deferasirox, denosumab, leflunomide: May enhance adverse effects of these drugs. Monitor patient.
Leflunomide: May increase risk of hematologic toxicity, such as pancytopenia, agranulocytosis, or thrombocytopenia. Consider not using leflunomide loading dose in patients receiving drug. Monitor patients receiving both leflunomide and flunisolide for bone marrow suppression at least monthly. Consider therapy modification.
Loop diuretics, thiazide diuretics: May enhance hypokalemic effect of these drugs. Monitor patient.
Moderate CYP3A4 inhibitors, tocilizumab: May decrease metabolism of CYP3A4 substrates. Monitor therapy.
Natalizumab, pimecrolimus, tacrolimus (topical): May enhance adverse effects of these drugs. Avoid using together.
Sipuleucel-T: May diminish therapeutic effect of this drug. Monitor therapy.
Strong CYP3A4 inhibitors: May decrease metabolism of CYP3A4 substrates. Consider therapy modification.
Telaprevir: May decrease telaprevir serum concentration. May increase serum concentration of corticosteroids. Concurrent use isn't recommended. If used together, employ extra caution and monitor patient closely.
Trastuzumab: May enhance neutropenic effect of immunosuppressants. Monitor therapy.
Vaccines (inactivated): May diminish therapeutic effect of vaccines. Monitor therapy.
Drug-herb. *Echinacea:* May diminish therapeutic effect of immunosuppressants. Consider therapy modification.

EFFECTS ON LAB TEST RESULTS
None reported.

CONTRAINDICATIONS & CAUTIONS
• Contraindicated in patients hypersensitive to drug and in those with status asthmaticus or respiratory tract infections.
• Drug isn't recommended in patients with nonasthmatic bronchial diseases or with

asthma controlled by bronchodilator or other noncorticosteroid alone.

NURSING CONSIDERATIONS
❸ *Alert:* All patients with asthma should have routine tests of adrenal cortical function, including measurement of early-morning resting cortisol levels to establish a baseline in the event of an emergency.
❸ *Alert:* There is an increased risk of death due to adrenal insufficiency in patients transferred from systematically active corticosteroids to flunisolide inhaler. Monitor patient carefully.
❸ *Alert:* Withdraw drug slowly in patients who have received long-term oral corticosteroid therapy.
❸ *Alert:* After withdrawing systemic corticosteroids, patient may need supplemental systemic corticosteroids if stress (trauma, surgery, or infection) causes adrenal insufficiency.
• Store drug at room temperature.
• *Look alike–sound alike:* Don't confuse flunisolide with fluocinonide.

PATIENT TEACHING
• Warn patient that drug doesn't relieve acute asthma attacks.
❸ *Alert:* Instruct patient to immediately contact prescriber if asthma episodes unresponsive to bronchodilators occur during treatment.
• Advise patient to ensure delivery of proper dose by gently warming the canister to room temperature before using. Some patients carry the canister in a pocket to keep it warm.
• Children should administer drug under adult supervision.
• Tell patient who also uses a bronchodilator to use it several minutes before beginning flunisolide treatment.
• Instruct patient to begin inhaling immediately before activating the canister to get the full dose.
• Instruct patient to allow 1 minute to elapse before repeating inhalations and to hold his breath for a few seconds to enhance drug action.
• Teach patient to keep inhaler clean and unobstructed. The HFA inhaler doesn't need cleaning during normal use.

• Teach patient to check mucous membranes frequently for signs and symptoms of fungal infection.

• Advise patient to prevent oral fungal infections by gargling or rinsing mouth with water after each inhaler use. Caution him not to swallow the water.

• Warn patient to avoid exposure to chickenpox or measles. If exposed, contact prescriber immediately.

• Advise parents of a child receiving long-term therapy that the child should have periodic growth measurements and be checked for evidence of hypothalamic-pituitary-adrenal axis suppression.

flunisolide (intranasal)
floo-NISS-oh-lide

Rhinalar†

Therapeutic class: Corticosteroids
Pharmacologic class: Corticosteroids
Pregnancy risk category: C

AVAILABLE FORMS
Nasal spray: 25 mcg/spray, 29 mcg/spray

INDICATIONS & DOSAGES
➤ **Symptoms of seasonal or perennial rhinitis**
Adults and children age 15 and older: Starting dose is 2 sprays in each nostril b.i.d. If needed, dosage may be increased to 2 sprays in each nostril t.i.d. Maximum total daily dose is 8 sprays in each nostril per day.
Children ages 6 to 14: Starting dose is 1 spray in each nostril t.i.d. or 2 sprays in each nostril b.i.d. Maximum total daily dose is 4 sprays in each nostril per day.

ADMINISTRATION
Intranasal
• Shake well before each use.
• Before first use, prime the nasal spray by pushing down on the pump five or six times until a fine mist appears. If the pump hasn't been used for 5 days or more, the spray must be primed again.

ACTION
Exact mechanism unknown. Decreases nasal inflammation, mainly by stabilizing leukocyte lysosomal membranes.

Route	Onset	Peak	Duration
Intranasal	Unknown	Unknown	Unknown

Half-life: 1 to 2 hours.

ADVERSE REACTIONS
CNS: dizziness, headache.
EENT: mild, transient nasal burning and stinging; epistaxis; nasal dryness; nasal congestion; pharyngitis; sneezing; watery eyes.
GI: nausea, vomiting.
Respiratory: cough.
Other: aftertaste, hypersensitivity reaction, loss of taste and smell.

INTERACTIONS
None significant.

EFFECTS ON LAB TEST RESULTS
None reported.

CONTRAINDICATIONS & CAUTIONS
• Contraindicated in patients hypersensitive to drug and in those with untreated localized infection involving nasal mucosa.
• Use cautiously, if at all, in patients with active or quiescent respiratory tract tuberculous infections or untreated fungal, bacterial, or systemic viral or ocular herpes simplex infections.
🔴 *Alert:* Drug is absorbed into the circulation and excessive doses may suppress hypothalamic-pituitary-adrenal (HPA) axis function.
• Use cautiously in patients who have recently had nasal septal ulcers, nasal surgery, or nasal trauma.

NURSING CONSIDERATIONS
• Drug isn't effective for acute exacerbations of rhinitis. Decongestants or antihistamines may be needed.
• Don't give drug for more than 3 weeks unless there is significant symptom improvement.
• *Look alike–sound alike:* Don't confuse flunisolide with fluocinonide, fluticasone, or Flumadine.

PATIENT TEACHING
• Tell patient to avoid exposure to chickenpox or measles.
• Advise patient or parent to read package instructions for drug use.
• Instruct patient to shake container before use, blow nose to clear nasal passages, tilt head slightly forward, and insert nozzle into nostril, pointing away from septum. Tell him to hold other nostril closed and inhale gently while spraying. Have him repeat procedure in other nostril. Tell him to clean nosepiece with warm water daily.
• Explain that drug doesn't work right away. Most patients notice improvement within a few days, but some may need 2 to 3 weeks.
• Advise patient to use drug regularly, as prescribed.
• Warn patient not to exceed recommended dosage to avoid HPA axis suppression.
• Tell patient to stop drug and notify prescriber if signs and symptoms don't diminish in 3 weeks or if nasal irritation persists.

---

fluocinolone acetonide
floo-oh-SIN-oh-lone

Capex, Derma-Smoothe/FS, Dermotic, Synalar

Therapeutic class: Corticosteroids
Pharmacologic class: Corticosteroids
Pregnancy risk category: C

AVAILABLE FORMS
Cream: 0.01%, 0.025%
Oil: 0.01%
Oil/drops (otic): 0.01%
Ointment: 0.025%
Shampoo: 0.01%
Topical solution: 0.01%

INDICATIONS & DOSAGES
➤ **Inflammation from corticosteroid-responsive dermatoses**
Adults and children: Clean area; apply product sparingly t.i.d. to q.i.d.
➤ **Atopic dermatitis**
Adults: Apply thin film of topical oil t.i.d.
Children age 3 months and older: Apply thin film of topical oil b.i.d. for maximum of 4 weeks. Avoid face and diaper area.

➤ **Scalp psoriasis**
Adults: Wet or dampen hair and scalp thoroughly. Apply a thin film of topical oil and massage into scalp. Cover with supplied shower cap overnight or for a minimum of 4 hours before washing thoroughly with regular shampoo and then rinsing thoroughly with water.
➤ **Seborrheic dermatitis of the scalp**
Adults: Apply no more than 30 mL of 0.01% shampoo to the scalp once daily, lather, and rinse thoroughly with water after 5 minutes.
➤ **Eczematous external otitis**
Adults and children age 2 and older: Apply 5 drops of oil (otic) into affected ear b.i.d. for 7 to 14 days.

ADMINISTRATION
Otic
• Tilt head to one side so the affected ear is facing up. Gently pull earlobe backward and upward and apply 5 drops of oil into the ear. Keep head tilted for at least 1 minute.
Topical
• Gently wash skin before applying. To prevent skin damage, rub in gently, leaving a thin coat. When treating hairy sites, part hair and apply directly to lesions.
• Avoid application near eyes or mucous membranes; in armpits, groin, or rectal area; or in ear canal if eardrum is perforated.
• Do not use occlusive dressing unless ordered.
• For patients with eczematous dermatitis whose skin may be irritated by adhesive material, hold dressing in place with gauze, elastic bandages, stockings, or stockinette.
• Change dressing as prescribed. Stop drug and notify prescriber if skin infection, striae, or atrophy occur.
• Shake shampoo well prior to use.

ACTION
Unclear. Is diffused across cell membranes to form complexes with receptors. Shows anti-inflammatory, antipruritic, vasoconstrictive, and antiproliferative activity. Considered a medium-potency to low-potency drug, according to vasoconstrictive properties.

Route	Onset	Peak	Duration
Otic, topical	Unknown	Unknown	Unknown

Half-life: Unknown.

ADVERSE REACTIONS
GU: glycosuria.
Metabolic: hyperglycemia.
Skin: burning, pruritus, irritation, dryness, erythema, folliculitis, hypertrichosis, hypopigmentation, acneiform eruptions, perioral dermatitis, allergic contact dermatitis, maceration, secondary infection, atrophy, striae, miliaria with occlusive dressings.
Other: *hypothalamic-pituitary-adrenal axis (HPA) suppression,* Cushing syndrome.

INTERACTIONS
None significant.

EFFECTS ON LAB TEST RESULTS
● May increase glucose level.

CONTRAINDICATIONS & CAUTIONS
● Contraindicated in patients hypersensitive to drug or its components.
● Don't use as monotherapy in primary bacterial infections (impetigo, paronychia, erysipelas, cellulitis, angular cheilitis), treatment of rosacea, perioral dermatitis, or acne.
● Drug isn't for ophthalmic use.
● Use cautiously in patients with peanut sensitivity.
● Use cautiously in pregnant or breast-feeding women.
⚠ *Overdose S&S:* Systemic effects.

NURSING CONSIDERATIONS
● If an occlusive dressing has been applied and a fever develops, notify prescriber and remove dressing.
● If antifungal or antibiotic combined with corticosteroid fails to provide prompt improvement, stop corticosteroid until infection is controlled.
● Systemic absorption is likely with use of occlusive dressings, prolonged treatment, or extensive body surface treatment. Watch for symptoms, such as hyperglycemia, glycosuria, HPA axis suppression, or Cushing syndrome.
● Avoid using plastic pants or tight-fitting diapers on treated areas in young children.

Children may absorb larger amounts of drug and be more susceptible to systemic toxicity.
🚫 *Alert:* Body oil and scalp oil formulations contain peanut oil.
● *Look alike–sound alike:* Don't confuse fluocinolone with fluocinonide or fluticasone.

PATIENT TEACHING
● Teach patient or family how to apply drug using gloves or sterile applicator.
● Tell patient to wash hands after application.
● If an occlusive dressing is used, advise patient to leave it in place for no longer than 12 hours each day and not to use dressing on infected or weeping lesions.
● Tell patient to stop using solution and notify prescriber if he develops signs of systemic absorption, skin irritation or ulceration, hypersensitivity, or infection.
● Advise patient using the shampoo not to bandage, cover, or wrap the treated scalp area unless directed.

---

fluocinonide
floo-oh-SIN-oh-nide

Lidex, Lidex-E, Vanos

Therapeutic class: Corticosteroids
Pharmacologic class: Corticosteroids
Pregnancy risk category: C

AVAILABLE FORMS
Cream: 0.05%, 0.1%
Gel: 0.05%
Ointment: 0.05%
Topical solution: 0.05%

INDICATIONS & DOSAGES
➤ **Inflammation from corticosteroid-responsive dermatoses**
Adults and children: Clean area; apply cream, gel, ointment, or topical solution sparingly b.i.d. to q.i.d. In children, use lowest dosage that promotes healing. If using Vanos 0.1% cream in adults and children age 12 and older, apply a thin layer once daily or b.i.d. for up to 2 weeks. Don't use more than 60 g/week.

ADMINISTRATION
Topical
• Gently wash skin before applying. To prevent skin damage, rub in gently, leaving a thin coat. When treating hairy sites, part hair and apply directly to lesion.
• Avoid applying near eyes or mucous membranes or in ear canal.
• Occlusive dressings may be used in severe or resistant dermatoses.
• For patients with eczematous dermatitis whose skin may be irritated by adhesive material, hold dressing in place with gauze, elastic bandages, stockings, or stockinette.
• Change dressing as prescribed. Stop drug and notify prescriber if skin infection, striae, or atrophy occur.
• Continue treatment for a few days after lesions clear.

ACTION
Unclear. Diffuses across cell membranes to form complexes with cytoplasmic receptors, showing anti-inflammatory, antipruritic, vasoconstrictive, and antiproliferative activity. Considered a high-potency drug, according to vasoconstrictive properties.

Route	Onset	Peak	Duration
Topical	Unknown	Unknown	Unknown

Half-life: Unknown.

ADVERSE REACTIONS
GU: glycosuria.
Metabolic: hyperglycemia.
Skin: burning, pruritus, irritation, dryness, erythema, folliculitis, hypertrichosis, hypopigmentation, acneiform eruptions, perioral dermatitis, allergic contact dermatitis, maceration, secondary infection, atrophy, striae, miliaria with occlusive dressings.
Other: *hypothalamic-pituitary-adrenal axis (HPA) suppression,* Cushing syndrome.

INTERACTIONS
None significant.

EFFECTS ON LAB TEST RESULTS
• May increase glucose level.

CONTRAINDICATIONS & CAUTIONS
• Contraindicated in patients hypersensitive to drug or its components.

• Don't use as monotherapy in primary bacterial infections (impetigo, paronychia, erysipelas, cellulitis, angular cheilitis), treatment of rosacea, perioral dermatitis, or acne.
• Don't use very-high-potency or high-potency agents on the face, groin, or armpits.
• Drug isn't for ophthalmic use.
• Use cautiously in pregnant or breast-feeding women.
⚠ Overdose S&S: Systemic effects.

NURSING CONSIDERATIONS
• If an occlusive dressing has been applied and a fever develops, notify prescriber and remove dressing.
• If antifungal or antibiotic combined with corticosteroid fails to provide prompt improvement, stop corticosteroid until infection is controlled.
• Systemic absorption is likely with use of occlusive dressings, prolonged treatment, or extensive body surface treatment. Watch for such symptoms as hyperglycemia, glycosuria, and HPA axis suppression.
• Avoid using plastic pants or tight-fitting diapers on treated areas in young children. Children may absorb larger amounts of drug and be more susceptible to systemic toxicity.
• *Look alike–sound alike:* Don't confuse fluocinonide with fluocinolone or fluticasone.

PATIENT TEACHING
• Teach patient and family how to apply drug using careful hand washing and gloves or sterile applicator.
• If an occlusive dressing is ordered, advise patient to leave it in place no more than 12 hours each day and not to use the dressing on infected or weeping lesions.
• Tell patient to stop drug and report signs of systemic absorption, skin irritation or ulceration, hypersensitivity, or infection.

fluorouracil (5-fluorouracil, 5-FU)

flure-oh-YOOR-a-sill

Carac, Efudex, Fluoroplex

Therapeutic class: Antineoplastics
Pharmacologic class: Pyrimidine analogues
Pregnancy risk category: D (injection); X (topical form)

AVAILABLE FORMS
Cream: 0.5%, 1%, 5%
Injection: 50 mg/mL
Topical solution: 2%, 5%

INDICATIONS & DOSAGES
➤ **Colon, rectal, breast, stomach, and pancreatic cancers**
Adults: Initially, 12 mg/kg I.V. daily for 4 days (daily dose shouldn't exceed 800 mg); if no toxicity, give 6 mg/kg on days 6, 8, 10, and 12; then give a single weekly maintenance dose of 10 to 15 mg/kg I.V. begun after toxicity (if any) from first course has subsided. (Recommended dosages are based on actual body weight unless patient is obese or retaining fluid.)
➤ **Multiple actinic (solar) keratoses**
Adults: Apply Carac cream once daily for up to 4 weeks. Or, apply Efudex or Fluoroplex cream or topical solution b.i.d. for 2 to 6 weeks.
➤ **Superficial basal cell carcinoma**
Adults: Apply 5% Efudex cream or topical solution b.i.d. usually for 3 to 6 weeks; maximum, 12 weeks.

ADMINISTRATION
I.V.
▼ Preparing and giving parenteral drug may be mutagenic, teratogenic, or carcinogenic. Follow facility policy to reduce risks.
▼ To reduce nausea, give antiemetic before 5-FU.
▼ Don't use cloudy solution. If crystals form, redissolve by warming.
▼ Drug may be given by direct injection without dilution.

▼ For infusion, dilute drug with D_5W, sterile water for injection, or normal saline solution for injection.
▼ For continuous infusion, use plastic I.V. containers. Solution is more stable in plastic than in glass bottles.
▼ Don't refrigerate. Protect drug from sunlight.
▼ Discard unused portion of vial after 1 hour.
▼ **Incompatibilities:** Aldesleukin, amphotericin B cholesteryl sulfate complex, carboplatin, cisplatin, cytarabine, diazepam, doxorubicin, droperidol, epirubicin, fentanyl citrate, filgrastim, gallium nitrate, leucovorin calcium, metoclopramide, morphine sulfate, ondansetron, topotecan, vinorelbine tartrate.

Topical
● Apply topical form cautiously near patient's eyes, nose, and mouth.
● Avoid occlusive dressings with topical form because they increase risk of inflammatory reactions in adjacent normal skin.
● Apply topical form with nonmetal applicator or suitable gloves. Wash hands immediately after handling topical form.
● The 1% topical strength is used on patient's face. Higher strengths, such as 5%, are used for thicker skinned areas or resistant lesions, such as superficial basal cell carcinoma.

ACTION
May interfere with DNA and RNA synthesis, leading to a thymine deficiency that provokes unbalanced growth and death of the cell.

Route	Onset	Peak	Duration
I.V., topical	Unknown	Unknown	Unknown

Half-life (I.V.): 16 minutes.

ADVERSE REACTIONS
CNS: acute cerebellar syndrome, confusion, disorientation, euphoria, ataxia, headache, weakness, malaise.
CV: *myocardial ischemia,* angina, thrombophlebitis.
EENT: epistaxis, photophobia, lacrimation, lacrimal duct stenosis, nystagmus, visual changes, eye irritation.

Reactions in bold italics are *life-threatening*. Interactions may have a *rapid onset* or a *delayed onset*.

GI: stomatitis, GI ulcer, nausea, vomiting, diarrhea, anorexia, *GI bleeding.*
Hematologic: *leukopenia, thrombocytopenia, agranulocytosis,* anemia.
Skin: dermatitis, erythema, scaling, pruritus, nail changes, pigmented palmar creases, erythematous contact dermatitis, desquamative rash of hands and feet, hand-foot syndrome with long-term use, photosensitivity reactions, reversible alopecia, pain, burning, soreness, suppuration, swelling, dryness, erosion with topical use.
Other: *anaphylaxis.*

INTERACTIONS
Drug-drug. *Leucovorin calcium:* May increase cytotoxicity and toxicity of fluorouracil. Monitor patient closely.
Live-virus vaccines: May increase risk of vaccine-induced adverse reactions. Concomitant use isn't recommended.
Drug-lifestyle. *Sun exposure:* May cause photosensitivity reactions. Advise patient to avoid excessive sunlight exposure.

EFFECTS ON LAB TEST RESULTS
● May increase alkaline phosphatase, AST, ALT, bilirubin, 5-hydroxyindoleacetic acid (in urine), and LDH levels. May decrease hemoglobin and plasma albumin levels.
● May decrease granulocyte, platelet, RBC, and WBC counts.

CONTRAINDICATIONS & CAUTIONS
● Contraindicated in patients hypersensitive to drug and in those with bone marrow suppression (WBC counts of 3,500/mm^3 or less or platelet counts of 100,000/mm^3 or less) or potentially serious infections.
● Contraindicated in patients in a poor nutritional state and those who have had major surgery within previous month.
● Topical formulations contraindicated in pregnant women.
🔴 **Alert:** Discontinue I.V. drug at first sign of stomatitis or esophagopharyngitis, WBC count less than 3,500/mm^3 or a rapidly falling WBC count, intractable vomiting, diarrhea, GI ulceration and bleeding, platelet count less than 100,000/mm^3 or hemorrhage from any site.
● Use cautiously in patients who have received high-dose pelvic radiation or

alkylating drugs and in those with impaired hepatic or renal function or widespread neoplastic infiltration of bone marrow.
⚠ **Overdose S&S:** Nausea, vomiting, diarrhea, GI ulceration and bleeding, bone marrow depression (thrombocytopenia, leukopenia, agranulocytosis).

NURSING CONSIDERATIONS
Black Box Warning I.V. drug should be administered under the supervision of a physician experienced in cancer chemotherapy. ∎
Black Box Warning Patient should be hospitalized at least during the initial course of I.V. drug therapy. ∎
● Ingestion and systemic absorption of topical form may cause leukopenia, thrombocytopenia, stomatitis, diarrhea, or GI ulceration, bleeding, and hemorrhage. Application to large ulcerated areas may cause systemic toxicity.
● Watch for stomatitis or diarrhea (signs of toxicity). Consider using topical oral anesthetic to soothe lesions. Stop drug and notify prescriber if diarrhea occurs.
● Encourage diligent oral hygiene to prevent superinfection of denuded mucosa.
● Monitor WBC and platelet counts. WBC counts with differential are recommended before each dose. Watch for ecchymoses, petechiae, easy bruising, and anemia.
● Monitor fluid intake and output, CBC, and renal and hepatic function tests.
● Long-term use may cause erythematous, desquamative rash of the hands and feet, which may be treated with pyridoxine 50 to 150 mg P.O. daily for 5 to 7 days.
● Dermatologic adverse effects are reversible when drug is stopped.
● To prevent bleeding, avoid I.M. injections when platelet count is below 50,000/mm^3.
● Anticipate blood transfusions because of cumulative anemia.
🔴 **Alert:** Toxicity may be delayed for 1 to 3 weeks.
● The WBC count nadir occurs 9 to 14 days after first dose; the platelet count nadir occurs in 7 to 14 days.
🔴 **Alert:** Drug may be ordered as "5-fluorouracil" or "5-FU." The numeral "5" is part of the drug name and shouldn't be confused with dosage units.

● *Look alike–sound alike:* Don't confuse fluorouracil with floxuridine, fludarabine, or flucytosine.

PATIENT TEACHING

● Warn patient that hair loss may occur but is reversible.

● Caution patient to avoid prolonged exposure to sunlight or ultraviolet light when topical form is used.

● Tell patient to use highly protective sunblock to avoid inflammatory skin irritation.

● Warn patient that topically treated area may be unsightly during therapy and for several weeks afterward. Complete healing may take 1 or 2 months.

● Caution women of childbearing age to consult prescriber before becoming pregnant.

● Advise women to stop breast-feeding during therapy because of risk of toxicity to infant.

fluoxetine hydrochloride
floo-OX-e-teen

Prozac✒, Prozac Weekly✒,
Sarafem✒

Therapeutic class: Antidepressants
Pharmacologic class: SSRIs
Pregnancy risk category: C

AVAILABLE FORMS

Capsules (delayed-release): 90 mg
Capsules (pulvules): 10 mg, 20 mg, 40 mg
Oral solution: 20 mg/5 mL
Tablets: 10 mg, 20 mg, 60 mg

INDICATIONS & DOSAGES

Adjust-a-dose (for all indications): For patients with renal or hepatic impairment and those taking several drugs at the same time, reduce dose or increase dosing interval.

➤ **Depression, obsessive-compulsive disorder (OCD) (excluding Sarafem)**
Adults: Initially, 20 mg P.O. in the morning; increase dosage based on patient response. Maximum daily dose is 80 mg.
Children ages 7 to 17 (OCD): 10 mg P.O. daily. After 2 weeks, increase to 20 mg daily. Dosage is 20 to 60 mg daily.

Children ages 8 to 18 (depression): 10 mg P.O. once daily for 1 week; then increase to 20 mg daily.

➤ **Maintenance therapy for depression (excluding Sarafem) in stabilized patients (not for newly diagnosed depression)**
Adults: 90 mg Prozac Weekly P.O. once weekly. Start once-weekly doses 7 days after the last daily dose of Prozac 20 mg.

➤ **Short-term and long-term treatment of bulimia nervosa (excluding Sarafem)**
Adults: 60 mg P.O. daily in the morning.

➤ **Short-term treatment of panic disorder with or without agoraphobia (excluding Sarafem)**
Adults: 10 mg P.O. once daily for 1 week; then increase dose as needed to 20 mg daily. Maximum daily dose is 60 mg.

➤ **Depressive episodes associated with bipolar I disorder (with olanzapine)**
Adults: 20 mg P.O. with 5 mg P.O. olanzapine once daily in the evening. Dosage adjustments can be made based on efficacy and tolerability within ranges of fluoxetine 20 to 50 mg and olanzapine 5 to 12.5 mg.

➤ **Treatment-resistant depression**
Adults: 20 mg P.O. with 5 mg P.O. olanzapine once daily in the evening. Dosage adjustments can be made based on efficacy and tolerability within ranges of fluoxetine 20 to 50 mg and olanzapine 5 to 20 mg.

➤ **Posttraumatic stress disorder (PTSD)** ◆
Adults, children, and adolescents: 10 to 20 mg P.O. daily. Evaluate response every 1 to 2 weeks. Average target daily dose is 20 to 50 mg (20 mg in older adults). Maximum target dose is 80 mg/day. Recommended therapy duration is 6 to 12 months for acute PTSD, 12 to 24 months for chronic PTSD with excellent response, and at least 24 months for chronic PTSD with residual symptoms. Tapering dosage over 2 weeks to 1 month is recommended.

➤ **Premenstrual dysphoric disorder**
Adults: 20 mg Sarafem P.O. daily continuously (every day of the menstrual cycle) or intermittently (daily dose starting 14 days before the anticipated onset of menstruation through the first full day of menses and repeating with each new cycle). Maximum daily dose is 80 mg P.O.

Reactions in bold italics are *life-threatening*. Interactions may have a *rapid onset* or a *delayed onset*.

> **Raynaud phenomenon** ◆
Adults: 20 to 60 mg P.O. daily.
> **Borderline personality disorder** ◆
Adults: 20 to 80 mg P.O. daily. A reasonable trial period for treatment is at least 12 weeks.
> **Irritable bowel syndrome** ◆
Adults: 10 to 20 mg P.O. daily after failure of laxatives, loperamide, or antispasmodics. May be used as maintenance therapy for 6 to 12 months.

ADMINISTRATION
P.O.
● Give drug without regard for food.
● Avoid giving drug in the afternoon, whenever possible, because doing so commonly causes nervousness and insomnia.
● Delayed-release capsules must be swallowed whole; don't crush or open.

ACTION
Thought to be linked to drug's inhibition of CNS neuronal uptake of serotonin.

Route	Onset	Peak	Duration
P.O.	Unknown	6–8 hr	Unknown

Half-life: Acute administration, 2 to 3 days; long-term administration, 4 to 6 days.

ADVERSE REACTIONS
CNS: nervousness, somnolence, anxiety, insomnia, headache, drowsiness, tremor, dizziness, asthenia, *suicidal behavior,* fatigue, fever.
CV: palpitations, hot flashes.
EENT: nasal congestion, pharyngitis, sinusitis.
GI: nausea, diarrhea, dry mouth, anorexia, dyspepsia, constipation, abdominal pain, vomiting, flatulence, increased appetite.
GU: sexual dysfunction.
Metabolic: weight loss, hyponatremia.
Musculoskeletal: muscle pain.
Respiratory: upper respiratory tract infection, cough, *respiratory distress.*
Skin: rash, pruritus, diaphoresis.
Other: flulike syndrome.

INTERACTIONS
Drug-drug. *Amphetamines, buspirone, dextromethorphan, dihydroergotamine, lithium salts, meperidine, other SSRIs or SSNRIs (duloxetine, venlafaxine), TCAs,* **tramadol,**

trazodone, tryptophan: May increase the risk of serotonin syndrome. Avoid combinations of drugs that increase the availability of serotonin in the CNS; monitor patient closely if used together.
Aspirin, NSAIDs: May increase risk of GI bleeding. Use together cautiously.
Benzodiazepines, lithium, TCAs: May increase CNS effects. Monitor patient closely.
Beta blockers, carbamazepine, flecainide, vinblastine: May increase levels of these drugs. Monitor drug levels and monitor patient for adverse reactions.
Cyclosporine: May increase renal toxicity of cyclosporine. Monitor patient carefully for cyclosporine toxicity.
Cyproheptadine: May reverse or decrease fluoxetine effect. Monitor patient closely.
Dextromethorphan: May cause unusual side effects such as visual hallucinations. Advise use of cough suppressant that doesn't contain dextromethorphan while taking fluoxetine.
Highly protein-bound drugs: May increase level of fluoxetine or other highly protein-bound drugs. Monitor patient closely.
Insulin, oral antidiabetics: May alter glucose level and antidiabetic requirements. Adjust dosage.
Linezolid, methylene blue: May cause serotonin syndrome. Use extreme caution and monitor closely.
MAO inhibitors (phenelzine, selegiline, tranylcypromine): May cause serotonin syndrome and signs and symptoms resembling neuroleptic malignant syndrome. Avoid using at the same time and for at least 5 weeks after stopping.
Phenytoin: May increase phenytoin level and risk of toxicity. Monitor phenytoin level and adjust dosage.
Pimozide, thioridazine: May increase levels of these drugs, increasing risk of serious ventricular arrhythmias and sudden death. Avoid using at the same time and for at least 5 weeks after stopping.
Tamoxifen: May decrease tamoxifen plasma level, leading to breast cancer recurrence. Monitor patient carefully.
Triptans: May cause weakness, hyperreflexia, incoordination, rapid changes in blood pressure, nausea, and diarrhea. Monitor patient closely, especially at

F

the start of treatment and when dosage increases.

Warfarin: May increase risk for bleeding. Monitor PT and INR.

Drug-herb. *St. John's wort:* May increase sedative and hypnotic effects; may cause serotonin syndrome. Discourage use together.

Drug-lifestyle. *Alcohol use:* May increase CNS depression. Discourage use together.

EFFECTS ON LAB TEST RESULTS
● May decrease sodium level.

CONTRAINDICATIONS & CAUTIONS
● Contraindicated in patients hypersensitive to drug and within 14 days of stopping an MAO inhibitor intended to treat psychiatric disorders. MAO inhibitors shouldn't be started within 5 weeks of stopping fluoxetine. Avoid using thioridazine with fluoxetine or within 5 weeks after stopping fluoxetine.

۞ Alert: Concomitant use with linezolid or methylene blue can cause serotonin syndrome (fever, mental status changes, muscle twitching, excessive sweating, shivering or shaking, diarrhea, loss of coordination). Use drug with linezolid or methylene blue only for life-threatening or urgent conditions when the potential benefits outweigh the risks of toxicity.

● Use cautiously in patients at high risk for suicide and in those with history of diabetes mellitus, seizures, mania, or hepatic, renal, or CV disease.

● Use in third trimester of pregnancy may be associated with neonatal complications at birth. Consider the risk versus benefit of treatment during this time.

Black Box Warning Fluoxetine is approved for use in children with major depressive disorder and OCD. Fluoxetine isn't approved for use in children younger than age 7. Sarafem isn't approved for use in children. ▌

⚠ Overdose S&S: Nausea, seizures, somnolence, tachycardia, vomiting, coma, delirium, ECG abnormalities, hypotension, mania, neuroleptic malignant syndrome–like reactions, pyrexia, stupor, syncope.

NURSING CONSIDERATIONS
۞ Alert: If linezolid or methylene blue must be given, fluoxetine must be stopped and the patient monitored for serotonin toxicity for 5 weeks or until 24 hours after the last dose of linezolid or methylene blue, whichever comes first. Treatment with fluoxetine may be resumed 24 hours after the last dose of linezolid or methylene blue.

● Use antihistamines or topical corticosteroids to treat rashes or pruritus.

● Watch for weight change during therapy, particularly in underweight or bulimic patients.

● Record mood changes. Watch for suicidal tendencies.

Black Box Warning Drug may increase the risk of suicidal thinking and behavior in children, adolescents, and young adults with major depressive disorder or other psychiatric disorder. ▌

● Drug has a long half-life; monitor patient for adverse effects for up to 2 weeks after drug is stopped.

۞ Alert: Combining triptans with an SSRI or an SSNRI may cause serotonin syndrome or neuroleptic malignant syndrome–like reactions. Serotonin syndrome may be more likely to occur when starting or increasing the dose of triptan, SSRI, or SSNRI.

● When discontinuing drug, taper dosage over 2 weeks to 1 month to avoid withdrawal syndrome.

● *Look alike–sound alike:* Don't confuse fluoxetine with fluvoxamine or fluvastatin. Don't confuse Prozac with Proscar, Prilosec, or ProSom.

PATIENT TEACHING
۞ Alert: Teach patient to recognize and immediately report symptoms of serotonin toxicity (fever, mental status changes, muscle twitching, excessive sweating, shivering or shaking, diarrhea, loss of coordination).

● Tell patient to avoid taking drug in the afternoon whenever possible because doing so commonly causes nervousness and insomnia.

● Drug may cause dizziness or drowsiness. Warn patient to avoid driving and other hazardous activities that require alertness and good psychomotor coordination until effects of drug are known.

Reactions in bold italics are *life-threatening*. Interactions may have a *rapid onset* or a *delayed onset*.

• Tell patient to consult prescriber before taking other prescription or OTC drugs.
• Advise patient that full therapeutic effect may not be seen for 4 weeks or longer.
Black Box Warning Advise families and caregivers to carefully observe patient for worsening suicidal thinking or behavior. ∎

fluphenazine decanoate
floo-FEN-a-zeen

Modecate†, Modecate Concentrate†

fluphenazine hydrochloride

Therapeutic class: Antipsychotics
Pharmacologic class: Phenothiazines
Pregnancy risk category: C

AVAILABLE FORMS
fluphenazine decanoate
Depot injection: 25 mg/mL*, 100 mg/mL†
fluphenazine hydrochloride
Elixir: 2.5 mg/5 mL*
I.M. injection: 2.5 mg/mL
Oral concentrate: 5 mg/mL*
Tablets: 1 mg, 2.5 mg, 5 mg, 10 mg

INDICATIONS & DOSAGES
➤ **Psychotic disorders**
Adults: Initially, 2.5 to 10 mg fluphenazine hydrochloride P.O. daily in divided doses every 6 to 8 hours; may increase cautiously to 20 mg. Maximum daily dose is 40 mg. Maintenance dose is 1 to 5 mg P.O. daily. I.M. doses are one-third to one-half of P.O. doses. Usual I.M. dose is 1.25 mg. Give more than 10 mg daily with caution.
  Or, 12.5 to 25 mg of fluphenazine decanoate I.M. or subcutaneously every 1 to 6 weeks; maintenance dose is 25 to 100 mg, as needed.
Elderly patients: 1 to 2.5 mg fluphenazine hydrochloride P.O. daily.

ADMINISTRATION
P.O.
• Oral liquid forms can cause contact dermatitis. Wear gloves when preparing solutions, and avoid contact with skin and clothing.

• Protect drug from light. Slight yellowing of concentrate is common and doesn't affect potency. Discard markedly discolored solutions.
• Dilute liquid concentrate with water, fruit juice, milk, or semisolid food just before administration.
I.M.
• Parenteral forms can cause contact dermatitis. Wear gloves when preparing solutions, and avoid contact with skin and clothing.
• Protect drug from light. Slight yellowing of injection is common and doesn't affect potency. Discard markedly discolored solutions.
• For long-acting form (decanoate), which is an oil preparation, use a dry needle of at least 21G.
Subcutaneous
• Long-acting form (decanoate) is indicated for subcutaneous administration.
• Use a dry syringe and needle of at least 21G.
• Don't use if solution is cloudy or contains particulate matter.

ACTION
A piperazine phenothiazine that probably blocks postsynaptic dopamine receptors in the brain.

Route	Onset	Peak	Duration
P.O.	<1 hr	30 min	6–8 hr
I.M. (decanoate)	24–72 hr	Unknown	1–6 wk
I.M. (hydrochloride)	<1 hr	90–120 min	6–8 hr
Subcut.	Unknown	Unknown	Unknown

Half-life: Hydrochloride, 15 hours; decanoate, 7 to 10 days.

ADVERSE REACTIONS
CNS: extrapyramidal reactions, tardive dyskinesia, pseudoparkinsonism, *seizures, neuroleptic malignant syndrome,* sedation, EEG changes, drowsiness, dizziness.
CV: orthostatic hypotension, tachycardia, ECG changes.
EENT: blurred vision, ocular changes, nasal congestion.
GI: dry mouth, constipation, increased appetite.

GU: urine retention, dark urine, menstrual irregularities, inhibited ejaculation.
Hematologic: *leukopenia, agranulocytosis, aplastic anemia, thrombocytopenia,* eosinophilia, hemolytic anemia.
Hepatic: cholestatic jaundice.
Metabolic: weight gain.
Skin: mild photosensitivity reactions, allergic reactions.
Other: gynecomastia, galactorrhea.

INTERACTIONS
Drug-drug. *Antacids:* May inhibit absorption of oral phenothiazines. Separate antacid and phenothiazine doses by at least 2 hours.
Anticholinergics: May increase anticholinergic effects. Use together cautiously.
Barbiturates, lithium: May decrease phenothiazine effect and increase neurologic adverse effects. Monitor patient.
Centrally acting antihypertensives: May decrease antihypertensive effect. Monitor blood pressure.
CNS depressants: May increase CNS depression. Use together cautiously.
Drug-herb. *St. John's wort:* May increase risk of photosensitivity reactions. Advise patient to avoid excessive sunlight exposure.
Drug-lifestyle. *Alcohol use:* May increase CNS depression, especially that involving psychomotor skills. Strongly discourage alcohol use.
Sun exposure: May increase risk of photosensitivity reactions. Advise patient to avoid excessive sunlight exposure.

EFFECTS ON LAB TEST RESULTS
● May increase LFT values. May decrease hemoglobin level and hematocrit.
● May increase eosinophil count. May decrease granulocyte, platelet, and WBC counts.
● May cause false-positive results for amylase, 5-hydroxyindoleacetic acid, urinary porphyrin, and urobilinogen tests and for urine pregnancy tests that use human chorionic gonadotropin.

CONTRAINDICATIONS & CAUTIONS
● Contraindicated in patients hypersensitive to drug and in those with coma, CNS depression, bone marrow suppression or other blood dyscrasia, subcortical damage, or liver damage.
● Use cautiously in elderly or debilitated patients and in those with pheochromocytoma, severe CV disease (may cause sudden drop in blood pressure), peptic ulcer, respiratory disorder, hypocalcemia, seizure disorder (may lower seizure threshold), severe reactions to insulin or electroconvulsive therapy, mitral insufficiency, glaucoma, or prostatic hyperplasia.
❸ Alert: Neonates exposed to antipsychotic drug during the third trimester of pregnancy are at risk for developing extrapyramidal signs and symptoms (repetitive muscle movements of the face and body) and withdrawal symptoms (agitation, abnormally increased or decreased muscle tone, tremors, sleepiness, severe difficulty breathing, difficulty feeding) following delivery. Use in pregnancy only if the potential benefit to the mother justifies the risk to the fetus.
● Use cautiously in those exposed to extreme heat or cold (including antipyretic therapy) or phosphorus insecticides.
● Use parenteral form cautiously in patients who have asthma or are allergic to sulfites.
⚠ Overdose S&S: Stupor, coma, seizures in children.

NURSING CONSIDERATIONS
● Monitor patient for tardive dyskinesia, which may occur after prolonged use. It may not appear until months or years later and may disappear spontaneously or persist for life, despite ending drug.
❸ Alert: Watch for signs and symptoms of neuroleptic malignant syndrome (extrapyramidal effects, hyperthermia, autonomic disturbance), which is rare but often fatal. It may not be related to length of drug use or type of neuroleptic; more than 60% of affected patients are men.
● Withhold dose and notify prescriber if patient, especially child or pregnant woman, develops signs or symptoms of blood dyscrasia (fever, sore throat, infection, cellulitis, weakness) or extrapyramidal reactions persisting longer than a few hours.
Black Box Warning Elderly patients with dementia-related psychosis treated with atypical or conventional antipsychotics are at increased risk for death. Antipsychotics

aren't approved for the treatment of dementia-related psychosis. ∎

• Don't withdraw drug abruptly unless serious adverse reactions occur.

• Abrupt withdrawal of long-term therapy may cause gastritis, nausea, vomiting, dizziness, tremor, feeling of warmth or cold, diaphoresis, tachycardia, headache, or insomnia.

PATIENT TEACHING

• Warn patient to avoid activities that require alertness and good coordination until effects of drug are known. Drowsiness and dizziness usually subside after first few weeks.

• Warn patient to avoid alcohol while taking drug.

• Tell patient to relieve dry mouth with sugarless gum or hard candy.

• Have patient report signs of urine retention or constipation.

• Advise patient to use sunblock and wear protective clothing to avoid sensitivity to the sun.

• Tell patient that drug may discolor urine.

SAFETY ALERT!

flutamide
FLOO-ta-mide

Euflex†

Therapeutic class: Antineoplastics
Pharmacologic class: Nonsteroidal antiandrogens
Pregnancy risk category: D

AVAILABLE FORMS
Capsules: 125 mg, 250 mg†

INDICATIONS & DOSAGES
➤ **Metastatic locally confined prostate cancer (stages B_2, C, D_2), combined with luteinizing hormone–releasing hormone analogues such as leuprolide acetate or goserelin**
Men: 250 mg P.O. every 8 hours.
➤ **Hirsutism in women with polycystic ovary syndrome** ◆
Women: 125 to 500 mg P.O. daily in one or two divided doses.

ADMINISTRATION
P.O.
• Drug is a hormonal agent and considered a potential teratogen. Follow safe handling procedures.
• Give drug with a full glass of water.
• Give drug without regard for food.

ACTION
Inhibits androgen uptake or prevents binding of androgens in nucleus of cells in target tissues.

Route	Onset	Peak	Duration
P.O.	Unknown	2 hr	Unknown

Half-life: For steady-state metabolite, about 8 hours.

ADVERSE REACTIONS
CNS: drowsiness, confusion, depression, anxiety, nervousness, paresthesia.
CV: peripheral edema, hypertension, hot flashes.
GI: diarrhea, nausea, vomiting, anorexia.
GU: erectile dysfunction, urine discoloration.
Hematologic: anemia, *leukopenia, thrombocytopenia,* hemolytic anemia.
Hepatic: *hepatic encephalopathy, liver failure.*
Skin: rash, photosensitivity reactions.
Other: loss of libido, gynecomastia.

INTERACTIONS
Drug-drug. *Warfarin:* May increase PT. Monitor PT and INR.
Drug-lifestyle. *Sun exposure:* May cause photosensitivity reactions. Advise patient to avoid excessive sunlight exposure.

EFFECTS ON LAB TEST RESULTS
• May increase BUN, creatinine, hemoglobin, and liver enzyme levels.
• May decrease platelet and WBC counts.
• May alter pituitary-gonadal system tests during therapy and for 12 weeks after.

CONTRAINDICATIONS & CAUTIONS
• Contraindicated in patients hypersensitive to drug and in those with severe liver dysfunction.
⚠ ***Overdose S&S:*** Gynecomastia, breast tenderness, increased AST level.

NURSING CONSIDERATIONS

Black Box Warning Drug may cause liver failure. Obtain LFTs before the start of therapy, monthly for the first 4 months of therapy, periodically thereafter, and at the first signs and symptoms suggesting liver dysfunction (nausea, vomiting, anorexia, fatigue). Immediately stop drug if jaundice occurs or AST level rises above 2 times upper limit of normal. ∎

• Monitor CBC periodically.

• Flutamide must be taken continuously with drug used for medical castration (such as leuprolide) to allow full therapeutic benefit. Leuprolide suppresses testosterone production, whereas flutamide inhibits testosterone action at cellular level; together, they can impair growth of androgen-responsive tumors.

PATIENT TEACHING

• Advise patient not to stop drug without consulting prescriber.

• Tell patient to take drug with a full glass of water.

• Tell patient drug may be taken without food, but if stomach irritation occurs, to take with food.

• Instruct patient to report adverse reactions promptly, especially dark yellow or brown urine, vomiting, or yellowing of the eyes or skin.

fluticasone furoate
floo-TIK-a-sone

Veramyst

fluticasone propionate
Flonase, Flovent Diskus, Flovent HFA

Therapeutic class: Corticosteroids
Pharmacologic class: Corticosteroids
Pregnancy risk category: C

AVAILABLE FORMS

Nasal spray (furoate): 27.5 mcg/spray
Nasal spray (propionate): 50 mcg/metered spray
Oral inhalation aerosol: 44 mcg, 110 mcg, 220 mcg

Oral inhalation powder: 50 mcg, 100 mcg, 250 mcg

INDICATIONS & DOSAGES

➤ **As preventative in maintenance of chronic asthma in patients requiring oral corticosteroid**

Flovent Diskus

Adults and children age 12 and older: In patients previously taking bronchodilators alone, initially, inhaled dose of 100 mcg b.i.d. to maximum of 500 mcg b.i.d.

Adults and children age 12 and older previously taking inhaled corticosteroids: Initially, inhaled dose of 100 to 250 mcg b.i.d. to maximum of 500 mcg b.i.d.

Adults and children age 12 and older previously taking oral corticosteroids: Inhaled dose of 500 to 1,000 mcg b.i.d. Maximum dose, 1,000 mcg b.i.d.

Children ages 4 to 11: For patients previously on bronchodilators alone or on inhaled corticosteroids, initially, inhaled dose of 50 mcg b.i.d. to maximum of 100 mcg b.i.d.

Flovent HFA

Adults and children age 12 and older: In those previously taking bronchodilators alone, initially, inhaled dose of 88 mcg b.i.d. to maximum of 440 mcg b.i.d.

Adults and children age 12 and older previously taking inhaled corticosteroids: Initially, inhaled dose of 88 to 220 mcg b.i.d. to maximum of 440 mcg b.i.d.

Adults and children age 12 and older previously taking oral corticosteroids: Initially, inhaled dose of 440 mcg b.i.d. to maximum of 880 mcg b.i.d.

Children ages 4 to 11: 88 mcg inhaled b.i.d. regardless of prior therapy.

➤ **Nasal symptoms of seasonal and perennial allergic and nonallergic rhinitis**

Flonase

Adults: Initially, 2 sprays (100 mcg) in each nostril daily or 1 spray b.i.d. Once symptoms are controlled, decrease to 1 spray in each nostril daily. Or, for seasonal allergic rhinitis, 2 sprays in each nostril once daily, as needed, for symptom control.

Adolescents and children age 4 and older: Initially, 1 spray (50 mcg) in each nostril daily. If not responding, increase to 2 sprays in each nostril daily. Once symptoms are controlled, decrease to 1 spray in each nostril daily. Maximum dose is 2 sprays in each nostril daily.

Veramyst
Adults and children age 12 and older:
110 mcg once daily administered as 2 sprays (27.5 mcg/spray) in each nostril.
Children ages 2 to 11: 55 mcg once daily administered as 1 spray (27.5 mcg/spray) in each nostril.

ADMINISTRATION
Inhalational
• For best results, aerosol canister should be at room temperature.
• Prime and shake well before each use.
• Patients should rinse mouth after inhalation.
Intranasal
• Prime and shake well before use.

ACTION
Anti-inflammatory and vasoconstrictor that may decrease inflammation by inhibiting mast cells, macrophages, and mediators such as leukotrienes.

Route	Onset	Peak	Duration
Inhalation (nasal)	12 hr	Several days	1–2 wk
Inhalation (oral)	24 hr	Several days	1–2 wk

Half-life: 3 hours.

ADVERSE REACTIONS
CNS: headache, dizziness, fever, migraine, nervousness.
EENT: pharyngitis, blood in nasal mucus, cataracts, conjunctivitis, dry eye, dysphonia, epistaxis, eye irritation, hoarseness, laryngitis, nasal burning or irritation, nasal discharge, rhinitis, sinusitis.
GI: oral candidiasis, abdominal discomfort, abdominal pain, diarrhea, mouth irritation, nausea, viral gastroenteritis, vomiting.
GU: UTI.
Hematologic: eosinophilia.
Metabolic: cushingoid features, growth retardation in children, hyperglycemia, weight gain.
Musculoskeletal: aches and pains, disorder or symptoms of neck sprain or strain, joint pain, muscular soreness, osteoporosis.

Respiratory: upper respiratory tract infection, *bronchospasm,* asthma symptoms, bronchitis, chest congestion, cough, dyspnea.
Skin: dermatitis, urticaria.
Other: *angioedema,* influenza, viral infections.

INTERACTIONS
Drug-drug. *Ketoconazole and other CYP3A4 inhibitors:* May increase mean fluticasone level. Use together cautiously.
Ritonavir: May cause systemic corticosteroid effects, such as Cushing syndrome and adrenal suppression. Avoid using together.

EFFECTS ON LAB TEST RESULTS
• Abnormal response to the 6-hour cosyntropin stimulation test may occur in patients taking high doses of fluticasone.

CONTRAINDICATIONS & CAUTIONS
• Contraindicated in patients hypersensitive to ingredients in these preparations.
• Contraindicated as primary treatment of patients with status asthmaticus or other acute, intense episodes of asthma.
• Use cautiously in breast-feeding women.
⚠ *Overdose S&S:* Hypercorticism.

NURSING CONSIDERATIONS
• Because of risk of systemic absorption of inhaled corticosteroids, observe patient carefully for evidence of systemic corticosteroid effects.
❸ *Alert:* Monitor patient, especially postoperatively, during periods of stress or severe asthma attack for evidence of inadequate adrenal response.
❸ *Alert:* During withdrawal from oral corticosteroids, some patients may experience signs and symptoms of systemically active corticosteroid withdrawal, such as joint or muscle pain, lassitude, and depression, despite maintenance or even improvement of respiratory function. Deaths due to adrenal insufficiency have occurred with transfer from active corticosteroids to fluticasone propionate inhaler.
• For patients starting therapy who are currently receiving oral corticosteroid therapy, reduce dose of prednisone to no more than 2.5 mg/day on a weekly basis, beginning

after at least 1 week of therapy with fluticasone.

🔸 **Alert:** As with other inhaled asthma drugs, bronchospasm may occur with an immediate increase in wheezing after a dose. If bronchospasm occurs after a dose of inhalation aerosol, treat immediately with a fast-acting inhaled bronchodilator.

PATIENT TEACHING

• Tell patient that drug isn't indicated for the relief of acute bronchospasm.

• For proper use of drug and to attain maximal improvement, tell patient to carefully follow the accompanying patient instructions.

• Advise patient to use drug at regular intervals, as directed.

• Instruct patient to contact prescriber if nasal spray doesn't improve condition after 4 days of treatment.

• Instruct patient to immediately contact prescriber if asthma episodes unresponsive to bronchodilators occur during treatment with fluticasone. During such episodes, patient may need therapy with oral corticosteroids.

• Warn patient to avoid exposure to chickenpox or measles and, if exposed, to consult prescriber immediately.

• Tell patient to carry or wear medical identification indicating that he may need supplementary corticosteroids during stress or a severe asthma attack.

🔸 **Alert:** During periods of stress or a severe asthma attack, instruct patient who has been withdrawn from systemic corticosteroids to resume prescribed oral corticosteroids immediately and to contact prescriber for further instruction.

• Tell patient to prime inhaler with 4 test sprays (away from his face) before first use, shaking well before each spray. Also, prime with 1 spray if inhaler has been dropped or has not been used for 1 week or longer.

• Advise patient to avoid spraying inhalation aerosol into eyes.

• Instruct patient to shake canister well before using inhalation aerosol.

• Instruct patient to rinse his mouth and spit water out after inhalation.

• Advise patient to store fluticasone powder in a dry place.

Flonase nasal spray

• Tell patient to prime the nasal inhaler before first use or after 1 week or longer of nonuse.

• Have patient clear nasal passages before use.

• Advise patient to follow manufacturer's recommendations for use and cleaning.

• Advise patient to use at regular intervals for full benefit.

• Tell patient to contact provider if signs or symptoms don't improve within 4 days or if signs or symptoms worsen.

• Tell patient that the correct amount of spray can't be guaranteed after 120 sprays, even though the bottle may not be completely empty.

✱ NEW DRUG

fluticasone furoate–vilanterol trifenatate
floo-TIK-a-sone–vye-LAN-ter-ol

Breo Ellipta

Therapeutic class: Corticosteroids–bronchodilators
Pharmacologic class: Corticosteroids–beta-2 adrenergic agonists
Pregnancy risk category: C

AVAILABLE FORMS
Powder for inhalation: Inhaler containing two double-foil blister strips of powder formulation; one strip contains fluticasone furoate 100 mcg/blister and the other contains vilanterol 25 mcg/blister

INDICATIONS & DOSAGES
➤ **Long-term, once-daily maintenance treatment of airflow obstruction; reducing exacerbations in patients with COPD**
Adults: 1 inhalation of 100 mcg fluticasone furoate–25 mcg vilanterol trifenatate once daily.

ADMINISTRATION
Inhalational

• After use, have patient rinse mouth with water without swallowing to help reduce the risk of oropharyngeal candidiasis.

• Give at the same time every day and not more than one time every 24 hours.

- Store at room temperature between 68° F and 77° F (20° C and 25° C).
- Keep drug stored inside the unopened moisture-protective foil tray; remove from tray immediately before initial use.
- Discard drug 6 weeks after opening foil tray or when the counter reads "0" (after all blisters have been used).
- Inhaler isn't reusable.
- Don't attempt to take the inhaler apart.

ACTION

Fluticasone furoate: Exact mechanism unknown. Anti-inflammatory and vasoconstrictor that may decrease inflammation by inhibiting mast cells, macrophages, and mediators such as leukotrienes. Vilanterol trifenatate: Relaxes bronchial smooth muscle and inhibits inflammatory mediators, especially mast cells.

Route	Onset	Peak	Duration
Inhalation (fluticasone)	Unknown	30–60 min	Unknown
Inhalation (vilanterol)	Unknown	10 min	Unknown

Half-life: Fluticasone, 24 hours; vilanterol, 21 hours.

ADVERSE REACTIONS

CNS: headache, pyrexia.
CV: hypertension, peripheral edema.
EENT: nasopharyngitis, oropharyngeal candidiasis, oropharyngeal pain, pharyngitis.
GI: diarrhea.
Musculoskeletal: back pain, arthralgia.
Respiratory: upper respiratory tract infection, COPD, pneumonia, bronchitis, sinusitis, cough.
Other: flulike symptoms.

INTERACTIONS

Drug-drug. *CYP3A4 inhibitors (clarithromycin, conivaptan, indinavir, itraconazole, ketoconazole, lopinavir, nefazodone, nelfinavir, ritonavir, saquinavir, telithromycin, troleandomycin, voriconazole):* May increase systemic effects of corticosteroids and increased CV adverse effects may occur. Use together cautiously.
Loop or thiazide diuretics (furosemide, hydrochlorothiazide, torsemide): May increase risk of hypokalemia or ECG changes.

Monitor patient closely with concurrent use.
MAO inhibitors, TCAs, other drugs known to prolong QTc interval: May increase adrenergic effects or risk of ventricular arrhythmias. Don't use together or within 2 weeks of discontinuation.
Nonselective beta blockers (carvedilol, propranolol, sotalol): May increase risk of bronchospasm. Use cardioselective agents only if absolutely needed.
Other long-acting beta-agonist drugs (arformoterol tartrate, formoterol fumarate, indacaterol, salmeterol): May increase risk of overdose. Don't use together.

EFFECTS ON LAB TEST RESULTS

- May increase glucose level. May decrease potassium level.

CONTRAINDICATIONS & CAUTIONS

- Contraindicated in patients with severe hypersensitivity to milk proteins and in those who have demonstrated hypersensitivity to fluticasone furoate, vilanterol, or their components.

Black Box Warning Long-acting beta-2 adrenergic agonists such as vilanterol increase risk of asthma-related death. Safety and efficacy of vilanterol in patients with asthma haven't been established; vilanterol isn't indicated for the treatment of asthma. ■

- Contraindicated in patients with acute bronchospasm, asthma, and acutely deteriorating COPD.

🕒 Alert: Don't exceed recommended dosage; serious adverse events, including fatalities, have been associated with excessive use of inhaled sympathomimetics.

- Use cautiously in patients with existing tuberculosis; fungal, bacterial, viral, or parasitic infections; or ocular herpes simplex. Drug may suppress the immune system and infection may worsen.
- Use cautiously in patients with thyrotoxicosis, diabetes mellitus, ketoacidosis, or CV disorders (coronary insufficiency, arrhythmias, hypertension).
- Use cautiously in patients with increased intraocular pressure (IOP), cataracts, or glaucoma. Increased IOP, glaucoma, and cataracts have occurred with prolonged use.

• Use cautiously in patients with seizure disorders; beta agonists may cause CNS stimulation.

• Use cautiously in pregnant women and only if benefit outweighs risk to fetus.

• Use cautiously in breast-feeding women; drug hasn't been studied in this population.

NURSING CONSIDERATIONS

• If not already prescribed, initiate an inhaled, short-acting beta-2 agonist in patients taking this drug.

• Patients who have been taking oral or inhaled short-acting beta-2 agonists on a regular basis (four times a day) should discontinue regular use of these drugs and use them only for relief of acute respiratory symptoms.

• Monitor short-acting beta-2 agonist rescue use. Increased use signals disease deterioration.

• Slowly wean patients requiring oral corticosteroids from systemic corticosteroid use after switch to an inhaler. Reduce daily prednisone dosage by 2.5 mg on a weekly basis during therapy with inhaled drug.

• Patients may require supplemental corticosteroid during times of stress when weaning from systemic corticosteroids.

• Monitor lung function and watch for COPD signs and symptoms and adrenal insufficiency (fatigue, lassitude, weakness, nausea, vomiting, hypotension).

• Discontinue drug slowly if hypercortisolism or adrenal suppression is suspected.

• Monitor patient periodically for candidal infections of the mouth. Have patient rinse mouth after inhalation without swallowing to help reduce the risk.

• Monitor patient for signs and symptoms of pneumonia.

• If paradoxical bronchospasm occurs, discontinue drug and institute alternative therapy.

• Monitor patient for increased IOP and for development or worsening of glaucoma or cataracts.

• Monitor patient for hypokalemia and hyperglycemia.

• Serious or even fatal courses of chickenpox or measles can occur in susceptible patients.

• Monitor patient for CV effects (tachycardia, hypertension, supraventricular tachycardia, extrasystoles).

• Monitor patient for reduction in bone mineral density (BMD) initially and periodically with long-term use. Patients who use tobacco and those with prolonged immobilization, family history of osteoporosis, postmenopausal status, advanced age, poor nutrition, or long-term use of other drugs that can reduce BMD (anticonvulsants, oral corticosteroids) are at increased risk.

PATIENT TEACHING

• Teach patient to rinse mouth without swallowing after inhalation to help reduce the risk of candidal infections.

• Caution patient not to use drug for acute symptoms or asthma.

• Warn patient not to use drug with other long-acting beta-2 agonists.

• Instruct patient to immediately notify health care provider if symptoms worsen, more inhalations than usual of rescue medication are needed, or a significant decrease in lung function occurs.

• Instruct patient not to discontinue drug without the guidance of health care provider.

• Advise patient to obtain regular eye examinations.

• Caution female patient to report pregnancy to health care provider as soon as possible.

fluticasone propionate (topical)
floo-TIK-a-sone

Cutivate

Therapeutic class: Corticosteroids
Pharmacologic class: Corticosteroids
Pregnancy risk category: C

AVAILABLE FORMS
Cream: 0.05%
Lotion: 0.05%
Ointment: 0.005%

INDICATIONS & DOSAGES

➤ **Inflammation and pruritus from dermatoses responsive to corticosteroids**
Adults: Apply sparingly to affected area b.i.d.; rub in gently and completely.
Children age 3 months and older: Apply a thin film of cream (0.05%) to affected areas b.i.d. Rub in gently. Don't use for longer than 4 weeks. If using lotion (0.05%) in adults and children age 1 year and older, apply once daily.

➤ **Inflammation and pruritus from atopic dermatitis**
Children age 3 months and older: Apply thin film (0.05%) to affected areas once daily or b.i.d. Rub in gently. Don't use for longer than 4 weeks.

ADMINISTRATION
Topical
• Don't use drug with an occlusive dressing or in diaper area.

ACTION
Unclear. Is diffused across cell membranes to form complexes with cytoplasmic receptors. Shows anti-inflammatory, antipruritic, vasoconstrictive, and antiproliferative activity. Considered a medium-potency drug, according to vasoconstrictive properties.

Route	Onset	Peak	Duration
Topical	Rapid	Unknown	10 hr

Half-life: About 7½ hours.

ADVERSE REACTIONS
CNS: light-headedness.
GU: glycosuria.
Metabolic: hyperglycemia.
Skin: urticaria, burning, hypertrichosis, pruritus, irritation, erythema, hives, dryness.
Other: *hypothalamic-pituitary-adrenal axis (HPA) suppression,* Cushing syndrome.

INTERACTIONS
None significant.

EFFECTS ON LAB TEST RESULTS
• May increase glucose level.

CONTRAINDICATIONS & CAUTIONS
• Contraindicated in patients hypersensitive to drug or its components.
• Don't use as monotherapy in primary bacterial, viral, fungal, herpetic, or tubercular skin infections or for treatment of rosacea, perioral dermatitis, or acne.
• Drug isn't for ophthalmic use.
• Use cautiously in pregnant or breast-feeding women.
⚠ ***Overdose S&S:*** Systemic effects (including reversible HPA axis suppression, Cushing syndrome, hyperglycemia, glycosuria).

NURSING CONSIDERATIONS
• Don't mix drug with other bases or vehicles because doing so may affect potency.
• If adverse reactions occur, prescriber may order less potent drug.
• Stop drug if local irritation or systemic infection, absorption, or hypersensitivity occurs.
• Absorption of corticosteroid is increased when drug is applied to inflamed or damaged skin, eyelids, or scrotal area; it's lowest when applied to intact normal skin, palms of hands, or soles of feet.
• *Look alike–sound alike:* Don't confuse fluticasone with fluconazole, fluocinolone, or fluocinonide.

PATIENT TEACHING
• Teach patient or family member how to apply drug using gloves, sterile applicator, or after careful hand washing.
• Tell patient to wash hands after application.
• Tell patient to avoid prolonged use and contact with eyes. Warn him not to apply to face, in skin creases, or around eyes, genitals, underarms, or rectum.
• Instruct patient to notify prescriber if condition persists or worsens or if burning or irritation develops.

fluticasone propionate–salmeterol inhalation powder

floo-TIK-a-sone–sal-MEE-ter-ol

Advair Diskus 100/50, Advair Diskus 250/50, Advair Diskus 500/50, Advair HFA 45/21, Advair HFA 115/21, Advair HFA 230/21

Therapeutic class: Antiasthmatics
Pharmacologic class: Corticosteroids–long-acting beta$_2$-adrenergic agonists
Pregnancy risk category: C

AVAILABLE FORMS

Inhalation powder: 100 mcg fluticasone and 50 mcg salmeterol, 250 mcg fluticasone and 50 mcg salmeterol, 500 mcg fluticasone and 50 mcg salmeterol
Aerosol spray: 45 mcg fluticasone propionate and 21 mcg salmeterol, 115 mcg fluticasone propionate and 21 mcg salmeterol, 230 mcg fluticasone propionate and 21 mcg salmeterol

INDICATIONS & DOSAGES

➤ **Long-term maintenance of asthma**
Adults and children age 12 and older:
1 inhalation of Advair Diskus b.i.d., at least 12 hours apart; or 2 inhalations of Advair HFA b.i.d. Starting doses are dependent on the patient's current asthma therapy. Maximum dose of Advair Diskus is 1 inhalation of fluticasone 500 mcg/salmeterol 50 mcg b.i.d. Maximum dose of Advair HFA is 2 inhalations of fluticasone 230 mcg/salmeterol 21 mcg b.i.d.
Children age 12 and older: 1 inhalation of Advair Diskus b.i.d. about 12 hours apart. Starting doses are based on patient's asthma severity. Or, 2 inhalations of Advair HFA b.i.d. about 12 hours apart. Starting dose is based on patient's current asthma therapy. Maximum dose for Advair HFA is 2 inhalations of fluticasone 230 mcg/21 mcg salmeterol.
Children ages 4 to 11 (Advair Diskus): 1 inhalation of fluticasone 100 mcg/salmeterol 50 mcg b.i.d. about 12 hours apart.

➤ **Maintenance therapy for airflow obstruction in patients with COPD from chronic bronchitis; to reduce exacerbations of COPD in patients with a history of exacerbations**
Adults: 1 inhalation of Advair Diskus 250/50 only, b.i.d., about 12 hours apart.

ADMINISTRATION

Inhalational
• Prime Advair HFA before first use by releasing 4 test sprays into the air, away from the face, shaking well for 5 seconds before each spray. If inhaler hasn't been used for 4 weeks or has been dropped, prime inhaler again by shaking well before each spray and releasing 2 test sprays into the air.
• Discard Advair HFA canister when counter reads "000."
• After administration, have the patient rinse his mouth without swallowing.

ACTION

Fluticasone is a synthetic corticosteroid with potent anti-inflammatory activity.

Salmeterol xinafoate, a long-acting beta agonist, relaxes bronchial smooth muscle and inhibits release of mediators.

Route	Onset	Peak	Duration
Inhalation (fluticasone)	Unknown	1–2 hr	Unknown
Inhalation (salmeterol)	Unknown	5 min	Unknown

Half-life: Fluticasone: 8 hours; salmeterol: 5½ hours.

ADVERSE REACTIONS

CNS: headache, compressed nerve syndromes, hypnagogic effects, sleep disorders, tremors, pain.
CV: palpitations.
EENT: pharyngitis, blood in nasal mucosa, congestion, conjunctivitis, dental discomfort and pain, eye redness, hoarseness or dysphonia, keratitis, nasal irritation, rhinorrhea, rhinitis, sinusitis, sneezing, viral eye infections.
GI: abdominal pain and discomfort, appendicitis, constipation, diarrhea, gastroenteritis, nausea, oral candidiasis, oral discomfort and pain, oral erythema and rashes, oral ulcerations, unusual taste, vomiting.

Reactions in bold italics are *life-threatening*. Interactions may have a *rapid onset* or a *delayed onset*.

Musculoskeletal: arthralgia, articular rheumatism, bone and cartilage disorders, muscle pain, muscle stiffness, rigidity, tightness.
Respiratory: upper respiratory tract infection, bronchitis, cough, lower respiratory tract infections, pneumonia.
Skin: disorders of sweat and sebum, infection, skin flakiness, sweating, urticaria.
Other: allergic reactions, chest symptoms, fluid retention, viral or bacterial infections.

INTERACTIONS
Drug-drug. *Beta blockers:* Blocked pulmonary effect of salmeterol may produce severe bronchospasm in patients with asthma. Avoid using together. If necessary, use a cardioselective beta blocker cautiously.
Ketoconazole, other inhibitors of CYP450: May increase fluticasone level and adverse effects. Use together cautiously.
Loop diuretics, thiazide diuretics: Potassium-wasting diuretics may cause or worsen ECG changes or hypokalemia. Use together cautiously.
MAO inhibitors, TCAs: May potentiate the action of salmeterol on the vascular system. Separate doses by 2 weeks.

EFFECTS ON LAB TEST RESULTS
• May increase liver enzyme levels.

CONTRAINDICATIONS & CAUTIONS
• Contraindicated in patients hypersensitive to drug or its components.
Black Box Warning When treating asthma, use only for patients not adequately controlled on a long-term asthma-controller medication. ∎
• Contraindicated as primary treatment of status asthmaticus or other acute asthmatic episodes.
① Alert: Don't use drug for transferring patients from systemic corticosteroid therapy. Deaths from adrenal insufficiency have occurred in patients with asthma during and after transfer from systemic corticosteroids to less systemically available inhaled corticosteroids.
• Use cautiously, if at all, in patients with active or quiescent respiratory tuberculosis infection; untreated systemic fungal,

bacterial, viral, or parasitic infection; or ocular herpes simplex.
• Use cautiously in patients with CV disorders, seizure disorders, or thyrotoxicosis; in patients unusually responsive to sympathomimetic amines; and in patients with hepatic impairment.
⚠ Overdose S&S: Hypercorticism, angina, arrhythmias, dizziness, dry mouth, fatigue, headache, hypertension, hypotension, insomnia, malaise, muscle cramps, nausea, nervousness, palpitations, seizures, tachycardia, prolonged QTc interval, hypokalemia, hyperglycemia, cardiac arrest, death.

NURSING CONSIDERATIONS
① Alert: Patient shouldn't be switched from systemic corticosteroids to Advair Diskus or Advair HFA because of hypothalamic-pituitary-adrenal (HPA) axis suppression. Death from adrenal insufficiency can occur. Several months are required for recovery of HPA function after withdrawal of systemic corticosteroids.
• Don't start therapy during rapidly deteriorating or potentially life-threatening episodes of asthma. Serious acute respiratory events, including fatality, can occur.
• The benefit of Advair 250/50 in treating patients with COPD for more than 6 months is unknown. If drug is used for longer than 6 months, periodically reevaluate patient to assess for benefits or risks of therapy.
• Monitor patient for urticaria, angioedema, rash, bronchospasm, or other signs of hypersensitivity.
• Don't use this drug to stop an asthma attack. Patients should carry an inhaled, short-acting beta$_2$ agonist (such as albuterol) for acute symptoms.
• If drug causes paradoxical bronchospasm, treat immediately with a short-acting inhaled bronchodilator (such as albuterol), and notify prescriber.
Black Box Warning Rare, serious asthma episodes or asthma-related deaths have occurred in patients taking salmeterol. Don't use for patients whose asthma is adequately controlled on low or medium-dose inhaled corticosteroids. ∎
• Monitor patient for increased use of inhaled short-acting beta$_2$ agonist. The dose of Advair may need to be increased.

• Closely monitor children for growth suppression.

PATIENT TEACHING

• Instruct patient on proper use of the prescribed inhaler to provide effective treatment.

• Tell patient to avoid exhaling into the dry-powder multidose inhaler; to activate and use the dry-powder multidose inhaler in a level, horizontal position; and not to use Advair Diskus with a spacer device.

• Instruct patient to keep the dry-powder multidose inhaler in a dry place, away from direct heat or sunlight, and to avoid washing the mouthpiece or other parts of the device. Patient should discard device 1 month after removal from the moisture-protective overwrap pouch or after every blister has been used, whichever comes first. He shouldn't attempt to take device apart.

• Instruct patient to rinse mouth after inhalation to prevent oral candidiasis.

• Inform patient that improvement may occur within 30 minutes after dose, but the full benefit may not occur for 1 week or more.

• Advise patient not to exceed recommended prescribing dose.

• Instruct patient not to relieve acute symptoms with Advair. Treat acute symptoms with an inhaled short-acting beta$_2$ agonist.

• Instruct patient to report decreasing effects or use of increasing doses of the short-acting inhaled beta$_2$ agonist.

• Tell patient to report palpitations, chest pain, rapid heart rate, tremor, or nervousness.

• Instruct patient to call immediately if exposed to chickenpox or measles.

fluvastatin sodium

flue-va-STA-tin

Lescol✧, Lescol XL

Therapeutic class: Antilipemics
Pharmacologic class: HMG-CoA reductase inhibitors
Pregnancy risk category: X

AVAILABLE FORMS

Capsules: 20 mg, 40 mg
Tablets (extended-release): 80 mg

INDICATIONS & DOSAGES

➤ **To reduce LDL and total cholesterol levels in patients with primary hypercholesterolemia (types IIa and IIb); to slow progression of coronary atherosclerosis in patients with coronary artery disease; to reduce elevated triglyceride and apolipoprotein B (apo B) levels in patients with primary hypercholesterolemia and mixed dyslipidemia whose response to dietary restriction and other nonpharmacologic measures has been inadequate**
Adults: Initially, 20 to 40 mg P.O. at bedtime, increasing if needed to maximum of 80 mg daily in divided doses or 80 mg Lescol XL P.O. at bedtime.

➤ **Adjunct to diet to reduce LDL, total cholesterol, and apo B levels in pediatric patients with heterozygous familial hypercholesterolemia whose response to dietary restriction hasn't been adequate and for whom the following findings are present: LDL-C remains at 190 mg/dL or more; or LDL-C remains at 160 mg/dL or more and there's a positive family history of premature CV disease or two or more other CV disease risk factors are present**
Adolescent boys and girls (who are at least 1 year postmenarche) ages 10 to 16: 20 mg P.O. once daily at bedtime. Dosage adjustments may be made at 6-week intervals up to maximum of 40 mg (capsule) P.O. b.i.d. or 80 mg extended-release tablet P.O. once daily.

➤ **To reduce the risk of undergoing coronary revascularization procedures**
Adults: In patients who must reduce LDL-C level by at least 25%, initially, 40 mg P.O. once daily or b.i.d.; or one 80-mg extended-release tablet as a single dose in the evening. In patients who must reduce LDL-C level by less than 25%, initially, 20 mg P.O. daily. Dosages range from 20 to 80 mg daily.

ADMINISTRATION

P.O.

• Give drug without regard for meals.
• For once-daily dosage, give immediate-release capsules in the evening.
• Don't crush or break tablets; don't open capsules.
• Administer extended-release tablet as a single dose at any time of the day.

Reactions in bold italics are *life-threatening*. Interactions may have a *rapid onset* or a *delayed onset*.

ACTION
Inhibits HMG-CoA reductase, an early (and rate-limiting) step in the cholesterol synthesis pathway.

Route	Onset	Peak	Duration
P.O.	Unknown	1 hr	Unknown

Half-life: About 3 hours.

ADVERSE REACTIONS
CNS: dizziness, fatigue, headache, insomnia.
EENT: pharyngitis, rhinitis, sinusitis.
GI: abdominal pain, constipation, diarrhea, dyspepsia, flatulence, nausea, vomiting.
GU: UTI.
Hematologic: *leukopenia, thrombocytopenia,* hemolytic anemia.
Musculoskeletal: *rhabdomyolysis,* arthralgia, back pain, myalgia, arthropathy.
Respiratory: upper respiratory tract infection, bronchitis, cough.
Other: hypersensitivity reactions, accidental trauma, flulike illness.

INTERACTIONS
Drug-drug. *Cholestyramine, colestipol:* May bind with fluvastatin in the GI tract and decrease absorption. Separate doses by at least 4 hours.
Cimetidine, omeprazole, ranitidine: May decrease fluvastatin metabolism. Monitor patient for enhanced effects.
Cyclosporine and other immunosuppressants, erythromycin, niacin: May increase risk of polymyositis and rhabdomyolysis. Avoid using together.
Digoxin: May alter digoxin pharmacokinetics. Monitor digoxin level carefully.
Erythromycin, nicotinic acid: May increase risk of myopathy and rhabdomyolysis. Don't use together.
Fibric acids (fenofibrate, gemfibrozil): May cause severe myopathy or rhabdomyolysis. If coadministration can't be avoided, monitor CK closely.
Fluconazole, itraconazole, ketoconazole: May increase fluvastatin level and adverse effects. Use cautiously together or, if given together, reduce dose of fluvastatin.
Glyburide: May increase levels of both drugs. Monitor serum glucose and signs and symptoms of toxicity.

Phenytoin: May increase phenytoin levels. Monitor phenytoin levels.
Protease inhibitors (atazanavir, darunavir, fosamprenavir, indinavir, nelfinavir, ritonavir, saquinavir, tipranavir): May increase fluvastatin level and risk of myopathy and rhabdomyolysis. Use together cautiously.
Rifampin: May enhance fluvastatin metabolism and decrease levels. Monitor patient for lack of effect.
Warfarin: May increase anticoagulant effect with bleeding. Monitor PT and INR.
Drug-herb. *Eucalyptus, jin bu huan, kava:* May increase risk of hepatotoxicity. Discourage use together.
Red yeast rice: May increase risk of adverse reactions because herb contains compounds similar to those in drug. Discourage use together.
Drug-lifestyle. *Alcohol use:* May increase risk of hepatotoxicity. Discourage use together.

EFFECTS ON LAB TEST RESULTS
● May increase ALT, AST, and CK levels. May decrease hemoglobin level and hematocrit.
● May decrease platelet and WBC counts.

CONTRAINDICATIONS & CAUTIONS
● Contraindicated in patients hypersensitive to drug and in those with active liver disease or unexplained persistent elevations of transaminase levels; also contraindicated in pregnant and breast-feeding women and in women of childbearing age.
● Drug may cause rhabdomyolysis in patients with renal function impairment.
● Use cautiously in patients with severe renal impairment and history of liver disease or heavy alcohol use.
⚠ Overdose S&S: GI complaints, elevated AST and ALT levels.

NURSING CONSIDERATIONS
● Patient should follow a diet restricted in saturated fat and cholesterol during therapy.
● Exercise caution when giving to patients with a history of liver disease or heavy alcohol ingestion. Closely monitor these patients.

• Perform LFTs before initiating therapy and if signs and symptoms of liver injury occur.
• Monitor lipid levels before starting therapy, at 4 weeks, at times of dosage changes, and periodically thereafter.
• Watch for signs of myositis.
• *Look alike–sound alike:* Don't confuse fluvastatin with fluoxetine.

PATIENT TEACHING

• Tell patient that drug may be taken without regard for meals; if taken once daily, immediate-release capsules are taken in the evening.
• Advise the patient who is also taking a bile acid sequestrant such as cholestyramine to take fluvastatin at bedtime, at least 4 hours after taking the sequestrant.
• Teach patient about proper dietary management, weight control, and exercise. Explain their importance in controlling elevated cholesterol and triglyceride levels.
• Warn patient to avoid alcohol.
• Tell patient to notify prescriber of adverse reactions, especially muscle aches and pains.
• Advise patient that it may take up to 4 weeks for the drug to be completely effective.
❸ *Alert:* Tell woman of childbearing age to stop drug and notify prescriber immediately if she is or may be pregnant or if she's breast-feeding.

fluvoxamine maleate
floo-VOX-a-meen

Luvox, Luvox CR

Therapeutic class: Antidepressants
Pharmacologic class: SSRIs
Pregnancy risk category: C

AVAILABLE FORMS
Capsules (extended-release): 100 mg, 150 mg
Tablets: 25 mg, 50 mg, 100 mg

INDICATIONS & DOSAGES
Adjust-a-dose (for all indications): In elderly patients and those with hepatic impairment, give lower first dose and adjust dose more slowly. When using Luvox CR capsules, titrate dosage more slowly after initial 100-mg dose.
➤ **Obsessive-compulsive disorder (OCD)**
Adults: Initially, 50 mg (tablet) P.O. daily at bedtime; increase by 50 mg every 4 to 7 days. Maximum, 300 mg daily. Give total daily amounts above 100 mg in two divided doses. Or, 100-mg extended-release capsule P.O. once per day as a single daily dose at bedtime. Increase in 50-mg increments every week, as tolerated, until maximum therapeutic benefit is achieved. Maximum dose is 300 mg/day.
Children ages 8 to 17: Initially, 25 mg P.O. daily at bedtime; increase by 25 mg every 4 to 7 days. Maximum, 200 mg daily for children ages 8 to less than 11 and 300 mg daily for children ages 11 to 17. Give total daily amounts over 50 mg in two divided doses.
➤ **Social anxiety disorder (capsules only)**
Adults: Initially, 100-mg extended-release capsule P.O. once per day as a single daily dose at bedtime. Increase in 50-mg increments every week, as tolerated, until maximum therapeutic benefit is achieved. Maximum dose is 300 mg/day.
➤ **Bulimia nervosa** ◆
Adults: 50 mg P.O. daily. May titrate dosage based on therapeutic response to 200 mg/day for up to 12 weeks.
➤ **Panic disorder** ◆
Adults: Initially, 50 mg P.O. daily. Maintain dosage for several days; then gradually increase to 150 mg daily. Further dosage increases up to 300 mg daily may be considered for patients without response after several weeks. Continue treatment for 1 to 2 years after response. When discontinuing drug, slowly taper dosage over 2 to 6 months with close supervision.
➤ **Posttraumatic stress disorder (PTSD)** ◆
Adults, children, and adolescents: Initially, 50 mg P.O. daily. Average daily target doses are 50 mg P.O. daily in children and younger adolescents, 100 to 250 mg P.O. daily for adults, and 100 mg P.O. daily for older adults. Maximum dosage is 300 mg/day for adults. Consider tapering dosage after 6 to 12 months in patients with acute PTSD,

---

after 12 to 24 months in patients with chronic PTSD who have had an excellent response to treatment, and after at least 24 months in patients with chronic PTSD and residual symptoms. Tapering should take place over 2 weeks to 1 month and over 4 to 12 weeks in patients at risk for relapse.
➤ **Migraine prevention** ◆
Adults: 50 mg P.O. at bedtime for 12 weeks.

ADMINISTRATION
P.O.
- Give drug without regard for food.
- Capsules shouldn't be crushed or chewed.
- Give extended-release capsules at bedtime.

ACTION
Unknown. Selectively inhibits the presynaptic neuronal uptake of serotonin, which may improve OCD.

Route	Onset	Peak	Duration
P.O. (capsules)	Unknown	Unknown	Unknown
P.O. (tablets)	Unknown	3–8 hr	Unknown

Half-life: 15 to 17 hours.

ADVERSE REACTIONS
CNS: agitation, headache, asthenia, somnolence, insomnia, nervousness, dizziness, tremor, anxiety, hypertonia, depression, CNS stimulation.
CV: palpitations, vasodilation.
EENT: amblyopia.
GI: nausea, diarrhea, constipation, dyspepsia, vomiting, dry mouth, anorexia, flatulence, dysphagia, taste perversion.
GU: abnormal ejaculation, urinary frequency, erectile dysfunction, anorgasmia, urine retention.
Respiratory: upper respiratory tract infection, dyspnea.
Skin: sweating.
Other: tooth disorder, flulike syndrome, chills, decreased libido, yawning.

INTERACTIONS
Drug-drug. *Benzodiazepines, theophylline, warfarin:* May reduce clearance of these drugs. Use together cautiously (except for diazepam, which shouldn't be used with fluvoxamine). Adjust dosage as needed.

Carbamazepine, clozapine, methadone, metoprolol, propranolol, TCAs, theophylline: May increase levels of these drugs. Use together cautiously, and monitor patient closely for adverse reactions. Dosage adjustments may be needed.
Diltiazem: May cause bradycardia. Monitor heart rate.
Linezolid, methylene blue: May cause serotonin syndrome. Use extreme caution and monitor closely.
Lithium, tryptophan: May enhance effects of fluvoxamine. Use together cautiously.
MAO inhibitors (phenelzine, selegiline, tranylcypromine): May cause serotonin syndrome (CNS irritability, shivering, and altered consciousness) or neuroleptic malignant syndrome. Avoid using within 2 weeks of MAO inhibitor.
Pimozide, thioridazine: May prolong QTc interval. Avoid using together.
Sumatriptan: May cause weakness, hyperreflexia, and incoordination. Monitor patient closely. May cause serotonin syndrome. Avoid using within 2 weeks of MAO inhibitor.
Tramadol: May cause serotonin syndrome. Monitor patient closely.
Drug-herb. *St. John's wort:* May increase sedative-hypnotic effects. Avoid use together.
Drug-lifestyle. *Alcohol use:* May increase CNS effects. Discourage use together.
Smoking: May decrease drug's effectiveness. Urge patient to stop smoking.

EFFECTS ON LAB TEST RESULTS
None reported.

CONTRAINDICATIONS & CAUTIONS
- Contraindicated in patients hypersensitive to drug or to other phenyl piperazine antidepressants; in those receiving pimozide, alosetron, tizanidine, or thioridazine therapy; and within 2 weeks of MAO inhibitor.
⊘ Alert: Concomitant use with linezolid or methylene blue can cause serotonin syndrome (fever, mental status changes, muscle twitching, excessive sweating, shivering or shaking, diarrhea, loss of coordination). Use drug with linezolid or methylene blue only for life-threatening or urgent conditions

when the potential benefits outweigh the risks of toxicity.

● Use cautiously in patients with hepatic dysfunction, other conditions that may affect hemodynamic responses or metabolism, or history of mania or seizures.

Black Box Warning Fluvoxamine tablets aren't approved for use in children, except for those with OCD. Fluvoxamine extended-release capsules shouldn't be used in children. ∎

⚠ Overdose S&S: Nausea, vomiting, diarrhea, coma, hypokalemia, hypotension, respiratory difficulties, somnolence, tachycardia, ECG abnormalities, seizures, dizziness, liver function disturbances, tremor, increased reflexes.

NURSING CONSIDERATIONS

Black Box Warning Don't use for the treatment of major depressive disorders in children younger than age 18 because of an increased risk of suicidal behavior. ∎

Black Box Warning Drug may increase the risk of suicidal thinking and behavior in young adults ages 18 to 24, especially during the first few months of treatment. ∎

● Record mood changes. Monitor patient for suicidal tendencies.

⟲ Alert: Combining an SSRI with a triptan may cause serotonin syndrome or neuroleptic malignant syndrome–like reactions. Serotonin syndrome is more likely to occur when starting or increasing the dose of a triptan.

⟲ Alert: If linezolid or methylene blue must be given, fluvoxamine must be stopped and the patient should be monitored for serotonin toxicity for 2 weeks or until 24 hours after the last dose of linezolid or methylene blue, whichever comes first. Treatment with fluvoxamine may be resumed 24 hours after the last dose of linezolid or methylene blue.

● Patients shouldn't stop drug without first consulting prescriber; abruptly stopping drug may cause withdrawal syndrome, including headache, muscle ache, and flulike symptoms.

● **Look alike–sound alike:** Don't confuse fluvoxamine with fluoxetine.

PATIENT TEACHING

Black Box Warning Advise families and caregivers to closely observe patient for increased suicidal thinking or behavior. ∎

⟲ Alert: Teach patient to recognize and immediately report symptoms of serotonin toxicity (fever, mental status changes, muscle twitching, excessive sweating, shivering or shaking, diarrhea, loss of coordination).

● Warn patient to avoid hazardous activities until CNS effects of drug are known.

● Tell women to notify prescriber about planned, suspected, or known pregnancy.

● Tell patient who develops a rash, hives, or a related allergic reaction to notify prescriber.

● Inform patient that several weeks of therapy may be needed to obtain full therapeutic effect. Once improvement occurs, advise patient not to stop drug until directed by prescriber.

● Suggest that patient keep a diary of changes in mood or behavior. Tell patient to report suicidal thoughts immediately.

● Advise patient to check with prescriber before taking OTC drugs; drug interactions can occur.

● Tell patient drug can be taken with or without food.

SAFETY ALERT!

fondaparinux sodium
fon-dah-PEAR-ah-nucks

Arixtra

Therapeutic class: Anticoagulants
Pharmacologic class: Activated factor X inhibitors
Pregnancy risk category: B

AVAILABLE FORMS
Injection: 2.5 mg/0.5 mL, 5 mg/0.4 mL, 7.5 mg/0.6 mL, 10 mg/0.8 mL single-dose prefilled syringe

INDICATIONS & DOSAGES
➤ **To prevent DVT, which may lead to PE, in patients undergoing surgery for hip fracture, hip replacement, knee replacement, or abdominal surgery**
Adults: 2.5 mg subcutaneously once daily for 5 to 9 days. Give first dose after

---

hemostasis is established, 6 to 8 hours after surgery. Giving the dose earlier than 6 hours after surgery increases the risk of major bleeding. Patients undergoing hip fracture surgery should receive an extended prophylaxis course of up to 24 additional days; a total of 32 days (perioperative and extended prophylaxis) has been tolerated.

➤ **Acute DVT (with warfarin); acute PE (with warfarin) when treatment is started in the hospital**
Adults weighing more than 100 kg (220 lb): 10 mg subcutaneously daily for 5 to 9 days (drug has been given for up to 26 days in clinical trials) and until INR is 2 to 3. Begin warfarin therapy as soon as possible, usually within 72 hours.
Adults weighing 50 to 100 kg: 7.5 mg subcutaneously daily for 5 to 9 days (drug has been given for up to 26 days in clinical trials) and until INR is 2 to 3. Begin warfarin therapy as soon as possible, usually within 72 hours.
Adults weighing less than 50 kg: 5 mg subcutaneously daily for 5 to 9 days (drug has been given for up to 26 days in clinical trials) and until INR is 2 to 3. Begin warfarin therapy as soon as possible, usually within 72 hours.

ADMINISTRATION
Subcutaneous
● Give subcutaneously only, never I.M. Inspect the single-dose, prefilled syringe for particulate matter and discoloration before giving.
● Give the drug in fatty tissue, rotating injection sites. If the drug has been properly injected, the needle will pull back into the syringe security sleeve and the white safety indicator will appear above the blue upper body. A soft click may be heard or felt when the syringe plunger is fully released. After injection of the syringe contents, the plunger automatically rises while the needle withdraws from the skin and retracts into the security sleeve. Don't recap the needle.
● **Incompatibilities:** Other injections or infusions.

ACTION
Binds to antithrombin III (AT-III) and potentiates the neutralization of factor Xa by AT-III, which interrupts coagulation and inhibits formation of thrombin and blood clots.

Route	Onset	Peak	Duration
Subcut.	Unknown	2–3 hr	Unknown

Half-life: 17 to 21 hours.

ADVERSE REACTIONS
CNS: fever, insomnia, dizziness, confusion, headache, pain.
CV: hypotension, edema.
GI: nausea, constipation, vomiting, diarrhea, dyspepsia.
GU: UTI, urine retention.
Hematologic: *hemorrhage,* anemia, hematoma, *postoperative hemorrhage, thrombocytopenia.*
Metabolic: hypokalemia.
Skin: mild local irritation (injection-site bleeding, rash, pruritus), bullous eruption, purpura, rash, increased wound drainage.

INTERACTIONS
Drug-drug. *Drugs that increase risk of bleeding (anticoagulants, NSAIDs, platelet inhibitors):* May increase risk of hemorrhage. Stop these drugs before starting fondaparinux. If use together is unavoidable, monitor patient closely.
Drug-herb. *Angelica (dong quai), boldo, bromelains, capsicum, chamomile, dandelion, danshen, devil's claw, fenugreek, feverfew, garlic, ginger, ginkgo, ginseng, horse chestnut, licorice, meadowsweet, onion, passion flower, red clover, willow:* May increase risk of bleeding. Discourage use together.

EFFECTS ON LAB TEST RESULTS
● May increase AST, ALT, and bilirubin levels. May decrease potassium and hemoglobin levels and hematocrit.
● May decrease platelet count.

CONTRAINDICATIONS & CAUTIONS
● Contraindicated in patients with CrCl less than 30 mL/minute and in those who are hypersensitive to the drug.
● Contraindicated for venous thromboembolism prophylaxis in patients weighing less than 50 kg who are undergoing hip

fracture, hip replacement, knee replacement, or abdominal surgery.

• Contraindicated in patients with active major bleeding, bacterial endocarditis, or thrombocytopenia with a positive test result for antiplatelet antibody after taking fondaparinux.

• Use cautiously in patients being treated with platelet inhibitors; in those at increased risk for bleeding, such as those with congenital or acquired bleeding disorders; in those with active ulcerative and angiodysplastic GI disease; in those with hemorrhagic stroke; and in patients shortly after brain, spinal, or ophthalmologic surgery.

• Use cautiously in elderly patients, in patients with CrCl of 30 to 50 mL/minute, and in those with a history of heparin-induced thrombocytopenia, a bleeding diathesis, uncontrolled arterial hypertension, or a history of recent GI ulceration, diabetic retinopathy, or hemorrhage.

❸ *Alert:* Use cautiously in latex-sensitive patients; the packaging (needle guard) contains dry natural rubber.

⚠ *Overdose S&S:* Hemorrhagic complications.

NURSING CONSIDERATIONS

• Don't use interchangeably with heparin, low–molecular-weight heparins, or heparinoids.

❸ *Alert:* To avoid loss of drug, don't expel air bubble from the syringe.

Black Box Warning Patients who receive epidural or spinal anesthesia, epidural catheters, or spinal puncture or have a history of spine deformity or surgery are at increased risk for developing an epidural or spinal hematoma, which may result in long-term or permanent paralysis. Monitor these patients closely for neurologic impairment and treat urgently. ∎

• Monitor renal function periodically and stop drug in patients who develop unstable renal function or severe renal impairment while receiving therapy.

• Routinely assess patient for signs and symptoms of bleeding, and regularly monitor CBC, platelet count, creatinine level, and stool occult blood test results. Stop use if platelet count is less than 100,000/mm^3.

• Anticoagulant effects may last for 2 to 4 days after stopping drug in patients with normal renal function.

• PT and activated PTT aren't suitable monitoring tests to measure drug activity. If coagulation parameters change unexpectedly or patient develops major bleeding, stop drug.

PATIENT TEACHING

• Tell patient to report signs and symptoms of bleeding or neurologic impairment.

• Instruct patient to avoid OTC products that contain aspirin or other salicylates.

• Advise patient to consult with prescriber before starting herbal therapy; many herbs have anticoagulant, antiplatelet, or fibrinolytic properties.

• Teach patient the correct technique for subcutaneous use, if needed.

formoterol fumarate
for-MOH-te-rol

Foradil Aerolizer, Perforomist

Therapeutic class: Bronchodilators
Pharmacologic class: Selective beta$_2$-adrenergic agonists
Pregnancy risk category: C

AVAILABLE FORMS
Capsules for inhalation: 12 mcg
Inhalation solution: 20 mcg/2-mL vial

INDICATIONS & DOSAGES
➤ **Maintenance treatment and prevention of bronchospasm in patients with reversible obstructive airway disease or nocturnal asthma, who usually require treatment with short-acting inhaled beta$_2$ agonists**
Adults and children age 5 and older: One 12-mcg capsule by inhalation via Aerolizer inhaler every 12 hours. Total daily dosage shouldn't exceed 1 capsule b.i.d. (24 mcg/day). If symptoms occur between doses, use a short-acting beta$_2$ agonist for immediate relief.
➤ **To prevent exercise-induced bronchospasm**
Adults and children age 5 and older: One 12-mcg capsule by inhalation via Aerolizer

---

Reactions in bold italics are *life-threatening*. Interactions may have a *rapid onset* or a *delayed onset*.

inhaler at least 15 minutes before exercise p.r.n. Don't give additional doses within 12 hours of first dose.

➤ **Maintenance treatment of bron-choconstriction in patients with COPD (chronic bronchitis, emphysema)**

Adults: One 20 mcg/2-mL vial (Performist) by oral inhalation through a jet nebulizer every 12 hours. Maximum dose, 40 mcg/day. Or, one 12-mcg capsule (Foradil) by inhalation via Aerolizer inhaler every 12 hours; total daily dosage shouldn't exceed 24 mcg/day.

ADMINISTRATION
Inhalational
Foradil
● Give Foradil capsules only by oral inhalation and only with the Aerolizer inhaler. They aren't for oral ingestion. Patient shouldn't exhale into the device. Capsules should remain in the unopened blister until administration time and be removed immediately before use.
● Pierce Foradil capsules only once. In rare instances, the gelatin capsule may break into small pieces and get delivered to the mouth or throat upon inhalation. The Aerolizer contains a screen that should catch any broken pieces before they leave the device. To minimize the possibility of shattering the capsule, strictly follow storage and use instructions.
Performist
● Give Performist inhalational solution through a standard jet nebulizer connected to an air compressor.

ACTION
Long-acting selective beta$_2$ agonist that causes bronchodilation. It ultimately increases cAMP, leading to relaxation of bronchial smooth muscle and inhibition of mediator release from mast cells.

Route	Onset	Peak	Duration
Inhalation powder	5 min	1–3 hr	12 hr
Inhalation solution	12 min	1–3 hr	12 hr

Half-life: 10 hours for Foradil; 7 hours for Performist.

ADVERSE REACTIONS
CNS: tremor, dizziness, insomnia, nervousness, headache, fatigue, malaise.
CV: *arrhythmias,* chest pain, angina, hypertension, hypotension, tachycardia, palpitations.
EENT: dry mouth, tonsillitis, dysphonia, nasopharyngitis.
GI: nausea, vomiting, diarrhea.
Metabolic: *metabolic acidosis,* hypokalemia, hyperglycemia.
Musculoskeletal: muscle cramps.
Respiratory: bronchitis, chest infection, dyspnea.
Skin: rash.
Other: viral infection.

INTERACTIONS
Drug-drug. *Adrenergics:* May potentiate sympathetic effects of formoterol. Use together cautiously.
Beta blockers: May antagonize effects of beta agonists, causing bronchospasm in asthmatic patients. Avoid use except when benefit outweighs risks. Use cardioselective beta blockers with caution to minimize risk of bronchospasm.
Diuretics, steroids, xanthine derivatives: May increase hypokalemic effect of formoterol. Use together cautiously.
MAO inhibitors, TCAs, other drugs that prolong QT interval: May increase risk of ventricular arrhythmias. Use together cautiously.
Non–potassium-sparing diuretics, such as loop or thiazide diuretics: May worsen ECG changes or hypokalemia. Use together cautiously, and monitor patient for toxicity.

EFFECTS ON LAB TEST RESULTS
● May increase glucose level. May decrease potassium level.

CONTRAINDICATIONS & CAUTIONS
● Contraindicated in patients hypersensitive to drug or its components, or with other long-acting beta$_2$ agonists.
● Use cautiously in patients with CV disease, especially coronary insufficiency, cardiac arrhythmias, and hypertension, and in those who are unusually responsive to sympathomimetic amines.

• Use cautiously in patients with diabetes mellitus because hyperglycemia and ketoacidosis have occurred rarely with the use of beta agonists.

• Use cautiously in patients with seizure disorders or thyrotoxicosis and in breast-feeding women.

• Use for asthma only as additional therapy for patients whose condition is not adequately controlled with other asthma-controller medications.

⚠ **Overdose S&S:** Exaggeration of adverse reactions, hypotension, cardiac arrest.

NURSING CONSIDERATIONS

• Drug isn't indicated for patients who can control asthma symptoms with just occasional use of inhaled, short-acting beta$_2$ agonists or for treatment of acute bronchospasm requiring immediate reversal with short-acting beta$_2$ agonists or in patients with rapidly deteriorating or significantly worsening asthma.

• Drug may be used along with short-acting beta agonists, inhaled corticosteroids, and theophylline therapy for asthma management.

❸ **Alert:** Drug isn't a substitute for short-acting beta$_2$ agonists for immediate relief of bronchospasm or as substitute for inhaled or oral corticosteroids.

• Patients using drug twice daily shouldn't take additional doses to prevent exercise-induced bronchospasm.

• For patients formerly using regularly scheduled short-acting beta$_2$ agonists, decrease use of the short-acting drug to an as-needed basis when starting long-acting formoterol.

Black Box Warning Drug may increase the risk of asthma-related death. Use only as additional therapy for patients not adequately controlled on low to medium dose of inhaled corticosteroids or in patients whose disease is severe and requires treatment with two maintenance therapies. ■

Black Box Warning For children and adolescents with asthma who require the addition of a long-acting beta$_2$ agonist to an inhaled corticosteroid, a fixed-dose combination product containing an inhaled corticosteroid and long-acting beta$_2$ agonist

should be considered to ensure adherence to both drugs. ■

❸ **Alert:** As with all beta$_2$ agonists, drug may produce life-threatening paradoxical bronchospasm. If bronchospasm occurs, notify prescriber immediately.

❸ **Alert:** If patient develops tachycardia, hypertension, or other CV adverse effects, drug may need to be stopped.

• Watch for immediate hypersensitivity reactions, such as anaphylaxis, urticaria, angioedema, rash, and bronchospasm.

• **Look alike–sound alike:** Don't confuse Foradil with Toradol.

PATIENT TEACHING

• Tell patient not to increase the dosage or frequency of use without medical advice.

• Warn patient not to stop or reduce other medication taken for asthma.

• Advise patient that drug isn't to be used for acute asthmatic episodes. Prescriber should give a short-acting beta$_2$ agonist for this use.

• Advise patient to report worsening symptoms, treatment that becomes less effective, or increased use of short-acting beta agonists.

• Tell patient to report nausea, vomiting, shakiness, headache, fast or irregular heartbeat, or sleeplessness.

• Tell patient using drug for exercise-induced bronchospasm to take it at least 15 minutes before exercise and to wait 12 hours before taking additional doses.

• Tell patient not to use the Foradil Aerolizer with a spacer device or to exhale or blow into the Aerolizer.

• Advise patient to avoid washing the Aerolizer and to always keep it dry. Each refill contains a new device to replace the old one.

• Tell patient to avoid exposing capsules to moisture and to handle them only with dry hands.

• Advise woman to notify prescriber if she becomes pregnant or is breast-feeding.

---

fosamprenavir calcium
foss-am-PREN-ah-ver

Lexiva

Therapeutic class: Antiretrovirals
Pharmacologic class: Protease inhibitors
Pregnancy risk category: C

AVAILABLE FORMS
Oral suspension: 50 mg/mL
Tablets: 700 mg

INDICATIONS & DOSAGES
➤ HIV infection, with other antiretrovirals

Adults: In patients not previously treated, 1,400 mg P.O. b.i.d. (without ritonavir). Or, 1,400 mg P.O. once daily and ritonavir 200 mg P.O. once daily. Or, 1,400 mg P.O. once daily and ritonavir 100 mg P.O. once daily. Or, 700 mg P.O. b.i.d. and ritonavir 100 mg P.O. b.i.d. In patients previously treated with a protease inhibitor, 700 mg P.O. b.i.d. plus ritonavir 100 mg P.O. b.i.d.

Adjust-a-dose: If the patient has mild hepatic impairment (Child-Pugh score of 5 to 6), reduce dosage to 700 mg P.O. b.i.d. without ritonavir (in therapy-naive patients) or 700 mg b.i.d. plus ritonavir 100 mg once daily (in therapy-naive or protease inhibitor–experienced patients). If the patient has moderate hepatic impairment (Child-Pugh score of 7 to 9), reduce dosage to 700 mg b.i.d. (in therapy-naive patients) without ritonavir or 450 mg b.i.d. plus ritonavir 100 mg once daily (in therapy-naive or protease inhibitor–experienced patients). If the patient has severe hepatic impairment (Child-Pugh score of 10 to 15), reduce dosage to 350 mg b.i.d. without ritonavir (in therapy-naive patients). Or, in therapy-naive or protease inhibitor–experienced patients, 300 mg P.O. b.i.d. plus ritonavir 100 mg once daily.

➤ HIV infection with other antiretrovirals for protease inhibitor–naive children age 4 weeks and older

Children ages 4 weeks to 18 years weighing 20 kg (44 lb) or more: 18 mg/kg P.O. with ritonavir 3 mg/kg b.i.d.

Children ages 4 weeks to 18 years weighing 15 kg (33 lb) to less than 20 kg: 23 mg/kg P.O. with ritonavir 3 mg/kg b.i.d.
Children ages 4 weeks to 18 years weighing 11 kg (24 lb) to less than 15 kg: 30 mg/kg P.O. with ritonavir 3 mg/kg b.i.d.
Children ages 4 weeks to 18 years weighing less than 11 kg: 45 mg/kg P.O. with ritonavir 7 mg/kg b.i.d.

Adjust-a-dose: There are no dosing recommendations for pediatric patients with hepatic impairment. Dosage for pediatric patients shouldn't exceed recommended adult dosage of 700 mg fosamprenavir with ritonavir 100 mg b.i.d. Drug isn't approved for once-daily dosing in pediatric patients.

➤ HIV infection with other antiretrovirals for protease inhibitor–experienced children age 6 months and older

Children ages 6 months to 18 years weighing 20 kg (44 lb) or more: 18 mg/kg P.O. with ritonavir 3 mg/kg b.i.d.
Children ages 6 months to 18 years weighing 15 kg (33 lb) to less than 20 kg: 23 mg/kg P.O. with ritonavir 3 mg/kg b.i.d.
Children ages 6 months to 18 years weighing 11 kg (24 lb) to less than 15 kg: 30 mg/kg P.O. with ritonavir 3 mg/kg b.i.d.
Children ages 6 months to 18 years weighing less than 11 kg: 45 mg/kg P.O. with ritonavir 7 mg/kg b.i.d.

Adjust-a-dose: There are no dosing recommendations for pediatric patients with hepatic impairment. Dosage for pediatric patients shouldn't exceed recommended adult dosage of 700 mg fosamprenavir with ritonavir 100 mg b.i.d. Drug isn't approved for once-daily dosing in pediatric patients.

➤ HIV infection without ritonavir in protease inhibitor–naive children

Children age 2 years and older: 30 mg/kg P.O. b.i.d.

Adjust-a-dose: There are no dosing recommendations for pediatric patients with hepatic impairment. Drug isn't approved for once-daily dosing in pediatric patients.

ADMINISTRATION
P.O.
- Give drug with other antiretrovirals.
- Tablets may be taken with or without food.

F

• Adults should take oral suspension without food. Children should take oral suspension with food. If patient vomits within 30 minutes after taking medication, dose should be repeated.
• Shake oral suspension before using.

ACTION

Converts rapidly to amprenavir, which binds to the active site of HIV-1 protease and forms immature noninfectious viral particles.

Route	Onset	Peak	Duration
P.O.	Unknown	1½–4 hr	Unknown

Half-life: 7¼ hours.

ADVERSE REACTIONS

CNS: depression, fatigue, headache, oral paresthesia.
CV: *MI.*
GI: abdominal pain, diarrhea, nausea, vomiting.
Metabolic: hyperglycemia, hypercholesterolemia.
Skin: rash, pruritus.

INTERACTIONS

Drug-drug. *Amitriptyline, cyclosporine, imipramine, rapamycin, tacrolimus:* May increase levels of these drugs. Monitor drug levels.
Antiarrhythmics (amiodarone, quinidine, systemic lidocaine): May increase antiarrhythmic level. Use together cautiously and monitor antiarrhythmic levels.
Atorvastatin: May increase atorvastatin level and risk of myopathy and rhabdomyolysis. Give 20 mg/day or less of atorvastatin and monitor patient carefully. Or, consider other HMG-CoA reductase inhibitors, such as fluvastatin, pravastatin, or rosuvastatin.
Benzodiazepines (alprazolam, clorazepate, diazepam, flurazepam): May increase benzodiazepine level. Decrease benzodiazepine dosage as needed.
Bepridil: May increase bepridil level, possibly leading to arrhythmias. Use together cautiously.
Calcium channel blockers (amlodipine, diltiazem, felodipine, isradipine, nifedipine, nicardipine, nimodipine, nisoldipine,

verapamil): May increase calcium channel blocker level. Use together cautiously.
Carbamazepine, dexamethasone, H₂-receptor antagonists, phenobarbital, phenytoin, proton pump inhibitors: May decrease amprenavir level. Use together cautiously.
Delavirdine: May cause loss of virologic response and resistance to delavirdine. Avoid using together.
Dihydroergotamine, ergonovine, ergotamine, flecainide, methylergonovine, midazolam, pimozide, propafenone, triazolam: May cause serious adverse reactions. Avoid using together.
Efavirenz, nevirapine, saquinavir: May decrease amprenavir level. Appropriate combination doses haven't been established.
Efavirenz with ritonavir: May decrease amprenavir level. Increase ritonavir by 100 mg/day (300 mg total) when giving efavirenz, fosamprenavir, and ritonavir once daily. No change needed in ritonavir when giving efavirenz, fosamprenavir, and ritonavir twice daily.
Ethinyl estradiol–norethindrone: May increase ethinyl estradiol–norethindrone levels. Recommend nonhormonal contraception.
Indinavir, nelfinavir: May increase amprenavir level. Appropriate combination doses haven't been established.
Ketoconazole, itraconazole: May increase ketoconazole and itraconazole levels. Reduce ketoconazole or itraconazole dosage as needed if patient receives more than 400 mg/day. (More than 200 mg/day isn't recommended.)
Lopinavir–ritonavir: May decrease amprenavir and lopinavir levels. Appropriate combination doses haven't been established.
Lovastatin, simvastatin: May increase statin level and risk of myopathy, including rhabdomyolysis. Use together is contraindicated.
Methadone: May decrease methadone level. Increase methadone dosage as needed.
Rifabutin: May increase rifabutin level. Obtain CBC weekly to watch for neutropenia, and decrease rifabutin dosage by at least half. If patient receives ritonavir, decrease dosage by at least 75% from the usual 300 mg/day (maximum, 150 mg every other day or three times weekly).

Reactions in bold italics are *life-threatening*. Interactions may have a *rapid onset* or a *delayed onset*.

Rifampin: May decrease amprenavir level and drug effects. Avoid using together.

Sildenafil, tadalafil, vardenafil: May increase levels of these drugs. Recommend cautious use of sildenafil at 25 mg every 48 hours, tadalafil at 10 mg every 72 hours, or vardenafil at no more than 2.5 mg every 24 hours. If patient receives ritonavir, advise no more than 2.5 mg vardenafil every 72 hours, and tell patient to report adverse events.

Warfarin: May alter warfarin level. Monitor INR.

Drug-herb. *St. John's wort:* May cause loss of virologic response and resistance to drug or its class of protease inhibitors. Discourage use together.

EFFECTS ON LAB TEST RESULTS
• May increase ALT, AST, glucose, lipase, and triglyceride levels.
• May decrease neutrophil count.

CONTRAINDICATIONS & CAUTIONS
۞ Alert: For pediatric patients, drug is only for use in infants born at 38 weeks' gestation or more and in those who have attained a postnatal age of 28 days.
۞ Alert: Drug isn't approved for once-daily dosing in pediatric patients.
• Contraindicated in patients hypersensitive to drug or its components.
• Contraindicated with dihydroergotamine, ergonovine, ergotamine, flecainide, lovastatin, methylergonovine, midazolam, pimozide, propafenone, simvastatin, and triazolam.
• Use cautiously in patients allergic to sulfonamides and those with hepatic impairment or cardiac disease.
• Use in pregnant woman only when benefit to mother justifies risk to fetus.
• Tell woman not to breast-feed during therapy.
⚠ Overdose S&S: Increased ALT and AST levels.

NURSING CONSIDERATIONS
• Patients with hepatitis B or C or marked increase in transaminases before treatment may have increased risk of transaminase elevation. Monitor patient closely.

• Monitor cholesterol, triglyceride, lipase, ALT, AST, and glucose levels before starting therapy and periodically throughout treatment.
• Assess and manage lipid disorders as clinically appropriate.
• Ask patient if he's allergic to sulfa drugs.
• Monitor patient with hemophilia for spontaneous bleeding.
• During first treatment, monitor patient for opportunistic infections, such as *Mycobacterium avium* complex, CMV, *Pneumocystis jiroveci (carinii)* pneumonia, and tuberculosis.
• Assess patient for redistribution or accumulation of body fat, as in central obesity, dorsocervical fat enlargement (buffalo hump), peripheral wasting, facial wasting, breast enlargement, and a cushingoid appearance.

PATIENT TEACHING
• Tell patient that drug doesn't reduce the risk of transmitting HIV to others.
• Inform patient that the drug may reduce the risk of progression to AIDS.
• Explain that fosamprenavir must be used with other antiretrovirals.
• Tell patient not to alter the dose or stop taking drug without consulting prescriber.
• Drug interacts with many other drugs; urge patient to tell prescriber about any prescription, OTC, or herbal medicines he's taking (especially St. John's wort).
• Explain that body fat may redistribute or accumulate.

---

foscarnet sodium (PFA, phosphonoformic acid)
foss-CAR-net

Foscavir

Therapeutic class: Antivirals
Pharmacologic class: Pyrophosphate analogues
Pregnancy risk category: C

AVAILABLE FORMS
Injection: 24 mg/mL in 250- and 500-mL bottles

F

INDICATIONS & DOSAGES
Adjust-a-dose (for all indications): Adjust dosage when CrCl is less than 1.4 mL/minute/kg. If CrCl falls below 0.4 mL/minute/kg, stop drug. Consult manufacturer's package insert for specific dosage adjustments.

Black Box Warning Drug is only indicated for use in immunocompromised patients with CMV retinitis and mucocutaneous acyclovir-resistant herpes simplex virus (HSV) infections. ▮

➤ **CMV retinitis in patients with AIDS**
Adults: Initially, for induction, 60 mg/kg I.V. over a minimum of 1 hour every 8 hours or 90 mg/kg I.V. over 1½ to 2 hours every 12 hours for 2 to 3 weeks, depending on patient response. Follow with a maintenance infusion of 90 to 120 mg/kg over 2 hours daily.

➤ **Acyclovir-resistant HSV infections**
Adults: 40 mg/kg I.V. over 1 hour every 8 to 12 hours for 2 to 3 weeks or until healed.

ADMINISTRATION
I.V.
Black Box Warning To minimize renal toxicity, make sure patient is adequately hydrated before and during infusion. ▮

▼ Don't exceed the recommended dosage, rate, or frequency of infusion. Doses must be individualized according to patient's renal function.

▼ Drug may be infused via a central or peripheral vein with enough blood flow for rapid distribution and dilution. If infusing into a central vein, don't dilute the commercially available form (24 mg/mL). If infusing into a peripheral vein, dilute to 12 mg/mL with D₅W or normal saline solution to decrease risk of local irritation. Use an infusion pump.

▼ Give induction treatment over 1 to 2 hours, depending on the dose, and maintenance infusions over 2 hours.

▼ **Incompatibilities:** Acyclovir, amphotericin B, dextrose 30%, diazepam, digoxin, diphenhydramine, dobutamine, droperidol, ganciclovir, haloperidol, lactated Ringer solution, leucovorin, lorazepam, midazolam, pentamidine, phenytoin, prochlorperazine, promethazine, solutions containing calcium (such as total parenteral nutrition), trimetrexate, sulfamethoxazole–trimethoprim, vancomycin.

ACTION
Inhibits herpes virus replication in vitro by blocking the pyrophosphate-binding site on DNA polymerases and reverse transcriptases.

Route	Onset	Peak	Duration
I.V.	Unknown	Immediate	Unknown

Half-life: 3 hours.

ADVERSE REACTIONS
CNS: asthenia, dizziness, fatigue, fever, headache, hypoesthesia, malaise, neuropathy, paresthesia, *seizures,* abnormal coordination, agitation, aggression, amnesia, anxiety, aphasia, ataxia, cerebrovascular disorder, confusion, dementia, depression, EEG abnormalities, generalized spasms, hallucinations, insomnia, meningitis, nervousness, pain, sensory disturbances, somnolence, stupor, tremor.
CV: ECG abnormalities, first-degree AV block, flushing, hypertension, hypotension, palpitations, sinus tachycardia, chest pain, edema.
EENT: conjunctivitis, eye pain, pharyngitis, rhinitis, sinusitis, visual disturbances.
GI: abdominal pain, anorexia, diarrhea, nausea, vomiting, *pancreatitis,* constipation, dysphagia, dry mouth, dyspepsia, flatulence, melena, rectal hemorrhage, taste perversion, ulcerative stomatitis.
GU: *acute renal failure,* abnormal renal function, albuminuria, candidiasis, dysuria, polyuria, urethral disorder, urine retention, UTI.
Hematologic: anemia, *bone marrow suppression, granulocytopenia, leukopenia, thrombocytopenia,* thrombocytosis.
Hepatic: abnormal hepatic function.
Metabolic: hyperphosphatemia, hypocalcemia, hypokalemia, *hypomagnesemia,* hypophosphatemia, hyponatremia.
Musculoskeletal: arthralgia, back pain, leg cramps, myalgia.
Respiratory: *bronchospasm,* cough, dyspnea, hemoptysis, pneumonitis, *pneumothorax,* pulmonary infiltration, *respiratory insufficiency,* stridor.

Reactions in bold italics are *life-threatening*. Interactions may have a *rapid onset* or a *delayed onset*.

Skin: diaphoresis, rash, erythematous rash, facial edema, pruritus, seborrhea, skin discoloration, skin ulceration.
Other: *sarcoma, sepsis,* abscess, bacterial or fungal infections, flulike symptoms, inflammation and pain at infusion site, lymphadenopathy, lymphoma-like disorder, rigors.

INTERACTIONS
Drug-drug. *Calcium:* May decrease serum level of ionized calcium. Avoid concurrent use.
Nephrotoxic drugs (such as aminoglycosides, amphotericin B): May increase risk of nephrotoxicity. Avoid using together.
Pentamidine: May increase risk of nephrotoxicity; severe hypocalcemia also has been reported. Monitor renal function tests and electrolytes.
Zidovudine: May increase risk or severity of anemia. Monitor blood counts.

EFFECTS ON LAB TEST RESULTS
• May increase alkaline phosphatase, ALT, AST, bilirubin, creatinine, and phosphate levels. May decrease calcium, hemoglobin, magnesium, phosphate, potassium, and sodium levels.
• May increase platelet count. May decrease granulocyte, platelet, and WBC counts.

CONTRAINDICATIONS & CAUTIONS
• Contraindicated in patients hypersensitive to drug.
Black Box Warning In patients with abnormal renal function, use cautiously, maintain adequate hydration, and reduce dosage. Drug is nephrotoxic and can worsen renal impairment. Some degree of nephrotoxicity occurs in most patients. ∎
⚠ Overdose S&S: Seizures, renal impairment, paresthesia (limb or perioral), calcium and phosphate electrolyte disturbances.

NURSING CONSIDERATIONS
⊕ Alert: Because drug is highly toxic, which is probably dose-related, always use the lowest effective maintenance dose.
Black Box Warning Frequent monitoring of serum creatinine, with dosage adjustment for changes in renal function, is imperative. ∎

• Monitor CrCl frequently during therapy because of drug's adverse effects on renal function. Obtain a baseline 24-hour CrCl. Monitor level two to three times weekly during induction and at least once every 1 to 2 weeks during maintenance.
Black Box Warning Drug can cause seizures related to altered mineral and electrolyte levels; monitor levels using a schedule similar to that established for monitoring of CrCl. Assess patient for tetany and seizures and treat with supplementation if necessary. ∎
• Monitor patient's hemoglobin level and hematocrit. Anemia occurs in about one-third of patients and may be severe enough to require transfusions.
• Drug may cause a dose-related transient decrease in ionized calcium, which may not always show up in patient's laboratory values.

PATIENT TEACHING
• Explain the importance of adequate hydration throughout therapy.
• Advise patient to report tingling around the mouth, numbness in the arms and legs, and pins-and-needles sensations.
• Tell patient to alert nurse about discomfort at I.V. insertion site.

fosinopril sodium
foh-SIN-oh-pril

Therapeutic class: Antihypertensives
Pharmacologic class: ACE inhibitors
Pregnancy risk category: C; D in 2nd and 3rd trimesters

AVAILABLE FORMS
Tablets: 10 mg, 20 mg, 40 mg

INDICATIONS & DOSAGES
➤ **Hypertension**
Adults: Initially, 10 mg P.O. daily; adjust dosage based on blood pressure response at peak and trough levels. Usual dosage is 20 to 40 mg daily; maximum is 80 mg daily. Dosage may be divided.
Children weighing more than 50 kg (110 lb): Initially, 5 to 10 mg P.O. once daily. Maximum dosage is 40 mg/day.

➤ **Adjunctive therapy for heart failure with diuretics and/or digoxin**
Adults: Initially, 10 mg P.O. once daily. Increase dosage over several weeks to a maximum of 40 mg P.O. daily, if needed.

ADMINISTRATION
P.O.
● Give drug without regard for meals.

ACTION
Inhibits ACE, preventing conversion of angiotensin I to angiotensin II, a potent vasoconstrictor. Less angiotensin II decreases peripheral arterial resistance, thus decreasing aldosterone secretion, which reduces sodium and water retention and lowers blood pressure.

Route	Onset	Peak	Duration
P.O.	1 hr	3 hr	24 hr

Half-life: 11½ hours.

ADVERSE REACTIONS
CNS: dizziness, *stroke,* headache, fatigue, syncope, paresthesia, sleep disturbance.
CV: *MI,* chest pain, angina pectoris, rhythm disturbances, palpitations, hypotension, orthostatic hypotension.
EENT: tinnitus, sinusitis.
GI: *pancreatitis,* nausea, vomiting, diarrhea, dry mouth, abdominal distention, abdominal pain, constipation.
GU: sexual dysfunction, renal insufficiency.
Hepatic: *hepatitis.*
Metabolic: *hyperkalemia.*
Musculoskeletal: arthralgia, musculoskeletal pain, myalgia.
Respiratory: dry, persistent, tickling, nonproductive cough; *bronchospasm.*
Skin: urticaria, rash, photosensitivity reactions, pruritus.
Other: *angioedema,* decreased libido, gout.

INTERACTIONS
Drug-drug. *Antacids:* May impair absorption. Separate dosage times by at least 2 hours.
Azathioprine: May increase risk of anemia or leukopenia. Monitor hematologic studies if used together.

Diuretics, other antihypertensives: May cause excessive hypotension. Stop diuretic or lower fosinopril dosage.
Lithium: May increase lithium level and lithium toxicity. Monitor lithium level.
Nesiritide: May increase hypotensive effects. Monitor blood pressure.
NSAIDs: May decrease antihypertensive effects. Monitor blood pressure.
Potassium-sparing diuretics, potassium supplements: May cause risk of hyperkalemia. Monitor patient closely.
Drug-herb. *Capsaicin:* May cause cough. Discourage use together.
Ma huang: May decrease antihypertensive effects. Discourage use together.
Drug-food. *Salt substitutes containing potassium:* May cause hyperkalemia. Discourage use together.

EFFECTS ON LAB TEST RESULTS
● May increase BUN, creatinine, potassium, and hemoglobin levels and hematocrit.
● May increase LFT values.
● May cause falsely low digoxin level with the Digi-Tab radioimmunoassay kit for digoxin.

CONTRAINDICATIONS & CAUTIONS
● Contraindicated in patients hypersensitive to drug or other ACE inhibitors and in breast-feeding women.
● Use cautiously in patients with impaired renal or hepatic function.
Black Box Warning Use during pregnancy can cause injury and death to the developing fetus. When pregnancy is detected, stop drug as soon as possible. ∎
⚠ *Overdose S&S:* Hypotension.

NURSING CONSIDERATIONS
● Monitor blood pressure for drug effect.
● Black patients who take ACE inhibitors as monotherapy for hypertension have a smaller reduction in blood pressure than non-Black patients. Black patients taking ACE inhibitors have a higher incidence of angioedema than non-Blacks.
● Monitor potassium intake and potassium level. Diabetic patients, those with impaired renal function, and those receiving drugs that can increase potassium level may develop hyperkalemia.

Reactions in bold italics are *life-threatening*. Interactions may have a *rapid onset* or a *delayed onset*.

• Other ACE inhibitors may cause agranulocytosis and neutropenia. Monitor CBC with differential counts before therapy and periodically thereafter.

• Assess renal and hepatic function before and periodically throughout therapy.

• *Look alike–sound alike:* Don't confuse fosinopril with lisinopril. Don't confuse Monopril with Monurol.

PATIENT TEACHING

• Tell patient to avoid salt substitutes; these products may contain potassium, which can cause high potassium level in patients taking drug.

• Instruct patient to contact prescriber if light-headedness or fainting occurs.

• Advise patient to report evidence of infection, such as fever and sore throat.

• Instruct patient to call prescriber if he develops easy bruising or bleeding; swelling of tongue, lips, face, eyes, mucous membranes, arms, or legs; difficulty swallowing or breathing; cough; or hoarseness.

• Urge patient to use caution in hot weather and during exercise. Inadequate fluid intake, vomiting, diarrhea, and excessive perspiration can lead to light-headedness and fainting.

• Tell women of childbearing age to notify prescriber if pregnancy occurs. Drug will need to be stopped.

---

fosphenytoin sodium
faws-FEN-i-toe-in

Therapeutic class: Anticonvulsants
Pharmacologic class: Hydantoin derivatives
Pregnancy risk category: D

AVAILABLE FORMS

Injection: 2 mL (150 mg fosphenytoin sodium equivalent to 100 mg phenytoin sodium), 10 mL (750 mg fosphenytoin sodium equivalent to 500 mg phenytoin sodium)

INDICATIONS & DOSAGES

Adjust-a-dose (for all indications): Phenytoin clearance is decreased slightly in elderly patients; lower or less frequent dosing may be required.

➤ **Seizures**
Adults: 15 to 20 mg phenytoin sodium equivalent/kg I.V. at infusion rate of 100 to 150 mg phenytoin sodium equivalent/minute as loading dose; then 4 to 6 mg phenytoin sodium equivalent/kg daily I.V. as maintenance dose.

➤ **To prevent and treat seizures during neurosurgery (nonemergent loading or maintenance dosing)**
Adults: Loading dose of 10 to 20 mg phenytoin sodium equivalent/kg I.M. or I.V. at infusion rate not exceeding 150 mg phenytoin sodium equivalent/minute. Maintenance dose is 4 to 6 mg phenytoin sodium equivalent/kg daily I.V. or I.M.

➤ **Short-term substitution for oral phenytoin therapy**
Adults: Same total daily dose equivalent as oral phenytoin sodium therapy given as a single daily dose I.M. or I.V. at infusion rate not exceeding 150 mg phenytoin sodium equivalent/minute. Some patients may need more frequent dosing.

ADMINISTRATION

I.V.
▼ If rapid phenytoin loading is a main goal, this form is preferred.

▼ For status epilepticus, give I.V. rather than I.M. because therapeutic phenytoin level occurs more rapidly.

▼ For infusion, dilute in D_5W or normal saline solution for injection to yield 1.5 to 25 mg phenytoin sodium equivalent/mL.

Black Box Warning Don't give more than 150 mg phenytoin sodium equivalent/minute because of risk of severe hypotension and cardiac arrhythmias. For a 50-kg (110-lb) patient, infusion should take 5 to 7 minutes. (Infusion of identical molar dose of phenytoin takes at least 15 minutes, because giving phenytoin I.V. at more than 50 mg/minute causes adverse CV effects.) ■

▼ Patients receiving 20 mg phenytoin sodium equivalent/kg at 150 mg phenytoin sodium equivalent/minute typically feel discomfort, usually in the groin. To reduce discomfort, slow or temporarily stop infusion.

▼ Monitor patient's ECG, blood pressure, and respirations continuously during maximum phenytoin level—about 10 to 20 minutes after end of fosphenytoin infusion. Severe CV complications are most common in elderly or gravely ill patients. If needed, decrease rate or stop infusion.

▼ Store drug under refrigeration. Don't store at room temperature longer than 48 hours. Discard vials that develop particulate matter.

▼ **Incompatibilities:** Other I.V. drugs.

I.M.

● Depending on dose ordered, may require two separate I.M. injections.

● I.M. administration generates systemic phenytoin levels similar enough to oral phenytoin sodium to allow essentially interchangeable use.

● Store drug under refrigeration. Don't store at room temperature longer than 48 hours. Discard vials that develop particulate matter.

ACTION

May stabilize neuronal membranes and limit seizure activity either by increasing efflux or decreasing influx of sodium ions across cell membranes in the motor cortex during generation of nerve impulses.

Route	Onset	Peak	Duration
I.V.	Unknown	End of infusion	Unknown
I.M.	Unknown	30 min	Unknown

Half-life: 15 minutes (fosphenytoin); 12 to 29 hours (phenytoin).

ADVERSE REACTIONS

CNS: ataxia, dizziness, somnolence, ***brain edema, intracranial hypertension,*** agitation, asthenia, dysarthria, extrapyramidal syndrome, fever, headache, hypesthesia, incoordination, increased or decreased reflexes, nervousness, paresthesia, speech disorders, stupor, thinking abnormalities, tremor, vertigo.

CV: hypertension, hypotension, tachycardia, vasodilation.

EENT: nystagmus, amblyopia, deafness, diplopia, tinnitus.

GI: constipation, dry mouth, taste perversion, tongue disorder, vomiting.

GU: pelvic pain.

Metabolic: *hypokalemia.*

Musculoskeletal: back pain, myasthenia.

Respiratory: pneumonia.

Skin: pruritus, ecchymoses, injection-site reaction and pain, rash.

Other: accidental injury, chills, facial edema, infection.

INTERACTIONS

Drug-drug. *Amiodarone, chloramphenicol, chlordiazepoxide, cimetidine, diazepam, disulfiram, estrogens, ethosuximide, fluoxetine, H2-receptor antagonists, halothane, isoniazid, methylphenidate, phenothiazines, phenylbutazone, salicylates, succinimides, sulfonamides, tolbutamide, trazodone:* May increase phenytoin level and effect. Use together cautiously.

Carbamazepine, reserpine: May decrease phenytoin level. Monitor patient.

Corticosteroids, doxycycline, estrogens, furosemide, hormonal contraceptives, quinidine, rifampin, theophylline, vitamin D, warfarin: May decrease effects of these drugs because of increased hepatic metabolism. Monitor patient closely.

Lithium: May increase lithium toxicity. Monitor patient's neurologic status closely. Marked neurologic symptoms have been reported despite normal lithium level.

Phenobarbital, valproate sodium, valproic acid: May increase or decrease phenytoin level. May increase or decrease levels of these drugs. Monitor patient.

TCAs: May lower seizure threshold and require adjustments in phenytoin dosage. Use together cautiously.

Drug-lifestyle. *Alcohol use:* Acute intoxication may increase phenytoin level and effect. Discourage use together.

Long-term alcohol use: May decrease phenytoin level. Monitor patient and strongly discourage use together.

EFFECTS ON LAB TEST RESULTS

● May increase alkaline phosphatase, GGT, and glucose levels. May decrease folate, potassium, and T4 levels.

● May cause falsely low dexamethasone and metyrapone test results.

CONTRAINDICATIONS & CAUTIONS

• Contraindicated in patients hypersensitive to drug or its components, phenytoin, or other hydantoins.

• Contraindicated in those with sinus bradycardia, SA block, second- or third-degree AV block, or Adams-Stokes syndrome.

Black Box Warning There is an increased risk of severe hypotension and cardiac arrhythmia (bradycardia, heart block, QT-interval prolongation, ventricular tachycardia, ventricular fibrillation) with I.V. infusion rate of greater than 150 mg phenytoin sodium equivalent/minute. CV effects can also occur at lower infusion rates; therefore, cardiac monitoring is needed during and after infusion. Reduce rate or discontinue drug as clinically necessary. ∎

• Use cautiously in patients with porphyria and in those with history of hypersensitivity to similarly structured drugs, such as barbiturates, oxazolidinediones, and succinimide.

☻ Alert: If patient develops acute hepatotoxicity, discontinue drug and don't readminister.

⚠ Overdose S&S: Asystole, bradycardia, cardiac arrest, hypocalcemia, hypotension, lethargy, metabolic acidosis, nausea, syncope, tachycardia, vomiting, death.

NURSING CONSIDERATIONS

☻ Alert: Because of risk of cardiac and local toxicity with I.V. fosphenytoin administration, use oral phenytoin whenever possible.

• Most significant drug interactions are those commonly seen with phenytoin.

☻ Alert: Drug should always be prescribed and dispensed in phenytoin sodium equivalent units. Don't make adjustments in the recommended doses when substituting fosphenytoin for phenytoin, and vice versa.

• In status epilepticus, phenytoin may be used as maintenance instead of fosphenytoin, using the appropriate dose.

• Phosphate load provided by fosphenytoin (0.0037 millimole phosphate/mg phenytoin sodium equivalent) must be taken into consideration when treating patients who need phosphate restriction, such as those with severe renal impairment. Monitor laboratory values.

• Asian patients who have tested positive for the allele HLA-B*1502 have a potentially increased risk of serious skin reactions, including Stevens-Johnson syndrome and toxic epidermal necrolysis. Monitor these patients carefully.

• If patient gets exfoliative, purpuric, or bullous rash or signs and symptoms of lupus erythematosus, Stevens-Johnson syndrome, or toxic epidermal necrolysis, stop drug and notify prescriber. If rash is mild (measleslike or scarlatiniform), therapy may resume after rash disappears. If rash recurs when therapy is resumed, further fosphenytoin or phenytoin administration is contraindicated. Document that patient is allergic to drug.

• Stop drug in patients with acute hepatotoxicity.

• After administration, phenytoin levels shouldn't be monitored until conversion to phenytoin is essentially complete—about 2 hours after the end of an I.V. infusion or 4 hours after I.M. administration.

• Interpret total phenytoin levels cautiously in patients with renal or hepatic disease or hypoalbuminemia caused by an increased fraction in unbound phenytoin. It may be more useful to monitor unbound phenytoin levels in these patients. When giving drug I.V., monitor patients with renal and hepatic disease because they are at increased risk for more frequent and severe adverse reactions.

• Monitor glucose level closely in diabetic patients; drug may cause hyperglycemia.

• Abrupt withdrawal of drug may precipitate status epilepticus.

• **Look alike–sound alike:** Don't confuse Cerebyx with Cerezyme, Celexa, or Celebrex.

PATIENT TEACHING

• Warn patient that sensory disturbances may occur with I.V. administration.

• Instruct patient to immediately report adverse reactions, especially rash.

• Warn patient not to stop drug abruptly or adjust dosage without discussing with prescriber.

• Advise women of childbearing age to discuss drug therapy with prescriber if considering pregnancy.

• Advise women of childbearing age that breast-feeding isn't recommended during therapy.

frovatriptan succinate
frow-vah-TRIP-tan

Frova◆

Therapeutic class: Antimigraine drugs
Pharmacologic class: Serotonin 5-HT₁ receptor agonists
Pregnancy risk category: C

AVAILABLE FORMS
Tablets: 2.5 mg

INDICATIONS & DOSAGES
➤ **Acute treatment of migraine attacks with or without aura**
Adults: 2.5 mg P.O. taken at the first sign of migraine attack. If the headache recurs, a second tablet may be taken at least 2 hours after the first dose. The total daily dose shouldn't exceed 7.5 mg.

ADMINISTRATION
P.O.
• Give drug without regard for food.
• Give drug with a full glass of water.
• If headache returns after first dose, give a second dose after 2 hours. Don't give more than 3 tablets in 24 hours.

ACTION
May cause vasoconstriction in response to excessive dilation of extracerebral and intracranial arteries during migraine headaches.

Route	Onset	Peak	Duration
P.O.	Unknown	2–4 hr	Unknown

Half-life: 26 hours.

ADVERSE REACTIONS
CNS: dizziness, headache, fatigue, paresthesia, insomnia, anxiety, somnolence, dysesthesia, hypoesthesia, hot or cold sensation, pain.
CV: *coronary artery vasospasm, transient myocardial ischemia, MI, ventricular tachycardia, ventricular fibrillation,* chest pain, palpitations, flushing.

EENT: abnormal vision, tinnitus, sinusitis, rhinitis.
GI: dry mouth, dyspepsia, vomiting, abdominal pain, diarrhea, nausea.
Musculoskeletal: skeletal pain.
Skin: increased sweating.

INTERACTIONS
Drug-drug. *5-HT₁ agonists:* May cause additive effects. Separate doses by 24 hours.
Ergotamine-containing or ergot-type drugs (such as dihydroergotamine or methysergide): May cause prolonged vasospastic reactions. Separate doses by 24 hours.
SSRIs (such as citalopram, fluoxetine, fluvoxamine, paroxetine, sertraline): May cause weakness, hyperreflexia, and incoordination. Monitor patient closely.

EFFECTS ON LAB TEST RESULTS
None reported.

CONTRAINDICATIONS & CAUTIONS
• Contraindicated in patients hypersensitive to drug or any of its components.
• Contraindicated in patients with history or symptoms of ischemic heart disease or coronary artery vasospasm, including Prinzmetal variant angina; in those with cerebrovascular or peripheral vascular disease, including ischemic bowel disease; in those with uncontrolled hypertension; and in those with hemiplegic or basilar migraine.
• Contraindicated within 24 hours of another triptan, drug containing ergotamine, or ergot-type drug.
• Contraindicated in patients with risk factors for coronary artery disease (CAD), such as hypertension, hypercholesterolemia, smoking, obesity, diabetes, strong family history of CAD, postmenopausal women, or men older than age 40, unless patient is free from cardiac disease. If drug is used in such a patient, monitor patient closely and consider obtaining an ECG after the first dose. Intermittent, long-term users of triptans or those with risk factors should undergo periodic cardiac evaluation while using drug.
• Use cautiously in breast-feeding women. It's unknown if drug appears in breast milk.

• The safety of treating an average of more than four migraine headaches in a 30-day period hasn't been established.

NURSING CONSIDERATIONS
❸ Alert: Serious cardiac events, including acute MI, life-threatening cardiac arrhythmias, and death, may occur within a few hours of taking a triptan.

• Use drug only when patient has a clear diagnosis of migraine. If a patient has no response for the first migraine attack treated with frovatriptan, reconsider the diagnosis of migraine.

❸ Alert: Combining a triptan with an SSRI or an SSNRI may cause serotonin syndrome. Symptoms may include restlessness, hallucinations, loss of coordination, fast heartbeat, rapid changes in blood pressure, increased body temperature, hyperreflexia, nausea, vomiting, and diarrhea. Serotonin syndrome is more likely to occur when starting or increasing the dose of a triptan, SSRI, or SSNRI.

PATIENT TEACHING
• Instruct patient to take dose at first sign of migraine headache. If headache comes back after first dose, he may take a second dose after 2 hours. Tell patient not to take more than 3 tablets in 24 hours.

• Caution patient to take extra care or avoid driving and operating machinery if dizziness or fatigue develops after taking drug.

• Stress importance of immediately reporting pain, tightness, heaviness, or pressure in chest, throat, neck, or jaw, or rash or itching after taking drug.

• Instruct the patient not to take drug within 24 hours of taking another serotonin-receptor agonist or ergot-type drug.

• Tell patient dose may be taken with or without food, but to take with a full glass of fluid.

SAFETY ALERT!

fulvestrant
full-VES-trant

Faslodex

Therapeutic class: Antineoplastics
Pharmacologic class: Estrogen antagonists
Pregnancy risk category: D

AVAILABLE FORMS
Injection: 50 mg/mL in 2.5-mL and 5-mL prefilled syringes

INDICATIONS & DOSAGES
➤ **Hormone receptor–positive metastatic breast cancer with disease progression after antiestrogen therapy**
Postmenopausal women: 500 mg I.M. slowly into buttocks over 1 to 2 minutes as two 5-mL injections, one in each buttock on days 1, 15, 29, and then once monthly thereafter.

Adjust-a-dose: For patients with moderate hepatic impairment (Child-Pugh class B), give 250 mg I.M. as one 5-mL injection on days 1, 15, 29, and then monthly thereafter.

ADMINISTRATION
I.M.
• Drug is a potential teratogen. Follow safe handling procedures.
• Drug may be warmed before use by storing at room temperature for 1 hour or rolling injection gently in hands.
• Expel gas bubble from syringe before giving.
• When using the 2.5-mL syringes, both must be given to obtain full dose.
• Give slowly into buttocks.

ACTION
Competitively binds estrogen receptors and downregulates estrogen-receptor protein in human breast cancer cells. It's effective in treating estrogen receptor–positive breast tumors.

Route	Onset	Peak	Duration
I.M.	Unknown	7 days	1 mo

Half-life: About 40 days.

ADVERSE REACTIONS

CNS: asthenia, headache, pain, dizziness, insomnia, fever, paresthesia, depression, anxiety.
CV: hot flashes, chest pain, peripheral edema, vasodilation.
EENT: pharyngitis.
GI: nausea, vomiting, constipation, abdominal pain, diarrhea, anorexia.
GU: UTI.
Hematologic: anemia.
Musculoskeletal: bone pain, back pain, pelvic pain, arthritis.
Respiratory: dyspnea, cough.
Skin: injection-site pain, rash, sweating.
Other: accidental injury, flulike syndrome.

INTERACTIONS

None reported.

EFFECTS ON LAB TEST RESULTS

- May decrease hemoglobin level and hematocrit.

CONTRAINDICATIONS & CAUTIONS

- Contraindicated in pregnant women and in patients allergic to drug or any of its components.
- Use cautiously in patients with moderate or severe hepatic impairment.

NURSING CONSIDERATIONS

- Because drug is given I.M., don't use in patients with bleeding diatheses or thrombocytopenia, or in those taking anticoagulants.
- Make sure woman isn't pregnant before starting drug.

PATIENT TEACHING

- Caution women to avoid pregnancy and to report suspected pregnancy immediately.
- Inform patient of the most common side effects, including pain at injection site, headache, GI symptoms, back pain, hot flashes, and sore throat.

furosemide
fur-OH-se-mide

Lasix◇, Lasix Special†

Therapeutic class: Antihypertensives
Pharmacologic class: Loop diuretics
Pregnancy risk category: C

AVAILABLE FORMS

Injection: 10 mg/mL
Oral solution: 10 mg/mL, 40 mg/5 mL
Tablets: 20 mg, 40 mg, 80 mg, 500 mg†

INDICATIONS & DOSAGES

➤ **Acute pulmonary edema**
Adults: 40 mg I.V. injected slowly over 1 to 2 minutes; then 80 mg I.V. in 60 to 90 minutes if needed.
➤ **Edema**
Adults: 20 to 80 mg P.O. daily in the morning. If response is inadequate, give a second dose, and each succeeding dose, every 6 to 8 hours. Carefully increase dose in 20- to 40-mg increments up to 600 mg daily. Once effective dose is attained, may give once daily or b.i.d. Or, 20 to 40 mg I.V. or I.M., increased by 20 mg 2 hours after previous dose until desired effect achieved.
Infants and children: 2 mg/kg P.O. daily, increased by 1 to 2 mg/kg in 6 to 8 hours if needed; carefully adjusted up to 6 mg/kg daily if needed. Or, 1 mg/kg slowly I.V. or I.M. Dosage may be increased by 1 mg/kg 2 hours after previous dose if needed up to 6 mg/kg/day.
➤ **Hypertension**
Adults: 40 mg P.O. b.i.d. Dosage adjusted based on response. May be used as adjunct to other antihypertensives if needed.

ADMINISTRATION
P.O.
- To prevent nocturia, give in the morning. Give second dose if ordered in early afternoon, 6 to 8 hours after morning dose.
- Give drug with food to prevent GI upset.
- Store tablets in light-resistant container to prevent discoloration (doesn't affect potency). Refrigerate oral solution to ensure drug stability.

Reactions in bold italics are *life-threatening*. Interactions may have a *rapid onset* or a *delayed onset*.

I.V.
▼ If discolored yellow, don't use.
▼ For direct injection, give over 1 to 2 minutes.
▼ For infusion, dilute with D_5W, normal saline solution, or lactated Ringer solution.
◐ *Alert:* To avoid ototoxicity, infuse no more than 4 mg/minute.
▼ Use prepared infusion solution within 24 hours.
▼ **Incompatibilities:** Acidic solutions, aminoglycosides, amiodarone, ascorbic acid, azithromycin, bleomycin, buprenorphine, chlorpromazine, ciprofloxacin, diazepam, diltiazem, dobutamine, doxapram, doxorubicin, droperidol, epinephrine, erythromycin, esmolol, filgrastim, fluconazole, fructose 10% in water, gentamicin, hydralazine, idarubicin, invert sugar 10% in electrolyte #2, isoproterenol, levofloxacin, mannitol, meperidine, methocarbamol, metoclopramide, midazolam, milrinone, morphine, netilmicin, norepinephrine, ondansetron, oxytetracycline, prochlorperazine, promethazine, protamine, quinidine, tetracycline, thiamine, vinblastine, vincristine, vitamins B and C.

I.M.
● To prevent nocturia, give in the morning. Give second dose if ordered in early afternoon, 6 to 8 hours after morning dose.
● Record administration site.

ACTION
Inhibits sodium and chloride reabsorption at the proximal and distal tubules and the ascending loop of Henle.

Route	Onset	Peak	Duration
P.O.	20–60 min	1–2 hr	6–8 hr
I.V.	Within 5 min	30 min	2 hr
I.M.	Unknown	30 min	2 hr

Half-life: 2 hours.

ADVERSE REACTIONS
CNS: vertigo, headache, dizziness, paresthesia, weakness, restlessness, fever.
CV: orthostatic hypotension, thrombophlebitis with I.V. administration.
EENT: transient deafness, blurred or yellowed vision, tinnitus.

GI: abdominal discomfort and pain, diarrhea, anorexia, nausea, vomiting, constipation, *pancreatitis.*
GU: azotemia, nocturia, polyuria, frequent urination, oliguria.
Hematologic: *agranulocytosis, aplastic anemia, leukopenia, thrombocytopenia,* anemia.
Hepatic: hepatic dysfunction, jaundice.
Metabolic: volume depletion and dehydration, asymptomatic hyperuricemia, impaired glucose tolerance, *hypokalemia,* hypochloremic alkalosis, hyperglycemia, dilutional hyponatremia, *hypocalcemia, hypomagnesemia.*
Musculoskeletal: muscle spasm.
Skin: dermatitis, purpura, photosensitivity reactions, transient pain at I.M. injection site.
Other: gout.

INTERACTIONS
Drug-drug. *Aminoglycoside antibiotics, cisplatin:* May increase ototoxicity. Use together cautiously.
Amphotericin B, corticosteroids, corticotropin, metolazone: May increase risk of hypokalemia. Monitor potassium level closely.
Antidiabetics: May decrease hypoglycemic effects. Monitor glucose level.
Antihypertensives: May increase risk of hypotension. Use together cautiously. Decrease antihypertensive dose if needed.
Cardiac glycosides, neuromuscular blockers: May increase toxicity of these drugs from furosemide-induced hypokalemia. Monitor potassium level.
Chlorothiazide, chlorthalidone, hydrochlorothiazide, indapamide, metolazone: May cause excessive diuretic response, causing serious electrolyte abnormalities or dehydration. Adjust doses carefully, and monitor patient closely for signs and symptoms of excessive diuretic response.
Ethacrynic acid: May increase risk of ototoxicity. Avoid using together.
Lithium: May decrease lithium excretion, resulting in lithium toxicity. Monitor lithium level.
NSAIDs: May inhibit diuretic response. Use together cautiously.

Phenytoin: May decrease diuretic effects of furosemide. Use together cautiously.

Propranolol: May increase propranolol level. Monitor patient closely.

Salicylates: May cause salicylate toxicity. Use together cautiously.

Sucralfate: May reduce diuretic and antihypertensive effect. Separate doses by 2 hours.

Drug-herb. *Aloe:* May increase drug effect. Discourage use together.

Dandelion: May interfere with drug activity. Discourage use together.

Ginseng: May decrease drug effect. Discourage use together.

Licorice: May cause unexpected rapid potassium loss. Discourage use together.

Drug-lifestyle. *Sun exposure:* May increase risk for photosensitivity reactions. Advise patient to avoid excessive sunlight exposure.

EFFECTS ON LAB TEST RESULTS

● May increase cholesterol, glucose, BUN, creatinine, and uric acid levels. May decrease calcium, hemoglobin, magnesium, potassium, and sodium levels.

● May decrease granulocyte, platelet, and WBC counts.

CONTRAINDICATIONS & CAUTIONS

● Contraindicated in patients hypersensitive to drug and in those with anuria.

● Use cautiously in patients with hepatic cirrhosis and in those allergic to sulfonamides. Use during pregnancy only if potential benefits to mother clearly outweigh risks to fetus.

⬥ Alert: Drug may cause tinnitus and reversible or irreversible hearing loss. Ototoxicity is associated with rapid injection, severe renal impairment, use of higher-than-recommended doses, hypoproteinemia, or use with other ototoxic drugs.

● Use cautiously in breast-feeding women. Drug appears in breast milk and may inhibit lactation.

● Premature infants may be at increased risk for persistent patent ductus arteriosus with furosemide treatment during first weeks of life.

⚠ Overdose S&S: Dehydration, blood volume reduction, hypotension, electrolyte imbalance.

NURSING CONSIDERATIONS

⬥ Alert: Monitor weight, blood pressure, and pulse rate routinely with long-term use.

Black Box Warning Drug is potent diuretic and can cause severe diuresis with water and electrolyte depletion. Monitor patient closely. ▌

● If oliguria or azotemia develops or increases, drug may need to be stopped.

● Monitor fluid intake and output and electrolyte, BUN, and carbon dioxide levels frequently.

● Watch for signs of hypokalemia, such as muscle weakness and cramps.

● Consult prescriber and dietitian about a high-potassium diet or potassium supplements. Foods rich in potassium include citrus fruits, tomatoes, bananas, dates, and apricots.

● Monitor glucose level in diabetic patients.

● Drug may not be well absorbed orally in patient with severe heart failure. Drug may need to be given I.V. even if patient is taking other oral drugs.

● Monitor uric acid level, especially in patients with a history of gout.

● Monitor elderly patients, who are especially susceptible to excessive diuresis, because circulatory collapse and thromboembolic complications are possible.

● Monitor patients with severe symptoms of urine retention due to bladder emptying disorders, prostate enlargement, or urethral narrowing or worsening of symptoms, especially during initial treatment.

● Drug may increase fetal birth weight. Monitor fetal growth during pregnancy.

● Nephrocalcinosis and nephrolithiasis have occurred in premature infants and in children younger than age 4 on long-term furosemide therapy. Monitor renal function and renal ultrasounds.

● *Look alike–sound alike:* Don't confuse furosemide with torsemide. Don't confuse Lasix with Lonox, Lidex, or Luvox.

PATIENT TEACHING

● Advise patient to take drug with food to prevent GI upset, and to take drug in morning to prevent need to urinate at night. If patient needs second dose, tell him to take it in early afternoon, 6 to 8 hours after morning dose.

• Inform patient of possible need for potassium or magnesium supplements.

• Instruct patient to stand slowly to prevent dizziness and to limit alcohol intake and strenuous exercise in hot weather to avoid worsening dizziness upon standing quickly.

• Advise patient to immediately report ringing in ears, severe abdominal pain, or sore throat and fever; these symptoms may indicate toxicity.

🜲 *Alert:* Discourage patient from storing different types of drugs in the same container, increasing the risk of drug errors. The most popular strengths of this drug and digoxin are white tablets about equal in size.

• Tell patient to check with prescriber or pharmacist before taking OTC drugs.

• Teach patient to avoid direct sunlight and to use protective clothing and a sunblock because of risk of photosensitivity reactions.

gabapentin
gab-ah-PEN-tin

Gralise, Neurontin✐

gabapentin enacarbil
Horizant

Therapeutic class: Anticonvulsants
Pharmacologic class: GABA structural analogues
Pregnancy risk category: C

AVAILABLE FORMS
Capsules: 100 mg, 300 mg, 400 mg
Oral solution: 250 mg/5 mL
Tablets: 100 mg, 300 mg, 400 mg, 600 mg, 800 mg
Tablets (extended-release): 300 mg, 600 mg

INDICATIONS & DOSAGES
Adjust-a-dose (for all indications): For patients age 12 and older with CrCl of 30 to 59 mL/minute, give 400 to 1,400 mg daily divided into two doses. For CrCl of 15 to 29 mL/minute, give 200 to 700 mg daily in a single dose. For CrCl of less than 15 mL/minute, give 100 to 300 mg daily in a single dose. Reduce daily dosage in proportion to CrCl (patients with a CrCl of 7.5 mL/minute should receive one-half the daily dosage of those with a CrCl of 15 mL/minute). For patients receiving hemodialysis, maintenance dosage is based on estimates of CrCl. Give supplemental dose of 125 to 350 mg after each 4 hours of hemodialysis.

➤ **Adjunctive treatment of partial seizures with or without secondary generalization in patients with epilepsy**
Adults and children older than age 12: Initially, 300 mg P.O. t.i.d. Increase dosage as needed and tolerated to 1,800 mg daily in divided doses. Dosages up to 3,600 mg daily have been well tolerated.

➤ **Adjunctive treatment to control partial seizures in children**
Starting dosage, children ages 3 to 12: 10 to 15 mg/kg daily P.O. in three divided doses, adjusting over 3 days to reach effective dosage.
Effective dosage, children ages 5 to 12: 25 to 35 mg/kg daily P.O. in three divided doses.
Effective dosage, children ages 3 to 4: 40 mg/kg daily P.O. in three divided doses.

➤ **Moderate to severe primary restless legs syndrome (Horizant)**
Adults: 600 mg extended-release tablet P.O. daily at about 5 p.m. If dose isn't taken at the recommended time, the next dose should be taken the following day as prescribed.
Adjust-a-dose: If CrCl is 30 to 59 mL/minute, give 600 mg on day 1, day 3, and then daily thereafter. Don't give to patients with CrCl of less than 30 mL/minute or to those receiving hemodialysis.

➤ **Postherpetic neuralgia (immediate-release)**
Adults: 300 mg P.O. once daily on first day, 300 mg b.i.d. on day 2, and 300 mg t.i.d. on day 3. Adjust as needed for pain to a maximum daily dose of 1,800 mg in three divided doses.

➤ **Postherpetic neuralgia (Gralise)**
Adults: Titrate dosage to 1,800 mg P.O. once daily with the evening meal. On day 1, give 300 mg; on day 2, 600 mg; on days 3 to 6, 900 mg; on days 7 to 10, 1,200 mg; on days 11 to 14, 1,500 mg; and on day 15 and thereafter, 1,800 mg.

G

Adjust-a-dose: For patients with reduced renal function, initiate Gralise at a daily dose of 300 mg. For patients with CrCl of 30 to 60 mL/minute, titrate dosage to 600 to 1,800 mg daily as tolerated. Don't give Gralise to patients with CrCl of less than 30 mL/minute or to those receiving hemodialysis.

➤ **Pain from diabetic neuropathy ◆**
Adults: 900 mg to 3.6 g P.O. daily in three divided doses.

➤ **Vasomotor symptoms in women with breast cancer and in postmenopausal women ◆**
Women: For cancer-related symptoms, 200 to 1,600 mg P.O. once daily to q.i.d. for 4 to 8 weeks. For postmenopausal symptoms, 200 to 2,700 mg P.O. once daily to q.i.d. for up to 12 weeks.

ADMINISTRATION
P.O.
● Give immediate-release forms without regard for food.
● Give extended-release tablets with food.
● Give drug 2 hours after an antacid.
● Refrigerate oral solution.
● Patient should swallow extended-release tablets whole and shouldn't cut, crush, or chew them.
● Gralise, Horizant, and other gabapentin products aren't interchangeable.

ACTION
Unknown. Structurally related to GABA but doesn't interact with GABA receptors, isn't converted into GABA or GABA agonist, doesn't inhibit GABA reuptake, and doesn't prevent degradation.

Route	Onset	Peak	Duration
P.O. (gabapentin immediate-release)	Unknown	2 hr	Unknown
P.O. (gabapentin extended-release)	Unknown	8 hr	Unknown
P.O. (gabapentin enacarbil)	Unknown	5–7 hr	Unknown

Half-life: 5 to 7 hours (gabapentin); 5 to 6 hours (gabapentin enacarbil).

ADVERSE REACTIONS
CNS: ataxia, dizziness, fatigue, somnolence, abnormal thinking, amnesia, depression, dysarthria, incoordination, nervousness, tremor.
CV: peripheral edema, vasodilation.
EENT: amblyopia, diplopia, dry throat, pharyngitis, rhinitis.
GI: constipation, dry mouth, dyspepsia, increased appetite, nausea, vomiting; diarrhea (Gralise).
GU: erectile dysfunction; UTI (Gralise).
Hematologic: *leukopenia.*
Metabolic: weight gain.
Musculoskeletal: back pain, fractures, myalgia.
Respiratory: coughing.
Skin: abrasion, pruritus.
Other: dental abnormalities.

INTERACTIONS
Drug-drug. *Antacids:* May decrease absorption of gabapentin. Separate dosage times by at least 2 hours.
Hydrocodone: May increase gabapentin level and decrease hydrocodone level. Monitor patient for increased adverse effects or loss of clinical effect.

EFFECTS ON LAB TEST RESULTS
● May decrease WBC count.
● May cause false-positive results with the Ames N-Multistix SG dipstick test for urine protein when used with other anticonvulsants.

CONTRAINDICATIONS & CAUTIONS
● Contraindicated in patients hypersensitive to drug.
● Use during pregnancy only if the potential benefit justifies the potential risk to the fetus.
● In elderly patients, adjust dosage based on CrCl values due to potentially decreased renal function.
● Gabapentin enacarbil isn't recommended for patients who must sleep during the day and remain awake at night.
⚠ ***Overdose S&S:*** Double vision, slurred speech, drowsiness, lethargy, diarrhea.

NURSING CONSIDERATIONS
● Give first dose at bedtime to minimize drowsiness, dizziness, fatigue, and ataxia.

> *Alert:* Closely monitor all patients taking or starting antiepileptic drugs for changes in behavior indicating worsening of suicidal thoughts or behavior or depression. Symptoms such as anxiety, agitation, hostility, mania, and hypomania may be precursors to emerging suicidality.

• If drug is to be stopped or an alternative drug substituted, do so gradually over at least 1 week to minimize risk of precipitating seizures.

> *Alert:* Don't suddenly withdraw other anticonvulsants in patients starting gabapentin therapy.

• Routine monitoring of drug levels isn't necessary. Drug doesn't appear to alter levels of other anticonvulsants.

• *Look alike–sound alike:* Don't confuse Neurontin with Noroxin.

PATIENT TEACHING
• Advise patient that drug may be taken without regard for meals.
• Advise patient to take extended-release tablets with food.
• Instruct patient to take first dose at bedtime to minimize adverse reactions.
• Tell patient with seizures that the maximum time interval between doses shouldn't exceed 12 hours.
• Warn patient that extended-release formulas can cause significant dizziness and sleepiness.
• Warn patient to avoid driving and operating heavy machinery until drug's CNS effects are known.
• Advise patient not to take extended-release formulas with alcohol or other drugs that may cause sleepiness or dizziness.
• Advise patient not to stop drug abruptly.
• Advise women to discuss drug therapy with prescriber if considering pregnancy.
• Tell patient to keep oral solution refrigerated.

galantamine hydrobromide
gah-LAN-tah-meen

Razadyne, Razadyne ER

Therapeutic class: Anti-Alzheimer drugs
Pharmacologic class: Cholinesterase inhibitors
Pregnancy risk category: B

AVAILABLE FORMS
Capsules (extended-release): 8 mg, 16 mg, 24 mg
Oral solution: 4 mg/mL
Tablets: 4 mg, 8 mg, 12 mg

INDICATIONS & DOSAGES
➤ **Mild to moderate Alzheimer dementia**
Adults: Initially, 4 mg b.i.d., preferably with morning and evening meals. If dose is well tolerated after minimum of 4 weeks of therapy, increase dosage to 8 mg b.i.d. A further increase to 12 mg b.i.d. may be attempted, but only after at least 4 weeks of therapy at the previous dosage. Dosage range is 16 to 24 mg daily in two divided doses.

Or, 8 mg extended-release capsule P.O. once daily in the morning with food. Increase to 16 mg P.O. once daily after a minimum of 4 weeks. May further increase to 24 mg once daily after a minimum of 4 weeks, based on patient response and tolerability.

Adjust-a-dose: For patients with Child-Pugh score of 7 to 9, dosage usually shouldn't exceed 16 mg daily. Drug isn't recommended for patients with Child-Pugh score of 10 to 15. For patients with moderate renal impairment, dosage usually shouldn't exceed 16 mg daily. For patients with CrCl less than 9 mL/minute, drug isn't recommended.

ADMINISTRATION
P.O.
> *Alert:* Give Razadyne tablets twice daily; give Razadyne ER capsules once daily. To avoid dosing errors, verify any prescription that suggests a different dosing schedule.

• Give drug with food and antiemetics, and ensure adequate fluid intake to decrease the risk of nausea and vomiting.
• Use proper technique when dispensing the oral solution with the pipette. Dispense measured amount into a beverage and give to patient right away.

ACTION

Thought to enhance cholinergic function by increasing acetylcholine level in brain.

Route	Onset	Peak	Duration
P.O.	Unknown	1 hr	Unknown

Half-life: About 7 hours.

ADVERSE REACTIONS

CNS: depression, dizziness, headache, tremor, insomnia, somnolence, fatigue, syncope, tremor.
CV: *bradycardia, AV block.*
EENT: rhinitis.
GI: diarrhea, nausea, vomiting, abdominal pain, dyspepsia, anorexia.
GU: UTI, hematuria, urinary incontinence.
Hematologic: anemia.
Metabolic: weight loss.

INTERACTIONS

Drug-drug. *Amitriptyline, fluoxetine, fluvoxamine, quinidine:* May decrease galantamine clearance. Monitor patient closely.
Anticholinergics: May antagonize anticholinergic activity. Monitor patient.
Cholinergics (such as bethanechol, succinylcholine): May have synergistic effect. Monitor patient closely. May need to avoid use before procedures using general anesthesia with succinylcholine-type neuromuscular blockers.
Cimetidine, clarithromycin, erythromycin, ketoconazole, paroxetine: May increase galantamine bioavailability. Monitor patient closely.
NSAIDs: May increase risk of bleeding due to increased gastric acid secretion. Monitor patient for symptoms of active or occult GI bleeding.

EFFECTS ON LAB TEST RESULTS

None reported.

CONTRAINDICATIONS & CAUTIONS

• Contraindicated in patients hypersensitive to drug or its components.
• Use cautiously in patients with supraventricular cardiac conduction disorders and in those taking other drugs that significantly slow heart rate.
• Use cautiously during or before procedures involving anesthesia using succinylcholine-type or similar neuromuscular blockers.
• Use cautiously in patients with history of peptic ulcer disease and in those taking NSAIDs. Because of the potential for cholinomimetic effects, use cautiously in patients with bladder outflow obstruction, seizures, asthma, or COPD.
⚠ *Overdose S&S:* Muscle weakness, muscle fasciculations, nausea, vomiting, GI cramping, excessive salivation, excessive lacrimation, sweating, bradycardia, hypotension, respiratory depression, syncope, seizures, QT-interval prolongation, hallucinations.

NURSING CONSIDERATIONS

❸ *Alert:* Drug may cause bradycardia and heart block. Consider all patients at risk for adverse effects on cardiac conduction.
• If drug is stopped for 3 days or longer, restart at the lowest dose and gradually increase, at 4-week or longer intervals, to the previous dosage level.
• Because of the risk of increased gastric acid secretion, monitor patients closely for symptoms of active or occult GI bleeding, especially those with an increased risk of developing ulcers.
• Monitor patient's weight during therapy.
• Monitor patients closely for seizures.

PATIENT TEACHING

• Advise caregiver to give drug with morning and evening meals (for the conventional form), or only in the morning (for the extended-release form) and with food.
• Inform patient that nausea and vomiting are common adverse effects.
• Teach caregiver the proper technique when measuring the oral solution with the pipette. Tell her to place measured amount in a nonalcoholic beverage and have patient drink right away.

- Urge patient or caregiver to report slow heartbeat immediately.
- Advise patient and caregiver that although drug may improve cognitive function, it doesn't alter the underlying disease process.

ganciclovir (DHPG)
gan-SYE-kloe-vir

Cytovene, Zirgan

Therapeutic class: Antivirals
Pharmacologic class: Nucleosides–nucleotides
Pregnancy risk category: C

AVAILABLE FORMS
Injection: 500 mg/vial
Ophthalmic gel: 0.15%

INDICATIONS & DOSAGES
Black Box Warning Ganciclovir I.V. is indicated only for the treatment of CMV retinitis in immunocompromised patients and for the prevention of CMV disease in transplant patients at risk for CMV disease. ∎

➤ **CMV retinitis in immunocompromised patients, including those with AIDS and normal renal function**
Adults: Induction treatment is 5 mg/kg I.V. every 12 hours for 14 to 21 days. Maintenance treatment is 5 mg/kg I.V. daily 7 days per week or 6 mg/kg I.V. daily five times weekly.

➤ **To prevent CMV disease in transplant recipients with normal renal function**
Adults: 5 mg/kg I.V. (given at a constant rate over 1 hour) every 12 hours for 7 to 14 days; then 5 mg/kg daily 7 days per week or 6 mg/kg daily five times weekly. Duration of therapy depends on degree of immunosuppression.

Initial I.V. therapy

CrCl (mL/min)	Dose (mg/kg)	Interval
50–69	2.5	12 hr
25–49	2.5	24 hr
10–24	1.25	24 hr
<10	1.25	3 times weekly after hemodialysis

Maintenance I.V. therapy

CrCl (mL/min)	Dose (mg/kg)	Interval
50–69	2.5	24 hr
25–49	1.25	24 hr
10–24	0.625	24 hr
<10	0.625	3 times weekly after hemodialysis

Adjust-a-dose: Adjust dosage in patients with renal impairment according to the table. If patient is receiving hemodialysis, give dose shortly after session is complete.

➤ **Acute herpetic keratitis**
Adults: 1 drop in affected eye five times daily (approximately every 3 hours while awake) until the corneal ulcer heals; then 1 drop t.i.d. for 7 days.

ADMINISTRATION
I.V.
▼ To reconstitute, add 10 mL sterile water for injection to 500-mg vial. Shake vial well to dissolve drug.
▼ Further dilute in 50 to 250 mL (usually 100 mL) of compatible I.V. solution.
▼ If fluids are being restricted, dilute to no more than 10 mg/mL.
▼ Don't give as bolus.
▼ Use an infusion pump.
▼ Infuse over at least 1 hour.
▼ Infusing drug too rapidly has toxic effects.
▼ Use caution when preparing solution, which is alkaline.
🕭 *Alert:* Don't give subcutaneously or I.M.
▼ **Incompatibilities:** Aldesleukin, amifostine, aztreonam, cefepime, cytarabine, doxorubicin hydrochloride, fludarabine, foscarnet, ondansetron, other I.V. drugs, paraben (bacteriostatic agent), piperacillin sodium–tazobactam, sargramostim, vinorelbine.

Ophthalmic
- Store at 59° to 77° F (15° to 20° C). Don't freeze.

ACTION
Inhibits binding of deoxyguanosine triphosphate to DNA polymerase, resulting in inhibition of DNA synthesis.

Route	Onset	Peak	Duration
I.V.	Unknown	Immediate	Unknown
Ophthalmic	Unknown	Unknown	Unknown

Half-life: About 4 hours (I.V.); ophthalmic, unknown.

ADVERSE REACTIONS

CNS: fever, *coma, seizures,* abnormal thinking, agitation, altered dreams, amnesia, anxiety, asthenia, ataxia, confusion, dizziness, headache, somnolence, tremor, neuropathy, paresthesia.
EENT: retinal detachment in CMV retinitis patients.
GI: abdominal pain, anorexia, diarrhea, nausea, vomiting, dry mouth, dyspepsia, flatulence.
Hematologic: anemia, *agranulocytosis, leukopenia, thrombocytopenia.*
Respiratory: pneumonia.
Skin: rash, sweating, inflammation, pruritus, pain and phlebitis at injection site.
Other: *sepsis,* chills, infection.

INTERACTIONS

Drug-drug. *Amphotericin B, cyclosporine, other nephrotoxic drugs:* May increase risk of nephrotoxicity. Monitor renal function.
Cytotoxic drugs: May increase toxic effects, especially hematologic effects and stomatitis. Monitor patient closely.
Imipenem–cilastatin: May increase seizure activity. Use together only if potential benefits outweigh risks.
Immunosuppressants (such as azathioprine, corticosteroids, cyclosporine): May enhance immune and bone marrow suppression. Use together cautiously.
Probenecid: May increase ganciclovir level. Monitor patient closely.
Zidovudine: May increase risk of agranulocytosis. Use together cautiously; monitor hematologic function closely.

EFFECTS ON LAB TEST RESULTS

● May increase alkaline phosphatase, ALT, AST, creatinine, and GGT levels. May decrease hemoglobin level.
● May decrease granulocyte, neutrophil, platelet, and WBC counts.

CONTRAINDICATIONS & CAUTIONS

Black Box Warning Contraindicated in patients hypersensitive to drug or acyclovir and in those with an absolute neutrophil count below 500/mm^3 or a platelet count below 25,000/mm^3. ∎
● Use cautiously and reduce dosage in patients with renal dysfunction. Monitor renal function tests.
Black Box Warning Ganciclovir caused aspermatogenesis and was carcinogenic and teratogenic in animal studies. ∎
⚠ *Overdose S&S:* Persistent bone marrow suppression, reversible neutropenia or granulocytopenia, hepatitis, renal toxicity, seizures (all with I.V. form).

NURSING CONSIDERATIONS

Black Box Warning Because of the frequency of agranulocytosis and thrombocytopenia, obtain neutrophil and platelet counts every 2 days during twice-daily dosing and at least weekly thereafter. ∎

PATIENT TEACHING

● Explain importance of drinking plenty of fluids during therapy.
● Instruct patient to report adverse reactions promptly.
● Tell patient to report discomfort at I.V. insertion site.
● Advise patient that drug causes birth defects. Instruct women to use effective birth control; men should use barrier contraception during and for at least 90 days after I.V. therapy.
● Advise patient using gel not to let dropper touch any surface because dropper is sterile.
● Advise patient not to wear contact lenses while undergoing ophthalmic treatment.
● Advise patient undergoing ophthalmic treatment to notify prescriber if eye pain, redness, itching, or inflammation becomes aggravated.

Reactions in bold italics are *life-threatening*. Interactions may have a *rapid onset* or a *delayed onset.*

gatifloxacin
ga-ti-FLOKS-a-sin

Zymar, Zymaxid

Therapeutic class: Antibiotics
Pharmacologic class: Fluoroquinolones
Pregnancy risk category: C

AVAILABLE FORMS
Solution: 0.3%, 0.5%

INDICATIONS & DOSAGES
➤ **Bacterial conjunctivitis caused by** *Corynebacterium propinquum, Streptococcus mitis, Staphylococcus aureus, Staphylococcus epidermidis, Streptococcus pneumoniae,* **or** *Haemophilus influenzae*
Adults and children age 1 and older: Instill 1 drop into affected eye every 2 hours while patient is awake, up to eight times daily for 2 days. Then instill 1 drop up to q.i.d. for 5 more days.
➤ **Bacterial conjunctivitis caused by** *S. mitis, S. aureus, S. epidermidis, S. pneumoniae,* **or** *H. influenzae*
Adults and children age 1 and older: Instill 1 drop Zymaxid into affected eye every 2 hours while patient is awake, up to eight times on day 1. Then instill 1 drop b.i.d. to q.i.d. while patient is awake on days 2 to 7.

ADMINISTRATION
Ophthalmic
● Apply gentle pressure to the inside corner of the eyelid for 1 to 2 minutes after instilling drop.

ACTION
Inhibits DNA gyrase and topoisomerase, preventing cell replication and division.

Route	Onset	Peak	Duration
Ophthalmic	Unknown	Unknown	Unknown

Half-life: Unknown.

ADVERSE REACTIONS
CNS: headache.
EENT: conjunctival irritation, increased lacrimation, keratitis, papillary conjunctivitis, chemosis, conjunctival hemorrhage, discharge, dry eyes, eye irritation, eyelid edema, pain, red eyes, reduced visual acuity.
GI: taste disturbance.

INTERACTIONS
None reported.

EFFECTS ON LAB TEST RESULTS
None reported.

CONTRAINDICATIONS & CAUTIONS
● Contraindicated in patients hypersensitive to drug or other quinolones.
● Safety and effectiveness in infants younger than age 1 year have not been established.
● Use cautiously in pregnant or breast-feeding women.

NURSING CONSIDERATIONS
● Solution isn't for injection subconjunctivally or into the anterior chamber of the eye.
● Systemic drug may cause serious hypersensitivity reactions. If allergic reaction occurs, stop drug and treat symptoms.
● Monitor patient for superinfection.
● Growth of resistant organisms, including fungi, may occur with prolonged use. Monitor patient carefully.

PATIENT TEACHING
● Urge patient to immediately stop drug and seek medical treatment if evidence of a serious allergic reaction, such as itching, rash, swelling of the face or throat, or difficulty breathing, develops.
● Instruct patient to apply gentle pressure to inside corner of eyelid for 1 to 2 minutes after instilling drop.
● Tell patient not to wear contact lenses during treatment.
● Warn patient to avoid touching the applicator tip to anything, including eyes and fingers.
● Teach patient that prolonged use may encourage infections with nonsusceptible bacteria.

G

gemcitabine hydrochloride
jem-SITE-ah-been

Gemzar

Therapeutic class: Antineoplastics
Pharmacologic class: Pyrimidine analogues
Pregnancy risk category: D

AVAILABLE FORMS
Powder for injection: 200-mg, 1-g vials
Solution for injection: 200-mg, 1-g, 2-g vials

INDICATIONS & DOSAGES
➤ **Locally advanced or metastatic adenocarcinoma of pancreas**
Adults: 1,000 mg/m^2 I.V. over 30 minutes once weekly for up to 7 weeks, unless toxicity occurs. Monitor CBC with differential and platelet count before giving each dose.
Adjust-a-dose: If bone marrow suppression is detected, adjust therapy. If absolute granulocyte count (AGC) is 1,000/mm^3 or more and platelet count is 100,000/mm^3 or more, give full dose. If AGC is 500 to 999/mm^3 or platelet count is 50,000 to 99,000/mm^3, give 75% of dose. If AGC is below 500/mm^3 or platelet count is below 50,000/mm^3, withhold dose. Course of 7 weeks is followed by 1 week of rest. Subsequent dosage cycles consist of one infusion weekly for 3 consecutive weeks out of every 4 weeks. Dosage adjustments for subsequent cycles are based on AGC and platelet count nadirs and degree of nonhematologic toxicity.
➤ **With cisplatin, first-line treatment of inoperable, locally advanced, or metastatic non–small-cell lung cancer**
Adults: For 4-week schedule, 1,000 mg/m^2 I.V. over 30 minutes on days 1, 8, and 15 of each 28-day cycle. 100 mg/m^2 cisplatin on day 1 after gemcitabine infusion.

For 3-week schedule, 1,250 mg/m^2 I.V. over 30 minutes on days 1 and 8 of each 21-day cycle. 100 mg/m^2 cisplatin on day 1 after gemcitabine infusion.

Adjust-a-dose: If bone marrow suppression is detected, adjust therapy. If AGC is 1,000/mm^3 or more and platelet count is 100,000/mm^3 or more, give full dose. If AGC is 500 to 999/mm^3 or platelet count is 50,000 to 99,000/mm^3, give 75% of dose. If AGC is below 500/mm^3 or platelet count is below 50,000/mm^3, withhold dose.
➤ **With carboplatin, for treatment of advanced ovarian cancer that relapsed at least 6 months after platinum-based therapy**
Adults: 1,000 mg/m^2 I.V. over 30 minutes on days 1 and 8 of each 21-day cycle. Give carboplatin (area under the curve 4) I.V. on day 1 after gemcitabine. Check CBC with differential and platelet count before each dose. The AGC should be 1,500/mm^3 or higher and platelet count 100,000/mm^3 or higher before each cycle.
Adjust-a-dose: Base adjustment on AGC and platelet count results on day 8 of cycle. If AGC is 1,000 to 1,499/mm^3, give 50% of dose. If AGC is below 1,000/mm^3 or platelet count is below 75,000/mm^3, hold dose. Adjustments for subsequent cycles based on observed toxicities.
➤ **With paclitaxel, first-line therapy for metastatic breast cancer after failure of other adjuvant chemotherapy with an anthracycline**
Adults: 1,250 mg/m^2 I.V. over 30 minutes on days 1 and 8 of each 21-day cycle, with 175 mg/m^2 paclitaxel I.V. as a 3-hour infusion given before gemcitabine dose on day 1 of the cycle. Adjust dosage based on total AGC and platelet counts taken on day 8 of the cycle.
Adjust-a-dose: If AGC is 1,000 to 1,199/mm^3 or platelet count is 50,000 to 75,000/mm^3, give 75% of dose. If AGC is 700 to 999/mm^3 and platelet count is 50,000/mm^3 or above, give 50% of dose. If AGC is below 700/mm^3 or platelet count is below 50,000/mm^3, withhold dose.

ADMINISTRATION
I.V.
▼ Preparing and giving parenteral drug may be mutagenic, teratogenic, or carcinogenic. Follow facility policy to reduce risks.

▼ To prepare solution, add 5 mL of unpreserved normal saline solution for injection to 200-mg vial or 25 mL to 1-g vial. Shake to dissolve.

▼ Resulting concentration is 40 mg/mL; reconstitution at higher concentrations isn't recommended.

▼ If needed, dilute to as little as 0.1 mg/mL by adding normal saline solution for injection.

▼ Make sure solution is clear to light straw-colored and free of particles.

▼ Don't extend infusion time beyond 60 minutes or give drug more often than once weekly; doing so may increase toxicity.

▼ Drug is stable 24 hours at room temperature.

▼ Don't refrigerate reconstituted drug because it may crystallize.

▼ **Incompatibilities:** Acyclovir, amphotericin B, cefoperazone, cefotaxime, furosemide, ganciclovir, imipenem–cilastatin, irinotecan, methotrexate, methylprednisolone, mitomycin, piperacillin, piperacillin–tazobactam sodium, prochlorperazine, sodium succinate.

ACTION

Cytotoxic and specific to cell cycle; inhibits DNA synthesis and blocks progression of cells.

Route	Onset	Peak	Duration
I.V.	Unknown	Unknown	Unknown

Half-life: About 2 to 19½ hours.

ADVERSE REACTIONS

CNS: somnolence, paresthesia, pain, fever.
CV: edema, peripheral edema.
GI: stomatitis, nausea, vomiting, constipation, diarrhea.
GU: proteinuria, hematuria.
Hematologic: anemia, *leukopenia, neutropenia, thrombocytopenia, hemorrhage.*
Hepatic: *hepatotoxicity.*
Respiratory: dyspnea, *bronchospasm, pneumonitis.*
Skin: alopecia, rash, pain at injection site.
Other: flulike syndrome, infection.

INTERACTIONS

Doxorubicin: May increase risk of hemolytic-uremic syndrome. Closely monitor patient.
Hydantoins (phenytoin): May decrease GI absorption of hydantoins. Monitor levels and adjust dosage as needed.
Live-virus vaccines: May increase risk of vaccine-induced adverse reactions. Defer use of live-virus vaccines.
Palmiferin: May increase toxic effects of gemcitabine. Don't administer within 24 hours before, during, or 24 hours after gemcitabine administration.
Warfarin: May increase the anticoagulant effect of warfarin. Monitor patient and INR.

EFFECTS ON LAB TEST RESULTS

● May increase ALT, AST, BUN, and creatinine levels. May decrease hemoglobin level.
● May decrease neutrophil, platelet, and WBC counts.

CONTRAINDICATIONS & CAUTIONS

● Contraindicated in patients hypersensitive to drug and in pregnant or breast-feeding women.
● Use cautiously in patients with renal or hepatic impairment.
● Use cautiously when given within 7 days of radiation therapy.
● In children, safety and effectiveness haven't been determined.
⚠ **Overdose S&S:** Myelosuppression, paresthesia, severe rash.

NURSING CONSIDERATIONS

● Monitor patient closely. Expect dosage modification according to toxicity and degree of myelosuppression. Age, gender, and presence of renal impairment may predispose patient to toxicity.
● Carefully monitor hematologic values, especially neutrophil and platelet counts.
● Obtain baseline and periodic renal and hepatic laboratory tests.

PATIENT TEACHING

● Advise patient to watch for evidence of infection (fever, sore throat, fatigue) and bleeding (easy bruising, nosebleeds, bleeding gums, tarry stools). Tell patient to take temperature daily.

G

• Advise patient to promptly report flulike symptoms or breathing problems.
• Tell patient that adverse effects may continue after treatment ends.
• Caution women to avoid pregnancy or breast-feeding during therapy.

gemfibrozil
jem-FI-broe-zil

Lopid✦

Therapeutic class: Antilipemics
Pharmacologic class: Fibric acid derivatives
Pregnancy risk category: C

AVAILABLE FORMS
Tablets: 600 mg

INDICATIONS & DOSAGES
➤ **Types IV and V hyperlipidemia unresponsive to diet and other drugs; to reduce risk of coronary artery disease in patients with type IIb hyperlipidemia who can't tolerate or who are refractory to treatment with bile acid sequestrants or niacin**
Adults: 1,200 mg P.O. daily in two divided doses, 30 minutes before morning and evening meals.

ADMINISTRATION
P.O.
• Give drug 30 minutes before breakfast and dinner.

ACTION
Inhibits peripheral lipolysis and reduces triglyceride synthesis in the liver; lowers triglyceride levels and increases HDL cholesterol levels.

Route	Onset	Peak	Duration
P.O.	2–5 days	4 wk	Unknown

Half-life: 1¼ hours.

ADVERSE REACTIONS
CNS: fatigue, headache, vertigo.
CV: atrial fibrillation.

GI: abdominal and epigastric pain, dyspepsia, acute appendicitis, constipation, diarrhea, nausea, vomiting.
Hematologic: *leukopenia, thrombocytopenia,* anemia, eosinophilia.
Hepatic: bile duct obstruction.
Metabolic: *hypokalemia.*
Skin: dermatitis, eczema, pruritus, rash.

INTERACTIONS
Drug-drug. *Colestipol:* May decrease colestipol effects. Separate administration times by 2 hours.
Cyclosporine: May decrease cyclosporine levels. Monitor cyclosporine levels and adjust dose as needed.
Glyburide, pioglitazone: May increase hypoglycemic effects. Monitor glucose level, and watch for signs of hypoglycemia.
HMG-CoA reductase inhibitors: May cause myopathy with rhabdomyolysis. Avoid using together.
Montelukast: May increase montelukast level and effects. Monitor clinical response and adjust montelukast dosage.
Oral anticoagulants: May enhance effects of oral anticoagulants. Monitor patient closely.
Repaglinide: May increase repaglinide level. Avoid using together if possible. If already taking both drugs, monitor glucose levels and adjust repaglinide dosage.

EFFECTS ON LAB TEST RESULTS
• May increase ALT, AST, and CK levels. May decrease potassium and hemoglobin levels and hematocrit.
• May decrease eosinophil, WBC, and platelet counts.

CONTRAINDICATIONS & CAUTIONS
• Contraindicated in patients hypersensitive to drug and in those with hepatic or severe renal dysfunction (including primary biliary cirrhosis) or gallbladder disease.

NURSING CONSIDERATIONS
• Check CBC and LFTs periodically during the first 12 months of therapy.
• If drug has no benefits after 3 months of therapy, stop drug.
• Patient shouldn't take drug together with repaglinide or itraconazole.

Reactions in bold italics are *life-threatening*. Interactions may have a *rapid onset* or a *delayed onset.*

PATIENT TEACHING

● Instruct patient to take drug 30 minutes before breakfast and dinner.

● Teach patient about proper dietary management of cholesterol and triglycerides. When appropriate, recommend weight control, exercise, and smoking cessation programs.

● Because of possible dizziness and blurred vision, advise patient to avoid driving and other hazardous activities until effects of drug are known.

● Tell patient to observe bowel movements and to report evidence of excess fat in feces or other signs of bile duct obstruction.

● Advise patient to report muscle pain to prescriber if occurs during therapy.

gemifloxacin mesylate
jem-ah-FLOX-a-sin

Factive

Therapeutic class: Antibiotics
Pharmacologic class: Fluoroquinolones
Pregnancy risk category: C

AVAILABLE FORMS
Tablets: 320 mg

INDICATIONS & DOSAGES
Adjust-a-dose (for all indications): If CrCl is 40 mL/minute or less, or if patient receives routine hemodialysis or continuous ambulatory peritoneal dialysis, reduce dosage to 160 mg P.O. once daily.

➤ **Acute bacterial worsening of chronic bronchitis caused by** *Streptococcus pneumoniae, Haemophilus influenzae, H. parainfluenzae,* **or** *Moraxella catarrhalis*
Adults: 320 mg P.O. once daily for 5 days.

➤ **Mild to moderate community-acquired pneumonia caused by** *S. pneumoniae* **(including multidrug-resistant strains),** *H. influenzae, M. catarrhalis, Mycoplasma pneumoniae, Chlamydia pneumoniae,* **or** *Klebsiella pneumoniae*
Adults: 320 mg P.O. once daily for 5 to 7 days.

ADMINISTRATION
P.O.
● Give drug with or without food; however, it must be given 2 hours before or 3 hours after an antacid.

● Give plenty of fluids during treatment.

ACTION
Prevents cell growth by inhibiting DNA gyrase and topoisomerase IV, which interferes with DNA synthesis.

Route	Onset	Peak	Duration
P.O.	Unknown	½–2 hr	Unknown

Half-life: 4 to 12 hours.

ADVERSE REACTIONS
CNS: headache, dizziness.
GI: diarrhea, nausea, abdominal pain, vomiting.
Musculoskeletal: ruptured tendons.
Skin: rash.
Other: *hypersensitivity reactions.*

INTERACTIONS
Drug-drug. *Antacids (magnesium or aluminum), didanosine (chewable tablets, buffered tablets, or pediatric powder for oral solution), ferrous sulfate, multivitamins containing metal cations (such as zinc), sucralfate:* May decrease gemifloxacin level. Give these drugs at least 3 hours before or 2 hours after gemifloxacin.
Antiarrhythmics of class IA (procainamide, quinidine) or class III (amiodarone, sotalol): May increase risk of prolonged QTc interval. Avoid using together.
Antipsychotics, erythromycin, TCAs: May increase risk of prolonged QTc interval. Use together cautiously.
Probenecid: May increase gemifloxacin level. May use with probenecid for this reason.
Black Box Warning *Steroids:* May increase risk of tendinitis and tendon rupture. Monitor patient for tendon pain or inflammation. ∎
Sucralfate: May decrease gemifloxacin level. Use together cautiously.
Warfarin: May increase anticoagulation effect. Monitor PT and INR.
Drug-lifestyle. *Sun exposure:* May increase risk of photosensitivity. Advise patient to avoid excessive sunlight exposure.

G

EFFECTS ON LAB TEST RESULTS

• May increase alkaline phosphatase, ALT, AST, bilirubin, BUN, CK, creatinine, GGT, and potassium levels. May decrease albumin, protein, and sodium levels. May increase or decrease calcium and hemoglobin levels and hematocrit.

• May increase or decrease neutrophil, platelet, and RBC counts.

CONTRAINDICATIONS & CAUTIONS

Black Box Warning Drug is associated with increased risk of tendinitis and tendon rupture, especially in patients older than age 60 and those with heart, kidney, or lung transplants. ▪

Black Box Warning Drug may exacerbate muscle weakness in patients with myasthenia gravis. Avoid using fluoroquinolones in patients with a known history of myasthenia gravis. ▪

۞ Alert: Oral or parenteral fluoroquinolones may increase the risk of peripheral neuropathy of the arms or legs. Symptoms can occur anytime during treatment and can last for months or years or be permanent. Stop drug immediately if patient develops symptoms and switch to a non-fluoroquinolone antibacterial drug unless the benefit of continued treatment outweighs the risk.

• Contraindicated in patients hypersensitive to fluoroquinolones, gemifloxacin, or their components.

• Contraindicated in patients with a history of prolonged QTc interval, those with uncorrected electrolyte disorders (such as hypokalemia or hypomagnesemia), and those taking a drug that could prolong the QTc interval.

• Use cautiously in patients with a proarrhythmic condition, epilepsy, or a predisposition to seizures.

• Safety and effectiveness haven't been established for children younger than age 18.

NURSING CONSIDERATIONS

• Use drug only for infections caused by susceptible bacteria.

۞ Alert: Don't exceed recommended dosage because this increases the risk of prolonging the QTc interval.

۞ Alert: Monitor the patient for symptoms of peripheral neuropathy (pain, burning, tingling, numbness, weakness, or a change in sensation to light touch, pain or temperature, or the sense of body position) and report them immediately to the practitioner.

• Mild to moderate maculopapular rash may appear, usually 8 to 10 days after therapy starts. It's more likely in women younger than age 40 and postmenopausal women taking hormone therapy. Stop drug if rash appears.

۞ Alert: Serious, occasionally fatal, hypersensitivity reactions may occur. Stop drug immediately if hypersensitivity reaction occurs.

Black Box Warning Fluoroquinolones may cause tendon rupture, arthropathy, or osteochondrosis; stop drug if patient reports pain or inflammation or ruptures a tendon. ▪

• Stop drug if patient has a photosensitivity reaction.

• Fluoroquinolones may cause CNS effects, such as tremors and anxiety. Monitor patient carefully.

• Serious diarrhea may reflect pseudomembranous colitis; drug may need to be stopped.

• Keep patient adequately hydrated to avoid concentration of urine.

PATIENT TEACHING

۞ Alert: Warn patient to contact practitioner immediately if symptoms of peripheral neuropathy occur.

• Urge patient to finish full course of treatment, even if symptoms improve.

• Tell patient that drug may be taken with or without food, but that it shouldn't be taken within 3 hours after or 2 hours before an antacid.

• Tell patient to stop drug and seek medical care if evidence of hypersensitivity reaction develops.

• Instruct patient to drink fluids liberally.

• Warn patient against taking OTC drugs or dietary supplements without consulting prescriber.

• Tell patient to avoid excessive exposure to sunlight or ultraviolet light.

• Urge patient to report pain, inflammation, or rupture of tendons.

Reactions in bold italics are *life-threatening*. Interactions may have a *rapid onset* or a *delayed onset*.

- Warn patient to avoid driving or other hazardous activities until effects of drug are known.

gentamicin sulfate (injection)
jen-ta-MYE-sin

Therapeutic class: Antibiotics
Pharmacologic class: Aminoglycosides
Pregnancy risk category: D

AVAILABLE FORMS
Injection: 40 mg/mL (adults), 10 mg/mL (children)
I.V. infusion (premixed): 40 mg, 60 mg, 70 mg, 80 mg, 90 mg, 100 mg, 120 mg in 100 mL normal saline solution

INDICATIONS & DOSAGES
➤ **Serious infections caused by sensitive strains of *Pseudomonas aeruginosa, Escherichia coli, Proteus, Klebsiella, Serratia,* or *Staphylococcus***
Adults: 3 mg/kg daily I.M. or I.V. infusion in three divided doses every 8 hours. For life-threatening infections, may give up to 5 mg/kg daily in three or four divided doses; reduce dosage to 3 mg/kg daily as soon as patient improves.
Children: 2 to 2.5 mg/kg I.M. or I.V. infusion every 8 hours.
Neonates older than 1 week and infants: 2.5 mg/kg I.M. or I.V. infusion every 8 hours.
Neonates younger than 1 week and preterm infants: 2.5 mg/kg I.M. or I.V. infusion every 12 hours.
Adjust-a-dose: For adults with impaired renal function, doses and frequency are determined by drug level and renal function. To maintain therapeutic levels, adults should receive 1 to 1.7 mg/kg I.M. or I.V. infusion after each dialysis session, and children should receive 2 to 2.5 mg/kg I.M. or I.V. infusion after each dialysis session.
➤ **Confirmed or presumed pelvic inflammatory disease (with clindamycin)** ◆
Women: Initial loading dose of 2 mg/kg I.V. or I.M., followed by 1.5 mg/kg every 8 hours or 3 to 5 mg/kg once daily. Continue gentamicin until 24 hours after noted clinical improvement. Administration of P.O. clindamycin or doxycycline should follow for a total of 14 days of treatment.
➤ **Patients undergoing surgery for which antibiotic prophylaxis is indicated for susceptible bacteria** ◆
Adults: 1.5 mg/kg I.V. over 30 to 60 minutes, 1 hour before incision. Base redosing on serum drug levels with discontinuation within 24 hours postoperatively.

ADMINISTRATION
I.V.
▼ Obtain specimen for culture and sensitivity tests before giving. Begin therapy while awaiting results.
▼ For intermittent infusion, dilute with 50 to 200 mL of D_5W or normal saline solution for injection.
▼ Infuse over 30 minutes to 2 hours.
▼ After completing infusion, flush the line with normal saline solution or D_5W.
▼ **Incompatibilities:** Allopurinol, amphotericin B, ampicillin, azithromycin, cefazolin, cefepime, cefotaxime, ceftazidime, ceftriaxone sodium, cefuroxime, certain parenteral nutrition formulations, cytarabine, dopamine, fat emulsions, furosemide, heparin, hetastarch, idarubicin, indomethacin sodium trihydrate, nafcillin, propofol, ticarcillin, warfarin.
I.M.
- Obtain specimen for culture and sensitivity tests before giving. Begin therapy while awaiting results.
- Obtain blood for peak level 1 hour after I.M. injection or 30 minutes after I.V. infusion finishes; for trough levels, draw blood just before next dose. Don't collect blood in a heparinized tube; heparin is incompatible with aminoglycosides.

ACTION
Inhibits protein synthesis by binding directly to the 30S ribosomal subunit; bactericidal.

Route	Onset	Peak	Duration
I.V.	Immediate	30–60 min	Unknown
I.M.	Unknown	30–60 min	Unknown

Half-life: 2 to 3 hours.

ADVERSE REACTIONS

CNS: *encephalopathy, seizures,* fever, headache, lethargy, confusion, dizziness, numbness, peripheral neuropathy, vertigo, ataxia, tingling.
CV: hypotension.
EENT: ototoxicity, blurred vision, tinnitus.
GI: vomiting, nausea.
GU: *nephrotoxicity,* possible increase in urinary excretion of casts.
Hematologic: *agranulocytosis, leukopenia, thrombocytopenia,* anemia, eosinophilia.
Musculoskeletal: muscle twitching, myasthenia gravis–like syndrome.
Respiratory: *apnea.*
Skin: rash, urticaria, pruritus, injection-site pain.
Other: *anaphylaxis.*

INTERACTIONS

Drug-drug. Black Box Warning *Acyclovir, amphotericin B, cephalosporins, cidofovir, cisplatin, methoxyflurane, vancomycin, other aminoglycosides:* May increase ototoxicity and nephrotoxicity. Monitor hearing and renal function test results. ∎
Atracurium, pancuronium, rocuronium, vecuronium: May increase effects of nondepolarizing muscle relaxants, including prolonged respiratory depression. Use together only when necessary, and expect to reduce dosage of nondepolarizing muscle relaxant.
Dimenhydrinate: May mask ototoxicity symptoms. Monitor patient's hearing.
General anesthetics: May increase neuromuscular blockade. Monitor patient closely.
Indomethacin: May increase peak and trough levels of gentamicin. Monitor gentamicin level.
Black Box Warning *I.V. loop diuretics (such as furosemide):* May increase risk of ototoxicity. Monitor patient's hearing. ∎
Nondepolarizing muscle relaxants (pancuronium, vecuronium): May increase neuromuscular-blocking effects of these drugs and cause prolonged respiratory depression and apnea. Use together with caution.
Parenteral penicillins (such as ampicillin and ticarcillin): May inactivate gentamicin in vitro. Don't mix together.

EFFECTS ON LAB TEST RESULTS

• May increase ALT, AST, bilirubin, BUN, creatinine, LDH, and nonprotein nitrogen levels. May decrease hemoglobin level.
• May increase eosinophil count. May decrease platelet and WBC counts.

CONTRAINDICATIONS & CAUTIONS

• Contraindicated in patients hypersensitive to drug or other aminoglycosides.
• Use cautiously in neonates, infants, elderly patients, and patients with impaired renal function or neuromuscular disorders.
⚠ *Overdose S&S:* Nephrotoxicity, neurotoxicity, ototoxicity.

NURSING CONSIDERATIONS

Black Box Warning Evaluate patient's hearing before and during therapy. Notify prescriber if patient complains of tinnitus, vertigo, or hearing loss. ∎
• Weigh patient and review renal function studies before therapy begins.
✪ *Alert:* Use preservative-free form when intrathecal route is used adjunctively for serious CNS infections, such as meningitis and ventriculitis.
Black Box Warning Maintain peak levels at 4 to 12 mcg/mL and trough levels at 1 to 2 mcg/mL. The maximum peak level is usually 8 mcg/mL, except in patients with cystic fibrosis, who need increased lung penetration. Prolonged peak levels of 10 to 12 mcg/mL or prolonged trough levels greater than 2 mcg/mL may increase risk of toxicity. ∎
Black Box Warning Nephrotoxicity risk is greater in patients with renal impairment and in those who receive high-dosage or prolonged therapy. Monitor renal function: urine output, specific gravity, urinalysis, BUN and creatinine levels, and CrCl. Report to prescriber evidence of declining renal function. ∎
Black Box Warning High-risk patients should have serial audiograms, especially if they show signs and symptoms of ototoxicity (dizziness, vertigo, ataxia, tinnitus, hearing loss). ∎
• Hemodialysis for 8 hours may remove up to 50% of drug from blood.
• Watch for signs and symptoms of superinfection (especially of upper respiratory

tract), such as continued fever, chills, and increased pulse rate.
● Therapy usually continues for 7 to 10 days. If no response occurs in 3 to 5 days, stop therapy and obtain new specimens for culture and sensitivity testing.

PATIENT TEACHING
● Instruct patient to promptly report adverse reactions, such as dizziness, vertigo, unsteady gait, ringing in the ears, hearing loss, numbness, tingling, or muscle twitching.
● Encourage patient to drink plenty of fluids.
● Warn patient to avoid hazardous activities if adverse CNS reactions occur.

gentamicin sulfate (ophthalmic)
jen-ta-MYE-sin

Genoptic, Gentak, Pred-G

Therapeutic class: Antibiotics
Pharmacologic class: Aminoglycosides
Pregnancy risk category: C

AVAILABLE FORMS
Ophthalmic ointment: 0.3% (base)
Ophthalmic solution: 0.3% (base)

INDICATIONS & DOSAGES
➤ **External ocular infections (conjunctivitis, keratoconjunctivitis, corneal ulcers, blepharitis, blepharoconjunctivitis, meibomianitis, and dacryocystitis) caused by susceptible organisms, especially** *Pseudomonas aeruginosa, Proteus, Klebsiella pneumoniae, Escherichia coli,* **and other gram-negative organisms**
Adults and children: 1 to 2 drops in affected eye every 4 hours. In severe infections, up to 2 drops every hour. Or, apply ointment (approximately ½ inch) to lower conjunctival sac b.i.d. or t.i.d.

ADMINISTRATION
Ophthalmic
● Store drug away from heat.
● Apply light finger pressure on lacrimal sac for 1 minute after drops are instilled.
● Wait at least 10 minutes before instilling other eyedrops.

ACTION
Thought to inhibit protein synthesis; usually bactericidal.

Route	Onset	Peak	Duration
Ophthalmic	Unknown	Unknown	Unknown

Half-life: Unknown.

ADVERSE REACTIONS
EENT: burning, stinging, or blurred vision with ointment; conjunctival hyperemia, transient irritation from solution, bacterial and fungal corneal ulcers.
Other: overgrowth of nonsusceptible organisms with long-term use.

INTERACTIONS
None significant.

EFFECTS ON LAB TEST RESULTS
None reported.

CONTRAINDICATIONS & CAUTIONS
● Contraindicated in patients hypersensitive to drug.
● Use cautiously in patients with history of sensitivity to aminoglycosides because cross-sensitivity may occur.

NURSING CONSIDERATIONS
● Obtain culture before giving drug. Therapy may begin before culture results are known.
● Solution isn't for injection into conjunctiva or anterior chamber of eye.
● If ophthalmic gentamicin is given together with systemic gentamicin, monitor gentamicin level.
● Systemic absorption from excessive use may cause toxicities.

PATIENT TEACHING
● Tell patient to clean eye area of excessive discharge before instilling drug.
● Teach patient how to instill drops or apply ointment. Advise him to wash hands before and after applying ointment or solution and not to touch tip of dropper or tube to eye or surrounding tissues.
● Instruct patient to apply light finger pressure on lacrimal sac for 1 minute after drops are instilled.

• Tell patient to wait at least 10 minutes before instilling other eyedrops.

• Instruct patient to stop drug and notify prescriber if signs and symptoms of sensitivity (itching lids, swelling, or constant burning) occur.

• Advise patient not to share drug, washcloths, or towels with family members and to notify prescriber if anyone develops same signs or symptoms.

• Tell patient that vision may be blurred for a few minutes after application of ointment.

🕃 **Alert:** Stress importance of following recommended therapy. *Pseudomonas* infections can cause complete vision loss within 24 hours if infection isn't controlled.

gentamicin sulfate (topical)
jen-ta-MYE-sin

Therapeutic class: Antibiotics
Pharmacologic class: Aminoglycosides
Pregnancy risk category: C

AVAILABLE FORMS
Cream: 0.1%
Ointment: 0.1%

INDICATIONS & DOSAGES
➤ **To treat or prevent superficial infections and superficial burns of the skin caused by susceptible bacteria**
Adults and children older than age 1: Rub in small amount gently t.i.d. or q.i.d., with or without gauze dressing.

ADMINISTRATION
Topical
• Topical forms are for dermatologic use only; not for ophthalmic use.
• Clean affected area and remove crusts of impetigo before applying to increase absorption.
• Wash hands after each application.
• Store drug in cool place.

ACTION
Exact mechanism unknown. An aminoglycoside that disrupts bacterial protein synthesis by binding to ribosomes. Susceptible bacteria include sensitive strains of streptococci and *Staphylococcus aureus*

and gram-negative bacteria, including *Pseudomonas aeruginosa, Aerobacter aerogenes, Escherichia coli, Proteus vulgaris,* and *Klebsiella pneumoniae.*

Route	Onset	Peak	Duration
Topical	Unknown	Unknown	Unknown

Half-life: Unknown.

ADVERSE REACTIONS
Skin: allergic contact dermatitis, erythema, minor skin irritation, photosensitivity.

INTERACTIONS
None significant.

EFFECTS ON LAB TEST RESULTS
None reported.

CONTRAINDICATIONS & CAUTIONS
• Contraindicated in patients hypersensitive to drug or its components and in those who may have cross-sensitivity with other aminoglycosides, such as neomycin.

NURSING CONSIDERATIONS
🕃 **Alert:** Avoid use on large skin lesions or over a wide area because of possible systemic toxic effects.
• Restrict use of drug to selected patients; widespread use may lead to resistant organisms.
• Prolonged use may result in overgrowth of nonsusceptible organisms.

PATIENT TEACHING
• Tell patient to clean affected area and to remove crusts of impetigo before applying to increase absorption.
• Tell patient to wash hands after each application.
• Instruct patient to store drug in cool place.
• Tell patient to stop using drug and notify prescriber immediately if no improvement occurs or if condition worsens.

glatiramer acetate
glah-TEER-ah-mer

Copaxone

Therapeutic class: MS drugs
Pharmacologic class: Biological
response modifiers
Pregnancy risk category: B

AVAILABLE FORMS
Injection: 20 mg glatiramer acetate and
40 mg mannitol, USP, in a single-use prefilled syringe

INDICATIONS & DOSAGES
➤ **For first clinical episode and to reduce
frequency of relapse in patients with
relapsing-remitting MS**
Adults: 20 mg subcutaneously daily.

ADMINISTRATION
Subcutaneous
• Give drug only subcutaneously.
• Drug doesn't contain preservatives; discard if solution contains particulate matter.
• Don't try to expel the air bubble from the
prefilled syringe. This may lead to loss of
drug and an incorrect dose.
• Store drug in refrigerator (36° to 46° F
[2° to 8° C]), allow drug to warm to room
temperature for 20 minutes before use. If
refrigeration is not available, may store at
room temperature for up to 1 month.

ACTION
May modify immune processes responsible
for the pathogenesis of MS.

Route	Onset	Peak	Duration
Subcut.	Unknown	Unknown	Unknown

Half-life: Unknown.

ADVERSE REACTIONS
CNS: anxiety, asthenia, abnormal dreams,
agitation, confusion, emotional lability,
fever, migraine, nervousness, pain, speech
disorder, stupor, syncope, tremor, vertigo.
CV: chest pain, palpitations, vasodilation,
hypertension, tachycardia.

EENT: rhinitis, ear pain, eye disorder,
laryngismus, nystagmus.
GI: diarrhea, nausea, anorexia, bowel
urgency, gastroenteritis, GI disorder, oral
candidiasis, salivary gland enlargement,
ulcerative stomatitis, vomiting.
GU: urinary urgency, *vaginal hemorrhage,*
abnormal Papanicolaou smear, amenorrhea,
dysmenorrhea, hematuria, erectile dysfunction, menorrhagia, vaginal candidiasis.
Hematologic: lymphadenopathy, ecchymosis.
Metabolic: weight gain.
Musculoskeletal: arthralgia, back pain,
hypertonia, footdrop, neck pain.
Respiratory: dyspnea, bronchitis, hyperventilation.
Skin: diaphoresis, injection-site reaction,
pruritus, rash, eczema, erythema or hemorrhage, nodule, skin atrophy, urticaria,
warts.
Other: flulike syndrome, infection, bacterial infection, chills, cyst, dental caries,
herpes simplex and zoster, peripheral and
facial edema.

INTERACTIONS
None significant.

EFFECTS ON LAB TEST RESULTS
None reported.

CONTRAINDICATIONS & CAUTIONS
• Contraindicated in patients hypersensitive
to drug or mannitol.

NURSING CONSIDERATIONS
• Immediate postinjection reactions may
occur; symptoms include flushing, chest
pain, palpitations, anxiety, dyspnea, constriction of the throat, and urticaria. They
typically are transient and self-limiting
and don't need specific treatment. Onset of
postinjection reaction may occur several
months after treatment starts, and patients
may have more than one episode.
• Patient may experience at least one
episode of transient chest pain, which usually begins at least 1 month after treatment
starts; it isn't accompanied by other signs
or symptoms and doesn't appear to be clinically important.

PATIENT TEACHING
- Instruct patient how to self-inject drug. Supervise first injection. Injection sites include arms, abdomen, hips, and thighs.
- Tell patient to rotate injection sites daily.
- Explain need for aseptic self-injection techniques and warn patient against reuse of needles and syringes. Periodically review proper disposal of needles, syringes, drug containers, and unused drug.
- Tell patient to notify prescriber about planned, suspected, or known pregnancy.
- Tell women to notify prescriber if breast-feeding.
- Advise patient not to change drug or dosage schedule or to stop drug without medical approval.
- Tell patient to notify prescriber immediately if dizziness, hives, profuse sweating, chest pain, difficulty breathing, or severe pain occurs after drug injection.

SAFETY ALERT!

glimepiride
glye-MEH-per-ide

Amaryl✒

Therapeutic class: Antidiabetics
Pharmacologic class: Sulfonylureas
Pregnancy risk category: C

AVAILABLE FORMS
Tablets: 1 mg, 2 mg, 3 mg, 4 mg, 6 mg, 8 mg

INDICATIONS & DOSAGES
Adjust-a-dose (for all indications): For patients with renal or hepatic impairment, initially, 1 mg P.O. once daily, then adjust to appropriate dosage, if needed.
➤ **Adjunct to diet and exercise to lower glucose level in patients with type 2 diabetes whose hyperglycemia can't be managed by diet and exercise alone**
Adults: Initially, 1 or 2 mg P.O. once daily; usual maintenance dose is 1 to 4 mg P.O. once daily. After reaching 2 mg, dosage is increased in increments not exceeding 2 mg every 1 to 2 weeks, based on patient's glucose level response. Maximum dose is 8 mg daily.

➤ **Adjunct to diet and exercise in conjunction with insulin or metformin therapy in patients with type 2 diabetes whose hyperglycemia can't be managed with the maximum dosage of glimepiride alone**
Adults: 8 mg P.O. once daily; used with low-dose insulin. Increase insulin dosage weekly, if needed, based on patient's glucose level response. Or, if patients do not respond adequately to maximum dose of glimepiride, addition of metformin may be considered.

ADMINISTRATION
P.O.
- Give drug with first meal of the day.

ACTION
Lowers glucose level, possibly by stimulating release of insulin from functioning pancreatic beta cells, and may lead to increased sensitivity of peripheral tissues to insulin.

Route	Onset	Peak	Duration
P.O.	1 hr	2–3 hr	>24 hr

Half-life: 9 hours.

ADVERSE REACTIONS
CNS: dizziness, asthenia, headache.
EENT: changes in accommodation.
GI: nausea.
Hematologic: *leukopenia,* hemolytic anemia, *agranulocytosis, thrombocytopenia, aplastic anemia, pancytopenia.*
Metabolic: *hypoglycemia,* dilutional hyponatremia.

INTERACTIONS
Drug-drug. *Beta blockers:* May mask symptoms of hypoglycemia. Monitor glucose level.
Drugs that tend to produce hyperglycemia (such as corticosteroids, estrogens, fosphenytoin, hormonal contraceptives, isoniazid, nicotinic acid, phenothiazines, phenytoin, thyroid products): May lead to loss of glucose control. Adjust dosage.
Insulin: May increase risk of hypoglycemia. Use together cautiously.

Reactions in bold italics are *life-threatening*. Interactions may have a *rapid onset* or a *delayed onset*.

NSAIDs, other drugs that are highly protein-bound (such as beta blockers, chloramphenicol, coumarin, MAO inhibitors, probenecid, sulfonamides): May increase hypoglycemic action of sulfonylureas such as glimepiride. Monitor glucose level carefully.

Rifamycins, thiazide diuretics: May increase risk of hyperglycemia. Monitor glucose level.

Salicylates: May increase hypoglycemic effects of sulfonylurea. Monitor glucose level.

Drug-herb. *Burdock, dandelion, eucalyptus, marshmallow:* May increase drug effects. Discourage use together.

Drug-lifestyle. *Alcohol use:* May alter glycemic control, most commonly causing hypoglycemia. May also cause disulfiram-like reaction. Discourage use together.

EFFECTS ON LAB TEST RESULTS

• May increase alkaline phosphatase, AST, BUN, and creatinine levels. May decrease glucose, hemoglobin, and sodium levels.
• May decrease granulocyte, platelet, RBC, and WBC counts.

CONTRAINDICATIONS & CAUTIONS

• Contraindicated in patients hypersensitive to drug and in those with diabetic ketoacidosis, which should be treated with insulin.
• Contraindicated as sole therapy for type 1 diabetes.
• Contraindicated in breast-feeding women because it may cause hypoglycemia in breast-fed infants.
• Use cautiously in debilitated or malnourished patients and in those with adrenal, pituitary, hepatic, or renal insufficiency; these patients are more susceptible to the hypoglycemic action of glucose-lowering drugs.
• Use cautiously with drugs that can cause hypoglycemia.
• Use cautiously in elderly patients and in patients allergic to sulfonamides.
• In children, safety and effectiveness haven't been established.
△ Overdose S&S: Hypoglycemia.

NURSING CONSIDERATIONS

• Glimepiride and insulin may be used together in patients who lose glucose control after first responding to therapy.
• Monitor fasting glucose level periodically to determine therapeutic response. Also monitor glycosylated hemoglobin level, usually every 3 to 6 months, to precisely assess long-term glycemic control.
⊘ Alert: Use of oral hypoglycemics may carry higher risk of CV mortality than use of diet alone or of diet and insulin therapy.
• When changing patient from other sulfonylureas to glimepiride, a transition period isn't needed. Monitor patient carefully for 1 to 2 weeks when changing from longer half-life sulfonylureas, such as chlorpropamide.
• **Look alike–sound alike:** Don't confuse glimepiride with glyburide or glipizide. Don't confuse Amaryl with Altace.

PATIENT TEACHING

• Tell patient to take drug with first meal of the day.
• Make sure patient understands that therapy relieves symptoms but doesn't cure the disease. He should also understand potential risks and advantages of taking drug and of other treatment methods.
• Stress importance of adhering to diet, weight reduction, exercise, and personal hygiene programs. Explain to patient and family how and when to monitor glucose level, and teach recognition of and intervention for signs and symptoms of high and low glucose levels.
• Advise patient to wear or carry medical identification at all times.
• Advise woman to consult prescriber before planning pregnancy. Insulin may be needed during pregnancy and breast-feeding.
• Advise patient to consult prescriber before taking any OTC products.
• Teach patient to carry candy or other simple sugars to treat mild episodes of low glucose level. Patient experiencing severe episode may need hospital treatment.
• Advise patient to avoid alcohol, which lowers glucose level.

SAFETY ALERT!

glipiZIDE
GLIP-i-zide

Glucotrol◆, Glucotrol XL◆

Therapeutic class: Antidiabetics
Pharmacologic class: Sulfonylureas
Pregnancy risk category: C

AVAILABLE FORMS
Tablets (extended-release): 2.5 mg, 5 mg, 10 mg
Tablets (immediate-release): 5 mg, 10 mg

INDICATIONS & DOSAGES
➤ **Adjunct to diet to lower glucose level in patients with type 2 diabetes**
Immediate-release tablets
Adults: Initially, 5 mg P.O. daily 30 minutes before breakfast. Maximum once-daily dose is 15 mg. Divide doses of more than 15 mg. Maximum daily dose is 40 mg.
Adjust-a-dose: Initially, for patients with hepatic insufficiency or patients older than age 65, give 2.5 mg P.O. daily.
Extended-release tablets
Adults: Initially, 5 mg P.O. with breakfast daily. Increase by 5 mg every 3 months, depending on level of glycemic control. Maximum daily dose is 20 mg.
➤ **To replace insulin therapy**
Adults: If insulin dosage is more than 20 units daily, start patient at usual dosage in addition to 50% of insulin. If insulin dosage is less than or equal to 20 units daily, insulin may be stopped when glipizide starts.

ADMINISTRATION
P.O.
● Give immediate-release tablet about 30 minutes before meals.
● Give extended-release tablet with breakfast.
● Don't split or crush extended-release tablets.

ACTION
Unknown. Probably stimulates insulin release from pancreatic beta cells, reduces glucose output by the liver, and increases peripheral sensitivity to insulin.

Route	Onset	Peak	Duration
P.O. (immediate-release)	15–30 min	1–3 hr	24 hr
P.O. (extended-release)	2–3 hr	6–12 hr	24 hr

Half-life: 2 to 4 hours.

ADVERSE REACTIONS
CNS: dizziness, drowsiness, headache, syncope, asthenia, nervousness, tremor.
GI: nausea, dyspepsia, flatulence, constipation, diarrhea.
GU: polyuria.
Hematologic: *leukopenia,* hemolytic anemia, *agranulocytosis, thrombocytopenia, aplastic anemia.*
Metabolic: *hypoglycemia.*
Musculoskeletal: arthralgia, leg cramps.
Respiratory: rhinitis.
Skin: pruritus, photosensitivity reactions.

INTERACTIONS
Drug-drug. *Amantadine, anabolic steroids, antifungals, chloramphenicol, clofibrate, guanethidine, MAO inhibitors, NSAIDs, probenecid, quinolones,* **salicylates,** *sulfonamides:* May increase hypoglycemic activity. Monitor glucose level.
Beta blockers: May prolong hypoglycemic effect and mask symptoms of hypoglycemia. Use together cautiously.
Corticosteroids, glucagon, phenytoin, **rifamycins,** **thiazide diuretics:** May decrease hypoglycemic response. Monitor glucose level.
Oral anticoagulants: May increase hypoglycemic activity or enhance anticoagulant effect. Monitor glucose level, PT, and INR.
Drug-herb. *Burdock, dandelion, eucalyptus, marshmallow:* May increase drug effects. Discourage use together.
Drug-lifestyle. *Alcohol use:* May alter glycemic control, most commonly causing hypoglycemia. May cause disulfiram-like reaction. Discourage use together.

EFFECTS ON LAB TEST RESULTS
● May increase alkaline phosphatase, AST, LDH, BUN, cholesterol, and creatinine levels. May decrease glucose and hemoglobin levels.
● May decrease granulocyte, platelet, and WBC counts.

Reactions in bold italics are *life-threatening*. Interactions may have a *rapid onset* or a *delayed onset*.

CONTRAINDICATIONS & CAUTIONS
• Contraindicated in patients hypersensitive to drug and in those with diabetic ketoacidosis with or without coma.
• Contraindicated in pregnant or breast-feeding women and as sole therapy in type 1 diabetes.
• Use cautiously in patients with severe GI narrowing, or renal or hepatic disease, in those allergic to sulfonamides, and in debilitated, malnourished, or elderly patients.
⚠ **Overdose S&S:** Hypoglycemia.

NURSING CONSIDERATIONS
• Some patients may attain effective control on a once-daily regimen, whereas others respond better with divided dosing.
• Patient may switch from immediate-release dose to extended-release tablets at the nearest equivalent total daily dose.
• Glipizide is a second-generation sulfonylurea. The frequency of adverse reactions appears to be lower than with first-generation drugs such as chlorpropamide.
🕃 **Alert:** Use of oral antidiabetic drugs may carry a higher risk of CV mortality than use of diet alone or of diet and insulin therapy.
• During periods of increased stress, patient may need insulin therapy. Monitor patient closely for hyperglycemia in these situations.
• Patient switching from insulin therapy to an oral antidiabetic should check glucose level at least three times a day before meals. Patient may need hospitalization during transition.
• **Look alike–sound alike:** Don't confuse glipizide with glyburide or glimepiride.

PATIENT TEACHING
• Instruct patient about disease and importance of following therapeutic regimen, adhering to diet, losing weight, getting exercise, following personal hygiene programs, and avoiding infection. Explain how and when to monitor glucose level, and teach recognition of episodes of low and high glucose levels.
• Tell patient to carry candy or other simple sugars to treat mild low-glucose episodes. Patient experiencing severe episode may need hospital treatment.

• Instruct patient not to change drug dosage without prescriber's consent and to report abnormal blood or urine glucose test results.
• Tell patient not to take other drugs, including OTC drugs, without first checking with prescriber.
• Advise patient to wear or carry medical identification at all times.
• Advise women planning pregnancy to first consult prescriber. Insulin may be needed during pregnancy and breast-feeding.
• Advise patient to avoid alcohol, which lowers glucose level.
• Tell patient that he may occasionally notice something in stool that looks like a tablet and that it's the nonabsorbable shell of the extended-release tablet.

SAFETY ALERT!

glyBURIDE (glibenclamide)
GLYE-byoor-ide

DiaBeta𝒫, Euglucon†, Glynase

Therapeutic class: Antidiabetics
Pharmacologic class: Sulfonylureas
Pregnancy risk category: B (Glynase);
C (DiaBeta)

AVAILABLE FORMS
Tablets: 1.25 mg, 2.5 mg, 5 mg
Tablets (micronized): 1.5 mg, 3 mg, 4.5 mg, 6 mg

INDICATIONS & DOSAGES
➤ **Adjunct to diet to lower glucose level in patients with type 2 diabetes**
Nonmicronized form
Adults: Initially, 2.5 to 5 mg P.O. once daily with breakfast or first main meal. Adjust to maintenance dose at no more than 2.5-mg increments at weekly intervals. Usual daily maintenance dose is 1.25 to 20 mg, in single dose or divided doses. Maximum daily dose is 20 mg P.O.
Micronized form
Adults: Initially, 1.5 to 3 mg P.O. daily with breakfast or first main meal. Adjust to maintenance dose at no more than 1.5-mg increments at weekly intervals. Usual daily maintenance dose is 0.75 to 12 mg. Dosages

exceeding 6 mg daily may have better response with b.i.d. dosing. Maximum dose is 12 mg P.O. daily.

Adjust-a-dose: For elderly patients, patients who are more sensitive to antidiabetics, and for those with renal, hepatic, adrenal, or pituitary insufficiency, start with 1.25 mg (nonmicronized) or 0.75 mg (micronized) daily. When using micronized tablets, patients who are more sensitive to antidiabetics should start with 0.75 mg daily.

➤ **To replace insulin therapy**
Adults: If insulin dosage is less than 40 units/day, patient may be switched directly to glyburide when insulin is stopped. If insulin dose is less than 20 units/day, initial dose is 2.5 to 5 mg (1.5 to 3 mg micronized) P.O. daily. If insulin dose is 20 to 40 units/day, initial dose is 5 mg (3 mg micronized) P.O. daily. If insulin dosage is 40 or more units/day, initially, 5 mg (3 mg micronized) P.O. once daily in addition to 50% of insulin dose.

ADMINISTRATION
P.O.
● Give drug with breakfast or first main meal.

ACTION
Unknown. Probably stimulates insulin release from pancreatic beta cells, reduces glucose output by the liver, and increases peripheral sensitivity to insulin.

Route	Onset	Peak	Duration
P.O. (micronized)	1 hr	2–3 hr	12–24 hr
P.O. (nonmicronized)	2–4 hr	2–4 hr	16–24 hr

Half-life: 10 hours.

ADVERSE REACTIONS
EENT: changes in accommodation or blurred vision.
GI: nausea, epigastric fullness, heartburn.
Hematologic: *leukopenia,* hemolytic anemia, *agranulocytosis, thrombocytopenia, aplastic anemia.*
Hepatic: cholestatic jaundice, *hepatitis.*
Metabolic: *hypoglycemia, hyponatremia.*
Musculoskeletal: arthralgia, myalgia.
Skin: rash, pruritus, other allergic reactions.
Other: *angioedema.*

INTERACTIONS
Drug-drug. *Anabolic steroids, chloramphenicol, clofibrate, fluoroquinolones, guanethidine, MAO inhibitors, miconazole, NSAIDs, probenecid, phenylbutazone,* **salicylates,** *sulfonamides:* May increase hypoglycemic activity. Monitor glucose level.
Beta blockers: May prolong hypoglycemic effect and mask symptoms of hypoglycemia. Use together cautiously.
Carbamazepine, corticosteroids, glucagon, **rifamycins, thiazide diuretics:** May decrease hypoglycemic response. Monitor glucose level.
Oral anticoagulants: May increase hypoglycemic activity or enhance anticoagulant effect. Monitor glucose level, PT, and INR.
Drug-herb. *Burdock, dandelion, eucalyptus, marshmallow:* May increase hypoglycemic effect. Discourage use together.
Drug-lifestyle. Alcohol use: May alter glycemic control, most commonly causing hypoglycemia. May cause disulfiram-like reaction. Discourage use together.

EFFECTS ON LAB TEST RESULTS
● May increase alkaline phosphatase, AST, ALT, bilirubin, BUN, and cholesterol levels. May decrease glucose, sodium, and hemoglobin levels.
● May decrease granulocyte, platelet, and WBC counts.

CONTRAINDICATIONS & CAUTIONS
● Contraindicated in patients hypersensitive to drug and in those with diabetic ketoacidosis with or without coma.
● Contraindicated as sole therapy for type 1 diabetes and in pregnant or breast-feeding women.
● Use cautiously in patients with hepatic or renal impairment; in debilitated, malnourished, or elderly patients; and in patients allergic to sulfonamides.
⚠ **Overdose S&S:** Hypoglycemia.

NURSING CONSIDERATIONS
⚠ **Alert:** Micronized glyburide (Glynase) contains drug in a smaller particle size and isn't bioequivalent to regular glyburide tablets. In patients who have been taking DiaBeta, adjust dosage.

- Although most patients may take drug once daily, those taking more than 10 mg daily may achieve better results with twice-daily dosage.
- Drug is a second-generation sulfonylurea. Adverse effects are less common with second-generation drugs than with first-generation drugs such as chlorpropamide.
- **❸ Alert:** Use of oral antidiabetic drugs may carry a higher risk of CV mortality than use of diet alone or of diet and insulin therapy.
- During periods of increased stress, such as infection, fever, surgery, or trauma, patient may need insulin therapy. Monitor patient closely for hyperglycemia in these situations.
- Patient switching from insulin therapy to an oral antidiabetic should check glucose level at least three times a day before meals. Patient may need hospitalization during transition.
- **Look alike–sound alike:** Don't confuse glyburide with glimepiride or glipizide.

PATIENT TEACHING

- Teach patient about diabetes and the importance of following therapeutic regimen, adhering to specific diet, losing weight, getting exercise, following personal hygiene programs, and avoiding infection. Explain how and when to monitor glucose level, and teach recognition of and intervention for low and high glucose levels.
- Tell patient not to change drug dosage without prescriber's consent and to report abnormal blood or urine glucose test results.
- Teach patient to carry candy or other simple sugars for mild low-glucose level. Patient experiencing severe episode may need hospital treatment.
- Advise patient not to take other drugs, including OTC drugs, without first checking with prescriber.
- Advise patient to wear or carry medical identification at all times.
- **❸ Alert:** Instruct patient to report episodes of low glucose to prescriber immediately; a severely low glucose level is sometimes fatal in patients receiving as little as 2.5 to 5 mg daily.
- Advise patient to avoid alcohol, which may lower glucose level.

golimumab
go-LIM-myoo-mab

Simponi, Simponi Aria

Therapeutic class: Antiarthritics
Pharmacologic class: TNF blockers
Pregnancy risk category: B

AVAILABLE FORMS
Injection: 50 mg/0.5-mL, 100 mg/mL prefilled syringe; 50 mg/0.5-mL, 100 mg/mL prefilled autoinjector
Injection: 50 mg/4-mL single-use vial

INDICATIONS & DOSAGES
➤ **Moderate to severe active rheumatoid arthritis in combination with methotrexate; active psoriatic arthritis alone or in combination with methotrexate; active ankylosing spondylitis**
Adults: 50 mg subcutaneously monthly.
✳ NEW INDICATION: **Moderate to severe ulcerative colitis in patients who have demonstrated an inadequate response or intolerance to prior treatment or who require continuous steroid therapy**
Adults: Initially, 200 mg subcutaneously, followed by 100 mg subcutaneously at week 2, then 100 mg subcutaneously every 4 weeks.
➤ **Moderate to severe rheumatoid arthritis in combination with methotrexate (Simponi Aria)**
Adults: 2 mg/kg I.V. infusion at weeks 0, and 4 and then every 8 weeks thereafter.

ADMINISTRATION
I.V.
▼ Dilute with 0.9% sodium chloride to a final volume of 100 mL.
▼ Administer over 30 minutes. Use a 0.22-μm low protein binding filter.
▼ Don't infuse with other drugs in the same I.V. line.
Subcutaneous
- Remove drug from refrigerator 30 minutes before administration and allow it to reach room temperature.

• Inspect solution before administration. Don't use solution if discolored or cloudy or if foreign particles are present. Drug is normally colorless to slightly opalescent to light yellow.

• Prefilled syringe and prefilled autoinjector contain latex. Don't handle if sensitive to latex.

• Don't use any leftover product remaining in prefilled syringe or prefilled autoinjector.

• Rotate injection sites. Don't inject drug into areas where skin is tender, bruised, red, or hard.

• If multiple injections are required, administer injections at different sites on the body.

ACTION

Binds to human TNF-alpha to neutralize its activity and inhibit its binding with receptors, thereby reducing the infiltration of inflammatory cells.

Route	Onset	Peak	Duration
I.V.	Unknown	12 weeks	Unknown
Subcut.	Unknown	2–6 days	Unknown

Half-life: 2 weeks.

ADVERSE REACTIONS

CNS: dizziness, paresthesia, fever.
CV: hypertension.
EENT: nasopharyngitis, oral herpes, pharyngitis, rhinitis, sinusitis.
GI: constipation.
Respiratory: bronchitis, upper respiratory tract infection.
Skin: injection-site reactions, superficial fungal infections.
Other: influenza.

INTERACTIONS

Drug-drug. *Abatacept, anakinra, other immunosuppressants:* May increase risk of serious infection. Avoid using together.
CYP450 substrates (such as cyclosporine, theophylline, warfarin): May alter levels of these drugs. Monitor patient closely and adjust dosages as needed.
Live-virus vaccines: May increase risk of infection. Postpone live-virus vaccine until therapy has ended.

EFFECTS ON LAB TEST RESULTS

• May increase LFT values.
• May decrease platelet, WBC, and neutrophil counts.

CONTRAINDICATIONS & CAUTIONS

• Use cautiously in patients with malignancies; invasive fungal infection; chronic infection (hepatitis B, tuberculosis [TB]); history of recurrent infection, hematologic abnormalities, or heart failure; or preexisting or recent onset of CNS demyelination.

• Use in pregnant women only if benefit outweighs risk to fetus. It isn't known if drug appears in breast milk. Women shouldn't breast-feed while taking drug.

• Safe use in children hasn't been established.

NURSING CONSIDERATIONS

Black Box Warning Monitor patient closely for signs and symptoms of infection before and after treatment. TB, invasive fungal infection, and other opportunistic infections, which are sometimes fatal, may occur in patients receiving golimumab. Stop drug if serious infection or sepsis develops during treatment. ∎

Black Box Warning Evaluate patient for latent TB with tuberculin skin test before initiating treatment. Treat latent TB before therapy with golimumab. Monitor all patients for active TB during treatment even if initial latent TB test is negative. ∎

• Monitor patient for new or worsening heart failure; stop drug if signs and symptoms occur.

Black Box Warning Lymphoma and other malignancies, some fatal, have been reported in children and adolescents treated with TNF blockers, including golimumab. ∎

• Monitor patient for lymphomas and other malignancies.

• Monitor CBC regularly during therapy.

PATIENT TEACHING

• Teach patient how to give subcutaneous injection. First self-injection should be under supervision of qualified health care practitioner.

• Advise patient that prefilled syringes and prefilled autoinjectors contain latex or a latex derivative.

• Instruct patient to report signs and symptoms of infection, new or worsening heart failure, or liver or nervous system problems.
• Advise women to report pregnancy, possible pregnancy, or plans to become pregnant.
• Tell patient to avoid live-virus vaccines while taking this drug.
• Advise breast-feeding women to stop breast-feeding during therapy.

granisetron
gran-IZ-e-tron

Sancuso

granisetron hydrochloride

Therapeutic class: Antiemetics
Pharmacologic class: Selective serotonin receptor antagonists
Pregnancy risk category: B

AVAILABLE FORMS
Injection: 0.1 mg/mL in 1-mL single-use vials; 1 mg/mL in 1-mL, single-dose, preservative-free vials and 4-mL multidose vials containing benzyl alcohol
Oral solution: 1 mg/5 mL
Tablets: 1 mg
Transdermal patch: 3.1 mg per 24 hours

INDICATIONS & DOSAGES
➤ **To prevent nausea and vomiting from emetogenic cancer chemotherapy**
Adults and children age 2 and older:
10 mcg/kg I.V. undiluted and given by direct injection over 30 seconds, or diluted and infused over 5 minutes. Start giving at least 30 minutes before chemotherapy. Or, for adults, 1 mg P.O. up to 1 hour before chemotherapy and repeated 12 hours later. Or, for adults, 2 mg P.O. daily given up to 1 hour before chemotherapy. Or, for adults, apply a single patch to the upper outer arm 24 to 48 hours before chemotherapy. Remove the patch a minimum of 24 hours after completion of chemotherapy or a maximum of 7 days.
➤ **To prevent nausea and vomiting from radiation, including total body irradiation and fractionated abdominal radiation**
Adults: 2 mg P.O. once daily within 1 hour of radiation.
➤ **Postoperative nausea and vomiting**
Adults: 1 mg I.V. undiluted and given over 30 seconds. For prevention, give before anesthesia induction or immediately before reversal.

ADMINISTRATION
P.O.
• Store bottle of oral solution in an upright position.
• Keep bottle of oral solution tightly closed; protect from light.
I.V.
▼ For direct injection, give drug undiluted over 30 seconds.
▼ For intermittent infusion, dilute with normal saline solution for injection or D_5W to a volume of 20 to 50 mL.
▼ Infuse over 5 minutes, starting within 30 minutes before chemotherapy and only on days chemotherapy is given.
▼ Diluted solutions are stable 24 hours at room temperature.
▼ Don't freeze vials.
▼ Once the multiuse vial is penetrated, use contents within 30 days.
▼ **Incompatibilities:** Other I.V. drugs.
Transdermal
• Apply patch to intact, healthy skin.
• Each patch is packed in a pouch and should be applied directly after the pouch has been opened.
• Do not cut the patch into pieces.

ACTION
May block 5-HT_3 in the CNS in the chemoreceptor trigger zone and in the peripheral nervous system on nerve terminals of the vagus nerve.

Route	Onset	Peak	Duration
P.O., I.V.	Unknown	Unknown	Unknown
Transdermal	Unknown	48 hr	Unknown

Half-life: 5 to 9 hours.

ADVERSE REACTIONS
CNS: asthenia, headache, fever, agitation, anxiety, CNS stimulation, dizziness, insomnia, somnolence, pain.
CV: *bradycardia,* hypertension, hypotension.

G

GI: constipation, nausea, vomiting, abdominal pain, decreased appetite, diarrhea, dyspepsia, flatulence, taste disorder.
GU: oliguria, UTI.
Hematologic: anemia, *leukocytosis, leukopenia, thrombocytopenia.*
Respiratory: cough, increased sputum.
Skin: alopecia, rash, dermatitis.
Other: hypersensitivity reactions (*anaphylaxis,* urticaria, dyspnea, hypotension), infection.

INTERACTIONS
Drug-drug. *Apomorphine:* May increase risk of profound hypotension and loss of consciousness. Use together is contraindicated.
Drug that prolong QT interval: May increase risk of life-threatening cardiac arrhythmias, including torsades de pointes. Use together cautiously and monitor patient.

EFFECTS ON LAB TEST RESULTS
● May increase ALT and AST levels. May decrease hemoglobin level and hematocrit. May alter fluid and electrolyte levels with prolonged use.
● May decrease platelet and WBC counts.

CONTRAINDICATIONS & CAUTIONS
● Contraindicated in patients hypersensitive to drug.
⚠ *Overdose S&S:* Headache.

NURSING CONSIDERATIONS
● Drug regimen is given only on days when chemotherapy is given. Treatment at other times isn't useful.

PATIENT TEACHING
● Stress importance of taking second dose of oral drug 12 hours after the first for maximum effectiveness.
● Tell patient to report adverse reactions immediately.

guaifenesin (glyceryl guaiacolate)
gwye-FEN-e-sin

Altarussin ◊, Balminil† ◊, Benylin E† ◊, Diabetic Tussin ◊, Fenesin IR ◊, Geri-Tussin ◊, Liquibid, Liquituss GG ◊, Mucinex ◊, Mucinex Mini-Melts ◊, Mucosa ◊, Mucus Relief ◊, Naldecon Senior EX ◊, Organ-I NR ◊, Q-Tussin ◊, Refenesen ◊, Robafen ◊, Robitussin ◊, Scot-Tussin Expectorant ◊, Siltussin ◊, Tussin ◊, Xpect ◊

Therapeutic class: Expectorants
Pharmacologic class: Propanediol derivatives
Pregnancy risk category: C

AVAILABLE FORMS
Capsules: 200 mg ◊
Granules: 50 mg ◊, 100 mg ◊
Liquid: 100 mg/5 mL ◊*, 200 mg/5 mL ◊
Syrup: 100 mg/5 mL ◊
Tablets: 100 mg ◊, 200 mg ◊, 400 mg
Tablets (extended-release): 600 mg ◊, 1,200 mg ◊

INDICATIONS & DOSAGES
➤ **Expectorant**
Adults and children age 12 and older: 200 to 400 mg P.O. every 4 hours, or 600 to 1,200 mg extended-release capsules or tablets P.O. every 12 hours. Maximum, 2,400 mg daily.
Children ages 6 to 11: 100 to 200 mg P.O. every 4 hours. Maximum, 1,200 mg daily.
Children ages 2 to 5: 50 to 100 mg (immediate-release) P.O. every 4 hours. Maximum, 600 mg daily.

ADMINISTRATION
P.O.
● Don't break or crush extended-release products.
● Empty entire contents of granule packet on the patient's tongue. Tell patient to swallow without chewing for best taste.

Reactions in bold italics are *life-threatening*. Interactions may have a *rapid onset* or a *delayed onset*.

ACTION
Increases production of respiratory tract fluids to help liquefy and reduce the viscosity of tenacious secretions.

Route	Onset	Peak	Duration
P.O.	Unknown	Unknown	Unknown

Half-life: 1 hour.

ADVERSE REACTIONS
CNS: dizziness, headache.
GI: vomiting, nausea.
Skin: rash, urticaria.

INTERACTIONS
None significant.

EFFECTS ON LAB TEST RESULTS
• May interfere with uric acid level determination and with 5-hydroxyindoleacetic acid and vanillylmandelic tests.

CONTRAINDICATIONS & CAUTIONS
• Contraindicated in patients hypersensitive to drug.

NURSING CONSIDERATIONS
• Some liquid formulations contain alcohol.
• Drug is used to liquefy thick, tenacious sputum. Evidence suggests that guaifenesin is effective as an expectorant, but no evidence exists to support its role as an antitussive.
• Monitor cough type and frequency.
• Stop use 48 hours before 5-hydroxyindoleacetic acid and vanillylmandelic tests.
• *Look alike–sound alike:* Don't confuse guaifenesin with guanfacine.

PATIENT TEACHING
• Tell patient to contact his health care provider if cough lasts longer than 1 week, recurs frequently, or is accompanied by high fever, rash, or severe headache.
• Inform patient that drug shouldn't be used for chronic or persistent cough, such as with smoking, asthma, chronic bronchitis, or emphysema.
• Advise patient to take each dose with one glass of water; increasing fluid intake may prove beneficial.

• Tell patient to empty entire contents of granule packet onto the tongue and to swallow without chewing for best taste.
• Encourage deep-breathing exercises.

guanfacine hydrochloride
GWAHN-fa-seen

Intuniv, Tenex

Therapeutic class: Antihypertensives
Pharmacologic class: Centrally acting antiadrenergics
Pregnancy risk category: B

AVAILABLE FORMS
Tablets: 1 mg, 2 mg
Tablets (extended-release): 1 mg, 2 mg, 3 mg, 4 mg

INDICATIONS & DOSAGES
➤ **Hypertension**
Adults: Initially, 1 mg immediate-release tablet P.O. once daily at bedtime. If response isn't adequate after 3 to 4 weeks, increase dosage to 2 mg daily. Dosage may be further increased to 3 mg P.O. after an additional 3 to 4 weeks.
➤ **Pediatric hypertension**
Children age 12 and older: Initially, 1 mg immediate-release tablet P.O. daily at bedtime. May increase to 2 mg after 3 to 4 weeks as needed.
➤ **Attention deficit hyperactivity disorder**
Children age 6 and older: Extended-release form only. Initially, 1 mg P.O. once daily in a.m. Adjust dosage in increments of 1 mg/week as needed. Dosage range is 1 to 4 mg/day. Or, initially, 0.05 to 0.08 mg/kg P.O. once daily. Adjust dosage up to 0.12 mg/kg once daily if well tolerated and necessary. Maximum total dose is 4 mg/day.
➤ **Tourette syndrome ◆**
Children and adolescents: Initially, 0.5 mg (immediate-release) P.O. daily. Maximum dose is 4 mg P.O. daily in three divided doses.

ADMINISTRATION
P.O.
• When given with another antihypertensive, give dose at bedtime to reduce somnolence.

- Don't give extended-release tablet with high-fat meal; give with water, milk, or other liquid.
- Don't crush, break, or allow patient to chew extended-release tablets.

ACTION

Reduces sympathetic outflow from the vasomotor center to the heart and blood vessels, resulting in a decrease in peripheral vascular resistance and a reduction in heart rate.

Route	Onset	Peak	Duration
P.O.	Unknown	1–4 hr	24 hr
P.O. (extended-release)	Unknown	4–8 hr	Unknown

Half-life: About 17 hours; for extended-release tablet, about 18 hours.

ADVERSE REACTIONS

CNS: dizziness, somnolence, fatigue, headache, insomnia, asthenia.
CV: *bradycardia.*
GI: constipation, dry mouth, diarrhea, nausea
GU: erectile dysfunction.
Skin: dermatitis, pruritus.

INTERACTIONS

Drug-drug. *Alpha-2 adrenergic agonists (tizanidine):* May cause additive hypotension. Avoid use together if possible.
Antihypertensives (lisinopril, metoprolol): May increase risk of hypotension and syncope. Use together cautiously.
CNS depressants: May increase sedation. Use together cautiously.
CYP3A4 inducers (phenytoin, rifampin): May reduce guanfacine efficacy. Consider increasing guanfacine dosage within recommended range.
CYP3A4/5 strong inhibitors (ketoconazole): May increase effects and adverse reactions of guanfacine. Monitor patient and adjust guanfacine dosage as needed.
TCAs: May inhibit antihypertensive effects. Monitor blood pressure.
Valproic acid: May increase valproic acid concentration. Monitor patient for additive CNS effects (sedation) and adjust valproic acid dosage as needed.
Drug-lifestyle. *Alcohol:* May increase sedation. Discourage alcohol use.

EFFECTS ON LAB TEST RESULTS

None reported.

CONTRAINDICATIONS & CAUTIONS

- Contraindicated in patients hypersensitive to drug.
- Use cautiously in patients with severe coronary insufficiency, recent MI, cerebrovascular disease, or chronic renal or hepatic insufficiency.
- **⚠ *Overdose S&S:*** Drowsiness, lethargy, bradycardia, hypotension.

NURSING CONSIDERATIONS

- Monitor blood pressure frequently.
- Risk and severity of adverse reactions increase with higher dosages.
- Drug may be used alone or with a diuretic.
- Rebound hypertension may occur and, if it occurs, will be noticeable within 2 to 4 days after therapy ends.
- Children on long-term treatment require periodic reassessment.
- Don't substitute immediate-release for extended-release form or vice versa, or use together.
- Immediate-release form may be used as monotherapy or in combination with other antihypertensives.
- ***Look alike–sound alike:*** Don't confuse guanfacine with guanidine, guaifenesin, or guanabenz. Don't confuse Tenex with Xanax, Entex, or Ten-K.

PATIENT TEACHING

- Tell patient not to stop therapy abruptly and to follow tapering instructions from provider.
- Advise patient to avoid activities that require alertness before drug's effects are known; drowsiness may occur.
- Warn patient that he may have a lower tolerance to alcohol and other CNS depressants during therapy.
- Caution patient that drug may decrease saliva and contribute to dental caries, periodontal disease, oral candidiasis, and discomfort. Advise patient to have routine dental examinations.
- Advise patient not to take extended-release form with a high-fat meal because of increase in drug exposure. Tablet may be taken with water, milk, or other liquid.
- Tell patient not to crush, chew, or break extended-release tablets.

Reactions in bold italics are *life-threatening*. Interactions may have a *rapid onset* or a *delayed onset*.

haloperidol
ha-loe-PER-i-dole

Haldol, Novo-Peridol†

haloperidol decanoate
Haldol Decanoate, Haloperidol LA†

haloperidol lactate
Haldol

Therapeutic class: Antipsychotics
Pharmacologic class: Phenylbutyl-
piperadine derivatives
Pregnancy risk category: C

AVAILABLE FORMS
haloperidol
Tablets: 0.5 mg, 1 mg, 2 mg, 5 mg, 10 mg,
20 mg
haloperidol decanoate
Injection: 50 mg/mL, 100 mg/mL
haloperidol lactate
Injection: 5 mg/mL
Oral solution: 2 mg/mL

INDICATIONS & DOSAGES
Adjust-a-dose (for all indications): For indications with oral dosing and for oral dosing
in elderly and debilitated patients, initially,
0.5 to 2 mg P.O. b.i.d. or t.i.d.; increase
gradually, as needed.
➤ **Psychotic disorders**
Adults and children older than age 12:
Dosage varies for each patient. Initially,
0.5 to 5 mg P.O. b.i.d. or t.i.d. Maximum,
100 mg P.O. daily. Or, 2 to 5 mg lactate
I.M. every 4 to 8 hours, although hourly
administration may be needed until control
is obtained.
*Children ages 3 to 12 weighing 15 to
40 kg (33 to 88 lb):* Initially, 0.5 mg P.O.
in two or three divided doses daily. May
increase dose by 0.5 mg at 5- to 7-day intervals, depending on therapeutic response and
patient tolerance. Maintenance dose, 0.05 to
0.15 mg/kg P.O. daily given in two or three
divided doses. Severely disturbed children
may need higher doses.
➤ **Chronic psychosis requiring
prolonged therapy**
Adults: 50 to 100 mg decanoate I.M. every
4 weeks.

Adjust-a-dose: For elderly or debilitated
patients, lower initial dose and gradual ad-
justments are recommended. Recommended
initial and maintenance dosage is 10 to
15 times the daily oral dose, administered
I.M. every 4 weeks.
➤ **Nonpsychotic behavior disorders**
Children ages 3 to 12: 0.05 to 0.075 mg/kg
P.O. daily, in two or three divided doses.
Maximum, 6 mg daily.
➤ **Tourette syndrome**
Adults: Initially, 0.5 to 2 mg P.O. b.i.d., t.i.d.,
or as needed. Up to about 100 mg/day may
be needed.
Children ages 3 to 12: 0.05 to 0.075 mg/kg
P.O. daily, in two or three divided doses.
Elderly patients: 0.5 to 2 mg P.O. b.i.d. or
t.i.d.; increase gradually, as needed.
➤ **Hiccups** ◆
Adults: 0.5 to 2 mg P.O. daily, b.i.d., or t.i.d.
Or, 2.5 to 5 mg I.M. daily to t.i.d. Or, 5 to
10 mg/day as subcutaneous injection.
➤ **Prevention of chemotherapy-induced
nausea and vomiting** ◆
Adults: 1 to 2 mg P.O. every 4 to 6 hours
given on a set schedule.

ADMINISTRATION
P.O.
◑ *Alert:* Haloperidol isn't approved for I.V.
use.
• Protect drug from light. Slight yellowing of concentrate is common and doesn't
affect potency. Discard very discolored
solutions.
• Dilute oral solution dose with water or a
beverage, such as orange juice, apple juice,
tomato juice, or cola, immediately before
administration.
I.M.
• Protect drug from light. Slight yellowing
of solution is common and doesn't affect
potency. Discard very discolored solutions.
• When switching from tablets to I.M.
decanoate injection, give 10 to 15 times the
oral dose once a month (maximum 100 mg).
Subcutaneous
• Protect drug from light. Slight yellowing
of solution is common and doesn't affect
potency. Discard very discolored solutions.

H

---

†Canada   ◇OTC   ◆Off-label use   ✿Photoguide   *Liquid contains alcohol.

ACTION
A butyrophenone that probably exerts antipsychotic effects by blocking postsynaptic dopamine receptors in the brain.

Route	Onset	Peak	Duration
P.O.	Unknown	3–6 hr	Unknown
I.M. (decanoate)	Unknown	3–9 days	Unknown
I.M. (lactate)	Unknown	10–20 min	Unknown
Subcut.	Unknown	Unknown	Unknown

Half-life: P.O., 18 hours; I.M. lactate, 21 hours; I.M. decanoate, 3 weeks.

ADVERSE REACTIONS
CNS: severe extrapyramidal reactions, tardive dyskinesia, *neuroleptic malignant syndrome, seizures,* sedation, drowsiness, lethargy, headache, insomnia, confusion, vertigo.
CV: tachycardia, hypotension, hypertension, *QT-interval prolongation* and other ECG changes, *torsades de pointes* with high doses.
EENT: blurred vision.
GI: dry mouth, anorexia, constipation, diarrhea, nausea, vomiting, dyspepsia.
GU: urine retention, menstrual irregularities, priapism.
Hematologic: *leukopenia,* leukocytosis.
Hepatic: jaundice.
Skin: rash, other skin reactions, diaphoresis.
Other: gynecomastia.

INTERACTIONS
Drug-drug. *Anticholinergics:* May increase anticholinergic effects and glaucoma. Use together cautiously.
Azole antifungals, buspirone, macrolides: May increase haloperidol level. Monitor patient for increased adverse reactions; haloperidol dose may need to be adjusted.
Carbamazepine: May decrease haloperidol level. Monitor patient.
CNS depressants: May increase CNS depression. Use together cautiously.
Lithium: May cause lethargy and confusion after high doses. Monitor patient.
Methyldopa: May cause dementia. Monitor patient closely.
Rifampin: May decrease haloperidol level. Monitor patient for clinical effect.
Drug-lifestyle. *Alcohol use:* May increase CNS depression. Discourage use together.

EFFECTS ON LAB TEST RESULTS
● May increase LFT values.
● May increase or decrease WBC count.

CONTRAINDICATIONS & CAUTIONS
● Contraindicated in patients hypersensitive to drug and in those with parkinsonism, coma, or CNS depression.
● Use cautiously in elderly and debilitated patients; in patients with history of seizures or EEG abnormalities, prolonged QT interval and other severe CV disorders, allergies, glaucoma, or urine retention; and in those taking anticonvulsants, anticoagulants, antiparkinsonians, or lithium.
◑ Alert: Neonates exposed to antipsychotic drugs during the third trimester of pregnancy are at risk for developing extrapyramidal signs and symptoms (repetitive muscle movements of the face and body) and withdrawal symptoms (agitation, abnormally increased or decreased muscle tone, tremors, sleepiness, severe difficulty breathing, difficulty feeding) following delivery. Use in pregnancy only if the potential benefit to the mother justifies the risk to the fetus.
⚠ Overdose S&S: Severe extrapyramidal reactions, hypotension, sedation.

NURSING CONSIDERATIONS
● Monitor patient for tardive dyskinesia, which may occur after prolonged use. It may not appear until months or years later and may disappear spontaneously or persist for life, despite ending drug.
◑ Alert: Watch for signs and symptoms of neuroleptic malignant syndrome (extrapyramidal effects, hyperthermia, autonomic disturbance), which is rare but commonly fatal.
◑ Alert: Monitor ECG when drug is given in high doses because of the increased risk of QT-interval prolongation and torsades de pointes.
Black Box Warning Elderly patients with dementia-related psychosis treated with atypical or conventional antipsychotics are at increased risk for death. Antipsychotics aren't approved for the treatment of dementia-related psychosis. ▮
● Don't withdraw drug abruptly unless required by severe adverse reactions.

Reactions in bold italics are *life-threatening*. Interactions may have a *rapid onset* or a *delayed onset*.

⊙ Alert: Haldol may contain tartrazine.
● **Look alike–sound alike:** Don't confuse Haldol with Halcion or Halog.

PATIENT TEACHING

● Although drug is the least sedating of the antipsychotics, warn patient to avoid activities that require alertness and good coordination until effects of drug are known. Drowsiness and dizziness usually subside after a few weeks.
● Warn patient to avoid alcohol during therapy.
● Tell patient to relieve dry mouth with sugarless gum or hard candy.

SAFETY ALERT!

heparin sodium
HEP-ah-rin

Heparin Lock Flush Solution (with Tubex), Heparin Sodium Injection

Therapeutic class: Anticoagulants
Pharmacologic class: Anticoagulants
Pregnancy risk category: C

AVAILABLE FORMS
Products are derived from beef lung or pork intestinal mucosa.

heparin sodium
Carpuject: 5,000 units/mL
Premixed I.V. solutions: 1,000 units in 500 mL (2 units/mL) of normal saline solution; 2,000 units in 1,000 mL (2 units/mL) of normal saline solution; 12,500 units in 250 mL (50 units/mL) of half-normal saline solution; 25,000 units in 250 mL (100 units/mL) of half-normal saline solution; 25,000 units in 500 mL (50 units/mL) of half-normal saline solution; 10,000 units in 100 mL (100 units/mL) of D$_5$W; 12,500 units in 250 mL (50 units/mL) of D$_5$W; 20,000 units in 500 mL (40 units/mL) of D$_5$W; 25,000 units in 250 mL (100 units/mL) of D$_5$W; 25,000 units in 500 mL (50 units/mL) of D$_5$W
Single-dose ampules and vials: 1,000 units/mL, 5,000 units/mL, 10,000 units/mL, 20,000 units/mL, 40,000 units/mL

Syringes: 1,000 units/mL, 2,500 units/mL, 5,000 units/mL, 7,500 units/mL, 10,000 units/mL, 20,000 units/mL
Unit-dose vials: 1,000 units/mL, 2,500 units/mL, 5,000 units/mL, 7,500 units/mL, 10,000 units/mL, 20,000 units/mL
Vials (multidose): 1,000 units/mL, 2,000 units/mL, 2,500 units/mL, 5,000 units/mL, 10,000 units/mL, 20,000 units/mL, 40,000 units/mL
heparin sodium flush
Syringes: 1 unit/mL, 10 units/mL, 100 units/mL
Vials: 10 units/mL, 100 units/mL

INDICATIONS & DOSAGES
➤ **Full-dose continuous I.V. infusion therapy for DVT, MI, or PE**
Adults: Initially, 5,000 units by I.V. bolus; then 20,000 to 40,000 units/day by I.V. infusion with pump. Titrate hourly rate based on PTT results (every 4 to 6 hours in the early stages of treatment).
Children: Initially, 50 units/kg I.V.; then 100 units/kg I.V. infusion every 4 hours or 20,000 units/m^2 daily by I.V. infusion pump. Titrate dosage based on PTT.
➤ **Full-dose subcutaneous therapy for DVT, MI, or PE**
Adults: Initially, 5,000 units I.V. bolus and 10,000 to 20,000 units in a concentrated solution subcutaneously; then 8,000 to 10,000 units subcutaneously every 8 hours or 15,000 to 20,000 units in a concentrated solution every 12 hours.
➤ **Full-dose intermittent I.V. therapy for DVT, MI, or PE**
Adults: Initially, 10,000 units by I.V. bolus; then titrated according to PTT, and 5,000 to 10,000 units I.V. every 4 to 6 hours.
➤ **Fixed low-dose therapy for prevention of venous thrombosis, PE, embolism associated with atrial fibrillation, and postoperative DVT**
Adults: 5,000 units subcutaneously every 12 hours. In surgical patients, give first dose 2 hours before procedure; then 5,000 units subcutaneously every 8 to 12 hours for 5 to 7 days or until patient can walk.
➤ **Open-heart surgery**
Adults: For total body perfusion, 150 to 400 units/kg continuous I.V. infusion.

H

Frequently, a dose of 300 units/kg for procedures estimated to last less than 60 minutes, or 400 units/kg for those estimated to last more than 60 minutes, is used.

ADMINISTRATION

I.V.

▼ Draw blood to establish baseline coagulation parameters before therapy.

▼ Use an infusion pump to provide maximum safety. Check continuous infusions regularly, even when pumps are in good working order, to ensure correct dosing. Place notice above patient's bed to caution I.V. team or laboratory personnel to apply pressure dressings after taking blood.

▼ During intermittent infusion, always draw blood 30 minutes before next scheduled dose to avoid falsely elevated PTT. Blood for PTT may be drawn 4 hours after continuous I.V. heparin therapy starts. Never draw blood for PTT from the tubing of the heparin infusion or from the infused vein, because falsely elevated PTT will result. Always draw blood from the opposite arm.

▼ Don't skip a dose or try to "catch up" with a solution containing heparin. If solution runs out, restart it as soon as possible, and reschedule bolus dose immediately. Monitor PTT.

▼ Concentrated heparin solutions (more than 100 units/mL) can irritate blood vessels.

▼ Never piggyback other drugs into an infusion line while heparin infusion is running. Never mix another drug and heparin in same syringe when giving a bolus.

▼ **Incompatibilities:** Alteplase; amikacin; amiodarone; amphotericin B cholesteryl sulfate complex; ampicillin sodium; atracurium; caspofungin; chlorpromazine; ciprofloxacin; codeine phosphate; cytarabine; dacarbazine; dantrolene; daunorubicin; dextrose 4.3% in sodium chloride solution 0.18%; diazepam; diltiazem; dobutamine; doxorubicin; doxycycline hyclate; droperidol; ergotamine; erythromycin glucoheptate or lactobionate; filgrastim; gentamicin; haloperidol lactate; hydrocortisone sodium succinate; hydroxyzine hydrochloride; idarubicin; kanamycin; labetalol; levofloxacin; levorphanol; meperidine; methadone; methylprednisolone sodium succinate; morphine sulfate; nesiritide; netilmicin; nicardipine; penicillin G potassium; penicillin G sodium; pentazocine lactate; phenytoin sodium; polymyxin B sulfate; prochlorperazine edisylate; promethazine hydrochloride; quinidine gluconate; reteplase; 1/6 M sodium lactate; solutions containing a phosphate buffer, sodium carbonate, or sodium oxalate; streptomycin; sulfamethoxazole–trimethoprim; tobramycin sulfate; trifluoperazine; triflupromazine; vancomycin; vinblastine; warfarin.

Subcutaneous

● Give low-dose injections sequentially between iliac crests in lower abdomen deep into subcutaneous fat. Inject drug subcutaneously slowly into fat pad.

● Don't massage injection site; watch for signs of bleeding there.

● Alternate sites every 12 hours—right for morning, left for evening. Record location.

ACTION

Accelerates formation of antithrombin III–thrombin complex and deactivates thrombin, preventing conversion of fibrinogen to fibrin.

Route	Onset	Peak	Duration
I.V.	Immediate	Unknown	Variable
Subcut.	20–60 min	2–4 hr	Variable

Half-life: 1 to 2 hours. Half-life is dose-dependent and nonlinear and may be disproportionately prolonged at higher doses.

ADVERSE REACTIONS

CNS: fever.
EENT: rhinitis.
Hematologic: *hemorrhage, overly prolonged clotting time, thrombocytopenia, white clot syndrome.*
Metabolic: *hyperkalemia,* hypoaldosteronism.
Skin: irritation, mild pain, hematoma, ulceration, cutaneous or subcutaneous necrosis, pruritus, urticaria.
Other: hypersensitivity reactions, including chills; *anaphylactoid reactions.*

INTERACTIONS
Drug-drug. *Antihistamines, digoxin, quinine, tetracycline:* May interfere with anticoagulant effect of heparin. Monitor patient for therapeutic effect.
Antiplatelet drugs, salicylates: May increase anticoagulant effect. Use together cautiously. Monitor coagulation studies and patient closely.
Cephalosporins, penicillins: May increase risk of bleeding. Monitor patient closely.
Nitroglycerin: May decrease effects of heparin. Monitor patient closely.
Oral anticoagulants: May increase additive anticoagulation. Monitor PT, INR, and PTT.
Thrombolytics: May increase risk of hemorrhage. Monitor patient closely.
Drug-herb. *Angelica (dong quai), boldo, bromelains, capsicum, chamomile, dandelion, danshen, devil's claw, fenugreek, feverfew, garlic, ginger, ginkgo, ginseng, horse chestnut, licorice, meadowsweet, motherwort, onion, passion flower, red clover, white willow:* May increase risk of bleeding. Discourage herb use.
Drug-lifestyle. *Smoking:* May interfere with anticoagulant effect of heparin. Discourage smoking.

EFFECTS ON LAB TEST RESULTS
• May increase ALT, AST, and potassium levels.
• May increase INR, PT, and PTT. May decrease platelet count.
• Drug may cause false elevations in some tests for thyroxine level.

CONTRAINDICATIONS & CAUTIONS
• Contraindicated in patients hypersensitive to drug. Conditionally contraindicated in patients with active bleeding, blood dyscrasia, or bleeding tendencies, such as hemophilia, thrombocytopenia, history of heparin-induced thrombocytopenia (HIT), or hepatic disease with hypoprothrombinemia; suspected intracranial hemorrhage; suppurative thrombophlebitis; inaccessible ulcerative lesions (especially of GI tract) and open ulcerative wounds; extensive denudation of skin; ascorbic acid deficiency; and other conditions that cause increased capillary permeability.

• Conditionally contraindicated during or after brain, eye, or spinal cord surgery; during spinal tap or spinal anesthesia; during continuous tube drainage of stomach or small intestine; and in subacute bacterial endocarditis, shock, advanced renal disease, threatened abortion, or severe hypertension.
• Use cautiously in women during menses or after childbirth and in patients with mild hepatic or renal disease, alcoholism, occupations with high risk of physical injury, or history of allergies, asthma, or GI ulcerations.
• Use cautiously in women older than age 60 because of an increased risk of bleeding.
⚠ **Overdose S&S:** Bleeding, nosebleeds, hematuria, tarry stools, easy bruising, petechial formations.

NURSING CONSIDERATIONS
• Although heparin use is clearly hazardous in certain conditions, its risks and benefits must be evaluated.
• If a woman needs anticoagulation during pregnancy, most prescribers use heparin.
🛈 **Alert:** Some commercially available heparin injections contain benzyl alcohol. Avoid using these products in neonates and pregnant women if possible.
• Drug requirements are higher in early phases of thrombogenic diseases and febrile states; they are lower when patient's condition stabilizes.
• Elderly patients should usually start at lower dosage.
🛈 **Alert:** Check order and vial carefully; heparin comes in various concentrations. It's now required that the label clearly state the strength of the entire container followed by how much medication is in 1 mL. Products with both the old and new labels will be available during a transition period.
🛈 **Alert:** USP and international units aren't equivalent for heparin.
🛈 **Alert:** Heparin, low–molecular-weight heparins, and danaparoid aren't interchangeable.
🛈 **Alert:** Don't change concentrations of infusions unless absolutely necessary. This is a common source of dosage errors.
🛈 **Alert:** There is the potential for delayed onset of HIT, a serious antibody-mediated

H

reaction resulting from irreversible aggregation of platelets. HIT may progress to the development of venous and arterial thromboses, a condition referred to as heparin-induced thrombocytopenia and thrombosis (HITT). Thrombotic events may be the initial presentation for HITT, which can occur up to several weeks after stopping heparin therapy. Evaluate patients presenting with thrombocytopenia or thrombosis after stopping heparin for HIT and HITT.

• Draw blood for PTT 4 to 6 hours after dose given subcutaneously.

• Avoid I.M. injections of other drugs to prevent or minimize hematoma.

• Measure PTT carefully and regularly. Anticoagulation is present when PTT values are 1½ to 2 times the control values.

• Monitor platelet count regularly. When new thrombosis accompanies thrombocytopenia (white clot syndrome), stop heparin.

• Regularly inspect patient for bleeding gums, bruises on arms or legs, petechiae, nosebleeds, melena, tarry stools, hematuria, and hematemesis.

• Monitor vital signs.

❸ **Alert:** To treat severe overdose, use protamine sulfate (1% solution), a heparin antagonist. Dosage is based on the dose of heparin, its route of administration, and the time since it was given. Generally, 1 to 1.5 mg of protamine per 100 units of heparin is given if only a few minutes have elapsed; 0.5 to 0.75 mg protamine per 100 units heparin, if 30 to 60 minutes have elapsed; and 0.25 to 0.375 mg protamine per 100 units heparin, if 2 hours or more have elapsed. Don't give more than 50 mg protamine in a 10-minute period.

• Abrupt withdrawal may cause increased coagulability; warfarin therapy usually overlaps heparin therapy for continuation of prophylaxis or treatment.

• **Look alike–sound alike:** Don't confuse heparin with Hespan.

• **Look alike–sound alike:** Don't confuse heparin sodium injection 10,000 units/mL and Hep-Lock 10 units/mL.

PATIENT TEACHING

• Instruct patient and family to watch for signs of bleeding or bruising and to notify prescriber immediately if any occur.

• Tell patient to avoid OTC drugs containing aspirin, other salicylates, or drugs that may interact with heparin unless ordered by prescriber.

• Advise patient to consult with prescriber before starting herbal therapy; many herbs have anticoagulant, antiplatelet, or fibrinolytic properties.

hydrALAZINE hydrochloride
hye-DRAL-a-zeen

Apresoline†, Novo-Hylazin†, Nu-Hydral†

Therapeutic class: Antihypertensives
Pharmacologic class: Peripheral dilators
Pregnancy risk category: C

AVAILABLE FORMS
Injection: 20 mg/mL in 1-mL vial
Tablets: 10 mg, 25 mg, 50 mg, 100 mg

INDICATIONS & DOSAGES
➤ **Essential hypertension**
Adults: Initially, 10 mg P.O. q.i.d.; gradually increase over 2 weeks to 50 mg q.i.d., based on patient tolerance and response. Recommended range is 12.5 to 50 mg b.i.d.
Children: Initially, 0.75 mg/kg daily P.O. divided into four doses; gradually increased over 3 to 4 weeks to maximum of 7.5 mg/kg or 200 mg daily. Maximum first P.O. dose is 25 mg.
➤ **Severe essential hypertension**
Adults: 20 to 40 mg I.M. or I.V. slowly; repeat as needed. Switch to oral form as soon as possible.
Children: 1.7 to 3.5 mg/kg/day I.M. or I.V. divided into four to six doses.

ADMINISTRATION
P.O.
• Give drug with food to increase absorption.
I.V.
▼ Give drug slowly and repeat p.r.n., generally every 4 to 6 hours. Hydralazine changes color in most infusion solutions; these color changes don't indicate loss of potency.

Reactions in bold italics are *life-threatening*. Interactions may have a *rapid onset* or a *delayed onset*.

▼ Drug is compatible with normal saline, Ringer, lactated Ringer, and several other common I.V. solutions.

▼ Replace parenteral therapy with oral therapy as soon as possible.

▼ **Incompatibilities:** Aminophylline, ampicillin sodium, chlorothiazide, D₅W, dextrose 10% in lactated Ringer solution, dextrose 10% in normal saline solution, diazoxide, doxapram, edetate calcium disodium, ethacrynate, fructose 10% in normal saline solution, fructose 10% in water, furosemide, hydrocortisone sodium succinate, mephentermine, metaraminol bitartrate, methohexital, nitroglycerin, phenobarbital sodium, verapamil.

I.M.

● Switch to oral form as soon as possible.

ACTION

Unknown. A direct-acting peripheral vasodilator that relaxes arteriolar smooth muscle.

Route	Onset	Peak	Duration
P.O.	20–30 min	1–2 hr	2–4 hr
I.V.	5–20 min	10–80 min	2–6 hr
I.M.	10–30 min	1 hr	2–6 hr

Half-life: 3 to 7 hours (P.O.); unknown (I.V., I.M.).

ADVERSE REACTIONS

CNS: headache, peripheral neuritis, dizziness.

CV: angina pectoris, palpitations, tachycardia, orthostatic hypotension, edema, flushing.

EENT: nasal congestion.

GI: nausea, vomiting, diarrhea, anorexia, constipation.

Hematologic: *neutropenia, leukopenia, agranulocytopenia, agranulocytosis, thrombocytopenia with or without purpura.*

Skin: rash.

Other: lupuslike syndrome.

INTERACTIONS

Drug-drug. *Diazoxide, MAO inhibitors:* May cause severe hypotension. Use together cautiously.

Diuretics, other hypotensive drugs: May cause excessive hypotension. Dosage adjustment may be needed.

Indomethacin: May decrease effects of hydralazine. Monitor blood pressure.

Metoprolol, propranolol: May increase levels and effects of these beta blockers. Monitor patient closely. May need to adjust dosage of either drug.

Drug-food. *Any food:* Food may increase drug absorption. Encourage patient to take with food.

EFFECTS ON LAB TEST RESULTS

● May decrease hemoglobin level.

● May decrease neutrophil, WBC, granulocyte, platelet, and RBC counts.

● May cause positive ANA titers.

CONTRAINDICATIONS & CAUTIONS

● Contraindicated in patients hypersensitive to drug.

● Contraindicated in those with coronary artery disease or mitral valvular rheumatic heart disease.

● Use cautiously in patients with suspected cardiac disease, stroke, or severe renal impairment and in those taking other antihypertensives.

⚠ **Overdose S&S:** Hypotension, tachycardia, headache, flushing.

NURSING CONSIDERATIONS

● Monitor patient's blood pressure, pulse rate, and body weight frequently. Drug may be given with diuretics and beta blockers to decrease sodium retention and tachycardia and to prevent angina attacks.

● Elderly patients may be more sensitive to drug's hypotensive effects.

● Obtain CBC, lupus erythematosus cell preparation, and ANA titer determination before therapy and periodically during long-term therapy.

🛈 **Alert:** Monitor patient closely for signs and symptoms of lupuslike syndrome (sore throat, fever, muscle and joint aches, rash), and notify prescriber immediately if they develop.

● Improve patient compliance by giving drug b.i.d. Check with prescriber.

● *Look alike–sound alike:* Don't confuse hydralazine with hydroxyzine.

H

PATIENT TEACHING

● Instruct patient to take oral form with meals to increase absorption.

● Inform patient that low blood pressure and dizziness upon standing can be minimized by rising slowly and avoiding sudden position changes.

● Tell woman of childbearing age to notify prescriber if she suspects pregnancy. Drug will need to be stopped.

● Tell patient to notify prescriber of unexplained prolonged general tiredness or fever, muscle or joint aching, or chest pain.

hydrochlorothiazide

hye-droe-klor-oh-THYE-a-zide

Apo-Hydro†, Microzide, Nu-hydro†, Oretic, Urozide†

Therapeutic class: Diuretics
Pharmacologic class: Thiazide diuretics
Pregnancy risk category: B

AVAILABLE FORMS

Capsules: 12.5 mg
Tablets: 12.5 mg, 25 mg, 50 mg, 100 mg†

INDICATIONS & DOSAGES

Adjust-a-dose (for all indications): In patients older than age 65 initially, 12.5 mg daily. Adjust in increments of 12.5 mg, if needed.

➤ **Edema**

Adults: 25 to 100 mg P.O. daily or intermittently; up to 200 mg initially for several days until nonedematous weight is attained.

Children ages 6 months to 12 years: Initially, 1 to 2 mg/kg/day P.O. in a single dose or two divided doses. May increase to a maximum of 37.5 mg/day for children ages 6 months to 2 years and 100 mg/day for children ages 2 to 12 years.

Children younger than age 6 months: May give up to 3 mg/kg/day P.O. in two divided doses.

➤ **Hypertension**

Adults: 12.5 to 50 mg P.O. once daily. Increase or decrease daily dose based on blood pressure.

Children ages 6 months to 12 years: Initially, 1 to 2 mg/kg/day P.O. in a single dose or two divided doses. May increase to a maximum of 37.5 mg/day for children ages 6 months to 2 years and 100 mg/day for children ages 2 to 12 years.

Children younger than age 6 months: May give up to 3 mg/kg/day P.O. in two divided doses.

ADMINISTRATION

P.O.

● To prevent nocturia, give drug in morning. If second dose is needed, give in early afternoon.

ACTION

Increases sodium and water excretion by inhibiting sodium and chloride reabsorption in distal segment of the nephron.

Route	Onset	Peak	Duration
P.O.	2 hr	4–6 hr	6–12 hr

Half-life: 5½ to 15 hours.

ADVERSE REACTIONS

CNS: dizziness, vertigo, headache, paresthesia, weakness, restlessness.

CV: orthostatic hypotension, allergic myocarditis, vasculitis.

GI: *pancreatitis,* anorexia, nausea, epigastric distress, vomiting, abdominal pain, diarrhea, constipation.

GU: *renal failure,* polyuria, frequent urination, interstitial nephritis, erectile dysfunction.

Hematologic: *aplastic anemia, agranulocytosis, leukopenia, thrombocytopenia,* hemolytic anemia.

Hepatic: jaundice.

Metabolic: asymptomatic hyperuricemia; hypokalemia; hyperglycemia and impaired glucose tolerance; fluid and electrolyte imbalances, including dilutional hyponatremia and hypochloremia; metabolic alkalosis; hypercalcemia; volume depletion and dehydration.

Musculoskeletal: muscle cramps.

Respiratory: *respiratory distress,* pneumonitis.

Skin: dermatitis, photosensitivity reactions, rash, purpura, alopecia.

Other: *anaphylactic reactions,* hypersensitivity reactions, gout.

INTERACTIONS

Drug-drug. *Amphotericin B, corticosteroids:* May increase risk of hypokalemia. Monitor potassium level closely.

Antidiabetics: May decrease hypoglycemic effects. Adjust dosage if needed. Monitor glucose level.

Antihypertensives: May have additive antihypertensive effect. Use together cautiously.

Barbiturates, opioids: May increase orthostatic hypotensive effect. Monitor patient closely.

Bumetanide, ethacrynic acid, furosemide, torsemide: May cause excessive diuretic response, causing serious electrolyte abnormalities or dehydration. Adjust doses carefully, and monitor patient closely for signs and symptoms of excessive diuretic response.

Cardiac glycosides: May increase risk of digoxin toxicity from diuretic-induced hypokalemia. Monitor potassium and digoxin levels.

Cholestyramine, colestipol: May decrease intestinal absorption of thiazides. Separate doses by 2 hours.

Diazoxide: May increase antihypertensive, hyperglycemic, and hyperuricemic effects. Use together cautiously.

Lithium: May decrease lithium excretion, increasing risk of lithium toxicity. Monitor lithium level.

NSAIDs: May increase risk of renal failure. May decrease diuretic and antihypertensive effects. Monitor renal function and blood pressure.

Drug-herb. *Dandelion:* May interfere with diuretic activity. Discourage use together.

Licorice: May cause unexpected rapid potassium loss. Discourage use together.

Drug-lifestyle. *Alcohol use:* May increase orthostatic hypotensive effect. Discourage use together.

EFFECTS ON LAB TEST RESULTS

• May increase glucose, cholesterol, triglyceride, calcium, and uric acid levels. May decrease potassium, sodium, chloride, and hemoglobin levels.

• May decrease granulocyte, WBC, and platelet counts.

CONTRAINDICATIONS & CAUTIONS

• Contraindicated in patients with anuria and patients hypersensitive to other thiazides or other sulfonamide derivatives.

• Use cautiously in children and in patients with severe renal disease, impaired hepatic function, or progressive hepatic disease.

⚠ **Overdose S&S:** Electrolyte imbalance, dehydration.

NURSING CONSIDERATIONS

• Monitor fluid intake and output, weight, blood pressure, and electrolyte levels.

• Watch for signs and symptoms of hypokalemia, such as muscle weakness and cramps.

• Drug may be used with potassium-sparing diuretic to prevent potassium loss.

• Consult prescriber and dietitian about a high-potassium diet or potassium supplement. Foods rich in potassium include citrus fruits, tomatoes, bananas, dates, and apricots.

• Monitor creatinine and BUN levels regularly. Cumulative effects of drug may occur with impaired renal function.

• Monitor uric acid level, especially in patients with history of gout.

• Monitor glucose level, especially in diabetic patients.

• Monitor elderly patients, who are especially susceptible to excessive diuresis.

• Stop thiazides and thiazide-like diuretics before parathyroid function tests.

• In patients with hypertension, therapeutic response may be delayed several weeks.

PATIENT TEACHING

• Instruct patient to take drug with food to minimize GI upset.

• Advise patient to take drug in morning to avoid need to urinate at night; if patient needs second dose, have him take it in early afternoon.

• Advise patient to avoid sudden posture changes and to rise slowly to avoid dizziness upon standing quickly.

• Encourage patient to use a sunblock to prevent photosensitivity reactions.

• Tell patient to check with prescriber or pharmacist before using OTC drugs.

SAFETY ALERT!

hydrocodone bitartrate–acetaminophen
hye-droe-KOE-done/a-seet-a-MIN-a fen

Anexsia, Co-gesic, Lortab&, Norco, Zydone

Therapeutic class: Analgesics
Pharmacologic class: Opioid analgesics–para-aminophenol derivatives
Pregnancy risk category: C
Controlled substance schedule: III

AVAILABLE FORMS
Capsules: 5 mg hydrocodone/500 mg acetaminophen
Oral solution*: 5 mg hydrocodone/500 mg acetaminophen per 15 mL, 7.5 mg hydrocodone/325 mg acetaminophen per 15 mL, 7.5 mg hydrocodone/500 mg acetaminophen per 15 mL, 10 mg hydrocodone/300 mg acetaminophen per 15 mL, 10 mg hydrocodone/325 mg acetaminophen per 15 mL, 10 mg hydrocodone/500 mg acetaminophen per 15 mL
Tablets: 2.5 mg hydrocodone/325 mg acetaminophen, 2.5 mg hydrocodone/500 mg acetaminophen, 5 mg hydrocodone/300 mg acetaminophen, 5 mg hydrocodone/325 mg acetaminophen, 5 mg hydrocodone/400 mg acetaminophen, 5 mg hydrocodone/500 mg acetaminophen, 5 mg hydrocodone/650 mg acetaminophen, 7.5 mg hydrocodone/300 mg acetaminophen, 7.5 mg hydrocodone/325 mg acetaminophen, 7.5 mg hydrocodone/400 mg acetaminophen, 7.5 mg hydrocodone/500 mg acetaminophen, 7.5 mg hydrocodone/650 mg acetaminophen, 7.5 mg hydrocodone/750 mg acetaminophen, 10 mg hydrocodone/300 mg acetaminophen, 10 mg hydrocodone/325 mg acetaminophen, 10 mg hydrocodone/400 mg acetaminophen, 10 mg hydrocodone/500 mg acetaminophen, 10 mg hydrocodone/650 mg acetaminophen, 10 mg hydrocodone/750 mg acetaminophen

INDICATIONS & DOSAGES
➤ **Moderate to moderately severe pain**
Adults: Adjust dosage according to severity of pain and patient response. Give 1 to 2 tablets or capsules (hydrocodone 2.5 to 10 mg/acetaminophen 300 to 750 mg) every 4 to 6 hours or 15 mL every 4 to 6 hours P.O. as needed. Maximum dosage is 60 mg hydrocodone/4,000 mg acetaminophen.
Children ages 2 to 14: 0.27 mL/kg (for hydrocodone 2.5 mg/acetaminophen 108 mg per 5 mL oral solution) every 4 to 6 hours as needed.
Adjust-a-dose: For patients with chronic alcoholism, limit acetaminophen to 2,000 mg daily. Acetaminophen intake shouldn't exceed 4,000 mg/day in adults and children age 13 and older; 3,200 mg/day for children age 12; 2,400 mg/day for children age 11; 2,000 mg/day for children ages 9 to 10; 1,600 mg/day for children ages 6 to 8; 1,200 mg/day for children ages 4 to 5; and 800 mg/day for children ages 2 to 3.

ADMINISTRATION
P.O.
• Give drug with food or milk.
• Administered oral solution by a calibrated device such as syringe or dropper.
• Only oral solution is approved for pediatric use.

ACTION
Inhibits synthesis of prostaglandins and binds to opiate receptors in CNS and peripherally blocks pain impulse generation; produces antipyresis by direct action on hypothalamic heat-regulating center; causes cough suppression by direct central action in medulla; may produce generalized CNS depression.

Route	Onset	Peak	Duration
P.O. (hydrocodone)	Unknown	1⅓ hr	Unknown
P.O. (acetaminophen)	Unknown	½–2 hr	3–4 hr

Half-life: Hydrocodone, 3.8 hours; acetaminophen, 1 to 4 hours.

ADVERSE REACTIONS
CNS: light-headedness, dizziness, sedation, drowsiness, mental clouding, lethargy, impairment of mental and physical

---

Reactions in bold italics are *life-threatening*. Interactions may have a *rapid onset* or a *delayed onset*.

performance, anxiety, fear, dysphoria, psychological dependence, mood changes, *stupor, coma.*
CV: *bradycardia, cardiac arrest, circulatory collapse,* hypotension.
EENT: hearing impairment, permanent hearing loss.
GI: nausea, vomiting, constipation, abdominal pain, gastric distress, heartburn, peptic ulcer.
GU: urethral spasms, spasm of vesical sphincters, urine retention, *renal tubular necrosis,* renal toxicity.
Hematologic: *thrombocytopenia, agranulocytosis,* occult blood loss, hemolytic anemia, iron deficiency anemia, prolonged bleeding time.
Hepatic: *hepatic necrosis, hepatitis,* increased LFT values.
Metabolic: *hypoglycemia, hypoglycemic coma.*
Musculoskeletal: muscle flaccidity.
Respiratory: *respiratory depression, acute airway obstruction.*
Skin: rash, pruritus, cold clammy skin, diaphoresis.
Other: allergic reaction.

INTERACTIONS
Drug-drug. *Anticholinergics:* May increase risk of paralytic ileus. Avoid use together.
Antidepressants, antihistamines, antipsychotics, anxiolytics, barbiturates or other CNS depressants, other opioids: May produce additive effects. Avoid use together.
Carbamazepine, hydantoins, isoniazid, sulfinpyrazone: May increase risk of hepatotoxicity from acetaminophen. Use cautiously together.
MAO inhibitors: May decrease blood pressure or cause additive effects. Avoid use together.
Phenothiazines, TCAs: May increase effect of either antidepressant or hydrocodone. Avoid use together.
Sodium oxybate: May increase sleep duration and CNS depression. Use together is contraindicated.
Drug-lifestyle. *Alcohol use:* May produce additive CNS effects and increase risk of hepatotoxicity. Discourage use together.

EFFECTS ON LAB TEST RESULTS
● May increase amylase and lipase levels.
● Acetaminophen may produce false-positive urinary 5-hydroxyindoleacetic acid test.

CONTRAINDICATIONS & CAUTIONS
Black Box Warning Acetaminophen has been associated with acute liver failure, at times resulting in liver transplant and death. Most liver injury has been associated with the use of acetaminophen at doses exceeding 4,000 mg/day, and often involves more than one acetaminophen-containing product. ■
◑ **Alert:** May cause serious, potentially fatal skin reactions, including Stevens-Johnson syndrome, toxic epidermal necrolysis, and acute generalized exanthematous pustulosis. Reaction may occur with first or subsequent use when acetaminophen is used as monotherapy or when it's one component of combination drug therapy. Monitor patient for reddening of the skin, rash, blisters, and detachment of the upper surface of the skin. Stop drug immediately if skin reaction is suspected.
● Contraindicated in patients hypersensitive to drug or its components and in breast-feeding women.
● Use cautiously in patients who are allergic to other opioids as cross-sensitivity may occur.
● Use cautiously in patients with a history of respiratory depression, drug abuse, head injury or increased intracranial pressure, acute abdominal conditions, liver disease, recent anesthesia, pulmonary disease, renal impairment, hypothyroidism, Addison disease, or BPH and urethral stricture, and in elderly or debilitated patients and those sensitive to CNS depressants.
● Use cautiously in patients with sulfite sensitivity; drug may contain sodium bisulfite.
● Use cautiously in pregnant women only if benefits outweigh risks. May increase risk of respiratory depression and physical dependence in neonate.
⚠ **Overdose S&S:** Hydrocodone: Loss of consciousness, pinpoint pupils, respiratory depression, stupor, coma, skeletal muscle flaccidity, cold clammy skin, bradycardia, hypotension, apnea, circulatory collapse,

H

cardiac arrest, death. Acetaminophen: Fatal hepatic necrosis, renal tubular necrosis, hypoglycemic coma, thrombocytopenia, nausea, vomiting, diaphoresis, general malaise.

NURSING CONSIDERATIONS

• Monitor patients closely for an allergic reaction, particularly those who are allergic to other opioids.

• Monitor patients for signs and symptoms of drug dependence or abuse.

• Monitor respiratory status.

• Monitor patients who have had a head injury.

• Use of opioids in patients with acute abdominal disorders may mask symptoms.

• Constipation is a very common adverse effect. Treat constipation aggressively.

• Monitor liver and kidney function. Acetaminophen elimination may be increased in patients with hepatic impairment.

• Monitor patient's ability to urinate; report urine retention.

• Monitor blood pressure and pulse regularly.

• Make sure to use a calibrated measuring device to administer oral solution.

Black Box Warning Keep track of the amount of acetaminophen given on a daily basis. Be sure it's less than 4,000 mg daily. ∎

PATIENT TEACHING

• For best results, instruct patient to take drug before pain becomes severe.

• Inform patient that it's very important to take this medication only as prescribed and, if oral solution is prescribed, to make sure to measure doses accurately using a calibrated device, such as a dropper or a syringe.

• Caution patient that this medication can be habit forming, and a tolerance to the dose may develop. Explain that drug is for short-term use only.

• Advise patient that this medication may impair judgment and not to operate heavy machinery or drive until the drug's effects are known.

• Instruct patient to avoid alcohol while taking this medication.

Black Box Warning Warn patient that this medicine contains acetaminophen (or Tylenol). Caution patient not to take more

than 4,000 mg of acetaminophen on a daily basis (including from all medications being taken). Instruct patient to contact health care provider if he has taken more than 4,000 mg in a day, even if he is feeling well. ∎

• Teach patient to eat a high-fiber diet, drink plenty of fluids, and use a stool softener or bulk laxative to prevent constipation.

• Tell patient to stop drug and immediately report blurred vision, rash, or yellowing of the skin.

🛈 *Alert:* Warn patient to stop drug and seek medical attention immediately if rash or reaction occurs while using acetaminophen.

hydrocortisone (oral; injection; rectal)
hye-droe-KOR-ti-sone

Cortef, Cortenema

hydrocortisone cypionate
Cortef

hydrocortisone sodium succinate
A-Hydrocort, Solu-Cortef

Therapeutic class: Corticosteroids
Pharmacologic class: Glucocorticoids
Pregnancy risk category: C

AVAILABLE FORMS
hydrocortisone
Enema: 100 mg/60 mL
Tablets: 5 mg, 10 mg, 20 mg
hydrocortisone cypionate
Tablets: 5 mg, 10 mg, 20 mg
hydrocortisone sodium succinate
Injection: 100-mg vial, 250-mg vial, 500-mg vial, 1,000-mg vial

INDICATIONS & DOSAGES
➤ **Severe inflammation, adrenal insufficiency**
Adults: 20 to 240 mg P.O. daily. Or, initially, 100 to 500 mg succinate I.M. or I.V.; repeat every 2, 4, or 6 hours as needed.
➤ **Shock**
Adults: Initially, 50 mg/kg succinate I.V., repeated in 4 hours. Repeat dosage every 24 hours as needed. Or, 0.5 to 2 g every 2 to

6 hours, continued until patient is stabilized (usually not longer than 48 to 72 hours).

➤ **Adjunct treatment for ulcerative colitis and proctitis**

Adults: 1 enema (100 mg) P.R. nightly for 21 days. Or, 1 applicatorful (90-mg foam) P.R. daily or b.i.d. for 14 to 21 days.

ADMINISTRATION
P.O.

● Give drug with milk or food when possible. Patient may need another drug to prevent GI irritation.

I.V.

▼ Don't use acetate form for I.V. route.

▼ Reconstitute hydrocortisone sodium succinate with bacteriostatic water or bacteriostatic saline solution before adding to I.V. solutions. For direct injection, inject over 30 seconds to 10 minutes. For infusion, dilute with D_5W, normal saline solution, or dextrose 5% in normal saline solution to 1 mg/mL or less.

▼ **Incompatibilities:** Amobarbital, ampicillin sodium, bleomycin, ciprofloxacin, colistimethate, cytarabine, dacarbazine, diazepam, dimenhydrinate, ephedrine, ergotamine, furosemide, heparin sodium, hydralazine, idarubicin, Ionosol B with invert sugar 10%, kanamycin, methylprednisolone sodium succinate, midazolam, nafcillin, pentobarbital sodium, phenobarbital sodium, phenytoin, prochlorperazine edisylate, promethazine hydrochloride, sargramostim, vancomycin, vitamin B complex with C.

I.M.

● Inject deep into gluteal muscle. Rotate injection sites to prevent muscle atrophy. Avoid subcutaneous injection because atrophy and sterile abscesses may occur.

● Injectable forms aren't used for alternate-day therapy.

Rectal

● Have the patient lie on his left side during administration and for 30 minutes afterward to allow fluid to distribute throughout the left colon. Have patient try to retain the enema for at least 1 hour but preferably all night.

ACTION

Not clearly defined. Decreases inflammation, mainly by stabilizing leukocyte lysosomal membranes; suppresses immune response; stimulates bone marrow; and influences protein, fat, and carbohydrate metabolism.

Route	Onset	Peak	Duration
P.O., I.V., I.M., P.R.	Variable	Variable	Variable

Half-life: 8 to 12 hours.

ADVERSE REACTIONS

CNS: euphoria, insomnia, psychotic behavior, *pseudotumor cerebri,* vertigo, headache, paresthesia, *seizures.*

CV: *heart failure,* hypertension, edema, *arrhythmias,* thrombophlebitis, *thromboembolism.*

EENT: cataracts, glaucoma.

GI: peptic ulceration, GI irritation, increased appetite, *pancreatitis,* nausea, vomiting.

GU: menstrual irregularities, increased urine calcium levels.

Hematologic: easy bruising.

Metabolic: *hypokalemia,* hyperglycemia, carbohydrate intolerance, hypercholesterolemia, *hypocalcemia.*

Musculoskeletal: growth suppression in children, muscle weakness, osteoporosis, tendon rupture.

Skin: hirsutism, delayed wound healing, acne, skin eruptions.

Other: cushingoid state, susceptibility to infections, *acute adrenal insufficiency after increased stress or abrupt withdrawal after long-term therapy.*

After abrupt withdrawal: rebound inflammation, fatigue, weakness, arthralgia, fever, dizziness, lethargy, depression, fainting, orthostatic hypotension, dyspnea, anorexia, *hypoglycemia. After prolonged use, sudden withdrawal may be fatal.*

INTERACTIONS

Drug-drug. *Aspirin, indomethacin, other NSAIDs:* May increase risk of GI distress and bleeding. Use together cautiously.

H

Barbiturates, carbamazepine, fosphenytoin, phenytoin, rifampin: May decrease corticosteroid effect. Increase corticosteroid dosage.

Cyclosporine: May increase toxicity. Monitor patient closely.

Live attenuated virus vaccines, other toxoids and vaccines: May decrease antibody response and increase risk of neurologic complications. Avoid using together.

Oral anticoagulants: May alter dosage requirements. Monitor PT and INR closely.

Potassium-depleting drugs such as thiazide diuretics: May enhance potassium-wasting effects of hydrocortisone. Monitor potassium level.

Skin-test antigens: May decrease response. Postpone skin testing until after therapy.

Drug-herb. *Echinacea:* May increase immune-stimulating effects. Discourage use together.

Ginseng: May increase immune-modulating response. Discourage use together.

EFFECTS ON LAB TEST RESULTS
• May increase glucose and cholesterol levels. May decrease T_3, T_4, potassium, and calcium levels.
• May cause decreased ^{131}I uptake and protein-bound iodine levels in thyroid function tests. May cause false-negative results in nitroblue tetrazolium test for systemic bacterial infections. May alter reactions to skin tests.

CONTRAINDICATIONS & CAUTIONS
• Contraindicated in patients hypersensitive to drug or its ingredients, in those with systemic fungal infections, in those receiving immunosuppressive doses together with live-virus vaccines, and in premature infants (succinate).
• Use with caution in patients with recent MI.
• Use cautiously in patients with GI ulcer, renal disease, hypertension, osteoporosis, diabetes mellitus, hypothyroidism, cirrhosis, diverticulitis, nonspecific ulcerative colitis, active hepatitis, recent intestinal anastomoses, thromboembolic disorders, seizures, myasthenia gravis, heart failure, tuberculosis, ocular herpes simplex, emotional instability, and psychotic tendencies and in women who are breast-feeding.

NURSING CONSIDERATIONS
• Determine whether patient is sensitive to other corticosteroids.
• Most adverse reactions to corticosteroids are dose- or duration-dependent.
• For better results and less toxicity, give a once-daily dose in morning.
🔕 *Alert:* Salts aren't interchangeable.
🔕 *Alert:* Only hydrocortisone sodium succinate can be given I.V.
• Enema may produce same systemic effects as other forms of hydrocortisone. If enema therapy must exceed 21 days, taper off by giving every other night for 2 to 3 weeks.
• High-dose therapy usually isn't continued beyond 48 hours.
• Always adjust to lowest effective dose.
• Monitor patient's weight, blood pressure, and electrolyte level.
• Monitor patient for cushingoid effects, including moon face, buffalo hump, central obesity, thinning hair, hypertension, and increased susceptibility to infection.
• Unless contraindicated, give a low-sodium diet that's high in potassium and protein. Give potassium supplements.
• Drug may mask or worsen infections, including latent amebiasis.
• Stress (fever, trauma, surgery, and emotional problems) may increase adrenal insufficiency. Increase dosage.
• Watch for depression or psychotic episodes, especially during high-dose therapy.
• Inspect patient's skin for petechiae.
• Diabetic patient may need increased insulin; monitor glucose level.
• Periodic measurement of growth and development may be needed during high-dose or prolonged therapy in children.
• Elderly patients may be more susceptible to osteoporosis with prolonged use.
• Gradually reduce dosage after long-term therapy.
• *Look alike–sound alike:* Don't confuse Solu-Cortef with Solu-Medrol (methylprednisolone sodium succinate). Don't confuse hydrocortisone with hydroxychloroquine.

Reactions in bold italics are *life-threatening*. Interactions may have a *rapid onset* or a *delayed onset*.

PATIENT TEACHING
• Tell patient not to stop drug abruptly or without prescriber's consent.
• Instruct patient to take oral form of drug with milk or food.
• Warn patient on long-term therapy about cushingoid effects (moon face, buffalo hump) and the need to notify prescriber about sudden weight gain or swelling.
• Teach patient signs and symptoms of early adrenal insufficiency: fatigue, muscle weakness, joint pain, fever, anorexia, nausea, shortness of breath, dizziness, and fainting.
• Instruct patient to carry a card with his prescriber's name and name and dosage of drug, indicating his need for supplemental systemic glucocorticoids during stress.
• Warn patient about easy bruising.
• Urge patient receiving long-term therapy to consider exercise or physical therapy. Also, tell him to ask prescriber about vitamin D or calcium supplement.
• Advise patient receiving long-term therapy to have periodic eye examinations.
• Caution patient to avoid exposure to infections (such as chickenpox or measles) and to notify prescriber if such exposure occurs.

hydrocortisone (topical)
hye-droo KOR ti-sone

Ala-Cort, Ala-Scalp, Anusol HC, Cortizone-5 ◇, Cortizone-10 ◇, Cortizone-10 Quickshot ◇, Dermolate ◇, Nutra-cort, Procort ◇, Scalpicin ◇, Synacort, Tegrin-HC ◇, Texacort, T/Scalp

hydrocortisone acetate (topical; rectal)
Anusol HC ◇, Cortaid ◇, Cortef Feminine Itch ◇, Corticaine ◇, Gynecort ◇, Lanacort-5 ◇, Lanacort-10 ◇, Micort-HC, Orabase HCA, ProctoFoam-HC, U-cort

hydrocortisone butyrate
Locoid, Locoid Lipocream

hydrocortisone probutate
Pandel

hydrocortisone valerate
Westcort

Therapeutic class: Corticosteroids
Pharmacologic class: Corticosteroids
Pregnancy risk category: C

AVAILABLE FORMS
hydrocortisone
Cream: 0.5% ◇, 1% ◇, 2.5%
Gel: 1%, 2%
Lotion: 0.25%, 0.5% ◇, 1% ◇, 1%, 2%, 2.5%
Ointment: 0.5% ◇, 1% ◇, 2.5%
Paste: 0.5%
Rectal cream: 1% ◇
Rectal ointment: 1%
Topical solution: 1%, 2.5%
hydrocortisone acetate
Cream: 0.5% ◇, 1% ◇, 1%, 2%, 2.5%
Lotion: 0.5%
Ointment: 0.5% ◇, 1% ◇
Rectal foam: 90 mg per application
Rectal suppositories: 25 mg
hydrocortisone butyrate
Cream: 0.1%
Ointment: 0.1%
Solution: 0.1%
hydrocortisone probutate
Cream: 0.1%
hydrocortisone valerate
Cream: 0.2%
Ointment: 0.2%

INDICATIONS & DOSAGES
➤ **Inflammation and pruritus from corticosteroid-responsive dermatoses, adjunctive topical management of seborrheic dermatitis of scalp**
Adults and children: Clean area; apply cream, gel, lotion, ointment, or topical solution sparingly daily to q.i.d. until acute phase is controlled; then reduce dosage to one to three times weekly as needed. Give children lowest dose that provides positive results.

H

➤ **Inflammation from proctitis; adjunctive treatment of chronic ulcerative colitis, cryptitis**
Adults: 1 applicatorful of rectal foam P.R. daily or b.i.d. for 2 to 3 weeks; then every other day as needed. Or, 1 suppository P.R. b.i.d. to t.i.d. or 2 suppositories P.R. b.i.d. for 2 weeks. In factitial proctitis, recommended duration of therapy is 6 to 8 weeks.

ADMINISTRATION
Rectal
● Refer to manufacturer's instructions to properly fill applicator barrel.
● Once applicator is properly filled, gently insert tip into anus. Once in place, push plunger to expel foam; then withdraw applicator.
● Thoroughly clean all applicator parts after each use.
● Avoid excessive handling of suppository, which is designed to melt at body temperature.
● Insert suppository, pointed end first, into rectum using gentle pressure.
Topical
● Gently wash skin before applying. To prevent skin damage, rub in gently, leaving a thin coat. When treating hairy sites, part hair and apply directly to lesions.
● Check individual products for frequency of administration.
● Avoid applying near eyes or mucous membranes or in ear canal; may be safely used on face, groin, armpits, and under breasts.
● Change dressing as prescribed. Stop drug and tell prescriber if skin infection, striae, or atrophy occurs.
● Continue treatment for a few days after lesions clear.

ACTION
Unclear. Diffuses across cell membranes to form complexes with cytoplasmic receptors, showing anti-inflammatory, antipruritic, vasoconstrictive, and antiproliferative activity. Considered a low-potency (hydrocortisone, hydrocortisone acetate) and a medium-potency (hydrocortisone butyrate, hydrocortisone probutate, hydrocortisone valerate) drug, according to vasoconstrictive properties.

Route	Onset	Peak	Duration
Topical, P.R.	Unknown	Unknown	Unknown

Half-life: Unknown.

ADVERSE REACTIONS
Topical
GU: glycosuria.
Metabolic: hyperglycemia.
Skin: burning, pruritus, irritation, dryness, erythema, folliculitis, hypertrichosis, hypopigmentation, acneiform eruptions, allergic contact dermatitis, atrophy, maceration, secondary infection, striae, miliaria with occlusive dressings.
Other: *hypothalamic-pituitary-adrenal (HPA) axis suppression,* Cushing syndrome.
Rectal
CNS: *seizures, increased intracranial pressure,* vertigo, headache.
CV: hypertension.
EENT: cataracts, glaucoma.
GI: peptic ulcer, *pancreatitis,* abdominal distention.
GU: menstrual irregularities.
Metabolic: fluid or electrolyte disturbances, decreased carbohydrate tolerance.
Musculoskeletal: muscle weakness, osteoporosis, necrosis and fractures in bone.
Skin: impaired wound healing, fragile skin, petechiae, erythema, sweating.

INTERACTIONS
None significant.

EFFECTS ON LAB TEST RESULTS
● May increase glucose level.

CONTRAINDICATIONS & CAUTIONS
● Contraindicated in patients hypersensitive to drug or its components.
● Don't use as monotherapy in primary bacterial infections (impetigo, paronychia, erysipelas, cellulitis, angular cheilitis), treatment of rosacea, perioral dermatitis, or acne.
● Drug isn't for ophthalmic use.
● Use cautiously in pregnant or breast-feeding women.
⚠ *Overdose S&S:* Systemic effects.

NURSING CONSIDERATIONS

• If an occlusive dressing is applied and a fever develops, notify prescriber and remove dressing.

• If antifungal or antibiotic combined with corticosteroid fails to provide prompt improvement, stop corticosteroid until infection is controlled.

• Systemic absorption is likely with use of occlusive dressings, prolonged treatment, or extensive body surface treatment. Watch for symptoms, such as hyperglycemia, glycosuria, and HPA axis suppression.

• Avoid using plastic pants or tight-fitting diapers on treated areas in young children. Children may absorb larger amounts of drug and be more susceptible to systemic toxicity.

• Monitor patient for fluid or electrolyte disturbances (sodium and fluid retention, potassium loss, hypokalemic alkalosis, negative nitrogen balance from catabolism of protein).

• Drug may suppress skin reaction testing.

• **Look alike–sound alike:** Don't confuse hydrocortisone with hydroxychloroquine.

PATIENT TEACHING

• Teach patient or family member how to apply drug.

• Tell patient to wash hands after application.

• If an occlusive dressing is ordered, advise patient to leave it in place for no longer than 12 hours each day and not to use the dressing on infected or weeping lesions.

• Teach patient how to use rectal foam applicator or suppository if needed.

• Tell patient to stop drug and report signs of systemic absorption, skin irritation or ulceration, hypersensitivity, infection, or lack of improvement.

• For perianal application, instruct patient to place small amount of drug on a tissue and gently rub in.

• Tell patient to disassemble applicator and clean with warm water after each use.

• Tell patient to stop using this product if condition worsens or if symptoms persist for more than 7 days.

SAFETY ALERT!

hydromorphone hydrochloride (dihydromorphinone hydrochloride)
hye-droe-MOR-fone

Dilaudid, Dilaudid-HP, Exalgo

Therapeutic class: Opioid analgesics
Pharmacologic class: Opioids
Pregnancy risk category: C
Controlled substance schedule: II

AVAILABLE FORMS

Injection: 1 mg/mL, 2 mg/mL, 4 mg/mL, 10 mg/mL
Liquid: 5 mg/5 mL
Lyophilized powder for injection: 10 mg/mL
Tablets: 2 mg, 4 mg, 8 mg
Tablets (extended-release): 8 mg, 12 mg, 16 mg

INDICATIONS & DOSAGES

➤ **Moderate to severe pain**
Adults: 2 to 4 mg P.O. every 4 to 6 hours p.r.n. Or, 1 to 4 mg I.M., subcutaneously, or I.V. (slowly over at least 2 to 5 minutes) every 4 to 6 hours p.r.n. Or, 2.5 to 10 mg oral liquid every 3 to 6 hours p.r.n. Or, for adults currently on immediate-release hydromorphone who require continuous analgesia for an extended period, starting dose of extended-release form is equivalent to total daily dose of immediate-release form. May increase every 3 to 4 days. Maximum dose is 64 mg (extended-release form) P.O. once daily.

Adjust-a-dose: For elderly patients and those with renal or hepatic impairment, reduce initial starting dose.

ADMINISTRATION

P.O.
• Give drug with food if GI upset occurs.

Black Box Warning Patient should swallow extended-release tablets whole; don't break, chew, dissolve, crush, or inject them. ∎

Black Box Warning Don't give extended-release tablets with other extended-release opioids. ∎

I.V.

▼ For infusion, drug may be mixed in D_5W, normal saline solution, dextrose 5% in normal saline solution, dextrose 5% in half-normal saline solution, or Ringer or lactated Ringer solutions.

▼ Give by direct injection over no less than 2 minutes.

▼ Respiratory depression and hypotension can occur. Give slowly, and monitor patient constantly. Keep resuscitation equipment available.

▼ **Incompatibilities:** Alkalies, amphotericin B cholesteryl complex, ampicillin sodium, bromides, cefazolin, dexamethasone, diazepam, gallium nitrate, haloperidol, heparin sodium, iodides, minocycline, phenobarbital sodium, phenytoin sodium, prochlorperazine edisylate, sargramostim, sodium bicarbonate, sodium phosphate, thiopental.

I.M.

● Document administration site.

Subcutaneous

● Rotate injection sites to avoid induration with subcutaneous injection.

ACTION

Unknown. Binds with opioid receptors in the CNS, altering perception of and emotional response to pain. Also suppresses the cough reflex by direct action on the cough center in the medulla.

Route	Onset	Peak	Duration
P.O.	15–30 min	30–60 min	4–5 hr
P.O. (extended-release)	15–30 min	12–16 hr	18–24 hr
I.V.	10–15 min	15–30 min	2–3 hr
I.M.	15 min	30–60 min	4–5 hr
Subcut.	15 min	30–90 min	4 hr

Half-life: 2½ to 4 hours; P.O. (extended-release), 11 hours.

ADVERSE REACTIONS

CNS: sedation, somnolence, clouded sensorium, dizziness, euphoria, light-headedness, insomnia, drug withdrawal syndrome (extended-release form), fever, asthenia, headache, pain.

CV: hypotension, flushing, ***bradycardia,*** chest discomfort, edema.

EENT: blurred vision, diplopia, nystagmus.

GI: nausea, vomiting, constipation, anorexia, weight loss, diarrhea, ileus, dry mouth.

GU: urine retention.

Musculoskeletal: arthralgia, muscle spasms.

Respiratory: *respiratory depression, bronchospasm.*

Skin: diaphoresis, pruritus, hyperhydrosis.

Other: induration with repeated subcutaneous injections, physical dependence, pain.

INTERACTIONS

Drug-drug. *Anticholinergics:* May increase risk of urine retention or severe constipation. Use together cautiously.

CNS depressants, general anesthetics, hypnotics, MAO inhibitors, neuromuscular blockers, other opioid analgesics, sedatives, TCAs, tranquilizers: May cause additive effects. Use together with caution; reduce hydromorphone dose and monitor patient response.

Drug-lifestyle. *Alcohol use:* May cause additive effects. Discourage use together.

EFFECTS ON LAB TEST RESULTS

● May increase amylase and lipase levels.

● May interfere with hepatobiliary imaging studies because delayed gastric emptying and contraction of sphincter of Oddi may increase biliary tract pressure.

CONTRAINDICATIONS & CAUTIONS

● Contraindicated in patients hypersensitive to drug; in those with intracranial lesions that cause increased intracranial pressure; in those with paralytic ileus or narrowed or obstructed GI tract; and in those with depressed ventilation, such as in status asthmaticus, COPD, cor pulmonale, emphysema, and kyphoscoliosis.

Black Box Warning Extended-release form is contraindicated in opioid-naive patients. It isn't indicated for acute pain or postoperative pain or as a p.r.n. analgesic. Fatal respiratory depression may occur in patients who aren't opioid-tolerant. Accidental intake, especially in children, can cause fatal hydromorphone overdose. ∎

Black Box Warning Hydromorphone is an opioid agonist with an abuse liability similar to other opioid agonists, legal or illicit. Risk of abuse is increased in patients with a personal or family history of substance abuse or mental illness. ■

• Use with caution in elderly or debilitated patients and in those with hepatic or renal disease, hypothyroidism, Addison disease, prostatic hyperplasia, or urethral stricture.

⚠ **Overdose S&S:** Constricted pupils, cold clammy skin, extreme somnolence progressing to stupor or coma, respiratory depression, skeletal muscle flaccidity, bradycardia, hypotension, apnea, cardiac arrest, circulatory collapse, death.

NURSING CONSIDERATIONS

• Reassess patient's level of pain at least 15 and 30 minutes after administration.

• For better analgesic effect, give drug on a regular schedule, before patient has intense pain.

Black Box Warning Routinely monitor all patients for signs and symptoms of misuse, abuse, and addiction during treatment.

Black Box Warning Dilaudid-HP, a highly concentrated form (10 mg/mL), may be given in smaller volumes to prevent the discomfort of large-volume I.M. or subcutaneous injections. Don't confuse Dilaudid-HP with standard parenteral formulations. Check dosage carefully. ■

• Discontinue all other extended-release opioids before giving extended-release form of hydromorphone.

• Monitor respiratory and circulatory status and bowel function.

• Keep opioid antagonist (naloxone) available.

• Don't use extended-release form within 14 days of stopping MAO inhibitor.

• Discontinue use of extended-release form if stopped for more than 3 days.

• Drug may worsen or mask gallbladder pain.

• Drug is a commonly abused opioid.

• Drug may cause constipation. Assess bowel function and need for stool softeners and stimulant laxatives.

🌓 **Alert:** Cough syrup may contain tartrazine.

• **Look alike–sound alike:** Don't confuse hydromorphone with morphine or oxymorphone. Don't confuse Dilaudid with Dilantin.

PATIENT TEACHING

• Instruct patient to request or take drug before pain becomes intense.

Black Box Warning Warn patient that extended-release tablets must be taken whole. Caution patient not to cut, chew, crush, dissolve, or inject them. ■

• Advise patient to take drug with food if GI upset occurs.

• When drug is used after surgery, encourage patient to turn, cough, and breathe deeply to avoid lung problems.

• Caution patient about getting out of bed or walking. Warn outpatient to avoid hazardous activities that require mental alertness until drug's CNS effects are known.

• Advise patient to avoid alcohol during therapy.

hydroxychloroquine sulfate
hye-drox-ee-KLOR-oh-kwin

Plaquenil

Therapeutic class: Antimalarials
Pharmacologic class: Aminoquinolines
Pregnancy risk category: C

AVAILABLE FORMS

Tablets: 200 mg (equivalent to 155 mg base)

INDICATIONS & DOSAGES

Black Box Warning Prescribers should be completely familiar with this drug before prescribing. ■

➤ **Suppressive prevention of malaria attacks caused by** *Plasmodium vivax, P. malariae, P. ovale,* **and susceptible strains of** *P. falciparum*

Adults: 310 mg base P.O. weekly on the same day each week, beginning 1 to 2 weeks before entering malaria-endemic area and continuing for 4 weeks after leaving area. If not started before exposure, double first dose to 620 mg base in two divided doses 6 hours apart.

Children: 5 mg/kg base P.O. weekly on the same day each week, beginning 1 to 2 weeks before entering malaria-endemic area and continuing for 4 weeks after leaving area. Don't exceed adult dose. If not started before exposure, double first dose to 10 mg/kg base in two divided doses, 6 hours apart.

➤ **Acute malarial attacks**

Adults: Initially, 620 mg base P.O., followed by 310 mg base 6 hours after first dose; then 310 mg base daily for 2 days.

Children: Initially, 10 mg/kg base P.O.; then 5 mg/kg base at 6 hours, 24 hours, and 48 hours after the first dose.

➤ **Lupus erythematosus**

Adults: Initially, 310 mg base P.O. daily or b.i.d., continued for several weeks or months, depending on response. For prolonged maintenance dose, 155 to 310 mg base daily.

➤ **Rheumatoid arthritis**

Adults: Initially, 310 to 465 mg base P.O. daily. When good response occurs, usually in 4 to 12 weeks, cut dosage in half. If objective improvement doesn't occur within 6 months, discontinue drug.

ADMINISTRATION

P.O.

🚱 *Alert:* Drug dosage may be discussed in "mg" or "mg base"; be aware of the difference.

● Give drug with food or milk to minimize GI upset.

● To improve compliance when drug is used for prevention, advise patient to take drug immediately before or after a meal on the same day each week.

ACTION

May bind to and alter the properties of DNA in susceptible organisms.

Route	Onset	Peak	Duration
P.O.	Unknown	2–4½ hr	Unknown

Half-life: 32 to 50 days.

ADVERSE REACTIONS

CNS: *seizures,* irritability, nightmares, ataxia, psychosis, vertigo, dizziness, hypoactive deep tendon reflexes, lassitude, headache.

CV: *cardiomyopathy.*

EENT: blurred vision, difficulty in focusing, reversible corneal changes, typically irreversible nystagmus, sometimes progressive or delayed retinal changes such as narrowing of arterioles, macular lesions, pallor of optic disk, optic atrophy.

GI: anorexia, abdominal cramps, diarrhea, nausea, vomiting.

Hematologic: *agranulocytosis, leukopenia, thrombocytopenia, hemolysis in patients with G6PD deficiency, aplastic anemia.*

Metabolic: weight loss.

Musculoskeletal: skeletal muscle weakness.

Skin: pruritus, lichen planus eruptions, skin and mucosal pigmentary changes, pleomorphic skin eruptions, worsened psoriasis, alopecia, bleaching of hair.

INTERACTIONS

Drug-drug. *Aluminum salts (kaolin), magnesium:* May decrease GI absorption. Separate dose times.

Beta blockers: May increase CV effects of certain beta blockers (metoprolol). Carefully monitor patient. Consider using alternative beta blocker (atenolol).

Cimetidine: May decrease hepatic metabolism of hydroxychloroquine. Monitor patient for toxicity.

Cyclosporine: May increase cyclosporine level, which can result in nephrotoxicity. Monitor cyclosporine and serum creatinine levels. Reduce cyclosporine dosage as needed.

Digoxin: May increase digoxin level. Monitor drug levels; monitor patient for toxicity.

Magnesium salts: May decrease antacid activity of magnesium salts. May reduce effect of hydroxychloroquine. Separate dosage times by 2 to 4 hours.

Mefloquine: May increase seizure risk when used concurrently. Monitor patient carefully.

EFFECTS ON LAB TEST RESULTS

● May decrease hemoglobin level.

● May decrease granulocyte, WBC, and platelet counts.

CONTRAINDICATIONS & CAUTIONS

● Contraindicated in patients hypersensitive to drug and in those with retinal or visual field changes or porphyria.

● Contraindicated for long-term therapy for children.

Reactions in bold italics are *life-threatening*. Interactions may have a *rapid onset* or a *delayed onset*.

• Use with caution in patients with severe GI, neurologic, or blood disorders.
• Use with caution in patients with hepatic disease or alcoholism because drug concentrates in liver.
• Use with caution in those with G6PD deficiency or psoriasis because drug may worsen these conditions.
⚠ **Overdose S&S:** Headache, drowsiness, visual disturbances, CV collapse, seizures, sudden and early respiratory and cardiac arrest, atrial standstill, nodal rhythm, prolonged intraventricular conduction time, progressive bradycardia leading to ventricular fibrillation or arrest.

NURSING CONSIDERATIONS
• Ensure that baseline and periodic ophthalmic examinations are performed. Check periodically for ocular muscle weakness after long-term use.
• Make sure patient is examined with an audiometer before, during, and after therapy, especially in long-term therapy.
• Monitor CBC and LFTs periodically during long-term therapy; if severe blood disorder—not caused by disease—develops, drug may need to be stopped.
• Monitor cyclosporine and serum creatinine levels when drug is used concurrently.
🔔 **Alert:** Monitor patient for possible overdose, which can quickly lead to toxic signs or symptoms. Children are extremely susceptible to toxicity.

PATIENT TEACHING
• Advise patient taking drug for prevention to take drug immediately before or after a meal on the same day each week, to improve compliance.
• Instruct patient to report adverse reactions promptly.
• Tell patient that dizziness may occur and to use caution while driving or performing other tasks that require alertness, coordination, or physical dexterity.

hydroxyprogesterone caproate
hye-drox-ee-proh-JESS-te-rone

Makena

Therapeutic class: Hormones
Pharmacologic class: Progestins
Pregnancy risk category: B

AVAILABLE FORMS
Injection: 250-mg/mL multidose vial*

INDICATIONS & DOSAGES
➤ **To reduce risk of preterm birth in women with singleton pregnancy and history of singleton spontaneous preterm birth**
Pregnant adolescents and women age 16 and older: 250 mg I.M. once weekly starting between 16 weeks, 0 days and 20 weeks, 6 days of gestation and continuing until week 37 (through 36 weeks, 6 days) of gestation or delivery, whichever occurs first.

ADMINISTRATION
I.M.
• Visually inspect solution for particulates and discoloration before injection. Solution should be clear and yellow.
• With an 18G needle, draw up 1 mL of drug into a 3-mL syringe. Switch to a 21G 1½-inch needle for the injection.
• Administer injection into the upper outer quadrant of the gluteus maximus. The solution is viscous and oily; inject slowly over a minute or longer.
• After injection, apply pressure to minimize bruising and swelling.
• Store vial upright in its box at a controlled room temperature. Protect from light.
• Discard unused product 5 weeks after first use.

ACTION
Unknown.

Route	Onset	Peak	Duration
I.M.	Unknown	3–7 days	Unknown

Half-life: 8 days.

ADVERSE REACTIONS

CV: preeclampsia, hypertension.
GI: nausea, diarrhea.
Metabolic: gestational diabetes.
Skin: urticaria, pruritus, injection-site reactions (pain, swelling, nodule, itching).
Other: *miscarriage, stillbirth,* oligohydramnios.

INTERACTIONS

Drug-drug. *Drugs metabolized by CYP1A2 (clozapine, theophylline), CYP2A6 (acetaminophen, halothane, nicotine), CYP2B6 (bupropion, efavirenz, methadone):* May decrease levels of drugs metabolized by these pathways. Monitor patient for diminished therapeutic response to these drugs.

EFFECTS ON LAB TEST RESULTS

• May increase serum glucose level.

CONTRAINDICATIONS & CAUTIONS

• Contraindicated in patients hypersensitive to drug or its components and in those with multiple gestations or other risk factors for preterm birth; current thromboembolic disorder or history of thrombosis; known, suspected, or history of breast cancer or other hormone-sensitive cancer; undiagnosed abnormal vaginal bleeding not related to pregnancy; cholestatic jaundice of pregnancy; benign or malignant liver tumors or active liver disease; or uncontrolled hypertension.
• Contraindicated during the first trimester of pregnancy or to stop active labor.
• Discontinue drug if depression recurs in patient with history of depression.

NURSING CONSIDERATIONS

• Monitor blood glucose level in prediabetic and diabetic patients and blood pressure in all patients.
• Allergic reactions to the castor oil component of the solution have occurred. Discontinue drug if reactions occur.
• Progestins may cause fluid retention. Monitor patients with conditions that may be influenced by fluid status (such as preeclampsia, asthma, cardiac or renal dysfunction, hypertension, epilepsy, and migraines).

• Monitor patient for jaundice (indicating hepatic dysfunction) or worsening of clinical depression.
• Monitor patient for signs and symptoms of clots (extremity swelling, pain, dyspnea). Discontinue drug if thrombosis or thromboembolism occurs.

PATIENT TEACHING

• Inform patient that injection may cause pain, swelling, bruising, or itching. Instruct patient to report oozing of blood or fluids, allergic reaction (inflammation, rash), or increased discomfort or soreness over time at the injection site.
• Remind diabetic or prediabetic patient to check her blood glucose level regularly.
• Tell patient to immediately report extremity swelling, pain, dyspnea, allergic reaction, depression, or jaundice.
• Stress importance of keeping all appointments and not missing any doses during treatment.

SAFETY ALERT!

hydroxyurea

hye-drox-ee-yoor-EE-a

Droxia, Hydrea

Therapeutic class: Antineoplastics
Pharmacologic class: Antimetabolites
Pregnancy risk category: D

AVAILABLE FORMS

Capsules: 200 mg, 300 mg, 400 mg, 500 mg

INDICATIONS & DOSAGES

Adjust-a-dose (for all indications): Base dosage on patient's actual or ideal weight, whichever is less. Dosage adjustment is recommended in renal impairment. According to manufacturer, if CrCl is less than 59 mL/minute, give 50% of the usual dose. If patient is on hemodialysis, give 50% of usual dose after dialysis on dialysis days.
➤ **Carcinoma of the head and neck (with radiation) (Hydrea)**
Adults: 80 mg/kg P.O. as a single dose every third day beginning at least 7 days before starting irradiation and continuing during and after radiotherapy.

➤ **Resistant chronic myelocytic leukemia (Hydrea)**
Adults: 20 to 30 mg/kg P.O. as a single daily dose.

Adjust-a-dose: Interrupt therapy if WBC count drops below 2,500/mm³ or if platelet count is below 100,000/mm³. Reevaluate counts after 3 days and resume therapy when counts return to acceptable levels. Correct severe anemia without interrupting hydroxyurea, if possible.

➤ **Solid tumors**
Adults: 80 mg/kg P.O. as a single daily dose every third day. Or, 20 to 30 mg/kg P.O. as a single daily dose.

Adjust-a-dose: Withhold intermittent therapy for WBC count below 2,500/mm³ or platelet count below 100,000/mm³.

➤ **To reduce frequency of painful crises and need for blood transfusions in adult patients with sickle cell anemia with recurrent moderate to severe painful crises**
Adults: 15 mg/kg Droxia P.O. once daily. If blood counts are in acceptable range, dose may be increased by 5 mg/kg daily every 12 weeks until maximum tolerated dose or 35 mg/kg daily has been reached. If blood counts are considered toxic, withhold drug until counts recover. Resume treatment after reducing dose by 2.5 mg/kg daily. Every 12 weeks, drug may then be adjusted up or down in 2.5-mg/kg daily increments until patient is at a stable, nontoxic dose for 24 weeks.

➤ **Thrombocytopenia ◆**
Adults: 15 to 20 mg/kg P.O. daily. Titrate to maintain platelet count of 400,000/mm³ or less and ANC of greater than 1,000 cells/mm³.

➤ **Psoriasis ◆**
Adults: 500 mg P.O. b.i.d. Increase up to 3 g/day as tolerated.

ADMINISTRATION
P.O.
• Wear gloves when handling drug or its container, and wash hands before and after contact with bottle or capsule. If powder from capsule is spilled, wipe up immediately with a damp towel. Dispose of towel in a closed container such as a plastic bag.

ACTION
May inhibit DNA synthesis.

Route	Onset	Peak	Duration
P.O.	Unknown	2 hr	24 hr

Half-life: 3 to 4 hours.

ADVERSE REACTIONS
CNS: malaise, fever, drowsiness.
GI: anorexia, nausea, vomiting, diarrhea, stomatitis, constipation.
Hematologic: *leukopenia, thrombocytopenia,* anemia, megaloblastosis, *bone marrow suppression.*
Metabolic: hyperuricemia, weight gain.
Skin: rash, itching, alopecia, cutaneous vasculitic toxicities (including vasculitic ulcerations and gangrene).
Other: chills.

INTERACTIONS
Drug-drug. ⊙ *Alert: Antiretrovirals (such as didanosine, stavudine):* May cause hepatotoxicity and hepatic failure, resulting in death. When given with didanosine to HIV-infected patients, severe peripheral neuropathy or fatal pancreatitis may occur. Avoid using with didanosine and stavudine.
Cytotoxic drugs, radiation therapy: May enhance toxicity of hydroxyurea. Use together cautiously.
Interferon: May increase the risk of cutaneous vasculitic toxicities, including vasculitic ulcerations and gangrene. Stop drug.
Uricosuric agents (probenecid): Increases uric acid levels. Adjust dosage of uricosuric agent as needed.

EFFECTS ON LAB TEST RESULTS
• May increase BUN, creatinine, hepatic enzyme, and uric acid levels. May decrease hemoglobin level.
• May decrease WBC, RBC, and platelet counts.

CONTRAINDICATIONS & CAUTIONS
• Contraindicated in patients hypersensitive to drug and in those with WBC count less than 2,500/mm³, platelet count less than 100,000/mm³, or severe anemia.
• Use cautiously in patients with renal dysfunction and in the elderly.

H

⚠ **Overdose S&S:** Acute mucocutaneous toxicity; soreness, violet erythema on palms and soles followed by scaling of hands and feet; severe generalized hyperpigmentation of the skin; stomatitis.

NURSING CONSIDERATIONS

Black Box Warning Droxia may cause severe, sometimes life-threatening adverse effects. Administer under the supervision of a physician experienced with the use of this medication for the treatment of sickle cell anemia. ∎

Black Box Warning Hydroxyurea is mutagenic, clastogenic, and genotoxic. Secondary leukemias have occurred after long-term use. Carefully consider the potential benefits relative to the undefined risk of developing secondary malignancies. ∎

• Routinely measure BUN, uric acid, liver enzyme, and creatinine levels; monitor blood counts every 2 weeks.

• Acceptable blood counts during dosage adjustment for sickle cell anemia are neutrophil count of $2,500/mm^3$ or more, platelet count of $95,000/mm^3$ or more, hemoglobin level more than 5.3 g/dL, and reticulocyte count (if hemoglobin level is below 9 g/dL) at least $95,000/mm^3$. Toxic levels are neutrophil count less than $2,000/mm^3$, platelet count less than $80,000/mm^3$, hemoglobin level less than 4.5 g/dL, and reticulocyte count (if hemoglobin level is below 9 g/dL) less than $80,000/mm^3$.

• Hydroxyurea may dramatically lower WBC count in 24 to 48 hours.

🕙 **Alert:** Patients who have received or are currently receiving interferon may be at a greater risk for developing cutaneous vasculitic toxicities. Monitor closely.

🕙 **Alert:** Patients with HIV infection who are also receiving didanosine may be at increased risk for severe peripheral neuropathy and fatal pancreatitis. Monitor closely.

• Monitor fluid intake and output; keep patient hydrated.

• To prevent bleeding, avoid all I.M. injections when platelet count is less than $50,000/mm^3$.

• Blood transfusions may be necessary for cumulative anemia.

• Dosage change may be needed after chemotherapy or radiation therapy.

• Auditory and visual hallucinations and hematologic toxicity increase when renal function decreases.

• Drug crosses blood-brain barrier.

• Radiation therapy may increase risk or severity of GI distress or stomatitis.

PATIENT TEACHING

• Tell patient and caregiver to wear gloves when handling drug or its container and to wash their hands before and after contact with the bottle or capsule. If powder from capsule is spilled, wipe up immediately with a damp towel and dispose of the towel in a closed container such as a plastic bag.

• Tell patient who can't swallow capsules that he may empty contents into water, drink immediately, and rinse mouth with water afterward. Inform patient that some inert material may not dissolve.

• Advise patient to watch for signs and symptoms of infection (fever, sore throat, fatigue) and bleeding (easy bruising, nosebleeds, bleeding gums, tarry stools). He also should take his temperature daily.

• Caution women of childbearing age to consult prescriber before becoming pregnant.

hydrOXYzine hydrochloride
hye-DROX-i-zeen

Atarax†, Vistaril

hydrOXYzine pamoate
Vistaril

Therapeutic class: Anxiolytics
Pharmacologic class: Piperazine derivatives
Pregnancy risk category: NR

AVAILABLE FORMS
hydroxyzine hydrochloride
Capsules: 25 mg, 50 mg
Injection: 25 mg/mL, 50 mg/mL
Syrup: 2 mg/mL†, 10 mg/5 mL
Tablets: 10 mg, 25 mg, 50 mg
hydroxyzine pamoate
Capsules: 25 mg, 50 mg, 100 mg
Oral suspension: 25 mg/5 mL

INDICATIONS & DOSAGES
➤ **Anxiety**
Adults: 50 to 100 mg P.O. q.i.d. Or, 50 to 100 mg I.M. q.i.d.
Children age 6 and older: 50 to 100 mg P.O. daily in divided doses.
Children younger than age 6: 50 mg P.O. daily in divided doses.
➤ **Preoperative and postoperative adjunctive therapy for sedation**
Adults: 50 to 100 mg P.O. or I.M.
Children: 0.6 mg/kg P.O or I.M.
➤ **Pruritus**
Adults: 25 mg P.O. or I.M. t.i.d. or q.i.d.
Children age 6 and older: 50 to 100 mg P.O. daily in divided doses.
Children younger than age 6: 50 mg P.O. daily in divided doses.

ADMINISTRATION
P.O.
● Give drug without regard for meals.
● Shake suspension well before giving.
I.M.
● Parenteral form (hydroxyzine hydrochloride) is for I.M. use only, preferably by Z-track injection.
۞ Alert: Never give drug I.V., subcutaneously, or intra-arterially.
● Aspirate I.M. injection carefully to prevent inadvertent I.V. injection. Inject deeply into a large muscle.

ACTION
Suppresses activity in certain essential regions of the subcortical area of the CNS.

Route	Onset	Peak	Duration
P.O.	15–30 min	2 hr	4–6 hr
I.M.	Unknown	Unknown	4–6 hr

Half-life: 3 hours.

ADVERSE REACTIONS
CNS: drowsiness, involuntary motor activity.
GI: dry mouth, constipation.
Skin: pain at I.M. injection site.
Other: hypersensitivity reactions.

INTERACTIONS
Drug-drug. *Anticholinergics:* May cause additive anticholinergic effects. Use together cautiously.

CNS depressants: May increase CNS depression. Use together cautiously; dosage adjustments may be needed.
Epinephrine: May inhibit and reverse vasopressor effect of epinephrine. Avoid using together.
Drug-lifestyle. *Alcohol use:* May increase CNS depression. Discourage use together.

EFFECTS ON LAB TEST RESULTS
● May cause false increase in urinary 17-hydroxycorticosteroid level.
● May cause false-negative skin allergen tests by reducing or inhibiting the cutaneous response to histamine.

CONTRAINDICATIONS & CAUTIONS
● Contraindicated in patients hypersensitive to drug, patients in early pregnancy, and breast-feeding women.
● Use cautiously in elderly patients.
⚠ Overdose S&S: Hypersedation.

NURSING CONSIDERATIONS
● If patient takes other CNS drugs, watch for oversedation.
● Elderly patients may be more sensitive to adverse anticholinergic effects; monitor these patients for dizziness, excessive sedation, confusion, hypotension, and syncope.
● **Look alike–sound alike:** Don't confuse hydroxyzine with hydroxyurea, Hydrogesic, or hydralazine. Don't confuse Vistaril with Restoril.

PATIENT TEACHING
● Warn patient to avoid hazardous activities that require alertness and good coordination until effects of drug are known.
● Tell patient to avoid use of alcohol while taking drug.
● Advise patient to use sugarless hard candy or gum to relieve dry mouth.
● Warn women of childbearing age to avoid use during pregnancy and breast-feeding.

ibandronate sodium
eh-BAN-drow-nate

Boniva◆

Therapeutic class: Antiosteoporotics
Pharmacologic class: Bisphosphonates
Pregnancy risk category: C

AVAILABLE FORMS
Injection: 3 mg/3-mL prefilled syringe
Tablets: 150 mg

INDICATIONS & DOSAGES
➤ **To treat or prevent postmenopausal osteoporosis**
Women: 150 mg P.O. once monthly, taken first thing in the morning, with a large glass of plain water, 1 hour before any food or other drugs. Or, for treatment, 3 mg I.V. bolus once every 3 months.
➤ **Bone metastases ◆**
Adults: 2 mg I.V. bolus or 6 mg I.V. infusion over 1 to 2 hours every 3 to 4 weeks for up to 2 years.
➤ **Hypercalcemia of malignancy ◆**
Adults: 2 to 6 mg as a single I.V. infusion over 15 minutes to 4 hours every 4 weeks. May give additional infusions up to 6 mg (including initial dose) if the albumin-corrected serum calcium level hasn't normalized by day 4 after the initial infusion.
➤ **Prevention of bone loss after kidney transplantation ◆**
Adults: 1 mg as an I.V. bolus immediately before kidney transplantation and 2 mg as an I.V. bolus at 3, 6, and 9 months after kidney transplantation.

ADMINISTRATION
P.O.
● Give drug first thing in the morning 1 hour before eating or drinking and before any other drugs.
● Make sure patient doesn't lie down for at least 1 hour after receiving drug.
● Give drug with plain water only.
I.V.
▼ Prefilled syringes are for single use only.
▼ Give undiluted using needle provided with the syringe.
▼ Give by I.V. bolus over 15 to 30 seconds.

▼ Don't use if drug is discolored or contains particulate matter.
▼ Store at room temperature.
▼ **Incompatibilities:** Calcium-containing solutions and other I.V. drugs.

ACTION
Inhibits bone breakdown and removal to reduce bone loss and increase bone mass.

Route	Onset	Peak	Duration
P.O.	Unknown	½–2 hr	Unknown
I.V.	Rapid	Unknown	Unknown

Half-life: 1½ to 6½ days for the 150-mg oral dose.

ADVERSE REACTIONS
CNS: asthenia, dizziness, headache, insomnia, nerve root lesion, vertigo.
CV: hypertension.
EENT: nasopharyngitis, pharyngitis.
GI: dyspepsia, abdominal pain, constipation, diarrhea, gastritis, nausea, vomiting.
GU: cystitis, UTI.
Musculoskeletal: back pain, arthralgia, arthritis, joint disorder, limb pain, localized osteoarthritis, muscle cramps, myalgia.
Respiratory: bronchitis, upper respiratory tract infection, pneumonia.
Skin: rash.
Other: allergic reaction, infection, influenza, tooth disorder.

INTERACTIONS
Drug-drug. *Aspirin, NSAIDs:* May increase GI irritation. Use together cautiously.
Products containing aluminum, calcium, magnesium, or iron: May decrease ibandronate absorption. Give oral ibandronate 1 hour before vitamins, minerals, or antacids.
Drug-food. *Food, milk, beverages (except water):* May decrease drug absorption. Give oral drug on an empty stomach with plain water.
Drug-lifestyle. *Alcohol use:* May decrease drug absorption and increase risk of esophageal irritation. Discourage use together.

EFFECTS ON LAB TEST RESULTS
● May increase cholesterol level.

Reactions in bold italics are *life-threatening*. Interactions may have a *rapid onset* or a *delayed onset*.

• May decrease total alkaline phosphatase level. May interfere with bone-imaging agents.

CONTRAINDICATIONS & CAUTIONS

• Contraindicated in patients hypersensitive to drug and in those with uncorrected hypocalcemia. Oral form is contraindicated in those who can't stand or sit upright for 60 minutes.

❸ **Alert:** There may be an increased risk of atypical fractures of the thigh in patients treated with bisphosphonates.

• Don't give to patients with severe renal impairment (CrCl less than 30 mL/minute).

• Use cautiously in patients with a history of GI disorders.

⚠ **Overdose S&S:** Hypocalcemia, hypophosphatemia, hypomagnesemia.

NURSING CONSIDERATIONS

• Correct hypocalcemia or other disturbances of bone and mineral metabolism before therapy.

• Make sure patient has adequate intake of calcium and vitamin D.

• Obtain serum creatinine level and perform an oral examination before each dose in patients receiving I.V. ibandronate.

• Watch for signs or symptoms of esophageal irritation, including dysphagia, painful swallowing, retrosternal pain, and heartburn.

• Monitor patient for bone, joint, and muscle pain, which may be severe and incapacitating and may occur within days, months, or years of start of therapy. When drug is stopped, symptoms may resolve partially or completely.

• Watch for signs and symptoms of uveitis and scleritis.

❸ **Alert:** Drug may lead to osteonecrosis, mainly in the jaw. Dental surgery may worsen condition.

• Use during pregnancy only if benefit outweighs risk to fetus.

• Use cautiously in breast-feeding women.

PATIENT TEACHING

• Tell patient receiving I.V. form, if she misses a dose, to reschedule the missed dose as soon as possible. Subsequent injections should be rescheduled once every 3 months from that dose. She shouldn't receive more than one dose in a 3-month time frame.

• Tell patient taking monthly dose to take it on same date each month and to wait at least 7 days between doses if she misses a scheduled dose.

• Instruct patient to take oral drug first thing in the morning 1 hour before eating or drinking and before any other drugs, including OTC drugs such as calcium, antacids, and vitamins.

• Advise patient to swallow drug whole with a full glass of plain water while standing or sitting and to remain upright for at least 1 hour after taking drug.

• Caution patient to take only with plain water.

• Instruct patient not to chew or suck on the tablet.

• Advise patient to take calcium and vitamin D supplements as directed by prescriber.

• Tell patient to report any bone, joint, or muscle pain.

• Advise patient to stop drug and immediately report to prescriber signs and symptoms of esophageal irritation, such as dysphagia, painful swallowing, retrosternal pain, or heartburn.

• Advise patient to have periodic dental examinations for signs and symptoms of osteonecrosis of the jaw.

---

ibuprofen
eye-byoo-PROH-fen

Advil ◇, Caldolor, Excedrin IB ◇, Ibuprohm ◇, Ibutab ◇, Midol ◇, Motrin IB Cramp Formula Maximum Strength ◇, Motrin Migraine Pain ◇, Pamprin Ibuprofen Formula† ◇, Profen ◇, Tab-Profen ◇

ibuprofen lysine
NeoProfen

Therapeutic class: NSAIDs
Pharmacologic class: NSAIDs
Pregnancy risk category: C; D in 3rd trimester

AVAILABLE FORMS
ibuprofen
Capsules: 200 mg ◇

Injection: 800 mg/8-mL (100 mg/mL) single-dose vials
Oral drops: 40 mg/mL ◊
Oral suspension: 40 mg/mL ◊, 100 mg/5 mL ◊
Tablets: 100 mg ◊, 200 mg ◊, 300 mg, 400 mg, 600 mg, 800 mg
Tablets (chewable): 50 mg ◊, 100 mg ◊
ibuprofen lysine
Injection: EQ 20 mg base/2 mL (EQ 10 mg base/mL)

INDICATIONS & DOSAGES
➤ **Rheumatoid arthritis, osteoarthritis, arthritis**
Adults: 300 to 800 mg P.O. t.i.d. or q.i.d. Maximum daily dose is 3.2 g.
➤ **Mild to moderate pain**
Adults: 400 mg P.O. every 4 to 6 hours p.r.n. Or, 400 to 800 mg I.V. every 6 hours p.r.n.
➤ **Fever**
Adults and children age 12 and older: 200 to 400 mg P.O. every 4 to 6 hours, for no longer than 3 days. Maximum daily dose is 1.2 g. Or, 400 mg I.V. followed by 400 mg I.V. every 4 to 6 hours or 100 to 200 mg I.V. every 4 hours p.r.n.
Children age 11 weighing 33 to 43 kg (72 to 95 lb): 300 mg chewable tablets or 15 mL (300 mg) oral suspension P.O. every 6 to 8 hours up to q.i.d.
Children ages 9 to 10 weighing 27 to 32 kg (60 to 71 lb): 250 mg chewable tablets or 12.5 mL (250 mg) oral suspension P.O. every 6 to 8 hours up to q.i.d.
Children ages 6 to 8 weighing 22 to 27 kg (48 to 59 lb): 200 mg chewable tablets or 10 mL (200 mg) oral suspension P.O. every 6 to 8 hours up to q.i.d.
Children ages 4 to 5 weighing 16 to 21 kg (36 to 47 lb): 150 mg chewable tablets or 7.5 mL (150 mg) oral suspension P.O. every 6 to 8 hours up to q.i.d.
Children ages 2 to 3 weighing 11 to 16 kg (24 to 35 lb): 100 mg (5 mL) oral suspension every 6 to 8 hours up to q.i.d.
Children ages 12 to 23 months weighing 8 to 10 kg (18 to 23 lb): 75 mg (1.875 mL) oral drops every 6 to 8 hours up to q.i.d.
Children ages 6 to 11 months weighing 5 to 8 kg (12 to 17 lb): 50 mg (1.25 mL) oral drops every 6 to 8 hours up to q.i.d.

Adjust-a-dose: For children ages 6 months to 11 years, use weight to determine dosage if possible; otherwise, use age. If needed, dose may be repeated every 6 to 8 hours but no more than q.i.d. or a maximum of 30 mg/kg in 24 hours. Consult a health care provider before giving ibuprofen 100 mg chewable tablets to children younger than age 6 or those weighing less than 22 kg (48 lb), 50 mg chewable tablets to children younger than age 4 or those weighing less than 16 kg (36 lb), 50 mg oral suspension to children younger than age 2 or those weighing less than 11 kg (24 lb), or 50 mg oral drops to infants younger than age 6 months or those weighing less than 5 kg (12 lb). Ibuprofen oral drops should be dosed at 7.5 mg/kg of body weight.
➤ **Migraine**
Adults: 400 mg (2 capsules) P.O. in 24 hours.
➤ **Clinically significant patent ductus arteriosus (ibuprofen lysine)**
Premature infants weighing between 500 and 1,500 g who are no more than 32 weeks' gestational age: 10 mg/kg I.V. followed by 5 mg/kg I.V. 24 hours later followed by a third dose of 5 mg/kg I.V. 24 hours after second dose.
➤ **Juvenile arthritis ◆**
Children: 30 to 50 mg/kg P.O. daily in three or four divided doses. Maximum daily dose is 2,400 mg/day.

ADMINISTRATION
P.O.
● Give drug with milk or meals.
● Shake oral suspension and drops well before using.
I.V.
▼ Dilute drug with normal saline solution, 5% dextrose, or lactated Ringer solution. For 800-mg dose, use at least 200 mL of diluent. Give over at least 30 minutes.
▼ Diluted solutions are stable for 24 hours at room temperature.
▼ Correct dehydration before administering drug.

ACTION
May inhibit prostaglandin synthesis, to produce anti-inflammatory, analgesic, and antipyretic effects.

Reactions in bold italics are *life-threatening*. Interactions may have a *rapid onset* or a *delayed onset*.

Route	Onset	Peak	Duration
P.O.	Variable	1–2 hr	4–6 hr
I.V.	Unknown	Unknown	Unknown

Half-life: 2 to 4 hours.

ADVERSE REACTIONS

CNS: dizziness, headache, nervousness.
CV: edema, fluid retention.
EENT: tinnitus.
GI: abdominal pain, bloating, constipation, decreased appetite, diarrhea, dyspepsia, epigastric distress, flatulence, heartburn, nausea, nonnecrotizing enterocolitis, vomiting.
GU: *acute renal failure,* azotemia, cystitis, hematuria.
Hematologic: *agranulocytosis, aplastic anemia, leukopenia, neutropenia, pancytopenia, thrombocytopenia,* anemia, prolonged bleeding time.
Metabolic: *hyperkalemia, hypoglycemia.*
Skin: pruritus, rash.

INTERACTIONS

Drug-drug. *Anticoagulants (warfarin):* May increase risk of serious GI bleeding. Use with extreme caution if concomitant use can't be avoided. Monitor patient closely.
Antihypertensives, furosemide, thiazide diuretics: May decrease the effectiveness of diuretics or antihypertensives. Monitor patient closely.
Aspirin: May negate the antiplatelet effect of low-dose aspirin therapy. Advise patient on the appropriate spacing of doses.
Aspirin, corticosteroids: May cause adverse GI reactions. Avoid using together.
Bisphosphonates: May increase risk of gastric ulceration. Monitor patient for signs of gastric irritation or bleeding.
Cyclosporine: May increase nephrotoxicity of both drugs. Avoid using together.
Digoxin, lithium, oral anticoagulants: May increase levels or effects of these drugs. Monitor patient toxicity.
Methotrexate: May decrease methotrexate clearance and increases toxicity. Use together cautiously.
Drug-herb. *Dong quai, feverfew, garlic, ginger, ginkgo biloba, horse chestnut, red clover:* May increase risk of bleeding, based on the known effects of components. Discourage use together.
White willow: Herb and drug contain similar components. Discourage use together.
Drug-lifestyle. *Alcohol use:* May cause adverse GI reactions. Discourage use together.
Sun exposure: May cause photosensitivity reactions. Advise patient to avoid excessive sunlight exposure.

EFFECTS ON LAB TEST RESULTS

• May increase BUN, creatinine, ALT, AST, and potassium levels.
• May decrease glucose and hemoglobin levels and hematocrit.
• May decrease neutrophil, WBC, RBC, platelet, and granulocyte counts.

CONTRAINDICATIONS & CAUTIONS

• Contraindicated in patients hypersensitive to drug and in those with angioedema, syndrome of nasal polyps, or bronchospastic reaction to aspirin or other NSAIDs. **Black Box Warning** Contraindicated for the treatment of perioperative pain after CABG surgery. ■
• Contraindicated in pregnant women.
• Use cautiously in elderly patients and in patients with GI disorders, history of peptic ulcer disease, hepatic or renal disease, cardiac decompensation, hypertension, asthma, or intrinsic coagulation defects.
⚠ *Overdose S&S:* Abdominal pain, nausea, vomiting, lethargy, drowsiness, headache, tinnitus, nystagmus, CNS depression, seizures, hypotension, bradycardia, tachycardia, atrial fibrillation, metabolic acidosis, coma, acute renal failure, hyperkalemia, respiratory depression and failure.

NURSING CONSIDERATIONS

• Check renal and hepatic function periodically in patients on long-term therapy. Stop drug if abnormalities occur and notify prescriber.
• Because of their antipyretic and anti-inflammatory actions, NSAIDs may mask signs and symptoms of infection.
• Blurred or diminished vision and changes in color vision may occur.

• Full anti-inflammatory effects may take 1 or 2 weeks to develop.

Black Box Warning NSAIDs cause an increased risk of serious GI adverse events, including bleeding, ulceration, and perforation of the stomach or intestines, which can be fatal. Elderly patients are at greater risk. ∎

• Monitor patients for signs and symptoms of GI ulceration and bleeding.

Black Box Warning NSAIDs may increase the risk of serious thrombotic events, MI, or stroke, which can be fatal. The risk may be greater with longer use or in patients with CV disease or risk factors for CV disease. ∎

• If patient consumes three or more alcoholic drinks per day, drug may cause stomach bleeding.

PATIENT TEACHING

• Tell patient to take with meals or milk to reduce adverse GI reactions.

🜂 *Alert:* Drug is available OTC. Instruct patient not to exceed 1.2 g daily for adults and children age 12 and older or 30 mg/kg for children ages 6 months to 11 years, not to give to children younger than age 6 months, and not to take for extended periods (longer than 3 days for fever or longer than 10 days for pain) without consulting prescriber.

• Tell patient that full therapeutic effect for arthritis may be delayed for 2 to 4 weeks. Although pain relief occurs at low dosage levels, inflammation doesn't improve at dosages less than 400 mg q.i.d.

• Caution patient that use with aspirin, alcohol, or corticosteroids may increase risk of GI adverse reactions.

• Teach patient to watch for and report to prescriber immediately signs and symptoms of GI bleeding, including blood in vomit, urine, or stool; coffee-ground vomit; and black, tarry stool.

• Tell patient to contact prescriber before using this drug if fluid intake hasn't been adequate or if fluids have been lost as a result of vomiting or diarrhea.

• Warn patient to avoid hazardous activities that require mental alertness until effects on CNS are known.

• Advise patient to wear sunscreen to avoid hypersensitivity to sunlight.

SAFETY ALERT!

ibutilide fumarate
eye-BYOO-ti-lyed

Corvert

Therapeutic class: Antiarrhythmics
Pharmacologic class: Methanesulfonanilide derivatives
Pregnancy risk category: C

AVAILABLE FORMS
Injection: 0.1 mg/mL in 10-mL vials

INDICATIONS & DOSAGES
➤ **Rapid conversion of recent onset atrial fibrillation or atrial flutter to sinus rhythm**
Adults weighing 60 kg (132 lb) or more: 1 mg I.V. infusion over 10 minutes. May repeat dose if arrhythmia doesn't respond 10 minutes after completing first dose.
Adults weighing less than 60 kg: 0.01 mg/kg I.V. infusion over 10 minutes. May repeat dose if arrhythmia doesn't respond 10 minutes after completing first dose.

ADMINISTRATION
I.V.
▼ Give drug undiluted or diluted in 50 mL of diluent, and add to normal saline solution for injection or D₅W before infusion. Add contents of 10-mL vial (0.1 mg/mL) to 50-mL infusion bag to form admixture of about 0.017 mg/mL ibutilide. Use drug with polyvinyl chloride plastic bags or polyolefin bags.
▼ Give drug over 10 minutes.
▼ Stop infusion if arrhythmia is terminated or patient develops ventricular tachycardia or marked prolongation of QT or QTc interval. If arrhythmia doesn't respond 10 minutes after infusion ends, may repeat dose.
▼ Admixtures with approved diluents are stable for 24 hours at room temperature; 48 hours if refrigerated.
▼ Don't infuse parenteral products that contain particulate matter or are discolored.
▼ **Incompatibilities:** None reported.

Reactions in bold italics are *life-threatening*. Interactions may have a *rapid onset* or a *delayed onset*.

ACTION
Prolongs action potential in isolated cardiac myocyte and increases atrial and ventricular refractoriness, namely class III electrophysiologic effects.

Route	Onset	Peak	Duration
I.V.	Unknown	Unknown	Unknown

Half-life: Averages about 6 hours.

ADVERSE REACTIONS
CNS: headache.
CV: *sustained polymorphic ventricular tachycardia, AV block, bradycardia, heart failure,* ventricular extrasystoles, *nonsustained ventricular tachycardia,* hypotension, bundle-branch block, hypertension, *prolonged QT interval,* palpitations, tachycardia.
GI: nausea.

INTERACTIONS
Drug-drug. *Class IA antiarrhythmics (disopyramide, procainamide, quinidine), other class III drugs (amiodarone, sotalol):* May increase potential for prolonged refractoriness. Don't give these drugs for at least five half-lives before and 4 hours after ibutilide dose.
Digoxin: Supraventricular arrhythmias may mask cardiotoxicity from excessive digoxin level. Use with caution in patients who may have an increased digoxin therapeutic range.
H$_1$-receptor antagonists, phenothiazines, TCAs, tetracyclic antidepressants, other drugs that prolong QT interval: May increase risk for proarrhythmia. Monitor patient closely.

EFFECTS ON LAB TEST RESULTS
None reported.

CONTRAINDICATIONS & CAUTIONS
Black Box Warning Administer drug only when the benefits of maintaining sinus rhythm outweigh the immediate risks of ibutilide administration and the risks of maintenance therapy. ■
● Contraindicated in patients hypersensitive to drug or its components.
● Contraindicated in patients with history of polymorphic ventricular tachycardia. Use not recommended in breast-feeding women.

● Use cautiously in patients with hepatic or renal dysfunction.
● Safety and effectiveness of drug haven't been established in children.
⚠ Overdose S&S: Ventricular ectopy, ventricular tachycardia, third-degree AV block.

NURSING CONSIDERATIONS
Black Box Warning Drug can cause potentially fatal arrhythmias. Only skilled personnel trained in identification and treatment of acute ventricular arrhythmias, particularly polymorphic ventricular tachycardia, should give drug. Cardiac monitor, intracardiac pacing, cardioverter or defibrillator, and drugs to treat sustained ventricular tachycardia must be available. ■
● Before therapy, correct hypokalemia and hypomagnesemia to reduce risk of proarrhythmia.
Black Box Warning Patients with atrial fibrillation lasting longer than 2 to 3 days must be adequately anticoagulated, generally over at least 2 weeks. ■
● Monitor ECG continuously during administration and for at least 4 hours afterward or until QTc interval returns to baseline; drug can induce or worsen ventricular arrhythmias. Longer monitoring is required if ECG shows arrhythmia or patient has hepatic insufficiency.
● Don't give class IA or other class III antiarrhythmics with infusion or for 4 hours afterward.

PATIENT TEACHING
● Tell patient to report adverse reactions promptly.
● Instruct patient to alert nurse of discomfort at injection site.

SAFETY ALERT!

idarubicin hydrochloride
eye-duh-ROO-bi-sin

Idamycin PFS

Therapeutic class: Antineoplastics
Pharmacologic class: Semisynthetic anthracyclines
Pregnancy risk category: D

AVAILABLE FORMS
Injection: 1 mg/mL in 5-, 10-, and 20-mL single-dose vials

INDICATIONS & DOSAGES
Dosages vary. Check treatment protocol with prescriber.
➤ **Acute myeloid leukemia, including French-American-British classifications M1 through M7, with other approved antileukemic drugs**
Adults: 12 mg/m^2 daily for 3 days by slow I.V. injection (over 10 to 15 minutes) with 100 mg/m^2 daily of cytarabine for 7 days by continuous I.V. infusion. Or, the cytarabine may be given as 25-mg/m^2 bolus; then 200 mg/m^2 daily for 5 days by continuous infusion. A second course may be given, if needed.
Adjust-a-dose: If patient experiences severe mucositis, delay second course of therapy until recovery is complete and reduce dosage by 25%. If serum creatinine level is greater than 2 mg/dL, reduce dosage by 25%. If serum bilirubin level is 2.6 to 5 mg/dL, give 50% of usual dose. If AST level is between 60 and 80 units/L, give 50% of usual dose.
Black Box Warning Reduce dosage in patients with hepatic or renal impairment. Don't give idarubicin if bilirubin level exceeds 5 mg/dL. ■

ADMINISTRATION
I.V.
▼ Preparing and giving parenteral drug may be mutagenic, teratogenic, or carcinogenic. Follow facility policy to reduce risks.
▼ Reconstitute to final concentration of 1 mg/mL using normal saline solution

for injection without preservatives. Add 5 mL to 5-mg vial, 10 mL to 10-mg vial, or 20 mL to 20-mg vial. Don't use bacteriostatic saline solution. Vial is under negative pressure.
Black Box Warning Give drug over 10 to 15 minutes into a free-flowing I.V. infusion of normal saline or D$_5$W solution running into a large vein. Do not give I.M. or subcutaneously. ■
Black Box Warning Drug is a vesicant; tissue necrosis may result. ■
▼ If extravasation occurs, stop infusion immediately and notify prescriber. Treat with intermittent ice packs for ½ hour immediately and then for ½ hour q.i.d. for 4 days.
▼ Reconstituted solutions are stable for 72 hours at 59° to 86° F (15° to 30° C); 7 days if refrigerated and protected from light. Label unused solutions with chemotherapy hazard label.
▼ **Incompatibilities:** Acyclovir sodium, alkaline solutions, allopurinol, ampicillin sodium–sulbactam, cefazolin, cefepime, ceftazidime, clindamycin phosphate, dexamethasone sodium phosphate, etoposide, furosemide, gentamicin, heparin, hydrocortisone sodium succinate, lorazepam, meperidine, methotrexate sodium, piperacillin sodium–tazobactam, sodium bicarbonate, teniposide, vancomycin, vincristine.

ACTION
Unknown. Probably inhibits nucleic acid synthesis and interacts with the enzyme topoisomerase II. Drug is highly lipophilic, which increases rate of cellular uptake.

Route	Onset	Peak	Duration
I.V.	Unknown	Few min	Unknown

Half-life: 20 to 22 hours.

ADVERSE REACTIONS
CNS: headache, changed mental status, peripheral neuropathy, *seizures,* fever.
CV: *hemorrhage, heart failure, MI, myocardial insufficiency, arrhythmias, myocardial toxicity,* atrial fibrillation, chest pain, asymptomatic decline in LVEF.
GI: nausea, vomiting, cramps, diarrhea, mucositis.

Reactions in bold italics are *life-threatening*. Interactions may have a *rapid onset* or a *delayed onset*.

GU: renal dysfunction, red urine.
Hematologic: *myelosuppression.*
Hepatic: changes in hepatic function.
Metabolic: hyperuricemia.
Skin: alopecia, rash, urticaria, bullous erythrodermatous rash on palms and soles, erythema at previously irradiated sites, tissue necrosis if extravasation occurs.
Other: *infection,* hypersensitivity reactions.

INTERACTIONS
Drug-drug. *Alkaline solutions, heparin:* These combinations are incompatible. Don't mix idarubicin with other drugs unless specific compatibility data are known.
Live-virus vaccines: May increase risk of vaccine-induced adverse reactions. Avoid using together.

EFFECTS ON LAB TEST RESULTS
• May increase uric acid level. May decrease hemoglobin level.
• May decrease WBC, neutrophil, and platelet counts.

CONTRAINDICATIONS & CAUTIONS
Black Box Warning Don't give idarubicin if serum bilirubin level exceeds 5 mg/dL. ∎
• Use cautiously in patients with bone marrow suppression induced by previous drug therapy or radiotherapy, impaired hepatic or renal function, previous treatment with anthracyclines or cardiotoxic drugs, or a cardiac condition.
⚠ *Overdose S&S:* Severe and prolonged myelosuppression, increased severity of GI toxicity, severe arrhythmia, acute cardiac toxicity, increased incidence of delayed heart failure.

NURSING CONSIDERATIONS
Black Box Warning Drug should be given only under the supervision of a physician experienced in the use of cancer chemotherapeutic agents. ∎
Black Box Warning Cardiotoxicity is the dose-limiting toxicity of drug. It is more common in those who have received prior anthracyclines or who have preexisting cardiac disease. No maximum cumulative lifetime dose for cardiotoxicity has been determined. ∎

• Cardiovascular side effects occur with greater frequency in older patients.
• Make sure patient is adequately hydrated before treatment. Hyperuricemia may result from rapid lysis of leukemic cells. Allopurinol may be ordered.
• Assess patient for systemic infection and ensure that it's controlled before therapy begins.
• Give antiemetics to prevent or treat nausea and vomiting.
• Monitor hepatic and renal function tests and CBC frequently.
• To prevent bleeding, avoid all I.M. injections when platelet count is below 50,000/mm^3.
Black Box Warning Severe myelosuppression may occur. ∎
• Anticipate need for blood transfusions for anemia.
• Notify prescriber if signs or symptoms of heart failure occur.
• *Look alike–sound alike:* Don't confuse idarubicin with daunorubicin or doxorubicin.

PATIENT TEACHING
• Teach patient to recognize signs and symptoms of leakage of drug into surrounding tissue, and tell him to report them if they occur.
• Warn patient to watch for signs and symptoms of infection (fever, sore throat, fatigue) and bleeding (easy bruising, nosebleeds, bleeding gums, tarry stools).
• Advise patient that red urine for several days is normal and doesn't indicate presence of blood.
• Caution woman of childbearing age to avoid becoming pregnant during therapy. Recommend that she consult prescriber before becoming pregnant.

ifosfamide
eye-FOSS-fa-mide

Ifex

Therapeutic class: Antineoplastics
Pharmacologic class: Nitrogen mustards
Pregnancy risk category: D

AVAILABLE FORMS
Powder for injection: 1-g, 3-g vials

INDICATIONS & DOSAGES
➤ **Germ cell testicular cancer**
Adults: 1.2 g/m^2 daily I.V. for 5 consecutive
days. Repeat treatment every 3 weeks or
after patient recovers from hematologic
toxicity. Don't repeat doses until WBC
count exceeds 4,000/mm^3 and platelet count
exceeds 100,000/mm^3.
Adjust-a-dose: For patients with renal
insufficiency, reduce dosage as follows:
If GFR is 30 to 60 mL/minute, give 75% of
usual dose; if GFR is 10 to 30 mL/minute,
give 50% of usual dose. Don't give dose if
GFR is less than 10 mL/minute. For patients
with hepatic dysfunction, consider decreasing dosage to 25% of usual dose if serum
AST level is greater than 300 units/L or if
bilirubin level is greater than 3 mg/dL.

ADMINISTRATION
I.V.
▼ Preparing and giving drug may be mutagenic, teratogenic, or carcinogenic. Follow
facility policy to reduce risks.
▼ Give a protective drug such as mesna to
prevent hemorrhagic cystitis. Ifosfamide
and mesna are physically compatible and
may be mixed in the same I.V. solution.
▼ Obtain urinalysis before each dose. If
microscopic hematuria occurs, notify
prescriber. Adjust dosage of mesna, if
needed. Adequate fluid intake (2 L daily,
either P.O. or I.V.) is essential before, and
72 hours after, therapy.
▼ Reconstitute each gram of drug with
20 mL of diluent to yield a solution of
50 mg/mL. Use sterile water for injection
or bacteriostatic water for injection. Solutions may then be further diluted with

sterile water, dextrose 2.5% or 5% in water,
half-normal or normal saline solution for
injection, dextrose 5% and normal saline
solution for injection, or lactated Ringer
injection.
▼ Infuse each dose over at least 30 minutes.
▼ Reconstituted solution is stable for
1 week at room temperature or 6 weeks if
refrigerated. However, use solution within
6 hours if drug was reconstituted with
sterile water without a preservative (such
as benzyl alcohol or parabens).
▼ **Incompatibilities:** Cefepime, mesna
with epirubicin, methotrexate sodium.

ACTION
Cross-links strands of cellular DNA and
interferes with RNA transcription, causing
an imbalance of growth that leads to cell
death. Not specific to cell cycle.

Route	Onset	Peak	Duration
I.V.	Unknown	Unknown	Unknown

Half-life: About 14 hours.

ADVERSE REACTIONS
CNS: somnolence, confusion, hallucinations,
depressive psychosis, fever, *seizures, coma.*
GI: nausea, vomiting.
GU: hemorrhagic cystitis, hematuria.
Hematologic: *leukopenia, thrombocytope-
nia, myelosuppression.*
Skin: alopecia.
Other: infection, phlebitis.

INTERACTIONS
Drug-drug. *Anticoagulants, aspirin,
NSAIDs:* May increase risk of bleeding.
Avoid using together.
*Barbiturates, chloral hydrate, fospheny-
toin, phenytoin:* May increase ifosfamide
toxicity. Monitor patient closely.
Corticosteroids: May inhibit hepatic
enzymes, reducing ifosfamide's effect.
Monitor patient for increased ifosfamide
toxicity if corticosteroid dosage is suddenly
reduced or stopped.
Cyclophosphamide: May increase risk of
cardiac tamponade in patients with thalassemia. Monitor patient closely.
Live-virus vaccines: May increase risk of
vaccine-induced adverse reactions. Avoid
using together.

Reactions in bold italics are *life-threatening*. Interactions may have a *rapid onset* or a *delayed onset*.

Myelosuppressives: May enhance hematologic toxicity. Dosage adjustment may be needed.

EFFECTS ON LAB TEST RESULTS
● May increase liver enzyme levels.
● May decrease WBC and platelet counts.

CONTRAINDICATIONS & CAUTIONS
● Contraindicated in patients hypersensitive to drug and in those with severe bone marrow suppression.
● Use cautiously in patients with renal impairment or compromised bone marrow reserve as indicated by leukopenia, granulocytopenia, extensive bone marrow metastases, previous radiation therapy, or previous therapy with cytotoxic drugs.
● Don't give drug if CrCl is less than 10 mL/minute.

NURSING CONSIDERATIONS
▄Black Box Warning▄ Drug should be administered under the supervision of a physician experienced in the use of cancer chemotherapeutic agents. ▮
▄Black Box Warning▄ Urotoxic side effects, especially hemorrhagic cystitis, and CNS toxicities, such as confusion and coma, may require cessation of ifosfamide therapy. ▮
▄Black Box Warning▄ Severe myelosuppression has been reported. ▮
● Give antiemetic before drug, to reduce nausea.
● Ensure that patient is adequately hydrated during therapy.
● Patients are at increased risk for hemorrhagic cystitis. Obtain urinalysis before each dose. Withhold drug for microscopic hematuria (greater than 10 RBCs per high power field) until completely resolved.
● Don't give drug at bedtime; infrequent urination during the night may increase possibility of cystitis. If cystitis develops, stop drug and notify prescriber.
● Bladder irrigation with normal saline solution may be done to treat cystitis.
● Monitor CBC, renal function, and LFT values.
● To prevent bleeding, avoid all I.M. injections when platelet count is less than 50,000/mm³.

● Anticipate blood transfusions because of cumulative anemia.
● Assess patient for mental status changes; dosage may have to be decreased.
● *Look alike–sound alike:* Don't confuse ifosfamide with cyclophosphamide.

PATIENT TEACHING
● Remind patient to urinate frequently to minimize contact of drug and its metabolites with the lining of the bladder.
● Advise patient to watch for signs and symptoms of infection (fever, sore throat, fatigue) and bleeding (easy bruising, nosebleeds, bleeding gums, tarry stools). Tell patient to take temperature daily.
● Instruct patient to avoid OTC products that contain aspirin.
● Advise women to stop breast-feeding during therapy because of possible risk of toxicity to infant.
● Caution woman of childbearing age to avoid becoming pregnant during therapy. Recommend that she consult prescriber before becoming pregnant.

---

iloperidone
ill-oh-PER-ih-done

Fanapt

Therapeutic class: Antipsychotics
Pharmacologic class: Dopamine–
serotonin antagonists
Pregnancy risk category: C

AVAILABLE FORMS
Tablets: 1 mg, 2 mg, 4 mg, 6 mg, 8 mg, 10 mg, 12 mg

INDICATIONS & DOSAGES
➤ **Schizophrenia**
Adults: Initially, 1 mg P.O. b.i.d. Increase dosage daily as needed according to the following dosing schedule: 2 mg P.O. b.i.d. on day 2; 4 mg P.O. b.i.d. on day 3; 6 mg P.O. b.i.d. on day 4; 8 mg P.O. b.i.d. on day 5; 10 mg P.O. b.i.d. on day 6; 12 mg P.O. b.i.d. on day 7. Maximum dosage is 12 mg P.O. b.i.d.
Adjust-a-dose: For patients taking CYP2D6 inhibitors (fluoxetine, paroxetine) and

CYP3A4 inhibitors (clarithromycin, ketoconazole), reduce dosage by half.

ADMINISTRATION
P.O.
• Give drug with or without food.

ACTION
May antagonize dopamine type 2 and serotonin type 2.

Route	Onset	Peak	Duration
P.O.	Unknown	2–4 hr	Unknown

Half-life: 18 to 37 hours.

ADVERSE REACTIONS
CNS: aggression, delusion, dizziness, extrapyramidal effects, fatigue, lethargy, restlessness, somnolence, tremor.
CV: hypotension, orthostatic hypotension, palpitations, tachycardia.
EENT: blurred vision, conjunctivitis, dry mouth, nasal congestion, nasopharyngitis.
GI: abdominal discomfort, diarrhea, nausea.
GU: ejaculation failure, erectile dysfunction, urinary incontinence.
Hematologic: hyperprolactinemia.
Metabolic: weight gain, weight loss.
Musculoskeletal: arthralgia, muscle spasm, musculoskeletal stiffness, myalgia.
Respiratory: dyspnea, upper respiratory tract infection.
Skin: rash.

INTERACTIONS
Drug-drug. *Alpha₁ blockers:* May enhance antihypertensive effects. Use together cautiously.
Centrally acting drugs: May increase CNS effects. Use together cautiously.
CYP3A4 or CYP2D6 inhibitors (clarithromycin, fluoxetine, ketoconazole, paroxetine): May increase iloperidone level. Reduce dosage by half.
Dextromethorphan: May increase dextromethorphan level. Avoid use together.
Drugs that prolong QT interval: May cause lethal arrhythmias. Avoid use together.
Drug-lifestyle. *Alcohol:* May increase CNS effects. Discourage use together.

EFFECTS ON LAB TEST RESULTS
• May decrease hematocrit.

CONTRAINDICATIONS & CAUTIONS
• Contraindicated in patients hypersensitive to drug or its components.
• Avoid use with other drugs known to prolong QT interval and in elderly patients with dementia-related psychosis.
• Use cautiously in patients with history of stroke, transient ischemic attack, arrhythmia, QT-interval prolongation, diabetes, seizures, orthostatic hypotension, neuroleptic malignant syndrome, tardive dyskinesia, leukopenia, neutropenia, agranulocytosis, suicidal ideation, or priapism.
• Use in patients with hepatic impairment isn't recommended.
❂ **Alert:** Neonates exposed to antipsychotics during the third trimester are at risk for developing extrapyramidal symptoms (repetitive muscle movements of the face and body) and withdrawal symptoms (agitation, abnormally increased or decreased muscle tone, tremors, sleepiness, severe difficulty breathing, difficulty feeding) following delivery. Use in pregnancy only if the potential benefit to the mother justifies the risk to the fetus.
• It isn't known if drug appears in breast milk. Patient shouldn't breast-feed during therapy.
⚠ **Overdose S&S:** Prolonged QT interval, drowsiness, sedation, tachycardia, hypotension.

NURSING CONSIDERATIONS
Black Box Warning Fatal CV events may occur in elderly patients with dementia. Drug isn't approved for use in patients with dementia-related psychosis. ∎
❂ **Alert:** Obtain baseline blood pressure measurements before starting therapy, and monitor blood pressure regularly. Watch for orthostatic hypotension, especially during first dosage adjustments.
❂ **Alert:** Watch for evidence of neuroleptic malignant syndrome (hyperthermia, muscle rigidity, altered mental status, and autonomic instability), which is rare but can be fatal.
❂ **Alert:** Life-threatening hyperglycemia may occur in patients taking atypical antipsychotics. Monitor patients with diabetes regularly. Monitor fasting blood glucose level at drug initiation and periodically

during therapy in patients with risk factors for diabetes.

• Monitor patient for tardive dyskinesia, which may occur with prolonged use of drug. If tardive dyskinesia occurs, discontinue drug unless patient's condition warrants continued use.

• Monitor patient for suicidal thinking and behavior.

• Dispense lowest appropriate quantity of drug to reduce the risk of overdose.

• Monitor patient for weight gain.

• Periodically reassess patient to determine continued need for therapy.

• Monitor CBC frequently during the first few months of therapy and discontinue drug if WBC count drops with no other underlying cause.

• Monitor potassium and magnesium levels at baseline and periodically in patients at risk for electrolyte imbalance.

• Drug may lower seizure threshold in patients with a history of seizures; monitor these patients closely.

PATIENT TEACHING

• Warn patient to avoid driving and other hazardous activities that require mental alertness until the drug's effects are known.

• Tell patient drug can be taken with or without food.

• Warn patient to rise slowly, avoid hot showers, and use other precautions to avoid fainting when starting therapy.

• Advise patient to avoid becoming overheated or dehydrated.

• Tell women of childbearing age to notify prescriber about planned, suspected, or known pregnancy.

• Advise breast-feeding women not to breast-feed during therapy.

• Instruct patient to report symptoms of dizziness, palpitations, or fainting to prescriber.

• Advise patient to avoid alcohol use while taking drug.

• Tell male patient to seek emergency medical care if an erection lasts more than 4 hours.

• Warn patient and caregiver about the risk of neuroleptic malignant syndrome, and advise them to seek emergency medical care if symptoms occur.

• Tell patient to notify prescriber about other prescription or OTC drugs he's taking or plans to take.

iloprost
EYE-loe-prost

Ventavis

Therapeutic class: Pulmonary vasodilators
Pharmacologic class: Prostacyclin analogues
Pregnancy risk category: C

AVAILABLE FORMS
Inhalation solution: 10 mcg/mL, 20 mcg/mL in single-dose ampules

INDICATIONS & DOSAGES
➤ **Pulmonary arterial hypertension in patients with New York Heart Association (NYHA) Class III or IV symptoms**
Adults: Initially, 2.5 mcg inhaled using the I-neb Adaptive Aerosol Delivery (AAD) or Prodose AAD systems. As tolerated, increase to 5 mcg inhaled six to nine times daily while patient is awake, as needed, but to no more than every 2 hours. Maximum, 5 mcg nine times daily.
Adjust-a-dose: For patients with hepatic impairment (Child-Pugh class B or C), consider increasing dosing interval to every 3 to 4 hours depending on patient response.
➤ **Raynaud phenomenon ◆**
Adults: 0.5 to 2 ng/kg/minute I.V. for 6 to 8 hours/day for 3 to 5 days every 6 to 8 weeks.

ADMINISTRATION
Inhalational
• Use only I-neb AAD or Prodose AAD delivery devices, per manufacturer's instructions.

ACTION
Lowers pulmonary arterial pressure by dilating systemic and pulmonary arterial beds. Drug also affects platelet aggregation, although effect in pulmonary hypertension treatment isn't known.

Route	Onset	Peak	Duration
Inhalation	Unknown	Within 5 min	30–60 min

Half-life: 20 to 30 minutes.

ADVERSE REACTIONS
CNS: headache, insomnia, syncope.
CV: hypotension, vasodilation, chest pain, *heart failure, supraventricular tachycardia,* palpitations, peripheral edema.
GI: nausea, tongue pain, vomiting.
GU: *renal failure.*
Musculoskeletal: trismus, back pain, muscle cramps.
Respiratory: cough, dyspnea, hemoptysis, pneumonia.
Other: flulike syndrome.

INTERACTIONS
Drug-drug. *Anticoagulants:* May increase risk of bleeding. Monitor patient closely.
Antihypertensives, vasodilators: May increase effects of these drugs. Monitor patient's blood pressure.

EFFECTS ON LAB TEST RESULTS
● May increase alkaline phosphatase and GGT levels.

CONTRAINDICATIONS & CAUTIONS
● No contraindications known. Avoid using in patients whose systolic blood pressure is less than 85 mm Hg.
● Use cautiously in elderly patients, patients with hepatic or renal impairment, and patients with COPD, severe asthma, or acute pulmonary infection.
⚠ **Overdose S&S:** Diarrhea, flushing, headache, hypotension, nausea, vomiting.

NURSING CONSIDERATIONS
● Keep drug away from skin and eyes.
● The 2-mL ampule must be used with the Prodose AAD and may be used with the I-neb AAD. The 1-mL ampule must be used only with the I-neb AAD.
● Take care not to inhale drug while providing treatment.
● Monitor patient's vital signs carefully at start of treatment.
● Watch for syncope.
● If patient develops evidence of pulmonary edema, stop treatment immediately.

PATIENT TEACHING
● Advise patient to take drug exactly as prescribed and using Prodose AAD or I-neb AAD.
● Urge patient to follow manufacturer's instructions for preparing and inhaling drug.
● Advise patient to keep a backup Prodose AAD or I-neb AAD in case the original malfunctions.
● Tell patient to keep drug away from skin and eyes and to rinse the area immediately if contact occurs.
● Caution patient not to ingest drug solution.
● Inform patient that drug may cause dizziness and fainting. Urge him to stand up slowly from a sitting or lying position and to report to prescriber worsening of symptoms.
● Tell patient to take drug before physical exertion but no more often than every 2 hours.
● Tell patient not to expose others, especially pregnant women and infants, to drug.
● Teach patient how to clean equipment and safely dispose of used ampules after each treatment. Caution patient not to save or use leftover solution.

SAFETY ALERT!

imatinib mesylate
eh-MAT-eh-nib

Gleevec

Therapeutic class: Antineoplastics
Pharmacologic class: Protein–tyrosine kinase inhibitors
Pregnancy risk category: D

AVAILABLE FORMS
Tablets: 100 mg, 400 mg

INDICATIONS & DOSAGES
Adjust-a-dose (for all indications): For patients with CrCl of 40 to 59 mL/minute, don't exceed 600 mg daily; if CrCl is 20 to 39 mL/minute, decrease starting dose by 50% and don't exceed 400 mg daily; if CrCl is less than 20 mL/minute, don't exceed 100 mg daily. For patients with severe hepatic failure, reduce dosage by 25%. See

Reactions in bold italics are *life-threatening*. Interactions may have a *rapid onset* or a *delayed onset*.

manufacturer's package insert for full details on dosage adjustments for children; patients with neutropenia, thrombocytopenia, or hepatotoxicity; and those with adverse reactions.

➤ **Relapsed or refractory Philadelphia chromosome–positive (Ph+) acute lymphoblastic leukemia (ALL)**
Adults: 600 mg P.O. daily.

✴ *NEW INDICATION:* **Newly diagnosed Ph+ ALL in pediatric patients in combination with chemotherapy**
Children age 1 and older: 340 mg/m^2 P.O. daily. Maximum dosage is 600 mg daily.

➤ **Aggressive systemic mastocytosis (ASM) without the D816V c-Kit mutation or with c-Kit mutational status unknown**
Adults: 400 mg P.O. daily.

Adjust-a-dose: For patients with ASM associated with eosinophilia, a clonal hematologic disease related to the fusion kinase FIP1L1-PDGFRα, initial dose is 100 mg/day. Increase dose from 100 mg to 400 mg/day if no adverse drug reactions and if insufficient response to therapy.

➤ **Hypereosinophilic syndrome (HES) or chronic eosinophilic leukemia (CEL), or both**
Adults: 400 mg P.O. daily.

Adjust-a-dose: In HES/CEL patients with demonstrated FIP1L1-PDGFRα fusion kinase, initial dose is 100 mg/day. Increase dose from 100 mg to 400 mg/day if no adverse drug reactions and if insufficient response to therapy.

➤ **Myelodysplastic (MDS) or myeloproliferative (MPD) disease with *PDGFR* gene rearrangements**
Adults: 400 mg P.O. daily.

➤ **Unresectable, recurrent, or metastatic dermatofibrosarcoma protuberans (DFSP)**
Adults: 800 mg P.O. daily.

➤ **Chronic myeloid leukemia (CML) in blast crisis, in accelerated phase, or in chronic phase after failure of alfa interferon therapy; newly diagnosed Ph+ chronic-phase CML**
Adults: For chronic-phase CML, 400 mg P.O. daily as single dose with a meal and large glass of water. For accelerated-phase CML or blast crisis, 600 mg P.O. daily as single dose with a meal and large glass

of water. Continue treatment as long as patient continues to benefit. May increase daily dose to 600 mg P.O. in chronic phase or to 800 mg P.O. (400 mg P.O. b.i.d.) in accelerated phase or blast crisis.
Children age 2 and older: For newly diagnosed Ph+ chronic-phase CML only, give 340 mg/m^2 daily P.O. Don't exceed 600 mg/day.

➤ **Kit (CD117)-positive or GI stromal tumors (GISTs) after resection**
Adults: 400 mg P.O. daily.

➤ **Kit-positive unresectable or metastatic malignant GISTs**
Adults: 400 mg P.O. daily or b.i.d.

ADMINISTRATION
P.O.
• For daily dosing of 800 mg and above, use the 400-mg tablet to reduce exposure to iron.
• For patients unable to swallow tablets, disperse the tablets in water or apple juice (50 mL for 100-mg tablet or 200 mL for 400-mg tablet). Stir and have patient drink immediately.

ACTION
Inhibits the abnormal tyrosine kinase created by the Philadelphia chromosome abnormality in CML; it inhibits tumor growth of murine myeloid cells and leukemia lines from CML patients in blast crisis.

Route	Onset	Peak	Duration
P.O.	Unknown	2–4 hr	Unknown

Half-life: Within 7 days.

ADVERSE REACTIONS
CNS: *cerebral hemorrhage,* fatigue, headache, pyrexia, weakness, depression, dizziness, insomnia.
CV: edema.
EENT: epistaxis, nasopharyngitis.
GI: *GI hemorrhage,* abdominal pain, anorexia, constipation, diarrhea, dyspepsia, nausea, vomiting.
Hematologic: *hemorrhage, neutropenia, thrombocytopenia,* anemia.
Metabolic: hypokalemia, weight increase.
Musculoskeletal: arthralgia, myalgia, muscle cramps, musculoskeletal pain, growth suppression in children.

Respiratory: cough, dyspnea, pneumonia.
Skin: petechiae, rash, pruritus.
Other: night sweats.

INTERACTIONS
Drug-drug. *Acetaminophen:* May increase risk of hepatotoxicity. Monitor patient closely.
CYP3A4 inducers (carbamazepine, dexamethasone, phenobarbital, phenytoin, rifampin): May increase metabolism and decrease imatinib level. Use together cautiously.
CYP3A4 inhibitors (clarithromycin, erythromycin, itraconazole, ketoconazole): May decrease metabolism and increase imatinib level. Monitor patient for toxicity.
Dihydropyridine–calcium channel blockers, certain HMG-CoA reductase inhibitors (simvastatin), cyclosporine, pimozide, triazolo-benzodiazepines: May increase levels of these drugs. Monitor patient for toxicity, and obtain drug levels, if appropriate.
Levothyroxine: May increase levothyroxine clearance, causing increased thyroid-stimulating hormone levels and symptoms of hypothyroidism. Monitor thyroid function.
Warfarin: May alter metabolism of warfarin. Avoid using together; use standard heparin or a low–molecular-weight heparin.
Drug-herb. *St. John's wort:* May decrease drug effects. Discourage use together.

EFFECTS ON LAB TEST RESULTS
● May increase creatinine, bilirubin, alkaline phosphatase, AST, and ALT levels. May decrease potassium and hemoglobin levels.
● May decrease neutrophil and platelet counts.

CONTRAINDICATIONS & CAUTIONS
● Contraindicated in patients hypersensitive to drug or its components.
● Use cautiously in elderly patients and in those with hepatic impairment.
● Severe congestive heart failure and left ventricular dysfunction have occurred in patients taking imatinib. Use cautiously in patients with cardiac disease or risk factors for heart failure.

● Growth retardation has occurred in children and preadolescents receiving imatinib; long-term effects of prolonged treatment are unknown.
● Safety and effectiveness in children younger than age 1 haven't been established.
⚠ Overdose S&S: Muscle cramps; ascites; vomiting; diarrhea; GI pain; elevated creatinine, AST, ALT, and bilirubin levels.

NURSING CONSIDERATIONS
● Monitor patient closely for possibly severe fluid retention. Elderly patients may have an increased risk of edema.
● Monitor weight daily. Report unexpected, rapid weight gain.
● Monitor CBC weekly for first month, every other week for second month, and periodically thereafter.
● Monitor LFTs carefully because hepatotoxicity (occasionally severe) may occur; decrease dosage as needed.
● Monitor growth of children being treated with imatinib.
● May increase dose if no severe adverse reactions or severe non–leukemia-related neutropenia or thrombocytopenia in the following circumstances: disease progression, failure to achieve a satisfactory hematologic response after at least 3 months of treatment, or loss of a previously achieved hematologic response.
● In patients with HES and cardiac involvement, cases of cardiogenic shock/left ventricular dysfunction have been associated with the initiation of imatinib therapy. The condition is reversible with administration of systemic steroids and circulatory support measures, and by temporarily withholding imatinib. Monitor echocardiogram and serum troponin in patients with HES/CEL and in patients with MDS/MPD or ASM associated with high eosinophil levels.
● Grade 3/4 hemorrhage has been reported in patients with newly diagnosed CML and with GIST. GI tumor sites may be the source of GI bleeds in GIST.
● GI perforations, some fatal, have been reported.

PATIENT TEACHING
● Tell patient to take drug with food and a large glass of water.

- Advise patient unable to swallow tablets to mix them in water or apple juice (50 mL for 100-mg tablet or 200 mL for 400-mg tablet). Tell him to stir and drink immediately.
- Advise patient to report to prescriber any adverse effects, such as fluid retention.
- Advise patient to obtain periodic LFTs and kidney function tests and blood work to determine blood counts.
- Tell patient to avoid or limit the use of acetaminophen in OTC or prescription products because of potential toxic effects on the liver.
- Inform patient and caregivers that growth retardation has occurred in children and preadolescents receiving imatinib, and that long-term effects of prolonged treatment are unknown. Monitor growth closely.
- Advise patient of the risk of dizziness, blurred vision, or somnolence during treatment and to use caution when driving a car or operating machinery.

imipenem–cilastatin sodium
im-ih-PEN-em and sye-luh-STAT-in

Primaxin

Therapeutic class: Antibiotics
Pharmacologic class: Carbapenems–beta-lactams
Pregnancy risk category: C

AVAILABLE FORMS
Powder for injection: 250 mg, 500 mg

INDICATIONS & DOSAGES
Adjust-a-dose (for all indications): If CrCl is less than 70 mL/minute, adjust dosage and monitor renal function test results. Consult manufacturer's package insert for specific dosage adjustments. For patients on hemodialysis, administer dose after hemodialysis and at 12-hour intervals timed from the end of that dialysis session. Dosage regimen for adults with normal renal function is based on type and severity of infection. Consult manufacturer's package insert for dosing.

➤ **Serious lower respiratory tract, bone, intra-abdominal, gynecologic, joint, skin, and soft-tissue infections; UTIs; endocarditis; and bacterial septicemia, caused by *Acinetobacter, Enterococcus, Staphylococcus aureus, Streptococcus, Escherichia coli, Haemophilus, Klebsiella, Morganella, Proteus, Enterobacter, Pseudomonas aeruginosa,* and *Bacteroides,* including *B. fragilis***
Adults weighing more than 70 kg (154 lb): 250 to 1,000 mg by I.V. infusion every 6 to 8 hours. Maximum daily dose is 50 mg/kg/day or 4 g/day, whichever is less.
Adults weighing less than 70 kg: 125 to 1,000 mg by I.V. infusion every 6 to 8 hours. Maximum daily dosage is 50 mg/kg/day or 4 g/day, whichever is less.
Children age 3 months and older (except for CNS infections): 15 to 25 mg/kg I.V. every 6 hours. Maximum daily dose is 2 to 4 g.
Infants ages 4 weeks to 3 months weighing 1.5 kg (3 lb) or more (except for CNS infections): 25 mg/kg I.V. every 6 hours.
Neonates ages 1 to 4 weeks weighing 1.5 kg or more (except for CNS infections): 25 mg/kg I.V. every 8 hours.
Neonates younger than age 1 week weighing 1.5 kg or more (except for CNS infections): 25 mg/kg I.V. every 12 hours.
➤ **Catheter-related bloodstream infections ◆**
Children and infants older than age 3 months: 60 to 100 mg/kg/day I.V. in divided doses every 6 hours.
Infants younger than age 3 months: 100 mg/kg/day I.V. in divided doses every 6 hours.
Neonates older than age 7 days weighing more than 1,500 g: 75 mg/kg/day I.V. in divided doses every 8 hours.
Neonates older than age 7 days weighing 1,200 to 1,500 g: 40 mg/kg/day I.V. in divided doses every 12 hours.
Neonates age 7 days and younger weighing more than 1,500 g: 50 mg/kg/day I.V. in divided doses every 12 hours.
Neonates age 7 days and younger weighing 1,200 to 1,500 g: 40 mg/kg/day I.V. in divided doses every 12 hours.
Neonates age 0 to 4 weeks weighing less than 1,200 g: 20 mg/kg I.V. every 18 to 24 hours.

➤ **Infective endocarditis due to *Enterococcus faecalis* infections resistant to penicillin, aminoglycosides, and vancomycin** ◆

Adults: 2 g I.V. every 24 hours in four divided doses in combination with ampicillin for at least 8 weeks.

Children and adolescents: 15 to 25 mg/kg I.V. every 6 hours in combination with ampicillin for at least 8 weeks.

ADMINISTRATION

I.V.

▼ Obtain specimens for culture and sensitivity testing before giving first dose. Begin therapy while awaiting results.

▼ Reconstitute piggyback units with 100 mL of compatible I.V. solution to provide solution containing 2.5 to 5 mg/mL.

▼ When reconstituting powder, shake until the solution is clear. Solutions may be colorless to yellow; variations of color within this range don't affect drug's potency.

▼ After reconstitution, solution is stable for 4 hours at room temperature and for 24 hours when refrigerated.

▼ Don't give by direct I.V. bolus injection.

▼ For adults, give each 250- or 500-mg dose by I.V. infusion over 20 to 30 minutes. Infuse each 750-mg to 1-g dose over 40 to 60 minutes. ◆

▼ For children, infuse doses of 500 mg or less over 15 to 30 minutes. Infuse doses greater than 500 mg over 40 to 60 minutes. If nausea occurs, the infusion may be slowed.

▼ **Incompatibilities:** Allopurinol, antibiotics, amiodarone, amphotericin B cholesteryl sulfate complex, azithromycin, dextrose 5% in lactated Ringer injection, etoposide, fluconazole, gemcitabine, lorazepam, meperidine, midazolam, milrinone, sargramostim, sodium bicarbonate.

I.M.

● Obtain specimen culture and sensitivity tests before giving first dose. Begin therapy while awaiting results.

🛈 **Alert:** Don't give I.M. solution by I.V. route.

ACTION

Inhibits bacterial cell-wall synthesis. Cilastatin prevents metabolism of imipenem, resulting in increased urinary recovery and decreased renal toxicity.

Route	Onset	Peak	Duration
I.V.	Immediate	Immediate	Unknown
I.M.	Unknown	1–2 hr	Unknown

Half-life: 1 hour after I.V. dose; 2 to 3 hours after I.M. dose.

ADVERSE REACTIONS

CNS: *seizures,* dizziness, fever, somnolence.

CV: hypotension, thrombophlebitis.

GI: *pseudomembranous colitis,* diarrhea, nausea, vomiting.

Hematologic: *leukopenia, thrombocytopenia,* eosinophilia.

Skin: injection-site pain, pruritus, rash, urticaria.

Other: *anaphylaxis,* hypersensitivity reactions.

INTERACTIONS

Drug-drug. *Cyclosporine:* May increase CNS adverse effects. Use together cautiously.

Ganciclovir: May cause seizures. Avoid using together.

Probenecid: May increase cilastatin level. May be used together for this effect.

EFFECTS ON LAB TEST RESULTS

● May increase BUN, creatinine, ALT, AST, alkaline phosphatase, bilirubin, and LDH levels.

● May increase eosinophil count. May decrease WBC and platelet counts.

● May interfere with glucose determination by Benedict solution or Clinitest.

CONTRAINDICATIONS & CAUTIONS

● Contraindicated in patients hypersensitive to drug, in those with a history of hypersensitivity to local anesthetics of the amide type, and in those with severe shock or heart block.

● Use cautiously in patients allergic to penicillins or cephalosporins because drug has similar chemical structure.

Reactions in bold italics are *life-threatening*. Interactions may have a *rapid onset* or a *delayed onset*.

• Use cautiously in patients with history of seizure disorders, especially if they also have compromised renal function.
• Use cautiously in children younger than age 3 months.

NURSING CONSIDERATIONS
☉ Alert: Don't use for CNS infections in children because drug increases the risk of seizures.
☉ Alert: If seizures develop and persist despite anticonvulsant therapy, stop drug and notify prescriber.
• For patients receiving hemodialysis, drug is recommended only when benefits outweigh possible risk of seizures.
• Monitor patient for bacterial or fungal superinfections and resistant infections during and after therapy.

PATIENT TEACHING
• Instruct patient to report adverse reactions promptly.
• Tell patient to report discomfort at I.V. insertion site.
• Urge patient to notify prescriber about loose stools or diarrhea.

imipramine hydrochloride
im-IP-ra-meen

Novo-pramine†, Tofranil

imipramine pamoate
Tofranil-PM

Therapeutic class: Antidepressants
Pharmacologic class: Tricyclic antidepressants
Pregnancy risk category: D

AVAILABLE FORMS
imipramine hydrochloride
Tablets: 10 mg, 25 mg, 50 mg
imipramine pamoate
Capsules: 75 mg, 100 mg, 125 mg, 150 mg

INDICATIONS & DOSAGES
➤ **Depression**
Adults: 75 to 100 mg P.O. daily in divided doses, increased by 25 to 50 mg. Maximum daily dose is 200 mg for outpatients and

300 mg for hospitalized patients. Give entire dose at bedtime.
Adolescents: 30 to 40 mg P.O. once daily, preferably at bedtime, or in divided doses if necessary. Dosage increases above 100 mg daily are generally unnecessary.
Elderly patients: Initially, 30 to 40 mg daily; maximum shouldn't exceed 100 mg daily.
➤ **Childhood enuresis**
Children age 6 and older: Initially, 25 mg P.O. 1 hour before bedtime. If patient doesn't improve within 1 week, increase dose to a maximum of 50 mg if child is younger than age 12; increase dose to a maximum of 75 mg for children age 12 and older.
➤ **Prevention of migraine ◆**
Adults: 10 to 25 mg P.O. t.i.d.
➤ **Attention deficit hyperactivity disorder ◆**
Children and adolescents: Initially, 1 mg/kg/day P.O. titrated to maximum dosage of 4 mg/kg/day or 200 mg/day, whichever is smaller.

ADMINISTRATION
P.O.
• Give drug without regard for food.
• Give full dose at bedtime if possible.

ACTION
Unknown. Increases norepinephrine, serotonin, or both in the CNS by blocking their reuptake by the presynaptic neurons.

Route	Onset	Peak	Duration
P.O.	Unknown	1–2 hr	Unknown

Half-life: 11 to 25 hours.

ADVERSE REACTIONS
CNS: drowsiness, dizziness, *seizures, stroke,* excitation, tremor, confusion, hallucinations, anxiety, ataxia, paresthesia, nervousness, EEG changes, extrapyramidal reactions.
CV: orthostatic hypotension, tachycardia, ECG changes, *MI, arrhythmias, heart block,* hypertension, *precipitation of heart failure.*
EENT: blurred vision, tinnitus, mydriasis.
GI: dry mouth, constipation, nausea, vomiting, anorexia, paralytic ileus, abdominal cramps.

GU: urine retention.
Hematologic: *bone marrow depression.*
Metabolic: *hypoglycemia,* hyperglycemia.
Skin: rash, urticaria, photosensitivity reactions, pruritus, diaphoresis.
Other: hypersensitivity reactions.

INTERACTIONS

Drug-drug. *Barbiturates, CNS depressants:* May enhance CNS depression. Avoid using together.
Cimetidine, fluoxetine, fluvoxamine, paroxetine, sertraline: May increase imipramine level. Monitor drug levels and patient for signs of toxicity.
Clonidine: May cause life-threatening hypertension. Avoid using together.
Epinephrine, norepinephrine: May increase hypertensive effect. Use together cautiously.
Linezolid, methylene blue: May cause serotonin syndrome. Use with extreme caution and monitor patient closely.
MAO inhibitors: May cause hyperpyretic crisis, severe seizures, and death. Avoid using within 14 days of MAO inhibitor therapy.
Quinolones: May increase the risk of life-threatening arrhythmias. Avoid using together.
Drug-herb. *Evening primrose oil:* May cause additive or synergistic effect, lowering the seizure threshold and increasing the risk of seizure. Discourage use together.
St. John's wort, SAM-e, yohimbe: May cause serotonin syndrome. Discourage use together.
Drug-lifestyle. *Alcohol use:* May enhance CNS depression. Discourage use together.
Smoking: May lower level of drug. Monitor patient for lack of effect.
Sun exposure: May increase risk of photosensitivity reactions. Advise patient to avoid excessive sunlight exposure.

EFFECTS ON LAB TEST RESULTS

• May increase or decrease glucose level.
• May increase LFT values.

CONTRAINDICATIONS & CAUTIONS

• Contraindicated in patients hypersensitive to drug and in those receiving MAO inhibitors; also contraindicated during acute recovery phase of MI.

❻ Alert: Concomitant use with linezolid or methylene blue can cause serotonin syndrome (fever, mental status changes, muscle twitching, excessive sweating, shivering or shaking, diarrhea, and loss of coordination). Use imipramine with linezolid or methylene blue only for life-threatening or urgent conditions when the potential benefits outweigh the risks of toxicity.

• Use with extreme caution in patients at risk for suicide; in elderly patients and in patients with history of urine retention, angle-closure glaucoma, or seizure disorders; in patients with increased intraocular pressure, CV disease, impaired hepatic function, hyperthyroidism, or impaired renal function; and in patients receiving thyroid drugs.

• Injectable form contains sulfites, which may cause allergic reactions in hypersensitive patients.

❻ Alert: Imipramine isn't approved for use in children except for those with nocturnal enuresis. Imipramine pamoate shouldn't be used in children of any age because of increased risk of acute overdosage.

⚠ Overdose S&S: Cardiac arrhythmias, severe hypotension, seizures, CNS depression, coma, ECG changes, drowsiness, stupor, ataxia, restlessness, agitation, hyperactive reflexes, muscle rigidity, athetoid and choreiform movements, tachycardia, congestive heart failure, respiratory depression, cyanosis, shock, vomiting, hyperpyrexia, mydriasis, diaphoresis.

NURSING CONSIDERATIONS

❻ Alert: If linezolid or methylene blue must be given, discontinue imipramine and monitor patient for serotonin toxicity for 2 weeks (5 weeks if fluoxetine was taken) or until 24 hours after the last dose of methylene blue or linezolid, whichever comes first. May resume imipramine 24 hours after last dose of methylene blue or linezolid.

• Monitor WBC count during therapy, and monitor patient for fever and sore throat. Discontinue drug if pathologic neutrophil depression occurs.

• Monitor patient for nausea, headache, and malaise after abrupt withdrawal of long-term therapy; these symptoms don't indicate addiction.

Reactions in bold italics are *life-threatening*. Interactions may have a *rapid onset* or a *delayed onset*.

- Don't withdraw drug abruptly.
- Because of hypertensive episodes during surgery in patients receiving TCAs, stop drug gradually several days before surgery.
- If signs or symptoms of psychosis occur or increase, expect prescriber to reduce dosage. Record mood changes. Monitor patient for suicidal tendencies, and allow only a minimum supply of drug.

Black Box Warning Drug may increase the risk of suicidal thinking and behavior in children, adolescents, and young adults with major depressive disorder or other psychiatric disorder. ∎

- To prevent relapse in children receiving drug for enuresis, withdraw drug gradually.
- Recommend sugarless hard candy or gum to relieve dry mouth. Saliva substitutes may be useful.
- **Alert:** Tofranil and Tofranil-PM may contain tartrazine.
- **Look alike–sound alike:** Don't confuse imipramine with desipramine.

PATIENT TEACHING

Black Box Warning Advise families and caregivers to closely observe patient for increased suicidal thinking and behavior. ∎

- **Alert:** Teach patient to recognize and immediately report symptoms of serotonin toxicity (fever, mental status changes, muscle twitching, excessive sweating, shivering or shaking, diarrhea, and loss of coordination).
- Tell patient to take full dose at bedtime whenever possible, but warn him of possible morning dizziness upon standing up quickly.
- If child is an early-night bed-wetter, tell parents it may be more effective to divide dose and give the first dose earlier in day.
- Tell patient to avoid alcohol while taking this drug.
- Advise patient to consult prescriber before taking other prescription or OTC drugs.
- Warn patient to avoid hazardous activities that require alertness and good coordination until effects of the drug are known. Drowsiness and dizziness usually subside after a few weeks.
- Warn patient not to stop drug suddenly.
- To prevent oversensitivity to the sun, advise patient to use sunblock, wear protective clothing, and avoid prolonged exposure to strong sunlight.

---

imiquimod
ih-mih-KWI-mahd

Aldara, Zyclara

Therapeutic class: Immunosuppressants (topical)
Pharmacologic class: Immune response modifiers
Pregnancy risk category: C

AVAILABLE FORMS
Cream: 2.5%, 3.75%, 5% in single-use packets containing 12.5 mg imiquimod

INDICATIONS & DOSAGES
➤ **External genital and perianal warts**
Adults and adolescents age 12 and older: Apply thin layer of 3.75% or 5% cream to affected area three times weekly before normal sleeping hours and leave on skin for 6 to 10 hours. Continue treatment until genital or perianal warts clear completely or maximum of 16 weeks.

➤ **Typical, nonhyperkeratotic, nonhypertrophic actinic keratoses on the face or scalp in immunocompetent adults**
Adults: Wash area with mild soap and water and dry at least 10 minutes. Apply Aldara cream to face or scalp, but not both concurrently, twice weekly at bedtime, and wash off after about 8 hours. Treat for 16 weeks. Or, apply Zyclara 3.75% once daily at bedtime for two 2-week cycles. Separate cycles by 2-week no-treatment period.

➤ **Superficial basal cell carcinoma**
Adults: Wash area with mild soap and water and allow to dry thoroughly. Apply a thin layer of 5% cream to the biopsy-confirmed area, including 1 cm of skin surrounding tumor, five times a week at bedtime; wash off after about 8 hours. Treat for 6 weeks.

ADMINISTRATION
Topical
- Wash area with mild soap and water and dry completely before applying cream.
- Discard unused portion of single-use packet.

ACTION

Has no direct antiviral activity in cell culture. Drug induces mRNA-encoding cytokines, including interferon alfa, at the treatment site.

Route	Onset	Peak	Duration
Topical	Unknown	Unknown	Unknown

Half-life: About 20 hours.

ADVERSE REACTIONS

CNS: dizziness, headache.
Musculoskeletal: myalgia.
Skin: local itching, burning, pain, soreness, erythema, ulceration, edema, erosion, induration, flaking, excoriation.
Other: fungal infection, flulike symptoms.

INTERACTIONS

None significant.

EFFECTS ON LAB TEST RESULTS

None reported.

CONTRAINDICATIONS & CAUTIONS

• The 5% cream hasn't been evaluated for treatment of urethral, intravaginal, cervical, rectal, or intra-anal human papillomavirus disease.
• Safety of drug in breast-feeding women is unknown.
⚠ *Overdose S&S:* Severe local skin reactions.

NURSING CONSIDERATIONS

• Don't use until genital or perianal tissue is healed from previous drug or surgical treatment.
• Patient usually experiences local skin reactions at site of application or surrounding areas. Use nonocclusive dressings, such as cotton gauze, or cotton undergarments in management of skin reactions. Patient's discomfort or severity of the local skin reaction may require a rest period of several days. Resume treatment once reaction subsides.
🖐 *Alert:* Women with a local inflammatory reaction that causes severe vulvar swelling may be at risk for urine retention. If symptoms of urine retention occur, interrupt or discontinue drug, and monitor patient carefully.

• Drug isn't a cure; new warts may develop during therapy.
• Maximum tumor diameter of superficial basal cell carcinoma should be 2 cm or smaller. Cream may be applied to neck, trunk, or arms and legs (excluding hands and feet).
• Assess treatment site for clearance 12 weeks after treatment.

PATIENT TEACHING

• Advise patient that effect of cream on transmission of genital or perianal warts is unknown. New warts may develop during therapy; drug isn't a cure.
• Tell patient to use cream only as directed and to avoid contact with eyes, lips, or nostrils.
• Tell patient to wash hands before and after applying cream.
• Tell patient to wash the area with mild soap and water and dry completely before applying cream.
• Advise patient to apply cream in thin layer over affected area and rub in until cream isn't visible. Advise patient to avoid excessive use of cream. Tell him not to occlude area after applying cream and to wash with mild soap and water 6 to 10 hours after application of cream.
• Advise patient that mild local skin reactions, such as redness, erosion, excoriation, flaking, and swelling at site of application or surrounding areas, are common. Tell him that most skin reactions are mild to moderate. Advise him to report severe skin reactions promptly.
• Instruct uncircumcised man being treated for warts under the foreskin to retract foreskin and clean area daily.
• Advise patient that drug can weaken condoms and vaginal diaphragms and that use together isn't recommended.
• Advise patient to avoid sexual contact while cream is on the skin.
• Advise patient to minimize or avoid exposure to sunlight and other UV light; encourage sunscreen use.
• Tell patient to store drug at temperatures below 86° F (30° C) and to avoid freezing.
• Tell patient to discard partially used packets and not to reuse.

Reactions in bold italics are *life-threatening*. Interactions may have a *rapid onset* or a *delayed onset*.

immune globulin intramuscular (gamma globulin, IG, IGIM)
GamaSTAN S/D

immune globulin intravenous (IGIV)
Carimune NF, Flebogamma, Gammagard Liquid, Gammagard S/D, Gamunex-C, Octagam, Privigen

immune globulin subcutaneous (IGSC, SCIG)
Gammagard, Gamunex-C, Hizentra, Vivaglobin

Therapeutic class: Antibodies
Pharmacologic class: Immune serums
Pregnancy risk category: C

AVAILABLE FORMS
immune globulin intramuscular
Injection: 15% to 18% in vials and single-dose syringes
immune globulin intravenous
Injection: 5% in 10-mL, 50-mL, 100-mL, 200-mL vials (Flebogamma); 5% in 1-g, 2.5-g, 5-g, 10-g single-use bottles (Octagam)
Injection: 5% single-use vials
Injection (preservative-free): 5%, 10% single-use vials
Powder for injection: 0.5-g, 3-g, 6-g, 12-g vials (Carimune NF)
immune globulin subcutaneous
Injection: 10%, 16%, 20% single-use vials

INDICATIONS & DOSAGES
➤ **Primary immunodeficiency**
Carimune NF
Adults and children: 400 to 800 mg/kg I.V. every 3 to 4 weeks. First infusion in previously untreated patients must be given as a 3% immunoglobulin solution at initial infusion rate of 0.5 mg/kg/minute. If tolerated, after 30 minutes the rate may be increased to 1 mg/kg/minute for the next 30 minutes, then gradually increased in a stepwise manner up to a maximum of 3 mg/kg/minute as tolerated. See package insert for infusion rates in mL/kg/minute.

Flebogamma
Adults: 300 to 600 mg/kg I.V. every 3 to 4 weeks. Infuse at 0.5 mg/kg/minute and increase after 30 minutes to 5 mg/kg/minute.
Gammagard Liquid
Adults and children age 2 and older: 300 to 600 mg/kg I.V. every 3 to 4 weeks. Infuse at 0.8 mg/kg/minute and increase every 30 minutes to 8 mg/kg/minute. Maintenance therapy may be given subcutaneously starting 1 week after last IGIV infusion. Initial subcutaneous dose is 1.37 × current I.V. dose in mg/kg ÷ number of weeks between I.V. doses.
Gammagard S/D
Adults and children age 2 and older: 300 to 600 mg/kg I.V. every 3 to 4 weeks depending on patient response, initially infused in a 5% solution at 0.5 mL/kg/hour that may be increased gradually if patient doesn't experience distress to a maximum rate of 4 mL/kg/hour for patients with no history of adverse reactions to IGIV and no significant risk factors for renal dysfunction or thrombotic complications. See package insert for subsequent solution concentration and infusion-rate increases.
Gamunex
Adults: 300 to 600 mg/kg I.V. every 3 to 4 weeks. Maintenance therapy may be given subcutaneously starting 1 week after last IGIV infusion. Initial subcutaneous dose is 1.37 × current I.V. dose in mg/kg ÷ number of weeks between I.V. doses.
Hizentra
Adults and children: Initial dose is 1.53 times previous IGIV dose in grams divided by number of weeks between IGIV doses. Multiply dose in grams by 5 to obtain dose in milliliters. Adjust dose based on clinical response and IgG trough levels to goal of 1.3 times trough level before last IGIV treatment. Give by subcutaneous infusion weekly. See package insert for full dosage adjustment guidelines.
Octagam
Adults and children: 300 to 600 mg/kg I.V. every 3 to 4 weeks. Start infusion at 30 mg/kg/hour for 30 minutes. If no discomfort is experienced, increase rate to 60 mg/kg/hour for 30 minutes. Rate can then be increased to maximum of 200 mg/kg/hour.

Privigen
Adults: 200 to 800 mg/kg every 3 to
4 weeks. Start infusion at 0.5 mg/kg/minute
and increase slowly to 8 mg/kg/minute.
Vivaglobin
Adults and children: Initial dose is
1.37 times previous IGIV dose divided
by number of weeks between IGIV doses.
Recommended weekly dose is 100 to
200 mg/kg by subcutaneous infusion.
Adjust dosage based on clinical response
and serum IgG trough levels. See package
insert for full dosage adjustment guidelines.
➤ **Chronic inflammatory demyelinating
polyneuropathy**
Adults: 2,000 mg/kg I.V. Gamunex in
divided doses over 2 to 4 days every
3 weeks. Or, 1,000 mg/kg I.V. over 1 day
every 3 weeks or 500 mg/kg I.V. on 2 consecutive days every 3 weeks.
➤ **Idiopathic thrombocytopenic purpura
(ITP)**
Carimune NF
Adults and children: 400 mg/kg I.V. for 2 to
5 consecutive days, depending on platelet
count and immune response.
Gammagard S/D
Adults: 1,000 mg/kg I.V. May give up to
three separate doses on alternate days, if
needed, as determined by clinical response
and platelet count.
Gamunex-C
Adults: 2,000 mg/kg I.V. in divided doses
over 2 days or 400 mg/kg I.V. in 5 doses over
5 days.
Privigen
Adults: 1,000 mg/kg I.V. for 2 days.
➤ **Kawasaki syndrome**
Children: 400 mg/kg I.V. daily over 2 hours
for 4 consecutive days, or a single dose of
1,000 mg/kg over 10 hours. Start within
10 days of disease onset. Give with aspirin
(100 mg/kg P.O. daily through day 14; then
3 to 5 mg/kg P.O. daily for 5 weeks).
➤ **Hepatitis A exposure (IGIM)**
Adults and children: 0.02 mL/kg I.M. as
soon as possible after exposure. Up to
0.06 mL/kg may be given for prolonged
or intense exposure.
➤ **Measles exposure (IGIM)**
Adults and children: 0.25 mL/kg I.M. within
6 days after exposure.

➤ **Measles postexposure prophylaxis
(IGIM)**
Immunocompromised children: 0.5 mL/kg
I.M. (maximum 15 mL) immediately after
exposure.
➤ **Chickenpox exposure (IGIM)**
Adults and children: 0.6 to 1.2 mL/kg I.M.
as soon as possible after exposure.
➤ **Rubella exposure in first trimester of
pregnancy (IGIM)**
Women: 0.55 mL/kg I.M. as soon as possible
after exposure (within 72 hours).
✳ **NEW INDICATION: B-cell chronic lympho-
cytic leukemia**
Adults and children: 400 mg/kg I.V. Gam-
magard S/D every 3 to 4 weeks for patients
with hypogammaglobulinemia or recurrent
bacterial infections.
➤ **Guillain-Barré syndrome (IGIV)** ◆
Adults: 2,000 mg/kg I.V. over 2 to 5 days
within 2 to 4 weeks of onset.
Children: 2,000 mg/kg I.V. over 2 days
within 2 to 4 weeks of onset.
➤ **Severe exacerbation of myasthenia
gravis (IGIV)** ◆
Adults: 1,000 to 2,000 mg/kg I.V. over 2 to
5 days.

ADMINISTRATION
I.M.
🕭 *Alert:* Verify drug, route, and dose carefully before administration.
● Give in the anterolateral aspects of the
upper thigh and the deltoid muscle of the
upper arm. Divide doses larger than 10 mL
and inject into several muscle sites to reduce
pain and discomfort.
● Don't administer I.V. or subcutaneously
because of risk of serious reactions.
● Give drug soon after reconstitution.
● The gluteal region should not routinely
be used. If necessary, only the upper outer
quadrant should be used.
I.V.
▼ After reconstitution, Carimune NF
contains at least 96% IgG; Octagam
contains about 50 mg of protein/mL and at
least 96% IgG.
▼ Most adverse reactions are related to a
rapid infusion rate. If they occur, decrease
infusion rate or stop infusion until reaction
subsides. Resume infusion at a rate the
patient can tolerate.

Reactions in bold italics are *life-threatening*. Interactions may have a *rapid onset* or a *delayed onset*.

▼ Store Octagam at 36° to 46° F (2° to 8° C) for 24 months or at no higher than 77° F (25° C) for up to 18 months from the date of manufacture.

Carimune NF

▼ Use 15-micron in-line filter when giving. Reconstitute with normal saline solution, D_5W, or sterile water. Don't shake vial. Infusion rate is 0.5 to 1 mL/minute for 3% solution. After 15 to 30 minutes, increase rate to 1.5 to 2.5 mL/minute.

Gammagard Liquid

▼ Drug should be at room temperature during administration.

▼ Normal saline solution should not be used as a diluent. If dilution is preferred, D_5W may be used.

▼ The use of an in-line filter is optional.

▼ Begin infusion at 0.5 mL/kg/hour. If tolerated, gradually increase every 30 minutes to 5 mL/kg/hour.

Gammagard S/D

▼ If refrigerated, allow diluent and immune globulin I.V. to reach room temperature before reconstitution and administration.

▼ Reconstitute according to manufacturer's instructions.

▼ Do not use if particulate matter or discoloration is visible.

▼ Use antecubital veins to infuse 10% solutions.

▼ Initially infuse 5% solution at 0.5 mL/kg/hour. Infusion rate may be gradually increased to maximum rate of 4 mL/kg/hour for those with no history of adverse reactions to immune globulin I.V., renal dysfunction, or thrombotic complications.

▼ Patients who tolerate 5% concentration at 4 mL/kg/hour can be infused with 10% concentration starting at 0.5 mL/kg/hour and increased to a maximum of 8 mL/kg/hour if no adverse effects occur.

▼ **Incompatibilities:** Other I.V. drugs and I.V. solutions. Don't mix with immune globulin from other manufacturers.

Gamunex-C

▼ Incompatible with saline solutions. Compatible with D_5W, if needed.

▼ Infuse I.V. at a rate of 0.01 mL/kg/minute for first 30 minutes. If no problems, rate can be slowly increased to maximum of 0.08 mL/kg/minute.

▼ Store vials at 36° to 46° F (2° to 8° C). During first 18 months from the date of manufacture, store vials for up to 5 months at room temperature not exceeding 77° F (25° C); then vials must be used immediately or discarded. Don't freeze vials.

Octagam

▼ Octagam should be at room temperature during infusion. If using an infusion set (not mandatory), the filter size must be 0.2 to 200 microns. Initially, infuse at 30 mg/kg/hour for the first 30 minutes; if tolerated, infuse at 60 mg/kg/hour for the second 30 minutes; if further tolerated, infuse at 120 mg/kg/hour for the third 30 minutes. If tolerated, infusion can be maintained at less than 200 mg/kg/hour. Adverse reactions usually disappear with slowing or stopping the infusion. For patients at risk for renal dysfunction, reduce infusion to less than 200 mg/kg/hour.

Privigen

▼ Don't shake vial.

▼ If necessary dilute with D_5W.

▼ Begin infusion at 0.5 mg/kg/minute. If well tolerated, may increase gradually to 8 mg/kg/minute.

▼ For chronic ITP, maximum infusion rate is 4 mg/kg/minute.

▼ Infusion line may be flushed with D_5W or normal saline solution.

▼ **Incompatibilities:** Other I.V. drugs.

Subcutaneous

● IGSC is given by subcutaneous infusion.

● Infusion sites include abdomen, thighs, upper arms, and lateral hip.

● Up to four infusion sites may be used at the same time, with at least 2 inches (5 cm) between sites.

● Give up to 15 mL per site with initial infusion. May increase to 20 mL per site after fourth infusion and to maximum of 25 mL per site as tolerated.

● Initially infuse at 15 mL/hour. May increase to maximum of 25 mL/hour per site as tolerated. Total infusion rate for all sites combined must not exceed 50 mL/hour.

● Gammagard I: For patients weighing 40 kg (88 lb) or more, give up to 30 mL per site at 20 mL/hour per site; may increase to maximum rate of 30 mL/hour per site as tolerated. For patients weighing less than 40 kg, give up to 20 mL per site at 15 mL/hour per site; may increase to maximum rate of 20 mL/hour per site as tolerated.

• Don't mix with other products.
• Gammagard, Hizentra, Vivaglobin: Don't shake vial.

ACTION

Provides passive immunity by increasing antibody titer. The primary component is IgG. It's unknown how it works for ITP.

Route	Onset	Peak	Duration
I.V.	Immediate	Immediate	Unknown
I.M.	Unknown	2–5 hr	Unknown
Subcut.	Unknown	2.9 days	Unknown

Half-life: 21 to 24 days in immunocompromised patients.

ADVERSE REACTIONS

CNS: severe headache requiring hospitalization, faintness, fever, headache, malaise.
CV: chest pain, chest tightness, *heart failure, MI.*
GI: diarrhea, abdominal pain, nausea, vomiting.
Musculoskeletal: back pain, arthralgia, hip pain, muscle stiffness at injection site.
Respiratory: *PE, transfusion-related acute lung injury,* dyspnea.
Skin: erythema, urticaria, pain, local infusion-site reactions, rash.
Other: *anaphylaxis, angioedema,* chills.

INTERACTIONS

Drug-drug. *Live-virus vaccines:* Length of time to wait before giving live-virus vaccinations varies with dose of immune globulin given. Check the recommendations of the American Academy of Pediatrics.

EFFECTS ON LAB TEST RESULTS

• May falsely elevate serum glucose level (for IGIV preparations containing maltose, such as Octagam).
• May cause positive Coombs test.

CONTRAINDICATIONS & CAUTIONS

• Contraindicated in patients hypersensitive to drug or its components.
• Hizentra is contraindicated in patients hypersensitive to polysorbate 80, patients

with hyperprolinemia, and IgA-deficient patients with antibodies against IgA and history of hypersensitivity.
• Use IGIV cautiously in patients with a history of CV disease or thrombotic episodes.

Black Box Warning Use IGIV cautiously in patients with renal dysfunction or a predisposition to renal failure, including patients with preexisting renal insufficiency, diabetes mellitus, volume depletion, sepsis, or paraproteinemia; those older than age 65; and those receiving nephrotoxic drugs. Give at minimum concentration and infuse as slowly as practicable. ■

NURSING CONSIDERATIONS

Black Box Warning Drug causes an increased risk of thrombosis, especially in elderly patients, in those with prolonged immobilization, hypercoagulable conditions, history of venous or arterial thrombosis, hyperviscosity, CV risk factors, or indwelling central venous catheters, and in patients using estrogens. Thrombosis may also occur without these risk factors. ■

Black Box Warning For patients at increased risk for thrombosis, give minimum concentration available at minimum rate of infusion practicable. ■

Black Box Warning Ensure adequate hydration before administration. ■

Black Box Warning Monitor patients for signs or symptoms of thrombosis (pain or swelling of the extremity with warmth over affected area, discoloration, unexplained dyspnea, chest pain or discomfort that worsens on deep inspiration, tachycardia, chest pain, numbness or weakness on one side of the body), and assess blood viscosity in patients at risk for hyperviscosity. ■

• Obtain history of allergies and reactions to immunizations. Keep epinephrine 1:1,000 available to treat anaphylaxis.
• IGIV administration may be linked to thrombotic events.
• If patient is at risk for a thrombotic event, make sure infusion concentration is no more than 5% and start infusion rate no faster than 0.5 mL/kg/hour. Advance rate slowly only if well tolerated, to a maximum rate of 4 mL/kg/hour.

• Don't give as prophylaxis against hepatitis A if 6 weeks or more have passed since exposure or onset of symptoms.
• Products made from human plasma may contain infectious agents, such as viruses and, potentially, the Creutzfeldt-Jakob disease agent.

PATIENT TEACHING
◑ Alert: Warn patient of risk of thrombosis. Instruct patient to report signs or symptoms immediately.
• Explain to patient and family how drug will be given.
• Tell patient that local reactions may occur at injection site. Instruct him to notify prescriber promptly if adverse reactions persist or become severe.
• Inform patient of possible need for therapy more than once monthly to maintain adequate IgG levels.

indacaterol maleate
in-da-KAT-er-ol

Arcapta Neohaler

Therapeutic class: Bronchodilators
Pharmacologic class: Beta₂-adrenergic agonists
Pregnancy risk category: C

AVAILABLE FORMS
Capsules (powder for inhalation): 75 mcg

INDICATIONS & DOSAGES
➤ **Long-term maintenance therapy for COPD**
Adults: 75 mcg (1 capsule) daily by oral inhalation.

ADMINISTRATION
Inhalational
• Patient shouldn't swallow capsules.
• Use inhalation capsules with the Neohaler device only. Always use the new Neohaler device that comes with each prescription. Administer inhaled capsules using the Neohaler device according to the package instructions.
• Don't wash the Neohaler device. The inhaler may be wiped between uses with a

clean, dry, lint-free cloth or a clean, dry, soft brush.
• Don't use other inhaler devices from other inhaled medications to administer indacaterol capsules.
• Always store capsules in the blister packaging and remove just before using. Don't keep or store capsules in the Neohaler device. Protect capsules from light and moisture.
• Administer indacaterol at the same time each day; patient shouldn't use more than once in 24 hours.

ACTION
Binds to beta₂ receptors in the lung and increases cAMP levels, resulting in relaxation of bronchial smooth muscle.

Route	Onset	Peak	Duration
Inhalation	Rapid	15 min	Unknown

Half-life: 46 to 126 hours.

ADVERSE REACTIONS
CNS: headache.
CV: peripheral edema.
EENT: nasopharyngitis, sinusitis, oropharyngeal pain.
GI: nausea.
Metabolic: hyperglycemia.
Musculoskeletal: muscle spasm, musculoskeletal pain.
Respiratory: cough, upper respiratory tract infection, dyspnea.

INTERACTIONS
Drug-drug. *Adrenergics (such as dobutamine, dopamine):* May increase risk of additive effects and adverse reactions. Use together cautiously.
Beta blockers: May block therapeutic effects of beta-adrenergic agonists and cause severe bronchospasm. If beta blocker use can't be avoided, administer indacaterol with extreme caution.
Drugs that prolong QTc interval, MAO inhibitors, tricyclic antidepressants: May increase risk of ventricular arrhythmias. Monitor patient carefully.
Xanthine derivatives (caffeine, theophylline), non-potassium-sparing diuretics, steroids: May cause hypokalemia. Monitor electrolyte levels closely.

EFFECTS ON LAB TEST RESULTS
● May increase glucose level. May decrease potassium level.

CONTRAINDICATIONS & CAUTIONS
Black Box Warning Long-acting beta$_2$-adrenergic agonists increase the risk of asthma-related death. The safety and effectiveness of indacaterol in patients with asthma haven't been established. Inhaled indacaterol isn't indicated for the treatment of asthma. ∎
● Contraindicated in patients with acutely deteriorating COPD, when used more than once daily, when used at higher doses than prescribed, or in addition to medications containing other long-acting beta$_2$-adrenergic agonists.
● Use cautiously in patients with a history of CV disorders (coronary insufficiency, arrhythmias, hypertension), seizures, thyrotoxicosis, diabetes, or abnormal electrolyte levels and in patients abnormally responsive to sympathomimetic amines.
● Use cautiously during labor because drug may interfere with uterine contractions. It isn't known if drug appears in breast milk.
⚠ **Overdose S&S:** Angina, hypertension or hypotension, tachycardia, cardiac arrest, arrhythmias, nervousness, headache, tremor, dry mouth, palpitations, muscle cramps, nausea, dizziness, fatigue, malaise, hypokalemia, hyperglycemia, metabolic acidosis, insomnia, death.

NURSING CONSIDERATIONS
❂ **Alert:** Drug may produce paradoxical bronchospasm that may be life-threatening. If paradoxical bronchospasm occurs, discontinue drug immediately and institute alternative therapy.
● Discontinue routine use of short-acting beta$_2$-adrenergic agonists when indacaterol therapy is begun. Short-acting beta$_2$-adrenergic agonists should be used only for symptomatic relief of acute respiratory symptoms.
● As long as the capsule is empty after inhalation, the full dose of medication has been received even if patient coughs. Monitor patient for worsening of symptoms, decreased effectiveness, or increased need for short-acting rescue inhaler.

PATIENT TEACHING
Black Box Warning Inform patient that indacaterol isn't for use in asthma and can increase the risk of asthma-related death. ∎
● Instruct patient on the proper administration, use, and storage of the Neohaler device and capsules. Remind patient to use only the Neohaler device and no other inhaler to administer the medication.
● Warn patient that indacaterol isn't to be used for acute exacerbations of COPD and that acute symptoms should be treated with a short-acting inhaler such as albuterol.
● Advise patient not to use indacaterol with other long-acting beta-adrenergic agonists because of the risk of significant CV effects (palpitations, arrhythmias, chest pain, increased heart rate, tremor, and nervousness).
● Advise patient to notify prescriber of worsening symptoms, decreased effectiveness of drug, or the need for more frequent use of a short-acting inhaler.
● Warn patient not to stop therapy without first discussing with health care provider.

indapamide
in-DAP-a-mide

Lozide†

Therapeutic class: Diuretics
Pharmacologic class: Thiazide-like diuretics
Pregnancy risk category: B

AVAILABLE FORMS
Tablets: 1.25 mg, 2.5 mg

INDICATIONS & DOSAGES
➤ **Edema of heart failure**
Adults: Initially, 2.5 mg P.O. daily in the morning. Increased to 5 mg daily after 1 week, if needed.
➤ **Hypertension**
Adults: Initially, 1.25 mg P.O. daily in the morning. Increased to 2.5 mg daily after 4 weeks, if needed. Increased to 5 mg daily after 4 more weeks, if needed. If response is inadequate, a second antihypertensive, given at 50% of the usual starting dose, may be needed.

ADMINISTRATION
P.O.
• Give drug with food to minimize GI upset.
• To prevent nocturia, give drug in the morning.

ACTION
Enhances excretion of sodium chloride and water by interfering with sodium transport in the distal tubule.

Route	Onset	Peak	Duration
P.O.	1–2 hr	Within 2 hr	Up to 36 hr

Half-life: About 14 hours.

ADVERSE REACTIONS
CNS: headache, nervousness, dizziness, light-headedness, weakness, vertigo, restlessness, drowsiness, fatigue, anxiety, depression, numbness of limbs, irritability, agitation, lethargy.
CV: orthostatic hypotension, palpitations, PVCs, irregular heartbeat, vasculitis, flushing, chest pain, edema.
EENT: rhinorrhea, blurred vision, pharyngitis, sinusitis, conjunctivitis.
GI: anorexia, nausea, epigastric distress, vomiting, abdominal pain or cramps, diarrhea, constipation.
GU: nocturia, polyuria, frequent urination, erectile dysfunction.
Metabolic: asymptomatic hyperuricemia; fluid and electrolyte imbalances, including dilutional hyponatremia, hypochloremia, metabolic alkalosis, and hypokalemia; weight loss; volume depletion and dehydration; hyperglycemia.
Musculoskeletal: muscle cramps and spasms.
Respiratory: cough.
Skin: rash, pruritus, urticaria.
Other: gout, infection.

INTERACTIONS
Drug-drug. *Amphotericin B, corticosteroids:* May increase risk of hypokalemia. Monitor potassium level closely.
Antidiabetics: May decrease hypoglycemic effect of sulfonylureas, causing elevated glucose levels. Adjust dosage, if needed. Monitor glucose level.
Barbiturates, opioids: May increase orthostasis. Monitor patient closely.

Bumetanide, ethacrynic acid, furosemide, torsemide: May cause excessive diuretic response, causing serious electrolyte abnormalities or dehydration. Adjust doses carefully, and monitor patient closely for signs and symptoms of excessive diuretic response.
Cardiac glycosides: May increase risk of digoxin toxicity from indapamide-induced hypokalemia. Monitor potassium and digoxin levels.
Cholestyramine, colestipol: May decrease absorption of thiazides. Separate doses by 2 hours.
Diazoxide: May increase antihypertensive, hyperglycemic, and hyperuricemic effects. Use together cautiously.
Lithium: May decrease lithium clearance, which may increase lithium toxicity. Avoid using together.
NSAIDs: May increase risk of NSAID-induced renal failure. Monitor patient for signs and symptoms of renal failure.
Drug-herb. *Dandelion:* May interfere with drug activity. Discourage use together.
Licorice: May cause unexpected rapid potassium loss. Discourage use together.
Drug-lifestyle. *Alcohol use:* May increase orthostatic hypotensive effect. Discourage use together.

EFFECTS ON LAB TEST RESULTS
• May increase BUN, creatinine, glucose, cholesterol, triglyceride, calcium, and uric acid levels. May decrease potassium, sodium, phosphate, and chloride levels.

CONTRAINDICATIONS & CAUTIONS
• Contraindicated in patients hypersensitive to other sulfonamide-derived drugs and in those with anuria.
• Use cautiously in patients with severe renal disease, impaired hepatic function, or progressive hepatic disease.
⚠ Overdose S&S: Nausea, vomiting, GI disorders, weakness, electrolyte imbalance, hypotension, depressed respirations.

NURSING CONSIDERATIONS
• Monitor fluid intake and output, weight, blood pressure, and electrolyte levels.
• Watch for signs of hypokalemia, such as muscle weakness and cramps. Drug may

be used with potassium-sparing diuretic to prevent potassium loss.
• Consult prescriber and dietitian about a high-potassium diet or potassium supplement. Foods rich in potassium include citrus fruits, tomatoes, bananas, dates, and apricots.
• Monitor creatinine and BUN levels regularly. Cumulative effects of drug may occur in patients with impaired renal function.
• Monitor uric acid level, especially in patients with history of gout.
• Monitor glucose level, especially in diabetic patients.
• Monitor elderly patients, who are especially susceptible to excessive diuresis.
• Stop thiazides and thiazide-like diuretics before parathyroid function tests.
• Therapeutic response may be delayed several weeks in hypertensive patients.

PATIENT TEACHING
• Instruct patient to take drug in morning to prevent need to urinate at night.
• Tell patient to take drug with food to minimize GI upset.
• Advise patient to avoid sudden posture changes and to rise slowly to avoid dizziness upon standing quickly.

indinavir sulfate
in-DIN-ah-ver

Crixivan◆

Therapeutic class: Antiretrovirals
Pharmacologic class: Protease inhibitors
Pregnancy risk category: C

AVAILABLE FORMS
Capsules: 100 mg, 200 mg, 400 mg

INDICATIONS & DOSAGES
➤ **HIV infection, with other antiretrovirals, when antiretrovirals are warranted**
Adults: 800 mg P.O. every 8 hours. Consider reducing indinavir to 600 mg every 8 hours when patient is taking delaviridine 400 mg t.i.d. Reduce indinavir to 600 mg every 8 hours when patient is taking itraconazole 200 mg b.i.d. or ketoconazole. When patient

is taking indinavir and rifabutin, decrease rifabutin to one-half the standard dosage and increase indinavir to 1,000 mg every 8 hours.
Adjust-a-dose: For patients with mild to moderate hepatic insufficiency from cirrhosis, reduce dosage to 600 mg P.O. every 8 hours.

ADMINISTRATION
P.O.
• Give drug on an empty stomach with water 1 hour before or 2 hours after a meal. Or, give it with other liquids (such as skim milk, juice, coffee, or tea) or a light meal. A meal high in fat, calories, and protein reduces drug absorption.
• Store capsules in the original container and keep desiccant in the bottle; capsules are sensitive to moisture.

ACTION
Inhibits HIV protease by binding to the protease-active site and inhibiting activity of the enzyme, preventing cleavage of the viral polyproteins and forming immature noninfectious viral particles.

Route	Onset	Peak	Duration
P.O.	Unknown	<1 hr	Unknown

Half-life: 2 hours.

ADVERSE REACTIONS
CNS: asthenia, dizziness, fatigue, headache, insomnia, malaise, somnolence.
GI: nausea, abdominal pain, acid regurgitation, anorexia, diarrhea, dry mouth, taste perversion, vomiting.
GU: hematuria, nephrolithiasis, dysuria.
Hematologic: *neutropenia, thrombocytopenia,* anemia.
Metabolic: hyperbilirubinemia, hyperglycemia.
Musculoskeletal: back pain.
Skin: pruritus, rash.
Other: flank pain.

INTERACTIONS
Drug-drug. *Atorvastatin, lovastatin, rosuvastatin, simvastatin:* May increase level of statin and risk of myopathy and rhabdomyolysis. Use together cautiously and use the lowest appropriate statin dose.

Reactions in bold italics are *life-threatening*. Interactions may have a *rapid onset* or a *delayed onset*.

Carbamazepine: May decrease indinavir concentration and effectiveness. Use with caution.

Clarithromycin: May alter clarithromycin level. Dosage adjustments not needed.

Delavirdine, itraconazole, ketoconazole: May increase indinavir level. Consider reducing indinavir to 600 mg every 8 hours.

Didanosine: May alter absorption of indinavir. Separate doses by 1 hour and give on an empty stomach.

Efavirenz, nevirapine: May decrease indinavir level. Closely monitor clinical response.

HMG-CoA reductase inhibitors: May increase levels of these drugs and increase risk of myopathy and rhabdomyolysis. Avoid using together.

Lopinavir–ritonavir: May increase indinavir level. Adjust indinavir dosage to 600 mg b.i.d.

Nelfinavir: May increase indinavir level. Monitor patient closely.

Proton pump inhibitors (lansoprazole, omeprazole, pantoprazole, rabeprazole): May reduce the antiviral activity of indinavir. Monitor clinical response and adjust indinavir dosage as needed.

Rifabutin: May increase rifabutin level and decrease indinavir level. Avoid using together.

Rifampin: May decrease indinavir level. Avoid using together.

Ritonavir: May increase indinavir level twofold to fivefold. Monitor clinical response and adjust dosage if needed.

Sildenafil, tadalafil, vardenafil: May increase levels of these drugs and increase adverse effects (hypotension, visual changes, and priapism). Tell patient not to exceed prescribed dosage. Sildenafil dosage shouldn't exceed 25 mg in a 48-hour period. Tadalafil dosage shouldn't exceed 10 mg in a 72-hour period. Vardenafil dosage shouldn't exceed 2.5 mg in a 24-hour period.

Drug-herb. St. John's wort: May reduce drug level by more than half. Coadministration isn't recommended.

Drug-food. *Grapefruit and grapefruit juice:* May decrease drug level and therapeutic effect. Discourage use together.

EFFECTS ON LAB TEST RESULTS
● May increase ALT, AST, bilirubin, amylase, hemoglobin, and glucose levels.
● May decrease neutrophil and platelet counts.

CONTRAINDICATIONS & CAUTIONS
● Contraindicated in patients hypersensitive to drug or its components.
● Contraindicated with alfuzosin, alprazolam, amiodarone, dihydroergotamine, ergonovine, ergotamine, lovastatin, methylergonovine, midazolam, sildenafil (when used to treat pulmonary hypertension), simvastatin, triazolam, and pimozide.
● Use cautiously in patients with hepatic insufficiency from cirrhosis.
● Safety and effectiveness in children haven't been established.
⚠ Overdose S&S: Nephrolithiasis/urolithiasis, flank pain, hematuria, nausea, vomiting, diarrhea.

NURSING CONSIDERATIONS
● Drug must be taken at 8-hour intervals.
● Drug may cause nephrolithiasis. If signs and symptoms of nephrolithiasis occur, prescriber may stop drug for 1 to 3 days during acute phases.
● To prevent nephrolithiasis, patient should maintain adequate hydration (at least 48 ounces or 1.5 L of fluids every 24 hours while taking indinavir).

PATIENT TEACHING
● Tell patient that drug doesn't cure HIV infection and that he may continue to develop opportunistic infections and other complications of HIV infection. Drug hasn't been shown to reduce the risk of HIV transmission.
● Advise patient to use barrier protection during sexual intercourse.
● Caution patient not to adjust dosage or stop therapy without first consulting prescriber.
● Advise patient that if a dose is missed, he should take the next dose at the regularly scheduled time and shouldn't double the dose.
● Instruct patient to take drug on an empty stomach with water 1 hour before or 2 hours after a meal. Or, he may take it with other

liquids (such as skim milk, juice, coffee, or tea) or a light meal.

• Instruct patient to store capsules in the original container and to keep desiccant in the bottle; capsules are sensitive to moisture.

• Tell patient to drink at least 48 ounces (1.5 L) of fluid daily.

• Advise women to avoid breast-feeding because drug may appear in breast milk. Also, to prevent transmitting virus to infant, advise HIV-positive women not to breast-feed.

indomethacin
in-doe-METH-a-sin

Indocin, Novo-Methacin†, Pro-Indo†

indomethacin sodium trihydrate
Indocin I.V.

Therapeutic class: NSAIDs
Pharmacologic class: NSAIDs
Pregnancy risk category: C

AVAILABLE FORMS
indomethacin
Capsules: 25 mg, 50 mg
Capsules (extended-release): 75 mg
Injection: 1 mg/vial
Oral suspension: 25 mg/5 mL*
Suppositories: 50 mg
indomethacin sodium trihydrate
Injection: 1-mg vials

INDICATIONS & DOSAGES
➤ **Moderate to severe rheumatoid arthritis or osteoarthritis, ankylosing spondylitis**
Adults and children age 15 and older: 25 mg P.O. b.i.d. or t.i.d. with food or antacids or 25 mg P.R. b.i.d. or t.i.d.; increase daily dose by 25 or 50 mg every 7 days, up to 200 mg daily. Or, 75 mg extended-release capsules P.O. to start, in morning or at bedtime, followed by 75 mg extended-release capsules b.i.d. if needed.
➤ **Acute gouty arthritis**
Adults and children age 15 and older: 50 mg P.O. or P.R. t.i.d. Reduce dose as soon as possible; then stop therapy. Don't use extended-release form.

➤ **Acute painful shoulders (bursitis or tendinitis)**
Adults and children age 15 and older: 75 to 150 mg P.O. or P.R. daily in divided doses t.i.d. or q.i.d. for 7 to 14 days. Or, 150 mg (extended-release) P.O. b.i.d. for 7 to 14 days.
➤ **To close a hemodynamically significant patent ductus arteriosus in premature neonates**
Neonates older than age 7 days: 0.2 mg/kg I.V.; then two doses of 0.25 mg/kg at 12- to 24-hour intervals.
Neonates ages 2 to 7 days: 0.2 mg/kg I.V.; then two doses of 0.2 mg/kg at 12- to 24-hour intervals.
Neonates younger than 48 hours: 0.2 mg/kg I.V.; then two doses of 0.1 mg/kg I.V. at 12- to 24-hour intervals.

ADMINISTRATION
P.O.
• Give drug with food, milk, or antacid.
I.V.
▼ Reconstitute powder for injection with sterile water or normal saline solution. For each 1-mg vial, add 1 or 2 mL of diluent for a solution containing 1 mg/mL or 0.5 mg/mL, respectively. Give over 20 to 30 minutes.
▼ Use only preservative-free sterile saline solution or sterile water to prepare. Never use diluents containing benzyl alcohol because it has been linked to toxicity in newborns.
▼ Because injection contains no preservatives, reconstitute drug immediately before use and discard unused solution.
▼ If anuria or marked oliguria is evident, withhold administration of second or third scheduled I.V. dose and notify prescriber.
▼ Watch carefully for bleeding and for reduced urine output.
▼ **Incompatibilities:** Amino acid injection, calcium gluconate, cimetidine, dextrose injection, dobutamine, dopamine, gentamicin, levofloxacin, solutions with pH less than 6, tobramycin sulfate, tolazoline.
Rectal
• If suppository is too soft, place in refrigerator for 15 minutes or run under cold water in wrapper.

ACTION

May inhibit prostaglandin synthesis, to produce anti-inflammatory, analgesic, and antipyretic effects.

Route	Onset	Peak	Duration
P.O.	30 min	1–4 hr	4–6 hr
I.V.	Immediate	Immediate	4–6 hr
P.R.	Unknown	Unknown	4–6 hr

Half-life: 4¼ hours.

ADVERSE REACTIONS

P.O. and rectal

CNS: headache, dizziness, depression, fatigue, somnolence, syncope, vertigo.
CV: edema, hypertension.
EENT: hearing loss, tinnitus.
GI: *pancreatitis,* abdominal pain, anorexia, constipation, diarrhea, dyspepsia, *GI bleeding,* nausea, peptic ulceration.
Other: hypersensitivity reactions.
I.V.
GU: hematuria, interstitial nephritis, proteinuria.

INTERACTIONS

Drug-drug. *ACE inhibitors (benazepril, enalaprilat), angiotensin II receptor blockers (candesartan, valsartan):* May reduce antihypertensive effects; may worsen renal function in those with impaired renal function. Monitor patient closely.
Aminoglycosides, cyclosporine, methotrexate: May enhance toxicity of these drugs. Avoid using together.
Anticoagulants: May cause bleeding. Monitor patient closely.
Antihypertensives: May decrease antihypertensive effect. Monitor patient closely.
Antihypertensives, furosemide, thiazide diuretics: May impair response to both drugs. Avoid using together, if possible.
Aspirin: May increase adverse reactions. Avoid using together.
Aspirin, corticosteroids: May increase risk of GI toxicity. Avoid using together.
Bisphosphonates: May increase risk of gastric ulceration. Monitor patient for symptoms of gastric irritation or GI bleeding.
Cyclosporine: May increase cyclosporine toxicity. Use cautiously and monitor renal function.

Diflunisal, probenecid: May decrease indomethacin excretion. Watch for increased indomethacin adverse effects.
Digoxin: May prolong half-life of digoxin. Use together cautiously.
Dipyridamole: May enhance fluid retention. Avoid using together.
Lithium: May increase lithium level. Monitor patient for toxicity.
Methotrexate: May increase methotrexate toxicity. Use together cautiously.
Penicillamine: May increase bioavailability of penicillamine. Monitor patient closely.
Phenytoin: May increase phenytoin level. Monitor patient closely.
SSRIs: May increase risk of GI bleeding. Adjust dosage as needed.
Triamterene: May cause nephrotoxicity. Avoid using together.
Drug-herb. *Dong quai, feverfew, garlic, ginger, horse chestnut, red clover:* May cause bleeding. Discourage use together.
Senna: May inhibit diarrheal effects. Discourage use together.
White willow: Herb and drug contain similar components. Discourage use together.
Drug-lifestyle. *Alcohol use:* May cause GI toxicity. Discourage use together.

EFFECTS ON LAB TEST RESULTS

• May increase potassium level.
• May decrease hemoglobin level and hematocrit.
• May increase LFT values.

CONTRAINDICATIONS & CAUTIONS

• Contraindicated in patients hypersensitive to drug and in those with a history of aspirin- or NSAID-induced asthma, rhinitis, or urticaria.
• Contraindicated in pregnant or breast-feeding women and in neonates with untreated infection, active bleeding, coagulation defects or thrombocytopenia, congenital heart disease needing patency of the ductus arteriosus, necrotizing enterocolitis, or significant renal impairment.
• Suppositories are contraindicated in patients with history of proctitis or recent rectal bleeding.
Black Box Warning Contraindicated for the treatment of perioperative pain after CABG surgery. ∎

• Use cautiously in elderly patients, those with history of GI disease, and those with epilepsy, parkinsonism, hepatic or renal disease, CV disease, infection, and mental illness or depression.

⚠ **Overdose S&S:** Drowsiness, lethargy, confusion, nausea, vomiting, paresthesia, numbness, aggressive behavior, disorientation, seizures, headache, dizziness, GI bleeding.

NURSING CONSIDERATIONS

• Because of the high risk of adverse effects from long-term use, drug shouldn't be used routinely as an analgesic or antipyretic.
• If ductus arteriosus reopens, a second course of one to three doses may be given. If ineffective, surgery may be needed.
• Watch for bleeding in patients receiving anticoagulants, patients with coagulation defects, and neonates.
• Because NSAIDs impair synthesis of renal prostaglandins, they can decrease renal blood flow and lead to reversible renal impairment, especially in patients with renal failure, heart failure, or liver dysfunction; in elderly patients; and in those taking diuretics. Monitor these patients closely.
• Drug causes sodium retention; watch for weight gain (especially in elderly patients) and increased blood pressure in patients with hypertension.
• Monitor patient for rash and respiratory distress, which may indicate a hypersensitivity reaction.
• Because of their antipyretic and antiinflammatory actions, NSAIDs may mask signs and symptoms of infection.

Black Box Warning NSAIDs cause an increased risk of serious GI adverse events, including bleeding, ulceration, and perforation of the stomach or intestines, which can be fatal. Elderly patients are at greater risk. ▮

Black Box Warning NSAIDs may increase the risk of serious thrombotic events, MI, or stroke, which can be fatal. The risk may be greater with longer use or in patients with CV disease or risk factors for CV disease. ▮

• Monitor patient on long-term oral therapy for toxicity by conducting regular eye examinations, hearing tests, CBCs, and kidney function tests.

PATIENT TEACHING

• Tell patient to take oral dose with food, milk, or antacid to prevent GI upset.
• Alert patient that using oral form with aspirin, alcohol, other NSAIDs, or corticosteroids may increase risk of adverse GI reactions.
• Teach patient signs and symptoms of GI bleeding, including blood in vomit, urine, or stool; coffee-ground vomit; and black, tarry stool. Tell him to notify prescriber immediately if any of these occurs.
• Tell patient to immediately report signs or symptoms of cardiac events, such as chest pain, shortness of breath, weakness, and slurred speech.
• Warn patient to avoid hazardous activities that require mental alertness until CNS effects are known.
• Tell patient to notify prescriber immediately if visual or hearing changes occur.

infliximab
in-FLICKS-ih-mab

Remicade

Therapeutic class: Anti-inflammatory drugs
Pharmacologic class: TNF blockers
Pregnancy risk category: B

AVAILABLE FORMS
Lyophilized powder for injection: 100-mg vial

INDICATIONS & DOSAGES
➤ **Moderately to severely active Crohn disease; reduction in the number of draining enterocutaneous and rectovaginal fistulas and maintenance of fistula closure in patients with fistulizing Crohn disease**
Adults: 5 mg/kg I.V. infusion over at least 2 hours. Repeat at 2 and 6 weeks, then every 8 weeks thereafter. For patients who respond and then lose their response, consider 10 mg/kg. Patients who don't respond by week 14 are unlikely to respond with continued therapy. In those patients, consider stopping drug.
Children ages 6 to 17: For Crohn disease, 5 mg/kg I.V. infusion over at least 2 hours.

Reactions in bold italics are *life-threatening*. Interactions may have a *rapid onset* or a *delayed onset*.

Repeat at 2 and 6 weeks, then every 8 weeks thereafter.

➤ **Moderately to severely active rheumatoid arthritis**

Adults: 3 mg/kg I.V. infusion over at least 2 hours. Repeat at 2 and 6 weeks after first infusion and every 8 weeks thereafter. Dose may be increased up to 10 mg/kg, or doses may be given every 4 weeks if response is inadequate. Use with methotrexate.

➤ **Moderate to severe ulcerative colitis**

Adults: Induction dose, 5 mg/kg I.V. over at least 2 hours. Repeat at 2 and 6 weeks, then every 8 weeks thereafter.

➤ **Moderate to severe ulcerative colitis in children who have had an inadequate response to conventional therapy**

Children age 6 and older: Initially, 5 mg/kg I.V. infusion over at least 2 hours at 0, 2, and 6 weeks, followed by a maintenance regimen of 5 mg/kg I.V. infusion over at least 2 hours every 8 weeks.

➤ **Ankylosing spondylitis**

Adults: 5 mg/kg I.V. infusion over at least 2 hours. Repeat at 2 and 6 weeks, then every 6 weeks thereafter.

➤ **Psoriatic arthritis, with or without methotrexate**

Adults: 5 mg/kg I.V. infusion over at least 2 hours. Repeat at 2 and 6 weeks after first infusion, then every 8 weeks thereafter.

➤ **Chronic severe plaque psoriasis**

Adults: 5 mg/kg I.V. infusion over at least 2 hours. Repeat dose in 2 and 6 weeks, then give 5 mg/kg every 8 weeks thereafter.

➤ **Behçet syndrome uveitis; uveitis ♦**

Adults: 3 to 5 mg/kg I.V. infusion over 2 hours. Repeat dose at 2 and 6 weeks, then every 6 to 8 weeks. For uveitis, 3 to 10 mg/kg I.V. over 2 hours. Repeat dose at 2- to 8-week intervals.

ADMINISTRATION

I.V.

▼ Reconstitute with 10 mL sterile water for injection, using syringe with 21G or smaller needle. Don't shake; gently swirl to dissolve powder. Solution should be colorless to light yellow and opalescent. It may also develop a few translucent particles; don't use if other types of particles develop or discoloration occurs.

▼ Dilute total volume of reconstituted drug to 250 mL with normal saline solution for injection. Infusion concentration range is 0.4 to 4 mg/mL.

▼ Use an in-line, sterile, nonpyrogenic, low–protein-binding filter with a pore size less than 1.2 micrometer.

▼ Begin infusion within 3 hours of preparation and give over at least 2 hours.

▼ **Incompatibilities:** Other I.V. drugs. Do not infuse with other drugs.

ACTION

Binds to human TNF-alpha to neutralize its activity and inhibit its binding with receptors, thereby reducing the infiltration of inflammatory cells and TNF-alpha production in inflamed areas of the intestine.

Route	Onset	Peak	Duration
I.V.	Unknown	Unknown	Unknown

Half-life: 9½ days.

ADVERSE REACTIONS

CNS: fatigue, fever, headache, dizziness, depression, insomnia, malaise, pain, systemic and cutaneous vasculitis.

CV: hypertension, chest pain, flushing, hypotension, pericardial effusion, tachycardia.

EENT: pharyngitis, rhinitis, sinusitis, conjunctivitis.

GI: abdominal pain, diarrhea, dyspepsia, nausea, *intestinal obstruction,* constipation, flatulence, oral pain, ulcerative stomatitis, vomiting.

GU: UTI, dysuria, increased urinary frequency.

Hematologic: *leukopenia, neutropenia, pancytopenia, thrombocytopenia,* anemia, hematoma.

Musculoskeletal: arthralgia, back pain, arthritis, myalgia.

Respiratory: coughing, upper respiratory tract infections, bronchitis, dyspnea, respiratory tract allergic reaction.

Skin: rash, acne, alopecia, candidiasis, dry skin, eczema, erythema, erythematous rash, increased sweating, maculopapular rash, papular rash, urticaria.

Other: abscess, chills, ecchymosis, flulike syndrome, hot flashes, peripheral edema, toothache.

INTERACTIONS

Drug-drug. *TNF blockers (abatacept, anakinra, golimumab, rilonacept):* May increase the risk of serious infections and neutropenia. Avoid using together.

Vaccines (live): May affect normal immune response. Postpone live-virus vaccine until therapy stops.

EFFECTS ON LAB TEST RESULTS

• May increase liver enzyme levels. May decrease hemoglobin level and hematocrit.
• May decrease WBC and platelet counts.
• May cause false-positive ANA test result.

CONTRAINDICATIONS & CAUTIONS

• Contraindicated in patients hypersensitive to murine proteins or other components of drug. Doses greater than 5 mg/kg are contraindicated in patients with moderate to severe heart failure.

Black Box Warning Lymphoma and other malignancies, some fatal, have occurred in children and adolescents treated with TNF blockers, including infliximab. ∎

Black Box Warning Hepatosplenic T-cell lymphoma, a rare type of lymphoma, has occurred in adolescents and young adults with inflammatory bowel disease treated with TNF blockers, including infliximab. ∎

• Use cautiously in elderly patients; in patients with active infection, history of chronic or recurrent infections, a history of hematologic abnormalities, or preexisting or recent-onset CNS demyelinating or seizure disorders; or in those who have lived in regions where histoplasmosis is endemic.

NURSING CONSIDERATIONS

❸ Alert: Watch for infusion-related reactions, including fever, chills, pruritus, urticaria, dyspnea, hypotension, hypertension, and chest pain during administration and for 2 hours afterward. If an infusion-related reaction occurs, stop drug, notify prescriber, and give acetaminophen, antihistamines, corticosteroids, and epinephrine.

• Give for Crohn disease and ulcerative colitis only after patient has an inadequate response to conventional therapy.

• Consider stopping treatment in patient who develops significant hematologic abnormalities or CNS adverse reactions.

• Notify prescriber for symptoms of new or worsening heart failure.

❸ Alert: Histoplasmosis, coccidioidomycosis, blastomycosis, and other opportunistic infections may develop with use of this drug.

Black Box Warning Watch for development of lymphoma and infection. A patient with chronic Crohn disease and long-term exposure to immunosuppressants is more likely to develop lymphoma and infection. ∎

• Drug may affect normal immune responses. Patient may develop autoimmune antibodies and lupus-like syndrome; stop drug if this happens. Symptoms should resolve.

Black Box Warning Drug may cause disseminated or extrapulmonary tuberculosis (TB) and fatal opportunistic infections. ∎

Black Box Warning Evaluate patient for latent TB infection with a tuberculin skin test. Treat latent TB infection before therapy. ∎

• **Look alike–sound alike:** Don't confuse Remicade with Renacidin. Don't confuse infliximab with rituximab.

PATIENT TEACHING

• Tell patient about infusion-reaction symptoms and adverse effects and the need to report them promptly.
• Advise patient to seek immediate medical attention for signs and symptoms of infection, including persistent fever, cough, shortness of breath, or fatigue, or unusual bleeding or bruising.
• Tell women to stop breast-feeding during therapy.
• Tell patient that before he receives vaccines, he should alert prescriber to therapy.
• Advise parent to get child up-to-date for all vaccines before therapy.

ingenol mebutate

IN-je-nol

Picato

Therapeutic class: Immunosuppressants (topical)
Pharmacologic class: Immune response modifiers
Pregnancy risk category: C

AVAILABLE FORMS
Topical gel: 0.015%, 0.05%

INDICATIONS & DOSAGES
➤ **Actinic keratosis on the face and scalp**
Adults: Apply 0.015% strength gel to affected area once daily for 3 consecutive days.
➤ **Actinic keratosis on the trunk and extremities**
Adults: Apply 0.05% strength gel to affected area once daily for 2 consecutive days.

ADMINISTRATION
Topical
• Store gel in refrigerator. Don't freeze.
• Spread evenly over treatment area using 1 unit-dose tube, and allow to dry for 15 minutes.
• Wash hands after application to avoid transferring gel to other areas of the body.
• Avoid washing and touching treated area for 6 hours after application; after 6 hours, area may be washed with a mild soap.
• One unit-dose tube covers about a 2-inch × 2-inch (5 cm × 5 cm) area. Use each tube only once; throw away open tube after use even if it still contains gel.

ACTION
Unknown. Thought to induce cell death.

Route	Onset	Peak	Duration
Topical	Unknown	Unknown	Unknown

Half-life: Unknown.

ADVERSE REACTIONS
CNS: headache.
EENT: nasopharyngitis, periorbital edema.
Skin: erythema, flaking, scaling, crusting, swelling, vesiculation, pustulation, erosion, ulceration, pain, pruritus, infection at treatment site, irritation.

INTERACTIONS
None reported.

EFFECTS ON LAB TEST RESULTS
None reported.

CONTRAINDICATIONS & CAUTIONS
• Contraindicated in patients hypersensitive to drug.
• Use cautiously in pregnant women; safety and effectiveness haven't been established. Use only if potential benefit to the mother outweighs potential risk to the fetus.
• It's unknown if drug appears in breast milk.

NURSING CONSIDERATIONS
• Monitor skin for serious adverse effects.
• Gel is for external use only; don't use via oral, ophthalmic, or intravaginal route.
• Don't use gel if skin hasn't healed from previous drug therapy, sunburn, or surgical treatment.
• Don't apply bandages or closed dressings to the treated area.

PATIENT TEACHING
• Warn patient that gel is for external use only and not to apply in mouth, eyes, or vagina.
• Teach patient proper application technique.
• Tell patient to store gel in refrigerator and not to freeze.
• Advise patient to wash hands well after applying drug to prevent transferring drug to eye area. If exposure occurs, tell patient to flush area with water and seek medical attention immediately.
• Instruct patient to use gel only after skin has healed from previous drug therapy, sunburn, or surgical treatment.
• Caution patient not to use gel immediately after showering or less than 2 hours before bedtime, and not to perform activities that cause increased sweating for 6 hours after applying gel.
• Tell patient to report serious adverse skin effects.
• Instruct patient to use each tube only once and to throw away the open tube after use even if there is still gel in it.

insulin (regular)
IN-su-lin

Humulin R ◊, Humulin R Regular
U-500 (concentrated), Novolin R ◊

insulin (lispro)
Humalog

insulin lispro protamine–insulin lispro
Humalog Mix 75/25, Humalog Mix 50/50

isophane insulin suspension (NPH)
Humulin N ◊, Novolin N ◊

isophane insulin suspension–insulin injection combinations
Humulin 70/30 ◊, Novolin 70/30 ◊

Therapeutic class: Antidiabetics
Pharmacologic class: Human insulin analogues
Pregnancy risk category: B

AVAILABLE FORMS
Available without a prescription
insulin (regular)
Injection (human): 100 units/mL
(Humulin R, Novolin R)
isophane insulin suspension (NPH)
Injection (human): 100 units/mL
(Humulin N, Novolin N)
isophane insulin suspension–insulin injection combinations
Injection (human): 100 units/mL (Humulin 70/30, Novolin 70/30)
Available by prescription only
insulin (regular)
Injection (human): 500 units/mL
(Humulin R Regular U-500 [concentrated])
insulin (lispro)
Injection (human): 100 units/mL (Humalog)
insulin lispro protamine–insulin lispro
Injection (human): 100 units/mL (Humalog Mix 75/25, Humalog Mix 50/50)

INDICATIONS & DOSAGES
➤ **Moderate to severe diabetic keto-acidosis or hyperosmolar hyperglycemia**
regular insulin
Adults older than age 20: Loading dose of 0.15 units/kg I.V. by direct injection, followed by 0.1 unit/kg/hour as a continuous infusion. If glucose level doesn't fall by 50 mg/dL in the first hour, double the insulin infusion rate every hour until glucose level decreases steadily by 50 to 75 mg/dL/hour. Decrease rate of insulin infusion to 0.05 to 0.1 unit/kg/hour when glucose level reaches 250 to 300 mg/dL. Start infusion of D_5W in half-normal saline solution separately from the insulin infusion when glucose level is 150 to 200 mg/dL in patients with diabetic ketoacidosis or 250 to 300 mg/dL in those with hyperosmolar hyperglycemia. Give dose of insulin subcutaneously 1 to 2 hours before stopping insulin infusion (intermediate-acting insulin is recommended).
Adults and children age 20 and younger: Loading dose isn't recommended. Begin therapy at 0.1 unit/kg/hour I.V. infusion. After condition improves, decrease rate of insulin infusion to 0.05 unit/kg/hour. Start infusion of D_5W in half-normal saline solution separately from the insulin infusion when glucose level is 250 mg/dL.
➤ **Mild diabetic ketoacidosis**
regular insulin
Adults older than age 20: Loading dose of 0.4 to 0.6 unit/kg divided in two equal parts, with half the dose given by direct I.V. injection and half given I.M. or subcutaneously. Subsequent doses can be based on 0.1 unit/kg/hour I.M. or subcutaneously.
➤ **Newly diagnosed diabetes, type 1**
regular insulin
Adults older than age 20: Individualize therapy. Initially, 0.5 to 1 unit/kg/day subcutaneously as part of a regimen with short-acting and long-acting insulin therapy.
Adults and children age 20 and younger: Individualize therapy. Initially, 0.1 to 0.25 unit/kg subcutaneously every 6 to 8 hours for the first 24 hours to determine insulin requirements; then adjust accordingly.

➤ **Control of hyperglycemia with Humalog and longer-acting insulin in patients with type 1 diabetes**
Adults: Dosage varies among patients and must be determined by prescriber familiar with patient's metabolic needs, eating habits, and other lifestyle variables. Inject subcutaneously within 15 minutes before or after a meal.

➤ **Control of hyperglycemia with Humalog and sulfonylureas in patients with type 2 diabetes**
Adults and children older than age 3: Dosage varies among patients and must be determined by prescriber familiar with patient's metabolic needs, eating habits, and other lifestyle variables. Inject subcutaneously within 15 minutes before or after a meal.

➤ **Hyperkalemia**
Adults: 50 mL of dextrose 50% given over 5 minutes, followed by 5 to 10 units of regular insulin by I.V. push.

ADMINISTRATION

I.V.
▼ Give only regular or lispro insulin I.V.
▼ Inject directly into vein or into a port close to I.V. access site. Intermittent infusion isn't recommended.
▼ For continuous infusion, dilute drug in normal saline solution and give at prescribed rate.
▼ **Incompatibilities:** Aminophylline, amobarbital, chlorothiazide, cytarabine, digoxin, diltiazem, dobutamine, dopamine, levofloxacin, methylprednisolone sodium succinate, nafcillin, norepinephrine, pentobarbital sodium, phenobarbital sodium, phenytoin sodium, ranitidine, sodium bicarbonate, thiopental.

Subcutaneous
● Injection dosage is expressed in USP units. Use only the syringes calibrated for that concentration of insulin.
● To mix insulin suspension, swirl vial gently or rotate between palms or between palm and thigh. Don't shake vigorously, to avoid bubbling and air in syringe.
● Regular insulin may be mixed with NPH insulin in any proportion. When mixing regular insulin with NPH, always draw up regular insulin into syringe first.

● Switching from separate injections to a prepared mixture may alter patient response. When NPH is mixed with regular insulin in the same syringe, give immediately to avoid loss of potency.
● Lispro insulin may be mixed with Humulin N; give within 15 minutes before a meal to prevent a hypoglycemic reaction.
● Don't use insulin that changes color or becomes clumped or granular in appearance.
● Check expiration date on vial before using contents.
● Drug is usually given subcutaneously. To give, pinch a fold of skin with fingers at least 3 inches (7.5 cm) apart and insert needle at a 45- to 90-degree angle.
● Press, don't rub, site after injection. Rotate injection sites to avoid overuse of one area. Diabetic patients may achieve better control if injection site is rotated within same anatomic region.
● Store injectable insulin in cool area. Refrigeration is desirable. Don't freeze.
● Drug may also be stored at room temperature (below 86° F [30° C]). See package insert for specific information and storage duration.
● After administering the first dose from the Humalog cartridge or prefilled pen, don't return to the refrigerator.

ACTION

Increases glucose transport across muscle and fat cell membranes to reduce glucose level. Helps convert glucose to glycogen; triggers amino acid uptake and conversion to protein in muscle cells; stimulates triglyceride formation and inhibits release of free fatty acids from adipose tissue; and stimulates lipoprotein lipase activity, which converts circulating lipoproteins to fatty acids.

Route	Onset	Peak	Duration
I.V. (regular)	Immediate	Unknown	Unknown
Subcut. (rapid)	½–1½ hr	2–3 hr	5–7 hr
Subcut. (intermediate)	1–2½ hr	4–15 hr	24 hr
Subcut. (long-acting)	4–8 hr	10–30 hr	36 hr

Half-life: About 9 minutes after I.V. use.

ADVERSE REACTIONS

EENT: blurred vision.
GI: dry mouth.
Metabolic: *hypoglycemia,* hyperglycemia, *hypomagnesemia,* hypokalemia.
Skin: rash, urticaria, pruritus, swelling, redness, stinging, warmth at injection site.
Respiratory: increased cough, respiratory tract infection, dyspnea, reduced pulmonary function.
Other: lipoatrophy, lipohypertrophy, *anaphylaxis,* hypersensitivity reactions.

INTERACTIONS

Drug-drug. *ACE inhibitors, anabolic steroids, antidiabetics, calcium, chloroquine, clonidine, disopyramide, fibrates, fluoxetine, guanethidine, lithium, MAO inhibitors, mebendazole, octreotide, pentamidine, propoxyphene, pyridoxine, salicylates, sulfinpyrazone, sulfonamides, tetracyclines:* May enhance hypoglycemic effects of insulin. Monitor glucose level.
Acetazolamide, adrenocorticosteroids, albuterol, antiretrovirals, asparaginase, calcitonin, cyclophosphamide, danazol, diazoxide, diltiazem, diuretics, dobutamine, epinephrine, estrogens, ethacrynic acid, hormonal contraceptives containing estrogen, isoniazid, lithium, morphine, niacin, nicotine, phenothiazines, phenytoin, progestogens, somatropin, terbutaline, thyroid hormones: May diminish insulin response. Monitor glucose level.
Bronchodilators and other inhaled drugs: May alter the absorption of inhaled insulin. Consistently time doses of other inhaled drugs with inhaled insulin, and monitor glucose level closely.
Carteolol, nadolol, pindolol, propranolol, timolol: May mask symptoms of hypoglycemia as a result of beta blockade (such as tachycardia). May delay recovery from hypoglycemic episodes. Use together cautiously in patients with diabetes.
Thiazolidinediones (pioglitazone, rosiglitazone): May cause fluid retention that may lead to or worsen heart failure. Monitor patient closely.
Drug-herb. *Basil, bay, bee pollen, burdock, ginseng, glucomannan, horehound, marshmallow, myrrh, sage:* May affect glycemic

control. Discourage use together, and monitor glucose level carefully.
Drug-food. *Unregulated diet:* May cause hyperglycemia or hypoglycemia. Urge caution and monitor patient's diet.
Drug-lifestyle. *Alcohol use:* May cause hypoglycemic effect. Discourage use together.
Marijuana use: May increase glucose level. Inform patient of this interaction.
Smoking: May increase glucose level and decrease response to drug. Monitor glucose level.

EFFECTS ON LAB TEST RESULTS

● May decrease glucose, magnesium, and potassium levels.

CONTRAINDICATIONS & CAUTIONS

● Contraindicated in patients with history of systemic allergic reaction to pork when porcine-derived products are used or hypersensitivity to any component of preparation.
● Contraindicated during episodes of hypoglycemia.
⚠ **Overdose S&S:** Hypoglycemia.

NURSING CONSIDERATIONS

🕄 **Alert:** Regular insulin is for patients with circulatory collapse, diabetic ketoacidosis, or hyperkalemia. Don't use Humulin Regular U-500 (concentrated) I.V. Don't use intermediate- or long-acting insulins for coma or other emergencies requiring rapid drug action. Also, ketosis-prone type 1, severely ill, and newly diagnosed diabetic patients with very high glucose levels may need hospitalization and I.V. treatment with regular fast-acting insulin.
🕄 **Alert:** Some patients may develop insulin resistance and need large insulin doses to control symptoms of diabetes. U-500 insulin is available as Humulin Regular U-500 (concentrated) for such patients. Give pharmacy sufficient notice when requesting refill prescription. Never store U-500 insulin in same area with other insulin preparations because of the risk of severe overdose if accidentally given to the wrong patient.
● Monitor patient for hyperglycemia (rebound, or Somogyi, effect).

• Monitor patient's weight and assess for signs and symptoms of fluid retention that may lead to or worsen heart failure.

PATIENT TEACHING
• Make sure patient knows that drug relieves symptoms but doesn't cure disease.
• Instruct patient about the disease and importance of following therapeutic regimen, adhering to specific diet, losing weight, getting exercise, following personal hygiene program, and avoiding infection. Emphasize importance of timing injections with eating and of not skipping meals.
• Stress that accuracy of measurement is important, especially with concentrated regular insulin. A magnifying sleeve or dose magnifier may improve accuracy. Show patient and caregivers how to measure and give insulin.
• Advise patient not to change order in which insulins are mixed or model or brand of insulin, syringe, or needle. Be sure patient knows when mixing two insulins to always draw the regular insulin into the syringe first.
• Teach patient that glucose level and urine ketone tests provide essential guides to dosage and success of therapy. It's important for patient to recognize symptoms of high and low glucose levels. Insulin-induced low glucose level is hazardous and may cause brain damage if prolonged; most adverse effects are temporary. Instruct patient on insulin peak times and their importance.
• Instruct patient on proper use of equipment for monitoring glucose level.
• Advise patient not to smoke within 30 minutes after insulin injection because smoking decreases amount of insulin absorbed subcutaneously.
• Advise patient to avoid vigorous exercise immediately after insulin injection, especially of the area where injection was given, because it increases absorption and risk of low glucose episodes.
• Teach patient to avoid alcohol because it lowers glucose level.
• Advise patient to wear or carry medical identification at all times, to carry ample insulin and syringes on trips, to keep carbohydrates (lump of sugar or candy) on hand for emergencies, and to note time zone changes for dosage schedule when traveling.
• Advise woman planning pregnancy to first consult prescriber.
• Advise patient to store injectable insulin at 36° to 46° F (2° to 8° C) or at room temperature (below 86° F [30° C]). Tell him not to freeze or expose vials to excessive heat or sunlight.
• Instruct patient using Humalog cartridge or prefilled pen not to store it in the refrigerator after it has been opened.

SAFETY ALERT!

insulin aspart (rDNA origin) injection
IN-su-lin AS-part

NovoLog, NovoRapid†

insulin aspart (rDNA origin) protamine suspension–insulin aspart (rDNA origin) injection
NovoLog Mix 70/30

Therapeutic class: Antidiabetics
Pharmacologic class: Human insulin analogues
Pregnancy risk category: B

AVAILABLE FORMS
PenFill cartridges: 3 mL (100 units/mL)
Prefilled syringes: 3 mL (100 units/mL)
Vial: 10 mL, containing 100 units of insulin aspart per mL (U-100)

INDICATIONS & DOSAGES
➤ **Control of hyperglycemia in patients with diabetes**
NovoLog
Adults and children age 2 and older:
Dosage is highly individualized. Typical daily insulin requirement is 0.5 to 1 unit/kg/day, divided in a meal-related treatment regimen. About 50% to 70% of dose is provided with NovoLog and the remainder by an intermediate- or long-acting insulin. Give 5 to 10 minutes before start of meal by subcutaneous injection in the abdominal wall, thigh, or upper arm.

External insulin infusion pumps (adults and children age 4 and older): Initially, based on the total daily insulin dose of the previous regimen. Usually 50% of the total dose is given as meal-related boluses, and the remainder as basal infusion. Adjust dose if needed.

NovoLog Mix 70/30

Adults: Dosage is individualized based on the needs of the patient. Doses are usually given b.i.d. within 15 minutes of meals. Each dose is intended to cover two meals or a meal and a snack.

ADMINISTRATION

Subcutaneous

• Inspect insulin vials before use. NovoLog is a clear, colorless solution. It should not contain particulate matter or be cloudy, viscous, or discolored. NovoLog Mix 70/30 should be uniformly white and cloudy and should not contain particulate matter or be discolored.

• Give NovoLog 5 to 10 minutes before start of meal. Give NovoLog Mix 70/30 up to 15 minutes before start of meal. Because of its rapid onset of action and short duration of action, patients also may need longer-acting insulins to prevent hyperglycemia.

• Let insulin warm to room temperature before giving to minimize discomfort. Give by subcutaneous injection into the abdominal wall, thigh, or upper arm. Rotate sites to minimize lipodystrophies.

• When giving and mixing NovoLog with NPH human insulin, draw up NovoLog into syringe first and give immediately after dose is drawn up.

• Store drug between 36° and 46° F (2° and 8° C). Don't freeze. Don't expose vials to excessive heat or sunlight. Opened vials of NovoLog Mix 70/30 and opened vials and cartridges of NovoLog are stable at room temperature for 28 days. Punctured cartridges of NovoLog Mix 70/30 may be stored at room temperature up to 14 days; don't refrigerate punctured cartridges.

Subcutaneous

External insulin pump

• Don't dilute or mix insulin aspart with any other insulin when using an external insulin pump.

• Insulin aspart is recommended for use with Disetronic H-TRON plus V100 with Disetronic 3.15 plastic cartridges and Classic or Tender infusion sets, Polyfin or Sof-set infusion sets, and MiniMed Models 505, 506, and 507 with MiniMed 3-mL syringes.

• Replace infusion sets, and choose a new infusion site every 48 hours or less. Insulin may be stored and used in the pump for up to 6 days.

• Discard insulin exposed to temperatures higher than 98.6° F (37° C). The temperature of the insulin may exceed ambient temperature when the pump housing, cover, tubing, or sport case is exposed to sunlight or radiant heat.

I.V.

▼ NovoLog may also be given as an I.V. infusion with close medical monitoring of glucose and potassium levels. Using a polypropylene bag, dilute insulin aspart to a concentration of 0.05 to 1 unit/mL in normal saline solution, D_5W, or 10% dextrose injection with 40 mEq/L of potassium chloride.

❸ *Alert:* Don't give 70/30 form I.V. and don't mix it with other insulin products.

ACTION

Regulates glucose metabolism. It has the same glucose-lowering effect as regular human insulin, but its effect is more rapid and of shorter duration.

Route	Onset	Peak	Duration
I.V.	Immediate	Unknown	3–5 hr
Subcut.	15 min	1–3 hr	3–5 hr
Subcut. (70/30)	Rapid	1–4 hr	≤24 hr

Half-life: 81 minutes.

ADVERSE REACTIONS

Metabolic: *hypoglycemia,* hypokalemia.
Skin: injection-site reactions, lipodystrophy, pruritus, rash.
Other: *allergic reactions.*

INTERACTIONS

Drug-drug. *ACE inhibitors, disopyramide, fibrates, fluoxetine, oral antidiabetics, propoxyphene, salicylates, somatostatin analogue (octreotide), sulfonamide antibiotics:* May enhance the glucose-lowering

---

Reactions in bold italics are *life-threatening*. Interactions may have a *rapid onset* or a *delayed onset*.

effect of insulin and may potentiate hypoglycemia. Monitor glucose level, and watch for signs and symptoms of hypoglycemia. May need insulin dose adjustment.

Beta blockers, clonidine: May increase or decrease the glucose-lowering effect of insulin and cause hypoglycemia or hyperglycemia. May reduce or mask symptoms of hypoglycemia. Monitor glucose level.

Corticosteroids, danazol, diuretics, estrogens, isoniazid, niacin, phenothiazine derivatives, progestins (as in hormonal contraceptives), somatropin, sympathomimetics (epinephrine, salbutamol, terbutaline), thyroid hormones: May decrease the glucose-lowering effect of insulin and cause hyperglycemia. Monitor glucose level. May require insulin dose adjustment.

Crystalline zinc preparations: May be incompatible with NovoLog. Don't mix together.

Guanethidine, reserpine: May reduce or mask symptoms of hypoglycemia. Monitor glucose level.

Lithium salts, pentamidine: May increase or decrease glucose-lowering effect of insulin and may cause hypoglycemia or hyperglycemia. Pentamidine may cause hypoglycemia, sometimes followed by hyperglycemia. Monitor glucose level.

MAO inhibitors: May increase insulin's effects. Monitor patient and glucose level closely.

Thiazolidinediones (pioglitazone, rosiglitazone): May cause fluid retention that may lead to or worsen heart failure. Monitor patient closely.

Drug-herb. *Burdock, dandelion, eucalyptus, marshmallow:* May increase drug's effects. Discourage use together.

Drug-lifestyle. *Alcohol use:* May increase or decrease drug effect, causing hypoglycemia or hyperglycemia. Advise patient to monitor glucose level.

Exercise: May alter the need for drug, requiring dose adjustment. Advise patient to report changes in physical activity.

Marijuana use: May increase glucose level. Inform patient of this interaction.

Smoking: May increase glucose level and decrease response to insulin. Monitor glucose level.

EFFECTS ON LAB TEST RESULTS
● May increase alkaline phosphatase level. May decrease glucose and potassium levels.

CONTRAINDICATIONS & CAUTIONS
● Contraindicated during episodes of hypoglycemia and in patients hypersensitive to NovoLog or one of its components.
● Use cautiously in patients susceptible to hypoglycemia and hypokalemia, such as those who have autonomic neuropathy or are fasting, taking potassium-lowering drugs, or taking drugs sensitive to potassium level.

⚠ Overdose S&S: Hypoglycemia, hypokalemia.

NURSING CONSIDERATIONS
● The time course of NovoLog action may vary among people or at different times in the same person and depends on the site of injection, blood supply, temperature, and physical activity.
● Adjustments in the dose of NovoLog or of any insulin may be needed with changes in physical activity or meal routine. Insulin requirements also may be altered during emotional disturbances, illness, or other stresses.
● Adjust dose regularly, according to patient's glucose measurements. Monitor glucose level regularly.
● Periodically monitor glycosylated hemoglobin level.
● Assess patient for rash (including pruritus) over whole body, shortness of breath, wheezing, hypotension, rapid pulse, or sweating, which may signify a generalized allergy to insulin. Severe cases, including anaphylactic reactions, may be life-threatening.
● Patients with renal dysfunction and hepatic impairment may need close glucose monitoring and dose adjustments of NovoLog.
● Observe injection sites for reactions, such as redness, swelling, itching, or burning. These reactions should resolve within a few days to a few weeks.
● Assess patient and notify prescriber for signs and symptoms of hypoglycemia (sweating, shaking, trembling, confusion, headache, irritability, hunger, rapid

pulse, nausea) and hyperglycemia (drowsiness, fruity breath odor, frequent urination, thirst).
• Monitor patient's weight and assess for signs and symptoms of fluid retention that may lead to or worsen heart failure.
• Symptoms of hypoglycemia may occur in patients with diabetes, regardless of glucose value.
• Patients with long duration of diabetes, diabetic nerve disease, or intensified diabetes control may have different or less-pronounced early-warning symptoms of hypoglycemia; severe hypoglycemia may occur in such patients with virtually no warning.

For external pump use with NovoLog
• Monitor patient with an external insulin pump for erythematous, pruritic, or thickened skin at injection site.
◊ Alert: Pump or infusion set malfunctions or insulin degradation can lead to hyperglycemia and ketosis in a short time because there's a subcutaneous depot of fast-acting insulin.
• Teach patient how to properly use the external insulin pump.
• **Look alike–sound alike:** Don't confuse NovoLog Mix 70/30 with Novolin 70/30.

PATIENT TEACHING
• Tell patient not to stop insulin therapy without medical approval.
• Advise patient of the warning signs of low glucose level (shaking, sweating, moodiness, irritability, confusion, or agitation). Tell patient to carry sugar (candy, sugar packets) to counteract low glucose level.
• Instruct patient to roll the cartridge or pen between his palms 10 times before inserting the NovoLog Penfill cartridge into a compatible delivery device or using the NovoLog FlexPen. Then, to turn the device upside down so the glass ball inside the cartridge or pen travels the length of the cartridge and to repeat this rolling and turning technique at least 10 times until the suspension is uniformly white and cloudy.
• Teach patient proper insulin injection technique and importance of timing dose to meals and adhering to meal plans.
• Tell patient to report swelling, redness, and itching at injection site, and instruct

patient on the importance of rotating injection sites to avoid lipodystrophies.
• Instruct patient on correct use of injection pen, if indicated.
• Instruct patient to use the same brand of insulin, especially if mixing insulin. Changing brands of insulin may necessitate dosage changes.
• Tell patient not to dilute or mix insulin aspart with any other insulin when using an external insulin pump.
• Instruct patient to monitor glucose level regularly.
• Advise patient to avoid vigorous exercise immediately after insulin injection, especially of the area where injection was given; it causes increased absorption and increased risk of low glucose level.
• Advise patient to store insulin at 36° to 46° F (2° to 8° C), and avoid freezing or excessive heat or sunlight.
• Advise women to notify prescriber about planned, suspected, or known pregnancy.
• Urge patient to carry medical identification at all times.
• Instruct patient about the importance of diet and exercise. Explain long-term complications of diabetes and the importance of yearly eye and foot examinations.

SAFETY ALERT!

insulin detemir (rDNA origin) injection
IN-su-lin DEH-teh-meer

Levemir

Therapeutic class: Antidiabetics
Pharmacologic class: Human insulin analogues
Pregnancy risk category: C

AVAILABLE FORMS
Injection: 100 units/mL in 10-mL vials, 3-mL prefilled syringes (FlexPen)

INDICATIONS & DOSAGES
➤ **Hyperglycemia in patients with diabetes mellitus who need basal (long-acting) insulin**
Adults and children age 2 and older: Base dosage on patient response and glucose

level. In insulin-naive patients with type 2 diabetes, start with 0.1 to 0.2 units/kg subcutaneously once daily in the evening or 10 units once daily or b.i.d. based on glucose level. Patients with type 1 or 2 diabetes already receiving basal-bolus treatment or basal insulin may switch to this drug on a unit-for-unit basis, adjusted to glycemic target.

ADMINISTRATION
Subcutaneous
⊘ Alert: Don't give I.V. or I.M.
⊘ Alert: Don't mix or dilute with other insulins.
• Give by subcutaneous injection in the thigh, abdominal wall, or upper arm. Rotate injection sites within the same region.
• Store unused insulin detemir between 36° and 46° F (2° and 8° C). Don't freeze. Don't use insulin detemir if it has been frozen.
• After initial use, store vials in a refrigerator, never in a freezer. If refrigeration isn't possible, keep in-use vial unrefrigerated at room temperature, below 86° F (30° C), for up to 42 days. Keep vial as cool as possible, away from direct heat and light.
• After initial use, a prefilled syringe may be used for up to 42 days if kept at room temperature, below 86° F (30° C). Don't store in-use prefilled syringes in a refrigerator or with the needle in place. Keep prefilled syringes away from direct heat and sunlight. Unopened prefilled syringes can be used until the expiration date printed on the label if they're stored in a refrigerator. Keep unused prefilled syringes in the carton so they'll stay clean and protected from light.

ACTION
Regulates glucose metabolism by binding to insulin receptors, facilitating cellular uptake of glucose into muscle and fat, and inhibiting release of glucose from liver.

Route	Onset	Peak	Duration
Subcut.	Unknown	6–8 hr	6–23 hr

Half-life: 5 to 7 hours.

ADVERSE REACTIONS
CV: edema.
Metabolic: *hypoglycemia,* sodium retention, weight gain.

Skin: injection-site reactions, lipodystrophy, pruritus, rash.
Other: *allergic reactions.*

INTERACTIONS
Drug-drug. *ACE inhibitors, antidiabetic drugs, disopyramide, fibrates, fluoxetine,* **MAO inhibitors,** *octreotide, propoxyphene, salicylates, sulfonamides:* May increase the glucose-lowering effect of insulin and risk of hypoglycemia. Monitor glucose level carefully.
Beta blockers, clonidine, guanethidine, reserpine: May decrease or conceal signs of hypoglycemia. Avoid using together, if possible.
Clonidine, lithium salts: May increase or decrease glucose-lowering effect of insulin. Monitor glucose level carefully.
Corticosteroids, danazol, diuretics, estrogens, isoniazid, phenothiazines, progestogens, somatropin, sympathomimetics, thyroid hormones: May decrease glucose-lowering effect of insulin. Monitor glucose level carefully.
Other insulins: May alter the action of one or both insulins if mixed together. Don't mix or dilute insulin detemir with other insulins.
Pentamidine: May cause initial hypoglycemia followed by hyperglycemia. Use together cautiously.
Thiazolidinediones (pioglitazone, rosiglitazone): May cause fluid retention that may lead to or worsen heart failure. Monitor patient closely.
Drug-lifestyle. *Alcohol use:* May increase or decrease effect of drug. Discourage use together.

EFFECTS ON LAB TEST RESULTS
• May decrease glucose level.

CONTRAINDICATIONS & CAUTIONS
• Contraindicated in patients hypersensitive to drug or its components. Don't give drug with an insulin infusion pump.
• Use cautiously in patients with hepatic or renal impairment; they may need dosage adjustment.
• Drug isn't recommended for treatment of diabetic ketoacidosis.
⚠ Overdose S&S: Hypoglycemia.

NURSING CONSIDERATIONS

- Monitor glucose level routinely in all patients receiving insulin.
- Measure patient's glycosylated hemoglobin level periodically.
- Watch for hyperglycemia, especially if patient's diet or exercise pattern changes.
- Assess patient for signs and symptoms of hypoglycemia. Insulin doses may need adjustment.
- Monitor patient's weight and assess for signs and symptoms of fluid retention that may lead to or worsen heart failure.
- Early warning symptoms of hypoglycemia may be less pronounced in patients who take beta blockers and those with longstanding diabetes, diabetic nerve disease, or intensified diabetes control. Monitor glucose level closely in these patients because severe hypoglycemia could develop before symptoms do.
- Insulin requirements may be altered during illness, emotional disturbance, or stress, or if patient changes his usual meal plan or exercise level.
- Starting dosage, increments of change, and maintenance dosage should be conservative in elderly patients because hypoglycemia may be harder to recognize.

PATIENT TEACHING

- Teach diabetes management, including glucose monitoring, injection techniques, and continuous rotation of injection sites.
- ☼ **Alert:** Urge patient not to mix with any other insulin or solution.
- Instruct patient to use only solution that's clear and colorless, with no visible particles.
- Tell patient to recognize and report signs and symptoms of hyperglycemia, such as nausea, vomiting, drowsiness, flushed dry skin, dry mouth, increased urination, thirst, and loss of appetite.
- Teach patient to recognize and report signs and symptoms of hypoglycemia, such as sweating, dizziness, light-headedness, headache, drowsiness, and irritability.
- Urge patient to check glucose level often to achieve control and avoid hyperglycemia and hypoglycemia.
- Advise patient to carry a quick source of simple sugar, such as hard candy or glucose tablets, in case of hypoglycemia.

- Caution patient not to stop insulin abruptly or change the amount or type of insulin used without consulting prescriber.
- Advise patient to avoid alcohol because it lowers the glucose level.
- Caution women to consult prescriber before trying to become pregnant.
- Tell patient to store unused vials and prefilled syringes in the refrigerator at 36° to 46° F (2° to 8° C).
- After initial use, vials may be refrigerated or stored at room temperature, below 86° F (30° C), away from direct heat and light, for up to 42 days. Prefilled syringes may be stored at room temperature, below 86° F (30° C). Tell patient not to store or refrigerate insulin with a needle in place.
- Caution against freezing drug and against using drug that has been frozen.

SAFETY ALERT!

insulin glargine (rDNA origin) injection
IN-su-lin GLAR-gene

Lantus

Therapeutic class: Antidiabetics
Pharmacologic class: Human insulin analogues
Pregnancy risk category: C

AVAILABLE FORMS
Injection: 100 units/mL in 10-mL vials, 3-mL cartridge system for use in OptiClik delivery device, 3-mL disposable insulin device (SoloStar)

INDICATIONS & DOSAGES
➤ **To manage type 1 diabetes in patients who need basal (long-acting) insulin to control hyperglycemia**
Adults and children age 6 and older: Individualize dosage, and give subcutaneously once daily at the same time each day. Maintenance dosage is 2 to 100 units daily.
➤ **To manage type 2 diabetes in patients who need basal (long-acting) insulin to control hyperglycemia**
Adults: Individualize dosage, and give subcutaneously once daily at the same time

each day. If patient is insulin-naive, start with 10 units subcutaneously daily. Adjust dose to patient response. Maintenance dosage is 2 to 100 units daily.

ADMINISTRATION
Subcutaneous
🕭 *Alert:* Don't give I.V. or with an insulin pump.

🕭 *Alert:* Don't mix or dilute with other insulins or solutions.

• Rotate injection sites with each dose.

• Store unopened insulin vials and 3-mL cartridge system in the refrigerator; opened vials may be stored at 86° F (30° C) or less and away from direct heat. Discard opened vials or cartridge system after 28 days whether refrigerated or not.

• Use only if clear and colorless.

ACTION
Reduces glucose level by stimulating peripheral glucose uptake, especially by skeletal muscle and fat, and by inhibiting hepatic glucose production.

Route	Onset	Peak	Duration
Subcut.	1 hr	None	24 hr

Half-life: Unknown.

ADVERSE REACTIONS
Metabolic: *hypoglycemia.*
Skin: lipodystrophy, pruritus, rash.
Other: allergic reactions, pain at injection site.

INTERACTIONS
Drug-drug. *ACE inhibitors, disopyramide, exenatide, fibrates, fluoxetine, MAO inhibitors, octreotide, oral antidiabetics, salicylates, sulfonamide antibiotics:* May cause hypoglycemia and increase insulin effect. Monitor glucose level. May need to adjust dosage of insulin glargine.

Beta blockers, clonidine: May mask signs of hypoglycemia and may either increase or reduce insulin's glucose-lowering effect. Avoid using together, if possible. If used together, monitor glucose level carefully.

Corticosteroids, danazol, diuretics, estrogens, isoniazid, phenothiazines (such as prochlorperazine, promethazine hydrochloride), progestins (such as hormonal contraceptives), somatropin, sympathomimetics (such as albuterol, epinephrine, terbutaline), thyroid hormones: May reduce the glucose-lowering effect of insulin. Monitor glucose level. May need to adjust dosage of insulin glargine.

Guanethidine, reserpine: May mask the signs of hypoglycemia. Avoid using together, if possible. Monitor glucose level carefully.

Lithium: May either increase or decrease the glucose-lowering effect of insulin. Monitor glucose level. May require dosage adjustments of insulin glargine.

Pentamidine: May cause hypoglycemia, which may be followed by hyperglycemia. Avoid using together, if possible.

Drug-herb. *Burdock, dandelion, eucalyptus, marshmallow:* May increase hypoglycemic effects. Discourage use together.

Licorice root: May increase dosage requirements of insulin. Discourage use together.

Drug-lifestyle. *Alcohol use, emotional stress:* May increase or decrease the glucose-lowering effect of insulin. Advise patient to self-monitor glucose level.

EFFECTS ON LAB TEST RESULTS
• May decrease glucose level.

CONTRAINDICATIONS & CAUTIONS
• Contraindicated during hypoglycemic episodes and in patients hypersensitive to drug or its components.

• Use cautiously in patients with renal or hepatic impairment.

⚠ *Overdose S&S:* Hypoglycemia, severe hypoglycemia (coma, neurologic impairment, seizures).

NURSING CONSIDERATIONS
• Because of prolonged duration of action, this isn't the insulin of choice for diabetic ketoacidosis.

• The rate of absorption, onset, and duration of action may be affected by exercise and other variables, such as illness and emotional stress.

• As with any insulin therapy, lipodystrophy may occur at the injection site and delay insulin absorption. Reduce this risk by rotating the injection site with each injection.

• Hypoglycemia is the most common adverse effect of insulin. Early symptoms may be different or less pronounced in patients with long duration of diabetes, diabetic nerve disease, or intensified diabetes control. Monitor glucose level closely in these patients because severe hypoglycemia may result before the patient develops symptoms.

• **Look alike–sound alike:** Don't confuse Lantus with Lente.

PATIENT TEACHING

• Teach proper glucose monitoring, injection techniques, and diabetes management.
• Tell patient to take dose once daily at the same time each day.
• **Alert:** Educate diabetic patients about signs and symptoms of low glucose level, such as fatigue, weakness, confusion, headache, pallor, and profuse sweating.
• Urge patient to wear or carry medical identification at all times.
• Advise patient to treat mild hypoglycemia with oral glucose tablets. Encourage patient to always carry glucose tablets in case of a low-glucose episode.
• Educate patients on the importance of maintaining prescribed diet, and explain that adjustments in drug dosage, meal patterns, and exercise may be needed to regulate glucose.
• **Alert:** Advise patient not to dilute or mix any other insulin or solution with insulin glargine. If the solution is cloudy, urge patient to discard the vial. Use solution only if it's clear and colorless.
• **Alert:** Make any change of insulin cautiously and only under medical supervision. Changes in insulin strength, manufacturer, type (such as regular, NPH, or insulin analogues), species (animal, human), or method of manufacturer (rDNA versus animal source insulin) may require a change in dosage. Oral antidiabetic treatment taken at the same time may need to be adjusted.
• Tell patient to consult prescriber before using OTC medications.
• Inform patient to avoid alcohol, which lowers glucose level.
• Advise patient to avoid vigorous exercise immediately after insulin injection, especially of the area where injection was given;

it causes increased absorption and increased risk of low glucose.
• Advise woman planning pregnancy to first consult prescriber.
• Advise patient on proper drug storage: store unopened insulin vials and 3-mL cartridge system in the refrigerator; opened vials may be stored at 86° F (30° C) or less and away from direct heat; discard opened vials or cartridge system after 28 days whether refrigerated or not.

SAFETY ALERT!

insulin glulisine (rDNA origin) injection
IN-su-lin GLUE-lih-seen

Apidra, Apidra SoloStar

Therapeutic class: Antidiabetics
Pharmacologic class: Human insulin analogues
Pregnancy risk category: C

AVAILABLE FORMS
Injection: 100 units/mL in 10-mL vial, 3-mL cartridge (OptiClik), or 3-mL prefilled pen

INDICATIONS & DOSAGES
➤ **Diabetes mellitus**
Adults and children age 4 and older:
Individualize dosage. Give 0.5 to 1 unit/kg/day subcutaneous injection within 15 minutes before a meal. If regimen also includes a longer-acting insulin or basal insulin analogue, give within 20 minutes after meal starts. Or, give drug as continuous subcutaneous infusion using an external infusion pump. Or, drug may be given I.V. under strict medical supervision with close monitoring of blood glucose and potassium levels.

ADMINISTRATION
Subcutaneous
• **Alert:** Drug has a more rapid onset and shorter duration of action than regular human insulin. Give within 15 minutes before or within 20 minutes after the start of a meal.
• Don't mix drug in a syringe with any other insulin except NPH. Draw insulin glulisine into syringe first.

Reactions in bold italics are *life-threatening*. Interactions may have a *rapid onset* or a *delayed onset*.

• When used in an external subcutaneous infusion pump, don't mix drug with any other insulin or diluent.

• Store unopened vials in the refrigerator or at room temperature for no longer than 28 days; store opened vials in the refrigerator or at room temperature below 77° F (25° C). Use opened vials within 28 days. Infusion bags are stable at room temperature for 48 hours. Protect from direct heat and light.

• Store opened cartridge and SoloStar at room temperature; discard after 28 days.

I.V.

▼ Use at a concentration of insulin glulisine 0.05 to 1 unit/mL in infusion systems with the infusion fluid, sterile normal saline solution, using polyvinyl chloride (PVC) Viaflex infusion bags and PVC tubing (Clearlink system Continu-Flo solution set) with a dedicated infusion line. The use of other bags and tubing hasn't been studied.

ACTION

Lowers glucose level by increasing peripheral glucose uptake and decreasing hepatic glucose production. When drug is given by subcutaneous injection, onset of action is more rapid and duration of action shorter than those of regular human insulin.

Route	Onset	Peak	Duration
I.V.	Immediate	Unknown	Unknown
Subcut.	15 min	55 min	Unknown

Half-life: 13 minutes (I.V.), 42 minutes (subcutaneous).

ADVERSE REACTIONS

CNS: headache, *seizures.*
CV: hypertension, peripheral edema.
EENT: nasopharyngitis.
Metabolic: *hypoglycemia,* weight gain, hypokalemia.
Respiratory: upper respiratory tract infection.
Skin: injection-site reactions, lipodystrophy, pruritus, rash.
Other: allergic reactions, *anaphylaxis,* insulin antibody production, influenza.

INTERACTIONS

Drug-drug. *ACE inhibitors, disopyramide, fibrates, fluoxetine,* **MAO inhibitors,** *oral antidiabetics, pentoxifylline, propoxyphene, salicylates, sulfonamide antibiotics:* May increase glucose-lowering effects. Monitor glucose level, and watch for evidence of hypoglycemia.

Beta blockers, clonidine, lithium, pentamidine: May cause unpredictable response to insulin. Use together cautiously; monitor patient closely.

Clozapine, corticosteroids, danazol, diazoxide, diuretics, estrogens, glucagons, isoniazid, olanzapine, phenothiazines, progestogens, protease inhibitors, somatropin, sympathomimetics (epinephrine, albuterol, terbutaline), thyroid hormone: May decrease glucose-lowering effects. Monitor glucose level carefully.

Drug-lifestyle. *Alcohol use:* May potentiate or reduce insulin effects, resulting in either hypoglycemia or hyperglycemia. Discourage alcohol use.

EFFECTS ON LAB TEST RESULTS

• May decrease glucose level.

CONTRAINDICATIONS & CAUTIONS

• Contraindicated during periods of hypoglycemia and in patients hypersensitive to insulin glulisine or one of its ingredients.

• Use cautiously in patients with impaired renal or hepatic function and in pregnant or breast-feeding women.

⚠ Overdose S&S: Hypoglycemia, hypokalemia.

NURSING CONSIDERATIONS

• Use with a longer-acting or basal insulin analogue.

• Changes in insulin strength, manufacturer, type, or species may cause a need for dosage adjustment.

• Changes in physical activity or usual meal plan may cause a need for dosage adjustment.

• Insulin requirements may be altered during illness, emotional disturbances, or stress.

• Early warning signs of hypoglycemia may be different or less pronounced in patients who take beta blockers, who have had an oral antidiabetic added to the regimen, or

who have long-term diabetes or diabetic nerve disease.
• Monitor patient for lipodystrophy at injection site; it may delay insulin absorption.
• Redness, swelling, or itching may occur at injection site.
• Give I.V. infusion only under strict medical supervision with close monitoring of glucose and potassium levels.

PATIENT TEACHING
• Tell patient to take drug within 15 minutes before starting a meal to 20 minutes after starting a meal, depending on regimen.
• Teach patient how to give subcutaneous insulin injections.
• Tell patient not to mix insulin glulisine in a syringe with any insulin other than NPH.
• If patient is mixing insulin glulisine with NPH, tell patient to use U-100 syringes, to draw insulin glulisine into the syringe first, followed by NPH insulin, and to inject the mixture immediately.
• Instruct patient to rotate injection sites to avoid injection-site reactions.
• If patient is using an external infusion pump, teach proper use of the device. Tell patient not to mix insulin glulisine with any other insulin or diluents. Instruct patient to change the infusion set, reservoir with insulin, and infusion site at least every 48 hours.
• Teach patient the signs and symptoms of hypoglycemia (sweating, rapid pulse, trembling, confusion, headache, irritability, and nausea). Advise the patient to treat these symptoms by eating or drinking something containing sugar.
• Instruct the patient to contact a health care provider for possible dosage adjustments if hypoglycemia occurs frequently.
• Show patient how to monitor and log glucose levels to evaluate diabetes control.
• Explain the possible long-term complications of diabetes and the importance of regular preventive therapy. Urge patient to follow prescribed diet and exercise regimen. To further reduce the risk of heart disease, encourage patient to stop smoking and lose weight.
• Instruct patient to carry medical identification showing that he has diabetes.
• Tell patient to store unopened vials in the refrigerator or at room temperature and

opened vials in the refrigerator or at room temperature below 77° F (25° C). Opened vials and those stored at room temperature should be used within 28 days.
• Opened cartridge and SoloStar must be stored at room temperature and discarded after 28 days. Protect from direct heat and light.

SAFETY ALERT!

interferon alfa-2b (recombinant) (IFN-alpha 2b)
in-ter-FEER-on

Intron A

Therapeutic class: Antivirals
Pharmacologic class: Biological response modifiers
Pregnancy risk category: C; X in combination with ribavirin

AVAILABLE FORMS
Solution for injection: 3, 5, and 10 million international units/dose in multidose pens; 18 and 25 million international units in multidose vials
Powder for injection: 10, 18, and 50 million international units/vial with diluent

INDICATIONS & DOSAGES
Adjust-a-dose (for all indications): (Applies to all indications except condylomata acuminata): If adverse effects occur, stop drug until they abate; then resume drug at 50% of the previous dose. If intolerance persists, stop drug. See package insert for specific guidance.
➤ **Hairy cell leukemia**
Adults: 2 million international units/m² I.M. or subcutaneously, three times weekly for 6 months or more if patient is responding to treatment.
➤ **AIDS-related Kaposi sarcoma**
Adults: 30 million international units/m² subcutaneously or I.M. three times weekly. Maintain dose unless disease progresses rapidly or intolerance occurs.
➤ **Chronic hepatitis B**
Adults: 30 to 35 million international units I.M. or subcutaneously weekly, given as 5 million international units daily or

10 million international units three times weekly for 16 weeks.

Children ages 1 to 17: 3 million international units/m^2 subcutaneously three times weekly for first week; then increase to 6 million international units/m^2 subcutaneously three times weekly (maximum is 10 million international units three times weekly) for total of 16 to 24 weeks.

Adjust-a-dose: If WBC count is less than 1.5×10^9/L, granulocyte count is less than 0.75×10^9/L, or platelet count is less than 50×10^9/L, reduce dose by 50%. Permanently discontinue drug if WBC count is less than 1×10^9/L, granulocyte count is less than 0.5×10^9/L, or platelet count is less than 25×10^9/L.

➤ **Chronic hepatitis C**

Adults: 3 million international units I.M. or subcutaneously three times weekly. In patients tolerating therapy with normalization of ALT at 16 weeks of therapy, continue for 18 to 24 months. In patients who haven't normalized the ALT, consider stopping therapy.

➤ **Adjunct to surgical treatment in patients with malignant melanoma who are asymptomatic after surgery but at high risk for systemic recurrence for up to 8 weeks after surgery**

Adults: Initially, 20 million international units/m^2 by I.V. infusion 5 consecutive days weekly for 4 weeks; then maintenance dose of 10 million international units/m^2 subcutaneously three times weekly for 48 weeks.

➤ **First treatment of clinically aggressive follicular non-Hodgkin lymphoma with chemotherapy containing anthracycline**

Adults: 5 million international units subcutaneously three times weekly for up to 18 months.

Adjust-a-dose: For neutrophil count of more than 1,000/mm^3 but less than 1,500/mm^3, decrease dosage by 50%. May resume starting dose if neutrophil count returns to more than 1,500/mm^3. Withhold drug if neutrophil count is less than 1,000/mm^3 or platelet count is less than 50,000/mm^3.

➤ **Condylomata acuminata (genital or venereal warts)**

Adults: 1 million international units for each lesion (maximum five lesions in a single course) intralesionally three times weekly for 3 weeks. Additional course may be given at 12 to 16 weeks.

ADMINISTRATION

I.V.

▼ Prepare infusion solution immediately before use.

▼ Based on desired dose, reconstitute appropriate vial strength of drug with diluent provided. Withdraw dose and inject into a 100-mL bag of normal saline solution. Final yield of drug shouldn't be less than 10 million international units/ 100 mL.

▼ Infuse over 20 minutes.

▼ Store solution in refrigerator. Store powder before and after reconstitution in refrigerator. Use within 24 hours.

▼ **Incompatibilities:** Dextrose solutions.

I.M.

● Carefully monitor injection sites in patient with thrombocytopenia. Avoid I.M. injections if possible.

● In patients whose platelet count is below 50,000/mm^3, give subcutaneously.

● Give drug at bedtime to minimize daytime drowsiness.

Subcutaneous

● For condylomata acuminata intralesional injection, use only 10 million-international unit vial because dilution of other strengths for intralesional use results in a hypertonic solution.

● Don't reconstitute drug in 10 million-international unit vial with more than 1 mL of diluent.

● Use tuberculin or similar syringe and 25G to 30G needle.

● Don't inject too deep beneath lesion or too superficially. As many as five lesions can be treated at one time.

● To ease discomfort, give in evening with acetaminophen.

ACTION

Unknown. May inhibit tumor or viral cell replication and modulate host immune response by enhancing macrophage activity and improving specific lymphocytes' cytotoxicity for target cells.

Route	Onset	Peak	Duration
I.V.	Unknown	15–60 min	4 hr
I.M., subcut.	Unknown	3–12 hr	16 hr

Half-life: I.V., 2 hours; I.M., 2 to 3 hours.

ADVERSE REACTIONS

CNS: apathy, amnesia, asthenia, depression, difficulty in thinking or concentrating, dizziness, fatigue, insomnia, paresthesia, somnolence, anxiety, lethargy, nervousness, weakness, headache.
CV: chest pain, *cyanosis,* edema, hypotension.
EENT: conjunctivitis, earache, rhinorrhea, sinusitis, pharyngitis, rhinitis.
GI: anorexia, diarrhea, dry mouth, dyspepsia, nausea, vomiting, abdominal pain, constipation, esophagitis, flatulence, stomatitis.
GU: decreased libido, impotence.
Hematologic: *leukopenia, thrombocytopenia, anemia, neutropenia.*
Hepatic: *hepatitis.*
Respiratory: coughing, dyspnea.
Skin: alopecia, dryness, increased diaphoresis, pruritus, rash, dermatitis.
Other: flulike syndrome, injection-site reaction.

INTERACTIONS

Drug-drug. *Aminophylline, theophylline:* May reduce theophylline clearance. Monitor theophylline level.
CNS depressants: May increase CNS effects. Avoid using together.
Live-virus vaccines: May increase adverse reactions to vaccine or decrease antibody response. Postpone immunization.
Zidovudine: May cause synergistic adverse effects (higher risk of neutropenia). Carefully monitor WBC count.

EFFECTS ON LAB TEST RESULTS

● May increase calcium, phosphate, AST, ALT, LDH, alkaline phosphatase, triglyceride, and fasting glucose levels. May decrease hemoglobin level.
● May increase PT, INR, and PTT. May decrease WBC and platelet counts.
● May increase or decrease thyroid-stimulating hormone level.

CONTRAINDICATIONS & CAUTIONS

● Contraindicated in patients hypersensitive to drug or its components and in those with autoimmune hepatitis or decompensated liver disease.
۞ Alert: Combination therapy with ribavirin is contraindicated in pregnant women and in men whose female partners are pregnant.
● Use cautiously in elderly patients and in those with history of CV disease, pulmonary disease, diabetes mellitus, coagulation disorders, renal impairment, and severe myelosuppression.
● Depression and suicidal behavior have been linked to drug use; patients with psychotic disorders, especially depression, shouldn't continue drug treatment.
۞ Alert: Neurotoxicity and cardiotoxicity are more common in elderly patients, especially those with underlying CNS or cardiac impairment.
⚠ Overdose S&S: Abnormal liver enzyme levels, renal failure, hemorrhage, MI.

NURSING CONSIDERATIONS

Black Box Warning Alpha interferons cause or aggravate fatal or life-threatening neuropsychiatric, autoimmune, ischemic, and infectious disorders. Monitor patients closely with periodic clinical and laboratory evaluations. Withdraw patients with persistently severe or worsening signs or symptoms of these conditions from therapy. ■
۞ Alert: Not all dosage forms are appropriate for all indications. Read package insert for approved indications before use.
● Ensure patient is well hydrated, especially at beginning of treatment.
● At start of treatment, monitor patient for flulike signs and symptoms, which tend to diminish with continued therapy. Premedicate patient with acetaminophen to minimize these symptoms.
● Periodically check for adverse CNS reactions, such as decreased mental status and dizziness, during therapy.
● Monitor CBC with differential, platelet count, blood chemistry and electrolyte studies, and LFTs. Monitor ECG before and during treatment if patient has cardiac disorder or advanced stages of cancer.
● For patients who develop thrombocytopenia, exercise extreme care in performing

---

invasive procedures; inspect injection site and skin frequently for signs and symptoms of bruising; limit frequency of I.M. injections; test urine, emesis fluid, stool, and secretions for occult blood.

• Severe adverse reactions may need dosage reduction to one-half or stoppage of drug until reactions subside.

• Use with blood dyscrasia–causing drugs, bone marrow suppressants, or radiation therapy may increase bone marrow suppression. Dosage reduction may be needed.

• For condylomata acuminata, maximum response usually occurs in 4 to 8 weeks. If results are not satisfactory after 12 to 16 weeks, a second course may be started. Patients with 6 to 10 condylomata may receive a second course of treatment; patients with more than 10 condylomata may receive additional courses.

PATIENT TEACHING

• Advise patient to avoid contact with persons with viral illness; patient is at increased risk for infection during therapy.

• Advise patient that laboratory tests will be performed before and periodically during therapy.

• Teach patient proper oral hygiene during treatment because bone marrow suppressant effects of interferon may lead to microbial infection, delayed healing, and bleeding gums. Drug also may decrease salivary flow.

• Advise patient to check with prescriber for instructions after missing a dose.

• Stress need to follow prescriber's instructions about taking and recording temperature and how and when to take acetaminophen.

• If patient will give drug to himself, teach him how to prepare injection and to use disposable syringe. Give him information on drug stability.

• Tell patient that drug may cause temporary partial hair loss; hair should return after drug is stopped.

• Advise patient to notify prescriber if signs or symptoms of depression occur.

⚠ **Alert:** Because of fetal risk, warn women of childbearing age and male patients with partners of childbearing age who are receiving combination therapy with ribavirin to use two forms of contraception.

SAFETY ALERT!

interferon alfacon-1
in-ter-FEER-on

Infergen

Therapeutic class: Immune response modifiers
Pharmacologic class: Biological response modifiers
Pregnancy risk category: C; X in combination with ribavirin

AVAILABLE FORMS
Injection: 9 mcg/0.3-mL, 15 mcg/0.5-mL vials

INDICATIONS & DOSAGES
➤ **Chronic hepatitis C viral infection in patients with compensated liver disease**
Adults: 9 mcg subcutaneously three times weekly for 24 weeks; for patients who don't respond or who relapse, 15 mcg subcutaneously three times weekly for up to 48 weeks. Allow at least 48 hours between doses.

Adjust-a-dose: For patients intolerant to higher doses, dose may be reduced to 7.5 mcg. Don't give doses below 7.5 mcg because decreased efficacy may result.
➤ **Chronic hepatitis C viral infection in patients with compensated liver disease (in combination with ribavirin)**
Adults weighing more than 75 kg (165 lb): 15 mcg daily subcutaneously with ribavirin 1,000 to 1,200 mg P.O. daily in two divided doses for up to 48 weeks.

Adults weighing less than 75 kg: 15 mcg daily subcutaneously with ribavirin 1,000 mg P.O. daily for up to 48 weeks.

Adjust-a-dose: For patients intolerant to starting dose, may decrease to 9 mcg daily, and then to 6 mcg daily as necessary. For patients with hematologic toxicities: If ANC is less than 0.75×10^9/L or platelet count is less than 50×10^9/L, reduce interferon alfacon-1 dose from 15 to 9 mcg, or from 9 to 6 mcg, and maintain ribavirin dose at 1,200 or 1,000 mg; if ANC is less than 50×10^9/L, stop interferon alfacon-1 and ribavirin until ANC values return to more than 1,000/mm³; if platelet count is less

---

than 25×10^9/L, discontinue interferon alfacon-1 and ribavirin.

ADMINISTRATION
Subcutaneous
● Store drug in refrigerator at 36° to 46° F (2° to 8° C); don't freeze. Injection may be allowed to reach room temperature just before use.
● Avoid vigorous shaking.
● Discard unused portion.

ACTION
Induces gene-mediated biological responses that include antiviral, antiproliferative, and immunomodulatory effects and cytokine regulation.

Route	Onset	Peak	Duration
Subcut.	Unknown	24–36 hr	Unknown

Half-life: Unknown.

ADVERSE REACTIONS
CNS: amnesia, anxiety, depression, dizziness, emotional lability, headache, insomnia, malaise, nervousness, paresthesia, *suicidal ideation,* agitation, confusion.
CV: hypertension, palpitations, tachycardia, chest pain.
EENT: pharyngitis, retinal hemorrhages, rhinitis, sinusitis, conjunctivitis, ear pain, epistaxis, loss of visual acuity or visual field, tinnitus.
GI: abdominal pain, anorexia, diarrhea, dyspepsia, nausea, vomiting, constipation, decreased saliva, flatulence, hemorrhoids, taste perversion.
GU: dysmenorrhea, vaginitis.
Hematologic: *anemia, granulocytopenia, leukopenia, thrombocytopenia,* ecchymosis, lymphadenopathy, *lymphocytosis, neutropenia.*
Metabolic: hypothyroidism.
Respiratory: congestion, cough, infection, bronchitis, dyspnea.
Skin: alopecia, erythema at injection site, pruritus, rash, dry skin.
Other: body pain, flulike symptoms, hypersensitivity reactions, decreased libido, toothache.

INTERACTIONS
Drug-drug. *Drugs metabolized by CYP450:* May alter drug levels. Monitor changes in levels of these drugs.
Myelosuppressives: May cause added hematologic toxicities; use cautiously together. Monitor CBC and therapeutic or toxic level of myelosuppressive.

EFFECTS ON LAB TEST RESULTS
● May increase triglyceride and thyroid-stimulating hormone (TSH) levels. May decrease T_4 level.
● May increase PT and INR. May decrease granulocyte, WBC, and platelet counts. May decrease hemoglobin and hematocrit levels.

CONTRAINDICATIONS & CAUTIONS
● Contraindicated in patients hypersensitive to alpha interferons, to *Escherichia coli–* derived products, or to any component of product; and in patients with history of severe psychiatric disorders or depression, autoimmune hepatitis, or decompensated hepatic disease.
● Use with caution in patients with history of cardiac disease and other autoimmune or endocrine disorders, in those with abnormally low peripheral blood cell counts, in those receiving drugs that cause myelosuppression, and in patients with mild to moderate depression.
● Use of monotherapy isn't recommended unless patient is intolerant to ribavirin.
● Use of combination therapy is contraindicated in patients with CrCl of less than 50 mL/minute.
● Use of combination therapy in treatment-naive patients and in patients with human papilloma virus or HIV-1 hasn't been evaluated for safety and efficacy.
● Patients with limited response to prior therapy; those with genotype 1 hepatitis C, high viral load, or cirrhosis; and African-Americans are less likely to benefit from combination therapy.
⚠ *Overdose S&S:* Anorexia, chills, fever, myalgia, elevated liver enzyme levels.

NURSING CONSIDERATIONS
Black Box Warning Alpha interferons may cause or aggravate fatal or life-threatening neuropsychiatric, autoimmune, ischemic,

and infectious disorders. Monitor patients closely with periodic clinical and laboratory evaluations. Withdraw patients with persistently severe or worsening signs or symptoms of these conditions from therapy. ■

Black Box Warning Use with ribavirin may cause birth defects or fetal death. Female patients and female partners of male patients should avoid pregnancy. ■

Black Box Warning Use with ribavirin may cause hemolytic anemia and worsen cardiac disease. ■

⊕ Alert: Drug is genotoxic and mutagenic and is considered a potential carcinogen.

• Discontinue ribavirin if interferon alfacon-1 is stopped, even temporarily.

• Obtain the following laboratory tests before therapy, 2 weeks after it starts, and periodically during therapy: CBC with platelet count and creatinine, albumin, bilirubin, TSH, and T₄ levels.

⊕ Alert: If hypersensitivity reaction occurs, stop drug immediately and treat. Premedication with acetaminophen or ibuprofen may decrease adverse effects.

• Allow at least 48 hours to elapse between doses.

• Dosages and adverse reactions vary among different subtypes of drug. Don't use different subtypes in a single treatment regimen.

PATIENT TEACHING

• If drug is to be used at home, instruct patient on appropriate use, dosage, and administration. Give the patient information leaflet available from the manufacturer to the patient. Also teach patient proper disposal procedures for needles, syringes, drug containers, and unused drug.

• Instruct patient not to reuse needles or syringes or reenter vial.

• Urge patient not to use vial that's discolored or contains particulates.

• Tell patient that nonnarcotic analgesics and bedtime administration may be used to prevent or lessen flulike symptoms (headache, fever, malaise, muscle pain) related to therapy.

• Instruct patient to immediately report symptoms of depression.

⊕ Alert: Tell patient to use at least two forms of contraception during treatment and for at least 6 months after treatment ends and to have monthly pregnancy tests.

SAFETY ALERT!

interferon beta-1a
in-ter-FEER-on

Avonex, Rebif

Therapeutic class: Antivirals
Pharmacologic class: Biological response modifiers
Pregnancy risk category: C

AVAILABLE FORMS
Avonex
Lyophilized powder for injection: 33 mcg (6.6 million international units)
Prefilled syringe or autoinjector: 30 mcg (6 million international units)/0.5 mL
Rebif
Parenteral: 8.8 mcg (2.4 million international units), 22 mcg (6 million international units), 44 mcg (12 million international units) in prefilled syringe or autoinjector

INDICATIONS & DOSAGES
➤ **To slow accumulation of physical disability and decrease frequency of clinical worsening in patients with relapsing forms of MS**
Adults age 18 and older: 30 mcg Avonex I.M. once weekly. Or, initially, 4.4 or 8.8 mcg Rebif subcutaneously three times weekly for 2 weeks; then increase dose to 11 or 22 mcg three times weekly for another 2 weeks. Then increase to a maintenance dose of 22 or 44 mcg subcutaneously three times weekly.
Adjust-a-dose: For Rebif, in patients with leukopenia or elevated LFT values (ALT greater than 5 times upper limit of normal), reduce dosage by 20% to 50% until toxicity is resolved. Stop treatment if jaundice or other signs of hepatic injury occur.
➤ **First MS attack if brain magnetic resonance imaging shows abnormalities consistent with MS**
Adults: 30 mcg Avonex I.M. once weekly.

ADMINISTRATION

Subcutaneous

● Visually inspect Rebif for particulate matter and discoloration before administration.

● Rotate sites of injection.

● Administer Rebif at same time on same 3 days at least 48 hours apart each week (late afternoon or evening on Monday, Wednesday, and Friday).

● Use only prefilled syringes for titration to 22 mcg prescribed dose of Rebif.

● Store Rebif in the refrigerator between 36° and 46° F (2° and 8° C). Don't freeze. Rebif may be stored at or below 77° F (25° C) for up to 30 days if away from heat and light.

I.M.

● To reconstitute lyophilized Avonex, inject 1.1 mL of supplied diluent (sterile water for injection) into vial and gently swirl to dissolve drug. Don't shake.

● Use drug as soon as possible; may be used up to 6 hours after being reconstituted if stored at 36° to 46° F.

● Rotate sites of injection.

● The Avonex and diluent vials are for single use only; discard unused portions.

● Store Avonex prefilled syringes and autoinjectors in the refrigerator at 36° to 46° F. If refrigeration is unavailable, may store at 77°F for up to 7 days. Once refrigerated, syringes and autoinjectors must not be stored above 77°F. Once removed from refrigerator, warm to room temperature (about 30 minutes). Don't use external heat sources, such as hot water, to warm syringe, or expose to high temperatures. Don't freeze. Protect from light.

● After giving each dose, discard any remaining product in the syringe or autoinjector.

ACTION

Unknown. Interacts with specific cell receptors found on the surface of cells. Binding of these receptors causes the expression of a number of interferon-induced gene products believed to mediate the biological actions of interferon beta-1a.

Route	Onset	Peak	Duration
Subcut.	Unknown	16 hr	Unknown
I.M.	Unknown	3–15 hr	Unknown

Half-life: I.M., 10 hours; subcutaneous, 69 hours.

ADVERSE REACTIONS

CNS: asthenia, dizziness, fatigue, fever, headache, pain, sleep difficulty, depression, *seizures, suicidal ideation or attempt, suicidal tendency,* abnormal coordination, ataxia, hypertonia, malaise, speech disorder, syncope.

CV: chest pain, vasodilation.

EENT: abnormal vision, sinusitis, decreased hearing, otitis media.

GI: abdominal pain, diarrhea, dyspepsia, nausea, anorexia, dry mouth.

GU: increased urinary frequency, ovarian cyst, urinary incontinence, vaginitis.

Hematologic: lymphadenopathy, *leukopenia, pancytopenia, thrombocytopenia,* anemia.

Hepatic: abnormal hepatic function, *autoimmune hepatitis,* bilirubinemia, hepatic injury, *hepatitis.*

Metabolic: hyperthyroidism, hypothyroidism.

Musculoskeletal: back pain, muscle ache, skeletal pain, arthralgia, muscle spasm.

Respiratory: upper respiratory tract infection, dyspnea.

Skin: injection-site reaction, alopecia, ecchymosis at injection site, nevus, urticaria.

Other: chills, flulike syndrome, infection, hypersensitivity reactions, herpes simplex, herpes zoster, neutralizing antibodies.

INTERACTIONS

Drug-drug. *Myelosuppressants:* May cause added hematologic toxicities; use cautiously together. Monitor CBC.

Drug-lifestyle. *Sun exposure:* May cause photosensitivity reactions. Advise patient to take precautions against sun exposure.

EFFECTS ON LAB TEST RESULTS

● May increase liver enzyme levels. May decrease hemoglobin level and hematocrit. May increase or decrease thyroid function test levels.

● May increase eosinophil count. May decrease WBC and platelet counts.

Reactions in bold italics are *life-threatening*. Interactions may have a *rapid onset* or a *delayed onset*.

CONTRAINDICATIONS & CAUTIONS
• Contraindicated in patients hypersensitive to natural or recombinant interferon beta, human albumin, or other components of drug.
• Use cautiously in patients with depression, seizure disorders, or severe cardiac conditions.
• It's unknown if drug appears in breast milk; a breast-feeding woman must either stop breast-feeding or stop drug.
• Safety and effectiveness of drug in chronic progressive MS or in children younger than age 18 haven't been established.

NURSING CONSIDERATIONS
• Monitor patient closely for depression and suicidal ideation. It isn't known if these symptoms are related to the underlying neurologic basis of MS or to the drug.
• Monitor WBC count, platelet count, and blood chemistries, including LFTs. Rare but severe liver injury, including liver failure, may occur in patients taking Avonex.
• Give analgesics or antipyretics to decrease flulike symptoms.

PATIENT TEACHING
• Advise patient to read medication guide that comes with drug.
• Teach patient and family member how to reconstitute drug and give Avonex I.M.
• Caution patient not to change dosage or schedule of administration. If a dose is missed, tell him to take it as soon as he remembers. He may then resume his regular schedule. Tell patient not to take two injections within 48 hours of each other.
• Show patient how to store drug.
• Inform patient that flulike signs and symptoms, such as fever, fatigue, muscle aches, headache, chills, and joint pain, are not uncommon at start of therapy. Acetaminophen 650 mg P.O. may be taken immediately before injection and for another 24 hours after each injection, to lessen severity of flulike signs and symptoms.
• Advise patient to report depression, suicidal thoughts, or other adverse reactions.
• Instruct patient to keep syringes and needles away from children. Also, instruct him not to reuse needles or syringes and to discard them in a syringe-disposal unit.

• Caution women not to become pregnant during therapy because of the potential risk of spontaneous abortion. If pregnancy occurs, instruct patient to notify prescriber immediately and to stop drug.
• Advise patient to use sunscreen and avoid sun exposure while taking drug because photosensitivity may occur.
• Tell patient to store drug in the refrigerator between 36° and 46° F (2° and 8° C) and not to freeze. Drug may also be stored at or below 77° F (25° C) for up to 30 days and away from heat and light.

SAFETY ALERT!

interferon beta-1b (recombinant)
in-ter-FEER-on

Betaseron, Extavia

Therapeutic class: Antivirals
Pharmacologic class: Biological response modifiers
Pregnancy risk category: C

AVAILABLE FORMS
Powder for injection: 9.6 million international units (0.3 mg)

INDICATIONS & DOSAGES
➤ **To reduce frequency of exacerbations in relapsing forms of MS**
Adults: 0.0625 mg subcutaneously every other day for weeks 1 and 2; then 0.125 mg subcutaneously every other day for weeks 3 and 4; then 0.1875 mg subcutaneously every other day for weeks 5 and 6; then 0.25 mg subcutaneously every other day thereafter.

ADMINISTRATION
Subcutaneous
• To reconstitute, inject 1.2 mL of supplied diluent (half-normal saline solution for injection) into vial and gently swirl to dissolve drug.
• Reconstituted solution contains 8 million international units (0.25 mg)/mL.
• Don't shake. Discard vial that contains particulates or discolored solution.
• Inject immediately after preparation.

• Rotate injection sites to minimize local reactions and observe site for necrosis.
• Store at room temperature. After reconstitution, if not used immediately, drug may be refrigerated for up to 3 hours.

ACTION

A naturally occurring antiviral and immunoregulatory drug derived from human fibroblasts. Drug attaches to membrane receptors and causes cellular changes, including increased protein synthesis.

Route	Onset	Peak	Duration
Subcut.	Unknown	1–8 hr	Unknown

Half-life: 8 minutes to 4¼ hours.

ADVERSE REACTIONS

CNS: depression, anxiety, emotional lability, depersonalization, *suicidal tendencies,* confusion, hypertonia, asthenia, migraine, *seizures,* headache, pain, dizziness, malaise, fever, chills, insomnia.
CV: chest pain, peripheral edema, palpitations, hypertension, tachycardia, peripheral vascular disorder.
EENT: laryngitis, sinusitis, conjunctivitis, abnormal vision.
GI: diarrhea, constipation, abdominal pain, vomiting, dyspepsia.
GU: menstrual bleeding or spotting, early or delayed menses, fewer days of menstrual flow, menorrhagia, urgency, impotence, prostate disorder, frequency.
Hematologic: *leukopenia,* lymphadenopathy.
Musculoskeletal: myasthenia, arthralgia, myalgia, leg cramps.
Respiratory: dyspnea.
Skin: inflammation, pain, necrosis at injection site, diaphoresis, alopecia, rash, skin disorder.
Other: breast pain, flulike syndrome, pelvic pain, generalized edema.

INTERACTIONS

None significant.

EFFECTS ON LAB TEST RESULTS

• May increase ALT and bilirubin levels.
• May decrease WBC and neutrophil counts.

CONTRAINDICATIONS & CAUTIONS

• Contraindicated in patients hypersensitive to interferon beta, human albumin, or components of drug.
• Use cautiously in women of childbearing age. Evidence is inconclusive about teratogenic effects, but drug may be an abortifacient.

NURSING CONSIDERATIONS

❸ *Alert:* Serious liver damage, including hepatic failure requiring transplant, can occur. Monitor liver function at 1, 3, and 6 months after therapy starts and periodically thereafter.
• Monitor patient for signs of depression.
• Monitor CBC.
• Monitor thyroid function tests every 6 months in patients being treated for thyroid disorder.

PATIENT TEACHING

• Warn woman about dangers to fetus. If pregnancy occurs during therapy, tell her to notify prescriber and stop taking drug.
• Advise patient to read medication guide that comes with drug.
• Teach patient how to perform subcutaneous injections, including solution preparation, aseptic technique, injection-site rotation, and equipment disposal. Periodically reevaluate patient's technique.
• Tell patient to take drug at bedtime to minimize mild flulike signs and symptoms that commonly occur.
• Advise patient to report suicidal thoughts or depression.
• Urge patient to immediately report signs or symptoms of tissue death at injection site.
• Advise patient of importance of obtaining routine blood tests.

Reactions in bold italics are *life-threatening*. Interactions may have a *rapid onset* or a *delayed onset*.

SAFETY ALERT!

interferon gamma-1b
in-ter-FEER-on

Actimmune

Therapeutic class: Immune response modifiers
Pharmacologic class: Biological response modifiers
Pregnancy risk category: C

AVAILABLE FORMS
Injection: 100 mcg (2 million international units)/0.5-mL vial

INDICATIONS & DOSAGES
➤ **Chronic granulomatous disease, severe malignant osteopetrosis**
Adults and children with BSA greater than $0.5\ m^2$: Give 50 mcg/m^2 (1 million international units/m^2) subcutaneously three times weekly, preferably at bedtime.
Adults and children with a BSA of 0.5 m^2 or less: 1.5 mcg/kg subcutaneously three times weekly.
Adjust-a-dose: If patient has severe reaction, decrease dosage by 50% or stop drug until reaction subsides.

ADMINISTRATION
Subcutaneous
● Discard unused drug. Each vial is for single use only and doesn't contain a preservative.
● Don't mix with other drugs in the same syringe.
● Optimum injection sites are the right and left deltoid and anterior thigh.
● Store in refrigerator before use. Discard unpunctured vials left at room temperature for more than 12 hours.

ACTION
Interleukin-type lymphokine. Drug has potent phagocyte-activating properties and increases the oxidative metabolism of tissue macrophages.

Route	Onset	Peak	Duration
Subcut.	Unknown	7 hr	Unknown

Half-life: 6 hours.

ADVERSE REACTIONS
CNS: fatigue, chills, dizziness, fever, headache.
GI: diarrhea, nausea, vomiting.
Hematologic: *neutropenia, thrombocytopenia.*
Musculoskeletal: arthralgia, myalgia.
Skin: erythema and tenderness at injection site, rash.
Other: flulike syndrome.

INTERACTIONS
Drug-drug. *Myelosuppressants:* May increase myelosuppression. Use together with caution. Monitor patient closely.
Rotavirus live-virus vaccine: May increase risk of infection by live-virus vaccine. Don't use together.

EFFECTS ON LAB TEST RESULTS
● May increase liver enzyme levels.
● May decrease neutrophil and platelet counts.

CONTRAINDICATIONS & CAUTIONS
● Contraindicated in patients hypersensitive to drug or to genetically engineered products derived from *Escherichia coli.*
● Use cautiously in patients with cardiac disease, including arrhythmias, ischemia, or heart failure. The flulike syndrome commonly seen with high doses of drug can worsen these conditions.
● Use cautiously in patients with compromised CNS function or seizure disorders. CNS adverse reactions that may occur at high doses of drug can worsen these conditions.
⚠ **Overdose S&S:** Decreased mental status, dizziness, gait disturbance, elevated liver enzyme and triglyceride levels, neutropenia, thrombocytopenia.

NURSING CONSIDERATIONS
● Administer in the deltoid or anterior thigh muscle.
🕔 **Alert:** The drug's activity is expressed in international units (1 million international units/50 mcg). This is equal to what was previously expressed as units (1.5 million units/50 mcg).
● Premedicate patient with acetaminophen to minimize signs and symptoms at start

of therapy; these tend to diminish with continued therapy.
• Before beginning therapy and at 3-month intervals, monitor CBC, platelet count, renal function tests and LFTs, and urinalysis.

PATIENT TEACHING

• If patient will give drug to himself, teach him how to give it and how to dispose of used needles, syringes, containers, and unused drug.
• Instruct patient how to manage flulike signs and symptoms (fever, fatigue, muscle aches, headache, chills, joint pain) that commonly occur.
• Advise use of acetaminophen to treat fever and headache.

SAFETY ALERT!

ipilimumab
IP-ih-LIM-yoo-mab

Yervoy

Therapeutic class: Antineoplastics
Pharmacologic class: Monoclonal antibodies
Pregnancy risk category: C

AVAILABLE FORMS
Injection: 50 mg/10 mL (5 mg/mL), 200 mg/40 mL (5 mg/mL)

INDICATIONS & DOSAGES
➤ **Treatment of unresectable or metastatic melanoma**
Adults: 3 mg/kg I.V. infusion over 90 minutes every 3 weeks for a total of four doses.
Adjust-a-dose: Withhold dose in patients with moderate immune-mediated adverse reactions or symptomatic endocrinopathy. For patient with grade 0 to 1 reactions that completely or partially resolve and if patient was receiving less than 7.5 mg prednisone or equivalent daily, resume drug at 3 mg/kg every 3 weeks for four doses or 16 weeks from first dose, whichever occurs first. Permanently discontinue drug in patients with persistent moderate adverse reactions or the inability to reduce corticosteroid dosage to 7.5 mg prednisone or equivalent daily.

Black Box Warning For patients with severe immune-mediated reactions, initiate systemic corticosteroids (prednisone or equivalent) at 1 to 2 mg/kg/day and permanently discontinue ipilimumab. ∎

ADMINISTRATION
I.V.
▼ Store vials in refrigerator at 36° to 46° F (2° to 8° C). Don't freeze or shake vials. Protect from light.
▼ Visually inspect solution. Solution may be clear to pale yellow. Discard if cloudy or discolored or if particles (other than translucent-to-white, amorphous particles) are present.
▼ Allow vials to come to room temperature for 5 minutes before preparing infusion.
▼ Withdraw required volume of drug and transfer into I.V. bag of normal saline solution or D$_5$W. Final concentration should range from 1 to 2 mg/mL. Invert bag gently to mix.
▼ Store diluted solution up to 24 hours under refrigeration or at room temperature (68° to 77° F [20° to 25° C]).
▼ Administer diluted solution over 90 minutes through I.V. line containing a sterile, nonpyrogenic, low–protein-binding in-line filter.
▼ After each dose, flush I.V. line with normal saline solution or D$_5$W.
▼ Discard unused portion of vial.
▼ **Incompatibilities:** Other I.V. drugs and solutions other than normal saline solution or D$_5$W.

ACTION
Binds to the cytotoxic T-lymphocyte–associated antigen 4; this blockade has been shown to augment T-cell–mediated antitumor immune responses.

Route	Onset	Peak	Duration
I.V.	Rapid	Unknown	Unknown

Half-life: 15 days.

ADVERSE REACTIONS
CNS: fatigue, neuropathy.
GI: diarrhea, colitis, enterocolitis.
GU: nephritis.
Hepatic: *hepatotoxicity.*

Reactions in bold italics are *life-threatening*. Interactions may have a *rapid onset* or a *delayed onset*.

Metabolic: endocrinopathy, hypopituitarism.
Skin: pruritus, rash, dermatitis, urticaria.
Other: *adrenal insufficiency.*

INTERACTIONS
None reported.

EFFECTS ON LAB TEST RESULTS
● May increase liver enzyme levels.
● May increase eosinophil count.
● May increase or decrease thyroid hormone levels.

CONTRAINDICATIONS & CAUTIONS
● Contraindicated in patients hypersensitive to drug or its components.
● Use during pregnancy only if potential benefit to the mother outweighs potential risk to the fetus.
● Drug may appear in breast milk. Because of the risk of serious adverse reactions in breast-feeding infants, the mother should discontinue either ipilimumab or breast-feeding, with consideration of the importance of the drug to the mother.
Black Box Warning Ipilimumab can cause severe and fatal immune-mediated adverse reactions involving any organ system, especially such reactions as enterocolitis, hepatitis, dermatitis (including toxic epidermal necrolysis), neuropathy, and endocrinopathy. Reactions usually occur during treatment, but may present weeks to months after therapy ends. If severe immune-mediated reactions occur, permanently discontinue ipilimumab and initiate systemic high-dose corticosteroid therapy. Assess patient for these reactions. ∎
● Permanently discontinue drug for any of the following: persistent moderate adverse reactions or inability to reduce corticosteroid dose to 7.5 mg of prednisone or equivalent daily; failure to complete full treatment course within 16 weeks from administration of first dose; severe or life-threatening adverse reactions, including colitis with abdominal pain, fever, ileus, or peritoneal signs and symptoms; increase in stool frequency (seven or more over baseline); fecal incontinence; need for I.V. hydration for more than 24 hours; GI hemorrhage; GI perforation; AST or ALT level

more than 5 times the upper limit of normal (ULN) or total bilirubin level more than 3 times ULN; Stevens-Johnson syndrome; toxic epidermal necrolysis; rash complicated by full-thickness dermal ulceration or necrotic, bullous, or hemorrhagic manifestations; severe motor or sensory neuropathy; Guillain-Barré syndrome; myasthenia gravis; severe immune-mediated reactions involving any organ system (nephritis, pneumonitis, pancreatitis, noninfectious myocarditis); or immune-mediated ocular disease unresponsive to topical immunosuppressive therapy.

NURSING CONSIDERATIONS
Black Box Warning Monitor patients for signs and symptoms of immune-mediated adverse reactions and withhold or discontinue drug as necessary. ∎
Black Box Warning Obtain clinical chemistry values, including liver function and thyroid function test results, at baseline and before each dose. ∎
● Review LFT results and assess patient for signs and symptoms of hepatotoxicity (jaundice, dark urine, nausea, vomiting, right upper quadrant pain, abnormal bleeding or bruising) before each dose. For patients with hepatotoxicity (AST or ALT level more than 5 times ULN or total bilirubin level more than 3 times ULN), rule out infectious or malignant causes and increase frequency of LFT monitoring until resolution. When LFT results show sustained improvement or return to baseline, initiate corticosteroid tapering and continue to taper over 1 month. Withhold ipilimumab in patients with grade 2 hepatotoxicity.
● Monitor patients for signs and symptoms of enterocolitis and bowel perforation (abdominal pain, fever, ileus, or peritoneal signs and symptoms; increase in stool frequency to seven or more over patient's baseline; fecal incontinence; need for I.V. hydration for more than 24 hours; GI hemorrhage; GI perforation). Rule out infection and consider endoscopic evaluation for persistent or severe symptoms. With improvement to grade 1 or less, taper corticosteroid dosage over at least 1 month. If moderate symptoms occur, administer antidiarrheal and, if persistent for more than 1 week, start systemic

corticosteroids (prednisone or equivalent) at 0.5 mg/kg/day.
- Monitor patients for signs and symptoms of motor or sensory neuropathy. Withhold ipilimumab in patients with moderate neuropathy. Permanently discontinue drug in patients with severe neuropathy that interferes with daily activities, such as Guillain-Barré–like syndromes (unilateral or bilateral weakness, sensory changes, paresthesia). Consider systemic corticosteroids (1 to 2 mg/kg/day prednisone or equivalent) for severe neuropathies.
- Monitor patients for signs and symptoms of dermatitis (rash, pruritus) and consider these symptoms immune-mediated unless an alternative cause is identified. Permanently discontinue ipilimumab in patients with Stevens-Johnson syndrome, toxic epidermal necrolysis, or rash complicated by full-thickness dermal ulceration or necrotic, bullous, or hemorrhagic manifestations. When dermatitis is controlled, taper corticosteroids over at least 1 month. For patients with mild to moderate dermatitis, treat symptomatically; give topical or systemic corticosteroids if there is no improvement within 1 week. Withhold ipilimumab in patients with moderate to severe signs and symptoms.
- Monitor patients for signs and symptoms of hypophysitis, adrenal insufficiency (including adrenal crisis), and hyperthyroidism or hypothyroidism (headaches, fatigue, feeling cold, weight gain, changes in mood or behavior, dizziness, or fainting). Endocrinopathies should be considered immune-mediated unless an alternative cause is identified. Withhold drug in symptomatic patients. Give corticosteroids and hormone replacement as appropriate.
- Monitor patients for ocular symptoms (vision changes, eye pain or redness). Administer corticosteroid eyedrops to patients who develop uveitis, iritis, or episcleritis. Permanently discontinue drug in patients with immune-mediated ocular disease unresponsive to local immunosuppressive therapy.

PATIENT TEACHING
- Instruct patient to report history of immune system disorders, such as ulcerative

colitis, Crohn disease, lupus, or sarcoidosis; organ transplant; or liver damage.
- Teach patient the signs and symptoms of serious immune-mediated adverse reactions and advise him to immediately report them to prescriber.
- Advise patient that blood chemistry studies will be needed before start of therapy and before each dose.
- Instruct patient to read the Yervoy Medication Guide before taking each dose.
- Warn women that ipilimumab may cause fetal harm and to report pregnancy immediately.
- Tell breast-feeding patients not to breast-feed while taking drug.

ipratropium bromide
ih-pra-TROE-pee-um

Atrovent, Atrovent HFA

Therapeutic class: Bronchodilators
Pharmacologic class: Anticholinergics
Pregnancy risk category: B

AVAILABLE FORMS
Inhaler: 17 mcg/metered dose (Atrovent HFA)
Nasal spray: 0.03% (21 mcg/metered dose), 0.06% (42 mcg/metered dose)
Solution (for inhalation): 0.02% (500 mcg/vial)

INDICATIONS & DOSAGES
➤ **Bronchospasm in chronic bronchitis and emphysema**
Adults: Usually, 2 inhalations q.i.d.; patient may take additional inhalations as needed but shouldn't exceed 12 inhalations in 24 hours. Or, 250 to 500 mcg every 6 to 8 hours via oral nebulizer.
➤ **Rhinorrhea caused by allergic and nonallergic perennial rhinitis**
Adults and children age 6 and older: Two 0.03% nasal sprays (42 mcg) per nostril b.i.d. or t.i.d.
➤ **Rhinorrhea caused by the common cold**
Adults and children age 12 and older: Two 0.06% nasal sprays (84 mcg) per nostril t.i.d. or q.i.d.

Children ages 5 to 11: Two 0.06% nasal sprays (84 mcg) per nostril t.i.d.
➤ **Rhinorrhea caused by seasonal allergic rhinitis**
Adults and children age 5 and older: Two 0.06% nasal sprays (84 mcg) per nostril q.i.d. Total dose is 672 mcg/day.
➤ **Acute asthma in patients who are currently using a beta-2 agonist or who are intolerant of beta-2 agonists** ◆
Adults: 2 to 3 inhalations of a 17-mcg/metered-dose inhaler (MDI) or 250 mcg of nebulizer solution every 6 hours for quick relief. Or, 500 mcg of nebulizer solution or 8 inhalations via MDI every 20 minutes for three doses for exacerbations.
Children: 250 to 500 mcg of nebulizer solution or 4 to 8 inhalations via MDI every 20 minutes for three doses for exacerbations.

ADMINISTRATION
Inhalational
• Shake canister before use, except for HFA aerosol.
• If more than 1 inhalation is ordered, wait at least 2 minutes between inhalations.
• Use spacer device to improve drug delivery, if appropriate.
Intranasal
• Prime nasal spray before first use and after it has not been used for more than 24 hours.
• Tilt patient's head backward after dose to allow drug to spread to back of nose.

ACTION
Inhibits vagally mediated reflexes by antagonizing acetylcholine at muscarinic receptors on bronchial smooth muscle.

Route	Onset	Peak	Duration
Inhalation	5–15 min	1–2 hr	3–6 hr

Half-life: About 2 hours.

ADVERSE REACTIONS
CNS: dizziness, pain, headache.
CV: palpitations, chest pain.
EENT: blurred vision, rhinitis, pharyngitis, sinusitis, epistaxis.
GI: nausea, GI distress, dry mouth.
Musculoskeletal: back pain.
Respiratory: upper respiratory tract infection, bronchitis, *bronchospasm,* cough, dyspnea, increased sputum.

Skin: rash.
Other: flulike symptoms, hypersensitivity reactions.

INTERACTIONS
Drug-drug. *Anticholinergics:* May increase anticholinergic effects. Avoid using together.
Drug-herb. *Pill-bearing spurge:* May decrease effect of drug. Advise patient to use cautiously.

EFFECTS ON LAB TEST RESULTS
None reported.

CONTRAINDICATIONS & CAUTIONS
• Contraindicated in patients hypersensitive to drug, atropine, or its derivatives.
• Use cautiously in patients with angle-closure glaucoma, prostatic hyperplasia, or bladder-neck obstruction.
• Safety and effectiveness of nebulization or inhaler in children younger than age 12 haven't been established.

NURSING CONSIDERATIONS
• If patient uses a face mask for a nebulizer, take care to prevent leakage around the mask because eye pain or temporary blurring of vision may occur.
• Safety and effectiveness of use beyond 4 days in patients with a common cold haven't been established.
• *Look alike–sound alike:* Don't confuse Atrovent with Alupent or Natru-Vent.

PATIENT TEACHING
• Warn patient that drug isn't effective for treating acute episodes of bronchospasm when rapid response is needed.
• Teach patient to perform oral inhalation correctly. Give the following instructions for using an MDI:
– Shake canister. The HFA form doesn't need to be shaken.
– Clear nasal passages and throat.
– Breathe out, expelling as much air from lungs as possible.
– Place mouthpiece well into mouth, and inhale deeply as you release dose from inhaler. (Patient should close his eyes.)
– Hold breath for several seconds, remove mouthpiece, and exhale slowly.

• Inform patient that use of a spacer device with an MDI may improve drug delivery to lungs.

• Warn patient to avoid accidentally spraying drug into eyes. Temporary blurring of vision may result.

• If more than 1 inhalation is prescribed, tell patient to wait at least 2 minutes before repeating procedure.

• Instruct patient to remove canister and wash inhaler in warm, soapy water at least once weekly.

• If patient is also using a corticosteroid inhaler, instruct him to use ipratropium first and then to wait about 5 minutes before using the corticosteroid. This lets the bronchodilator open air passages for maximal effectiveness of the corticosteroid.

• Instruct patient to prime nasal spray by pumping seven times before first use or after it has not been used for 1 week. Prime with two pumps after it has not been used for 1 day.

• Instruct patient to sniff deeply after each spray and to breathe out through mouth. Tell him to tilt head backward to allow drug to spread to back of nose.

irbesartan
er-bah-SAR-tan

Avapro♦

Therapeutic class: Antihypertensives
Pharmacologic class: Angiotensin II receptor antagonists
Pregnancy risk category: D

AVAILABLE FORMS
Tablets: 75 mg, 150 mg, 300 mg

INDICATIONS & DOSAGES
➤ **Hypertension**
Adults: Initially, 150 mg P.O. daily, increased to maximum of 300 mg daily, if needed.
Adjust-a-dose: For volume- and sodium-depleted patients, initially, 75 mg P.O. daily.

➤ **Nephropathy in patients with type 2 diabetes**
Adults: Target maintenance dose is 300 mg P.O. once daily.

ADMINISTRATION
P.O.
• Give drug without regard for meals.

ACTION
Produces antihypertensive effect by competitive antagonist activity at the angiotensin II receptor.

Route	Onset	Peak	Duration
P.O.	Unknown	1½–2 hr	24 hr

Half-life: 11 to 15 hours.

ADVERSE REACTIONS
CNS: fatigue, anxiety, dizziness, headache.
CV: chest pain, edema, tachycardia.
EENT: pharyngitis, rhinitis, sinus abnormality.
GI: diarrhea, dyspepsia, abdominal pain, nausea, vomiting.
GU: UTI.
Musculoskeletal: musculoskeletal trauma or pain.
Respiratory: upper respiratory tract infection, cough.
Skin: rash.

INTERACTIONS
ACE inhibitors: May increase risk of renal dysfunction and hyperkalemia. Use together cautiously; closely monitor renal function and potassium level.
⚠ Alert: *Aliskiren:* May increase risk of renal impairment, hypotension, and hyperkalemia in diabetic patients and those with moderate to severe renal impairment (GFR less than 60 mL/minute). Concomitant use is contraindicated in diabetic patients. Avoid concomitant use in those with moderate to severe renal impairment.
Lithium: May increase lithium concentration, possibly causing toxicity. Monitor lithium serum concentration, and observe patient's clinical response. Adjust lithium dosage as needed.
NSAIDs, selective cyclooxygenase-2 inhibitors (celecoxib): May result in deterioration of renal function, including possible

---

acute renal failure, in patients who are elderly, volume-depleted (including those on diuretic therapy), or have compromised renal function. May decrease antihypertensive effect of irbesartan. Periodically monitor renal function during coadministration.

Potassium-sparing diuretics, potassium supplements, trimethoprim: May increase risk of hyperkalemia. Closely monitor serum potassium concentration and adjust treatment as needed.

EFFECTS ON LAB TEST RESULTS
None reported.

CONTRAINDICATIONS & CAUTIONS
• Contraindicated in patients hypersensitive to drug or its components.
• Use cautiously in patients with impaired renal function, heart failure, and renal artery stenosis and in breast-feeding women.
Black Box Warning Use during pregnancy can cause injury and death to the developing fetus. When pregnancy is detected, stop drug as soon as possible. ▪
⚠ *Overdose S&S:* Hypotension, tachycardia, bradycardia.

NURSING CONSIDERATIONS
• Drug may be given with a diuretic or other antihypertensive, if needed, for control of hypertension.
• Symptomatic hypotension may occur in volume- or sodium-depleted patients (vigorous diuretic use or dialysis). Correct the cause of volume depletion before administration or before a lower dose is used.
• If hypotension occurs, place patient in a supine position and give an I.V. infusion of normal saline solution, if needed. Once blood pressure has stabilized after a transient hypotensive episode, drug may be continued.
• Dizziness and orthostatic hypotension may occur more frequently in patients with type 2 diabetes and renal disease.

PATIENT TEACHING
• Warn woman of childbearing age of consequences of drug exposure to fetus. Tell her to notify prescriber immediately if pregnancy is suspected.

• Tell patient that drug may be taken without regard to food.
• Tell patient to inform prescriber of other prescription and OTC drugs and supplements he's taking.

SAFETY ALERT!

irinotecan hydrochloride
eh-rin-OH-te-kan

Camptosar

Therapeutic class: Antineoplastics
Pharmacologic class: DNA topoisomerase inhibitors
Pregnancy risk category: D

AVAILABLE FORMS
Injection: 20 mg/mL in 2-, 5-, and 15-mL vials

INDICATIONS & DOSAGES
➤ **Metastatic carcinoma of the colon or rectum that has recurred or progressed after 5-FU therapy**
Adults: Initially, 125 mg/m^2 by I.V. infusion over 90 minutes on days 1, 8, 15, and 22; then 2-week rest period. Thereafter, additional courses of treatment may be repeated every 6 weeks with 4 weeks on and 2 weeks off. Subsequent doses may be adjusted to low of 50 mg/m^2 or maximum of 150 mg/m^2 in 25- to 50-mg/m^2 increments based on patient's tolerance. Or, 350 mg/m^2 by I.V. infusion over 90 minutes once every 3 weeks. Additional courses may continue indefinitely in patients who respond favorably and in those whose disease remains stable, provided intolerable toxicity doesn't occur.
Adjust-a-dose: Consider reducing starting dose in patients age 65 and older, in those who have received pelvic or abdominal radiation, or in those who have a performance status of 2 or increased bilirubin level. Give 300 mg/m^2 by I.V. infusion over 90 minutes once every 3 weeks. Or, give 100 mg/m^2 by I.V. infusion over 90 minutes once weekly.

➤ **First-line therapy for metastatic colorectal cancer with 5-FU and leucovorin**

Regimen 1
Adults: 125 mg/m^2 I.V. over 90 minutes on days 1, 8, 15, and 22; then leucovorin 20 mg/m^2 I.V. bolus on days 1, 8, 15, and 22 and 5-FU 500 mg/m^2 I.V. bolus on days 1, 8, 15, and 22. Courses are repeated every 6 weeks.

Regimen 2
Adults: 180 mg/m^2 I.V. over 90 minutes on days 1, 15, and 29; then leucovorin 200 mg/m^2 I.V. over 2 hours on days 1, 2, 15, 16, 29, and 30; then 5-FU 400 mg/m^2 I.V. bolus on days 1, 2, 15, 16, 29, and 30 and 5-FU 600 mg/m^2 I.V. infusion over 22 hours on days 1, 2, 15, 16, 29, and 30.

Adjust-a-dose: See manufacturer's package insert for details on dosage adjustment.

ADMINISTRATION

I.V.
▼ Drug packaged in plastic blister to protect against inadvertent breakage and leakage. Inspect vial for damage and signs of leakage before removing blister.
▼ Wear gloves while handling and preparing infusion solutions. If drug contacts skin, wash thoroughly with soap and water. If drug contacts mucous membranes, flush thoroughly with water.
▼ Dilute drug in D$_5$W injection (preferred) or normal saline solution for injection before infusion to yield 0.12 to 2.8 mg/mL.
▼ Solution is stable for up to 24 hours at 77° F (25° C) in ambient fluorescent lighting. Solutions diluted in D$_5$W, stored at 36° to 46° F (2° to 8° C), and protected from light are stable for 48 hours. However, because microbial contamination may occur during dilution, use admixture within 24 hours if refrigerated or 6 hours if kept at room temperature. Refrigerating admixtures using normal saline solution isn't recommended because of low and sporadic risk of visible particulate. Don't freeze admixture because drug may precipitate.
▼ Premedicate patient with antiemetic drugs on day of treatment starting at least 30 minutes before giving irinotecan.

▼ Watch for irritation and infiltration; extravasation can cause tissue damage. If extravasation occurs, flush site with sterile water and apply ice. Notify prescriber.
▼ Store vial at 59° to 86° F (15° to 30° C). Protect from light.
▼ **Incompatibilities:** Other I.V. drugs.

ACTION

Interacts with topoisomerase I, inducing reversible single-strand DNA breaks. Drug binds to the topoisomerase I–DNA complex and prevents religation of these single-strand breaks.

Route	Onset	Peak	Duration
I.V.	Unknown	1 hr	Unknown

Half-life: About 6 to 12 hours.

ADVERSE REACTIONS

CNS: asthenia, dizziness, fever, headache, insomnia, pain, akathisia.
CV: edema, vasodilation, orthostatic hypotension.
EENT: rhinitis.
GI: *diarrhea,* abdominal cramping, abdominal pain and enlargement, anorexia, constipation, dyspepsia, flatulence, nausea, stomatitis, vomiting.
Hematologic: anemia, *leukopenia, neutropenia, thrombocytopenia.*
Metabolic: dehydration, weight loss.
Musculoskeletal: back pain.
Respiratory: dyspnea, increased cough.
Skin: alopecia, rash, sweating.
Other: chills, infection.

INTERACTIONS

Drug-drug. *CYP3A4 enzyme-inducing anticonvulsants (phenytoin, phenobarbital, or carbamazepine), rifampin, rifabutin:* May significantly decrease irinotecan levels. For patients requiring anticonvulsant treatment, consider substituting non–enzyme-inducing anticonvulsants at least 2 weeks before start of irinotecan therapy.
Diuretics: May increase risk of dehydration and electrolyte imbalance. Consider stopping diuretic during active periods of nausea and vomiting.
Ketoconazole: May increase irinotecan levels, leading to drug toxicity. Stop ketoconazole at least 1 week before starting

---

Reactions in bold italics are *life-threatening*. Interactions may have a *rapid onset* or a *delayed onset*.

irinotecan therapy. Ketoconazole is contraindicated during irinotecan therapy.

Laxatives: May increase risk of diarrhea. Avoid using together.

Neuromuscular blockers: May prolong the neuromuscular-blocking effects of succinylcholine, and the neuromuscular blockade of nondepolarizing drugs may be antagonized. Monitor patient for prolonged effects of succinylcholine if given together.

Other antineoplastics: May cause additive adverse effects, such as myelosuppression and diarrhea. Monitor patient closely.

Prochlorperazine: May increase risk of akathisia. Monitor patient closely.

Vaccines (killed or inactivated virus): May diminish response to vaccine. Avoid use together.

Vaccines (live-virus): May cause serious or fatal infection. Don't give together.

Drug-herb. *St. John's wort:* May decrease drug levels by about 40%. Use together is contraindicated.

EFFECTS ON LAB TEST RESULTS
- May increase alkaline phosphatase, AST, and bilirubin levels. May decrease hemoglobin level.
- May decrease WBC and neutrophil counts.

CONTRAINDICATIONS & CAUTIONS
- Contraindicated in patients hypersensitive to drug.
- Safety and effectiveness of drug in children haven't been established.
- Use cautiously in elderly patients.
- **⚠ Overdose S&S:** Severe neutropenia, severe diarrhea.

NURSING CONSIDERATIONS
Black Box Warning Administer drug under the supervision of a physician experienced with cancer chemotherapy. ∎

Black Box Warning Drug may cause severe myelosuppression. ∎

- Pelvic or abdominal irradiation may increase risk of severe myelosuppression. Avoid use of drug in patients undergoing irradiation.
- Patients with UGT1A1*28 allele or UGT1A1 7/7 genotype are at increased risk for neutropenia. Patient should be

considered for initial minus 1 level dosage adjustment; monitor patient closely.

- If neutropenic fever occurs or if ANC drops below 500/mm³, temporarily stop therapy. Reduce dosage, especially if WBC count is below 2,000/mm³, neutrophil count is below 1,000/mm³, hemoglobin level is below 8 g/dL, or platelet count is below 100,000/mm³.
- A colony-stimulating factor may be helpful in patients with significant neutropenia.
- Monitor WBC count with differential, hemoglobin level, and platelet count before each dose.

Black Box Warning Drug can cause severe diarrhea. Treat diarrhea occurring within 24 hours of drug administration with 0.25 to 1 mg atropine I.V., unless contraindicated. Treat late diarrhea (more than 24 hours after irinotecan administration) promptly with loperamide. Monitor patient for dehydration, electrolyte imbalance, or sepsis, and treat appropriately. ∎

- Delay subsequent doses until normal bowel function returns for at least 24 hours without antidiarrheal. If grade 2, 3, or 4 late diarrhea occurs, decrease subsequent doses within the current cycle.
- To decrease risk of dehydration, withhold diuretic during treatment and periods of active vomiting or diarrhea.
- **Look alike–sound alike:** Don't confuse irinotecan with topotecan.

PATIENT TEACHING
- Inform patient about risk of diarrhea and methods to treat it; tell him to avoid laxatives.
- Instruct patient to contact prescriber if any of the following occur: diarrhea for the first time during treatment; black or bloody stools; symptoms of dehydration such as light-headedness, dizziness, or faintness; inability to drink fluids due to nausea or vomiting; inability to control diarrhea within 24 hours; or fever or infection.
- Warn patient that hair loss may occur.
- Caution women to avoid pregnancy or breast-feeding during therapy.

iron dextran
DexFerrum, InFeD, Proferdex

Therapeutic class: Iron supplements
Pharmacologic class: Hematinics
Pregnancy risk category: C

AVAILABLE FORMS
1 mL iron dextran provides 50 mg elemental iron.
Injection: 50 mg elemental iron/mL in 1-mL and 2-mL single-dose vials

INDICATIONS & DOSAGES
➤ **Iron deficiency anemia**
Adults and children weighing more than 15 kg (33 lb): I.V. or I.M. test dose is required. (See manufacturer's instructions.) Total dose may be calculated using dosage table in package insert or by using the following formula:

$$\text{Dose (mL)} = 0.0442 \text{ (desired Hb} - \text{observed Hb)} \times \text{LBW} + (0.26 \times \text{LBW})$$

Note: LBW = lean body weight in kg. For males, LBW = 50 kg + 2.3 kg for each inch of patient's height over 5 feet. For females, LBW = 45.5 kg + 2.3 kg for each inch of patient's height over 5 feet.
Children weighing 5 to 15 kg (11 to 33 lb): Use dosage table in package insert or calculate dose as follows:

$$\text{Dose (mL)} = 0.0442 \text{ (desired Hb} - \text{observed Hb)} \times \text{weight in kg} + (0.26 \times \text{weight in kg})$$

I.V.
Adults and children: Inject 0.5-mL test dose over at least 5 minutes. If no reaction occurs in 1 hour, give remainder of therapeutic I.V. dose. Repeat therapeutic I.V. dose daily. Single daily dose shouldn't exceed 100 mg. Give slowly (1 mL/minute). Don't give drug in the first 4 months of life.
I.M. (by Z-track method)
Adults and children: Inject 0.5-mL test dose. If no reaction occurs in 1 hour, give remainder of dose. Daily dose ordinarily shouldn't exceed 0.5 mL (25 mg) for infants weighing less than 5 kg (11 lb); 1 mL (50 mg) for those weighing less than 10 kg (22 lb); and 2 mL (100 mg) for heavier children and adults. Don't give drug in the first 4 months of life.
➤ **Iron replacement for blood loss**
Adults: Replacement iron (in mg) = blood loss (in mL) × hematocrit.
Note: This formula is based on the approximation that 1 mL of normocytic, normochromic red cells contains 1 mg of elemental iron.

ADMINISTRATION
I.V.
▼ Check hospital policy before giving I.V.
▼ After completing I.V. dose, flush the vein with 10 mL of normal saline solution.
▼ Patient should rest for 15 to 30 minutes after I.V. administration.
▼ **Incompatibilities:** Other I.V. drugs, parenteral nutrition solutions for I.V. infusion.
I.M.
● Inject I.M. deep into upper outer quadrant of buttock—never into the arm or other exposed area—with a 2″ to 3″ 19G or 20G needle.
● Use Z-track method to avoid leakage into subcutaneous tissue and staining of skin.
● After drawing up drug, use a new sterile needle to give injection.

ACTION
Provides elemental iron, an essential component in the formation of hemoglobin.

Route	Onset	Peak	Duration
I.V.	Unknown	Unknown	Unknown
I.M.	72 hr	Unknown	3–4 wk

Half-life: 5 to 20 hours.

ADVERSE REACTIONS
CNS: headache, transitory paresthesia, dizziness, malaise, fever, chills, *seizures,* disorientation.
CV: chest pain, tachycardia, *bradycardia,* hypotensive reaction, peripheral vascular flushing.
GI: nausea, anorexia, abdominal pain, diarrhea.
GU: hematuria.
Hematologic: leukocytosis, lymphadenopathy.
Musculoskeletal: arthralgia, myalgia.

Reactions in bold italics are *life-threatening*. Interactions may have a *rapid onset* or a *delayed onset*.

Respiratory: *bronchospasm,* dyspnea, wheezing, *respiratory arrest.*
Skin: rash, urticaria, soreness, inflammation, brown skin discoloration at I.M. injection site, local phlebitis at I.V. injection site, sterile abscess, necrosis, atrophy.
Other: fibrosis, *anaphylaxis, delayed sensitivity reactions.*

INTERACTIONS
Drug-drug. *ACE inhibitors:* Increases risk of adverse systemic reactions. Stop one of the agents if interaction occurs.
Chloramphenicol: May increase iron level. Monitor patient closely.

EFFECTS ON LAB TEST RESULTS
• May cause false increase in bilirubin level and false decrease in calcium level. Use of more than 250 mg iron may color the serum brown. Drug may alter measurement of iron level and total iron-binding capacity for up to 3 weeks; I.M. injection may cause dense areas of activity for 1 to 6 days on bone scans using technetium-99m diphosphonate.

CONTRAINDICATIONS & CAUTIONS
Black Box Warning Fatal anaphylactic reactions have been reported. Fatal reactions have occurred when the test dose was tolerated. Give only when indications have been clearly established and for iron deficiencies not amenable to oral iron therapy. Keep emergency equipment readily available. ■
• Contraindicated in patients hypersensitive to drug, in those with acute infectious renal disease, and in those with any anemia except iron deficiency anemia.
• Use cautiously in patients who have serious hepatic impairment, rheumatoid arthritis, or other inflammatory diseases because these patients may be at higher risk for certain delays and reactions.
• Use cautiously in patients with history of significant allergies or asthma.
⚠ Overdose S&S: Hemosiderosis.

NURSING CONSIDERATIONS
Black Box Warning Observe for signs and symptoms of anaphylactic-type reactions with every dose given. Have epinephrine

immediately available in event of acute hypersensitivity reaction. ■
• Don't give iron dextran with oral iron preparations.
• I.V. or I.M. injections of iron are advisable only for patients in whom oral administration is impossible or ineffective.
• Monitor hemoglobin level, hematocrit, and reticulocyte count.
• Maximum daily dose should not exceed 2 mL undiluted iron dextran.

PATIENT TEACHING
• Teach patient signs and symptoms of hypersensitivity and iron toxicity, and tell him to report them to prescriber.
• Inform patient that drug may stain skin.

iron sucrose injection
Venofer

Therapeutic class: Iron supplements
Pharmacologic class: Hematinics
Pregnancy risk category: B

AVAILABLE FORMS
Injection: 20 mg/mL of elemental iron in 2.5-mL, 3.25-mL, 5-mL, and 10-mL single-dose vials

INDICATIONS & DOSAGES
➤ **Iron deficiency anemia in patients who are hemodialysis dependent and are receiving erythropoietin therapy**
Adults: 100 mg (5 mL) of elemental iron I.V. directly in the dialysis line, either by slow injection over 2 to 5 minutes or by infusion over 15 minutes during the dialysis session one to three times a week to a total of 1,000 mg in 10 doses; repeat as needed.
➤ **Iron deficiency anemia in chronic kidney disease patients not on dialysis**
Adults: 200 mg by undiluted slow I.V. injection over 2 to 5 minutes on five separate occasions in a 14-day period to a total cumulative dose of 1,000 mg.
➤ **Iron deficiency anemia in peritoneal dialysis-dependent chronic kidney disease patients**
Adults: 300 mg I.V. infusion over 90 minutes on two separate occasions 14 days

apart, followed by one 400-mg infusion over 2½ hours 14 days later.

➤ **Maintenance treatment in pediatric patients with hemodialysis-dependent chronic kidney disease, non-dialysis-dependent chronic kidney disease who are receiving erythropoietin, or peritoneal dialysis–dependent chronic kidney disease who are receiving erythropoietin** *Children ages 2 and older:* 0.5 mg/kg I.V. every 2 weeks for 12 weeks. Give undiluted by slow I.V. injection over 5 minutes or diluted in 25 mL normal saline solution and administered over 5 to 60 minutes. May repeat treatment if necessary. Don't give more than 100 mg per dose.

ADMINISTRATION

I.V.

▼ Inspect drug for particulate matter and discoloration before giving.

▼ For infusion, dilute 100 mg elemental iron in a maximum of 100 mL normal saline solution immediately before infusion, and infuse over at least 15 minutes. Dilute dose 300 mg or greater in a maximum of 250 mL normal saline solution.

▼ **Incompatibilities:** Other I.V. drugs, parenteral nutrition solutions.

ACTION

Exogenous source of iron that replenishes depleted body iron stores and is essential for hemoglobin synthesis.

Route	Onset	Peak	Duration
I.V.	Unknown	Unknown	Variable

Half-life: 6 hours.

ADVERSE REACTIONS

CNS: headache, asthenia, malaise, dizziness, fever.
CV: *heart failure,* hypotension, chest pain, hypertension, fluid retention.
GI: nausea, vomiting, diarrhea, abdominal pain, taste perversion.
Metabolic: gout, *hypoglycemia,* hyperglycemia.
Musculoskeletal: leg cramps, bone and muscle pain.
Respiratory: dyspnea, wheezing, pneumonia, cough.
Skin: rash, pruritus, injection-site reaction.

Other: accidental injury, pain, *sepsis, hypersensitivity reactions.*

INTERACTIONS

Drug-drug. *Oral iron preparations:* May reduce absorption of oral iron preparations. Avoid using together.

EFFECTS ON LAB TEST RESULTS

None reported.

CONTRAINDICATIONS & CAUTIONS

• Contraindicated in patients with hypersensitivity to drug or its components, evidence of iron overload, or anemia not caused by iron deficiency.

• Use cautiously in breast-feeding women.

⚠ *Overdose S&S:* Hypotension, dyspnea, headache, vomiting, nausea, dizziness, joint aches, paresthesia, abdominal pain, muscle pain, edema, CV collapse.

NURSING CONSIDERATIONS

⊕ *Alert:* Rare but fatal hypersensitivity reactions, characterized by anaphylactic shock, loss of consciousness, collapse, hypotension, dyspnea, or seizures, may occur. Have epinephrine readily available.

• Mild to moderate hypersensitivity reactions, with wheezing, dyspnea, hypotension, rash, or pruritus, may occur.

• Giving drug by infusion may reduce the risk of hypotension.

• Transferrin saturation level increases rapidly after I.V. administration of drug. Obtain iron level 48 hours after I.V. use.

• Monitor ferritin level, transferrin saturation, hemoglobin level, and hematocrit.

• Withhold dose in patient with signs and symptoms of iron overload.

• Keep dose selection in elderly patients conservative because of decreased hepatic, renal, or cardiac function; other disease; and other drug therapy.

PATIENT TEACHING

• Instruct patient to notify prescriber if symptoms of overdose or allergic reaction occur.

Reactions in bold italics are *life-threatening*. Interactions may have a *rapid onset* or a *delayed onset*.

isoniazid (INH, isonicotinic acid hydrazide)

eye-soe-NYE-a-zid

Isotamine†

Therapeutic class: Antituberculotics
Pharmacologic class: Isonicotinic acid hydrazines
Pregnancy risk category: C

AVAILABLE FORMS
Injection: 100 mg/mL
Oral solution: 50 mg/5 mL
Tablets: 50 mg†, 100 mg, 300 mg

INDICATIONS & DOSAGES
Adjust-a-dose (for all indications): For patients with CrCl of less than 10 mL/minute, give 50% of usual dose. For patients undergoing continuous ambulatory peritoneal dialysis, give 50% of usual dose every 24 hours.

➤ **Actively growing tubercle bacilli**
Adults and children age 15 and older:
5 mg/kg daily P.O. or I.M. in a single daily dose, up to 300 mg/day, with other drugs, continued for 6 months to 2 years. For intermittent multiple-drug regimen, 15 mg/kg (up to 900 mg) P.O. or I.M. up to three times a week.
Infants and children: 10 to 15 mg/kg P.O. or I.M. in a single daily dose, up to 300 mg/day, continued long enough to prevent relapse. Give with at least one other antituberculotic. For intermittent multidrug regimen, 20 to 30 mg/kg (up to 900 mg) P.O. or I.M. two or three times weekly.

➤ **To prevent tubercle bacilli in those exposed to tuberculosis (TB) or those with positive skin test results whose chest X-rays and bacteriologic study results indicate nonprogressive TB**
Adults: 300 mg P.O. daily in a single dose, continued for 6 months to 1 year.
Infants and children: 10 mg/kg P.O. daily in a single dose, up to 300 mg/day, continued for up to 1 year.

➤ **Actively growing tubercle bacilli (once weekly)** ◆
Adults: 15 mg/kg P.O. once/week (not to exceed 900 mg), with other drugs, for a 2-month initial phase and a 4- to 7-month continuation phase.

ADMINISTRATION
P.O.
● Always give drug with other antituberculotics to prevent development of resistant organisms.
● Give drug 1 hour before or 2 hours after meals.
I.M.
● Solution may crystallize at a low temperature. Warm vial to room temperature before use to redissolve crystals.

ACTION
May inhibit cell-wall biosynthesis by interfering with lipid and DNA synthesis; bactericidal.

Route	Onset	Peak	Duration
P.O., I.M.	Unknown	1–2 hr	Unknown

Half-life: 1 to 4 hours.

ADVERSE REACTIONS
CNS: peripheral neuropathy, *seizures, toxic encephalopathy,* memory impairment, toxic psychosis.
EENT: optic neuritis and atrophy.
GI: epigastric distress, nausea, vomiting.
Hematologic: *agranulocytosis, aplastic anemia, thrombocytopenia,* eosinophilia, hemolytic anemia, sideroblastic anemia.
Hepatic: *hepatitis,* bilirubinemia, jaundice.
Metabolic: hyperglycemia, hypocalcemia, hypophosphatemia, *metabolic acidosis.*
Skin: irritation at injection site.
Other: gynecomastia, hypersensitivity reactions, pyridoxine deficiency, rheumatic and lupuslike syndromes.

INTERACTIONS
Drug-drug. *Acetaminophen:* May inhibit acetaminophen metabolism. Monitor patient closely for hepatotoxicity.
Antacids and laxatives containing aluminum: May decrease isoniazid absorption. Give isoniazid at least 1 hour before antacid or laxative.
Benzodiazepines, such as diazepam, triazolam: May inhibit metabolic clearance of benzodiazepines that undergo oxidative metabolism, possibly increasing benzodiazepine activity. Monitor patient for adverse reactions.

Carbamazepine: May increase carbamazepine levels. Monitor drug levels closely.

Cycloserine: May increase CNS adverse reactions. Use safety precautions.

Disulfiram: May cause neurologic symptoms, including changes in behavior and coordination. Avoid using together.

Enflurane: In rapid acetylators of isoniazid, may cause high-output renal failure because of nephrotoxic inorganic fluoride level. Monitor renal function.

Ketoconazole: May decrease ketoconazole level. Monitor patient for lack of efficacy.

Meperidine: May increase CNS adverse reactions and hypotension. Use safety precautions.

Oral anticoagulants: May enhance anticoagulant activity. Monitor PT and INR.

Phenytoin: May inhibit phenytoin metabolism and increase phenytoin level. Monitor patient for phenytoin toxicity.

Rifampin: May increase the risk of hepatotoxicity. Monitor LFTs closely.

Drug-food. *Foods containing tyramine (such as aged cheese, beer, and chocolate):* May cause hypertensive crisis. Tell patient to avoid such foods or eat in small quantities.

Drug-lifestyle. *Alcohol use:* May increase risk of drug-related hepatitis. Discourage use of alcohol.

EFFECTS ON LAB TEST RESULTS

● May increase transaminase, glucose, and bilirubin levels. May decrease calcium, phosphate, and hemoglobin levels.

● May increase eosinophil count. May decrease granulocyte and platelet counts.

● May alter result of urine glucose tests that use cupric sulfate method, such as Benedict reagent and Diastix.

CONTRAINDICATIONS & CAUTIONS

Black Box Warning Contraindicated in patients with acute hepatic disease or isoniazid-related liver damage. Severe and sometimes fatal hepatitis associated with isoniazid therapy may occur even after months of treatment. If signs or symptoms suggest hepatic damage, discontinue isoniazid because a more severe form of liver damage can occur. ∎

● Use cautiously in elderly patients, in those with chronic non–isoniazid-related liver disease or chronic alcoholism, in those with seizure disorders (especially if taking phenytoin), and in those with severe renal impairment.

⚠ *Overdose S&S:* Nausea, vomiting, dizziness, slurring of speech, blurring of vision, visual hallucinations, respiratory distress, CNS depression progressing from stupor to coma, seizures, severe metabolic acidosis, acetonuria, hyperglycemia.

NURSING CONSIDERATIONS

Black Box Warning Drug's pharmacokinetics vary among patients because drug is metabolized in the liver by genetically controlled acetylation. Fast acetylators metabolize drug up to 5 times faster than slow acetylators. About 50% of blacks and whites are fast acetylators; more than 80% of Chinese, Japanese, and Inuits are fast acetylators. A report suggests the risk of fatal hepatitis increases in black and Hispanic women and in the postpartum period. The risk of hepatitis increases with daily alcohol use and with age. ∎

● Peripheral neuropathy is more common in patients who are slow acetylators, malnourished, alcoholic, or diabetic. Give pyridoxine to prevent peripheral neuropathy.

Black Box Warning Monitor and interview patients monthly. For those patients older than age 35, also measure hepatic enzyme levels before and periodically throughout treatment. Elevated LFT results occur in about 15% of patients; most abnormalities are mild and transient, but some may persist throughout treatment and progressive liver dysfunction may occur. ∎

PATIENT TEACHING

● Instruct patient to take drug exactly as prescribed; warn against stopping drug without prescriber's consent.

● Advise patient to take drug 1 hour before or 2 hours after meals.

Black Box Warning Tell patient to notify prescriber immediately if signs and symptoms of liver impairment occur, such as appetite loss, fatigue, malaise, yellow skin or eye discoloration, and dark urine. ∎

Reactions in bold italics are *life-threatening*. Interactions may have a *rapid onset* or a *delayed onset*.

• Advise patient to avoid alcoholic beverages while taking drug. Also tell him to avoid certain foods: fish, such as skipjack tuna, and products containing tyramine, such as aged cheese, beer, and chocolate, because drug has some MAO inhibitor activity.

• Encourage patient to comply fully with treatment, which may take months or years.

isoproterenol hydrochloride
eye-soe-proe-TER-e-nole

Isuprel

Therapeutic class: Bronchodilators
Pharmacologic class: Nonselective beta-adrenergic agonists
Pregnancy risk category: C

AVAILABLE FORMS
Injection: 200 mcg/mL in 1- and 5-mL ampules

INDICATIONS & DOSAGES
➤ **Bronchospasm during anesthesia**
Adults: Dilute 1 mL (0.2 mg) with 10 mL of normal saline solution or D_5W. Give 0.01 to 0.02 mg I.V. and repeat as necessary.
➤ **Heart block, ventricular arrhythmias**
Adults: Initially, 0.02 to 0.06 mg I.V.; then 0.01 to 0.2 mg I.V. or 5 mcg/minute I.V. Or, initially, 0.2 mg I.M.; then 0.02 to 1 mg I.M., as needed.
Children ◆ *:* Initial I.V. infusion of 0.1 mcg/kg/minute. Adjust dosage based on patient's response. Usual dosage range is 0.1 to 1 mcg/kg/minute.
➤ **Shock**
Adults: 0.5 to 5 mcg/minute by continuous I.V. infusion. Usual concentration is 1 mg in 500 mL D_5W. Titrate infusion rate according to heart rate, central venous pressure, blood pressure, and urine flow.

ADMINISTRATION
I.V.
▼ For infusion, dilute with most common I.V. solutions, but don't use with sodium bicarbonate injection; drug decomposes rapidly in alkaline solutions.

▼ Don't use solution if it's discolored or contains precipitate.
▼ Give by direct injection or I.V. infusion.
▼ For shock, closely monitor blood pressure, central venous pressure, ECG, arterial blood gas measurements, and urine output. Carefully titrate infusion rate according to these measurements. Use a continuous infusion pump to regulate flow rate.
▼ Store at room temperature. Protect from light.
▼ **Incompatibilities:** Alkalies, aminophylline, furosemide, metals, sodium bicarbonate.

ACTION
Relaxes bronchial smooth muscle by stimulating $beta_2$ receptors. As a cardiac stimulant, acts on $beta_1$ receptors in the heart.

Route	Onset	Peak	Duration
I.V.	Immediate	Unknown	< 60 min

Half-life: Unknown.

ADVERSE REACTIONS
CNS: headache, mild tremor, weakness, dizziness, nervousness, insomnia, anxiety.
CV: palpitations, rapid rise and fall in blood pressure, tachycardia, angina, *arrhythmias, cardiac arrest, pulmonary edema.*
GI: nausea, vomiting.
Metabolic: hyperglycemia.
Skin: diaphoresis, pallor.
Other: swelling of parotid glands with prolonged use.

INTERACTIONS
Drug-drug. *Aminophylline (I.V.), corticosteroids (I.V.), theophylline:* May cause cardiotoxic effects leading to myocardial necrosis and death. Use together cautiously.
Epinephrine, other sympathomimetics: May increase risk of arrhythmias. Use together cautiously. If used together, give at least 4 hours apart.
Halogenated general anesthetics or cyclopropane: May increase risk of arrhythmias. Avoid using together.
Propranolol, other beta blockers: May block bronchodilating effect of isoproterenol. Monitor patient carefully.

EFFECTS ON LAB TEST RESULTS
• May increase glucose level.

CONTRAINDICATIONS & CAUTIONS
• Contraindicated in patients with tachycardia or AV block caused by digoxin intoxication, arrhythmias other than those that may respond to drug, angina pectoris, or angle-closure glaucoma.
• Contraindicated when used with general anesthetics with halogenated drugs or cyclopropane.
• Use cautiously in elderly patients and in those with renal or CV disease, coronary insufficiency, diabetes, hyperthyroidism, or history of sensitivity to sympathomimetic amines.
⚠ Overdose S&S: Hypotension, hypertension, tachycardia, ventricular tachycardia or fibrillation, palpitations, angina, sudden death.

NURSING CONSIDERATIONS
• Correct volume deficit before giving vasopressors.
❸ Alert: If heart rate exceeds 110 beats/minute during I.V. infusion, notify prescriber. Doses that increase the heart rate to more than 130 beats/minute may induce ventricular arrhythmias.
• Drug may cause a slight increase in systolic blood pressure and a slight to marked decrease in diastolic blood pressure.
• Monitor patient for adverse reactions.
• **Look alike–sound alike:** Don't confuse Isuprel with Isordil.

PATIENT TEACHING
• Tell patient to report chest pain, fluttering in chest, or other adverse reactions.
• Remind patient to report pain at the I.V. injection site.

---

isosorbide dinitrate
eye-soe-SOR-bide

ISDN†, Dilatrate-SR, Isordil

isosorbide mononitrate
Apo-ISMN†, Imdur†, Monoket, PMS-ISMN†, PRO-ISMN†

Therapeutic class: Antianginals
Pharmacologic class: Nitrates
Pregnancy risk category: C; B for mononitrate

AVAILABLE FORMS
isosorbide dinitrate
Capsules (sustained-release): 40 mg
Tablets: 5 mg, 10 mg, 20 mg, 30 mg, 40 mg
Tablets (S.L.): 2.5 mg, 5 mg
Tablets (sustained-release): 40 mg
isosorbide mononitrate
Tablets: 10 mg, 20 mg
Tablets (extended-release): 30 mg, 60 mg, 120 mg

INDICATIONS & DOSAGES
➤ **Acute anginal attacks (S.L. isosorbide dinitrate only); to prevent situations that may cause anginal attacks**
Adults: 2.5 to 5 mg S.L. tablets for prompt relief of angina, repeated every 5 to 10 minutes (maximum of three doses for each 30-minute period). For prevention, 2.5 to 5 mg 15 minutes before anticipated activity likely to cause angina. Or, 5 to 40 mg isosorbide dinitrate P.O. b.i.d. or t.i.d. for prevention only (use smallest effective dose). Or, 20 mg isosorbide mononitrate tablets b.i.d., with the two doses given 7 hours apart. Or, 30 or 60 mg isosorbide mononitrate extended-release tablets once daily. May increase to 120 mg once daily after several days.
➤ **Prevention of variceal rebleeding in combination with a beta-adrenergic blocker (isosorbide mononitrate)** ◆
Adults: In combination with a beta-adrenergic blocker, titrate isosorbide mononitrate dosage up to a maximum of 40 mg P.O. b.i.d.

Reactions in bold italics are *life-threatening*. Interactions may have a *rapid onset* or a *delayed onset*.

ADMINISTRATION
P.O.
● Give patient S.L. tablet at first sign of attack. Tell him to wet tablet with saliva and place under his tongue until absorbed. Dose may be repeated every 10 to 15 minutes for a maximum of three doses.
● Tell patient taking P.O. form of isosorbide dinitrate to swallow oral tablet whole on an empty stomach either 30 minutes before or 1 to 2 hours after meals.
● Store drug in a cool place, in a tightly closed container, and away from light.
● Don't crush or allow patient to chew tablets or capsules.

ACTION
Thought to reduce cardiac oxygen demand by decreasing preload and afterload. Drug also may increase blood flow through the collateral coronary vessels.

Route	Onset	Peak	Duration
P.O.	15–40 min	Unknown	4–8 hr
P.O. (extended-release)	½–4 hr	Unknown	6–12 hr
P.O. (S.L.)	2–5 min	Unknown	1–4 hr

Half-life: dinitrate P.O., 5 to 6 hours; S.L., 2 hours; mononitrate, about 5 hours.

ADVERSE REACTIONS
CNS: headache, dizziness, weakness.
CV: orthostatic hypotension, tachycardia, palpitations, ankle edema, flushing, fainting.
EENT: sublingual burning.
GI: nausea, vomiting.
Skin: cutaneous vasodilation, rash.

INTERACTIONS
Drug-drug. *Antihypertensives:* May increase hypotensive effects. Monitor patient closely during initial therapy.
Sildenafil, tadalafil, vardenafil: May cause life-threatening hypotension. Use of nitrates in any form with these drugs is contraindicated.
Drug-lifestyle. *Alcohol use:* May increase hypotension. Discourage use together.

EFFECTS ON LAB TEST RESULTS
● May falsely reduce value in cholesterol tests using the Zlatkis-Zak color reaction.

CONTRAINDICATIONS & CAUTIONS
● Contraindicated in patients with hypersensitivity or idiosyncrasy to nitrates and in those with severe hypotension, angle-closure glaucoma, increased intracranial pressure, shock, or acute MI with low left ventricular filling pressure.
● Use cautiously in patients with blood volume depletion (such as from diuretic therapy) or mild hypotension.
⚠ Overdose S&S: Venous pooling, decreased cardiac output, hypotension, methemoglobinemia.

NURSING CONSIDERATIONS
● To prevent tolerance, a nitrate-free interval of 10 to 14 hours per day is recommended. The regimen for isosorbide mononitrate (1 tablet on awakening with the second dose in 7 hours, or 1 extended-release tablet daily) is intended to minimize nitrate tolerance by providing a substantial nitrate-free interval.
● Monitor blood pressure and heart rate and intensity and duration of drug response.
● Drug may cause headaches, especially at beginning of therapy. Dosage may be reduced temporarily, but tolerance usually develops. Treat headache with aspirin or acetaminophen.
● Methemoglobinemia has been seen with nitrates. Symptoms are those of impaired oxygen delivery despite adequate cardiac output and adequate arterial partial pressure of oxygen.
● **Look alike–sound alike:** Don't confuse Isordil with Plendil, Isuprel, or Inderal.

PATIENT TEACHING
● Caution patient to take drug regularly, as prescribed, and to keep it accessible at all times.
🟊 Alert: Advise patient that stopping drug abruptly may cause spasm of the coronary arteries with increased angina symptoms and potential risk of heart attack.
● Tell patient to take S.L. tablet at first sign of attack. He should wet tablet with saliva and place under his tongue until absorbed; he should sit down and rest. Dose may be repeated every 10 to 15 minutes for a maximum of three doses. If drug doesn't

provide relief, tell patient to seek medical help promptly.

• Advise patient who complains of tingling sensation with S.L. drug to try holding tablet in cheek.

• Warn patient not to confuse S.L. with P.O. form.

• Advise patient taking P.O. form of isosorbide dinitrate to take oral tablet on an empty stomach either 30 minutes before or 1 to 2 hours after meals and to swallow oral tablets whole.

• Tell patient to minimize dizziness upon standing up by changing to upright position slowly. Advise him to go up and down stairs carefully and to lie down at first sign of dizziness.

• Caution patient to avoid alcohol because it may worsen low blood pressure effects.

• Advise patient that use of sildenafil, tadalafil, or vardenafil with any nitrate may cause severe low blood pressure. Patient should talk to his prescriber before using these drugs together.

• Instruct patient to store drug in a cool place, in a tightly closed container, and away from light.

isotretinoin
eye-so-TRET-i-noyn

Absorica, Amnesteem, Claravis, Myorisan, Sotret, Zenatane

Therapeutic class: Antiacne drugs
Pharmacologic class: Retinoic acid derivatives
Pregnancy risk category: X

AVAILABLE FORMS
Capsules: 10 mg, 20 mg, 30 mg, 40 mg

INDICATIONS & DOSAGES
➤ **Severe nodular acne that's unresponsive to conventional therapy**
Adults and adolescents: 0.5 to 2 mg/kg P.O. daily in two divided doses with food for 15 to 20 weeks.

ADMINISTRATION
P.O.
• Before use, have patient read patient information and sign accompanying consent form.

• Give drug with or shortly after meals to facilitate absorption.

ACTION
May normalize keratinization, reversibly decrease size of sebaceous glands, and make sebum less viscous and less likely to plug follicles.

Route	Onset	Peak	Duration
P.O.	Unknown	3 hr	Unknown

Half-life: 21 to 24 hours.

ADVERSE REACTIONS
CNS: pseudotumor cerebri, depression, *psychosis, suicidal ideation or attempts, suicide, aggressive and violent behavior,* emotional instability, headache, fatigue.
EENT: conjunctivitis, epistaxis, drying of mucous membranes, dry nose, corneal deposits, dry eyes, hearing impairment (sometimes irreversible), decreased night vision, visual disturbances.
GI: nonspecific GI symptoms, nausea, vomiting, abdominal pain, dry mouth, anorexia, gum bleeding and inflammation, *acute pancreatitis,* inflammatory bowel disease.
Hematologic: increased erythrocyte sedimentation rate, anemia, *thrombocytosis.*
Hepatic: *hepatitis.*
Metabolic: hypertriglyceridemia, hyperglycemia.
Musculoskeletal: *rhabdomyolysis,* skeletal hyperostosis, tendon and ligament calcification, premature epiphyseal closure, decreased bone mineral density and other bone abnormalities, back pain, arthralgia, arthritis, tendinitis.
Skin: cheilitis, cheilosis, fragility, rash, dry skin, facial skin desquamation, petechiae, pruritus, nail brittleness, thinning of hair, skin infection, peeling of palms and toes, photosensitivity reaction.

INTERACTIONS
Drug-drug. *Corticosteroids:* May increase risk of osteoporosis. Use together cautiously.
Medicated soaps, cleansers, and coverups; preparations containing alcohol; topical resorcinol peeling agents (benzoyl peroxide): May have cumulative drying effect. Use together cautiously.
Micro-dose progesterone hormonal contraceptives ("minipills") that don't contain estrogen: May decrease effectiveness of contraceptive. Advise patient to use different contraceptive method.
Phenytoin: May increase risk of osteomalacia. Use together cautiously.
Products containing vitamin A, vitamin A: May increase toxic effects of isotretinoin. Avoid using together.
Tetracyclines: May increase risk of pseudotumor cerebri. Avoid using together.
Drug-food. *Any food:* May increase absorption of drug. Advise patient to take drug with milk, a meal, or shortly after a meal.
Drug-lifestyle. *Alcohol use:* May increase risk of hypertriglyceridemia. Discourage use together.
Sun exposure: May increase photosensitivity reaction. Advise patient to avoid excessive sunlight exposure.

EFFECTS ON LAB TEST RESULTS
• May increase AST, ALT, alkaline phosphatase, triglyceride, glucose, and uric acid levels.
• May decrease serum HDL levels.
• May increase platelet count and erythrocyte sedimentation rate.

CONTRAINDICATIONS & CAUTIONS
• Contraindicated in patients hypersensitive to parabens (used as preservatives), vitamin A, or other retinoids.
Black Box Warning Because of an extremely high risk of severe birth defects, drug is contraindicated in woman of childbearing potential, unless patient has had two negative pregnancy test results before beginning therapy, will begin drug therapy on second or third day of next menstrual period, and will comply with stringent contraceptive measures for 1 month before

therapy, during therapy, and for at least 1 month after therapy. ■
• Use cautiously in patients with a history of mental illness or a family history of psychiatric disorders, asthma, liver disease, diabetes, heart disease, osteoporosis, genetic predisposition for age-related osteoporosis, history of childhood osteoporosis, weak bones, anorexia nervosa, osteomalacia, or other disorders of bone metabolism.
⚠ Overdose S&S: Vomiting, facial flushing, abdominal pain, headache, dizziness, ataxia.

NURSING CONSIDERATIONS
• Patient must have negative results from two urine or serum pregnancy tests; one is performed in the office when the patient is qualified for therapy, the second during the first 5 days of the next normal menstrual period immediately preceding the beginning of therapy. For patients with amenorrhea, the second test should be done at least 11 days after the last unprotected act of sexual intercourse. A pregnancy test must be repeated every month before the patient receives the prescription.
Black Box Warning If pregnancy does occur during treatment, discontinue drug immediately and refer patient to an obstetrician-gynecologist experienced in reproductive toxicity. ■
• Monitor baseline lipid studies, LFTs, and pregnancy tests before therapy and at monthly intervals.
• Regularly monitor glucose level and CK levels in patients who participate in vigorous physical activity.
• Most adverse reactions occur at doses exceeding 1 mg/kg daily. Reactions are generally reversible when therapy is stopped or dosage is reduced.
◆ Alert: If patient experiences headache, nausea and vomiting, or visual disturbances, screen for papilledema. Signs and symptoms of pseudotumor cerebri require stopping the drug immediately and beginning neurologic interventions promptly.
Black Box Warning To minimize the risk of fetal exposure, the drug is only available through a restricted FDA-approved distribution program called iPLEDGE. ■

• A second course of therapy may begin 8 weeks after completion of the first course, if necessary. Improvements may continue after first course is complete.

• Patients may be at increased risk of bone fractures or injury when participating in sports with repetitive impact.

• Spontaneous reports of osteoporosis, osteopenia, bone fractures, and delayed healing of bone fractures have occurred in patients taking drug. To decrease this risk, don't exceed recommended doses and duration.

• **Look alike–sound alike:** Don't confuse Accutane with Accupril or Accolate.

PATIENT TEACHING

Black Box Warning Warn woman of childbearing age that, if this drug is used during pregnancy, severe fetal abnormalities may occur. Advise her to either abstain from sex or use two reliable forms of contraception simultaneously for 1 month before, during, and for 1 month after treatment. An isotretinoin medication guide must be given to the patient each time isotretinoin is dispensed, as required by law. ■

• Advise patient to take drug with or shortly after meals to facilitate absorption.

• Tell patient to immediately report visual disturbances and bone, muscle, or joint pain.

• Warn patient that contact lenses may feel uncomfortable during therapy.

• Advise patient not to drive at night until effect on vision is known. Drug may decrease night vision.

• Warn patient against using abrasives, medicated soaps and cleansers, acne preparations containing peeling drugs, and topical products containing alcohol (including cosmetics, aftershave, cologne) because they may cause cumulative irritation or excessive drying of skin.

• Tell patient to avoid prolonged sun exposure and to use sunblock. Drug may have additive effect if used with other drugs that cause photosensitivity reaction.

• Warn patient that transient exacerbations may occur during therapy.

• Warn patient not to donate blood during therapy and for 1 month after stopping drug because drug could harm fetus of a pregnant recipient.

• Tell patient to report adverse reactions immediately, especially depression, suicidal thoughts, persistent headaches, and persistent GI pain.

• Advise patient to read iPLEDGE carefully and to fully understand all information before signing it.

itraconazole
eye-tra-KON-a-zole

Onmel, Sporanox

Therapeutic class: Antifungals
Pharmacologic class: Synthetic triazoles
Pregnancy risk category: C

AVAILABLE FORMS
Capsules: 100 mg
Oral solution: 10 mg/mL
Tablets: 200 mg

INDICATIONS & DOSAGES

➤ **Pulmonary and extrapulmonary blastomycosis, nonmeningeal histoplasmosis**
Adults: 200 mg P.O. daily; increase as needed and tolerated by 100 mg to maximum of 400 mg daily. Give dosages exceeding 200 mg P.O. daily in two divided doses. Continue treatment for at least 3 months. In life-threatening illness, give a loading dose of 200 mg P.O. t.i.d. for 3 days.

➤ **Aspergillosis**
Adults: 200 to 400 mg P.O. daily.

➤ **Onychomycosis of the toenail (with or without fingernail involvement)**
Adults: 200 mg P.O. once daily for 12 consecutive weeks.

➤ **Onychomycosis of the fingernail**
Adults: 200 mg P.O. b.i.d. for 1 week, followed by 3 weeks drug-free. Repeat dosage.

➤ **Oropharyngeal candidiasis**
Adults: 200 mg oral solution swished in mouth vigorously and swallowed daily, for 1 to 2 weeks.

➤ **Oropharyngeal candidiasis in patients unresponsive to fluconazole tablets**
Adults: 100 mg oral solution swished in mouth vigorously and swallowed b.i.d., for 2 to 4 weeks.

Reactions in bold italics are *life-threatening*. Interactions may have a *rapid onset* or a *delayed onset*.

➤ Esophageal candidiasis

Adults: 100 to 200 mg oral solution swished in mouth vigorously and swallowed daily, for at least 3 weeks. Treatment should continue for 2 weeks after symptoms resolve.

ADMINISTRATION

P.O.

• Before starting therapy, confirm diagnosis of onychomycosis by sending nail specimens for testing.
• Don't interchange capsules and oral solution.
• Give capsules and tablets with a full meal.
• Give oral solution on an empty stomach if possible.

ACTION

Interferes with fungal cell-wall synthesis by inhibiting ergosterol formation and increasing cell-wall permeability, leading to osmotic instability.

Route	Onset	Peak	Duration
P.O.	Unknown	3–4 hr	Unknown

Half-life: 32 to 96 hours.

ADVERSE REACTIONS

CNS: headache, fever, dizziness, somnolence, fatigue, malaise, asthenia, pain, tremor, abnormal dreams, anxiety, depression.
CV: *heart failure,* hypertension, edema, orthostatic hypotension.
EENT: rhinitis, sinusitis, pharyngitis.
GI: nausea, vomiting, diarrhea, abdominal pain, anorexia, dyspepsia, flatulence, increased appetite, constipation, gastritis, gastroenteritis, ulcerative stomatitis, gingivitis.
GU: albuminuria.
Hematologic: *neutropenia.*
Hepatic: *hepatotoxicity, liver failure,* impaired hepatic function.
Metabolic: hypokalemia, hypertriglyceridemia.
Musculoskeletal: myalgia.
Respiratory: *pulmonary edema,* upper respiratory tract infection.
Skin: rash, pruritus.
Other: decreased libido, injury, herpes zoster, hypersensitivity reactions (urticaria, *angioedema, Stevens-Johnson syndrome*).

INTERACTIONS

Drug-drug. *Alprazolam:* May increase and prolong drug levels, CNS depression, and psychomotor impairment. Avoid using together.
*Antacids, carbamazepine, H₂-receptor antagonists, isoniazid, phenobarbital, **phenytoin**, rifabutin, rifampin:* May decrease itraconazole level. Avoid using together.
Chlordiazepoxide, clonazepam, clorazepate, diazepam, estazolam, flurazepam, quazepam: May increase and prolong drug levels, CNS depression, and psychomotor impairment. Avoid using together.
Clarithromycin, erythromycin: May increase itraconazole levels. Monitor patient for signs of itraconazole toxicity.
*Cyclosporine, **digoxin**, tacrolimus:* May increase levels of these drugs. Monitor drug levels.
Black Box Warning *Dofetilide, ergometrine, ergot alkaloids, ergotamine, felodipine, levacetylmethadol, lovastatin, methadone, methylergotamine, midazolam (oral), nisoldipine, pimozide, quinidine, simvastatin, triazolam:* May increase levels of these drugs by CYP450 metabolism, causing serious CV events, including torsades de pointes, QT-interval prolongation, ventricular tachycardia, cardiac arrest, and sudden death. Use together is contraindicated. ■
HMG-CoA reductase inhibitors (atorvastatin, fluvastatin, pravastatin): May increase levels and adverse effects of these drugs. Avoid using together, or reduce dose of HMG-CoA reductase inhibitor.
NNRTIs (nevirapine): May decrease itraconazole level. Use together isn't recommended.
Oral anticoagulants: May enhance anticoagulant effect. Monitor PT and INR.
Oral antidiabetics: May cause hypoglycemia, similar to effect of other antifungals. Monitor glucose level. Avoid using together.
PDE5 inhibitors (sildenafil, tadalafil, vardenafil): May increase levels of these drugs, increasing adverse effects. Give PDE5 inhibitors with caution and in reduced doses.

Protease inhibitors (boceprevir, indinavir, ritonavir, saquinavir, telaprevir): May increase levels of these drugs; indinavir and ritonavir may increase itraconazole levels. Monitor patient for toxicity.

EFFECTS ON LAB TEST RESULTS
● May increase alkaline phosphatase, ALT, AST, bilirubin, triglyceride, and GGT levels. May decrease potassium level.

CONTRAINDICATIONS & CAUTIONS
Black Box Warning Contraindicated in patients hypersensitive to drug; in those receiving alprazolam, dofetilide, ergometrine, ergot alkaloids, ergotamine, felodipine, levacetylmethadol, lovastatin, methadone, methylergotamine, midazolam (oral), nisoldipine, pimozide, quinidine, simvastatin, or triazolam; and in those with ventricular dysfunction or a history of heart failure. If signs and symptoms of heart failure occur, stop itraconazole. ∎
● Use cautiously in patients with hypochlorhydria; they may not absorb drug readily.
● Use cautiously in HIV-infected patients because hypochlorhydria can accompany HIV infection.
● Use cautiously in patients receiving other highly bound drugs.
● Don't use to treat onychomycosis in pregnant women or those contemplating pregnancy.
● Drug appears in breast milk. If patient is breast-feeding, weigh expected benefits of therapy for the mother against potential risk to the infant.

NURSING CONSIDERATIONS
❸ *Alert:* Oral solution isn't interchangeable with other forms.
● Perform baseline LFTs and monitor results periodically. In patients with baseline hepatic impairment, give drug only if patient's condition is life threatening. If liver dysfunction occurs during therapy, notify prescriber immediately.

PATIENT TEACHING
● Teach patient to recognize and report signs and symptoms of liver disease

(anorexia, dark urine, pale stools, unusual fatigue, and jaundice).
● Instruct patient not to use oral solution interchangeably with capsules or tablets.
● For the oral solution, tell patient to take 10 mL at a time.
● Advise patient to take solution without food and to take capsules or tablets with a full meal.
● Urge patient to list the other drugs he's taking for prescriber to avoid drug interactions.
● Advise women of childbearing age that an effective form of contraception must be used during therapy and for two menstrual cycles after stopping therapy with capsules or tablets.

SAFETY ALERT!

ixabepilone
ecks-ah-BEH-pill-own

Ixempra

Therapeutic class: Antineoplastics
Pharmacologic class: Microtubule inhibitors
Pregnancy risk category: D

AVAILABLE FORMS
Injection: 15-mg, 45-mg vials

INDICATIONS & DOSAGES
➤ **With capecitabine for metastatic or locally advanced breast cancer, after failure of anthracycline and a taxane; or alone for metastatic or locally advanced breast cancer, after failure of anthracycline, taxanes, and capecitabine**
Adults: 40 mg/m^2 I.V. over 3 hours every 3 weeks. Doses for patients with BSA greater than 2.2 m^2 should be calculated based on 2.2 m^2. Premedicate with an H$_1$-receptor antagonist, such as diphenhydramine 50 mg P.O., and an H$_2$-receptor antagonist, such as ranitidine 150 to 300 mg P.O., 1 hour before ixabepilone infusion. For patients who experienced a prior hypersensitivity reaction, premedicate with corticosteroids (such as dexamethasone 20 mg I.V. 30 minutes before infusion or

P.O. 60 minutes before infusion) in addition to the H_1- and H_2-receptor antagonists.

Adjust-a-dose: If toxicities occur, refer to package insert for adjustments for monotherapy and combination therapy.

In patients with hepatic impairment receiving combination therapy who have an AST or ALT up to 2.5 times the upper limit of normal (ULN) or bilirubin up to 1 × ULN, the standard dose may be given. Treatment is contraindicated with higher AST, ALT, or bilirubin levels. Patients with moderate hepatic impairment receiving monotherapy should be started at 20 mg/m². The dosage in subsequent cycles may be increased to 30 mg/m² if tolerated. Use in patients with AST or ALT greater than 10 × ULN or bilirubin greater than 2 × ULN isn't recommended. Refer to package insert for additional guidance.

ADMINISTRATION

I.V.

▼ Protect drug from light.

▼ Keep refrigerated. Let stand at room temperature for 30 minutes before administration.

▼ The white precipitate in diluent will clear at room temperature.

▼ Drug may be a contact irritant; handle and give with care. Wear gloves and avoid inhaling vapors.

▼ Reconstitute drug before use, using supplied diluent, to a concentration of 15 mg/8 mL or 45 mg/23.5 mL. Gently swirl and invert vial.

▼ Before giving drug, further dilute with lactated Ringer solution supplied in di(2-ethylhexyl) phthalate (DEHP)–free bags. Final concentration should yield 0.2 to 0.6 mg/mL.

▼ Infuse within 6 hours of preparation.

▼ Administer through a 0.2- to 1.2-micron in-line filter, using a DEHP-free administration set.

▼ **Incompatibilities:** Unknown. Don't give with other I.V. drugs.

ACTION

Causes cell death by inhibiting cell division.

Route	Onset	Peak	Duration
I.V.	Rapid	3 hr	3 wk

Half-life: 52 hours.

ADVERSE REACTIONS

CNS: insomnia, peripheral neuropathy, headache, fatigue, asthenia, dizziness, fever, pain.

CV: edema, chest pain.

EENT: increased lacrimation.

GI: anorexia, taste disorder, nausea, vomiting, stomatitis, mucositis, diarrhea, constipation, abdominal pain, GERD.

Hematologic: *febrile neutropenia, leukopenia,* anemia, *thrombocytopenia.*

Hepatic: *acute hepatic failure,* jaundice.

Metabolic: dehydration, weight loss.

Musculoskeletal: myalgia, arthralgia, skeletal pain.

Respiratory: upper respiratory tract infection, dyspnea, cough.

Skin: alopecia, rash, nail disorder, palmar-plantar erythrodysesthesia disorder, pruritus, exfoliation, hyperpigmentation.

Other: hypersensitivity reactions, hot flush.

INTERACTIONS

Drug-drug. *CYP3A4 inducers (carbamazepine, dexamethasone, phenobarbital, phenytoin, rifabutin, rifampicin, rifampin):* May decrease ixabepilone level, causing treatment failure. Avoid using together.

CYP3A4 inhibitors (amprenavir, atazanavir, clarithromycin, delavirdine, indinavir, itraconazole, ketoconazole, nefazodone, nelfinavir, ritonavir, saquinavir, telithromycin, voriconazole): May increase ixabepilone level. Avoid using together. If use together is necessary, decrease ixabepilone dose according to manufacturer's instructions.

Drug-herb. *St. John's wort:* May decrease drug level. Discourage use together.

Drug-food. *Grapefruit juice:* May increase drug level. Discourage use together.

EFFECTS ON LAB TEST RESULTS

● May increase bilirubin, AST, and ALT levels.

● May decrease neutrophil, WBC, RBC, and platelet counts.

CONTRAINDICATIONS & CAUTIONS
• Contraindicated in patients hypersensitive to drug or its components.
• Contraindicated in patients with neutrophil counts less than 1,500 cells/mm^3 or platelet count less than 100,000 cells/mm^3.

Black Box Warning Contraindicated in patients with AST or ALT greater than 2.5 × ULN or bilirubin greater than 1 × ULN in combination with capecitabine because of increased risk of toxicity and neutropenia-related death. ∎

• Use cautiously in patients with cardiac disease.
• Drug may cause fetal harm if taken during pregnancy.

NURSING CONSIDERATIONS
• Monitor baseline and periodic CBC and liver enzymes and adjust dose as needed.
• Premedicate with H$_1$- and H$_2$-receptor antagonists 1 hour before infusion to avoid hypersensitivity reaction. If patient experiences a hypersensitivity reaction, also premedicate with corticosteroids.
• Monitor cardiac function. Discontinue drug in those who develop cardiac ischemia or impaired cardiac function.
• In patients with CNS changes, be aware that drug contains dehydrated alcohol.
• Monitor for signs of peripheral neuropathy, hypersensitivity reactions, or infections.
• Peripheral neuropathy is generally reversible and should be managed by dose adjustment and delays.
• Drug may cause fetal harm. Tell patient to avoid becoming pregnant.
• Because of drug's potential risk, breast-feeding should be stopped or drug should be stopped. ∎
• Elderly patients have a greater risk of grade 3 or 4 adverse effects when used with capecitabine.

PATIENT TEACHING
• Tell patient to report numbness or tingling of hands or feet.
• Advise patient to call prescriber for temperature above 100.5° F (38° C) or signs of infections such as chills, cough, or pain or burning on urination.

• Advise patient to call prescriber for skin rash, itching, flushing, swelling, difficulty breathing, or chest tightness.
• Tell patient that he will need periodic blood testing during treatment.
• Tell patient not to drink grapefruit juice while taking drug.
• **🛈 Alert:** Advise patient that ixabepilone contains alcohol. Avoid dangerous activities such as driving or operating machinery if dizzy or drowsy.
• Caution women of childbearing age to avoid pregnancy and breast-feeding during therapy.

ketoconazole (oral)
kee-toe-KOE-na-zole

Nizoral

Therapeutic class: Antifungals
Pharmacologic class: Imidazole derivatives
Pregnancy risk category: C

AVAILABLE FORMS
Tablets: 200 mg

INDICATIONS & DOSAGES
Black Box Warning Drug should only be used when other effective antifungal therapy isn't available or tolerated and the potential benefits outweigh the potential risks. ∎
➤ **Fungal infections (coccidioidomycosis, blastomycosis, histoplasmosis, chromomycosis, and paracoccidioidomycosis)**
Adults: Initially, 200 mg P.O. daily in a single dose. May increase dosage to 400 mg once daily in patients who don't respond. Maximum dosage is 400 mg once daily.
Children age 2 and older: 3.3 to 6.6 mg/kg P.O. daily in a single dose. Maximum dosage is 400 mg once daily.

ADMINISTRATION
P.O.
• For patient with achlorhydria, dissolve each tablet in 4 mL aqueous solution of 0.2 N hydrochloric acid and have patient sip solution through a glass or plastic straw. Then have patient drink a glass of water

---

because drug needs gastric acidity for dissolution and absorption.

• Patient should wait at least 2 hours after dose before taking antacids, anticholinergics, and H_2-receptor antagonists.

ACTION

Interferes with fungal cell-wall synthesis by inhibiting formation of ergosterol and increasing cell-wall permeability that makes the fungus susceptible to osmotic instability.

Route	Onset	Peak	Duration
P.O.	Unknown	1–2 hr	Unknown

Half-life: 8 hours.

ADVERSE REACTIONS

CNS: *suicidal tendencies,* severe depression.

GI: nausea, vomiting, abdominal pain, diarrhea.

Hematologic: *leukopenia, thrombocytopenia.*

Hepatic: *fatal hepatotoxicity.*

Skin: pruritus.

INTERACTIONS

Drug-drug. *Aliskiren:* May increase aliskiren level. Monitor therapy.

Alosetron: May increase alosetron serum concentration. Monitor therapy.

Amphotericin B: May decrease therapeutic effect of amphotericin B. Monitor therapeutic effect.

Antacids, anticholinergics, H_2-receptor antagonists: May decrease ketoconazole absorption. Wait at least 2 hours after ketoconazole dose before giving these drugs.

Bosentan: May increase risk of bosentan-related adverse effects. Monitor patient closely.

Buspirone: May increase buspirone level and risk of adverse effects. Reduce initial dosage of buspirone and adjust dosage as needed.

Calcium channel blockers metabolized by CYP3A4 pathway (amlodipine, felodipine, nicardipine, nifedipine): May increase plasma concentrations of calcium channel blockers and risk of adverse effects. Monitor plasma concentrations; reduce dosage of calcium channel blockers if needed.

Carbamazepine: May increase carbamazepine level. Closely monitor carbamazepine plasma level.

Chlordiazepoxide, clonazepam, clorazepate, diazepam, estazolam, flurazepam, midazolam, quazepam, triazolam: May increase and prolong levels of these drugs. May cause CNS depression and psychomotor impairment. Avoid using together.

Cilostazol: May increase cilostazol level and risk of cilostazol-related adverse effects such as headache. Consider reducing cilostazol dosage by 50%.

Cyclosporine, methylprednisolone, tacrolimus: May increase levels of these drugs. Monitor drug levels, if appropriate.

Digoxin: May increase digoxin level. Monitor digoxin level.

Docetaxel: May prolong clearance of docetaxel by 50%. Consider reducing docetaxel dosage.

Eplerenone: May cause hyperkalemia and hypotension. Use together is contraindicated.

Ergot alkaloids: May cause severe vasospasm and cerebral or extremity ischemia. Use together is contraindicated.

Fentanyl: May increase fentanyl level. Monitor fentanyl-related adverse effects and reduce fentanyl dosage if needed.

HMG-CoA reductase inhibitors (atorvastatin, fluvastatin, lovastatin, pravastatin, simvastatin): May increase levels and adverse effects of these drugs. Use together is contraindicated.

Indinavir: May increase indinavir plasma concentration. Reduce indinavir dosage if needed.

Isoniazid, rifampin, rifabutin: May decrease ketoconazole level. Use together isn't recommended.

Methylprednisolone: May alter methylprednisolone metabolism and methylprednisolone level. Adjust methylprednisolone dosage if needed.

Nevirapine: May alter nevirapine metabolism. Use together isn't recommended.

Nisoldipine: May increase nisoldipine level. Use together is contraindicated.

Oral antidiabetics: May cause hypoglycemia. Monitor glucose level.

K

Paclitaxel: May increase paclitaxel level. Monitor patient carefully.

PDE5 inhibitors (sildenafil, tadalafil, vardenafil): May increase levels of these drugs. Use together cautiously and reduce dosage of PDE5 inhibitor.

Phenytoin: May alter metabolism of one or both drugs. Monitor patient for adverse effects.

Ritonavir: May increase bioavailability of ketoconazole. When used together, maximum dosage of ketoconazole is 200 mg/day.

Sirolimus: May increase sirolimus level. Use together isn't recommended.

Telithromycin: May alter telithromycin metabolism. Use cautiously and monitor patient for telithromycin-related adverse effects.

Theophylline: May decrease theophylline level. Monitor theophylline level.

Tolterodine: May increase tolterodine level. Consider reducing tolterodine dosage by 50%.

Verapamil: May increase verapamil serum concentration. Use together cautiously.

Vinca alkaloids (vinblastine, vincristine, vinorelbine): May inhibit metabolism of vinca alkaloids. Monitor patient closely for vinca alkaloid–related toxicities.

Warfarin: May enhance effects of anticoagulant. Monitor PT and INR and adjust dosage as needed.

Drug-herb. *Yew:* May inhibit drug metabolism. Discourage use together.

Drug-lifestyle. *Alcohol use:* May cause disulfiram-like reaction (flushing, rash, peripheral edema, nausea, headache). Don't use together.

EFFECTS ON LAB TEST RESULTS

● May increase lipid, alkaline phosphatase, ALT, and AST levels.

● May decrease hemoglobin level and platelet and WBC counts.

CONTRAINDICATIONS & CAUTIONS

● Contraindicated in patients hypersensitive to drug or its components.

Black Box Warning Administration with dofetilide, pimozide, quinidine, or cisapride is contraindicated because ketoconazole can cause elevated levels of these drugs

and prolong the QT interval, resulting in life-threatening ventricular arrhythmias. ∎

Black Box Warning Drug can cause serious hepatotoxicity that may be fatal or require liver transplantation, even in patients with no obvious risk factors for liver disease. Drug is contraindicated in patients with acute or chronic liver disease. ∎

● Neuropsychiatric disturbances, including suicidal tendency and depression, have occurred rarely in patients taking drug.

● Drug decreases adrenal corticosteroid secretions at doses of 400 mg. Don't exceed recommended dose of 400 mg.

● Women taking ketoconazole shouldn't breast-feed.

NURSING CONSIDERATIONS

🛈 *Alert:* Because of risk of hepatotoxicity, drug shouldn't be used for less serious conditions, such as fungal infections of the skin or nails.

Black Box Warning Because of increased risk of hepatotoxicity, monitor patient for signs and symptoms of hepatotoxicity, including elevated liver enzyme levels, nausea that doesn't subside, unusual fatigue, jaundice, dark urine, or pale stool. ∎

🛈 *Alert:* Drug is a potent inhibitor of the CYP450 enzyme system. Giving this drug with drugs metabolized by CYP3A4 may lead to increased drug levels, which could increase or prolong therapeutic and adverse effects.

● Monitor adrenal function in patients with adrenal insufficiency or borderline adrenal function and in those experiencing prolonged periods of stress (such as major surgery).

● Assess liver function status (AST, ALT, total bilirubin, alkaline phosphatase, PT, and INR) before starting drug.

● Measure ALT level weekly for duration of treatment. If ALT levels increase above the upper limit of normal or 30% above baseline, or if patient develops signs and symptoms of hepatotoxicity, obtain a full set of LFTs. Repeat LFTs to ensure normalization of values. If drug is restarted, monitor patient frequently.

Reactions in bold italics are *life-threatening*. Interactions may have a *rapid onset* or a *delayed onset*.

• Review all medications patient is receiving for potential drug interactions with ketoconazole.

PATIENT TEACHING

• Instruct patient with achlorhydria to dissolve each tablet in 4 mL aqueous solution of 0.2 N hydrochloric acid, sip mixture through a glass or plastic straw, and then drink a glass of water because drug needs gastric acidity for dissolution and absorption.

• Instruct patient to wait at least 2 hours after dose before taking antacids, anticholinergics, or H$_2$-receptor antagonists.

• Make sure patient understands that treatment should continue until all tests indicate that active fungal infection has subsided. If drug is stopped too soon, infection will recur. Treatment for systemic fungal infections may last 6 months.

• Reassure patient that nausea is common early in therapy but will subside. To minimize nausea, instruct patient to divide daily amount into two doses or to take drug with meals.

• Review signs and symptoms of hepatotoxicity with patient; instruct him to stop drug and notify prescriber if they occur.

• Instruct patient to immediately report irregular heartbeats, palpitations, feeling faint, dizziness, or light-headedness.

• Advise patient to discuss any new drugs or herbal supplements he may be taking with prescriber.

ketoconazole (topical)

kee-toe-KOE-na-zole

Extina, Ketoderm†, Ketozole, Nizoral, Nizoral A-D ◊, Xolegel

Therapeutic class: Antifungals
Pharmacologic class: Imidazoles
Pregnancy risk category: C

AVAILABLE FORMS

Cream: 2%
Foam: 2%
Gel: 2%
Shampoo: 1% ◊, 2%

INDICATIONS & DOSAGES

➤ **Seborrheic dermatitis in immunocompetent patients**
Adults and children age 12 and older: Apply foam to affected area b.i.d. for 4 weeks. Apply gel to affected area once daily for 2 weeks.

➤ **Tinea corporis, tinea cruris, tinea pedis, tinea versicolor from susceptible organisms; seborrheic dermatitis; cutaneous candidiasis**
Adults: Cover affected and immediate surrounding areas daily for at least 2 weeks. For seborrheic dermatitis, apply b.i.d. for 4 weeks. Patients with tinea pedis need 6 weeks of treatment.

➤ **Scaling caused by dandruff**
Adults: Using shampoo, wet hair, lather, and massage for 1 minute. Rinse hair thoroughly with warm water, then repeat. Leave drug on scalp for 3 minutes, then rinse and dry hair with towel or warm air flow. Shampoo twice weekly for 4 weeks, with at least 3 days between shampoos and then intermittently, as needed, to maintain control.

ADMINISTRATION

Topical
• Don't let drug come in contact with eyes.

ACTION

Probably inhibits yeast growth by altering the permeability of the cell membrane.

Route	Onset	Peak	Duration
Topical	Unknown	Unknown	Unknown

Half-life: Unknown.

ADVERSE REACTIONS

Skin: abnormal hair texture; increase in normal hair loss; irritation, pruritus, oiliness, or dryness of hair and scalp with shampoo use; scalp pustules; severe irritation, pruritus, and stinging with cream.

INTERACTIONS

None known.

EFFECTS ON LAB TEST RESULTS

None reported.

K

CONTRAINDICATIONS & CAUTIONS
• Contraindicated in patients hypersensitive to drug or its components.
• Use cautiously in pregnant and breast-feeding women.
• Ketoconazole cream contains sulfites that may cause allergic reactions, including anaphylaxis, in susceptible patients.

NURSING CONSIDERATIONS
• Most patients show improvement soon after treatment begins.
• Treatment of tinea corporis or tinea cruris should continue for at least 2 weeks to reduce possibility of recurrence.
⚠ Alert: Product contains sodium sulfite anhydrous, which may cause severe or life-threatening allergic reactions, including anaphylaxis, in patients with asthma.

PATIENT TEACHING
• Tell patient to stop drug and notify prescriber if hypersensitivity reaction occurs.
• Advise patient to check with prescriber if condition worsens; drug may have to be stopped and diagnosis reevaluated.
• Tell patient to avoid using shampoo on scalp if skin is broken or inflamed.
• Warn patient that shampoo applied to permanent-waved hair removes curl.
• Warn patient to avoid drug contact with eyes.
• Tell patient to continue drug for intended duration of therapy, even if signs and symptoms improve soon after starting treatment.
• Tell patient not to store drug above room temperature (77° F [25° C]) and to protect from light.

ketoprofen
kee-toe-PROE-fen

Therapeutic class: NSAIDs
Pharmacologic class: NSAIDs
Pregnancy risk category: C; D in 3rd trimester

AVAILABLE FORMS
Capsules: 25 mg, 50 mg, 75 mg
Capsules (extended-release): 100 mg, 150 mg, 200 mg

INDICATIONS & DOSAGES
Adjust-a-dose (for all indications): For patients age 75 and older, reduce dosage. For patients with mildly impaired renal function, maximum daily dose is 150 mg. For patients with GFR of less than 25 mL/minute/1.73 m^2, ESRD, or impaired liver function and serum albumin level less than 3.5 g/dL, maximum daily dose is 100 mg.
➤ **Rheumatoid arthritis, osteoarthritis**
Adults: 75 mg P.O. t.i.d. or 50 mg P.O. q.i.d., or 200 mg as an extended-release capsule once daily. Maximum dose is 300 mg daily, or 200 mg daily for extended-release capsules.
➤ **Mild to moderate pain, dysmenorrhea**
Adults: 25 to 50 mg P.O. every 6 to 8 hours p.r.n. Maximum dose is 300 mg daily.

ADMINISTRATION
P.O.
• Give drug 30 minutes before or 2 hours after meals with a full glass of water. If adverse GI reactions occur, drug may be given with milk or meals.
• Don't open extended-release capsules.

ACTION
Unknown. Produces anti-inflammatory, analgesic, and antipyretic effects, possibly by inhibiting prostaglandin synthesis.

Route	Onset	Peak	Duration
P.O.	1–2 hr	30–120 min	3–4 hr
P.O. (extended-release)	2–3 hr	6–7 hr	Unknown

Half-life: 2 to 5½ hours for extended-release forms.

ADVERSE REACTIONS
CNS: headache, dizziness, CNS excitation (insomnia, nervousness, and dreams) or CNS depression (somnolence and malaise).
CV: peripheral edema.
EENT: tinnitus, visual disturbances.
GI: dyspepsia, abdominal pain, anorexia, constipation, diarrhea, flatulence, nausea, stomatitis, vomiting.
GU: *nephrotoxicity,* UTI signs and symptoms.
Skin: photosensitivity reactions, rash.

Reactions in bold italics are *life-threatening*. Interactions may have a *rapid onset* or a *delayed onset*.

INTERACTIONS

Drug-drug. *Aspirin, corticosteroids:* May increase risk of adverse GI reactions. Avoid using together.

Aspirin, probenecid: May increase ketoprofen level. Avoid using together.

Cyclosporine: May increase nephrotoxicity. Avoid using together.

Hydrochlorothiazide, other diuretics: May decrease diuretic effectiveness. Monitor patient for lack of effect.

Lithium, methotrexate, phenytoin: May increase levels of these drugs, leading to toxicity. Monitor patient closely.

Warfarin: May increase risk of bleeding. Monitor patient closely.

Drug-herb. *Dong quai, feverfew, garlic, ginger, horse chestnut, red clover:* May cause bleeding based on the known effects of components. Discourage use together.

White willow: Herb and drug contain similar components. Discourage use together.

Drug-lifestyle. *Alcohol use:* May cause GI toxicity. Discourage use together.

Sun exposure: May cause photosensitivity reactions. Advise patient to avoid excessive sunlight exposure.

EFFECTS ON LAB TEST RESULTS

● May increase creatinine, BUN, ALT, and AST levels.
● May increase bleeding time.
● May increase or decrease iron test results.
● May falsely increase bilirubin level.

CONTRAINDICATIONS & CAUTIONS

● Contraindicated in patients hypersensitive to drug and in those with history of aspirin- or NSAID-induced asthma, urticaria, or other allergic reactions.

Black Box Warning Contraindicated for the treatment of perioperative pain after CABG surgery. ∎

● Use during pregnancy only if potential benefit outweighs the risk. Avoid use during last trimester.

● Drug isn't recommended for children or breast-feeding women.

● Use cautiously in patients with history of peptic ulcer disease, renal dysfunction, hypertension, heart failure, or fluid retention.

⚠ **Overdose S&S:** Lethargy, drowsiness, nausea, vomiting, epigastric pain, respiratory depression, coma, seizures, GI bleeding, hypotension, hypertension, acute renal failure.

NURSING CONSIDERATIONS

● Don't use sustained-release form for patients in acute pain.

● Because NSAIDs impair synthesis of renal prostaglandins, they can decrease renal blood flow and lead to reversible renal impairment, especially in patients with renal or heart failure or liver dysfunction, in elderly patients, and in those taking diuretics. Monitor these patients closely.

● Check renal and hepatic function every 6 months or as indicated.

● Drug decreases platelet adhesion and aggregation, and can prolong bleeding time about 3 to 4 minutes from baseline.

Black Box Warning NSAIDs cause an increased risk of serious GI adverse events, including bleeding, ulceration, and perforation of the stomach or intestines, which can occur at any time during use and without warning signs and symptoms and can be fatal. Elderly patients are at greater risk. ∎

Black Box Warning NSAIDs may increase the risk of serious thrombotic events, MI, or stroke, which can be fatal. The risk may be greater with longer use or in patients with CV disease or risk factors for CV disease. ∎

● NSAIDs may mask signs and symptoms of infection because of their antipyretic and anti-inflammatory actions.

PATIENT TEACHING

● Tell patient to take drug 30 minutes before or 2 hours after meals with a full glass of water. If adverse GI reactions occur, patient may take drug with milk or meals.

● Tell patient not to open extended-release capsules.

● Tell patient that full therapeutic effect may be delayed for 2 to 4 weeks.

● Teach patient signs and symptoms of GI bleeding, including blood in vomit, urine, or stool; coffee-ground vomit; and black, tarry stools. Tell him to notify prescriber immediately if any of these occurs.

K

• Alert patient that using with aspirin, alcohol, other NSAIDs, or corticosteroids may increase risk of adverse GI reactions.
• Warn patient to avoid hazardous activities that require mental alertness until CNS effects are known.
• Because of possibility of sensitivity to the sun, advise patient to use a sunblock, wear protective clothing, and avoid prolonged exposure to sunlight.
• Instruct patient to report problems with vision or hearing immediately.
• Tell patient to protect drug from direct light and excessive heat and humidity.

ketorolac tromethamine (ophthalmic)
KEE-toe-role-ak

Acular, Acular LS, Acuvail

Therapeutic class: Anti-inflammatory drugs (ophthalmic)
Pharmacologic class: NSAIDs
Pregnancy risk category: C

AVAILABLE FORMS
Acular
Ophthalmic solution: 0.5%
Acular LS
Ophthalmic solution: 0.4%
Acuvail
Ophthalmic solution: 0.45%

INDICATIONS & DOSAGES
➤ **Relief from ocular itching caused by seasonal allergic conjunctivitis (Acular)**
Adults and children age 3 and older: 1 drop into conjunctival sac in each eye q.i.d.
➤ **Relief of postoperative inflammation in patients who have had cataract extraction (Acular)**
Adults and children age 3 and older: 1 drop to affected eye q.i.d. beginning 24 hours after cataract surgery and continuing through first 2 weeks of postoperative period.
➤ **Reduce ocular pain, burning, and stinging after corneal refractive surgery (Acular LS)**
Adults and children age 3 and older: 1 drop q.i.d. to affected eye, as needed, for up to 4 days after surgery.

➤ **Reduce pain and inflammation after cataract surgery (Acuvail)**
Adults: 1 drop b.i.d. to affected eye beginning 1 day before surgery, continuing on day of surgery, and through first 2 weeks after surgery.

ADMINISTRATION
Ophthalmic
• Apply light finger pressure on lacrimal sac for 1 minute after instillation.
• Store drug away from heat in a dark, tightly closed container and protect from freezing.

ACTION
Thought to inhibit the action of cyclo-oxygenase, an enzyme responsible for prostaglandin synthesis. Prostaglandins mediate the inflammatory response and cause miosis.

Route	Onset	Peak	Duration
Ophthalmic	Unknown	Unknown	Unknown

Half-life: 4 hours.

ADVERSE REACTIONS
CNS: headache (Acular LS).
EENT: transient stinging and burning on instillation, conjunctival hyperemia, corneal edema, corneal infiltrates, iritis, ocular edema and ocular pain (Acular LS), ocular inflammation (Acular), ocular irritation, ocular pain, superficial keratitis, superficial ocular infections.
Other: hypersensitivity reactions.

INTERACTIONS
None significant.

EFFECTS ON LAB TEST RESULTS
None reported.

CONTRAINDICATIONS & CAUTIONS
• Contraindicated in patients hypersensitive to components of drug and in those wearing soft contact lenses.
• Use cautiously in patients with bleeding disorders, in those receiving other drugs that may prolong bleeding time, and in those hypersensitive to other NSAIDs or aspirin.
• Use cautiously in breast-feeding women.

Nursing2015
DRUG
HANDBOOK®

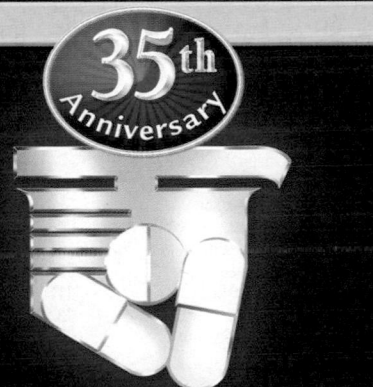

35th Anniversary

Photoguide to tablets and capsules

This photoguide includes over 450 tablets and capsules, representing the most commonly prescribed generic and trade name drugs. These drugs, organized alphabetically by generic name, are shown in actual size and color with cross-references to drug information. Each product is labeled with its trade name and its strength.

INDEX OF TRADE NAMES IN PHOTOGUIDE TO TABLETS AND CAPSULES

ACAMPROSATE CALCIUM

Campral
(Page 72)

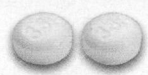

333 mg

ALENDRONATE SODIUM

Fosamax
(Page 95)

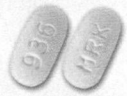 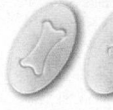

10 mg   40 mg   70 mg

ALFUZOSIN HYDROCHLORIDE

Uroxatral
(Page 97)

10 mg

ALPRAZOLAM

Xanax
(Page 105)

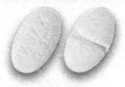 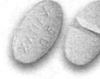 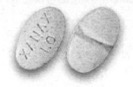

0.25 mg   0.5 mg   1 mg

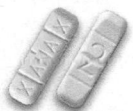

2 mg

AMLODIPINE BESYLATE

Norvasc
(Page 124)

 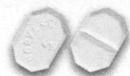

2.5 mg   5 mg

ANASTROZOLE

Arimidex
(Page 139)

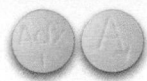

1 mg

ARIPIPRAZOLE

Abilify
(Page 148)

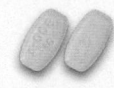 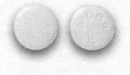 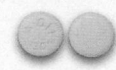

| 10 mg | 15 mg | 30 mg |

ATAZANAVIR SULFATE

Reyataz
(Page 158)

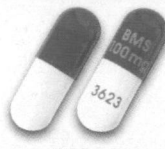 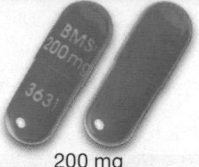

| 100 mg | 200 mg |

ATENOLOL

Tenormin
(Page 164)

 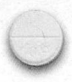 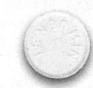

| 25 mg | 50 mg | 100 mg |

ATOMOXETINE HYDROCHLORIDE

Strattera
(Page 165)

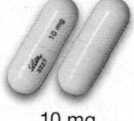 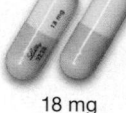 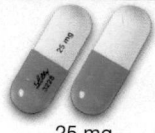

| 10 mg | 18 mg | 25 mg |

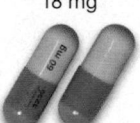

| 40 mg | 60 mg |

ATORVASTATIN CALCIUM

Lipitor
(Page 167)

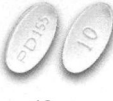 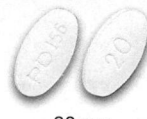 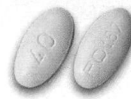

| 10 mg | 20 mg | 40 mg |

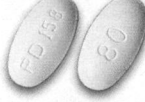

| 80 mg |

AZITHROMYCIN

Zithromax
(Page 187)

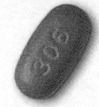 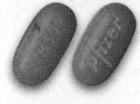 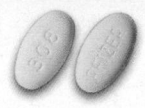

| 250 mg | 500 mg | 600 mg |

BENAZEPRIL HYDROCHLORIDE

Lotensin
(Page 201)

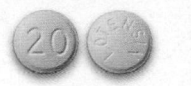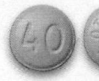

20 mg   40 mg

BUPROPION HYDROCHLORIDE

Wellbutrin
(Page 244)

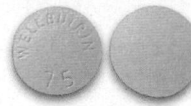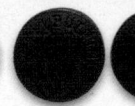

75 mg   100 mg

Wellbutrin SR
(Page 244)

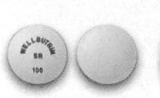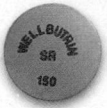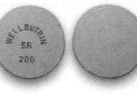

100 mg   150 mg   200 mg

Zyban
(Page 244)

150 mg

CARISOPRODOL

Soma
(Page 272)

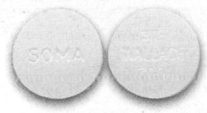

350 mg

CELECOXIB

Celebrex
(Page 303)

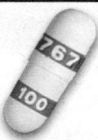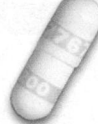

100 mg   200 mg

CIPROFLOXACIN

Cipro
(Page 329)

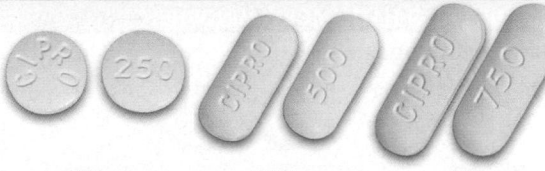

250 mg   500 mg   750 mg

CITALOPRAM HYDROBROMIDE

Celexa
(Page 338)

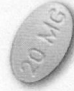

20 mg   40 mg

CLARITHROMYCIN

Biaxin
(Page 341)

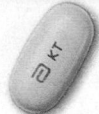   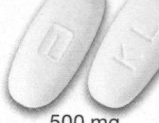

250 mg   500 mg

Biaxin XL
(Page 341)

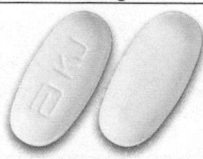

500 mg

CLONAZEPAM

Klonopin
(Page 354)

                    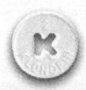

0.5 mg   1 mg   2 mg

CLOPIDOGREL BISULFATE

Plavix
(Page 359)

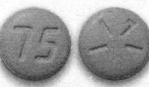

75 mg

CLOZAPINE

Clozaril
(Page 362)

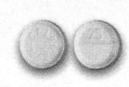   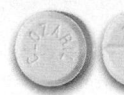

25 mg   100 mg

CODEINE PHOSPHATE—ACETAMINOPHEN

Tylenol with Codeine #3
(Page 367)

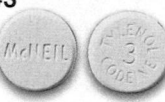

30 mg/300 mg

COLCHICINE

Colcrys
(Page 369)

0.6 mg

COLESEVELAM HYDROCHLORIDE

Welchol
(Page 370)

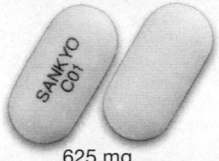

625 mg

DABIGATRAN ETEXILATE MESYLATE

Pradaxa
(Page 385)

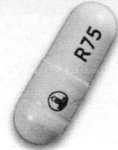

75 mg   150 mg

DARIFENACIN HYDROBROMIDE

Enablex
(Page 397)

7.5 mg   15 mg

DESLORATADINE

Clarinex
(Page 418)

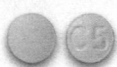

5 mg

DESVENLAFAXINE SUCCINATE

Pristiq
(Page 422)

50 mg   100 mg

DEXLANSOPRAZOLE

Dexilant
(Page 428)

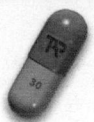   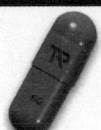

30 mg   60 mg

DEXMETHYLPHENIDATE HYDROCHLORIDE

Focalin XR
(Page 429)

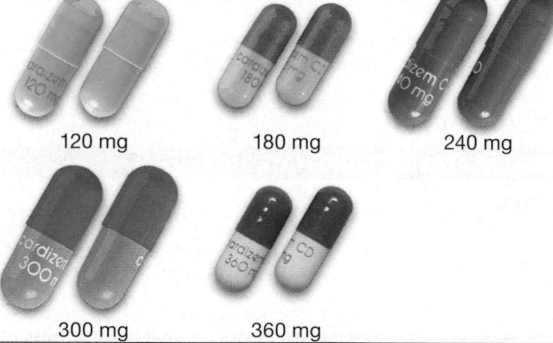

5mg   10 mg   15 mg

20 mg   30 mg   40 mg

DIAZEPAM

Valium
(Page 435)

2 mg   5 mg   10 mg

DILTIAZEM HYDROCHLORIDE

Cardizem
(Page 450)

30 mg   90 mg

Cardizem CD
(Page 450)

120 mg   180 mg   240 mg

300 mg   360 mg

Cardizem LA
(Page 450)

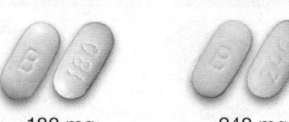

180 mg   240 mg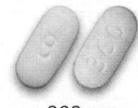

360 mg

DIVALPROEX SODIUM

Depakote
(Page 1437)

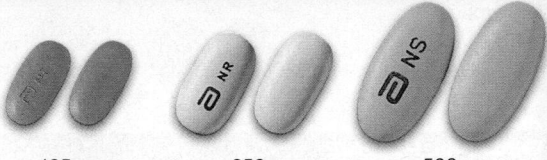

125 mg   250 mg   500 mg

Depakote Sprinkle
(Page 1437)

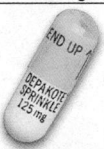

125 mg

DONEPEZIL HYDROCHLORIDE

Aricept
(Page 469)

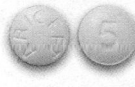

5 mg   10 mg

DOXAZOSIN MESYLATE

Cardura
(Page 474)

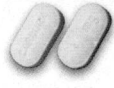   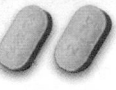   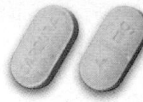

1 mg   2 mg   4 mg

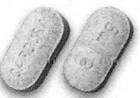

8 mg

DULOXETINE HYDROCHLORIDE

Cymbalta
(Page 494)

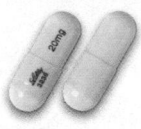   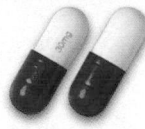   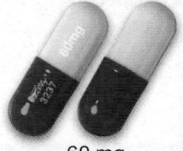

20 mg   30 mg   60 mg

DUTASTERIDE

Avodart
(Page 496)

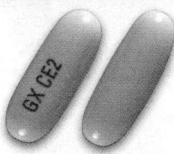

0.5 mg

ELETRIPTAN HYDROBROMIDE

Relpax
(Page 501)

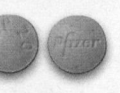

20 mg   40 mg

ENALAPRIL MALEATE

Vasotec
(Page 507)

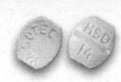   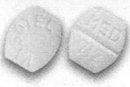   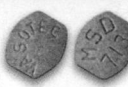

2.5 mg   5 mg   10 mg

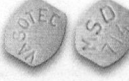

20 mg

ERYTHROMYCIN BASE

Eryc
(Page 537)

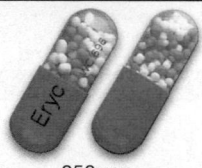

250 mg

Ery-Tab
(Page 537)

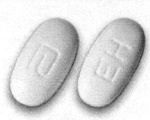

333 mg

ESCITALOPRAM OXALATE

Lexapro
(Page 540)

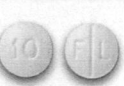   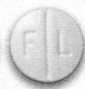

10 mg   20 mg

ESOMEPRAZOLE MAGNESIUM

Nexium
(Page 544)

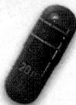   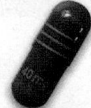

20 mg   40 mg

ESTROGENS (CONJUGATED)

Premarin
(Page 559)

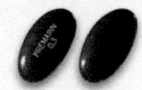   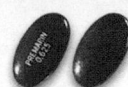

0.3 mg   0.45 mg   0.625 mg

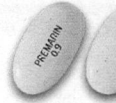   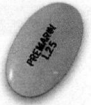

0.9 mg   1.25 mg

ESZOPICLONE

Lunesta
(Page 564)

      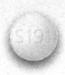

1 mg   2 mg   3 mg

EZETIMIBE

Zetia
(Page 589)

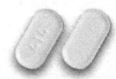

10 mg

EZETIMIBE—SIMVASTATIN

Vytorin
(Page 1535)

          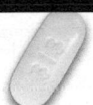

10 mg/10 mg   10 mg/20 mg   10 mg/40 mg

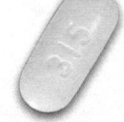

10 mg/80 mg

FAMCICLOVIR

Famvir
(Page 592)

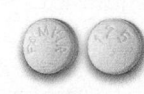   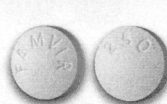   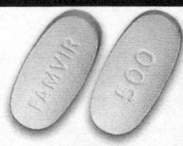

125 mg   250 mg   500 mg

FAMOTIDINE

Pepcid
(Page 593)

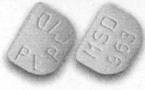

20 mg   40 mg

FENOFIBRATE

TriCor
(Page 597)

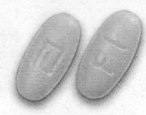

48 mg   145 mg

FINASTERIDE

Proscar
(Page 613)

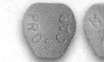

5 mg

FLUCONAZOLE

Diflucan
(Page 618)

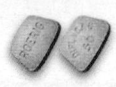   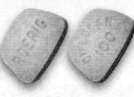   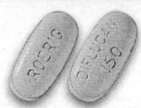

50 mg   100 mg   150 mg

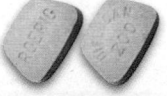

200 mg

FLUOXETINE HYDROCHLORIDE

Prozac
(Page 630)

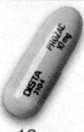   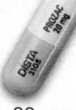   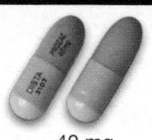

10 mg   20 mg   40 mg

Prozac Weekly
(Page 630)

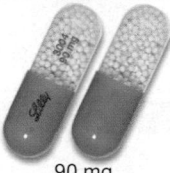

90 mg

Sarafem
(Page 630)

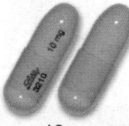   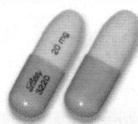

10 mg   20 mg

FLUVASTATIN SODIUM

Lescol
(Page 644)

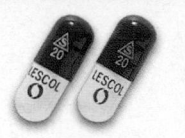 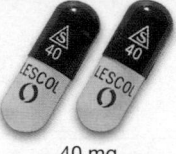

20 mg   40 mg

FROVATRIPTAN SUCCINATE

Frova
(Page 662)

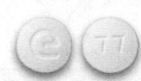

2.5 mg

FUROSEMIDE

Lasix
(Page 664)

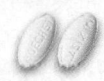   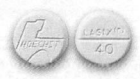   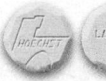

20 mg   40 mg   80 mg

GABAPENTIN

Neurontin
(Page 667)

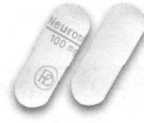   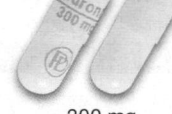   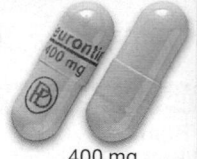

100 mg   300 mg   400 mg

GEMFIBROZIL

Lopid
(Page 676)

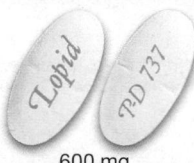

600 mg

GLIMEPIRIDE

Amaryl
(Page 684)

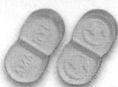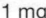   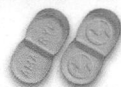   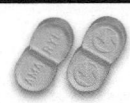

1 mg   2 mg   4 mg

GLIPIZIDE

Glucotrol
(Page 686)

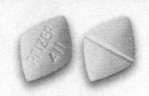 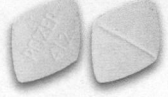

5 mg   10 mg

Glucotrol XL
(Page 686)

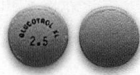   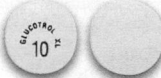

2.5 mg   5 mg   10 mg

GLYBURIDE

DiaBeta
(Page 687)

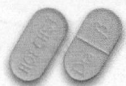 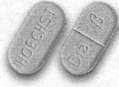 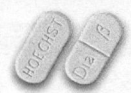

1.25 mg   2.5 mg   5 mg

HYDROCODONE BITARTRATE—ACETAMINOPHEN

Lortab
(Page 704)

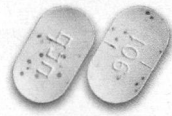

5 mg/500 mg

IBANDRONATE SODIUM

Boniva
(Page 720)

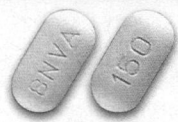

150 mg

INDINAVIR SULFATE

Crixivan
(Page 748)

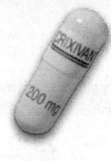 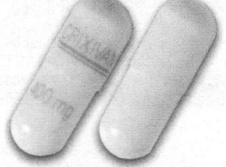

200 mg   400 mg

IRBESARTAN

Avapro
(Page 782)

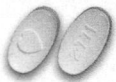 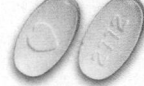 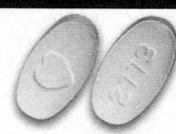

75 mg   150 mg   300 mg

LAMIVUDINE—ZIDOVUDINE

Combivir
(Page 1532)

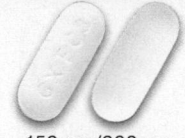

150 mg/300 mg

LANSOPRAZOLE

Prevacid
(Page 821)

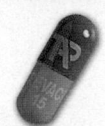

15 mg

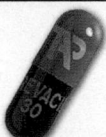

30 mg

LEVODOPA— CARBIDOPA

Sinemet
(Page 835)

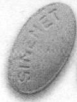

100 mg/10 mg

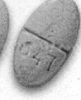

250 mg/25 mg

Sinemet CR
(Page 835)

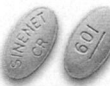

100 mg/25 mg

LEVODOPA—CARBIDOPA—ENTACAPONE

Stalevo
(Page 837)

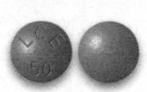

50 mg/12.5 mg/
200 mg

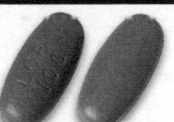

100 mg/25 mg/
200 mg

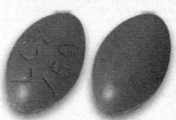

150 mg/37.5 mg/
200 mg

LEVOFLOXACIN

Levaquin
(Page 839)

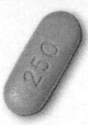

250 mg

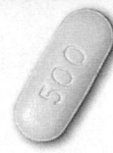

500 mg

LEVOTHYROXINE SODIUM

Levoxyl
(Page 845)

25 mcg

50 mcg

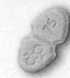
75 mcg

88 mcg

100 mcg

112 mcg

125 mcg

137 mcg

150 mcg

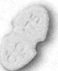
175 mcg

200 mcg

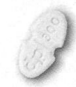
300 mcg

Synthroid
(Page 845)

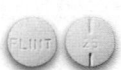
25 mcg

50 mcg

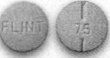
75 mcg

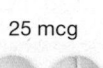
88 mcg

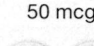
100 mcg

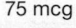
112 mcg

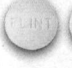
125 mcg

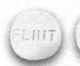
150 mcg

175 mcg

200 mcg

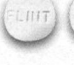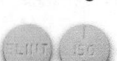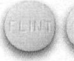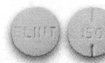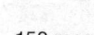
300 mcg

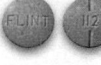

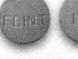

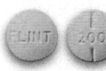
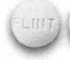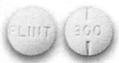

LISDEXAMFETAMINE DIMESYLATE

Vyvanse
(Page 857)

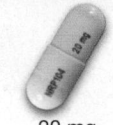 20 mg

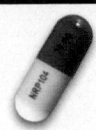 30 mg

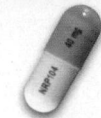 40 mg

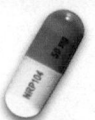 50 mg

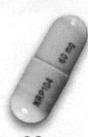 60 mg

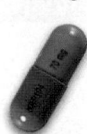 70 mg

LISINOPRIL

Prinivil
(Page 859)

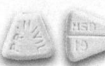 5 mg

 10 mg

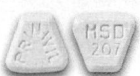 20 mg

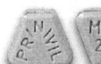 40 mg

Zestril
(Page 859)

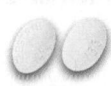 2.5 mg

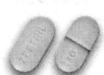 5 mg

 10 mg

 20 mg

 40 mg

LOPINAVIR – RITONAVIR

Kaletra
(Page 869)

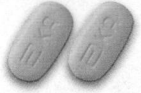 200 mg/50 mg

LORAZEPAM

Ativan
(Page 874)

 0.5 mg

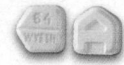 1 mg

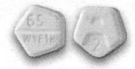 2 mg

LOSARTAN POTASSIUM

Cozaar
(Page 877)

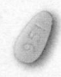 

25 mg   50 mg

LUBIPROSTONE

Amitiza
(Page 1559)

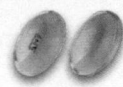

24 mcg

MEDROXYPROGESTERONE ACETATE

Provera
(Page 894)

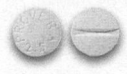   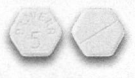   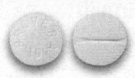

2.5 mg   5 mg   10 mg

MEMANTINE HYDROCHLORIDE

Namenda
(Page 902)

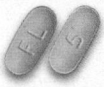   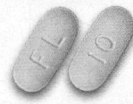

5 mg   10 mg

MEPERIDINE HYDROCHLORIDE

Demerol
(Page 903)

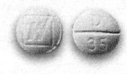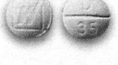

50 mg   100 mg

METFORMIN HYDROCHLORIDE

Glucophage
(Page 911)

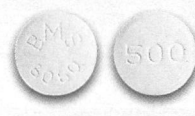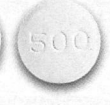   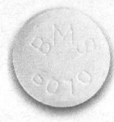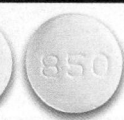

500 mg   850 mg

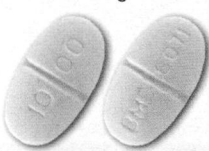

1,000 mg

Glucophage XR
(Page 911)

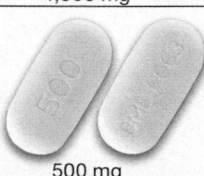

500 mg

METHYLPHENIDATE HYDROCHLORIDE

Concerta
(Page 925)

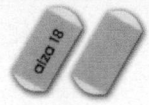 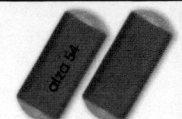

18 mg   36 mg   54 mg

Ritalin
(Page 925)

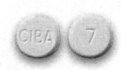 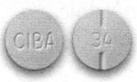

5 mg   10 mg   20 mg

Ritalin-SR
(Page 925)

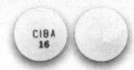

20 mg

METHYLPREDNISOLONE

Medrol
(Page 929)

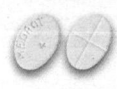

4 mg   16 mg

METOPROLOL SUCCINATE

Toprol-XL
(Page 937)

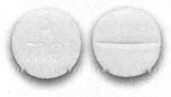  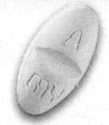

50 mg   100 mg   200 mg

METOPROLOL TARTRATE

Lopressor
(Page 937)

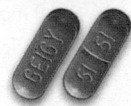 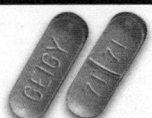

50 mg   100 mg

MILNACIPRAN HYDROCHLORIDE

Savella
(Page 843)

 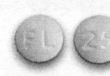 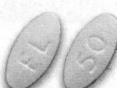

12.5 mg   25 mg   50 mg

MODAFANIL

Provigil
(Page 964)

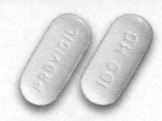
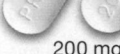

100 mg   200 mg

MONTELUKAST SODIUM

Singulair
(Page 970)

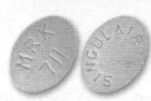

4 mg   5 mg   10 mg

MOXIFLOXACIN HYDROCHLORIDE

Avelox
(Page 978)

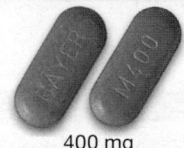

400 mg

NAPROXEN

Naprosyn
(Page 991)

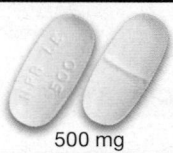

500 mg

NEBIVOLOL HYDROCHLORIDE

Bystolic
(Page 997)

2.5 mg   5 mg   10 mg

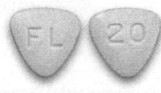

20 mg

NIFEDIPINE

Procardia XL
(Page 1007)

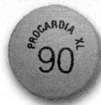

30 mg   60 mg   90 mg

NITROFURANTOIN MACROCRYSTALS

Macrodantin
(Page 1015)

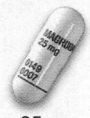 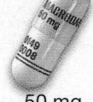 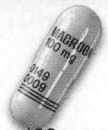

25 mg   50 mg   100 mg

NITROGLYCERIN

Nitrostat
(Page 1016)

0.4 mg

NORTRIPTYLINE HYDROCHLORIDE

Pamelor
(Page 1026)

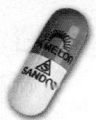 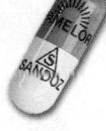 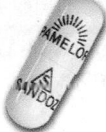

10 mg   25 mg   50 mg

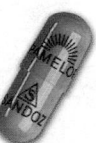

75 mg

OLANZAPINE

Zyprexa
(Page 1037)

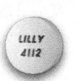 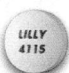

2.5 mg   5 mg   7.5 mg

 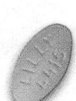

10 mg   15 mg   20 mg

OLMESARTAN MEDOXOMIL

Benicar
(Page 1040)

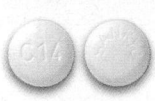 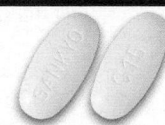

20 mg   40 mg

OLMESARTAN MEDOXOMIL—HYDROCHLOROTHIAZIDE

Benicar HCT
(Page 1527)

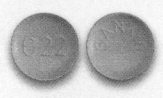

20 mg/12.5 mg   40 mg/12.5 mg   40 mg/25 mg

OMEGA-3-ACID ETHYL ESTERS

Lovaza
(Page 1045)

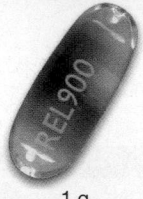

1 g

OMEPRAZOLE

Prilosec
(Page 1046)

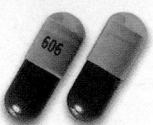   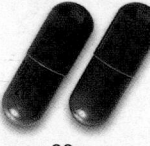   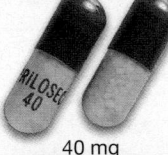

10 mg   20 mg   40 mg

OXYCODONE HYDROCHLORIDE

OxyContin
(Page 1069)

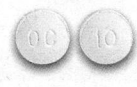   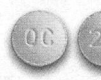   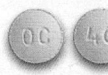

10 mg   20 mg   40 mg

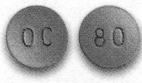

80 mg

PANTOPRAZOLE SODIUM

Protonix
(Page 1094)

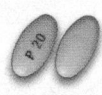   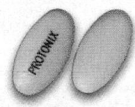

20 mg   40 mg

PENTOXIFYLLINE

Trental
(Page 1576)

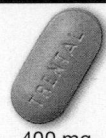

400 mg

PIOGLITAZONE HYDROCHLORIDE

Actos
(Page 1145)

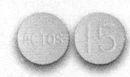

15 mg

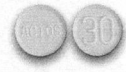

30 mg

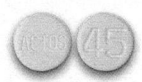

45 mg

PRASUGREL

Effient
(Page 1166)

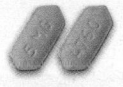

5 mg

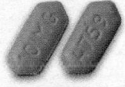

10 mg

PRAVASTATIN SODIUM

Pravachol
(Page 1167)

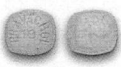

10 mg

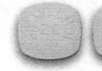

20 mg

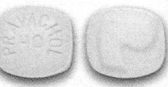

40 mg

PREGABALIN

Lyrica
(Page 1176)

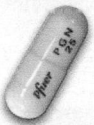

25 mg

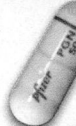

50 mg

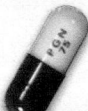

75 mg

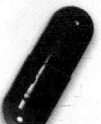

100 mg

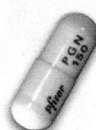

150 mg

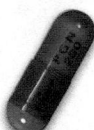

200 mg

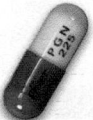

225 mg

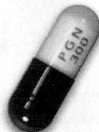

300 mg

PROPRANOLOL HYDROCHLORIDE

Inderal
(Page 1193)

    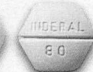

40 mg	60 mg	80 mg

Inderal LA
(Page 1193)

 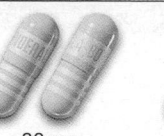 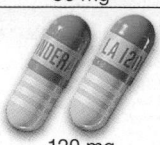

60 mg	80 mg	120 mg

160 mg

QUETIAPINE FUMARATE

Seroquel
(Page 1204)

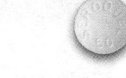 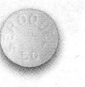

25 mg	50 mg	100 mg

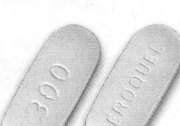 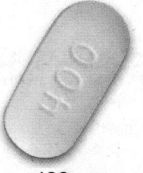

200 mg	300 mg	400 mg

QUINAPRIL HYDROCHLORIDE

Accupril
(Page 1207)

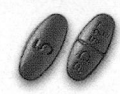   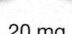

5 mg	10 mg	20 mg

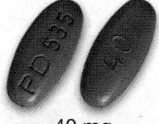

40 mg

RABEPRAZOLE SODIUM

Aciphex
(Page 1212)

20 mg

RALOXIFENE HYDROCHLORIDE

Evista
(Page 1213)

60 mg

RANITIDINE HYDROCHLORIDE

Zantac
(Page 1221)

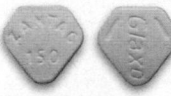   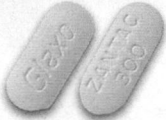

150 mg   300 mg

RANOLAZINE

Ranexa
(Page 1223)

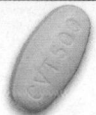

500 mg

RASAGILINE MESYLATE

Azilect
(Page 1224)

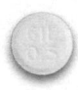

0.5 mg   1 mg

RISEDRONATE SODIUM

Actonel
(Page 1241)

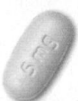   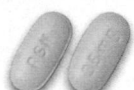

5 mg   35 mg

RISPERIDONE

Risperdal
(Page 1243)

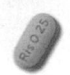   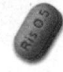

0.25 mg   0.5 mg   1 mg

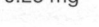

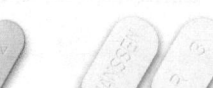   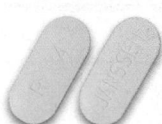

2 mg   3 mg   4 mg

RIVASTIGMINE TARTRATE

(Page 1254)

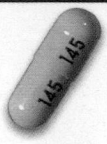

1.5 mg

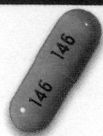

3 mg

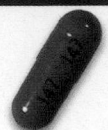

4.5 mg

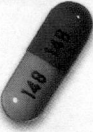

6 mg

ROSIGLITAZONE MALEATE

Avandia
(Page 1261)

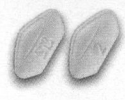

2 mg

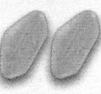

4 mg

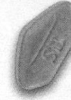

8 mg

ROSUVASTATIN CALCIUM

Crestor
(Page 1263)

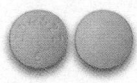

5 mg

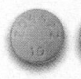

10 mg

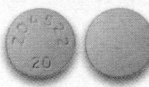

20 mg

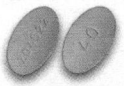

40 mg

SAXAGLIPTIN

Onglyza
(Page 1271)

2.5 mg

5 mg

SERTRALINE HYDROCHLORIDE

Zoloft
(Page 1275)

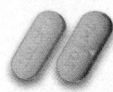

50 mg

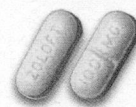

100 mg

SILDENAFIL CITRATE

Viagra
(Page 1278)

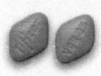 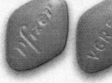 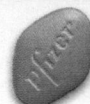 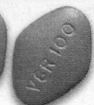

25 mg 50 mg 100 mg

SIMVASTATIN

Zocor
(Page 1284)

 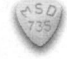 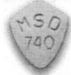

5 mg 10 mg 20 mg

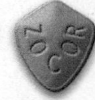

40 mg

SITAGLIPTIN PHOSPHATE

Januvia
(Page 1289)

100 mg

SOLIFENACIN SUCCINATE

VESIcare
(Page 1298)

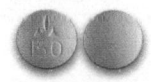 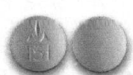

5 mg 10 mg

SPIRONOLACTONE

Aldactone
(Page 1306)

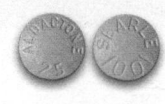 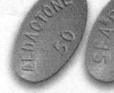 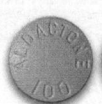 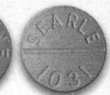

25 mg 50 mg 100 mg

SUCRALFATE

Carafate
(Page 1311)

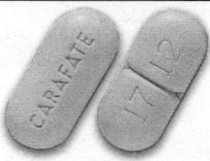

1 g

SULFAMETHOXAZOLE—TRIMETHOPRIM

Bactrim DS
(Page 1314)

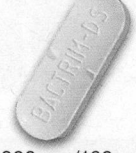

800 mg/160 mg

SUMATRIPTAN SUCCINATE

Imitrex
(Page 1318)

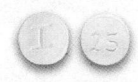

25 mg   50 mg

SUNITINIB MALATE

Sutent
(Page 1320)

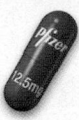 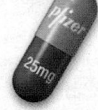 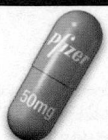

12.5 mg   25 mg   50 mg

TADALAFIL

Cialis
(Page 1326)

2.5 mg   5 mg   10 mg

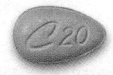

20 mg

TAMSULOSIN HYDROCHLORIDE

Flomax
(Page 1331)

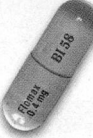

0.4 mg

TELMISARTAN

Micardis
(Page 1342)

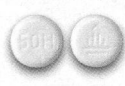 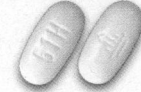 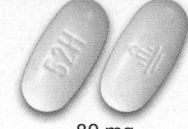

20 mg   40 mg   80 mg

TEMAZEPAM

Restoril
(Page 1343)

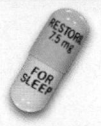 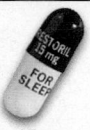

7.5 mg   15 mg   30 mg

TENOFOVIR DISOPROXIL FUMARATE

Viread
(Page 1348)

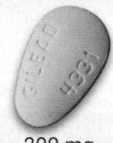

300 mg

TERAZOSIN HYDROCHLORIDE

Hytrin
(Page 1350)

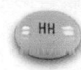   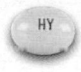

1 mg   2 mg   5 mg

10 mg

TOLTERODINE TARTRATE

Detrol
(Page 1396)

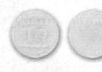

1 mg   2 mg

TOPIRAMATE

Topamax
(Page 1399)

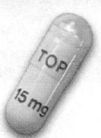   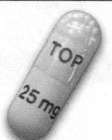   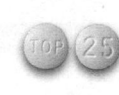

15 mg   25 mg   25 mg

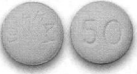

50 mg   100 mg   200 mg

TORSEMIDE

Demadex
(Page 1405)

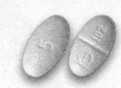 5 mg

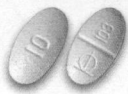 10 mg

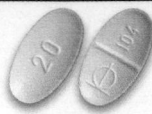 20 mg

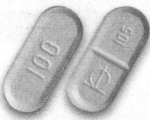 100 mg

TRAMADOL HYDROCHLORIDE—ACETAMINOPHEN

Ultracet
(Page 1523)

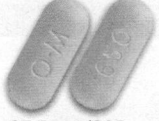 37.5 mg/325 mg

TRANDOLAPRIL

Mavik
(Page 1408)

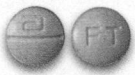 1 mg

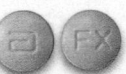 2 mg

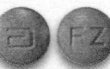 4 mg

VALACYCLOVIR HYDROCHLORIDE

Valtrex
(Page 1433)

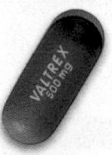 500 mg

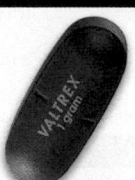 1,000 mg

VALSARTAN

Diovan
(Page 1440)

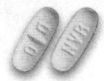 40 mg

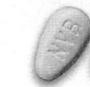 80 mg

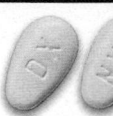 160 mg

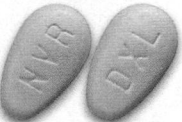 320 mg

VALSARTAN—HYDROCHLOROTHIAZIDE

Diovan HCT
(Page 1528)

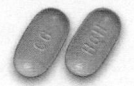 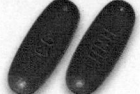 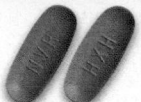

80 mg/12.5 mg   160 mg/12.5 mg   160 mg/25 mg

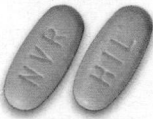 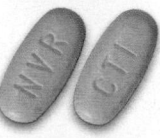

320 mg/12.5 mg   320 mg/25 mg

VARDENAFIL HYDROCHLORIDE

Levitra
(Page 1443)

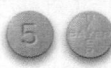 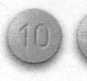 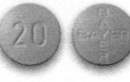

5 mg   10 mg   20 mg

VARENICLINE TARTRATE

Chantix
(Page 1445)

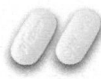 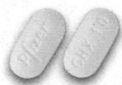

0.5 mg   1 mg

VENLAFAXINE HYDROCHLORIDE

Effexor XR
(Page 1446)

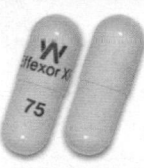 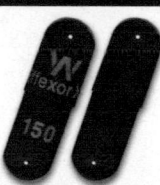

75 mg   150 mg

VERAPAMIL HYDROCHLORIDE

Calan
(Page 1449)

 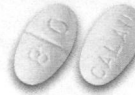 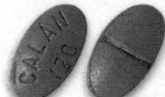

40 mg   80 mg   120 mg

Verelan
(Page 1449)

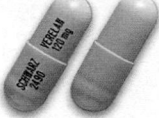 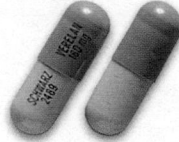 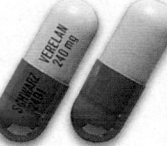

120 mg   180 mg   240 mg

WARFARIN SODIUM

Coumadin
(Page 1467)

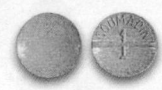

1 mg

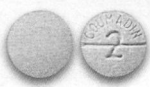

2 mg

2.5 mg

3 mg

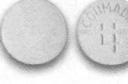

4 mg

5 mg

6 mg

7.5 mg

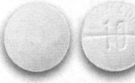

10 mg

ZIDOVUDINE

Retrovir
(Page 1473)

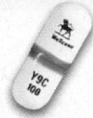

100 mg

300 mg

ZIPRASIDONE HYDROCHLORIDE

Geodon
(Page 1475)

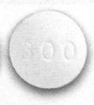

20 mg

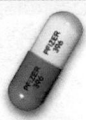

40 mg

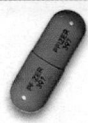

60 mg

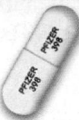

80 mg

ZOLPIDEM TARTRATE

Ambien
(Page 1481)

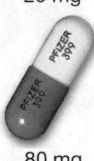

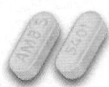

5 mg

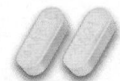

10 mg

• May slow or delay healing, especially when used with other topical NSAIDs or topical steroids.

NURSING CONSIDERATIONS

• Acuvail may be used with other topical ophthalmics when given at least 5 minutes apart.

• *Look alike–sound alike:* Don't confuse Acular with Acthar.

PATIENT TEACHING

• Teach patient how to instill drops. Advise him to wash hands before and after instilling solution, and warn him not to touch tip of dropper to eye or surrounding tissue.

• Advise patient to apply light finger pressure on lacrimal sac for 1 minute after instillation.

• Stress importance of compliance with recommended therapy.

• Tell patient not to instill drops while wearing contact lenses.

• Advise patient to report excessive bleeding or bruising to prescriber.

• Remind patient to discard drug when it's no longer needed.

---

ketorolac tromethamine (oral; injection)
KEE-toe-role-ak

Sprix, Toradol†

Therapeutic class: NSAIDs
Pharmacologic class: NSAIDs
Pregnancy risk category: C; D in 3rd trimester

AVAILABLE FORMS

Injection: 15 mg/mL in 1- and 2-mL vials and 1-mL Tubex syringes; 30 mg/mL in 1- and 2-mL single-dose vials, 1- and 2-mL Tubex syringes, and 10-mL multiple-dose vials
Nasal spray: 15.75 mg/spray
Tablets: 10 mg

INDICATIONS & DOSAGES

➤ **Short-term management of moderately severe, acute pain for single-dose treatment**
Adults younger than age 65: 60 mg I.M. or 30 mg I.V.
Adults age 65 and older: 30 mg I.M. or 15 mg I.V.
Adjust-a-dose: For renally impaired patients or those who weigh less than 50 kg (110 lb), 30 mg I.M. or 15 mg I.V.

➤ **Short-term management of moderately severe, acute pain for multiple-dose treatment**
Adults younger than age 65: 30 mg I.M. or I.V. every 6 hours for maximum of 5 days. Maximum daily dose is 120 mg. Or, 31.5 mg (one 15.75-mg spray in each nostril) every 6 to 8 hours; maximum daily dose is 126 mg.
Adults age 65 and older: 15 mg I.M. or I.V. every 6 hours for maximum of 5 days. Maximum daily dose is 60 mg. Or, 15.75 mg (one spray in only one nostril) every 6 to 8 hours; maximum daily dose is 63 mg.
Adjust-a-dose: For renally impaired patients or those who weigh less than 50 kg, 15 mg I.M. or I.V. every 6 hours. Maximum daily dose is 60 mg. Or, 15.75 mg (one spray in only one nostril) every 6 to 8 hours; maximum daily dose is 63 mg.
➤ **Short-term management of moderately severe, acute pain when switching from parenteral to oral administration (oral therapy is indicated only as continuation of parenterally given drug and should never be given without patient first having received parenteral therapy)**
Adults younger than age 65: 20 mg P.O. as single dose; then 10 mg P.O. every 4 to 6 hours for maximum of 5 days. Maximum daily dose is 40 mg.
Adults age 65 and older: 10 mg P.O. as single dose; then 10 mg P.O. every 4 to 6 hours for maximum of 5 days. Maximum daily dose is 40 mg.
Adjust-a-dose: For renally impaired patients or those who weigh less than 50 kg, give 10 mg P.O. as single dose; then 10 mg P.O. every 4 to 6 hours. Maximum daily dose is 40 mg.

K

ADMINISTRATION

P.O.
• Give drug with food if GI upset occurs.

I.V.
▼ Dilute with normal saline solution, D_5W, 5% dextrose and normal saline solution, Ringer solution, lactated Ringer solution, or Plasma-Lyte A.
▼ Give injection over at least 15 seconds.
▼ Protect from light.
▼ **Incompatibilities:** Azithromycin; fenoldopam mesylate; haloperidol lactate; nalbuphine; solutions that result in a relatively low pH, such as hydroxyzine, meperidine, morphine sulfate, and prochlorperazine; thiethylperazine.

I.M.
• When appropriate, give by deep I.M. injection.
• Patient may feel pain at injection site.
• Put pressure on site for 15 to 30 seconds after injection to minimize local effects.

Intranasal
• Discard nasal spray within 24 hours of first dose, even if bottle still contains medication.
• Each 1.7-g bottle contains eight sprays.
• Activate pump before first use by pumping five times.
• Have patient blow his nose before use, sit upright or stand, and tilt his head slightly forward.
• Insert tip into the nostril, point away from the septum, and spray once.

ACTION

May inhibit prostaglandin synthesis, to produce anti-inflammatory, analgesic, and antipyretic effects.

Route	Onset	Peak	Duration
P.O.	30–60 min	30–60 min	6–8 hr
I.V.	Immediate	1–3 min	6–8 hr
I.M.	10 min	30–60 min	6–8 hr
Intranasal	Unknown	½–2 hr	6–8 hr

Half-life: 4 to 6 hours.

ADVERSE REACTIONS

CNS: headache, dizziness, drowsiness, sedation.
CV: *arrhythmias,* edema, hypertension, palpitations.
EENT: (nasal spray only) increased lacrimation, nasal discomfort, rhinalgia, rhinitis, throat irritation.
GI: dyspepsia, GI pain, nausea, constipation, diarrhea, flatulence, peptic ulceration, stomatitis, vomiting.
GU: *renal failure.*
Hematologic: decreased platelet adhesion, prolonged bleeding time, purpura.
Skin: diaphoresis, pruritus, rash.
Other: pain at injection site.

INTERACTIONS

Drug-drug. *ACE inhibitors, angiotensin II receptor blockers:* May cause renal impairment, particularly in volume-depleted patients. Avoid using together in volume-depleted patients.
Anticoagulants: May increase anticoagulant levels in the blood. Use together with extreme caution and monitor patient closely.
Anticonvulsants (carbamazepine, phenytoin): May increase seizure activity. Use together cautiously.
Antihypertensives, diuretics: May decrease effectiveness. Monitor patient closely.
Lithium: May increase lithium level. Monitor patient closely.
Methotrexate: May decrease methotrexate clearance and increase toxicity. Avoid using together.
Pentoxifylline: May increase risk of bleeding. Avoid use together.
Probenecid: May increase level and toxicity of ketorolac. Avoid using together.
Salicylates: May increase the risk of serious ketorolac adverse effects. Avoid using together.
SSRIs: May increase risk of GI bleeding. Use together cautiously.
Drug-herb. *Dong quai, feverfew, garlic, ginger, horse chestnut, red clover:* May cause bleeding. Discourage use together.
White willow: Herb and drug contain similar components. Discourage use together.

EFFECTS ON LAB TEST RESULTS

• May increase ALT and AST levels.
• May increase bleeding time.

Reactions in bold italics are *life-threatening*. Interactions may have a *rapid onset* or a *delayed onset*.

CONTRAINDICATIONS & CAUTIONS

Black Box Warning Contraindicated in patients hypersensitive to drug and in those with active peptic ulcer disease, recent GI bleeding or perforation, advanced renal impairment, cerebrovascular bleeding, hemorrhagic diathesis, or incomplete hemostasis; in women during labor and delivery and while breast-feeding; and in those at risk for renal impairment from volume depletion or at risk for bleeding. ■

Black Box Warning Contraindicated in pediatric patients and in patients with history of peptic ulcer disease or GI bleeding or past allergic reactions to aspirin or other NSAIDs. ■

Black Box Warning Contraindicated as prophylactic analgesic before major surgery or intraoperatively when hemostasis is critical. ■

Black Box Warning Contraindicated for treatment of perioperative pain in patients requiring CABG surgery. ■

Black Box Warning Contraindicated in patients currently receiving aspirin, probenecid, or NSAIDs. ■

• Use cautiously in patients who are elderly or have hepatic or renal impairment or cardiac decompensation.

⚠ **Overdose S&S:** Abdominal pain, nausea, vomiting, peptic ulcers, GI bleeding, hyperventilation, renal dysfunction, metabolic acidosis, hypertension, lethargy, drowsiness, respiratory depression, coma, anaphylaxis.

NURSING CONSIDERATIONS

• Correct hypovolemia before giving.

Black Box Warning Oral therapy is only indicated as a continuation of I.V./I.M. therapy. The maximum combined duration of parenteral, nasal, and oral therapy is 5 days. ■

Black Box Warning Sprix isn't indicated for minor or chronic painful conditions. ■

• Don't give drug epidurally or intrathecally because of alcohol content.

• Carefully observe patients with coagulopathies and those taking anticoagulants. Drug inhibits platelet aggregation and can prolong bleeding time. This effect disappears within 48 hours of stopping drug and doesn't alter platelet count, INR, PTT, or PT.

Black Box Warning NSAIDs may increase the risk of serious thrombotic events, MI, or stroke, which can be fatal. The risk may be greater with longer use or in patients with CV disease or risk factors for CV disease. ■

Black Box Warning NSAIDs cause an increased risk of serious GI adverse events, including bleeding, ulceration, and perforation of the stomach or intestines, which can be fatal. Elderly patients are at greater risk. ■

• Don't give drug concomitantly with other forms of ketorolac or other NSAIDs.

• NSAIDs may mask signs and symptoms of infection because of their antipyretic and anti-inflammatory actions.

• **Look alike–sound alike:** Don't confuse ketorolac with Ketalar or methadone.

PATIENT TEACHING

• Tell patient to discard nasal spray within 24 hours of the first dose, even if medication remains in the bottle.

• Warn patient using nasal spray that he may experience transient, mild to moderate nasal irritation that lasts for a few minutes and won't worsen with next dose.

• Advise patient to take a sip of water after using nasal spray to decrease throat sensation.

• Teach patient to read package insert and full directions for use of nasal spray bottle.

• Warn patient not to take ketorolac with other NSAIDs.

• Advise patient to maintain adequate fluid intake.

• Advise patient to be alert for signs and symptoms of CV events (chest pain, shortness of breath, weakness, slurred speech) and to seek medical attention immediately if they occur.

• Tell patient to promptly report edema and weight gain.

• Teach patient the warning signs and symptoms of hepatotoxicity (nausea, fatigue, lethargy, pruritus, jaundice, right upper quadrant abdominal tenderness, flulike symptoms), and advise him to stop drug and seek medical help immediately if they occur.

• Instruct patient to notify prescriber immediately if she is pregnant.

K

• Warn patient receiving drug I.M. that pain may occur at injection site.
• Teach patient signs and symptoms of GI bleeding, including blood in vomit, urine, or stool; coffee-ground vomit; and black, tarry stool. Tell him to notify prescriber immediately if any of these occurs.
• Tell patient not to take drug for more than 5 days in a row.

ketotifen fumarate
kee-toe-TYE-fen

Alaway ◇, Zaditor ◇

Therapeutic class: Antihistamines (ophthalmic)
Pharmacologic class: H₁-receptor antagonists–mast cell stabilizers
Pregnancy risk category: C

AVAILABLE FORMS
Ophthalmic solution: 0.025%

INDICATIONS & DOSAGES
➤ **To temporarily prevent eye itching from allergic conjunctivitis or temporarily relieve itchy eyes due to pollen, ragweed, grass, animal hair, and dander**
Adults and children age 3 and older: Instill 1 drop in each affected eye every 8 to 12 hours but not more than b.i.d.

ADMINISTRATION
Ophthalmic
• Drug is for ophthalmic use only. Don't inject or give orally.
• Close bottle tightly when not in use.
• Don't touch tip of dropper to any surface.

ACTION
Stabilizes mast cells to inhibit release of mediators involved in hypersensitivity reactions and blocks action of histamine at the H₁ receptor, temporarily preventing itching of the eye.

Route	Onset	Peak	Duration
Ophthalmic	Within min	Unknown	Unknown

Half-life: Unknown.

ADVERSE REACTIONS
CNS: headache.
EENT: conjunctival infection, rhinitis, burning or stinging of eyes, conjunctivitis, dry eyes, eye discharge, eye pain, eyelid disorder, itching of eyes, keratitis, lacrimation disorder, mydriasis, ocular allergic reactions, ocular rash, pharyngitis, photophobia.
Other: flulike syndrome.

INTERACTIONS
None significant.

EFFECTS ON LAB TEST RESULTS
None reported.

CONTRAINDICATIONS & CAUTIONS
• Contraindicated in patients hypersensitive to components of drug.
• Contraindicated for irritation related to contact lenses.

NURSING CONSIDERATIONS
• Soft contact lenses may absorb the preservative benzalkonium. Contact lenses shouldn't be inserted until 10 minutes after drug is instilled.
• To prevent contaminating dropper tip and solution, don't touch eyelids or surrounding areas with dropper tip of bottle.

PATIENT TEACHING
• Teach patient the proper technique for instilling drops.
• Advise patient not to wear contact lens if eye is red. Warn him not to use drug to treat contact lens–related irritation.
• Instruct patient who wears soft contact lenses and whose eyes aren't red to wait at least 10 minutes after instilling drug before inserting contact lenses.
• Advise patient to report adverse reactions.
• Advise patient to keep bottle tightly closed when not in use.

labetalol hydrochloride
la-BET-ah-loll

Therapeutic class: Antihypertensives
Pharmacologic class: Alpha–beta blockers
Pregnancy risk category: C

AVAILABLE FORMS
Injection: 5 mg/mL in 20- and 40-mL multiple-dose vials
Tablets: 100 mg, 200 mg, 300 mg

INDICATIONS & DOSAGES
➤ **Hypertension**
Adults (inpatients): 200 mg P.O., followed by 200 to 400 mg P.O. in 6 to 12 hours depending on blood pressure response. May increase by 200 mg P.O. b.i.d.
Adults (outpatients): 100 mg P.O. b.i.d. with or without a diuretic. If needed, dosage is increased to 200 mg b.i.d. after 2 days. Further increases may be made every 2 to 3 days until optimal response is reached. Usual maintenance dosage is 100 to 400 mg b.i.d. Maximum dose is 2.4 g daily in two divided doses given alone or with a diuretic.
➤ **Severe hypertension, hypertensive emergencies**
Adults: 200 mg diluted in 160 mL of D₅W, infused at 2 mg/minute I.V. until satisfactory response is obtained; then infusion is stopped. Maximum dose is 300 mg.
Or, give by repeated I.V. injection; initially, 20 mg I.V. slowly over 2 minutes. Repeat injections of 40 to 80 mg every 10 minutes until maximum dose of 300 mg is reached, as needed.
➤ **Pediatric hypertension ◆**
Children ages 1 to 17: Initially, 1 to 3 mg/kg/day P.O. in two divided doses. Titrate until target blood pressure is reached, the child has adverse reactions, or the highest recommended dosage is reached. Maximum dose is 10 to 12 mg/kg/day up to 1,200 mg/day.
➤ **Pediatric hypertensive emergency ◆**
Children ages 1 to 17: Initially, 0.2 to 1 mg/kg I.V. over 2 minutes every 10 minutes as needed with a maximum of 40 mg/dose.

Or, 0.25 to 3 mg/kg/hour as a continuous I.V. infusion.

ADMINISTRATION
P.O.
● When switching from I.V. to P.O. form, begin P.O. regimen at 200 mg after blood pressure begins to rise; repeat dose with 200 to 400 mg in 6 to 12 hours. Adjust dosage according to blood pressure response.
● If dizziness occurs, give dose at bedtime or in smaller doses t.i.d.
I.V.
▼ Give by slow, direct I.V. injection over 2 minutes at 10-minute intervals.
▼ For I.V. infusion, prepare by diluting with D₅W or normal saline solutions; for example, 200 mg of drug to 160 mL D₅W to yield 1 mg/mL.
▼ Give labetalol infusion with an infusion-control device.
▼ Monitor blood pressure closely every 5 minutes for 30 minutes; then every 30 minutes for 2 hours. Then, monitor hourly for 6 hours.
▼ Patient should remain supine for 3 hours after infusion. When given I.V. for hypertensive emergencies, drug produces a rapid, predictable fall in blood pressure within 5 to 10 minutes.
▼ Store at room temperature. Protect from light.
▼ **Incompatibilities:** Alkali solutions, amphotericin B, cefoperazone, ceftriaxone, furosemide, heparin, nafcillin, sodium bicarbonate, thiopental, warfarin.

ACTION
May be related to reduced peripheral vascular resistance, as a result of alpha and beta blockade.

Route	Onset	Peak	Duration
P.O.	20 min	2–4 hr	8–12 hr
I.V.	2–5 min	5 min	2–4 hr

Half-life: About 5½ hours after I.V. use; 6 to 8 hours after P.O. use.

ADVERSE REACTIONS
CNS: dizziness, vivid dreams, fatigue, headache, paresthesia, transient scalp tingling, syncope, vertigo, asthenia.

L

CV: orthostatic hypotension, *ventricular arrhythmias.*
EENT: nasal congestion.
GI: nausea, vomiting.
GU: sexual dysfunction, urine retention.
Respiratory: *bronchospasm,* dyspnea.
Skin: rash.

INTERACTIONS

Drug-drug. *Beta agonists:* May blunt bronchodilator effect of these drugs in patients with bronchospasm. May need to increase dosages of these drugs.
Cimetidine: May enhance labetalol's effect. Use together cautiously.
Diuretics, CV drugs: May increase hypotensive effects. Monitor blood pressure.
Halothane: May increase hypotensive effect. Monitor blood pressure closely.
Insulin, oral antidiabetics: May alter dosage requirements in previously stabilized diabetic patient. Monitor patient closely.
Nitroglycerin: May blunt reflex tachycardia produced by nitroglycerin but not the hypotension. Monitor blood pressure if used together.
NSAIDs: May decrease antihypertensive effects. Monitor blood pressure.
TCAs: May increase incidence of tremor. Monitor patient for tremor.
Drug-herb. *Ma huang:* May decrease antihypertensive effects. Discourage use together.

EFFECTS ON LAB TEST RESULTS

• May increase transaminase and urea levels.
• May cause false-positive increase of urine free and total catecholamine levels when measured by a nonspecific trihydroxyindole fluorometric method. May cause false-positive test result for amphetamines when screening urine for drugs.

CONTRAINDICATIONS & CAUTIONS

• Contraindicated in patients hypersensitive to drug or its components and in those with bronchial asthma, overt cardiac failure, greater than first-degree heart block, cardiogenic shock, severe bradycardia, and other conditions that may cause severe and prolonged hypotension.
• Use cautiously in patients with heart failure, hepatic failure, chronic bronchitis,

emphysema, peripheral vascular disease, and pheochromocytoma.
⚠ *Overdose S&S:* Orthostatic hypotension, bradycardia, heart failure, bronchospasm, seizures.

NURSING CONSIDERATIONS

• Monitor blood pressure frequently. Drug masks common signs and symptoms of shock.
• In diabetic patients, monitor glucose level closely because beta blockers may mask certain signs and symptoms of hypoglycemia.

PATIENT TEACHING

🔴 *Alert:* Tell patient that stopping drug abruptly can worsen chest pain and trigger a heart attack.
• Advise patient that dizziness is the most troublesome adverse reaction and tends to occur in the early stages of treatment, in patients taking diuretics, and with higher dosages. Inform patient that dizziness can be minimized by rising slowly and avoiding sudden position changes.
• Warn patient that occasional, harmless scalp tingling may occur, especially when therapy begins.

lacosamide
lah-COSS-ah-mide

Vimpat

Therapeutic class: Anticonvulsants
Pharmacologic class: Functionalized amino acids
Pregnancy risk category: C
Controlled substance schedule: V

AVAILABLE FORMS
Injection: 200 mg/20-mL vial
Oral solution: 10 mg/mL
Tablets: 50 mg, 100 mg, 150 mg, 200 mg

INDICATIONS & DOSAGES
➤ **Adjunctive therapy for partial-onset seizures**
Adults and adolescents age 17 and older:
Initially, 50 mg P.O. b.i.d.; increase at weekly intervals to a maximum daily dosage

of 100 to 200 mg P.O. b.i.d. May administer I.V. at an equivalent daily dosage and frequency when P.O. administration is temporarily not feasible.

Adjust-a-dose: In patients with mild or moderate hepatic impairment or severe renal impairment (CrCl of 30 mL/minute or less), maximum recommended daily dosage is 300 mg. Withhold drug in patients with severe hepatic impairment. Dosage supplementation of up to 50% should be considered following a 4-hour hemodialysis treatment.

ADMINISTRATION
P.O.
● Give drug with or without food.
I.V.
▼ Reconstitute with normal saline solution, D_5W, or lactated Ringer solution. Discard solution if discolored or if particulate matter is present. Solution is stable for 24 hours at room temperature.
▼ Infuse over 30 to 60 minutes.
▼ Discard unused solution in vial.
▼ **Incompatibilities:** None known.

ACTION
May selectively enhance slow inactivation of sodium channels, stabilizing hyperexcitable neuronal membranes and inhibiting repetitive neuronal firing.

Route	Onset	Peak	Duration
P.O.	Unknown	1–4 hr	Unknown
I.V.	Unknown	30–60 min	Unknown

Half-life: Approximately 13 hours.

ADVERSE REACTIONS
CNS: asthenia, ataxia, balance disorder, depression, dizziness, fatigue, gait disturbance, headache, memory impairment, somnolence, tremor.
EENT: blurred vision, diplopia, nystagmus, vertigo.
GI: diarrhea, nausea, vomiting.
Skin: pruritus, skin laceration.
Other: contusion.

INTERACTIONS
Drug-drug. *Carbamazepine, phenobarbital, phenytoin:* May decrease lacosamide level. Adjust dosage as needed.

Drug-lifestyle. *Alcohol use:* May cause additive drowsiness. Don't use together.

EFFECTS ON LAB TEST RESULTS
● May increase LFT values.

CONTRAINDICATIONS & CAUTIONS
● Lacosamide isn't recommended for patients with severe hepatic impairment.
● Use cautiously in patients with known cardiac conduction problems, depression, myocardial ischemia, or heart failure and in those with a history of suicidal thoughts.
● Use lacosamide during pregnancy only if potential benefit to the mother justifies potential risk to the fetus.
● It isn't known if drug appears in breast milk. Patient should either stop breast-feeding or stop drug.
● Safety and effectiveness in children younger than age 17 haven't been established.
⚠ Overdose S&S: Coma.

NURSING CONSIDERATIONS
● Monitor patient for signs and symptoms of multiorgan hypersensitivity reaction, including fever, rash, eosinophilia, hepatitis, nephritis, lymphadenopathy, and myocarditis. If reaction is suspected, discontinue drug and begin alternative treatment.
● Obtain an ECG in patients with severe cardiac disease or known conduction defects before starting drug.
⊙ Alert: Withdraw drug gradually over 1 week to minimize potential for increased seizure activity.
● Encourage pregnant patients to enroll in the North American AED Pregnancy Registry at 1-888-233-2334. Registry information can also be found at www. aedpregnancyregistry.org.
⊙ Alert: Drug may increase risk of suicidal thinking and behavior. Monitor patient closely for worsening depression, suicidal thoughts or behavior, and unusual changes in mood or behavior.
● Closely observe patients with mild to moderate hepatic impairment during dosage titration.

PATIENT TEACHING
• Inform patient that drug may be taken without regard to meals.
• Tell patient to report mood changes or suicidal thoughts immediately.
• Warn patient to avoid driving and operating heavy machinery until drug's CNS effects are known.
• Advise woman to notify prescriber if she suspects or is considering pregnancy or plans to breast-feed.
• Warn patient not to stop drug abruptly.
• Tell patient to avoid alcohol while taking drug.
• Advise patient to report blurred vision, dizziness, double vision, nausea, uncoordinated movement, or vertigo.

lactulose
LAK-tyoo-lose

Cholac, Constilac, Constulose, Enulose, Euro-lac†, Generlac

Therapeutic class: Laxatives
Pharmacologic class: Disaccharides
Pregnancy risk category: B

AVAILABLE FORMS
Oral solution: 10 g/15 mL
Packets: 10 g, 20 g
Rectal solution: 10 g/15 mL

INDICATIONS & DOSAGES
➤ **Constipation**
Adults: 10 to 20 g or 15 to 30 mL P.O. daily, increased to 60 mL/day, if needed.
➤ **To prevent and treat hepatic encephalopathy, including hepatic precoma and coma in patients with severe hepatic disease**
Adults: Initially, 20 to 30 g or 30 to 45 mL P.O. t.i.d. or q.i.d., until two or three soft stools are produced daily. Usual dose is 60 to 100 g daily in divided doses. Or, 200 g or 300 mL diluted with 700 mL of water or normal saline solution and given as retention enema P.R. every 4 to 6 hours, as needed.
Infants: Initially, 2.5 to 10 mL/day P.O. in divided doses to produce two or three soft stools daily.

Older children and adolescents: 40 to 90 mL/day P.O. in divided doses to produce two or three soft stools daily.
➤ **Treatment of subclinical hepatic encephalopathy** ◆
Adults: 30 to 60 mL/day P.O. in two to three divided doses to maintain two or three daily bowel movements for up to 3 months. If diarrhea develops, stop drug and reinstitute at a lower dosage.

ADMINISTRATION
P.O.
• Dissolve packet contents (crystals) in ½ glass of water (120 mL). Resulting solution may be clear to pale yellow.
• To minimize sweet taste, dilute with water or fruit juice or give with food.
Rectal
• Prepare enema (not commercially available) by adding 200 g (300 mL) to 700 mL of water or normal saline solution. The diluted solution is given as retention enema for 30 to 60 minutes. Use a rectal balloon.
• If enema isn't retained for at least 30 minutes, repeat dose.

ACTION
Produces an osmotic effect in colon; resulting distention promotes peristalsis. Also decreases ammonia, probably as a result of bacterial degradation, which lowers the pH of colon contents.

Route	Onset	Peak	Duration
P.O.	24–48 hr	Variable	Variable
P.R.	Unknown	Unknown	Unknown

Half-life: Unknown.

ADVERSE REACTIONS
GI: abdominal cramps, belching, diarrhea, flatulence, gaseous distention, nausea, vomiting.

INTERACTIONS
Drug-drug. *Antacids:* May decrease lactulose effectiveness. Avoid using together.

EFFECTS ON LAB TEST RESULTS
None reported.

Reactions in bold italics are *life-threatening*. Interactions may have a *rapid onset* or a *delayed onset*.

CONTRAINDICATIONS & CAUTIONS
• Contraindicated in patients on a low-galactose diet.
• Use cautiously in patients with diabetes mellitus.
⚠ **Overdose S&S:** Diarrhea, abdominal cramps.

NURSING CONSIDERATIONS
• Monitor sodium level for hypernatremia, especially when giving in higher doses to treat hepatic encephalopathy.
• Monitor mental status and potassium levels when giving to patients with hepatic encephalopathy.
• Replace fluid loss.
• **Look alike–sound alike:** Don't confuse lactulose with lactose.

PATIENT TEACHING
• Show home care patient how to mix and use drug.
• Inform patient about adverse reactions, and tell him to notify prescriber if reactions become bothersome or if diarrhea occurs.
• Instruct patient not to take other laxatives during lactulose therapy.

lamivudine (3TC)
lam-ah-VEW-den

Epivir, Epivir-HBV, Heptovir†

Therapeutic class: Antiretrovirals
Pharmacologic class: Nucleoside–nucleotide reverse transcriptase inhibitors
Pregnancy risk category: C

AVAILABLE FORMS
Epivir
Oral solution: 10 mg/mL
Tablets: 150 mg, 300 mg
Epivir-HBV
Oral solution: 5 mg/mL
Tablets: 100 mg

INDICATIONS & DOSAGES
Black Box Warning Epivir tablets and oral solution (used to treat HIV infection) contain a higher dose of the active ingredient than Epivir-HBV tablets and oral solution (used to treat chronic hepatitis B virus [HBV] infection). Patient with HIV infection should receive only dosing forms appropriate for HIV treatment. ■

➤ **HIV infection, with other antiretrovirals**
Adults and children older than age 16: 300 mg Epivir P.O. once daily or 150 mg P.O. b.i.d.
Children ages 3 months to 16 years: 4 mg/kg Epivir solution P.O. b.i.d. Maximum dose is 150 mg b.i.d.
Children weighing 14 kg (31 lb) or more who can reliably swallow tablets: Weighing 14 to 21 kg (46 lb), give ½ tablet (75 mg) P.O. b.i.d.; 21 to less than 30 kg (66 lb), give ½ tablet (75 mg) P.O. in morning and 1 tablet (150 mg) P.O. in evening; 30 kg or more, give 150 mg P.O. b.i.d.
Adjust-a-dose: For patients with HIV infection and CrCl of 30 to 49 mL/minute, give 150 mg Epivir P.O. daily. If CrCl is 15 to 29 mL/minute, give 150 mg P.O. on day 1 and then 100 mg daily; if CrCl is 5 to 14 mL/minute, give 150 mg on day 1 and then 50 mg daily; if CrCl is less than 5 mL/minute, give 50 mg on day 1 and then 25 mg daily.

➤ **Chronic hepatitis B with evidence of HBV replication and active liver inflammation**
Adults: 100 mg Epivir-HBV P.O. once daily.
Children ages 2 to 17 years: 3 mg/kg Epivir-HBV P.O. once daily, up to a maximum dose of 100 mg daily. Optimum duration of treatment isn't known; safety and effectiveness of treatment beyond 1 year haven't been established.
Adjust-a-dose: For adult patients with chronic hepatitis B and CrCl of 30 to 49 mL/minute, give first dose of 100 mg Epivir-HBV; then give 50 mg P.O. once daily. If CrCl is 15 to 29 mL/minute, give first dose of 100 mg; then give 25 mg P.O. once daily. If CrCl is 5 to 14 mL/minute, give first dose of 35 mg; then give 15 mg P.O. once daily. If CrCl is less than 5 mL/minute, give first dose of 35 mg; then give 10 mg P.O. once daily.

ADMINISTRATION
P.O.
• Give without regard for food.

L

ACTION

A synthetic nucleoside analogue that inhibits HIV and HBV reverse transcription via viral DNA chain termination. RNA- and DNA-dependent DNA polymerase activities.

Route	Onset	Peak	Duration
P.O.	Unknown	1–3 hr	Unknown

Half-life: Adults, 5 to 7 hours; children, 2 hours.

ADVERSE REACTIONS

Adverse reactions pertain to the combination therapy of lamivudine and zidovudine.
CNS: dizziness, fatigue, fever, headache, insomnia and other sleep disorders, malaise, neuropathy, depressive disorders.
EENT: nasal symptoms.
GI: anorexia, diarrhea, nausea, vomiting, *pancreatitis,* abdominal cramps, abdominal pain, dyspepsia.
Hematologic: *neutropenia, thrombocytopenia,* anemia.
Hepatic: *hepatotoxicity.*
Metabolic: *lactic acidosis.*
Musculoskeletal: musculoskeletal pain, arthralgia, myalgia.
Respiratory: cough.
Skin: rash.
Other: chills.

INTERACTIONS

Drug-drug. *Sulfamethoxazole–trimethoprim:* May increase lamivudine level because of decreased clearance of drug. Monitor patient for toxicity.

EFFECTS ON LAB TEST RESULTS

• May increase ALT and bilirubin levels. May decrease hemoglobin level.
• May decrease neutrophil and platelet counts.

CONTRAINDICATIONS & CAUTIONS

Black Box Warning Lactic acidosis and severe hepatomegaly with steatosis, including fatal cases, have been reported. ∎
• Contraindicated in patients hypersensitive to drug.
• Use cautiously in patients with renal impairment.
❸ Alert: Use drug cautiously, if at all, in children with history of pancreatitis or other

significant risk factors for development of pancreatitis.
• The Antiretroviral Pregnancy Registry monitors maternal-fetal outcomes of pregnant women exposed to lamivudine. To register a pregnant woman, call the Antiretroviral Pregnancy Registry at 1-800-258-4263.

NURSING CONSIDERATIONS

❸ Alert: Stop treatment immediately and notify prescriber if signs, symptoms, or laboratory abnormalities suggest pancreatitis. Monitor amylase level.
❸ Alert: Lactic acidosis and hepatotoxicity have been reported. Notify prescriber if signs of lactic acidosis or hepatotoxicity occur.
Black Box Warning Hepatitis may recur in some patients with chronic HBV infection when they stop taking drug. Monitor hepatic function closely. ∎
• Safety and effectiveness of Epivir-HBV for longer than 1 year haven't been established; optimum duration of treatment isn't known.
Black Box Warning Test patients for HIV before starting treatment and during therapy because form and dosage of lamivudine in Epivir-HBV aren't appropriate for those infected with both HBV and HIV. If lamivudine is given to patients with HBV and HIV, use the higher dosage indicated for HIV therapy as part of an appropriate combination regimen. ∎
• Because of a high rate of early virologic resistance, don't use triple antiretroviral therapy with abacavir or didanosine, lamivudine, and tenofovir as new treatment for never-treated or pretreated patients. Monitor patients currently taking this therapy and those who take it with other antiretrovirals, and consider a different therapy.
• Monitor patient's CBC, platelet count, and renal and liver function studies. Report abnormalities.

PATIENT TEACHING

• Inform patient that long-term effects of drug aren't known.
• Stress importance of taking drug exactly as prescribed.

Black Box Warning Offer HIV counseling and testing to all patients before beginning treatment with lamivudine-HBV and periodically during treatment because lamivudine-HBV contains a lower dose of the same active ingredient as in lamivudine tablets and oral solution used to treat HIV. If treatment with lamivudine-HBV is prescribed for chronic hepatitis B in a patient with unrecognized or untreated HIV infection, rapid emergence of HIV resistance is likely because of the subtherapeutic dose and inappropriate monotherapy. ■

• Inform patient that drug doesn't cure HIV infection, that opportunistic infections and other complications of HIV infection may still occur, and that transmission of HIV to others through sexual contact or blood contamination is still possible.

• Teach parents or guardians the signs and symptoms of pancreatitis. Advise them to report signs and symptoms immediately.

lamotrigine
la-MO-tri-geen

Lamictal, Lamictal CD, Lamictal ODT, Lamictal XR

Therapeutic class: Anticonvulsants
Pharmacologic class: Phenyltriazines
Pregnancy risk category: C

AVAILABLE FORMS
Tablets: 25 mg, 100 mg, 150 mg, 200 mg
Tablets (chewable dispersible): 2 mg, 5 mg, 25 mg
Tablets (extended-release): 25 mg, 50 mg, 100 mg, 200 mg, 250 mg, 300 mg
Tablets (orally disintegrating): 25 mg, 50 mg, 100 mg, 200 mg

INDICATIONS & DOSAGES
⊙ Alert: Extended-release formula isn't for use as initial monotherapy or for conversion to monotherapy from two or more concomitant antiepileptic drugs (AEDs).
➤ **Conversion to monotherapy using extended-release formula in patients with partial seizures who are receiving treatment with a single enzyme-inducing AED**

Adults and children age 13 and older: Add lamotrigine (extended-release tablet) 50 mg P.O. daily to current drug regimen for 2 weeks, followed by 100 mg P.O. daily. Then, increase by 100 mg every week until maintenance dosage of 500 mg P.O. daily is reached. The concomitant enzyme-inducing AED can then be gradually reduced by 20% decrements each week over a 4-week period. Two weeks after completing withdrawal of the enzyme-inducing AED, decrease lamotrigine (extended-release tablet) no faster than 100 mg/day each week to achieve the monotherapy maintenance dosage of 250 to 300 mg/day.
➤ **Conversion to monotherapy using extended-release formula in patients with partial seizures who are receiving adjunctive treatment with valproate**

Adults and children age 13 and older: Add lamotrigine (extended-release tablet) 25 mg P.O. every other day for 2 weeks; then increase to 25 mg P.O. daily for weeks 3 and 4. Increase to 50 mg P.O. daily for week 5, 100 mg P.O. daily for week 6, and 150 mg P.O. daily for week 7. Maintain dosage at 150 mg P.O. daily while decreasing valproate dosage by no more than 500 mg/day each week until 500 mg/day is achieved; maintain for 1 week. Then, simultaneously increase lamotrigine (extended-release tablet) to 200 mg/day while decreasing valproate to 250 mg/day; maintain for 1 week. Increase lamotrigine (extended-release tablet) to 250 or 300 mg P.O. daily as maintenance dosage and discontinue valproate.
➤ **Conversion to monotherapy using extended-release formula in patients with partial seizures who are receiving treatment with a single drug other than an enzyme-inducing AED or valproate**

Adults and children age 13 and older: Add lamotrigine (extended-release tablet) 25 mg P.O. daily for 2 weeks; then increase to 50 mg P.O. daily for weeks 3 and 4. Increase to 100 mg P.O. daily for week 5, 150 mg P.O. daily for week 6, and 200 mg P.O. daily for week 7. In week 8, increase to maintenance dosage of 250 to 300 mg P.O. daily. After achieving maintenance dosage, withdraw concomitant AED therapy by 20% decrements each week over a 4-week period.

No additional lamotrigine (extended-release tablet) adjustment is needed.

▶ **Adjunctive treatment of partial seizures or primary generalized tonic-clonic seizures caused by epilepsy or generalized seizures of Lennox-Gastaut syndrome**

Adults and children older than age 12 taking valproate: 25 mg (immediate-release) P.O. every other day for 2 weeks; then 25 mg P.O. daily for 2 weeks. Continue to increase, as needed, by 25 to 50 mg daily every 1 to 2 weeks until an effective maintenance dosage of 100 to 400 mg daily given in one or two divided doses is reached. When added to valproate alone, the usual daily maintenance dose is 100 to 200 mg. Or, 25 mg (extended-release) P.O. every other day for 2 weeks; then 25 mg P.O. daily for 2 weeks; then 50 mg P.O. daily for 1 week; then 100 mg P.O. daily for 1 week; then 150 mg P.O. daily for 1 week. Daily maintenance dose is 200 to 250 mg.

Adults and children older than age 12 not taking carbamazepine, phenytoin, phenobarbital, primidone, or valproate: 25 mg (extended-release) P.O. daily for 2 weeks; then 50 mg P.O. daily for 2 weeks; then 100 mg P.O. daily for 1 week; then 150 mg P.O. daily for 1 week; then 200 mg P.O. daily for 1 week. Daily maintenance dose is 300 to 400 mg.

Adults and children older than age 12 taking anticonvulsant drugs but not carbamazepine, phenytoin, phenobarbital, primidone, or valproate: 25 mg (immediate-release) P.O. daily for 1 to 2 weeks; then 50 mg P.O. daily for another 2 weeks. Continue to increase by 50 mg/day every 1 to 2 weeks until an effective maintenance dose is reached. Daily maintenance dose is 225 to 375 mg P.O. daily in two divided doses.

Adults and children older than age 12 taking carbamazepine, phenytoin, phenobarbital, or primidone but not valproate: 50 mg (immediate-release) P.O. daily for 2 weeks; then 100 mg P.O. daily in two divided doses for 2 weeks. Increase, as needed, by 100 mg daily every 1 to 2 weeks. Usual maintenance dosage is 300 to 500 mg P.O. daily in two divided doses. Or, 50 mg (extended-release) P.O. daily for 2 weeks; then 100 mg P.O. daily for 2 weeks; then 200 mg P.O. daily for 1 week; then 300 mg P.O. daily for 1 week; then 400 mg P.O. daily for 1 week. Daily maintenance dose is 400 to 600 mg.

Children ages 2 to 12 weighing 7 to 40 kg (15 to 88 lb) taking valproate: 0.15 mg/kg P.O. daily in one or two divided doses (rounded down to nearest whole tablet) for 2 weeks, followed by increasing the daily dose with an additional 0.3 mg/kg daily in one or two divided doses for every 1 to 2 weeks. Thereafter, usual maintenance dosage is 1 to 5 mg/kg daily (maximum, 200 mg daily in one to two divided doses).

Children ages 2 to 12 weighing 7 to 40 kg (15 to 88 lb) taking anticonvulsant drugs but not carbamazepine, phenytoin, phenobarbital, primidone, or valproate: 0.3 mg/kg (immediate-release) P.O. daily in one or two divided doses (rounded down to the nearest whole tablet) for 2 weeks; then 0.6 mg/kg P.O. daily in two divided doses for another 2 weeks; then increase the daily dose with an additional 0.6 mg/kg P.O. daily in two divided doses every 1 to 2 weeks. Thereafter, usual maintenance dose is 4.5 to 7.5 mg/kg P.O. daily. Maximum dose is 300 mg daily in two divided doses.

Children ages 2 to 12 weighing 7 to 40 kg (15 to 88 lb) taking carbamazepine, phenytoin, phenobarbital, or primidone but not valproate: 0.6 mg/kg P.O. daily in two divided doses (rounded down to nearest whole tablet) for 2 weeks; then increase the daily dose with an additional 1.2 mg/kg daily in two divided doses every 1 to 2 weeks. Usual maintenance dosage is 5 to 15 mg/kg P.O. daily (maximum 400 mg daily in two divided doses).

▶ **To convert patients from therapy with a hepatic enzyme-inducing AED alone to lamotrigine therapy**

Adults and children age 16 and older: Add lamotrigine (immediate-release) 50 mg P.O. once daily to current drug regimen for 2 weeks, followed by 100 mg P.O. daily in two divided doses for 2 weeks. Then increase daily dosage by 100 mg every 1 to 2 weeks until maintenance dose of 500 mg daily in two divided doses is reached. The concomitant hepatic enzyme-inducing AED can then be gradually reduced by 20% decrements weekly for 4 weeks.

Adjust-a-dose: For patients with severe renal impairment, use lower maintenance dosage.

➤ **To convert patients with partial seizures from adjunctive therapy with valproate to therapy with lamotrigine alone**

Adults and children age 16 and older: Add lamotrigine (immediate-release) until 200 mg daily is achieved; then gradually decrease valproate to 500 mg daily by decrements of no more than 500 mg daily per week. Maintain these dosages for 1 week, then increase lamotrigine to 300 mg daily while decreasing valproate to 250 mg daily. Maintain these dosages for 1 week, then stop valproate completely while increasing lamotrigine by 100 mg daily every week until a dose of 500 mg daily is reached.

➤ **Bipolar disorder**

Adults: Initially, 25 mg (immediate-release) P.O. once daily for 2 weeks; then 50 mg P.O. once daily for 2 weeks. Dosage may then be doubled at weekly intervals, to maintenance dosage of 200 mg daily.

Adults taking carbamazepine or other hepatic enzyme-inducing drugs without valproate: Initially, 50 mg (immediate-release) P.O. once daily for 2 weeks; then 100 mg daily in two divided doses for 2 weeks. Dosage is then increased by 100 mg weekly to maintenance dosage of 400 mg daily, given in two divided doses.

Adults taking valproate: Initially, 25 mg (immediate-release) P.O. every other day for 2 weeks; then 25 mg P.O. once daily for 2 weeks. Dosage may then be doubled at weekly intervals to maintenance dosage of 100 mg daily.

ADMINISTRATION

P.O.

• Chewable dispersible tablets may be swallowed whole, chewed, or dispersed in water or diluted fruit juice.

• If tablets are chewed, give a small amount of water or diluted fruit juice to aid in swallowing.

• Orally disintegrating tablets should be placed on the tongue and moved around in the mouth.

• Orally disintegrating tablets may be swallowed with or without water and without regard to food.

• Give extended-release tablets once daily with or without food. Patient must swallow tablets whole and must not chew, crush, or divide them.

ACTION

Unknown. May inhibit release of glutamate and aspartate (excitatory neurotransmitters) in the brain via action at voltage-sensitive sodium channels.

Route	Onset	Peak	Duration
P.O.	Unknown	1–5 hr	Unknown

Half-life: 14½ to 70¼ hours, depending on dosage schedule and use of other anticonvulsants.

ADVERSE REACTIONS

CNS: ataxia, dizziness, headache, somnolence, *seizures,* aggravated reaction, anxiety, concentration disturbance, decreased memory, depression, dysarthria, emotional lability, fever, incoordination, insomnia, irritability, malaise, mind racing, speech disorder, sleep disorder, tremor, vertigo.

CV: palpitations.

EENT: blurred vision, diplopia, rhinitis, nystagmus, pharyngitis, vision abnormality.

GI: nausea, vomiting, abdominal pain, anorexia, constipation, diarrhea, dry mouth, dyspepsia.

GU: amenorrhea, dysmenorrhea, vaginitis.

Musculoskeletal: muscle spasm, neck pain.

Respiratory: cough, dyspnea.

Skin: rash, *Stevens-Johnson syndrome, toxic epidermal necrolysis,* acne, alopecia, hot flashes, pruritus.

Other: chills, flulike syndrome, infection, tooth disorder.

INTERACTIONS

Drug-drug. *Acetaminophen:* May decrease therapeutic effects of lamotrigine. Monitor patient.

Carbamazepine: May decrease effects of lamotrigine while increasing toxicity of carbamazepine. Adjust doses and monitor patient.

Ethosuximide, oxcarbazepine, phenobarbital, phenytoin, primidone: May decrease lamotrigine level. Monitor patient closely.

Folate inhibitors (methotrexate, sulfamethoxazole–trimethoprim): May have additive effect because lamotrigine inhibits dihydrofolate reductase, an enzyme involved in folic acid synthesis. Monitor patient.

Hormonal contraceptives containing estrogen, rifampin: May decrease lamotrigine levels. Adjust dosage. By the end of the "pill-free" week, lamotrigine levels may double.

Valproate: May decrease clearance of lamotrigine, which increases lamotrigine level; also decreases valproate level. Monitor patient for toxicity.

Drug-lifestyle. *Sun exposure:* May cause photosensitivity reactions. Advise patient to avoid excessive sun exposure.

EFFECTS ON LAB TEST RESULTS
None reported.

CONTRAINDICATIONS & CAUTIONS
• Contraindicated in patients hypersensitive to drug or its components.
• Use cautiously in patients with renal, hepatic, or cardiac impairment.

⚠ **Overdose S&S:** Ataxia, nystagmus, increased seizures, decreased level of consciousness, coma, intraventricular conduction delay.

NURSING CONSIDERATIONS
❸ **Alert:** Closely monitor all patients taking or starting AEDs for changes in behavior indicating worsening of suicidal thoughts or behavior or depression. Symptoms such as anxiety, agitation, hostility, mania, and hypomania may be precursors to emerging suicidality

• Don't stop drug abruptly because this may increase seizure frequency. Instead, taper drug over at least 2 weeks.

Black Box Warning Serious rashes requiring hospitalization and discontinuation of treatment have been reported in association with lamotrigine therapy. Don't exceed initial dose or recommended dosage escalation, or maintain coadministration with valproate. Stop drug at first sign of rash, unless rash is clearly not drug-related. ■

❸ **Alert:** Drug may cause aseptic meningitis. Monitor patient for symptoms such

as headache, fever, neck stiffness, nausea, vomiting, rash, and photophobia. Discontinue drug if no other cause of meningitis is found.

• Reduce lamotrigine dose if drug is added to a multidrug regimen that includes valproic acid.

• Evaluate patients for changes in seizure activity. Check adjunct anticonvulsant level.

• Enroll patients in Lamotrigine Pregnancy Registry (1-800-336-2176). Encourage patients to enroll in the North American Antiepileptic Drug Pregnancy Registry (1-888-233-2334).

• **Look alike–sound alike:** Don't confuse lamotrigine with lamivudine or levothyroxine. Don't confuse Lamictal with Lamisil, Ludiomil, labetalol, or Lomotil.

PATIENT TEACHING
• Inform patient that drug may cause rash. Combination therapy of valproic acid and lamotrigine may cause a serious rash. Tell patient to report rash or signs or symptoms of hypersensitivity promptly to prescriber because they may warrant stopping drug.

• Warn patient not to engage in hazardous activity until drug's CNS effects are known.

• Advise patient or caregiver to immediately report headache, fever, neck stiffness, nausea, vomiting, rash, drowsiness, confusion, or light sensitivity to his health care provider.

• Warn patient that the drug may trigger sensitivity to the sun and to take precautions until tolerance is determined.

• Warn patient not to stop drug abruptly.

❸ **Alert:** Advise women of childbearing age to discuss drug therapy with prescriber if considering pregnancy. Babies exposed to drug during the first trimester have a greater risk of cleft lip or palate.

• Advise women of childbearing age that breast-feeding isn't recommended during therapy.

Reactions in bold italics are *life-threatening*. Interactions may have a *rapid onset* or a *delayed onset*.

lansoprazole

lanz-AH-pray-zol

Prevacid✔, Prevacid SoluTab

Therapeutic class: Antiulcer drugs
Pharmacologic class: Proton pump inhibitors
Pregnancy risk category: B

AVAILABLE FORMS
Capsules (delayed-release): 15 mg, 30 mg
Orally disintegrating tablets (ODTs) (delayed-release): 15 mg, 30 mg

INDICATIONS & DOSAGES
➤ **Short-term treatment of active duodenal ulcer**
Adults: 15 mg P.O. daily before eating for 4 weeks.
➤ **Maintenance of healed duodenal ulcers**
Adults: 15 mg P.O. daily.
➤ **Short-term treatment of active benign gastric ulcer**
Adults: 30 mg P.O. once daily for up to 8 weeks.
➤ **Short-term treatment of erosive esophagitis**
Adults: 30 mg P.O. daily before eating for up to 8 weeks. If healing doesn't occur, 8 more weeks of therapy may be given. Maintenance dosage for healing is 15 mg P.O. daily.
Children ages 12 to 17: 30 mg P.O. once daily for up to 8 weeks.
Children ages 1 to 11 weighing more than 30 kg (66 lb): 30 mg P.O. once daily for up to 12 weeks. Increase dosage up to 30 mg b.i.d. in patients who remain symptomatic after 2 weeks.
Children ages 1 to 11 weighing 30 kg or less: 15 mg P.O. once daily for up to 12 weeks. Increase dosage up to 30 mg b.i.d. in patients who remain symptomatic after 2 weeks.
➤ **Long-term treatment of pathologic hypersecretory conditions, including Zollinger-Ellison syndrome**
Adults: Initially, 60 mg P.O. once daily. Increase dosage, as needed. Give daily

amounts above 120 mg in evenly divided doses.
➤ *Helicobacter pylori* **eradication to reduce risk of duodenal ulcer recurrence**
Adults: For patients receiving dual therapy, 30 mg P.O. lansoprazole with 1 g P.O. amoxicillin, each given t.i.d. for 14 days. For patients receiving triple therapy, 30 mg P.O. lansoprazole with 1 g P.O. amoxicillin and 500 mg P.O. clarithromycin, all given b.i.d. for 10 to 14 days.
➤ **Short-term treatment of symptomatic GERD**
Adults: 15 mg P.O. once daily for up to 8 weeks.
Children ages 12 to 17: 15 mg P.O. once daily for up to 8 weeks.
Children ages 1 to 11 weighing more than 30 kg (66 lb): 30 mg P.O. once daily for up to 12 weeks. Dosage can be increased up to 30 mg b.i.d. in patients who remain symptomatic after 2 weeks.
Children ages 1 to 11 weighing 30 kg or less: 15 mg P.O. once daily for up to 12 weeks. Dosage can be increased up to 30 mg b.i.d. in patients who remain symptomatic after 2 weeks.
➤ **NSAID-related ulcer in patients who continue NSAID use**
Adults: 30 mg P.O. daily for 8 weeks.
➤ **To reduce risk of NSAID-related ulcer in patients with history of gastric ulcer who need NSAIDs**
Adults: 15 mg P.O. daily for up to 12 weeks.
➤ **Stress ulcer prophylaxis (depending on risk factors and clinical situation of patient); GI bleeding prophylaxis in severely septic patients; reduction of gastric acid production in critically ill neurosurgical patients** ♦
Adults: 30 mg P.O. or via nasogastric (NG) or nasojejunal tube once daily.

ADMINISTRATION
P.O.
● Give 30 to 60 minutes before a meal.
● Don't crush or allow patient to chew capsules.
● For patients who have difficulty swallowing capsules, the capsules can be opened and the intact granules sprinkled on 1 tablespoon of applesauce, Ensure pudding, cottage cheese, yogurt, or strained pears

L

and swallowed immediately. Or, capsule contents may be emptied into a small volume (60 mL) of apple, orange, or tomato juice and swallowed.

• Contents of capsule can be mixed with 40 mL of apple juice in a syringe and given within 3 to 5 minutes via an NG or nasojejunal tube. Flush with additional apple juice to give entire dose and maintain patency of the tube.

• Place ODT on patient's tongue and allow it to disintegrate with or without water until the particles can be swallowed.

• To give ODTs using an oral syringe, dissolve a 15-mg tablet in 4 mL water or a 30-mg tablet in 10 mL water and give within 15 minutes. Refill syringe with about 2 mL (15-mg tablet) or 5 mL (30-mg tablet) of water, shake gently, and give any remaining contents.

• To give ODTs through an NG tube 8 French or larger, dissolve a 15-mg tablet in 4 mL water or a 30-mg tablet in 10 mL water and give within 15 minutes. Refill syringe with about 5 mL of water, shake gently, and flush the NG tube.

• ODTs contain 2.5 mg phenylalanine/15-mg tablet and 5.1 mg phenylalanine/30-mg tablet.

ACTION
Inhibits proton pump activity by binding to hydrogen-potassium adenosine triphosphates, located at secretory surface of gastric parietal cells, to suppress gastric acid secretions.

Route	Onset	Peak	Duration
P.O.	1–3 hr	Unknown	24 hr

Half-life: Less than 2 hours.

ADVERSE REACTIONS
GI: abdominal pain, constipation, diarrhea, nausea.

INTERACTIONS
Drug-drug. *Ampicillin esters, digoxin, iron salts, ketoconazole:* May inhibit absorption of these drugs. Monitor patient closely.
Atazanavir: May reduce GI absorption of atazanavir, reducing antiviral activity. Don't use together.

Clarithromycin: May increase lansoprazole levels and adverse effects. Monitor patient.
Clopidogrel: May interfere with conversion of clopidogrel to its active metabolite. Avoid use together.
Methotrexate: May increase methotrexate serum level. Monitor methotrexate concentration and adjust dosage as needed.
Sucralfate: May cause delayed lansoprazole absorption. Give lansoprazole at least 30 minutes before sucralfate.
Theophylline: May mildly increase theophylline clearance. Adjust theophylline dosage when lansoprazole is started or stopped. Use together cautiously.
Warfarin: May increase bleeding risk. Monitor INR and PT.
Drug-herb. *Male fern:* May inactivate herb. Discourage use together.
St. John's wort: May increase risk of sun sensitivity. Advise patient to avoid excessive sunlight exposure.
Drug-food. *Food:* May decrease rate and extent of GI absorption. Advise patient to take before meals.

EFFECTS ON LAB TEST RESULTS
None reported.

CONTRAINDICATIONS & CAUTIONS
• Contraindicated in patients hypersensitive to drug.
❸ **Alert:** Prolonged use of proton pump inhibitors may cause low magnesium levels that may require magnesium supplementation and possible discontinuation of drug. Monitor magnesium levels before starting treatment and periodically thereafter.
❸ **Alert:** There may be an increased risk of hip, wrist, and spine fractures associated with proton pump inhibitors.
• It's unknown if drug appears in breast milk. Breast-feeding women should either stop breast-feeding or stop drug.

NURSING CONSIDERATIONS
❸ **Alert:** Monitor patient for signs and symptoms of low magnesium level, such as abnormal heart rate or rhythm, palpitations, muscle spasms, tremor, or seizures. In children, abnormal heart rate may present as fatigue, upset stomach, dizziness, and lightheadedness.

Reactions in bold italics are *life-threatening*. Interactions may have a *rapid onset* or a *delayed onset*.

❸ *Alert:* May increase risk of *Clostridium difficile*–associated diarrhea (CDAD). Evaluate for CDAD in patients who develop diarrhea that doesn't improve.

• Patients with severe liver disease may need dosage adjustment, but don't adjust dosage for elderly patients or those with renal insufficiency.

• Just because symptoms respond to therapy, gastric malignancy shouldn't be ruled out.

• *Look alike–sound alike:* Don't confuse Prevacid with Pepcid, Prilosec, or Prevpac.

PATIENT TEACHING

• For best effect, instruct patient to take drug 30 to 60 minutes before eating.

• Teach patient how to take drug and alternative methods if needed.

• Teach patient to recognize and report signs and symptoms of low magnesium levels.

latanoprost
lah-TAN-oh-prost

Xalatan

Therapeutic class: Antiglaucoma drugs
Pharmacologic class: Prostaglandin analogues
Pregnancy risk category: C

AVAILABLE FORMS
Ophthalmic solution: 0.005% (50 mcg/mL)

INDICATIONS & DOSAGES
➤ **Increased intraocular pressure (IOP) in patients with ocular hypertension or open-angle glaucoma who are intolerant or who had insufficient response to other IOP-lowering medications**
Adults: Instill 1 drop in conjunctival sac of each affected eye once daily at bedtime.

ADMINISTRATION
Ophthalmic

• Don't allow tip of dispenser to contact eye or surrounding tissue. Serious damage to eye and subsequent vision loss may be caused by contaminated solutions.

• Apply light finger pressure on lacrimal sac for 1 minute after instilling drug to minimize systemic absorption.

• If more than one ophthalmic drug is being used, give at least 5 minutes apart.

ACTION
Thought to increase outflow of aqueous humor, thereby lowering IOP.

Route	Onset	Peak	Duration
Ophthalmic	3–4 hr	8–12 hr	Unknown

Half-life: 3 hours (from aqueous humor).

ADVERSE REACTIONS
CV: angina pectoris.
EENT: blurred vision, burning, foreign body sensation, increased brown pigmentation of the iris, itching, stinging, conjunctival hyperemia, dry eye, excessive tearing, eye pain, eyelash changes, lid crusting or edema, lid discomfort, photophobia, punctate epithelial keratopathy.
Musculoskeletal: muscle, joint, or back pain.
Respiratory: upper respiratory tract infection.
Skin: allergic skin reaction, rash.
Other: cold, flulike syndrome.

INTERACTIONS
Drug-drug. *Eyedrops that contain thimerosal:* May cause precipitation of eyedrops. Give at least 5 minutes apart.

EFFECTS ON LAB TEST RESULTS
None reported.

CONTRAINDICATIONS & CAUTIONS
• Contraindicated in patients hypersensitive to drug, benzalkonium chloride, or other components of drug.

• Use cautiously in patients with impaired renal or hepatic function.

• Use cautiously in breast-feeding women; it's unknown if drug appears in breast milk.

• Safety and effectiveness of drug in children haven't been established.

⚠ *Overdose S&S:* Ocular irritation, conjunctival or episcleral congestion.

NURSING CONSIDERATIONS

• Don't give drug while patient is wearing contact lenses.
• Giving drug more frequently than recommended may decrease its IOP-lowering effects; don't exceed once-daily dosing.
• Drug may gradually change eye color, increasing amount of brown pigment in iris. This change in iris color occurs slowly and may not be noticeable for months or years. Increased pigmentation may be permanent.

PATIENT TEACHING

• Inform patient of risk that iris color may change in treated eye.
• Teach patient how to instill drops, and advise him to wash hands before and after instilling solution. Warn him not to touch tip of dropper to eye or surrounding tissue.
• Advise patient to apply light finger pressure on lacrimal sac for 1 minute after instillation to minimize systemic absorption.
• Instruct patient to report reactions in the eye, especially eye inflammation and lid reactions.
• Tell patient who wears contact lenses to remove them before instilling solution and not to reinsert the lenses until 15 minutes have elapsed.
• If patient is using more than one topical ophthalmic drug, tell him to apply them at least 5 minutes apart.
• If patient develops another eye condition (such as trauma or infection) or needs eye surgery, advise him to contact prescriber about continued use of multidose container.
• Stress importance of compliance with recommended therapy.

leflunomide
leh-FLEW-no-mide

Arava

Therapeutic class: Antiarthritics
Pharmacologic class: Pyrimidine synthesis inhibitors
Pregnancy risk category: X

AVAILABLE FORMS
Tablets: 10 mg, 20 mg, 100 mg

INDICATIONS & DOSAGES

➤ **To reduce signs and symptoms of active rheumatoid arthritis; to slow structural damage as shown by erosions and joint space narrowing seen on X-ray; to improve physical function**
Adults: 100 mg P.O. loading dose every 24 hours for 3 days; then 20 mg (maximum daily dose) P.O. every 24 hours. Eliminating loading dose may decrease risk of adverse reactions, especially in patients at risk for hematologic or hepatic toxicity. Dose may be decreased to 10 mg daily if higher dose isn't well tolerated.
Adjust-a-dose: For confirmed ALT elevations between 2 and 3 times the upper limit of normal (ULN), reduce dose to 10 mg/day; if elevations persist despite dose reduction or if ALT elevations of greater than 3 × ULN are present, stop drug and give cholestyramine or charcoal.
➤ **Psoriasis in patients refractory to or intolerant of standard systemic psoriasis therapies ♦**
Adults: 100 mg P.O. daily for 3 days, followed by 20 mg P.O. daily as needed for long-term therapy.

ADMINISTRATION
P.O.
• Give drug without regard for food.

ACTION

An immunomodulatory drug that inhibits dihydro-orotate dehydrogenase, an enzyme involved in pyrimidine synthesis that has antiproliferative activity and anti-inflammatory effects.

Route	Onset	Peak	Duration
P.O.	Unknown	6–12 hr	Unknown

Half-life: 15 to 18 days.

ADVERSE REACTIONS

CNS: anxiety, asthenia, depression, dizziness, fever, headache, insomnia, malaise, migraine, neuralgia, neuritis, pain, paresthesia, sleep disorder, vertigo.
CV: hypertension, angina pectoris, chest pain, palpitations, peripheral edema, tachycardia, varicose veins, vasculitis, vasodilation.

Reactions in bold italics are *life-threatening*. Interactions may have a *rapid onset* or a *delayed onset*.

EENT: blurred vision, cataracts, conjunctivitis, epistaxis, eye disorder, pharyngitis, rhinitis, sinusitis.

GI: diarrhea, abdominal pain, anorexia, cholelithiasis, colitis, constipation, dry mouth, dyspepsia, enlarged salivary glands, esophagitis, flatulence, gastritis, gastroenteritis, gingivitis, melena, mouth ulcer, nausea, oral candidiasis, stomatitis, taste perversion, vomiting.

GU: albuminuria, cystitis, dysuria, hematuria, menstrual disorder, pelvic pain, prostate disorder, urinary frequency, UTI, vaginal candidiasis.

Hematologic: anemia.

Hepatic: *hepatotoxicity.*

Metabolic: *diabetes mellitus,* hyperglycemia, hyperlipidemia, hyperthyroidism, hypokalemia, weight loss.

Musculoskeletal: arthralgia, arthrosis, back pain, bone necrosis, bone pain, bursitis, joint disorder, leg cramps, muscle cramps, myalgia, neck pain, synovitis, tendon rupture, tenosynovitis.

Respiratory: respiratory infection, *asthma,* bronchitis, dyspnea, increased cough, lung disorder, pneumonia.

Skin: alopecia, rash, acne, contact dermatitis, dry skin, eczema, fungal dermatitis, hair discoloration, hematoma, maculopapular rash, nail disorder, pruritus, skin discoloration, skin disorder, skin nodule, skin ulcer, subcutaneous nodule.

Other: abscess, allergic reaction, cyst, ecchymoses, flulike syndrome, hernia, herpes simplex, herpes zoster, increased sweating, injury or accident, tooth disorder.

INTERACTIONS

Drug-drug. *Charcoal, cholestyramine:* May decrease leflunomide level. Sometimes used for this effect in overdose.

Methotrexate, other hepatotoxic drugs: May increase risk of hepatotoxicity. Monitor liver enzyme levels.

NSAIDs (diclofenac, ibuprofen): May increase NSAID level. Monitor patient.

Rifampin: May increase active leflunomide metabolite level. Use together cautiously.

Tolbutamide: May increase tolbutamide level. Monitor patient.

EFFECTS ON LAB TEST RESULTS

● May increase AST, ALT, glucose, lipid, and CK levels.

● May decrease potassium level.

CONTRAINDICATIONS & CAUTIONS

● Contraindicated in patients hypersensitive to drug or its components.

Black Box Warning Contraindicated in pregnant women and women of childbearing potential who are not using reliable contraception. Pregnancy must be excluded before start of therapy. ■

● Drug isn't recommended for patients with evidence of infection with hepatitis B or C viruses, severe immunodeficiency, bone marrow dysplasia, or severe uncontrolled infections; in women who are breast-feeding; in patients younger than age 18; or in men attempting to father a child.

Black Box Warning Drug isn't recommended for patients with preexisting liver disease or ALT more than $2\times$ ULN. ■

Black Box Warning Use cautiously in patients taking other drugs that can cause liver damage. ■

● Use cautiously in patients with renal insufficiency.

⚠ Overdose S&S: Diarrhea, abdominal pain, leukopenia, anemia, elevated LFT results.

NURSING CONSIDERATIONS

● Vaccination with live-virus vaccines isn't recommended. Consider the long half-life of drug when contemplating giving a live-virus vaccine after stopping drug treatment.

۞ Alert: Men planning to father a child should stop drug therapy and follow recommended leflunomide removal protocol (cholestyramine 8 g P.O. t.i.d. for 11 days). In addition to cholestyramine, verify drug levels are less than 0.02 mg/L by two separate tests at least 14 days apart. If level is greater than 0.02 mg/L, consider additional cholestyramine treatment.

● Risk of malignancy, particularly lymphoproliferative disorders, is increased with use of some immunosuppressants, including leflunomide.

Black Box Warning Liver enzyme levels should be monitored at least monthly for 6 months after beginning therapy and every 6 to 8 weeks thereafter. If ALT rises to more than 2× ULN, discontinue drug and monitor LFTs until ALT returns to normal. ■

❸ Alert: Monitor platelet and WBC counts and hemoglobin level or hematocrit at baseline and monthly for 6 months after starting therapy and every 6 to 8 weeks thereafter.

❸ Alert: Monitor AST, ALT, and serum albumin levels monthly if treatment includes methotrexate or other potential immunosuppressives.

• Stop drug and start cholestyramine or charcoal therapy if bone marrow suppression occurs.

• Watch for overlapping hematologic toxicity when switching to another antirheumatic.

❸ Alert: Rare cases of severe liver injury, including cases with fatal outcome, have occurred during leflunomide therapy. Most cases occur within 6 months of therapy and in a setting of multiple risk factors for hepatotoxicity (liver disease, other hepatotoxins).

• Carefully monitor patient after dose reduction. Because the active metabolite of leflunomide has a prolonged half-life, it may take several weeks for levels to decline.

PATIENT TEACHING
• Explain need for and frequency of required blood tests and monitoring.

Black Box Warning Instruct patient to use birth control during course of treatment and until it's been determined that drug is no longer active. ■

• Warn patient to immediately notify prescriber if signs or symptoms of pregnancy (such as late menstrual periods or breast tenderness) occur because of risk of fetal birth defects.

• Advise women to stop breast-feeding during therapy.

• Instruct patient to immediately report rash or mucous membrane lesions, unusual tiredness, abdominal pain, jaundice, easy bruising, bleeding, fever, recurrent infections, or pallor, which may be warnings of infrequent but serious adverse reactions.

• Inform patient he may continue taking aspirin, other NSAIDs, and low-dose corticosteroids during treatment.

• Inform patient that it may take 4 weeks to begin to see improvement from therapy.

letrozole
LE-tro-zol

Femara

Therapeutic class: Antineoplastics
Pharmacologic class: Aromatase inhibitors
Pregnancy risk category: X

AVAILABLE FORMS
Tablets: 2.5 mg

INDICATIONS & DOSAGES
➤ **Metastatic breast cancer with disease progression after antiestrogen therapy (such as tamoxifen)**
Postmenopausal women: 2.5 mg P.O. as single daily dose.
➤ **First-line treatment of hormone receptor–positive or hormone receptor–unknown, locally advanced, or metastatic breast cancer**
Postmenopausal women: 2.5 mg P.O. once daily until tumor progression is evident.
➤ **Adjuvant treatment of hormone-sensitive early breast cancer**
Postmenopausal women: 2.5 mg P.O. daily.
➤ **Extended adjuvant treatment of early breast cancer following 5 years of adjuvant tamoxifen therapy**
Postmenopausal women: 2.5 mg P.O. once daily for 5 years.

ADMINISTRATION
P.O.
• Drug is a hormonal agent and considered a potential teratogen. Follow safe handling procedures.
• Give drug without regard for meals.

ACTION
Inhibits conversion of androgens to estrogens, which decreases tumor mass or delays progression of tumor growth in some women.

Route	Onset	Peak	Duration
P.O.	Unknown	2 days	Unknown

Half-life: About 2 days.

ADVERSE REACTIONS
CNS: headache, somnolence, dizziness, fatigue, mood changes.
CV: hot flashes, *MI, thromboembolism,* chest pain, edema, hypertension.
GI: nausea, vomiting, constipation, diarrhea, abdominal pain, anorexia.
Metabolic: hypercholesterolemia, weight gain.
Musculoskeletal: bone pain, limb pain, back pain, arthralgia, fractures.
Respiratory: dyspnea, cough.
Skin: rash, pruritus, alopecia, diaphoresis.
Other: viral infections, breast pain.

INTERACTIONS
Drug-drug. *Tamoxifen:* May reduce plasma letrozole levels. Give letrozole immediately after tamoxifen course is completed.

EFFECTS ON LAB TEST RESULTS
• May increase cholesterol level.

CONTRAINDICATIONS & CAUTIONS
• Contraindicated in patients hypersensitive to drug or its components.
• Use cautiously in patients with severe liver impairment; dosage adjustment isn't needed in those with mild to moderate liver dysfunction.

NURSING CONSIDERATIONS
• Dosage adjustment isn't needed in patients with CrCl of 10 mL/minute or more.
• Use drug only in postmenopausal women. Rule out pregnancy before starting drug.
• *Look alike–sound alike:* Don't confuse Femara with FemHRT.

PATIENT TEACHING
• Instruct patient to take drug exactly as prescribed.
• Tell patient to take drug with a small glass of water, with or without food.
• Inform patient about potential adverse effects.
• Advise patient to use caution performing tasks that require alertness, coordination, or dexterity, such as driving, until effects are known.

leuprolide acetate
loo-PROE-lide

Eligard, Lupron, Lupron Depot, Lupron Depot-Ped, Lupron Depot–3 Month, Lupron Depot–4 Month, Lupron Depot–6 Month

Therapeutic class: Antineoplastics
Pharmacologic class: Gonadotropin-releasing hormone analogues
Pregnancy risk category: X

AVAILABLE FORMS
Depot injection: 3.75 mg, 7.5 mg, 11.25 mg, 15 mg, 22.5 mg, 30 mg, 45 mg
Injection: 5 mg/mL in 2.8-mL multiple-dose vials

INDICATIONS & DOSAGES
➤ **Advanced prostate cancer**
Adults: 1 mg subcutaneously daily. Or, 7.5 mg I.M. depot injection monthly. Or, 7.5 mg subcutaneous Eligard once monthly. Or, 22.5 mg I.M. depot injection every 3 months. Or, 22.5 mg subcutaneous Eligard every 3 months. Or, 30 mg I.M. depot injection every 4 months. Or, 30 mg subcutaneous Eligard every 4 months. Or, 45 mg subcutaneous Eligard every 6 months. Or, 45 mg I.M. depot injection every 6 months.
➤ **Endometriosis**
Adults: 3.75 mg I.M. depot injection as single injection once monthly for up to 6 months. Or, 11.25 mg I.M. every 3 months for up to 6 months.
➤ **Central precocious puberty**
Children: Initially, 0.3 mg/kg (minimum 7.5 mg) I.M. depot injection as single injection every 4 weeks. May increase in increments of 3.75 mg every 4 weeks, if needed. Stop drug before girl reaches age 11 or boy reaches age 12.
➤ **Anemia related to uterine fibroids (with iron therapy)**
Adults: 3.75 mg I.M. depot injection once monthly for up to 3 consecutive months. Or 11.25 mg I.M. depot injection for 1 dose.

L

ADMINISTRATION

• Products have specific mixing and administration instructions. Read manufacturer's directions closely.

I.M.

• Never give by I.V. injection.
• Give depot injections under medical supervision.
• Use supplied diluent to reconstitute drug (extra diluent is provided; discard remainder).
• Inject into vial; shake well. Suspension will appear milky. Use immediately.
• Draw appropriate amount into a syringe with a 22G needle.
• When using prefilled dual-chamber syringes, prepare for injection according to manufacturer's instructions.
• Gently shake syringe to form a uniform milky suspension. If particles adhere to stopper, tap syringe against your finger.
• Remove needle guard and advance plunger to expel air from syringe. Inject entire contents I.M. as with a normal injection.

Subcutaneous

• For the two-syringe mixing system, connect the syringes and inject the liquid contents according to manufacturer's instructions.
• Mix product by pushing contents back and forth between syringes for about 45 seconds; shaking the syringes won't mix the contents enough.
• Attach the needle provided in the kit and inject subcutaneously.
• Suspension settles very quickly. Remix if settling occurs. Must be given within 30 minutes.
• Never give by I.V. injection.

ACTION

Stimulates and then inhibits release of follicle-stimulating hormone and luteinizing hormone, which suppresses testosterone and estrogen levels.

Route	Onset	Peak	Duration
I.M., subcut.	Variable	1–2 mo	60–90 days
Implant	Unknown	4 hr	12 mo

Half-life: Unknown.

ADVERSE REACTIONS

CNS: dizziness, depression, headache, pain, insomnia, paresthesia, asthenia.
CV: *arrhythmias,* angina, *MI,* peripheral edema, ECG changes, hypotension, hypertension, murmur, hot flashes.
GI: nausea, vomiting, anorexia, constipation.
GU: impotence, vaginitis, urinary frequency, hematuria, UTI, amenorrhea.
Hematologic: anemia.
Metabolic: weight gain or loss.
Musculoskeletal: transient bone pain during first week of treatment, joint disorder, myalgia, neuromuscular disorder, bone loss.
Respiratory: dyspnea, sinus congestion, *pulmonary fibrosis.*
Skin: injection-site reactions, dermatitis, acne.
Other: gynecomastia, androgen-like effects.

INTERACTIONS

None significant.

EFFECTS ON LAB TEST RESULTS

• May increase albumin, alkaline phosphatase, bilirubin, BUN, calcium, creatinine, glucose, LDH, phosphorus, and uric acid levels. May decrease hemoglobin level.
• May alter results of pituitary-gonadal system tests during therapy and for 12 weeks after.

CONTRAINDICATIONS & CAUTIONS

• Contraindicated in patients hypersensitive to drug or other gonadotropin-releasing hormone analogues, in women with undiagnosed vaginal bleeding, and in pregnant or breast-feeding women.
• The 30- and 45-mg depot injections are contraindicated in women and children.
• Use cautiously in patients hypersensitive to benzyl alcohol.

NURSING CONSIDERATIONS

• A fractional dose of drug formulated to give every 3, 4, or 6 months isn't equivalent to same dose of once-a-month formulation.
• After starting treatment for central precocious puberty, monitor patient response

---

Reactions in bold italics are *life-threatening*. Interactions may have a *rapid onset* or a *delayed onset*.

every 1 to 2 months with a gonadotropin-releasing hormone stimulation test and sex corticosteroid level determinations. Measure bone age for advancement every 6 to 12 months.

🌑 *Alert:* During first few weeks of treatment for prostate cancer, signs and symptoms of disease may temporarily worsen or additional signs and symptoms may occur (tumor flare).

• May increase risk of diabetes and CV events. Monitor patient closely.

• *Look alike–sound alike:* Don't confuse Lupron Depot–3 Month with Lupron Depot-Ped.

PATIENT TEACHING

• Before starting child on treatment for central precocious puberty, make sure parents understand importance of continuous therapy.

• Carefully instruct patient who will give himself subcutaneous injection about the proper technique, and advise him to use only the syringes provided by manufacturer.

• Advise patient that, if another syringe must be substituted, a low-dose insulin syringe (U-100, 0.5 mL) may be an appropriate choice but that needle gauge should be no smaller than 22G (except when using Lupron Depot–3 Month 22.5 mg).

• Instruct patient to store leuprolide acetate powder (depot) and diluent at room temperature, to refrigerate unopened vials of leuprolide acetate injection, and to protect leuprolide acetate injection from heat and light.

• Inform patient with history of undesirable effects from other endocrine therapies that leuprolide is easier to tolerate.

• Reassure patient that adverse effects disappear after about 1 week. Explain that symptoms of prostate cancer or central precocious puberty may worsen at first.

• Advise women of childbearing age to use a nonhormonal form of contraception during treatment.

levalbuterol hydrochloride
lev-al-BYOO-ter-ol

Xopenex

levalbuterol tartrate
Xopenex HFA

Therapeutic class: Bronchodilators
Pharmacologic class: Beta$_2$ agonists
Pregnancy risk category: C

AVAILABLE FORMS

Inhalation aerosol: 45 mcg per actuation
Solution for inhalation: 0.31 mg, 0.63 mg, or 1.25 mg in 3-mL vials; 1.25 mg/0.5-mL vials (concentrate)

INDICATIONS & DOSAGES

➤ **To prevent or treat bronchospasm in patients with reversible obstructive airway disease**

Adults and adolescents age 12 and older: 0.63 mg given t.i.d. every 6 to 8 hours, by oral inhalation via a nebulizer. Patients with more severe asthma who don't respond adequately to 0.63 mg t.i.d. may benefit from 1.25 mg t.i.d.

Children ages 6 to 11: 0.31 mg inhaled by nebulizer t.i.d. Routine dosage shouldn't exceed 0.63 mg t.i.d.

Adults and children age 4 and older: 2 inhalations Xopenex HFA (90 mcg) every 4 to 6 hours. In some patients, 1 inhalation every 4 hours is sufficient.

➤ **To provide quick relief and treatment for asthma exacerbation ◆**

Children younger than age 4: For quick relief, 0.31 to 1.25 mg in 3 mL nebulizer solution every 4 to 6 hours as needed. Or, for asthma exacerbation, 0.075 mg/kg (minimum dose, 1.25 mg) nebulizer solution every 20 minutes for three doses; then 0.075 to 0.15 mg/kg, up to 5 mg every 1 to 4 hours as needed.

ADMINISTRATION
Inhalational

• Keep unopened vial in foil pouch. After opened, vial must be used within 2 weeks and protected from light.

L

- Release four test sprays before first use of inhaler or after inhaler has not been used for more than 3 days.
- Shake canister well before use.
- Use a spacer device to improve inhalation, as appropriate.
- Dilute concentrated solution (1.25 mg/ 0.5 mL) with sterile normal saline solution before administration by nebulization.

ACTION

Relaxes bronchial smooth muscle by stimulating beta$_2$ receptors; also inhibits release of mediators from mast cells in the airway.

Route	Onset	Peak	Duration
Inhalation	5–15 min	1 hr	3–4 hr

Half-life: 3¼ to 4 hours.

ADVERSE REACTIONS

CNS: dizziness, migraine, nervousness, pain, tremor, anxiety, asthenia, fever, headache.
CV: tachycardia.
EENT: rhinitis, sinusitis, turbinate edema, pharyngitis.
GI: dyspepsia, diarrhea.
Musculoskeletal: leg cramps.
Respiratory: increased cough, asthma.
Other: viral infection, flulike syndrome, accidental injury, lymphadenopathy.

INTERACTIONS

Drug-drug. *Beta blockers:* May block pulmonary effect of the drug and cause severe bronchospasm. Avoid using together, if possible. If use together is unavoidable, consider a cardioselective beta blocker, but use cautiously.
Digoxin: May decrease digoxin level up to 22%. Monitor digoxin level.
Loop or thiazide diuretics: May cause ECG changes and hypokalemia. Use together cautiously.
MAO inhibitors, TCAs: May potentiate action of levalbuterol on the vascular system. Avoid using within 2 weeks of MAO inhibitor or TCA therapy.
Other short-acting sympathomimetic aerosol bronchodilators, epinephrine: May increase adrenergic adverse effects. Use together cautiously.

EFFECTS ON LAB TEST RESULTS

None reported.

CONTRAINDICATIONS & CAUTIONS

- Contraindicated in patients hypersensitive to drug or to racemic albuterol.
- Use cautiously in patients with CV disorders (especially coronary insufficiency, hypertension, and arrhythmias), seizure disorders, hyperthyroidism, or diabetes mellitus, and in those who are unusually responsive to sympathomimetic amines.
⚠ Overdose S&S: Exaggeration of adverse reactions, hypokalemia, seizures, angina, hypertension, hypotension, arrhythmias, muscle cramps, dry mouth, palpitations, nausea, insomnia, cardiac arrest, sudden death.

NURSING CONSIDERATIONS

❸ Alert: As with other inhaled beta agonists, drug can produce paradoxical bronchospasm or life-threatening CV effects. If this occurs, stop drug immediately and notify prescriber.
- Drug may worsen diabetes mellitus and ketoacidosis.
- Drug may temporarily decrease potassium level, but potassium supplementation is usually unnecessary.
- The compatibility of levalbuterol mixed with other drugs in a nebulizer hasn't been established.

PATIENT TEACHING

- Warn patient that he may experience worsened breathing. Tell him to stop drug and contact prescriber immediately if this occurs.
- Tell patient not to increase dosage without consulting prescriber.
- Urge patient to seek medical attention immediately if levalbuterol becomes less effective, if signs and symptoms become worse, or if he's using drug more frequently than usual.
- Tell patient that the effects of levalbuterol may last up to 8 hours.
- Tell patient not to double the next dose if he misses one. Tell him to take doses at least 6 hours apart.

Reactions in bold italics are *life-threatening*. Interactions may have a *rapid onset* or a *delayed onset*.

• Advise patient to use other inhalational drugs and antiasthmatics only as directed while taking levalbuterol.
• Inform patient that common adverse reactions include palpitations, rapid heart rate, headache, dizziness, tremor, and nervousness.
• Encourage woman to contact prescriber if she becomes pregnant or is breast-feeding.
• Tell patient to keep unopened vials in foil pouch. After the foil pouch is opened, vials must be used within 2 weeks. Inform patient that vials removed from the pouch, if not used immediately, should be protected from light and excessive heat and used within 1 week.
• Teach patient to use drug correctly when inhaling by nebulizer.
• Instruct patient to breathe as calmly, deeply, and evenly as possible until no more mist is formed in the nebulizer reservoir (5 to 15 minutes).
• Tell patient using the inhaler to release four test sprays into the air away from the face before the first use or if it hasn't been used for more than 3 days.
• Instruct patient to thoroughly wash and dry plastic actuator of inhaler at least once a week to prevent medication build-up and blockage. If actuator becomes blocked, washing actuator will remove blockage.

levetiracetam
lee-vah-tih-RACE-ah-tam

Keppra, Keppra XR

Therapeutic class: Anticonvulsants
Pharmacologic class: Pyrrolidine derivatives
Pregnancy risk category: C

AVAILABLE FORMS
Injection: 500 mg/5 mL single-use vial
Oral solution: 100 mg/mL
Tablets: 250 mg, 500 mg, 750 mg, 1,000 mg
Tablets (extended-release): 500 mg, 750 mg

INDICATIONS & DOSAGES
Adjust-a-dose (for all indications): For immediate-release and oral solution, in

adults with CrCl of 50 to 80 mL/minute, give 500 to 1,000 mg every 12 hours; if CrCl is 30 to 50 mL/minute, give 250 to 750 mg every 12 hours; if CrCl is less than 30 mL/minute, give 250 to 500 mg every 12 hours. For dialysis patients, give 500 to 1,000 mg every 24 hours. Give a 250- to 500-mg dose after dialysis.
   For extended-release tablets, if CrCl is 50 to 80 mL/minute, give 1,000 to 2,000 mg every 24 hours. If CrCl is 30 to 50 mL/minute, give 500 to 1,500 mg every 24 hours. If CrCl is less than 30 mL/minute, give 500 to 1,000 mg every 24 hours.
➤ **Adjunctive therapy for myoclonic seizures of juvenile myoclonic epilepsy**
Adults and adolescents age 12 and older: Initially, 500 mg P.O. b.i.d. Increase by 1,000 mg/day every 2 weeks to a dose of 3,000 mg/day.
➤ **Adjunctive therapy for primary generalized tonic-clonic seizures**
Adults and adolescents age 16 and older: Initially, 500 mg P.O. b.i.d. Increase dose by 500 mg b.i.d. every 2 weeks to dose of 1,500 mg b.i.d.
Children ages 6 to 16: Initially, 10 mg/kg P.O. b.i.d. Increase dose by 10 mg/kg b.i.d. at 2-week intervals to dose of 30 mg/kg b.i.d. For children who weigh more than 20 kg (44 lb), use either tablets or oral solution. For children who weigh 20 kg or less, use the oral solution.
➤ **Adjunctive treatment for partial-onset seizures in patients with epilepsy**
Adults and adolescents age 16 or older: Initially, 500 mg P.O. or I.V. b.i.d. Increase dosage by 500 mg b.i.d., as needed, for seizure control at 2-week intervals to maximum of 1,500 mg b.i.d. Or, give extended-release tablets 1,000 mg P.O. daily. May increase in increments of 1,000 mg every 2 weeks to maximum recommended dosage of 3,000 mg P.O. daily.
Children ages 4 to 16: Initially, 10 mg/kg P.O. b.i.d. Increase dose by 10 mg/kg b.i.d. at 2-week intervals to recommended dose of 30 mg/kg b.i.d. If patient can't tolerate this dose, reduce it. For children who weigh 20 kg or less, use the oral solution.

L

Children ages 6 months to 4 years: Initially, 10 mg/kg P.O. b.i.d. Increase by 10 mg/kg b.i.d. at 2-week intervals to recommended dosage of 25 mg/kg b.i.d. Reduce dosage if patient can't tolerate total daily dose of 50 mg/kg.

Children ages 1 month to 6 months: Initially, 7 mg/kg P.O. b.i.d. Increase by 7 mg/kg b.i.d. at 2-week intervals to recommended dosage of 21 mg/kg b.i.d.

ADMINISTRATION
P.O.
- Give drug without regard for food.
- P.O. and I.V. forms are bioequivalent.
- Tablets should be swallowed whole and shouldn't be chewed, broken, or crushed.

I.V.
▼ Dilute drug before giving.
▼ Dilute 500-mg, 1,000-mg, or 1,500-mg dose in 100 mL normal saline solution, D_5W, or lactated Ringer injection and infuse over 15 minutes.
▼ Drug is compatible with diazepam, lorazepam, and valproate sodium for 24 hours at a controlled room temperature.
▼ **Incompatibilities:** Unknown with other antiepileptics besides diazepam, lorazepam, and valproate sodium.

ACTION
May act by inhibiting simultaneous neuronal firing that leads to seizure activity.

Route	Onset	Peak	Duration
P.O., I.V.	1 hr	1 hr	12 hr

Half-life: About 7 hours in patients with normal renal function.

ADVERSE REACTIONS
CNS: asthenia, headache, somnolence, amnesia, anxiety, ataxia, depression, dizziness, emotional lability, hostility, nervousness, paresthesia, pain, vertigo.
EENT: diplopia, pharyngitis, rhinitis, sinusitis.
GI: anorexia.
Hematologic: *leukopenia, neutropenia.*
Respiratory: cough.
Other: infection.

INTERACTIONS
Drug-drug. *Antihistamines, benzodiazepines, opioids, other drugs that cause drowsiness, TCAs:* May lead to severe sedation. Avoid using together.
Drug-lifestyle. *Alcohol use:* May lead to severe sedation. Discourage use together.

EFFECTS ON LAB TEST RESULTS
- May alter LFT results. May decrease hemoglobin and hematocrit.
- May decrease WBC, RBC, and neutrophil counts.

CONTRAINDICATIONS & CAUTIONS
- Contraindicated in patients hypersensitive to drug.
- Use cautiously in immunocompromised patients, such as those with cancer or HIV infection. Leukopenia and neutropenia have been reported with drug use.
- Use cautiously in patients with history of psychiatric symptoms, especially psychotic symptoms and behaviors.
- Drug's effect in pregnant women is unknown. Use during pregnancy only if the potential benefit outweighs the potential risk to the fetus.
⚠ *Overdose S&S:* Drowsiness, aggression, agitation, coma, depressed level of consciousness, respiratory depression, somnolence.

NURSING CONSIDERATIONS
- Use drug only with other anticonvulsants; it's not recommended for monotherapy.
- Seizures can occur if drug is stopped abruptly. Tapering is recommended.
- Monitor patients closely for such adverse reactions as dizziness, which may lead to falls.
🟡 *Alert:* Closely monitor all patients taking or starting antiepileptic drugs for changes in behavior indicating worsening of suicidal thoughts or behavior or depression. Symptoms such as anxiety, agitation, hostility, mania, and hypomania may be precursors to emerging suicidality.
- *Look alike–sound alike:* Don't confuse levetiracetam with levofloxacin. Don't confuse Keppra with Kaletra or Keflex.

PATIENT TEACHING
• Tell patient to seek medical attention for emerging or worsening depression, suicidal thoughts or behavior, or unusual changes in mood or behavior and to report such symptoms as anxiety, agitation, hostility, mania, and hypomania, which may be precursors to emerging suicidality.
• Warn patient to use extra care when sitting or standing to avoid falling.
• Advise patient to call prescriber and not to stop drug suddenly if adverse reactions occur.
• Tell patient to take with other prescribed seizure drugs.
• For the oral solution, tell patient or parent to use a calibrated measuring device, not a household spoon.
• Warn patient that drug may cause dizziness and somnolence and that he should avoid driving, bike riding, or other hazardous activities until he knows how the drug will affect him.
• Inform patient that drug can be taken with or without food.
• Tell patient not to chew, crush, or break tablets.
• Advise patient not to stop drug abruptly because doing so may increase seizure frequency.

levobunolol hydrochloride
LEE-voe-BYOO-no-lahl

AKBeta, Betagan

Therapeutic class: Antiglaucoma drugs
Pharmacologic class: Nonselective beta blockers
Pregnancy risk category: C

AVAILABLE FORMS
Ophthalmic solution: 0.25%, 0.5%

INDICATIONS & DOSAGES
➤ **Chronic open-angle glaucoma, ocular hypertension**
Adults: One or two drops once daily (0.5%) or b.i.d. (0.25%).

ADMINISTRATION
Ophthalmic
• Don't let tip of dropper touch patient's eye or surrounding tissue.
• Apply light finger pressure on lacrimal sac for 1 minute after instilling drug to minimize systemic absorption.

ACTION
Thought to reduce formation, and possibly increase outflow, of aqueous humor.

Route	Onset	Peak	Duration
Ophthalmic	1 hr	2–6 hr	24 hr

Half-life: Unknown.

ADVERSE REACTIONS
CNS: syncope, depression, headache, insomnia.
CV: hypotension, *bradycardia, heart failure,* slight reduction in resting heart rate.
EENT: transient eye stinging and burning, blepharoconjunctivitis, corneal punctate staining, decreased corneal sensitivity, erythema, itching, keratitis, photophobia, tearing.
GI: nausea.
Respiratory: *bronchospasm.*
Skin: urticaria.

INTERACTIONS
Drug-drug. *Dipivefrin, epinephrine, systemically administered carbonic anhydrase inhibitors, topical miotics:* May further reduce intraocular pressure (IOP). Use together cautiously.
Metoprolol, propranolol, other oral beta blockers: May increase ocular and systemic effects. Use together cautiously.
Reserpine, other catecholamine-depleting drugs: May increase hypotensive and bradycardiac effects. Monitor blood pressure and heart rate closely.
Drug-lifestyle. *Sun exposure:* May cause photophobia. Advise patient to wear sunglasses.

EFFECTS ON LAB TEST RESULTS
None reported.

CONTRAINDICATIONS & CAUTIONS
• Contraindicated in patients hypersensitive to drug and in those with bronchial

L

asthma, sinus bradycardia, second- or third-degree AV block, cardiac failure, cardiogenic shock, or history of bronchial asthma or severe COPD.

• Use cautiously in patients with chronic bronchitis, emphysema, diabetes mellitus, hyperthyroidism, or myasthenia gravis.

• Safe use in pregnant or breast-feeding women hasn't been established.

⚠ **Overdose S&S:** Bradycardia, hypotension, bronchospasm, acute heart failure.

NURSING CONSIDERATIONS
• Normal IOP is 10 to 21 mm Hg.

PATIENT TEACHING
• Teach patient how to instill drug. Advise him to wash hands before and after instillation and to apply light finger pressure on lacrimal sac for 1 minute after drops are instilled.

• Warn patient not to touch tip of dropper to eye or surrounding tissue.

• Advise elderly patient to report shortness of breath, chest pain, or heart irregularities to prescriber. Drug may be absorbed systemically and produce signs and symptoms of beta blockade.

• Advise patient to carry medical identification at all times during therapy.

levocetirizine dihydrochloride
LEE-voe-se-TIR-a-zeen

Xyzal

Therapeutic class: Antihistamines
Pharmacologic class: H_1-receptor antagonists
Pregnancy risk category: B

AVAILABLE FORMS
Oral solution: 2.5 mg/5 mL
Tablets: 5 mg

INDICATIONS & DOSAGES
➤ **Seasonal and perennial allergic rhinitis; uncomplicated skin manifestations of chronic idiopathic urticaria**
Adults and children age 12 and older: 5 mg P.O. once daily in the evening.

Children ages 6 to 11: 2.5 mg P.O. once daily in the evening.
Children ages 6 months to 5 years: 1.25 mg (2.5 mL) P.O. daily in the evening. Don't exceed this dose.

Adjust-a-dose: For patients ages 12 and older with CrCl of 50 to 80 mL/minute, give 2.5 mg P.O. once daily; with CrCl of 30 to 50 mL/minute, give 2.5 mg P.O. every other day; and with CrCl 10 to 30 mL/minute, give 2.5 mg P.O. twice weekly (once every 3 to 4 days).

ADMINISTRATION
P.O.
• Give drug without regard for food.

ACTION
H_1-receptor inhibition creates antihistamine effect, relieving allergy symptoms.

Route	Onset	Peak	Duration
P.O.	Unknown	1 hr	24 hr

Half-life: 8 hours.

ADVERSE REACTIONS
CNS: fatigue, pyrexia, somnolence.
EENT: dry mouth, epistaxis, nasopharyngitis, pharyngitis.
Respiratory: cough.

INTERACTIONS
Drug-drug. *CNS depressants:* May have additive effects when taken together. Avoid using together.
Ritonavir: May increase serum concentration and increase half-life of levocetirizine. Use cautiously together.
Theophylline: May decrease the clearance of levocetirizine. Use cautiously together.
Drug-lifestyle. *Alcohol use:* May have additive effect when taken with levocetirizine. Discourage use together.

EFFECTS ON LAB TEST RESULTS
• May prevent, reduce, or mask positive result skin wheal in diagnostic skin test.

CONTRAINDICATIONS & CAUTIONS
• Contraindicated in patients hypersensitive to drug or to cetirizine.

Reactions in bold italics are *life-threatening*. Interactions may have a *rapid onset* or a *delayed onset*.

- Contraindicated in patients with CrCl of less than 10 mL/minute or those undergoing hemodialysis.
- Contraindicated in patients age 6 to 11 with impaired renal function.
- Use cautiously in patients with predisposing factors for urine retention, such as spinal cord lesion or prostatic hyperplasia. Discontinue drug if urine retention occurs.
⚠ **Overdose S&S:** Drowsiness; initial agitation and restlessness, then drowsiness (in children).

NURSING CONSIDERATIONS
- Monitor patient's renal function.
- Patient should avoid engaging in hazardous occupations requiring mental alertness and motor coordination, such as operating machinery or driving a motor vehicle.
- Drug is excreted in breast milk; avoid use in breast-feeding women.
- Safety and effectiveness in patients younger than age 6 months haven't been established.
- Use drug during pregnancy only if benefits to mother clearly outweigh risk to fetus.

PATIENT TEACHING
- Warn patient not to perform hazardous tasks or those requiring alertness and coordination until CNS effects are known.
- Advise patient to avoid use of alcohol and other CNS depressants while taking this drug.
- Advise patient not to take more than the recommended dose because of increased risk of somnolence at higher doses.

levodopa–carbidopa
lee-voe-DOE-pa and kar-bih-DOE-pa

Parcopa, Sinemet✐, Sinemet CR✐

Therapeutic class: Antiparkinsonians
Pharmacologic class: Decarboxylase inhibitors–dopamine precursors
Pregnancy risk category: C

AVAILABLE FORMS
Tablets: 100 mg levodopa with 10 mg carbidopa (Sinemet 10–100), 100 mg levodopa with 25 mg carbidopa (Sinemet 25–100), 250 mg levodopa with 25 mg carbidopa (Sinemet 25–250)
Tablets (extended-release): 200 mg levodopa with 50 mg carbidopa (Sinemet CR), 100 mg levodopa with 25 mg carbidopa
Tablets (orally disintegrating): 100 mg levodopa with 10 mg carbidopa, 100 mg levodopa with 25 mg carbidopa, 250 mg levodopa with 25 mg carbidopa

INDICATIONS & DOSAGES
➤ **Idiopathic Parkinson disease, postencephalitic parkinsonism, and symptomatic parkinsonism resulting from carbon monoxide or manganese intoxication**
Adults: 1 tablet of 100 mg levodopa with 25 mg carbidopa P.O. t.i.d.; then increased by 1 tablet daily or every other day, as needed, to maximum daily dose of 8 tablets. May use 250 mg levodopa with 25 mg carbidopa or 100 mg levodopa with 10 mg carbidopa tablets, as directed, to obtain maximal response. Optimum daily dose must be determined by careful adjustment for each patient.

Patients given conventional tablets may receive extended-release tablets; dosage is calculated on current levodopa intake. Extended-release tablets should provide 10% more levodopa daily, increased as needed and as tolerated to 30% more levodopa daily. Give in divided doses at intervals of 4 to 8 hours. Allow at least a 3-day interval between dosage adjustments.

ADMINISTRATION
P.O.
- Give drug with food to decrease GI upset, but avoid giving with high-protein meals, which can impair absorption and reduce effectiveness.
- Don't crush or break extended-release form.
- Give orally disintegrating tablet (ODT) immediately after removing from bottle. Place tablet on patient's tongue, where it will dissolve in seconds and be swallowed with saliva. No additional fluid is needed.

L

ACTION

Levodopa, a dopamine precursor, relieves parkinsonian symptoms by being converted to dopamine in the brain. Carbidopa inhibits the decarboxylation of peripheral levodopa, which allows more intact levodopa to travel to the brain.

Route	Onset	Peak	Duration
P.O.	Unknown	40–150 min	Unknown

Half-life: 1 to 2 hours.

ADVERSE REACTIONS

CNS: syncope, agitation, bradykinetic episodes, confusion, dementia, *suicidal tendencies,* dizziness, dream abnormalities, headache, insomnia, *neuroleptic malignant syndrome,* paresthesia, psychotic episodes, somnolence.
CV: cardiac irregularities, hypertension, hypotension, orthostatic hypotension, palpitations, phlebitis, *MI.*
GI: anorexia, constipation, dark saliva, duodenal ulcer, diarrhea, dry mouth, dyspepsia, *GI bleeding,* taste alterations, vomiting.
GU: dark urine, urinary frequency, UTI.
Hematologic: *agranulocytosis,* hemolytic and nonhemolytic anemia, *leukopenia, thrombocytopenia.*
Musculoskeletal: back pain, muscle cramps, shoulder pain.
Respiratory: dyspnea, upper respiratory tract infection.
Skin: alopecia, rash, diaphoresis, dark sweat.
Other: increased libido, hypersensitivity.

INTERACTIONS

Drug-drug. *Antihypertensives:* May cause additive hypotensive effects. Use together cautiously.
Iron salts: May reduce bioavailability of levodopa–carbidopa. Give iron 1 hour before or 2 hours after Sinemet.
MAO inhibitors: May cause risk of severe hypertension. Avoid using together.
Methylphenidate: May increase risk of adverse effects related to levodopa–carbidopa. Monitor patient carefully.
Metoclopramide: May decrease therapeutic effects of levodopa–carbidopa. Monitor therapeutic effects.

Papaverine, phenytoin: May antagonize antiparkinsonian actions. Avoid using together.
Phenothiazines, other antipsychotics: May antagonize antiparkinsonian actions. Use together cautiously. Therapy modification may be necessary.
Sapropterin: May increase risk of levodopa–related adverse effects. Monitor patient carefully.
Drug-herb. *Kava:* May decrease action of drug. Discourage kava use altogether.
Octacosanol: May worsen dyskinesias. Discourage use together.
Drug-food. *Foods high in protein:* May decrease levodopa absorption. Don't give levodopa with high-protein foods.

EFFECTS ON LAB TEST RESULTS

- May increase uric acid, ALT, AST, alkaline phosphatase, LDH, and bilirubin levels. May decrease hemoglobin level and hematocrit.
- May decrease WBC, granulocyte, and platelet counts.
- May falsely increase urinary cate-cholamine level and serum and urinary uric acid levels in colorimetric tests. May falsely decrease urinary vanillylmandelic acid level. May cause false-positive results in urine ketone tests using sodium nitroprus-side reagent and in urine glucose tests using cupric sulfate reagent. May cause false-negative urine glucose or false-positive urine acetone results in tests using glucose oxidase. May alter results of urine screening tests for phenylketonuria.

CONTRAINDICATIONS & CAUTIONS

- Contraindicated in patients hypersensitive to drug and in those with angle-closure glaucoma, melanoma, or undiagnosed skin lesions.
- Contraindicated within 14 days of MAO inhibitor therapy.
- Use cautiously in patients with severe CV, renal, hepatic, endocrine, or pulmonary disorders; history of peptic ulcer; psychiatric illness; MI with residual arrhythmias; bronchial asthma; emphysema; or well-controlled, chronic open-angle glaucoma.

Reactions in bold italics are *life-threatening*. Interactions may have a *rapid onset* or a *delayed onset*.

• May increase risk of impulse-control disorders, dyskinesia, melanoma, orthostatic hypotension, and sudden somnolence.

⚠ *Overdose S&S:* Muscle twitching, blepharospasm.

NURSING CONSIDERATIONS
• Observe patient and monitor vital signs, especially changes in blood pressure when changing positions and while adjusting dosage. Report significant changes.

🔵 *Alert:* Because of risk of precipitating a symptom complex resembling neuroleptic malignant syndrome, observe patient closely if levodopa dosage is reduced abruptly or stopped.

• Hallucinations may require reduction or withdrawal of drug.
• Test patients receiving long-term therapy regularly for diabetes and acromegaly, and periodically for hepatic, renal, and hematopoietic function.

PATIENT TEACHING
• Tell patient to take drug with food to minimize GI upset; however, high-protein meals can impair absorption and reduce effectiveness.
• Tell patient not to chew or crush extended-release form.
• Advise patient to have skin checks.
• Warn patient and caregivers not to increase dosage without prescriber's orders.
• Caution patient about possible dizziness when standing up quickly, especially at start of therapy. Tell him to change positions slowly and dangle his legs before getting out of bed.
• Instruct patient to report adverse reactions (such as somnolence, loss of impulse control) and therapeutic effects.
• Inform patient that pyridoxine (vitamin B_6) doesn't reverse beneficial effects of levodopa–carbidopa. Multivitamins can be taken without reversing levodopa's effects.
• Teach patient to take ODT immediately after taking from bottle and to place on top of tongue. Tablet will dissolve in seconds and will be swallowed with saliva. No additional fluid is needed.

levodopa–carbidopa–entacapone
lee-voe-DOE-pa, kar-bih-DOE-pa, and en-ta-KAP-own

Stalevo⊘

Therapeutic class: Antiparkinsonians
Pharmacologic class: Dopamine precursors–decarboxylase inhibitors–catecholamine-*O*-methyltransferase inhibitors
Pregnancy risk category: C

AVAILABLE FORMS
Tablets (film-coated): 50 mg levodopa, 12.5 mg carbidopa, and 200 mg entacapone; 75 mg levodopa, 18.75 mg carbidopa, and 200 mg entacapone; 100 mg levodopa, 25 mg carbidopa, and 200 mg entacapone; 125 mg levodopa, 31.25 mg carbidopa, and 200 mg entacapone; 150 mg levodopa, 37.5 mg carbidopa, and 200 mg entacapone; 200 mg levodopa, 50 mg carbidopa, and 200 mg entacapone

INDICATIONS & DOSAGES
➤ **Idiopathic Parkinson disease, to replace (with equivalent strengths) levodopa, carbidopa, and entacapone given individually or to replace immediate-release levodopa–carbidopa for a patient who has end-of-dose "wearing off," who's taking a total daily levodopa dose of 600 mg or less, and who has no dyskinesia**
Adults: 1 tablet P.O.; determine dose and interval by therapeutic response. Maximum, 8 tablets daily for all strengths except levodopa 200 mg, carbidopa 50 mg, and entacapone 200 mg; for these strengths, give 6 tablets/day.

ADMINISTRATION
P.O.
• Don't cut tablets.
• Give only 1 tablet at each dosing interval.
• Give drug with food to decrease GI upset, but avoid giving with high-protein meal, which can decrease absorption.

L

ACTION

Levodopa, a dopamine precursor, relieves parkinsonian symptoms by converting to dopamine in the brain. Carbidopa inhibits the decarboxylation of peripheral levodopa, which allows more intact levodopa to travel to the brain. Entacapone is a reversible catecholamine-*O*-methyltransferase (COMT) inhibitor that increases levodopa level.

Route	Onset	Peak	Duration
P.O.	Unknown	1½ hr	Unknown

Half-life: 1½ to 2 hours carbidopa, 1 to 5 hours levodopa, and 1 to 4 hours entacapone.

ADVERSE REACTIONS

levodopa and carbidopa
CNS: syncope, agitation, bradykinetic episodes, confusion, dementia, *suicidal tendencies,* dizziness, dream abnormalities, headache, insomnia, *neuroleptic malignant syndrome,* paresthesia, psychotic episodes, somnolence.
CV: cardiac irregularities, hypertension, hypotension, orthostatic hypotension, palpitations, phlebitis, *MI.*
GI: anorexia, constipation, dark saliva, duodenal ulcer, diarrhea, dry mouth, dyspepsia, *GI bleeding,* taste alterations, vomiting.
GU: dark urine, urinary frequency, UTI.
Hematologic: *agranulocytosis,* hemolytic and nonhemolytic anemia, *leukopenia, thrombocytopenia.*
Musculoskeletal: back pain, muscle cramps, shoulder pain.
Respiratory: dyspnea, upper respiratory tract infection.
Skin: alopecia, rash, diaphoresis, dark sweat.
Other: increased libido, hypersensitivity.
entacapone
CNS: dyskinesia, hyperkinesia, agitation, anxiety, asthenia, dizziness, fatigue, hypokinesia, somnolence.
GI: diarrhea, nausea, abdominal pain, constipation, dry mouth, dyspepsia, flatulence, gastritis, taste perversion, vomiting.
GU: urine discoloration.
Musculoskeletal: back pain.
Respiratory: dyspnea.
Skin: increased sweating, purpura.
Other: bacterial infection.

INTERACTIONS

Drug-drug. *Ampicillin, chloramphenicol, cholestyramine, erythromycin, probenecid, rifampin:* May interfere with entacapone excretion. Use together cautiously.
Antihypertensives: May cause orthostatic hypotension. Adjust antihypertensive dosage as needed.
CNS depressants: Additive effects. Use together cautiously.
Dopamine (D2) receptor antagonists such as butyrophenones, iron salts, isoniazid, metoclopramide, phenothiazines, phenytoin, risperidone: May decrease levodopa, carbidopa, and entacapone effects. Monitor patient for effectiveness.
Drugs metabolized by COMT, such as methyldopa, apomorphine, dobutamine, dopamine, epinephrine, isoproterenol, isoetharine, norepinephrine: May increase heart rate, arrhythmias, and excessive blood pressure changes. Use together cautiously.
Metoclopramide: May increase availability of levodopa and carbidopa by increasing gastric emptying. Monitor patient for adverse effects.
Nonselective MAO inhibitors: May disrupt catecholamine metabolism. Avoid using together.
Selegiline: May cause severe hypotension. Use together cautiously, and monitor blood pressure.
TCAs: May increase risk of hypertension and dyskinesia. Monitor patient closely.

EFFECTS ON LAB TEST RESULTS

● May increase alkaline phosphatase, AST, ALT, LDH, glucose, BUN, and bilirubin levels. May decrease hemoglobin level and hematocrit.
● May decrease platelet and WBC counts.
● May cause false-positive reaction for urinary ketone bodies on a test tape. May cause false-negative result for glucosuria with glucose oxidase testing methods.

CONTRAINDICATIONS & CAUTIONS

● Contraindicated in patients hypersensitive to drug or its ingredients.
❸ *Alert:* Drug may increase the risk for MI, stroke, and death. Monitor CV status closely.

Reactions in bold italics are *life-threatening*. Interactions may have a *rapid onset* or a *delayed onset*.

• Contraindicated in patients with angle-closure glaucoma, suspicious undiagnosed skin lesions, or a history of melanoma.
• Contraindicated within 2 weeks of MAO inhibitor therapy.
• Use cautiously in patients with past or current psychosis and in patients with severe CV or pulmonary disease; bronchial asthma; biliary obstruction; peptic ulcer; or renal, hepatic, or endocrine disease.
• Use cautiously in patients with chronic open-angle glaucoma, hepatic impairment, or a history of MI and residual atrial, nodal, or ventricular arrhythmias.
A Overdose S&S: CNS disturbances, hypotension, tachycardia, rhabdomyolysis, transient renal insufficiency, abdominal pain, loose stools.

NURSING CONSIDERATIONS
• Certain CNS effects, such as dyskinesia, may occur at lower dosages and sooner with levodopa–carbidopa–entacapone than with levodopa alone. Dyskinesia may require a reduced dosage.
• During the first adjustment period, monitor patient with CV disease carefully and in a facility equipped to provide intensive cardiac care.
• Neuroleptic malignant syndrome may develop when levodopa and carbidopa are reduced or stopped, especially in patients taking antipsychotic drugs. Watch patient carefully for fever, hyperthermia, muscle rigidity, involuntary movements, altered consciousness, mental status changes, and autonomic dysfunction.
• During extended therapy, periodically monitor hepatic, hematopoietic, CV, and renal function.
• Diarrhea is common; it usually develops 4 to 12 weeks after treatment starts but may appear as early as the first week or as late as many months after treatment starts.
◑ Alert: Monitor patient for hallucinations, depression, and suicidal tendencies.

PATIENT TEACHING
• Advise patient to take drug exactly as prescribed and not to split tablets.
• Tell patient to report a "wearing-off" effect, which may occur at the end of the dosing interval.

• Tell patient that urine, sweat, and saliva may turn dark (red, brown, or black) during treatment.
• Advise patient to notify the prescriber if problems making voluntary movements increase.
• Tell patient that diarrhea is common with this treatment.
• Inform patient that hallucinations may occur.
• Urge patient to immediately report depression or suicidal thoughts.
• Explain that he may become dizzy if he rises quickly. Urge patient to use caution when rising.
• Tell patient that a high-protein diet, excessive acidity, and iron salts may reduce the drug's effectiveness.
• Urge patient to avoid hazardous activities until the CNS effects of the drug are known.
• Advise patient to notify prescriber if she becomes pregnant.

levofloxacin
lee-voe-FLOX-a-sin

Levaquin✐

Therapeutic class: Antibiotics
Pharmacologic class: Fluoroquinolones
Pregnancy risk category: C

AVAILABLE FORMS
Infusion (premixed): 250 mg in 50 mL D₅W, 500 mg in 100 mL D₅W, 750 mg in 150 mL D₅W
Oral solution: 25 mg/mL*
Single-use vials: 500 mg, 750 mg
Tablets: 250 mg, 500 mg, 750 mg

INDICATIONS & DOSAGES
Adjust-a-dose (for all indications): For patients with CrCl of less than 50 mL/minute, adjust the oral or I.V. dosage regimen according to the manufacturer's instructions.
➤ **Acute bacterial sinusitis caused by susceptible strains of** *Streptococcus pneumoniae, Moraxella catarrhalis,* **or** *Haemophilus influenzae*
Adults: 500 mg P.O. or I.V. infusion over 60 minutes every 24 hours for 10 to 14 days

or 750 mg P.O. or I.V. every 24 hours for 5 days.

➤ **Mild to moderate skin and skin-structure infections caused by _Staphylococcus aureus_ or _Streptococcus pyogenes_**
Adults: 500 mg P.O. or I.V. infusion over 60 minutes every 24 hours for 7 to 10 days.

➤ **Acute bacterial worsening of chronic bronchitis caused by _S. aureus, S. pneumoniae, M. catarrhalis, H. influenzae,_ or _Haemophilus parainfluenzae_**
Adults: 500 mg P.O. or I.V. infusion over 60 minutes every 24 hours for 7 days.

➤ **To prevent inhalation anthrax after confirmed or suspected exposure to _Bacillus anthracis_**
Adults: 500 mg I.V. infusion or P.O. every 24 hours for 60 days.
Children age 6 months and older weighing at least 50 kg (110 lb): 500 mg by slow I.V. infusion every 24 hours for 60 days.
Children age 6 months and older weighing less than 50 kg (110 lb): 8 mg/kg (not to exceed 250 mg/dose) by slow I.V. infusion every 12 hours for 60 days.

➤ **Chronic bacterial prostatitis caused by _Escherichia coli, Enterococcus faecalis,_ or _Staphylococcus epidermidis_**
Adults: 500 mg P.O. or I.V. over 60 minutes every 24 hours for 28 days.

➤ **Community-acquired pneumonia from _S. pneumoniae_ (excluding multidrug-resistant strains), _H. influenzae, H. parainfluenzae,_ Mycoplasma pneumoniae, and _Chlamydia pneumoniae_**
Adults: 750 mg P.O. or I.V. over 90 minutes every 24 hours for 5 days.

➤ **Community-acquired pneumonia caused by methicillin-susceptible _S. aureus, S. pneumoniae, H. influenzae, H. parainfluenzae, Klebsiella pneumoniae, M. catarrhalis, C. pneumoniae, Legionella pneumophila,_ or _M. pneumoniae_**
Adults: 500 mg P.O. or I.V. every 24 hours for 7 to 14 days.

➤ **Complicated skin and skin-structure infections caused by methicillin-sensitive _S. aureus, E. faecalis, S. pyogenes,_ or _Proteus mirabilis_**
Adults: 750 mg P.O. or I.V. infusion over 90 minutes every 24 hours for 7 to 14 days.

➤ **Nosocomial pneumonia caused by methicillin-susceptible _S. aureus, Pseu-domonas aeruginosa, Serratia marcescens, E. coli, K. pneumoniae, H. influenzae,_ or _S. pneumoniae_**
Adults: 750 mg P.O. or I.V. infusion over 90 minutes every 24 hours for 7 to 14 days.

➤ **Complicated UTI caused by _E. faecalis, Enterobacter cloacae, E. coli, K. pneumoniae, P. mirabilis,_ or _Pseudomonas aeruginosa;_ acute pyelonephritis caused by _E. coli_**
Adults: 250 mg P.O. or I.V. over 60 minutes every 24 hours for 10 days.

➤ **Complicated UTI caused by _E. coli, K. pneumoniae,_ or _P. mirabilis;_ acute pyelonephritis caused by _E. coli_**
Adults: 750 mg P.O. or I.V. over 90 minutes daily for 5 days.

➤ **Mild to moderate uncomplicated UTI caused by _E. coli, K. pneumoniae,_ or _Staphylococcus saprophyticus_**
Adults: 250 mg P.O. daily for 3 days.

➤ **Prophylaxis or treatment of pneumonic and septicemic plague (_Yersinia pestis_)**
Adults: 500 mg P.O. or I.V. every 24 hours for 10 to 14 days.
Children age 6 months and older weighing 50 kg (110 lb) or more: 500 mg by slow I.V. infusion every 24 hours for 10 to 14 days.
Children age 6 months and older weighing less than 50 kg: 8 mg/kg (not to exceed 250 mg/dose) by slow I.V. infusion every 12 hours for 10 to 14 days.

➤ **Traveler's diarrhea ◆**
Adults: 500 mg P.O. daily for up to 3 days.

➤ **Epididymitis likely to be caused by enteric organisms or those confirmed negative for gonococcal infection ◆**
Adults: 500 mg P.O. once daily for 10 days.

➤ **Infection prophylaxis in neutropenia ◆**
Adults: 500 mg P.O. daily, initiated at time of stem cell infusion, first day of cytotoxic therapy, or day after last dose of cytotoxic therapy. Discontinue drug when recovery from neutropenia occurs or empirical antibiotic therapy for fever is initiated.

➤ **Drug-resistant tuberculosis caused by organisms known or presumed to be sensitive to fluoroquinolones or when first-line drugs can't be used because of intolerance ◆**
Adults: 500 to 1,000 mg P.O. daily.

Reactions in bold italics are _life-threatening_. Interactions may have a _rapid onset_ or a _delayed onset_.

ADMINISTRATION

P.O.

• Obtain specimen for culture and sensitivity tests before therapy and as needed to determine if bacterial resistance has occurred.

• Give drug with plenty of fluids.

• Give 2 hours before or 6 hours after antacids, sucralfate, and products containing iron or zinc.

• Give oral solution 1 hour before or 2 hours after a meal.

I.V.

▼ Obtain specimen for culture and sensitivity tests before therapy and as needed to determine if bacterial resistance has occurred.

▼ Give this form only by infusion.

▼ Dilute drug in single-use vials, according to manufacturer's instructions, with D₅W or normal saline solution for injection to a final concentration of 5 mg/mL.

▼ Infuse doses of 500 mg or less over 60 minutes and doses of 750 mg over 90 minutes.

▼ Reconstituted solution should be clear, slightly yellow, and free of particulate matter.

▼ Reconstituted drug is stable for 72 hours at room temperature, for 14 days when refrigerated in plastic containers, and for 6 months when frozen.

▼ Thaw at room temperature or in refrigerator.

▼ **Incompatibilities:** Acyclovir sodium, alprostadil, azithromycin, furosemide, heparin sodium, indomethacin sodium trihydrate, insulin, mannitol 20%, nitroglycerin, propofol, sodium bicarbonate, sodium nitroprusside. The manufacturer recommends not mixing or infusing other drugs with levofloxacin.

ACTION

Inhibits bacterial DNA gyrase and prevents DNA replication, transcription, repair, and recombination in susceptible bacteria.

Route	Onset	Peak	Duration
P.O., I.V.	Unknown	1–2 hr	Unknown

Half-life: About 6 to 8 hours.

ADVERSE REACTIONS

CNS: *encephalopathy, seizures,* dizziness, headache, insomnia.

GI: *pseudomembranous colitis,* abdominal pain, constipation, diarrhea, dyspepsia, nausea, vomiting.

GU: vaginitis.

Hematologic: *lymphopenia,* eosinophilia, hemolytic anemia.

Metabolic: *hypoglycemia.*

Musculoskeletal: back pain, tendon rupture.

Respiratory: allergic pneumonitis, dyspnea.

Skin: *erythema multiforme, Stevens-Johnson syndrome,* photosensitivity, pruritus, rash.

Other: *anaphylaxis, multisystem organ failure, hypersensitivity reactions.*

INTERACTIONS

Drug-drug. *Aluminum hydroxide, aluminum–magnesium hydroxide, calcium carbonate, didanosine, magnesium hydroxide, products containing zinc, sucralfate:* May interfere with GI absorption of levofloxacin. Give levofloxacin 2 hours before or 6 hours after these products.

Antiarrhythmics (Class IA [procainamide, quinidine] or Class III [amiodarone, dofetilide]), chlorpromazine, erythromycin, fluconazole, imipramine, ziprasidone: May increase risk of life-threatening cardiac arrhythmias. Avoid use together.

Antidiabetics: May alter glucose level. Monitor glucose level closely.

Iron salts: May decrease absorption of levofloxacin, reducing anti-infective response. Separate doses by at least 2 hours.

NSAIDs: May increase CNS stimulation. Monitor patient for seizure activity.

Black Box Warning *Steroids:* May increase risk of tendinitis and tendon rupture. Monitor patient for tendon pain or inflammation. ∎

Theophylline: May decrease clearance of theophylline. Monitor theophylline level.

Warfarin and derivatives: May increase effect of oral anticoagulant. Monitor PT and INR.

Drug-herb. *Dong quai, St. John's wort:* May cause photosensitivity reactions. Advise patient to avoid excessive sunlight exposure.

L

Drug-lifestyle. *Sun exposure:* May cause photosensitivity reactions. Advise patient to avoid excessive sunlight exposure.

EFFECTS ON LAB TEST RESULTS
● May decrease glucose and hemoglobin levels.
● May increase eosinophil count. May decrease WBC count.
● May produce false-positive opioid assay results.

CONTRAINDICATIONS & CAUTIONS
Black Box Warning Drug is associated with increased risk of tendinitis and tendon rupture, especially in patients older than age 60 and those with heart, kidney, or lung transplants. ■
Black Box Warning Drug may exacerbate muscle weakness in patients with myasthenia gravis. Avoid using fluoroquinolones in patients with a history of myasthenia gravis. ■
❸ Alert: Oral or parenteral fluoroquinolones may increase risk of peripheral neuropathy of the arms or legs. Signs and symptoms can occur at any time during treatment and can last for months or years or be permanent. Stop drug immediately if patient develops signs or symptoms and switch to a non-fluoroquinolone antibacterial unless benefit of continued treatment outweighs risk.
❸ Alert: Drug is associated with an in-creased incidence of musculoskeletal dis-orders (arthralgia, arthritis, tendinopathy, and gait abnormality) in pediatric patients. Testing of drug in immature animals has resulted in increased osteochondrosis, ero-sions in weight-bearing joints, and other signs and symptoms of arthropathy.
● Contraindicated in patients hypersensitive to drug, its components, or other fluoro-quinolones.
● Use cautiously in patients with history of seizure disorders or other CNS diseases, such as cerebral arteriosclerosis.
● Use cautiously and with dosage adjust-ment in patients with renal impairment.
● Safety and effectiveness of drug in preg-nant and breast-feeding women haven't been established.
● Drug is indicated in pediatric patients (age 6 months and older) only for postexpo-sure inhalational anthrax prevention and for plague.

NURSING CONSIDERATIONS
● If patient experiences symptoms of excessive CNS stimulation (restlessness, tremor, confusion, hallucinations), stop drug and notify prescriber. Begin seizure precautions.
● Patients with acute hypersensitivity reactions may need treatment with epinephrine, oxygen, I.V. fluids, antihis-tamines, corticosteroids, pressor amines, and airway management.
❸ Alert: Monitor patient for signs and symp-toms of peripheral neuropathy (pain, burn-ing, tingling, numbness, weakness, or a change in sensation to light touch, pain, temperature, or the sense of body position), and report them immediately to health care provider.
● Most antibacterials can cause pseu-domembranous colitis. If diarrhea occurs, notify prescriber; drug may be stopped.
● Drug may cause an abnormal ECG.
❸ Alert: If *P. aeruginosa* is a confirmed or suspected pathogen, use with a beta-lactam.
● Monitor glucose level and results of renal and hepatic function tests and blood counts.
● *Look alike–sound alike:* Don't confuse levofloxacin with levetiracetam. Don't confuse Levaquin with Lariam.

PATIENT TEACHING
❸ Alert: Warn patient to immediately report signs and symptoms of peripheral neuro-pathy.
● Tell patient to take drug as prescribed, even if signs and symptoms disappear.
● Advise patient to take drug with plenty of fluids and to space antacids, sucralfate, and products containing iron or zinc.
● Tell patient to take oral solution 1 hour before or 2 hours after eating.
● Warn patient to avoid hazardous tasks until adverse effects of drug are known.
● Advise patient to avoid excessive sunlight exposure.
● Instruct patient to stop drug and notify prescriber if rash or other signs or symptoms of hypersensitivity develop.

Black Box Warning Tell patient that tendon rupture may occur with drug and to notify prescriber if he experiences pain or inflammation. ∎
● Instruct diabetic patient to monitor glucose level and notify prescriber about low-glucose reaction.
● Instruct patient to notify prescriber of loose stools or diarrhea.

levomilnacipran hydrochloride
lee-voe-mil-NAY-sih-pran

Fetzima

milnacipran hydrochloride
Savella⌇

Therapeutic class: Antifibromyalgia drugs–antidepressants
Pharmacologic class: SSNRIs
Pregnancy risk category: C

AVAILABLE FORMS
Capsules (extended-release): 20 mg, 40 mg, 80 mg, 120 mg
Tablets: 12.5 mg, 25 mg, 50 mg, 100 mg

INDICATIONS & DOSAGES
➤ **Fibromyalgia (Savella)**
Adults: Initially, 12.5 mg P.O. once daily; increase dosage to 12.5 mg b.i.d. on days 2 and 3, followed by 25 mg b.i.d. on days 4 to 7. Increase to 50 mg b.i.d. after day 7. May increase to 100 mg P.O. b.i.d. based on individual response.
Adjust-a-dose: For patients with CrCl of 5 to 29 mL/minute, give 25 mg b.i.d.
➤ **Major depressive disorder (Fetzima)**
Adults: Initially, 20 mg P.O. once daily for 2 days; then increase to 40 mg once daily. May increase in increments of 40 mg at intervals of 2 or more days. Maximum dosage is 120 mg once daily.
Adjust-a-dose: For patients with CrCl of 30 to 59 mL/minute, maximum maintenance dosage is 80 mg once daily. If CrCl is 15 to 29 mL/minute, maximum maintenance dosage is 40 mg once daily. Don't use for patients with ESRD.

ADMINISTRATION
P.O.
● Give drug with or without food.
● Make sure patient swallows extended-release capsules whole and doesn't chew, crush, or open them.

ACTION
Unclear. Milnacipran is a potent inhibitor of neuronal norepinephrine and serotonin reuptake; however, it doesn't affect the uptake of dopamine or other transmitters.

Route	Onset	Peak	Duration
P.O. (immediate-release)	Unknown	2–4 hr	36–48 hr
P.O. (extended-release)	Unknown	6–8 hr	Unknown

Half-life: Immediate-release, 6 to 8 hours; active metabolite, 8 to 10 hours. Extended-release, 12 hours.

ADVERSE REACTIONS
CNS: anxiety, depression, dizziness, dysgeusia, falls, fatigue, fever, headache, hypoesthesia, irritability, insomnia, migraine, paresthesia, *seizures,* stress, somnolence, tension headache, tremors.
CV: chest discomfort, chest pain, flushing, hypertension, palpitations, peripheral edema, tachycardia.
EENT: blurred vision.
GI: abdominal distention, abdominal pain, constipation, decreased appetite, diarrhea, dry mouth, flatulence, GERD, dyspepsia, nausea, vomiting.
GU: cystitis, UTI; in men—dysuria, ejaculation disorder, ejaculation failure, erectile dysfunction, libido decrease, prostatitis, scrotal pain, testicular pain, testicular swelling, urethral pain, urinary hesitation, urine retention, urine flow decrease.
Metabolic: hypercholesterolemia, weight loss.
Respiratory: dyspnea, upper respiratory tract infection.
Skin: hyperhidrosis, pruritus, rash.
Other: chills, contusion, hot flush, night sweats, peripheral edema.

L

INTERACTIONS

Drug-drug. *Antipsychotics (risperidone), cyclobenzaprine, dopamine antagonists (metoclopramide):* May cause serotonin syndrome. If use together can't be avoided, closely monitor patient for signs and symptoms of serotonin syndrome. If these occur, discontinue milnacipran or levomilnacipran.

⚠ Alert: *Aspirin, NSAIDs, warfarin:* May increase risk of bleeding. Use together cautiously.

Clomipramine: May cause euphoria and orthostatic hypotension when switching from clomipramine to milnacipran. Monitor patient closely.

Clonidine: May inhibit clonidine's effects. Use together cautiously.

Digoxin: May cause orthostatic hypotension and tachycardia. Avoid use together.

Epinephrine, norepinephrine: May cause paroxysmal hypertension and arrhythmia. Avoid use together.

Lithium, other serotonergic drugs: May cause serotonin syndrome (diarrhea, dysreflexia, fever, hallucinations, loss of coordination, nausea, tachycardia). Avoid use together.

MAO inhibitors: May cause hyperthermia, rigidity, myoclonus, autonomic instability, rapid fluctuations of vital signs, agitation, delirium, and coma. Avoid using drug within 2 weeks after MAO inhibitor therapy; wait at least 5 days after stopping milnacipran or levomilnacipran before starting MAO inhibitor.

Methylene blue: May cause CNS toxicity and serotonin syndrome. Avoid use together.

Drug-lifestyle. *Alcohol use:* May enhance CNS depression and aggravate preexisting liver disease. Don't administer to patients with alcohol use or chronic liver disease.

EFFECTS ON LAB TEST RESULTS

- May increase LFT values.
- May decrease sodium level.

CONTRAINDICATIONS & CAUTIONS

- Contraindicated in patients hypersensitive to drug or its components, in those with uncontrolled angle-closure glaucoma, and within 14 days of discontinuing MAO inhibitor therapy. Extended-release form isn't approved for the treatment of fibromyalgia.

⚠ Alert: Serotonin syndrome, a potentially life-threatening condition, may occur, particularly with concomitant use of serotonergic drugs (including triptans and tramadol) and drugs that impair serotonin metabolism (including MAO inhibitors). Signs and symptoms of serotonin syndrome include mental status changes (agitation, coma, hallucinations), autonomic instability (hyperthermia, labile blood pressure, tachycardia), neuromuscular aberrations (hyperreflexia, incoordination), and diarrhea, nausea, and vomiting.

- Not recommended for use in patients with ESRD.
- Use cautiously in patients with a history of mania, seizures, severe hepatic impairment, or dysuria; in patients who consume substantial amounts of alcohol; and in those with hypertension or controlled angle-closure glaucoma.
- Use in pregnant women only if the benefit to the mother outweighs the risk to the fetus. It isn't known if drug appears in breast milk; discourage breast-feeding during therapy.

⚠ Overdose S&S: Hypertension, cardiac arrest, decreased level of consciousness, dizziness, elevated LFT results.

NURSING CONSIDERATIONS

Black Box Warning Drug may increase the risk of suicidal thinking and behavior in children, adolescents, and young adults with major depressive disorder or other psychiatric disorder. Drug isn't approved for use in children. ∎

- At least 14 days should elapse between discontinuation of an MAO inhibitor and initiation of milnacipran or levomilnacipran therapy. Allow at least 5 days after stopping milnacipran or levomilnacipran before starting an MAO inhibitor.
- Monitor patient closely for worsening depression or suicidal behavior, especially during the first few months of therapy and with dosage adjustments.
- To prevent withdrawal signs and symptoms, decrease dosage gradually, and watch for signs and symptoms that may arise when drug is stopped, such as dysphoria, irritability, agitation, dizziness, sensory disturbances, anxiety, confusion, headache,

---

lethargy, emotional lability, insomnia, hypomania, tinnitus, and seizures.
• Carefully monitor heart rate and blood pressure.
• Monitor patient for signs of hyponatremia (headache, difficulty concentrating, memory impairment, confusion, weakness, unsteadiness, hallucination, syncope, seizures, coma, respiratory arrest).
• Monitor LFT values and sodium level before and during therapy.

PATIENT TEACHING
Black Box Warning Warn families and caregivers to immediately report signs and symptoms of worsening depression (such as agitation, irritability, insomnia, hostility, and impulsivity) and suicidal behavior. ∎
• Advise patient to avoid taking NSAIDs and aspirin while taking drug to reduce the risk of bleeding.
• Tell patient to avoid alcohol while taking drug.
• Instruct patient to have frequent heart rate and blood pressure monitoring.
• Tell patient to report urinary hesitation or urine retention.
• Instruct woman of childbearing age to notify prescriber if she becomes pregnant, is planning pregnancy during therapy, or is breast-feeding.
• Warn patient not to stop drug suddenly.
• Tell patient to consult prescriber before taking other prescription or OTC drugs.
• Warn patient to avoid hazardous activities that require alertness and good coordination until drug's effects are known.
• Tell patient that drug may be taken with or without food but that food may increase tolerability.
• Instruct patient to swallow capsules whole and not to chew, crush, or open them.
• Advise patient to regularly monitor blood pressure and pulse while taking drug.

levothyroxine sodium (T₄, L-thyroxine sodium)

$\text{levothyroxine sodium (T}_4\text{, L-thyroxine sodium)}$

lee-voe-thye-ROX-een

Eltroxin†, Euthyrox†, Levo-T, Levothroid, Levoxyl𝒫, Synthroid𝒫, Tirosint, Unithroid

Therapeutic class: Thyroid hormone replacements
Pharmacologic class: Thyroid hormones
Pregnancy risk category: A

AVAILABLE FORMS
Capsules: 13 mcg, 25 mcg, 50 mcg, 75 mcg, 88 mcg, 100 mcg, 112 mcg, 125 mcg, 137 mcg, 150 mcg
Powder for injection: 100 mcg, 200 mcg, 500 mcg
Tablets: 25 mcg, 50 mcg, 75 mcg, 88 mcg, 100 mcg, 112 mcg, 125 mcg, 137 mcg, 150 mcg, 175 mcg, 200 mcg, 300 mcg

INDICATIONS & DOSAGES
➤ **Thyroid hormone replacement**
Adults: For patients younger than age 50 or those older than age 50 who have been recently treated for hyperthyroidism, or have been hypothyroid for a short time, 1.7 mcg/kg P.O. once daily. Monitor thyroid-stimulating hormone (TSH) levels every 6 to 8 weeks, making dosage adjustments in 12.5- to 25-mcg increments until patient is euthyroid and TSH level normalizes.
Adults: For patients age 50 or older or those younger than age 50 with underlying cardiac disease, 25 to 50 mcg P.O. daily. Adjust dose every 6 to 8 weeks, if needed, until patient is euthyroid and TSH level normalizes.
Children in whom growth and puberty are complete: 1.7 mcg/kg P.O. once daily.
Children older than age 12 in whom growth and puberty are incomplete: More than 150 mcg or 2 to 3 mcg/kg P.O. daily.
Children ages 6 to 12: 100 to 150 mcg or 4 to 5 mcg/kg P.O. daily.
Children ages 1 to 5: 75 to 100 mcg or 5 to 6 mcg/kg P.O. daily.
Children ages 6 months to 1 year: 50 to 75 mcg or 6 to 8 mcg/kg P.O. daily.

L

Children ages 3 to 6 months: 25 to 50 mcg or 8 to 10 mcg/kg P.O. daily.

Infants and neonates birth to 3 months: 10 to 15 mcg/kg P.O. daily. In neonates at risk for cardiac failure, use a lower initial dose (such as 25 mcg daily), and increase every 4 to 6 weeks as needed.

Elderly patients with underlying CV disease: 12.5 to 25 mcg P.O. daily; increase by 12.5 to 25 mcg every 4 to 6 weeks, depending on response.

➤ **Severe, long-standing hypothyroidism**
Adults: 12.5 to 25 mcg P.O. daily. Increase in increments of 25 mcg every 2 to 4 weeks as needed.

Children: 25 mcg P.O. daily. Increase in increments of 25 mcg every 2 to 4 weeks as needed.

➤ **Hypothyroidism (when rapid onset of effect is critical or when oral route is precluded for long periods of time)**
Adults and children: Approximately one-half of previously established oral dosage I.V. or I.M. Maintenance dosage is 50 to 100 mcg/day (0.05 to 0.1 mg/day) I.V. or I.M.

➤ **Myxedema coma or stupor without concomitant severe heart disease**
Adults and children: 200 to 500 mcg (0.2 to 0.5 mg) I.V. as solution containing 100 mcg/mL. May give additional 100 to 300 mcg or more on second day. Maintain continued daily administration of lesser amounts until patient can take daily oral dose.

ADMINISTRATION

P.O.
• Synthroid may contain tartrazine.
• Give drug at same time each day on an empty stomach, preferably ½ to 1 hour before breakfast.
• Give Levoxyl with a full glass of water to prevent choking, gagging, and difficulty swallowing.
• If necessary, crush tablet and suspend it in small amount of formula (except soy formula, which may decrease the absorption), breast milk, or water, and give by spoon or dropper. Crushed tablet can also be sprinkled over food, except foods containing large amounts of soybean, fiber, or iron.

I.V.
▼ Reconstitute by adding 5 mL normal saline injection only.
▼ Shake vial.
▼ Use immediately after reconstitution.
▼ Discard any unused portion.
▼ **Incompatibilities:** Don't mix or give with anything other than normal saline injection.

I.M.
• Reconstitute by adding 5 mL normal saline injection only.
• Shake vial.
• Use immediately after reconstitution.
• Discard any unused portion.

ACTION

Not completely defined. Stimulates metabolism of all body tissues by accelerating rate of cellular oxidation.

Route	Onset	Peak	Duration
P.O.	24 hr	Unknown	Unknown
I.V., I.M.	Unknown	Unknown	Unknown

Half-life: 3 to 4 days in hyperthyroidism; 9 to 10 days in hypothyroidism.

ADVERSE REACTIONS

CNS: nervousness, insomnia, tremor, headache, fever, fatigue.
CV: tachycardia, palpitations, *arrhythmias,* angina pectoris, *cardiac arrest.*
GI: diarrhea, vomiting.
GU: menstrual irregularities.
Metabolic: weight loss, increased appetite.
Musculoskeletal: decreased bone density, muscle weakness.
Respiratory: dyspnea.
Skin: allergic skin reactions, diaphoresis, hair loss.
Other: heat intolerance, impaired fertility.

INTERACTIONS

Drug-drug. *Amiodarone, iodide (including iodine-containing radiographic contrast agents), lithium:* May reduce thyroid hormone secretion. Monitor thyroid function studies if used together.
Antacids, calcium carbonate, cholestyramine, colestipol, ferrous sulfate, sucralfate: May impair levothyroxine absorption. Separate doses by 4 to 5 hours.

Reactions in bold italics are *life-threatening*. Interactions may have a *rapid onset* or a *delayed onset*.

Beta blockers: May reduce beta-blocker effects. Monitor patient.

Carbamazepine, hydantoins, phenobarbital, rifampin: May increase hepatic metabolism, resulting in hypothyroidism. Monitor patient.

Digoxin: May decrease cardiac glycoside effects. Monitor patient for clinical effect.

Estrogens: May decrease thyroid levels. Monitor levels after 12 weeks of therapy and adjust levothyroxine dosage as needed.

Fosphenytoin, phenytoin: May release free thyroid hormone. Monitor patient for tachycardia.

Insulin, oral antidiabetics: May alter glucose level. Monitor glucose level. Dosage adjustments may be needed.

Ketamine: May produce marked hypertension and tachycardia. Use together cautiously.

SSRIs: May increase levothyroxine requirements. Adjust dosage as needed.

Sympathomimetics such as epinephrine: May increase risk of coronary insufficiency. Monitor patient closely.

Tetracyclic antidepressants, TCAs: May increase therapeutic effects and toxicity of both drugs. Monitor patient closely.

Theophylline: May decrease theophylline clearance in hypothyroidism; clearance may return to normal when euthyroid state is achieved. Monitor theophylline level.

Warfarin: May increase anticoagulant effects. Monitor patient for bleeding and check PT and INR closely. Warfarin dosage adjustment may be needed.

Drug-herb. *Horseradish:* May cause abnormal thyroid function. Discourage use in patients undergoing thyroid function tests.

Lemon balm: May have antithyroid effects; may inhibit TSH. Discourage use together.

Drug-food. *Cottonseed meal, dietary fiber, soybean flour, walnuts:* May decrease absorption of drug. Dosage adjustments may be needed.

EFFECTS ON LAB TEST RESULTS
● May decrease thyroid function test results. May alter results of liothyronine, protein-bound iodine, and radioactive ^{131}I uptake studies.

CONTRAINDICATIONS & CAUTIONS
● Contraindicated in patients hypersensitive to drug and in those with acute MI uncomplicated by hypothyroidism, untreated subclinical or overt thyrotoxicosis, or uncorrected adrenal insufficiency.

Black Box Warning Don't use either alone or with other therapeutic agents for treatment of obesity or for weight loss. ■

● Use cautiously in elderly patients and in those with angina pectoris, hypertension, other CV disorders, renal insufficiency, or ischemia.

● Use cautiously in patients with diabetes mellitus, diabetes insipidus, or myxedema and during rapid replacement in those with arteriosclerosis.

⚠ ***Overdose S&S:*** Signs and symptoms of hyperthyroidism, confusion, disorientation, cerebral embolism, shock, coma, seizures, death.

NURSING CONSIDERATIONS
● Patients with diabetes mellitus may need increased antidiabetic doses when starting thyroid hormone replacement.

● Watch for angina, coronary occlusion, or stroke in patients with arteriosclerosis who are receiving rapid replacement.

● In patients with coronary artery disease who must receive thyroid hormone, observe carefully for possible coronary insufficiency.

● Patients with adult hypothyroidism are unusually sensitive to thyroid hormone. Start at lowest dosage, and adjust to higher dosages according to patient's symptoms and laboratory data until euthyroid state is reached.

● When changing from levothyroxine to liothyronine, stop levothyroxine and begin liothyronine. Increase dosage in small increments after residual effects of levothyroxine have disappeared. When changing from liothyronine to levothyroxine, start levothyroxine several days before withdrawing liothyronine to avoid relapse. Drugs aren't interchangeable.

● Long-term therapy causes bone loss in premenopausal and postmenopausal women. Consider a basal bone density measurement, and monitor patient closely for osteoporosis.

L

• Patients taking levothyroxine who need to have ^{131}I uptake studies performed must stop drug 4 weeks before test.

• Patients taking anticoagulants may need their dosage modified and require careful monitoring of coagulation status.

• Dosage may need to be increased in pregnant patients.

• Drug shouldn't be used for infertility (unless associated with hypothyroidism).
Black Box Warning Drug should not be used for the treatment of obesity or for weight loss. ▪

• *Look alike–sound alike:* Don't confuse levothyroxine with lamotrigine or Lanoxin.

PATIENT TEACHING

• Teach patient the importance of compliance. Tell him to take drug at same time each day, preferably ½ to 1 hour before breakfast, to maintain constant hormone levels and help prevent insomnia.

• Make sure patient understands that replacement therapy is usually for life. The drug should never be stopped unless directed by prescriber.

• Warn patient (especially elderly patient) to notify prescriber immediately about chest pain, palpitations, sweating, nervousness, shortness of breath, or other signals of overdose or aggravated CV disease.

• Tell caregiver of infant or child who can't swallow tablets to crush tablet and suspend in small amount of water and give by spoon or dropper. Crushed tablet can be sprinkled over food, except foods containing large amounts of soybean, fiber, or iron.

• Tell patient using Levoxyl to take pill with plenty of water to avoid choking, gagging, or getting the pill stuck in his throat.

• Advise patient who has achieved stable response not to change brands.

• Tell patient to report unusual bleeding and bruising.

• Advise patient not to take OTC or other prescription drugs without first consulting prescriber.

• Advise patient to report pregnancy to prescriber because dosage may need adjustment.

• Advise patient to protect tablets from light and moisture.

SAFETY ALERT!

lidocaine hydrochloride
LYE-doe-kane

LidoPen Auto-Injector, Xylocaine, Xylocard†

Therapeutic class: Antiarrhythmics
Pharmacologic class: Amide derivatives
Pregnancy risk category: B

AVAILABLE FORMS
Infusion (premixed): 0.2% (2 mg/mL), 0.4% (4 mg/mL), 0.8% (8 mg/mL)
Injection (for direct I.V. use): 1% (10 mg/mL), 2% (20 mg/mL)
Injection (for I.V. admixtures): 4% (40 mg/mL), 10% (100 mg/mL), 20% (200 mg/mL)

INDICATIONS & DOSAGES
➤ **Ventricular arrhythmias caused by MI, cardiac manipulation, or cardiac glycosides**
Adults: 50 to 100 mg (1 to 1.5 mg/kg) by I.V. bolus at 25 to 50 mg/minute. Bolus dose is repeated every 3 to 5 minutes until arrhythmias subside or adverse reactions develop. Don't exceed 300-mg total bolus during a 1-hour period. Simultaneously, constant infusion of 20 to 50 mcg/kg/minute (1 to 4 mg/minute) is begun. If single bolus has been given, smaller bolus dose may be repeated 15 to 20 minutes after start of infusion to maintain therapeutic level.
Children: 1 mg/kg by I.V. or intraosseous bolus. Start infusion at 30 mcg/kg/minute.
Elderly patients: Reduce dosage and rate of infusion by 50%.
Adjust-a-dose: For patients with heart failure, with renal or liver disease, or who weigh less than 50 kg (110 lb), reduce dosage.

ADMINISTRATION
I.V.
▼ Injections (additive syringes and single-use vials) containing 40, 100, or 200 mg/mL are for the preparation of I.V. infusion solutions only and must be diluted before use.
▼ Prepare I.V. infusion by adding 1 g (using 25 mL of 4% or 5 mL of 20% injection) to 1 L of D₅W injection to provide a solution containing 1 mg/mL.

Reactions in bold italics are *life-threatening*. Interactions may have a *rapid onset* or a *delayed onset*.

▼ Use a more concentrated solution of up to 8 mg/mL in fluid-restricted patient.
▼ Patients receiving infusions must be on a cardiac monitor and must be attended at all times. Use an infusion control device for giving infusion precisely. Don't exceed 4 mg/minute; faster rate greatly increases risk of toxicity.
▼ Avoid giving injections containing preservatives.
▼ **Incompatibilities:** Amphotericin, ampicillin, cefazolin, ceftriaxone, fentanyl citrate (higher pH brands), methohexital sodium, phenytoin sodium, sodium bicarbonate, thiopental sodium.

ACTION
A class IB antiarrhythmic that decreases the depolarization, automaticity, and excitability in the ventricles during the diastolic phase by direct action on the tissues, especially the Purkinje network.

Route	Onset	Peak	Duration
I.V.	Immediate	Immediate	10–20 min

Half-life: 1½ to 2 hours (may be prolonged in patients with heart failure or hepatic disease).

ADVERSE REACTIONS
CNS: confusion, tremor, stupor, restlessness, light-headedness, *seizures,* lethargy, somnolence, anxiety, hallucinations, nervousness, paresthesia, muscle twitching.
CV: hypotension, *bradycardia, new or worsened arrhythmias, cardiac arrest.*
EENT: tinnitus, blurred or double vision.
GI: vomiting.
Respiratory: *respiratory depression and arrest.*
Skin: soreness at injection site.
Other: *anaphylaxis,* sensation of cold.

INTERACTIONS
Drug-drug. *Atenolol, metoprolol, nadolol, pindolol, propranolol:* May reduce hepatic metabolism of lidocaine, increasing the risk of toxicity. Give bolus doses of lidocaine at a slower rate, and monitor lidocaine level and patient closely.
Cimetidine: May decrease clearance of lidocaine, increasing the risk of toxicity. Consider using a different H_2-receptor

antagonist if possible. Monitor lidocaine level closely.
Ergot-type oxytocic drugs: May cause severe, persistent hypertension or stroke. Avoid using together.
Mexiletine: May increase pharmacologic effects. Avoid using together.
Phenytoin, procainamide, propranolol, quinidine: May increase cardiac depressant effects. Monitor patient closely.
Succinylcholine: May prolong neuromuscular blockade. Monitor patient closely.
Drug-herb. *Pareira:* May increase the effects of neuromuscular blockade. Discourage use together.
Drug-lifestyle. *Smoking:* May increase metabolism of lidocaine. Monitor patient closely.

EFFECTS ON LAB TEST RESULTS
None.

CONTRAINDICATIONS & CAUTIONS
● Contraindicated in patients hypersensitive to amide-type local anesthetics.
● Contraindicated in those with Adams-Stokes syndrome, Wolff-Parkinson-White syndrome, and severe degrees of SA, AV, or intraventricular block in the absence of an artificial pacemaker.
● Use cautiously and at reduced dosages in patients with complete or second-degree heart block or sinus bradycardia, in elderly patients, in those with heart failure or renal or hepatic disease, and in those weighing less than 50 kg (110 lb).
⚠ *Overdose S&S:* Circulatory depression, change in level of consciousness, seizures, hypoventilation.

NURSING CONSIDERATIONS
● Monitor drug level. Therapeutic levels are 2 to 5 mcg/mL.
● *Alert:* Monitor patient for toxicity. In many severely ill patients, seizures may be the first sign of toxicity, but severe reactions are usually preceded by somnolence, confusion, tremors, and paresthesia. If signs of toxicity occur, stop drug at once and notify prescriber. Continuing could lead to seizures and coma. Give oxygen through a nasal cannula if not contraindicated. Keep

oxygen and cardiopulmonary resuscitation equipment available.

• Monitor patient's response, especially blood pressure and electrolytes, BUN, and creatinine levels. Notify prescriber promptly if abnormalities develop.

• If arrhythmias worsen or ECG changes (for example, QRS complex widens or PR interval substantially prolongs), stop infusion and notify prescriber.

PATIENT TEACHING
• Tell patient to report adverse reactions promptly because toxicity can occur.

SAFETY ALERT!

linagliptin
lin-a-GLIP-tin

Tradjenta

Therapeutic class: Antidiabetics
Pharmacologic class: DPP-4 inhibitors
Pregnancy risk category: B

AVAILABLE FORMS
Tablets: 5 mg

INDICATIONS & DOSAGES
➤ **Adjunct to diet and exercise to improve glycemic control in adults with type 2 diabetes as monotherapy or as combination therapy with an insulin secretagogue (such as a sulfonylurea) or insulin**
Adults: 5 mg P.O. daily.
Adjust-a-dose: When used in combination with an insulin secretagogue or insulin, use lower doses of those drugs to decrease the risk of hypoglycemia.

ADMINISTRATION
P.O.
• Give drug without regard for food.
• Store tablets at 77° F (25° C) with excursions permitted to 59° to 86° F (15° to 30° C).
• Store tablets out of reach of children.

ACTION
Inhibits DPP-4, an enzyme that rapidly inactivates incretin hormones, which play a part in the body's regulation of glucose.

Route	Onset	Peak	Duration
P.O.	Rapid	1½ hr	Unknown

Half-life: About 12 hours (accumulation).

ADVERSE REACTIONS
CNS: headache.
EENT: nasopharyngitis.
Metabolic: *hypoglycemia.*
Musculoskeletal: arthralgia, back pain, myalgia.

INTERACTIONS
Drug-drug. *CYP3A4 or P-glycoprotein inducers (such as rifampin):* May decrease linagliptin level. Avoid use together.
Ritonavir: May increase linagliptin effects and risk of adverse effects. Use with caution; monitor response, and adjust dosage as necessary.
Sulfonylureas (such as glyburide), insulin: May increase risk of hypoglycemia. Monitor glucose level carefully and adjust sulfonylurea or insulin dosage as necessary.

EFFECTS ON LAB TEST RESULTS
• May increase uric acid level.
• May decrease fasting glucose and glycosylated hemoglobin levels.

CONTRAINDICATIONS & CAUTIONS
• Contraindicated in patients hypersensitive to drug (with such signs and symptoms as urticaria, angioedema, and bronchial hyperactivity).
• Drug not for use in patients with type 1 diabetes or for treatment of diabetic ketoacidosis.
• Acute pancreatitis, including fatal pancreatitis, has occurred in patients taking linagliptin. It's unknown whether patients with a history of pancreatitis are at increased risk for development of pancreatitis while using linagliptin.
• It isn't known if drug appears in breast milk. Use cautiously in breast-feeding women.

NURSING CONSIDERATIONS
• Monitor glycosylated hemoglobin and fasting blood glucose levels periodically.
• Monitor patient for signs and symptoms of hypoglycemia (anxiety, confusion,

diaphoresis, tachycardia, paresthesia) and hyperglycemia (excess thirst, urination).
• Monitor patient for signs and symptoms of pancreatitis (persistent, severe abdominal pain, which may radiate to the back, and vomiting). If pancreatitis is suspected, promptly discontinue linagliptin and initiate appropriate management.

PATIENT TEACHING
• Inform patient of the potential risks and benefits of linagliptin and of alternative modes of therapy.
• Instruct patient to take drug only as prescribed. If a dose is missed, advise patient not to double the next dose.
• Explain the importance of proper diet, regular physical activity, and periodic blood glucose monitoring.
• Teach patient to recognize and manage hypoglycemia and hyperglycemia.
• Advise patient to notify the health care provider promptly during periods of stress (such as fever, trauma, infection, or surgery) because medication requirements may change.
• Teach patient signs and symptoms of pancreatitis and to immediately contact prescriber if they occur.

lindane
LIN-dayn

Therapeutic class: Scabicides–pediculicides
Pharmacologic class: Ectoparasiticides–ovicides
Pregnancy risk category: C

AVAILABLE FORMS
Lotion: 1%
Shampoo: 1%

INDICATIONS & DOSAGES
➤ **Parasitic infestation (scabies, pediculosis)**
Adults and children: Centers for Disease Control and Prevention recommend not bathing before applying on skin. If patient does bathe, let skin dry and cool thoroughly before using drug. For scabies, apply thin

layer of lotion over entire skin surface from the neck down (with special attention to skinfolds, creases, under fingernails, interdigital spaces, and genital area) and rub in thoroughly; for pediculosis, apply thin layer of lotion to hairy areas. After 8 to 12 hours, wash drug off.

Apply shampoo undiluted to dry hair and work into lather for 4 minutes; small amounts of water may increase lathering. Apply 30 mL of shampoo for short hair, 45 mL for medium-length hair, or 60 mL for long hair. Rinse thoroughly and rub dry with towel. Comb with a fine-tooth comb.
Elderly patients: May need to reduce dosage because of increased skin absorption.

ADMINISTRATION
Topical
• If patient bathes before application, make sure his skin is dry and cool before applying drug.
• Apply thin layer to cover body only once. Use 1 ounce for children younger than age 6 and 1 to 2 ounces for older children and adults.
• Don't leave drug on for longer than 12 hours; remove drug by washing thoroughly.

ACTION
May inhibit neuronal membrane function in arthropods, causing neuronal hyperactivity, seizures, and death after penetrating the parasite's exoskeleton.

Route	Onset	Peak	Duration
Topical	190 min	Unknown	Unknown

Half-life: About 18 hours.

ADVERSE REACTIONS
CNS: *seizures,* dizziness.
Skin: alopecia, dermatitis, pruritus, urticaria.

INTERACTIONS
Drug-drug. *Drugs that lower the seizure threshold (anticholinesterases, antidepressants, antipsychotics, cyclosporine, chloroquine sulfate, imipenem, isoniazid, methocarbamol, meperidine, mycophenolate mofetil, penicillins, pyrimethamine,*

quinolones, tacrolimus, theophylline): May precipitate seizure activity if used together. Monitor patient if used together.
Drug-lifestyle. *Alcohol use:* May lower seizure threshold. Discourage use together. *Oil-based hair products:* May increase absorption of drug. If oil-based hair products are used, urge patient to wash and dry hair before using drug.

EFFECTS ON LAB TEST RESULTS
None reported.

CONTRAINDICATIONS & CAUTIONS
Black Box Warning Contraindicated in premature infants and in those with seizure disorders. Use cautiously in infants, children, elderly patients, patients with skin conditions other than lice infestation, and those who weigh less than 50 kg (110 lb); all are at greater risk for CNS toxicity, including seizures and death. ▮
• Contraindicated in patients hypersensitive to drug or its components and in those with inflamed skin.
⚠ *Overdose S&S:* CNS excitation, seizures.

NURSING CONSIDERATIONS
Black Box Warning Use lindane products only as second-line treatment of lice infestation or in patients who can't tolerate treatment with safer medications. ▮
• Permethrin 1% cream rinse and pyrethrins with piperonyl butoxide are safer than lindane for pubic lice.
• Apply topical corticosteroids or give oral antihistamines, as prescribed, for pruritus.
• Make sure that hospitalized patients are placed in isolation, with special linen-handling precautions, until treatment is completed.
• Intact skin absorbs 6% to 13% of drug. Absorption is increased if applied to face, scalp, axillae, neck, scrotum, or irritated or broken skin.
• Avoid drug contact with eyes.
Black Box Warning When used correctly, drug is safe and effective. When overused, it can cause adverse reactions. Don't confuse prolonged itching with reinfestation. ▮
• Treat sexual partners simultaneously.

PATIENT TEACHING
• Teach patient or family member how to apply drug: Apply thin layer to cover body only once. Use 1 ounce for children younger than age 6 and 1 to 2 ounces for older children and adults. Don't leave drug on for longer than 12 hours; remove drug by washing thoroughly.
• If patient bathes before application, tell him to let skin dry thoroughly and cool before applying drug.
• Instruct patient to put lotion under fingernails after trimming nails short. A toothbrush can be used to apply lotion under fingernails. Tell patient to wrap toothbrush in paper and throw away immediately after use.
• Inform patient that drug can be poisonous when misused. Warn patient not to apply to open areas, acutely inflamed skin, or to face, eyes, mucous membranes, or urethral opening. If accidental contact with eyes occurs, advise patient to flush with water and notify prescriber.
• Tell patient to avoid inhaling vapors.
• Advise family member to wear gloves when applying drug.
• Tell patient to wash drug off skin and to notify prescriber immediately if skin irritation or hypersensitivity develops.
• Discourage repeated use, which can lead to skin irritation, systemic toxicity, or seizures. Advise patient to repeat use only if live lice or nits are found after 1 week.
• Warn patient not to use other creams or oils during treatment because of potential for increased absorption.
• Advise breast-feeding women to avoid a lot of skin-to-skin contact with infant while drug is present. Interrupt breast-feeding with expression and discarding of milk for at least 24 hours after use.
• Instruct patient to change all clothing and bed linens and launder them in hot water or dry clean after drug is washed off body.
• After application for lice infestation, tell patient to use fine-tooth comb or tweezers to remove nits from hairy areas.
• Advise patient to use shampoo form to clean combs or brushes and to wash them thoroughly afterward.
• Warn patient that itching may continue for several weeks after effective treatment, especially for scabies.

Reactions in bold italics are *life-threatening*. Interactions may have a *rapid onset* or a *delayed onset*.

• Instruct patient to reapply drug if it's washed off during treatment time.

• Tell patient to warn other family members and sexual partners about infestation.

Black Box Warning Advise patient to use product carefully and follow all directions. Overusing product will cause unwanted side effects. Tell him not to confuse prolonged itching with reinfestation. ∎

linezolid
lih-NEH-zoe-lid

Zyvox

Therapeutic class: Antibiotics
Pharmacologic class: Oxazolidinones
Pregnancy risk category: C

AVAILABLE FORMS
Injection: 2 mg/mL
Powder for oral suspension: 100 mg/5 mL when reconstituted
Tablets: 600 mg

INDICATIONS & DOSAGES
➤ **Vancomycin-resistant *Enterococcus faecium* infections, including those with concurrent bacteremia**
Adults and children age 12 and older: 600 mg I.V. or P.O. every 12 hours for 14 to 28 days.
Neonates age 7 days or older and infants and children through age 11: 10 mg/kg I.V. or P.O. every 8 hours for 14 to 28 days.
Neonates younger than age 7 days: 10 mg/kg I.V. or P.O. every 12 hours for 14 to 28 days. Increase to 10 mg/kg every 8 hours when patient is 7 days old. Consider this dosage increase if neonate has inadequate response.
➤ **Hospital-acquired pneumonia caused by *Staphylococcus aureus* (methicillin-susceptible [MSSA] and methicillin-resistant [MRSA] strains) or *Streptococcus pneumoniae* (including multidrug-resistant strains [MDRSP]); complicated skin and skin-structure infections, including diabetic foot infections without osteomyelitis caused by *S. aureus* (MSSA and MRSA), *Streptococcus pyogenes,* or *Streptococcus agalactiae;* community-**

acquired pneumonia caused by *S. pneumoniae* (including MDRSP), including those with concurrent bacteremia, or *S. aureus* (MSSA only)
Adults and children age 12 and older: 600 mg I.V. or P.O. every 12 hours for 10 to 14 days.
Neonates age 7 days or older, infants, and children through age 11: 10 mg/kg I.V. or P.O. every 8 hours for 10 to 14 days.
Neonates younger than age 7 days: 10 mg/kg I.V. or P.O. every 12 hours for 10 to 14 days. Increase to 10 mg/kg every 8 hours when patient is 7 days old. Consider this dosage increase if neonate has inadequate response.
➤ **Uncomplicated skin and skin-structure infections caused by *S. aureus* (MSSA only) or *S. pyogenes***
Adults: 400 mg P.O. every 12 hours for 10 to 14 days.
Children ages 12 to 18: 600 mg P.O. every 12 hours for 10 to 14 days.
Children ages 5 to 11: 10 mg/kg P.O. every 12 hours for 10 to 14 days.
Neonates age 7 days or older, infants, and children younger than age 5: 10 mg/kg P.O. every 8 hours for 10 to 14 days.
Neonates younger than age 7 days: 10 mg/kg P.O. every 12 hours for 10 to 14 days. Increase to 10 mg/kg every 8 hours when patient is 7 days old. Consider this dosage increase if neonate has inadequate response.
➤ **Treatment for endocarditis caused by *E. faecium* infections resistant to penicillin, aminoglycosides, and vancomycin ◆**
Adults: 1,200 mg P.O. or I.V. every 24 hours in two equally divided doses for at least 8 weeks.
Children and adolescents: 30 mg/kg/day P.O. or I.V. in three equally divided doses for at least 8 weeks.
➤ **Brain abscess, empyema, epidural abscess, or septic thrombosis of cavernous or dural venous sinus caused by MRSA in patients allergic to or who have experienced treatment failure with vancomycin ◆**
Adults: 600 mg P.O. or I.V. b.i.d. for at least 4 to 6 weeks.

L

➤ **MRSA-associated meningitis in patients allergic to vancomycin or in whom vancomycin with or without rifampin therapy has failed ◆**
Adults: 600 mg P.O. b.i.d. for at least 14 days.

ADMINISTRATION
P.O.
● Give tablets and suspension with or without meals.
● Reconstitute suspension according to manufacturer's instructions.
● Store reconstituted suspension at room temperature and use within 21 days.

I.V.
▼ Inspect solution for particulate matter and leaks.
▼ Drug is compatible with D_5W injection, normal saline solution for injection, and lactated Ringer injection.
▼ Don't inject additives into infusion bag. Give other I.V. drugs separately or via a separate I.V. line to avoid incompatibilities. If single I.V. line is used, flush line before and after infusion with a compatible solution.
▼ Infuse over 30 minutes to 2 hours. Don't infuse drug in a series connection.
▼ Store drug at room temperature in its protective overwrap. Solution may turn yellow over time, but this doesn't affect drug's potency.
▼ **Incompatibilities:** Amphotericin B, ceftriaxone sodium, chlorpromazine hydrochloride, diazepam, erythromycin lactobionate, pentamidine isethionate, phenytoin sodium, sulfamethoxazole–trimethoprim.

ACTION
Prevents bacterial protein synthesis by interfering with DNA translation in the ribosomes. Also prevents formation of a functional 70S ribosomal subunit by binding to a site on the bacterial 50S ribosomal subunit.

Route	Onset	Peak	Duration
P.O.	Unknown	1 hr	Unknown
I.V.	Unknown	30 min	Unknown

Half-life: 6¼ hours.

ADVERSE REACTIONS
CNS: headache, dizziness, fever, insomnia.
GI: diarrhea, nausea, *pseudomembranous colitis,* altered taste, constipation, oral candidiasis, tongue discoloration, vomiting.
GU: vaginal candidiasis.
Hematologic: *leukopenia, myelosuppression, neutropenia, thrombocytopenia,* anemia.
Skin: rash.
Other: fungal infection.

INTERACTIONS
Drug-drug. *Adrenergic drugs (such as dopamine, epinephrine, pseudoephedrine):* May cause hypertension. Monitor blood pressure and heart rate; start continuous infusions of dopamine and epinephrine at lower doses and titrate to response.
Insulin, oral hypoglycemic agents: May cause symptomatic hypoglycemia. Monitor patient closely.
Serotoninergic drugs: May cause serotonin syndrome, including confusion, delirium, restlessness, tremors, blushing, diaphoresis, and hyperpyrexia. Notify prescriber immediately of signs and symptoms of serotonin syndrome.
Drug-food. *Foods and beverages high in tyramine (such as aged cheeses, air-dried meats, red wines, sauerkraut, soy sauce, tap beers):* May increase blood pressure. Provide a list of foods containing tyramine and advise patient that tyramine content of meals shouldn't exceed 100 mg.

EFFECTS ON LAB TEST RESULTS
● May increase ALT, AST, bilirubin, alkaline phosphatase, creatinine, amylase, lipase, and BUN levels. May decrease hemoglobin level.
● May decrease glucose level and WBC, neutrophil, and platelet counts.

CONTRAINDICATIONS & CAUTIONS
● Contraindicated in patients hypersensitive to drug or its components.
◐ **Alert:** Concomitant use with psychiatric drugs that work through the serotonin system of the brain (SSRIs, selective serotonin and norepinephrine reuptake inhibitors, TCAs, MAO inhibitors, and others) can cause serotonin syndrome (fever, mental

---

status changes, muscle twitching, excessive sweating, shivering or shaking, diarrhea, and loss of coordination). Use linezolid with these drugs only for life-threatening or urgent conditions when the potential benefits outweigh the risks of toxicity.

NURSING CONSIDERATIONS
• No dosage adjustment is needed when switching from I.V. to P.O. forms.

🕓 *Alert:* Before giving linezolid, stop any serotonergic drug and monitor patient for serotonin toxicity for 2 weeks (5 weeks if fluoxetine was taken) or until 24 hours after the last dose of linezolid, whichever comes first. May resume serotonergic psychiatric drugs 24 hours after last dose of linezolid.

🕓 *Alert:* Nausea and vomiting may be symptoms of lactic acidosis. Monitor patient for unexplained acidosis or low bicarbonate level and notify prescriber immediately if these occur.

🕓 *Alert:* Drug may cause thrombocytopenia. In patients at increased risk for bleeding, those with existing thrombocytopenia, those taking other drugs that may cause thrombocytopenia, and those receiving this drug for longer than 14 days, monitor platelet count.

🕓 *Alert:* Drug may lead to myelosuppression. Monitor CBC weekly.

🕓 *Alert:* Pseudomembranous colitis or superinfection may occur. Consider these diagnoses and take appropriate measures in patients with persistent diarrhea or secondary infections.

🕓 *Alert:* Drug may cause symptomatic hypoglycemia in patients taking insulin or oral hypoglycemic agents. Monitor patient closely.

• Inappropriate use of antibiotics may lead to development of resistant organisms; carefully consider other drugs before starting therapy, especially in outpatient setting.

• *Look alike–sound alike:* Don't confuse Zyvox with Zovirax. Both come in a 400-mg strength.

PATIENT TEACHING
• Tell patient that tablets and oral suspension may be taken with or without meals.

• Stress importance of completing entire course of therapy, even if patient feels better.

• Tell patient to alert prescriber if he has high blood pressure; is taking cough or cold preparations, insulin, or oral hypoglycemic agents; or is being treated with SSRIs or other antidepressants.

🕓 *Alert:* Teach patient to recognize and immediately report signs and symptoms of serotonin toxicity (fever, mental status changes, muscle twitching, excessive sweating, shivering or shaking, diarrhea, and loss of coordination).

• Advise patient that he may need to stop taking prescribed psychiatric drugs while taking linezolid but that he shouldn't stop them without first speaking to the prescriber.

• Advise patient to avoid large quantities of tyramine-containing foods (such as aged cheeses, soy sauce, tap beers, red wine) during therapy.

• Inform patient with phenylketonuria that each 5 mL of oral suspension contains 20 mg of phenylalanine. Tablets and injection don't contain phenylalanine.

SAFETY ALERT!

liraglutide
leer-ah-GLOO-tide

Victoza

Therapeutic class: Antidiabetics
Pharmacologic class: Glucagon-like peptide-1 receptor agonists
Pregnancy risk category: C

AVAILABLE FORMS
Injection: Prefilled syringes that deliver 0.6 mg, 1.2 mg, 1.8 mg

INDICATIONS & DOSAGES
➤ **As adjunct to diet and exercise to improve glycemic control in patients with type 2 diabetes mellitus**
Adults: Initially, 0.6 mg subcutaneously daily; after 1 week, increase dosage to 1.2 mg subcutaneously daily. May increase dosage to 1.8 mg subcutaneously daily if needed to achieve glycemic control.

ADMINISTRATION
Subcutaneous
- Give drug once daily at any time of day, independently of meals. Inject into abdomen, thigh, or upper arm. Injection site and timing can be changed without dosage adjustment.
- Inspect solution before each injection. Use solution only if it is clear, colorless, and contains no particles.
- Before first use, store drug in refrigerator at between 36° and 46° F (2° and 8° C).
- After initial use of liraglutide pen, pen can be stored for 30 days at room temperature (59° to 86° F [15° to 30° C]) or in refrigerator (36° to 46° F). Keep pen cap on when not in use. Discard pen after 30 days.

ACTION
Stimulates insulin release in the presence of elevated glucose levels by increasing intracellular cAMP.

Route	Onset	Peak	Duration
Subcut.	Unknown	8–12 hr	Unknown

Half-life: 13 hours.

ADVERSE REACTIONS
CNS: dizziness, headache.
CV: hypertension.
EENT: nasopharyngitis, sinusitis.
GI: constipation, diarrhea, dyspepsia, nausea, vomiting.
GU: UTI.
Metabolic: hypoglycemia.
Musculoskeletal: back pain.
Respiratory: influenza, upper respiratory tract infection.
Skin: injection-site reactions.
Other: *thyroid cancer.*

INTERACTIONS
Drug-drug. *Insulin secretagogues (sulfonylureas):* May increase risk of hypoglycemia. Reduce dosage of insulin secretagogue before beginning drug.
Oral medications: May impair absorption of oral drugs because of delayed gastric emptying. Use together cautiously.

EFFECTS ON LAB TEST RESULTS
- May decrease blood glucose level.
- May increase serum bilirubin level.

CONTRAINDICATIONS & CAUTIONS
Black Box Warning Contraindicated in patients with personal or family history of medullary thyroid carcinoma and in those with multiple endocrine neoplasia syndrome type 2. ■
- Use cautiously in patients with renal or hepatic impairment and in those with history of pancreatitis.
- **Alert:** Acute pancreatitis, including fatal pancreatitis and nonfatal hemorrhagic or necrotizing pancreatitis, has occurred in patients taking liraglutide.
- Safe use in pregnancy hasn't been established. Use only if benefit outweighs risk to fetus. It isn't known if drug appears in breast milk. Patient should either stop breast-feeding or stop drug.
- Elderly adults may be more sensitive to drug. Use cautiously.
- **Overdose S&S:** Nausea, vomiting, hypoglycemia.

NURSING CONSIDERATIONS
Black Box Warning Drug may cause thyroid C-cell tumors, including medullary thyroid cancer. Monitor patient closely. ■
- Monitor patient closely for signs and symptoms of pancreatitis (persistent, severe abdominal pain, which may radiate to the back, and vomiting). Discontinue drug promptly if pancreatitis is suspected. Don't restart if pancreatitis is confirmed.
- **Alert:** Patients with thyroid nodules found on examination or with neck imaging or with elevated serum calcitonin levels should be evaluated by an endocrinologist.
- Drug isn't recommended for first-line therapy in patients who have inadequate glycemic control with diet and exercise.
- Drug isn't a substitute for insulin; it shouldn't be used for treatment of diabetic ketoacidosis or type 1 diabetes mellitus.
- Monitor blood glucose and glycosylated hemoglobin levels. Consider decreasing insulin dosage when initiating liraglutide.
- Monitor patient for signs and symptoms of hypoglycemia (tachycardia, palpitations, anxiety, hunger, nausea, diaphoresis, tremors, pallor, restlessness, headache, and speech and motor dysfunction).
- Monitor GI status; drug slows gastric emptying.

Reactions in bold italics are *life-threatening*. Interactions may have a *rapid onset* or a *delayed onset*.

PATIENT TEACHING
● Warn patient that drug may increase risk of thyroid tumor; tell him to report such signs and symptoms as hoarseness, difficulty swallowing, difficulty breathing, or lump in the neck.
● Advise patient to stop taking drug and notify health care provider if he experiences persistent, severe abdominal pain that may radiate to the back and may or may not be accompanied by vomiting.
● Warn patient to avoid sharing pen with another person, even if needle is changed.
● Tell patient that stress, such as fever, trauma, infection, or surgery, may change drug requirements and to seek medical advice promptly.
● Emphasize to patient importance of adhering to a diet and exercise program and monitoring glucose and glycosylated hemoglobin levels.
● Teach patient how to give subcutaneous injection; instruct patient to rotate sites to prevent injection-site reactions.
● Instruct patient to discard pen after 30 days.

---

lisdexamfetamine dimesylate
lis-DEX-am-FET-a-meen

Vyvanse⁄

Therapeutic class: CNS stimulants
Pharmacologic class: Amphetamines
Pregnancy risk category: C
Controlled substance schedule: II

AVAILABLE FORMS
Capsules: 20 mg, 30 mg, 40 mg, 50 mg, 60 mg, 70 mg

INDICATIONS & DOSAGES
➤ **Attention deficit hyperactivity disorder (ADHD)**
Adults and children ages 6 to 17: Initially, 30 mg P.O. once daily in the morning. Increase by 10 or 20 mg at weekly intervals to a maximum of 70 mg daily.

ADMINISTRATION
P.O.
● Give drug in the morning to prevent insomnia.
● Give drug without regard for meals.
● Capsules may be swallowed whole or the contents dissolved in a glass of water and taken immediately.

ACTION
May increase the release of norepinephrine and dopamine into extraneural spaces by blocking their reuptake into the presynaptic neuron.

Route	Onset	Peak	Duration
P.O.	Rapid	1 hr	Unknown

Half-life: Less than 1 hour.

ADVERSE REACTIONS
CNS: headache, insomnia, irritability, aggressive or hostile behavior, agitation, delusional thinking, dizziness, fever, hallucinations, labile affect, restlessness, somnolence, tic, tremor.
CV: *ventricular hypertrophy,* increased blood pressure, increased heart rate.
EENT: abnormal vision, blurred vision.
GI: abdominal pain, decreased appetite, dry mouth, nausea, vomiting.
Metabolic: slow growth, weight loss.
Respiratory: dyspnea.
Skin: hyperhidrosis, rash.

INTERACTIONS
Drug-drug. *Adrenergic blockers:* May inhibit adrenergic blocking effects. Monitor blood pressure and adjust adrenergic blocker dosage if necessary.
Antihistamines: May inhibit sedative effects of antihistamines. Monitor patient.
Antihypertensives, veratrum alkaloids: May inhibit antihypertensive effects of these drugs. If use together can't be avoided, closely monitor blood pressure when lisdex-amfetamine is started or stopped, and adjust antihypertensive dosage as needed.
Chlorpromazine, haloperidol: May decrease effectiveness of amphetamines. Monitor patient closely.
Ethosuximide: May delay absorption of this drug. Monitor patient closely.

L

Lithium: May inhibit anorectic and CNS stimulant effects of amphetamine. Monitor patient closely.

MAO inhibitors: May cause severe hypertension or hypertensive crisis. Avoid using within 14 days of MAO inhibitor therapy.

Meperidine: May increase the analgesic effect of meperidine. Use together cautiously.

Norepinephrine: May increase adrenergic effects of norepinephrine. Monitor patient closely.

Phenobarbital, phenytoin: May delay intestinal absorption of these drugs and enhance their anticonvulsant effects. Monitor patient closely.

TCAs: May cause adverse CV effects. Avoid using together.

Urine acidifiers (ammonium chloride, sodium acid phosphate), methenamine: May decrease serum level due to increased renal excretion of amphetamine. Monitor patient for decreased drug effects.

Urine alkalinizers (sodium bicarbonate): May increase lisdexamfetamine serum level because of decreased renal excretion of amphetamine. Monitor patient for increased drug effects and adjust dosage accordingly.

Drug-food. *Caffeine:* May increase CNS stimulation. Discourage use together.

EFFECTS ON LAB TEST RESULTS
• May increase corticosteroid level.
• May interfere with urinary steroid test.

CONTRAINDICATIONS & CAUTIONS
• Contraindicated in patients hypersensitive to sympathomimetic amines or in those with idiosyncratic reactions to them, in agitated patients, and in those with a history of drug abuse.
• Contraindicated in patients with advanced arteriosclerosis, hyperthyroidism, symptomatic CV disease, structural cardiac abnormalities, cardiomyopathy, serious heart arrhythmia, moderate to severe hypertension, or glaucoma, and those intolerant of changes in heart rate or blood pressure.
• Contraindicated within 14 days of MAO inhibitor therapy.
• Use cautiously in patients with a history of arrhythmias, MI, stroke, or seizures.

• Use cautiously in patients with preexisting psychosis, bipolar disorder, aggressive behavior, or Tourette syndrome.

⚠ *Overdose S&S:* Assaultiveness, confusion, hallucinations, hyperpyrexia, hyperreflexia, panic states, rapid respiration, restlessness, rhabdomyolysis, tremor, fatigue, depression, arrhythmias, circulatory collapse, hypertension, hypotension, abdominal cramps, diarrhea, nausea, vomiting, seizures, coma.

NURSING CONSIDERATIONS
• Diagnosis of ADHD must be based on complete history and evaluation of the child with consultation of psychological, educational, and social resources.
• Give the lowest effective dose in the morning. Afternoon doses may cause insomnia.

Black Box Warning Assess the risk of abuse before initiating therapy, and monitor patient for signs of drug dependence or abuse. Misuse may cause sudden death. ▋

☯ *Alert:* Periodically monitor patients for changes in heart rate or blood pressure.
• Abruptly stopping the drug can cause severe fatigue and depression.
• Monitor patient closely for adverse CV effects, new or worsening behavior (aggression, mania), vision problems, or seizures.
• Monitor blood pressure and pulse routinely.
• Carefully observe patient for digital changes because stimulants used to treat ADHD are associated with peripheral vasculopathy, including Raynaud phenomenon.
• Effectiveness of this drug when taken longer than 4 weeks isn't known. Periodically interrupt therapy to determine whether continuation is necessary.
• Growth may be suppressed with long-term stimulant use. Monitor the child for growth and weight gain. Stop treatment if growth is suppressed or if weight gain is lower than expected.
• The drug may trigger Tourette syndrome. Monitor patient, especially at the start of therapy.
• Monitor patient for the appearance or worsening of aggressive behavior or hostility, especially when treatment is initiated.

Reactions in bold italics are *life-threatening*. Interactions may have a *rapid onset* or a *delayed onset*.

PATIENT TEACHING

Black Box Warning Warn patient that the misuse of amphetamines can cause serious CV adverse events, including sudden death. ∎

◑ Alert: Instruct patient to immediately report chest pain, shortness of breath, or fainting.

• Tell patient or caregiver that drug should be taken in the morning to prevent insomnia.

• Advise patient to swallow capsule whole. If he's unable to do so, the contents may be dissolved in a glass of water and taken immediately. Once dissolved, don't store for later use.

• Tell patient or caregiver that abruptly stopping drug can cause severe fatigue, depression, or general withdrawal reaction.

• Caution patient to avoid activities that require alertness or good psychomotor coordination until CNS effects of drug are known.

• Warn patient with seizure disorder that drug may decrease seizure threshold. Urge him to notify his prescriber if a seizure occurs.

• Instruct patient or caregiver to report palpitations or visual disturbances.

• Tell patient or caregiver to report worsening aggression, hallucinations, delusions, or mania.

• Advise patient to avoid caffeine consumption while taking drug.

lisinopril
lye-SIN-oh-pril

Prinivil◈, Zestril◈

Therapeutic class: Antihypertensives
Pharmacologic class: ACE inhibitors
Pregnancy risk category: D

AVAILABLE FORMS
Tablets: 2.5 mg, 5 mg, 10 mg, 20 mg, 30 mg, 40 mg

INDICATIONS & DOSAGES
➤ **Hypertension**
Adults: Initially, 10 mg P.O. daily for patients not taking a diuretic. Most patients are well controlled on 20 to 40 mg daily as

a single dose. For patients taking a diuretic, initially, 5 mg P.O. daily.
Children age 6 and older: Initially, 0.07 mg/kg (up to 5 mg) P.O. once daily. Increase dosage based on patient response and tolerance. Maximum dose, 0.61 mg/kg (don't exceed 40 mg). Don't use in children with a CrCl of less than 30 mL/minute.
Adjust-a-dose: In adults, if CrCl is 10 to 30 mL/minute, give 5 mg P.O. daily; if CrCl is less than 10 mL/minute, give 2.5 mg P.O. daily.
➤ **Adjunctive treatment (with diuretics and cardiac glycosides) for heart failure**
Adults: Initially, 5 mg P.O. daily; increased as needed to maximum of 20 mg (40 mg for Zestril) P.O. daily.
Adjust-a-dose: If sodium level is less than 130 mEq/L, serum creatinine greater than 3 mg/dL, or CrCl less than 30 mL/minute, start treatment at 2.5 mg daily.
➤ **Hemodynamically stable patients within 24 hours of acute MI to improve survival**
Adults: Initially, 5 mg P.O.; then 5 mg after 24 hours, 10 mg after 48 hours, followed by 10 mg once daily for 6 weeks.
Adjust-a-dose: For patients with systolic blood pressure 120 mm Hg or less when treatment is started or during first 3 days after an infarct, decrease dosage to 2.5 mg P.O. If systolic blood pressure drops to 100 mm Hg or less, reduce daily maintenance dose of 5 mg to 2.5 mg, if needed. If prolonged systolic blood pressure stays under 90 mm Hg for longer than 1 hour, withdraw drug.

ADMINISTRATION
P.O.
• Give drug without regard for food.
• If made into a suspension by pharmacist, shake before each use.

ACTION
Causes decreased production of angiotensin II and suppression of the renin-angiotensin-aldosterone system.

Route	Onset	Peak	Duration
P.O.	1 hr	7 hr	24 hr

Half-life: 12 hours.

ADVERSE REACTIONS

CNS: dizziness, headache, fatigue, paresthesia.
CV: orthostatic hypotension, hypotension, chest pain.
EENT: nasal congestion.
GI: diarrhea, nausea, dyspepsia.
GU: impaired renal function, impotence.
Metabolic: *hyperkalemia.*
Respiratory: dyspnea; dry, persistent, tickling, nonproductive cough.
Skin: rash.
Other: *angioedema.*

INTERACTIONS

Drug-drug. *Aliskiren:* May increase risk of renal impairment, hypotension, and hyperkalemia in diabetic patients and those with moderate to severe renal impairment (GFR < 60 mL/minute). Concomitant use is contraindicated in diabetic patients. Avoid concomitant use in those with moderate to severe renal impairment.
Allopurinol: May cause hypersensitivity reaction. Use together cautiously.
Azathioprine: May increase risk of anemia or leukopenia. Monitor hematologic studies if used together.
Diuretics, thiazide diuretics: May cause excessive hypotension with diuretics. Monitor blood pressure closely.
Indomethacin, NSAIDs: May reduce hypotensive effects of drug. Adjust dose as needed.
Insulin, oral antidiabetics: May cause hypoglycemia, especially at start of lisinopril therapy. Monitor glucose level.
Lithium: May cause lithium toxicity. Monitor lithium levels.
Phenothiazines: May increase hypotensive effects. Monitor blood pressure closely.
Potassium-sparing diuretics, potassium supplements: May cause hyperkalemia. Monitor laboratory values.
Tizanidine: May cause severe hypotension. Monitor patient.
Drug-herb. *Capsaicin:* May cause ACE inhibitor-induced cough. Discourage use together.
Ma huang: May decrease antihypertensive effects. Discourage use together.

Drug-food. *Potassium-containing salt substitutes:* May cause hyperkalemia. Monitor laboratory values.

EFFECTS ON LAB TEST RESULTS

● May increase BUN, creatinine, potassium, and bilirubin levels.
● May increase LFT values.

CONTRAINDICATIONS & CAUTIONS

● Contraindicated in patients hypersensitive to ACE inhibitors and in those with a history of angioedema related to previous treatment with ACE inhibitor.
Black Box Warning Use during pregnancy can cause injury and death to the developing fetus. When pregnancy is detected, stop drug as soon as possible. ∎
● Use cautiously in patients with impaired renal function; adjust dosage.
● Use cautiously in patients at risk for hyperkalemia or hypotension and in those with aortic stenosis or hypertrophic cardiomyopathy. The safety and effectiveness of lisinopril on blood pressure in children younger than age 6 or in children with GFR less than 30 mL/minute hasn't been established.
⚠ **Overdose S&S:** Hypotension.

NURSING CONSIDERATIONS

● When using drug in acute MI, give patient the appropriate and standard recommended treatment, such as thrombolytics, aspirin, and beta blockers.
● Although ACE inhibitors reduce blood pressure in all races, blood pressure reduction is less in blacks taking an ACE inhibitor alone. Black patients should take drug with a thiazide diuretic for a more favorable response.
● ACE inhibitors appear to increase risk of angioedema in black patients.
● Monitor blood pressure frequently. If drug doesn't adequately control blood pressure, diuretics may be added.
● Monitor WBC with differential counts before therapy, every 2 weeks for first 3 months of therapy, and periodically thereafter.
● *Look alike–sound alike:* Don't confuse lisinopril with fosinopril or Lioresal. Don't confuse Zestril with Zostrix, Zetia,

---

Reactions in bold italics are *life-threatening*. Interactions may have a *rapid onset* or a *delayed onset*.

Zebeta, or Zyrtec. Don't confuse Prinivil with Proventil or Prilosec.

PATIENT TEACHING
◑ *Alert:* Rarely, facial and throat swelling (including swelling of the larynx) may occur, especially after first dose. Advise patient to report signs or symptoms of breathing problems or swelling of face, eyes, lips, or tongue.

• Inform patient that light-headedness can occur, especially during first few days of therapy. Tell him to rise slowly to minimize this effect and to report symptoms to prescriber. If he faints, advise patient to stop taking drug and call prescriber immediately.

• If unpleasant adverse reactions occur, tell patient not to stop drug suddenly but to notify prescriber.

• Advise patient to report signs and symptoms of infection, such as fever and sore throat.

• Tell women of childbearing age to notify prescriber if pregnancy occurs. Drug will need to be stopped.

• Instruct patient not to use salt substitutes that contain potassium without first consulting prescriber.

lisinopril–hydrochlorothiazide
lye-SIN-oh-pril/hye-droe-klor-oh-THYE-a-zide

Prinzide, Zestoretic

Therapeutic class: Antihypertensives
Pharmacologic class: ACE inhibitors–thiazide diuretics
Pregnancy risk category: D

AVAILABLE FORMS
Tablets: 10 mg lisinopril and 12.5 mg hydrochlorothiazide, 20 mg lisinopril and 12.5 mg hydrochlorothiazide, 20 mg lisinopril and 25 mg hydrochlorothiazide

INDICATIONS & DOSAGES
➤ **Hypertension in patients not adequately controlled on lisinopril or hydrochlorothiazide monotherapy**
Adults: Initially, 10 mg lisinopril and 12.5 mg hydrochlorothiazide or 20 mg lisinopril

and 12.5 mg hydrochlorothiazide P.O. once daily; titrate based on clinical response. Don't increase the hydrochlorothiazide component until 2 to 3 weeks have elapsed. In patients on adequate pressure control on single-agent hydrochlorothiazide 25 mg P.O. daily but with significant potassium loss, switch to 10 mg lisinopril and 12.5 mg hydrochlorothiazide tablets. Maximum dosage is 80 mg lisinopril and 50 mg hydrochlorothiazide P.O. once daily.
Adjust-a-dose: Not for use in patients with CrCl of less than 30 mL/minute/1.73 m^2. Dosage selection for elderly patients should be cautious, usually starting at low end of dosing range.

ADMINISTRATION
P.O.
• Store at controlled room temperature; protect from excessive light and humidity.
• May give without regard for food.

ACTION
Lisinopril inhibits ACE, leading to decreased angiotensin II production, decreased aldosterone secretion, and increased potassium level. Hydrochlorothiazide increases aldosterone secretion, increasing excretion of sodium, chloride, and water, and decreasing excretion of potassium.

Route	Onset	Peak	Duration
P.O. (lisinopril)	1 hr	7 hr	Unknown
P.O. (hydrochloro-thiazide)	2 hr	4 hr	6–12 hr

Half-life: Lisinopril, 12 hours; hydrochlorothiazide, 5.6 to 14.8 hours.

ADVERSE REACTIONS
CNS: dizziness, headache, fatigue, asthenia, paresthesia.
CV: orthostatic effects, hypotension.
GI: diarrhea, nausea, vomiting, dyspepsia.
GU: erectile dysfunction.
Musculoskeletal: muscle cramps.
Respiratory: cough, upper respiratory tract infection.
Skin: rash.

INTERACTIONS
Drug-drug. *Antidiabetic agents, insulin:* May increase blood glucose level.

L

Monitor patient carefully; adjust dosage of antidiabetic as needed.

Barbiturates, opioids: May increase risk of orthostatic hypotension. Avoid use together.

Colestipol resins, cholestyramine: May impair absorption of hydrochlorothiazide. Avoid use together.

Corticosteroids, corticotropin: May worsen electrolyte depletion, particularly hypokalemia. Monitor patient carefully.

Diuretics, other antihypertensives: May increase hypotensive effects. Monitor patient carefully.

Gold injections: May increase risk of nitritoid effects (flushing, nausea, vomiting, hypotension) Avoid use together.

Lithium: May increase lithium level. Monitor patient carefully.

Nondepolarizing skeletal muscle relaxants (tubocurarine): May increase response to muscle relaxant. Avoid use together.

NSAIDs: May diminish antihypertensive effects. Use cautiously together.

Potassium-sparing diuretics, potassium supplements: May increase risk of hyperkalemia. Avoid use together.

Pressor amines (norepinephrine): May decrease response to pressor amines. Use together cautiously.

Drug-food. *Potassium-containing salt substitutes:* May increase risk of hyperkalemia. Discourage use together.

Drug-lifestyle. *Alcohol use:* May increase risk of orthostatic hypotension. Discourage use together.

Sun exposure: May increase risk of photosensitivity. Discourage sun exposure.

EFFECTS ON LAB TEST RESULTS

● May increase glucose, cholesterol, triglyceride, BUN, creatinine, potassium, and bilirubin levels and LFT values.

● May decrease calcium, potassium, and magnesium levels and WBC count.

CONTRAINDICATIONS & CAUTIONS

Black Box Warning When used during the second and third trimesters of pregnancy, ACE inhibitors can cause injury to and even death of the developing fetus. When pregnancy is detected, discontinue lisinopril–hydrochlorothiazide tablets as soon as possible. ■

● Contraindicated in patients hypersensitive to either drug or sulfonamides and in those with history of angioedema related to previous treatment with an ACE inhibitor, hereditary or idiopathic angioedema, or anuria.

● Use cautiously in patients with a history or risk of angioedema, anaphylactoid reactions, salt or volume depletion, collagen vascular disease, obstruction in the outflow tract of the left ventricle, congestive heart failure, renal artery stenosis, renal disease, jaundice or hepatic disease, asthma, systemic lupus erythematosus, history of aortic stenosis, hypertrophic cardiomyopathy, existing hyperkalemia or other electrolyte imbalance, or hyperuricemia.

● It isn't known if lisinopril appears in breast milk; hydrochlorothiazide does appear in breast milk. Patient should either discontinue breast-feeding or discontinue drug.

⚠ Overdose S&S: Hypotension, dehydration, electrolyte imbalance.

NURSING CONSIDERATIONS

● Drug isn't to be used for initial therapy. Begin combination therapy only after patient has failed to achieve desired effect with monotherapy.

● Consider ACE inhibitor–induced cough if patient develops cough of unknown etiology.

● Correct lisinopril-induced hypotension before major surgery and anesthesia.

● If hypotension occurs, place patient in supine position and give I.V. normal saline solution if appropriate. May resume drug once blood pressure has increased.

● Monitor glucose, electrolyte, and lipid levels during therapy.

● Monitor WBC count in patients with collagen vascular disease or renal disease.

● Monitor patient for jaundice and elevated liver enzyme levels. Discontinue drug and treat appropriately if these occur.

● Drug may cause intestinal angioedema. Monitor patient for abdominal pain.

● Monitor patient for angioedema of the face, extremities, lips, tongue, glottis, or larynx, which may occur at any time during treatment. If symptoms occur, discontinue

---

drug, treat appropriately, and monitor patient until symptoms have resolved.

• If airway obstruction is likely, give subcutaneous epinephrine solution 1:1,000 or other appropriate treatment as necessary to ensure patent airway.

• Black patients and patients with a history of angioedema unrelated to ACE inhibitors may be at increased risk for angioedema from ACE inhibitors.

• Black patients may have a more limited response to lisinopril than non-black patients.

PATIENT TEACHING

• Instruct patient to stop drug and immediately report signs or symptoms suggesting angioedema (swelling of the face, extremities, eyes, lips, tongue; difficulty swallowing or breathing).

• Caution patient to report lightheadedness, especially during the first few days of therapy, and if syncope occurs, to discontinue drug and notify prescriber.

• Tell patient to consult prescriber if fluid losses occur (excessive perspiration, dehydration, vomiting, or diarrhea).

• Advise patient to immediately report signs and symptoms of fluid and electrolyte imbalance (dry mouth, thirst, weakness, lethargy, drowsiness, restlessness, confusion, seizures, muscle pains or cramps, muscle fatigue, decreased urination, rapid heartbeat, nausea, vomiting).

• Instruct patient to promptly report signs and symptoms of infection (sore throat, fever).

• Warn patient to avoid salt substitutes containing potassium.

Black Box Warning Counsel patient to report possible pregnancy to prescriber as soon as possible. ∎

lithium carbonate
LITH-ee-um

Carbolith†, Lithane†, Lithobid

lithium citrate

Therapeutic class: Antimanics
Pharmacologic class: Alkali metals
Pregnancy risk category: D

AVAILABLE FORMS
lithium carbonate
Capsules: 150 mg, 300 mg, 600 mg
Tablets: 300 mg
Tablets (extended-release): 300 mg, 450 mg
lithium citrate
Syrup (sugarless): 8 mEq lithium/5 mL;
5 mL lithium citrate liquid contains 8 mEq
lithium, equal to 300 mg lithium carbonate

INDICATIONS & DOSAGES
➤ **To prevent or control mania in bipolar disorder**
Adults and children age 12 and older:
600 mg P.O. t.i.d. Or, 900-mg extended-release tablets P.O. every 12 hours. Or, 10 mL (lithium 16 mEq) P.O. t.i.d. Increase dosage based on blood levels to achieve optimum dosage. Recommended therapeutic lithium levels are 1 to 1.5 mEq/L for acute mania and 0.6 to 1.2 mEq/L for maintenance therapy.
➤ **Borderline personality disorder** ◆
Adults: 900 to 2,400 mg P.O. daily in three to four divided doses or 900 to 1,800 mg (extended-release) P.O. daily in two divided doses, titrated to maintain serum levels of 0.8 to 1 mEq/L.

ADMINISTRATION
P.O.
• Give drug after meals with plenty of water to minimize GI upset.
• Don't crush extended-release tablets.

ACTION
Probably alters chemical transmitters in the CNS, possibly by interfering with ionic pump mechanisms in brain cells, and may compete with or replace sodium ions.

Route	Onset	Peak	Duration
P.O.	Unknown	30 min–3 hr	Unknown

Half-life: 18 hours (adolescents) to 36 hours (elderly).

ADVERSE REACTIONS

CNS: fatigue, lethargy, *coma, epileptiform seizures,* tremors, drowsiness, headache, confusion, restlessness, dizziness, psychomotor retardation, blackouts, EEG changes, worsened organic mental syndrome, impaired speech, ataxia, incoordination.

CV: *arrhythmias, bradycardia,* reversible ECG changes, *severe bradycardia,* hypotension.

EENT: tinnitus, blurred vision.

GI: vomiting, anorexia, diarrhea, thirst, nausea, metallic taste, dry mouth, abdominal pain, flatulence, indigestion.

GU: polyuria, *renal toxicity with long-term use,* glycosuria, decreased CrCl, albuminuria.

Hematologic: leukocytosis with leukocyte count of 14,000 to 18,000/mm^3.

Metabolic: transient hyperglycemia, goiter, hypothyroidism, hyponatremia.

Musculoskeletal: muscle weakness.

Skin: pruritus, rash, diminished or absent sensation, drying and thinning of hair, psoriasis, acne, alopecia.

Other: ankle and wrist edema.

INTERACTIONS

Drug-drug. *ACE inhibitors:* May increase lithium level. Monitor lithium level; adjust lithium dosage, as needed.

Aminophylline, sodium bicarbonate, urine alkalinizers: May increase lithium excretion. Avoid excessive salt, and monitor lithium levels.

Antiarrhythmics and other drugs that prolong QT interval: May increase risk of life-threatening arrhythmias. Avoid use together.

Calcium channel blockers (verapamil): May decrease lithium levels and may increase risk of neurotoxicity. Use together cautiously.

Carbamazepine, fluoxetine, methyldopa, NSAIDs, probenecid: May increase effect of lithium. Monitor patient for lithium toxicity.

Neuromuscular blockers: May cause prolonged paralysis or weakness. Monitor patient closely.

Thiazide diuretics: May increase reabsorption of lithium by kidneys, with possible toxic effect. Use with caution, and monitor lithium and electrolyte levels (especially sodium).

Drug-food. *Caffeine:* May decrease lithium level and drug effect. Advise patient who ingests large amounts of caffeine to tell prescriber before stopping caffeine. Adjust lithium dosage, as needed.

EFFECTS ON LAB TEST RESULTS

• May increase glucose and creatinine and TSH levels. May decrease sodium, T_3, T_4, and protein-bound iodine levels.

• May increase ^{131}I uptake and WBC and neutrophil counts.

CONTRAINDICATIONS & CAUTIONS

• Contraindicated if therapy can't be closely monitored.

• Avoid using in pregnant patient unless benefits outweigh risks.

• Use with caution in patients receiving neuromuscular blockers and diuretics; in elderly or debilitated patients; and in patients with thyroid disease, seizure disorder, infection, renal or CV disease, severe debilitation or dehydration, or sodium depletion.

⚠ *Overdose S&S:* Diarrhea, vomiting, drowsiness, muscular weakness, lack of coordination, giddiness, ataxia, blurred vision, confusion, tinnitus, large output of dilute urine, slurred speech, loss of consciousness, myoclonic limb movements, agitation, urinary or fecal incontinence, seizures, arrythmias, hypotension, peripheral vascular collapse, coma.

NURSING CONSIDERATIONS

Black Box Warning Lithium toxicity is closely related to serum lithium levels and can occur at doses close to therapeutic levels. Facilities for prompt and accurate serum lithium determinations should be available before initiation of therapy. ∎

• When drug level is less than 1.5 mEq/L, adverse reactions are usually mild.

Reactions in bold italics are *life-threatening*. Interactions may have a *rapid onset* or a *delayed onset*.

- Monitor baseline ECG, thyroid studies, renal studies, and electrolyte levels.
- Check fluid intake and output, especially when surgery is scheduled.
- Weigh patient daily; check for edema or sudden weight gain.
- Adjust fluid and salt ingestion to compensate if excessive loss occurs from protracted diaphoresis or diarrhea. Under normal conditions, patient fluid intake should be 2½ to 3 L daily, and he should follow a balanced diet with adequate salt intake.
- Check urine specific gravity and report level below 1.005, which may indicate diabetes insipidus.
- Drug alters glucose tolerance in diabetic patients. Monitor glucose level closely.
- Perform outpatient follow-up of thyroid and renal functions every 6 to 12 months. Palpate thyroid to check for enlargement.
- **Look alike–sound alike:** Don't confuse lithium carbonate with lanthanum carbonate. Don't confuse Lithobid with Levbid.

PATIENT TEACHING
- Tell patient to take drug with plenty of water and after meals to minimize GI upset.
- Explain the importance of having regular blood tests to determine drug levels; even slightly high values can be dangerous.
- Warn patient and caregivers to expect transient nausea, large amounts of urine, thirst, and discomfort during first few days of therapy and to watch for evidence of toxicity.
- Instruct patient to withhold one dose and call prescriber if signs and symptoms of toxicity appear, but not to stop drug abruptly.
- Warn patient to avoid hazardous activities that require alertness and good psychomotor coordination until CNS effects of drug are known.
- Tell patient not to switch brands or take other prescription or OTC drugs without prescriber's guidance.
- Tell patient to wear or carry medical identification at all times.

✳ NEW DRUG

lomitapide mesylate
lom-i-TA-pide

Juxtapid

Therapeutic class: Antilipemics
Pharmacologic class: Microsomal triglyceride transfer protein inhibitors
Pregnancy risk category: X

AVAILABLE FORMS
Capsules: 5 mg, 10 mg, 20 mg

INDICATIONS & DOSAGES
➤ **As an adjunct to low-fat diet and other lipid-lowering treatments, including LDL apheresis where available, to reduce LDL, total cholesterol, apolipoprotein B, and non-HDL cholesterol levels in patients with homozygous familial hypercholesterolemia**
Adults: 5 mg P.O. once daily. May increase to 10 mg daily after 2 weeks; may increase 4 weeks later to 20 mg, then 4 weeks later to 40 mg, then 4 weeks later to 60 mg. Maximum daily dosage is 60 mg.
Adjust-a-dose: Decrease maximum daily dosage to 30 mg daily with concomitant use of weak CYP3A4 inhibitors. In patients with ESRD receiving dialysis and in patients with mild hepatic impairment (Child-Pugh class A), don't exceed 40 mg P.O. daily. If ALT or AST level is 3 times to less than 5 times the upper limit of normal (ULN), confirm result within 1 week; reduce dosage and monitor liver enzyme levels weekly. May resume drug at a reduced dosage when transaminase levels are less than 3× ULN; monitor liver enzyme levels more frequently. If bilirubin level or INR increases, or transaminase levels rise above 5× ULN or don't fall below 3× ULN within 4 weeks, stop drug and obtain additional liver-related tests (alkaline phosphatase, total bilirubin, INR) and investigate for probable cause.

ADMINISTRATION
P.O.
- Give drug with a glass of water on an empty stomach at least 2 hours after evening meal.
- Don't crush or open capsules.

L

Black Box Warning Rule out pregnancy in women of childbearing potential before starting treatment. ■

Black Box Warning Check LFTs (ALT, AST, alkaline phosphatase, and total bilirubin) before starting and periodically during treatment. ■

● To reduce risk of developing a fat-soluble nutrient deficiency, patients should take drug with concurrent daily doses of vitamin E, 400 IU; linoleic acid, 200 mg; alpha-linolenic acid, 210 mg; eicosapentaenoic acid, 110 mg; and docosahexaenoic acid, 80 mg.

ACTION

Inhibits microsomal triglyceride transfer protein, stopping synthesis of chylomicrons and very low-density lipoprotein, leading to reduced levels of plasma LDL cholesterol.

Route	Onset	Peak	Duration
P.O.	Unknown	6 hr	Unknown

Half-life: 39.7 hours.

ADVERSE REACTIONS

CNS: headache, dizziness, fever, fatigue.
CV: chest pain, angina pectoris, palpitations.
EENT: nasopharyngitis, pharyngolaryngeal pain, nasal congestion.
GI: diarrhea, nausea, dyspepsia, vomiting, abdominal pain, abdominal discomfort, abdominal distention, constipation, flatulence, GERD, defecation urgency, rectal tenesmus, gastroenteritis.
Hepatic: increased ALT level, hepatic steatosis, *hepatotoxicity.*
Metabolic: weight loss.
Musculoskeletal: back pain.
Other: flulike symptoms.

INTERACTIONS

Drug-drug. *Bile acid sequestrants (cholestyramine, colesevelam, colesevelam hydrochloride, colestipol, colestipol hydrochloride):* May interfere with absorption of lomitapide. Separate doses by 4 hours.
Hepatotoxins (acetaminophen [more than 4 g/day for 3 days/week or more], amiodarone, isotretinoin, methotrexate,

tamoxifen, tetracyclines): May accelerate liver injury. Use together cautiously.
Lovastatin: May increase risk of myopathy. Use together cautiously; consider lower lovastatin dosage.
Moderate CYP3A4 inhibitors (amprenavir, aprepitant, atazanavir, ciprofloxacin, crizotinib, darunavir/ritonavir, diltiazem, erythromycin, fluconazole, fosamprenavir, imatinib, verapamil): May increase lomitapide concentration. Use together is contraindicated.
P-glycoprotein substrates (aliskiren, ambrisentan, colchicine, dabigatran, digoxin, everolimus, fexofenadine, imatinib, lapatinib, maraviroc, nilotinib, posaconazole, ranolazine, saxagliptin, sirolimus, sitagliptin, talinolol, tolvaptan, topotecan): May increase level of substrate. Use together cautiously; consider substrate dosage reduction.
Simvastatin: May increase risk of myopathy. Decrease simvastatin dosage to 20 mg daily, or to 40 mg for patients previously taking 80 mg daily with no muscle toxicity in last year.
Strong CYP3A4 inhibitors (boceprevir, clarithromycin, conivaptan, indinavir, itraconazole, ketoconazole, lopinavir–ritonavir, mibefradil, nefazodone, nelfinavir, posaconazole, ritonavir, saquinavir, telaprevir, telithromycin, voriconazole): May increase lomitapide level. Use together is contraindicated.
Warfarin: May increase INR. Use together cautiously. Monitor INR carefully, especially after lomitapide dosage adjustments.
Weak CYP3A4 inhibitors (alprazolam, amiodarone, amlodipine, atorvastatin, bicalutamide, cilostazol, cimetidine, cyclosporine, fluoxetine, fluvoxamine, isoniazid, lapatinib, nilotinib, oral contraceptives, pazopanib, ranitidine, ranolazine, tipranavir/ritonavir, ticagrelor, zileuton): Use together cautiously, with maximum lomitapide dosage of 30 mg P.O. daily.
Drug-herb. *Ginkgo biloba, goldenseal:* May increase lomitapide level. Use together cautiously, with maximum lomitapide dosage of 30 mg daily.
Drug-food. *Fat-soluble nutrients (alpha-linolenic acid, docosahexaenoic acid,*

eicosapentaenoic acid, linoleic acid, vitamin E): May decrease absorption of these nutrients. Supplements should be given. *Grapefruit juice:* May adversely affect absorption. Discourage use together.
Drug-lifestyle. *Alcohol use:* May exacerbate liver injury and increase hepatic fat levels. Discourage consumption of more than one alcoholic drink per day.

EFFECTS ON LAB TEST RESULTS
• May increase INR and transaminase, bilirubin, and alkaline phosphatase levels.

CONTRAINDICATIONS & CAUTIONS
Black Box Warning Because of risk of hepatotoxicity, lomitapide is available only through a restricted program under a Risk Evaluation and Mitigation Strategy (REMS) called the Juxtapid REMS program. ∎
• Contraindicated in patients hypersensitive to drug or its components, in those with moderate or severe hepatic impairment (Child-Pugh class B or C) or active liver disease, including unexplained persistent elevations of serum transaminases, and in pregnant women.
Black Box Warning Drug causes increased hepatic fat (steatosis), a risk factor for progressive liver disease, including steatohepatitis and cirrhosis. ∎
• Avoid use in patients with galactose intolerance, Lapp lactase deficiency, or glucose–galactose malabsorption; decreased absorption of concurrent drugs may result.
• It isn't known if drug appears in breast milk. Women who are breast-feeding should discontinue drug or discontinue breast-feeding.

NURSING CONSIDERATIONS
• Drug has restricted access through Juxtapid REMS program at 1-95-JUXTAPID and is available only from certified pharmacies.
Black Box Warning Drug may cause hepatic steatosis or transaminase elevations. Measure AST, ALT, alkaline phosphatase, and total bilirubin levels before treatment; then obtain AST and ALT levels periodically and with dosage changes. Adjust dosage if AST or ALT level is more than

$3 \times$ ULN. Discontinue drug for clinically significant liver toxicity. ∎
• Assess liver-related tests (ALT and AST, at a minimum) monthly or before each dosage increase, whichever occurs first during the first year; then assess at least every 3 months and before any dosage increase.
• If transaminase elevations are accompanied by clinical signs and symptoms of liver injury (such as nausea, vomiting, abdominal pain, fever, jaundice, lethargy, or flulike symptoms), increase in bilirubin level $2 \times$ ULN or more, or active liver disease, discontinue treatment and investigate probable cause.
• Obtain a negative pregnancy test before beginning therapy in women of childbearing potential.
• Women who become pregnant should stop drug immediately and notify their prescriber.
• Monitor patient for GI adverse effects. Absorption of oral medications, including oral contraceptives, may be affected in patients with diarrhea and vomiting.

PATIENT TEACHING
• Inform patient about participation in drug's registry program. Information is available at www.juxtapid.com.
• Advise patient to limit alcohol to one drink daily.
• Instruct patient to report severe stomach upset or other GI signs and symptoms, fever, jaundice, lethargy, or flulike symptoms.
• Teach female patient that drug may harm a fetus and to use effective contraception during therapy and to discontinue drug and immediately notify prescriber if she becomes pregnant.
• Teach female patient of childbearing potential who is taking oral contraceptives to use additional contraceptive methods if vomiting and diarrhea occur.
• Remind patient to take vitamin E and other supplements as required.
• Caution patient to adhere to low-fat diet (less than 20% of calories from fat) and to take drug at least 2 hours after evening meal to minimize GI adverse effects.

L

● Warn patient to contact health care provider if drug has been stopped for more than a week.

loperamide hydrochloride
loe-PER-a-mide

Diamode ◊, Imodium, Imodium A-D ◊

Therapeutic class: Antidiarrheals
Pharmacologic class: Piperidine derivatives
Pregnancy risk category: B

AVAILABLE FORMS
Capsules: 2 mg
Chewable tablets: 2 mg ◊
Oral liquid: 1 mg/5 mL ◊, 1 mg/7.5 mL ◊
Tablets: 2 mg ◊

INDICATIONS & DOSAGES
➤ **Acute, nonspecific diarrhea**
Adults and children older than age 12:
Initially, give 4 mg P.O.; then 2 mg after each unformed stool. Maximum, 16 mg daily, unless otherwise directed.
Children ages 8 to 12: 2 mg P.O. t.i.d. on first day. Maximum, 6 mg daily. If diarrhea persists, contact prescriber.
Children ages 6 to younger than 8: 2 mg P.O. b.i.d. on first day. If diarrhea persists, contact prescriber. Maximum, 4 mg daily.
Children ages 2 to 5: 1 mg P.O. t.i.d. on first day. Maximum, 3 mg daily. If diarrhea persists, contact prescriber.
➤ **Chronic diarrhea associated with chronic bowel disease**
Adults: Initially, give 4 mg P.O.; then 2 mg after each unformed stool until diarrhea subsides. Adjust dosage to individual response. Maximum dose is 16 mg/day.
➤ **Traveler's diarrhea** ◆
Adults: 4 mg P.O. followed by 2 mg after each unformed stool for a maximum of 16 mg/day.

ADMINISTRATION
P.O.
● Use the liquid formulation for children ages 2 to 5.

ACTION
Inhibits peristalsis.

Route	Onset	Peak	Duration
P.O.	Unknown	2½–5 hr	24 hr

Half-life: 9 to 14½ hours.

ADVERSE REACTIONS
CNS: dizziness, drowsiness, fatigue.
GI: constipation, abdominal pain, distention or discomfort, dry mouth, nausea, vomiting.
Skin: hypersensitivity reactions, rash.

INTERACTIONS
Drug-drug. *Saquinavir:* May increase loperamide levels and decrease saquinavir levels. Avoid using together.

EFFECTS ON LAB TEST RESULTS
None reported.

CONTRAINDICATIONS & CAUTIONS
● Contraindicated in patients hypersensitive to drug and in those who must avoid constipation.
● Contraindicated in patients with bloody diarrhea or diarrhea with fever greater than 101° F (38° C), in breast-feeding women, and in children younger than age 2.
● Use cautiously in patients with hepatic disease.
⚠ *Overdose S&S:* Paralytic ileus, CNS depression.

NURSING CONSIDERATIONS
● If symptoms don't improve within 48 hours, stop therapy and consider another drug.
● Drug produces antidiarrheal action similar to that of diphenoxylate but without as many adverse CNS effects.
✪ *Alert:* Monitor children closely for CNS effects; children may be more sensitive to these effects than adults.
● *Look alike–sound alike:* Don't confuse Imodium with Ionamin.

PATIENT TEACHING
● Advise patient not to exceed recommended dosage.
● Tell patient with acute diarrhea to stop drug and seek medical attention if no improvement occurs within 48 hours. In

---

chronic diarrhea, tell patient to notify prescriber and to stop drug if no improvement occurs after taking 16 mg daily for at least 10 days.
● Advise patient with acute colitis to stop drug immediately and notify prescriber about abdominal distention.
● Warn patient to avoid activities that require mental alertness until CNS effects of drug are known.
● Tell patient to report nausea, abdominal pain, or abdominal discomfort.
● Advise patient to relieve dry mouth with ice chips or sugarless gum.

lopinavir–ritonavir
low-PIN-ah-ver

Kaletra*✐

Therapeutic class: Antiretrovirals
Pharmacologic class: Protease inhibitors
Pregnancy risk category: C

AVAILABLE FORMS
Solution: lopinavir 400 mg and ritonavir 100 mg/5 mL (80 mg and 20 mg/mL)*
Tablets: lopinavir 100 mg and ritonavir 25 mg; lopinavir 200 mg and ritonavir 50 mg

INDICATIONS & DOSAGES
➤ **HIV infection, without other antiretrovirals (efavirenz, fosamprenavir, nevirapine, nelfinavir)**
Adults: 800 mg lopinavir and 200 mg ritonavir P.O. once daily (patients with less than 3 lopinavir resistance-associated substitutions) or in two evenly divided doses.
Children ages 6 months to 18 years: 230 mg lopinavir and 57.5 mg/m² ritonavir (oral solution) P.O. b.i.d. with food. Or, if patient weighs more than 35 kg (77 lb), give 4 tablets of lopinavir 100 mg and ritonavir 25 mg P.O. b.i.d. If patient weighs between 25 and 35 kg (55 and 77 lb), give 3 tablets of lopinavir 100 mg and ritonavir 25 mg P.O. b.i.d. If patient weighs 15 to 25 kg (33 to 55 lb), give 2 tablets of lopinavir 100 mg and ritonavir 25 mg P.O. b.i.d. Maximum dosage is lopinavir 400 mg and ritonavir 100 mg P.O. b.i.d.

Children ages 14 days to 6 months: 16 mg lopinavir and 4 mg ritonavir/kg P.O. b.i.d. Or, lopinavir 300 mg and ritonavir 75 mg/m² P.O. b.i.d.
➤ **HIV infection, with other antiretrovirals (efavirenz, fosamprenavir, nevirapine, nelfinavir)**
Adults: 500 mg lopinavir and 125 mg ritonavir (tablets) P.O. b.i.d., or 533 mg lopinavir and 133 mg ritonavir (oral solution) P.O. b.i.d.
Children ages 6 months to 18 years: 300 mg lopinavir and 75 mg/m² ritonavir (oral solution) P.O. b.i.d. with food. Maximum dosage is lopinavir 533 mg and ritonavir 133 mg (oral solution) P.O. b.i.d. Or, if patient weighs more than 45 kg (99 lb), give 5 tablets of lopinavir 100 mg and ritonavir 25 mg P.O. b.i.d. If patient weighs between 30 and 45 kg (66 and 99 lb), give 4 tablets of lopinavir 100 mg and ritonavir 25 mg P.O. b.i.d. If patient weighs 20 to 30 kg (44 to 66 lb), give 3 tablets of lopinavir 100 mg and ritonavir 25 mg P.O. b.i.d. If patient weighs 15 to 20 kg (33 to 44 lb), give 2 tablets of lopinavir 100 mg and ritonavir 25 mg P.O. b.i.d. Maximum dosage is lopinavir 500 mg and ritonavir 125 mg (tablets) P.O. b.i.d.

ADMINISTRATION
P.O.
⊕ *Alert:* Many drug interactions are possible. Review all drugs patient is taking.
● Give oral solution and capsules with food. Give tablets without regard for food.
● Tablets must be swallowed whole; don't crush or divide, and tell patient not to chew.
● Refrigerated solution remains stable until expiration date on package. If stored at room temperature, use drug within 2 months.

ACTION
Lopinavir is an HIV protease inhibitor, which produces immature, noninfectious viral particles. Ritonavir, also an HIV protease inhibitor, slows lopinavir metabolism, thereby increasing lopinavir level.

Route	Onset	Peak	Duration
P.O.	Unknown	4 hr	5–6 hr

Half-life: About 6 hours.

ADVERSE REACTIONS

CNS: *encephalopathy,* abnormal dreams, abnormal thinking, agitation, amnesia, anxiety, asthenia, ataxia, confusion, depression, dizziness, dyskinesia, emotional lability, fever, headache, hypertonia, insomnia, malaise, nervousness, neuropathy, pain, paresthesia, peripheral neuritis, somnolence, tremors.

CV: chest pain, *DVT,* edema, hypertension, palpitations, thrombophlebitis, vasculitis.

EENT: abnormal vision, eye disorder, otitis media, sinusitis, tinnitus.

GI: *hemorrhagic colitis, pancreatitis,* diarrhea, nausea, abdominal pain, abnormal stools, anorexia, cholecystitis, constipation, dry mouth, dyspepsia, dysphagia, enterocolitis, eructation, esophagitis, fecal incontinence, flatulence, gastritis, gastroenteritis, GI disorder, increased appetite, inflammation of the salivary glands, stomatitis, taste perversion, ulcerative stomatitis, vomiting.

GU: abnormal ejaculation, hypogonadism, renal calculus, urine abnormality.

Hematologic: *leukopenia, neutropenia, thrombocytopenia in children,* anemia.

Hepatic: hyperbilirubinemia in children.

Metabolic: Cushing syndrome, dehydration, decreased glucose tolerance, hyperglycemia, hyperuricemia, hyponatremia in children, hypothyroidism, *lactic acidosis,* weight loss.

Musculoskeletal: arthralgia, arthrosis, back pain, myalgia.

Respiratory: bronchitis, dyspnea, lung edema.

Skin: acne, alopecia, benign skin neoplasm, dry skin, exfoliative dermatitis, furunculosis, nail disorder, pruritus, rash, skin discoloration, sweating.

Other: chills, decreased libido, facial edema, flu syndrome, gynecomastia, immune reconstitution syndrome, lymphadenopathy, viral infection.

INTERACTIONS

Drug-drug. *Amiodarone, bepridil, lidocaine, quinidine:* May increase antiarrhythmic level. Use together cautiously. Monitor levels of these drugs, if possible.

Amprenavir, efavirenz, nelfinavir, nevirapine: May decrease lopinavir level. Consider increasing lopinavir–ritonavir combination dose. Don't use a once-daily regimen of lopinavir–ritonavir combination with these drugs.

Antiarrhythmics (flecainide, propafenone), pimozide: May increase risk of cardiac arrhythmias. Avoid using together.

Atorvastatin: May increase level of this drug and risk of myopathy and rhabdomyolysis. Use lowest possible dose and monitor patient carefully.

Atovaquone, methadone: May decrease levels of these drugs. Consider increasing doses of these drugs.

Bosentan: May increase bosentan level. Withhold bosentan for at least 36 hours before starting lopinavir–ritonavir, and decrease bosentan dosage and frequency.

Bupropion: May decrease bupropion level and antidepressant effect. Monitor patient for adequate clinical response and adjust bupropion dosage as needed.

Carbamazepine, dexamethasone, phenobarbital, phenytoin: May decrease lopinavir level. Use together cautiously.

Clarithromycin: May increase clarithromycin level in patients with renal impairment. Adjust clarithromycin dosage.

Colchicine: May increase colchicine level. Don't use together in patient with renal or hepatic impairment. Decrease colchicine dosage if used together in patient with normal renal and hepatic function.

Cyclosporine, rapamycin, tacrolimus: May increase levels of these drugs. Monitor therapeutic levels.

Dasatinib, nilotinib: May increase levels of these drugs and risk of adverse events. Adjust dasatinib and nilotinib dosages as needed.

Delavirdine: May increase lopinavir level. Avoid using together.

Didanosine: May decrease absorption of didanosine because lopinavir–ritonavir combination is taken with food. Give didanosine 1 hour before or 2 hours after lopinavir–ritonavir combination.

Disulfiram, metronidazole: May cause disulfiram-like reaction. Avoid using together.

Drugs that prolong PR interval (such as atazanavir, beta blockers, calcium channel blockers, digoxin): May further prolong PR interval. Use cautiously together.

Reactions in bold italics are *life-threatening*. Interactions may have a *rapid onset* or a *delayed onset*.

Drugs that prolong QT interval (such as amiodarone, flecainide, propafenone): May further prolong QT interval and increase risk of ventricular arrhythmias. Avoid use together.

Ergot derivatives (dihydroergotamine, ergonovine, ergotamine, methylergonovine): May increase risk of ergot toxicity characterized by peripheral vasospasm and ischemia. Avoid using together.

Felodipine, nicardipine, nifedipine: May increase levels of these drugs. Use together cautiously.

Fentanyl, triazolam: May increase or prolong sedation or cause respiratory depression. Monitor patient carefully.

Fluticasone: May increase fluticasone plasma concentration, leading to decreased serum cortisol level, Cushing syndrome, and adrenal suppression. Use together isn't recommended unless benefits outweigh risks.

Hormonal contraceptives (ethinyl estradiol): May decrease effectiveness of contraceptives. Recommend nonhormonal contraceptives.

Indinavir, saquinavir: May increase levels of these drugs. Avoid using together.

Itraconazole, ketoconazole: May increase levels of these drugs. Don't give more than 200 mg/day of these drugs.

Lovastatin, simvastatin: May increase risk of adverse reactions, such as myopathy and rhabdomyolysis. Use together is contraindicated.

Methadone: May decrease methadone level. Monitor clinical response and increase methadone dosage as needed.

Midazolam (parenteral), triazolam: May cause prolonged or increased sedation or respiratory depression. Avoid using together. Don't give with oral midazolam.

Pitavastatin, pravastatin: May increase statin level and risk of myopathy and rhabdomyolysis. Use together cautiously.

Rifabutin: May increase rifabutin level. Decrease rifabutin dosage by at least 75% or a maximum of 150 mg every other day or three times a week. Monitor patient carefully and adjust dosage as needed.

Rifampin: May decrease effectiveness of Kaletra. Avoid using together.

Rosuvastatin: May increase statin level and risk of myopathy and rhabdomyolysis. Rosuvastatin dosage shouldn't exceed 10 mg daily.

Salmeterol: May increase salmeterol level and risk of CV adverse reactions. Use together isn't recommended.

Sildenafil, tadalafil, vardenafil: May increase level of these drugs and adverse effects, such as hypotension and prolonged erection. Warn patient not to take more than 25 mg of sildenafil in 48 hours, more than 10 mg of tadalafil in 72 hours, or more than 2.5 mg vardenafil in 72 hours.

Trazodone: May increase trazodone level and risk of adverse reactions. Consider lower dosage of trazodone.

Vinblastine, vincristine: May increase levels of these drugs and risk of adverse reactions. Temporarily withhold antiretroviral regimen for hematologic or GI adverse reactions. If cancer treatment is prolonged, consider other antivirals.

Warfarin: May affect warfarin level. Monitor PT and INR.

Drug-herb. *St. John's wort:* Loss of virologic response and possible resistance to drug. Discourage use together.

Drug-food. *Any food:* May increase absorption of oral solution. Tell patient to take with food.

EFFECTS ON LAB TEST RESULTS

• May increase glucose, amylase, cholesterol, and triglyceride levels. May decrease hemoglobin level and hematocrit.
• May decrease RBC, WBC, neutrophil, and platelet counts.

CONTRAINDICATIONS & CAUTIONS

• Contraindicated in patients hypersensitive to drug or any of its components.
• Contraindicated with drugs metabolized by CYP3A, including dihydroergotamine, ergonovine, lovastatin, methylergonovine, midazolam, pimozide, rifampin, simvastatin, triazolam, and St. John's wort.
• Avoid use in patients with congenital long QT syndrome or hypokalemia and in those taking drugs that prolong QT interval. Correct potassium abnormalities before starting therapy.

L

• Use cautiously in patients with a history of pancreatitis or with hepatic impairment, hepatitis B or C, marked elevations in liver enzyme levels, or hemophilia.

• Use cautiously in elderly patients.

❸ **Alert:** Safety and effectiveness in neonates younger than age 14 days haven't been established. Use only if benefit outweighs risk. Monitor neonates for toxicity, such as hyperosmolality with or without lactic acidosis, renal toxicity, CNS depression (stupor, coma, apnea), seizures, hypotonia, cardiac arrhythmias, ECG changes, and hemolysis. Toxicity in preterm neonates can be severe or fatal.

• The Antiretroviral Pregnancy Registry monitors maternal-fetal outcomes of pregnant women taking Kaletra. Health care providers are encouraged to enroll women by calling 1-800-258-4263.

⚠ **Overdose S&S:** Alcohol-related toxicity.

NURSING CONSIDERATIONS

• Don't administer tablets, capsules, or oral solution as a once-daily dosing regimen when combined with efavirenz, nevirapine, amprenavir, or nelfinavir.

• Avoid once-daily dosing in pregnant women and in children younger than age 18.

• During initial phase of treatment, patients responding to antiretroviral therapy may develop an inflammatory response to indolent or residual opportunistic infections (CMV, *Mycobacterium avium* complex, *Pneumocystis jiroveci* pneumonia, tuberculosis), which may necessitate further evaluation and treatment. Autoimmune disorders (such as Graves disease, polymyositis, and Guillain-Barré syndrome) have also been reported in the setting of immune reconstitution; however, time to onset is more variable, and onset can occur many months after initiation of antiretroviral treatment.

• Monitor patient for signs of fat redistribution, including central obesity, buffalo hump, peripheral wasting, breast enlargement, and cushingoid appearance.

• Monitor glucose, total cholesterol, and triglyceride levels before starting therapy and periodically thereafter.

• Monitor patient for signs and symptoms of pancreatitis (nausea, vomiting, abdominal pain, or increased lipase and amylase values).

• Monitor patient for signs and symptoms of bleeding (hypotension, rapid heart rate).

• **Look alike–sound alike:** Don't confuse Kaletra with Keppra.

PATIENT TEACHING

• Tell patient to take oral solution with food. Tablets and capsules may be taken without regard to food.

❸ **Alert:** Tablets must be swallowed whole; don't crush or divide, and tell patient not to chew.

• Tell patient also taking didanosine to take it 1 hour before or 2 hours after lopinavir–ritonavir combination.

• Advise patient to report side effects to prescriber.

• Tell patient to immediately report severe nausea, vomiting, or abdominal pain.

• Inform patient that drug doesn't cure HIV infection, that opportunistic infections and other complications of HIV infection may still occur, and that transmission of HIV to others through sexual contact or blood contamination remains possible.

• Advise patient taking an erectile dysfunction drug of an increased risk of adverse effects, including low blood pressure, visual changes, and painful erections, and to promptly report any symptoms to his prescriber. Tell him not to take more often than directed.

• Warn patient to tell prescriber about any other prescription or nonprescription medicine that he's taking, including herbal supplements.

---

loratadine

lor-AT-a-deen

Alavert ◇, Alavert Children's ◇,
Children's Claritin Allergy ◇,
Claritin ◇, Claritin Hives Relief ◇,
Claritin 24-Hour Allergy ◇, Claritin
Liqui-Gels ◇, Claritin RediTabs ◇,
Clear-Atadine ◇, Dimetapp Children's
Non-Drowsy Allergy ◇, Triaminic
Allerchews ◇

Therapeutic class: Antihistamines
Pharmacologic class: Piperidines
Pregnancy risk category: B

AVAILABLE FORMS

Capsules: 10 mg ◇
Syrup: 1 mg/mL ◇
Tablets: 10 mg ◇
Tablets (chewable): 5 mg ◇
Tablets (orally disintegrating): 5 mg ◇,
10 mg ◇

INDICATIONS & DOSAGES

Adjust-a-dose (for all indications): In adults
and children age 6 and older with hepatic
impairment or GFR less than 30 mL/minute,
give 10 mg every other day. In children ages
2 to 5 years with hepatic or renal impairment, give 5 mg every other day.
➤ **Allergic rhinitis**
Adults and children age 6 and older:
10 mg P.O. daily. Or, 5 mg Claritin
RediTabs every 12 hours.
Children ages 2 to 5: 5 mg chewable tablets
or syrup P.O. daily.
✸ **NEW INDICATION: To relieve itching due
to hives (urticaria) (Claritin Hives Relief
only)**
Adults and children age 6 and older: 10 mg
P.O. daily.

ADMINISTRATION

P.O.
• Place Claritin RediTabs on the tongue,
where they disintegrate within a few seconds.
• Give drug with or without water.

ACTION

Blocks effects of histamine at H_1-receptor
sites. Drug is a nonsedating antihistamine;
its chemical structure prevents entry into the
CNS.

Route	Onset	Peak	Duration
P.O.	Rapid	1.3–2.5 hr	24 hr

Half-life: 8½ hours.

ADVERSE REACTIONS

CNS: headache, drowsiness, fatigue,
insomnia, nervousness.
GI: dry mouth.

INTERACTIONS

Drug-drug. *Cimetidine, ketoconazole,
macrolide antibiotics (clarithromycin,
erythromycin):* May increase loratadine
level. Monitor patient closely.
Drug-lifestyle. *Alcohol use:* May increase
CNS depression. Discourage use together.

EFFECTS ON LAB TEST RESULTS

• May prevent, reduce, or mask positive
result in diagnostic skin test.

CONTRAINDICATIONS & CAUTIONS

• Contraindicated in patients hypersensitive
to drug.
• Use cautiously in patients with hepatic
or renal impairment and in breast-feeding
women.
⚠ **Overdose S&S:** Somnolence, tachycardia, headache, extrapyramidal reactions,
palpitations.

NURSING CONSIDERATIONS

• Stop drug 4 days before patient undergoes
diagnostic skin tests because drug can prevent,
reduce, or mask positive skin test response.

PATIENT TEACHING

• Make sure patient understands to take
drug once daily. If symptoms persist or
worsen, tell him to contact prescriber.
• Tell patient taking Claritin RediTabs
to use tablet immediately after opening
individual blister.
• Advise patient taking Claritin RediTabs
to place tablet on the tongue, where it
disintegrates within a few seconds. It can
be swallowed with or without water.
• Warn patient to avoid alcohol and hazardous activities that require alertness until
CNS effects of drug are known.

● Tell patient that dry mouth can be relieved with sugarless gum, hard candy, or ice chips.

lorazepam
lor-AZ-e-pam

Ativan✦, Lorazepam Intensol, Novo-Lorazem†

Therapeutic class: Anxiolytics
Pharmacologic class: Benzodiazepines
Pregnancy risk category: D
Controlled substance schedule: IV

AVAILABLE FORMS
Injection: 2 mg/mL, 4 mg/mL
Oral solution: 2 mg/mL
Tablets: 0.5 mg, 1 mg, 2 mg

INDICATIONS & DOSAGES
➤ **Anxiety**
Adults: 2 to 6 mg P.O. daily in divided doses. Maximum, 10 mg daily.
Elderly patients: 1 to 2 mg P.O. daily in divided doses. Maximum, 10 mg daily.
➤ **Insomnia from anxiety**
Adults: 2 to 4 mg P.O. at bedtime.
➤ **Preoperative sedation**
Adults: 2 mg I.V. total or 0.044 mg/kg I.V., whichever is smaller. Larger doses up to 0.05 mg/kg I.V., to total of 4 mg, may be needed. Or, 0.05 mg/kg I.M. 2 hours before procedure. Total dose shouldn't exceed 4 mg.
➤ **Status epilepticus**
Adults: 4 mg I.V. at a rate of 2 mg/minute. If seizures continue or recur after 10 to 15 minutes, an additional 4-mg dose may be given. Drug may be given I.M. if I.V. access isn't available.

ADMINISTRATION
P.O.
● Mix oral solution with liquid or semisolid food, such as water, juices, carbonated beverages, applesauce, or pudding.
I.V.
▼ Keep emergency resuscitation equipment and oxygen available.
▼ Dilute with an equal volume of sterile water for injection, normal saline solution for injection, or D₅W. Give slowly at no more than 2 mg/minute.
▼ Monitor respirations every 5 to 15 minutes and before each I.V. dose.
▼ Contains benzyl alcohol. Avoid use in neonates.
▼ Refrigerate intact vials and protect from light.
▼ **Incompatibilities:** Aldesleukin, aztreonam, buprenorphine, caffeine citrate, floxacillin, foscarnet, idarubicin, imipenem–cilastatin sodium, omeprazole, ondansetron hydrochloride, sargramostim, sufentanil citrate, thiopental.
I.M.
● For status epilepticus, drug may be given I.M. if I.V. access isn't available.
● For I.M. use, inject deeply into a muscle. Don't dilute.
● Refrigerate parenteral form to prolong shelf life.

ACTION
May potentiate the effects of GABA, depress the CNS, and suppress the spread of seizure activity.

Route	Onset	Peak	Duration
P.O.	1 hr	2 hr	12–24 hr
I.V.	5 min	60–90 min	6–8 hr
I.M.	15–30 min	60–90 min	6–8 hr

Half-life: 10 to 20 hours.

ADVERSE REACTIONS
CNS: drowsiness, sedation, amnesia, insomnia, agitation, dizziness, weakness, unsteadiness, disorientation, depression, headache.
CV: hypotension.
EENT: visual disturbances, nasal congestion.
GI: abdominal discomfort, nausea, change in appetite.

INTERACTIONS
Drug-drug. *CNS depressants:* May increase CNS depression. Use together cautiously.
Digoxin: May increase digoxin level and risk of toxicity. Monitor patient and digoxin level closely.
Drug-herb. *Kava:* May increase sedation. Discourage use together.

Reactions in bold italics are *life-threatening*. Interactions may have a *rapid onset* or a *delayed onset*.

Drug-lifestyle. *Alcohol use:* May cause additive CNS effects. Discourage use together.
Smoking: May decrease drug's effectiveness. Monitor patient closely.

EFFECTS ON LAB TEST RESULTS
• May increase LFT values.

CONTRAINDICATIONS & CAUTIONS
• Contraindicated in patients hypersensitive to drug, other benzodiazepines, or the vehicle used in parenteral dosage form; in patients with acute angle-closure glaucoma; and in pregnant women, especially in the first trimester.
• Use cautiously in patients with pulmonary, renal, or hepatic impairment, or history of substance abuse.
• Use cautiously in elderly, acutely ill, or debilitated patients.
⚠ **Overdose S&S:** Drowsiness, confusion lethargy, ataxia, hypotonia, hypotension, hypnotic state, stage 1 to 3 coma, death.

NURSING CONSIDERATIONS
• Monitor hepatic, renal, and hematopoietic function periodically in patients receiving repeated or prolonged therapy.
🖐 **Alert:** Use of this drug may lead to abuse and addiction. Don't stop drug abruptly after long-term use because withdrawal symptoms may occur.
• **Look alike–sound alike:** Don't confuse lorazepam with alprazolam, clonazepam, or Lovaza. Don't confuse Ativan with Atgam.

PATIENT TEACHING
• When used before surgery, drug causes substantial preoperative amnesia. Patient teaching requires extra care to ensure adequate recall. Provide written materials or inform a family member, if possible.
• Warn patient to avoid hazardous activities that require alertness or good coordination until effects of drug are known.
• Tell patient to avoid use of alcohol while taking drug.
• Notify patient that smoking may decrease drug's effectiveness.
• Warn patient not to stop drug abruptly because withdrawal symptoms may occur.

• Advise women to avoid becoming pregnant while taking drug.

---

lorcaserin hydrochloride
lor-ca-SER-in

Belviq

Therapeutic class: Appetite suppressants
Pharmacologic class: Serotonin 2C receptor agonists
Pregnancy risk category: X

AVAILABLE FORMS
Tablets: 10 mg

INDICATIONS & DOSAGES
➤ **Weight management in patients with initial body mass index of 30 kg/m^2 or greater (obese) or 27 kg/m^2 or greater (overweight) in the presence of at least one weight-related comorbid condition as adjunct to reduced-calorie diet and increased physical activity**
Adults: 10 mg P.O. b.i.d.
Adjust-a-dose: If patient hasn't lost at least 5% of baseline body weight by week 12, discontinue drug.

ADMINISTRATION
P.O.
• Store at room temperature.
• May give without regard for food.

ACTION
Exact mechanism of action unknown. May decrease food consumption and promote satiety by selectively activating 5-HT$_{2C}$ receptors on anorexigenic pro-opiomelanocortin neurons located in the hypothalamus.

Route	Onset	Peak	Duration
P.O.	Unknown	1½–2 hr	Unknown

Half-life: 11 hours.

ADVERSE REACTIONS
CNS: headache, dizziness, fatigue, anxiety, insomnia, stress, depression, impaired memory and attention.

L

CV: hypertension, *valvulopathy,* peripheral edema.
EENT: eye disorder, nasopharyngitis, oropharyngeal pain, sinus congestion, toothache, dry mouth.
GI: nausea, vomiting, diarrhea, constipation, gastroenteritis.
GU: UTI.
Metabolic: *hypoglycemia,* worsening of diabetes mellitus, decreased appetite.
Musculoskeletal: back pain, musculoskeletal pain, muscle spasms.
Respiratory: upper respiratory tract infection, cough.
Skin: rash.

INTERACTIONS
Drug-drug. *Antipsychotics, bupropion, dextromethorphan, dopamine antagonists, linezolid, lithium, MAO inhibitors, serotonin–norepinephrine reuptake inhibitors (SNRIs), SSRIs, tramadol, TCAs, triptans:* May increase risk of serotonin syndrome or neuroleptic malignant syndrome (NMS)–like reactions. Use together cautiously.
CYP2D6 substrates (antipsychotics, dextromethorphan, metoclopramide, SNRIs, SSRIs, TCAs): May increase levels of CYP2D6 substrates. Use together cautiously.
Insulin, sulfonylureas: May increase risk of hypoglycemia in patients with type 2 diabetes. Monitor patient closely; adjust antidiabetic regimen as needed.
PDE5 inhibitors (sildenafil): May increase risk of priapism. Use together cautiously.
Potent 5-HT$_{2B}$ agonists (cabergoline): May increase risk of valvulopathy. Don't use together.
Drug-herb. *St. John's wort, tryptophan:* May increase risk of serotonin syndrome or NMS-like reactions. Discourage use together.

EFFECTS ON LAB TEST RESULTS
● May increase prolactin level. May decrease hemoglobin level and hematocrit.
● May decrease total WBC, lymphocyte, neutrophil, and total RBC counts.

CONTRAINDICATIONS & CAUTIONS
● Contraindicated in patients hypersensitive to drug or its components, in those with severe renal impairment or ESRD, and in pregnant or breast-feeding women.
● Contraindicated in combination with serotoninergic and dopaminergic drugs that are potent 5-HT$_{2B}$ receptor agonists and are known to increase risk of heart valvulopathy.
● Use cautiously in patients with moderate renal impairment, severe hepatic impairment, congestive heart failure, hemodynamically significant valvular disease, bradycardia, or heart block greater than first degree.
● Use cautiously in men who have conditions that might predispose them to priapism (sickle cell anemia, multiple myeloma, or leukemia) and in men with anatomic deformation of the penis (angulation, cavernosal fibrosis, or Peyronie disease).
⚠ **Overdose S&S:** Headache, nausea, abdominal discomfort, dizziness.

NURSING CONSIDERATIONS
● Safety and effectiveness of using drug with other products intended for weight loss, including prescription drugs, OTC drugs, and herbal preparations, haven't been established.
● Measure blood glucose levels before and during treatment in patients with type 2 diabetes.
● Monitor patient for dyspnea, dependent edema, heart failure, or new murmur. Effect on CV morbidity and mortality hasn't been established.
● Monitor CBC periodically.
● Measure prolactin level if gynecomastia or galactorrhea occurs.
● Monitor patient for serotonin syndrome (mental status changes, tachycardia, labile blood pressure, hyperthermia, hyperreflexia, incoordination, nausea, vomiting, diarrhea).
● Monitor patient for confusion or impaired attention and memory.
● Monitor patient for new or worsening depression, suicidal thoughts or behaviors, or unusual changes in mood or behavior. Discontinue drug if symptoms occur.

Reactions in bold italics are *life-threatening.* Interactions may have a *rapid onset* or a *delayed onset.*

PATIENT TEACHING

• Teach patient to use drug only in conjunction with a reduced-calorie diet and increased physical activity.

• Tell patient drug will be discontinued if 5% weight loss isn't achieved by 12 weeks of treatment.

• Warn patient to seek medical attention if signs or symptoms of valvular heart disease (dyspnea or dependent edema) occur.

• Advise patient to seek medical attention in the event of emerging or worsening depression, suicidal thoughts or behavior, or unusual changes in mood or behavior.

• Caution patient not to operate hazardous machinery, including automobiles, until drug's effects are known.

• Warn patient never to increase dosage.

• Advise men experiencing an erection lasting longer than 4 hours, whether painful or not, to immediately stop drug and seek emergency medical attention.

• Instruct patient to inform prescriber of all medications, nutritional supplements, and vitamins (including weight-loss products) they are using while taking this drug.

• Caution women to avoid pregnancy and not to breast-feed while taking this drug and to notify prescriber immediately if pregnancy occurs.

---

losartan potassium
low-SAR-tan

Cozaar✐

Therapeutic class: Antihypertensives
Pharmacologic class: Angiotensin II receptor antagonists
Pregnancy risk category: C; D in 2nd and 3rd trimesters

AVAILABLE FORMS
Tablets: 25 mg, 50 mg, 100 mg

INDICATIONS & DOSAGES
➤ **Hypertension**
Adults: Initially, 50 mg P.O. daily. Maximum daily dose is 100 mg in one or two divided doses.

Children age 6 and older: 0.7 mg/kg (up to 50 mg) P.O. daily, adjusted as needed up to 1.4 mg/kg/day (maximum 100 mg).

Adjust-a-dose: For adults with hepatic impairment or intravascular volume depletion (such as those taking diuretics), initially, 25 mg.

➤ **Nephropathy in type 2 diabetic patients**
Adults: 50 mg P.O. once daily. Increase dosage to 100 mg once daily based on blood pressure response.

➤ **To reduce risk of stroke in patients with hypertension and left ventricular hypertrophy**
Adults: Initially, 50 mg P.O. once daily. Adjust dosage based on blood pressure response, adding hydrochlorothiazide 12.5 mg once daily, increasing losartan to 100 mg daily, or both. If further adjustments are required, may increase the daily dosage of hydrochlorothiazide to 25 mg.

➤ **Heart failure in patients with current or prior symptoms and reduced LVEF who are intolerant of ACE inhibitors ◆**
Adults: Initially, 25 to 50 mg P.O. once daily, up to a maximum of 50 to 100 mg once daily. Within 1 or 2 weeks of starting drug, blood pressure, renal function, and potassium levels should be checked and reassessed after dosage adjustments.

ADMINISTRATION
P.O.
• Give drug without regard for meals.
• If made into suspension by pharmacist, store in refrigerator and shake well before each use.

ACTION
Inhibits vasoconstrictive and aldosterone-secreting action of angiotensin II by blocking angiotensin II receptor on the surface of vascular smooth muscle and other tissue cells.

Route	Onset	Peak	Duration
P.O.	Unknown	1 hr	Unknown

Half-life: 2 hours.

ADVERSE REACTIONS
Patients with hypertension or left ventricular hypertrophy
CNS: dizziness, asthenia, fatigue, headache, insomnia.
CV: edema, chest pain.
EENT: nasal congestion, sinusitis, pharyngitis, sinus disorder.
GI: abdominal pain, nausea, diarrhea, dyspepsia.
Musculoskeletal: muscle cramps, myalgia, back or leg pain.
Respiratory: cough, upper respiratory tract infection.
Other: *angioedema.*
Patients with nephropathy
CNS: asthenia, fatigue, fever, hypesthesia.
CV: chest pain, hypotension, orthostatic hypotension.
EENT: sinusitis, cataract.
GI: diarrhea, dyspepsia, gastritis.
GU: UTI.
Hematologic: anemia.
Metabolic: *hyperkalemia, hypoglycemia,* weight gain.
Musculoskeletal: back pain, leg or knee pain, muscle weakness.
Respiratory: cough, bronchitis.
Skin: cellulitis.
Other: flulike syndrome, *diabetic vascular disease, angioedema,* infection, trauma, diabetic neuropathy.

INTERACTIONS
Drug-drug. *Aliskiren:* May increase risk of renal impairment, hypotension, and hyperkalemia in diabetic patients and those with moderate to severe renal impairment (GFR less than 60 mL/minute). Concomitant use is contraindicated in diabetic patients. Avoid concomitant use in those with moderate to severe renal impairment.
Lithium: May increase lithium level. Monitor lithium level and patient for toxicity.
NSAIDs: May decrease antihypertensive effects. Monitor blood pressure.
Potassium-sparing diuretics, potassium supplements: May cause hyperkalemia. Monitor patient closely.
Drug-herb. *Ma huang:* May decrease antihypertensive effects. Discourage use together.

Drug-food. *Salt substitutes containing potassium:* May cause hyperkalemia. Monitor patient closely.

EFFECTS ON LAB TEST RESULTS
● May increase liver enzyme or bilirubin levels.

CONTRAINDICATIONS & CAUTIONS
● Contraindicated in patients hypersensitive to drug. Breast-feeding isn't recommended during losartan therapy.
● Use cautiously in patients with impaired renal or hepatic function.
Black Box Warning Drugs that act directly on the renin-angiotensin system can cause fetal and neonatal morbidity and death when given to women in the second or third trimester of pregnancy. These problems haven't been detected when exposure was limited to the first trimester. If pregnancy is suspected, notify prescriber because drug should be stopped. ▮
⚠ *Overdose S&S:* Hypotension, tachycardia, bradycardia.

NURSING CONSIDERATIONS
● Drug can be used alone or with other antihypertensives.
● If antihypertensive effect is inadequate using once-daily doses, a twice-daily regimen using the same or increased total daily dose may give a more satisfactory response.
● Monitor patient's blood pressure closely to evaluate effectiveness of therapy. When used alone, drug has less of an effect on blood pressure in black patients than in patients of other races.
● Monitor patients who are also taking diuretics for symptomatic hypotension.
● Regularly assess the patient's renal function (via creatinine and BUN levels).
● Patients with severe heart failure whose renal function depends on the angiotensin-aldosterone system may develop acute renal failure during therapy. Closely monitor patient's blood pressure, renal function, and potassium levels, especially during first few weeks of therapy and after dosage adjustments.
● *Look alike–sound alike:* Don't confuse Cozaar with Zocor or Colace.

Reactions in bold italics are *life-threatening*. Interactions may have a *rapid onset* or a *delayed onset.*

PATIENT TEACHING
● Tell patient to avoid salt substitutes; these products may contain potassium, which can cause high potassium level in patients taking losartan.

● Inform women of childbearing age about consequences of second- and third-trimester exposure to drug. Prescriber should be notified immediately if pregnancy is suspected.

● Advise patient to immediately report swelling of face, eyes, lips, or tongue or any breathing difficulty.

---

lovastatin (mevinolin)
loe-va-STA-tin

Altoprev

Therapeutic class: Antilipemics
Pharmacologic class: HMG-CoA reductase inhibitors
Pregnancy risk category: X

AVAILABLE FORMS
Tablets: 10 mg, 20 mg, 40 mg
Tablets (extended-release): 20 mg, 40 mg, 60 mg

INDICATIONS & DOSAGES
Adjust-a-dose (for all indications): Avoid use of lovastatin with fibrates or niacin at doses greater than 1 g daily. For patients also taking danazol, diltiazem, dronedarone, or verapamil, start lovastatin at 10 mg (immediate-release) and don't exceed 20 mg daily. For patients also taking amiodarone, lovastatin dosage shouldn't exceed 40 mg daily unless clinical benefit is likely to outweigh increased risk of myopathy or rhabdomyolysis. For elderly patients or patients with CrCl of less than 30 mL/minute, carefully consider dosage increase greater than 20 mg daily and implement cautiously if necessary. For patients requiring smaller reductions in cholesterol levels, use immediate-release lovastatin.
➤ **To prevent and treat coronary artery disease; hyperlipidemia**
Adults: Initially, 20 mg P.O. once daily with evening meal. Recommended range is 10 to 80 mg as a single dose or in two divided

doses; maximum daily recommended dose is 80 mg. Or, 20 to 60 mg extended-release tablets P.O. at bedtime.

Make dosage adjustments at intervals of 4 weeks or more.
➤ **Heterozygous familial hypercholesterolemia in adolescents**
Adolescents ages 10 to 17: Give 10 to 40 mg daily P.O. with evening meal. Patients requiring reductions in LDL cholesterol level of 20% or more should start with 20 mg daily.

ADMINISTRATION
P.O.
● Give immediate-release drug with evening meal, which improves absorption and cholesterol biosynthesis. Give extended-release drug at bedtime.
● Don't crush, split, or allow patient to chew extended-release tablets.

ACTION
Inhibits HMG-CoA reductase, an early (and rate-limiting) step in cholesterol biosynthesis.

Route	Onset	Peak	Duration
P.O.	Unknown	2–4 hr	Unknown
P.O. (extended-release)	Unknown	12–14 hr	Unknown

Half-life: 1.1 to 1.7 hours.

ADVERSE REACTIONS
CNS: headache, dizziness, insomnia, peripheral neuropathy.
EENT: blurred vision.
GI: abdominal pain or cramps, constipation, diarrhea, dyspepsia, flatulence, heartburn, nausea, vomiting.
Musculoskeletal: muscle cramps, myalgia, myositis, *rhabdomyolysis.*
Skin: alopecia, rash, pruritus.

INTERACTIONS
Drug-drug. *Amiodarone:* May decrease the metabolism of lovastatin. Avoid combining lovastatin at doses exceeding 40 mg daily with amiodarone unless clinical benefit is likely to outweigh increased risk of myopathy.
Azole antifungals: May cause myopathy and rhabdomyolysis. Avoid using together.

L

Colchicine: May increase risk of myopathy or rhabdomyolysis. If coadministration can't be avoided, monitor patient for unexplained muscle pain, tenderness, or weakness.

Cyclosporine, gemfibrozil: May cause severe myopathy and rhabdomyolysis. Avoid this combination.

Danazol, diltiazem, dronedarone, verapamil: May cause myopathy and rhabdomyolysis. Don't exceed 20 mg lovastatin daily.

Dronedarone: May increase lovastatin serum concentration. Limit lovastatin to maximum of 20 mg/day (in adults). Increase monitoring for signs and symptoms of lovastatin toxicity (such as myopathy and rhabdomyolysis). Consider therapy modification.

Erythromycin, protease inhibitors (atazanavir, boceprevir, darunavir, fosamprenavir, indinavir, nefazodone, nelfinavir, ritonavir, saquinavir, telaprevir, tipranavir), strong CYP3A inhibitors (such as clarithromycin, itraconazole, ketoconazole, posaconazole, telithromycin, voriconazole): Increase risk of myopathy and rhabdomyolysis. Use together is contraindicated.

Macrolides (azithromycin, clarithromycin, telithromycin), nefazodone: May decrease metabolism of HMG-CoA reductase inhibitor, increasing toxicity. Monitor patient for adverse effects and report unexplained muscle pain.

Mifepristone (CYP3A4 inhibitor): May increase lovastatin plasma level, increasing risk of toxicity. Use together is contraindicated.

Niacin, other fibrates: May increase the risk for adverse and toxic effects of lovastatin. Avoid use of lovastatin with fibrates or niacin at doses greater than 1 g daily.

Oral anticoagulants: May increase anticoagulant effect. Monitor patient closely.

Phenytoin: May decrease serum concentration of HMG-CoA reductase inhibitors. Consider therapy modification.

Ranolazine: May increase risk of myopathy and rhabdomyolysis. Consider lovastatin dosage adjustment.

Drug-herb. *Eucalyptus, jin bu huan, kava:* May increase risk of hepatotoxicity. Discourage use together.

Pectin: May decrease drug effect. Discourage use together.

Red yeast rice: May increase risk of adverse reactions because herb contains compounds similar to those in drug. Discourage use together.

Drug-food. *Grapefruit juice:* May increase drug level, increasing risk of adverse effects. Discourage use together.

Drug-lifestyle. *Alcohol use:* May increase risk of hepatotoxicity. Discourage use together.

EFFECTS ON LAB TEST RESULTS
● May increase ALT, AST, and CK levels.

CONTRAINDICATIONS & CAUTIONS
● Contraindicated in patients hypersensitive to drug and in those with active liver disease or unexplained persistently increased transaminase level.
● Contraindicated in patients also taking erythromycin, protease inhibitors (atazanavir, boceprevir, darunavir, fosamprenavir, indinavir, nefazodone, nelfinavir, ritonavir, saquinavir, telaprevir, or tipranavir), or strong CYP3A inhibitors (clarithromycin, itraconazole, ketoconazole, posaconazole, voriconazole, telithromycin) because of myopathy and rhabdomyolysis risk.
● Contraindicated in pregnant and breastfeeding women and in women of childbearing age.
● Use cautiously in patients who consume substantial quantities of alcohol or have a history of liver disease.

NURSING CONSIDERATIONS
● Have patient follow a diet restricted in saturated fat and cholesterol during therapy.
● Obtain LFT results at the start of therapy, at 6 and 12 weeks after the start of therapy, and when increasing dose; then monitor results periodically.
● Heterozygous familial hypercholesterolemia can be diagnosed in adolescent boys and in girls who are at least 1 year postmenarche and are 10 to 17 years old; if after an adequate trial of diet therapy LDL cholesterol level remains over 189 mg/dL or LDL cholesterol over 160 mg/dL and patient has a positive family history of premature CV disease or two or more other CV disease risk factors.

Reactions in bold italics are *life-threatening*. Interactions may have a *rapid onset* or a *delayed onset*.

• Obtain CK level in patients with unexplained muscle pain.
• Discontinue lovastatin immediately if markedly elevated CK levels occur or myopathy is diagnosed or suspected.
• Predisposing factors for skeletal muscle effects include advanced age (65 and older), female gender, uncontrolled hypothyroidism, and renal impairment.
• **Look alike–sound alike:** Don't confuse lovastatin with Lotensin, Leustatin, or Livostin.

PATIENT TEACHING

• Instruct patient to take immediate-release drug with the evening meal and extended-release drug at bedtime.
• Teach patient about proper dietary management of cholesterol and triglycerides. When appropriate, recommend weight control, exercise, and smoking cessation programs.
• Instruct patient to store tablets at room temperature in a light-resistant container.
• Advise patient of the risk of myopathy and rhabdomyolysis and tell him to promptly report unexplained muscle pain, tenderness, or weakness, particularly when accompanied by malaise or fever.
• Teach patient about substances that shouldn't be taken with lovastatin and tell him to inform other health care providers that he's taking lovastatin, especially if a new medication is being prescribed.
❸ Alert: Tell woman to stop drug and notify prescriber immediately if she is or may be pregnant or if she's breast-feeding.
❸ Alert: Advise patient not to crush or chew extended-release tablets.

lucinactant
LOO-sin-AK-tant

Surfaxin

Therapeutic class: Lung surfactants
Pharmacologic class: Synthetic lung surfactants
Pregnancy risk category: N/A

AVAILABLE FORMS

Intratracheal suspension: 30 mg phospholipids/mL in 8.5-mL single-use vial

INDICATIONS & DOSAGES
➤ **Prevention of respiratory distress syndrome in premature infants at high risk**
Neonates: 5.8 mL/kg birth weight intratracheally divided into four quarter-doses and given with infant in a different position to ensure even drug distribution. May give up to four doses in first 48 hours of life. Administer doses no more than every 6 hours.

ADMINISTRATION
Intratracheal
• Refrigerate at 36° to 46° F (2° to 8° C). Don't freeze.
• Protect from light.
• Before use, warm vial for 15 minutes in preheated dry block heater set at 111° F (44° C). Label date and time of warming.
• After warming, shake vigorously to form a uniform and free-flowing suspension that is opaque white to off-white. Inspect contents before administering.
• May store unopened vials that have been warmed at room temperature, protected from light (in carton), for up to 2 hours. Don't return drug to refrigerator after warming. Discard vial if not used within 2 hours of warming.
• Vials are for single use only. Discard unused drug.
• Use 16G or 18G needle to draw up drug. Give drug using a #5 French end-hole catheter.
• Ensure proper placement and patency of endotracheal (ET) tube; tube may be suctioned before drug is administered. Allow infant to stabilize before proceeding with dosing.
• Position infant on its right side with head and thorax upward 30 degrees. Thread catheter through a Bodai valve or equivalent device that allows maintenance of positive end-expiratory pressure. Advance tip of catheter into ET tube; position so that tip is slightly distal to the end of ET tube. Give each dose in four quarter-doses. Instill first quarter-dose while continuing positive-pressure mechanical ventilation and maintaining positive end-expiratory pressure of 4 to 5 cm H_2O. Adjust ventilator settings to maintain appropriate oxygenation and ventilation. Ventilate until infant is

L

stable (oxygen saturation of at least 90% and heart rate greater than 120 beats/minute).
● Between giving quarter-doses, pause to allow for evaluation of infant's respiratory status. Repeat procedure with infant on its left side while maintaining adequate positive-pressure ventilation. Repeat procedure with infant on its right side, then left side.
● Remove catheter after last quarter-dose and resume usual ventilator management and critical care while keeping head of infant's bed elevated at least 10 degrees for at least 1 to 2 hours.

ACTION
Lowers surface tension at the air–liquid interface of the alveolar surfaces during respiration and stabilizes alveoli against collapse at resting transpulmonary pressures.

Route	Onset	Peak	Duration
Intratracheal	Unknown	Unknown	Unknown

Half-life: Unknown.

ADVERSE REACTIONS
CNS: periventricular leukomalacia, ***intraventricular hemorrhage.***
CV: ***bradycardia,*** patent ductus arteriosus, hypotension.
EENT: retinopathy of prematurity.
GI: ***necrotizing enterocolitis.***
Hematologic: anemia.
Hepatic: jaundice.
Metabolic: ***metabolic acidosis,*** hyperglycemia, hyponatremia, ***respiratory acidosis.***
Respiratory: oxygen desaturation, ***apnea,*** pulmonary interstitial emphysema, ***pneumothorax,*** pneumonia, ***pulmonary hemorrhage,*** ET tube obstruction.
Skin: pallor.
Other: ***acquired sepsis.***

INTERACTIONS
None reported.

EFFECTS ON LAB TEST RESULTS
● May increase glucose level.
● May decreased sodium level and RBC count.

CONTRAINDICATIONS & CAUTIONS
● Contraindicated in patients hypersensitive to drug or its components.
● Contraindicated in adults with acute respiratory distress syndrome because of an increased incidence of death, multiorgan failure, sepsis, anoxic encephalopathy, renal failure, hypoxia, pneumothorax, hypotension, and PE.

NURSING CONSIDERATIONS
● Only staff experienced in intubation, ventilator management, and general care of premature infants should give drug.
● Accurate weight determination is essential for proper management of dosage.
● Monitor patient for bradycardia, oxygen desaturation, reflux of drug into ET tube, and airway or ET obstruction. Stop drug if reactions occur; stabilize patient. If airway obstruction persists or is severe, suctioning of ET tube or reintubation may be required.
● Frequently evaluate lung compliance and oxygenation status so that oxygen and ventilatory support can be modified to respond to changes in respiratory status.
● Don't suction infant for 1 hour after dosing unless there are other signs and symptoms of airway obstruction.

PATIENT TEACHING
● Inform parent or guardian of infant's need for drug and explain drug's action and use.
● Reassure parent or guardian that infant's heart and lung function will be constantly monitored.
● Notify parent or guardian that although infant may improve rapidly after treatment, intubation and mechanical ventilation may still be needed.
● Encourage parent or guardian to ask questions, and address their concerns.

---

lurasidone hydrochloride
loo-RAS-i-dohne

Latuda

Therapeutic class: Antipsychotics
Pharmacologic class: Dopamine–
serotonin receptor antagonists
Pregnancy risk category: B

AVAILABLE FORMS
Tablets: 20 mg, 40 mg, 80 mg, 120 mg

INDICATIONS & DOSAGES
Adjust-a-dose (for all indications): For patients with moderate (CrCl of 30 to less than 50 mL/minute) or severe (CrCl of less than 30 mL/minute) renal impairment or those concomitantly taking a moderate CYP3A4 inhibitor (such as diltiazem), the recommended starting dose is 20 mg and the maximum recommended dose is 80 mg. For patients with moderate (Child-Pugh score 7 to 9) or severe (Child-Pugh score 10 to 15) hepatic impairment, the recommended starting dose is 20 mg. The maximum recommended dose is 80 mg for patients with moderate hepatic impairment and 40 mg for those with severe hepatic impairment.
➤ **Schizophrenia**
Adults: Initially, 40 mg P.O. once daily. May increase to maximum dose of 160 mg daily.
✱ *NEW INDICATION:* **Depressive episodes associated with bipolar I disorder as monotherapy or as adjunctive therapy with lithium or valproate**
Adults: Initially, 20 mg P.O. once daily. May increase to maximum dosage of 120 mg daily.

ADMINISTRATION
P.O.
● Give with food (at least 350 calories).

ACTION
Exact mechanism is unknown. Drug's efficacy is mediated through antagonism at the dopamine type 2 and serotonin type 2 receptors.

Route	Onset	Peak	Duration
P.O.	Unknown	1–3 hr	Unknown

Half-life: 18 hours.

ADVERSE REACTIONS
CNS: somnolence, akathisia, parkinsonism (bradykinesia, cogwheel rigidity, drooling, extrapyramidal disorder, hypokinesia, muscle rigidity, psychomotor retardation, tremor), agitation, dystonia, dizziness, insomnia, anxiety, restlessness, seizures, fatigue.
CV: tachycardia.
EENT: blurred vision.
GI: nausea, vomiting, dyspepsia, abdominal pain, diarrhea, dysphagia, decreased appetite.
Metabolic: dyslipidemia, hyperglycemia, weight gain.
Musculoskeletal: back pain.
Skin: rash, pruritus.

INTERACTIONS
Drug-drug. *Antihypertensives:* May increase risk of hypotension. Monitor orthostatic vital signs and adjust antihypertensive dosage as needed.
Centrally acting drugs: May increase risk of adverse effects (such as increased cognitive impairment). Avoid use together.
Moderate inhibitors of CYP3A4 (such as diltiazem): May increase lurasidone level. Use together cautiously and limit lurasidone dosage.
Strong inducers of CYP3A4 (such as rifampin): May significantly reduce lurasidone level. Don't use together.
Strong inhibitors of CYP3A4 (such as ketoconazole): May significantly increase lurasidone level. Don't use together.
Drug-lifestyle. *Alcohol use:* May increase risk of adverse effects (such as increased cognitive impairment). Discourage use together.

EFFECTS ON LAB TEST RESULTS
● May increase prolactin, total cholesterol, triglyceride, glucose, serum creatinine, AST, ALT, and CK levels.
● May decrease WBC, neutrophil, and granulocyte counts.

L

CONTRAINDICATIONS & CAUTIONS

• Contraindicated in patients hypersensitive to drug or its components.

Black Box Warning Elderly patients with dementia-related psychosis treated with atypical or conventional antipsychotics are at increased risk for death. Antipsychotics aren't approved for the treatment of dementia-related psychosis. ▪

• Use cautiously in patients with hyperlipidemia, diabetes or risk factors for diabetes (family history, obesity), seizures or conditions that lower the seizure threshold (Alzheimer dementia), body temperature dysregulation, suicide attempts, dysphagia, or concomitant illness.

• Use cautiously in patients with known CV disease, cerebrovascular disease, and conditions that cause hypotension (dehydration, hypovolemia, antihypertensive use) and in antipsychotic-naive patients because of increased risk of dizziness, tachycardia or bradycardia, and syncope.

• Use cautiously in patients with preexisting low WBC count or a history of drug-induced neutropenia or leukopenia.

• Use cautiously in pregnant and breast-feeding women. Use only if benefit to mother outweighs risk to fetus.

• Safety and effectiveness in children haven't been established.

NURSING CONSIDERATIONS

Black Box Warning Antidepressants increase risk of suicidal thinking and behavior in children, adolescents, and young adults. Monitor patient for worsening or emergence of suicidal thoughts and behaviors. ▪

• Monitor patients for tardive dyskinesia. Risk increases in elderly patients and women and with long-term administration. Use the lowest dose for the shortest time possible to minimize risk. Discontinue drug if symptoms occur.

• Monitor patients for orthostatic hypotension, syncope, and excessive sedation.

• Monitor patients for signs and symptoms of neuroleptic malignant syndrome (NMS), such as fever, diaphoresis, muscle rigidity, altered mental status, irregular pulse or blood pressure, cardiac arrhythmias, increased CK level, rhabdomyolysis,

and acute renal failure. Discontinue drug immediately if NMS occurs.

• Monitor CBC, renal function, and prolactin level periodically; discontinue drug if severe neutropenia develops.

• Monitor patients for metabolic changes (such as weight gain and elevated blood glucose, triglyceride, or cholesterol levels), and treat appropriately.

• Psychotic illness predisposes patients to suicide. Assess patients for suicidal thoughts and prescribe drug in small quantities to reduce risk of overdose.

PATIENT TEACHING

Black Box Warning Advise family or caregivers to observe patient closely for suicidal thoughts and behaviors. Encourage them to report such behaviors to health care provider immediately. ▪

• Advise patient to take drug on a regular basis and not to skip doses.

• Inform patient that periodic blood tests will be needed to monitor tolerance to the drug.

• Tell patient to avoid overheating and to maintain adequate hydration.

• Teach patient to monitor weight and maintain a healthy diet because drug may increase weight and blood glucose and cholesterol levels.

• Instruct patient to immediately report sudden changes in temperature or blood pressure, irregular heart rate, or severe muscle rigidity.

• Counsel patient to tell her prescriber if she is pregnant or breast-feeding before taking drug.

• Tell patient to avoid alcohol during therapy.

• Warn patient to avoid driving or operating hazardous machinery until drug's effects are known.

---

lymphocyte immune globulin (antithymocyte globulin [equine], ATG, LIG)
LIM-foh-site

Atgam

Therapeutic class: Immunosuppressants
Pharmacologic class: Immunoglobulins
Pregnancy risk category: C

AVAILABLE FORMS
Injection: 50 mg of equine IgG/mL in 5-mL ampules

INDICATIONS & DOSAGES
➤ **To prevent acute renal allograft rejection**
Adults and children: 15 mg/kg I.V. daily for 14 days; then alternate-day therapy for 14 days. Give first dose within 24 hours of transplantation.
➤ **Acute renal allograft rejection**
Adults and children: 10 to 15 mg/kg I.V. daily for 14 days. Additional alternate-day therapy to total of 21 doses can be given. Start therapy when rejection is diagnosed.
➤ **Aplastic anemia**
Adults and children: 10 to 20 mg/kg I.V. daily for 8 to 14 days. Additional alternate-day therapy to total of 21 doses can be given.

ADMINISTRATION
I.V.
▼ Don't use solutions that are older than 24 hours, including actual infusion time.
▼ Dilute concentrated drug for injection before giving. Dilute required dose in 250 to 1,000 mL of half-normal or normal saline solution. Final concentration of drug shouldn't exceed 4 mg/mL.
▼ Allow diluted drug to reach room temperature before infusion.
▼ When adding drug to infusion solution, make sure container is inverted so drug doesn't contact air inside container. Gently rotate or swirl container to mix contents; don't shake because this may cause excessive foaming or denature the drug protein.

▼ Infuse with an in-line filter with a pore size of 0.2 to 1 micron over at least 4 hours (most institutions use 4 to 8 hours) into a vascular shunt, arteriovenous fistula, or high-flow central vein.
▼ Refrigerate at 36° to 46° F (2° to 8° C). Concentrate is heat sensitive. Don't freeze.
▼ **Incompatibilities:** Don't dilute with dextrose solutions or those with a low salt concentration because a precipitate may form. Proteins in drug can be denatured by air. Drug is unstable in acidic solutions.

ACTION
Unknown. Inhibits cell-mediated immune responses either by altering T-cell function or eliminating antigen-reactive T cells.

Route	Onset	Peak	Duration
I.V.	Immediate	5 days	Unknown

Half-life: About 6 days.

ADVERSE REACTIONS
CNS: *seizures,* headache, malaise.
CV: chest pain, hypotension, edema, iliac vein obstruction, tachycardia, thrombophlebitis.
EENT: *laryngospasm.*
GI: diarrhea, nausea, vomiting, abdominal distention, epigastric pain, hiccups, stomatitis.
GU: renal artery stenosis.
Hematologic: *leukopenia, thrombocytopenia, aplastic anemia,* hemolysis, lymphadenopathy.
Metabolic: hyperglycemia.
Musculoskeletal: arthralgia, myalgia.
Respiratory: dyspnea, *pulmonary edema.*
Skin: pruritus, rash, urticaria.
Other: *anaphylaxis,* chills, febrile reactions, hypersensitivity reactions, infections, night sweats, serum sickness.

INTERACTIONS
None significant.

EFFECTS ON LAB TEST RESULTS
● May increase liver enzyme and glucose levels. May decrease hemoglobin level.
● May decrease WBC and platelet counts.

CONTRAINDICATIONS & CAUTIONS
• Contraindicated in patients hypersensitive to drug.
• Use cautiously in patients receiving additional immunosuppressive therapy (such as corticosteroids or azathioprine) because of increased risk of infection.

NURSING CONSIDERATIONS
◑ *Alert:* Do an I.D. skin test at least 1 hour before first dose. Give an I.D. dose of 0.1 mL of a 1:1,000 lymphocyte immune globulin along with a contralateral normal saline control. Marked local swelling or erythema larger than 10 mm indicates increased risk of severe systemic reaction such as anaphylaxis. Severe reactions to skin test, such as hypotension, tachycardia, dyspnea, generalized rash, or anaphylaxis, usually preclude further use of drug. Anaphylaxis may still occur in patients with negative skin tests.
Black Box Warning Drug should only be used by physicians experienced in immunosuppressive therapy in the treatment of renal transplant or aplastic anemia patients. Patients receiving drug should be treated in facilities equipped and staffed with adequate laboratory and supportive medical resources. ∎
• Monitor patient for hypotension, respiratory distress, and chest, flank, or back pain, which may indicate anaphylaxis or hemolysis.
• Keep airway adjuncts and anaphylaxis drugs at bedside during administration.
• Watch for signs and symptoms of infection, such as fever, sore throat, malaise.

PATIENT TEACHING
• Instruct patient to report adverse drug reactions promptly, especially signs and symptoms of infection (fever, sore throat, fatigue).
• Tell patient to immediately report discomfort at I.V. insertion site because drug can cause a chemical phlebitis.
• Advise women to avoid pregnancy during therapy.

magnesium sulfate

Therapeutic class: Electrolyte replacements
Pharmacologic class: Minerals
Pregnancy risk category: D

AVAILABLE FORMS
Injectable: 4%, 8%, 50% in 2-, 10-, 20-, and 50-mL ampules, vials, and prefilled syringes
Injection solution: 1% in D_5W, 2% in D_5W

INDICATIONS & DOSAGES
Adjust-a-dose (for all indications): In severe renal impairment, reduce dosage and obtain frequent serum magnesium levels.
➤ **Mild hypomagnesemia**
Adults: 1 g I.M. every 6 hours for four doses, depending on magnesium level.
➤ **Symptomatic severe hypomagnesemia, with magnesium level of 0.8 mEq/L or less**
Adults: 5 g I.V. in 1 L of solution over 3 hours. Base subsequent doses on magnesium level.
➤ **Magnesium supplementation in total parenteral nutrition (TPN)**
Adults: 5 to 8 mEq I.V. daily added to TPN solution.
Children: 0.25 to 0.6 mEq/kg/day I.V. added to TPN solution.
➤ **Seizures associated with nephritis**
Children: 20 to 40 mg/kg of a 20% solution I.M. as needed to control seizures.
➤ **Seizures in preeclampsia or eclampsia**
Adults: 4 to 5 g I.V. in 250 mL of solution. Simultaneously, give 8 to 10 g I.M. (5 g or 10 mL of the undiluted 50% solution in each buttock.) Base subsequent doses on magnesium level. Do not exceed 30 to 40 g in a 24-hour period.

ADMINISTRATION
P.O.
• Store between 20° and 25° C (68° and 77° F).
I.V.
▼ Concentration should be 200 mg/mL or less.

▼ Inject bolus dose slowly at a rate of 150 mg/minute or less, or use infusion pump for continuous infusion to avoid respiratory or cardiac arrest. Maximum infusion rate is 150 mg/minute. Rapid drip causes feeling of heat.

▼ For severe hypomagnesemia, watch for respiratory depression and evidence of heart block. Respirations should be better than 16 breaths/minute before giving dose.

▼ **Incompatibilities:** Alcohol (in large amounts), alkali carbonates and bicarbonates, amiodarone, amphotericin B, calcium chloride, calcium gluconate, cefepime, ciprofloxacin, clindamycin, cyclosporine, dobutamine, drotrecogin alfa, heavy metals, hydralazine, hydrocortisone sodium succinate, I.V. fat emulsion 10%, phytonadione, polymyxin B, procaine, quinolones, salicylates, sodium bicarbonate, soluble phosphates, vitamin B complex.

I.M.
● Undiluted 50% solutions may be given by deep I.M. injection to adults. Dilute solutions to 20% or less for use in children.

ACTION
Replaces magnesium and maintains magnesium level; as an anticonvulsant, reduces muscle contractions by interfering with release of acetylcholine at myoneural junction.

Route	Onset	Peak	Duration
P.O.	Unknown	4 hr	4–6 hr
I.V.	Immediate	Unknown	30 min
I.M.	1 hr	Unknown	3–4 hr

Half-life: Unknown.

ADVERSE REACTIONS
CNS: toxicity, weak or absent deep tendon reflexes, flaccid paralysis, drowsiness, stupor.
CV: slow, weak pulse; *arrhythmias;* hypotension; *circulatory collapse;* flushing.
GI: diarrhea.
Metabolic: hypocalcemia.
Respiratory: *respiratory paralysis.*
Skin: diaphoresis.
Other: hypothermia.

INTERACTIONS
Drug-drug. *Alendronate, fluoroquinolones, nitrofurantoin, penicillamine, sodium polystyrene sulfonate, tetracyclines:* May decrease bioavailability with oral magnesium supplements. Separate doses by 2 to 3 hours.
Cardiac glycosides: May cause serious cardiac conduction changes. Use together with caution.
CNS depressants: May have additive effect. Use together cautiously.
Neuromuscular blockers: May cause increased neuromuscular blockage. Use together cautiously.
Nifedipine: May increase risk of neuromuscular blockade and hypotension. Closely monitor clinical response.

EFFECTS ON LAB TEST RESULTS
● May increase magnesium level. May decrease calcium level.

CONTRAINDICATIONS & CAUTIONS
● Contraindicated in patients with myocardial damage or heart block, coma, and in pregnant women in actively progressing labor.
● Use magnesium sulfate with caution in patients with impaired renal function.
۞ Alert: Using magnesium sulfate to stop preterm labor isn't an FDA-approved use of drug; safety and effectiveness of drug for this indication haven't been established. Continuous administration of magnesium sulfate injection beyond 5 to 7 days during pregnancy for treatment of preterm labor can cause low calcium levels and bone changes in the developing fetus.
۞ Alert: Pregnancy Risk Category has been changed to D, in which there is positive evidence of human fetal risk, but potential benefits of use in pregnant women may warrant use of drug despite potential risks in certain situations.
⚠ Overdose S&S: Hypotension, facial flushing, feeling of warmth, thirst, nausea, vomiting, lethargy, dysarthria, drowsiness, diminished deep tendon reflexes, shallow respirations, apnea, coma, cardiac arrest.

M

NURSING CONSIDERATIONS

• Keep I.V. calcium available to reverse magnesium intoxication.

• Test knee-jerk and patellar reflexes before each additional dose. If absent, notify prescriber and give no more magnesium until reflexes return; otherwise, patient may develop temporary respiratory failure and need cardiopulmonary resuscitation or I.V. administration of calcium.

• Check magnesium level after repeated doses. Monitor levels hourly in patients with severe hypomagnesemia.

• Monitor fluid intake and output. Output should be 100 mL or more during 4-hour period before dose.

• Monitor renal function.

• After giving to toxemic pregnant woman within 24 hours before delivery, watch neonate for signs and symptoms of magnesium toxicity, including neuromuscular and respiratory depression.

• *Look alike–sound alike:* Don't confuse magnesium sulfate with manganese sulfate.

PATIENT TEACHING

• Explain use and administration of drug to patient and family.

• Tell patient to report adverse effects.

mannitol
MAN-i-tole

Osmitrol

Therapeutic class: Diuretics
Pharmacologic class: Osmotic diuretics
Pregnancy risk category: B

AVAILABLE FORMS
Injection: 5%, 10%, 15%, 20%, 25%
Solution for irrigation: 5 g/100 mL

INDICATIONS & DOSAGES

➤ **Test dose for marked oliguria or suspected inadequate renal function**
Adults and children older than age 12:
200 mg/kg or 12.5 g as a 15% to 20% I.V. solution over 3 to 5 minutes. Response is adequate if 30 to 50 mL of urine/hour is excreted over 2 to 3 hours; if response is inadequate, a second test dose is given. If

still no response after second dose, stop drug.

➤ **Oliguria**
Adults and children older than age 12:
50 to 100 g I.V. as a 15% to 25% solution over 90 minutes to several hours.

➤ **To prevent oliguria or acute renal failure**
Adults and children older than age 12:
50 to 100 g I.V. of a 5% to 25% solution. Determine exact concentration by fluid requirements.

➤ **To reduce intraocular or intracranial pressure or cerebral edema**
Adults and children older than age 12:
1.5 to 2 g/kg as a 15%, 20%, or 25% I.V. solution over 30 to 60 minutes. For maximum intraocular pressure reduction before surgery, give 60 to 90 minutes preoperatively.

➤ **Diuresis in drug intoxication**
Adults and children older than age 12:
5% to 25% solution continuously up to 200 g I.V., while maintaining 100 to 500 mL urine output/hour and a positive fluid balance.

➤ **Irrigating solution during transurethral surgical procedures**
Adults: 2.5% to 5% solution.

ADMINISTRATION
I.V.

▼ Change I.V. administration apparatus every 24 hours.

▼ To redissolve crystallized solution (crystallization occurs at low temperatures or in concentrations higher than 15%), warm bottle or bag by appropriate means to approximately 140° F (60° C) with occasional shaking. Cool to body temperature before giving. Don't use solution with undissolved crystals.

▼ Give as intermittent or continuous infusion at prescribed rate, using an inline filter and an infusion pump. Don't give as direct injection.

▼ Check patency at infusion site before and during administration.

▼ Monitor patient for signs and symptoms of infiltration; if it occurs, watch for inflammation, edema, and necrosis.

▼ **Incompatibilities:** Blood products, cefepime, doxorubicin liposomal, filgrastim, imipenem–cilastatin, meropenem, potassium chloride, sodium chloride, strongly acidic or alkaline solutions.

ACTION

Increases osmotic pressure of glomerular filtrate, thus inhibiting tubular reabsorption of water and electrolytes. Drug elevates plasma osmolality and increases urine output.

Route	Onset	Peak	Duration
I.V.	30–60 min	1 hr	6–8 hr

Half-life: About 1½ hours.

ADVERSE REACTIONS

CNS: *seizures,* dizziness, headache, fever.
CV: edema, thrombophlebitis, hypotension, hypertension, *heart failure,* tachycardia, angina-like chest pain, vascular overload.
EENT: blurred vision, rhinitis.
GI: thirst, dry mouth, nausea, vomiting, diarrhea.
GU: urine retention.
Metabolic: dehydration.
Skin: local pain, urticaria.
Other: chills, thirst.

INTERACTIONS

Drug-drug. *Lithium:* May increase urinary excretion of lithium. Monitor lithium level closely.

EFFECTS ON LAB TEST RESULTS

• May increase or decrease electrolyte levels.
• May interfere with tests for inorganic phosphorus or ethylene glycol level.

CONTRAINDICATIONS & CAUTIONS

• Contraindicated in patients hypersensitive to drug.
• Contraindicated in patients with anuria; severe pulmonary congestion; frank pulmonary edema; active intracranial bleeding (except during craniotomy); severe dehydration; metabolic edema; previous progressive renal disease or dysfunction after starting drug, including increasing azotemia and oliguria; or previous progressive heart failure or pulmonary congestion after drug.
⚠ *Overdose S&S:* Increased electrolyte excretion, orthostatic tachycardia or hypotension, decreased central venous pressure, impaired neuromuscular function, intestinal dilation and ileus, pulmonary edema or water intoxication if urine output is inadequate.

NURSING CONSIDERATIONS

• Monitor vital signs, including central venous pressure and fluid intake and output hourly. Report increasing oliguria. Check weight, renal function, fluid balance, and serum and urine sodium and potassium levels daily.
• In comatose or incontinent patient, use urinary catheter because therapy is based on strict evaluation of fluid intake and output. If patient has urinary catheter, use an hourly urometer collection bag to evaluate output accurately and easily.
• To relieve thirst, give frequent mouth care or fluids.
• Drug is commonly used in chemotherapy regimens to enhance diuresis of renally toxic drugs.
• Don't give electrolyte-free solutions with blood. If blood is given simultaneously, add at least 20 mEq of sodium chloride to each liter of drug solution to avoid pseudoagglutination.

PATIENT TEACHING

• Tell patient that he may feel thirsty or have a dry mouth, and emphasize importance of drinking only the amount of fluids ordered.
• Instruct patient to promptly report adverse reactions and discomfort at I.V. site.

M

maraviroc
mahr-AY-vih-rok

Selzentry

Therapeutic class: Antiretrovirals
Pharmacologic class: CCR5 co-receptor antagonists
Pregnancy risk category: B

AVAILABLE FORMS
Tablets: 150 mg, 300 mg

INDICATIONS & DOSAGES
➤ **Combined with CYP3A4 inhibitors, including protease inhibitors (except tipranavir and ritonavir), to treat CCR5-tropic HIV-1 infection with evidence of viral replication or HIV-1 strains resistant to multiple antiretrovirals**
Adults and children age 16 and older: 150 mg P.O. b.i.d.
➤ **Combined with nucleoside reverse transcriptase inhibitors, tipranavir–ritonavir, nevirapine, or enfuvirtide to treat CCR5-tropic HIV-1 infection**
Adults and children age 16 and older: 300 mg P.O. b.i.d.
Adjust-a-dose: For patients with severe renal impairment (CrCl of less than 30 mL/minute) or ESRD on hemodialysis who experience orthostatic hypotension, reduce dosage to 150 mg P.O. b.i.d.
➤ **Combined with CYP3A inducers, without strong CYP3A inhibitors, to treat CCR5-tropic HIV-1 infection**
Adults and children age 16 and older: 600 mg P.O. b.i.d.

ADMINISTRATION
P.O.
● Give drug without regard for food.

ACTION
Blocks viral entry into cells by binding to chemokine receptor type 5 co-receptor and preventing the initiation of HIV replication cycle.

Route	Onset	Peak	Duration
P.O.	Unknown	½–4 hr	Unknown

Half-life: 14 to 18 hours.

ADVERSE REACTIONS
CNS: dizziness, paresthesia, sensory abnormalities, peripheral neuropathy, sleep disturbances, depressive disorders, pyrexia, pain, disturbances in consciousness, ***stroke.***
CV: unstable angina, ***acute cardiac failure,*** coronary artery disease, ***MI,*** myocardial ischemia, vascular hypertensive disorders.
GI: abdominal pain, constipation, dyspepsia, stomatitis, appetite disorders.
GU: urinary tract signs and symptoms.
Hepatic: ***cirrhosis, hepatic failure,*** cholestatic jaundice.
Metabolic: lipodystrophies.
Musculoskeletal: muscle pains, joint pain, myositis, osteonecrosis, ***rhabdomyolysis.***
Respiratory: upper respiratory tract infection, bronchitis, sinusitis, cough, pneumonia.
Skin: rash, pruritus, dermatitis, eczema, folliculitis, condyloma acuminatum.
Other: herpes infection, immune reconstitution syndrome, influenza.

INTERACTIONS
Drug-drug. *CYP3A inducers (carbamazepine, efavirenz, phenobarbital, phenytoin, rifampin):* May decrease levels of maraviroc. Increase dose of maraviroc.
CYP3A inhibitors (protease inhibitors except tipranavir and ritonavir), delavirdine, ketoconazole, itraconazole, clarithromycin, nefazodone, telithromycin: May increase levels of maraviroc. Decrease dose of maraviroc.
Drug-herb. *St. John's wort:* May decrease levels of maraviroc. Discourage use together.

EFFECTS ON LAB TEST RESULTS
● May increase AST, ALT, bilirubin, amylase, lipase, and CK levels.
● May decrease ANC.

CONTRAINDICATIONS & CAUTIONS
● Contraindicated in patients hypersensitive to drug or its components.
● Contraindicated in patients with severe renal impairment or ESRD (CrCl of less than 30 mL/minute) who are taking potent CYP3A inhibitors or inducers.
● Use cautiously in patients with pre-existing liver dysfunction or patients who are infected with viral hepatitis B or C.

Reactions in bold italics are *life-threatening*. Interactions may have a *rapid onset* or a *delayed onset*.

- Use cautiously in patients at risk for CV events, with a history of postural hypotension, or taking another medication known to lower blood pressure.
- During initial phase of treatment, patients treated with combination antiretroviral therapy may develop an inflammatory response to indolent or residual opportunistic infections (CMV, *Mycobacterium avium* complex, *Pneumocystis jiroveci* pneumonia, tuberculosis), which may necessitate further evaluation and treatment. Autoimmune disorders (such as Graves disease, polymyositis, and Guillain-Barré syndrome) have also been reported in the setting of immune reconstitution; however, time to onset is more variable, and onset can occur many months after initiation of antiretroviral treatment.
- Safety and effectiveness haven't been established in children younger than age 16.
- Patient shouldn't breast-feed while taking drug because of the potential for HIV transmission and serious drug side effects in infants.
- Pregnant women exposed to drug should be registered in the Antiretroviral Pregnancy Registry by calling 1-800-258-4263.

NURSING CONSIDERATIONS
- Effectiveness hasn't been established in patients with dual, mixed, or CXCR4–tropic HIV-1 infection.
- Monitor patient closely for signs and symptoms of infection.

Black Box Warning Due to increased risk of hepatotoxicity, monitor patient closely. Systemic allergic reaction with pruritic rash, eosinophilia, or elevated IgE may precede hepatotoxicity. Patients with signs or symptoms of hepatitis or allergic reaction should be evaluated immediately. ■

PATIENT TEACHING
- Instruct patient to immediately report signs or symptoms of hepatitis or allergic reaction (rash, yellow eyes or skins, dark urine, vomiting, and abdominal pain).
- Caution patients that drug doesn't cure HIV infection and that they may still develop HIV-related illness, including opportunistic infections.

- Caution patient that drug doesn't reduce risk of transmission of HIV to others.
- If patient feels dizzy while taking drug, advise him to avoid driving or operating machinery.
- Instruct woman to tell her prescriber if she's pregnant or planning to become pregnant while taking drug.
- Advise patient to take drug every day as prescribed with other antiretrovirals. Tell patient not to change the dose or dosing schedule or stop any antiretroviral without consulting prescriber.

mebendazole
me-BEN-da-zole

Therapeutic class: Anthelmintics
Pharmacologic class: Benzimidazoles
Pregnancy risk category: C

AVAILABLE FORMS
Tablets (chewable): 100 mg

INDICATIONS & DOSAGES
➤ **Pinworm**
Adults and children older than age 2: Give 100 mg P.O. as a single dose; repeat if infestation persists 3 weeks later.
➤ **Roundworm, whipworm, and hookworm**
Adults and children older than age 2: Give 100 mg P.O. b.i.d. for 3 days; repeat if infestation persists 3 weeks later.

ADMINISTRATION
P.O.
- Tablets may be chewed, swallowed whole, or crushed and mixed with food.

ACTION
Selectively and irreversibly inhibits uptake of glucose and other nutrients by susceptible helminths.

Route	Onset	Peak	Duration
P.O.	Unknown	2–4 hr	Variable

Half-life: 3 to 9 hours.

ADVERSE REACTIONS
GI: transient abdominal pain and diarrhea in massive infestation and during expulsion of worms.
Hematologic: *agranulocytosis, neutropenia.*
Skin: urticaria.

INTERACTIONS
Drug-drug. *Carbamazepine, hydantoin:* May decrease mebendazole level, which may decrease drug's effect. Monitor patient for drug effectiveness.
Cimetidine: May increase mebendazole level. Monitor patient for increased adverse effects.

EFFECTS ON LAB TEST RESULTS
• May increase LFT values with prolonged use.
• May decrease WBC count.

CONTRAINDICATIONS & CAUTIONS
• Contraindicated in patients hypersensitive to drug.
• Safe use in pregnant women and children younger than age 2 hasn't been established.
⚠ *Overdose S&S:* GI complaints.

NURSING CONSIDERATIONS
• Give drug to all family members to decrease risk of spreading the infestation.
• No dietary restrictions, laxatives, or enemas are needed.

PATIENT TEACHING
• Teach patient about personal hygiene, especially good hand-washing technique. Advise him to refrain from preparing food for others.
• To avoid reinfestation, teach patient to wash perianal area daily, change undergarments and bedclothes daily, and wash hands and clean fingernails before meals and after bowel movements.

mecasermin
meh-KAH-sur-men

Increlex

Therapeutic class: Growth factors
Pharmacologic class: Human insulin growth factors
Pregnancy risk category: C

AVAILABLE FORMS
Injection: 10 mg/mL*

INDICATIONS & DOSAGES
➤ **Growth failure in children with severe primary insulin growth factor-1 (IGF-1) deficiency or children with growth-hormone gene deletion who have developed neutralizing antibodies to growth hormone**
Children age 2 and older: Initially, 0.04 to 0.08 mg/kg subcutaneously b.i.d. If well tolerated for at least 1 week, may increase by 0.04 mg/kg per dose, to the maximum dose of 0.12 mg/kg b.i.d.

ADMINISTRATION
Subcutaneous
• Reduce dose if hypoglycemia occurs despite adequate food intake.
• Give dose about 20 minutes before or after a meal or snack.
• Hold dose if patient is unable to eat.
• Do not increase dose to make up for one or more omitted doses.
• Rotate sites for injection (thigh, abdomen, buttocks, or upper arm). New injections should be given at least 1 inch from previous injection site(s) and never into areas where the skin is tender, bruised, red, or hard or lacks fatty tissue.

ACTION
Promotes growth because synthetic drug is identical to endogenous insulin-like growth factor-binding protein-3 (IGFBP-3) and IGF-1.

Route	Onset	Peak	Duration
Subcut.	1 hr	2 hr	Unknown

Half-life: About 6 hours.

Reactions in bold italics are *life-threatening*. Interactions may have a *rapid onset* or a *delayed onset*.

ADVERSE REACTIONS

CNS: headache, dizziness, *seizures, intracranial hypertension,* pain.
CV: murmur.
EENT: tonsillar hypertrophy, otitis media, papilledema, fluid in middle ear, sensitivity to sound.
GI: vomiting.
GU: hematuria, ovarian cysts.
Hematologic: iron deficiency anemia, enlarged thymus, lymphadenopathy.
Metabolic: hyperglycemia, *hypoglycemia,* lipohypertrophy.
Musculoskeletal: muscle atrophy, arthralgia, bone pain, scoliosis.
Skin: injection-site reaction, bruising.
Other: snoring.

INTERACTIONS

None known.

EFFECTS ON LAB TEST RESULTS

• May increase AST, LDH, and transaminase levels. May increase or decrease glucose level.

CONTRAINDICATIONS & CAUTIONS

• Contraindicated in patients with closed epiphyses, known or suspected cancer, or allergy to drug or its components. I.V. use is also contraindicated. Don't use in place of growth hormone or for other causes of growth failure.
• Use cautiously in pregnant or breast-feeding women.
⚠ *Overdose S&S:* Hypoglycemia, acromegaly.

NURSING CONSIDERATIONS

• Make sure patient has had a baseline ophthalmic examination before therapy.
• Monitor glucose level before starting treatment and continue to monitor glucose level carefully, especially in small children, whose oral intake can be inconsistent.
• Check patient regularly for adenotonsillar enlargement. Ask parent or caregiver if the child has developed snoring, sleep apnea, or reduced hearing.
• Monitor patient for changes typical of acromegaly.
• Monitor child experiencing rapid growth closely for development of a limp or hip

or knee pain to check for slipped capital femoral epiphysis or progression of scoliosis (if present).
• Safety and effectiveness in adults and children younger than age 2 aren't known.

PATIENT TEACHING

• Explain that drug must be kept refrigerated and protected from direct light and freezing.
• Tell parent that vials are stable for 30 days after opening if kept refrigerated.
• Warn parent not to use cloudy drug.
• Tell parent to give drug 20 minutes before or after a meal or snack and to withhold dose if the child can't or won't eat.
• Teach parent how to inject drug and dispose of syringes properly.
• Tell parent to inject drug subcutaneously into child's upper arm, upper thigh, stomach area, or buttocks. Caution against injecting it into a muscle or vein.
• To decrease injection-site reactions, advise parent to rotate the injection site for each dose.
• Tell parent to regularly monitor the child's glucose level. Review signs and symptoms of hypoglycemia, including dizziness, tiredness, hunger, irritability, sweating, nausea, and a fast or irregular heartbeat.
• Advise parent and child to keep a quick source of sugar (such as orange juice, glucose gel, or candy) readily available in case hypoglycemia occurs.
• Explain that child should avoid hazardous activities while the dose is being adjusted. Hypoglycemia can cause unconsciousness, seizures, or death.
• Advise parent to have the child's tonsils checked regularly and to monitor child for enlarged tonsils and snoring or sleep apnea.
• Tell parent to notify prescriber if child develops nausea and vomiting with headache, hypoglycemic episodes, limping, hip or knee pain, snoring, trouble swallowing, earaches, or breathing problems.

M

meclizine hydrochloride (meclozine hydrochloride)
MEK-li-zeen

Antivert, Bonine ◊, Dramamine Less Drowsy Formula ◊

Therapeutic class: Antivertigo drugs
Pharmacologic class: Anticholinergics
Pregnancy risk category: B

AVAILABLE FORMS
Capsules: 25 mg
Tablets: 12.5 mg, 25 mg ◊, 50 mg
Tablets (chewable): 25 mg ◊

INDICATIONS & DOSAGES
➤ **Vertigo**
Adults: 25 to 100 mg P.O. daily in divided doses. Dosage varies with response.
➤ **Motion sickness**
Adults and children age 12 and older: 25 to 50 mg P.O. 1 hour before travel; then daily for duration of trip.

ADMINISTRATION
P.O.
● Chewable tablets may be chewed or swallowed with water.

ACTION
Unknown. May affect neural pathways originating in the labyrinth to inhibit nausea and vomiting.

Route	Onset	Peak	Duration
P.O.	1 hr	3 hr	8–24 hr

Half-life: About 5 hours.

ADVERSE REACTIONS
CNS: drowsiness, auditory and visual hallucinations, excitation, nervousness, restlessness.
CV: hypotension, palpitations, tachycardia.
EENT: blurred vision, diplopia, dry nose and throat, tinnitus.
GI: anorexia, constipation, diarrhea, dry mouth, nausea, vomiting.
GU: urinary frequency, urine retention.
Skin: rash, urticaria.

INTERACTIONS
Drug-drug. *CNS depressants:* May increase drowsiness. Use together cautiously.
Drug-lifestyle. *Alcohol use:* May increase drowsiness. Avoid use together.

EFFECTS ON LAB TEST RESULTS
● May prevent, reduce, or mask diagnostic skin test response.

CONTRAINDICATIONS & CAUTIONS
● Contraindicated in patients hypersensitive to drug.
● Use cautiously in patients with asthma, glaucoma, or prostatic hyperplasia.
⚠ *Overdose S&S:* Hyperexcitability alternating with drowsiness, seizures, hallucinations, respiratory paralysis.

NURSING CONSIDERATIONS
● Stop drug 4 days before diagnostic skin tests to avoid interference with test response.
● Drug may mask signs and symptoms of ototoxicity, brain tumor, or intestinal obstruction.
● *Look alike–sound alike:* Don't confuse Antivert with Axert. Don't confuse Dramamine Less Drowsy with other Dramamine formulations.

PATIENT TEACHING
● Advise patient to avoid hazardous activities that require alertness until CNS effects of drug are known.
● Urge patient to report persistent or serious adverse reactions promptly.

medroxyPROGESTERone acetate
me-DROX-ee-proe-JESS-te-rone

Depo-Provera, Depo-subQ Provera 104, Provera⌀

Therapeutic class: Estrogens
Pharmacologic class: Progestins
Pregnancy risk category: X

AVAILABLE FORMS
Injection (suspension): 104 mg/0.65 mL, 150 mg/mL, 400 mg/mL
Tablets: 2.5 mg, 5 mg, 10 mg

Reactions in bold italics are *life-threatening*. Interactions may have a *rapid onset* or a *delayed onset*.

INDICATIONS & DOSAGES

➤ **Abnormal uterine bleeding caused by hormonal imbalance**
Women: 5 to 10 mg P.O. daily for 5 to 10 days beginning on day 16 or 21 of menstrual cycle. If patient also has received estrogen, give 10 mg P.O. daily for 10 days beginning on day 16 or 21 of cycle.

➤ **Secondary amenorrhea**
Women: 5 to 10 mg P.O. daily for 5 to 10 days. Start at any time during menstrual cycle (usually during latter half of cycle).

➤ **Endometrial hyperplasia**
Postmenopausal women (intact uterus) receiving conjugated estrogen 0.625 mg: 5 or 10 mg P.O. daily for 12 to 14 consecutive days per month, beginning day 1 or 16 of cycle.

➤ **Endometrial or renal cancer**
Adults: 400 to 1,000 mg I.M. weekly. Dosage may be decreased to 400 mg/month when disease has stabilized.

➤ **Contraception**
Women: 150 mg (Depo-Provera) I.M. once every 3 months. Or, 104 mg Depo-subQ Provera subcutaneously once every 3 months. Give first dose during first 5 days of normal menstrual period; only within first 5 days postpartum if patient isn't breast-feeding; and, if patient is exclusively breast-feeding, only at sixth postpartum week.

➤ **Endometriosis-associated pain**
Women: 104 mg subcutaneously every 3 months (12 to 14 weeks).

ADMINISTRATION

P.O.
- Giving this drug immediately before or after a meal increases its bioavailability.

I.M.
- Shake vigorously before use.
- Give by deep I.M. injection in the gluteal or deltoid muscle.
- I.M. injection may be painful. Monitor sites for evidence of sterile abscess. Rotate injection sites to prevent muscle atrophy.
- For multidose vials, use a povidone-iodine solution or similar product to cleanse vial top before aspirating contents. Take special care to prevent contamination of vial's contents, especially when multidose vial is used for endometrial or renal carcinoma.

Subcutaneous
- Shake vigorously before use.
- Give subcutaneous injection into the anterior thigh or abdomen.

ACTION

Suppresses ovulation, possibly by inhibiting pituitary gonadotropin secretion, thus preventing follicular maturation and causing endometrial thinning.

Route	Onset	Peak	Duration
P.O.	Rapid	2–4 hr	3–5 days
I.M.	Slow	24 hr	3–4 mo
Subcut.	Unknown	Unknown	Unknown

Half-life: 2¼ to 9 hours P.O., 50 days I.M., 40 days subcutaneous.

ADVERSE REACTIONS

CNS: anxiety, depression, fatigue, insomnia, somnolence, dementia, *stroke,* pain, dizziness.
CV: thrombophlebitis, *PE,* edema, *thromboembolism,* syncope.
EENT: exophthalmos, diplopia.
GI: bloating, abdominal pain.
GU: breakthrough bleeding, dysmenorrhea, amenorrhea, cervical erosion, abnormal secretions.
Hepatic: cholestatic jaundice.
Metabolic: weight changes.
Musculoskeletal: loss of bone mineral density.
Skin: rash, induration, sterile abscesses, acne, pruritus, melasma, alopecia, hirsutism.
Other: breast tenderness, enlargement, or secretion; hot flashes.

INTERACTIONS

Drug-drug. *Aminoglutethimide, carbamazepine, fosphenytoin, phenobarbital, phenytoin, rifampin:* May decrease progestin effects. Monitor patient for diminished therapeutic response. Tell patient to use a nonhormonal contraceptive during therapy with these drugs.
Anticonvulsants, corticosteroids: These drugs can also reduce bone mass. Monitor patient.
Drug-food. *Caffeine:* May increase caffeine level. Advise caution.

M

Drug-lifestyle. *Smoking:* May increase risk of adverse CV effects. If smoking continues, may need alternative therapy.

EFFECTS ON LAB TEST RESULTS
● May increase LFT values, thyroid-binding globulin levels, HDL and triglyceride levels, coagulation tests, and prothrombin factors VII, VIII, IX, and X.
● May reduce metyrapone test results. May alter glucose level.

CONTRAINDICATIONS & CAUTIONS
Black Box Warning Estrogens with progestins shouldn't be used for prevention of CV disease or dementia. ■
● Contraindicated in patients hypersensitive to drug and in those with active thromboembolic disorders or history of thromboembolic disorders, cerebrovascular disease, stroke, breast cancer, history of breast cancer, undiagnosed abnormal vaginal bleeding, missed abortion, or hepatic dysfunction; also contraindicated during pregnancy. Tablets are contraindicated in patients with liver dysfunction or known or suspected malignant disease of genital organs.
Black Box Warning Injectable drug shouldn't be used for long-term birth control (more than 2 years) unless other forms of birth control are inadequate. ■
● Use cautiously in patients with diabetes, seizures, migraine, cardiac or renal disease, strong family history of breast cancer, asthma, depression, or breast nodules.
Black Box Warning The Women's Health Initiative (WHI) Estrogen Plus Progestin substudy reported increased risks of MI, stroke, invasive breast cancer, PE, and DVT in postmenopausal women (ages 50 to 79) during 5.6 years of treatment with daily oral conjugated estrogens 0.625 mg combined with medroxyprogesterone 2.5 mg relative to placebo. The WHI Memory Study, a substudy of the WHI study, reported increased risk of developing probable dementia in postmenopausal women age 65 and older during 4 years of treatment with daily conjugated estrogens 0.625 mg combined with medroxyprogesterone 2.5 mg relative to placebo. It's unknown whether this finding applies to younger postmenopausal women.

In the absence of comparable data, these risks should be assumed to be similar for other doses of conjugated estrogens and medroxyprogesterone and other combinations and dosage forms of estrogens and progestins. Because of these risks, estrogens with or without progestins should be prescribed at lowest effective doses and for shortest durations consistent with treatment goals and risks for the individual woman. ■

NURSING CONSIDERATIONS
● Drug shouldn't be used as test for pregnancy; it may cause birth defects and masculinization of female fetus.
Black Box Warning Depo-Provera and Depo-subQ Provera may cause a significant loss of bone mineral density. Loss is greater with increasing duration of use and may not be reversible. In adolescents and young adults, drug may reduce peak bone mass and increase risk of osteoporotic fractures in later life. ■
● Monitor patient for pain, swelling, warmth, or redness in calves; sudden, severe headaches; visual disturbances; numbness in extremities; signs of depression; and signs of liver dysfunction (abdominal pain, dark urine, jaundice).

PATIENT TEACHING
● According to FDA regulations, patient must read package insert explaining possible adverse effects of progestins before receiving first dose. Also, give patient verbal explanation.
Black Box Warning Teach patient that this product does not protect against HIV or other sexually transmitted diseases. ■
● Advise patient to take medication with food if GI upset occurs.
۞ Alert: Tell patient to report unusual symptoms immediately and to stop drug and notify prescriber about visual disturbances or migraine.
● Teach women how to perform routine breast self-examination.
● Advise patient to immediately report to prescriber any breast abnormalities, vaginal bleeding, swelling, yellowed skin or eyes, dark urine, clay-colored stools, shortness of breath, chest pain, or pregnancy.

• Advise patient that injection must be given every 3 months to maintain adequate contraceptive effects.

• Tell patient that because this is a long-acting method of birth control, it may take some time for fertility to return after the last injection.

• Tell women to immediately report a suspected pregnancy to prescriber.

• Advise patient that amenorrhea is possible with prolonged use.

• Encourage adequate intake of calcium and vitamin D.

mefloquine hydrochloride
MEH-flow-kwin

Therapeutic class: Antimalarials
Pharmacologic class: Quinine derivatives
Pregnancy risk category: B

AVAILABLE FORMS
Tablets: 250 mg

INDICATIONS & DOSAGES
➤ **Acute malaria infections caused by mefloquine-sensitive strains of *Plasmodium falciparum* or *P. vivax***
Adults: 1,250 mg (5 tablets) P.O. as a single dose with food and at least 8 ounces of water. Patients with *P. vivax* infections should receive further therapy with primaquine or other 8-aminoquinolines to avoid relapse after treatment of the initial infection.
Children: 20 to 25 mg/kg P.O. as a single dose with food and at least 8 ounces of water. Maximum dose 1,250 mg. Dosage may be divided into two doses given 6 to 8 hours apart to reduce the incidence and severity of adverse effects. Patients with *P. vivax* infections should receive further therapy with primaquine or other 8-aminoquinolines to avoid relapse after treatment of the initial infection.
➤ **To prevent malaria**
Adults and children weighing more than 45 kg (99 lb): 250 mg P.O. once weekly. Prevention therapy should start 1 week before entering endemic area and continue for 4 weeks after returning. If patient returns to an area without malaria after a prolonged stay in an endemic area, prevention therapy should end after three doses.
Children weighing 31 to 45 kg (68 to 99 lb): 187.5 mg (¾ of a 250-mg tablet) P.O. once weekly.
Children weighing 21 to 30 kg (46 to 66 lb): 125 mg (½ of a 250-mg tablet) P.O. once weekly.
Children weighing 11 to 20 kg (24 to 44 lb): 62.5 mg (¼ of a 250-mg tablet) P.O. once weekly.
Children weighing 5 to 10 kg (11 to 22 lb): 5 mg/kg (approximately ⅛ of a 250-mg tablet) P.O. once weekly.

ADMINISTRATION
P.O.
• Because giving quinine and mefloquine together poses a health risk, give mefloquine no sooner than 12 hours after the last dose of quinine or quinidine.
• Patient should avoid taking drug on empty stomach and should always take it with at least 8 ounces of water.

ACTION
May be caused by drug's ability to form complexes with hemin and to raise intravesicular pH in parasite acid vesicles.

Route	Onset	Peak	Duration
P.O.	Unknown	7–24 hr	Unknown

Half-life: About 21 days.

ADVERSE REACTIONS
CNS: *seizures, suicidal behavior,* fever, dizziness, syncope, headache, psychotic changes, hallucinations, confusion, anxiety, fatigue, vertigo, depression, tremor, ataxia, mood changes, panic attacks.
CV: chest pain, edema.
EENT: tinnitus, visual disturbances.
GI: vomiting, nausea, loose stools, diarrhea, abdominal discomfort or pain, dyspepsia.
Hematologic: *leukopenia, thrombocytopenia.*
Musculoskeletal: myalgia.
Skin: rash.
Other: chills.

M

INTERACTIONS

Drug-drug. *Beta blockers, quinidine, quinine:* May cause ECG abnormalities and cardiac arrest. Avoid using together.

Carbamazepine, phenytoin, valproic acid: May decrease drug levels and loss of seizure control at start of mefloquine therapy. Monitor anticonvulsant level.

Chloroquine, quinine: May increase risk of seizures and ECG abnormalities. Give mefloquine at least 12 hours after last dose.

Halofantrine: May cause fatal prolongation of the QTc interval if given with or subsequent to mefloquine. Do not use together.

Valproic acid: May decrease valproic acid level and loss of seizure control at start of mefloquine therapy. Monitor anticonvulsant level.

EFFECTS ON LAB TEST RESULTS

- May increase transaminase level.
- May decrease hematocrit.
- May decrease WBC and platelet counts.

CONTRAINDICATIONS & CAUTIONS

- Contraindicated in patients hypersensitive to mefloquine or related compounds.
- Other I.V. antimalarials should be used to initially treat life-threatening or serious malarial infections. Mefloquine may be used after I.V. treatment is completed.

Black Box Warning Contraindicated for prevention of malaria in patients with a history of seizures or an active or recent history of depression, generalized anxiety disorder, psychosis, schizophrenia, or other major psychiatric disorders. ∎

- If psychiatric symptoms occur with prophylactic treatment, discontinue drug.
- Use cautiously when treating patients with cardiac disease or seizure disorders.

⚠ Overdose S&S: Possibly more pronounced adverse reactions.

NURSING CONSIDERATIONS

- Patients with *P. vivax* infections are at high risk for relapse because drug doesn't eliminate the hepatic-phase exoerythrocytic parasites. Give follow-up therapy with primaquine.
- Monitor LFT results periodically.

- If patient vomits within 30 minutes of receiving dose, repeat full dose; if within 30 to 60 minutes, give a half dose.
- If overdose is suspected, induce vomiting or perform gastric lavage because of risk of cardiotoxicity. Mefloquine has produced cardiac reactions similar to those caused by quinidine and quinine.

Black Box Warning Monitor patient for neurologic signs and symptoms (dizziness, vertigo, tinnitus, seizures, insomnia) or psychiatric signs and symptoms (anxiety, paranoia, hallucinations, depression, restlessness, confusion, behavior changes). Signs and symptoms may be more difficult to detect in children. ∎

Black Box Warning During prophylactic use, if psychiatric or neurologic signs and symptoms occur, the drug should be discontinued and an alternative medication prescribed. ∎

PATIENT TEACHING

- Advise patient taking drug for prevention to take dose immediately before or after a meal on the same day each week, to improve compliance beginning 1 week before arrival at endemic area.
- Tell patient not to take drug on an empty stomach and always to take it with at least 8 ounces of water.
- Advise patient to use caution when performing activities that require alertness and coordination because dizziness, disturbed sense of balance, and neuropsychiatric reactions may occur.
- **⚠ Alert:** Inform patient that dizziness, vertigo, and tinnitus can occur during treatment, may continue for months or years after treatment, or may be permanent.
- **⚠ Alert:** Warn patient to contact prescriber immediately if neurologic or psychiatric signs or symptoms occur and not to stop drug until discussing with prescriber. Encourage patient to read the medication guide that comes with every prescription.
- Advise patient undergoing long-term therapy to have periodic ophthalmic exams because drug may cause ocular lesions.
- Advise women of childbearing age to use reliable contraception during treatment.

Reactions in bold italics are *life-threatening*. Interactions may have a *rapid onset* or a *delayed onset*.

megestrol acetate
me-JESS-trole

Megace, Megace ES, Megace OS†

Therapeutic class: Antineoplastics
Pharmacologic class: Progestins
Pregnancy risk category: D (tablets);
X (oral suspension)

AVAILABLE FORMS
Oral suspension: 40 mg/mL
Oral suspension (concentrated): 125 mg/mL
Tablets: 20 mg, 40 mg

INDICATIONS & DOSAGES
➤ **Breast cancer (palliative treatment)**
Adults: 40 mg P.O. q.i.d.
➤ **Endometrial cancer (palliative treatment)**
Adults: 40 to 320 mg P.O. daily in divided doses.
➤ **Anorexia, cachexia, or unexplained significant weight loss in patients with AIDS**
Adults: 800 mg P.O. (20 mL regular oral suspension) or 625 mg P.O. (5 mL concentrated oral suspension) once daily.

ADMINISTRATION
P.O.
• Drug is a hormonal agent and is considered a teratogen. Follow safe handling procedures.
• Give drug without regard for meals.
• Shake suspension well before pouring.

ACTION
Inhibits hormone-dependent tumor growth by inhibiting pituitary and adrenal steroidogenesis. Drug may also have direct cytotoxicity; its appetite-stimulating mechanism is unknown.

Route	Onset	Peak	Duration
P.O.	Unknown	1–5 hr	Unknown

Half-life: About 10 days.

ADVERSE REACTIONS
CV: thrombophlebitis, *heart failure,* hypertension, *thromboembolism.*
GI: nausea, vomiting, diarrhea, flatulence, constipation, dry mouth, increased appetite.
GU: breakthrough menstrual bleeding, impotence, vaginal bleeding or discharge, UTI.
Metabolic: hyperglycemia, weight gain.
Musculoskeletal: carpal tunnel syndrome.
Respiratory: *PE,* dyspnea, pneumonia.
Skin: alopecia, rash.
Other: gynecomastia, tumor flare.

INTERACTIONS
Dofetilide: May increase dofetilide plasma level, increasing risk of life-threatening cardiac arrhythmias, including torsades de pointes. Avoid use together.
Rifamycins (rifampin): May increase megestrol metabolism due to induction of CYP3A4 pathway, reducing pharmacologic effects. Consider increasing megestrol dosage.

EFFECTS ON LAB TEST RESULTS
• May increase glucose level.

CONTRAINDICATIONS & CAUTIONS
• Contraindicated in patients hypersensitive to drug.
• Contraindicated in known or suspected pregnancy. Patient shouldn't breast-feed while taking drug.
• Use cautiously in patients with history of thrombophlebitis or thromboembolism.

NURSING CONSIDERATIONS
• May increase glucose level in diabetic patients.
• Drug isn't intended for prophylactic use to avoid weight loss. Start treatment with megestrol acetate oral suspension only after treatable causes of weight loss are sought and addressed.
• Two months is an adequate trial period in patients with cancer.

PATIENT TEACHING
• Inform patient that therapeutic response isn't immediate. Drug must be taken for at least 2 months to determine effectiveness.
• Tell patient drug may be taken without regard for food.
• **Alert:** Tell patient that the ES oral suspension is more concentrated than the regular

oral suspension, so a smaller amount is needed if prescription is changed.

• Advise women to stop breast-feeding during therapy because of risk of toxicity to infant.

• Advise women of childbearing age to use an effective form of contraception while receiving drug.

SAFETY ALERT!

melphalan (L-PAM, phenylalanine mustard)
MEL-fa-lan

Alkeran

melphalan hydrochloride
Alkeran

Therapeutic class: Antineoplastics
Pharmacologic class: Nitrogen mustards
Pregnancy risk category: D

AVAILABLE FORMS
Lyophilized powder for injection: 50 mg
Tablets (scored): 2 mg

INDICATIONS & DOSAGES
➤ **Multiple myeloma**
Adults: Initially, 6 mg P.O. daily for 2 to 3 weeks; then stop drug for up to 4 weeks or until WBC and platelet counts stop dropping and begin to rise again; maintenance dose is 2 mg daily. Or, 10 mg/day for 7 to 10 days, followed by 2 mg/day when WBC is greater than 4,000 cells/mm^3 and platelet count is greater than 100,000 cells/mm^3; dosage is adjusted to between 1 and 3 mg/day depending on hematologic response. Or, 0.15 mg/kg P.O. daily for 7 days followed by a rest period of at least 14 days; maintenance dose is 0.05 mg/kg/day or less. Or 0.25 mg/kg/day for 4 days (or 0.2 mg/kg/day for 5 days); repeat every 4 to 6 weeks.

Or, give I.V. to patients who can't tolerate oral therapy, 16 mg/m^2 given by infusion over 15 to 20 minutes at 2-week intervals for four doses. After patient has recovered from toxicity, give drug at 4-week intervals.

➤ **Nonresectable advanced ovarian cancer**
Adults: 0.2 mg/kg P.O. daily for 5 days. Repeat every 4 to 5 weeks, depending on bone marrow recovery.

ADMINISTRATION
P.O.
• Give drug when patient has an empty stomach; food decreases drug absorption.
I.V.
▪ **Black Box Warning** Preparing and giving this form may be mutagenic, teratogenic, or carcinogenic. Follow facility policy to reduce risks. ▪

▼ Because drug isn't stable in solution, reconstitute immediately before giving with the 10 mL of sterile diluent supplied by manufacturer. Shake vigorously until solution is clear. The resulting solution will contain 5 mg/mL of melphalan. Immediately dilute required dose in normal saline solution for injection to no more than 0.45 mg/mL. Give infusion over 15 to 20 minutes.

▼ Monitor infusion carefully. Extravasation causes painful inflammation.

▼ Reconstituted product begins to degrade within 30 minutes. After final dilution, nearly 1% of drug degrades every 10 minutes. Administration must be finished within 60 minutes of reconstitution.

▼ Don't refrigerate reconstituted product because precipitate will form.

▼ **Incompatibilities:** Amphotericin B, chlorpromazine, D$_5$W, lactated Ringer injection. Compatibility with normal saline injection depends on the concentration; don't prepare solutions with a concentration exceeding 0.45 mg/mL.

ACTION
Cross-links strands of cellular DNA and interferes with RNA transcription, causing an imbalance of growth that leads to cell death. Not specific to cell cycle.

Route	Onset	Peak	Duration
P.O., I.V.	Unknown	Unknown	Unknown

Half-life: 2 hours.

Reactions in bold italics are *life-threatening*. Interactions may have a *rapid onset* or a *delayed onset*.

ADVERSE REACTIONS

CV: vasculitis.
GI: nausea, vomiting, diarrhea, oral ulceration, stomatitis.
Hematologic: *thrombocytopenia, leukopenia, bone marrow suppression,* hemolytic anemia.
Hepatic: *hepatotoxicity.*
Respiratory: *pneumonitis, pulmonary fibrosis.*
Skin: pruritus, alopecia, urticaria, ulceration at injection site.
Other: *anaphylaxis,* hypersensitivity reactions.

INTERACTIONS

Drug-drug (I.V. melphalan only). *Anticoagulants, aspirin, NSAIDs:* May increase risk of bleeding. Avoid using together.
Carmustine: May decrease threshold for pulmonary toxicity. Use together cautiously.
Cimetidine: May decrease melphalan level. Monitor patient closely.
Cisplatin: May increase renal impairment, decreasing melphalan clearance. Monitor patient closely.
Cyclosporine: May cause severe renal impairment. Monitor renal function closely.
Interferon alfa: May increase melphalan elimination. Monitor patient closely.
Myelosuppressives: May increase myelosuppression. Monitor patient.
Vaccines: May decrease effectiveness of killed-virus vaccines and increase risk of toxicity from live-virus vaccines. Postpone routine immunization for at least 3 months after last dose of melphalan.
Drug-food. *Any food:* May decrease oral drug absorption. Advise patient to take drug on an empty stomach.

EFFECTS ON LAB TEST RESULTS

● May increase urine urea level. May decrease hemoglobin level.
● May decrease RBC, WBC, and platelet counts.
● May cause a false-positive direct Coombs test.

CONTRAINDICATIONS & CAUTIONS

● Contraindicated in patients hypersensitive to drug and in those with disease resistant to drug. Patients hypersensitive to chlor-

ambucil may have cross-sensitivity to this drug.
● Contraindicated in patients with severe leukopenia, thrombocytopenia, or anemia and in those with chronic lymphocytic leukemia.
● Use cautiously in patients receiving radiation and chemotherapy.
● Drug is a vesicant and may cause local tissue damage if extravasation occurs. If signs or symptoms of extravasation develop, stop infusion immediately and notify prescriber.
⚠ Overdose S&S: Vomiting, ulceration of the mouth, diarrhea, GI hemorrhage, bone marrow suppression.

NURSING CONSIDERATIONS

Black Box Warning Administer drug only under the supervision of a physician experienced in the use of cancer chemotherapeutic agents. ■
Black Box Warning Severe bone marrow suppression with resulting bleeding or infection may occur. ■
Black Box Warning Drug is leukemogenic and potentially mutagenic. ■
Black Box Warning Hypersensitivity reactions, including anaphylaxis, have occurred with I.V. form. ■
● Dosage may need to be reduced in patients with renal impairment.
● Monitor uric acid level and CBC.
● To prevent bleeding, avoid all I.M. injections when platelet count is less than $50,000/mm^3$.
● Blood transfusions may be needed for cumulative anemia.
● Anaphylaxis may occur. Keep antihistamines and steroids readily available to give if needed.
● *Look alike–sound alike:* Don't confuse melphalan with Mephyton.

PATIENT TEACHING

● Advise patient to take tablets on empty stomach.
● Advise patient to report pain or redness at I.V. site.
● Advise patient to watch for signs and symptoms of infection (fever, sore throat, fatigue) and bleeding (easy bruising,

M

nosebleeds, bleeding gums, tarry stools). Tell patient to take temperature daily.
• Instruct patient to avoid OTC products that contain aspirin or NSAIDs.
• Advise women to stop breast-feeding during therapy because of risk of toxicity to infant.
• Advise women of childbearing age to avoid becoming pregnant while taking the drug. Advise patient that the drug can interfere with menstrual cycle in women and stop sperm production in men.

memantine hydrochloride
meh-MAN-teen

Namenda✧, Namenda XR

Therapeutic class: Anti-Alzheimer drugs
Pharmacologic class: N-methyl-D-aspartate receptor antagonists
Pregnancy risk category: B

AVAILABLE FORMS
Capsules (extended-release): 7 mg, 14 mg, 21 mg, 28 mg
Oral solution: 2 mg/mL
Tablets: 5 mg, 10 mg

INDICATIONS & DOSAGES
➤ **Moderate to severe Alzheimer dementia**
Adults: Initially, 5 mg P.O. once daily. Increase by 5 mg/day every week until target dose is reached. Maximum, 10 mg P.O. b.i.d. Doses greater than 5 mg should be given in two divided doses.

Or, for extended-release capsules, initial dose is 7 mg P.O. once daily. Increase as tolerated by 7-mg increments each week to target dosage of 28 mg P.O. once daily.
To convert from immediate-release to extended-release form: Patients taking immediate-release 10 mg b.i.d. may switch to extended-release 28 mg once daily the day following the last immediate-release tablet. Patients with severe renal failure taking immediate-release 5 mg b.i.d. may switch to extended-release 14 mg once daily the day following the last immediate-release tablet.

Adjust-a-dose: For immediate-release form, no dosage adjustment is recommended for patients with mild to moderate renal impairment; target dosage of 5 mg b.i.d. is recommended for patients with severe renal impairment (CrCl of 5 to 29 mL/minute). For extended-release form, no dosage adjustment is recommended for patients with mild to moderate renal impairment; a target dosage of 14 mg/day is recommended for patients with severe renal impairment (CrCl of 5 to 29 mL/minute).

ADMINISTRATION
P.O.
• Give drug without regard for food.
• Patients may take capsules intact or capsules may be opened, sprinkled on applesauce, then swallowed. Don't allow patients to divide, chew, or crush capsules.

ACTION
Antagonizes N-methyl-D-aspartate receptors, the persistent activation of which seems to increase Alzheimer symptoms.

Route	Onset	Peak	Duration
P.O.	Unknown	3–7 hr	Unknown

Half-life: 60 to 80 hours.

ADVERSE REACTIONS
CNS: *stroke,* aggressiveness, agitation, anxiety, ataxia, confusion, depression, dizziness, fatigue, hallucinations, headache, hypokinesia, insomnia, pain, somnolence, syncope, transient ischemic attack, vertigo.
CV: *heart failure,* edema, hypertension.
EENT: cataracts, conjunctivitis.
GI: anorexia, constipation, diarrhea, nausea, vomiting.
GU: incontinence, urinary frequency, UTI.
Hematologic: anemia.
Metabolic: weight loss.
Musculoskeletal: arthralgia, back pain.
Respiratory: bronchitis, coughing, dyspnea, flulike symptoms, pneumonia, upper respiratory tract infection.
Skin: rash.
Other: abnormal gait, falls, injury.

INTERACTIONS
Drug-drug. *Cimetidine, hydrochlorothiazide, quinidine, ranitidine, triamterene:*

Reactions in bold italics are *life-threatening*. Interactions may have a *rapid onset* or a *delayed onset*.

May alter levels of both drugs. Monitor patient.

NMDA antagonists (amantadine, dextromethorphan, ketamine): Effects of combined use unknown. Use together cautiously.

Urine alkalinizers (carbonic anhydrase inhibitors, sodium bicarbonate): May decrease memantine clearance. Monitor patient for adverse effects.

Drug-food. *Foods that alkalinize urine:* May increase drug level and adverse effects. Use together cautiously.

Drug-lifestyle. *Alcohol use:* May alter drug adherence, decrease its effectiveness, or increase adverse effects. Discourage use together.

Nicotine: May alter levels of drug and nicotine. Discourage use together.

EFFECTS ON LAB TEST RESULTS
● May increase alkaline phosphatase level. May decrease hemoglobin level and hematocrit.

CONTRAINDICATIONS & CAUTIONS
● Contraindicated in patients allergic to drug or its components.
● Contraindicated for mild Alzheimer disease or other types of dementia.
● Immediate-release form isn't recommended for patients with severe renal impairment.
● Use cautiously in patients with seizures, hepatic impairment, or moderate renal impairment.
● Use cautiously in patients who may have an increased urine pH (from drugs, diet, renal tubular acidosis, or severe UTI, for example).

⚠ *Overdose S&S:* Restlessness, psychosis, visual hallucinations, somnolence, stupor, loss of consciousness.

NURSING CONSIDERATIONS
● In elderly patients, even those with a normal creatinine level, use of this drug may impair renal function. Estimate CrCl; reduce dosage in patients with moderate renal impairment. Don't give drug to patients with severe renal impairment.
● Monitor patient carefully for adverse reactions as he may not be able to recognize changes or communicate effectively.

PATIENT TEACHING
● Explain that drug doesn't cure Alzheimer disease but may aid patient to maintain function for a longer period of time.
● Tell patient or caregiver to report adverse effects.
● Urge patient to avoid alcohol during treatment.
● To avoid possible interactions, advise patient not to take herbal or OTC products without consulting prescriber.

meperidine hydrochloride (pethidine hydrochloride)
me-PER-i-deen

Demerol◆, Pethidine†

Therapeutic class: Opioid analgesics
Pharmacologic class: Opioids
Pregnancy risk category: B; D if used for prolonged periods or in high doses at term
Controlled substance schedule: II

M

AVAILABLE FORMS
Injection: 10 mg/mL, 25 mg/mL, 50 mg/mL, 75 mg/mL, 100 mg/mL
Syrup: 50 mg/5 mL
Tablets: 50 mg, 100 mg

INDICATIONS & DOSAGES
➤ **Moderate to severe pain**
Adults: 50 to 150 mg P.O., I.M., or subcutaneously every 3 to 4 hours p.r.n. Or, 10 mg I.V. slowly by patient-controlled analgesia device, with range of 1 to 5 mg per dose; lockout interval is 6 to 10 minutes. Or, continuous I.V. infusion of 15 to 30 mg/hour.
Children: 1.1 to 1.8 mg/kg P.O., I.M., or subcutaneously every 3 to 4 hours. Maximum, 100 mg every 4 hours p.r.n.
Adjust-a-dose: Reduce meperidine doses by 25% to 50% when administered with phenothiazines and other tranquilizers because they potentiate the action of meperidine. Reduce dosage in elderly patients and in those with hepatic and renal impairment. If CrCl is 10 to 50 mL/minute, give

75% of normal dose. If CrCl is less than 10 mL/minute, give 25% to 50% of normal dose.

➤ **Preoperative analgesia**
Adults: 50 to 100 mg I.M. or subcutaneously 30 to 90 minutes before surgery.
Children: 1 to 2.2 mg/kg I.M. or subcutaneously up to the adult dose 30 to 90 minutes before surgery.
Adjust-a-dose: Reduce dosage in elderly patients and in those with hepatic or renal impairment. If CrCl is 10 to 50 mL/minute, give 75% of normal dose. If CrCl is less than 10 mL/minute, give 25% to 50% of normal dose.

➤ **Adjunct to anesthesia**
Adults: Repeated slow I.V. injections of fractional doses (10 mg/mL). Or, continuous I.V. infusion of a more dilute solution (1 mg/mL) titrated to patient's needs.

➤ **Obstetric analgesia**
Adults: 50 to 100 mg I.M. or subcutaneously when pain becomes regular; repeated at 1- to 3-hour intervals.

ADMINISTRATION
P.O.
• Syrup has local anesthetic effect on mucous membranes. Give with a half glass of water.
• Oral dose is less than half as effective as parenteral dose. Give I.M. if possible. When changing from parenteral to oral route, increase dosage.

I.V.
▼ Keep opioid antagonist (naloxone) available.
▼ Give drug slowly by direct injection.
▼ Drug may also be given by slow continuous infusion. Drug is compatible with most solutions, including D_5W, normal saline solution, and Ringer or lactated Ringer solutions.
▼ Protect from light and store at room temperature.
▼ **Incompatibilities:** Acyclovir, allopurinol, aminophylline, amobarbital, amphotericin B, cefepime, cefoperazone, doxorubicin liposomal, ephedrine, furosemide, heparin, hydrocortisone sodium succinate, idarubicin, imipenem–cilastatin sodium, methylprednisolone sodium succinate, morphine, pentobarbital, phenobarbital

sodium, phenytoin, sodium bicarbonate, sodium iodide, thiopental.
I.M.
• Inject into large muscle mess, taking care to avoid nerve trunks.
Subcutaneous
• Subcutaneous injection isn't recommended because it's very painful, but it may be suitable for occasional use. Monitor patient for pain at injection site, local tissue irritation, and induration after subcutaneous injection.

ACTION
Unknown. Binds with opioid receptors in the CNS, altering perception of and emotional response to pain.

Route	Onset	Peak	Duration
P.O.	15 min	60–90 min	2–4 hr
I.V.	1 min	5–7 min	2–4 hr
I.M., subcut.	10–15 min	30–50 min	2–4 hr

Half-life: 2½ to 4 hours.

ADVERSE REACTIONS
CNS: agitation, incoordination, clouded sensorium, dizziness, euphoria, lightheadedness, sedation, somnolence, *seizures,* hallucinations, headache, paradoxical anxiety, physical dependence, syncope, tremor.
CV: *bradycardia, cardiac arrest, shock,* hypotension, tachycardia.
GI: biliary tract spasms, constipation, dry mouth, ileus, nausea, vomiting.
GU: urine retention.
Musculoskeletal: muscle twitching.
Respiratory: *respiratory arrest, respiratory depression.*
Skin: diaphoresis, pruritus, urticaria.
Other: induration, local tissue irritation, pain at injection site, phlebitis after I.V. delivery.

INTERACTIONS
Drug-drug. *Aminophylline, barbiturates, heparin, methicillin, morphine sulfate, phenytoin, sodium bicarbonate, sulfonamides:* Incompatible when mixed in same I.V. container. Avoid using together.
Chlorpromazine: May cause excessive sedation and hypotension. Avoid using together.

Reactions in bold italics are *life-threatening*. Interactions may have a *rapid onset* or a *delayed onset*.

Cimetidine: May increase respiratory and CNS depression. Monitor patient closely.

CNS depressants, general anesthetics, hypnotics, other opioid analgesics, phenothiazines, sedatives, TCAs: May cause respiratory depression, hypotension, profound sedation, or coma. Use together with caution; reduce meperidine dosage.

MAO inhibitors: May increase CNS excitation or depression that can be severe or fatal. Use together is contraindicated.

Phenytoin: May decrease meperidine level. Watch for decreased analgesia.

Protease inhibitors: May increase respiratory and CNS depression. Avoid using together.

Ritonavir: May significantly increase level and toxic effects of meperidine. Avoid use together.

Drug-lifestyle. *Alcohol use:* May cause additive effects. Discourage use together.

EFFECTS ON LAB TEST RESULTS
● May increase amylase and lipase levels.

CONTRAINDICATIONS & CAUTIONS
● Contraindicated in patients hypersensitive to drug and in those who have received MAO inhibitors within past 14 days.
● Avoid use in patients with ESRD.
● Use with caution in elderly or debilitated patients and in those with increased intracranial pressure, head injury, asthma and other respiratory conditions, supraventricular tachycardias, seizures, acute abdominal conditions, hepatic or renal disease, hypothyroidism, Addison disease, urethral stricture, and prostatic hyperplasia.

⚠ Overdose S&S: Dry mouth, increased muscle activity, tremors, tachycardia, respiratory depression, delirium, hallucinations, tonic-clonic seizures, mydriasis, skeletal muscle flaccidity, circulatory collapse, death.

NURSING CONSIDERATIONS
● In elderly patients, patients using meperidine for longer than 48 hours, those with preexisting renal or CNS disease, and those taking more than 600 mg/day, the active metabolite may accumulate, causing increased adverse CNS reactions. Avoid prolonged use.

● Drug may be used in some patients who are allergic to morphine.
● Reassess patient's level of pain at least 15 and 30 minutes after administration.
● Because drug toxicity frequently appears after several days of treatment, drug isn't recommended for treatment of chronic pain.
● In neonates exposed to drug during labor, monitor respirations. Have resuscitation equipment and naloxone available.
● Monitor respiratory and CV status carefully. Don't give if respirations are below 12 breaths/minute, if respiratory rate or depth is decreased, or if change in pupils is noted.
● If drug is stopped abruptly after longterm use, monitor patient for withdrawal symptoms.
● In postoperative patients, monitor bladder function.
● Monitor bowel function. Patient may need a stimulant laxative and stool softener.
● **Look alike–sound alike:** Don't confuse Demerol with Demulen.

PATIENT TEACHING
● Encourage postoperative patient to turn, cough, deep-breathe, and use an incentive spirometer to prevent lung problems.
● Caution ambulatory patient about getting out of bed or walking. Warn outpatient to avoid driving and other potentially hazardous activities that require mental alertness until drug's CNS effects are known.
● Advise patient to avoid alcohol during therapy.
● Caution patient that drug isn't intended for long-term use.

SAFETY ALERT!

mercaptopurine
(6-mercaptopurine, 6-MP)
mer-kap-toe-PYOOR-een

Purinethol

Therapeutic class: Antineoplastics
Pharmacologic class: Purine antagonists
Pregnancy risk category: D

AVAILABLE FORMS
Tablets (scored): 50 mg

INDICATIONS & DOSAGES
➤ **Acute lymphatic leukemia**
Adults and children: 2.5 mg/kg P.O. once daily (rounded to nearest 25 mg). May increase to 5 mg/kg daily after 4 weeks if no improvement.

After remission is attained, usual maintenance dose for adults and children is 1.5 to 2.5 mg/kg once daily.

Adjust-a-dose: For patients with CrCl of less than 50 mL/minute, or patients receiving hemodialysis, continuous ambulatory peritoneal dialysis, or continuous renal replacement therapy, give dose every 48 hours. If given concurrently with allopurinol, reduce dosage to 25% to 33% of usual dose.

ADMINISTRATION
P.O.
● Give total daily dosage at one time, calculated to the nearest multiple of 25 mg.
● Give on an empty stomach.

ACTION
Inhibits RNA and DNA synthesis.

Route	Onset	Peak	Duration
P.O.	Unknown	Unknown	Unknown

Half-life: Children, 21 minutes; adults, 47 minutes.

ADVERSE REACTIONS
GI: nausea, vomiting, anorexia, painful oral ulcers, diarrhea, *pancreatitis,* GI ulceration.
Hematologic: *leukopenia, thrombocytopenia,* anemia.
Hepatic: jaundice, *hepatotoxicity, hepatic necrosis.*
Metabolic: hyperuricemia.
Skin: rash, hyperpigmentation.

INTERACTIONS
Drug-drug. *Allopurinol:* Slows inactivation of mercaptopurine. Decrease mercaptopurine to 25% or 33% of normal dose.
Azathioprine: Increased risk of severe myelosuppression. Avoid giving together.
Febuxostat: May increase risk of toxicity. Use together is contraindicated.
Hepatotoxic drugs: May enhance hepatotoxicity of mercaptopurine. Monitor patient for hepatotoxicity.

Nondepolarizing neuromuscular blockers: May antagonize muscle relaxant effect. Notify anesthesiologist that patient is receiving mercaptopurine.
Sulfamethoxazole–trimethoprim: May enhance bone marrow suppression. Monitor CBC with differential carefully.
Warfarin: May decrease or increase anticoagulant effect. Monitor PT and INR.

EFFECTS ON LAB TEST RESULTS
● May increase uric acid, transaminase, alkaline phosphatase, and bilirubin levels. May decrease hemoglobin level.
● May decrease WBC, RBC, and platelet counts.

CONTRAINDICATIONS & CAUTIONS
● Contraindicated in patients resistant or hypersensitive to drug.
● Drug may increase risk of neoplasia.
● Use cautiously in elderly patients.
⚠ *Overdose S&S:* Anorexia, nausea, vomiting, diarrhea, myelosuppression, hepatic dysfunction, gastroenteritis.

NURSING CONSIDERATIONS
☙ *Alert:* A diagnosis of acute lymphatic leukemia must be established before starting therapy. The supervising physician must be knowledgeable in assessing response to chemotherapy.
● Risk of relapse is lower with evening administration than with morning administration.
☙ *Alert:* Patients with thiopurine S-methyltransferase deficiency are at increased risk for severe mercaptopurine toxicity and generally require substantial dosage reduction.
● Consider modifying dosage after chemotherapy or radiation therapy in patients who have depressed neutrophil or platelet counts or impaired hepatic or renal function.
☙ *Alert:* Drug may be ordered as "6-mercaptopurine" or as "6-MP." The numeral 6 is part of drug name and doesn't refer to dosage.
● Monitor CBC and transaminase, alkaline phosphatase, and bilirubin levels weekly during induction and monthly during maintenance.

Reactions in bold italics are *life-threatening*. Interactions may have a *rapid onset* or a *delayed onset*.

• Leukopenia, thrombocytopenia, or anemia may persist for several days after drug is stopped.

• Watch for signs of bleeding and infection.

• Monitor fluid intake and output. Encourage 3 L fluid intake daily.

⊘ Alert: Watch for jaundice, clay-colored stools, and frothy, dark urine. Hepatic dysfunction is reversible when drug is stopped. If right-sided abdominal tenderness occurs, stop drug and notify prescriber.

• Monitor uric acid level. Use allopurinol cautiously.

• To prevent bleeding, avoid all I.M. injections when platelet count is below 100,000/mm^3.

• Anticipate need for blood transfusions because of cumulative anemia.

• GI adverse reactions are less common in children than in adults.

• **Look alike–sound alike:** Don't confuse Purinethol and propylthiouracil (PTU). Both are available in 50-mg strengths.

PATIENT TEACHING

• Instruct patient to watch for signs and symptoms of infection (fever, sore throat, fatigue) and bleeding (easy bruising, nosebleeds, bleeding gums, tarry stools). Tell patient to take temperature daily.

• Tell patient to take drug on an empty stomach in the evening.

• Caution women of childbearing age to consult prescriber before becoming pregnant.

• Advise women to stop breast-feeding during therapy because of risk of toxicity to infant.

---

meropenem
mare-oh-PEN-em

Merrem IV

Therapeutic class: Antibiotics
Pharmacologic class: Carbapenems
Pregnancy risk category: B

AVAILABLE FORMS
Powder for injection: 500 mg, 1 g

INDICATIONS & DOSAGES

Adjust-a-dose (for all indications): For adults with CrCl of 26 to 50 mL/minute, give usual dose every 12 hours. If CrCl is 10 to 25 mL/minute, give half usual dose every 12 hours; if CrCl is less than 10 mL/minute, give half usual dose every 24 hours.

➤ **Complicated skin and skin-structure infections from *Staphylococcus aureus* (beta-lactamase or non-beta-lactamase– producing, methicillin-susceptible isolates only), *Streptococcus pyogenes, S. agalactiae,* viridans group streptococci, *Enterococcus faecalis* (excluding vancomycin-resistant isolates), *Pseudomonas aeruginosa, Escherichia coli, Proteus mirabilis, Bacteroides fragilis,* and *Peptostreptococcus* species**

Adults and children weighing more than 50 kg (110 lb): 500 mg I.V. every 8 hours over 15 to 30 minutes as I.V. infusion.

Children age 3 months and older weighing 50 kg or less: 10 mg/kg I.V. every 8 hours over 15 to 30 minutes as I.V. infusion or over 3 to 5 minutes as I.V. bolus injection (5 to 20 mL); maximum dose is 500 mg I.V. every 8 hours.

➤ **Complicated appendicitis and peritonitis from viridans group streptococci, *E. coli, Klebsiella pneumoniae, Pseudomonas aeruginosa, B. fragilis, B. thetaiotaomicron,* and *Peptostreptococcus* species**

Adults and children weighing more than 50 kg: 1 g I.V. every 8 hours over 15 to 30 minutes as I.V. infusion or over 3 to 5 minutes as I.V. bolus injection (5 to 20 mL).

Children age 3 months and older weighing 50 kg or less: 20 mg/kg I.V. every 8 hours over 15 to 30 minutes as I.V. infusion or over 3 to 5 minutes as I.V. bolus injection (5 to 20 mL); maximum dose is 1 g I.V. every 8 hours.

➤ **Bacterial meningitis from *S. pneumoniae, Haemophilus influenzae,* and *Neisseria meningitidis***

Children weighing more than 50 kg: 2 g I.V. every 8 hours.

Children age 3 months and older weighing 50 kg or less: 40 mg/kg I.V. every 8 hours; maximum dose, 2 g I.V. every 8 hours.

M

➤ **Community-acquired pneumonia** ◆
Adults: 500 mg I.V. every 8 hours for at least 5 days in combination with a fluoro-quinolone.

➤ **Hospital-acquired pneumonia (uncomplicated)** ◆
Adults: 1 g I.V. every 8 hours for 7 to 8 days.

➤ **Catheter-related bloodstream infections** ◆
Adults: 1 g I.V. infused over 15 to 30 minutes every 8 hours.
Children age 3 months and older: 20 mg/kg I.V. infused over 15 to 30 minutes every 8 hours.
Neonates older than 7 days weighing more than 2 kg (4.5 lb): 20 mg/kg I.V. infused over 15 to 30 minutes every 8 hours.
Neonates older than 7 days weighing 1.2 to 2 kg (2.5 to 4.5 lb): 20 mg/kg I.V. infused over 15 to 30 minutes every 12 hours.
Neonates ages 0 to 7 days: 20 mg/kg I.V. infused over 15 to 30 minutes every 12 hours.

ADMINISTRATION

I.V.

▼ Obtain specimen for culture and sensitivity tests before giving first dose. Begin therapy while awaiting results.

🌙 *Alert:* Serious hypersensitivity reactions may occur in patients receiving beta-lactams. Before therapy begins, determine if patient has had previous hypersensitivity reactions to penicillins, cephalosporins, beta-lactams, or other allergens. If an allergic reaction occurs, stop drug and notify prescriber. Serious anaphylactic reactions require emergency treatment.

▼ Use freshly prepared solutions of drug immediately whenever possible. Stability of drug varies with form of drug used (injection vial, infusion vial, or ADD-Vantage container).

▼ For bolus, add 10 mL of sterile water for injection to 500 mg/20-mL vial or 20 mL to 1 g/30-mL vial. Shake to dissolve, and let stand until clear. Give over 3 to 5 minutes.

▼ For infusion, an infusion vial (500 mg/100 mL or 1 g/100 mL) may be directly reconstituted with a compatible infusion fluid. Or, an injection vial may be reconstituted and the resulting solution added to an I.V. container and further diluted with an appropriate infusion fluid. Don't use ADD-Vantage vials for this purpose. Give over 15 to 30 minutes.

▼ For ADD-Vantage vials, constitute only with half-normal saline solution for injection, normal saline solution for injection, or D₅W in 50-, 100-, or 250-mL Abbott ADD-Vantage flexible diluent containers. Follow manufacturer's guidelines closely when using ADD-Vantage vials.

▼ **Incompatibilities:** Other I.V. drugs.

ACTION

Inhibits cell-wall synthesis in bacteria. Readily penetrates cell wall of most gram-positive and gram-negative bacteria to reach penicillin-binding protein targets.

Route	Onset	Peak	Duration
I.V.	Unknown	1 hr	Unknown

Half-life: 1 hour.

ADVERSE REACTIONS

CNS: *seizures,* headache.
CV: phlebitis, thrombophlebitis.
GI: *Clostridium difficile–associated diarrhea,* constipation, diarrhea, glossitis, nausea, vomiting.
GU: RBCs in urine.
Respiratory: *apnea,* dyspnea, pneumonia.
Skin: injection-site inflammation, pruritus, rash.
Other: *anaphylaxis, sepsis,* hypersensitivity reactions, inflammation.

INTERACTIONS

Drug-drug. *Probenecid:* May decrease renal excretion of meropenem; probenecid competes with meropenem for active tubular secretion, which significantly increases elimination half-life of meropenem and extent of systemic exposure. Avoid using together.
Valproic acid: May decrease valproic acid levels, increasing the risk of breakthrough seizures. Monitor levels frequently and observe patient for seizure activity. Consider alternative antibiotic or supplemental anticonvulsant therapy.

Reactions in bold italics are *life-threatening*. Interactions may have a *rapid onset* or a *delayed onset*.

EFFECTS ON LAB TEST RESULTS

• May increase ALT, AST, bilirubin, alkaline phosphatase, LDH, creatinine, and BUN levels. May decrease hemoglobin level and hematocrit.

• May increase eosinophil count. May decrease WBC count. May increase or decrease PT, PTT, and INR, and platelet count.

CONTRAINDICATIONS & CAUTIONS

• Contraindicated in patients hypersensitive to components of drug or other drugs in same class and in patients who have had anaphylactic reactions to beta-lactams.

• Use cautiously in elderly patients and in those with a history of seizure disorders or impaired renal function.

• Safety and effectiveness of drug haven't been established for infants younger than age 3 months.

• Use drug cautiously in breast-feeding women; it's unknown if drug appears in breast milk.

⚠ *Overdose S&S:* Exaggerated adverse reactions.

NURSING CONSIDERATIONS

• In patients with CNS disorders, bacterial meningitis, and compromised renal function, drug may cause seizures and other CNS adverse reactions.

• If seizures occur during therapy, stop infusion and notify prescriber. Dosage adjustment may be needed.

• Monitor patient for signs and symptoms of superinfection. Drug may cause overgrowth of nonsusceptible bacteria or fungi.

• Periodic assessment of organ system functions, including renal, hepatic, and hematopoietic function, is recommended during prolonged therapy.

• Monitor patient's fluid balance and weight carefully.

PATIENT TEACHING

• Advise women not to breast-feed during therapy.

• Instruct patient to report adverse reactions or signs and symptoms of superinfection.

• Advise patient to report loose stools to prescriber.

mesalamine
me-SAL-a-meen

Apriso, Asacol, Asacol HD, Canasa, Lialda, Pentasa, Rowasa, sfRowasa

Therapeutic class: Anti-inflammatory drugs
Pharmacologic class: Salicylates
Pregnancy risk category: B (rectal, Apriso, Lialda, Pentasa); C (Asacol, Asacol HD)

AVAILABLE FORMS

Capsules (controlled-release): 250 mg, 375 mg, 500 mg
Rectal suspension: 4 g/60 mL
Suppositories: 1,000 mg
Tablets (delayed-release): 400 mg, 800 mg, 1.2 g

INDICATIONS & DOSAGES

➤ **Active mild to moderate distal ulcerative colitis, proctitis, or proctosigmoiditis**
Adults: Two 400-mg tablets (800 mg) P.O. t.i.d. for total dose of 2.4 g daily for 6 weeks. Or 1 g capsules P.O. q.i.d. for total dose of 4 g up to 8 weeks. Or 1,000 mg suppository P.R., retained in the rectum for 1 to 3 hours or longer, once daily at bedtime. Or 4 g retention enema once daily (preferably at bedtime).

➤ **Remission-induction of active, mild to moderate ulcerative colitis**
Lialda
Adults: Two to four 1.2-g tablets (2.4 to 4.8 g) P.O. once daily with a meal for up to 8 weeks.
Pentasa
Adults: Four 250-mg capsules or two 500-mg capsules (1 g) P.O. q.i.d. for a total dose of 4 g for up to 8 weeks.

➤ **Maintenance of remission of ulcerative colitis**
Adults: 1.5 g Apriso P.O. once daily in the morning. Or, 1.6 g Asacol daily in divided doses. Or, two 1.2-g tablets (Lialda) P.O. once daily.

M

ADMINISTRATION

P.O.

- Give Lialda with food.
- Don't administer drug with antacids.
- Don't crush or cut delayed-release or controlled-release forms.
- Intact or partially intact tablets may be seen in stool. Notify prescriber if this occurs repeatedly.

Rectal

- Patient should retain rectal dosage form overnight (for about 8 hours). Usual course of therapy for rectal form is 3 to 6 weeks.
- Shake suspension well before each use and remove sheath before inserting into rectum.

ACTION

An active metabolite of sulfasalazine, drug probably acts topically by inhibiting prostaglandin production in the colon.

Route	Onset	Peak	Duration
P.O., P.R.	Unknown	3–12 hr	Unknown

Half-life: About 5 to 10 hours.

ADVERSE REACTIONS

CNS: headache, dizziness, fever, fatigue, malaise, asthenia.
CV: chest pain.
EENT: pharyngitis.
GI: abdominal pain, cramps, discomfort, flatulence, diarrhea, rectal pain, bloating, nausea, pancolitis, vomiting, constipation, eructation.
GU: interstitial nephritis, nephropathy, *nephrotoxicity.*
Musculoskeletal: arthralgia, myalgia, back pain, hypertonia.
Respiratory: wheezing.
Skin: itching, rash, urticaria, hair loss.
Other: chills, acne.

INTERACTIONS

Drug-drug. *Azathioprine, mercaptopurine:* May cause blood disorders. Monitor blood cell counts and adjust therapy as needed.
Lactulose: May impair release of delayed- or extended-release products. Monitor patient closely.
Warfarin: May decrease anticoagulation effect. Monitor effectiveness of therapy closely.

EFFECTS ON LAB TEST RESULTS

- May increase BUN, creatinine, AST, ALT, alkaline phosphatase, LDH, amylase, and lipase levels.
- May decrease RBC and WBC counts.

CONTRAINDICATIONS & CAUTIONS

- Contraindicated in children and in patients allergic to mesalamine, sulfites (including sulfasalazine), any salicylates, or any component of the preparation.
- Use cautiously in elderly patients, in patients with renal or hepatic impairment, and in pregnant and breast-feeding patients.
⚠ Overdose S&S: Confusion, diarrhea, headache, hyperventilation, diaphoresis, tinnitus, vertigo, vomiting.

NURSING CONSIDERATIONS

- Monitor periodic renal function studies and blood cell counts in patients on long-term therapy.
- Because the mesalamine rectal suspension contains potassium metabisulfite, it may cause hypersensitivity reactions in patients sensitive to sulfites.
- Absorption of drug may be nephrotoxic.
- *Look alike–sound alike:* Don't confuse Asacol with Os-Cal.

PATIENT TEACHING

- Instruct patient to carefully follow instructions supplied with drug and to swallow tablets whole without crushing or chewing.
- Tell patient not to take drug with antacids.
- Advise patient to stop drug if fever or rash occurs. Patient intolerant of sulfasalazine may also be hypersensitive to mesalamine.
- Tell patient to remove foil wrapper from suppositories before inserting into rectum.
- Teach patient about proper use of retention enema.
- Tell patient that enema solution may stain bedsheets, clothing, and most floor coverings. Patient should use protective underpads and linens.

Reactions in bold italics are *life-threatening*. Interactions may have a *rapid onset* or a *delayed onset*.

SAFETY ALERT!

metformin hydrochloride
met-FORE-min

Fortamet, Glucophage✐,
Glucophage XR✐, Glumetza,
Riomet

Therapeutic class: Antidiabetics
Pharmacologic class: Biguanides
Pregnancy risk category: B

AVAILABLE FORMS
Oral solution: 500 mg/5 mL
Tablets: 500 mg, 850 mg, 1,000 mg
Tablets (extended-release): 500 mg,
750 mg, 1,000 mg

INDICATIONS & DOSAGES
Adjust-a-dose (for all indications): For elderly
or debilitated patients, use conservative
initial and maintenance dosage because of
potential decrease in renal function. Adjust
dosage carefully. Don't adjust to maximum
dosage.
➤ **Adjunct to diet to lower glucose level in
patients with type 2 diabetes**
Adults: If using regular-release tablets or
oral solution, initially 500 mg P.O. b.i.d.
given with morning and evening meals, or
850 mg P.O. once daily given with morning
meal. When 500-mg dose of regular-release
form is used, may increase dosage by 500 mg
weekly to maximum dose of 2,500 mg
P.O. daily in divided doses. When 850-mg
dose of regular-release form is used, may
increase dosage by 850 mg every other
week to maximum dose of 2,550 mg P.O.
daily in divided doses. If using extended-
release formulation, start therapy at 500 mg
(1,000 mg for Glumetza and Fortamet)
P.O. once daily with the evening meal.
May increase dose weekly in increments of
500 mg daily, up to a maximum dose of
2,000 mg once daily (2,500 mg for Fortamet). If higher doses are required, consider
a trial of 1,000 mg b.i.d. or using the regular-
release formulation up to its maximum dose.
Children ages 10 to 16: 500 mg P.O. b.i.d.
using the regular-release formulation only.
Increase dosage in increments of 500 mg

weekly up to a maximum of 2,000 mg daily
in divided doses.
➤ **Adjunct to diet and exercise in type
2 diabetes as monotherapy or with a
sulfonylurea or insulin (Fortamet)**
Adults age 17 and older: Initially, 500 mg
P.O. with evening meal for patients on insulin therapy. Increase dosage based on glucose level in increments of 500 mg weekly
to a maximum of 2,500 mg daily. Decrease
insulin dose by 10% to 25% when fasting
blood glucose level is less than 120 mg/dL.
    If patient has not responded to 4 weeks
of maximum dose Fortamet monotherapy,
consider the gradual addition of an oral
sulfonylurea.
➤ **Adjunct to diet and exercise in type
2 diabetes as monotherapy or with a
sulfonylurea or insulin (Glumetza)**
Adults: Initially, 500 mg P.O. once daily in
the evening with food for patients on insulin therapy. Increase as needed in weekly
increments of 500 mg, to a maximum of
2,000 mg daily. If glycemic control not
attained at this dose, give 1,000 mg b.i.d.
Decrease insulin dose by 10% to 25% when
fasting glucose level is less than 120 mg/dL.
    If patient has not responded to 4 weeks
of maximum dose Glumetza monotherapy,
consider the gradual addition of an oral
sulfonylurea.
➤ **Polycystic ovary syndrome ◆**
Adults: 1,500 to 2,000 mg P.O. daily in
divided doses as monotherapy or as part of a
combination.

ADMINISTRATION
P.O.
● Give drug with meals. Maximum doses
may be better tolerated if total dose is
divided and given in three doses with meals
(immediate-release tablets only).
● Don't cut or crush extended-release
tablets.
● Give Fortamet with full glass of water
with the evening meal.

ACTION
Decreases hepatic glucose production
and intestinal absorption of glucose and
improves insulin sensitivity (increases
peripheral glucose uptake and use).

M

Route	Onset	Peak	Duration
P.O. (conventional)	Unknown	2–4 hr	Unknown
P.O. (extended-release)	Unknown	4–8 hr	Unknown
P.O. (solution)	Unknown	2½ hr	Unknown

Half-life: About 6 hours.

ADVERSE REACTIONS

CNS: asthenia, headache, dizziness, chills, light-headedness.
GI: diarrhea, nausea, vomiting, abdominal bloating, flatulence, anorexia, taste disorder, abnormal stools, constipation, dyspepsia.
Hematologic: megaloblastic anemia.
Metabolic: *lactic acidosis, hypoglycemia.*
Respiratory: rhinitis, upper respiratory tract infection.
Other: accidental injury, infection.

INTERACTIONS

Drug-drug. *Beta blockers:* Hypoglycemia may be difficult to recognize in patients using beta blockers. Monitor patient and blood glucose.
Calcium channel blockers, corticosteroids, estrogens, fosphenytoin, hormonal contraceptives, isoniazid, nicotinic acid, phenothiazines, phenytoin, sympathomimetics, thiazide and other diuretics, thyroid drugs: May produce hyperglycemia. Monitor patient's glycemic control. Metformin dosage may need to be increased.
Cationic drugs (such as amiloride, cimetidine, digoxin, morphine, procainamide, quinidine, quinine, ranitidine, triamterene, trimethoprim, vancomycin): May compete for common renal tubular transport systems, which may increase metformin level. Monitor glucose level.
Nifedipine: May increase metformin level. Monitor patient closely. Metformin dosage may need to be decreased.
Radiologic contrast dye: May cause acute renal failure. Withhold metformin at the time of or prior to the procedure and 48 hours after the procedure. Restart drug only after renal function is evaluated and found to be normal.
Drug-herb. *Guar gum:* May decrease hypoglycemic effect. Discourage use together.
Drug-lifestyle. *Alcohol use:* May increase drug effects. Discourage use together.

EFFECTS ON LAB TEST RESULTS

● May decrease vitamin B_{12} and hemoglobin levels.

CONTRAINDICATIONS & CAUTIONS

● Contraindicated in patients hypersensitive to drug and in those with hepatic disease or metabolic acidosis.
● Contraindicated in patients with renal disease and in those with a serum creatinine level greater than or equal to 1.5 mg/dL (males) or greater than or equal to 1.4 mg/dL (females).
● Contraindicated in patients with acute heart failure requiring pharmacologic intervention and in patients with conditions predisposing to renal dysfunction, CV collapse, MI, hypoxia, and septicemia. Temporarily withhold from patients having radiologic studies involving use of contrast media containing iodine.
Black Box Warning Because of risk of lactic acidosis, drug is contraindicated in patients older than age 80, unless CrCl indicates normal renal function. ■
● Use caution when giving drug to elderly, debilitated, or malnourished patients and to those with adrenal or pituitary insufficiency because of increased risk of hypoglycemia.
⚠ Overdose S&S: Hypoglycemia, lactic acidosis.

NURSING CONSIDERATIONS

● Before therapy begins and at least annually thereafter, assess patient's renal function. If renal impairment is detected, a different antidiabetic may be indicated.
● When switching patients from chlorpropamide to metformin, take care during the first 2 weeks of metformin therapy because the prolonged retention of chlorpropamide increases the risk of hypoglycemia during this time.
● Monitor patient's glucose level regularly to evaluate effectiveness of therapy. Notify prescriber if glucose level increases despite therapy.
● If patient hasn't responded to 4 weeks of therapy with maximum dosage, an oral sulfonylurea can be added while keeping metformin at maximum dosage. If patient still doesn't respond after several months of therapy with both drugs at maximum

---

Reactions in bold italics are *life-threatening*. Interactions may have a *rapid onset* or a *delayed onset*.

dosage, prescriber may stop both and start insulin therapy.

• Monitor patient closely during times of increased stress, such as infection, fever, surgery, or trauma. Insulin therapy may be needed in these situations.

Black Box Warning Suspect lactic acidosis in diabetic patients with metabolic acidosis who don't have evidence of ketoacidosis. Lactic acidosis is a medical emergency and must be treated in a hospital setting. Risk of drug-induced lactic acidosis is very low; however, when it occurs, it is fatal in approximately 50% of cases. Reported cases have occurred primarily in diabetic patients with significant renal insufficiency; in those with other medical or surgical problems; and in those with other drug regimens. Risk increases with degree of renal impairment and patient age. Hemodialysis may be necessary. ■

Black Box Warning Stop drug immediately and notify prescriber if patient develops a condition related to hypoxemia or dehydration because of risk of lactic acidosis. ■

• Stop drug temporarily for surgical procedures (except minor procedures that don't restrict intake of food and fluids) and for patients undergoing radiologic studies involving use of contrast media containing iodine. Don't restart drug until patient's oral intake has resumed and renal function has been deemed normal by prescriber and at least 48 hours after contrast media.

• Monitor patient's hematologic status for evidence of megaloblastic anemia. Patients with inadequate vitamin B_{12} or calcium intake or absorption appear to be predisposed to developing subnormal vitamin B_{12} level. These patients should have routine vitamin B_{12} level determinations every 2 to 3 years.

• **Look alike–sound alike:** Don't confuse Glucophage with Glucovance or Glucotrol.

PATIENT TEACHING

• Instruct patient about nature of diabetes and importance of following therapeutic regimen, adhering to specific diet, losing weight, getting exercise, following personal hygiene programs, and avoiding infection. Explain how and when to monitor glucose level. Teach evidence of low and high glucose levels. Explain emergency measures.

Black Box Warning Instruct patient to stop drug and immediately notify prescriber about unexplained hyperventilation, muscle pain, malaise, dizziness, light-headedness, unusual sleepiness, unexplained stomach pain, feeling of coldness, slow or irregular heart rate, or other nonspecific symptoms of early lactic acidosis. ■

• Warn patient not to consume excessive alcohol while taking drug.

• Tell patient not to change drug dosage without prescriber's consent. Encourage patient to report abnormal glucose level test results.

• **Alert:** Advise patient not to cut, crush, or chew extended-release tablets; instead, he should swallow them whole.

• Tell patient that inactive ingredients may be eliminated in the stool as a soft mass resembling the original tablet.

• Advise patient not to take other drugs, including OTC drugs, without first checking with prescriber.

• Instruct patient to carry medical identification at all times.

• Tell patient that adverse effects of diarrhea, nausea, and upset stomach generally subside over time.

SAFETY ALERT!

methadone hydrochloride
METH-a-done

Dolophine, Methadose

Therapeutic class: Opioid analgesics
Pharmacologic class: Opioid agonists
Pregnancy risk category: C
Controlled substance schedule: II

AVAILABLE FORMS
Dispersible tablets (for methadone maintenance therapy): 40 mg
Injection: 10 mg/mL
Oral solution: 5 mg/5 mL, 10 mg/5 mL, 10 mg/mL (concentrate)
Tablets: 5 mg, 10 mg

M

INDICATIONS & DOSAGES
Adjust-a-dose (for all indications): For elderly patients and those with renal or hepatic impairment, reduce initial dose.
➤ **Severe pain in opioid nontolerant patients**
Adults: Initially, 2.5 to 10 mg P.O., I.M., or subcutaneously every 8 to 12 hours p.r.n. Titrate slowly and give more frequently as needed to maintain analgesia.
➤ **Opioid withdrawal syndrome**
Adults: Initially, 20 to 30 mg P.O. daily to suppress withdrawal symptoms (highly individualized; some patients may require a higher dose). Initial dose shouldn't exceed 30 mg. Maintenance dose is 20 to 120 mg P.O. daily. Dosage adjusted, as needed.

ADMINISTRATION
P.O.
● Oral form legally required in maintenance programs. Completely dissolve dispersible tablets in ½ cup of orange juice or powdered citrus drink.
● Oral dose is half as potent as injected dose.
I.M.
● For parenteral use, I.M. injection is preferred. Rotate injection sites.
Subcutaneous
● Monitor patient for pain at injection site, tissue irritation, and induration after injection.

ACTION
Unknown. Binds with opioid receptors in the CNS, altering perception of and emotional response to pain.

Route	Onset	Peak	Duration
P.O.	30–60 min	90–120 min	4–6 hr
I.M., subcut.	10–20 min	1–2 hr	4–5 hr

Half-life: 8 to 59 hours.

ADVERSE REACTIONS
CNS: clouded sensorium, hallucinations, dizziness, light-headedness, sedation, somnolence, *seizures,* agitation, choreic movements, euphoria, headache, insomnia, syncope.
CV: *arrhythmias, bradycardia, prolonged QT interval, cardiac arrest, shock, cardio-myopathy, heart failure,* flushing, phlebitis, edema, hypotension, palpitations.
EENT: visual disturbances.
GI: nausea, vomiting, abdominal pain, anorexia, biliary tract spasm, constipation, dry mouth, glossitis, ileus.
GU: urine retention.
Metabolic: hypokalemia, *hypomagnesemia,* weight gain.
Respiratory: *respiratory arrest, respiratory depression, pulmonary edema.*
Skin: diaphoresis, pruritus, urticaria.
Other: decreased libido, induration, pain at injection site, physical dependence, tissue irritation.

INTERACTIONS
Drug-drug. *Ammonium chloride, other urine acidifiers:* May reduce methadone effect. Watch for decreased pain control.
CNS depressants, general anesthetics, hypnotics, MAO inhibitors, sedatives, TCAs, tranquilizers: May cause respiratory depression, hypotension, profound sedation, or coma. Use together with caution. Monitor patient response.
CYP2C9 inhibitors (such as fluvoxamine), CYP3A4 inhibitors (such as clarithromycin, erythromycin, itraconazole, ketoconazole, telithromycin, voriconazole): May increase or prolong adverse drug effects and cause fatal respiratory depression. Monitor patient closely and reduce dosage if necessary.
CYP450 inducers (such as carbamazepine, phenytoin, rifampin): May decrease methadone effect and precipitate a withdrawal syndrome. Monitor patient closely.
NNRTIs (delavirdine, efavirenz, nevirapine), protease inhibitors (lopinavir and ritonavir, nelfinavir, ritonavir), rifamycins: May increase methadone metabolism, causing opioid withdrawal symptoms. Monitor patient and adjust dose as needed.
Protease inhibitors, cimetidine, fluvoxamine: May increase respiratory and CNS depression. Monitor patient closely.
Drug-herb. *St. John's wort:* May reduce methadone effect and precipitate a withdrawal syndrome. Monitor patient closely.
Drug-lifestyle. *Alcohol use:* May cause additive effects. Discourage use together.

Reactions in bold italics are *life-threatening*. Interactions may have a *rapid onset* or a *delayed onset*.

EFFECTS ON LAB TEST RESULTS

• May increase amylase level.

CONTRAINDICATIONS & CAUTIONS

• Contraindicated in patients hypersensitive to drug.

Black Box Warning Accidental ingestion of methadone, especially in children, can result in a fatal overdose of methadone. ■

• Use with caution in elderly or debilitated patients and in those with acute abdominal conditions, severe hepatic or renal impairment, hypothyroidism, Addison disease, prostatic hyperplasia, urethral stricture, head injury, increased intracranial pressure, asthma, and other respiratory conditions.

Black Box Warning Deaths have been reported during initiation of methadone therapy for opioid dependence. Exercise extreme caution when initiating treatment. ■

⚠ **Overdose S&S:** Miosis, respiratory depression, somnolence, coma, cool clammy skin, skeletal muscle flaccidity, hypotension, apnea, bradycardia, noncardiac pulmonary edema, death.

NURSING CONSIDERATIONS

Black Box Warning Methadone is an opioid agonist and Schedule II controlled substance with an abuse liability similar to that of other opioid agonists, legal or illicit. Assess each patient's risk of opioid abuse or addiction before prescribing methadone. Risk of opioid abuse increases in patients with personal or family history of substance abuse (including drug or alcohol abuse or addiction) or mental illness (such as major depressive disorder). Routinely monitor all patients receiving methadone for signs and symptoms of misuse, abuse, and addiction during treatment. ■

Black Box Warning Oral methadone can only be dispensed by certified treatment programs or during inpatient care for conditions other than concurrent opioid addiction. ■

Black Box Warning Respiratory depression, QT interval prolongation, and torsades de pointes have been observed during treatment. Be vigilant during treatment initiation and dose titration. ■

• Reassess patient's level of pain at least 15 and 30 minutes after parenteral administration and 30 minutes after oral administration.

Black Box Warning When used in opioid withdrawal syndrome, treatment products shall be dispensed only by opioid treatment programs. ■

• An around-the-clock regimen is needed to manage severe, chronic pain.

• Patient treated for opioid withdrawal syndrome usually needs an additional analgesic if pain control is needed.

• Monitor patient closely because drug has cumulative effect; marked sedation can occur after repeated doses.

• Monitor circulatory and respiratory status and bladder and bowel function. Patient may need a stool softener and stimulant laxative.

⟁ **Alert:** Respiratory depressant effects may last longer than analgesic effects. Monitor patient's respiratory status closely.

• When used as an adjunct in the treatment of opioid addiction (maintenance), withdrawal is usually delayed and mild.

⟁ **Alert:** Use caution when dosing. Confusion has occurred between mL and mg doses.

• **Look alike–sound alike:** Don't confuse methadone with ketorolac, methylphenidate (Metadate CD, Metadate ER), dexmethylphenidate, and Mephyton.

PATIENT TEACHING

• Caution ambulatory patient about getting out of bed or walking. Warn outpatient to avoid hazardous activities that require mental alertness until drug's CNS effects are known.

• Instruct patient to increase fluid and fiber in diet, if not contraindicated, to combat constipation.

• Advise patient to avoid alcohol during therapy.

Black Box Warning Caution patients not to use CNS depressants during initiation of treatment with methadone. ■

methimazole
meth-IM-a-zole

Tapazole

Therapeutic class: Antihyperthyroid drugs
Pharmacologic class: Thyroid hormone antagonists
Pregnancy risk category: D

AVAILABLE FORMS
Tablets: 5 mg, 10 mg, 20 mg

INDICATIONS & DOSAGES
➤ **Hyperthyroidism**
Adults: If mild, 15 mg P.O. daily in three divided doses given at 8-hour intervals. If moderately severe, 30 to 40 mg daily in three divided doses given at 8-hour intervals. If severe, 60 mg daily in three divided doses given at 8-hour intervals. Maintenance dosage is 5 to 15 mg daily.
Children: 0.4 mg/kg P.O. in three divided doses daily given at 8-hour intervals. Maintenance dosage is 0.2 mg/kg in divided doses daily.

ADMINISTRATION
P.O.
• Give drug with meals to minimize adverse GI effects.

ACTION
Inhibits synthesis of thyroid hormones.

Route	Onset	Peak	Duration
P.O.	Rapid	30–60 min	Unknown

Half-life: 5 to 13 hours.

ADVERSE REACTIONS
CNS: headache, drowsiness, vertigo, paresthesia, neuritis, neuropathies, CNS stimulation, fever.
CV: edema.
GI: nausea, vomiting, salivary gland enlargement, loss of taste, epigastric distress.
Hematologic: *agranulocytosis, leukopenia, thrombocytopenia, aplastic anemia.*
Hepatic: jaundice, hepatic dysfunction, *hepatitis.*

Metabolic: hypothyroidism.
Musculoskeletal: arthralgia, myalgia.
Skin: rash, urticaria, discoloration, pruritus, erythema nodosum, exfoliative dermatitis, lupuslike syndrome, abnormal hair loss.
Other: lymphadenopathy.

INTERACTIONS
Drug-drug. *Aminophylline, theophylline:* May decrease clearance of these drugs. Dosage may need to be adjusted.
Anticoagulants: May increase anticoagulant effect due to anti–vitamin K activity. Monitor patient closely.
Beta blockers: Beta-blocker clearance may be enhanced by hyperthyroidism. Dosage of beta blocker may need to be reduced when patient becomes euthyroid.
Cardiac glycosides: May increase cardiac glycoside level. Cardiac glycoside dosage may need to be reduced.
Potassium iodide: May decrease response to drug. Methimazole dosage may need to be increased.
Warfarin: May alter dosage requirements. Monitor PT, PTT, and INR.

EFFECTS ON LAB TEST RESULTS
• May decrease hemoglobin level.
• May decrease granulocyte, WBC, and platelet counts.
• May alter thyroid uptake of ^{123}I or ^{131}I.

CONTRAINDICATIONS & CAUTIONS
• Contraindicated in patients hypersensitive to drug and in breast-feeding women.
• Use cautiously in pregnant patients because drug can harm fetus.
⚠ Overdose S&S: Nausea, vomiting, epigastric distress, headache, fever, joint pain, pruritus, edema, aplastic anemia, agranulocytosis, hepatitis, nephrotic syndrome, exfoliative dermatitis, neuropathies, CNS stimulation or depression.

NURSING CONSIDERATIONS
• Pregnant women may need less drug as pregnancy progresses. Monitor thyroid function studies closely. Thyroid hormone may be added to regimen. Drug may be stopped during last few weeks of pregnancy.
• Monitor CBC periodically to detect impending leukopenia, thrombocytopenia,

---

Reactions in bold italics are *life-threatening*. Interactions may have a *rapid onset* or a *delayed onset*.

and agranulocytosis; also monitor hepatic function. Stop drug if liver abnormality occurs.

❸ **Alert:** Doses higher than 30 mg daily increase risk of agranulocytosis.

❸ **Alert:** Patients older than age 40 may have an increased risk of drug-induced agranulocytosis.

• Watch for evidence of hypothyroidism (mental depression, cold intolerance, and hard, nonpitting edema); notify prescriber because patient may need dosage adjustment.

❸ **Alert:** Stop drug and notify prescriber if severe rash or enlarged cervical lymph nodes develop.

• **Look alike–sound alike:** Don't confuse methimazole with mebendazole, methazolamide, metolazone, or metronidazole.

PATIENT TEACHING

• Tell patient to take drug with meals to reduce adverse GI reactions.
• Warn patient to report fever, sore throat, mouth sores, skin eruptions, anorexia, itching, right upper quadrant pain, or yellow skin or eyes.
• Tell patient to ask prescriber about using iodized salt and eating shellfish because the iodine in these foods may make the drug less effective.
• Warn patient that drug may cause drowsiness; advise patient to use caution when operating machinery or a vehicle.
• Instruct patient to store drug in light-resistant container.
• Teach patient to watch for evidence of hypothyroidism (unexplained weight gain, fatigue, cold intolerance) and to notify prescriber if it arises.
• Tell women not to use drug while breast-feeding.

SAFETY ALERT!

methotrexate (amethopterin, MTX)
meth-oh-TREX-ate

methotrexate sodium
Methotrexate LPF, Trexall

Therapeutic class: Antineoplastics
Pharmacologic class: Folate antagonists
Pregnancy risk category: X

AVAILABLE FORMS

Injection: 25 mg/mL in 2-mL, 4-mL, 8-mL, 10-mL, 20-mL, and 40-mL preservative-free single-use vials; 25 mg/mL in 2-mL and 10-mL vials containing benzyl alcohol
Lyophilized powder: 1,000-mg vials, preservative-free; 2.5-mg/mL, 25-mg/mL vials
Tablets (scored): 2.5 mg, 5 mg, 7.5 mg, 10 mg, 15 mg

INDICATIONS & DOSAGES

Adjust-a-dose (for all indications): Reduce dosage in patients with impaired renal function.

➤ **Trophoblastic tumors (choriocarcinoma, hydatidiform mole)**
Adults: 15 to 30 mg P.O. or I.M. daily for 5 days. Repeat after 1 or more weeks, based on response or toxicity. Number of courses is three to maximum of five.

➤ **Acute lymphocytic leukemia**
Adults and children: 3.3 mg/m^2 daily P.O., I.V., or I.M. with 60 mg/m^2 prednisone daily for 4 to 6 weeks or until remission occurs; then 30 mg/m^2 P.O. or I.M. weekly in two divided doses or 2.5 mg/kg I.V. every 14 days.

➤ **Meningeal leukemia**
Adults and children: 12 mg/m^2 or less (maximum 15 mg) intrathecally every 2 to 5 days until CSF is normal; then one additional dose. Or, for children, use dosages based on age.
Children age 3 and older: 12 mg intrathecally every 2 to 5 days.
Children ages 2 to 3: 10 mg intrathecally every 2 to 5 days.
Children ages 1 to 2: 8 mg intrathecally every 2 to 5 days.

M

Children younger than age 1: 6 mg intrathecally every 2 to 5 days.

➤ **Burkitt lymphoma (stage I, II)**
Adults: 10 to 25 mg P.O. daily for 4 to 8 days, with 1-week rest intervals.

➤ **Lymphosarcoma (stage III)**
Adults: 0.625 to 2.5 mg/kg daily P.O., I.M., or I.V.

➤ **Osteosarcoma**
Adults: Initially, 12 g/m² I.V. as 4-hour infusion. Give subsequent doses 15 g/m² I.V. as 4-hour I.V. infusion at postoperative weeks 4, 5, 6, 7, 11, 12, 15, 16, 29, 30, 44, and 45. Give with leucovorin, 15 mg P.O. every 6 hours for 10 doses, beginning 24 hours after start of methotrexate infusion.

➤ **Mycosis fungoides**
Adults: 5 to 50 mg P.O. or I.M. once weekly; or 15 to 37.5 mg I.M. twice weekly.

➤ **Psoriasis**
Adults: 10 to 25 mg P.O., I.M., or I.V. as single weekly dose; or 2.5 to 5 mg P.O. every 12 hours for three doses weekly. Dosage shouldn't exceed 30 mg per week.

➤ **Rheumatoid arthritis**
Adults: Initially, 7.5 mg P.O. weekly, either in single dose or divided as 2.5 mg P.O. every 12 hours for three doses once weekly. Dosage may be gradually increased to maximum of 30 mg weekly.

➤ **Polyarticular course, juvenile rheumatoid arthritis**
Children and adolescents age 2 to 16: 10 mg/m² P.O. or I.M. once weekly. Or, 20 to 30 mg/m²/week I.M. or subcutaneously.

➤ **Head and neck carcinomas**
Adults: 40 to 60 mg/m² I.V. weekly. Response to therapy is limited to 4 months.

➤ **Uveitis ◆**
Adults: 7.5 to 20 mg P.O. weekly either alone or in conjunction with other corticosteroids or immunosuppressants.

ADMINISTRATION
P.O.
● Give drug when patient has an empty stomach.
I.V.
▼ Preparing and giving parenteral drug may be mutagenic, teratogenic, or carcinogenic. Follow facility policy to reduce risks.

▼ Dilution of drug depends on product, and infusion guidelines vary, depending on dose.

▼ Reconstitute 20-mg vial to a concentration no greater than 25 mg/mL. Reconstitute 1-g vial to a concentration of 50 mg/mL.

▼ If giving infusion, dilute total dose in D_5W.

▼ Reconstitute solutions without preservatives with normal saline solution or D_5W immediately before use, and discard unused drug.

▼ **Incompatibilities:** Bleomycin, chlorpromazine, droperidol, gemcitabine, idarubicin, ifosfamide, midazolam, nalbuphine, promethazine, propofol.
I.M.
● Preparing and giving parenteral drug may be mutagenic, teratogenic, or carcinogenic. Follow facility policy to reduce risks.
Intrathecal
● Preparing and giving parenteral drug may be mutagenic, teratogenic, or carcinogenic. Follow facility policy to reduce risks.
Black Box Warning Use preservative-free form for intrathecal administration. ∎

ACTION
Reversibly binds to dihydrofolate reductase, blocking reduction of folic acid to tetrahydrofolate, a cofactor necessary for purine, protein, and DNA synthesis.

Route	Onset	Peak	Duration
P.O.	Unknown	1–2 hr	Unknown
I.V.	Immediate	Immediate	Unknown
I.M.	Unknown	30 min–1 hr	Unknown
Intrathecal	Unknown	Unknown	Unknown

Half-life: For doses below 30 mg/m², about 3 to 10 hours; for doses of 30 mg/m² and above, 8 to 15 hours.

ADVERSE REACTIONS
CNS: *arachnoiditis within hours of intrathecal use, leukoencephalopathy, seizures,* subacute neurotoxicity possibly beginning a few weeks later, demyelination, malaise, fatigue, dizziness, headache, aphasia, hemiparesis, fever, drowsiness.
EENT: pharyngitis, blurred vision.

GI: gingivitis, stomatitis, diarrhea, abdominal distress, anorexia, GI ulceration and *bleeding*, enteritis, nausea, vomiting.
GU: nephropathy, tubular necrosis, *renal failure*, hematuria, menstrual dysfunction, defective spermatogenesis, infertility, abortion, cystitis.
Hematologic: anemia, *leukopenia, thrombocytopenia.*
Hepatic: *acute toxicity, chronic toxicity,* including cirrhosis and *hepatic fibrosis*.
Metabolic: *diabetes,* hyperuricemia.
Musculoskeletal: arthralgia, myalgia, osteoporosis in children on long-term therapy.
Respiratory: *pulmonary fibrosis, pulmonary interstitial infiltrates,* pneumonitis; dry, nonproductive cough.
Skin: urticaria, pruritus, hyperpigmentation, erythematous rashes, ecchymoses, rash, photosensitivity reactions, alopecia, acne, psoriatic lesions aggravated by exposure to sun.
Other: chills, reduced resistance to infection, *septicemia, sudden death.*

INTERACTIONS
Drug-drug. *Acitretin:* May increase the risk of hepatitis. Avoid using together.
Acyclovir: Use with intrathecal methotrexate may cause neurologic abnormalities. Monitor patient closely.
Digoxin: May decrease digoxin level. Monitor digoxin level closely.
Folic acid derivatives: Antagonizes methotrexate effect. Avoid using together, except for leucovorin rescue with high-dose methotrexate therapy.
Fosphenytoin, phenytoin: May decrease phenytoin and fosphenytoin levels. Monitor drug levels closely.
Hepatotoxic drugs: May increase risk of hepatotoxicity. Monitor patient closely.
NSAIDs, phenylbutazone, salicylates: May increase methotrexate toxicity. Avoid using together.
Oral antibiotics: May decrease absorption of methotrexate. Monitor patient closely.
Penicillins, sulfonamides, trimethoprim: May increase methotrexate level. Monitor patient for methotrexate toxicity.
Probenecid: May impair excretion of methotrexate, causing increased level, effect, and toxicity of methotrexate. Monitor

methotrexate level closely and adjust dosage accordingly.
Procarbazine: May increase risk of nephrotoxicity. Monitor patient closely.
❸ *Alert: Proton pump inhibitors:* May cause methotrexate toxicity, especially when high doses of methotrexate are given. Use cautiously.
Theophylline: May increase theophylline level. Monitor theophylline level closely.
Thiopurines: May increase thiopurine level. Monitor patient closely.
Vaccines: May make immunizations ineffective; may cause risk of disseminated infection with live-virus vaccines. Postpone immunization, if possible.
Drug-food. *Any food:* May delay absorption and reduce peak level of methotrexate. Instruct patient to take drug on an empty stomach.
Drug-lifestyle. *Alcohol use:* May increase hepatotoxicity. Discourage use together.
Sun exposure: May cause photosensitivity reactions. Advise patient to avoid excessive sunlight exposure.

EFFECTS ON LAB TEST RESULTS
• May increase uric acid level. May decrease hemoglobin level.
• May decrease WBC, RBC, and platelet counts.
• May alter results of laboratory assay for folate, which interferes with detection of folic acid deficiency.

CONTRAINDICATIONS & CAUTIONS
• Contraindicated in patients hypersensitive to drug and in those with psoriasis or rheumatoid arthritis who also have alcoholism, alcoholic liver, chronic liver disease, immunodeficiency syndromes, or blood dyscrasias.
Black Box Warning Methotrexate given with radiotherapy may increase the risk of soft-tissue necrosis and osteonecrosis. ■
Black Box Warning When high doses of drug are used to treat osteosarcoma, don't give NSAIDs before or with drug. Use together may elevate and prolong serum methotrexate level, resulting in severe bone marrow suppression, aplastic anemia, and GI toxicity. ■

M

Black Box Warning Contraindicated in pregnancy; do not use in women of childbearing potential unless benefits outweigh risks. ∎

• Contraindicated in breast-feeding women.

Black Box Warning Use cautiously and at modified dosage in patients with impaired hepatic or renal function, bone marrow suppression, aplasia, leukopenia, thrombocytopenia, or anemia. ∎

• Use cautiously in very young, elderly, or debilitated patients and in those with infection, peptic ulceration, or ulcerative colitis.

⚠ **Overdose S&S:** Leukopenia, thrombocytopenia, anemia, pancytopenia, bone marrow suppression, mucositis, stomatitis, oral ulceration, nausea, vomiting, GI ulceration, GI bleeding, sepsis or septic shock, renal failure, aplastic anemia, headache, seizures, acute toxic encephalopathy, cerebellar herniation associated with increased intracranial pressure, death.

NURSING CONSIDERATIONS

Black Box Warning Methotrexate-induced lung disease is a potentially dangerous lesion that may occur at any time during therapy. It isn't always fully reversible. Pulmonary symptoms (especially a dry, nonproductive cough) may require interruption of treatment and careful investigation. ∎

Black Box Warning Diarrhea and ulcerative stomatitis require interruption of therapy; hemorrhagic enteritis and death from intestinal perforation may occur. ∎

Black Box Warning Malignant lymphomas may occur in patients receiving low-dose methotrexate. ∎

Black Box Warning Methotrexate may induce tumor lysis syndrome in patients with rapidly growing tumors. ∎

Black Box Warning Severe, occasionally fatal skin reactions have been reported following single or multiple doses of methotrexate. Reactions have occurred within days of methotrexate administration. Recovery has been reported with discontinuation of therapy. ∎

Black Box Warning Potentially fatal opportunistic infections, especially *Pneumocystis*

jiroveci (carinii) pneumonia, may occur with methotrexate therapy. ∎

Black Box Warning The high-dose regimens for osteosarcoma require meticulous care. ∎

❸ **Alert:** Drug may be given daily or once weekly, depending on the disease. To avoid administration errors, know your patient's dosing schedule.

• Monitor pulmonary function tests periodically and fluid intake and output daily. Encourage fluid intake of 2 to 3 L daily.

• Monitor uric acid level.

• Drug distributes readily into pleural effusions and other third-space compartments, such as ascites, leading to prolonged systemic level and risk of toxicity. Use drug cautiously in these patients.

❸ **Alert:** Alkalinize urine by giving sodium bicarbonate tablets or fluids to prevent precipitation of drug, especially at high doses. Maintain urine pH above 7. If BUN level is 20 to 30 mg/dL or creatinine level is 1.2 to 2 mg/dL, reduce dosage. If BUN level exceeds 30 mg/dL or creatinine level is higher than 2 mg/dL, stop drug and notify prescriber.

Black Box Warning Watch for increases in AST, ALT, and alkaline phosphatase levels, which may signal hepatic dysfunction. Periodic liver biopsies are recommended for psoriatic patients who are receiving long-term treatment. ∎

• Watch for signs and symptoms of bleeding (especially GI) and infection.

• To prevent bleeding, avoid all I.M. injections when platelet count is below $50,000/mm^3$.

• Give blood transfusions for cumulative anemia. Patient may receive injections of RBC colony-stimulating factors to promote RBC production and decrease need for blood transfusions.

• Leucovorin rescue is needed with doses of more than 100 mg and starts 24 hours after therapy starts. Leucovorin is continued until methotrexate level falls below 5×10^{-8} M. Consult specialized references for specific recommendations for leucovorin dosage. Monitor methotrexate level and adjust leucovorin dose.

• The WBC and platelet count nadirs usually occur on day 7.

PATIENT TEACHING
• Advise patient to watch for signs and symptoms of infection (fever, sore throat, fatigue) and bleeding (easy bruising, nosebleeds, bleeding gums, tarry stools). Tell patient to take temperature daily.

Black Box Warning Fully inform patient of the risks involved with methotrexate therapy. ■

• Teach and encourage diligent mouth care to reduce risk of superinfection in the mouth.
• Instruct patient how to take leucovorin. Stress the importance of taking as prescribed until instructed by prescriber to stop.
• Tell patient to use highly protective sunblock when exposed to sunlight.
• Warn both men and women to avoid conception during and for at least 12 weeks after therapy because of risk of abortion, birth defects, or fetal death.
• Advise women to stop breast-feeding during therapy.

SAFETY ALERT!

methyldopa
meth-ill-DOE-pa

Novo-Medopa†

methyldopate hydrochloride

Therapeutic class: Antihypertensives
Pharmacologic class: Centrally acting antiadrenergics
Pregnancy risk category: B for P.O.; C for I.V.

AVAILABLE FORMS
methyldopa
Tablets: 125 mg†, 250 mg, 500 mg
methyldopate hydrochloride
Injection: 50 mg/mL

INDICATIONS & DOSAGES
➤ **Hypertension, hypertensive crisis**
Adults: Initially, 250 mg P.O. b.i.d. to t.i.d. in first 48 hours. Increase if needed every 2 days. May give entire daily dose in evening or at bedtime. Adjust dosages if other antihypertensives are added to or deleted from therapy. Adjust dosage at 48-hour intervals. Maintenance dosage is 500 mg to 2 g daily in two to four divided doses. Maximum recommended P.O. daily dose is 3 g. Or, 250 to 500 mg I.V. every 6 hours. Maximum I.V. dosage is 1 g every 6 hours. Switch to oral antihypertensives as soon as possible.
Children: Initially, 10 mg/kg P.O. daily in two to four divided doses; or, 20 to 40 mg/kg I.V. daily in four divided doses. Increase dose daily until desired response occurs. Maximum daily dose is 65 mg/kg or 3 g, whichever is less.

ADMINISTRATION
P.O.
• If unpleasant adverse reactions occur, patient shouldn't suddenly stop taking drug but should notify his prescriber.

I.V.
▼ Dilute appropriate dose in 100 mL D₅W. Infuse slowly over 30 to 60 minutes.
▼ **Incompatibilities:** Amphotericin B; drugs with poor solubility in acidic media, such as barbiturates and sulfonamides; methohexital; some total parenteral nutrition solutions.

ACTION
May inhibit the central vasomotor centers, decreasing sympathetic outflow to the heart, kidneys, and peripheral vasculature.

Route	Onset	Peak	Duration
P.O.	4–6 hr	Unknown	12–48 hr
I.V.	4–6 hr	Unknown	10–16 hr

Half-life: About 2 hours.

ADVERSE REACTIONS
CNS: decreased mental acuity, sedation, headache, weakness, dizziness, paresthesia, parkinsonism, involuntary choreoathetoid movements, psychic disturbances, depression, nightmares.
CV: orthostatic hypotension, edema, *bradycardia, myocarditis,* aggravated angina, paradoxical pressor response with I.V. use.
EENT: nasal congestion.
GI: dry mouth, *pancreatitis,* nausea, vomiting, diarrhea, constipation.
GU: galactorrhea, dark urine.
Hematologic: *thrombocytopenia, leukopenia, bone marrow depression,* hemolytic anemia.

M

Hepatic: *hepatic necrosis, hepatitis.*
Musculoskeletal: arthralgia.
Skin: rash.
Other: drug-induced fever, gynecomastia.

INTERACTIONS
Drug-drug. *Amphetamines, nonselective beta blockers, norepinephrine, phenothiazines, TCAs:* May cause hypertensive effects. Monitor patient closely.
Anesthetics: May need lower doses of anesthetics. Use together cautiously.
Barbiturates: May decrease actions of methyldopa. Monitor patient closely.
Ferrous sulfate: May decrease bioavailability of methyldopa. Separate doses.
Haloperidol: May increase antipsychotic effects of haloperidol or cause psychosis. Use together cautiously.
Levodopa: May increase hypotensive effects, which may increase adverse CNS reactions. Monitor patient closely.
Lithium: May increase lithium level. Watch for increased lithium level and signs and symptoms of toxicity.
MAO inhibitors: May cause excessive sympathetic stimulation. Avoid using together.
Drug-herb. *Capsicum:* May reduce antihypertensive effect. Discourage use together.

EFFECTS ON LAB TEST RESULTS
● May increase creatinine level. May decrease hemoglobin level and hematocrit.
● May increase LFT values. May decrease platelet and WBC counts.
● May interfere with results of urinary uric acid testing, serum creatinine test, and AST test. May cause positive Coombs test result. May falsely increase urine catecholamine level, interfering with the diagnosis of pheochromocytoma.

CONTRAINDICATIONS & CAUTIONS
● Contraindicated in patients hypersensitive to drug and in those with active hepatic disease (such as acute hepatitis) or active cirrhosis.
● Contraindicated in those whose previous methyldopa therapy caused liver problems and in those taking MAO inhibitors.
● Use cautiously in patients with history of impaired hepatic function or sulfite sensitivity and in breast-feeding women.

⚠ *Overdose S&S:* Sedation, acute hypotension, weakness, bradycardia, dizziness, constipation, abdominal distention, flatus, diarrhea, nausea, vomiting.

NURSING CONSIDERATIONS
● Monitor patient's blood pressure regularly. Elderly patients are more likely to experience hypotension and sedation.
● Occasionally, tolerance may occur, usually between the second and third months of therapy. Adding a diuretic or adjusting dosage may be needed. If patient's response changes significantly, notify prescriber.
● After dialysis, monitor patient for hypertension and notify prescriber, if needed. Patient may need an extra dose of drug.
● Monitor CBC with differential counts before therapy and periodically thereafter.
● Patients who need blood transfusions should have direct and indirect Coombs tests to prevent crossmatching problems.
● Monitor patient's Coombs test results. In patients who have received drug for several months, positive reaction to direct Coombs test may indicate hemolytic anemia.
● Report involuntary choreoathetoid movements. Drug may be stopped.

PATIENT TEACHING
● If unpleasant adverse reactions occur, advise patient not to suddenly stop taking drug but to notify prescriber.
● Instruct patient to report signs and symptoms of infection, yellowing of the skin, flulike symptoms, and muscle aches.
● Tell patient to check his weight daily and to notify prescriber if he gains 2 or more pounds in 1 day or 5 pounds in 1 week. Sodium and water retention may occur but can be relieved with diuretics.
● Warn patient that, particularly at the start of therapy, drug may impair ability to perform tasks that require mental alertness. A once-daily dose at bedtime minimizes daytime drowsiness.
● Inform patient that low blood pressure and dizziness upon rising can be minimized by rising slowly and avoiding sudden position changes and that dry mouth can be relieved by chewing gum or sucking on hard candy or ice chips.

• Tell patient that urine may turn dark if left sitting in toilet bowl or if toilet bowl has been treated with bleach.

methylergonovine maleate
meth-ill-er-goe-NOE-veen

Methergine

Therapeutic class: Oxytocics
Pharmacologic class: Ergot alkaloids
Pregnancy risk category: C

AVAILABLE FORMS
Injection: 0.2 mg/mL in 1-mL ampules
Tablets: 0.2 mg

INDICATIONS & DOSAGES
➤ **To prevent and treat postpartum hemorrhage caused by uterine atony or subinvolution**
Adults: 0.2 mg I.V. every 2 to 4 hours to a maximum of five doses. For excessive uterine bleeding or other emergencies, 0.2 mg I.V. over at least 1 minute while monitoring blood pressure and uterine contractions. After first I.M. or I.V. dose, 0.2 mg P.O. every 6 to 8 hours for 2 to 7 days. Decrease dosage if severe cramping occurs.

ADMINISTRATION
P.O.
• Store tablets in tightly closed, light-resistant container. Discard if discolored.
I.V.
▼ Don't routinely use this form because of risk of severe hypertension and stroke.
▼ Dilute to 5 mL with normal saline solution.
▼ Administer only a clear and colorless solution.
▼ Give slowly over at least 1 minute while carefully monitoring blood pressure.
▼ Store solution below 46° F (8° C). Daily stock may be kept at room temperature for 60 to 90 days.
▼ **Incompatibilities:** None reported.
I.M.
• Store in refrigerator and protect from light.
• Drug may be given after delivery of the anterior shoulder, after delivery of the placenta, or during the puerperium.

ACTION
Increases motor activity of the uterus by direct stimulation of the smooth muscle, shortening the third stage of labor and reducing blood loss.

Route	Onset	Peak	Duration
P.O.	5–10 min	30 min	3 hr
I.V.	Immediate	Unknown	45 min
I.M.	2–5 min	Unknown	3 hr

Half-life: 1½ to 12¾ hours.

ADVERSE REACTIONS
CNS: *seizures, stroke with I.V. use,* dizziness, headache, hallucinations.
CV: hypertension, transient chest pain, palpitations, hypotension, thrombophlebitis.
EENT: tinnitus, nasal congestion.
GI: nausea, vomiting, diarrhea, foul taste.
GU: hematuria.
Musculoskeletal: leg cramps.
Respiratory: dyspnea.
Skin: diaphoresis.

INTERACTIONS
Drug-drug. *Clarithromycin, delavirdine, erythromycin, indinavir, itraconazole, ketoconazole, nelfinavir, ritonavir, telithromycin, troleandomycin, voriconazole:* May cause vasospasm, leading to ischemia. Avoid using together.
Clotrimazole, fluconazole, fluoxetine, fluvoxamine, nefazodone, saquinavir, zileuton: May increase risk of vasospasm. Use together cautiously.
Dopamine, ergot alkaloids, I.V. oxytocin, regional anesthetics, vasoconstrictors: May cause excessive vasoconstriction. Use together cautiously.

EFFECTS ON LAB TEST RESULTS
• May decrease prolactin level.

CONTRAINDICATIONS & CAUTIONS
• Contraindicated in pregnant patients, in patients sensitive to ergot preparations, and in patients with hypertension or toxemia.
• Use cautiously in patients with sepsis, obliterative vascular disease, or hepatic or renal disease.
• Use cautiously during last stage of labor.
⚠ *Overdose S&S:* Nausea, vomiting, abdominal pain, numbness, tingling of the

M

extremities, rise in blood pressure; in severe cases, followed by hypotension, respiratory depression, hypothermia, seizures, coma.

NURSING CONSIDERATIONS
• Monitor and record blood pressure, pulse rate, and uterine response; report sudden change in vital signs, frequent periods of uterine relaxation, and character and amount of vaginal bleeding.
• Monitor contractions, which may begin immediately. Contractions may continue for up to 45 minutes after I.V. use or for 3 hours or more after P.O. or I.M. use.
• *Look alike–sound alike:* Don't confuse Methergine with terbutaline.

PATIENT TEACHING
• Explain use of drug to patient and family.
• Instruct patient to report adverse reactions promptly.
• Tell patient to wait at least 12 hours after administration of last dose of methylergonovine maleate before initiating or resuming breast-feeding and to discard milk secreted during this time because drug may produce adverse effects in breast-feeding infant.

---

methylnaltrexone bromide
mehht-eel-NAHL-trek-zone

Relistor

Therapeutic class: GI drugs
Pharmacologic class: Peripherally acting mu-opioid receptor antagonists
Pregnancy risk category: B

AVAILABLE FORMS
Injection: 8 mg/0.4 mL, 12 mg/0.6 mL single-use vials

INDICATIONS & DOSAGES
➤ **Opioid-induced constipation in those receiving palliative care for advanced illness when response to laxatives is insufficient**
Adults weighing less than 38 kg (84 lb): 0.15 mg/kg subcutaneously every other day, as needed.

Adults weighing 38 to 61 kg (84 to 134 lb): 8 mg subcutaneously every other day, as needed.
Adults weighing 62 to 114 kg (136 to 251 lb): 12 mg subcutaneously every other day, as needed.
Adults weighing more than 114 kg (251 lb): 0.15 mg/kg subcutaneously every other day, as needed.
Adjust-a-dose: If CrCl is less than 30 mL/minute, reduce dose by one-half.

ADMINISTRATION
Subcutaneous
• Administer no more than one dose within 24 hours.
• To determine injection volume for the 0.15 mg/kg dose, multiply patient's weight in pounds by 0.0034 and round up to the nearest 0.1 mL, or multiply patient's weight in kilograms by 0.0075 and round up to the nearest 0.1 mL.
• Store drug at room temperature, away from light.
• After drawn into a syringe as directed, drug is stable at room temperature for 24 hours.
• Give injections subcutaneously into the abdomen, thighs, or upper arms.

ACTION
Antagonizes GI mu-opioid receptors, preventing opioid-induced slowing of GI motility and transit time.

Route	Onset	Peak	Duration
Subcut.	Unknown	30 min	Unknown

Half-life: About 8 hours.

ADVERSE REACTIONS
CNS: dizziness.
GI: abdominal pain, flatulence, nausea, diarrhea.

INTERACTIONS
None reported.

EFFECTS ON LAB TEST RESULTS
None reported.

Reactions in bold italics are *life-threatening*. Interactions may have a *rapid onset* or a *delayed onset*.

CONTRAINDICATIONS & CAUTIONS
• Contraindicated in patients hypersensitive to the drug and in those with known or suspected mechanical GI obstruction.
⊙ Alert: GI perforation has occurred rarely in patients with reduced GI tract integrity. Use cautiously.
• Use cautiously in patients with peritoneal catheters.
⚠ Overdose S&S: Orthostatic hypotension.

NURSING CONSIDERATIONS
• Drug will relieve opioid-induced constipation without affecting opioid-mediated analgesic effects.
• Don't use in pregnant women unless the benefits outweigh risk to fetus.
• It's unknown whether the drug is excreted in breast milk. Avoid use in breast-feeding women.
• Safety and effectiveness in children haven't been established.

PATIENT TEACHING
• Inform patient that drug may be effective within a few minutes to a few hours after administration.
• Instruct patient to discontinue therapy, and notify prescriber if severe or persistent diarrhea occurs.
• Tell patient that vial is for single-use only; remaining drug should be discarded.
• Advise patient to avoid injecting the drug into areas where the skin is tender, bruised, red, or hard, to avoid areas with scars or stretch marks, and to rotate injection sites.
• Warn patient that no more than one dose should be taken within a 24-hour period.
• Advise women of childbearing age to notify prescriber if pregnancy is desired or if it occurs.

---

methylphenidate hydrochloride
meth-ill-FEN-i-date

Concerta🖉, Metadate CD, Metadate ER, Methylin, Methylin ER, Quillivant XR, Ritalin🖉, Ritalin LA, Ritalin-SR🖉

methylphenidate transdermal system
Daytrana

Therapeutic class: CNS stimulants
Pharmacologic class: Piperidine derivatives
Pregnancy risk category: NR; C (for Concerta, Daytrana, Metadate CD, Quillivant XR, Ritalin LA)
Controlled substance schedule: II

AVAILABLE FORMS
Oral solution (Methylin): 5 mg/5 mL, 10 mg/5 mL
Tablets (chewable): 2.5 mg, 5 mg, 10 mg
Tablets (Ritalin): 5 mg, 10 mg, 20 mg
Extended-release
Capsules (Metadate CD): 10 mg, 20 mg, 30 mg, 40 mg, 50 mg, 60 mg
Capsules (Ritalin LA): 10 mg, 20 mg, 30 mg, 40 mg
Oral suspension: 25 mg/5 mL
Tablets (Concerta): 18 mg, 27 mg, 36 mg, 54 mg
Tablets (Metadate ER, Methylin ER): 10 mg, 20 mg
Sustained-release
Tablets (Ritalin-SR): 20 mg
Transdermal system
Patch: 10 mg, 15 mg, 20 mg, 30 mg

INDICATIONS & DOSAGES
➤ **Attention deficit hyperactivity disorder (ADHD)**
Adults: 10 mg (immediate-release) P.O. b.i.d. or t.i.d. Dosage varies; maximum dosage is 60 mg daily.
Children age 6 and older: Initially, 5 mg P.O. b.i.d. immediate-release form before breakfast and lunch, increasing by 5 to 10 mg at weekly intervals, as needed, until an optimum daily dose of 2 mg/kg is reached, not to exceed 60 mg/day.

To use Ritalin-SR, Metadate ER, and Methylin ER tablets in place of immediate-release methylphenidate tablets, calculate methylphenidate dosage in 8-hour intervals.

Concerta
Adults ages 18 to 65 not taking methylphenidate, or for patients taking other stimulants: Initially, 18 or 36 mg P.O. daily. May increase dosage in 18-mg increments at weekly intervals to maximum of 72 mg daily.

Adolescents ages 13 to 17 not currently taking methylphenidate, or for patients taking other stimulants: 18 mg P.O. extended-release Concerta once daily in the morning. Adjust dosage by 18 mg at weekly intervals to a maximum of 72 mg P.O. once daily in the morning.

Children ages 6 to 12 not currently taking methylphenidate, or for patients taking other stimulants: 18 mg extended-release P.O. once daily every morning. Adjust dosage by 18 mg at weekly intervals to a maximum of 54 mg daily every morning.

Adolescents and children age 6 and older currently taking methylphenidate: If previous methylphenidate dosage was 5 mg b.i.d. or t.i.d., give 18 mg P.O. every morning. If previous dosage was 10 mg b.i.d. or t.i.d., give 36 mg P.O. every morning. If previous dosage was 15 mg b.i.d. or t.i.d., give 54 mg P.O. every morning. Maximum conversion daily dose is 54 mg. Once conversion is complete, adjust maximum dose in adolescents ages 13 to 17 to 72 mg once daily.

Metadate CD
Adults and children age 6 and older: Initially, 20 mg P.O. daily before breakfast, increasing by 10 to 20 mg at weekly intervals to a maximum of 60 mg daily.

Ritalin LA
Adults and children age 6 and older: Initially, 10 to 20 mg P.O. once daily. Increase by 10 mg at weekly intervals to a maximum of 60 mg daily. If previous methylphenidate dosage was 5 mg P.O. b.i.d., give 10 mg P.O. once daily. If previous methylphenidate dosage was 10 mg b.i.d., give 20 mg P.O. once daily. If previous methylphenidate dosage was 15 mg b.i.d., give 30 mg P.O. once daily. If previous methylphenidate dosage was 20 mg b.i.d., give 40 mg P.O. once daily. If previous

methylphenidate dosage was 30 mg b.i.d., give 60 mg P.O. once daily.

Daytrana
Adults and children ages 6 to 17: Initially, apply one 10-mg patch to clean, dry, nonirritated skin on the hip, alternating sites daily. Apply 2 hours before desired effect and remove 9 hours later. Increase dose weekly as needed to a maximum of 30 mg daily. Base final dose and wear time on patient response.

Quillivant XR
Children age 6 and older: Initially, 20 mg P.O. once daily in a.m. May titrate weekly in dosages of 10 to 20 mg. Maximum dosage is 60 mg daily.

➤ **Narcolepsy**
Adults: 10 mg immediate-release, P.O. b.i.d. or t.i.d. 30 to 45 minutes before meals. Dosage varies; maximum dose is 60 mg/day.
Children age 6 and older: Initially, 5 mg immediate-release P.O. b.i.d. (before breakfast and lunch). Increase dosage, if needed, by 5 to 10 mg weekly. Maximum dose is 60 mg. To use Ritalin-SR, Metadate ER, or Methylin ER tablets in place of immediate-release methylphenidate tablets, calculate the dose of methylphenidate in 8-hour intervals.

ADMINISTRATION
P.O.
● Give chewable tablet with at least 8 oz (240 mL) of water.
● Give immediate-release tablets, chewable tablets, and oral solution in divided doses two or three times daily, preferably 30 to 45 minutes before meals. Give last daily dose at least 6 hours before bedtime to prevent insomnia.
● Metadate CD or Ritalin LA may be swallowed whole, or the contents of the capsule may be sprinkled onto a small amount of cool applesauce and taken immediately.
● Extended-release and sustained-release tablets (Metadate ER, Methylin ER, Ritalin-SR) must be swallowed whole and never crushed, chewed, or divided.
● Concerta may be taken with or without food and must be swallowed whole. Don't crush, divide, or allow patient to chew Concerta tablets.

• Vigorously shake oral suspension bottle for 10 seconds before administering dose. Use oral dosing dispenser to measure dose. May give with or without food.

Transdermal

• Avoid placing the patch on the waistline or where tight clothing may rub it off. If possible, alternate sides of the body daily.

ACTION

Releases nerve terminal stores of norepinephrine, promoting nerve impulse transmission. At high doses, effects are mediated by dopamine.

Route	Onset	Peak	Duration
P.O. (Methylin, Ritalin)	Unknown	2 hr	Unknown
P.O. (Methylin ER, Ritalin-SR)	Unknown	5 hr	8 hr
P.O. (Metadate CD)	Unknown	1½ hr; 4½ hr	Unknown
P.O. (Ritalin LA)	Unknown	1–3 hr; 4–7 hr	Unknown
P.O. (Concerta)	Unknown	6–8 hr	Unknown
P.O. (Quillivant XR)	Unknown	5 hr	Unknown
Transdermal	2 hr	Variable	14 hr

Half-life: Conventional, 3 to 6 hours; extended-release (Metadate ER, Methylin ER, Ritalin-SR), 3 to 8 hours, (Concerta, Metadate CD, Ritalin LA), 8 to 12 hours; (Quillivant XR), 6 hours; transdermal, 3 to 4 hours.

ADVERSE REACTIONS

CNS: nervousness, headache, insomnia, *seizures,* tics, dizziness, akathisia, dyskinesia, drowsiness, mood swings.
CV: palpitations, tachycardia, *arrhythmias,* hypertension.
EENT: pharyngitis, sinusitis.
GI: nausea, abdominal pain, anorexia, decreased appetite, vomiting.
Hematologic: *thrombocytopenia, thrombocytopenic purpura, leukopenia,* anemia.
Metabolic: weight loss.
Respiratory: cough, upper respiratory tract infection.
Skin: exfoliative dermatitis, *erythema multiforme,* rash, urticaria, application-site irritation (redness, swelling, papules).
Other: viral infection.

INTERACTIONS

Drug-drug. *Anticonvulsants (such as phenobarbital, phenytoin, primidone), SSRIs, TCAs (imipramine, clomipramine, desipramine), warfarin:* May increase levels of these drugs. Monitor patient for adverse reactions, and decrease dose of these drugs as needed. Monitor drug levels (or coagulation times if patient is also taking warfarin).
Centrally acting alpha$_2$ agonists, clonidine: May cause serious adverse events. Avoid using together.
Centrally acting antihypertensives: May decrease antihypertensive effect. Monitor blood pressure.
MAO inhibitors: May cause severe hypertension or hypertensive crisis. Avoid using within 14 days of MAO inhibitor therapy.
Drug-food. *Caffeine:* May increase amphetamine and related amine effects. Discourage use together.

EFFECTS ON LAB TEST RESULTS

• May decrease hemoglobin level and hematocrit.
• May decrease platelet and WBC counts.

CONTRAINDICATIONS & CAUTIONS

• Contraindicated in patients hypersensitive to drug and in those with glaucoma, motor tics, family history or diagnosis of Tourette syndrome, or history of marked anxiety, tension, or agitation. Also contraindicated within 14 days of MAO inhibitor therapy. Avoid use in patients with structural cardiac abnormalities.
• Because it doesn't dissolve, Concerta isn't recommended in patients with a history of peritonitis or with severe GI narrowing (such as small-bowel inflammatory disease, short-gut syndrome caused by adhesions or decreased transit time, cystic fibrosis, chronic intestinal pseudoobstruction, or Meckel diverticulum).
• Use cautiously in patients with a history of emotional disorder, seizures, EEG abnormalities, or hypertension, and in patients whose underlying medical conditions might be compromised by increases in blood pressure or heart rate, such as those with preexisting hypertension, heart failure, recent MI, or hyperthyroidism.

M

Black Box Warning Use cautiously in patients who have a history of drug dependence or alcoholism. Long-term abusive use can lead to tolerance and psychological dependence. Psychotic episodes can occur. Monitor patient for severe depression and the effects of chronic overactivity during drug withdrawal. ■

⚠ *Overdose S&S:* Agitation, cardiac arrhythmias, confusion, seizures, coma, delirium, dryness of mucous membranes, euphoria, flushing, hallucinations, headache, hyperpyrexia, hyperreflexia, hypertension, muscle twitching, mydriasis, palpitations, sweating, tachycardia, tremors, vomiting.

NURSING CONSIDERATIONS

- Chewable tablets contain phenylalanine.
- Don't use drug to prevent fatigue or treat severe depression.
- Drug may trigger Tourette syndrome in children. Monitor patient, especially at start of therapy.
- Observe patient for signs of excessive stimulation. Monitor blood pressure.
- Check CBC, differential, and platelet counts with long-term use, particularly if patient shows signs or symptoms of hematologic toxicity (fever, sore throat, easy bruising).
- Monitor height and weight in children on long-term therapy. Drug may delay growth spurt, but children will attain normal height when drug is stopped.
- Monitor patient for tolerance or psychological dependence.
- Carefully observe patient for digital changes because stimulants used to treat ADHD are associated with peripheral vasculopathy, including Raynaud phenomenon.
- *Look alike–sound alike:* Don't confuse methylphenidate with methadone. Don't confuse Ritalin with ritodrine or Rifadin. Don't confuse Ritalin SR with Ritalin LA.

PATIENT TEACHING

- Tell patient or caregiver to give drug 30 to 45 minutes before meals and to give last daily dose at least 6 hours before bedtime to prevent insomnia.
- Warn patient against chewing sustained-release tablets.
- Metadate CD or Ritalin LA may be swallowed whole, or the contents of the capsule may be sprinkled onto a small amount of cool applesauce and taken immediately.
- 🜋 *Alert:* Warn patient to take chewable tablet with at least 8 oz (240 mL) of water. Not using enough water to swallow tablet may cause the tablet to swell and block the throat, causing choking.
- Caution patient to avoid activities that require alertness or good psychomotor coordination until CNS effects of drug are known.
- Warn patient with seizure disorder that drug may decrease seizure threshold. Urge him to notify prescriber if seizure occurs.
- Advise patient to avoid beverages containing caffeine while taking drug.
- Teach parent to always use oral dosing dispenser to measure oral suspension dose.
- Tell parent to apply patch in morning immediately after opening; don't use if pouch seal is broken. Press firmly in place for about 30 seconds using the palm of your hand, being sure there is good contact with the skin, especially around the edges. Once the patch has been applied correctly, the child may shower, bathe, or swim as usual.
- Inform parent that, if patch comes off, a new one may be applied on a different site, but the total wear time for that day should be 9 hours. Upon removal, fold patch in half so the sticky sides adhere to itself, then flush down toilet or dispose of in a lidded container.
- If the applied patch is missing, have parent ask the child when or how the patch came off. Teach child that patch shouldn't be shared or removed except by parent or health care provider.
- Encourage parent to use the application chart provided with patch carton to keep track of application and removal.
- Tell parent to remove patch sooner than 9 hours if the child has decreased evening appetite or has difficulty sleeping.
- Tell parent the effects of the patch lasts for several hours after its removal.
- Warn parent and patient to avoid exposing patch to direct external heat sources, such as heating pads, electric blankets, and heated water beds.
- Tell parent to notify prescriber if the child develops bumps, swelling, or blistering at the application site or is experiencing blurred vision or other serious side effects.

methylPREDNISolone
meth-ill-pred-NISS-oh-lone

Medrol🖋

methylPREDNISolone acetate
Depo-Medrol

methylPREDNISolone sodium succinate
Solu-Medrol

Therapeutic class: Corticosteroids
Pharmacologic class: Glucocorticoids
Pregnancy risk category: C

AVAILABLE FORMS
methylprednisolone
Tablets: 4 mg, 8 mg, 16 mg, 32 mg
methylprednisolone acetate
Injection (suspension): 20 mg/mL,
40 mg/mL, 80 mg/mL
methylprednisolone sodium succinate
Injection: 40-mg vial, 125-mg vial, 500-mg
vial, 1,000-mg vial, 2,000-mg vial

INDICATIONS & DOSAGES
➤ **Severe inflammation or immunosuppression**
Adults and children: 4 to 48 mg P.O. daily
depending on the disease treated. After
favorable response is noted, determine
maintenance dosage by decreasing dosage
until lowest dosage that will maintain adequate clinical response is achieved. Or,
10 to 80 mg acetate I.M. daily, or 10 to
40 mg succinate I.M. or I.V., with subsequent doses dictated by patient's clinical
response and condition. Or, 4 to 40 mg
acetate into smaller joints or 20 to 80 mg
acetate into larger joints. Intralesional use is
usually 20 to 60 mg acetate. Repeat intralesional and intra-articular injections every
1 to 5 weeks.
Children: Not less than 0.5 mg/kg I.M.
every 24 hours.
➤ **Shock unresponsive to conventional therapy if adrenocortical insufficiency is suspected**
Adults: 100 to 250 mg succinate I.V. every
2 to 6 hours. Give over 3 to 15 minutes.
Continue therapy for 2 to 3 days or until
patient is stable. Or, 30 mg/kg I.V. initially

over at least 30 minutes; repeat every 4 to
6 hours for 48 hours as needed.

ADMINISTRATION
P.O.
● Give drug with milk or food when
possible. Critically ill patients may need
to take drug with an antacid or H_2-receptor
antagonist.
I.V.
▼ Use only methylprednisolone sodium
succinate, never the acetate form.
▼ Reconstitute according to manufacturer's
directions using supplied diluent, or use
bacteriostatic water for injection with
benzyl alcohol.
▼ Compatible solutions include D_5W,
normal saline solution, and dextrose 5% in
normal saline solution.
▼ For direct injection, inject diluted drug
into vein or free-flowing compatible I.V.
solution over at least 1 minute.
▼ For I.V. infusion, dilute solution according to manufacturer's instructions and give
over prescribed duration.
▼ For doses greater than 0.5 g, give I.V.
over at least 10 minutes to prevent arrhythmias and circulatory collapse. Recommended infusion rate is giving over at least
30 minutes.
▼ Discard reconstituted solution after
48 hours.
▼ **Incompatibilities:** Allopurinol, aminophylline, calcium gluconate, ciprofloxacin,
cytarabine, diltiazem, docetaxel, doxapram, etoposide, filgrastim, gemcitabine,
glycopyrrolate, nafcillin, ondansetron,
paclitaxel, penicillin G sodium, potassium chloride, propofol, sargramostim,
vinorelbine, vitamin B complex with C.
I.M.
● Give injection deeply into gluteal muscle.
Avoid subcutaneous injection because
atrophy and sterile abscesses may occur.
● Dermal atrophy may occur with large
doses of acetate form. Use several small
injections rather than a single large dose,
and rotate injection sites.

ACTION
Not clearly defined. Decreases inflammation, mainly by stabilizing leukocyte
lysosomal membranes; suppresses immune

M

response; stimulates bone marrow; and influences protein, fat, and carbohydrate metabolism.

Route	Onset	Peak	Duration
P.O.	Rapid	2–3 hr	30–36 hr
I.V.	Rapid	Immediate	1 wk
I.M.	6–48 hr	4–8 days	4–8 days
Intra-articular	Rapid	7 days	1–5 wk

Half-life: 18 to 36 hours.

ADVERSE REACTIONS

CNS: euphoria, insomnia, psychotic behavior, *pseudotumor cerebri,* vertigo, headache, paresthesia, *seizures.*
CV: *arrhythmias, heart failure,* hypertension, edema, thrombophlebitis, *thromboembolism, cardiac arrest, circulatory collapse after rapid use of large I.V. dose.*
EENT: cataracts, glaucoma, increased intraocular pressure.
GI: peptic ulceration, GI irritation, increased appetite, *pancreatitis,* nausea, vomiting.
GU: menstrual irregularities.
Metabolic: hypokalemia, hyperglycemia, sodium and water retention, carbohydrate intolerance, hypercholesterolemia, hypocalcemia.
Musculoskeletal: growth suppression in children, muscle weakness, osteoporosis.
Skin: hirsutism, delayed wound healing, acne, various skin eruptions.
Other: cushingoid state, susceptibility to infections, *acute adrenal insufficiency after increased stress or abrupt withdrawal after long-term therapy.*

INTERACTIONS

Drug-drug. *Aspirin, indomethacin, other NSAIDs:* May increase risk of GI distress and bleeding. Use together cautiously.
Barbiturates, carbamazepine, phenytoin, rifampin: May decrease corticosteroid effect. Increase corticosteroid dosage.
Cyclosporine: May increase toxicity. Monitor patient closely.
Ketoconazole and macrolide antibiotics: May decrease methylprednisolone clearance. Decreased dose may be required.
Oral anticoagulants: May alter dosage requirements. Monitor PT and INR closely.

Potassium-depleting drugs such as thiazide diuretics: May enhance potassium-wasting effects of methylprednisolone. Monitor potassium level.
Salicylates: May decrease salicylate levels. Monitor patient for lack of salicylate effectiveness.
Skin-test antigens: May decrease response. Postpone skin testing until after therapy.
Toxoids, vaccines: May decrease antibody response and may increase risk of neurologic complications. Avoid using together.
Drug-herb. *Echinacea:* May increase immune-stimulating effects. Discourage use together.
Ginseng: May increase immune-regulating response. Discourage use together.

EFFECTS ON LAB TEST RESULTS

● May increase glucose and cholesterol levels and ALT, AST, alkaline phosphatase, and urine calcium levels.
● May decrease T_3, T_4, potassium, and calcium levels.
● May decrease ^{131}I uptake and protein-bound iodine levels in thyroid function tests. May cause false-negative results in nitroblue tetrazolium test for systemic bacterial infections. May alter reactions to skin tests.

CONTRAINDICATIONS & CAUTIONS

● Contraindicated in patients hypersensitive to drug or its ingredients, in those with systemic fungal infections, in premature infants (acetate and succinate), and in patients receiving immunosuppressive doses together with live-virus vaccines.
● Use cautiously in patients with GI ulceration or renal disease, hypertension, osteoporosis, diabetes mellitus, hypothyroidism, cirrhosis, diverticulitis, nonspecific ulcerative colitis, recent intestinal anastomoses, thromboembolic disorders, seizures, active hepatitis, myasthenia gravis, heart failure, tuberculosis, ocular herpes simplex, emotional instability, and psychotic tendencies or in breast-feeding women.

NURSING CONSIDERATIONS

● Medrol may contain tartrazine. Watch for allergic reaction to tartrazine in patients with sensitivity to aspirin.

Reactions in bold italics are *life-threatening*. Interactions may have a *rapid onset* or a *delayed onset*.

• Drug may be used for alternate-day therapy.

• Most adverse reactions to corticosteroids are dose- or duration-dependent. For better results and less toxicity, give a once-daily dose in the morning.

⊙ *Alert:* Different salts aren't interchangeable.

⊙ *Alert:* Don't give Solu-Medrol intrathecally because severe adverse reactions may occur.

• If immediate onset of action is needed, don't use acetate form.

• Always adjust to lowest effective dose.

• Monitor patient's weight, blood pressure, electrolyte level, and sleep patterns. Euphoria may initially interfere with sleep, but patients typically adjust to therapy in 1 to 3 weeks.

• Monitor patient for cushingoid effects, including moon face, buffalo hump, central obesity, thinning hair, hypertension, and increased susceptibility to infection.

• Measure growth and development periodically in children during high-dose or prolonged treatment.

• Drug may mask or worsen infections, including latent amebiasis.

• Watch for depression or psychotic episodes, especially in high-dose therapy.

• Diabetic patient may need increased insulin; monitor glucose level.

• Watch for an enhanced response to drug in patients with hypothyroidism or cirrhosis.

• Unless contraindicated, give low-sodium diet that's high in potassium and protein. Give potassium supplements as needed.

• Elderly patients may be more susceptible to osteoporosis with prolonged use.

• Taper off dosage after long-term therapy.

• *Look alike–sound alike:* Don't confuse Solu-Medrol with Solu-Cortef. Don't confuse methylprednisolone with medroxyprogesterone or methyltestosterone.

PATIENT TEACHING

• Tell patient not to stop drug abruptly or without prescriber's consent.

• Instruct patient to take oral form of drug with milk or food.

• Teach patient signs and symptoms of early adrenal insufficiency: fatigue, muscle weakness, joint pain, fever, anorexia, nausea, shortness of breath, dizziness, and fainting.

• Instruct patient to carry or wear medical identification indicating his need for supplemental systemic glucocorticoids during stress. This card should contain prescriber's name, name of drug, and dosage taken.

• Warn patient on long-term therapy about cushingoid effects (moon face, buffalo hump) and the need to notify prescriber about sudden weight gain or swelling.

• Advise patient receiving long-term therapy to consider exercise or physical therapy. Also, tell patient to ask prescriber about vitamin D or calcium supplement.

• Instruct patient to avoid exposure to infections (such as chickenpox or measles) and to contact prescriber if such exposure occurs.

methylTESTOSTERone
meth-ill-tes-TOSS-ter-own

Android, Testred

Therapeutic class: Androgens
Pharmacologic class: Androgens
Pregnancy risk category: X
Controlled substance schedule: III

M

AVAILABLE FORMS
Capsules: 10 mg
Tablets: 10 mg, 25 mg

INDICATIONS & DOSAGES
➤ **Metastatic breast cancer**
Women 1 to 5 years after menopause: 50 to 200 mg P.O. daily.
➤ **Hypogonadism**
Men: 10 to 50 mg P.O. daily.

ADMINISTRATION
P.O.
• Give without regard for food.

ACTION
Stimulates target tissues to develop normally in androgen-deficient men. May have some antiestrogen properties, making it useful in treating certain estrogen-dependent breast cancers.

Route	Onset	Peak	Duration
P.O.	Unknown	2 hr	Unknown

Half-life: Varies from 10 to 100 minutes.

ADVERSE REACTIONS
CNS: headache, anxiety, depression, paresthesia.
CV: edema.
GI: irritation of oral mucosa with buccal administration, nausea.
GU: oligospermia, decreased ejaculatory volume, priapism, amenorrhea.
Hematologic: *suppression of clotting factors,* polycythemia.
Hepatic: reversible jaundice, *cholestatic hepatitis.*
Metabolic: hypernatremia, *hyperkalemia,* hyperphosphatemia, hypercholesterolemia, hypercalcemia.
Musculoskeletal: muscle cramps or spasms.
Skin: hypersensitivity reactions, acne.
Other: androgenic effects in women, altered libido, gynecomastia, hypoestrogenic effects in women, excessive hormonal effects in men, male pattern baldness.

INTERACTIONS
Drug-drug. *Cyclosporine:* May increase cyclosporine toxicity. Monitor cyclosporine levels.
Hepatotoxic drugs: May increase risk of hepatotoxicity. Monitor liver function closely.
Insulin, oral antidiabetics: May decrease glucose level; may alter dosage requirements. Monitor glucose level in diabetic patients.
Oral anticoagulants: May increase sensitivity to oral anticoagulants; may alter dosage requirements. Monitor PT and INR.

EFFECTS ON LAB TEST RESULTS
• May increase sodium, potassium, phosphate, liver enzyme, lipid, and calcium levels. May decrease thyroxine-binding globulin and total T_4 levels.
• May increase RBC count and resin uptake of T_3 and T_4.

CONTRAINDICATIONS & CAUTIONS
• Contraindicated in pregnant or breast-feeding women and in men with breast or prostate cancer.
• Use cautiously in elderly patients; patients with cardiac, renal, or hepatic disease; and healthy males with delayed puberty.
⚠ *Overdose S&S:* Nausea, edema.

NURSING CONSIDERATIONS
• Don't give to women of childbearing age until pregnancy is ruled out. Use during pregnancy may cause virilization of the female fetus.
• In children, obtain X-rays of wrist bones before therapy begins to establish bone maturation level. During treatment, bones may mature more rapidly than they grow in length. Periodically review X-rays to monitor bone maturation.
• Drug is typically used only for intermittent therapy. Because of potential hepatotoxicity, watch closely for jaundice.
• Promptly report evidence of virilization in women, such as deepening of the voice, increased hair growth, acne, or baldness.
• Watch for hypoestrogenic effects in women (flushing, diaphoresis, vaginal bleeding, nervousness, emotional lability, menstrual irregularities, and vaginitis, including itching, dryness, and burning).
• Watch for excessive hormonal effects in men. If patient is prepubertal, watch for premature epiphyseal closure, acne, priapism, growth of body and facial hair, and phallic enlargement. If he's postpubertal, watch for testicular atrophy, oligospermia, decreased ejaculatory volume, impotence, gynecomastia, and epididymitis.
• Unless contraindicated, use with high-calorie, high-protein diet. Give small, frequent meals.
• Periodically check cholesterol, calcium, and hemoglobin levels, hematocrit, and cardiac and LFT results.
• Check weight regularly. Control edema with sodium restriction or diuretics.
⚠ *Alert:* In breast cancer, therapeutic response usually occurs within 3 months. If disease appears to progress, stop drug.
• Report signs of hypercalcemia. In metastatic breast cancer, hypercalcemia may indicate progression of bone metastases.

Reactions in bold italics are *life-threatening*. Interactions may have a *rapid onset* or a *delayed onset*.

• Evaluate semen every 3 to 4 months, especially in adolescent boys.

⊗ Alert: Don't use to enhance athletic performance or physique.

• **Look alike–sound alike:** Testosterone and methyltestosterone aren't interchangeable. Don't confuse methyltestosterone with medroxyprogesterone.

PATIENT TEACHING
• Make sure patient understands importance of using effective contraception during therapy.
• Tell women of childbearing age to report menstrual irregularities and to stop drug while awaiting examination.
• Instruct patient to stop drug immediately and notify prescriber if pregnancy is suspected.
• Tell women to immediately report evidence of virilization, such as acne, swelling, weight gain, increased hair growth, hoarseness, clitoral enlargement, decreased breast size, deepening of voice, changes in libido, male pattern baldness, and oily skin or hair.
• Teach patient signs and symptoms of low glucose level (hypoglycemia) and method for checking glucose level; drug enhances hypoglycemia. Instruct patient to report signs or symptoms of hypoglycemia immediately.
• Advise women to wear cotton underwear and to wash after intercourse to decrease risk of vaginitis.

---

metoclopramide hydrochloride
met-oh-KLOE-pra-mide

Apo-Metoclop†, Metozolv ODT, Reglan

Therapeutic class: Antiemetics
Pharmacologic class: Dopamine antagonists
Pregnancy risk category: B

AVAILABLE FORMS
Injection: 5 mg/mL
Syrup: 5 mg/5 mL
Tablets: 5 mg, 10 mg
Tablets (orally disintegrating): 5 mg, 10 mg

INDICATIONS & DOSAGES
Adjust-a-dose (for all indications): For patients with CrCl below 40 mL/minute, decrease dosage by half.

➤ **To prevent or reduce nausea and vomiting from emetogenic cancer chemotherapy**
Adults: 1 to 2 mg/kg I.V. 30 minutes before chemotherapy; repeat every 2 hours for two doses, then every 3 hours for three doses.

➤ **To prevent or reduce postoperative nausea and vomiting**
Adults: 10 to 20 mg I.M. near end of surgical procedure; repeat every 4 to 6 hours, as needed.

➤ **To facilitate small-bowel intubation, to aid in radiologic examinations**
Adults and children older than age 14: 10 mg I.V. as a single dose over 1 to 2 minutes.
Children ages 6 to 14: 2.5 to 5 mg I.V. slowly over 1 to 2 minutes.
Children younger than age 6: 0.1 mg/kg I.V. slowly over 1 to 2 minutes.

➤ **Delayed gastric emptying secondary to diabetic gastroparesis**
Adults: 10 mg P.O. 30 minutes before each meal and at bedtime for mild symptoms. Or, give 10 mg by slow I.V. infusion over 1 to 2 minutes 30 minutes before each meal and at bedtime for up to 10 days for severe symptoms; then P.O. dose may be started and continued for 2 to 8 weeks.

➤ **GERD**
Adults: 10 to 15 mg P.O. q.i.d., as needed, 30 minutes before meals and at bedtime.

➤ **Gastroparesis ♦**
Adults: 10 to 20 mg P.O. 30 minutes before meals and at bedtime for up to 8 weeks.

➤ **Prevention or treatment of hiccups ♦**
Adults: 10 mg P.O. every 6 to 8 hours starting day of or 1 day before anticipated hiccup-precipitating event. For treatment, 10 mg P.O. every 6 to 8 hours. Initially, therapy may begin as 5 to 10 mg I.V. or I.M. every 8 hours and transition to oral dosing when hiccups are controlled. Usual treatment continues until drug can be stopped without provoking a recurrence.

M

ADMINISTRATION

P.O.
● Give drug before each meal and at bedtime.

P.O. (orally disintegrating tablet [ODT])
● Give drug at least 30 minutes before eating and at bedtime.
● Give immediately after opening sealed blister. If the tablet breaks or crumbles, throw it away and obtain a new one.
● Place tablet on patient's tongue. Tell him to let it melt and then swallow.

I.V.
▼ Drug is compatible with D₅W, normal saline solution for injection, dextrose 5% in half-normal saline solution, Ringer injection, and lactated Ringer injection. Normal saline solution is the preferred diluent; drug is most stable in this solution.
▼ Give doses of 10 mg or less by direct injection over 1 to 2 minutes. Dilute doses larger than 10 mg in 50 mL of compatible diluent, and infuse over at least 15 minutes. Monitor blood pressure closely.
▼ No need to protect drug from light if infusion mixture is given within 24 hours. If protected from light and refrigerated, it's stable for 48 hours.
▼ **Incompatibilities:** Allopurinol, ampicillin, amphotericin B, calcium gluconate, cefepime, chloramphenicol sodium succinate, cisplatin, doxorubicin liposomal, erythromycin lactobionate, 5-FU, furosemide, methotrexate sodium, penicillin G potassium, propofol, sodium bicarbonate.

I.M.
● Inspect for particulate matter and discoloration. If either is present, don't use.

ACTION

Stimulates motility of upper GI tract, increases lower esophageal sphincter tone, and blocks dopamine receptors at the chemoreceptor trigger zone.

Route	Onset	Peak	Duration
P.O.	30–60 min	1–2 hr	1–2 hr
I.V.	1–3 min	Unknown	1–2 hr
I.M.	10–15 min	Unknown	1–2 hr

Half-life: 4 to 6 hours.

ADVERSE REACTIONS

CNS: anxiety, drowsiness, dystonic reactions, fatigue, lassitude, restlessness, *neuroleptic malignant syndrome, seizures, suicidal ideation,* akathisia, confusion, depression, dizziness, extrapyramidal symptoms, fever, hallucinations, headache, insomnia, tardive dyskinesia.
CV: *bradycardia, supraventricular tachycardia,* hypotension, transient hypertension.
GI: bowel disorders, diarrhea, nausea.
GU: incontinence, urinary frequency.
Hematologic: *agranulocytosis, neutropenia.*
Skin: rash, urticaria.
Other: loss of libido, prolactin secretion.

INTERACTIONS

Drug-drug. *Anticholinergics, opioid analgesics:* May antagonize GI motility effects of metoclopramide. Use together cautiously.
CNS depressants: May cause additive CNS effects. Avoid using together.
Levodopa: Levodopa and metoclopramide have opposite effects on dopamine receptors. Avoid using together.
MAO inhibitors: May increase release of catecholamines in patients with hypertension. Use together cautiously.
Phenothiazines: May increase risk of extrapyramidal effects. Monitor patient closely.
Drug-lifestyle. *Alcohol use:* May cause additive CNS effects. Discourage use together.

EFFECTS ON LAB TEST RESULTS

● May increase LFT values, aldosterone levels, and prolactin levels.
● May decrease neutrophil and granulocyte counts.

CONTRAINDICATIONS & CAUTIONS

● Contraindicated in patients hypersensitive to drug and in those with pheochromocytoma, tardive dyskinesia, or seizure disorders.
● Contraindicated in patients for whom stimulation of GI motility might be dangerous (those with hemorrhage, obstruction, or perforation).

Reactions in bold italics are *life-threatening*. Interactions may have a *rapid onset* or a *delayed onset*.

Black Box Warning Long-term or high-dose drug use has been linked to possibly irreversible tardive dyskinesia, even after the drug was stopped, especially in older, female, and diabetic patients. Discontinue drug if signs and symptoms occur. Except in rare cases, avoid treatment for longer than 12 weeks. ∎

❸ Alert: Neuroleptic malignant syndrome has occurred rarely. If signs and symptoms develop (fever, CNS symptoms, irregular pulse, cardiac arrhythmias, or abnormal blood pressure), discontinue drug.

• Use cautiously in patients with history of depression, Parkinson disease, or hypertension.

⚠ Overdose S&S: Drowsiness, disorientation, extrapyramidal reactions; seizures, lethargy (in infants and children).

NURSING CONSIDERATIONS
• Monitor bowel sounds.
• Safety and effectiveness of drug haven't been established for therapy lasting longer than 12 weeks.
• Metozolv ODT contains acesulfame K and mannitol.

Black Box Warning Discontinue drug if signs and symptoms of tardive dyskinesia develop. Avoid treatment for longer than 12 weeks except in rare cases in which therapeutic benefit is thought to outweigh risk of tardive dyskinesia. ∎

• Monitor patient for involuntary movements of face, tongue, and extremities, which may indicate tardive dyskinesia.
• Monitor patient for fever, CNS symptoms, irregular pulse, cardiac arrhythmias, or abnormal blood pressure, which may indicate neuroleptic malignant syndrome.
• Monitor patient for dizziness, headache, or nervousness after metoclopramide is stopped; these may indicate withdrawal.
❸ Alert: Use 50 mg diphenhydramine I.M. or benztropine 1 to 2 mg I.M. to counteract extrapyramidal adverse effects from high doses.

PATIENT TEACHING
• Instruct patient to take ODTs 30 minutes before food and at bedtime and not to repeat dose if inadvertently taken with food.

• Tell patient taking ODTs to open blister pack with dry hands and immediately place tablet on tongue, let it melt completely, and then swallow. (Taking it with water isn't necessary.) If tablet breaks or crumbles, advise patient to throw it away and take a new tablet out of the blister pack.
• Tell patient to avoid activities that require alertness for 2 hours after doses.
• Urge patient to report persistent or serious adverse reactions promptly.
• Advise patient not to drink alcohol during therapy.
• Teach patient signs and symptoms of tardive dyskinesia and neuroleptic malignant syndrome and to report any signs and symptoms that develop.

metolazone
me TOLE-a-zone

Zaroxolyn

Therapeutic class: Diuretics
Pharmacologic class: Thiazide-like diuretics
Pregnancy risk category: B

M

AVAILABLE FORMS
Tablets: 2.5 mg, 5 mg, 10 mg

INDICATIONS & DOSAGES
➤ **Edema in heart failure or renal disease**
Adults: 5 to 20 mg P.O. once daily.
➤ **Hypertension**
Adults: 2.5 to 5 mg P.O. once daily. Base maintenance dosage on blood pressure.

ADMINISTRATION
P.O.
• Give drug without regard for meals.
• To prevent nocturia, give drug in the morning.
❸ Alert: Don't interchange Zaroxolyn tablets and other formulations of metolazone that share its slow and incomplete bioavailability.

ACTION
Increases sodium and water excretion by inhibiting sodium reabsorption in ascending loop of Henle.

Route	Onset	Peak	Duration
P.O.	1 hr	2–8 hr	12–24 hr

Half-life: About 14 hours.

ADVERSE REACTIONS

CNS: dizziness, headache, fatigue, vertigo, paresthesia, weakness, restlessness, drowsiness, anxiety, depression, nervousness, blurred vision.

CV: orthostatic hypotension, palpitations, chest pain, venous thrombosis.

GI: *pancreatitis,* anorexia, nausea, epigastric distress, vomiting, abdominal pain, diarrhea, constipation, dry mouth.

GU: nocturia, polyuria, impotence.

Hematologic: *aplastic anemia, agranulocytosis, leukopenia,* purpura.

Hepatic: jaundice, *hepatitis.*

Metabolic: hyperglycemia and impaired glucose tolerance; fluid and electrolyte imbalances, including hypokalemia, hypomagnesemia, dilutional hyponatremia and hypochloremia, metabolic alkalosis, and hypercalcemia; volume depletion and dehydration.

Musculoskeletal: muscle cramps.

Skin: dermatitis, photosensitivity reactions, rash, pruritus, urticaria.

INTERACTIONS

Drug-drug. *Amphotericin B, corticosteroids:* May increase risk of hypokalemia. Monitor potassium level closely.

Anticoagulants: May decrease anticoagulant response. Monitor PT and INR.

Antidiabetics: May alter glucose level and require dosage adjustment of antidiabetics. Monitor glucose level.

Barbiturates, opioids: May increase orthostatic hypotensive effect. Monitor patient closely.

Bumetanide, ethacrynic acid, furosemide, torsemide: May cause excessive diuretic response, causing serious electrolyte abnormalities or dehydration. Adjust doses carefully, and monitor patient closely for signs and symptoms of excessive diuretic response.

Cardiac glycosides: May increase risk of digoxin toxicity from metolazone-induced hypokalemia. Monitor potassium and digoxin levels.

Cholestyramine, colestipol: May decrease intestinal absorption of thiazides. Separate doses.

Diazoxide: May increase antihypertensive, hyperglycemic, and hyperuricemic effects. Use together cautiously.

Lithium: May decrease lithium clearance, increasing risk of lithium toxicity. Monitor lithium level.

NSAIDs: May increase risk of renal failure. May decrease diuretic and antihypertensive effects. Monitor renal function and blood pressure.

Other antihypertensives: May have additive effects. Use together cautiously.

Drug-herb. *Dandelion:* May interfere with diuretic activity. Discourage use together.

Licorice: May cause unexpected rapid potassium loss. Discourage use together.

Drug-lifestyle. *Alcohol use:* May increase orthostatic hypotensive effect. Discourage use together.

Sun exposure: May increase risk for photosensitivity reaction. Advise patient to avoid excessive sunlight exposure.

EFFECTS ON LAB TEST RESULTS

● May increase glucose, calcium, cholesterol, and triglyceride levels. May decrease potassium, sodium, magnesium, chloride, and hemoglobin levels.

● May decrease granulocyte and WBC counts.

CONTRAINDICATIONS & CAUTIONS

● Contraindicated in patients hypersensitive to thiazides or other sulfonamide-derived drugs and in those with anuria, hepatic coma, or precoma.

● Use cautiously in patients with impaired renal or hepatic function.

⚠ *Overdose S&S:* Orthostatic hypotension, dizziness, drowsiness, lethargy, syncope, CNS depression, electrolyte abnormalities, hemoconcentration, depressed respirations, GI irritation and hypermotility.

NURSING CONSIDERATIONS

● Monitor fluid intake and output, weight, blood pressure, and electrolyte levels.

● Watch for signs and symptoms of hypokalemia, such as muscle weakness and

---

Reactions in bold italics are *life-threatening*. Interactions may have a *rapid onset* or a *delayed onset*.

cramps. Drug may be used with potassium-sparing diuretic to prevent potassium loss.
• Consult dietitian about a high-potassium diet. Foods rich in potassium include citrus fruits, tomatoes, bananas, dates, and apricots.
• Monitor glucose level, especially in diabetic patients.
• Monitor uric acid level, especially in patients with history of gout.
• Monitor elderly patients, who are especially susceptible to excessive diuresis.
• In hypertensive patients, therapeutic response may be delayed several weeks.
• Monitor blood pressure. If response is inadequate, another antihypertensive may be added.
• Metolazone and furosemide may be used together to enhance diuretic effect.
• Unlike thiazide diuretics, metolazone is effective in patients with decreased renal function.
• Stop thiazides and thiazide-like diuretics before parathyroid function tests.
• *Look alike–sound alike:* Don't confuse Zaroxolyn with Zarontin.

PATIENT TEACHING
• Tell patient to take drug in morning to prevent need to urinate at night.
• Advise patient to avoid sudden posture changes and to rise slowly to avoid effects of dizziness upon standing quickly.
• Instruct patient to use a sunblock to prevent photosensitivity reactions.
• Instruct patient to increase dietary intake of potassium-containing foods.

metoprolol succinate
meh-TOH-pruh-lol

Toprol-XL✐

metoprolol tartrate
Betaloc†, Lopresor†, Lopresor SR†, Lopressor✐

Therapeutic class: Antihypertensives
Pharmacologic class: Selective beta-adrenergic blockers
Pregnancy risk category: C

AVAILABLE FORMS
metoprolol succinate
Tablets (extended-release): 25 mg, 50 mg, 100 mg, 200 mg
metoprolol tartrate
Injection: 1 mg/mL in 5-mL ampules
Tablets: 25 mg, 50 mg, 100 mg
Tablets (extended-release): 100 mg†, 200 mg†

INDICATIONS & DOSAGES
➤ **Hypertension**
Adults: Initially, 50 mg P.O. b.i.d. or 100 mg P.O. once daily; then up to 100 to 450 mg daily in two or three divided doses. Or, 50 to 100 mg extended-release tablets (tartrate equivalent) P.O. once daily. Adjust dosage as needed and tolerated at intervals of not less than 1 week to maximum of 400 mg daily.
Children ages 6 to 16: 1 mg/kg P.O. once daily, not to exceed 50 mg P.O. once daily.
➤ **Early intervention in acute MI**
Adults: 5 mg metoprolol tartrate I.V. bolus every 2 minutes for three doses. Then, starting 15 minutes after the last I.V. dose, 25 to 50 mg P.O. every 6 hours for 48 hours. Maintenance dosage is 100 mg P.O. b.i.d.
➤ **Angina pectoris**
Adults: Initially, 100 mg P.O. daily as a single dose or in two equally divided doses; increased at weekly intervals until an adequate response or a pronounced decrease in heart rate is seen. Effects of daily dose beyond 400 mg aren't known. Or, 100 mg extended-release tablets (tartrate equivalent) once daily. Adjust dosage as needed and tolerated at intervals of not less than 1 week to maximum of 400 mg daily.

M

➤ **Stable symptomatic heart failure (New York Heart Association class II) resulting from ischemia, hypertension, or cardiomyopathy**
Adults: 25 mg Toprol-XL P.O. once daily for 2 weeks. Double the dose every 2 weeks, as tolerated, to a maximum of 200 mg daily.
Adjust-a-dose: In patients with more severe heart failure, start with 12.5 mg Toprol-XL P.O. once daily for 2 weeks.
➤ **Cardiac risk reduction during surgery ◆**
Adults: Initially, 100 mg P.O. in a single or divided dose started well before planned procedure. Titrate according to heart rate. Continue for 7 to 30 days after procedure.

ADMINISTRATION
P.O.
● Give drug with or immediately after meal.
● Extended-release tablets may be cut in half on scored line, but never crushed or chewed.
I.V.
▼ Give drug undiluted by direct injection.
▼ Although best avoided, drug can be mixed with meperidine hydrochloride or morphine sulfate or given with an alteplase infusion at a Y-site connection.
▼ Store drug at room temperature and protect from light. Discard solution if it's discolored or contains particles.
▼ **Incompatibilities:** Amphotericin B.

ACTION
Unknown. A selective beta blocker that selectively blocks beta$_1$ receptors; decreases cardiac output, peripheral resistance, and cardiac oxygen consumption; and depresses renin secretion.

Route	Onset	Peak	Duration
P.O.	15 min	1 hr	6–12 hr
P.O. (extended-release)	15 min	6–12 hr	24 hr
I.V.	5 min	20 min	5–8 hr

Half-life: 3 to 7 hours.

ADVERSE REACTIONS
CNS: fatigue, dizziness, depression.
CV: hypotension, ***bradycardia, heart failure, AV block,*** edema.
GI: nausea, diarrhea, constipation, heartburn.
Respiratory: dyspnea, wheezing.
Skin: rash.

INTERACTIONS
Drug-drug. *Amobarbital, butabarbital, butalbital, pentobarbital, phenobarbital, primidone, secobarbital:* May reduce metoprolol effect. May need to increase metoprolol dose.
Cardiac glycosides, diltiazem: May cause excessive bradycardia and increased depressant effect on myocardium. Use together cautiously.
Catecholamine-depleting drugs such as MAO inhibitors, reserpine: May have additive effect. Monitor patient for hypotension and bradycardia.
Chlorpromazine: May decrease hepatic clearance. Watch for greater beta-blocking effect.
Cimetidine: May increase metoprolol effects. Monitor patient and adjust metoprolol dose as needed.
Fluoxetine, paroxetine, propafenone, quinidine: May increase metoprolol level. Monitor vital signs.
Hydralazine: May increase levels and effects of both drugs. Monitor patient closely. May need to adjust dosage.
Indomethacin, NSAIDs: May decrease antihypertensive effect. Monitor blood pressure and adjust dosage.
Insulin, oral antidiabetics: May alter dosage requirements in previously stabilized diabetic patients. Monitor patient closely.
I.V. lidocaine: May reduce hepatic metabolism of lidocaine, increasing risk of toxicity. Give bolus doses of lidocaine at a slower rate, and monitor lidocaine level closely.
Prazosin: May increase risk of orthostatic hypotension in the early phases of use together. Assist patient to stand slowly until effects are known.
Rifampin: May increase metoprolol metabolism. Watch for decreased effect.
Terbutaline: May antagonize bronchodilatory effects of terbutaline. Monitor patient.
Verapamil: May increase effects of both drugs. Monitor cardiac function closely, and decrease dosages as needed.

Reactions in bold italics are ***life-threatening***. Interactions may have a *rapid onset* or a ***delayed onset***.

Drug-herb. *Ma huang:* May decrease antihypertensive effects. Discourage use together.

Drug-food. *Any food:* May increase absorption. Encourage patient to take drug with food.

EFFECTS ON LAB TEST RESULTS
● May increase transaminase, alkaline phosphatase, LDH, and uric acid levels.

CONTRAINDICATIONS & CAUTIONS
● Contraindicated in patients hypersensitive to drug or other beta blockers.
● Contraindicated in patients with sinus bradycardia, greater than first-degree heart block, cardiogenic shock, or overt cardiac failure when used to treat hypertension or angina. When used to treat MI, drug is contraindicated in patients with heart rate less than 45 beats/minute, greater than first-degree heart block, PR interval of 0.24 second or longer with first-degree heart block, systolic blood pressure less than 100 mm Hg, or moderate to severe cardiac failure.
● Use cautiously in patients with heart failure, diabetes, or respiratory or hepatic disease.

⚠ **Overdose S&S:** Bradycardia, hypotension, bronchospasm, cardiac failure, cardiac arrest, coma, AV block, nausea, vomiting.

NURSING CONSIDERATIONS
● Always check patient's apical pulse rate before giving drug. If it's slower than 60 beats/minute, withhold drug and call prescriber immediately.
● In diabetic patients, monitor glucose level closely because drug masks common signs and symptoms of hypoglycemia.
● Monitor blood pressure frequently; drug masks common signs and symptoms of shock.
● Beta blockers may mask tachycardia caused by hyperthyroidism. In patients with suspected thyrotoxicosis, taper off beta blocker to avoid thyroid storm.
Black Box Warning When stopping therapy, taper dosage over 1 to 2 weeks. Abrupt discontinuation may cause exacerbations of angina or MI. Don't discontinue

therapy abruptly even in patients treated only for hypertension. ▮
● Beta selectivity is lost at higher doses. Watch for peripheral side effects.
● *Look alike–sound alike:* Don't confuse metoprolol succinate with metoprolol tartrate. Don't confuse metoprolol with metaproterenol, misoprostol, or metolazone. Don't confuse Toprol-XL with Topamax, Tegretol, or Tegretol-XR.

PATIENT TEACHING
● Instruct patient to take drug exactly as prescribed and with meals.
● Caution patient to avoid driving and other tasks requiring mental alertness until response to therapy has been established.
● Advise patient to inform dentist or prescriber about use of this drug before procedures or surgery.
● Tell patient to alert prescriber if shortness of breath occurs.
Black Box Warning Instruct patient not to stop drug suddenly but to notify prescriber about unpleasant adverse reactions. Inform him that drug must be withdrawn gradually over 1 or 2 weeks. ▮
● Inform patient that use isn't advisable in breast-feeding women.

metronidazole (oral; injection)
me-troe-NI-da-zole

Flagyl, Flagyl ER, Novo-Nidazol†

metronidazole hydrochloride
Flagyl IV RTU

Therapeutic class: Antiprotozoals
Pharmacologic class: Nitroimidazoles
Pregnancy risk category: B

AVAILABLE FORMS
Capsules: 375 mg
Injection: 500 mg/100 mL in vials or ready-to-use (RTU) minibags
Tablets: 250 mg, 500 mg
Tablets (extended-release): 750 mg

M

INDICATIONS & DOSAGES

Black Box Warning Use metronidazole only for the conditions for which it's indicated because it may be carcinogenic. Avoid unnecessary use. ∎

➤ **Amebic liver abscess**
Adults: 500 to 750 mg P.O. t.i.d. for 5 to 10 days; or 2.4 g P.O. once daily for 1 to 2 days. Or, 500 mg I.V. every 6 hours for 10 days if patient can't tolerate P.O. route.
Children: 35 to 50 mg/kg daily in three divided doses for 10 days. Maximum, 750 mg/dose.

➤ **Intestinal amebiasis**
Adults: 750 mg P.O. t.i.d. for 5 to 10 days; then treat with a luminal amebicide, such as iodoquinol or paromomycin.
Children: 35 to 50 mg/kg P.O. daily in three divided doses for 10 days; then treat with a luminal amebicide, such as iodoquinol or paromomycin.

➤ **Trichomoniasis**
Adults: 500 mg P.O. b.i.d. for 7 days, or 2 g P.O. in single dose (may give the 2-g dose in two 1-g doses, both on the same day); wait 4 to 6 weeks before repeating course.

➤ **Refractory trichomoniasis**
Adults: 500 mg P.O. b.i.d. for 7 days.

➤ **Bacterial infections caused by anaerobic microorganisms**
Adults: Loading dose is 15 mg/kg I.V. infused over 1 hour. Maintenance dose is 7.5 mg/kg I.V. or P.O. every 6 hours. Give first maintenance dose 6 hours after loading dose. Maximum dose shouldn't exceed 4 g daily.

➤ **To prevent postoperative infection in contaminated or potentially contaminated colorectal surgery**
Adults: Infuse 15 mg/kg I.V. over 30 to 60 minutes and complete about 1 hour before surgery. Then, infuse 7.5 mg/kg I.V. over 30 to 60 minutes at 6 and 12 hours after first dose.

➤ **Bacterial vaginosis**
Adults: 750 mg Flagyl ER P.O. daily for 7 days.

➤ *Clostridium difficile*–associated **diarrhea and colitis** ◆
Adults: Usually 250 mg P.O. q.i.d. or 500 mg P.O. t.i.d. for 10 days. Or, 500 mg to 750 mg I.V. every 6 to 8 hours when P.O. route isn't practical.

➤ **Pelvic inflammatory disease (PID)** ◆
Adults and adolescents: 500 mg P.O. b.i.d. with doxycycline and a third-generation cephalosporin or possibly a fluoroquinolone for 14 days.

ADMINISTRATION
P.O.
● Give tablets and capsules with food if GI upset occurs.
● Give extended-release tablets (750 mg) at least 1 hour before or 2 hours after meals.
I.V.
▼ Flagyl IV RTU minibags need no preparation.
▼ Don't use aluminum needles or hubs to reconstitute the drug or to transfer reconstituted drug. Equipment that contains aluminum will turn the solution orange; the potency isn't affected.
▼ To reconstitute lyophilized vials, add 4.4 mL of sterile water for injection, bacteriostatic water for injection, sterile normal saline solution for injection, or bacteriostatic normal saline solution for injection. Reconstituted drug contains 100 mg/mL. Add contents of vial to 100 mL of D_5W, lactated Ringer injection, or normal saline solution to yield 5 mg/mL. Neutralize this highly acidic solution by carefully adding 5 mEq sodium bicarbonate to each 500 mg; the carbon dioxide gas that forms may need to be vented.
▼ Don't give by I.V. push.
▼ Don't refrigerate the neutralized diluted solution; precipitation may occur. Refrigerated Flagyl IV RTU may form crystals, which disappear after the solution warms to room temperature.
▼ **Incompatibilities:** Aluminum, amino acid 10%, amoxicillin sodium–clavulanate potassium, amphotericin B, aztreonam, ceftriaxone, dopamine, filgrastim, meropenem, other I.V. drugs, warfarin.

ACTION
Direct-acting trichomonicide and amebicide that works inside and outside the intestines. It's thought to enter the cells of microorganisms that contain nitroreductase, forming unstable compounds that bind to

---

DNA and inhibit synthesis, causing cell death.

Route	Onset	Peak	Duration
P.O.	Unknown	2 hr	Unknown
I.V.	Immediate	1 hr	Unknown

Half-life: 6 to 8 hours.

ADVERSE REACTIONS

CNS: headache, *seizures,* fever, vertigo, ataxia, dizziness, syncope, incoordination, confusion, irritability, depression, weakness, insomnia, peripheral neuropathy.
CV: flattened T wave, edema, flushing, thrombophlebitis after I.V. infusion.
EENT: rhinitis, sinusitis, pharyngitis.
GI: nausea, abdominal cramping or pain, stomatitis, epigastric distress, vomiting, anorexia, diarrhea, constipation, proctitis, dry mouth, metallic taste.
GU: vaginitis, darkened urine, polyuria, dysuria, cystitis, dyspareunia, dryness of vagina and vulva, vaginal candidiasis, genital pruritus.
Hematologic: *transient leukopenia, neutropenia.*
Musculoskeletal: transient joint pains.
Respiratory: upper respiratory tract infection.
Skin: rash.
Other: decreased libido, overgrowth of nonsusceptible organisms, especially *Candida.*

INTERACTIONS

Drug-drug. *Busulfan:* May increase busulfan toxicity. Avoid using together.
Cimetidine: May increase risk of metronidazole toxicity because of inhibited hepatic metabolism. Monitor for toxicity.
Disulfiram: May cause acute psychosis and confusion. Avoid giving metronidazole within 2 weeks of disulfiram.
Lithium: May increase lithium level, which may cause toxicity. Monitor lithium level.
Phenobarbital, phenytoin: May decrease metronidazole effectiveness; may reduce total phenytoin clearance. Monitor patient.
Warfarin: May increase anticoagulant effects and risk of bleeding. Reduce warfarin as needed.
Drug-lifestyle. *Alcohol use:* May cause disulfiram-like reaction, including nausea,

vomiting, headache, cramps, and flushing. Warn patient to avoid alcohol during and for 3 days after completing drug therapy.

EFFECTS ON LAB TEST RESULTS

- May decrease WBC and neutrophil counts.
- May falsely decrease triglyceride and aminotransferase levels.

CONTRAINDICATIONS & CAUTIONS

- Contraindicated in patients hypersensitive to drug or other nitroimidazole derivatives and in patients in first trimester of pregnancy.
☉ Alert: If drug must be given to a pregnant woman for trichomoniasis, use the 7-day regimen, not the 2-g single-dose regimen. The 2-g dose produces a high level that's more likely to reach fetal circulation.
- Drug has been shown to be carcinogenic in animal studies. Use only for conditions for which it's indicated.
- Use cautiously in patients with history of blood dyscrasia, CNS disorder, or retinal or visual field changes.
- Use cautiously in patients who take hepatotoxic drugs or have hepatic disease or alcoholism.
⚠ Overdose S&S: Nausea, vomiting, ataxia, neurotoxicity.

NURSING CONSIDERATIONS

- Monitor LFT results carefully in elderly patients.
- Observe patient for edema, especially if he's receiving corticosteroids; Flagyl IV RTU may cause sodium retention.
- Record number and character of stools when drug is used to treat amebiasis. Give drug only after *Trichomonas vaginalis* infection is confirmed by wet smear or culture or *Entamoeba histolytica* is identified.
- Sexual partners of patients being treated for *T. vaginalis* infection, even if asymptomatic, must also be treated to avoid reinfection.
- **Look alike–sound alike:** Don't confuse metronidazole with metformin.

PATIENT TEACHING

- Instruct patient to take extended-release tablets at least 1 hour before or 2 hours after meals but to take all other oral forms with food to minimize GI upset.

M

• Inform patient of need for sexual partners to be treated simultaneously to avoid reinfection.

• Instruct patient in proper hygiene.

• Tell patient to avoid alcohol and alcohol-containing drugs during and for at least 3 days after treatment course.

• Tell patient he may experience a metallic taste and have dark or red-brown urine.

• Tell patient to report to prescriber symptoms of candidal overgrowth.

• Tell patient to report to prescriber immediately any neurologic symptoms (seizures, peripheral neuropathy).

metronidazole (topical; vaginal)
me-troe-NI-da-zole

MetroCream, MetroGel, MetroGel Vaginal, MetroLotion, Noritate, Vandazole

Therapeutic class: Antibacterials (topical)
Pharmacologic class: Nitroimidazoles
Pregnancy risk category: B

AVAILABLE FORMS
Topical cream: 0.75%, 1%
Topical gel: 0.75%, 1%
Topical lotion: 0.75%
Vaginal gel: 0.75%

INDICATIONS & DOSAGES
➤ **Inflammatory papules and pustules of acne rosacea**
Adults: If using a 0.75% preparation, apply thin film to affected area b.i.d., morning and evening. If using a 1% preparation, apply thin film to affected area once daily. After response is seen (usually within 3 weeks), adjust frequency and duration of therapy.
➤ **Bacterial vaginosis**
Adults: One applicatorful vaginally daily or b.i.d. for 5 days. For once-daily use, give at bedtime.

ADMINISTRATION
Topical
• Clean area thoroughly before use, and then wait 15 to 20 minutes before applying

drug to minimize risk of local irritation. Avoid contact with eyes.
Vaginal
• Screw the end of the applicator onto the tube and squeeze slowly. The plunger will stop when the applicator is full.
• Wash plunger and barrel in warm, soapy water and rinse thoroughly. Dry before reassembling.

ACTION
Unknown. May cause bactericidal effect by interacting with bacterial DNA. Drug is active against many anaerobic gram-negative bacilli, anaerobic gram-positive cocci, *Gardnerella vaginalis,* and *Campylobacter fetus.*

Route	Onset	Peak	Duration
Topical	Unknown	8–12 hr	Unknown
Vaginal	Unknown	6–12 hr	Unknown

Half-life: Unknown.

ADVERSE REACTIONS
Topical form
EENT: lacrimation if applied around eyes.
Skin: transient redness, dryness, mild burning, stinging, contact dermatitis, pruritus, rash.
Vaginal form
GI: cramps, nausea, loose stools, metallic or bad taste in mouth, pain.
GU: cervicitis, vaginitis, perineal and vulvovaginal itching, vaginal burning.
Skin: transient redness, dryness, mild burning, stinging.
Other: overgrowth of nonsusceptible organisms.

INTERACTIONS
Drug-drug. *Disulfiram:* May cause disulfiram-like reaction when used with vaginal form of metronidazole. Avoid using together, and wait 2 weeks after stopping disulfiram before starting metronidazole vaginal therapy.
Lithium: May increase lithium level. Monitor lithium level.
Oral anticoagulants: May increase anticoagulant effect. Monitor patient for adverse reactions.

Reactions in bold italics are *life-threatening*. Interactions may have a *rapid onset* or a *delayed onset*.

Drug-lifestyle. *Alcohol use:* May cause disulfiram-like reaction when used with vaginal form. Discourage use together.

EFFECTS ON LAB TEST RESULTS
• May interfere with AST, ALT, LDH, triglyceride, and glucose levels.
• May increase or decrease WBC count.

CONTRAINDICATIONS & CAUTIONS
• Contraindicated in patients hypersensitive to drug or its ingredients, such as parabens, and other nitroimidazole derivatives.
• Use cautiously in patients with history or evidence of blood dyscrasia and in those with hepatic impairment.
• Use vaginal gel cautiously in patients with history of CNS diseases. Oral form may cause seizures and peripheral neuropathy.
• Use in pregnant and breast-feeding women only if clearly needed.

NURSING CONSIDERATIONS
• Topical therapy hasn't been linked to the adverse effects observed with parenteral or oral therapy, but some drug may be absorbed after topical use.
• Don't use vaginal gel in patients who have taken disulfiram within past 2 weeks.

PATIENT TEACHING
• Instruct patient to avoid use of topical gel around eyes.
• Advise patient to clean area thoroughly before use and to wait 15 to 20 minutes after cleaning skin before applying drug to minimize risk of local irritation. Cosmetics may be used 5 minutes after medication has dried.
• If local reactions occur, advise patient to apply drug less frequently or stop using it and notify prescriber.
• Advise patient to avoid sexual intercourse while using vaginal preparation.
• Caution patient to avoid alcohol while being treated with vaginal preparation.

micafungin sodium
mick-a-FUN-gin

Mycamine

Therapeutic class: Antifungals
Pharmacologic class: Echinocandins
Pregnancy risk category: C

AVAILABLE FORMS
Lyophilized powder for injection: 50 mg, 100 mg single-use vial

INDICATIONS & DOSAGES
➤ **Candidemia, acute disseminated candidiasis, and *Candida* peritonitis and abscesses**
Adults: 100 mg I.V. daily for 10 to 47 days (mean duration, 15 days).
Children age 4 months and older: 2 mg/kg I.V. once daily. Maximum dosage is 100 mg daily.
➤ **Esophageal candidiasis**
Adults: 150 mg I.V. daily for 10 to 30 days (mean duration, 15 days).
Children age 4 months and older weighing more than 30 kg (66 lb): 2.5 mg/kg I.V. once daily. Maximum dosage is 150 mg daily.
Children age 4 months and older weighing 30 kg or less: 3 mg/kg I.V. once daily. Maximum dosage is 150 mg daily.
➤ **To prevent candidal infection in hematopoietic stem cell transplant recipients**
Adults: 50 mg I.V. daily for 6 to 51 days (mean duration, 19 days).
Children age 4 months and older: 1 mg/kg I.V. once daily. Maximum dosage is 50 mg daily.

ADMINISTRATION
I.V.
▼ Use aseptic technique when preparing drug.
▼ Reconstitute each 50-mg or 100-mg vial with 5 mL of normal saline solution or D_5W for injection. To minimize foaming, dissolve powder by swirling the vial; don't shake it.
▼ For adult, dilute dose in 100 mL of normal saline solution or D_5W for injection.

M

▼ For children's doses: Add reconstituted drug to normal saline solution or D₅W I.V. infusion bag or syringe. Ensure that final concentration of solution is between 0.5 and 4 mg/mL. To minimize risk of infusion reactions, administer concentrations of greater than 1.5 mg/mL via central catheter.

▼ Flush line with normal saline solution for injection before infusing drug.

▼ Infuse drug over 1 hour.

▼ Reconstituted product and diluted infusion may be stored for up to 24 hours at room temperature.

▼ Protect diluted solution from light.

▼ **Incompatibilities:** Drug may precipitate when mixed with commonly used drugs.

ACTION

Inhibits synthesis of an essential component of fungal cell walls. Drug is active against *Candida albicans, C. glabrata, C. krusei, C. parapsilosis,* and *C. tropicalis.*

Route	Onset	Peak	Duration
I.V.	Unknown	Unknown	Unknown

Half-life: 11 to 21 hours.

ADVERSE REACTIONS

CNS: headache, insomnia.
CV: atrial fibrillation, bradycardia, cardiac disorders, hypertension, hypotension, tachycardia, vascular disorders.
GI: abdominal pain, diarrhea, nausea, vomiting.
Hematologic: *leukopenia, neutropenia, thrombocytopenia,* anemia.
Metabolic: hypocalcemia, hypokalemia, *hypomagnesemia,* hypophosphatemia.
Skin: infusion-site inflammation, phlebitis, pruritus, rash.
Other: pyrexia, rigors.

INTERACTIONS

Drug-drug. *Cyclosporine:* May increase cyclosporine level. Monitor for adverse reactions, and decrease cyclosporine dose if needed.
Itraconazole: May increase itraconazole level. Monitor for itraconazole toxicity, and reduce itraconazole dose if needed.

Nifedipine: May increase nifedipine level. Monitor blood pressure, and decrease nifedipine dose if needed.
Sirolimus: May increase sirolimus level. Monitor patient for evidence of toxicity, and decrease sirolimus dose if needed.

EFFECTS ON LAB TEST RESULTS

● May increase alkaline phosphatase, ALT, AST, bilirubin, BUN, creatinine, and LDH levels.
● May decrease calcium, magnesium, phosphorus, potassium, and hemoglobin levels and hematocrit.
● May decrease neutrophil and platelet counts.

CONTRAINDICATIONS & CAUTIONS

● Contraindicated in patients hypersensitive to drug.
● Effects of micafungin are unknown in patients with severe hepatic disease.
● It isn't known if drug appears in breast milk. Use cautiously in breast-feeding women.

NURSING CONSIDERATIONS

● Injection-site reactions occur more often in patients receiving drug by peripheral I.V.
● To reduce the risk of histamine-mediated reactions, infuse drug over at least 1 hour.
❸ *Alert:* If patient develops signs of serious hypersensitivity reaction, including shock, stop infusion and notify prescriber.
● Monitor hepatic and renal function during therapy.
● Monitor patient for hemolysis and hemolytic anemia.
● Use drug in pregnant women only if clearly needed.

PATIENT TEACHING

● Advise patient to report pain or redness at infusion site.
● Tell patient he'll likely need laboratory tests to monitor his hematologic, renal, and hepatic function.

miconazole
mi-KON-a-zole

Oravig

miconazole nitrate
Desenex ◊, Femizol-M ◊, Fungoid
Tincture ◊, Lotrimin AF ◊, Micatin ◊,
Micozole† , Monistat 1 ◊,
Monistat 3 ◊, Monistat 7 ◊,
M-Zole 3 ◊, M-Zole 7 ◊, Tetterine† ◊,
Ting ◊, Vagistat-1 ◊, Zeasorb-AF ◊

Therapeutic class: Antifungals
Pharmacologic class: Imidazoles
Pregnancy risk category: C

AVAILABLE FORMS
Aerosol powder: 2% ◊
Aerosol spray: 2% ◊
Buccal tablets: 50 mg
Lotion: 2% ◊
Powder: 2% ◊
Topical cream: 2% ◊
Topical ointment: 2% ◊
Topical solution: 2% ◊
Vaginal cream: 2% ◊, 4% ◊
Vaginal suppositories: 100 mg ◊,
200 mg ◊, 1,200 mg ◊

INDICATIONS & DOSAGES
➤ **Tinea corporis, tinea cruris, tinea
pedis, cutaneous candidiasis, common
dermatophyte infections**
Adults and children older than age 2: Apply
sparingly b.i.d. for 2 to 4 weeks. Powder
or spray can be used liberally over affected
area. In children younger than age 2, use
only under the direction and supervision of a
physician.
➤ **Tinea versicolor**
Adults and children older than age 2: Apply
sparingly daily for 2 weeks. In children
younger than age 2, use only under the
direction and supervision of a physician.
➤ **Vulvovaginal candidiasis**
Adults and children age 12 and older: One
applicatorful or 100-mg Monistat 7 suppository vaginally at bedtime for 7 days; repeat
course, if needed. Or, 200-mg Monistat 3
suppository vaginally at bedtime for 3 days.
Or, one 1,200-mg suppository vaginally at

bedtime for 1 day. Or, apply topical cream
sparingly to affected area b.i.d. for 7 days.
➤ **Oropharyngeal candidiasis**
Adults and children age 16 and older: One
buccal tablet to the gum region once daily
for 14 consecutive days.

ADMINISTRATION
P.O.
● Apply buccal tablet to the gum in the
morning with dry hands after patient has
brushed teeth.
● Place the rounded surface of the tablet
against the gum just above the incisor.
Apply slight pressure over the upper lip for
30 seconds to ensure adhesion.
● Alternate sides of the mouth for each
dose.
● Instruct patient not to crush, chew, or
swallow buccal tablets.
Topical
● Don't use occlusive dressings.
● Lotion is preferred in skinfolds.
Vaginal
● Suppository is inserted high into vagina
with applicator provided.
● Store between 59° and 86° F (15° and
30° C).

ACTION
Fungicidal; disrupts fungal cell membrane
permeability.

Route	Onset	Peak	Duration
P.O.	Unknown	7 hr	Unknown
Topical, vaginal	Unknown	Unknown	Unknown

Half-life: Unknown.

ADVERSE REACTIONS
CNS: headache.
GI: diarrhea, nausea, dysgeusia, upper
abdominal pain, vomiting (buccal tablets).
GU: pelvic cramps, pruritus, and irritation
with vaginal cream; vulvovaginal burning.
Skin: allergic contact dermatitis, burning,
irritation, maceration, pain, edema.

INTERACTIONS
Drug-drug. *Warfarin:* Buccal form of
drug may enhance anticoagulant effect.
Monitor PT and INR, and observe patient
for bleeding.

M

EFFECTS ON LAB TEST RESULTS
None reported.

CONTRAINDICATIONS & CAUTIONS
• Contraindicated in patients hypersensitive to drug or its components. Cross-sensitivity to imidazole antifungals may occur.
• Safety and effectiveness of Oravig haven't been established for children younger than age 16.
• Don't use in children younger than age 2.
• Don't use vaginal preparation during the first trimester of pregnancy.
• Use cautiously in breast-feeding women.

NURSING CONSIDERATIONS
• Avoid using within 72 hours of certain vaginal and latex products, such as condoms or vaginal contraceptive diaphragms, because drug causes latex breakdown.

PATIENT TEACHING
• Advise patient that vaginal form of drug is for perineal or vaginal use only and to keep drug out of eyes.
• Caution patient that frequent or persistent yeast infections may suggest a more serious medical problem.
• Tell patient to cautiously insert vaginal form high into the vagina with applicator provided.
🔾 **Alert:** Vaginal preparation shouldn't be used during first trimester of pregnancy. Use vaginal preparation during pregnancy only if recommended by prescriber.
• Tell patient that drug may stain clothing.
• Warn patient to stop drug if sensitivity or chemical irritation occurs.
• Tell patient to use drug for full treatment period prescribed and to notify prescriber if symptoms persist or worsen despite therapy.
• Advise patient to avoid tampons and sexual intercourse during vaginal treatment.
• Instruct patient to apply sparingly in skinfolds and rub in well to prevent skin breakdown.
• Tell patient to store vaginal product between 59° and 86° F (15° and 30° C).
• Tell patient not to crush, chew, or swallow buccal tablets.
• Advise patient that he can eat and drink with the buccal tablet in place but to avoid chewing gum.

• Instruct patient how to use buccal tablet.
• Tell patient that if the tablet falls off or is swallowed after it is in place for at least 6 hours, he shouldn't apply a new tablet until the next regularly scheduled dose.

SAFETY ALERT!

midazolam hydrochloride
mid-AY-zoh-lam

Therapeutic class: Anxiolytics
Pharmacologic class: Benzodiazepines
Pregnancy risk category: D
Controlled substance schedule: IV

AVAILABLE FORMS
Injection: 1 mg/mL, 5 mg/mL
Syrup: 2 mg/mL

INDICATIONS & DOSAGES
➤ **Preoperative sedation (to induce sleepiness or drowsiness and relieve apprehension)**
Adults: 0.07 to 0.08 mg/kg I.M. about 1 hour before surgery.
➤ **Moderate sedation before short diagnostic or endoscopic procedures**
Adults younger than age 60: Initially, small dose not to exceed 2.5 mg I.V. given slowly; repeat in 2 minutes p.r.n., in small increments of first dose over at least 2 minutes to achieve desired effect. Total dose of up to 5 mg may be used. Additional doses to maintain desired level of sedation may be given by slow titration in increments of 25% of dose used to first reach the sedative end point.
Patients age 60 or older and debilitated patients: 0.5 to 1.5 mg I.V. over at least 2 minutes. Incremental doses shouldn't exceed 1 mg. A total dose of up to 3.5 mg is usually sufficient.
➤ **To induce sleepiness and amnesia and to relieve apprehension before anesthesia or before and during procedures**
P.O.
Children ages 6 to 16 who are cooperative: 0.25 to 0.5 mg/kg P.O. as a single dose, up to 20 mg.

Reactions in bold italics are *life-threatening*. Interactions may have a *rapid onset* or a *delayed onset*.

Infants and children ages 6 months to 5 years or less cooperative, older children: 0.25 to 1 mg/kg P.O. as a single dose, up to 20 mg.

I.V.

Children ages 12 to 16: Initially, no more than 2.5 mg I.V. given slowly; repeat in 2 minutes, if needed, in small increments of first dose over at least 2 minutes to achieve desired effect. Total dose of up to 10 mg may be used. Additional doses to maintain desired level of sedation may be given by slow titration in increments of 25% of dose used to first reach the sedative end point.

Children ages 6 to 12: 0.025 to 0.05 mg/kg I.V. over 2 to 3 minutes. Additional doses may be given in small increments after 2 to 3 minutes. Total dose of up to 0.4 mg/kg, not to exceed 10 mg, may be used.

Children ages 6 months to 5 years: 0.05 to 0.1 mg/kg I.V. over 2 to 3 minutes. Additional doses may be given in small increments after 2 to 3 minutes. Total dose of up to 0.6 mg/kg, not to exceed 6 mg, may be used.

I.M.

Children: 0.1 to 0.15 mg/kg I.M. Use up to 0.5 mg/kg in more anxious patients.

Adjust-a-dose: For obese children, base dose on ideal body weight; high-risk or debilitated children and children receiving other sedatives need lower doses.

➤ **To induce general anesthesia**

Adults older than age 55: 0.3 mg/kg I.V. over 20 to 30 seconds if patient hasn't received premedication, or 0.2 mg/kg I.V. over 20 to 30 seconds if patient has received a sedative or opioid premedication. Additional increments of 25% of first dose may be needed to complete induction.

Adults younger than age 55: 0.3 to 0.35 mg/kg I.V. over 20 to 30 seconds if patient hasn't received premedication, or 0.25 mg/kg I.V. over 20 to 30 seconds if patient has received a sedative or opioid premedication. Additional increments of 25% of first dose may be needed to complete induction.

Adjust-a-dose: For debilitated patients, initially, 0.2 to 0.25 mg/kg. As little as 0.15 mg/kg may be needed. Reduce doses in elderly patients.

➤ **As continuous infusion to sedate intubated patients in critical care unit**

Adults: Initially, 0.01 to 0.05 mg/kg may be given I.V. over several minutes, repeated at 10- to 15-minute intervals until adequate sedation is achieved. To maintain sedation, usual initial infusion rate is 0.02 to 0.1 mg/kg/hour. Higher loading dose or infusion rates may be needed in some patients. Use the lowest effective rate.

Children: Initially, 0.05 to 0.2 mg/kg may be given I.V. over 2 to 3 minutes or longer; then continuous infusion at rate of 0.06 to 0.12 mg/kg/hour. Increase or decrease infusion to maintain desired effect.

Neonates more than 32 weeks' gestational age: Initially, 0.06 mg/kg/hour. Adjust rate, as needed, using lowest possible rate.

Neonates less than 32 weeks' gestational age: Initially, 0.03 mg/kg/hour. Adjust rate, as needed, using lowest possible rate.

ADMINISTRATION

P.O.

Black Box Warning Midazolam syrup has been associated with respiratory depression and respiratory arrest, especially when used in noncritical-care settings. Midazolam syrup should only be used in hospital or ambulatory care settings that can provide continuous respiratory and cardiac function monitoring. Availability of appropriate resuscitative drugs and equipment and personnel trained in their use and skilled in airway management should be ensured. ▮

• Give drug without regard for food, but don't give with grapefruit juice or grapefruit.

I.V.

Black Box Warning I.V. midazolam should only be used in hospital or ambulatory care settings, including physicians' and dental offices, that can provide continuous monitoring of cardiac and respiratory function. Availability of appropriate resuscitative drugs and equipment and personnel trained in their use and skilled in airway management should be ensured. ▮

▼ Drug may be mixed in the same syringe with morphine sulfate, meperidine, atropine, or scopolamine.

M

▼ When mixing infusion, use 5-mg/mL vial and dilute to 0.5 mg/mL with D₅W or normal saline solution.

Black Box Warning Give slowly over at least 2 minutes, and wait at least 2 minutes when titrating doses to produce therapeutic effect. ∎

Black Box Warning Don't administer by rapid injection in the neonatal population. ∎

▼**Incompatibilities:** Albumin, amoxicillin sodium, amphotericin B, ampicillin sodium, bumetanide, butorphanol, ceftazidime, cefuroxime, clonidine, dexamethasone sodium phosphate, dimenhydrinate, dobutamine, foscarnet, fosphenytoin, furosemide, heparin sodium, hydrocortisone, imipenem–cilastatin sodium, lactated Ringer's injection, methotrexate sodium, nafcillin, omeprazole sodium, pentobarbital sodium, perphenazine, prochlorperazine edisylate, ranitidine hydrochloride, sodium bicarbonate, thiopental, some total parenteral nutrition formulations, sulfamethoxazole–trimethoprim.

I.M.
● Inject deeply into a large muscle.

ACTION

May potentiate the effects of GABA, depress the CNS, and suppress the spread of seizure activity.

Route	Onset	Peak	Duration
P.O.	10–20 min	45–60 min	2–6 hr
I.V.	90 sec–5 min	Rapid	2–6 hr
I.M.	15 min	15–60 min	2–6 hr

Half-life: 2 to 6 hours.

ADVERSE REACTIONS

CNS: oversedation, drowsiness, amnesia, headache, involuntary movements, nystagmus, paradoxical behavior or excitement.
CV: variations in blood pressure and pulse rate.
GI: nausea, vomiting.
Respiratory: *apnea,* decreased respiratory rate, hiccups.
Other: pain at injection site.

INTERACTIONS

Drug-drug. *Anticonvulsants (carbamazepine, phenytoin):* May decrease midazolam level. Monitor patient for midazolam effectiveness.
CNS depressants: May cause apnea. Use together cautiously. Adjust dosage of midazolam if used with opiates or other CNS depressants.
Diltiazem: May increase CNS depression and prolong effects of midazolam. Use lower dose of midazolam.
Erythromycin: May alter metabolism of midazolam. Use together cautiously.
Fluconazole, itraconazole, ketoconazole, miconazole: May increase and prolong midazolam level, CNS depression, and psychomotor impairment. Avoid using together. If must be given together, monitor patient closely.
Hormonal contraceptives: May prolong half-life of midazolam. Use together cautiously.
Protease inhibitors (ritonavir, saquinavir, telaprevir): May increase midazolam level. Use together cautiously.
Rifampin: May decrease midazolam level. Monitor for midazolam effectiveness.
Theophylline: May antagonize sedative effect of midazolam. Use together cautiously.
Verapamil: May increase midazolam level. Monitor patient closely.
Drug-herb. *St. John's wort:* May decrease drug level. Discourage use together.
Drug-food. *Grapefruit juice:* May increase bioavailability of oral drug. Discourage use together.
Drug-lifestyle. *Alcohol use:* May cause additive CNS effects. Discourage use together.

EFFECTS ON LAB TEST RESULTS
None reported.

CONTRAINDICATIONS & CAUTIONS
● Contraindicated in patients hypersensitive to drug and in those with acute angle-closure glaucoma, shock, coma, or acute alcohol intoxication.
● Use cautiously in patients with uncompensated acute illness and in elderly or debilitated patients.

Reactions in bold italics are *life-threatening*. Interactions may have a *rapid onset* or a *delayed onset*.

Black Box Warning Pediatric dosages must be calculated on a mg/kg basis, and all dosages should be titrated slowly. ■

◑ Alert: Midazolam should only be administered by persons specifically trained in the use of anesthetics and the management of respiratory effects of anesthetics, including resuscitation of patients in the age-group being treated.

⚠ Overdose S&S: Excessive sedation, somnolence, confusion, impaired coordination, diminished reflexes, coma, altered vital signs.

NURSING CONSIDERATIONS
Black Box Warning A qualified individual, other than the practitioner performing the procedure, should monitor patient throughout procedure. Have oxygen and resuscitation equipment available in case of severe respiratory depression. Excessive amounts and rapid infusion have been linked to respiratory arrest. Continuously monitor patient, including children taking syrup form, for life-threatening respiratory depression. ■
• Monitor blood pressure, heart rate and rhythm, respirations, airway integrity, and pulse oximetry during procedure.

PATIENT TEACHING
• Because drug diminishes patient's recall of events around the time of surgery, provide written information, family member instructions, and follow-up contact.
• Warn patient to avoid hazardous activities that require alertness or good coordination until effects of drug are known.

SAFETY ALERT!

miglitol
MIG-lah-tall

Glyset

Therapeutic class: Antidiabetics
Pharmacologic class: Alpha-glucosidase inhibitors
Pregnancy risk category: B

AVAILABLE FORMS
Tablets: 25 mg, 50 mg, 100 mg

INDICATIONS & DOSAGES
➤ **Adjunct to diet in patients with type 2 diabetes, alone or with a sulfonylurea**
Adults: 25 mg P.O. t.i.d. May start with 25 mg P.O. daily and increase gradually to t.i.d. to minimize GI upset; dosage may be increased after 4 to 8 weeks to 50 mg P.O. t.i.d. Dosage may then be further increased after 3 months, based on glycosylated hemoglobin (HbA_{1c}) level, to maximum of 100 mg P.O. t.i.d.

ADMINISTRATION
P.O.
• Give drug with first bite of each main meal.

ACTION
Lowers glucose level by inhibiting the alpha-glucosidases in the small intestine, which convert carbohydrates to glucose. Inhibiting these enzymes delays the digestion of carbohydrates after a meal, resulting in a smaller increase in postprandial glucose level.

Route	Onset	Peak	Duration
P.O.	Unknown	2–3 hr	Unknown

Half-life: About 2 hours.

ADVERSE REACTIONS
GI: abdominal pain, diarrhea, flatulence.
Skin: rash.

INTERACTIONS
Drug-drug. *Digoxin, propranolol, ranitidine:* May decrease bioavailability of these drugs. Monitor clinical response and adjust dosage.
Insulin, sulfonylureas: May increase risk of hypoglycemia. Consider decreasing dosages of miglitol, insulin, and sulfonylureas.
Intestinal absorbents (such as charcoal), digestive enzyme preparations (such as amylase, pancreatin): May reduce effect of miglitol. Avoid using together.

EFFECTS ON LAB TEST RESULTS
• May decrease iron level.

CONTRAINDICATIONS & CAUTIONS
• Contraindicated in patients hypersensitive to drug or its components and in those with

diabetic ketoacidosis, inflammatory bowel disease, colonic ulceration, partial intestinal obstruction, chronic intestinal diseases with marked disorders of digestion or absorption, or conditions that may deteriorate because of increased gas formation in the intestine.

• Contraindicated in those predisposed to intestinal obstruction and in those with creatinine level greater than 2 mg/dL.

⚠ **Overdose S&S:** Transient increases in flatulence, diarrhea, and abdominal discomfort.

NURSING CONSIDERATIONS

• In patients also taking insulin or a sulfonylurea, dosage adjustment of these drugs may be needed. Monitor patient for hypoglycemia.

• Diabetes management should include diet control, an exercise program, and regular testing of urine and glucose level.

• Monitor glucose level regularly, especially during situations of increased stress, such as infection, fever, surgery, or trauma.

• Monitor HbA$_{1c}$ level every 3 months to evaluate long-term glycemic control.

• Treat mild to moderate hypoglycemia with a ready form of sugar, such as glucose tablets or gel. Severe hypoglycemia may necessitate I.V. glucose or glucagon.

• Monitor patient for adverse GI effects.

PATIENT TEACHING

• Stress importance of adhering to diet, weight reduction, and exercise instructions. Urge patient to have glucose and HbA$_{1c}$ levels tested regularly.

• Inform patient that drug treatment relieves symptoms but doesn't cure diabetes.

• Teach patient how to recognize high and low glucose levels.

• Instruct patient to have a source of glucose readily available to treat hypoglycemia.

• Advise patient that sucrose (table sugar, cane sugar) or fruit juices shouldn't be used to treat low-glucose reactions with this drug. Oral glucose (dextrose) or glucagon is necessary to increase glucose.

• Advise patient to seek medical advice promptly during periods of stress, such as fever, trauma, infection, or surgery, because dosage may have to be adjusted.

• Instruct patient to take drug three times daily with first bite of each main meal.

• Show patient how and when to monitor glucose level.

• Advise patient that adverse GI effects are most common during first few weeks of therapy and should improve over time.

• Urge patient to carry medical identification at all times.

SAFETY ALERT!

milrinone lactate
MILL-ri-none

Therapeutic class: Inotropes
Pharmacologic class: Bipyridine phosphodiesterase inhibitors
Pregnancy risk category: C

AVAILABLE FORMS
Injection: 1 mg/mL
Injection (premixed): 200 mcg/mL in D$_5$W

INDICATIONS & DOSAGES
➤ **Short-term treatment of acutely decompensated heart failure**
Adults: Give first loading dose of 50 mcg/kg I.V. slowly over 10 minutes; then give continuous I.V. infusion of 0.375 to 0.75 mcg/kg/minute. Titrate infusion dose based on clinical and hemodynamic responses. Don't exceed 1.13 mg/kg/day.
Adjust-a-dose: If CrCl is 50 mL/minute, infusion rate is 0.43 mcg/kg/minute; if 40 mL/minute, infusion rate is 0.38 mcg/kg/minute; if 30 mL/minute, infusion rate is 0.33 mcg/kg/minute; if 20 mL/minute, infusion rate is 0.28 mcg/kg/minute; if 10 mL/minute, infusion rate is 0.23 mcg/kg/minute; and if 5 mL/minute, infusion rate is 0.2 mcg/kg/minute. Don't exceed 1.13 mg/kg/day.

ADMINISTRATION
I.V.
▼ Give loading dose undiluted as a direct injection over 10 minutes.
▼ Prepare I.V. infusion solution using half-normal saline solution, normal saline solution, or D$_5$W. Prepare the 100-mcg/mL solution by adding 180 mL of diluent per 20-mg (20-mL) vial, the 150-mcg/mL solution by adding 113 mL of diluent per

20-mg (20-mL) vial, and the 200-mcg/mL solution by adding 80 mL of diluent per 20-mg (20-mL) vial.

▼ **Incompatibilities:** Bumetanide, furosemide, imipenem–cilastatin sodium, procainamide, torsemide.

ACTION

Produces inotropic action by increasing cellular levels of cAMP and vasodilation by relaxing vascular smooth muscle.

Route	Onset	Peak	Duration
I.V.	5–15 min	1–2 hr	3–6 hr

Half-life: 2½ to 3¾ hours.

ADVERSE REACTIONS

CNS: headache.
CV: *ventricular arrhythmias,* ventricular ectopic activity, *sustained ventricular tachycardia, ventricular fibrillation,* hypotension, nonsustained ventricular tachycardia.

INTERACTIONS

None significant.

EFFECTS ON LAB TEST RESULTS

● May cause abnormal LFT results.

CONTRAINDICATIONS & CAUTIONS

● Contraindicated in patients hypersensitive to drug.
◑ **Alert:** Use of milrinone for more than 48 hours in patients with heart failure hasn't been shown to be safe or effective and may increase risk of hospitalization and death.
◑ **Alert:** Drug has been associated with increased frequency of ventricular arrhythmias, including nonsustained ventricular tachycardia and supraventricular and ventricular arrhythmias in the high-risk population. Closely monitor patient during infusion.
● Contraindicated in patients with severe aortic or pulmonic valvular disease in place of surgery and during acute phase of MI.
● Use cautiously in patients with atrial flutter or fibrillation because drug slightly shortens AV node conduction time and may increase ventricular response rate.
▲ **Overdose S&S:** Hypotension.

NURSING CONSIDERATIONS

● In patients with atrial flutter or fibrillation, give digoxin before milrinone therapy. Drug is typically given with digoxin and diuretics.
● Improved cardiac output may increase urine output. Reduce diuretic dosage when heart failure improves. Potassium loss may cause digitalis toxicity.
● Monitor fluid and electrolyte status, blood pressure, heart rate, and renal function during therapy. Excessive decrease in blood pressure requires stopping or slowing rate of infusion.
● Correct hypoxemia.

PATIENT TEACHING

● Instruct patient to report adverse reactions to prescriber promptly, especially angina.
● Tell patient that drug may cause headache, which can be treated with analgesics.
● Tell patient to report discomfort at I.V. insertion site.

minocycline hydrochloride
mi-noe-SYE-kleen

Dynacin, Minocin, Solodyn

Therapeutic class: Antibiotics
Pharmacologic class: Tetracyclines
Pregnancy risk category: D

M

AVAILABLE FORMS

Capsules: 50 mg, 75 mg, 100 mg
Capsules (pellet-filled): 50 mg, 100 mg
Injection: 100 mg
Tablets: 50 mg, 75 mg, 100 mg
Tablets (extended-release): 45 mg, 55 mg, 65 mg, 80 mg, 90 mg, 105 mg, 115 mg, 135 mg

INDICATIONS & DOSAGES

Adjust-a-dose (for all indications): Decrease dosage or increase dosing interval in patients with renal impairment. Don't exceed 200 mg Minocin in 24 hours.
➤ **Infections caused by susceptible gram-negative and gram-positive organisms (including *Haemophilus ducreyi, Yersinia pestis,* and *Campylobacter fetus*), Rickettsiae species, *Mycoplasma pneumoniae,***

and *Chlamydia trachomatis;* psittacosis;
granuloma inguinale
Adults: 200 mg P.O. or I.V. initially; then
100 mg P.O. or I.V. every 12 hours. May use
100 or 200 mg P.O. initially; then 50 mg
q.i.d.
Children older than age 8: Initially, 4 mg/kg
P.O. or I.V.; then, 2 mg/kg P.O. or I.V. every
12 hours.

➤ **Gonorrhea in patients allergic to
penicillin**
Adults: Initially, 200 mg P.O.; then 100 mg
every 12 hours for at least 4 days. Obtain
samples for follow-up cultures within 2 to
3 days after treatment.

➤ **Syphilis in patients allergic to
penicillin**
Adults: Initially, 200 mg P.O.; then 100 mg
every 12 hours for 10 to 15 days.

➤ **Meningococcal carrier state**
Adults: 100 mg P.O. every 12 hours for
5 days.

➤ **Uncomplicated urethral, endocervical,
or rectal infection caused by *C. trachomatis* or *Ureaplasma urealyticum***
Adults: 100 mg P.O. every 12 hours for at
least 7 days.

➤ **Uncomplicated gonococcal urethritis**
Men: 100 mg P.O. every 12 hours for 5 days.

➤ **Treatment of inflammatory lesions
of nonnodular moderate to severe acne
vulgaris**
Adults and children age 12 and older:
1 mg/kg extended-release tablets (Solodyn)
P.O. once daily for 12 weeks.

➤ **Rheumatoid arthritis ◆**
Adults: 100 mg P.O. b.i.d. for up to 2 years.

ADMINISTRATION
P.O.
• Obtain specimen for culture and sensitivity tests before first dose. Begin therapy
while awaiting results.
• Give pellet-filled capsules and tablets
1 hour before or 2 hours after a meal.
• Give drug with a full glass of water. Drug
may be taken with food.
• Drug shouldn't be given within 1 hour of
bedtime, to avoid esophageal irritation or
ulceration.
• Give capsules and extended-release tablets
at the same time each day, with or without
food.

• Capsules and extended-release tablets
must be swallowed whole and not crushed,
chewed, or split.

I.V.
▼ Reconstitute powder with 5 mL sterile
water for injection; further dilute to 500 to
1,000 mL with sodium chloride injection,
dextrose injection, dextrose and sodium
chloride injection, Ringer injection, or lactated Ringer injection. (Don't use solutions
containing calcium because a precipitate
may form.)
▼ Avoid rapid administration and don't
administer with other drugs.
▼ Parenteral therapy is indicated only when
oral therapy is inadequate or isn't tolerated.
Institute oral therapy as soon as possible.

ACTION
May be bacteriostatic by binding to
microorganism's ribosomal subunits, inhibiting protein synthesis; may also alter
the cytoplasmic membrane of susceptible
microorganisms.

Route	Onset	Peak	Duration
P.O.	Unknown	1–4 hr	Unknown
P.O. (extended-release)	Unknown	3½–4 hr	Unknown
I.V.	Unknown	Unknown	Unknown

Half-life: 11 to 26 hours P.O., 15 to 23 hours I.V.

ADVERSE REACTIONS
CNS: *intracranial hypertension,* headache,
light-headedness, dizziness, vertigo.
CV: thrombophlebitis, pericarditis.
EENT: tooth disorder, periodontitis, gingivitis, mouth ulceration, pharyngitis.
GI: anorexia, diarrhea, nausea, dysphagia,
glossitis, epigastric distress, oral candidiasis, vomiting.
Hematologic: *neutropenia, thrombocytopenia,* eosinophilia, hemolytic anemia.
Hepatic: *hepatotoxicity.*
Musculoskeletal: bone growth retardation
in children younger than age 8.
Skin: increased pigmentation, maculopapular and erythematous rashes, photosensitivity reactions, urticaria.
Other: *anaphylaxis,* enamel defects,
hypersensitivity reactions, permanent discoloration of teeth, superinfection.

Reactions in bold italics are *life-threatening*. Interactions may have a *rapid onset* or a *delayed onset*.

INTERACTIONS
Drug-drug. *Antacids (including sodium bicarbonate) and laxatives containing aluminum, magnesium, or calcium; antidiarrheals:* May decrease antibiotic absorption. Give antibiotic 1 hour before or 2 hours after these drugs.

Ferrous sulfate and other iron products, zinc: May decrease antibiotic absorption. Give drug 2 hours before or 3 hours after iron.

Hormonal contraceptives: May decrease contraceptive effectiveness and increase risk of breakthrough bleeding. Advise patient to use nonhormonal contraceptive.

Isotretinoin: May cause pseudomotor cerebri. Avoid giving shortly before, during, and shortly after minocycline therapy.

Methoxyflurane: May cause nephrotoxicity when given with tetracyclines. Avoid using together.

Oral anticoagulants: May increase anticoagulant effect. Monitor PT and INR, and adjust dosage.

Penicillins: May disrupt bactericidal action of penicillins. Avoid using together.

Drug-lifestyle. *Sun exposure:* May cause photosensitivity reactions. Advise patient to avoid excessive sunlight exposure.

EFFECTS ON LAB TEST RESULTS
● May increase BUN and liver enzyme levels. May decrease hemoglobin level.

● May increase eosinophil count. May decrease platelet and neutrophil counts.

● May falsely elevate fluorometric test results for urine catecholamines. Parenteral form may cause false-positive results of copper sulfate test (Clinitest). May cause false-negative results in urine glucose tests using glucose oxidase reagent (Diastix or Chemstrip uG).

CONTRAINDICATIONS & CAUTIONS
● Contraindicated in patients hypersensitive to drug or other tetracyclines, in pregnant and breast-feeding patients, and in persons of either gender attempting to conceive a child.

● Use cautiously in patients with impaired renal or hepatic function. Use of these drugs during last half of pregnancy and in children younger than age 8 may cause permanent discoloration of teeth, enamel defects, and bone growth retardation.

⚠ *Overdose S&S:* Dizziness, nausea, vomiting.

NURSING CONSIDERATIONS
● Monitor renal function and LFT results.

☼ *Alert:* Check expiration date. Outdated or deteriorated drug may cause reversible nephrotoxicity (Fanconi syndrome).

● Don't expose drug to light or heat. Keep cap tightly closed.

● If large doses are given, therapy is prolonged, or patient is at high risk, monitor patient for signs and symptoms of superinfection.

● Check patient's tongue for signs of candidal infection. Stress good oral hygiene.

● Drug may discolor teeth in older children and young adults, more commonly when used as long-term treatment. Watch for brown pigmentation, and notify prescriber if it occurs.

● Photosensitivity reactions may occur within a few minutes to several hours after exposure. Photosensitivity lasts after therapy ends.

● Monitor patient for drug rash with eosinophilia and systemic symptoms (DRESS syndrome). Discontinue drug immediately if syndrome occurs.

● *Look alike–sound alike:* Don't confuse Minocin with niacin or Mithracin.

PATIENT TEACHING
● Tell patient to take entire amount of drug exactly as prescribed, even after he feels better.

● Instruct patient to take drug with a full glass of water. Drug may be taken with food. Tell patient not to take within 1 hour of bedtime to avoid esophageal irritation or ulceration.

● Warn patient to avoid driving or other hazardous tasks because of possible adverse CNS effects.

● Caution patient to avoid direct sunlight and ultraviolet light, wear protective clothing, and use sunscreen.

● Tell patient to take Solodyn at the same time each day, with or without food.

● Tell patient to swallow Solodyn tablet whole and not to crush, chew, or split tablet.

M

• Warn patient not to take more than one extended-release tablet each day.
• Warn patient to avoid pregnancy because drug can cause fetal harm.

minoxidil (topical)
mi-NOX-i-dill

Men's Rogaine ◇, Minoxidil Extra Strength for Men ◇, Rogaine Extra Strength for Men ◇, Theroxidil ◇, Women's Rogaine ◇

Therapeutic class: Hair-growth stimulants
Pharmacologic class: Direct-acting vasodilators
Pregnancy risk category: C

AVAILABLE FORMS
Topical foam: 5% ◇
Topical solution: 2% ◇, 5% ◇

INDICATIONS & DOSAGES
➤ **Androgenetic alopecia**
Adults: 1 mL of solution or half a capful of foam applied to affected area b.i.d. Maximum daily dose is 2 mL of solution.

ADMINISTRATION
Topical
• Don't use 5% strength in women.
• Dry hair and scalp thoroughly before application.

ACTION
Stimulates hair growth, possibly by dilating arterial microcapillaries around hair follicles.

Route	Onset	Peak	Duration
Topical	Unknown	Unknown	Unknown

Half-life: Unknown.

ADVERSE REACTIONS
CNS: headache, dizziness, faintness, light-headedness.
CV: edema, chest pain, hypertension, hypotension, palpitations, increased or decreased pulse rate.
EENT: sinusitis.
GI: diarrhea, nausea, vomiting.

GU: UTI, renal calculi, urethritis.
Metabolic: weight gain.
Musculoskeletal: back pain, tendinitis.
Respiratory: bronchitis, upper respiratory infection.
Skin: irritant dermatitis, dry skin or scalp, flaking, local erythema, pruritus, allergic contact dermatitis, eczema, hypertrichosis, worsening of hair loss.

INTERACTIONS
Drug-drug. *Petroleum jelly, topical corticosteroids, topical retinoids, other drugs that may increase skin absorption:* May increase risk of systemic effects of minoxidil. Avoid using together.

EFFECTS ON LAB TEST RESULTS
None reported.

CONTRAINDICATIONS & CAUTIONS
• Contraindicated in patients hypersensitive to drug or components of solution.
• Use cautiously in patients older than age 50 and in those with cardiac, renal, or hepatic disease.
• Accidental ingestion could lead to adverse systemic effects.
• Don't use in pregnant or breast-feeding women.

NURSING CONSIDERATIONS
• Patient needs to have normal, healthy scalp before beginning therapy because absorption of drug through irritated skin may cause adverse systemic effects.
• Treatment will most likely succeed in patients with balding area smaller than 4 inches (10 cm) that developed within past 10 years.

PATIENT TEACHING
• Teach patient how to apply drug. Tell him to dry hair and scalp thoroughly before application and not to apply drug to other body areas. Tell patient not to use drug on irritated or sunburned scalp or with other drugs on scalp. Tell him to thoroughly wash hands after application.
• Warn patient to avoid inhaling any spray or mist from drug and to avoid spraying around eyes because solution contains alcohol and may be irritating.

Reactions in bold italics are *life-threatening*. Interactions may have a *rapid onset* or a *delayed onset*.

• Inform patient that more frequent applications or using more than 2 mL daily won't increase hair growth but instead may increase adverse reactions. Tell patient not to double the dose for missed applications.

• Advise patient to wait 4 hours after application to wash hair or go swimming.

• Teach patient to monitor pulse rate and body weight.

• Advise patient that therapy will be prolonged and will continue for at least 4 months before clinical effects appear. Tell him that drug must be used daily for optimal results. Almost half of patients will experience moderate to dense hair growth.

• Tell patient that stopping drug may cause loss of new hair growth. New hair growth is usually fine and may be colorless but will resemble existing hair after continued treatment.

✳ NEW DRUG

mipomersen sodium
MI-poe-MER-sen

Kynamro

Therapeutic class: Antilipemics
Pharmacologic class: Oligonucleotides
Pregnancy risk category: B

AVAILABLE FORMS
Injection: 200 mg/mL single-use vials or prefilled syringes

INDICATIONS & DOSAGES
➤ **As adjunctive treatment for homozygous familial hypercholesterolemia with lipid-lowering medications and diet to reduce LDL cholesterol, apolipoprotein B, total cholesterol, and non-HDL cholesterol**
Adults: 200 mg subcutaneously once weekly on same day each week.

Adjust-a-dose: If AST or ALT level is 3 times to less than 5 times the upper limit of normal (ULN), repeat measurement within 1 week; if elevations are confirmed, withhold drug. Perform additional LFTs if not already measured (such as total bilirubin, alkaline phosphatase, and INR) and investigate to identify probable cause of elevations.

Consider monitoring LFTs more frequently if resuming drug after transaminase levels resolve to less than 3× ULN. If AST or ALT is 5× ULN or greater, withhold drug. Perform additional liver-related tests to identify probable cause. If transaminase elevations are accompanied by clinical symptoms of liver injury (such as nausea, vomiting, abdominal pain, fever, jaundice, lethargy, and flulike symptoms), increases in bilirubin level at least 2× ULN, or active liver disease, discontinue treatment and identify probable cause.

ADMINISTRATION
Subcutaneous
• Store refrigerated at 36° to 46 °F (2° to 8°C). Protect from light and keep in original carton until time of use. If refrigeration isn't possible, store at or below 86°F (30°C), away from heat sources, for up to 14 days.

• Remove from refrigeration at least 30 minutes before use.

• Inspect solution for clarity or particulate matter; if solution is cloudy or contains particles, return product to pharmacy.

• Administer first dose under supervision of health care provider.

• Administration sites include the abdomen, thigh region, and outer area of the upper arm. Alternate sites.

• Don't inject in areas of active skin disease or injury (such as sunburn, rash, inflammation, skin infection, or active areas of psoriasis). Avoid tattooed and scarred skin.

• Vials and syringes are for single use only. Discard excess solution; product contains no preservatives.

• Don't give I.V. or I.M.

• Don't mix or administer this drug with other products.

• If a dose is missed, give missed dose at least 3 days from the next scheduled weekly dose.

ACTION
Inhibits synthesis of apolipoprotein B-100, a primary component of LDL cholesterol and its metabolic precursor, very low-density lipoprotein.

M

Route	Onset	Peak	Duration
Subcut.	Unknown	3–4 hr	Unknown

Half-life: 1 to 2 months.

ADVERSE REACTIONS

CNS: fatigue, headache, pyrexia, chills, insomnia.
CV: angina pectoris, palpitations, peripheral edema, hypertension.
GI: nausea, vomiting, abdominal pain.
GU: proteinuria.
Hepatic: *hepatotoxicity,* hepatic steatosis.
Musculoskeletal: extremity pain, musculoskeletal pain.
Skin: injection-site reactions (pain, hematoma, erythema, pruritus, swelling, discoloration).
Other: flulike symptoms, benign neoplasms, *malignant neoplasms.*

INTERACTIONS

Drug-drug. *Hepatotoxic drugs (acetaminophen, amiodarone, isotretinoin, methotrexate, tamoxifen, tetracyclines):* May increase risk of liver injury. Monitor LFTs frequently.
Other LDL-lowering agents (nicotinic acid, statins): No formal studies have been completed. Use together isn't recommended.
Drug-lifestyle. *Alcohol use:* May increase risk of hepatotoxicity. Limit alcohol intake to one drink per day.

EFFECTS ON LAB TEST RESULTS

• May increase AST, ALT, and urine protein levels.

CONTRAINDICATIONS & CAUTIONS

Black Box Warning Drug may cause elevated transaminase levels and may increase hepatic fat, with or without concomitant increases in transaminase levels. Hepatic steatosis is a risk factor for advanced liver disease, including steatohepatitis and cirrhosis. Measure ALT, AST, alkaline phosphatase, and total bilirubin levels before initiating treatment and monitor ALT and AST levels regularly as recommended. During treatment, withhold dose if ALT or AST level is 3× ULN or more. Discontinue drug for clinically significant liver toxicity. ∎

• Contraindicated in patients with known hypersensitivity to drug or its components and in those with moderate or severe hepatic impairment (Child-Pugh class B or C) or active liver disease, including unexplained, persistent serum transaminase elevations.
• Drug isn't recommended in patients with severe renal impairment or clinically significant proteinuria, or in patients on renal dialysis.
• Using mipomersen as an adjunct to LDL apheresis isn't recommended.
• Drug may cause fetal harm. Women of childbearing potential should use effective contraception during therapy. Use drug only if clearly needed.
• It isn't known if drug appears in breast milk. Patient should discontinue drug or discontinue breast-feeding.

NURSING CONSIDERATIONS

• If baseline LFT values are abnormal, consider treatment only after appropriate evaluation and resolution or explanation of any abnormalities.
• Obtain LFT values monthly for first year, then at least every 3 months thereafter. Discontinue drug if persistent or clinically significant increases occur.
• If transaminase elevations are accompanied by clinical signs and symptoms of liver injury (nausea, vomiting, abdominal pain, fever, jaundice, lethargy, flulike symptoms), increases in bilirubin to 2× ULN or more, or active liver disease, discontinue drug and identify probable cause.
• Measure lipid levels at least every 3 months for first year. Measure LDL levels after 6 months, since maximum LDL reduction occurs at that time. Assess whether drug is effective, taking into account possible hepatotoxicity.
Black Box Warning Because of hepatotoxicity, only providers and pharmacies certified through the Kynamro REMS (Risk Evaluation and Mitigation Strategy) program may prescribe and administer this medication. For more information, call 1-877-KYNAMRO (1-877-596-2676) or go to www.kynamrorems.com. ∎
• Drug's effect on CV morbidity and mortality hasn't been determined.

Reactions in bold italics are *life-threatening*. Interactions may have a *rapid onset* or a *delayed onset*.

• Proper injection technique may help decrease risk of injection-site reactions, which occur frequently.

PATIENT TEACHING
• Caution patient that there must be at least 3 days between a missed dose and the next regularly scheduled weekly dose.
• Instruct patient or caregiver on the proper technique for administering this drug, including use of aseptic technique. Needles or syringes may only be used once, and should be properly disposed of in a suitable puncture-resistant container. Proper administration technique may decrease risk of injection-site reactions.
• Advise patient to avoid or limit alcohol to one drink per day because of additive liver toxicity.
• Tell patient to report signs and symptoms of liver damage, including nausea, vomiting, fever, anorexia, fatigue, jaundice, dark urine, pruritus, and abdominal pain. Encourage compliance with follow-up blood tests to monitor safe use of drug.
• Advise patient that injection-site reactions (erythema, pain, tenderness, pruritus, or local swelling) may occur.
• Advise patient that flulike symptoms, typically appearing within 2 days after an injection, may occur and include flulike illness, pyrexia, chills, myalgia, arthralgia, malaise, and fatigue.

mirabegron
MIR-a-BEG ron

Myrbetriq

Therapeutic class: Bladder antispasmodics
Pharmacologic class: Beta-3 adrenergic agonists
Pregnancy risk category: C

AVAILABLE FORMS
Tablets: 25 mg, 50 mg

INDICATIONS & DOSAGES
➤ **Overactive bladder with symptoms of urge incontinence, urgency, and frequency**

Adults: Initially, 25 mg P.O. once daily. May increase to 50 mg after 8 weeks if necessary.
Adjust-a-dose: For patients with severe renal impairment (CrCl of 15 to 29 mL/minute) or moderate hepatic impairment (Child-Pugh class B), give no more than 25 mg daily. Drug isn't recommended for patients with ESRD (CrCl of less than 15 mL/minute) or for patients with severe hepatic impairment (Child-Pugh class C).

ADMINISTRATION
P.O.
• May give without regard to food.
• Patient should swallow tablets whole with water; don't crush or divide tablets.

ACTION
Relaxes the detrusor smooth muscle during storage phase of the urinary bladder fill-void cycle, increasing bladder capacity.

Route	Onset	Peak	Duration
P.O.	Unknown	3.5 hr	Unknown

Half-life: 50 hours.

ADVERSE REACTIONS
CNS: headache, fatigue, dizziness.
CV: *hypertension,* tachycardia.
EENT: nasopharyngitis, dry mouth, sinusitis.
GI: constipation, diarrhea, abdominal pain.
GU: UTI, cystitis, urine retention.
Musculoskeletal: arthralgia, back pain.
Respiratory: upper respiratory tract infection.
Other: flulike symptoms.

INTERACTIONS
Drug-drug. *Antimuscarinics (pirenzepine):* May increase risk of urine retention. Use cautiously together.
Digoxin: May increase digoxin level. Monitor digoxin level and titrate mirabegron to lowest effective dosage.
Drugs metabolized by CYP2D6 (desipramine, flecainide, metoprolol, propafenone, thioridazine): May increase levels of these drugs. Monitor patient for adverse events; adjust dosage as needed.
Warfarin: May increase warfarin level. Monitor INR; adjust warfarin dosage as necessary.

M

EFFECTS ON LAB TEST RESULTS
• May increase ALT, AST, GGT, LDH, and digoxin levels.
• May increase INR.

CONTRAINDICATIONS & CAUTIONS
• Contraindicated in patients hypersensitive to drug or its components and in those with severe, uncontrolled hypertension; ESRD; or severe hepatic impairment (Child-Pugh class C).
• Use cautiously in patients with hypertension, urine retention, or bladder outlet obstruction.
• Use cautiously in pregnant or breast-feeding women and only if benefits outweigh risks.
⚠ **Overdose S&S:** Palpitations, increased heart rate and blood pressure.

NURSING CONSIDERATIONS
• Monitor blood pressure and pulse regularly, especially in patients with hypertension or atrial fibrillation.
• Monitor patients closely for urine retention and bladder obstruction, especially in those already taking bladder antispasmodics.
• Monitor LFT values periodically.
• Monitor patients for rash or pruritus.

PATIENT TEACHING
• Warn patient not to crush, chew, or cut tablets.
• Tell patient that drug may be taken without regard to food.
• Warn patient that drug may cause an increase in blood pressure or pulse. Teach patient to monitor blood pressure and pulse at home and to report increases to the health care provider.
• Advise patient that he may experience difficulty in emptying his bladder and infrequent bladder infections and to report concerns to his health care provider.
• Tell patient to report rash or itching, which may indicate an allergy or a serious adverse reaction.
• Teach female patient to report pregnancy to her health care provider as soon as possible.

mirtazapine
mer-TAH-zah-peen

Remeron, Remeron Soltab

Therapeutic class: Antidepressants
Pharmacologic class: Tetracyclic antidepressants
Pregnancy risk category: C

AVAILABLE FORMS
Tablets: 7.5 mg, 15 mg, 30 mg, 45 mg
Tablets (orally disintegrating): 15 mg, 30 mg, 45 mg

INDICATIONS & DOSAGES
➤ **Major depressive disorder**
Adults: Initially, 15 mg P.O. at bedtime. Maintenance dose is 15 to 45 mg daily. Adjust dosage at intervals of at least 1 week.

ADMINISTRATION
P.O.
• Give drug without regard for food.
• Remove orally disintegrating tablet (ODT) from blister pack and immediately place on patient's tongue.
• ODT may be given with or without water.
• Don't split or crush ODT.

ACTION
Thought to enhance central noradrenergic and serotonergic activity.

Route	Onset	Peak	Duration
P.O.	Unknown	2 hr	Unknown

Half-life: About 20 to 40 hours.

ADVERSE REACTIONS
CNS: somnolence, *suicidal behavior,* dizziness, asthenia, abnormal dreams, abnormal thinking, tremors, confusion.
CV: edema, peripheral edema.
GI: increased appetite, dry mouth, constipation, nausea.
GU: urinary frequency.
Metabolic: weight gain.
Musculoskeletal: back pain, myalgia.
Respiratory: dyspnea.
Other: flulike syndrome.

Reactions in bold italics are *life-threatening*. Interactions may have a *rapid onset* or a *delayed onset*.

INTERACTIONS

Drug-drug. *Diazepam, other CNS depressants:* May cause additive CNS effects. Avoid using together.

Linezolid, methylene blue, rasagiline: May cause serotonin syndrome. Use extreme caution and monitor patient closely.

MAO inhibitors: May sometimes cause fatal reactions. Avoid using within 14 days of MAO inhibitor therapy.

Warfarin: May increase anticoagulant effect. Closely monitor INR when mirtazapine is started or stopped, and adjust warfarin dosage as needed.

Drug-herb. *St. John's wort:* May increase risk of serotonin syndrome. Coadminister cautiously and monitor patient closely for adverse reactions.

Drug-lifestyle. *Alcohol use:* May cause additive CNS effects. Discourage use together.

EFFECTS ON LAB TEST RESULTS

● May increase ALT, cholesterol, and triglyceride levels.

CONTRAINDICATIONS & CAUTIONS

● Contraindicated in patients hypersensitive to drug and within 14 days of MAO inhibitor therapy.

Black Box Warning Mirtazapine isn't approved for use in children. ∎

● **Alert:** Concomitant use with linezolid or methylene blue can cause serotonin syndrome (fever, mental status changes, muscle twitching, excessive sweating, shivering or shaking, diarrhea, or loss of coordination). Use mirtazapine with linezolid or methylene blue only for life-threatening or urgent conditions when the potential benefits outweigh the risks of toxicity.

● Use cautiously in patients with CV or cerebrovascular disease, seizure disorders, suicidal thoughts, hepatic or renal impairment, or history of mania or hypomania.

● Use cautiously in patients with conditions that predispose them to hypotension, such as dehydration, hypovolemia, or antihypertensive therapy.

● Give drug cautiously to elderly patients; decreased clearance has occurred in this age group.

⚠ Overdose S&S: Disorientation, drowsiness, impaired memory, tachycardia.

NURSING CONSIDERATIONS

● **Alert:** If linezolid or methylene blue must be given, mirtazapine must be stopped and the patient should be monitored for serotonin toxicity for 2 weeks, or until 24 hours after the last dose of methylene blue or linezolid, whichever comes first. Treatment with mirtazapine may be resumed 24 hours after last dose of methylene blue or linezolid.

● Don't use within 14 days of MAO inhibitor therapy.

● Record mood changes. Watch for suicidal tendencies.

Black Box Warning Drug may increase risk of suicidal thinking and behavior in children, adolescents, and young adults ages 18 to 24 with major depressive or other psychiatric disorder. ∎

● Although agranulocytosis occurs rarely, stop drug and monitor patient closely if he develops a sore throat, fever, stomatitis, or other signs and symptoms of infection with a low WBC count.

● Lower dosages tend to be more sedating than higher dosages.

PATIENT TEACHING

Black Box Warning Advise families and caregivers to closely observe patient for increasing suicidal thinking and behavior. ∎

● **Alert:** Teach patient to recognize and immediately report signs and symptoms of serotonin toxicity (fever, mental status changes, muscle twitching, excessive sweating, shivering or shaking, diarrhea, or loss of coordination).

● Instruct patient to take drug at bedtime. Caution patient not to perform hazardous activities if he gets too sleepy.

● Tell patient to report signs and symptoms of infection, such as fever, chills, sore throat, mucous membrane irritation, or flulike syndrome.

● Instruct patient not to use alcohol or other CNS depressants while taking drug.

● Stress importance of following prescriber's orders.

● Instruct patient not to take other drugs without prescriber's approval.

• Tell women of childbearing age to report suspected pregnancy immediately and to notify prescriber if breast-feeding.
• Instruct patient to remove ODTs from blister pack and place immediately on tongue. Tell the patient to be sure his hands are clean and dry if he touches the tablet.
• Advise patient not to break or split tablet.

misoprostol
mye-soe-PROST-ole

Cytotec

Therapeutic class: Antiulcer drugs
Pharmacologic class: Prostaglandin E₁ analogues
Pregnancy risk category: X

AVAILABLE FORMS
Tablets: 100 mcg, 200 mcg

INDICATIONS & DOSAGES
➤ **To prevent NSAID-induced gastric ulcer in patients at high risk for complications from gastric ulcer and in patients with history of NSAID-induced ulcer**
Adults: 200 mcg P.O. q.i.d. with food; if not tolerated, decrease to 100 mcg P.O. q.i.d. Give dosage for duration of NSAID therapy.

ADMINISTRATION
P.O.
• Give drug with food.
• Give last dose at bedtime.
• Drug is considered an abortifacient and a teratogen. Follow safe handling procedures when preparing or administering drug.

ACTION
A synthetic prostaglandin E₁ analogue that replaces gastric prostaglandins depleted by NSAID therapy, decreases basal and stimulated gastric acid secretion, and increases gastric mucus and bicarbonate production.

Route	Onset	Peak	Duration
P.O.	30 min	60–90 min	3 hr

Half-life: 20 to 40 minutes.

ADVERSE REACTIONS
CNS: headache.
GI: abdominal pain, diarrhea, constipation, dyspepsia, flatulence, nausea, vomiting.
GU: cramps, dysmenorrhea, hypermenorrhea, menstrual disorders, postmenopausal vaginal bleeding, spotting.

INTERACTIONS
Drug-drug. *Magnesium-containing antacids:* May enhance adverse or toxic effect of misoprostol. Monitor patient for increased adverse effects, such as diarrhea and dehydration, and consider therapy modification.
Drug-food. *Any food:* May decrease absorption rate of drug. However, manufacturer recommends that patient take drug with food.

EFFECTS ON LAB TEST RESULTS
None reported.

CONTRAINDICATIONS & CAUTIONS
• Contraindicated in those allergic to prostaglandins, pregnant women, or those who are breast-feeding.
• Use with caution in patients with inflammatory bowel disease.
⚠ **Overdose S&S:** Sedation, tremors, seizures, dyspnea, abdominal pain, fever, diarrhea, palpitations, hypotension, bradycardia.

NURSING CONSIDERATIONS
Black Box Warning Take special precautions to prevent use of drug during pregnancy. Uterine rupture is linked to certain risk factors, including later trimester pregnancies, higher doses of the drug, prior cesarean delivery or uterine surgery, and five or more previous pregnancies. Make sure woman understands dangers of drug to herself and her fetus and that she receives both oral and written warnings about these dangers. Also, make sure she can comply with effective contraception and that the result of a pregnancy test performed within 2 weeks of starting therapy is negative. ■
• Drug causes modest decrease in basal pepsin secretion.
• **Look alike–sound alike:** Don't confuse misoprostol with mifepristone.

Reactions in bold italics are *life-threatening*. Interactions may have a *rapid onset* or a *delayed onset*.

PATIENT TEACHING
• Instruct patient not to share drug.

Black Box Warning Remind pregnant woman that drug may cause miscarriage, often with potentially life-threatening bleeding. ■

Black Box Warning Advise woman not to begin therapy until second or third day of next normal menstrual period. ■

• Advise patient to take drug as prescribed for duration of NSAID therapy.

• Tell patient that diarrhea usually occurs early in the course of therapy and is usually self-limiting. Taking drug with food helps minimize the diarrhea.

SAFETY ALERT!

mitomycin (mitomycin-C)
mye-toe-MYE-sin

Therapeutic class: Antineoplastics
Pharmacologic class: Antineoplastic antibiotics
Pregnancy risk category: D

AVAILABLE FORMS
Powder for injection: 5-, 20-, 40-mg vials

INDICATIONS & DOSAGES
Dosage and indications vary. Check treatment protocol with prescriber.

➤ **Disseminated adenocarcinoma of stomach or pancreas in combination with other chemotherapeutic agents**
Adults: 20 mg/m^2 I.V. as a single dose at 6- to 8-week intervals if patient has full hematologic recovery. Fully evaluate patient after each cycle and reduce dosage if toxicities occur.

Adjust-a-dose: For patients with myelosuppression, if WBC count is 2,000 to 2,999/mm^3 and platelet count is 25,000 to 74,999/mm^3, give 70% of initial dose. If WBC count is less than 2,000/mm^3 and platelet count is less than 25,000/mm^3, give 50% of initial dose. Don't repeat full dosage until WBC count has returned to 4,000/mm^3 and platelet count to 100,000/mm^3.

ADMINISTRATION
I.V.

▼ Drug is a vesicant. Never give drug I.M. or subcutaneously.

▼ Preparing and giving drug may be mutagenic, teratogenic, or carcinogenic. Follow institutional policy to reduce risks.

▼ Using sterile water for injection, reconstitute drug in 5-mg vials with 10 mL, 20-mg vials with 40 mL, and 40-mg vials with 80 mL.

▼ Give drug into the side arm of a freeflowing I.V.

▼ When reconstituted with sterile water, solution is stable for 14 days under refrigeration and 7 days at room temperature. When diluted, drug is stable in D$_5$W for no more than 3 hours, in normal saline solution for no more than 12 hours, and in sodium lactate for no more than 24 hours.

▼ The combination of mitomycin (5 to 15 mg) and heparin (1,000 to 10,000 units) in 30 mL normal saline solution is stable for 48 hours at room temperature.

▼ Stop infusion immediately and notify prescriber if extravasation occurs because of potential for severe ulceration and necrosis.

▼ **Incompatibilities:** Aztreonam, bleomycin, cefepime, etoposide, filgrastim, gemcitabine, piperacillin sodium–tazobactam sodium, sargramostim, topotecan, vinorelbine.

ACTION
Similar to an alkylating drug, cross-linking strands of DNA and causing an imbalance of cell growth, leading to cell death.

Route	Onset	Peak	Duration
I.V.	Unknown	Unknown	Unknown

Half-life: About 50 minutes.

ADVERSE REACTIONS
CNS: headache, neurologic abnormalities, confusion, drowsiness, fatigue, fever, pain.
EENT: blurred vision.
GI: mucositis, nausea, vomiting, anorexia, diarrhea, stomatitis.
GU: *renal toxicity, hemolytic-uremic syndrome.*
Hematologic: *thrombocytopenia, leukopenia, microangiopathic hemolytic anemia.*

M

Respiratory: *interstitial pneumonitis, pulmonary edema,* dyspnea, nonproductive cough, *acute respiratory distress syndrome.* **Skin:** cellulitis, induration, desquamation, pruritus, pain at injection site, reversible alopecia, purple bands on nails, rash, sloughing with extravasation.
Other: *septicemia,* ulceration.

INTERACTIONS
Drug-drug. *Vinca alkaloids:* May cause acute respiratory distress when given together. Monitor patient closely.

EFFECTS ON LAB TEST RESULTS
● May increase BUN and creatinine levels. May decrease hemoglobin level.
● May decrease WBC and platelet counts.

CONTRAINDICATIONS & CAUTIONS
● Contraindicated in patients hypersensitive to drug and in those with thrombocytopenia, coagulation disorders, or an increased bleeding tendency from other causes.
● Don't give to patients with serum creatinine level greater than 1.7 mg/dL.

NURSING CONSIDERATIONS
Black Box Warning Administer drug under the supervision of a physician experienced with cancer chemotherapeutic agents. ■
Black Box Warning Bone marrow suppression is the most common and severe toxic effect. ■
● Reevaluate patient fully after each course of mitomycin, and reduce dosage if patient has experienced toxicities.
❸ Alert: Extravasation may occur, causing cellulitis, ulceration, and tissue slough. If signs or symptoms of these conditions occur, stop infusion immediately and notify prescriber. Withdraw 3 to 5 mL of blood; then remove infusion needle. Treatment may include ice compresses, application of dimethyl sulfoxide, limb elevation, and protecting site from friction. If skin necrosis develops, skin grafting may be necessary.
● Continue CBC and blood studies at least 8 weeks after therapy stops. Leukopenia and thrombocytopenia are cumulative. If WBC count falls below 2,000/mm³ or granulocyte count falls below 1,000/mm³,

follow institutional policy for infection control in immunocompromised patients.
● To prevent bleeding, avoid all I.M. injections when platelet count is less than 100,000/mm³.
● Anticipate need for blood transfusions to combat anemia.
● Monitor patient for dyspnea with nonproductive cough; chest X-ray may show infiltrates.
● Monitor renal function tests.
● Leukopenia may occur up to 8 weeks after therapy and may be cumulative with successive doses.
Black Box Warning Hemolytic-uremic syndrome is characterized by microangiopathic hemolytic anemia, thrombocytopenia, and renal failure. Most cases occur at doses of 60 mg or more. ■

PATIENT TEACHING
● Advise patient to report any pain or burning at site of injection during or after administration.
● Warn patient to watch for signs and symptoms of infection (fever, sore throat, fatigue) and bleeding (easy bruising, nosebleeds, bleeding gums, tarry stools). Tell patient to take temperature daily.
● Inform patient that hair loss may occur but that it's usually reversible.

SAFETY ALERT!

mitoxantrone hydrochloride
mye-toe-ZAN-trone

Therapeutic class: Antineoplastics
Pharmacologic class: DNA-reactive drugs–anthracenediones
Pregnancy risk category: D

AVAILABLE FORMS
Injection: 2 mg/mL

INDICATIONS & DOSAGES
➤ **Combination initial therapy for acute nonlymphocytic leukemia (ANLL)**
Adults: Induction begins with 12 mg/m² I.V. daily on days 1 to 3, with 100 mg/m² daily of cytarabine on days 1 to 7 as a continuous 24-hour infusion. A second induction may

---

be given if response isn't adequate. Maintenance therapy is 12 mg/m^2 on days 1 and 2, with cytarabine 100 mg/m^2 on days 1 to 5 as a continuous 24-hour infusion.

➤ **To reduce neurologic disability and frequency of relapse in chronic progressive, progressive relapsing, or worsening relapsing-remitting MS**

Adults: 12 mg/m^2 I.V. over 5 to 15 minutes every 3 months. Maximum cumulative lifetime dose is 140 mg/m^2.

➤ **Advanced hormone-refractory prostate cancer**

Men: 12 to 14 mg/m^2 as a short I.V. infusion every 21 days. Drug is given as an adjunct to corticosteroid therapy.

ADMINISTRATION

I.V.

▼ Preparing and giving drug may be mutagenic, teratogenic, or carcinogenic. Follow facility policy to reduce risks.

▼ Dilute dose in at least 50 mL of normal saline solution for injection or D$_5$W injection. Don't mix with other drugs.

Black Box Warning Give slowly into a free-flowing I.V. infusion of normal saline solution or D$_5$W injection over at least 3 minutes. ∎

Black Box Warning Never give subcutaneously, intra-arterially, intramuscularly, or intrathecally. ∎

Black Box Warning Severe local tissue damage may result if extravasation occurs. ∎

▼ If extravasation occurs, stop infusion immediately and notify prescriber. Place ice packs over the area intermittently.

▼ Once vial is penetrated, undiluted solution may be stored for 7 days at room temperature or 14 days in refrigerator. Don't freeze.

▼ **Incompatibilities:** Amphotericin B, aztreonam, cefepime, doxorubicin liposomal, heparin sodium, hydrocortisone, other I.V. drugs, paclitaxel, piperacillin sodium–tazobactam sodium, propofol, sargramostim.

ACTION

Reacts with DNA, producing cytotoxic effect. Probably not specific to cell cycle.

Route	Onset	Peak	Duration
I.V.	Unknown	Unknown	Unknown

Half-life: Terminal half-life, 23 to 215 hours.

ADVERSE REACTIONS

CNS: fever, headache, *seizures.*

CV: *arrhythmias,* ECG abnormalities, *heart failure,* tachycardia.

EENT: conjunctivitis, sinusitis.

GI: abdominal pain, bleeding, constipation, diarrhea, mucositis, nausea, stomatitis, vomiting.

GU: amenorrhea, menstrual disorder, UTI, *renal failure.*

Hematologic: *myelosuppression,* anemia.

Hepatic: jaundice.

Metabolic: hyperuricemia.

Musculoskeletal: back pain.

Respiratory: cough, dyspnea, upper respiratory tract infection, pneumonia.

Skin: alopecia, ecchymoses, local irritation or phlebitis, petechiae.

Other: fungal infections, *sepsis.*

INTERACTIONS

Cyclosporine: May increase effects of mitoxantrone. Monitor patient closely.

Digoxin: May decrease digoxin level. Monitor serum level and patient closely, and adjust digoxin dosage as needed.

Hydantoins (such as phenytoin): May decrease levels of these drugs, increasing risk of seizure. Monitor levels and adjust hydantoin dosage as needed.

Palifermin: May increase severity of oral mucositis. Don't give palifermin within 24 hours before or after mitoxantrone dose.

Trastuzumab: May increase risk of trastuzumab-induced cardiac dysfunction. Monitor patient closely for signs and symptoms of cardiac dysfunction.

Vaccines (live-virus): May increase risk of vaccine-induced adverse reactions. Defer vaccination until mitoxantrone therapy has been completed.

EFFECTS ON LAB TEST RESULTS

● May increase ALT, AST, bilirubin, GGT, and uric acid levels. May decrease hemoglobin level and hematocrit.

● May decrease leukocyte and granulocyte counts.

M

CONTRAINDICATIONS & CAUTIONS
● Contraindicated in patients hypersensitive to drug.

[Black Box Warning] Evaluate LVEF before initiating treatment and before administering each dose of mitoxantrone to patients with MS. All patients with MS who have finished treatment should receive yearly, quantitative LVEF evaluation to detect late-occurring cardiotoxicity. ▪

● Use cautiously in patients with previous exposure to anthracyclines or other cardiotoxic drugs, previous radiation therapy to mediastinal area, or heart disease. Significantly myelosuppressed patients shouldn't receive drug unless benefits outweigh risks.

⚠ **Overdose S&S:** Severe leukopenia.

NURSING CONSIDERATIONS
[Black Box Warning] Administer under the supervision of a physician experienced with cytotoxic chemotherapy. ▪

[Black Box Warning] Except when used to treat ANLL, mitoxantrone should generally not be given to patients with baseline neutrophil counts less than 1,500 cells/mm^3. Frequently monitor peripheral blood cell counts for all patients using drug. ▪

● Closely monitor hematologic and laboratory chemistry parameters, including LFTs. Obtain CBC and platelet count before each course of treatment. Patient may require blood transfusion or RBC or WBC colony-stimulating factors.

● Avoid all I.M. injections if platelet count falls below 50,000/mm^3.

[Black Box Warning] Use of drug has been associated with cardiotoxicity. Monitor LVEF before initiating therapy and prior to each dose; risk of cardiotoxicity increases with cumulative dose of 140 mg/m^2, although toxicities may occur at any dose. Continue ongoing cardiac monitoring to detect late occurring cardiotoxicity. ▪

● If severe nonhematologic toxicity occurs during first course, delay second course until patient recovers.

[Black Box Warning] Secondary acute myelocytic leukemia has been reported with mitoxantrone therapy. ▪

☙ **Alert:** Women with MS who are biologically capable of becoming pregnant should

have a pregnancy test even if they are using birth control. The results should be known before receiving each dose.

PATIENT TEACHING
● Advise patient to report any pain or burning at site of injection during or after administration.

● Tell patient that urine may appear blue-green within 24 hours after receiving drug and that the whites of his eyes may turn blue. These effects are not harmful but may persist during therapy.

● Advise patient to watch for signs and symptoms of bleeding and infection.

● Advise patient to use appropriate method of birth control to avoid pregnancy while receiving drug.

---

modafinil
moe-DAFF-in-ill

Alertec†, Provigil✐

Therapeutic class: CNS stimulants
Pharmacologic class: Analeptics
Pregnancy risk category: C
Controlled substance schedule: IV

AVAILABLE FORMS
Tablets: 100 mg, 200 mg

INDICATIONS & DOSAGES
➤ **To improve wakefulness in patients with excessive daytime sleepiness caused by narcolepsy, obstructive sleep apnea-hypopnea syndrome, and shift-work sleep disorder**
Adults and adolescents age 16 and older: 200 mg P.O. daily, as a single dose in the morning. Patients with shift-work sleep disorder should take dose about 1 hour before the start of their shift. Maximum dose is 400 mg P.O. daily as a single dose.
Adjust-a-dose: In patients with severe hepatic impairment, give 100 mg P.O. daily, as a single dose in the morning.
➤ **MS-related fatigue ◆**
Adults: 100 mg P.O. once daily in the morning. Titrate by 100 mg weekly to a maximum of 400 mg P.O. daily.

ADMINISTRATION
P.O.
• Give drug without regard for food; however, food may delay effect of drug.

ACTION
Unknown. Similar to action of sympathomimetics, including amphetamines, but drug is structurally distinct from amphetamines and doesn't alter release of dopamine or norepinephrine to produce CNS stimulation.

Route	Onset	Peak	Duration
P.O.	Unknown	2–4 hr	Unknown

Half-life: 15 hours.

ADVERSE REACTIONS
CNS: headache, nervousness, dizziness, insomnia, fever, depression, anxiety, cataplexy, paresthesia, dyskinesia, hypertonia, confusion, syncope, amnesia, emotional lability, ataxia, tremor, mania, hallucination, *suicidal ideation.*
CV: *arrhythmias,* hypotension, hypertension, vasodilation, chest pain.
EENT: rhinitis, pharyngitis, epistaxis, amblyopia, abnormal vision.
GI: nausea, diarrhea, dry mouth, anorexia, vomiting, mouth ulcer, gingivitis, thirst.
GU: abnormal urine, urine retention, abnormal ejaculation, albuminuria.
Hematologic: eosinophilia.
Metabolic: hyperglycemia.
Musculoskeletal: joint disorder, neck pain, neck rigidity.
Respiratory: *asthma,* dyspnea, lung disorder.
Skin: sweating.
Other: herpes simplex, chills.

INTERACTIONS
Drug-drug. *Carbamazepine, phenobarbital, rifampin, other inducers of CYP3A4:* May alter modafinil level. Monitor patient closely.
Cyclosporine, theophylline: May reduce levels of these drugs. Use together cautiously.
Diazepam, phenytoin, propranolol, other drugs metabolized by CYP2C19: May inhibit CYP2C19 and lead to higher levels of drugs metabolized by this enzyme. Use together cautiously; adjust dosage as needed.

Hormonal contraceptives: May reduce contraceptive effectiveness. Advise patient to use alternative or additional method of contraception during modafinil therapy and for 1 month after drug is stopped.
Itraconazole, ketoconazole, other inhibitors of CYP3A4: May alter modafinil level. Monitor patient closely.
Methylphenidate: May cause 1-hour delay in modafinil absorption. Separate dosage times.
Phenytoin, warfarin: May inhibit CYP2C9 and increase phenytoin and warfarin levels. Monitor patient closely for toxicity.
TCAs (such as clomipramine, desipramine): May increase TCA level. Reduce dosage of these drugs.
Drug-lifestyle. *Alcohol use:* Coadministration hasn't been studied. Avoid using together.

EFFECTS ON LAB TEST RESULTS
• May increase glucose, GGT, and AST levels.
• May increase eosinophil count.

CONTRAINDICATIONS & CAUTIONS
• Contraindicated in patients hypersensitive to drug and in those with a history of left ventricular hypertrophy or ischemic ECG changes, chest pain, arrhythmias, or other evidence of mitral valve prolapse linked to CNS stimulant use.
• Use cautiously in patients with recent MI or unstable angina and in those with history of psychosis.
• Use cautiously and give reduced dosage to patients with severe hepatic impairment, with or without cirrhosis.
• Use cautiously in patients taking MAO inhibitors.
• Safety and effectiveness in patients with severe renal impairment haven't been determined.
• Modafinil isn't approved for use in children younger than age 16 for any indication.
⚠ Overdose S&S: Agitation or excitation, insomnia, slight or moderate elevations in hemodynamic parameters, aggressiveness, anxiety, confusion, decreased PT, diarrhea, irritability, nausea, nervousness, palpitations, sleep disturbances, tremor,

M

bradycardia, chest pain, hypertension, tachycardia, hallucination, restlessness.

NURSING CONSIDERATIONS
• Monitor patient for rash or emergence or exacerbation of psychiatric signs and symptoms.
• Monitor hypertensive patients closely.
• Although single daily 400-mg doses have been well tolerated, the larger dose is no more beneficial than the 200-mg dose.
• **Look alike–sound alike:** Don't confuse Provigil with Nuvigil.

PATIENT TEACHING
❶ **Alert:** Advise patient to stop drug and notify prescriber if rash, peeling skin, trouble swallowing or breathing, or other symptoms of allergic reaction occur. Rare cases of serious rash, including Stevens-Johnson syndrome, toxic epidermal necrolysis, and drug rash with eosinophilia and hypersensitivity, have been reported.
• Advise woman to notify prescriber about planned, suspected, or known pregnancy, or if she's breast-feeding.
• Caution patient that use of hormonal contraceptives (including depot or implantable contraceptives) together with modafinil tablets may reduce contraceptive effectiveness. Recommend an alternative method of contraception during modafinil therapy and for 1 month after drug is stopped.
• Instruct patient to confer with prescriber before taking prescription or OTC drugs to avoid drug interactions.
• Tell patient to avoid alcohol while taking drug.
• Warn patient to avoid activities that require alertness or good coordination until CNS effects of drug are known.

---

moexipril hydrochloride
moe-EX-eh-pril

Univasc

Therapeutic class: Antihypertensives
Pharmacologic class: ACE inhibitors
Pregnancy risk category: D

AVAILABLE FORMS
Tablets: 7.5 mg, 15 mg

INDICATIONS & DOSAGES
➤ **Hypertension, alone or in combination with thiazide diuretics**
Adults: Initially, 7.5 mg P.O. once daily as monotherapy, given 1 hour before a meal. Or initially, 3.75 mg if diuretic therapy can't be discontinued. Increase dosage incrementally according to blood pressure response. Maximum dosage is 30 mg daily in one or two divided doses.
Adjust-a-dose: For patients currently being treated with a diuretic, if possible stop diuretic 2 to 3 days before therapy is initiated to reduce likelihood of hypotension. If blood pressure isn't adequately controlled with moexipril alone, may reinstitute diuretic therapy. For patients with CrCl of 40 mL/minute/1.73 m^2 or less, cautiously give initial dose of 3.75 mg once daily. May titrate dosage upward to a maximum daily dosage of 15 mg.

ADMINISTRATION
P.O.
• Give 1 hour before meal on empty stomach.
• Check blood pressure before next dose to evaluate effectiveness.
• Store, tightly closed, at controlled room temperature. Protect from excessive moisture.

ACTION
Decreases angiotensin II formation, leading to decreased vasoconstriction, increased plasma renin activity, and decreased aldosterone secretion.

Route	Onset	Peak	Duration
P.O.	1 hr	1½ hr	Unknown

Half-life: 2 to 9 hours.

ADVERSE REACTIONS
CNS: dizziness, fatigue, headache, pain.
CV: flushing, chest pain, peripheral edema.
EENT: pharyngitis, rhinitis, sinusitis.
GI: diarrhea, dyspepsia, nausea.
GU: urinary frequency.
Musculoskeletal: myalgia.
Respiratory: cough, upper respiratory tract infections.
Skin: rash.
Other: flulike syndrome.

INTERACTIONS

❷ *Alert: Aliskiren:* May increase risk of renal impairment, hypotension, and hyperkalemia in diabetic patients and in those with moderate to severe renal impairment (GFR less than 60 mL/minute). Concomitant use is contraindicated in diabetic patients. Avoid concomitant use in those with moderate to severe renal impairment.

Diuretics: May increase risk of hypotension. Discontinue diuretic therapy for several days or cautiously increase salt intake before initiation of moexipril. If this isn't an option, decrease moexipril starting dose.

Gold: May cause rare nitritoid reaction (facial flushing, nausea, vomiting, and hypotension). Monitor patient closely.

Lithium: May increase serum lithium level and risk of lithium toxicity. Use cautiously together and monitor lithium level frequently. If concomitant diuretic is prescribed, risk of lithium toxicity may increase.

Potassium-sparing diuretics, potassium supplements: May increase serum potassium level. Use together cautiously; monitor potassium level periodically.

NSAIDs: May increase risk of renal dysfunction and acute renal failure in patients who are elderly or volume-depleted (including those on diuretics) or have compromised renal function. Monitor renal function. These drugs may increase moexipril's antihypertensive effect. Use cautiously together.

Drug-food. *Potassium-containing salt substitutes:* May increase risk of hyperkalemia. Discourage use together.

EFFECTS ON LAB TEST RESULTS

• May increase potassium, BUN, creatinine, AST, ALT, and uric acid levels.
• May decrease WBC count.

CONTRAINDICATIONS & CAUTIONS

• Contraindicated in patients hypersensitive to drug and in those with a history of angioedema related to previous treatment with an ACE inhibitor.

Black Box Warning Contraindicated in pregnant women. When pregnancy is detected, discontinue moexipril as soon as possible. Drugs that act directly on the renin-angiotensin system can cause injury and death to a developing fetus. ■

• Use cautiously in patients with salt and volume depletion as a result of prolonged diuretic therapy, dietary salt restriction, dialysis, diabetes, diarrhea, or vomiting.

• Use cautiously in patients with congestive heart failure, ischemic heart disease, aortic stenosis or cerebrovascular disease, renal stenosis, or renal impairment.

• Use cautiously in patients who are to undergo surgery or anesthesia.

⚠ *Overdose S&S:* Hypotension.

NURSING CONSIDERATIONS

• Before starting drug, correct fluid volume and salt depletion and stop diuretics.
• After initial dose of moexipril, monitor patients currently being treated with a diuretic for symptomatic hypotension.
• Begin therapy under close supervision and monitor patient closely with each adjustment in dosage of moexipril or accompanying diuretic.
• If hypotension occurs, place patient in a supine position and treat with I.V. normal saline if needed. May restart moexipril once patient is stable.
• In controlled trials, ACE inhibitors were shown to have less effect on blood pressure and cause a higher risk of angioedema in black patients than in non-black patients.
• Monitor patients for anaphylactoid or possible related reactions, which can be serious. If facial edema occurs, discontinue drug and monitor patient carefully until swelling disappears. Swelling usually resolves without treatment or with antihistamines and glucocorticoids. Angioedema involving the tongue, glottis, or larynx may be fatal due to airway obstruction; therapy with subcutaneous epinephrine solution 1:1,000 (0.3 to 0.5 mL) or measures to ensure an open airway should be provided.
• Monitor patients for neutropenia and signs and symptoms of infection.
• Monitor WBC count in patients with collagen vascular disease, especially if it's affecting renal function.
• Monitor patients for signs and symptoms of liver injury (jaundice, increased LFT values). If necessary, stop drug and provide appropriate medical management.

M

• Monitor renal function and potassium level before and periodically during treatment.

PATIENT TEACHING

• Advise patient to take moexipril 1 hour before meals, on an empty stomach, for best results.

• Tell patient to stop drug and immediately report signs or symptoms of angioedema (swelling of the face, extremities, eyes, lips, or tongue and difficulty breathing).

• Caution patient that light-headedness may occur, especially during first few days of therapy. If fainting occurs, patient should stop moexipril and consult prescriber.

• Warn patient to contact health care provider if excessive perspiration, dehydration, or vomiting occurs, which may decrease blood pressure to an unsafe level.

• Tell patient to avoid potassium supplements or salt substitutes containing potassium.

• Instruct patient to report signs and symptoms of infection (sore throat, fever).

Black Box Warning Tell female patient of childbearing age to stop drug and report possible pregnancy promptly. ▮

• Advise patient to inform health care provider if a persistent cough develops during therapy.

mometasone furoate
moe-MEH-tah-zone

Asmanex Twisthaler

mometasone furoate monohydrate
Nasonex

Therapeutic class: Antiasthmatics
Pharmacologic class: Glucocorticoids
Pregnancy risk category: C

AVAILABLE FORMS
Inhalation powder: 110 mcg/inhalation, 220 mcg/inhalation
Nasal spray: 50 mcg/spray

INDICATIONS & DOSAGES
➤ **Maintenance therapy for asthma; asthma in patients who take an oral corticosteroid**
Adults and children age 12 and older who previously used a bronchodilator or inhaled corticosteroid: Initially, 220 mcg by oral inhalation every day in the evening. Maximum, 440 mcg/day.
Adults and children age 12 and older who take an oral corticosteroid: 440 mcg b.i.d. by oral inhalation. Maximum, 880 mcg/day. Reduce oral corticosteroid dosage by no more than 2.5 mg/day at weekly intervals, beginning at least 1 week after starting mometasone. After stopping oral corticosteroid, reduce mometasone dose to lowest effective amount.
Children ages 4 to 11: 110 mcg by oral inhalation once daily in the evening.
➤ **Allergic rhinitis**
Adults and children age 12 and older: 2 sprays (50 mcg/spray) in each nostril once daily.
Children ages 2 to 11: 1 spray (50 mcg/spray) in each nostril once daily.
➤ **Nasal polyps**
Adults: 2 sprays (50 mcg/spray) in each nostril once daily to b.i.d.

ADMINISTRATION
Inhalational
• Have patient breathe deeply and rapidly during administration.
• Have patient rinse his mouth after administration.
Intranasal
• Before initial use, prime nasal spray pump 10 times or until fine spray appears.
• Pump may be stored for 1 week without repriming. If unused for more than 1 week, reprime two times or until a fine spray appears.

ACTION
Unknown, although corticosteroids inhibit many cells and mediators involved in inflammation and the asthmatic response.

Route	Onset	Peak	Duration
Inhalation	Unknown	1–2½ hr	Unknown
Intranasal	Unknown	Unknown	Unknown

Half-life: 5 hours (oral); 5.8 hours (nasal).

Reactions in bold italics are *life-threatening*. Interactions may have a *rapid onset* or a *delayed onset*.

ADVERSE REACTIONS

CNS: headache, depression, fatigue, insomnia, pain.
EENT: allergic rhinitis, pharyngitis, dry throat, dysphonia, earache, epistaxis, nasal irritation, sinus congestion, sinusitis, oral candidiasis.
GI: abdominal pain, anorexia, dyspepsia, flatulence, gastroenteritis, nausea, vomiting.
GU: dysmenorrhea, menstrual disorder, UTI.
Musculoskeletal: arthralgia, back pain, myalgia.
Respiratory: upper respiratory tract infection, respiratory disorder.
Other: flulike symptoms, infection.

INTERACTIONS

Drug-drug. *Ketoconazole:* May increase mometasone level. Use together cautiously.

EFFECTS ON LAB TEST RESULTS

None reported.

CONTRAINDICATIONS & CAUTIONS

• Contraindicated in patients hypersensitive to drug or its ingredients and in those with status asthmaticus or other acute forms of asthma or bronchospasm (as primary treatment).
• Use cautiously in patients at high risk for decreased bone mineral content (those with a family history of osteoporosis, prolonged immobilization, long-term use of drugs that reduce bone mass), patients switching from a systemic to an inhaled corticosteroid, and patients with active or dormant tuberculosis, untreated systemic infections, ocular herpes simplex, or immunosuppression.
• Use cautiously in breast-feeding women.
⚠ **Overdose S&S:** Hypercorticism.

NURSING CONSIDERATIONS

🔶 **Alert:** Don't use for acute bronchospasm.
• Wean patient slowly from a systemic corticosteroid after he switches to mometasone. Monitor lung function tests, beta-agonist use, and asthma symptoms.
🔶 **Alert:** If patient is switching from an oral corticosteroid to an inhaled form, watch closely for evidence of adrenal insufficiency, such as fatigue, lethargy, weakness, nausea, vomiting, and hypotension.

• After an oral corticosteroid is withdrawn, hypothalamic-pituitary-adrenal (HPA) function may not recover for months. If patient has trauma, stress, infection, or surgery during this HPA recovery period, he is particularly vulnerable to adrenal insufficiency or adrenal crisis.
• Because an inhaled corticosteroid can be systemically absorbed, watch for cushingoid effects.
• Assess patient for bone loss during long-term use.
• Watch for evidence of localized mouth infections, glaucoma, and immunosuppression.
• Use drug only if benefits to mother justify risks to fetus. If a woman takes a corticosteroid during pregnancy, monitor neonate for hypoadrenalism.
• Monitor elderly patients for increased sensitivity to drug effects.

PATIENT TEACHING

• Instruct patient on proper use and routine care of the inhaler or nasal spray pump.
• Tell patient to use drug regularly and at the same time each day. If he uses it only once daily, tell him to do so in the evening.
• Caution patient not to use drug for immediate relief of an asthma attack or bronchospasm.
• Inform patient that maximal benefits might not occur for 1 to 2 weeks or longer after therapy starts; instruct him to notify his prescriber if his condition fails to improve or worsens.
• Tell patient that if he has bronchospasm after taking drug, he should immediately use a fast-acting bronchodilator. Urge him to contact prescriber immediately if bronchospasm doesn't respond to the fast-acting bronchodilator.
🔶 **Alert:** If patient has been weaned from an oral corticosteroid, urge him to contact prescriber immediately if an asthma attack occurs or if he is experiencing a period of stress. The oral corticosteroid may need to be resumed.
• Warn patient to avoid exposure to chickenpox or measles and to notify prescriber if such contact occurs.
• Long-term use of an inhaled corticosteroid may increase the risk of cataracts

M

or glaucoma; tell patient to report vision changes.

● Advise patient to write the date on a new inhaler on the day he opens it and to discard the inhaler after 45 days or when the dose counter reads "00."

montelukast sodium
mon-tell-OO-kast

Singulair✦

Therapeutic class: Antiasthmatics
Pharmacologic class: Leukotriene-receptor antagonists
Pregnancy risk category: B

AVAILABLE FORMS
Oral granules: 4-mg packet
Tablets (chewable): 4 mg, 5 mg
Tablets (film-coated): 10 mg

INDICATIONS & DOSAGES
➤ **Asthma, seasonal allergic rhinitis, perennial allergic rhinitis**
Adults and children age 15 and older:
10 mg P.O. once daily in evening.
Children ages 6 to 14: 5 mg chewable tablet P.O. once daily in evening.
Children ages 2 to 5: 4 mg chewable tablet or 1 packet of 4-mg oral granules P.O. once daily in the evening.
Children ages 12 to 23 months (asthma only): 1 packet of 4-mg oral granules P.O. once daily in the evening.
Children ages 6 to 23 months (perennial allergic rhinitis only): 1 packet of 4-mg oral granules P.O. once daily in the evening.
➤ **Prevention of exercise-induced bronchoconstriction**
Adults and children age 15 and older:
10 mg P.O. at least 2 hours before exercise. Patients already taking a daily dose shouldn't take an additional dose. Also, an additional dose shouldn't be taken within 24 hours of a previous dose.
Children ages 6 to 14: 5 mg P.O. at least 2 hours before exercise (1 chewable tablet). An additional dose shouldn't be taken within 24 hours of a previous dose.

ADMINISTRATION
P.O.
● Give oral granules directly in the mouth, dissolved in 5 mL of cold or room-temperature baby formula or breast milk, or mixed with a spoonful of cold or room-temperature soft foods (use only applesauce, carrots, rice, or ice cream).

ACTION
Reduces early and late-phase bronchoconstriction from antigen challenge.

Route	Onset	Peak	Duration
P.O. (chewable, granules)	Unknown	2–2½ hr	24 hr
P.O. (film-coated)	Unknown	3–4 hr	24 hr

Half-life: 2¾ to 5½ hours.

ADVERSE REACTIONS
CNS: headache, asthenia, dizziness, fatigue, fever.
EENT: dental pain, nasal congestion.
GI: abdominal pain, dyspepsia, infectious gastroenteritis.
GU: pyuria.
Hematologic: systemic eosinophilia.
Respiratory: cough.
Skin: rash.
Other: influenza, trauma.

INTERACTIONS
Drug-drug. *Phenobarbital, rifampin:* May decrease bioavailability of montelukast because of hepatic metabolism induction. Monitor patient for effectiveness.

EFFECTS ON LAB TEST RESULTS
● May increase ALT and AST levels.

CONTRAINDICATIONS & CAUTIONS
● Contraindicated in patients hypersensitive to drug or its ingredients.
● Use cautiously and with appropriate monitoring in patients whose dosages of systemic corticosteroids are reduced.
⚠ ***Overdose S&S:*** Headache, vomiting, psychomotor hyperactivity, thirst, somnolence, mydriasis, hyperkinesia, abdominal pain.

NURSING CONSIDERATIONS
● Assess patient's underlying condition, and monitor him for effectiveness.

⟩ Alert: Don't abruptly substitute drug for inhaled or oral corticosteroids. Dose of inhaled corticosteroids may be reduced gradually.

⟩ Alert: Drug isn't indicated for use in patients with acute asthmatic attacks, status asthmaticus, or as monotherapy for management of exercise-induced bronchospasm. Continue appropriate rescue drug for acute worsening.

• Drug may cause behavior and mood changes. Monitor patient and consider discontinuing drug if neuropsychiatric symptoms develop.

PATIENT TEACHING

• Inform caregiver that the oral granules may be given directly into the child's mouth, dissolved in 1 teaspoon of cold or room-temperature baby formula or breast milk, or mixed in a spoonful of applesauce, carrots, rice, or ice cream.

• Tell caregiver not to open packet until ready to use and, after opening, to give the full dose within 15 minutes. Tell her that if she's mixing the drug with food, not to store excess for future use and to discard the unused portion.

• Advise patient to take drug daily, even if asymptomatic, and to contact his prescriber if asthma isn't well controlled.

• Warn patient not to reduce or stop taking other prescribed antiasthmatics without prescriber's approval.

• Advise patient to seek medical attention if short-acting inhaled bronchodilators are needed more often than usual during drug therapy.

• Warn patient that drug isn't beneficial in acute asthma attacks or in exercise-induced bronchospasm, and advise him to keep appropriate rescue drugs available.

• Warn patient that drug may cause behavior and mood changes, and to report development of these symptoms to prescriber.

• Advise patient with known aspirin sensitivity to continue to avoid using aspirin and NSAIDs during drug therapy.

⟩ Alert: Advise patient with phenylketonuria that chewable tablet contains phenylalanine.

morphine hydrochloride
MOR-feen

Doloral†, M.O.S†, M.O.S.-S.R†

morphine sulfate
Astramorph PF, Avinza, Duramorph PF, Infumorph, Kadian, M-Eslon†, Morphine LP Epidural†, M.O.S. Sulphate†, MS Contin, Statex†

Therapeutic class: Opioid analgesics
Pharmacologic class: Opioids
Pregnancy risk category: C
Controlled substance schedule: II

AVAILABLE FORMS
morphine hydrochloride
Suppositories: 10 mg†, 20 mg†, 30 mg†
Syrup: 1 mg/mL†*, 5 mg/mL†*, 10 mg/mL†*, 20 mg/mL†*, 50 mg/mL†*
Tablets: 10 mg†, 20 mg†, 40 mg†, 60 mg†
Tablets (extended-release): 30 mg†, 60 mg†
morphine sulfate
Capsules (extended-release microgranules [M-Eslon]): 10 mg†, 15 mg†, 30 mg†, 60 mg†, 100 mg†, 200 mg†
Capsules (extended-release pellets [Avinza]): 30 mg, 45 mg, 60 mg, 75 mg, 90 mg, 120 mg
Capsules (extended-release pellets [Kadian]): 10 mg, 20 mg, 30 mg, 40 mg, 50 mg, 60 mg, 70 mg, 80 mg, 100 mg, 130 mg, 150 mg, 200 mg
Drops: 20 mg/mL†, 50 mg/mL†
Injection (epidural): 0.5 mg/mL, 1 mg/mL, 10 mg/mL, 25 mg/mL
Injection (with preservative): 0.5 mg/mL, 1 mg/mL, 2 mg/mL, 5 mg/mL, 10 mg/mL, 15 mg/mL, 25 mg/mL, 50 mg/mL
Injection (without preservative): 0.5 mg/mL, 1 mg/mL, 5 mg/mL, 10 mg/mL, 25 mg/mL
Injection (without preservative [Carpuject and prefilled syringes]): 2 mg/mL, 4 mg/mL, 8 mg/mL, 10 mg/mL, 15 mg/mL
Oral solution: 10 mg/5 mL, 20 mg/5 mL, 20 mg/mL (concentrate), 100 mg/5 mL (concentrate)
Suppositories: 5 mg, 10 mg, 20 mg, 30 mg
Syrup: 1 mg/mL†, 5 mg/mL†, 10 mg/mL

M

Tablets: 5 mg†, 10 mg†, 15 mg, 25 mg,
30 mg†, 50 mg†
Tablets (extended-release): 15 mg, 30 mg,
60 mg, 100 mg, 200 mg

INDICATIONS & DOSAGES
➤ **Moderate to severe pain**
Adults: 5 to 20 mg subcutaneously or I.M.
or 5 to 15 mg I.V. every 4 hours p.r.n. Or,
5 to 30 mg (immediate-release tablets) P.O.,
or 10 to 20 mg (oral solution) P.O., or 10 to
20 mg P.R. every 4 hours p.r.n.

For extended-release tablet, give 15 or
30 mg P.O. every 8 to 12 hours.

For epidural injection, give 5 mg by
epidural catheter; then, if pain isn't relieved
adequately in 1 hour, give supplementary
doses of 1 to 2 mg at intervals sufficient to
assess effectiveness. Maximum total epidural
dose shouldn't exceed 10 mg/24 hours.

For intrathecal injection, a single dose
of 0.2 to 1 mg may provide pain relief for
24 hours (only in the lumbar area). Don't
repeat injections.
Children: 0.1 to 0.2 mg/kg subcutaneously
or I.M. every 4 hours p.r.n. Maximum single
dose, 15 mg.
➤ **Moderate to severe pain requiring
continuous, around-the-clock oral opioid**
Adults: For patients receiving other oral
morphine formulations: May convert to
extended-release capsules by administering patient's total daily oral morphine dose
as extended-release capsules once daily or
by administering one-half of patient's total
daily oral morphine dose as Kadian b.i.d.
Don't give Avinza more frequently than
every 24 hours; don't give Kadian more
frequently than every 12 hours. Supplemental pain medication may be required until
response to patient's daily Avinza dosage
has stabilized (up to 4 days). For controlled-
release tablets, patient may convert in one of
two ways: by administering one-half of patient's 24-hour requirement as MS Contin on
an every-12-hour schedule or by administering one-third of patient's daily requirement
as MS Contin on an every-8-hour schedule.
➤ **Severe, chronic pain associated with
terminal cancer**
Adults: Prior to initiating continuous morphine infusion, a loading dose of 15 mg of
morphine by I.V. push may be necessary.

Then give continuous infusion of 0.8 to
80 mg/hour via infusion pump.

ADMINISTRATION
P.O.
Black Box Warning Take care when administering morphine oral solution to avoid
dosing errors because of confusion among
different concentrations and between milligrams and milliliters, which could result in
accidental overdose and death. Take care to
ensure the proper dose is communicated and
dispensed. ■
• Oral solutions of various concentrations
and an intensified oral solution (20 mg/mL)
are available. Carefully note the strength
given.
Black Box Warning The 20-mg/mL concentration is indicated for use only in
opioid-tolerant patients because of the risk
of fatal respiratory depression in opioid-
naive patients. It's packaged with a calibrated oral syringe for accurate dosing. ■
• Give morphine sulfate without regard to
food.
• Oral capsules may be carefully opened
and the entire contents poured into cool,
soft foods, such as water, orange juice,
applesauce, or pudding; patient should
consume mixture immediately.
Black Box Warning Don't crush, break,
or allow patient to chew extended-release
forms. ■
I.V.
▼ For direct injection, dilute 2.5 to 15 mg
in 4 or 5 mL of sterile water for injection
and give slowly over 4 to 5 minutes.
▼ For continuous infusion, mix drug with
D_5W to yield 0.1 to 1 mg/mL, and give by
a continuous infusion device.
▼ In adults with severe, chronic pain,
maintenance I.V. infusion is 0.8 to
80 mg/hour; sometimes higher doses are
needed.
▼ Make sure an opioid antagonist is
immediately available before administering I.V.
▼ **Incompatibilities:** Aminophylline,
amobarbital, cefepime, chlorothiazide,
5-FU, haloperidol, heparin sodium,
meperidine, pentobarbital, phenobarbital
sodium, phenytoin sodium, prochlorperazine, sodium bicarbonate, thiopental.

Reactions in bold italics are *life-threatening*. Interactions may have a *rapid onset* or a *delayed onset*.

I.M.
• Document injection site.
• Store injection solution at room temperature and protect from light.
• Solution may darken with age. Don't use if injection is darker than pale yellow, discolored, or contains precipitate.

Subcutaneous
• Document injection site.
• Store injection solution at room temperature and protect from light.
• Solution may darken with age. Don't use if injection is darker than pale yellow, discolored, or contains precipitate.

Epidural
• Document injection site.
• Verify proper placement of needle or catheter in the epidural space before injecting drug.
• Inspect for particulate matter and discoloration before administration. Don't use if color is darker than pale yellow, if it's discolored in any other way, or if it contains a precipitate.
• Store injection solution at room temperature until ready to use; discard unused portion.
• Protect from light; don't freeze or heat sterilize.

Rectal
• Refrigeration of rectal suppository isn't needed.

ACTION
Unknown. Binds with opioid receptors in the CNS, altering perception of and emotional response to pain.

Route	Onset	Peak	Duration
P.O.	30 min	1–2 hr	4–12 hr
P.O. (extended-release)	1–2 hr	3–4 hr	12–24 hr
I.V.	5 min	20 min	4–5 hr
I.M.	10–30 min	30–60 min	4–5 hr
Subcut.	10–30 min	50–90 min	4–5 hr
P.R.	20–60 min	20–60 min	4–5 hr
Epidural	15–60 min	15–60 min	24 hr
Intrathecal	15–60 min	30–60 min	24 hr

Half-life: 2 to 3 hours.

ADVERSE REACTIONS
CNS: dizziness, euphoria, light-headedness, nightmares, sedation, somnolence, *seizures,* depression, hallucinations, nervousness, physical dependence, syncope.

CV: *bradycardia, cardiac arrest, shock,* hypertension, hypotension, tachycardia.
GI: constipation, nausea, vomiting, anorexia, biliary tract spasms, dry mouth, ileus.
GU: urine retention.
Hematologic: *thrombocytopenia.*
Respiratory: *apnea, respiratory arrest, respiratory depression.*
Skin: diaphoresis, edema, pruritus, skin flushing.
Other: decreased libido.

INTERACTIONS
Drug-drug. *Cimetidine:* May increase respiratory and CNS depression when given with morphine sulfate. Monitor patient closely.
CNS depressants, general anesthetics, hypnotics, MAO inhibitors, other opioid analgesics, sedatives, TCAs, tranquilizers: May cause respiratory depression, hypotension, profound sedation, or coma. Use together with caution, reduce morphine dose, and monitor patient response.
Drug-lifestyle. *Alcohol use:* May cause additive CNS effects. Warn patient to avoid alcohol.

EFFECTS ON LAB TEST RESULTS
• May increase amylase level. May decrease hemoglobin level (morphine sulfate).
• May decrease platelet count.
• May cause abnormal LFT values (morphine sulfate).

CONTRAINDICATIONS & CAUTIONS
• Contraindicated in patients hypersensitive to drug and in those with conditions that would preclude I.V. administration of opioids (acute bronchial asthma or upper airway obstruction).
• Contraindicated in patients with GI obstruction.
• Use with caution in elderly or debilitated patients and in those with head injury, increased intracranial pressure, seizures, chronic pulmonary disease, prostatic hyperplasia, severe hepatic or renal disease, acute abdominal conditions, hypothyroidism, Addison disease, and urethral stricture.
• Use with caution in patients with circulatory shock, biliary tract disease, CNS depression, toxic psychosis, acute alcoholism, delirium tremens, and seizure disorders.

M

• Use with caution in breast-feeding patients. Limit use and supplement with non-opioid agents. Monitor infant for increased sleepiness, difficulty feeding or breathing, and limpness.

⚠ *Overdose S&S:* Miosis, CNS depression, respiratory depression, apnea, flaccid skeletal muscles, bradycardia, hypotension, circulatory collapse, cardiac arrest, respiratory arrest, death.

NURSING CONSIDERATIONS

• Reassess patient's level of pain at least 15 and 30 minutes after giving parenterally and 30 minutes after giving orally.

☸ *Alert:* Keep opioid antagonist (naloxone) and resuscitation equipment available.

• Monitor circulatory, respiratory, bladder, and bowel functions carefully. Drug may cause hypotension, urine retention, nausea, vomiting, ileus, or altered level of consciousness regardless of the route.

Black Box Warning Life-threatening respiratory depression may occur with morphine use, even when drug has been used as recommended and not misused or abused. Proper dosing and titration are essential and morphine should only be prescribed by health care providers knowledgeable in the use of potent opioids for management of long-term pain. Monitor patients for respiratory depression, especially during initiation of morphine or after a dosage increase. Instruct patients to swallow morphine capsule whole or to sprinkle contents of capsule on applesauce and swallow without chewing. Crushing, dissolving, or chewing pellets within the capsule can cause rapid release and absorption of a potentially fatal dose of morphine. ∎

• If respirations drop below 12 breaths/minute, withhold dose and notify prescriber.

Black Box Warning Morphine has an abuse liability similar to other opioid analgesics and may be misused, abused, or diverted. ∎

☸ *Alert:* Extended-release tablets and capsules aren't for use on an as-needed basis for mild or acute pain or for postoperative pain, unless patient has already been receiving long-term opioid therapy before surgery or if postoperative pain is expected to be moderate to severe and persist for an extended period.

• Preservative-free preparations are available for epidural and intrathecal use.

Black Box Warning When the epidural or intrathecal route is used, observe patients in a fully equipped and staffed environment for at least 24 hours after the initial dose. ∎

Black Box Warning Infumorph isn't recommended for single-dose I.V., I.M., or subcutaneous administration. ∎

• When drug is given epidurally, monitor patient closely for respiratory depression up to 24 hours after the injection. Check respiratory rate and depth every 30 to 60 minutes for 24 hours. Watch for pruritus and skin flushing.

• Morphine is drug of choice in relieving MI pain; may cause transient decrease in blood pressure.

• An around-the-clock regimen best manages severe, chronic pain.

• Morphine may worsen or mask gallbladder pain.

• Constipation is commonly severe with maintenance dose. Ensure that stool softener or stimulant laxative is ordered.

• Taper morphine sulfate therapy gradually when stopping therapy.

Black Box Warning Accidental consumption of morphine, especially by children, can result in a fatal overdose of morphine. ∎

• *Look alike–sound alike:* Don't confuse morphine with hydromorphone. Don't confuse MS Contin with Oxycontin. Don't confuse Avinza with Invanz or Evista.

PATIENT TEACHING

• When drug is used after surgery, encourage patient to turn, cough, deep-breathe, and use incentive spirometer to prevent lung problems.

• Caution ambulatory patient about getting out of bed or walking. Warn outpatient to avoid driving and other potentially hazardous activities that require mental alertness until drug's adverse CNS effects are known.

Black Box Warning Drinking alcohol or taking drugs containing alcohol while taking extended-release capsules may cause additive CNS effects. Warn patient to read labels on OTC drugs carefully and not to use alcohol in any form. ∎

• Tell patient to swallow morphine sulfate whole or to open capsule and sprinkle beads

---

or pellets on a small amount of applesauce immediately before taking.

Black Box Warning Tell patient to keep morphine oral preparations out of the reach of children. In case of accidental ingestion, advise patient to seek emergency medical help immediately. ∎

❸ *Alert:* Warn patient not to crush, break, or chew extended-release forms.

SAFETY ALERT!

morphine sulfate–naltrexone hydrochloride
MOR-feen and nal-TREX-own

Embeda

Therapeutic class: Opioid analgesics
Pharmacologic class: Opioid agonist-antagonists
Pregnancy risk category: C
Controlled substance schedule: II

AVAILABLE FORMS
Capsules: 20 mg morphine and 0.8 mg naltrexone, 30 mg morphine and 1.2 mg naltrexone, 50 mg morphine and 2 mg naltrexone, 60 mg morphine and 2.4 mg naltrexone, 80 mg morphine and 3.2 mg naltrexone, 100 mg morphine and 4 mg naltrexone

INDICATIONS & DOSAGES
➤ **Moderate to severe pain when a continuous, around-the-clock opioid analgesic is needed for an extended period of time**
Adults: Individualize dosage according to patient's previous analgesic treatment, general condition, concurrent medication, type and severity of pain, and degree of opioid tolerance. Initially, give lowest dose possible; titrate no more frequently than every other day to allow for stabilization before escalating dosage. If pain relief is inadequate, administer every 12 hours. The 100-mg morphine/4-mg naltrexone capsules are for use only in opioid-tolerant patients. First dose of Embeda may be taken with last dose of any immediate-release (short-acting) opioid medication because of extended-release characteristics of Embeda.

Adjust-a-dose: For patients receiving other morphine preparations, convert by administering half of patient's daily morphine dose as Embeda every 12 hours or by administering total morphine dose as Embeda every 24 hours.

ADMINISTRATION
P.O.
Black Box Warning If patient has difficulty swallowing whole capsule, open capsule, sprinkle pellets onto small amount of applesauce, and administer immediately. Caution patient not to chew pellets. Have patient rinse mouth to make sure all pellets are swallowed. ∎

• Black Box Warning Crushing, chewing, or dissolving morphine–naltrexone capsules can cause rapid release and absorption of a potentially fatal dose of morphine. ∎

• Don't administer pellets through a nasogastric or gastric tube.

ACTION
Morphine is a selective mu agonist that produces analgesia and sedation by binding with the mu opioid receptor. Naltrexone is a centrally acting mu agonist that reverses subjective and analgesic effects of morphine by competing for mu receptor sites.

Route	Onset	Peak	Duration
P.O.	Unknown	7½ hr	Days

Half-life: 29 hours.

ADVERSE REACTIONS
CNS: anxiety, depression, dizziness, fatigue, headache, insomnia, irritability, lethargy, restlessness, sedation, somnolence, tremor.
CV: *cardiac arrest,* flushing, hypotension, peripheral edema, *shock.*
EENT: dry mouth.
GI: abdominal pain, anorexia, constipation, decreased appetite, diarrhea, dyspepsia, flatulence, nausea, stomach discomfort, vomiting.
Musculoskeletal: arthralgia, muscle spasms.
Respiratory: *apnea, respiratory arrest, respiratory depression.*
Skin: hyperhidrosis, pruritus.
Other: hot flush, chills.

M

INTERACTIONS

Drug-drug. *Anticholinergics:* May cause urine retention, severe constipation, or paralytic ileus. Use together cautiously and monitor patient closely.

Cimetidine: May cause confusion and severe respiratory depression. Avoid use together.

CNS depressants (antiemetics, general anesthetics, phenothiazines, sedative-hypnotics, other tranquilizers): May cause respiratory depression, hypotension, profound sedation, or coma. Use together cautiously; reduce initial dosage of one or both agents by at least 50% and monitor patient closely.

Diuretics: May cause antidiuretic hormone release, rendering diuretics ineffective, and urine retention due to bladder sphincter spasm. Use together cautiously.

MAO inhibitors: May cause anxiety, confusion, significant respiratory depression, or coma. Avoid use together and within 14 days of stopping treatment with MAO inhibitors.

Mixed agonist-antagonist opioid analgesics (butorphanol, nalbuphine, pentazocine): May reduce analgesic effects and precipitate withdrawal symptoms. Use together cautiously.

Muscle relaxants: May enhance neuromuscular blocking action of skeletal muscle relaxants, causing respiratory depression. Use together cautiously.

P-glycoprotein inhibitors (such as quinidine): May increase morphine level and risk of adverse effects. Use together cautiously.

Rifamycins (rifampin): May reduce morphine level and analgesic effects. Monitor response and increase morphine–naltrexone dosage if necessary.

Drug-lifestyle. *Alcohol use:* May cause additive CNS effects. Warn patient to avoid alcohol.

EFFECTS ON LAB TEST RESULTS

● May interfere with tests that use enzymes to detect opioids.

CONTRAINDICATIONS & CAUTIONS

● Contraindicated in patients hypersensitive to drug or its components and in those with significant respiratory depression, acute or severe bronchial asthma, or hypercapnia in unmonitored settings without resuscitative equipment.

● Contraindicated in patients with known or suspected paralytic ileus.

● Use cautiously in patients with COPD, cor pulmonale, decreased respiratory reserve, hypoxia, hypercapnia, head injury, increased intracranial pressure, shock, biliary tract disease including pancreatitis, CNS depression, toxic psychosis, acute alcoholism, or delirium tremens.

● Use caution in elderly and debilitated patients and in those with severe renal or hepatic insufficiency, Addison disease, myxedema, hypothyroidism, prostatic hypertrophy, and urethral stricture.

⚠ *Overdose S&S:* Respiratory depression, somnolence progressing to stupor or coma, skeletal muscle flaccidity, cold and clammy skin, constricted pupils, pulmonary edema, bradycardia, hypotension, death.

NURSING CONSIDERATIONS

Black Box Warning Capsules contain pellets of morphine sulfate. The pellets shouldn't be crushed, dissolved, or chewed because drug will be released and absorbed rapidly; resulting dose may be fatal, especially in opioid-naive patients. ∎

Black Box Warning Drug has an abuse liability similar to that of other opioid agonists, legal or illicit. Assess each patient's risk of opioid abuse or addiction before prescribing. Risk of opioid abuse increases in patients with personal or family history of substance abuse (including drug or alcohol abuse or addiction) or mental illness (such as major depressive disorder). Routinely monitor all patients receiving drug for signs and symptoms of misuse, abuse, and addiction during treatment. ∎

● *Alert:* Don't use for mild or acute pain, on an as-needed basis, or for postoperative pain, unless patient has already been receiving long-term opioid therapy before surgery or if postoperative pain is expected to be moderate to severe and persist for an extended period.

Black Box Warning Morphine 100 mg/naltrexone 4 mg is for use in opioid-tolerant patients only. ∎

Black Box Warning Respiratory depression, including fatal cases, may occur with morphine–naltrexone, even when drug has been used as recommended and not misused or abused. Proper dosing and titration are essential, and drug should only be prescribed by health care professionals knowledgeable in the use of potent opioids for management of chronic pain. Monitor patient for respiratory depression, especially during initiation of drug or after a dosage increase. ■

• Monitor circulatory, respiratory, bladder, and bowel functions carefully. Drug may cause hypotension, urine retention, nausea, vomiting, constipation, ileus, or altered level of consciousness.

• Taper drug gradually when stopping therapy to avoid withdrawal symptoms.

Black Box Warning Accidental ingestion of drug can result in fatal overdose of morphine, especially in children. ■

• Keep opioid antagonist (naloxone) and resuscitation equipment available.

PATIENT TEACHING
Black Box Warning Warn patient taking Embeda that consuming alcoholic beverages or prescription or nonprescription drugs containing alcohol may cause dose to be fatal. ■

Black Box Warning Tell patient to swallow capsules whole or open capsule and sprinkle pellets on small amount of applesauce immediately before taking; instruct patient that capsules shouldn't be crushed, dissolved, or chewed. ■

• Caution patient that drug has potential for abuse and should be protected from theft.

Black Box Warning Tell patient to keep morphine oral preparations out of the reach of children. In case of accidental ingestion, advise patient to seek emergency medical help immediately. ■

• Warn patient to avoid driving and other potentially hazardous activities that require mental alertness until drug's effects are known.

• Caution ambulatory patient about getting out of bed or walking because drug may cause a drop in blood pressure with position change.

• Tell patient the importance of dietary changes, stool softeners, and laxatives to prevent constipation, a common adverse effect of drug.

moxifloxacin hydrochloride (ophthalmic)
mocks-ah-FLOX-a-sin

Moxeza, Vigamox

Therapeutic class: Antibiotics
Pharmacologic class: Fluoroquinolones
Pregnancy risk category: C

AVAILABLE FORMS
Solution: 0.5%

INDICATIONS & DOSAGES
➤ **Bacterial conjunctivitis caused by susceptible strains of aerobic gram-positive and gram-negative organisms and *Chlamydia trachomatis***
Adults and children age 1 and older (Vigamox): 1 drop into affected eye t.i.d. for 7 days.
Adults and children age 4 months and older (Moxeza): 1 drop into affected eye b.i.d. for 7 days.

ADMINISTRATION
Ophthalmic
• Place gentle pressure on lacrimal duct for 1 to 2 minutes after instilling drop.

ACTION
Inhibits DNA gyrase and topoisomerase, preventing cell replication and division.

Route	Onset	Peak	Duration
Ophthalmic	Unknown	Unknown	Unknown

Half-life: 13 hours.

ADVERSE REACTIONS
CNS: fever.
EENT: conjunctivitis; dry eyes; increased lacrimation; keratitis; ocular discomfort, pain, or pruritus; otitis media; pharyngitis; reduced visual acuity; rhinitis; subconjunctival hemorrhage.
Respiratory: increased cough.
Skin: rash.
Other: infection.

INTERACTIONS
None reported.

EFFECTS ON LAB TEST RESULTS
None reported.

CONTRAINDICATIONS & CAUTIONS
• Contraindicated in patients hypersensitive to drug or other fluoroquinolones.
• Use cautiously in pregnant or breast-feeding women.

NURSING CONSIDERATIONS
• Systemic drug may cause serious hypersensitivity reactions. If allergic reaction occurs, stop drug and treat symptoms.
• Monitor patient for superinfection.
• Solution isn't for injection subconjunctivally or into anterior chamber of the eye.

PATIENT TEACHING
• Tell patient to stop drug and seek medical treatment immediately if evidence of hypersensitivity reaction develops, such as itching, rash, swelling of the face or throat, or difficulty breathing.
• Tell patient not to wear contact lenses during treatment.
• Instruct patient not to touch dropper tip to anything, including eyes and fingers.

---

moxifloxacin hydrochloride (oral; injection)
mocks-ah-FLOX-a-sin

Avelox✲, Avelox I.V.

Therapeutic class: Antibiotics
Pharmacologic class: Fluoroquinolones
Pregnancy risk category: C

AVAILABLE FORMS
Injection: 400 mg/250 mL
Tablets (film-coated): 400 mg

INDICATIONS & DOSAGES
➤ **Acute bacterial sinusitis caused by** *Streptococcus pneumoniae, Haemophilus influenzae,* **or** *Moraxella catarrhalis*
Adults: 400 mg P.O. or I.V. every 24 hours for 10 days.
➤ **Complicated skin and skin-structure infections caused by methicillin-susceptible** *Staphylococcus aureus, Escherichia coli, Klebsiella pneumoniae,* **or** *Enterobacter cloacae*

Adults: 400 mg P.O. or I.V. every 24 hours for 7 to 21 days.
➤ **Complicated intra-abdominal infection caused by** *E. coli, Bacteroides fragilis, Streptococcus anginosus, Streptococcus constellatus, Enterococcus faecalis, Proteus mirabilis, Clostridium perfringens, Bacteroides thetaiotaomicron,* **or** *Peptostreptococcus* **species**
Adults: 400 mg P.O. or I.V. every 24 hours for 5 to 14 days. Start with the I.V. form; switch to P.O. when appropriate.
➤ **Community-acquired pneumonia from multidrug-resistant** *S. pneumoniae* **(resistance to two or more of the following antibiotics: penicillin, second-generation cephalosporins, macrolides, sulfamethoxazole–trimethoprim, tetracyclines),** *S. aureus, M. catarrhalis, H. influenzae, H. parainfluenzae, K. pneumoniae, Chlamydia pneumoniae, Legionella pneumophila,* **or** *Mycoplasma pneumoniae*
Adults: 400 mg P.O. or I.V. every 24 hours for 7 to 14 days.
➤ **Acute bacterial worsening of chronic bronchitis caused by** *S. pneumoniae, H. influenzae, H. parainfluenzae, K. pneumoniae, S. aureus,* **or** *M. catarrhalis*
Adults: 400 mg P.O. or I.V. every 24 hours for 5 days.
➤ **Uncomplicated skin-structure or skin infection caused by** *S. aureus* **or** *S. pyogenes*
Adults: 400 mg P.O. or I.V. every 24 hours for 7 days.
➤ **Hospital-acquired pneumonia ◆**
Adults: 400 mg I.V. once daily over 60 minutes, followed by switch to 400 mg P.O. once daily. Recommended duration of treatment is 7 to 8 days.
➤ **Tuberculosis ◆**
Adults: 400 mg P.O. or I.V. daily.

ADMINISTRATION
P.O.
• Give drug without regard for food. Give at same time each day.
• Space doses of antacids, sucralfate, multivitamins, and products containing aluminum, magnesium, iron, and zinc to avoid decreasing drug's therapeutic effects.
• Store drug at controlled room temperature.

Reactions in bold italics are *life-threatening*. Interactions may have a *rapid onset* or a *delayed onset*.

I.V.
▼ Don't refrigerate. Product precipitates if refrigerated.

▼ Don't use if particulate matter is visible.

▼ Flush I.V. line with a compatible solution such as D_5W, normal saline, or lactated Ringer solution before and after use.

▼ Give only by infusion over 1 hour. Avoid rapid or bolus infusion.

▼ **Incompatibilities:** Other I.V. drugs.

ACTION
Interferes with action of enzymes needed for bacterial replication. Inhibits topoisomerases I (DNA gyrase) and IV, impairing bacterial DNA replication, transcription, repair, and recombination.

Route	Onset	Peak	Duration
P.O., I.V.	Unknown	1–3 hr	Unknown

Half-life: About 12 hours.

ADVERSE REACTIONS
CNS: dizziness, headache, malaise, insomnia, nervousness, anxiety, somnolence, tremor, vertigo.

CV: *prolonged QT interval,* palpitations, tachycardia.

GI: *pseudomembranous colitis,* abdominal pain, anorexia, constipation, diarrhea, dyspepsia, nausea.

GU: vaginal candidiasis, vaginitis.

Hematologic: *leukopenia, thrombocytopenia, thrombocytosis,* eosinophilia.

Hepatic: abnormal liver function, cholestatic jaundice.

Musculoskeletal: tendon rupture.

Respiratory: dyspnea.

Skin: injection-site reaction, pruritus, rash (maculopapular, purpuric, pustular), sweating.

Other: allergic reaction.

INTERACTIONS
Drug-drug. *Aluminum hydroxide, aluminum–magnesium hydroxide, calcium carbonate, didanosine, magnesium hydroxide, multivitamins, products containing zinc:* May interfere with GI absorption of moxifloxacin. Give moxifloxacin 4 hours before or 8 hours after these products.

Class IA antiarrhythmics (such as procainamide, quinidine), class III antiarrhythmics (such as amiodarone, sotalol): May increase risk of cardiac arrhythmias. Avoid using together.

Drugs that prolong QT interval (such as antipsychotics, erythromycin, TCAs): May have additive effect. Avoid using together.

NSAIDs: May increase risk of CNS stimulation and seizures. Avoid using together.

Black Box Warning *Steroids:* May increase risk of tendinitis and tendon rupture. Monitor patient for tendon pain or inflammation. ■

Sucralfate: May decrease absorption of moxifloxacin, reducing anti-infective response. If use together can't be avoided, give at least 6 hours apart.

Warfarin: May increase anticoagulant effects. Monitor PT and INR closely.

Drug-lifestyle. *Sun exposure:* May cause photosensitivity reactions. Advise patient to avoid excessive sunlight exposure.

EFFECTS ON LAB TEST RESULTS
● May increase liver enzyme, creatinine, uric acid, triglyceride, ionized calcium, chloride, and albumin levels.

● May decrease hematocrit and hemoglobin, potassium, and glucose levels.

● May increase or decrease bilirubin and amylase levels and PT ratio.

● May increase WBC count. May decrease RBC, eosinophil, and basophil counts. May increase or decrease neutrophil count.

CONTRAINDICATIONS & CAUTIONS
Black Box Warning Drug is associated with increased risk of tendinitis and tendon rupture, especially in patients older than age 60 and those with heart, kidney, or lung transplants. ■

❸ *Alert:* Oral or parenteral fluoroquinolones may increase the risk of peripheral neuropathy of the arms or legs. Symptoms can occur at any time during treatment and can last for months or years or be permanent. Stop drug immediately if patient develops symptoms and switch to a non-fluoroquinolone antibacterial drug unless the benefit of continued treatment outweighs the risk.

● Contraindicated in patients hypersensitive to drug or other fluoroquinolones and in those with prolonged QT interval or uncorrected hypokalemia.

M

• Use cautiously in patients with ongoing proarrhythmic conditions, such as clinically significant bradycardia or acute myocardial ischemia.

• Use cautiously in patients who may have CNS disorders or risk factors for seizures.

Black Box Warning Drug may exacerbate muscle weakness in patients with myasthenia gravis. Avoid use of fluoroquinolones in patients with known history of myasthenia gravis. ∎

• Safety and effectiveness in children, adolescents younger than age 18, and pregnant or breast-feeding women haven't been established.

NURSING CONSIDERATIONS

⚠ *Alert:* Monitor patient for adverse CNS effects, including seizures, dizziness, confusion, tremors, hallucinations, depression, and suicidal thoughts. If these occur, stop drug and notify prescriber.

⚠ *Alert:* Monitor the patient for symptoms of peripheral neuropathy (pain, burning, tingling, numbness, weakness, or a change in sensation to light touch, pain or temperature, or the sense of body position) and report them immediately to the health care provider.

• Monitor patient for hypersensitivity reactions, including anaphylaxis.

• If diarrhea develops during therapy, send stool specimen for *Clostridium difficile* test.

Black Box Warning Rupture of the Achilles and other tendons is linked to fluoroquinolone use. If pain, inflammation, or tendon rupture occurs, stop drug and notify prescriber. ∎

• *Look alike–sound alike:* Don't confuse Avelox with Avonex.

PATIENT TEACHING

• Instruct patient to take drug once daily, at the same time each day, without regard to meals.

• Tell patient to finish entire course of therapy, even if symptoms are relieved.

• Advise patient to drink plenty of fluids.

• Tell patient to space antacids, sucralfate, multivitamins, and products containing aluminum, magnesium, iron, and zinc to avoid decreasing drug's therapeutic effects.

⚠ *Alert:* Warn patient to contact his health care provider immediately if symptoms of peripheral neuropathy occur.

• Instruct patient to contact prescriber and stop drug if he experiences allergic reaction, rash, heart palpitations, fainting, or persistent diarrhea.

• Direct patient to contact prescriber, stop drug, rest, and refrain from exercise if he experiences pain, inflammation, or tendon rupture.

• Warn patient that drug may cause dizziness and light-headedness. Tell patient to avoid hazardous activities, such as driving or operating machinery, until effects of drug are known.

• Instruct patient to avoid excessive sunlight exposure and ultraviolet light and to report photosensitivity reactions to prescriber.

mupirocin
myoo-PIHR-oh-sin

Bactroban, Centany

Therapeutic class: Antibacterials (topical)
Pharmacologic class: Antibiotics
Pregnancy risk category: B

AVAILABLE FORMS
Intranasal ointment: 2%
Topical cream: 2%
Topical ointment: 2%

INDICATIONS & DOSAGES
➤ **Impetigo**
Adults and children age 2 months and older: Apply to affected areas t.i.d. for 1 to 2 weeks. Reevaluate patient in 3 to 5 days; may cover affected area with dressing.

➤ **Traumatic skin lesions infected with** *Staphylococcus aureus* **or** *Streptococcus pyogenes*
Adults and children age 2 months and older: Apply thin film t.i.d. for 10 days; may cover with gauze dressing, if needed. Reevaluate patient if improvement doesn't occur in 3 to 5 days.

➤ **To eradicate nasal colonization by methicillin-resistant** *S. aureus* **in adult patients and health care workers**
Adults and children age 12 and older: Divide ointment in single-use tube between

nostrils (½ tube per nostril) b.i.d. for 5 days. After application, close nostrils by pressing together and releasing sides of nose repeatedly for 1 minute to spread ointment throughout nares.

ADMINISTRATION
Topical
• Cosmetics and other skin products shouldn't be used on treated area.
Intranasal
• Other nasal products shouldn't be used with intranasal ointment.

ACTION
Inhibits bacterial protein synthesis by reversibly and specifically binding to bacterial isoleucyl transfer-RNA synthetase.

Route	Onset	Peak	Duration
Topical	Unknown	Unknown	Unknown

Half-life: Unknown.

ADVERSE REACTIONS
CNS: headache.
EENT: rhinitis, pharyngitis, burning or stinging with intranasal use.
GI: taste perversion, nausea.
Respiratory: upper respiratory tract congestion, cough with intranasal use.
Skin: burning, erythema with topical use, pain, pruritus, rash, stinging.

INTERACTIONS
Drug-drug. *Other nasal products:* May interfere with absorption of other nasal drugs. Don't use together.

EFFECTS ON LAB TEST RESULTS
None reported.

CONTRAINDICATIONS & CAUTIONS
• Contraindicated in patients hypersensitive to drug or its components.
• Use cautiously in patients with burns or large open wounds and in those with impaired renal function because serious renal toxicity may occur.

NURSING CONSIDERATIONS
• Drug isn't for ophthalmic or internal use.
• Prolonged use may cause overgrowth of nonsusceptible bacteria and fungi.

• **Look alike–sound alike:** Don't confuse Bactroban with bacitracin, baclofen, or Bactrim.

PATIENT TEACHING
• Tell patient to notify prescriber immediately if condition doesn't improve or gets worse in 3 to 5 days.
• Tell patient not to use other nasal products with intranasal ointment.
• Warn patient about local adverse reactions related to drug use.
• Caution patient not to use cosmetics or other skin products on treated area.

---

mycophenolate mofetil
my-koe-FIN-oh-late

CellCept

mycophenolate mofetil hydrochloride
CellCept Intravenous

mycophenolic acid (mycophenolate sodium)
Myfortic

Therapeutic class: Immunosuppressants
Pharmacologic class: Mycophenolic acid derivatives
Pregnancy risk category: D

M

AVAILABLE FORMS
mycophenolate mofetil
Capsules: 250 mg
Powder for oral suspension: 200 mg/mL
Tablets: 500 mg
mycophenolate mofetil hydrochloride
Injection: 500 mg/vial
mycophenolic acid
Tablets (extended-release): 180 mg, 360 mg

INDICATIONS & DOSAGES
➤ **To prevent organ rejection in patients receiving allogeneic renal transplants**
Adults: 1 g I.V. or P.O. (regular-release) b.i.d. with corticosteroids and cyclosporine. Or, 720 mg extended-release tablets P.O. b.i.d. 1 hour before or 2 hours after food.
Children ages 5 to 16 (extended-release): 400 mg/m^2 P.O. b.i.d. Maximum dose, 720 mg P.O. b.i.d. Or, for patients with body

surface area (BSA) of 1.19 to 1.58 m², give 540 mg P.O. b.i.d. If BSA is greater than 1.58 m², give 720 mg P.O. b.i.d. Extended-release formulation isn't recommended for BSA of less than 1.19 m².

Children ages 3 months to 18 years: For oral suspension, give 600 mg/m² P.O. b.i.d.; maximum dose is 1 g b.i.d. Or, for patients with BSA of 1.25 to 1.5 m², give 750 mg (tablets or capsules) P.O. b.i.d. If BSA is greater than 1.5 m², give 1 g (tablets or capsules) P.O. b.i.d.

Adjust-a-dose: For patients with severe chronic renal impairment outside of immediate posttransplant period, avoid doses above 1 g b.i.d. If neutropenia develops, interrupt or reduce dosage.

➤ **To prevent organ rejection in patients receiving allogeneic cardiac transplant**
Adults: 1.5 g P.O. or I.V. b.i.d. with cyclosporine and corticosteroids.

➤ **To prevent organ rejection in patients receiving allogeneic hepatic transplants**
Adults: 1 g I.V. b.i.d. over no less than 2 hours or 1.5 g P.O. b.i.d. with cyclosporine and corticosteroids.

Adjust-a-dose: If neutropenia develops, stop or reduce dosage.

ADMINISTRATION
P.O.
• Don't crush tablets; don't open or crush capsules.
• Avoid inhaling powder in capsule or having it contact skin or mucous membranes. If contact occurs, wash skin thoroughly with soap and water, and rinse eyes with water.
• The extended-release tablets are not interchangeable with other forms.

I.V.
▼ Reconstitute and dilute to 6 mg/mL using 14 mL of D₅W.
▼ Never give by rapid or bolus I.V. injection. Infuse drug over at least 2 hours.
▼ Use within 4 hours of reconstitution and dilution.
▼ **Incompatibilities:** Other I.V. drugs or solutions.

ACTION
Inhibits proliferative response of T and B lymphocytes, suppresses antibody formation by B lymphocytes, and may inhibit recruitment of leukocytes into sites of inflammation and graft rejection.

Route	Onset	Peak	Duration
P.O.	Unknown	30–75 min	7–18 hr
P.O. (extended-release)	Unknown	1½–2¾ hr	8–17 hr
I.V.	Unknown	Unknown	10–17 hr

Half-life: About 18 hours.

ADVERSE REACTIONS
CNS: asthenia, fever, headache, pain, tremor, dizziness, insomnia, *progressive multifocal leukoencephalopathy.*
CV: chest pain, edema, hypertension.
EENT: pharyngitis.
GI: abdominal pain, constipation, diarrhea, dyspepsia, nausea, oral candidiasis, vomiting, *hemorrhage.*
GU: hematuria, UTI, *renal tubular necrosis.*
Hematologic: anemia, *leukopenia, thrombocytopenia,* hypochromic anemia, leukocytosis.
Metabolic: hypercholesterolemia, hyperglycemia, *hyperkalemia,* hypokalemia, hypophosphatemia.
Musculoskeletal: back pain.
Respiratory: cough, dyspnea, infection, bronchitis, pneumonia.
Skin: acne, rash.
Other: infection, *sepsis.*

INTERACTIONS
Drug-drug. *Acyclovir, ganciclovir, other drugs that undergo renal tubular secretion:* May increase risk of toxicity for both drugs. Monitor patient closely.
Antacids with magnesium and aluminum hydroxides: May decrease mycophenolate absorption. Separate dosing times.
Azathioprine: May increase risk of bone marrow suppression. Don't use together.
Cholestyramine: May interfere with enterohepatic recirculation, reducing mycophenolate bioavailability. Avoid using together.
Cyclosporine, drugs that alter normal GI flora, rifamycins (rifampin): May decrease mycophenolate level. Monitor response to therapy and increase dosage if necessary.
Hormonal contraceptives: May decrease effectiveness of contraceptive. Recommend

addition of barrier form of contraception during treatment.

Immunosuppressants (sirolimus, tacrolimus): May increase mycophenolate level. Monitor patient closely.

Phenytoin, theophylline: May increase both drug levels. Monitor drug levels closely.

Probenecid, salicylates: May increase mycophenolate level. Monitor patient closely.

Vaccines (live-virus): May decrease vaccine effectiveness. Avoid using together.

Drug-herb. *Cat's claw, echinacea:* May increase immunostimulation. Discourage use together.

Drug-food. *Any food:* May delay absorption of extended-release form. Advise patient to take on an empty stomach 1 hour before or 2 hours after a meal.

EFFECTS ON LAB TEST RESULTS

• May increase cholesterol and glucose levels. May decrease phosphorus and hemoglobin levels. May increase or decrease potassium level.

• May decrease platelet count. May increase or decrease WBC count.

CONTRAINDICATIONS & CAUTIONS

• Contraindicated in patients hypersensitive to drug, its ingredients, or mycophenolic acid and in patients sensitive to polysorbate 80.

• Use cautiously in patients with GI disorders.

• Oral suspension contains aspartame; use cautiously in patients with phenylketonuria or those who restrict intake of phenylalanine.

⚠ Overdose S&S: Nausea, vomiting, diarrhea, neutropenia.

NURSING CONSIDERATIONS

Black Box Warning Increased risk of infection and lymphoma may result from immunosuppression. ∎

Black Box Warning Drug should only be used by health care providers experienced in immunosuppressive therapy and management of renal, cardiac, or hepatic transplant patients and in facilities equipped and staffed with adequate laboratory and supportive medical resources. ∎

Black Box Warning Use during pregnancy is associated with increased risk of first-trimester pregnancy loss and congenital malformations. Women of childbearing potential must be counseled regarding pregnancy prevention and planning. ∎

• Start drug therapy within 24 hours after transplantation. Use I.V. form in patients unable to take oral forms.

• I.V. form can be given for up to 14 days; switch patient to capsules or tablets as soon as oral drugs can be tolerated.

❸ Alert: Drug may cause progressive multifocal leukoencephalopathy (PML). Consider PML in patients reporting neurologic symptoms.

❸ Alert: Drugs causing immunosuppression increase the risk of opportunistic infections, including activation of latent viral infections such as BK virus–associated neuropathy, which may lead to serious outcomes, including kidney graft loss.

❸ Alert: Pure red cell aplasia (PRCA) has occurred in patients treated with this drug in combination with other immunosuppressants. Patients may experience fatigue, lethargy, or pallor. PRCA may be reversible with dose reduction or stopping drug. However, this may put graft at risk.

PATIENT TEACHING

• Warn patient not to open or crush capsules nor to cut, crush, or chew extended-release tablets, but to swallow them whole on an empty stomach 1 hour before or 2 hours after a meal.

• Stress importance of following treatment as prescribed.

• Inform patient of the importance of follow-up visits and ongoing laboratory tests during therapy.

• Tell women to have a pregnancy test 1 week before therapy begins.

Black Box Warning Instruct woman to use two forms of contraception during therapy and for 6 weeks afterward, even if she has a history of infertility. Tell her to notify prescriber immediately if she suspects pregnancy. ∎

Black Box Warning Warn patient of the increased risk of lymphoma and other malignancies. ∎

nadolol
nay-DOE-lol

Apo-Nadol†, Corgard

Therapeutic class: Antihypertensives
Pharmacologic class: Nonselective beta blockers
Pregnancy risk category: C

AVAILABLE FORMS
Tablets: 20 mg, 40 mg, 80 mg

INDICATIONS & DOSAGES
Adjust-a-dose (for all indications): If CrCl is 31 to 50 mL/minute, change dosing interval to every 24 to 36 hours; if CrCl is 10 to 30 mL/minute, every 24 to 48 hours; and if CrCl is less than 10 mL/minute, every 40 to 60 hours.

➤ **Angina pectoris**
Adults: 40 mg P.O. once daily. Increase in 40- to 80-mg increments at 3- to 7-day intervals until optimal response occurs. Usual maintenance dose is 40 to 80 mg once daily; up to 240 mg once daily may be needed.

➤ **Hypertension**
Adults: 40 mg P.O. once daily. Increase in 40- to 80-mg increments until optimal response occurs. Usual maintenance dose is 40 to 80 mg once daily. Doses of 320 mg daily may be needed.

➤ **Prevention of migraine** ◆
Adults: 80 to 240 mg P.O. daily.

ADMINISTRATION
P.O.
● Give drug without regard for food.
● Check apical pulse before giving drug. If slower than 60 beats/minute, withhold drug and call prescriber.

Black Box Warning Abruptly stopping drug may worsen angina and cause an MI. Reduce dosage gradually over 1 to 2 weeks. ■

ACTION
Reduces cardiac oxygen demand by blocking catecholamine-induced increases in heart rate, blood pressure, and force of myocardial contraction. Depresses renin secretion.

Route	Onset	Peak	Duration
P.O.	Unknown	2–4 hr	24 hr

Half-life: About 20 to 24 hours.

ADVERSE REACTIONS
CNS: fatigue, dizziness, fever.
CV: *bradycardia, heart failure,* hypotension, peripheral vascular disease, rhythm and conduction disturbances.
Skin: rash.

INTERACTIONS
Drug-drug. *Antihypertensives:* May increase antihypertensive effect. Monitor blood pressure closely.
Cardiac glycosides: May cause excessive bradycardia and additive effects on AV conduction. Use together cautiously.
Epinephrine: May decrease the patient response to epinephrine for treatment of an allergic reaction. Monitor patient closely for decreased clinical effect.
General anesthetics: May increase hypotensive effects. Consider stopping nadolol before surgery.
Insulin: May mask symptoms of hypoglycemia (such as tachycardia), as a result of beta blockade. Use with caution in patients with diabetes.
I.V. lidocaine: May reduce hepatic metabolism of lidocaine, increasing the risk of toxicity. Give bolus doses of lidocaine at a slower rate and monitor lidocaine level closely.
MAO inhibitors: May enhance orthostatic hypotensive effect. Monitor patient.
NSAIDs: May decrease antihypertensive effect. Monitor blood pressure and adjust dosage.
Oral antidiabetics: May alter dosage requirements in previously stabilized diabetic patients. Monitor glucose closely.
Phenothiazines: May increase hypotensive effects. Monitor blood pressure.
Prazosin: May increase risk of orthostatic hypotension in the early phases of use together. Assist patient to stand slowly until effects are known.
Reserpine: May increase hypotension or bradycardia. Monitor patient for adverse effects, such as dizziness, syncope, and postural hypotension.

Reactions in bold italics are *life-threatening*. Interactions may have a *rapid onset* or a *delayed onset*.

Verapamil: May increase effects of both drugs. Monitor cardiac function closely and decrease dosages as necessary.

Drug-herb. *Dong quai, ephedra, garlic, ginseng, licorice, yohimbe:* May worsen hypertension or affect fluid and electrolytes. Avoid use.

EFFECTS ON LAB TEST RESULTS
None reported.

CONTRAINDICATIONS & CAUTIONS
● Contraindicated in patients with bronchial asthma, sinus bradycardia and greater than first-degree heart block, cardiogenic shock, and overt heart failure.
● Use cautiously in patients with heart failure, chronic bronchitis, emphysema, or renal or hepatic impairment and in patients undergoing major surgery involving general anesthesia.
● Use cautiously in diabetic patients because beta blockers may mask certain signs and symptoms of hypoglycemia.
Black Box Warning Exacerbation of ischemic heart disease may occur following abrupt withdrawal of drug. Exacerbation of angina and, in some cases, MI have occurred after abrupt discontinuation of therapy. ■
● Drug appears in breast milk. Discontinue breast-feeding or discontinue therapy.
⚠ Overdose S&S: Bradycardia, cardiac failure, hypotension, bronchospasm.

NURSING CONSIDERATIONS
● Monitor blood pressure frequently. If patient develops severe hypotension, give a vasopressor, as prescribed.
● Drug masks signs and symptoms of shock and hyperthyroidism.
Black Box Warning If nadolol is to be discontinued after long-term administration, particularly in patients with ischemic heart disease, dosage should be gradually reduced over a period of 1 to 2 weeks and the patient carefully monitored. If angina markedly worsens or acute coronary insufficiency develops after drug cessation, nadolol should be temporarily restarted and other measures taken to appropriately manage unstable angina. Because coronary artery disease is common and may be unrecognized, don't

discontinue nadolol therapy abruptly, even in patients treated only for hypertension. ■

PATIENT TEACHING
● Explain importance of taking drug as prescribed, even when patient feels well.
● Teach patient how to check pulse rate and tell him to check it before each dose. If pulse rate is below 60 beats/minute, tell patient to notify prescriber.
Black Box Warning Warn patient not to stop drug suddenly. ■

nafcillin sodium
naf-SIL-in

Therapeutic class: Antibiotics
Pharmacologic class: Penicillinase-resistant penicillins
Pregnancy risk category: B

AVAILABLE FORMS
Infusion: 1 g, 2 g premixed or Add-Vantage vials

INDICATIONS & DOSAGES
Adjust-a-dose (for all indications): In patients with renal failure or hepatic insufficiency, measure nafcillin serum levels and adjust dosage accordingly. For adults receiving continuous renal replacement therapy, give 2 g I.V. every 4 to 6 hours (assuming ultrafiltration and dialysis flow rates of 1 to 2 L/hour). For adults receiving intermittent hemodialysis (IHD), give 2 g every 4 to 6 hours (assuming patient is receiving IHD three times per week and completes full dialysis sessions).
➤ **Systemic infection caused by susceptible organisms (methicillin-sensitive *Staphylococcus aureus*)**
Adults: 500 mg to 1 g I.V. every 4 hours, depending on severity of infection. Duration depends on the type and severity of the infection and overall condition of the patient. In severe infection, continue for at least 14 days. Continue for at least 48 hours after patient is afebrile and asymptomatic and cultures are negative. Treatment of endocarditis and osteomyelitis may require a longer duration of therapy.

N

➤ **Catheter-related bloodstream infections** ◆

Infants and children: 100 to 200 mg/kg/day I.V. in divided doses every 4 to 6 hours for a minimum of 14 days.

Neonates: 50 to 100 mg/kg/day I.V. in divided doses every 6 to 12 hours for a minimum of 14 days.

ADMINISTRATION

I.V.

▼ Before giving drug, ask patient about allergic reactions to penicillin.

▼ Obtain specimen for culture and sensitivity tests before giving. Begin therapy while awaiting results.

▼ Check container for leaks, cloudiness, or precipitate before use. Discard if present.

▼ Give drug over 30 to 60 minutes.

▼ Change site every 48 hours to prevent vein irritation.

▼ Reconstituted vials of 10 to 40 mg/mL are stable for 24 hours at room temperature.

▼ **Incompatibilities:** Aminoglycosides, aminophylline, ascorbic acid, aztreonam, bleomycin, cytarabine, diltiazem, droperidol, gentamicin, hydrocortisone sodium succinate, insulin, labetalol, meperidine, methylprednisolone sodium succinate, midazolam, nalbuphine, pentazocine lactate, promazine, vancomycin, verapamil hydrochloride, vitamin B complex with C.

ACTION

Inhibits cell-wall synthesis during bacterial multiplication.

Route	Onset	Peak	Duration
I.V.	Immediate	Immediate	Unknown

Half-life: 30 to 90 minutes.

ADVERSE REACTIONS

CNS: *neurotoxicity.*

CV: thrombophlebitis, vein irritation.

GI: nausea, *pseudomembranous colitis,* diarrhea, vomiting.

Hematologic: *agranulocytosis, leukopenia, neutropenia, thrombocytopenia,* anemia, eosinophilia.

Skin: severe tissue necrosis.

Other: *anaphylaxis,* hypersensitivity reactions.

INTERACTIONS

Drug-drug. *Aminoglycosides:* May have synergistic effect; drugs are chemically and physically incompatible. Don't combine in same I.V. solution.

Cyclosporine: May cause subtherapeutic cyclosporine levels. Monitor cyclosporine levels.

Hormonal contraceptives: May decrease contraceptive effectiveness. Advise use of additional form of contraception during therapy.

Live-virus vaccines: May reduce effectiveness of live-virus vaccine. Don't use concurrently.

Methotrexate: May cause methotrexate toxicity. Monitor patient closely.

Probenecid: May increase nafcillin level. Probenecid may be used for this purpose.

Rifampin: May cause dose-dependent antagonism. Monitor patient closely.

Tetracycline: May decrease nafcillin's effectiveness. Avoid concurrent use.

Warfarin: May decrease effects of warfarin. Monitor PT and INR closely.

EFFECTS ON LAB TEST RESULTS

● May decrease hemoglobin level and hematocrit.

● May decrease neutrophil, WBC, eosinophil, granulocyte, and platelet counts.

CONTRAINDICATIONS & CAUTIONS

● Contraindicated in patients hypersensitive to drug or other penicillins.

● Safety and effectiveness in children haven't been established. There are no approved pediatric dosage regimens.

● Use cautiously in patients with GI distress and in those with other drug allergies (especially to cephalosporins) because of possible cross-sensitivity.

● Skin sloughing from subcutaneous extravasation has been reported.

⚠ **Overdose S&S:** Neuromuscular hyperexcitability, seizures.

NURSING CONSIDERATIONS

● If large doses are given or if therapy is prolonged, bacterial or fungal superinfection may occur, especially in elderly, debilitated, or immunosuppressed patients.

Reactions in bold italics are *life-threatening*. Interactions may have a *rapid onset* or a *delayed onset*.

• Monitor sodium level because each gram of drug contains 2.9 mEq of sodium.
• Monitor WBC counts twice weekly in patients receiving drug for longer than 2 weeks. Neutropenia commonly occurs in the third week.
• An abnormal urinalysis result may indicate drug-induced interstitial nephritis.

PATIENT TEACHING

• Tell patient to report burning or irritation at the I.V. site.
• Advise patient to notify prescriber if a rash develops or if signs and symptoms of superinfection appear, such as recurring fever, chills, and malaise.

SAFETY ALERT!

nalbuphine hydrochloride
NAL-byoo-feen

Nubain†

Therapeutic class: Opioid analgesics
Pharmacologic class: Opioid agonist-antagonists–opioid partial agonists
Pregnancy risk category: B

AVAILABLE FORMS
Injection: 10 mg/mL, 20 mg/mL

INDICATIONS & DOSAGES
Adjust-a-dose (for all indications): In patients with renal or hepatic impairment, decrease dosage.
➤ **Moderate to severe pain**
Adults: For a patient of about 70 kg (154 lb), 10 to 20 mg subcutaneously, I.M., or I.V. every 3 to 6 hours p.r.n. Maximum, 160 mg daily.
➤ **Adjunct to balanced anesthesia**
Adults: 0.3 to 3 mg/kg I.V. over 10 to 15 minutes; then maintenance doses of 0.25 to 0.50 mg/kg in single I.V. dose p.r.n.

ADMINISTRATION
I.V.
▼ Inject slowly over at least 2 to 3 minutes into a vein or into an I.V. line containing a compatible, free-flowing I.V. solution, such as D_5W, normal saline solution, or lactated Ringer solution.

▼ Respiratory depression can be reversed with naloxone. Keep resuscitation equipment available, particularly when giving I.V.
▼ **Incompatibilities:** Allopurinol, amphotericin B, cefepime, diazepam, docetaxel, ketorolac, methotrexate sodium, nafcillin, pentobarbital sodium, piperacillin–tazobactam sodium, promethazine, sargramostim, sodium bicarbonate, thiethylperazine.
I.M.
• Document injection site.
• Store vial in carton to protect from light.
Subcutaneous
• Document injection site.
• Store vial in carton to protect from light.

ACTION
Unknown. Binds with opioid receptors in the CNS, altering perception of and emotional response to pain.

Route	Onset	Peak	Duration
I.V.	2–3 min	30 min	3–6 hr
I.M.	15 min	1 hr	3–6 hr
Subcut.	15 min	Unknown	3–6 hr

Half-life: 5 hours.

ADVERSE REACTIONS
CNS: dizziness, headache, sedation, vertigo.
CV: *bradycardia.*
EENT: dry mouth.
GI: nausea, vomiting.
Respiratory: *respiratory depression.*
Skin: clamminess, diaphoresis.

INTERACTIONS
Drug-drug. *CNS depressants, general anesthetics, hypnotics, MAO inhibitors, sedatives, tranquilizers, TCAs:* May cause respiratory depression, hypertension, profound sedation, or coma. Use together with caution, and monitor patient response. *Opioid analgesics:* May decrease analgesic effect. Avoid using together.
Drug-lifestyle. *Alcohol use:* May cause additive effects. Discourage use together.

EFFECTS ON LAB TEST RESULTS
None reported.

CONTRAINDICATIONS & CAUTIONS
● Contraindicated in patients hypersensitive to drug.
۞ Alert: Drug should only be administered as a supplement to general anesthesia by those specifically trained in the use of I.V. anesthetics and management of respiratory effects of potent opioids. Naloxone hydrochloride and emergency resuscitative equipment should be readily available.
● Use cautiously in patients with history of drug abuse and in those with emotional instability, head injury, increased intracranial pressure, impaired ventilation, MI accompanied by nausea and vomiting, upcoming biliary surgery, and hepatic or renal disease.
۞ Alert: Certain commercial preparations contain sodium metabisulfite.
⚠ Overdose S&S: Sleepiness, mild dysphoria.

NURSING CONSIDERATIONS
● Reassess patient's level of pain at least 15 and 30 minutes after parenteral administration.
● Drug acts as an opioid antagonist and may cause withdrawal syndrome. For patients who have received long-term opioids, give 25% of the usual dose initially. Watch for signs of withdrawal.
۞ Alert: Drug causes respiratory depression, which at 10 mg is equal to respiratory depression produced by 10 mg of morphine.
● Monitor circulatory and respiratory status and bladder and bowel function. If respirations are shallow or rate is below 12 breaths/minute, withhold dose and notify prescriber.
● Constipation is commonly severe with maintenance therapy. Make sure stool softener or other stimulant laxative is ordered.
● Psychological and physical dependence may occur with prolonged use.
● **Look alike–sound alike:** Don't confuse Nubain with Navane.

PATIENT TEACHING
● Caution ambulatory patient about getting out of bed or walking. Warn outpatient to avoid driving and other hazardous activities that require mental alertness until drug's CNS effects are known.

● Teach patient how to manage troublesome adverse effects such as constipation.

---

naltrexone
nal-TREX-one

Vivitrol

naltrexone hydrochloride
ReVia

Therapeutic class: Opioid cessation drugs
Pharmacologic class: Opioid antagonists
Pregnancy risk category: C

AVAILABLE FORMS
naltrexone
Injection: 380-mg vial dose kit
naltrexone hydrochloride
Tablets: 50 mg

INDICATIONS & DOSAGES
➤ **Adjunct for maintaining opioid-free state in detoxified patients**
Adults: Initially, 25 mg P.O. If no withdrawal signs occur within 1 hour, the patient may be started on 50 mg every 24 hours the following day. From 50 to 150 mg may be given daily, depending on schedule prescribed. Or, 380 mg I.M. every 4 weeks or once a month.
➤ **Alcohol dependence**
Adults: 50 mg P.O. once daily or 380 mg I.M. in the gluteal muscle once monthly.
➤ **Cholestatic pruritus ◆**
Adults: 12.5 mg P.O. daily. Increase by 12.5 mg every 3 to 7 days until pruritus is eliminated.
➤ **Severe pruritus ◆**
Adults who are refractory to traditional treatment: 50 mg P.O. daily.

ADMINISTRATION
P.O.
● Keep container tightly closed and protect from light.
● Give without regard to meals; give with food if GI upset occurs.

I.M.
• Use only the diluent, needles, and other components supplied with the dose kit. Don't substitute.
• Administer I.M. into gluteal muscle. Avoid giving I.V., subcutaneously, or inadvertently into fatty tissue. Monitor the injection site.

ACTION
Probably reversibly blocks the effects of I.V. opioids by competitively occupying opiate receptors in the brain.

Route	Onset	Peak	Duration
P.O.	15–30 min	1 hr	24 hr
I.M.	Unknown	2–3 days	>30 days

Half-life: About 4 hours.

ADVERSE REACTIONS
CNS: insomnia, anxiety, nervousness, headache, depression, dizziness, fatigue, somnolence, syncope.
CV: hypertension.
GI: nausea, vomiting, abdominal pain, anorexia, constipation, increased thirst.
GU: delayed ejaculation, decreased potency.
Hepatic: *hepatotoxicity.*
Musculoskeletal: muscle and joint pain.
Skin: injection-site reaction, rash.
Other: chills.

INTERACTIONS
Drug-drug. *Products that contain opioids:* May decrease effect of opioid. Avoid using together.
Thioridazine: May increase somnolence and lethargy. Monitor patient closely.

EFFECTS ON LAB TEST RESULTS
• May increase AST, ALT, and LDH levels.
• May increase lymphocyte count.

CONTRAINDICATIONS & CAUTIONS
• Contraindicated in patients hypersensitive to drug or dependent on opioids, those receiving opioid analgesics, those who fail the naloxone challenge test or who have a positive urine screen for opioids, or those in acute opioid withdrawal.
Black Box Warning Contraindicated in patients with acute hepatitis or liver failure. Use cautiously in patients with mild he-patic disease or history of recent hepatic disease. ■

⚠ *Overdose S&S:* Injection-site reaction, nausea, abdominal pain, somnolence, dizziness.

NURSING CONSIDERATIONS
Black Box Warning Discontinue drug if patient develops symptoms or signs of acute hepatitis. ■
• Don't begin treatment for opioid dependence until patient receives naloxone challenge, a test of opioid dependence. If signs and symptoms of opioid withdrawal persist after naloxone challenge, don't give drug.
• Patient must be completely free from opioids before taking naltrexone or severe withdrawal symptoms may occur. Patients who have been addicted to short-acting opioids, such as heroin and meperidine, must wait at least 7 days after last opioid dose before starting drug. Patients who have been addicted to longer-acting opioids such as methadone should wait at least 10 days.
• In an emergency, patient may be given an opioid analgesic, but dose must be higher than usual to overcome naltrexone's effect. Watch for respiratory depression from the opioid; it may be longer and deeper.
• For patients expected to be noncompliant because of history of opioid dependence, use a flexible maintenance-dose regimen of 100 mg on Monday and Wednesday and 150 mg on Friday.
• Use drug only as part of a comprehensive rehabilitation program.
• *Look alike–sound alike:* Don't confuse naltrexone with naloxone.

PATIENT TEACHING
• Advise patient to carry medical identification and to tell medical personnel that he takes naltrexone.
• Tell patient that drug can block the effects of opioids or opioid-like drugs, including heroin, pain medicine, antidiarrheals, or cough medicine.
• **Alert:** Warn patient if he uses large doses of heroin or any other opioid that serious injury, coma, or death can occur.
• Advise patient who previously used opioids that he may be more sensitive to

N

lower doses of opioids once naltrexone therapy is stopped.

Black Box Warning Tell patient to report adverse effects, especially those related to liver injury, to prescriber immediately. ■

❸ *Alert:* Tell caregiver of alcohol-dependent patient to monitor him closely for signs of depression or suicide ideation and to report this immediately to prescriber.

• Give patient the names of nonopioid drugs that he can continue to take for pain, diarrhea, or cough.

• Tell patient to report pain, swelling, tenderness, induration, bruising, pruritis, or redness at the injection site.

naphazoline hydrochloride
naf-AZ-oh-leen

Advanced Eye Relief: Redness Maximum Relief ◇, AK-Con, Albalon, All Clear ◇, Clear Eyes ◇, Naphcon Forte†

Therapeutic class: Vasoconstrictors
Pharmacologic class: Sympathomimetics
Pregnancy risk category: C

AVAILABLE FORMS
Ophthalmic solution: 0.012% ◇, 0.03% ◇, 0.1%

INDICATIONS & DOSAGES
➤ **Ocular congestion, irritation, itching**
Adults: Instill 1 or 2 drops into the conjunctival sac of affected eye(s) every 3 to 4 hours, up to q.i.d.

ADMINISTRATION
Ophthalmic
• Store drug in tightly closed container.

ACTION
Thought to cause vasoconstriction by local adrenergic action on the blood vessels of the conjunctiva.

Route	Onset	Peak	Duration
Ophthalmic	10 min	Unknown	2–6 hr

Half-life: Unknown.

ADVERSE REACTIONS
CNS: dizziness, headache, nervousness, weakness.
EENT: blurred vision, eye irritation, increased intraocular pressure, keratitis, lacrimation, photophobia, pupillary dilation, transient eye stinging.
GI: nausea.
Skin: diaphoresis.

INTERACTIONS
Drug-drug. *Anesthetics:* Cyclopropane and halothane may sensitize the myocardium to sympathomimetics; local anesthetics may increase the absorption of topical drugs. Monitor patient for increased adverse effects.
Beta blockers: May cause more systemic adverse effects. Monitor patient for adverse systemic effects.
MAO inhibitors, maprotiline, TCAs: May cause hypertensive crisis if naphazoline is systemically absorbed. Use together cautiously.

EFFECTS ON LAB TEST RESULTS
None reported.

CONTRAINDICATIONS & CAUTIONS
• Contraindicated in patients hypersensitive to drug's ingredients and in those with acute angle-closure glaucoma.
• Use of 0.1% solution is contraindicated in infants and small children.
• Use cautiously in patients with hyperthyroidism, cardiac disease, hypertension, or diabetes mellitus.

NURSING CONSIDERATIONS
• Drug is most widely used ocular decongestant.
• Rebound congestion and conjunctivitis may occur with frequent or prolonged use.

PATIENT TEACHING
• Teach patient how to instill drug. Advise him to wash hands before and after instillation and to apply light finger pressure on lacrimal sac for 1 minute after drops are instilled. Warn him not to touch tip of dropper to eye or surrounding tissue.

Reactions in bold italics are *life-threatening*. Interactions may have a *rapid onset* or a *delayed onset*.

- Warn patient not to exceed recommended dosage to avoid rebound congestion and conjunctivitis.
- Tell patient to notify prescriber if sun sensitivity, blurred vision, pain, or lid swelling develops.
- Instruct patient not to use OTC preparations for longer than 72 hours without consulting prescriber.

naproxen
na-PROX-en

EC-Naprosyn, Naprosyn🖉,
Novo-Naprox†, Nu-Naprox†

naproxen sodium
Aleve ◇, Anaprox, Anaprox DS,
Apo-Napro-Na† ◇, Flanax Pain
Relief ◇, Mediproxen ◇, Midol
Extended Relief ◇, Naprelan,
Novo-Naprox Sodium†, Pamprin
All Day Relief ◇, TH Naproxen ◇

Therapeutic class: NSAIDs
Pharmacologic class: NSAIDs
Pregnancy risk category: B; D in
3rd trimester

AVAILABLE FORMS
naproxen
Oral suspension: 125 mg/5 mL
Tablets: 250 mg, 375 mg, 500 mg
Tablets (delayed-release): 375 mg, 500 mg
naproxen sodium
Capsules: 200 mg ◇
Tablets (extended-release): 375 mg,
500 mg, 750 mg
Tablets (film-coated): 220 mg ◇, 275 mg,
550 mg
Note: 275 mg of naproxen sodium contains
250 mg of naproxen.

INDICATIONS & DOSAGES
Adjust-a-dose (for all indications): Consider lower dosage in elderly patients and patients with renal or hepatic impairment. Not recommended for patients with moderate to severe renal impairment (CrCl less than 30 mL/minute).
➤ **Acute gout**
Adults: 750 mg naproxen P.O.; then 250 mg every 8 hours until attack subsides. Or,

825 mg naproxen sodium P.O.; then 275 mg every 8 hours until attack subsides. Or, 1,000 to 1,500 mg extended-release tablets P.O. on day 1, followed by 1,000 mg daily until attack subsides.
➤ **Acute tendinitis, bursitis, pain, primary dysmenorrhea**
Adults: 550 mg naproxen sodium P.O., then 550 mg P.O. every 12 hours or 275 mg every 6 to 8 hours. Initial total daily dose shouldn't exceed 1,375 mg; thereafter, total daily dose shouldn't exceed 1,100 mg. Or, 500 mg naproxen P.O. followed by 500 mg P.O. every 12 hours or 250 mg P.O. every 6 to 8 hours. Or, 1,000 mg extended-release tablets P.O. once daily for a limited time.
➤ **Ankylosing spondylitis, osteoarthritis, rheumatoid arthritis**
Adults: 275 to 550 mg naproxen sodium P.O. b.i.d. Or, 250 to 500 mg naproxen tablet or suspension P.O. b.i.d. Or, 375 or 500 mg naproxen delayed-release tablet P.O. b.i.d. Or, 750 to 1,000 mg extended-release tablets P.O. once daily. During long-term administration, the dose of naproxen may be adjusted up or down depending on the patient's clinical response. In patients who tolerate lower doses well, the dose may be increased to 1,500 mg/day when a higher level of anti-inflammatory/analgesic activity is required.
➤ **Juvenile arthritis**
Children age 2 and older: 10 mg/kg naproxen suspension P.O. daily given in two divided doses. Don't exceed 15 mg/kg/day.
➤ **Episodic migraine prevention** ◆
Adults: 250 to 500 mg P.O. b.i.d.

ADMINISTRATION
P.O.
- Give drug with food or milk to minimize GI upset. Have patient drink a full glass of water or other liquid with each dose.
- Shake suspension well.
- Make sure patient swallows tablets whole and doesn't break, crush, or chew them.

ACTION
May inhibit prostaglandin synthesis to produce anti-inflammatory, analgesic, and antipyretic effects.

N

Route	Onset	Peak	Duration
P.O.	1 hr	2–4 hr	7 hr

Half-life: 10 to 20 hours.

ADVERSE REACTIONS
CNS: dizziness, drowsiness, headache, vertigo.
CV: edema, palpitations.
EENT: tinnitus, auditory disturbances, visual disturbances.
GI: abdominal pain, constipation, diarrhea, dyspepsia, epigastric pain, heartburn, nausea, occult blood loss, peptic ulceration, stomatitis, thirst.
Hematologic: ecchymoses, increased bleeding time.
Respiratory: dyspnea.
Skin: diaphoresis, pruritus, purpura.

INTERACTIONS
Drug-drug. *ACE inhibitors:* May cause renal impairment. Use together cautiously.
Antihypertensives, diuretics: May decrease effect of these drugs. Monitor patient closely.
Aspirin, corticosteroids: May cause adverse GI reactions. Avoid using together.
Digoxin: May increase serum digoxin level. Monitor levels.
Lithium: May increase lithium level. Observe patient for toxicity and monitor level. Adjustment of lithium dosage may be required.
Loop diuretics, thiazide diuretics: May reduce diuretic effects. Monitor patient and consider therapy modification.
Methotrexate: May cause toxicity. Monitor patient closely.
Oral anticoagulants, NSAIDs, SSRIs, other sulfonylureas, highly protein-bound drugs: May cause toxicity. Monitor patient closely.
Potassium-sparing diuretics: May reduce antihypertensive effects and enhance hyperkalemic effects. Monitor patient closely.
Probenecid: May decrease elimination of naproxen. Monitor patient for toxicity.
Drug-herb. *Alfalfa, anise, bilberry, dong quai, feverfew, garlic, ginger, ginkgo, horse chestnut, red clover:* May cause bleeding, based on the known effects of components. Discourage use together.
White willow: Herb and drug contain similar components. Discourage use together.

Drug-lifestyle. *Alcohol use:* May cause GI irritation. Discourage use together.

EFFECTS ON LAB TEST RESULTS
• May increase BUN, creatinine, ALT, AST, and potassium levels.
• May increase bleeding time.
• May interfere with urinary 5-hydroxyindoleacetic acid and 17-hydroxycorticosteroid determinations.

CONTRAINDICATIONS & CAUTIONS
• Contraindicated in patients hypersensitive to drug and in those with the syndrome of asthma, rhinitis, and nasal polyps.
Black Box Warning Naproxen is contraindicated for the treatment of perioperative pain after CABG surgery. ∎
• Patient should avoid drug during last trimester of pregnancy and while breast-feeding.
• Use cautiously in elderly patients and in patients with renal disease, CV disease, GI disorders, hepatic disease, or history of peptic ulcer disease.
⚠ **Overdose S&S:** Drowsiness, heartburn, indigestion, nausea, vomiting, seizures.

NURSING CONSIDERATIONS
• Because NSAIDs impair synthesis of renal prostaglandins, they can decrease renal blood flow and lead to reversible renal impairment, especially in patients with renal failure, heart failure, or liver dysfunction; in elderly patients; and in those taking diuretics. Monitor these patients closely.
• Monitor CBC and renal and hepatic function every 4 to 6 months during long-term therapy.
Black Box Warning NSAIDs cause an increased risk of serious GI adverse events, including bleeding, ulceration, and perforation of the stomach or intestines, which can be fatal. Elderly patients are at greater risk. ∎
Black Box Warning NSAIDs may increase the risk of serious thrombotic events, MI, or stroke, which can be fatal. The risk may be greater with longer use or in patients with CV disease or risk factors for CV disease. ∎

• Because of their antipyretic and anti-inflammatory actions, NSAIDs may mask signs and symptoms of infection.
• Drug may have a heart benefit, similar to aspirin, in preventing blood clotting.

PATIENT TEACHING
🛈 **Alert:** Drug is available without prescription (naproxen sodium, 220 mg). Instruct adult not to take more than 440 mg of naproxen sodium in any 8- to 12-hour period or 660 mg of naproxen sodium in a 24-hour period.
• Advise patient to take drug with food or milk to minimize GI upset. Tell him to drink a full glass of water or other liquid with each dose.
• Tell patient taking prescription doses for arthritis that full therapeutic effect may be delayed 2 to 4 weeks.
• Warn patient against taking naproxen and naproxen sodium at the same time.
• Teach patient signs and symptoms of GI bleeding, including blood in vomit, urine, or stool; coffee-ground vomit; and black, tarry stools. Tell him to notify prescriber immediately if any of these occurs.
• Caution patient that use with aspirin, alcohol, other NSAIDs, or corticosteroids may increase risk of adverse GI reactions.
• Warn patient against hazardous activities that require mental alertness until CNS effects are known.

naratriptan hydrochloride
nar-ah-TRIP-tan

Amerge

Therapeutic class: Antimigraine drugs
Pharmacologic class: Serotonin 5-HT₁ receptor agonists
Pregnancy risk category: C

AVAILABLE FORMS
Tablets: 1 mg, 2.5 mg

INDICATIONS & DOSAGES
➤ **Acute migraine attacks with or without aura**
Adults: 1 or 2.5 mg P.O. as a single dose. If headache returns or responds only par-

tially, dose may be repeated after 4 hours. Maximum, 5 mg in 24 hours.
Adjust-a-dose: For patients with mild to moderate renal or hepatic impairment, reduce dosage. Maximum, 2.5 mg in 24 hours.

ADMINISTRATION
P.O.
• Give drug with fluid without regard for food.
• Give drug whole; don't split or crush tablet.
• If no response occurs with first tablet, prescriber should be consulted before giving second tablet. If more relief is needed after first tablet (if a partial response occurs or headache returns), and prescriber has approved a second dose, give a second tablet (but not sooner than 4 hours after first tablet).

ACTION
May act as an agonist at serotonin receptors on extracerebral intracranial blood vessels, which constricts the affected vessels, inhibits neuropeptide release, and reduces pain transmission in the trigeminal pathways.

Route	Onset	Peak	Duration
P.O.	Unknown	2–3 hr	Unknown

Half-life: 6 hours.

ADVERSE REACTIONS
CNS: paresthesia, dizziness, drowsiness, malaise, fatigue, vertigo.
CV: *tachyarrhythmias, abnormal ECG changes, coronary artery vasospasm, transient myocardial ischemia, MI, ventricular tachycardia, ventricular fibrillation,* palpitations, hypertension.
EENT: ear, nose, and throat infections; photophobia.
GI: nausea, hyposalivation, vomiting.
Other: sensations of warmth, cold, pressure, tightness, or heaviness.

INTERACTIONS
Drug-drug. *Drugs that prolong QT interval (antiarrhythmics, arsenic trioxide, chlorpromazine, dolasetron, droperidol, mefloquine, mesoridazine, moxifloxacin, pentamidine, pimozide, tacrolimus, thioridazine, ziprasidone):* May cause an additive

N

effect and prolong QT interval. Monitor patient closely.

Ergot-containing or ergot-type drugs (dihydroergotamine, methysergide), other 5-HT$_1$ agonists: May prolong vasospastic reactions. Avoid using within 24 hours of naratriptan.

Hormonal contraceptives: May slightly increase naratriptan level. Monitor patient.

MAO inhibitors: May decrease metabolic elimination of naratriptan. Don't use together.

SSRIs (fluoxetine, fluvoxamine, paroxetine, sertraline): May cause weakness, hyperreflexia, and incoordination. Monitor patient.

Drug-herb. *St. John's wort:* May increase serotonergic effect. Discourage use together.

Drug-lifestyle. *Smoking:* May increase naratriptan clearance. Discourage smoking.

EFFECTS ON LAB TEST RESULTS
None reported.

CONTRAINDICATIONS & CAUTIONS
• Contraindicated in patients hypersensitive to drug or its components and in those with prior or current cardiac ischemia, cerebrovascular or peripheral vascular syndromes, hemiplegic or basilar migraines, or uncontrolled hypertension.

• Contraindicated in elderly patients, patients with severe renal impairment (CrCl below 15 mL/minute), patients with severe hepatic impairment (Child-Pugh class C), and patients who have used ergot-containing, ergot-type, or other 5-HT$_1$ agonists within 24 hours.

• Use cautiously in patients with risk factors for coronary artery disease (CAD), such as hypertension, hypercholesterolemia, obesity, diabetes, smoking, strong family history of CAD, postmenopausal women, and men older than age 40, unless patient is free from cardiac disease. Monitor patient closely after first dose.

• Use cautiously in patients with renal or hepatic impairment.

• Safety and effectiveness when treating cluster headaches or more than four headaches in a 30-day period haven't been established.

⚠ *Overdose S&S:* Chest pain, ischemic ECG changes.

NURSING CONSIDERATIONS
• Assess cardiac status in patients who develop risk factors for CAD.

⚠ *Alert:* Drug can cause coronary artery vasospasm and increased risk of cerebrovascular events.

• Drug isn't intended to prevent migraines or manage hemiplegic or basilar migraine.

• Use drug only when patient has a clear diagnosis of migraine.

⚠ *Alert:* Combining drug with an SSRI or an SSNRI may cause serotonin syndrome. Symptoms include restlessness, hallucinations, loss of coordination, fast heartbeat, rapid changes in blood pressure, increased body temperature, hyperreflexia, nausea, vomiting, and diarrhea. Serotonin syndrome is more likely to occur when starting or increasing the dose of naratriptan, the SSRI, or the SSNRI.

• *Look alike–sound alike:* Don't confuse Amerge with Altace or Amaryl.

PATIENT TEACHING
• Instruct patient to take drug only as prescribed and to read the accompanying patient instruction leaflet before using drug.

• Tell patient that drug is intended to relieve, not prevent, migraines.

• Instruct patient to take dose soon after headache starts. If no response occurs with first tablet, tell him to seek medical approval before taking second tablet. Tell patient that if more relief is needed after first tablet (if a partial response occurs or headache returns), and prescriber has approved a second dose, he may take a second tablet (but not sooner than 4 hours after first tablet). Tell him not to exceed 2 tablets within 24 hours.

• Advise patient to increase fluid intake.

• Advise patient not to use drug if she suspects or knows that she's pregnant.

• Tell patient to alert prescriber about bothersome adverse effects.

• Tell patient to swallow tablet whole, and not to split, crush, or chew tablet.

Reactions in bold italics are *life-threatening*. Interactions may have a *rapid onset* or a *delayed onset*.

natalizumab
nah-tah-LIZ-yoo-mab

Tysabri

Therapeutic class: Immune response modifiers
Pharmacologic class: Monoclonal antibodies
Pregnancy risk category: C

AVAILABLE FORMS
Injection: 300 mg/15 mL single-use vials

INDICATIONS & DOSAGES
➤ **To slow the accumulation of physical disabilities and reduce the frequency of clinical exacerbations in relapsing forms of multiple sclerosis (MS) for patients who failed to respond or were unable to tolerate other therapies; moderate to severe Crohn disease in patients with inadequate response or intolerance to conventional therapy**
Adults: 300 mg I.V. over 1 hour every 4 weeks.

ADMINISTRATION
I.V.
▼ Dilute 300 mg in 100 mL normal saline solution.
▼ Invert I.V. bag gently to mix solution; don't shake.
▼ Infuse over 1 hour; don't give by I.V. push or bolus.
▼ Flush I.V. line with normal saline solution after infusion is complete.
▼ Refrigerate solution and use within 8 hours if not used immediately. Protect from light.
▼ **Incompatibilities:** Don't mix or infuse with other drugs. Don't use any diluent other than normal saline solution.

ACTION
May block interaction between adhesion molecules on inflammatory cells and receptors on endothelial cells of vessel walls.

Route	Onset	Peak	Duration
I.V.	Unknown	Unknown	Unknown

Half-life: 7 to 15 days.

ADVERSE REACTIONS
CNS: *progressive multifocal leukoencephalopathy (PML),* depression, fatigue, headache, somnolence, vertigo.
CV: chest discomfort, peripheral edema.
EENT: tonsillitis.
GI: abdominal discomfort, diarrhea, gastroenteritis.
GU: UTI, vaginitis, amenorrhea, dysmenorrhea, irregular menstruation, urinary frequency, urinary urgency, ovarian cyst.
Metabolic: weight increase or decrease.
Musculoskeletal: arthralgia, extremity pain, muscle cramps, swollen joints.
Respiratory: lower respiratory tract infection.
Skin: rash, dermatitis, pruritus, urticaria, night sweats.
Other: hypersensitivity reaction, infusion-related reaction, tooth infections, herpes, infection, rigors, seasonal allergy, cholelithiasis.

INTERACTIONS
Drug-drug. *Corticosteroids, immunosuppressants, TNF inhibitors:* May increase risk of infection. Avoid using together.
Live-virus vaccines: May cause reduced effectiveness of the vaccine. Defer vaccine administration until immune function has returned.
Drug-herb. *Echinacea:* May decrease effectiveness of natalizumab. Consider therapy modification.

EFFECTS ON LAB TEST RESULTS
• May increase LFT values and lymphocyte, monocyte, eosinophil, basophil, and nucleated RBC counts.
• May cause transient decrease in hemoglobin.

CONTRAINDICATIONS & CAUTIONS
• Contraindicated in patients hypersensitive to drug or its components or in those with current or past history of PML. Use with other immunosuppressants isn't recommended.
⊘ *Alert:* Patients who test positively for anti-JC virus antibodies are at increased risk for developing PML. Consider testing for anti-JC virus antibodies before or during treatment if antibody status is unknown. Use drug cautiously in patients who are anti-JC

N

virus antibody–positive and especially in those with one or more additional PML risk factors.
● Safety and effectiveness in patients with chronic progressive MS haven't been established.

NURSING CONSIDERATIONS

Black Box Warning Only prescribers registered in the TOUCH Prescribing Program may prescribe drug. Contact the TOUCH Prescribing Program at 1-800-456-2255. ■
● Report serious opportunistic and atypical infections to Biogen Idec at 1-800-456-2255 and to the FDA's MedWatch Program at 1-800-FDA-1088.
● The safety and effectiveness of natalizumab treatment beyond 2 years are unknown.

Black Box Warning Drug may cause PML. Withhold drug immediately at the first signs or symptoms suggestive of PML. Symptoms include clumsiness; progressive weakness; and visual, speech, and sometimes personality changes. ■
● The risk of PML increases with the number of infusions and if the patient has taken immunosuppressants in the past.
● Obtain a brain magnetic resonance imaging scan before starting therapy.
● **Alert:** Watch for evidence of hypersensitivity reaction during and for 1 hour after infusion, which may include dizziness, urticaria, fever, rash, rigors, pruritus, nausea, flushing, hypotension, dyspnea, and chest pain.
● If hypersensitivity reaction occurs, stop drug and notify prescriber.
● Patients who develop antibodies to drug have an increased risk of infusion-related reaction.
● Discontinue drug in patients with jaundice or other evidence of significant liver injury. Elevated serum hepatic enzymes and elevated total bilirubin levels may occur as early as 6 days after the first dose.

PATIENT TEACHING

● Tell patient to read the "Medication Guide for Tysabri" before each infusion.
● Urge patient to immediately report progressively worsening symptoms persisting

over several days, including changes in thinking, eyesight, balance, or strength.
● Advise patient to inform all health care providers caring for him that he's receiving this drug.
● Tell patient to schedule follow-up appointments with prescriber at 3 and 6 months after the first infusion, then at least every 6 months thereafter.
● Urge patient to immediately report rash, hives, dizziness, fever, shaking chills, or itching while drug is infusing or up to 1 hour afterward.
● Tell patient about the potential for liver injury.

SAFETY ALERT!

nateglinide
nah-TEG-lah-nyde

Starlix

Therapeutic class: Antidiabetics
Pharmacologic class: Meglitinide derivatives
Pregnancy risk category: C

AVAILABLE FORMS
Tablets: 60 mg, 120 mg

INDICATIONS & DOSAGES
➤ **Type 2 diabetes, as monotherapy, or with metformin or a thiazolidinedione**
Adults: 120 mg P.O. t.i.d. taken 1 to 30 minutes before meals. Patients near goal glycosylated hemoglobin (HbA_{1c}) level when treatment is started may receive 60 mg P.O. t.i.d.

ADMINISTRATION
P.O.
● Give drug 1 to 30 minutes before a meal.
● If a meal is skipped, dose should be skipped to reduce risk of hypoglycemia.

ACTION
Lowers glucose level by stimulating insulin secretion from pancreatic beta cells.

Route	Onset	Peak	Duration
P.O.	20 min	1 hr	4 hr

Half-life: About 1½ hours.

ADVERSE REACTIONS
CNS: dizziness.
GI: diarrhea.
Metabolic: *hypoglycemia.*
Musculoskeletal: back pain, arthropathy.
Respiratory: upper respiratory tract infection, bronchitis, coughing.
Other: flulike symptoms, accidental trauma.

INTERACTIONS
Drug-drug. *Corticosteroids, rifamycins, sympathomimetics, thiazides, thyroid products:* May reduce hypoglycemic action of nateglinide. Monitor glucose level closely.
MAO inhibitors, nonselective beta blockers, NSAIDs, salicylates: May increase hypoglycemic action of nateglinide. Monitor glucose level closely.

EFFECTS ON LAB TEST RESULTS
• May increase uric acid level.

CONTRAINDICATIONS & CAUTIONS
• Contraindicated in patients hypersensitive to drug, in those with type 1 diabetes or diabetic ketoacidosis, and in pregnant or breast-feeding patients.
• Use cautiously in patients with moderate to severe liver dysfunction or adrenal or pituitary insufficiency, and in elderly and malnourished patients.
⚠ **Overdose S&S:** Hypoglycemic symptoms.

NURSING CONSIDERATIONS
• Don't use with glyburide or other oral antidiabetics; may use with metformin or a thiazolidinedione.
• Monitor glucose level regularly to evaluate drug's effectiveness.
• Observe patient for signs and symptoms of hypoglycemia. To minimize risk of hypoglycemia, make sure that patient has a meal immediately after dose. If hypoglycemia occurs and patient remains conscious, give him an oral form of glucose. If he's unconscious, treat with I.V. glucose.
• Risk of hypoglycemia increases with strenuous exercise, alcohol ingestion, or insufficient caloric intake.
• Symptoms of hypoglycemia may be masked in patients with autonomic neuropathy and in those who use beta blockers.

• Insulin therapy may be needed for glycemic control in patients with fever, infection, or trauma and in those undergoing surgery.
• Monitor glucose level closely when other drugs are started or stopped, to detect possible drug interactions.
• Periodically monitor HbA$_{1c}$ level.
• Drug's effectiveness may decrease over time.
• Usually, no special dosage adjustments are necessary in elderly patients, but some elderly patients may have greater sensitivity to glucose-lowering effect.

PATIENT TEACHING
• Tell patient to take drug 1 to 30 minutes before a meal.
• Advise patient to skip the scheduled dose if he skips a meal to reduce risk of hypoglycemia.
• Instruct patient on risk of hypoglycemia, its signs and symptoms (sweating, rapid pulse, trembling, confusion, headache, irritability, and nausea), and ways to treat these symptoms by eating or drinking something containing sugar.
• Teach patient how to monitor and log glucose levels to evaluate diabetes control.
• Advise patient to notify prescriber for persistent low or high glucose level.
• Instruct patient to adhere to prescribed diet and exercise regimen.
• Explain possible long-term complications of diabetes and importance of regular preventive therapy.
• Encourage patient to wear a medical identification bracelet.

N

nebivolol hydrochloride
neh-BIH-voh-lawl

Bystolic⚘

Therapeutic class: Antihypertensives
Pharmacologic class: Beta blockers
Pregnancy risk category: C

AVAILABLE FORMS
Tablets: 2.5 mg, 5 mg, 10 mg, 20 mg

INDICATIONS & DOSAGES
➤ **Hypertension**
Adults: Initially, 5 mg P.O. once daily. Increase at 2-week intervals to a maximum dose of 40 mg, if needed.
Adjust-a-dose: For patients with severe renal impairment (CrCl less than 30 mL/minute) or moderate hepatic impairment, start with 2.5 mg P.O. once daily. Increase dose cautiously, if needed.

ADMINISTRATION
P.O.
● May give drug without regard to food.

ACTION
Selectively blocks beta$_1$-adrenergic receptors, reducing heart rate, myocardial contractility, and sympathetic tone. Nebivolol also reduces blood pressure by suppressing renin activity and decreasing peripheral vascular resistance.

Route	Onset	Peak	Duration
P.O.	Unknown	1½–4 hr	Unknown

Half-life: 12 to 19 hours.

ADVERSE REACTIONS
CNS: asthenia, dizziness, fatigue, headache, insomnia, paresthesia.
CV: *bradycardia,* chest pain, peripheral edema.
GI: abdominal pain, diarrhea, nausea.
Metabolic: hypercholesterolemia, hyperuricemia.
Respiratory: dyspnea.
Skin: rash.

INTERACTIONS
Drug-drug. *Alpha-1 blockers:* May enhance severity and duration of hypotension. A smaller starting dose of alpha-1 blocker may be necessary.
Antidiabetic agents (insulin, sulfonylureas): May mask signs of hypoglycemia. Monitor blood glucose level.
Beta agonists (dobutamine, isoproterenol): May reverse nebivolol effects or cause protracted, severe hypotension. Avoid concomitant use.
Beta blockers (atenolol, nadolol): May increase synergistic activity and bradycardia. Don't use together.

Catecholamine-depleting drugs (such as guanethidine, reserpine): May cause bradycardia or severe hypotension. Monitor patient closely.
Clonidine: May cause further decrease in blood pressure. Simultaneous withdrawal may cause life-threatening rebound hypertension. Discontinue nebivolol for several days before gradual tapering of clonidine.
CYP2D6 inhibitors (such as fluoxetine, paroxetine, propafenone, quinidine): May increase nebivolol level. Monitor blood pressure closely, and adjust nebivolol dose as needed.
Digoxin, diltiazem, disopyramide, verapamil: May increase the risk of bradycardia. Monitor patient's ECG and vital signs.
Fingolimod: May increase risk of bradycardia. Monitor patient closely.
Mefloquine: May cause CV toxicity. Consider an alternative drug.
NSAIDs: May decrease antihypertensive effect. Monitor blood pressure; adjust nebivolol dosage as needed.

EFFECTS ON LAB TEST RESULTS
● May increase BUN, uric acid, and triglyceride levels. May decrease HDL and cholesterol levels.
● May decrease platelet count.

CONTRAINDICATIONS & CAUTIONS
● Contraindicated in patients hypersensitive to drug and those with decompensated heart failure, severe bradycardia, second- or third-degree AV block, sick sinus syndrome (unless a permanent pacemaker is in place), cardiogenic shock, bronchial asthma or related bronchospastic conditions, or severe hepatic impairment (greater than Child-Pugh class B).
● Use cautiously in patients with compensated heart failure, in perioperative patients receiving anesthetics that depress myocardial function (such as cyclopropane and trichloroethylene), in diabetic patients receiving insulin or oral antidiabetics or subject to spontaneous hypoglycemia, in patients with severe renal impairment, and in patients with thyroid disease (use may mask hyperthyroidism and withdrawal may worsen it), pheochromocytoma, or

---

peripheral vascular disease (may cause or worsen symptoms of arterial insufficiency).
⚠ *Overdose S&S:* Bradycardia, hypotension, cardiac failure, fatigue, dizziness, hypoglycemia, vomiting, bronchospasm, heart block.

NURSING CONSIDERATIONS
⟩ *Alert:* Patients with a history of severe anaphylactic reaction to several allergens may be more reactive to repeated exposure to nebivolol (accidental, diagnostic, or therapeutic), and they may not respond to amounts of epinephrine typically used to treat allergic reactions.
• Check patient's blood pressure and heart rate often.
• Monitor hepatic and renal function test results.
• If nebivolol must be stopped, do so gradually over 1 to 2 weeks.
• Because beta blockers may mask tachycardia caused by hyperthyroidism, be sure to withdraw nebivolol gradually in patients with suspected thyrotoxicosis to avoid thyroid storm.
• Observe a diabetic patient closely because drug may mask evidence of hypoglycemia.
• If patient has heart failure, watch for worsening symptoms, renal dysfunction, or fluid retention. His diuretic dosage may need to be increased.
• Store drug at room temperature in a light-resistant container.

PATIENT TEACHING
• Instruct patient not to stop drug suddenly but to notify prescriber about unpleasant adverse reactions. Explain that drug must be withdrawn gradually over 1 or 2 weeks.
• Caution patient to avoid driving and other tasks requiring alertness until his response to therapy is known.
• Tell patient to alert prescriber if he develops shortness of breath.
• Caution patient with diabetes or spontaneous hypoglycemia that drug may mask symptoms of low blood glucose level, especially increased heart rate.
• Urge women not to breast-feed during therapy.

nelfinavir mesylate
nell-FIN-ah-veer

Viracept

Therapeutic class: Antiretrovirals
Pharmacologic class: Protease inhibitors
Pregnancy risk category: B

AVAILABLE FORMS
Tablets: 250 mg, 625 mg

INDICATIONS & DOSAGES
➤ **HIV infection**
Adults and children age 13 and older:
1,250 mg P.O. b.i.d. or 750 mg P.O. t.i.d. in combination with other antiretrovirals. Maximum dosage is 2,500 mg/day.
Children ages 2 to 12: 45 to 55 mg/kg P.O. b.i.d. or 25 to 35 mg/kg P.O. t.i.d. in combination with other antiretrovirals; don't exceed 2,500 mg/day (b.i.d. dosing) or 2,250 mg/day (t.i.d. dosing).

ADMINISTRATION
P.O.
• Give tablets with a meal.
• May dissolve tablets in a small amount of water. The cloudy liquid should then be given immediately and the glass rinsed and given to patient to ensure entire dose is consumed.

ACTION
An HIV-1 protease inhibitor, which prevents cleavage of the viral polyprotein, resulting in the production of immature, noninfectious virus.

Route	Onset	Peak	Duration
P.O.	Unknown	2–4 hr	Unknown

Half-life: 3½ to 5 hours.

ADVERSE REACTIONS
CNS: *seizures, suicidal ideation.*
CV: *QTc prolongation, torsades de pointes.*
GI: diarrhea, *pancreatitis,* flatulence, nausea.
Hematologic: *leukopenia, thrombocytopenia.*
Hepatic: *hepatitis.*

N

Metabolic: *hypoglycemia,* dehydration, *diabetes mellitus,* hyperlipidemia, hyperuricemia.
Skin: rash.
Other: redistribution or accumulation of body fat.

INTERACTIONS

Drug-drug. *Amiodarone, ergot derivatives, midazolam, pimozide, quinidine, triazolam:* May increase levels of these drugs, causing increased risk of life-threatening adverse events. Avoid using together.

❸ *Alert:* **Atorvastatin:** May increase statin level and risk of myopathy and rhabdomyolysis. Atorvastatin dosage shouldn't exceed 40 mg/day.

Azithromycin: May increase azithromycin level. Monitor patient for liver impairment.

Carbamazepine, phenobarbital: May reduce the effectiveness of nelfinavir. Use together cautiously.

Cyclosporine, sirolimus, tacrolimus: May increase levels of these immunosuppressants. Use together cautiously.

Delavirdine, HIV protease inhibitors (indinavir, saquinavir): May increase levels of protease inhibitors. Use together cautiously.

Didanosine: May decrease didanosine absorption. Take nelfinavir with food at least 2 hours before or 1 hour after didanosine.

Drugs that prolong QT interval: May increase risk of life-threatening cardiac arrhythmias such as torsades de pointes. Monitor patient and ECG closely.

Ethinyl estradiol: May decrease contraceptive level and effectiveness. Advise patient to use alternative contraceptive measures during therapy.

❸ *Alert:* **Lovastatin, simvastatin:** May increase statin level and risk of myopathy and rhabdomyolysis. Use together is contraindicated.

Methadone, phenytoin: May decrease levels of these drugs. Adjust dosage of these drugs accordingly.

Rifabutin: May increase rifabutin level and decrease nelfinavir level. Reduce dosage of rifabutin to half the usual dose and increase nelfinavir to 1,250 mg b.i.d.

Sildenafil: May increase adverse effects of sildenafil. Caution patient not to exceed 25 mg of sildenafil in a 48-hour period.
Drug-herb. *St. John's wort:* May decrease drug level. Discourage use together.

EFFECTS ON LAB TEST RESULTS

• May increase ALT, AST, alkaline phosphatase, bilirubin, GGT, amylase, CK, and lipid levels. May decrease hemoglobin level. May increase or decrease glucose level.
• May decrease WBC and platelet counts.

CONTRAINDICATIONS & CAUTIONS

• Contraindicated in patients hypersensitive to drug or its components, in those with moderate or severe hepatic impairment, and in patients receiving amiodarone, ergot derivatives, lovastatin, midazolam, pimozide, quinidine, simvastatin, or triazolam.
• Use cautiously in patients with hepatic dysfunction or hemophilia types A or B. Monitor LFT results.
• It's not known if drug appears in breast milk. Because safety hasn't been established, advise HIV-infected women not to breast-feed, to avoid transmitting virus to the infant.

NURSING CONSIDERATIONS

• Drug dosage is the same whether drug is used alone or with other antiretrovirals.
• *Look alike–sound alike:* Don't confuse nelfinavir with nevirapine. Don't confuse Viracept with Viramune or Viramune XR.

PATIENT TEACHING

• Advise patient to take drug with food.
• Inform patient that drug doesn't cure HIV infection.
• Tell patient that long-term effects of drug are unknown and that there are no data stating that nelfinavir reduces risk of HIV transmission.
• Advise patient to take drug daily as prescribed and not to alter dose or stop drug without medical approval.
• If patient misses a dose, tell him to take it as soon as possible and then return to his normal schedule. Advise patient not to double the dose.

- Tell patient that diarrhea is the most common adverse effect and that it can be controlled with loperamide, if needed.
- Instruct patient taking hormonal contraceptives to use alternative or additional contraceptive measures while taking nelfinavir.

⊙ **Alert:** Advise patient taking sildenafil about an increased risk of sildenafil-related adverse events, including low blood pressure, visual changes, and painful erections. Tell him to promptly report any symptoms. Tell him not to exceed 25 mg of sildenafil in a 48-hour period.

- Advise patient to report use of other prescribed or OTC drugs because of possible drug interactions.

neomycin sulfate
nee-o-MYE-sin

Neo-Fradin

Therapeutic class: Antibiotics
Pharmacologic class: Aminoglycosides
Pregnancy risk category: D

AVAILABLE FORMS
Oral solution: 125 mg/5 mL
Tablets: 500 mg

INDICATIONS & DOSAGES
➤ **To suppress intestinal bacteria before surgery**
Adults: After saline cathartic, 1 g neomycin with 1 g erythromycin base P.O. at 1 p.m., 2 p.m., and 11 p.m. on day before 8 a.m. surgery.
➤ **Adjunctive treatment for hepatic coma**
Adults: 4 to 12 g P.O. daily in divided doses for 5 to 6 days.

ADMINISTRATION
P.O.
- For preoperative disinfection, provide a low-residue diet and a cathartic immediately before therapy.

ACTION
Inhibits protein synthesis by binding directly to the 30S ribosomal subunit; bactericidal.

Route	Onset	Peak	Duration
P.O.	Unknown	1–4 hr	8 hr

Half-life: 2 to 3 hours.

ADVERSE REACTIONS
CNS: *neuromuscular blockade.*
EENT: ototoxicity.
GI: nausea, vomiting, diarrhea, malabsorption syndrome, *Clostridium difficile*–related colitis.
GU: *nephrotoxicity,* possible increase in urinary excretion of casts.

INTERACTIONS
Drug-drug. ▉Black Box Warning▉ *Acyclovir, amphotericin B, cephalosporins, cidofovir, cisplatin, methoxyflurane, vancomycin, other aminoglycosides:* May increase nephrotoxicity. Monitor renal function test results. ▉

▉Black Box Warning▉ *Atracurium, pancuronium, rocuronium, vecuronium:* May increase effects of nondepolarizing muscle relaxants, including prolonged respiratory depression. Use together only when necessary, and expect to reduce dosage of nondepolarizing muscle relaxants. ▉
Digoxin: May decrease digoxin absorption. Monitor digoxin level.
▉Black Box Warning▉ *I.V. loop diuretics (such as furosemide):* May increase ototoxicity. Monitor patient's hearing. ▉
Oral anticoagulants: May inhibit vitamin K–producing bacteria; may increase anticoagulant effect. Monitor PT and INR.

EFFECTS ON LAB TEST RESULTS
- May increase BUN, creatinine, and non-protein nitrogen levels.

CONTRAINDICATIONS & CAUTIONS
- Contraindicated in patients hypersensitive to other aminoglycosides, in those with intestinal obstruction or inflammatory or ulcerative GI disease, and in patients who are breast-feeding.
- Use cautiously in elderly patients and in those with impaired renal function or neuromuscular disorders.

⚠ **Overdose S&S:** Neurotoxicity, ototoxicity, nephrotoxicity.

N

NURSING CONSIDERATIONS

Black Box Warning Due to increased risk of nephrotoxicity, monitor renal function: urine output, specific gravity, urinalysis, BUN and creatinine levels, and creatinine clearance. Report to prescriber evidence of declining renal function. ■

Black Box Warning Due to increased risk of ototoxicity, evaluate patient's hearing before and during prolonged therapy. Notify prescriber if patient has tinnitus, vertigo, or hearing loss. Deafness may start several weeks after drug is stopped. ■

• Watch for signs and symptoms of superinfection, such as fever, chills, and increased pulse rate.

Black Box Warning Neuromuscular blockade and respiratory paralysis have been reported after administration of aminoglycosides. Monitor patient closely. ■

• For adjunctive treatment for hepatic coma, decrease patient's dietary protein and assess neurologic status frequently during therapy.

• The ototoxic and nephrotoxic properties of drug limit its usefulness.

PATIENT TEACHING

• Instruct patient to report adverse reactions promptly.

• Encourage patient to maintain adequate fluid intake.

SAFETY ALERT!

nesiritide
neh-SIR-ih-tide

Natrecor

Therapeutic class: Vasodilators
Pharmacologic class: Human B-type natriuretic peptides
Pregnancy risk category: C

AVAILABLE FORMS

Injection: Single-dose vials of 1.5 mg sterile, lyophilized powder

INDICATIONS & DOSAGES

➤ **Acutely decompensated heart failure in patients with dyspnea at rest or with minimal activity**

Adults: 2 mcg/kg by I.V. bolus over 60 seconds, followed by continuous infusion of 0.01 mcg/kg/minute. Maximum dosage is 0.03 mcg/kg/minute.

Adjust-a-dose: If hypotension develops during administration, reduce dosage or stop drug. Restart drug at dosage reduced by 30% with no bolus doses.

ADMINISTRATION

I.V.

▼ Reconstitute one 1.5-mg vial with 5 mL of diluent (such as D_5W, normal saline solution, 5% dextrose and 0.2% saline solution injection, or 5% dextrose and half-normal saline solution) from a prefilled 250-mL I.V. bag.

▼ Gently rock (don't shake) vial until solution becomes clear and colorless.

▼ Withdraw contents of vial and add back to the 250-mL I.V. bag to yield 6 mcg/mL. Invert the bag several times to ensure complete mixing, and use the solution within 24 hours.

▼ Use the formulas below to calculate bolus volume (2 mcg/kg) and infusion flow rate (0.01 mcg/kg/minute):

$$\text{Bolus volume (mL)} = 0.33 \times \text{patient weight (kg)}$$

$$\text{Infusion flow rate (mL/hr)} = 0.1 \times \text{patient weight (kg)}$$

▼ Before giving bolus dose, prime the I.V. tubing. Withdraw the bolus and give over 60 seconds through an I.V. port in the tubing.

▼ Immediately after giving bolus, infuse drug at 0.1 mL/kg/hour to deliver 0.01 mcg/kg/minute.

▼ Store drug at 68° to 77° F (20° to 25° C). Protect from light. May store reconstituted vials at 36° to 77° F (2° to 25° C) for up to 24 hours.

▼ **Incompatibilities:** Bumetanide, enalaprilat, ethacrynate sodium, furosemide, heparin, hydralazine, insulin, sodium metabisulfite.

ACTION

Increases cyclic guanosine monophosphate (cGMP) level, relaxes smooth muscle, and dilates veins and arteries. Drug reduces pulmonary capillary wedge pressure and systemic arterial pressure in patients with heart failure.

Route	Onset	Peak	Duration
I.V.	15 min	1 hr	3 hr

Half-life: 18 minutes.

ADVERSE REACTIONS
CNS: anxiety, confusion, dizziness, fever, headache, insomnia, paresthesia, somnolence, tremor.
CV: hypotension, *bradycardia, ventricular tachycardia,* angina, atrial fibrillation, AV node conduction abnormalities, ventricular extrasystoles.
GI: abdominal pain, nausea, vomiting.
Hematologic: anemia.
Musculoskeletal: back pain, leg cramps.
Respiratory: *apnea,* cough, hemoptysis.
Skin: injection-site reactions, rash, pruritus, sweating.

INTERACTIONS
Drug-drug. *ACE inhibitors:* May increase hypotension symptoms. Monitor blood pressure closely.

EFFECTS ON LAB TEST RESULTS
• May increase creatinine level more than 0.5 mg/dL above baseline. May decrease hemoglobin level and hematocrit.

CONTRAINDICATIONS & CAUTIONS
• Contraindicated in patients hypersensitive to drug or its components.
• Contraindicated in patients with cardiogenic shock, systolic blood pressure below 100 mm Hg, low cardiac filling pressures, conditions in which cardiac output depends on venous return, or conditions that make vasodilators inappropriate, such as valvular stenosis, restrictive or obstructive cardiomyopathy, constrictive pericarditis, and pericardial tamponade.
⚠ **Overdose S&S:** Excessive hypotension.

NURSING CONSIDERATIONS
• Don't start drug at higher-than-recommended dosage because this may cause hypotension and may increase creatinine level.

⟳ **Alert:** This drug may cause hypotension. Monitor patient's blood pressure closely, particularly if he also takes an ACE inhibitor.
⟳ **Alert:** Drug binds to heparin, including the heparin lining of a coated catheter, decreasing the amount of nesiritide delivered. Don't give nesiritide through a central heparin-coated catheter.
• Drug may affect renal function. In patients with severe heart failure whose renal function depends on the renin-angiotensin-aldosterone system, treatment may lead to azotemia.
• There is limited experience with giving this drug for longer than 96 hours.

PATIENT TEACHING
• Tell patient to report discomfort at I.V. site.
• Urge patient to report to prescriber symptoms of hypotension, such as dizziness, light-headedness, blurred vision, or sweating.
• Tell patient to report other adverse effects to prescriber promptly.

---

nevirapine
neh-VEER-ah-pine

Auro-Nevirapine†, Viramune, Viramune XR

Therapeutic class: Antiretrovirals
Pharmacologic class: Nonnucleoside reverse transcriptase inhibitors
Pregnancy risk category: B

AVAILABLE FORMS
Oral suspension: 50 mg/5 mL
Tablets: 200 mg
Tablets (extended-release): 100 mg, 400 mg

INDICATIONS & DOSAGES
➤ **Adjunctive treatment in HIV-infected adults who have experienced clinical or immunologic deterioration; used with nucleoside analogue antiretrovirals**
Black Box Warning Adhere strictly to 14-day lead-in period with nevirapine 200-mg-daily dosing. ∎
Adults: 200 mg (immediate-release) P.O. daily for the first 14 days; then 200 mg P.O.

N

b.i.d. Or, 400 mg (extended-release) P.O. once daily after 14-day lead-in period with 200-mg daily dosing.

Children age 6 to less than 18 years: Initially 150 mg/m^2 (immediate-release) P.O. once daily for 14 days. Maximum dose is 200 mg per day. Then if BSA is 0.58 to 0.83 m^2, increase to 200 mg (extended-release) once daily; if BSA is 0.84 to 1.16 m^2, increase to 300 mg (extended-release) once daily; if BSA is greater than or equal to 1.17 m^2, increase to 400 mg (extended-release) once daily.

Children age 15 days and older: 150 mg/m^2 (immediate-release) P.O. once daily for 14 days. Then, 150 mg/m^2 P.O. b.i.d. maintenance dosage. Maximum dosage is 100 mg daily.

Adjust-a-dose: For patients on dialysis, give an additional 200-mg (immediate-release) dose after each dialysis treatment. Patients with a CrCl equal to or greater than 20 mL/minute don't require dosage adjustment. Extended-release formula hasn't been studied in patients with renal impairment.

ADMINISTRATION
P.O.
● Use drug with at least one other antiretroviral.
● Administer with or without food.
● Extended-release tablets must be swallowed whole and shouldn't be crushed, chewed, or divided.
● Shake the suspension gently before administering. An oral dosing syringe is recommended.

ACTION
Binds directly to reverse transcriptase and blocks RNA-dependent and DNA-dependent DNA polymerase activities by disrupting the enzyme's catalytic site.

Route	Onset	Peak	Duration
P.O.	Unknown	4 hr	Unknown

Half-life: 25 to 30 hours.

ADVERSE REACTIONS
CNS: fever, headache, paresthesia, fatigue.
GI: nausea, abdominal pain, diarrhea.
Hematologic: *neutropenia.*

Hepatic: *hepatitis.*
Musculoskeletal: myalgia.
Skin: blistering, rash, *Stevens-Johnson syndrome.*

INTERACTIONS
Drug-drug. *Drugs extensively metabolized by CYP450:* May lower levels of these drugs. Dosage adjustment of these drugs may be needed.
Efavirenz: May decrease efavirenz concentration and increase adverse reactions. Concurrent use isn't recommended.
Ketoconazole: May decrease ketoconazole level. Avoid using together.
Protease inhibitors or hormonal contraceptives: May decrease levels of these drugs. Use together cautiously.
Rifabutin, rifampin: Dosage adjustment may be needed. Monitor patient closely.
Warfarin: May increase anticoagulant effect of warfarin. Monitor INR and adjust warfarin dose as needed.
Drug-herb. *St. John's wort:* May decrease drug level. Discourage use together.

EFFECTS ON LAB TEST RESULTS
● May increase ALT, AST, GGT, and bilirubin levels. May decrease hemoglobin level.
● May decrease neutrophil count.

CONTRAINDICATIONS & CAUTIONS
● Contraindicated in patients hypersensitive to drug.
● If rash is present beyond 14-day lead-in period with immediate-release formulation, don't begin extended-release drug. The lead-in period prior to switching to extended-release formula isn't required if the patient is already taking twice daily immediate-release formulation in combination with other antiretroviral drugs.
● Don't give to patients with moderate or severe hepatic impairment or use as part of occupational and nonoccupational postexposure prophylaxis regimens.
● In patients with mild hepatic impairment, use cautiously; pharmacokinetics haven't been evaluated in these patients.
● Drug appears in breast milk. Don't use drug in breast-feeding women.
▲ **Overdose S&S:** Edema, erythema nodosum, fatigue, fever, headache, insomnia,

---

nausea, pulmonary infiltrates, rash, vertigo, vomiting, weight decrease.

NURSING CONSIDERATIONS
• Perform laboratory tests, including renal function tests, before therapy and regularly throughout.
• Increased AST or ALT levels or coinfection with hepatitis B or C at the start of therapy suggest a greater risk of hepatic adverse events.

Black Box Warning Severe and, in some cases, fatal hepatotoxicity, particularly in the first 18 weeks of treatment, has been reported and may occur in all patients, including those receiving the drug for postexposure prophylaxis, an approved use. Hepatotoxicity is often linked with rash and fever. Women and patients with higher CD4 $^+$ cell counts are at increased risk. Women with CD4 $^+$ cell counts greater than 250/mm^3, including pregnant women receiving long-term treatment for HIV infection, are at considerably higher risk for hepatotoxicity. ■

• Monitor patient for signs and symptoms of hepatitis, including rash. Closely monitor LFTs at baseline and during the first 18 weeks of treatment; then monitor frequently thereafter.
• Perform LFTs immediately if hepatitis or hypersensitivity reactions are suspected.
Alert: If hepatitis occurs, permanently stop drug and don't restart after recovery. In some cases, hepatic injury progresses anyway.

Black Box Warning Severe, life-threatening skin reactions, including fatalities, have occurred. The greatest risk of reaction is within the first 6 weeks of therapy. Monitor patient for blistering, oral lesions, conjunctivitis, muscle or joint aches, or general malaise. Especially look for a severe rash or rash accompanied by fever. Report these signs and symptoms to prescriber. Patients who experience a rash or hypersensitivity reactions must discontinue nevirapine and seek medical evaluation immediately. ■

Alert: If mild to moderate rash occurs during 14-day lead-in period with immediate-release nevirapine, don't increase dosage until the rash has resolved. Total duration of the once-daily lead-in dosing shouldn't

exceed 28 days, at which point an alternative regimen should be sought.
Alert: Patients who have stopped therapy for more than 7 days should restart therapy as if receiving drug for the first time.
• Antiretroviral therapy may be changed if disease progresses while patient is receiving this drug.
• *Look alike–sound alike:* Don't confuse nevirapine with nelfinavir. Don't confuse Viramune with Viracept.

PATIENT TEACHING
• Inform patient that drug doesn't cure HIV and that illnesses from advanced HIV infection still may occur. Explain that drug doesn't reduce risk of HIV transmission.
• Instruct patient to report rash immediately and to stop drug until told to resume.
• Tell patient with signs or symptoms of hepatitis (such as fatigue, malaise, anorexia, nausea, jaundice, liver tenderness or hepatomegaly, with or without initially abnormal transaminase levels) to stop drug and seek medical evaluation immediately.
• Stress importance of taking drug exactly as prescribed. If a dose is missed, tell patient to take the next dose as soon as possible and not to double next dose.
• Tell patient not to use other drugs unless approved by prescriber.
• Advise women of childbearing age that hormonal contraceptives and other hormonal methods of birth control shouldn't be used with this drug.

---

niCARdipine hydrochloride
nye-KAR-de-peen

Cardene, Cardene I.V., Cardene SR

Therapeutic class: Antihypertensives
Pharmacologic class: Calcium channel blockers
Pregnancy risk category: C

AVAILABLE FORMS
Capsules: 20 mg, 30 mg
Capsules (sustained-release): 30 mg, 45 mg, 60 mg
Injection: 2.5-mg/mL vial; 20 mg/200-mL, 40 mg/200-mL premixed bag

INDICATIONS & DOSAGES
➤ **Chronic stable angina (used alone or with other antianginals)**
Adults: Initially, 20 mg immediate-release capsule P.O. t.i.d. Adjust dosage every 3 days based on patient response. Usual range, 20 to 40 mg t.i.d.
➤ **Hypertension**
Adults: Initially, 20 mg immediate-release capsule P.O. t.i.d.; range, 20 to 40 mg t.i.d. Or, 30 mg sustained-release capsule b.i.d.; range, 30 to 60 mg b.i.d. Adjust dosage every 3 days based on patient response. Or, for patient who can't take oral form, 5 mg/hour I.V. infusion initially; then, increase by 2.5 mg/hour every 5 minutes for rapid control or every 15 minutes for gradual control to maximum of 15 mg/hour. After achieving blood pressure goal, decrease infusion rate to 3 mg/hour.
➤ **Pediatric hypertensive urgency or emergency ◆**
Children and adolescents ages 1 to 17: 1 to 3 mcg/kg/minute by I.V. infusion. Goal is to reduce blood pressure by up to 25% over the first 8 hours from presentation, then gradually normalize pressure over 26 to 48 hours.

ADMINISTRATION
P.O.
● Give drug with or without food, but avoid giving with high-fat meal.
● Patient should avoid grapefruit juice during therapy.
● Don't break or crush sustained-release capsules; they must be swallowed whole.
I.V.
▼ Dilute to a concentration of 0.1 mg/mL with D₅W, dextrose 5% in normal saline solution or half-normal saline solution, and normal saline solution or half-normal saline solution.
▼ Check premixed bags for leaks, solution clarity, and intact seal. Don't add other drugs to bag.
▼ Give by slow infusion.
▼ Closely monitor blood pressure during and after completion of infusion.
▼ If hypotension or tachycardia occurs, titrate infusion rate.

▼ Change peripheral infusion site every 12 hours to minimize risk of venous irritation.
▼ When switching to oral form, give first dose of t.i.d. regimen 1 hour before stopping infusion. If using a different oral drug, start it when infusion ends.
▼ If solution is kept at room temperature, use within 24 hours.
▼ **Incompatibilities:** Ampicillin sodium, ampicillin–sulbactam sodium, cefoperazone, ceftazidime, furosemide, heparin sodium, lactated Ringer's solution, sodium bicarbonate, thiopental.

ACTION
Inhibits calcium ion influx across cardiac and smooth muscle cells but is more selective to vascular smooth muscle than cardiac muscle. Drug also dilates coronary arteries and arterioles.

Route	Onset	Peak	Duration
P.O. (immediate-release)	20 min	1–2 hr	Unknown
P.O. (sustained-release)	20 min	1–4 hr	12 hr
I.V.	Immediate	Immediate	Unknown

Half-life: 2 to 4 hours.

ADVERSE REACTIONS
CNS: headache, dizziness, light-headedness, asthenia.
CV: peripheral edema, palpitations, flushing, angina, tachycardia.
GI: nausea, vomiting, abdominal discomfort, dry mouth.
Skin: rash.

INTERACTIONS
Drug-drug. *Antihypertensives, protease inhibitors:* May increase antihypertensive effect. Monitor blood pressure closely.
Cimetidine: May decrease metabolism of calcium channel blockers. Monitor patient for increased pharmacologic effect.
Cyclosporine: May increase plasma level of cyclosporine. Monitor patient for toxicity.
Digoxin: May increase digoxin level. Monitor digoxin level.
Drugs that prolong QT interval: May have an additive effect. Monitor patient and ECG.

Reactions in bold italics are *life-threatening*. Interactions may have a *rapid onset* or a *delayed onset*.

Fentanyl: May cause severe hypotension. Closely monitor blood pressure.

Drug-food. *Grapefruit and grapefruit juice:* May increase bioavailability of nicardipine. Discourage use together.

High-fat foods: May decrease absorption of nicardipine. Discourage use together.

EFFECTS ON LAB TEST RESULTS
• May decrease potassium level (I.V. form).

CONTRAINDICATIONS & CAUTIONS
• Contraindicated in patients hypersensitive to drug and in those with advanced aortic stenosis.

• Use cautiously in patients with hypotension, heart failure, or impaired hepatic and renal function.

⚠ **Overdose S&S:** Hypotension, bradycardia, palpitations, flushing, drowsiness, confusion, slurred speech.

NURSING CONSIDERATIONS
• Measure blood pressure frequently during initial therapy. Maximal response occurs about 1 hour after giving the immediate-release form and 2 to 4 hours after giving the sustained-release form. Check for orthostatic hypotension. Because large swings in blood pressure may occur based on drug level, assess antihypertensive effect 8 hours after dosing.

🔂 **Alert:** Only immediate-release form is approved for treatment of angina.

• Extended-release form is preferred because of improved compliance, fewer fluctuations in blood pressure, and less risk of death than with shorter-acting drugs.

• **Look alike–sound alike:** Don't confuse Cardene with Cardura or codeine.

PATIENT TEACHING
• Tell patient to take oral form exactly as prescribed.

• Advise patient to report chest pain immediately. Some patients may experience increased frequency, severity, or duration of chest pain at beginning of therapy or during dosage adjustments.

• Tell patient to get up from a sitting or lying position slowly to avoid dizziness caused by a decrease in blood pressure.

• Tell patient drug may be taken with or without food but shouldn't be taken with high-fat foods.

• Tell patient to swallow sustained-release capsules whole; don't crush, break, or chew.

NIFEdipine
nye-FED-i-peen

Adalat CC, Adalat XL†, Afeditab CR, Apo-Nifed†, Nifediac CC, Nifedical XL, Nu-Nifed†, Nu-Nifedipine-PA†, Procardia, Procardia XL✐

Therapeutic class: Antihypertensives
Pharmacologic class: Calcium channel blockers
Pregnancy risk category: C

AVAILABLE FORMS
Capsules: 10 mg, 20 mg
Tablets (extended-release): 20 mg†, 30 mg, 60 mg, 90 mg

INDICATIONS & DOSAGES
Adjust-a-dose (for all indications): For elderly patients and patients with renal and hepatic impairment, initiate drug at the low end of the dosing range.

➤ **Vasospastic angina (Prinzmetal or variant angina), classic chronic stable angina pectoris**
Adults: Initially, 10 mg short-acting capsule P.O. t.i.d. Usual effective dosage range is 10 to 20 mg t.i.d. Some patients may require up to 30 mg q.i.d. Maximum daily dose is 180 mg. Adjust dosage over 7 to 14 days to evaluate response. Or, 30 to 60 mg (extended-release tablets, except Adalat CC, Afeditab CR, or Nifediac CC) P.O. once daily. Maximum daily dose is 120 mg. Adjust dosage over 7 to 14 days to evaluate response.

➤ **Hypertension**
Adults: 30 or 60 mg extended-release tablet (Adalat CC, Afeditab CR, or Nifediac CC) P.O. once daily, adjusted over 7 to 14 days. Doses larger than 90 mg aren't recommended.

N

➤ **Raynaud phenomenon** ◆
Adults: 5 to 20 mg P.O. t.i.d. or 20 mg extended-release form P.O. b.i.d. for up to 12 weeks.

➤ **Pediatric hypertension** ◆
Children ages 1 to 17: 0.25 to 0.5 mg/kg/day extended-release form P.O. once daily or in two divided doses. Maximum dose is 3 mg/kg/day (up to 120 mg/day).

ADMINISTRATION
P.O.
● Don't give immediate-release capsules within 1 week of acute MI or in acute coronary syndrome.

❸ *Alert:* Don't use capsules S.L. to rapidly reduce severe high blood pressure because the result may be fatal.

● Give extended-release tablets whole; don't break or crush tablet.
● Don't give drug with grapefruit juice.
● Protect capsules from direct light and moisture and store at room temperature.

ACTION
Thought to inhibit calcium ion influx across cardiac and smooth muscle cells, decreasing contractility and oxygen demand. Drug may also dilate coronary arteries and arterioles.

Route	Onset	Peak	Duration
P.O.	20 min	30–60 min	4–8 hr
P.O. (extended)	20 min	6 hr	24 hr

Half-life: 2 to 5 hours.

ADVERSE REACTIONS
Immediate-release
CNS: dizziness, light-headedness, giddiness, headache, weakness, nervousness, mood changes, shakiness, sleep disturbances, fever.
CV: flushing, heat sensation, peripheral edema, palpitations, transient hypotension.
EENT: nasal congestion, sore throat, blurred vision.
GI: nausea, heartburn, diarrhea, constipation, cramps, flatulence.
Musculoskeletal: muscle cramps, tremor, inflammation, joint stiffness.
Respiratory: dyspnea, cough, wheezing, chest congestion, shortness of breath.

Skin: dermatitis, pruritus, urticaria, sweating.
Other: difficulties in balance, chills, sexual difficulties.
Extended-release
CNS: dizziness, headache, fatigue, insomnia, nervousness, paresthesia, somnolence, asthenia, pain.
CV: palpitations, chest pain, flushing.
GI: nausea, constipation, abdominal pain, diarrhea, dry mouth, dyspepsia, flatulence.
GU: erectile dysfunction, polyuria.
Musculoskeletal: arthralgia, leg cramps.
Respiratory: dyspnea.
Skin: pruritus, rash.

INTERACTIONS
Drug-drug. *ACE inhibitors (benazepril):* May increase hypotensive effects. Monitor blood pressure and adjust nifedipine dosage as needed.
Alpha-1 blockers (doxazosin): May increase nifedipine plasma concentration. Monitor blood pressure and adjust nifedipine dosage as needed.
Antiretrovirals, cimetidine, verapamil: May decrease nifedipine metabolism. Monitor blood pressure closely and adjust nifedipine dosage as needed.
Azole antifungals, erythromycin, nefazodone, quinupristin–dalfopristin, valproic acid: May increase the effects of nifedipine. Monitor blood pressure closely and decrease nifedipine dosage as needed.
Cyclosporine, tacrolimus: May increase serum levels of these drugs and increase risk of toxicity. Monitor serum levels and adjust dosage as needed.
Digoxin: May cause elevated digoxin level. Monitor digoxin level.
Diltiazem: May increase the effects of nifedipine. Monitor patient closely.
Diuretics, fentanyl: May increase hypotensive effects. Monitor blood pressure.
PDE5 inhibitors (such as sildenafil): Increases risk of hypotension. Monitor blood pressure and adjust nifedipine dosage if needed.
Phenytoin: May reduce nifedipine metabolism. Monitor patient and adjust nifedipine dosage as needed.

Reactions in bold italics are *life-threatening*. Interactions may have a *rapid onset* or a *delayed onset*.

Propranolol, other beta blockers: May cause hypotension and heart failure. Use together cautiously.

Quinidine: May decrease levels and effects of quinidine while increasing effects of nifedipine. Monitor heart rate and adjust nifedipine dose as needed.

Strong CYP3A4 inducers (carbamazepine, dexamethasone, phenytoin, rifabutin, rifampin): May decrease nifedipine level. Use together is contraindicated.

Warfarin: May increase PT. Monitor coagulation parameters and adjust warfarin dosage as needed.

Drug-herb. *Ginkgo:* May increase effects of drug. Discourage use together.

Ginseng: May increase drug levels with possible toxicity. Discourage use together.

Melatonin, St. John's wort: May interfere with antihypertensive effect. Discourage use together.

Drug-food. *Grapefruit juice:* May increase bioavailability of drug. Discourage use together.

EFFECTS ON LAB TEST RESULTS
● May increase ALT, AST, alkaline phosphatase, and LDH levels.

CONTRAINDICATIONS & CAUTIONS
● Contraindicated in patients hypersensitive to drug, in those taking strong CYP450 inducers (rifampin), and in patients with cardiogenic shock.
● Use cautiously in patients with heart failure or hypotension and in elderly patients. Use extended-release tablets cautiously in patients with severe GI narrowing.
● **Alert:** Use extended-release form cautiously because of an increased risk of serious GI obstruction in patients both with and without risk factors. (Risk factors for GI obstruction include altered GI anatomy, GI hypomotility related to gastroesophageal reflux disease, colon cancer, ileus, obesity, hypothyroidism, diabetes, and concomitant use of H_2 blockers, NSAIDs, laxatives, anticholinergic agents, and levothyroxine.)
▲ **Overdose S&S:** Hypotension, dizziness, palpitations, flushing, nervousness.

NURSING CONSIDERATIONS
● Monitor blood pressure and heart rate regularly, especially in patients who take beta blockers or antihypertensives.
● Watch for symptoms of heart failure.
● **Look alike–sound alike:** Don't confuse nifedipine with nimodipine or nicardipine.

PATIENT TEACHING
● If patient is kept on nitrate therapy while nifedipine dosage is being adjusted, urge continued compliance. Patient may take S.L. nitroglycerin, as needed, for acute chest pain.
● Tell patient that chest pain may worsen briefly as therapy starts or dosage increases.
● Instruct patient to swallow extended-release tablets without breaking, crushing, or chewing them.
● Advise patient to avoid taking drug with grapefruit juice.
● Reassure patient taking the extended-release tablet that the wax mold may be passed in the stools. Assure him that drug has already been completely absorbed.
● Tell patient to protect capsules from direct light and moisture and to store at room temperature.

SAFETY ALERT!

nilotinib
nye-low-TIH-nibb

Tasigna

Therapeutic class: Antineoplastics
Pharmacologic class: Kinase inhibitors
Pregnancy risk category: D

AVAILABLE FORMS
Capsules: 150 mg, 200 mg

INDICATIONS & DOSAGES
Adjust-a-dose (for all indications): If QTcF interval exceeds 480 msec, withhold drug; if it returns to less than 450 msec and within 20 msec of baseline within 2 weeks, resume therapy at previous dose. If QTcF interval is 450 to 480 msec after 4 weeks, reduce dose to 400 mg once daily; if QTcF interval returns to more than 480 msec, stop therapy. If neutrophil count is less than 1,000/mm³

or platelet count is less than 50,000/mm³, stop therapy. If neutrophil count exceeds 1,000/mm³ and platelet count exceeds 50,000/mm³ within 2 weeks, resume therapy at previous dose. If blood counts stay low for more than 2 weeks, reduce dose to 400 mg P.O. once daily. If serum amylase, lipase, bilirubin, or hepatic transaminase levels are grade 3 or greater, withhold drug; when levels return to grade 1 or less, resume therapy. Withhold drug with other clinically significant moderate or severe toxicity. When toxicity resolves, resume at 400 mg P.O. once daily; increase to 400 mg P.O. b.i.d. when clinically appropriate.

Black Box Warning Dosage reduction is recommended in patients with hepatic impairment. For mild to moderate impairment at baseline, initially give 300 mg b.i.d. If tolerated, may increase to 400 mg b.i.d. For severe hepatic impairment at baseline, initially give 200 mg b.i.d. May titrate to 300 mg b.i.d., then 400 mg b.i.d. as tolerated. ∎

➤ **Newly diagnosed, chronic-phase Philadelphia chromosome–positive chronic myelogenous leukemia (CML)**
Adults: 300 mg P.O. b.i.d.

➤ **Chronic and accelerated-phase Philadelphia chromosome–positive CML in patients resistant to or intolerant of imatinib**
Adults: 400 mg P.O. b.i.d., 12 hours apart.

ADMINISTRATION
P.O.
Black Box Warning Give with water on an empty stomach. Restrict food intake for at least 2 hours before and 1 hour after dose. Give capsule whole. ∎

• For patients unable to swallow capsules, mix contents of each capsule with one teaspoon of applesauce. Administer this mixture within 15 minutes. Don't store for future use.

ACTION
Stops leukemic cell lines by inhibiting Bcr-Abl kinase.

Route	Onset	Peak	Duration
P.O.	Unknown	3 hr	Unknown

Half-life: 17 hours.

ADVERSE REACTIONS
CNS: asthenia, fatigue, fever, headache, insomnia, dizziness, paresthesia, vertigo.
CV: flushing, hypertension, palpitations, peripheral edema, ***prolonged QT interval.***
EENT: nasopharyngitis.
GI: abdominal discomfort, abdominal pain, anorexia, constipation, diarrhea, dyspepsia, flatulence, nausea, vomiting.
Hematologic: anemia, ***febrile neutropenia, thrombocytopenia, neutropenia, pancytopenia.***
Hepatic: elevated lipase level.
Metabolic: hyperglycemia, ***hyperkalemia, hypocalcemia, hypokalemia, hypomagnesemia,*** hyponatremia, hypophosphatemia, weight gain or loss.
Musculoskeletal: arthralgia, myalgia, back pain, bone pain, limb pain, muscle spasms, musculoskeletal chest pain, pain in extremities.
Respiratory: cough, dysphonia, dyspnea, exertional dyspnea.
Skin: alopecia, dry skin, eczema, erythema, hyperhidrosis, night sweats, pruritus, rash, urticaria.

INTERACTIONS
Drug-drug. **Black Box Warning** *Antiarrhythmics and other drugs that prolong QTc interval:* May further prolong QTc interval. Avoid using together. ∎
CYP2C8, CYP2C9, CYP2D6, CYP3A4, UGT1A1 substrates, warfarin: May increase levels of these drugs. Avoid using together.
CYP3A4 inducers (carbamazepine, dexamethasone, phenobarbital, phenytoin, rifabutin, rifampin, rifapentin): May decrease nilotinib level. Avoid using together, or consider increasing dosage.
Black Box Warning *CYP3A4 inhibitors (atazanavir, clarithromycin, indinavir, itraconazole, ketoconazole, nefazodone, nelfinavir, ritonavir, saquinavir, telithromycin, voriconazole):* May increase nilotinib level. Avoid using together. If a strong CYP3A4 inhibitor must be given, reduce nilotinib dosage to 300 mg once daily in patients with resistant or intolerant Philadelphia chromosome–positive CML or 200 mg once daily in patients with newly

---

Reactions in bold italics are *life-threatening*. Interactions may have a *rapid onset* or a *delayed onset*.

diagnosed Philadelphia chromosome–positive CML in chronic phase. Closely monitor patient for prolonged QTc interval. ∎

Midazolam: May increase midazolam level. Avoid using together.

P-glycoprotein substrates: May increase nilotinib levels. Avoid using together.

Drug-herb. *St. John's wort:* May decrease nilotinib level. Avoid using together.

Drug-food. *Any food:* May increase drug level. Avoid eating 2 hours before and 1 hour after taking dose.

Grapefruit: May increase drug level. Avoid using together.

EFFECTS ON LAB TEST RESULTS

• May increase lipase, bilirubin, alkaline phosphatase, AST, ALT, potassium, and creatinine levels. May decrease albumin, sodium, potassium, calcium, phosphate, and hemoglobin levels.

• May decrease neutrophil and platelet counts.

CONTRAINDICATIONS & CAUTIONS

Black Box Warning Contraindicated in patients with prolonged QT-interval syndrome, hypokalemia, and hypomagnesemia. Avoid use in patients with galactose intolerance, severe lactose deficiency, or glucose-galactose malabsorption. ∎

Black Box Warning Obtain ECG to monitor the QTc at baseline, 7 days after initiation, and periodically thereafter, as well as following any dose adjustments. ∎

• Use cautiously in patients with hepatic impairment, elevated lipase levels, or a history of pancreatitis.

NURSING CONSIDERATIONS

• Monitor patient's phosphate, potassium, calcium, and sodium levels before and during therapy. Monitor the complete blood count every 2 weeks for the first 2 months and then monthly thereafter.

• Assess patient for evidence of fluid retention, such as shortness of breath and swelling of hands, ankles, feet, or face.

• Check lipase, amylase, ALT, AST, and alkaline phosphatase levels periodically during therapy.

• If stopping a CYP3A4 inhibitor, allow an appropriate washout period before escalating the nilotinib dose.

• Caution women to avoid becoming pregnant during therapy because of the risk of fetal harm.

• It isn't known whether drug appears in breast milk. Advise women to avoid breast-feeding during therapy.

• Safety and effectiveness in children haven't been established.

PATIENT TEACHING

• Instruct patient to immediately report an irregular heartbeat, shortness of breath, or swelling of the hands, ankles, feet, or face.

• Urge patient to immediately notify prescriber about a sudden onset of abdominal pain, nausea, and vomiting.

• Tell patient to avoid grapefruit during therapy.

Black Box Warning Instruct patient to take drug with water, and to restrict food intake for at least 2 hours before and 1 hour after taking the drug. ∎

• Advise women of childbearing age to use an effective form of contraception while taking nilotinib and to notify prescriber immediately if pregnancy occurs.

• Advise women to stop breast-feeding during therapy because of the risk of toxicity to infant.

N

---

nimodipine
nye-MOE-dih-peen

Nymalize

Therapeutic class: Vasodilators
Pharmacologic class: Calcium channel blockers
Pregnancy risk category: C

AVAILABLE FORMS
Capsules: 30 mg
Oral solution: 60 mg/20 mL

INDICATIONS & DOSAGES
➤ **To improve neurologic deficits after subarachnoid hemorrhage from ruptured intracranial berry aneurysm**

Adults: 60 mg P.O. every 4 hours for 21 days. Begin therapy within 96 hours after subarachnoid hemorrhage.
Adjust-a-dose: For patients with hepatic failure, 30 mg P.O. every 4 hours for 21 days.

ADMINISTRATION
P.O.
[Black Box Warning] Don't give drug I.V. or by other parenteral routes. Death and serious, life-threatening adverse reactions have occurred. ▪
• For administration via nasogastric (NG) or gastric tube, use the oral syringe labeled "ORAL USE ONLY" supplied with the oral solution. After each dose, refill the syringe with 20 mL of saline solution and flush any remaining contents from NG or gastric tube into the stomach.
• Administer drug not less than 1 hour before or 2 hours after a meal.
• Protect capsules from light; don't freeze. Don't refrigerate oral solution.

ACTION
Inhibits calcium ion influx across cardiac and smooth-muscle cells, decreasing my-ocardial contractility and oxygen demand; also dilates coronary and cerebral arteries and arterioles.

Route	Onset	Peak	Duration
P.O.	Unknown	1 hr	Unknown

Half-life: 8 to 9 hours; may be 1 to 2 hours.

ADVERSE REACTIONS
CNS: headache, depression.
CV: *bradycardia, ECG abnormalities,* hypotension, edema, tachycardia.
GI: nausea, diarrhea, GI symptoms.
Musculoskeletal: muscle cramps, muscle pain.
Respiratory: dyspnea.
Skin: acne, rash.

INTERACTIONS
Drug-drug. *Alpha-1 blockers:* May enhance nimodipine hypotensive effects. Monitor therapy.
Amifostine: May enhance amifostine hy-potensive effect. When amifostine is used at chemotherapy doses, withhold nimodipine for 24 hours before amifostine administra-tion. If antihypertensive therapy can't be withheld, don't give amifostine. Consider therapy modification.
Antifungals: May enhance nimodipine adverse or toxic effects. Concurrent use with itraconazole is contraindicated. Consider therapy modification.
Antihypertensives: May enhance hypoten-sive effects. Monitor therapy.
Atosiban: May increase risk of pulmonary edema or dyspnea. Monitor therapy.
Barbiturates: May increase nimodipine metabolism. Observe for decreased thera-peutic effect of nimodipine; dosage adjust-ments may be needed.
Calcium channel blockers (nondihydropy-ridine, such as verapamil): May enhance hypotensive effects of nimodipine. Monitor patient closely.
Calcium salts: May diminish nimodipine's therapeutic effect. Monitor therapy.
Carbamazepine: May increase nimodipine metabolism. Consider dosage adjustments or alternative therapy.
Cimetidine: May increase nimodipine serum concentration. Consider alternatives to cimetidine. If no suitable alternative exists, monitor patient for increased effects of nimodipine.
Clopidogrel: May diminish clopidogrel therapeutic effect. Monitor therapy.
Conivaptan: May increase nimodipine serum concentration. Avoid combination.
Cyclosporine, fluconazole: May decrease nimodipine metabolism. Monitor therapy.
CYP3A4 inducers (strong): May increase nimodipine metabolism. Consider alter-native therapies. Some combinations may be specifically contraindicated. Consult appropriate manufacturer labeling.
CYP3A4 inhibitors (moderate, strong): May decrease nimodipine metabolism. Monitor therapy; consider therapy modification if needed.
Dasatinib, fluoxetine: May increase ni-modipine serum concentration. Monitor therapy.
Deferasirox: May decrease nimodipine serum concentration. Monitor therapy.
Diazoxide: May enhance hypotensive ef-fects. Monitor therapy.

Fosphenytoin: May increase fosphenytoin serum concentration. Monitor patient for phenytoin toxicity with concomitant use or decreased phenytoin effects with nimodipine discontinuation. Monitor patient for decreased nimodipine therapeutic effects.

Hypotensive agents: May enhance adverse or toxic effect of other hypotensive agents. Monitor patient.

Ivacaftor: May increase nimodipine serum concentration. Monitor therapy.

Macrolide antibiotics: May decrease nimodipine metabolism. Consider using a noninteracting macrolide. Monitor patient for increased nimodipine therapeutic effects if interacting macrolide antibiotic is initiated, or decreased effects if macrolide is discontinued.

Magnesium salts: May enhance adverse or toxic effect of magnesium salts. Magnesium salts may enhance nimodipine hypotensive effect. Monitor therapy.

MAO inhibitors: May enhance nimodipine hypotensive effect. Monitor therapy.

Melatonin: May decrease nimodipine antihypertensive effect. Monitor therapy.

Methylphenidate: May decrease nimodipine antihypertensive effect. Monitor blood pressure.

Mifepristone: May increase nimodipine serum concentration. Minimize nimodipine doses, and monitor patient for increased concentration or toxicity during and for 2 weeks after treatment with mifepristone.

Nafcillin: May increase nimodipine metabolism. Consider therapy modification.

Neuromuscular blockers (nondepolarizing): May enhance neuromuscular-blocking effects. Monitor patient.

Nitroprusside: May enhance hypotensive effect of nitroprusside. Monitor blood pressure.

Pentoxifylline: May enhance hypotensive effect. Monitor therapy.

Phenytoin: May increase phenytoin serum concentration. Monitor patient for phenytoin toxicity with concomitant use or decreased phenytoin effects with nimodipine discontinuation. Monitor patient for decreased nimodipine therapeutic effects.

PDE5 inhibitors: May enhance nimodipine antihypertensive effect. Monitor therapy.

Prostacyclin analogues: May enhance nimodipine hypotensive effect. Monitor blood pressure.

Protease inhibitors: May decrease nimodipine metabolism. Consider therapy modification.

Quinidine: May increase or decrease quinidine serum concentration and increase nimodipine serum concentration. Monitor therapy.

Rifamycin derivatives: May increase nimodipine metabolism. Consult labeling. Consider therapy modification.

Rituximab: May enhance rituximab hypotensive effect. Consider therapy modification.

Tacrolimus: May increase tacrolimus serum concentration. Monitor therapy.

Tocilizumab: May decrease nimodipine serum concentration. Monitor therapy.

Drug-herb. *Dong quai, ephedra, garlic, ginseng, St. John's wort, yohimbe:* Interactions possible. Avoid concomitant use.

Drug-food. *Grapefruit:* May increase nimodipine serum concentration. Avoid combination.

EFFECTS ON LAB TEST RESULTS
None reported.

CONTRAINDICATIONS & CAUTIONS
• No known contraindications.
• Use cautiously in patients with hepatic failure.
⚠ **Overdose S&S:** Marked hypotension.

NURSING CONSIDERATIONS
• Monitor blood pressure and heart rate in all patients, especially at start of therapy.

PATIENT TEACHING
• Explain use of drug and review administration schedule with patient and family. Stress importance of compliance for maximum drug effectiveness.
• Instruct patient to report persistent or severe adverse reactions promptly.
• Tell patient not to drink grapefruit juice while taking this drug.

N

nisoldipine
nye-SOHL-di-peen

Sular

Therapeutic class: Antihypertensives
Pharmacologic class: Calcium channel blockers
Pregnancy risk category: C

AVAILABLE FORMS
Tablets (extended-release): 8.5 mg, 17 mg, 20 mg, 25.5 mg, 30 mg, 34 mg, 40 mg

INDICATIONS & DOSAGES
➤ **Hypertension**
Adults: Initially, 17 mg P.O. once daily, increased by 8.5 mg/week or at longer intervals, as needed. Usual maintenance dose is 17 to 34 mg daily. Doses of more than 34 mg daily aren't recommended. Or, initially, 20 mg P.O. once daily, increased by 10 mg per week or at longer intervals as needed. Usual maintenance dose is 20 to 40 mg daily. Doses of more than 40 mg daily aren't recommended.
Patients older than age 65: Initially, 8.5 or 10 mg P.O. once daily; adjust dosage as for other adults.
Adjust-a-dose: For patients with impaired liver function, initially, 8.5 or 10 mg P.O. once daily; dosage is adjusted as for adults.

ADMINISTRATION
P.O.
● Give drug whole; don't crush or split tablet.
● Give on an empty stomach (1 hour before or 2 hours after a meal).

ACTION
Prevents calcium ions from entering vascular smooth muscle cells, causing dilation of arterioles, which decreases peripheral vascular resistance.

Route	Onset	Peak	Duration
P.O.	Unknown	6–12 hr	24 hr

Half-life: 13.7 ± 4.3 hours.

ADVERSE REACTIONS
CNS: headache, dizziness.
CV: peripheral edema, vasodilation, palpitations, chest pain.
EENT: sinusitis, pharyngitis.
GI: nausea.
Skin: rash.

INTERACTIONS
Drug-drug. *Azole antifungals (such as ketoconazole):* May increase nisoldipine levels. Monitor patient closely for adverse effects.
Cimetidine: May increase bioavailability and peak nisoldipine level. Monitor blood pressure closely.
CYP3A4 inducers such as phenytoin: May decrease nisoldipine level. Avoid using together; consider alternative antihypertensive therapy.
Quinidine: May decrease bioavailability of nisoldipine. Adjust dosage accordingly.
Drug-herb. *Ma huang:* May decrease antihypertensive effects. Discourage use together.
Peppermint oil: May decrease drug effect. Discourage use together.
Drug-food. *Grapefruit products:* May increase drug level, increasing adverse reactions. Discourage use together.
High-fat foods: May increase peak drug level. Discourage use together.

EFFECTS ON LAB TEST RESULTS
None reported.

CONTRAINDICATIONS & CAUTIONS
● Contraindicated in patients hypersensitive to dihydropyridine calcium channel blockers.
● Use cautiously in patients with heart failure or compromised ventricular function, particularly those receiving beta blockers and those with severe hepatic dysfunction.
● It isn't known if drug appears in breast milk. Patient should avoid breast-feeding or use an alternative drug.
⚠ *Overdose S&S:* Hypotension.

NURSING CONSIDERATIONS
● Monitor frequency, duration, or severity of angina after starting calcium channel

---

Reactions in bold italics are *life-threatening*. Interactions may have a *rapid onset* or a *delayed onset*.

blocker therapy or at time of dosage increase. Report worsening of symptoms to prescriber immediately.
• Monitor blood pressure regularly, especially when starting therapy and during dosage adjustment.
• *Look alike–sound alike:* Don't confuse nisoldipine with nifedipine or nimodipine.

PATIENT TEACHING
• Tell patient to take drug as prescribed, even if he feels better.
• Advise patient to swallow tablet whole and not to chew, divide, or crush it.
• Remind patient not to take drug with a high-fat meal or with grapefruit products. Both may increase drug level in the body beyond intended amount.

nitrofurantoin macrocrystals
nye-troh-fyoo-RAN-toyn

Macrobid, Macrodantin🖊

nitrofurantoin microcrystals
Furadantin, Novo-Furantoin†

Therapeutic class: Antibiotics
Pharmacologic class: Nitrofurans
Pregnancy risk category: B

AVAILABLE FORMS
nitrofurantoin macrocrystals
Capsules: 25 mg, 50 mg, 100 mg
nitrofurantoin microcrystals
Oral suspension: 25 mg/5 mL

INDICATIONS & DOSAGES
➤ **UTIs caused by susceptible *Escherichia coli, Staphylococcus aureus,* enterococci, or certain strains of *Klebsiella* and *Enterobacter* species**
Adults and children older than age 12: 50 to 100 mg P.O. q.i.d. with meals and at bedtime. Continue for 1 week or for at least 3 days after sterility of urine is obtained. Or, 100 mg Macrobid P.O. every 12 hours for 7 days.
Children ages 1 month to 12 years: 5 to 7 mg/kg P.O. daily in four divided doses. Continue for 1 week or for at least 3 days after sterility of urine is obtained.

➤ **Long-term suppression therapy**
Adults: 50 to 100 mg P.O. daily at bedtime.
Children: 1 mg/kg P.O. daily in a single dose at bedtime or divided into two doses given every 12 hours.

ADMINISTRATION
P.O.
• Obtain urine specimen for culture and sensitivity tests before giving. Repeat as needed. Begin therapy while awaiting results.
• Give drug with food or milk to minimize GI distress and improve absorption.

ACTION
May interfere with bacterial enzyme systems and bacterial cell-wall formation.

Route	Onset	Peak	Duration
P.O.	Unknown	Unknown	Unknown

Half-life: 15 minutes to 1 hour.

ADVERSE REACTIONS
CNS: *ascending polyneuropathy with high doses or renal impairment,* dizziness, drowsiness, headache, peripheral neuropathy.
GI: anorexia, diarrhea, nausea, vomiting, abdominal pain.
GU: overgrowth of nonsusceptible organisms in urinary tract.
Hematologic: *agranulocytosis, hemolysis in patients with G6PD deficiency, thrombocytopenia.*
Hepatic: *hepatic necrosis, hepatitis.*
Metabolic: *hypoglycemia.*
Respiratory: *asthmatic attacks, pulmonary sensitivity reactions.*
Skin: *Stevens-Johnson syndrome;* exfoliative dermatitis; maculopapular, erythematous, or eczematous eruption; pruritus; transient alopecia; urticaria.
Other: *anaphylaxis,* drug fever, hypersensitivity reactions.

INTERACTIONS
Drug-drug. *Antacids containing magnesium:* May decrease nitrofurantoin absorption. Separate dosage times by 1 hour.
Probenecid, sulfinpyrazone: May inhibit excretion of nitrofurantoin, increasing drug levels and risk of toxicity. The resulting

decreased urinary levels could lessen antibacterial effects. Avoid using together.
Drug-food. *Any food:* May increase absorption. Advise patient to take drug with food or milk.

EFFECTS ON LAB TEST RESULTS
• May increase bilirubin and alkaline phosphatase levels. May decrease glucose level.
• May decrease granulocyte and platelet counts.
• May cause false-positive results in urine glucose tests using cupric sulfate (such as Benedict reagent, Fehling solution, or Chemstrip uG).

CONTRAINDICATIONS & CAUTIONS
• Contraindicated in infants age 1 month and younger; in patients with anuria, oliguria, or CrCl less than 60 mL/minute; and in patients with a history of cholestatic jaundice or hepatic dysfunction associated with nitrofurantoin use. Also contraindicated in pregnant patients at 38 to 42 weeks' gestation and during labor and delivery.
• Use cautiously in patients with renal impairment, asthma, anemia, diabetes mellitus, electrolyte abnormalities, vitamin B deficiency, debilitating disease, and G6PD deficiency.
⚠ *Overdose S&S:* Vomiting.

NURSING CONSIDERATIONS
• Drug may cause an asthma attack in patients with a history of asthma.
• Monitor fluid intake and output carefully. Treatment may turn urine brown or dark yellow.
• Monitor CBC, renal function, and pulmonary status regularly.
☼ *Alert:* Monitor patient for signs and symptoms of superinfection. Use of nitrofurantoin may result in growth of nonsusceptible organisms, especially *Pseudomonas* species.
• Monitor patient for pulmonary sensitivity reactions, including cough, chest pain, fever, chills, dyspnea, and pulmonary infiltration with consolidation or effusions.
☼ *Alert:* Hypersensitivity may develop when drug is used for long-term therapy.
• Some patients may experience fewer adverse GI effects with nitrofurantoin macrocrystals.

• Dual-release capsules (25 mg nitrofurantoin macrocrystals combined with 75 mg nitrofurantoin monohydrate) enable patients to take drug only twice daily.
• Continue treatment for 3 days after sterile urine specimens have been obtained.
• Store drug in amber container. Don't store in metals other than stainless steel or aluminum to avoid precipitation.

PATIENT TEACHING
• Instruct patient to take drug for as long as prescribed, exactly as directed, even after he feels better.
• Tell patient to take drug with food or milk to minimize stomach upset.
• Instruct patient to report adverse reactions, especially peripheral neuropathy, which can become severe or irreversible.
• Alert patient that drug may turn urine dark yellow or brown.
• Warn patient not to store drug in metals other than stainless steel or aluminum.
• Advise patient not to use antacid preparations containing magnesium trisilicate.

SAFETY ALERT!

nitroglycerin (glyceryl trinitrate)
nye-troe-GLIH-ser-in

Minitran, Nitro-Dur, Nitrolingual, NitroMist, Nitrostat◆, Rectiv, Trinipatch†

Therapeutic class: Vasodilators
Pharmacologic class: Nitrates
Pregnancy risk category: C

AVAILABLE FORMS
Aerosol (translingual): 0.4 mg/metered spray
Capsules (sustained-release): 2.5 mg, 6.5 mg, 9 mg
Injection: 5 mg/mL, 100 mcg/mL, 200 mcg/mL, 400 mcg/mL
Tablets (S.L.): 0.3 mg (1/200 grain), 0.4 mg (1/150 grain), 0.6 mg (1/100 grain)
Topical: 0.4% ointment, 2% ointment
Transdermal: 0.1 mg/hour, 0.2 mg/hour, 0.3 mg/hour, 0.4 mg/hour, 0.6 mg/hour, 0.8 mg/hour release rate

---

Reactions in bold italics are *life-threatening*. Interactions may have a *rapid onset* or a *delayed onset*.

INDICATIONS & DOSAGES
➤ **To prevent chronic anginal attacks**
Adults: 2.5 or 6.5 mg sustained-release capsule P.O. every 8 to 12 hours. Increase to an effective dose in 2.5- or 6.5-mg increments b.i.d. to q.i.d. Or, use 2% ointment: Start dosage with ½ inch ointment, increasing by ½ inch increments until desired results are achieved. Range of dosage with ointment is ½ inch to 5 inches. Usual dose is 1 inch to 2 inch every 6 to 8 hours. Or, transdermal patch 0.2 to 0.4 mg/hour once daily.
➤ **Acute angina pectoris; to prevent or minimize anginal attacks before stressful events**
Adults: 1 S.L. tablet (¹/₂₀₀ grain, ¹/₁₅₀ grain, ¹/₁₀₀ grain) dissolved under the tongue or in the buccal pouch as soon as angina begins. Repeat every 5 minutes, if needed, for 15 minutes. Or, one or two metered-dose sprays Nitrolingual into mouth, preferably onto or under the tongue. Repeat every 3 to 5 minutes, if needed, to a maximum of three doses within a 15-minute period.
➤ **Hypertension from surgery, heart failure after MI, angina pectoris in acute situations; to produce controlled hypotension during surgery (by I.V. infusion)**
Adults: Initially, infuse at 5 mcg/minute, increasing as needed by 5 mcg/minute every 3 to 5 minutes until response occurs. If a 20-mcg/minute rate doesn't produce a response, increase dosage by as much as 20 mcg/minute every 3 to 5 minutes. Up to 100 mcg/minute may be needed.
➤ **Moderate to severe pain from chronic anal fissure**
Adults: 1 inch of ointment P.R. every 12 hours for up to 3 weeks.

ADMINISTRATION
P.O.
• Give 30 minutes before or 1 to 2 hours after meals.
• Drug must be swallowed whole and not chewed.
I.V.
▼ Dilute with D₅W or normal saline solution for injection. Concentration shouldn't exceed 400 mcg/mL.
▼ Always give with an infusion control device and titrate to desired response.

▼ Regular polyvinyl chloride tubing can bind up to 80% of drug, making it necessary to infuse higher dosages. A special nonabsorbent polyvinyl chloride tubing is available from the manufacturer. Always mix in glass bottles and avoid using a filter.
▼ Use the same type of infusion set when changing lines.
▼ When changing the concentration of infusion, flush the administration set with 15 to 20 mL of the new concentration before use. This will clear the line of the old drug solution.
▼ **Incompatibilities:** Alteplase, bretylium, hydralazine, levofloxacin, phenytoin sodium.
Topical
• To apply ointment, measure the prescribed amount on the application paper; then place the paper on any nonhairy area. Don't rub in. Cover with plastic film to aid absorption and to protect clothing. Remove all excess ointment from previous site before applying the next dose. Avoid getting ointment on fingers.
P.R.
• Cover a finger with plastic wrap, disposable surgical glove, or a finger cot.
• Apply 1 inch of ointment onto the covered finger.
• Gently insert the ointment into the anal canal using the covered finger no further than the first finger joint.
Transdermal
• Patch can be applied to any nonhairy part of the skin except distal parts of the arms or legs. (Absorption won't be maximal at distal sites.) Patch may cause contact dermatitis.
• A cardioverter-defibrillator shouldn't be discharged through a paddle electrode that overlies a nitroglycerin patch.
• Remove patch before defibrillation. Because of the aluminum backing on the patch, the electric current may cause arcing that can damage the paddles and burn the patient.
• When stopping transdermal treatment of angina, gradually reduce the dosage and frequency of application over 4 to 6 weeks.
S.L.
• Give tablet at first sign of attack. Patient should wet the tablet with saliva and place it under tongue until absorbed. Dose may be

N

repeated every 5 minutes for a maximum of three doses. If drug doesn't provide relief, obtain prompt medical attention.

Buccal

• The tablet should be placed between the lip and gum above the incisors or between the cheek and gum. Tablets shouldn't be swallowed or chewed.

Translingual

• Patient using translingual aerosol form shouldn't inhale the spray but should release it onto or under the tongue. He should wait about 10 seconds or so before swallowing.

ACTION

Reduces cardiac oxygen demand by decreasing left ventricular end-diastolic pressure (preload) and, to a lesser extent, systemic vascular resistance (afterload). Also increases blood flow through the collateral coronary vessels.

Route	Onset	Peak	Duration
P.O.	20–45 min	Unknown	3–8 hr
I.V.	Immediate	Immediate	3–5 min
Topical	30 min	Unknown	2–12 hr
Transdermal	30 min	Unknown	24 hr
S.L.	1–3 min	Unknown	30–60 min
Buccal	3 min	Unknown	3–5 hr
Translingual	2–4 min	Unknown	30–60 min
P.R.	Immediate	Unknown	Unknown

Half-life: About 1 to 4 minutes.

ADVERSE REACTIONS

CNS: headache, dizziness, syncope, weakness.
CV: orthostatic hypotension, tachycardia, flushing, palpitations.
EENT: S.L. burning.
GI: nausea, vomiting.
Skin: cutaneous vasodilation, contact dermatitis, rash.
Other: hypersensitivity reactions.

INTERACTIONS

Drug-drug. *Alteplase:* May decrease tissue plasminogen activator-antigen level. Avoid using together; if unavoidable, use lowest effective dose of nitroglycerin.
Antihypertensives: May increase hypotensive effect. Monitor blood pressure closely.

Heparin: I.V. nitroglycerin may interfere with anticoagulant effect of heparin. Monitor PTT.
Sildenafil, tadalafil, vardenafil: May cause severe hypotension. Use of nitrates in any form with these drugs is contraindicated.
Drug-lifestyle. *Alcohol use:* May increase hypotension. Discourage use together.

EFFECTS ON LAB TEST RESULTS

• May falsely decrease values in cholesterol determination tests using the Zlatkis-Zak color reaction.

CONTRAINDICATIONS & CAUTIONS

• Contraindicated in patients hypersensitive to drug.
• Contraindicated in patients with early MI (oral and sublingual), severe anemia, increased intracranial pressure, angle-closure glaucoma, orthostatic hypotension, allergy to adhesives (transdermal), or hypersensitivity to nitrates.
• I.V. nitroglycerin is contraindicated in patients hypersensitive to I.V. form, with cardiac tamponade, restrictive cardiomyopathy, or constrictive pericarditis.
• Use cautiously in patients with hypotension or volume depletion.

⚠ **Overdose S&S:** Vasodilation, decreased cardiac output, venous pooling, hypotension, methemoglobinemia.

NURSING CONSIDERATIONS

• Closely monitor vital signs, particularly blood pressure, during infusion, especially in a patient with an MI. Excessive hypotension can worsen ischemia.
• Monitor blood pressure and intensity and duration of drug response.
• Drug may cause headaches, especially at beginning of therapy. Dosage may be reduced temporarily, but tolerance usually develops. Treat headache with aspirin or acetaminophen.
• Tolerance to drug can be minimized with a 10- to 12-hour nitrate-free interval. To achieve this, remove the transdermal system in the early evening and apply a new system the next morning or omit the last daily dose of a buccal, sustained-release, or ointment form. Check with the prescriber

---

for alterations in dosage regimen if toler-ance is suspected.

• Wipe off nitroglycerin paste or remove patch before defibrillation to avoid patient burns.

• *Look alike–sound alike:* Don't confuse nitroglycerin with nitroprusside.

PATIENT TEACHING

• Caution patient to take nitroglycerin regularly, as prescribed, and to have it accessible at all times.

⑤ *Alert:* Advise patient that stopping drug abruptly causes spasm of the coronary arteries.

• Teach patient how to give the prescribed form of nitroglycerin.

• Tell patient to take S.L. tablet at first sign of attack. Patient should wet the tablet with saliva, place it under tongue until absorbed, and then sit down and rest. Dose may be repeated every 5 minutes for a maximum of three doses. If drug doesn't provide relief, he should obtain medical help promptly.

• Advise patient who complains of a tingling sensation with S.L. drug to try holding tablet in cheek.

• Tell patient to take oral tablets on an empty stomach either 30 minutes before or 1 to 2 hours after meals, to swallow oral tablets whole, and not to chew tablets.

• Remind patient using translingual aerosol form that he shouldn't inhale the spray but should release it onto or under the tongue. Tell him to wait about 10 seconds or so before swallowing.

• Tell patient to place the buccal tablet between the lip and gum above the incisors or between the cheek and gum. Tablets shouldn't be swallowed or chewed.

• Tell patient to take an additional dose before anticipated stress or at bedtime if chest pain occurs at night.

• Urge patient using skin patches to dispose of them carefully because enough medication remains after normal use to be hazardous to children and pets.

• If patients using skin patches are sched-uled for a magnetic resonance imaging scan, advise them to notify the facility that they are wearing a patch.

• Advise patient to avoid alcohol.

• To minimize dizziness when standing up, tell patient to rise slowly. Advise him to go up and down stairs carefully and to lie down at the first sign of dizziness.

⑤ *Alert:* Advise patient that use of sildenafil, tadalafil, or vardenafil with any nitrate may cause life-threatening low blood pressure. Use together is contraindicated.

• Tell patient to store drug in cool, dark place in a tightly closed container. Tell him to remove cotton from container because it absorbs drug.

• Tell patient to store S.L. tablets in original container or other container specifically approved for this use and to carry the container in a jacket pocket or purse, not in a pocket close to the body.

SAFETY ALERT!

nitroprusside sodium
nye-troe-PRUSS-ide

Nipride†, Nitropress

Therapeutic class: Antihypertensives
Pharmacologic class: Vasodilators
Pregnancy risk category: C

N

AVAILABLE FORMS
Injection: 25 mg/mL

INDICATIONS & DOSAGES
➤ **To lower blood pressure quickly in hypertensive emergencies, to produce controlled hypotension during anesthe-sia, to reduce preload and afterload in cardiac pump failure or cardiogenic shock (may be used with or without dopamine)**

Adults and children: Begin infusion at 0.3 mcg/kg/minute I.V. and gradually titrate every few minutes to a maximum infusion rate of 10 mcg/kg/minute.

Adjust-a-dose: Patients also taking other antihypertensives are extremely sensitive to nitroprusside. Titrate dosage accordingly. Use with caution in patients with severe renal impairment or hepatic insufficiency; use minimum effective dose.

ADMINISTRATION

I.V.

▼ Prepare solution by dissolving 50 mg in 2 to 3 mL of D_5W injection or according to manufacturer's instructions.

Black Box Warning Further dilute concentration in 250, 500, or 1,000 mL of D_5W to provide solutions with 200, 100, or 50 mcg/mL, respectively. ■

▼ Reconstitute ADD-Vantage vials labeled as containing 50 mg of drug according to manufacturer's directions.

▼ Because drug is sensitive to light, wrap solution in foil or other opaque material; it's not necessary to wrap the tubing. Fresh solution has a faint brownish tint. Discard if highly discolored after 24 hours.

▼ Use an infusion pump. Drug is best given via piggyback through a peripheral line with no other drug. Don't titrate rate of main I.V. line while drug is being infused. Even a small bolus can cause severe hypotension.

▼ Check blood pressure every 5 minutes during titration at start of infusion and every 15 minutes thereafter.

▼ If severe hypotension occurs, stop infusion; effects of drug quickly reverse. Notify prescriber.

▼ If possible, start an arterial pressure line. Regulate drug flow to desired blood pressure response.

▼ **Incompatibilities:** Amiodarone, atracurium besylate, bacteriostatic water for injection, cisatracurium, drotrecogin alfa, haloperidol lactate, levofloxacin, pantoprazole. Don't mix with other I.V. drugs or preservatives.

ACTION

Relaxes arteriolar and venous smooth muscle.

Route	Onset	Peak	Duration
I.V.	Immediate	1–2 min	10 min

Half-life: 2 minutes.

ADVERSE REACTIONS

CNS: headache, dizziness, *increased intracranial pressure,* loss of consciousness, apprehension, restlessness.

CV: *bradycardia,* hypotension, tachycardia, palpitations, ECG changes, flushing.

GI: nausea, abdominal pain, ileus.

Hematologic: *methemoglobinemia.*

Metabolic: acidosis, hypothyroidism.

Musculoskeletal: muscle twitching.

Skin: diaphoresis, pink color, rash.

Other: *thiocyanate toxicity, cyanide toxicity,* venous streaking, irritation at infusion site.

INTERACTIONS

Drug-drug. *Antihypertensives:* May cause sensitivity to nitroprusside. Adjust dosage. *Ganglionic-blocking drugs, general anesthetics, negative inotropic drugs, other antihypertensives:* May cause additive effects. Monitor blood pressure closely. *Sildenafil, vardenafil:* May increase hypotensive effects. Avoid use together.

EFFECTS ON LAB TEST RESULTS

● May increase creatinine level.
● May decrease RBC and WBC counts.

CONTRAINDICATIONS & CAUTIONS

● Contraindicated in patients hypersensitive to drug.

● Contraindicated in those with compensatory hypertension (such as in arteriovenous shunt or coarctation of the aorta), inadequate cerebral circulation, acute heart failure with reduced peripheral vascular resistance, congenital optic atrophy, or tobacco-induced amblyopia.

● Use with extreme caution in patients with increased intracranial pressure.

● Use cautiously in patients with hypothyroidism, hepatic or renal disease, hyponatremia, or low vitamin B level.

⚠ *Overdose S&S:* Hypotension, acidosis, cyanide or thiocyanate toxicity.

NURSING CONSIDERATIONS

Black Box Warning Drug may cause rapid decrease in blood pressure. Use drug only when available equipment and personnel allow blood pressure to be continuously monitored. ■

● Obtain baseline vital signs before giving drug; find out parameters prescriber wants to achieve. Monitor blood pressure continuously.

● Keep patient in supine position when starting therapy or titrating drug.

Reactions in bold italics are *life-threatening*. Interactions may have a *rapid onset* or a *delayed onset*.

Black Box Warning Giving excessive doses of 500 mcg/kg delivered faster than 2 mcg/kg/minute or using maximum infusion rate of 10 mcg/kg/minute for more than 10 minutes can cause cyanide toxicity. ■

Black Box Warning Although acid-base balance and venous oxygen concentration should be monitored and may indicate cyanide toxicity, these laboratory tests provide imperfect guidance. ■

☉ *Alert:* If patient is at risk, check thiocyanate level every 72 hours. Level higher than 100 mcg/mL may be toxic. If profound hypotension, metabolic acidosis, dyspnea, headache, loss of consciousness, ataxia, or vomiting occurs, stop drug immediately and notify prescriber.

● *Look alike–sound alike:* Don't confuse nitroprusside with nitroglycerin.

PATIENT TEACHING

● Instruct patient to report adverse reactions promptly.
● Tell patient to alert nurse if discomfort occurs at I.V. insertion site.

---

norelgestromin–ethinyl estradiol transdermal system
nor-el-JES-troe-min and ETH-i-nill

Ortho Evra

Therapeutic class: Contraceptives
Pharmacologic class: Estrogen–progestin combinations
Pregnancy risk category: X

AVAILABLE FORMS

Transdermal patch: norelgestromin 6 mg and ethinyl estradiol 0.75 mg per patch, delivering 150 mcg norelgestromin and 20 mcg ethinyl estradiol daily

INDICATIONS & DOSAGES

➤ **Contraception**
Women of childbearing age: Apply 1 patch weekly for 3 weeks. Apply each new patch on the same day of the week. Week 4 is patch-free and withdrawal bleeding is expected. On the day after week 4 ends, apply a new patch to start a new 4-week cycle. The patch-free interval between cycles should never be longer than 7 days.

ADMINISTRATION

Transdermal
● Apply patch to a clean, dry area of the skin on the buttocks, abdomen, upper outer arm, or upper torso. Don't apply to the breasts or to skin that is red, irritated, or cut.

ACTION

Combination hormonal contraceptives act by suppressing gonadotropins. The primary mechanism of this action is ovulation inhibition. However, changes in cervical mucus increase the difficulty of sperm entry into the uterus, and changes in the endometrium decrease the likelihood of implantation.

Route	Onset	Peak	Duration
Transdermal	Rapid	2 days	Unknown

Half-life: Ethinyl estradiol, 6 to 45 hours; norelgestromin, 28 hours.

ADVERSE REACTIONS

CNS: headache, emotional lability, dizziness, fatigue.
CV: *thromboembolic events, MI,* hypertension, edema, *cerebral hemorrhage.*
EENT: contact lens intolerance, changes in corneal curvature.
GI: nausea, abdominal pain, vomiting, gallbladder disease, cholestatic jaundice.
GU: dysmenorrhea, changes in menstrual flow, vaginal candidiasis.
Hepatic: *hepatic adenomas,* benign liver tumors.
Metabolic: weight changes.
Skin: application-site reaction, melasma, pruritus, acne.
Other: breast tenderness, enlargement, or secretion.

INTERACTIONS

Drug-drug. *Acetaminophen, clofibric acid, morphine, salicylic acid, temazepam:* May decrease levels or increase clearance of these drugs. Monitor patient for lack of effect.
Ampicillin, barbiturates, carbamazepine, felbamate, griseofulvin, oxcarbazepine, phenylbutazone, phenytoin, rifampin, tetracyclines, topiramate: May reduce contraceptive effectiveness, resulting in unintended

N

pregnancy or breakthrough bleeding. Encourage backup method of contraception if used together.

Anticoagulants: May increase or decrease effect of anticoagulant. Monitor patient and laboratory values.

Ascorbic acid, atorvastatin, itraconazole, ketoconazole: May increase hormone levels. Use together cautiously.

Cyclosporine, prednisolone, theophylline: May increase levels of these drugs. Monitor patient for adverse reactions.

HIV protease inhibitors: May affect contraceptive effectiveness and safety. Use together cautiously.

Drug-herb. *St. John's wort:* May reduce effectiveness of drug and cause breakthrough bleeding. Discourage use together.

Drug-lifestyle. *Smoking:* May increase risk of CV adverse effects, related to age and smoking 15 or more cigarettes daily. Urge patient not to smoke.

EFFECTS ON LAB TEST RESULTS

• May increase circulating total thyroid hormone, triglyceride, other binding protein, sex hormone–binding globulin, total circulating endogenous sex steroid, corticoid, and factor VII, VIII, IX, and X levels. May decrease antithrombin III and folate levels.

• May decrease free T_3 resin uptake and glucose tolerance.

CONTRAINDICATIONS & CAUTIONS

Black Box Warning Cigarette smoking increases the risk of serious adverse cardiac effects from hormonal contraceptive use. Risk increases with age, especially in women older than age 35, and with the number of cigarettes smoked. Hormonal contraceptives are contraindicated in women older than age 35 who smoke. ∎

Black Box Warning There is an increased risk of venous thromboembolism in women ages 15 to 44 using the norelgestromin–ethinyl estradiol transdermal system compared to women using oral contraceptives containing 30 to 35 mcg of ethinyl estradiol and either levonorgestrel or norgestimate. ∎

• Contraindicated in patients hypersensitive to any component of this drug and in those with past history of deep vein thrombosis or

related disorder; current or past history of cerebrovascular or coronary artery disease; past or current known or suspected breast cancer, endometrial cancer, or other known or suspected estrogen-dependent neoplasia; hepatic adenoma or cancer; and in those who are or may be pregnant.

• Contraindicated in patients with thrombophlebitis, thromboembolic disorders, valvular heart disease with complications, severe hypertension, diabetes with vascular involvement, headaches with focal neurologic symptoms, major surgery with prolonged immobilization, undiagnosed abnormal genital bleeding, cholestatic jaundice of pregnancy or jaundice with previous hormonal contraceptive use, or acute or chronic hepatocellular disease with abnormal liver function.

• Use cautiously in patients with CV disease risk factors, with conditions that might be aggravated by fluid retention, or with a history of depression.

⚠ Overdose S&S: Nausea, vomiting, withdrawal uterine bleeding.

NURSING CONSIDERATIONS

❸ Alert: Patients taking combination hormonal contraceptives may be at increased risk for thrombophlebitis, venous thrombosis with or without embolism, pulmonary embolism, MI, cerebral hemorrhage, cerebral thrombosis, hypertension, gallbladder disease, hepatic adenomas, benign liver tumors, mesenteric thrombosis, and retinal thrombosis.

• Increased risk of MI occurs primarily in smokers and women with hypertension, hypercholesterolemia, morbid obesity, and diabetes.

• Encourage women with a history of hypertension or renal disease to use a different contraceptive. If this drug is used, monitor blood pressure closely and stop use if hypertension occurs.

• Drug may be less effective in women who weigh 90 kg (198 lb) or more.

• The risk of thromboembolic disease increases if therapy is used postpartum or postabortion.

Black Box Warning Birth control patch users may be at higher risk for developing serious blood clots versus birth control pill users. ∎

• Rule out pregnancy if withdrawal bleeding fails to occur for two consecutive cycles.

• If skin becomes irritated, the patch may be removed and a new patch applied at a different site.

• Stop drug and notify prescriber at least 4 weeks before and for 2 weeks after an elective surgery that increases the risk of thromboembolism, and during and after prolonged immobilization. Teach the patient about alternative methods of contraception during this time.

• Stop drug and notify prescriber if patient has headaches, vision loss, proptosis, diplopia, papilledema, retinal vascular lesions, jaundice, or depression.

PATIENT TEACHING

• Emphasize the importance of having regular annual physical examinations to check for adverse effects or developing contraindications.

• Tell patient that drug doesn't protect against HIV and other sexually transmitted diseases.

• Advise women to initiate and apply patch on the first day of menstrual cycle and then on the same day each week.

• Advise patient to use a backup method of contraception for the first 7 days.

• Tell patient switching from estrogen–progestin oral contraceptives to apply first patch on the first day of withdrawal bleeding. If no bleeding within 5 days of last hormonally active pill, advise patient to obtain a pregnancy test.

• Advise patient to immediately apply a new patch once the used patch is removed, on the same day of the week every 7 days for 3 weeks. Week 4 is patch-free. Withdrawal bleeding is expected to occur during this time.

• Tell patient to apply each patch to a clean, dry area of the skin on the buttocks, abdomen, upper outer arm, or upper torso. Tell patient not to apply to the breasts or to skin that's red, irritated, or cut.

• Tell patient to carefully fold the used patch in half so that it sticks to itself before discarding.

• Tell women to immediately stop use if pregnancy is confirmed.

• Tell patient who wears contact lenses to report visual changes or changes in lens tolerance.

• Advise patient not to smoke while using the patch.

• Tell patient that if a patch becomes detached for less than 1 day, to reapply it or replace it immediately and continue the schedule. If the patch is detached for more than 1 day, a new cycle should be started and back-up contraception should be used for the first week.

• Stress that if patient isn't sure what to do about mistakes with patch use, she should use a backup method of birth control and contact her health care provider.

• Tell patient undergoing a magnetic resonance imaging scan to alert facility that she's using a transdermal patch.

SAFETY ALERT!

norepinephrine bitartrate (levarterenol bitartrate, noradrenaline acid tartrate)
nor-ep-i-NEF-rin

Levophed

Therapeutic class: Vasopressors
Pharmacologic class: Direct-acting adrenergics
Pregnancy risk category: C

AVAILABLE FORMS
Injection: 1 mg/mL

INDICATIONS & DOSAGES
➤ **To restore blood pressure in acute hypotension; severe hypotension during cardiac arrest**
Adults: Initially, 8 to 12 mcg/minute by I.V. infusion; then titrate to maintain systolic blood pressure at 80 to 100 mm Hg in previously normotensive patients and 40 mm Hg below preexisting systolic blood pressure in previously hypertensive patients. Average maintenance dose is 2 to 4 mcg/minute.

N

ADMINISTRATION

I.V.

▼ Use a central venous catheter or large vein, such as the antecubital fossa, to minimize risk of extravasation. Give in D_5W alone or D_5W in normal saline solution for injection. Use continuous infusion pump to regulate infusion flow rate and a piggyback setup so I.V. line stays open if norepinephrine is stopped.

▼ Never leave patient unattended during infusion. Check blood pressure every 2 minutes until stabilized; then check every 5 minutes.

▼ During infusion, frequently monitor ECG, cardiac output, central venous pressure, pulmonary artery wedge pressure, pulse rate, urine output, and color and temperature of limbs. Titrate infusion rate based on findings and prescriber guidelines.

Black Box Warning Check site frequently for signs and symptoms of extravasation. If they appear, stop infusion immediately and call prescriber. To prevent sloughing and necrosis, use a fine hypodermic needle to infiltrate area with 5 to 10 mg phentolamine in 10 to 15 mL of normal saline solution. Also, check for blanching along course of infused vein, which may progress to superficial sloughing. ■

▼ Protect drug from light. Discard discolored solution or solution that contains precipitate. Solution will deteriorate after 24 hours.

▼ If prolonged therapy is needed, change injection site frequently.

▼ Avoid mixing with alkaline solutions, oxidizing drugs, or iron salts. The use of normal saline solution alone isn't recommended because of the lack of oxidation protection.

▼ **Incompatibilities:** Alkaline-buffered antibiotics, aminophylline, amobarbital, chlorothiazide, chlorpheniramine, insulin, lidocaine, pentobarbital sodium, phenobarbital sodium, phenytoin sodium, ranitidine hydrochloride, sodium bicarbonate, streptomycin, thiopental, whole blood.

ACTION

Stimulates alpha and $beta_1$ receptors in the sympathetic nervous system, causing vasoconstriction and cardiac stimulation.

Route	Onset	Peak	Duration
I.V.	Immediate	Immediate	1–2 min after infusion

Half-life: About 1 minute.

ADVERSE REACTIONS

CNS: headache, anxiety.
CV: *bradycardia, severe hypertension, arrhythmias.*
Respiratory: *asthma attacks,* respiratory difficulties.
Skin: irritation with extravasation, necrosis and gangrene secondary to extravasation.
Other: *anaphylaxis.*

INTERACTIONS

Drug-drug. *Alpha blockers:* May antagonize drug effects. Avoid using together.
Antihistamines, atropine, ergot alkaloids, guanethidine, MAO inhibitors, methyldopa, oxytocics: When given with sympathomimetics, may cause severe hypertension (hypertensive crisis). Avoid using together.
Inhaled anesthetics: May increase risk of arrhythmias. Monitor ECG.
TCAs: May potentiate the pressor response and cause arrhythmias. Use together cautiously.

EFFECTS ON LAB TEST RESULTS

None reported.

CONTRAINDICATIONS & CAUTIONS

● Contraindicated in patients with mesenteric or peripheral vascular thrombosis, profound hypoxia, hypercarbia, or hypotension resulting from blood volume deficit.
● Contraindicated during cyclopropane and halothane anesthesia.
● Use cautiously in patients taking MAO inhibitors, TCAs, or imipramine-type antidepressants.
● Use cautiously in patients with sulfite sensitivity.
⚠ *Overdose S&S:* Headache, severe hypertension, reflex bradycardia, increased peripheral resistance, decreased cardiac output.

Reactions in bold italics are *life-threatening*. Interactions may have a *rapid onset* or a *delayed onset*.

NURSING CONSIDERATIONS

• Drug isn't a substitute for blood or fluid replacement therapy. If patient has volume deficit, replace fluids before giving vasopressors.

• Keep emergency drugs on hand to reverse effects of drug: atropine for reflex bradycardia, phentolamine to decrease vasopressor effects, and propranolol for arrhythmias.

• Notify prescriber immediately of decreased urine output.

• When stopping drug, gradually slow infusion rate. Continue monitoring vital signs, watching for possible severe drop in blood pressure.

• *Look alike–sound alike:* Don't confuse norepinephrine with epinephrine.

PATIENT TEACHING

• Tell patient to report adverse reactions promptly.

• Advise patient to report discomfort at I.V. insertion site.

---

norethindrone

nor-ETH-in-drone

Camila, Errin, Heather, Jencycla, Micronor, Nor-QD

norethindrone acetate

Aygestin

Therapeutic class: Contraceptives
Pharmacologic class: Progestins
Pregnancy risk category: X

AVAILABLE FORMS

norethindrone
Tablets: 0.35 mg
norethindrone acetate
Tablets: 5 mg

INDICATIONS & DOSAGES

➤ **Amenorrhea, abnormal uterine bleeding**

Women: 2.5 to 10 mg norethindrone acetate P.O. daily for 5 to 10 days, beginning in the assumed latter half of the menstrual cycle.

➤ **Endometriosis**

Women: 5 mg norethindrone acetate P.O. daily for 14 days; then increased by 2.5 mg daily every 2 weeks, up to 15 mg daily.

Therapy may continue for 6 to 9 months or until breakthrough bleeding warrants temporary termination.

➤ **Contraception**

Women of childbearing age and menarchal girls: Initially, 0.35 mg norethindrone P.O. on first day of menstruation; then 0.35 mg daily.

ADMINISTRATION

P.O.

• Give drug at same time every day, continuously, with no interruption between pill packs.

• Give norethindrone acetate without regard to meals. May give with food if GI upset occurs.

ACTION

Suppresses ovulation, possibly by inhibiting pituitary gonadotropin secretion, and forms thick cervical mucus.

Route	Onset	Peak	Duration
P.O.	Unknown	Unknown	Unknown

Half-life: 5 to 14 hours.

ADVERSE REACTIONS

CNS: depression, *stroke,* headache, mood swings.
CV: thrombophlebitis, *pulmonary embolism,* edema, *thromboembolism.*
GI: bloating, abdominal pain or cramping.
GU: breakthrough bleeding, dysmenorrhea, amenorrhea, cervical erosion, abnormal secretions.
Hepatic: cholestatic jaundice.
Metabolic: weight changes.
Skin: melasma, rash, acne, pruritus, alopecia, hirsutism, hemorrhagic skin eruptions.
Other: breast tenderness, enlargement, or secretion; premenstrual-like syndrome, *anaphylactic reactions.*

INTERACTIONS

Drug-drug. *Barbiturates, carbamazepine, fosphenytoin, phenytoin, rifampin:* May decrease progestin effects. Monitor patient for diminished therapeutic response.
Drug-food. *Caffeine:* May increase caffeine level. Urge caution.

N

Drug-lifestyle. *Smoking:* May increase risk of adverse CV effects. If smoking continues, may need alternative therapy.

EFFECTS ON LAB TEST RESULTS
• May increase LFT values. May alter coagulation factors and thyroid function tests.
• May decrease metyrapone test results and HDL levels. May increase LDL/HDL ratio.

CONTRAINDICATIONS & CAUTIONS
• Contraindicated in pregnant women, patients hypersensitive to drug, and patients with breast cancer, undiagnosed abnormal vaginal bleeding, severe hepatic disease, missed abortion, or current or previous thromboembolic disorders.
• Use cautiously in patients with diabetes, seizures, migraines, cardiac or renal disease, asthma, and depression.
۞ Alert: Norethindrone acetate may cause papilledema or retinal vascular lesions. If these occur, discontinue drug.

NURSING CONSIDERATIONS
• If switching from combined oral contraceptives to progestin-only pills (POPs), take the first POP the day after the last active combined pill.
• If switching from POPs to combined pills, take the first active combined pill on the first day of menstruation, even if the POP pack isn't finished.
۞ Alert: Norethindrone acetate is twice as potent as norethindrone. Norethindrone acetate shouldn't be used for contraception.
• Patients with menstrual disorders usually need preliminary estrogen treatment.
• Watch patient closely for signs of edema.
• Monitor blood pressure.
• **Look alike–sound alike:** Don't confuse Micronor with Micro-K or Micronase.

PATIENT TEACHING
• According to FDA regulations, patient must read package insert explaining possible adverse effects before receiving first dose. Also, give patient verbal explanation.
• Tell patient to take drug at the same time every day when used as a contraceptive. If she's more than 3 hours late taking the pill

or if she has missed a pill, she should take the pill as soon as she remembers, and then continue the normal schedule. Also tell her to use a backup method of contraception for the next 48 hours.
۞ Alert: Tell patient to report unusual symptoms immediately and to stop drug and notify prescriber about visual disturbances or migraine, or pain or numbness in her arms or legs.
• Teach women how to perform routine breast self-examination.
• Tell women to report suspected pregnancy to prescriber.
• Encourage patient to stop or reduce smoking because of the risk of CV complications.
• Tell patient with diabetes that glucose levels may be affected and to closely monitor her levels.
• Advise patient to immediately report sudden partial or complete loss of vision, diplopia, migraine, or bulging of the eye.
• Tell patient that drug does not protect against HIV or other sexually transmitted diseases.
• Tell patient that if she vomits soon after taking a pill to use a back-up method of birth control for 48 hours.

nortriptyline hydrochloride
nor-TRIP-ti-leen

Aventyl, Pamelor๗*

Therapeutic class: Antidepressants
Pharmacologic class: Tricyclic antidepressants
Pregnancy risk category: D

AVAILABLE FORMS
Capsules: 10 mg, 25 mg, 50 mg, 75 mg
Oral solution: 10 mg/5 mL*

INDICATIONS & DOSAGES
➤ **Depression**
Adults: 25 mg P.O. t.i.d. or q.i.d., gradually increased to maximum of 150 mg daily. Give entire dose at bedtime. Monitor level when doses above 100 mg daily are given.
Adolescents and elderly patients: 30 to 50 mg P.O. daily given once or in divided doses.

Reactions in bold italics are ***life-threatening***. Interactions may have a *rapid onset* or a ***delayed onset***.

➤ **Postherpetic neuralgia** ◆
Adults: Mean dosage is between 58 and
89 mg P.O. for at least 5 weeks.
➤ **Irritable bowel syndrome** ◆
Adults: 10 to 50 mg/day P.O. as a maintenance dosage. Can be used as long-term
maintenance therapy for 3 or more months.

ADMINISTRATION
P.O.
- Give drug without regard for food.
- Whenever possible, give full dose at
bedtime.

ACTION
Unknown. Increases the amount of norepinephrine, serotonin, or both in the CNS
by blocking reuptake by the presynaptic
neurons.

Route	Onset	Peak	Duration
P.O.	Unknown	7–8½ hr	Unknown

Half-life: 18 to 24 hours.

ADVERSE REACTIONS
CNS: *stroke,* numbness, tingling, paresthesia of extremities, incoordination, ataxia,
tremors, peripheral neuropathy, extrapyramidal symptoms, *seizures,* alteration in
EEG, confusional states, anxiety, restlessness, agitation, insomnia, nightmares,
hypomania, exacerbation of psychosis,
drowsiness, dizziness, weakness, fatigue,
headache.
CV: edema, hypotension, hypertension,
tachycardia, palpitations, *MI,* arrhythmias,
heart block, flushing.
EENT: blurred vision, disturbance of accommodation, mydriasis, tinnitus.
GI: dry mouth, constipation, paralytic ileus,
nausea and vomiting, anorexia, epigastric
distress, diarrhea, peculiar taste, stomatitis,
abdominal cramps, black tongue.
GU: urine retention, delayed micturition, dilation of the urinary tract, erectile dysfunction, testicular swelling, urinary frequency,
nocturia.
Hematologic: bone marrow depression,
eosinophilia, purpura, *thrombocytopenia.*
Hepatic: jaundice, altered liver function.
Metabolic: weight gain or loss.
Skin: rash, petechiae, urticaria, itching,
photosensitivity, alopecia.

Other: drug fever, gynecomastia, breast
enlargement and galactorrhea in women,
increased or decreased libido, SIADH,
diaphoresis.

INTERACTIONS
Drug-drug. *Barbiturates, CNS depressants:*
May enhance CNS depression. Avoid using
together.
Cimetidine, **fluoxetine, fluvoxamine, paroxetine, sertraline:** May increase nortriptyline
level. Monitor drug levels and patient for
signs of toxicity.
Clonidine: May cause life-threatening hypertension. Avoid using together.
Drugs that prolong QT interval: May
increase risk of life-threatening cardiac
arrhythmias, including torsades de pointes.
Monitor patient and ECG.
Epinephrine, norepinephrine: May increase
hypertensive effect. Use together cautiously.
Linezolid, methylene blue: May cause serotonin syndrome. Use extreme caution and
monitor patient closely.
MAO inhibitors: May cause severe excitation, hyperpyrexia, or seizures, usually with
high doses. Avoid using within 14 days of
MAO inhibitor therapy.
Quinolones: May increase the risk of life-
threatening arrhythmias. Avoid using
together.
Drug-herb. *Evening primrose oil:* May
cause additive or synergistic effect, lowering
seizure threshold and increasing the risk of
seizure. Discourage use together.
St. John's wort, SAM-e, yohimbe: May cause
serotonin syndrome and reduced drug level.
Discourage use together.
Drug-lifestyle. *Alcohol use:* May enhance
CNS depression. Discourage use together.
Smoking: May decrease drug level. Monitor
patient for lack of effect.
Sun exposure: May increase risk of photosensitivity reactions. Advise patient to avoid
excessive sunlight exposure.

EFFECTS ON LAB TEST RESULTS
- May increase or decrease glucose level.
- May increase eosinophil count and LFT
values. May decrease WBC, RBC, granulocyte, and platelet counts.

N

CONTRAINDICATIONS & CAUTIONS
• Contraindicated in patients hypersensitive to drug and during acute recovery phase of MI; also contraindicated within 14 days of MAO inhibitor therapy.

Black Box Warning Nortriptyline isn't approved for use in children. ▮

☉ Alert: Concomitant use with linezolid or methylene blue can cause serotonin syndrome (fever, mental status changes, muscle twitching, excessive sweating, shivering or shaking, diarrhea, loss of coordination). Use drug with linezolid or methylene blue only for life-threatening or urgent conditions when the potential benefits outweigh the risks of toxicity.

• Use with extreme caution in patients with glaucoma, suicidal tendency, history of urine retention or seizures, CV disease, or hyperthyroidism and in those receiving thyroid drugs.

⚠ Overdose S&S: Cardiac arrhythmias, severe hypotension, shock, congestive heart failure, pulmonary edema, seizures, CNS depression, coma, ECG changes, confusion, restlessness, disturbed concentration, transient visual hallucinations, dilated pupils, agitation, hyperactive reflexes, stupor, drowsiness, muscle rigidity, vomiting, hypothermia, hyperpyrexia.

NURSING CONSIDERATIONS
☉ Alert: If linezolid or methylene blue must be given, stop nortriptyline and monitor patient for serotonin toxicity for 2 weeks or until 24 hours after the last dose of methylene blue or linezolid, whichever comes first. Treatment with nortriptyline may resume 24 hours after the last dose of methylene blue or linezolid.

• Monitor patient for nausea, headache, and malaise after abrupt withdrawal of long-term therapy; these symptoms don't indicate addiction.

• Because patients using TCAs may suffer hypertensive episodes during surgery, stop drug gradually several days before surgery.

• If signs or symptoms of psychosis occur or increase, expect to reduce dosage. Record mood changes. Monitor patient for suicidal tendencies and allow him only a minimum supply of drug.

Black Box Warning Drug may increase the risk of suicidal thinking and behavior in children, adolescents, and young adults with major depressive disorder or other psychiatric disorder. ▮

• **Look alike–sound alike:** Don't confuse nortriptyline with amitriptyline.

PATIENT TEACHING
Black Box Warning Advise families and caregivers to closely observe patient for increased suicidal thinking or behavior. ▮

• Teach patient to recognize and immediately report signs and symptoms of serotonin syndrome (fever, mental status changes, muscle twitching, excessive sweating, shivering or shaking, diarrhea, loss of coordination).

• Advise patient to take full dose at bedtime whenever possible to reduce risk of dizziness upon standing quickly.

• Warn patient to avoid activities that require alertness and good coordination until effects of drug are known. Drowsiness and dizziness usually subside after a few weeks.

• Recommend use of sugarless hard candy or gum to relieve dry mouth. Saliva substitutes may be needed.

• Tell patient to consult prescriber before taking other prescription or OTC drugs.

• Warn patient not to stop drug suddenly.

• To prevent oversensitivity to the sun, advise patient to use sunblock, wear protective clothing, and avoid prolonged exposure to strong sunlight.

---

nystatin
nye-STAT-in

Nystop

Therapeutic class: Antifungals
Pharmacologic class: Polyene macrolides
Pregnancy risk category: C

AVAILABLE FORMS
Ointment: 100,000 units/g
Oral suspension: 100,000 units/mL
Powder: 100,000 units/g
Powder (bulk): 50, 150, or 500 million units; 1, 2, or 5 billion units

---

Reactions in bold italics are *life-threatening*. Interactions may have a *rapid onset* or a *delayed onset*.

Tablets: 500,000 units
Vaginal tablets: 100,000 units

INDICATIONS & DOSAGES
➤ **Intestinal candidiasis**
Adults: 500,000 to 1 million units P.O. as
tablets t.i.d.
➤ **Mycotic infections**
Adults: Apply ointment liberally to affected
areas b.i.d. Or, apply powder to lesions b.i.d.
to t.i.d. until lesions have healed.
➤ **Oral candidiasis (thrush)**
Adults and children: 400,000 to 600,000
units P.O. as oral suspension q.i.d. for up to
14 days.
Infants: 200,000 units P.O. as oral suspen-
sion q.i.d.
Low-birth-weight and premature infants:
100,000 units P.O. oral suspension q.i.d.
➤ **Vaginal candidiasis**
Adults: 100,000 units, as vaginal tablets,
inserted high into vagina, daily at bedtime
for 14 days.

ADMINISTRATION
P.O.
● To treat oral candidiasis, after the patient's
mouth is clean of food debris, have him hold
suspension in mouth for several minutes
before swallowing. When treating infants,
swab medication on oral mucosa.
● Suspension made with bulk powder
contains no preservatives. Use immediately,
don't store.
● Prescriber may instruct immunosuppressed patient to suck on vaginal tablets
(100,000 units) because this provides
prolonged contact with oral mucosa.
Topical
● Store at room temperature.
Vaginal
● Vaginal tablets can be used by pregnant
patients up to 6 weeks before term to treat
maternal infection that may cause oral
candidiasis in neonates.

ACTION
Probably binds to sterols in fungal cell
membrane, altering cell permeability and
allowing leakage of intracellular components.

Route	Onset	Peak	Duration
P.O., vaginal	Unknown	Unknown	Unknown

Half-life: Unknown.

ADVERSE REACTIONS
GI: transient nausea, vomiting, diarrhea.
GU: irritation, sensitization, vulvovaginal
burning (vaginal form).
Skin: rash.

INTERACTIONS
None significant.

EFFECTS ON LAB TEST RESULTS
None reported.

CONTRAINDICATIONS & CAUTIONS
● Contraindicated in patients hypersensitive
to drug.
⚠ *Overdose S&S:* Nausea, GI upset.

NURSING CONSIDERATIONS
● Drug isn't effective against systemic
infections.

PATIENT TEACHING
● Advise patient to continue taking drug
for at least 2 days after signs and symptoms
disappear. Consult prescriber for exact
length of therapy.
● Instruct patient to continue therapy during
menstruation.
● Explain that factors predisposing
women to vaginal infection include use of
antibiotics, hormonal contraceptives, and
corticosteroids; diabetes; reinfection by
sexual partner; and tight-fitting pantyhose.
Encourage woman to wear cotton underwear.
● Instruct woman in careful hygiene for
affected areas, including cleaning perineal
area from front to back.
● Advise patient to report redness, swelling,
or irritation.
● Tell patient, especially an older patient, that overusing mouthwash or wearing poorly fitting dentures may promote
infection.
● For fungal foot infections, teach patient to
dust powder freely on the feet as well as in
shoes and socks.

N

octreotide acetate
ok-TREE-oh-tide

Sandostatin, Sandostatin LAR
Depot

Therapeutic class: Growth hormones
Pharmacologic class: Synthetic
octapeptides
Pregnancy risk category: B

AVAILABLE FORMS
Injection ampules: 50 mcg/mL, 100 mcg/
mL
Injection (single-dose vials): 50 mcg/mL,
100 mcg/mL
Injection (multidose vials): 200 mcg/mL,
500 mcg/mL, 1,000 mcg/mL
Injection for LAR (powder for suspension):
10 mg/5 mL, 20 mg/5 mL, 30 mg/5 mL

INDICATIONS & DOSAGES
➤ **Flushing and diarrhea from carcinoid
tumors**
Adults: 100 to 600 mcg subcutaneously or
I.V. daily in two to four divided doses for
first 2 weeks of therapy. Usual daily dosage
is 450 mcg. Base subsequent dosage on individual response. If Sandostatin LAR Depot is used, give 20 mg I.M. (intragluteally)
at 4-week intervals for 2 months. Patients
should continue to receive octreotide solution subcutaneously for 2 weeks at same
dosage they were taking before the switch.
After 2 months, adjust dosage based on
symptoms.
➤ **Watery diarrhea from vasoactive
intestinal polypeptide–secreting tumors
(VIPomas)**
Adults: 200 to 300 mcg subcutaneously or
I.V. daily in two to four divided doses for
first 2 weeks of therapy. Base subsequent
dosage on individual response, but usually
shouldn't exceed 450 mcg daily. If Sandostatin LAR Depot is used, give 20 mg
I.M. (intragluteally) at 4-week intervals for
2 months. Patients should continue to receive octreotide solution subcutaneously for
2 weeks at same dosage they were taking
before the switch. After 2 months, adjust
dosage based on symptoms.

➤ **Acromegaly**
Adults: Initially, 50 mcg subcutaneously or
I.V. t.i.d.; then adjust based on somatomedin
C levels every 2 weeks. Usual dosage is
100 mcg t.i.d. subcutaneously or I.V.;
some patients require up to 500 mcg t.i.d.
If Sandostatin LAR Depot is used, give
20 mg I.M. (intragluteally) at 4-week inter-
vals for 3 months; then adjust dosage based
on growth hormone and somatomedin C
levels and symptoms.
➤ **Dumping syndrome** ◆
Adults: 50 to 100 mcg subcutaneously daily
to t.i.d. before meals. Or, 10 to 20 mg LAR
depot I.M. monthly.
➤ **Chemotherapy-induced diarrhea** ◆
Adults: 0.1 to 0.5 mg subcutaneously
b.i.d. to t.i.d. Or, 0.15 to 2.4 mg I.V. in
24 hours.
➤ **Orthostatic hypotension** ◆
Adults: 25 to 50 mcg subcutaneously
30 minutes before a meal.
➤ **Pancreatic endocrine tumors** ◆
Adults: 25 to 50 mcg subcutaneously
30 minutes before a meal.

ADMINISTRATION
I.V.
▼ For other uses, dilute in 50 to 200 mL
D₅W or normal saline solution and infuse
over 15 to 30 minutes.
▼ Solution is stable for 24 hours.
▼ **Incompatibilities:** Total parenteral
nutrition.
I.M.
● Don't use if particulates or discoloration
are observed.
● Follow the mixing instructions included
in the packaging and give immediately after
mixing.
● Rotate injection sites.
● Avoid deltoid muscle injections. May
cause significant discomfort.
🛈 *Alert:* Never give the injectable suspen-
sion by I.V. or subcutaneous routes.
Subcutaneous
● Don't use if particulates or discoloration
are observed.

ACTION
Mimics action of naturally occurring
somatostatin.

Route	Onset	Peak	Duration
I.V.	Rapid	30 min	<12 hr
I.M.	Unknown	2–3 wk	Unknown
Subcut.	30 min	30 min	<12 hr

Half-life: About 1½ hours; long-acting, unknown.

ADVERSE REACTIONS

CNS: dizziness, fatigue, headache, light-headedness, depression, weakness.
CV: *arrhythmias, bradycardia,* conduction abnormalities, edema.
EENT: blurred vision.
GI: abdominal pain or discomfort, diarrhea, gallbladder abnormalities, loose stools, nausea, *pancreatitis,* constipation, fat malabsorption, flatulence, vomiting.
GU: urinary frequency, UTI.
Metabolic: *hypoglycemia,* hyperglycemia, hypothyroidism, suppressed secretion of growth hormone and gastroenterohepatic peptides (gastrin, VIP, insulin, glucagon, secretin, motilin, and pancreatic polypeptide).
Musculoskeletal: backache, joint pain.
Skin: alopecia, erythema or pain at injection site, flushing, wheal, bruising, hair loss.
Other: cold symptoms, flulike symptoms, pain or burning at subcutaneous injection site.

INTERACTIONS

Drug-drug. *Beta blockers (such as propranolol):* May have additive effect and further lower heart rate. Decrease beta blocker dosage as needed.
Bromocriptine: May decrease bromocriptine availability. Monitor patient for effectiveness.
Cyclosporine: May decrease cyclosporine level. Monitor patient closely.
CYP3A4-metabolized drugs (such as quinidine, terfenadine): May decrease excretion of these drugs. Use with caution and reduce dosage as needed.
Drugs that prolong QT interval: May increase risk of life-threatening cardiac arrhythmias, including torsades de pointes. Monitor patient and ECG.
Insulin, oral antidiabetics: May have decreased effectiveness from octreotide. Monitor patient and adjust dosage of antidiabetics as needed.

EFFECTS ON LAB TEST RESULTS
• May decrease vitamin B_{12} level. May increase or decrease glucose level.
• May alter LFT values.

CONTRAINDICATIONS & CAUTIONS
• Contraindicated in patients hypersensitive to drug or its components.
• Use cautiously in elderly patients, who may be more sensitive to drug.
⚠ **Overdose S&S:** Hypoglycemia, flushing, dizziness, nausea.

NURSING CONSIDERATIONS
• Monitor baseline thyroid function tests.
• Monitor somatomedin C levels every 2 weeks. Dosage adjustments are based on this level.
• Periodically monitor laboratory tests, such as thyroid function, glucose, urine 5-hydroxyindoleacetic acid, plasma serotonin, and plasma substance P (for carcinoid tumors).
• Monitor patient regularly for gallbladder disease. Therapy may be related to the development of cholelithiasis because of its effect on gallbladder motility or fat absorption.
• Monitor patient closely for signs and symptoms of glucose imbalance. Patients with type 1 diabetes mellitus and those receiving oral antidiabetics or oral diazoxide may need dosage adjustments during therapy. Monitor glucose level.
• Drug may alter fluid and electrolyte balance; other therapies may need adjusting.
• Half-life may be altered in patients with ESRD who are receiving dialysis.
• *Look alike–sound alike:* To avoid giving drug by the wrong route, don't confuse octreotide acetate injection with injectable depot suspension product.
• *Look alike–sound alike:* Don't confuse Sandostatin with Sandimmune or Sandoglobulin.

PATIENT TEACHING
• Urge patient to report signs and symptoms of abdominal discomfort immediately.
• Stress importance of the need for periodic laboratory testing during octreotide therapy.
• Advise patient that drug may restore fertility in some women with acromegaly

and that she should use effective birth control if pregnancy isn't desired.

● Tell patient that drug may cause dizziness, drowsiness, or vision changes and that these symptoms may increase with alcohol use or certain other medications. Advise patient not to drive or perform hazardous tasks until drug's effects are known.

● Warn diabetic patient to monitor blood glucose level closely and to discuss results with prescriber before making dosage changes.

SAFETY ALERT!

ofatumumab
oh-fuh-TOO-moo-mab

Arzerra

Therapeutic class: Antineoplastics
Pharmacologic class: Monoclonal antibodies
Pregnancy risk category: C

AVAILABLE FORMS
Injection: 100 mg/5-mL single-use vials

INDICATIONS & DOSAGES
➤ **Chronic lymphocytic leukemia (CLL) refractory to fludarabine and alemtuzumab**
Adults: Initially, 300 mg I.V. infusion (dose 1), followed 1 week later by 2,000 mg I.V. weekly for 7 weeks (doses 2 through 8); then 4 weeks later give 2,000 mg I.V. weekly for 4 weeks (doses 9 through 12). Give acetaminophen 1,000 mg, an oral or I.V. antihistamine (cetirizine 10 mg or equivalent), and an I.V. corticosteroid (prednisolone 100 mg or equivalent) 30 minutes to 2 hours before treatment. May reduce corticosteroid dosage for doses 3 through 8 if a grade 3 or greater infusion reaction didn't occur with preceding dose. For doses 10 through 12, give prednisolone 50 to 100 mg or equivalent if a grade 3 or greater infusion reaction didn't occur with dose 9.
Adjust-a-dose: For grade 1, 2, or 3 infusion reaction, interrupt infusion. If reaction resolves or remains grade 2 or less, infuse at half the previous infusion rate; if grade 3, infuse at 12 mL/hour. If tolerated, may

increase infusion rate after resuming infusion. For grade 4 infusion reaction, discontinue therapy.

ADMINISTRATION
I.V.
▼ To prepare 300-mg dose, withdraw and discard 15 mL from 1,000-mL bag of normal saline solution. Withdraw 5 mL of drug from each of three vials and add to normal saline solution. Gently invert bag to mix solution.
▼ To prepare 2,000-mg dose, withdraw and discard 100 mL from 1,000-mL bag of normal saline solution. Withdraw 5 mL of drug from each of 20 vials and add to normal saline solution. Gently invert bag to mix solution.
▼ Inspect solution; discard if discolored or cloudy, or if particulate matter is present.
▼ Administer using infusion pump, in-line filter provided by manufacturer, and administration set containing polyvinyl chloride.
▼ Flush I.V. line with normal saline solution before and after each dose.
▼ Begin infusion within 12 hours of preparation; discard prepared solution after 24 hours.
▼ Begin dose 1 at 3.6 mg/hour (12 mL/hour) and dose 2 at 24 mg/hour (12 mL/hour) for 30 minutes; then, if no signs of toxicity, increase dose every 30 minutes to 25 mL/hour, 50 mL/hour, 100 mL/hour, and 200 mL/hour, respectively. For doses 3 through 12, begin infusion at 50 mg/hour (25 mL/hour). If no signs of toxicity, increase dose every 30 minutes to 50 mL/hour, 100 mL/hour, 200 mL/hour, and 400 mL/hour, respectively.
▼ **Incompatibilities:** Other I.V. medications.

ACTION
Binds to normal and CLL B lymphocytes, causing cell lysis.

Route	Onset	Peak	Duration
I.V.	Unknown	Unknown	Unknown

Half-life: 14 days.

Reactions in bold italics are *life-threatening*. Interactions may have a *rapid onset* or a *delayed onset*.

ADVERSE REACTIONS

CNS: fatigue, fever, headache, insomnia.
CV: hypertension, hypotension, peripheral edema, tachycardia.
EENT: nasopharyngitis, sinusitis.
GI: diarrhea, nausea.
Hematologic: anemia, *neutropenia, thrombocytopenia.*
Hepatic: *hepatitis B reactivation.*
Musculoskeletal: back pain, muscle spasm.
Respiratory: bronchitis, cough, dyspnea, pneumonia, upper respiratory tract infection.
Skin: hyperhidrosis, rash, urticaria.
Other: chills, herpes zoster infection, infusion reactions, *sepsis.*

INTERACTIONS

None reported.

EFFECTS ON LAB TEST RESULTS

• May decrease neutrophil and platelet counts.

CONTRAINDICATIONS & CAUTIONS

Black Box Warning HBV reactivation (including fulminant hepatitis), hepatic failure, and death may occur in patients treated with ofatumumab. ∎

☙ Alert: Screen all patients for HBV infection before treatment by measuring hepatitis B surface antigen (HBsAg) and hepatitis B core antibody (anti-HBc). Monitor patients with evidence of current or prior HBV infection during and for several months after therapy. In event of HBV reactivation, discontinue ofatumumab and concomitant chemotherapy and begin appropriate treatment.

☙ Alert: Consult hepatitis expert when screening identifies patients at risk for HBV reactivation due to prior HBV infection.

• Use cautiously in patients with history of COPD, serious infusion reaction, neutropenia, or thrombocytopenia.

• Live-virus vaccines are contraindicated during and following treatment.

• Use in pregnancy only if benefit outweighs risk to fetus.

• It isn't known if drug appears in breast milk. Because of the risk of adverse effects, women shouldn't breast-feed while taking drug.

• Safety and effectiveness in children haven't been established.

NURSING CONSIDERATIONS

☙ Alert: Don't administer live-virus vaccines during or after treatment.

• Drug has been associated with small-intestine obstruction; perform a diagnostic evaluation if suspected.

☙ Alert: Monitor neurologic status closely for signs and symptoms of progressive multifocal leukoencephalopathy, a potentially fatal condition. Discontinue drug and consult neurologist if condition is suspected.

☙ Alert: Drug may cause serious infusion reactions (bronchospasm, dyspnea, laryngeal edema, pulmonary edema, flushing, hypertension, hypotension, syncope, cardiac ischemia, MI, back pain, abdominal pain, fever, rash, urticaria, and angioedema); monitor patient closely. Discontinue infusion and institute symptomatic treatment if reactions occur.

• Screen patients at high risk for hepatitis B infection before starting drug. Monitor patients with history of hepatitis B for signs and symptoms of active infection. Discontinue drug and administer appropriate treatment if active infection is suspected.

• Monitor CBC regularly during therapy; increase frequency of monitoring if grade 3 or 4 cytopenias develop.

PATIENT TEACHING

• Instruct patient to watch for signs and symptoms of infection (fever, sore throat, fatigue) and bleeding (easy bruising, pallor, petechiae, nosebleeds, bleeding gums, worsening weakness, tarry stools) and to report them to prescriber.

• Teach the patient to take his temperature daily and to report any elevation to prescriber.

• Advise patient to report signs and symptoms of infusion reactions, including fever, chills, rash, or breathing problems within 24 hours of infusion.

• Tell patient to report signs and symptoms of hepatitis, including worsening fatigue and yellowing of skin or eyes.

• Advise patient to report new or worsening abdominal pain or nausea or new neurologic symptoms, such as dizziness, confusion, loss of balance, difficulty talking or walking, and vision problems.

• Warn patient to avoid live-virus vaccines during and after treatment.

• Inform patient that periodic blood testing will be necessary during therapy.

• Caution woman of childbearing age to avoid becoming pregnant and to use effective contraception during therapy. Advise her to consult prescriber before becoming pregnant.

ofloxacin (ophthalmic)
oh-FLOX-a-sin

Ocuflox

ofloxacin (otic)
Floxin Otic

Therapeutic class: Antibiotics
Pharmacologic class: Fluoroquinolones
Pregnancy risk category: C

AVAILABLE FORMS
Ophthalmic solution: 0.3%
Otic solution: 0.3%

INDICATIONS & DOSAGES
➤ **Conjunctivitis caused by** *Staphylococcus aureus, Staphylococcus epidermidis, Streptococcus pneumoniae, Enterobacter cloacae, Haemophilus influenzae, Proteus mirabilis,* **and** *Pseudomonas aeruginosa*
Adults and children older than age 1: Give 1 or 2 drops in conjunctival sac every 2 to 4 hours daily while patient is awake, for first 2 days; then q.i.d. for up to 5 additional days.
➤ **Bacterial corneal ulcer caused by** *S. aureus, S. epidermidis, S. pneumoniae, P. aeruginosa, Serratia marcescens,* **and** *Propionibacterium acnes*
Adults and children older than age 1: Give 1 or 2 drops every 30 minutes while patient is awake and 1 or 2 drops 4 and 6 hours after patient goes to bed on days 1 and 2. On day 3, 1 or 2 drops hourly while patient is awake; continue for 4 to 6 days. Then, 1 or 2 drops q.i.d. for an additional 3 days or until cured.

➤ **Chronic suppurative otitis media with perforated tympanic membrane**
Adults and children age 12 and older: 10 drops instilled into the affected ear b.i.d. for 14 days.
➤ **Otitis externa**
Adults and children age 13 and older: 10 drops instilled into the affected ear once daily for 7 days.
Children ages 6 months to 13 years: 5 drops into the affected ear once daily for 7 days.
➤ **Acute otitis media in children with tympanostomy tubes**
Children ages 1 to 12: 5 drops instilled into the affected ear b.i.d. for 10 days.

ADMINISTRATION
Ophthalmic
• Apply light finger pressure on lacrimal sac for 1 minute after drug instillation.
Otic
• Before instilling drops, warm the bottle by holding it in the hand for 1 to 2 minutes.
• Have patient lie with the affected ear upward, instill the drops, and have patient maintain this position for 5 minutes.

ACTION
Inhibits bacterial DNA gyrase, an enzyme needed for bacterial replication.

Route	Onset	Peak	Duration
Ophthalmic, otic	Unknown	Unknown	Unknown

Half-life: 4 to 8 hours.

ADVERSE REACTIONS
CNS: dizziness, vertigo.
EENT: transient ocular burning or discomfort, chemical conjunctivitis or keratitis, eye dryness, eye pain, itching, lacrimation, periocular or facial edema, photophobia, eye redness, stinging, earache, taste perversion.
Skin: rash.

INTERACTIONS
None significant.

EFFECTS ON LAB TEST RESULTS
None reported.

Reactions in bold italics are *life-threatening*. Interactions may have a *rapid onset* or a *delayed onset*.

CONTRAINDICATIONS & CAUTIONS

• Contraindicated in patients hypersensitive to drug or other fluoroquinolones and in breast-feeding women.

NURSING CONSIDERATIONS

• Stop drug if improvement doesn't occur within 7 days, and obtain cultures. Prolonged use may result in overgrowth of nonsusceptible organisms, including fungi.
• Ophthalmic solution isn't for injection into conjunctiva or anterior chamber of the eye.
• Otic solution isn't for ophthalmic use or injection.
• *Look alike–sound alike:* Don't confuse Ocuflox with Ocufen.

PATIENT TEACHING

• If an allergic reaction occurs, tell patient to stop drug and notify prescriber. Serious acute hypersensitivity reactions may need emergency treatment.
• Tell patient to clean excessive discharge from eye area before application.
• Teach patient how to instill drops. Advise him to wash hands before and after instilling solution, and warn him not to touch tip of ophthalmic dropper to eye or surrounding tissue.
• Advise patient to apply light finger pressure on lacrimal sac for 1 minute after drug instillation.
• Tell patient not to share drug, washcloths, or towels with family members and to notify prescriber if anyone develops same signs or symptoms.
• Stress importance of compliance with recommended therapy.
• Warn patient not to use leftover drug for new eye infection.
• Remind patient to discard drug when it's no longer needed.
• Warn patient not to touch the otic applicator.
• Teach patient to warm the bottle in his hand for 1 to 2 minutes to avoid dizziness from instilling cold eardrops, then to lie with the affected ear upward for instillation of the drops. This position should be maintained for 5 minutes.

ofloxacin (oral)
oh-FLOX-a-sin

Therapeutic class: Antibiotics
Pharmacologic class: Fluoroquinolones
Pregnancy risk category: C

AVAILABLE FORMS
Tablets: 200 mg, 300 mg, 400 mg

INDICATIONS & DOSAGES
Adjust-a-dose (for all indications): For patients with CrCl of 20 to 50 mL/minute, give first dose as recommended; then give usual maintenance dose every 24 hours. For patients with CrCl less than 20 mL/minute, give first dose as recommended; then give subsequent doses at 50% of recommended dose every 24 hours. For patients with hepatic impairment, don't exceed 400 mg/day.
➤ **Acute bacterial worsening of chronic bronchitis, uncomplicated skin and skin-structure infections, and community-acquired pneumonia**
Adults: 400 mg P.O. every 12 hours for 10 days.
➤ **Cystitis from *Escherichia coli*, *Klebsiella pneumoniae*, or other organisms**
Adults: 200 mg P.O. every 12 hours for 3 days (*E. coli* or *K. pneumoniae*) or 200 mg P.O. every 12 hours for 7 days (other organisms).
➤ **Complicated UTI**
Adults: 200 mg P.O. every 12 hours for 10 days.
➤ **Prostatitis from *E. coli***
Adults: 300 mg P.O. every 12 hours for 6 weeks.
➤ **Pelvic inflammatory disease**
Adults: 400 mg P.O. every 12 hours with metronidazole for 10 to 14 days.
➤ **Moderate to severe traveler's diarrhea ◆**
Adults: 200 mg P.O. b.i.d. for 3 days.
➤ **Epididymitis ◆**
Adults: 300 mg P.O. b.i.d. for 10 days.

O

ADMINISTRATION
P.O.
● Give drug without regard for meals but not at the same time as antacids and vitamins.
● Give drug with plenty of fluids.

ACTION
Interferes with DNA gyrase, which is needed for synthesis of bacterial DNA. Spectrum of action includes many gram-positive and gram-negative aerobic bacteria, including *Enterobacteriaceae* and *Pseudomonas aeruginosa.*

Route	Onset	Peak	Duration
P.O.	Unknown	15–120 min	Unknown

Half-life: 4 to 7½ hours.

ADVERSE REACTIONS
CNS: *seizures, increased intracranial pressure,* dizziness, drowsiness, fatigue, fever, headache, insomnia, lethargy, malaise, nervousness, sleep disorders, visual disturbances.
CV: chest pain, phlebitis.
GI: nausea, *pseudomembranous colitis,* abdominal pain or discomfort, anorexia, constipation, diarrhea, dry mouth, dysgeusia, flatulence, vomiting.
GU: external genital pruritus in women, glycosuria, hematuria, proteinuria, vaginal discharge, vaginitis.
Hematologic: *leukopenia, neutropenia,* anemia, eosinophilia, leukocytosis.
Metabolic: *hypoglycemia,* hyperglycemia.
Musculoskeletal: body pain, tendon rupture.
Skin: photosensitivity, pruritus, rash.
Other: *anaphylactoid reaction,* hypersensitivity reactions.

INTERACTIONS
Drug-drug. *Aluminum hydroxide, aluminum–magnesium hydroxide, calcium carbonate, magnesium hydroxide:* May decrease effects of ofloxacin. Give antacid at least 2 hours before or 2 hours after ofloxacin.
Antidiabetics: May affect glucose level, causing hypoglycemia or hyperglycemia. Monitor patient closely.
Didanosine (chewable or buffered tablets or pediatric powder for oral solution): May

interfere with GI absorption of ofloxacin. Separate doses by 2 hours.
Iron salts: May decrease absorption of ofloxacin, reducing anti-infective response. Separate doses by at least 2 hours.
Black Box Warning *Steroids:* May increase risk of tendinitis and tendon rupture. Monitor patient for tendon pain or inflammation. ■
Sucralfate: May decrease absorption of ofloxacin, reducing anti-infective response. If use together can't be avoided, separate doses by at least 6 hours.
Theophylline: May increase theophylline level. Monitor patient closely and adjust theophylline dosage as needed.
Warfarin: May prolong PT and INR. Monitor PT and INR.
Drug-lifestyle. *Sun exposure:* May cause photosensitivity reactions. Advise patient to avoid excessive sunlight exposure.

EFFECTS ON LAB TEST RESULTS
● May increase BUN, creatinine, and liver enzyme levels. May decrease hemoglobin level and hematocrit. May increase or decrease glucose level.
● May increase erythrocyte sedimentation rate and eosinophil count. May decrease neutrophil count. May increase or decrease WBC count.

CONTRAINDICATIONS & CAUTIONS
Black Box Warning Drug is associated with increased risk of tendinitis and tendon rupture, especially in patients older than age 60 and those with heart, kidney, or lung transplants. ■
Black Box Warning Drug may exacerbate muscle weakness in patients with myasthenia gravis. Avoid use in patients with a known history of myasthenia gravis. ■
۞ Alert: Oral or parenteral fluoroquinolones may increase the risk of peripheral neuropathy of the arms or legs. Symptoms can occur at any time during treatment and can last for months or years or be permanent. Stop drug immediately if patient develops symptoms, and switch to a non-fluoroquinolone antibacterial drug unless the benefit of continued treatment outweighs the risk.
● Contraindicated in patients hypersensitive to drug or other fluoroquinolones.

Reactions in bold italics are *life-threatening*. Interactions may have a *rapid onset* or a *delayed onset.*

• Use cautiously in pregnant patients and in those with seizure disorders, CNS diseases such as cerebral arteriosclerosis, hepatic disorders, or renal impairment.

• Ofloxacin appears in breast milk in levels similar to those found in plasma. Safety hasn't been established in breast-feeding or pregnant women.

• Safety and effectiveness in children younger than age 18 haven't been established.

⚠ **Overdose S&S:** Nausea, vomiting, seizures, vertigo, dysgeusia, psychosis, dizziness, drowsiness, hot and cold flushes, facial swelling and numbness, slurred speech, mild to moderate disorientation.

NURSING CONSIDERATIONS

Black Box Warning Rupture of tendons is linked to fluoroquinolone use. If pain, inflammation, or tendon rupture occurs, stop drug and notify prescriber. ▪

❸ Alert: Monitor the patient for symptoms of peripheral neuropathy (pain, burning, tingling, numbness, weakness, or a change in sensation to light touch, pain or temperature, or the sense of body position) and report them immediately to the health care provider.

❸ Alert: Patients treated for gonorrhea should be tested for syphilis. Drug isn't effective against syphilis, and treating gonorrhea may mask or delay syphilis symptoms.

• Periodically assess organ system functions during prolonged therapy.

• Monitor patient for overgrowth of nonsusceptible organisms.

• Monitor renal and hepatic studies and CBC in prolonged therapy.

• Monitor blood sugar closely.

• Monitor patient for adverse CNS effects, including dizziness, headache, seizures, or depression. Stop drug and notify prescriber if these effects occur.

• Monitor patient for hypersensitivity reactions. Stop drug and initiate supportive therapy, as indicated.

PATIENT TEACHING

• Tell patient to drink plenty of fluids during drug therapy and to finish the entire prescription, even if he starts feeling better.

• Tell patient drug may be taken without regard to meals, but he shouldn't take antacids and vitamins at the same time as ofloxacin.

❸ Alert: Warn patient to contact his health care provider immediately if symptoms of peripheral neuropathy occur.

• Warn patient that dizziness and lightheadedness may occur. Advise caution when driving or operating hazardous machinery until effects of drug are known.

• Warn patient that hypersensitivity reactions may follow first dose; he should stop drug at first sign of rash or other allergic reaction and call prescriber immediately.

• Advise patient to avoid prolonged exposure to direct sunlight and to use a sunscreen when outdoors.

---

olanzapine
oh-LAN-za-peen

Zyprexa✓, Zyprexa Zydis

olanzapine pamoate
Zyprexa Relprevv

Therapeutic class: Antipsychotics
Pharmacologic class: Dibenzapine derivatives
Pregnancy risk category: C

AVAILABLE FORMS
Injection: 10 mg
Injection (extended-release): 210-mg base/vial, 300-mg base/vial, 405-mg base/vial
Tablets: 2.5 mg, 5 mg, 7.5 mg, 10 mg, 15 mg, 20 mg
Tablets (orally disintegrating): 5 mg, 10 mg, 15 mg, 20 mg

INDICATIONS & DOSAGES
➤ **Schizophrenia**
Adults: Initially, 5 to 10 mg P.O. once daily with the goal to be at 10 mg daily within several days of starting therapy. Adjust dose in 5-mg increments at intervals of 1 week or more. Most patients respond to 10 to 15 mg daily. Safety of dosages greater than 20 mg daily hasn't been established. Or, 150 to 300 mg (extended-release) I.M. every 2 weeks or 405 mg (extended-release) I.M. every 4 weeks.

Children age 13 and older: 2.5 or 5 mg P.O. once daily. Adjust dose as needed in increments of 2.5 or 5 mg. Maintenance dose is 10 mg/day.

➤ **Short-term treatment of acute manic episodes linked to bipolar I disorder**
Adults: Initially, 10 to 15 mg P.O. daily. Adjust dosage as needed in 5-mg daily increments at intervals of 24 hours or more. Maximum, 20 mg P.O. daily. Duration of treatment is 3 to 4 weeks.
Children age 13 and older: 2.5 or 5 mg P.O. once daily. Adjust dose as needed in increments of 2.5 or 5 mg. Maintenance dose is 10 mg/day.

➤ **Short-term treatment, with lithium or valproate, of acute mixed or manic episodes linked to bipolar I disorder**
Adults: 10 mg P.O. once daily. Dosage range is 5 to 20 mg daily. Duration of treatment is 6 weeks.

➤ **Long-term treatment of bipolar I disorder**
Adults: 5 to 20 mg P.O. daily.
Adjust-a-dose: In elderly or debilitated patients, those predisposed to hypotensive reactions, patients who may metabolize olanzapine more slowly than usual (non-smoking women older than age 65) or may be more pharmacodynamically sensitive to olanzapine, initially, 5 mg P.O. Increase dose cautiously.

➤ **Agitation caused by schizophrenia and bipolar I mania**
Adults: 10 mg I.M. (short-acting) (range 2.5 to 10 mg). Subsequent doses of up to 10 mg may be given 2 hours after the first dose or 4 hours after the second dose, up to 30 mg I.M. daily. If maintenance therapy is required, convert patient to 5 to 20 mg P.O. daily.
Adjust-a-dose: In elderly patients, give 5 mg I.M. In debilitated patients, in those predisposed to hypotension, and in patients sensitive to effects of drug, give 2.5 mg I.M.

➤ **Depressive episodes associated with bipolar I disorder**
Adults: 5 mg P.O. with fluoxetine 20 mg P.O. once daily in the evening. Dosage adjustments can be made based on efficacy and tolerability within ranges of olanzapine 5 to 12.5 mg and fluoxetine 20 to 50 mg.

➤ **Treatment-resistant depression**
Adults: 5 mg P.O. with 20 mg fluoxetine P.O. once daily in the evening. Dosage adjustments can be made based on efficacy and tolerability within ranges of olanzapine 5 to 20 mg and fluoxetine 20 to 50 mg.

➤ **Obsessive-compulsive disorder ♦**
Adults: 5 mg P.O. daily. Increase based on therapeutic effect and tolerance. Once therapeutic management has been achieved, continue for 1 to 2 years before tapering is attempted.

➤ **Tourette syndrome ♦**
Adults: 5 mg P.O. daily titrated to a maximum of 20 mg daily for 6 to 8 weeks.

ADMINISTRATION
P.O.
● Give drug without regard for food.
● Don't crush or break orally disintegrating tablet (ODT).
● Place ODT on patient's tongue immediately after opening package.
● ODT may be given without water.
I.M.
● Inspect I.M. solution for particulate matter and discoloration before administration.
● To reconstitute I.M. injection, dissolve contents of one vial with 2.1 mL of sterile water for injection to yield a clear yellow 5 mg/mL solution. Store at room temperature and give within 1 hour of reconstitution. Discard any unused solution.
● Olanzapine extended-release formula is intended for deep gluteal I.M. injection only.

ACTION
May block dopamine and 5-HT$_2$ receptors.

Route	Onset	Peak	Duration
P.O.	Unknown	6 hr	Unknown
I.M.	Rapid	15–45 min	Unknown
I.M. (extended-release)	Unknown	6 hr	Months

Half-life: 21 to 54 hours; extended release, 30 days.

ADVERSE REACTIONS
CNS: somnolence, insomnia, parkinsonism, dizziness, ***neuroleptic malignant syndrome, suicide attempt,*** abnormal gait, asthenia, personality disorder, akathisia, tremor,

---

Reactions in bold italics are *life-threatening*. Interactions may have a *rapid onset* or a *delayed onset*.

articulation impairment, tardive dyskinesia, fever, extrapyramidal events (I.M.).
CV: orthostatic hypotension, tachycardia, chest pain, hypertension, ecchymosis, peripheral edema, hypotension (I.M.).
EENT: amblyopia, rhinitis, pharyngitis, conjunctivitis.
GI: constipation, dry mouth, dyspepsia, increased appetite, increased salivation, vomiting, thirst.
GU: hematuria, metrorrhagia, urinary incontinence, UTI, amenorrhea, vaginitis.
Hematologic: *leukopenia.*
Metabolic: hyperglycemia, weight gain.
Musculoskeletal: joint pain, extremity pain, back pain, neck rigidity, twitching, hypertonia.
Respiratory: increased cough, dyspnea.
Skin: sweating, injection-site pain (I.M.).
Other: flulike syndrome, injury.

INTERACTIONS
Drug-drug. *Antihypertensives:* May potentiate hypotensive effects. Monitor blood pressure closely.
Carbamazepine, omeprazole, rifampin: May increase clearance of olanzapine. Monitor patient.
Ciprofloxacin: May increase olanzapine level. Monitor patient for increased adverse effects.
Diazepam: May increase CNS effects. Monitor patient.
Dopamine agonists, levodopa: May antagonize activity of these drugs. Monitor patient.
Fluoxetine: May increase olanzapine level. Use together cautiously.
Fluvoxamine: May increase olanzapine level. May need to reduce olanzapine dose.
Drug-herb. *St. John's wort:* May decrease drug level. Discourage use together.
Drug-lifestyle. *Alcohol use:* May increase CNS effects. Discourage use together.
Smoking: May increase drug clearance. Urge patient to quit smoking.

EFFECTS ON LAB TEST RESULTS
• May increase AST, ALT, GGT, CK, triglyceride, and prolactin levels.
• May increase eosinophil count. May decrease WBC count.

CONTRAINDICATIONS & CAUTIONS
• Contraindicated in patients hypersensitive to drug.
Black Box Warning Sedation (including coma) or delirium have been reported following injections of olanzapine extended-release formula. This drug must be administered in a registered health care facility with ready access to emergency response services. After each injection, patient must be observed at the health care facility by a health care provider for at least 3 hours. Olanzapine extended-release is available only through the restricted Zyprexa Relprevv Patient Care Program (1-877-772-9390). ■
• Use cautiously in patients with heart disease, cerebrovascular disease, conditions that predispose patient to hypotension, history of seizures or conditions that might lower the seizure threshold, and hepatic impairment.
• Use cautiously in elderly patients, those with a history of paralytic ileus, and those at risk for aspiration pneumonia, prostatic hyperplasia, or angle-closure glaucoma.
❧ Alert: Neonates exposed to antipsychotics during the third trimester of pregnancy are at risk for developing extrapyramidal signs and symptoms (repetitive muscle movements of the face and body) and withdrawal signs and symptoms (agitation, abnormally increased or decreased muscle tone, tremors, sleepiness, severe difficulty breathing, difficulty feeding) following delivery. Use in pregnancy only if the potential benefit to the mother justifies the risk to the fetus.
⚠ Overdose S&S: Agitation, aggressiveness, dysarthria, tachycardia, extrapyramidal symptoms, reduced level of consciousness, aspiration, cardiopulmonary arrest, cardiac arrhythmias, delirium, neuroleptic malignant syndrome, respiratory depression or arrest, seizures, hypertension, hypotension.

NURSING CONSIDERATIONS
• ODTs contain phenylalanine.
• Monitor patient for abnormal body temperature regulation, especially if he exercises, is exposed to extreme heat, takes anticholinergics, or is dehydrated.

● Obtain baseline and periodic LFT results.

● Monitor patient for weight gain.

❸ **Alert:** Watch for evidence of neuroleptic malignant syndrome (hyperpyrexia, muscle rigidity, altered mental status, autonomic instability), which is rare but commonly fatal. Stop drug immediately; monitor and treat patient as needed.

❸ **Alert:** Drug may cause hyperglycemia. Monitor patients with diabetes regularly. In patients with risk factors for diabetes, obtain fasting blood glucose test results at baseline and periodically.

❸ **Alert:** Monitor patient for symptoms of metabolic syndrome (significant weight gain and increased body mass index, hypertension, hyperglycemia, hypercholesterolemia, and hypertriglyceridemia).

● Monitor patient for mental status changes, sedation, coma, or delirium.

● Monitor patient for tardive dyskinesia, which may occur after prolonged use. It may not appear until months or years later and may disappear spontaneously or persist for life, despite stopping drug.

● Periodically reevaluate the long-term usefulness of olanzapine.

Black Box Warning Drug may increase risk of CV or infection-related death in elderly patients with dementia. Olanzapine isn't approved to treat patients with dementia-related psychosis. ∎

● A patient who feels dizzy or drowsy after an I.M. injection should remain recumbent until he can be assessed for orthostatic hypotension and bradycardia. He should rest until the feeling passes.

❸ **Alert:** Drug may increase the risk of suicidal thinking and behavior in young adults ages 18 to 24 during the first 2 months of treatment.

● **Look alike–sound alike:** Don't confuse olanzapine with olsalazine. Don't confuse Zyprexa with Zyrtec.

PATIENT TEACHING

● Warn patient to avoid hazardous tasks until full effects of drug are known.

● Warn patient against exposure to extreme heat; drug may impair body's ability to reduce temperature.

● Inform patient that he may gain weight.

● Advise patient to avoid alcohol.

● Tell patient to rise slowly to avoid dizziness upon standing up quickly.

● Inform patient that ODTs contain phenylalanine.

● Tell patient to peel foil away from ODT, not to push tablet through. Have patient take tablet immediately, allowing tablet to dissolve on tongue and be swallowed with saliva; no additional fluid is needed.

● Tell patient to take drug with or without food.

● Urge woman of childbearing age to notify prescriber if she becomes pregnant or plans or suspects pregnancy. Tell her not to breast-feed during therapy.

---

olmesartan medoxomil
ol-ma-SAR-tan

Benicar⬧

Therapeutic class: Antihypertensives
Pharmacologic class: Angiotensin II receptor antagonists
Pregnancy risk category: D

AVAILABLE FORMS
Tablets: 5 mg, 20 mg, 40 mg

INDICATIONS & DOSAGES
➤ **Hypertension**
Adults: 20 mg P.O. once daily if patient has no volume depletion. May increase dosage to 40 mg P.O. once daily if blood pressure isn't reduced after 2 weeks of therapy.
Children ages 6 to 16: For children weighing 35 kg (77 lb) or more, initially, 20 mg P.O. daily, with maintenance dosage of 20 to 40 mg daily. For children weighing 20 to less than 35 kg (44 to less than 77 lb), initially, 10 mg P.O. daily, with maintenance dosage of 10 to 20 mg daily.
Adjust-a-dose: In patients with possible depletion of intravascular volume (those with impaired renal function who are taking diuretics), consider using lower starting dose.

ADMINISTRATION
P.O.
● Give drug without regard for food.
● Drug may be made into suspension by pharmacist if patient is unable to swallow pills.

Reactions in bold italics are *life-threatening*. Interactions may have a *rapid onset* or a *delayed onset*.

• Refrigerate suspension, which may be stored for up to 4 weeks.
• Shake suspension well before use.

ACTION

Blocks vasoconstrictor and aldosterone-secreting effects of angiotensin II by selectively blocking the binding of angiotensin II to the angiotensin I, or AT_1, receptor in the vascular smooth muscle.

Route	Onset	Peak	Duration
P.O.	Rapid	1–2 hr	24 hr

Half-life: 13 hours.

ADVERSE REACTIONS

CNS: headache, dizziness.
EENT: pharyngitis, rhinitis, sinusitis.
GI: diarrhea.
GU: hematuria.
Metabolic: hyperglycemia, hypertriglyceridemia.
Musculoskeletal: back pain.
Respiratory: bronchitis, upper respiratory tract infection.
Other: flulike symptoms.

INTERACTIONS

Drug-drug. *ACE inhibitors:* May increase risk of hyperkalemia and decrease renal function. Consider monotherapy; if coadministration can't be avoided, closely monitor renal function and serum potassium level.
❸ Alert: *Aliskiren:* May increase risk of renal impairment, hypotension, and hyperkalemia in diabetic patients and those with moderate to severe renal impairment (GFR less than 60 mL/minute). Concomitant use is contraindicated in diabetic patients. Avoid concomitant use in those with moderate to severe renal impairment.
Colesevelam: Reduces olmesartan level. Give olmesartan at least 4 hours before colesevelam.
Cyclo-oxygenase-2 inhibitors, NSAIDs: May decrease antihypertensive effects of olmesartan. Coadministration in elderly or volume-depleted patients or in those with compromised renal function may result in deterioration of renal function, including possible acute renal failure. Monitor blood pressure and renal function periodically.

Lithium: May increase serum lithium level and risk of toxicity. Closely monitor serum lithium level and adjust dosage as needed.
Potassium: May increase risk of hyperkalemia, possibly with cardiac arrhythmias or arrest. Closely monitor serum potassium level and renal function; adjust therapy as needed.
Trimethoprim: May increase risk of hyperkalemia, especially in elderly patients. If use together can't be avoided, closely monitor potassium level.
Drug-herb. *Ma huang:* May decrease antihypertensive effects. Discourage use together.

EFFECTS ON LAB TEST RESULTS

• May increase glucose, triglyceride, uric acid, liver enzyme, bilirubin, and CK levels.
• May decrease hemoglobin level and hematocrit.

CONTRAINDICATIONS & CAUTIONS

• Contraindicated in patients hypersensitive to the drug or any of its components and in patients who are pregnant.
Black Box Warning Drug may cause fetal and neonatal complications and death when given to pregnant women after the first trimester. If patient taking drug becomes pregnant, stop drug immediately. ∎
• Use cautiously in patients who are volume- or sodium-depleted, those whose renal function depends on the renin-angiotensin-aldosterone system (such as patients with severe heart failure), and those with unilateral or bilateral renal artery stenosis.
❸ Alert: Drug can cause spruelike enteropathy (severe chronic diarrhea with substantial weight loss).
• It's unknown if drug appears in breast milk. Patient should either stop breastfeeding or stop using drug.
⚠ Overdose S&S: Hypotension, tachycardia, bradycardia.

NURSING CONSIDERATIONS

• Symptomatic hypotension may occur in patients who are volume- or sodium-depleted, especially those being treated with high doses of a diuretic. If hypotension occurs, place patient supine and treat supportively. Treatment may continue once blood pressure is stabilized.

• If blood pressure isn't adequately controlled, a diuretic or other antihypertensive drugs also may be prescribed.

• Closely monitor patients with heart failure for oliguria, azotemia, and acute renal failure.

• Monitor BUN and creatinine level in patients with unilateral or bilateral renal artery stenosis.

• The antihypertensive effect is reduced in black patients, as has occurred with other angiotensin receptor blockers. Black patients may have a more favorable response if drug is taken with a thiazide diuretic.

PATIENT TEACHING

• Tell patient to take drug exactly as prescribed and not to stop taking it, even if he feels better.

• Tell patient to take drug without regard to meals.

• Tell patient to report any adverse reactions, especially light-headedness and fainting, to health care provider promptly.

ⓘ *Alert:* Tell patient to contact prescriber if severe chronic diarrhea with substantial weight loss develops, even if months to years have elapsed before symptoms occur.

• Advise women of childbearing age of the consequences of second- and third-trimester exposure to drug and to immediately report pregnancy to health care provider.

• Inform diabetic patients that glucose readings may rise and that the dosage of their diabetes drugs may need adjustment.

• Warn patients that inadequate fluid intake, excessive perspiration, diarrhea, or vomiting may lead to an excessive drop in blood pressure, light-headedness, and possibly fainting.

• Instruct patients that other antihypertensives can have additive effects. Patient should inform his prescriber of all medications he's taking, including OTC drugs.

olopatadine hydrochloride
oh-loh-PAT-ah-dine

Pataday, Patanase, Patanol

Therapeutic class: Antihistamines
Pharmacologic class: H_1-receptor antagonists
Pregnancy risk category: C

AVAILABLE FORMS
Nasal spray: 0.6%
Ophthalmic solution: 0.1%, 0.2%

INDICATIONS & DOSAGES
➤ **Seasonal allergic rhinitis (nasal)**
Adults and children age 12 and older: 2 sprays into each nostril b.i.d.
Children ages 6 to 11: 1 spray into each nostril b.i.d.
➤ **Allergic conjunctivitis**
Adults and children age 3 and older: 1 to 2 drops (0.1%) in each affected eye b.i.d. at an interval of 6 to 8 hours. Or, 1 drop (0.2%) in each affected eye once a day.

ADMINISTRATION
Intranasal
• Prime before use by releasing 5 sprays or until a fine mist appears.
• Reprime with 2 sprays when drug has not been used for more than 7 days.
Ophthalmic
• Before instilling drops, make sure patient has removed contact lenses.
• Don't touch eyelids and surrounding areas with dropper tip.

ACTION
Selectively antagonizes H_1-receptor activity.

Route	Onset	Peak	Duration
Intranasal	Rapid	¼–2 hr	Unknown
Ophthalmic	Unknown	2 hr	Unknown

Half-life: 8 to 12 hours, intranasal; 3 hours, ophthalmic.

ADVERSE REACTIONS
Intranasal
CNS: headache, fever.
EENT: nasal septum perforation, epistaxis, pharyngolaryngeal pain, postnasal drip.

Reactions in bold italics are *life-threatening*. Interactions may have a *rapid onset* or a *delayed onset*.

GI: bitter taste, dry mouth, diarrhea.
GU: UTI.
Respiratory: cough.
Ophthalmic
CNS: headache, asthenia.
EENT: burning or stinging eye, dry eye, sensation of foreign body in eye, hyperemia (eye), keratitis, lid edema, pruritus (eye), cold syndrome, pharyngitis, rhinitis, taste perversion.

INTERACTIONS
Drug-drug. *CNS depressants:* May cause additive sedative effects. Use together cautiously.
Drug-lifestyle. *Alcohol use:* May increase CNS depression. Discourage using together.

EFFECTS ON LAB TEST RESULTS
• May increase CK levels.

CONTRAINDICATIONS & CAUTIONS
• Contraindicated in patients hypersensitive to drug or its components.
⚠ *Overdose S&S:* Drowsiness (in adults), agitation and restlessness followed by drowsiness (in children).

NURSING CONSIDERATIONS
• Monitor nasal passages for ulceration before and during intranasal therapy.
• Monitor for somnolence.
• Give drug only if benefit to mother outweighs risk to fetus.
• Appearance of drug in breast milk isn't known. Use only if benefits to mother outweigh risk to child.
• Use cautiously in elderly patients because they may have impaired liver, renal, or cardiac function.

PATIENT TEACHING
• Advise patient or parent to read package instructions for drug use.
• Tell patient to prime the intranasal spray before initial use, and again when spray hasn't been used for more than 7 days.
• Caution patient to avoid hazardous activities until drug effects are known.
• Tell patient to notify prescriber if epistaxis or nasal ulcerations occur.
• Warn patient to avoid spraying intranasal drug into eyes.

• Warn patient not to instill ophthalmic drops while wearing contact lenses.
• Advise patient to avoid alcohol use while taking drug.

olsalazine sodium
ol-SAL-uh-zeen

Dipentum

Therapeutic class: Anti-inflammatory drugs
Pharmacologic class: Salicylates
Pregnancy risk category: C

AVAILABLE FORMS
Capsules: 250 mg

INDICATIONS & DOSAGES
➤ **Maintenance of remission of ulcerative colitis in patients intolerant of sulfasalazine**
Adults: 500 mg P.O. b.i.d. with meals.

ADMINISTRATION
P.O.
• Give drug with food.

ACTION
Unknown. After oral use, converts to 5-aminosalicylic acid (5-ASA, or mesalamine) in the colon, where it has local anti-inflammatory effect.

Route	Onset	Peak	Duration
P.O.	Unknown	1 hr	Unknown

Half-life: About 1 hour.

ADVERSE REACTIONS
CNS: headache, depression, vertigo, dizziness, fatigue.
GI: diarrhea, nausea, abdominal pain, dyspepsia, bloating, anorexia, stomatitis, vomiting.
Musculoskeletal: arthralgia.
Respiratory: upper respiratory tract infection.
Skin: rash, itching.

INTERACTIONS
Drug-drug. *Anticoagulants:* May prolong PT or INR. Monitor bleeding study results.

Drug-food. *Any food:* May decrease GI irritation. Advise patient to take drug with food.

EFFECTS ON LAB TEST RESULTS
• May increase ALT and AST levels.

CONTRAINDICATIONS & CAUTIONS
• Contraindicated in patients hypersensitive to salicylates.
• Use cautiously in patients with asthma, hepatic impairment, and renal disease.

NURSING CONSIDERATIONS
• Regularly monitor BUN and creatinine levels and urinalysis in patients with renal disease.
• Monitor liver enzyme levels in patients with hepatic impairment.
• Absorption of drug or its metabolites may cause renal tubular damage.
• Diarrhea sometimes occurs during therapy. Although diarrhea appears to be dose-related, it's difficult to distinguish from worsening of disease symptoms.
• Similar drugs have caused worsening of disease.
• *Look alike–sound alike:* Don't confuse olsalazine with olanzapine.

PATIENT TEACHING
• Teach patient to take drug in evenly divided doses and with food to minimize adverse GI reactions.
• Instruct patient to report persistent or severe adverse reactions promptly.

omalizumab
oh-mah-LIZ-uh-mab

Xolair

Therapeutic class: Antiasthmatics
Pharmacologic class: Monoclonal antibodies
Pregnancy risk category: B

AVAILABLE FORMS
Powder for injection: 150 mg in 5-mL vial

INDICATIONS & DOSAGES
➤ **Moderate to severe persistent asthma in patients with positive skin test or in vitro reactivity to a perennial aeroallergen and whose symptoms aren't adequately controlled by inhaled corticosteroids**
Adults and adolescents age 12 and older: 150 to 375 mg subcutaneously every 2 or 4 weeks. Dose and frequency vary with pretreatment immunoglobulin E (IgE) level (international units/mL) and patient weight. Divide doses larger than 150 mg among more than one injection site.

ADMINISTRATION
Subcutaneous
• Reconstitute with sterile water for injection only. Swirl gently, don't shake. Use 18G needle to draw medication into syringe, then replace with a 25G needle for administration.
• The lyophilized product takes 15 to 20 minutes to dissolve.
• The fully reconstituted product will appear clear or slightly opalescent and may have a few small bubbles or foam around the edge of the vial.
• Because the solution is slightly viscous, it may take 5 to 10 seconds to give.
• Use reconstituted solution within 4 hours if at room temperature or within 8 hours if refrigerated.

ACTION
Inhibits binding of IgE to high-affinity receptor on surface of mast cells and basophils, which limits release of allergic response mediators.

Route	Onset	Peak	Duration
Subcut.	Unknown	7–8 days	Unknown

Half-life: About 26 days.

ADVERSE REACTIONS
CNS: headache, dizziness, fatigue, pain.
EENT: pharyngitis, sinusitis, earache.
Musculoskeletal: arm pain, arthralgia, fracture, leg pain.
Respiratory: upper respiratory tract infection.

Skin: injection-site reaction, dermatitis, pruritus.
Other: viral infections.

INTERACTIONS
None reported.

EFFECTS ON LAB TEST RESULTS
• May increase IgE level.

CONTRAINDICATIONS & CAUTIONS
• Contraindicated in patients severely hypersensitive to drug.
• Safety and effectiveness haven't been established in children younger than age 12.
• Drug should be given only in a health care setting under direct medical supervision because of the risk of anaphylaxis.

NURSING CONSIDERATIONS
❸ Alert: Don't use this drug to treat acute bronchospasm or status asthmaticus.
• Don't abruptly stop systemic or inhaled corticosteroid when omalizumab therapy starts; taper the dose gradually and under supervision.
• Injection-site reactions, such as bruising, redness, warmth, burning, stinging, itching, hives, pain, induration, and inflammation, may occur, usually within 1 hour after the injection. These reactions last fewer than 8 days and decrease in frequency with subsequent injections.
Black Box Warning Observe patient for at least 2 hours after the injection, and keep drugs available to respond to anaphylactic reactions (such as bronchospasm, hypotension, syncope, urticaria, or angioedema of the throat or tongue). These reactions usually occur within 2 hours of subcutaneous injection; however, delayed reactions may occur up to 24 hours after administration. Anaphylaxis has also occurred beyond 1 year after beginning regularly administered treatment. If the patient has a severe hypersensitivity reaction, stop treatment. ∎
• Drug increases IgE level, so it can't be used to determine appropriate dosage during therapy or for 1 year after therapy ends.
• Patient medication guide must be given with each dose.

PATIENT TEACHING
• Tell patients not to stop or reduce the dosage of any other asthma drugs unless directed by the prescriber. Patient medication guide must be given with each dose.
• Explain that patient may not notice an immediate improvement in asthma after therapy starts.
Black Box Warning Teach patient the signs and symptoms of anaphylaxis and tell him to seek immediate medical care if symptoms occur. ∎

omega-3–acid ethyl esters
oh-may-gah-three-ASS-id

Lovaza⬦, Omacor

Therapeutic class: Antilipemics
Pharmacologic class: Ethyl esters
Pregnancy risk category: C

AVAILABLE FORMS
Capsules: 1 g

INDICATIONS & DOSAGES
➤ **Adjunct to diet to reduce triglyceride levels 500 mg/dL or higher**
Adults: 4 g P.O. once daily or divided as 2 g b.i.d.

ADMINISTRATION
P.O.
• Give drug with meals.
• Capsules must be swallowed whole. Do not extract contents of capsule.

ACTION
May reduce hepatic formation of triglycerides because two components of drug are poor substrates for the necessary enzymes. These components also block formation of other fatty acids.

Route	Onset	Peak	Duration
P.O.	Unknown	Unknown	Unknown

Half-life: Unknown.

ADVERSE REACTIONS
CNS: pain.
CV: angina pectoris.
GI: altered taste, belching, dyspepsia.

Musculoskeletal: back pain.
Skin: rash.
Other: flulike syndrome, infection.

INTERACTIONS
Drug-drug. *Anticoagulants:* May prolong bleeding time. Monitor patient.

EFFECTS ON LAB TEST RESULTS
• May increase ALT and LDL cholesterol levels.

CONTRAINDICATIONS & CAUTIONS
• Contraindicated in patients hypersensitive to drug or its components.
• Use cautiously in patients sensitive to fish.

NURSING CONSIDERATIONS
• Assess patient for conditions that contribute to increased triglycerides, such as diabetes and hypothyroidism, before treatment.
• Evaluate patient's current drug regimen for any drugs known to sharply increase triglyceride levels, including estrogen therapy, thiazide diuretics, and beta blockers. Stopping these drugs, if appropriate, may negate the need for drug.
• Continue diet and lifestyle modifications during treatment.
• Obtain baseline triglyceride levels to confirm that they're consistently abnormal before therapy; then recheck periodically during treatment. If patient has an inadequate response after 2 months, stop drug.
• Monitor LDL level to make sure it doesn't increase excessively during treatment.
• *Look alike–sound alike:* Don't confuse Lovaza with lorazepam or lovastatin.

PATIENT TEACHING
• Explain that taking drug doesn't reduce the importance of following the recommended diet and exercise plan.
• Remind patient of the need for follow-up blood work to evaluate progress.
• Advise patient to notify prescriber about bothersome side effects.
• Tell patient to report planned or suspected pregnancy.

omeprazole
oh-ME-pray-zole

Losec†, Prilosec⌀

omeprazole magnesium
Prilosec OTC ◊

Therapeutic class: Antiulcer drugs
Pharmacologic class: Proton pump inhibitors
Pregnancy risk category: C

AVAILABLE FORMS
Capsules (delayed-release): 10 mg, 20 mg, 40 mg
Powder for oral suspension: 2.5 mg/packet, 10 mg/packet
Tablets (delayed-release): 20 mg ◊

INDICATIONS & DOSAGES
➤ **Symptomatic GERD without esophageal lesions**
Adults: 20 mg P.O., as delayed-release form or oral suspension, daily for 4 weeks for patients who respond poorly to customary medical treatment, usually including an adequate course of H_2-receptor antagonists.
Children ages 1 to 16 weighing 20 kg (44 lb) or more: 20 mg P.O. daily.
Children ages 1 to 16 weighing 10 kg (22 lb) to less than 20 kg (44 lb): 10 mg P.O. daily.
Children ages 1 to 16 weighing 5 kg (11 lb) to less than 10 kg (22 lb): 5 mg P.O. daily.
➤ **Erosive esophagitis**
Adults: 20 mg P.O. daily. For symptoms caused by GERD, treat for 4 to 8 weeks.
Children ages 1 to 16 weighing 20 kg (44 lb) or more: 20 mg P.O. daily.
Children ages 1 to 16 weighing 10 kg (22 lb) to less than 20 kg (44 lb): 10 mg P.O. daily.
Children ages 1 to 16 weighing 5 kg (11 lb) to less than 10 kg (22 lb): 5 mg P.O. daily.
➤ **Pathologic hypersecretory conditions (such as Zollinger-Ellison syndrome)**
Adults: Initially, 60 mg P.O. daily; adjust dosage based on patient response. If daily dose exceeds 80 mg, give in divided doses. Doses up to 120 mg t.i.d. have been given. Continue therapy as long as clinically indicated.

➤ **Duodenal ulcer (short-term treatment)**
Adults: 20 mg P.O., as delayed-release form or oral suspension, daily for 4 to 8 weeks.
➤ *Helicobacter pylori* **infection and duodenal ulcer disease, to eradicate *H. pylori* with clarithromycin (dual therapy)**
Adults: 40 mg P.O. every morning with clarithromycin 500 mg P.O. t.i.d. for 14 days. For patients with an ulcer at start of therapy, give another 14 days of omeprazole 20 mg P.O. once daily.
➤ *H. pylori* **infection and duodenal ulcer disease, to eradicate *H. pylori* with clarithromycin and amoxicillin (triple therapy)**
Adults: 20 mg P.O. with clarithromycin 500 mg P.O. and amoxicillin 1,000 mg P.O., each given b.i.d. for 10 days. For patients with an ulcer at start of therapy, give another 18 days of omeprazole 20 mg P.O. once daily.
➤ **Short-term treatment of active benign gastric ulcer**
Adults: 40 mg P.O. once daily for 4 to 8 weeks.
➤ **Frequent heartburn (2 or more days a week)**
Adults: 20 mg Prilosec OTC P.O. once daily before breakfast for 14 days. May repeat the 14-day course every 4 months.
➤ **Laryngitis** ◆
Adults: 20 to 40 mg P.O. at bedtime for 6 to 24 weeks. Or, 20 mg P.O. b.i.d. for 4 to 12 weeks.
➤ **Stress ulcer prophylaxis** ◆
Adults: 40 mg loading dose P.O. or via nasogastric (NG) tube followed by 20 to 40 mg daily.

ADMINISTRATION
P.O.
• Don't crush tablets or capsules. Capsules may be opened for patients who have difficulty swallowing.
• Give drug at least 1 hour before meals.
• For oral suspension, empty contents of 2.5-mg packet into container containing 5 mL water; empty contents of 10-mg packet into container containing 15 mL water. Stir and leave for 2 to 3 minutes to thicken. Stir and administer within 30 minutes. If material remains after

drinking, add more water, stir, and give immediately.
• For patients with an NG or gastric tube in place, add 5 mL water to catheter-tipped syringe; then add contents of 2.5-mg packet (or 15 mL water for 10-mg packet). Immediately shake syringe and leave for 2 to 3 minutes to thicken. Shake syringe and inject through NG or gastric tube, #6 French or larger, into stomach within 30 minutes. Refill syringe with an equal amount of water. Shake and flush any remaining contents from NG or gastric tube into stomach.

ACTION
Inhibits proton pump activity by binding to hydrogen–potassium adenosine triphosphatase, located at secretory surface of gastric parietal cells, to suppress gastric acid secretion.

Route	Onset	Peak	Duration
P.O.	1 hr	30 min–2 hr	<3 days

Half-life: 30 to 60 minutes.

ADVERSE REACTIONS
CNS: asthenia, dizziness, headache.
GI: abdominal pain, constipation, diarrhea, flatulence, nausea, vomiting.
Musculoskeletal: back pain.
Respiratory: cough, upper respiratory tract infection.
Skin: rash.

INTERACTIONS
Drug-drug. *Ampicillin esters, azole antifungals (such as ketoconazole), iron derivatives:* May cause poor bioavailability of these drugs because they need a low gastric pH for optimal absorption. Avoid using together.
Benzodiazepines, diazepam, fosphenytoin, phenytoin, warfarin: May decrease hepatic clearance, possibly leading to increased levels of these drugs. Monitor drug levels.
Calcium salts: May decrease GI absorption of calcium salts. Closely monitor clinical response and increase calcium dosage if needed.
Cilostazol: May increase cilostazol level. Reduce cilostazol dosage.
Clopidogrel: May decrease antiplatelet activity. Avoid use together.

Fluvoxamine: May increase omeprazole level. Monitor patient for increased adverse reactions.

Iron salts: May interfere with iron absorption. Omeprazole may need to be temporarily stopped, or parenteral iron may be given as an alternative.

Methotrexate: May increase methotrexate level, causing toxicity. Monitor patient closely.

Rifampin: May substantially decrease omeprazole concentration. Avoid concomitant use.

Salicylates: Enteric-coated forms may dissolve faster, increasing risk of gastric adverse effects. Use together cautiously.

Tacrolimus: May increase tacrolimus level and risk of toxicity. Monitor tacrolimus trough concentration when omeprazole is started and stopped.

Drug-herb. *Ginkgo biloba, St. John's wort:* May decrease omeprazole level. Avoid use together.

EFFECTS ON LAB TEST RESULTS

● May increase LFT values and falsely elevate serum chromogranin A levels.

● May decrease magnesium, sodium, and glucose levels.

CONTRAINDICATIONS & CAUTIONS

● Contraindicated in patients hypersensitive to drug or its components.

❸ **Alert:** There may be an increased risk of hip, wrist, and spine fractures associated with proton pump inhibitors.

● Use cautiously in patients with hypokalemia and respiratory alkalosis and in patients on a low-sodium diet.

● Long-term administration of bicarbonate with calcium or milk can cause milk-alkali syndrome.

⚠ **Overdose S&S:** Confusion, drowsiness, blurred vision, tachycardia, nausea, vomiting, diaphoresis, flushing, headache, dry mouth.

NURSING CONSIDERATIONS

❸ **Alert:** May increase risk of *Clostridium difficile*–associated diarrhea (CDAD). Evaluate for CDAD in patients who develop diarrhea that doesn't improve.

● Dosage adjustments may be necessary in Asians and patients with hepatic impairment.

● Drug increases its own bioavailability with repeated doses. Drug is unstable in gastric acid; less drug is lost to hydrolysis because drug increases gastric pH.

● Gastrin level rises in most patients during the first 2 weeks of therapy.

❸ **Alert:** Prolonged use of proton pump inhibitors may cause low magnesium levels. Monitor magnesium levels before starting treatment and periodically thereafter.

❸ **Alert:** Monitor patients for signs and symptoms of low magnesium level, such as abnormal heart rate or rhythm, palpitations, muscle spasms, tremors, or seizures. In children, an abnormal heart rate may present as fatigue, upset stomach, dizziness, and lightheadedness. Magnesium supplementation or drug discontinuation may be required.

● **Look alike–sound alike:** Don't confuse Prilosec with Prozac, Prilocaine, or Prinivil.

PATIENT TEACHING

● Tell patient to swallow tablets whole and not to open, crush, or chew them.

● Give patient instructions on how to take oral suspension.

● Instruct patient to take drug at least 1 hour before meals.

● Caution patient to avoid hazardous activities if he gets dizzy.

● Advise patient that Prilosec OTC isn't intended to treat infrequent heartburn (one episode of heartburn a week or less), or for those who want immediate relief of heartburn.

● Inform patient that Prilosec OTC may take 1 to 4 days for full effect, although some patients may get complete relief of symptoms within 24 hours.

● Teach patient to recognize and report signs and symptoms of low magnesium levels.

---

onabotulinumtoxinA
OH-na-BOT-ue-LYE-num-TOX-in A

Botox

Therapeutic class: Neuromuscular transmission blockers
Pharmacologic class: Acetylcholine release inhibitors
Pregnancy risk category: C

AVAILABLE FORMS
Injection: 50 units/vial, 100 units/vial, 200 units/vial

INDICATIONS & DOSAGES
Adjust-a-dose (for all indications): When adults are being treated for one or more indications, maximum cumulative dose generally shouldn't exceed 360 units in a 3-month interval.

➤ **Overactive bladder signs and symptoms (urge urinary incontinence, urgency, and frequency) in patients with inadequate response to or intolerant of anticholinergic medication**
Adults: Recommended total dose is 100 units, given as 0.5 mL (5 units) I.M. across 20 sites into the detrusor muscle. Give prophylactic antibiotics (except aminoglycosides) 1 to 3 days before treatment, on treatment day, and 1 to 3 days after treatment to reduce likelihood of procedure-related UTI.

➤ **Urinary incontinence due to detrusor overactivity associated with a neurologic condition, such as spinal cord injury or MS, after inadequate response or intolerance to anticholinergic medication**
Adults: Recommended total dose is 200 units, given as 30 injections of 1 mL (6.7 units) each (total volume of 30 mL) I.M. across 30 sites into the detrusor muscle.

➤ **Prophylaxis of headaches in patients with chronic migraine (15 days per month or more, with headache lasting 4 hours a day or longer)**
Adults: Recommended total dose is 155 units, given as 0.1 mL (5 units) per site I.M. divided across seven head/neck muscles. Refer to manufacturer's instructions for injection-site diagrams.

➤ **Upper limb spasticity**
Adults: 12.5 to 50 units per site I.M. The lowest recommended starting dose should be used. Tailor dosing in initial and sequential treatment sessions to the individual based on the size, number, and location of muscles involved; severity of spasticity; presence of local muscle weakness; and patient's response to previous treatment or adverse event history with onabotulinumtoxinA. Administer no more than 50 units per site. Refer to manufacturer's instructions for specific sites and dosages.

➤ **Cervical dystonia to reduce severity of abnormal head position and neck pain**
Adults and children age 16 and older: Adjust initial and subsequent dosing based on patient's head and neck position, localization of pain, muscle hypertrophy, patient response, and adverse event history. Use lower initial dose in botulinum toxin–naive patients. Administer no more than 50 units per site.

➤ **Severe axillary hyperhidrosis inadequately managed by topical agents**
Adults: 50 units (2 mL) injected intradermally in 0.1- to 0.2-mL aliquots to each axilla, evenly distributed in 10 to 15 sites approximately 1 to 2 cm apart. May administer repeat injections when clinical effect of a previous injection diminishes.

➤ **Blepharospasm associated with dystonia**
Adults and children age 12 and older: 1.25 to 2.5 units (0.05 to 0.1 mL volume at each site) I.M. into medial and lateral pretarsal orbicularis oculi of upper lid and into lateral pretarsal orbicularis oculi of lower lid. Cumulative dose in a 30-day period shouldn't exceed 200 units.

➤ **Strabismus**
Adults and children age 12 and older: For vertical muscles, and for horizontal strabismus of less than 20 prism diopters: 1.25 to 2.5 units in any one muscle. For horizontal strabismus of 20 to 50 prism diopters: 2.5 to 5 units in any one muscle.

➤ **Persistent cranial nerve VI palsy of 1 month or longer duration**
Adults and children age 12 and older: 1.25 to 2.5 units I.M. in medial rectus muscle.

O

---

†Canada   ◇OTC   ◆Off-label use   ✐Photoguide   *Liquid contains alcohol.

ADMINISTRATION
I.M., intradermal
● Reconstitute each vial with sterile, non-preserved normal saline solution for injection by drawing up proper amount of diluent (see manufacturer's instructions) in appropriate-sized syringe (see manufacturer's instructions) and slowly injecting diluent into vial.

● Gently mix drug with the saline by rotating vial.

● Administer within 24 hours after reconstitution; store in refrigerator until administration.

ACTION
Blocks neuromuscular transmission by inhibiting release of acetylcholine. I.M. doses chemically denervate muscle, reducing muscular activity either temporarily or permanently. Intradermal administration causes temporary chemical denervation of sweat glands, resulting in local reduction in sweating. Intradetrusor injection affects detrusor muscle activity via inhibition of acetylcholine release.

Route	Onset	Peak	Duration
I.M.	Varies by site	Unknown	Varies by site
Intradermal	Varies by site	Unknown	Varies by site

Half-life: Unknown.

ADVERSE REACTIONS
Overactive bladder symptoms
GU: UTI, dysuria, urine retention, bacteriuria, residual urine volume, hematuria.
Other: injection-site soreness or ***hemorrhage***.
Urinary incontinence due to detrusor overactivity associated with a neurologic condition
GI: constipation.
GU: UTI, dysuria, urine retention, hematuria.
Musculoskeletal: weakness, muscle spasm, gait disturbance, falls.
Other: injection-site soreness or ***hemorrhage***.
Chronic migraine headache prophylaxis
CNS: headache, worsening migraine.
CV: hypertension.

EENT: ptosis, facial paresis.
Musculoskeletal: neck pain, weakness, stiffness, myalgia, muscle spasm.
Respiratory: bronchitis.
Other: injection-site pain.
Upper limb spasticity
CNS: fatigue.
GI: nausea.
Musculoskeletal: extremity pain, weakness.
Respiratory: bronchitis.
Other: injection-site soreness or ***hemorrhage***.
Cervical dystonia
CNS: headache, dizziness, drowsiness, fever, speech disorder, numbness, asthenia, drowsiness.
EENT: rhinitis, oral dryness, ptosis, diplopia.
GI: nausea, dysphagia.
Musculoskeletal: neck pain, back pain, stiffness, hypertonia.
Respiratory: upper respiratory tract infection, increased cough, dyspnea.
Other: flulike syndrome, injection-site soreness.
Severe axillary hyperhidrosis
CNS: headache, fever, anxiety.
EENT: pharyngitis.
Metabolic: nonaxillary sweating.
Musculoskeletal: neck or back pain.
Skin: pruritus.
Other: flulike syndrome, injection-site pain or ***hemorrhage***, infection.
Blepharospasm associated with dystonia
EENT: ptosis, superficial punctate keratitis, eye dryness, irritation, tearing, lagophthalmos, photophobia, ectropion, keratitis, diplopia, entropion, local swelling of eyelid skin.
Skin: diffuse rash.
Other: injection-site soreness or ***hemorrhage***.
Strabismus
EENT: vertical deviation due to effect on adjacent extraocular muscles, ptosis.
Other: injection-site soreness or ***hemorrhage***.
Persistent cranial nerve VI palsy
Other: injection-site soreness or ***hemorrhage***.

Reactions in bold italics are ***life-threatening***. Interactions may have a *rapid onset* or a ***delayed onset***.

INTERACTIONS

Drug-drug. *Aminoglycosides, neuromuscular blockers (curare or curare-like compounds):* May increase effect of toxin and risk of respiratory depression. Don't use together.

Anticholinergics: May increase systemic anticholinergic effects. Avoid use together.

Anticoagulants, antiplatelet drugs: May increase risk of bleeding. Discontinue antiplatelet therapy at least 3 days before injection procedure; monitor patients on anticoagulant therapy carefully.

Muscle relaxants, other botulinum neurotoxin products: May cause excessive neuromuscular weakness. Avoid use together.

EFFECTS ON LAB TEST RESULTS

None reported.

CONTRAINDICATIONS & CAUTIONS

Black Box Warning The effects of onabotulinumtoxinA and all botulinum toxin products may spread from injection area to produce signs and symptoms consistent with botulinum toxin effects. These may include asthenia, generalized muscle weakness, diplopia, ptosis, dysphagia, dysphonia, dysarthria, urinary incontinence, and breathing difficulties, which have reportedly occurred hours to weeks after injection. Swallowing and breathing difficulties can be life-threatening; deaths have been reported. Risk of symptoms developing is probably greatest in children treated for spasticity, but symptoms can also occur in adults treated for spasticity and other conditions, particularly in those with an underlying condition predisposing them to these symptoms. In unapproved uses (including spasticity in children), and in approved indications, cases of spread of effect have been reported at doses comparable to those used to treat cervical dystonia and at lower doses. ∎

◑ Alert: In the event of overdose, antitoxin raised against botulinum toxin is available from the Centers for Disease Control and Prevention (CDC). However, the antitoxin will not reverse botulinum toxin–induced effects already apparent by the time of antitoxin administration. In the event of suspected or actual cases of botulinum toxin poisoning, contact your local or state

health department to process a request for antitoxin through the CDC. If you don't receive a response within 30 minutes, contact the CDC directly at 1-770-488-7100. More information can be obtained at www.cdc.gov/mmwr/preview/mmwrhtml/mm5232a8.htm.

• Contraindicated in known hypersensitivity to botulinum toxin and in patient with infection at injection sites.

• Contraindicated in patients being treated for overactive bladder with UTIs and in patients with overactive bladder or detrusor overactivity associated with a neurologic condition who have post-void residual urine volume but don't catheterize routinely (patients with MS or diabetes mellitus).

• Use cautiously in patients with inflammation at the proposed injection site or when excessive weakness or atrophy is present in the target muscle.

• Use cautiously in patients with preexisting neuromuscular disorders, compromised respiratory function, or corneal exposure and ulceration due to reduced blinking.

• Use in pregnancy only if benefit outweighs fetal risk.

• Use cautiously in breast-feeding women. It isn't known if drug appears in breast milk.

⚠ Overdose S&S: Neuromuscular weakness, aspiration pneumonia, respiratory muscle paralysis, respiratory failure, death.

NURSING CONSIDERATIONS

◑ Alert: Signs and symptoms of overdose usually don't occur immediately after injection. Should accidental injection or oral ingestion occur or overdose be suspected, patient should be medically supervised for several weeks for signs and symptoms of systemic muscular weakness, which could be local or distant from the injection.

Black Box Warning Monitor patient for swallowing and breathing difficulties, which can lead to death. ∎

• Prescribers administering drug must understand the relevant neuromuscular or orbital anatomy of the area involved and any alterations to the anatomy due to prior surgical procedures.

• Understanding of standard electromyographic techniques is required for treatment of strabismus and upper limb spasticity, and

may be useful for the treatment of cervical dystonia.
- Drug isn't interchangeable with other preparations of botulinum toxin products and can't be converted into units of other botulinum toxin products.
- Start treatment at lowest recommended dosage.
- Watch for bronchitis and upper respiratory tract infection in patients being treated for upper limb spasticity.
- Discontinue antiplatelet therapy at least 3 days before the injection procedure; patients on anticoagulant therapy need to be managed appropriately to decrease bleeding risk.
- Repeat treatment may be administered when the effect of a previous injection has diminished, but generally no sooner than 12 weeks after previous injection.
- Follow indication-specific dosage and administration recommendations. Don't exceed a total dose of 360 units in a 3-month interval.
- Degree or pattern of muscle spasticity at the time of reinjection may necessitate alterations in dosage and of muscles to be injected.
- To prepare eye for injection, several drops of a local anesthetic and an ocular decongestant are instilled several minutes before injection.
- Monitor patient for retrobulbar hemorrhages and compromised retinal circulation after eye injections.

PATIENT TEACHING
Black Box Warning Caution patient to seek immediate medical attention if serious side effects occur, such as difficulty swallowing, speaking, or breathing. These side effects can occur hours, days, or even weeks after injection and can be fatal. ■
- Teach patient to report signs and symptoms of botulism toxicity (such as loss of strength or muscle weakness, double vision, blurred vision, drooping eyelids, hoarseness, change in or loss of voice, trouble speaking clearly, or loss of bladder control). Inform patient that, if these side effects occur, the patient should not drive a car, operate machinery, or perform other dangerous activities.

- Advise patient that onabotulinumtoxinA injections may cause reduced blinking or effectiveness of blinking, and to seek immediate medical attention if eye pain or irritation occurs after treatment.
- Instruct patient to report voiding difficulties after bladder injections for urinary incontinence.

ondansetron
on-DAN-sah-tron

Zuplenz

ondansetron hydrochloride
Zofran, Zofran ODT

Therapeutic class: Antiemetics
Pharmacologic class: Selective serotonin (5-HT$_3$) receptor antagonists
Pregnancy risk category: B

AVAILABLE FORMS
Injection: 2 mg/mL, 4 mg/2 mL
Orally disintegrating tablets (ODTs): 4 mg, 8 mg
Oral soluble film: 4 mg, 8 mg
Oral solution: 4 mg/5 mL
Premixed injection: 32 mg/50 mL
Tablets: 4 mg, 8 mg, 24 mg

INDICATIONS & DOSAGES
Adjust-a-dose (for all indications): For patients with severe hepatic impairment, total daily dose shouldn't exceed 8 mg.
➤ **To prevent nausea and vomiting from highly emetogenic chemotherapy**
Adults: 24 mg P.O. 30 minutes before chemotherapy. Or, three successive 8-mg doses of oral soluble film given 30 minutes before start of single-day highly emetogenic chemotherapy.
Children ages 6 months to 18 years: 0.15 mg/kg I.V. over 15 minutes beginning 30 minutes before chemotherapy. Give second dose of 0.15 mg/kg I.V. over 15 minutes 4 hours after first dose. Give third 0.15-mg/kg I.V. dose 8 hours after first dose. No single I.V. dose should exceed 16 mg.

Reactions in bold italics are *life-threatening*. Interactions may have a *rapid onset* or a *delayed onset*.

➤ **To prevent nausea and vomiting from moderately emetogenic chemotherapy**
Adults and children age 12 and older:
8 mg P.O. 30 minutes before chemotherapy. Then, 8 mg P.O. 8 hours after first dose. Then, 8 mg every 12 hours for 1 to 2 days. Or, three doses of 0.15 mg/kg I.V. For three-dose regimen, give first dose 30 minutes before chemotherapy and subsequent doses 4 and 8 hours after first dose. Infuse drug over 15 minutes. No single I.V. dose should exceed 16 mg. Or, 8 mg oral soluble film 30 minutes before chemotherapy, followed by 8 mg oral soluble film 8 hours after first dose. Then give 8 mg oral soluble film every 12 hours for 1 to 2 days after completing chemotherapy.
Children ages 4 to 11: 4 mg P.O. or oral soluble film 30 minutes before chemotherapy. Then, 4 mg P.O. 4 and 8 hours after first dose. Then, 4 mg every 8 hours for 1 to 2 days.
Infants and children ages 6 months to 11 years: Three doses of 0.15 mg/kg I.V. Give first dose 30 minutes before chemotherapy; give subsequent doses 4 and 8 hours after first dose. Infuse drug over 15 minutes. No single I.V. dose should exceed 16 mg.

➤ **To prevent postoperative nausea and vomiting**
Adults: 4 mg undiluted solution for injection I.M. or I.V. over 2 to 5 minutes immediately before induction of anesthesia. Or, 16 mg P.O. or two successive 8-mg oral soluble films 1 hour before induction of anesthesia.
Children ages 1 month to 12 years weighing more than 40 kg (88 lb): 4 mg I.V. as a single dose.
Children ages 1 month to 12 years weighing 40 kg or less: 0.1 mg/kg I.V. as a single dose.

➤ **To prevent nausea and vomiting from radiation therapy in patients receiving total body irradiation, single high-dose fraction radiation therapy to abdomen, or daily fractionated radiation therapy to abdomen**
Adults: 8 mg P.O. t.i.d. For patients receiving total body irradiation, give 8 mg P.O. or oral soluble film 1 to 2 hours before each fraction of radiation therapy each day. For patients receiving single high-dose fraction

radiation therapy to the abdomen, give 8 mg P.O. or oral soluble film 1 to 2 hours before therapy, then every 8 hours for 1 to 2 days after completion of therapy. For patients receiving daily fractionated radiation therapy, give 8 mg P.O. or oral soluble film 1 to 2 hours before therapy, then every 8 hours for each day therapy is given.

➤ **Nausea and vomiting of pregnancy ◆**
Adults: 8 mg I.V. over 15 minutes every 12 hours.

➤ **Postanesthetic shivering ◆**
Adults: 4 or 8 mg I.V. as a single dose during anesthesia induction.

➤ **Opioid-related pruritus ◆**
Adults: For prevention, 4 or 8 mg I.V. 20 to 30 minutes before spinal opioid administration. For treatment, 4 or 8 mg I.V.

ADMINISTRATION
P.O.
● Open blister of ODT just before use by peeling backing off. Don't push ODT through foil blister.
● For Zuplenz, open film pouch with dry hands and immediately place film on top of the tongue, where it will dissolve in 4 to 20 seconds. Then have patient swallow with or without liquid. Wash hands after giving Zuplenz.

I.V.
❸ *Alert:* No single I.V. dose should exceed 16 mg due to the risk of QT-interval prolongation.
▼ If precipitate is noted in vial, shake vigorously until dissolved.
▼ Dilute drug in 50 mL of D_5W injection or normal saline solution for injection.
▼ Drug is stable for up to 48 hours after dilution in D_5W, 5% dextrose in half-normal saline solution for injection, 5% dextrose in normal saline solution, and 3% sodium chloride solution for injection.
▼ Infuse over 15 minutes.
▼ **Incompatibilities:** Acyclovir sodium, allopurinol, aminophylline, amphotericin B, ampicillin sodium, ampicillin sodium–sulbactam sodium, cefepime, cefoperazone, dacarbazine with doxorubicin, dexamethasone sodium phosphate, droperidol, 5-FU, furosemide, ganciclovir, lorazepam, meropenem, methylprednisolone sodium

O

succinate, piperacillin sodium, sargramostim, sodium bicarbonate.

I.M.
• Document injection site.
• If precipitate is noted in vial, shake
vigorously until dissolved.

ACTION
May block 5-HT$_3$ in the CNS in the
chemoreceptor trigger zone and in the
peripheral nervous system on nerve
terminals of the vagus nerve.

Route	Onset	Peak	Duration
P.O.	Unknown	Unknown	Unknown
I.V.	Immediate	10 min	Unknown
I.M.	Unknown	41 min	Unknown

Half-life: 4 hours.

ADVERSE REACTIONS
CNS: dizziness, fatigue, headache, malaise,
sedation, extrapyramidal syndrome, fever,
pain.
CV: *arrhythmias,* chest pain.
GI: constipation, diarrhea, abdominal pain,
decreased appetite, xerostomia.
GU: gynecologic disorders, urine retention.
Respiratory: *hypoxia.*
Skin: pruritus, rash.
Other: chills, injection-site reaction.

INTERACTIONS
Drug-drug. *Apomorphine:* May cause
profound hypotension and loss of consciousness. Use together is contraindicated.
*Drugs such as cimetidine that alter hepatic
drug-metabolizing enzymes, phenobarbital,
rifampin:* May change pharmacokinetics of
ondansetron. No need to adjust dosage.
Drug-herb. *Horehound:* May enhance
serotoninergic effects. Discourage use
together.

EFFECTS ON LAB TEST RESULTS
• May increase ALT and AST levels.

CONTRAINDICATIONS & CAUTIONS
• Contraindicated in patients hypersensitive
to drug.
🟊 *Alert:* Contraindicated for use with apomorphine.

• ECG changes, including prolonged QT interval, have been reported. Monitor patient
carefully.
• Use cautiously in patients with hepatic
impairment.
⚠ *Overdose S&S:* Sudden transient blindness, severe constipation, hypotension.

NURSING CONSIDERATIONS
🟊 *Alert:* Drug may increase the risk of prolonged QT interval and torsades de pointes
(a potentially fatal heart rhythm). Monitor
ECG in patients with congenital long QT
syndrome, in those with heart failure or
bradyarrhythmias, and in those taking other
medications that can prolong the QT interval.
🟊 *Alert:* Correct electrolyte abnormalities
(hypokalemia or hypomagnesemia) before
infusing drug.
• Monitor LFT results. Don't exceed 8 mg
in patients with hepatic impairment.
• *Look alike–sound alike:* Don't confuse
Zofran with Zosyn, Zantac, or Zoloft.

PATIENT TEACHING
🟊 *Alert:* Caution patient to contact health
care provider immediately if he experiences
signs and symptoms of abnormal heart rate
or rhythm, such as palpitations, dyspnea, or
dizziness.
• Tell patient that an ECG may be necessary
to monitor his heart rate and rhythm.
• Instruct patient to immediately report
difficulty breathing after drug administration.
• Tell patient receiving drug I.V. to report
discomfort at insertion site.
• For patient taking ODTs, tell him to open
blister just before use by peeling backing
off and not by pushing through foil blister,
and tell him that taking it with liquid isn't
required.
• Teach patient to place ODTs on tongue,
allow to dissolve, then swallow with saliva.

---

oprelvekin
oh-PRELL-veh-kin

Neumega

Therapeutic class: Hematopoietics
Pharmacologic class: Recombinant
human interleukins
Pregnancy risk category: C

AVAILABLE FORMS
Injection: 5-mg single-dose vial with
diluent

INDICATIONS & DOSAGES
➤ **To prevent severe thrombocytopenia
and reduce need for platelet transfusions
after myelosuppressive chemotherapy
with nonmyeloid malignancies**
Adults: 50 mcg/kg as single daily subcutaneous injection until postnadir platelet
count is at least $50,000/mm^3$. Treatment
beyond 21 days per course isn't recommended. Begin dosing 6 to 24 hours after
completion of chemotherapy. Discontinue
drug at least 2 days before the start of the
next planned cycle of chemotherapy.
Adjust-a-dose: In patients with severe renal
impairment (CrCl less than 30 mL/minute),
the recommended dosage is 25 mcg/kg
daily.

ADMINISTRATION
Subcutaneous
• Give drug in the abdomen, thigh, hip, or
upper arm. Don't inject I.D. or intravascu-
larly.
• Reconstitute each single-dose vial with
1 mL of supplied diluent. Avoid excessive
or vigorous agitation. Discard unused
portions.
• Use reconstituted drug within 3 hours.
• Store drug and diluent in refrigerator until
ready to use. Don't freeze.

ACTION
Directly stimulates proliferation of
hematopoietic stem cells and megakaryocyte progenitor cells. Also induces
megakaryocyte maturation, resulting in
increased platelet production.

Route	Onset	Peak	Duration
Subcut.	Unknown	3–5 hr	Unknown

Half-life: 7 hours.

ADVERSE REACTIONS
CNS: asthenia, headache, insomnia, dizzi-
ness, paresthesia, syncope.
CV: *atrial flutter or fibrillation,* tachycar-
dia, palpitations, edema, vasodilation.
EENT: conjunctival injection, blurred
vision, eye hemorrhage, pharyngitis,
rhinitis.
GI: oral candidiasis, nausea, vomiting,
diarrhea.
Hematologic: anemia.
Metabolic: dehydration, *hypocalcemia.*
Respiratory: dyspnea, cough, pleural
effusions.
Skin: rash, skin discoloration, exfoliative
dermatitis.
Other: hypersensitivity reactions, allergic
reaction, *anaphylaxis,* neutropenic fever.

INTERACTIONS
Drug-drug. *Diuretics, ifosfamide:* May
cause life-threatening hypokalemia. Closely
monitor fluid and electrolyte status.

EFFECTS ON LAB TEST RESULTS
• May increase fibrinogen and von Willebrand factor.
• May decrease calcium and hemoglobin
levels and hematocrit.

CONTRAINDICATIONS & CAUTIONS
• Contraindicated in patients hypersensitive
to drug or its components.
• Use drug cautiously in patients with heart
failure because of fluid retention.
⚠ Overdose S&S: Increased incidence of
CV reactions.

NURSING CONSIDERATIONS
Black Box Warning Oprelvekin has caused
allergic or hypersensitivity reactions,
including anaphylaxis. Discontinue drug
permanently in patients who develop
allergic or hypersensitivity reaction. ∎
• Drug isn't indicated following myeloabla-
tive chemotherapy.

• Closely monitor fluid and electrolyte status in patients receiving long-term diuretic therapy.
• Fluid retention can be severe; monitor patient closely.
• Obtain a CBC before chemotherapy and at regular intervals during drug therapy.

PATIENT TEACHING
• Instruct patient about appropriate preparation and administration of drug if he is going to self-administer.
• Warn patient about potential adverse reactions. Tell him to report any occurrence.
• Tell patient to keep drug refrigerated and not to reconstitute until just before use.
• Urge patient to call prescriber immediately if swelling, rapid heartbeat, or difficulty breathing occurs.
• Tell patient to report signs and symptoms of increased bleeding or bruising.

orlistat
ORE-lah-stat

Alli ◇, Xenical

Therapeutic class: Antiobesity drugs
Pharmacologic class: Lipase inhibitors
Pregnancy risk category: X

AVAILABLE FORMS
Capsules: 60 mg ◇, 120 mg

INDICATIONS & DOSAGES
➤ **To manage obesity, including weight loss and weight maintenance with a reduced-calorie diet; to reduce risk of weight gain after previous weight loss**
Adults and children ages 12 to 16: 120 mg P.O. t.i.d. with or up to 1 hour after each main meal containing fat.
➤ **Weight loss (OTC formulation)**
Adults age 18 and older: One 60-mg capsule P.O. with each meal containing fat. Dosage shouldn't exceed 3 capsules a day.

ADMINISTRATION
P.O.
• Give drug with each main meal containing fat (during or up to 1 hour after the meal).

ACTION
Forms a bond with active site of gastric and pancreatic lipases, inactivating them. As a result, enzymes can't hydrolyze dietary triglycerides into absorbable free fatty acids and monoglycerides. The undigested triglycerides are not absorbed, resulting in caloric deficit.

Route	Onset	Peak	Duration
P.O.	Unknown	Unknown	Unknown

Half-life: 1 to 2 hours.

ADVERSE REACTIONS
CNS: headache, dizziness, fatigue, sleep disorder, anxiety, depression.
CV: pedal edema.
EENT: otitis.
GI: flatus with discharge, fecal urgency, fatty or oily stool, oily spotting, increased defecation, abdominal pain, fecal incontinence, nausea, infectious diarrhea, rectal pain, vomiting.
GU: menstrual irregularity, vaginitis, UTI.
Musculoskeletal: back pain, leg pain, arthritis, myalgia, joint disorder, tendinitis.
Respiratory: upper respiratory tract infection, lower respiratory tract infection.
Skin: rash, dry skin.
Other: tooth and gingival disorders, influenza.

INTERACTIONS
Drug-drug. *Cyclosporine:* May decrease cyclosporine levels, risking organ rejection in transplant patients. Avoid using together.
Fat-soluble vitamins (such as vitamins A and E and beta-carotene): May decrease absorption of vitamins. Separate doses by 2 hours.
Warfarin: May change coagulation values. Monitor INR.

EFFECTS ON LAB TEST RESULTS
None reported.

CONTRAINDICATIONS & CAUTIONS
• Contraindicated in patients hypersensitive to drug or its components and in those with chronic malabsorption syndrome or cholestasis.
• Use cautiously in patients with history of hyperoxaluria or calcium oxalate

---

nephrolithiasis or those at risk for anorexia nervosa or bulimia.

• Use cautiously in patients receiving cyclosporine therapy because of potential changes in cyclosporine absorption related to variations in dietary intake.

NURSING CONSIDERATIONS

• Exclude organic causes of obesity, such as hypothyroidism, before starting drug therapy.

• Drug is recommended for use in patients with an initial body mass index (BMI) of 30 or more or those with a BMI of 27 or more and other risk factors (such as hypertension, diabetes, or dyslipidemia).

❸ *Alert:* Drug may cause pancreatitis or, rarely, liver dysfunction, including liver failure. Monitor patient closely.

• In diabetic patients, dosage of oral antidiabetic or insulin may need to be reduced because improved metabolic control may accompany weight loss.

• As with other weight-loss drugs, potential for misuse exists in certain patients (such as those with anorexia nervosa or bulimia).

• *Look alike–sound alike:* Don't confuse Xenical with Xeloda.

PATIENT TEACHING

• Advise patient to follow a nutritionally balanced, reduced-calorie diet that derives only 30% of its calories from fat. Tell him to distribute daily intake of fat, carbohydrate, and protein over three main meals. If a meal is occasionally missed or contains no fat, tell patient that dose of drug can be omitted.

• Advise patient to adhere to dietary guidelines. GI effects may increase when patient takes drug with high-fat foods, specifically when more than 30% of total daily calories come from fat.

• Drug reduces absorption of some fat-soluble vitamins and beta-carotene.

• Tell patient with diabetes that weight loss may improve his glycemic control, so dosage of his oral antidiabetic (such as a sulfonylurea or metformin) or insulin may need to be reduced during drug therapy.

• Tell women of childbearing age to inform prescriber if pregnancy or breast-feeding is planned during therapy.

• Advise patient to report signs and symptoms of liver injury, such as loss of appetite, itching, yellowing of skin, dark urine, light-colored stools, or right upper quadrant abdominal pain.

oseltamivir phosphate
oz-el-TAM-ah-ver

Tamiflu

Therapeutic class: Antivirals
Pharmacologic class: Selective neuraminidase inhibitors
Pregnancy risk category: C

AVAILABLE FORMS
Capsules: 30 mg, 45 mg, 75 mg
Oral suspension: 6 mg/mL after reconstitution

INDICATIONS & DOSAGES
➤ **To prevent influenza during a community outbreak**
Adults and adolescents age 13 and older: 75 mg P.O. once daily for up to 6 weeks.
Children ages 1 to 12 weighing 41 kg (90 lb) or more: 75 mg (12.5 mL) P.O. once daily for 10 days.
Children ages 1 to 12 weighing 24 to 40 kg (53 to 88 lb): 60 mg (10 mL) P.O. once daily for 10 days.
Children ages 1 to 12 weighing 16 to 23 kg (35 to 51 lb): 45 mg (7.5 mL) P.O. once daily for 10 days.
Children ages 1 to 12 weighing 15 kg (33 lb) or less: 30 mg (5 mL) P.O. once daily for 10 days.
Adjust-a-dose: For adults and adolescents with CrCl of 10 to 30 mL/minute, reduce dosage to 75 mg P.O. every other day or 30 mg once daily.
➤ **To treat influenza**
Adults and adolescents age 13 and older: 75 mg P.O. b.i.d. for 5 days. Begin treatment within 2 days of onset of influenza symptoms.
Children ages 1 to 12 weighing 41 kg or more: 75 mg (12.5 mL) P.O. b.i.d. for 5 days.
Children ages 1 to 12 weighing 24 to 40 kg: 60 mg (10 mL) P.O. b.i.d. for 5 days.

Children ages 1 to 12 weighing 16 to 23 kg:
45 mg (7.5 mL) P.O. b.i.d. for 5 days.
*Children ages 1 to 12 weighing 15 kg or
less:* 30 mg (5 mL) P.O. b.i.d. for 5 days.
*Children ages 2 weeks to younger than
1 year:* 3 mg/kg P.O. b.i.d. for 5 days. Begin
treatment within 2 days of influenza onset.
Adjust-a-dose: For adults and adolescents
with CrCl of 10 to 30 mL/minute, reduce
dosage to 75 mg P.O. once daily for 5 days.

➤ **To prevent influenza after close contact
with infected person within 2 days of
exposure; to prevent H1N1 influenza A ◆**
Adults and adolescents age 13 and older:
75 mg P.O. once daily for at least 10 days.
*Children age 1 and older weighing more
than 40 kg:* 75 mg P.O. once daily for
10 days.
*Children age 1 and older weighing 23 to
40 kg:* 60 mg P.O. once daily for 10 days.
*Children age 1 and older weighing 15 to
23 kg:* 45 mg P.O. once daily for 10 days.
*Children age 1 and older weighing 15 kg or
less:* 30 mg oral suspension P.O. once daily
for 10 days.

➤ **To prevent H1N1 influenza A in
children younger than age 12 months ◆**
Children ages 6 to 11 months: 25 mg P.O.
once daily for 10 days.
Children ages 3 to 5 months: 20 mg P.O.
once daily for 10 days.

➤ **To treat H1N1 influenza A ◆**
Adults: 75 mg P.O. b.i.d. for 5 days.
*Children age 1 and older weighing more
than 40 kg:* 75 mg P.O. b.i.d. for 5 days.
*Children age 1 and older weighing more
than 23 kg to 40 kg:* 60 mg P.O. b.i.d. for
5 days.
*Children age 1 and older weighing more
than 15 kg to 23 kg:* 45 mg P.O. b.i.d. for
5 days.
*Children age 1 and older weighing less than
15 kg:* 30 mg P.O. b.i.d. for 5 days.
Children ages 6 to 11 months: 25 mg P.O.
b.i.d. for 5 days.
Children ages 3 to 5 months: 20 mg P.O.
b.i.d. for 5 days.
Children younger than age 3 months: 12 mg
P.O. b.i.d. for 5 days.

ADMINISTRATION
P.O.
● Give drug with meals to decrease GI
adverse effects.
● Store at controlled room temperature
(59° to 86° F [15° to 30° C]).
● Capsules may be opened and mixed with
sweetened liquids such as chocolate syrup.
● Shake oral suspension well before use.

ACTION
Inhibits influenza A and B virus enzyme
neuraminidase, which is thought to play a
role in viral particle aggregation and release
from the host cell and appears to interfere
with viral replication.

Route	Onset	Peak	Duration
P.O.	Unknown	Unknown	Unknown

Half-life: 1 to 10 hours.

ADVERSE REACTIONS
CNS: dizziness, fatigue, headache, insomnia, vertigo.
EENT: epistaxis, sinusitis, conjunctivitis,
ear disorder, otitis media, tympanic membrane disorder (children).
GI: abdominal pain, diarrhea, nausea,
vomiting.
Respiratory: bronchitis, cough, asthma
(children).
Skin: dermatitis (children).
Other: lymphadenopathy (children).

INTERACTIONS
None significant.

EFFECTS ON LAB TEST RESULTS
None reported.

CONTRAINDICATIONS & CAUTIONS
● Contraindicated in patients hypersensitive
to drug or its components.
● Use cautiously in patients with chronic
cardiac or respiratory diseases, or any
medical condition that may require imminent hospitalization. Also use cautiously
in patients with renal failure.
● Don't administer live attenuated influenza
vaccine within 2 weeks before or 48 hours
after oseltamivir administration unless
medically indicated.

• It's unknown if drug or its metabolite appears in breast milk. Use only if benefits to patient outweigh risks to infant.

⚠ Overdose S&S: Nausea, vomiting.

NURSING CONSIDERATIONS

• Drug must be given within 2 days of onset of symptoms.

• Safety and effectiveness of repeated treatment courses haven't been established.

⊙ Alert: Closely monitor patients with influenza for neuropsychiatric symptoms, such as hallucinations, delirium, and abnormal behavior. Risks and benefits of continuing drug should be evaluated.

PATIENT TEACHING

• Instruct patient to begin treatment as soon as possible after appearance of flu symptoms.

• Inform patient that drug may be taken with or without meals. If nausea or vomiting occurs, he can take drug with food or milk.

• Tell patient that, if a dose is missed, he should take it as soon as possible. However, if next dose is due within 2 hours, tell him to skip the missed dose and take the next dose on schedule.

• Advise patient to complete the full course of treatment, even if symptoms resolve.

• Alert patient that drug isn't a replacement for the annual influenza vaccination. Patients for whom vaccine is indicated should continue to receive the vaccine each fall.

✴ NEW DRUG

ospemifene
os-PEM-i-feen

Osphena

Therapeutic class: Selective estrogen receptor modulators
Pharmacologic class: Selective estrogen agonist/antagonists
Pregnancy risk category: X

AVAILABLE FORMS
Tablets: 60 mg

INDICATIONS & DOSAGES
➤ **Moderate to severe dyspareunia due to menopause**
Adults: 60 mg P.O. once daily.

ADMINISTRATION
P.O.
• Give with food.
• Store medication at room temperature.

ACTION
Binds to estrogen receptors, activating estrogenic pathways in some tissues (agonism) and blocking estrogenic pathways in others (antagonism).

Route	Onset	Peak	Duration
P.O.	Unknown	2 hr	Unknown

Half-life: 26 hours.

ADVERSE REACTIONS
CV: hot flush.
GU: vaginal or genital discharge.
Musculoskeletal: muscle spasms.
Skin: hyperhidrosis.

INTERACTIONS
Drug-drug. *CYP2C9, CYP2C19, CYP3A4 inducers (rifampin):* May decrease ospemifene level, decreasing therapeutic effect. Avoid use together.
CYP2C9, CYP2C19 , CYP3A4 inhibitors (fluconazole, ketoconazole, omeprazole): May increase ospemifene level, increasing risk of ospemifene-related adverse effects. Avoid use together.
Estrogen agonists–antagonists, estrogens: Safety of concomitant use hasn't been established. Don't use together.

EFFECTS ON LAB TEST RESULTS
None reported.

CONTRAINDICATIONS & CAUTIONS
• Contraindicated in women hypersensitive to drug or its components; in those with severe hepatic impairment, undiagnosed abnormal genital bleeding, or known or suspected estrogen-dependent neoplasm; in those with active or previous DVT or PE or active or previous arterial thromboembolic disease (stroke, MI); and in women who are pregnant or may become pregnant.

• Don't use in women with known or suspected breast cancer or in those with a history of breast cancer. Drug hasn't been studied in this population.
• Use cautiously in women with an increased risk of CV disorders, arterial vascular disease, or venous thromboembolism (obesity, systemic lupus erythematosus, family history, personal history).
• It isn't known if drug appears in breast milk.

NURSING CONSIDERATIONS

Black Box Warning Risk of endometrial cancer is increased in women with a uterus who use unopposed estrogens; consider adding a progestin in these women. Women without a uterus don't need a progestin. Evaluate patient for uterine cancer if patient experiences persistent abnormal genital bleeding. ■

Black Box Warning Postmenopausal women who received daily oral conjugated estrogens as part of the Women's Health Initiative experienced an increased risk of stroke and DVT. To reduce these risks, this drug should be used for the shortest period of time necessary. Periodically reevaluate the need to continue therapy. ■

• Discontinue drug immediately if a venous thromboembolism or thromboembolic or hemorrhagic stroke is suspected or occurs.
• Discontinue drug at least 4 to 6 weeks before surgery that's associated with an increased risk of thromboembolism or during periods of extended immobilization.

PATIENT TEACHING

• Instruct patient to take drug with food for better absorption.
• Inform patient that drug may initiate or worsen hot flashes.
• Advise patient to immediately report unusual vaginal discharge or bleeding.

SAFETY ALERT!

oxaliplatin
ox-ah-li-PLA-tin

Eloxatin

Therapeutic class: Antineoplastics
Pharmacologic class: Platinum-containing compounds
Pregnancy risk category: D

AVAILABLE FORMS
Solution for injection: 5 mg/mL in 10-mL, 20-mL, and 40-mL single-use vials

INDICATIONS & DOSAGES
➤ **First-line treatment of advanced colorectal cancer with 5-FU and leucovorin (5-FU/LV)**
Adults: On day 1, give 85 mg/m^2 oxaliplatin I.V. in 250 to 500 mL D$_5$W and leucovorin 200 mg/m^2 I.V. in D$_5$W simultaneously over 120 minutes, in separate bags using a Y-line, followed by 5-FU 400 mg/m^2 I.V. bolus over 2 to 4 minutes, followed by 600 mg/m^2 5-FU I.V. infusion in 500 mL D$_5$W over 22 hours.

On day 2, give 200 mg/m^2 leucovorin I.V. infusion over 120 minutes, followed by 400 mg/m^2 5-FU I.V. bolus over 2 to 4 minutes, followed by 600 mg/m^2 5-FU I.V. infusion in 500 mL D$_5$W over 22 hours.

Repeat cycle every 2 weeks.
Adjust-a-dose: In patients with unresolved and persistent grade 2 neurosensory events, reduce oxaliplatin to 65 mg/m^2. In those with persistent grade 3 neurosensory events, consider stopping drug. In patients recovering from grade 3 or 4 GI or hematologic events, reduce dose to 65 mg/m^2 and reduce dose of 5-FU by 20%. Delay dose until neutrophil count is 1.5×10^9/L or more and platelet count is 75×10^9/L or more.
➤ **With 5-FU/LV for the adjuvant treatment of stage III colon cancer in patients who have had complete resection of the primary tumor**
Adults: On day 1, give oxaliplatin, 85 mg/m^2 I.V. in 250 to 500 mL D$_5$W and 200 mg/m^2 leucovorin I.V. infusion in D$_5$W, both over 120 minutes at the same time, in separate bags, using a Y-line. Follow with 400 mg/m^2

Reactions in bold italics are *life-threatening*. Interactions may have a *rapid onset* or a *delayed onset*.

5-FU I.V. bolus over 2 to 4 minutes, then 600 mg/m^2 5-FU in 500 mL D$_5$W as a 22-hour continuous infusion.

On day 2, give leucovorin, 200 mg/m^2 I.V. infused over 120 minutes, followed by 400 mg/m^2 5-FU as an I.V. bolus over 2 to 4 minutes, then 600 mg/m^2 5-FU in 500 mL D$_5$W as a 22-hour infusion.

Repeat cycle every 2 weeks for a total of 6 months. Premedicate with antiemetics, with or without dexamethasone.

Adjust-a-dose: For patients with persistent grade 2 neurotoxicity, consider an oxaliplatin dose reduction to 75 mg/m^2. For patients who recovered from grade 4 neutropenia, grade 3 or 4 thrombocytopenia, or a grade 3 or 4 GI event, reduce oxaliplatin to 75 mg/m^2 and 5-FU to a 300 mg/m^2 bolus and 500 mg/m^2 22-hour infusion. Delay dose until neutrophils are 1.5×10^9/L or more and platelets are 75×10^9/L or more.

ADMINISTRATION

I.V.

▼ Preparing and giving drug may be mutagenic, teratogenic, or carcinogenic. Follow facility policy to reduce risks.

▼ Reconstitute powder using sterile water for injection or D$_5$W. Add 10 mL to a 50-mg vial or 20 mL to a 100-mg vial, for a yield of 5 mg/mL. Never reconstitute with sodium chloride solution or other solution containing chloride.

▼ Reconstituted solutions must be further diluted in an infusion solution of 250 to 500 mL of D$_5$W.

▼ Inspect bag for particulate matter and discoloration before giving, and discard if present.

▼ Don't use needles or I.V. administration sets that contain aluminum because it displaces the platinum, causing it to lose potency and form a black precipitate.

▼ Give oxaliplatin and leucovorin over 2 hours at the same time in separate bags, using a Y-line. Extend the infusion time to 6 hours to decrease acute toxicities.

▼ Store unopened vials at room temperature. Reconstituted solutions are stable if refrigerated (36° to 46° F [2° to 8° C]) for up to 24 hours. After final dilution, solutions are stable for 6 hours at room temperature and up to 24 hours under refrigeration.

▼ **Incompatibilities:** Alkaline solutions or drugs such as 5-FU. Flush infusion line with D$_5$W before giving any other drugs simultaneously.

ACTION

Probably inhibits cell replication and transcription by forming platinum complexes that cross-link with DNA molecules. Not specific to cell cycle.

Route	Onset	Peak	Duration
I.V.	Unknown	Unknown	Unknown

Half-life: 391 hours (gamma phase).

ADVERSE REACTIONS

CNS: pain, peripheral neuropathy, fatigue, headache, dizziness, insomnia, fever, anxiety, depression.

CV: chest pain, *thromboembolism,* edema, flushing, peripheral edema, hypotension.

EENT: rhinitis, pharyngolaryngeal dysesthesias, pharyngitis, epistaxis, abnormal lacrimation.

GI: nausea, vomiting, diarrhea, stomatitis, abdominal pain, anorexia, constipation, dyspepsia, taste perversion, gastroesophageal reflux, flatulence, mucositis.

GU: dysuria, hematuria.

Hematologic: *febrile neutropenia,* anemia, *leukopenia, thrombocytopenia.*

Hepatic: veno-occlusive disease.

Metabolic: *hypokalemia,* dehydration.

Musculoskeletal: back pain, arthralgia, myalgia.

Respiratory: dyspnea, cough, upper respiratory tract infection, hiccups, *pulmonary toxicity.*

Skin: injection-site reaction, rash, alopecia, dry skin, flushing, pruritus, sweating.

Other: *anaphylaxis,* hand-foot syndrome, allergic reaction, rigors.

INTERACTIONS

Drug-drug. *Clozapine:* May increase risk of agranulocytosis. Avoid use together.

Denosumab: May increase risk of serious infections. Monitor therapy.

Digoxin (oral): May decrease digoxin absorption. Monitor therapy.

Fosphenytoin, phenytoin: May decrease serum concentration of fosphenytoin and phenytoin. Monitor therapy.

Leflunomide: May increase risk of pancytopenia, agranulocytosis, or thrombocytopenia. Consider not using a leflunomide loading dose in patients receiving other immunosuppressants. Monitor patient for bone marrow suppression at least monthly. Consider therapy modification.

Live-virus vaccines, pimecrolimus, tacrolimus (topical): May enhance adverse or toxic effects of these drugs. Avoid combination.

Natalizumab: May enhance adverse or toxic effect of natalizumab; specifically, may increase risk of concurrent infection. Avoid combination.

Nephrotoxic drugs (such as gentamicin): May decrease elimination of these drugs and increase gentamicin level. Monitor patient for toxicity.

Roflumilast: May enhance immunosuppressive effect of roflumilast. Consider therapy modification.

Sipuleucel-T: May diminish sipuleucel-T therapeutic effect. Monitor therapy.

Taxane derivatives: May enhance myelosuppressive effect of taxane derivatives. Administer taxane derivative before platinum derivative when given as sequential infusions to limit toxicity. Consider therapy modification.

Tofacitinib: May enhance immunosuppressive effect of tofacitinib. Avoid combination.

Topotecan: May enhance adverse or toxic effect of topotecan. Consider therapy modification.

Trastuzumab: May increase neutropenia. Monitor therapy.

Vaccines (inactivated): May diminish therapeutic effect of inactivated vaccines. Monitor therapy.

Vitamin K antagonists (warfarin): May enhance anticoagulant effect of vitamin K antagonists. Monitor therapy and adjust vitamin K antagonist dosage as needed.

EFFECTS ON LAB TEST RESULTS

● May increase glucose, creatinine, bilirubin, AST, and ALT levels. May decrease potassium, albumin, calcium, sodium, and hemoglobin levels.

● May decrease neutrophil, WBC, and platelet counts.

CONTRAINDICATIONS & CAUTIONS

● Contraindicated in patients allergic to drug or other platinum-containing compounds and in pregnant or breast-feeding patients.

● Oxaliplatin may cause early-onset (occurs within hours or 1 to 2 days) or persistent (greater than 14 days) peripheral sensory neuropathy.

● Oxaliplatin has been associated with rare, sometimes fatal, pulmonary fibrosis.

● Extravasation of oxaliplatin can cause tissue necrosis. If extravasation occurs, stop infusion and notify health care provider immediately.

● Use cautiously in patients with renal impairment or peripheral sensory neuropathy.

⚠ *Overdose S&S:* Thrombocytopenia, dyspnea, wheezing, paresthesia, vomiting, chest pain, respiratory failure, bradycardia, dysesthesia, laryngospasm, myelosuppression, nausea, diarrhea, neurotoxicity.

NURSING CONSIDERATIONS

● Administer drug under the supervision of a physician experienced in the use of cancer chemotherapeutic agents.

● Premedication with antiemetics, including 5-HT$_3$ receptor antagonists with or without dexamethasone, is recommended.

● Drug doesn't require patient prehydration.

● Give antiemetic with or without dexamethasone before drug to reduce nausea.

● Drug clearance is reduced in patients with renal impairment. Dosage adjustment for patients with renal impairment hasn't been established.

● Monitor CBC, platelet count, and liver and kidney function before each chemotherapy cycle.

Black Box Warning Monitor patient for anaphylactic reactions, which may occur within minutes of administration. Keep epinephrine, corticosteroids, and antihistamines available. ■

● Monitor patient for injection-site reaction; extravasation may occur.

● Monitor patient for neuropathy and pulmonary toxicity. Peripheral neuropathy may be acute or persistent. Acute neuropathy is reversible; it occurs within 2 days of dosing and resolves within 14 days. Persistent peripheral neuropathy occurs more than 14 days after dosing and causes paresthesias, dysesthesias, hypoesthesias, and other neurologic impairment that can interfere with daily activities (such as walking or swallowing).

• Avoid ice and cold exposure during infusion of drug because cold temperatures can worsen acute neurologic symptoms. Cover patient with a blanket during infusion.

• Diarrhea, dehydration, hypokalemia, and fatigue may occur more frequently in elderly patients.

PATIENT TEACHING

• Inform patient of potential adverse reactions.

• Tell patient to avoid exposure to cold or cold objects (such as cold drinks or ice cubes), which can bring on or worsen acute symptoms of peripheral neuropathy. Advise patient to drink warm drinks, wear warm clothing, and cover any exposed skin (hands, face, and head).

• Tell patient to contact prescriber immediately if he has trouble breathing or experiences signs and symptoms of an allergic reaction, such as rash, hives, swelling of lips or tongue, or sudden cough.

• Tell patient to contact prescriber if fever, signs and symptoms of an infection, persistent vomiting, diarrhea, or signs and symptoms of dehydration (thirst, dry mouth, light-headedness, and decreased urination) occur.

• Caution women of childbearing age not to becoming pregnant during therapy.

SAFETY ALERT!

oxazepam
ox-AZ-e-pam

Novoxapam†, Oxpam†

Therapeutic class: Anxiolytics
Pharmacologic class: Benzodiazepines
Pregnancy risk category: D
Controlled substance schedule: IV

AVAILABLE FORMS
Capsules: 10 mg, 15 mg, 30 mg

INDICATIONS & DOSAGES
➤ **Alcohol withdrawal, severe anxiety**
Adults: 15 to 30 mg P.O. t.i.d. or q.i.d.
➤ **Mild to moderate anxiety**
Adults and children older than age 12: 10 to 15 mg P.O. t.i.d. or q.i.d.
Elderly patients: Initially, 10 mg P.O. t.i.d.; cautiously increase to 15 mg t.i.d. to q.i.d.
➤ **Severe anxiety syndromes; agitation; anxiety associated with depression**
Adults and children older than age 12: 15 to 30 mg P.O. t.i.d. or q.i.d.
➤ **Anxiety, tension, irritability, agitation**
Elderly patients: 10 mg P.O. t.i.d. May increase cautiously to 15 mg t.i.d. or q.i.d.

ADMINISTRATION
P.O.
• Give drug without regard for meals.

ACTION
May stimulate GABA receptors in the ascending reticular activating system.

Route	Onset	Peak	Duration
P.O.	Unknown	3 hr	Unknown

Half-life: 5 to 13 hours.

ADVERSE REACTIONS
CNS: drowsiness, lethargy, dizziness, vertigo, headache, syncope, tremor, slurred speech, changes in EEG patterns.
CV: edema.
GI: nausea.
Hepatic: *hepatic dysfunction.*
Skin: rash.
Other: altered libido.

INTERACTIONS
Drug-drug. *CNS depressants:* May increase CNS depression. Use together cautiously.
Digoxin: May increase digoxin level and risk of toxicity. Monitor patient closely.
Drug-herb. *Kava:* May increase sedation. Discourage use together.
Drug-lifestyle. *Alcohol use:* May cause additive CNS effects. Discourage use together.

EFFECTS ON LAB TEST RESULTS
• May increase LFT values.

CONTRAINDICATIONS & CAUTIONS

• Contraindicated in patients hypersensitive to drug; in pregnant women, especially in the first trimester; and in those with psychoses.

• Use cautiously in elderly patients and in those with history of substance abuse or in whom a decrease in blood pressure might lead to cardiac problems.

⚠ **Overdose S&S:** Drowsiness, confusion, lethargy, ataxia, hypotonia, hypotension, hypnotic state, stage 1 to 3 coma, death.

NURSING CONSIDERATIONS

• Monitor hepatic, renal, and hematopoietic function periodically in patients receiving repeated or prolonged therapy.

❸ **Alert:** Use of this drug may lead to abuse and addiction. Don't stop drug abruptly because withdrawal symptoms may occur.

• **Look alike–sound alike:** Don't confuse oxazepam with oxaprozin.

PATIENT TEACHING

• Warn patient to avoid hazardous activities that require alertness or good coordination until effects of drug are known.

• Tell patient to avoid use of alcohol while taking drug.

• Notify patient that smoking may decrease drug's effectiveness.

• Warn patient not to stop drug abruptly because withdrawal symptoms may occur.

• Warn women of childbearing age to avoid use during pregnancy.

oxcarbazepine
oks-car-BAZ-e-peen

Oxtellar XR, Trileptal

Therapeutic class: Anticonvulsants
Pharmacologic class: Carboxamide derivatives
Pregnancy risk category: C

AVAILABLE FORMS

Oral suspension: 300 mg/5 mL (60 mg/mL)
Tablets (extended-release): 150 mg, 300 mg, 600 mg
Tablets (film-coated): 150 mg, 300 mg, 600 mg

INDICATIONS & DOSAGES

Adjust-a-dose (for all indications): If CrCl is less than 30 mL/minute, start therapy at 150 mg P.O. b.i.d. (one-half usual starting dose) and increase slowly to achieve desired response.

➤ **Adjunctive treatment of partial seizures in patients with epilepsy**
Adults: Initially, 300 mg P.O. b.i.d. Increase by a maximum of 600 mg daily (300 mg P.O. b.i.d.) at weekly intervals. Recommended daily dose is 1,200 mg P.O. divided b.i.d. Or, 600 mg extended-release tablets P.O. daily. May increase at weekly intervals in 600-mg/day increments.

Children ages 4 to 16 (immediate-release): Initially, 8 to 10 mg/kg P.O. daily in two divided doses, not to exceed 600 mg daily. The target maintenance dose depends on patient's weight and should be divided in two doses. If patient weighs between 20 and 29 kg (44 and 64 lb), target maintenance dose is 900 mg daily. If patient weighs between 29 and 39 kg (64 and 86 lb), target maintenance dose is 1,200 mg daily. If patient weighs more than 39 kg (86 lb), target maintenance dose is 1,800 mg daily. Target doses should be achieved over 2 weeks.

Children ages 2 to 4 (immediate-release): Initially, 8 to 10 mg/kg P.O. daily in two divided doses, not to exceed 600 mg daily. If patient weighs less than 20 kg, a starting dose of 16 to 20 mg/kg may be considered. Maximum maintenance dosage should be achieved over 2 to 4 weeks and shouldn't exceed 60 mg/kg/day in a two-dose divided regimen.

Children ages 6 to 17 (extended-release): 8 to 10 mg/kg P.O. once daily, not to exceed 600 mg daily in first week. May increase at weekly intervals in 8- to 10-mg/kg increments once daily, not to exceed 600 mg. Target daily dose in patients weighing more than 39 kg is 1,800 mg/day; from 29.1 to 39 kg, 1,200 mg/day; and from 20 to 29 kg, 900 mg/day.

Elderly patients: When using extended-release tablets, consider a lower starting dose (300 or 450 mg/day). Dosage increases can be made at weekly intervals in increments of 300 to 450 mg/day.

➤ **To change from multidrug to single-drug treatment of partial seizures in patients with epilepsy**
Adults: Initially, 300 mg P.O. b.i.d., while reducing dose of concomitant anticonvulsant. Increase oxcarbazepine by a maximum of 600 mg daily at weekly intervals over 2 to 4 weeks. Recommended daily dose is 2,400 mg P.O. in two divided doses. Withdraw other anticonvulsant completely over 3 to 6 weeks.
Children ages 4 to 16: Initially, 8 to 10 mg/kg P.O. daily in two divided doses, while reducing dose of concomitant anticonvulsant. Increase oxcarbazepine by a maximum of 10 mg/kg daily at weekly intervals to achieve the recommended daily dose shown in the table. Withdraw other anticonvulsant completely over 3 to 6 weeks.
➤ **To start single-drug treatment of partial seizures in patients with epilepsy**
Adults: Initially, 300 mg P.O. b.i.d. Increase dosage by 300 mg daily every third day to a daily dose of 1,200 mg in two divided doses.
Children ages 4 to 16: Initially, 8 to 10 mg/kg P.O. daily in two divided doses, increasing the dosage by 5 mg/kg daily every third day to the recommended daily dose range shown in the table.

Recommended doses for monotherapy

Weight (kg)	Dose (mg/day)
20	600–900
25	900–1,200
30	900–1,200
35	900–1,500
40	900–1,500
45	1,200–1,500
50	1,200–1,800
55	1,200–1,800
60	1,200–2,100
65	1,200–2,100
70	1,500–2,100

➤ **Alcohol withdrawal syndrome ◆**
Adults: 600 to 1,800 mg P.O. in divided doses for 6 weeks to 6 months.

ADMINISTRATION
P.O.
● Shake suspension well.
● Mix suspension with water or give directly from syringe.

● Give immediate-release tablets without regard for food.
● Give extended-release tablets on an empty stomach (at least 1 hour before or 2 hours after a meal). Don't cut or crush tablets. For ease of swallowing, use multiple lower-strength tablets for appropriate dose.
● When converting from immediate-release to extended-release form, higher doses may be needed.

ACTION
Thought to prevent seizure spread in the brain by blocking voltage-sensitive sodium channels and to produce anticonvulsant effects by increasing potassium conduction and modulating high-voltage activated calcium channels.

Route	Onset	Peak	Duration
P.O.	Unknown	Variable	Unknown

Half-life: Immediate-release: About 2 hours for the drug; about 9 hours for the active metabolite. Children younger than age 8 have a 30% to 40% increase in clearance. Extended-release: 7 to 11 hours.

ADVERSE REACTIONS
CNS: abnormal gait, ataxia, dizziness, fatigue, headache, somnolence, tremor, vertigo, *aggravated seizures,* abnormal coordination, agitation, amnesia, anxiety, asthenia, confusion, emotional lability, feeling abnormal, fever, hypesthesia, impaired concentration, insomnia, nervousness, speech disorder.
CV: chest pain, edema, hypotension.
EENT: abnormal vision, diplopia, nystagmus, abnormal accommodation, ear pain, epistaxis, pharyngitis, rhinitis, sinusitis.
GI: abdominal pain, nausea, vomiting, *rectal hemorrhage,* anorexia, constipation, diarrhea, dry mouth, dyspepsia, gastritis, taste perversion, thirst.
GU: urinary frequency, UTI, vaginitis.
Metabolic: hyponatremia, weight increase.
Musculoskeletal: back pain, muscular weakness.
Respiratory: upper respiratory tract infection, bronchitis, chest infection, coughing.
Skin: acne, bruising, hot flashes, increased sweating, purpura, rash.

Other: allergic reaction, infection, lymphadenopathy, toothache.

INTERACTIONS

Drug-drug. *Carbamazepine, valproic acid, verapamil:* May decrease level of active metabolite of oxcarbazepine. Monitor patient and level closely.

Felodipine: May decrease felodipine level. Monitor patient closely.

Hormonal contraceptives: May decrease levels of ethinyl estradiol and levonorgestrel, reducing hormonal contraceptive effectiveness. Caution women of childbearing age to use alternative forms of contraception.

Phenobarbital: May decrease level of active metabolite of oxcarbazepine; may increase phenobarbital level. Monitor patient closely.

Phenytoin: May decrease level of active metabolite of oxcarbazepine; may increase phenytoin level in adults receiving high doses of oxcarbazepine. Monitor phenytoin level closely when starting therapy in these patients.

Drug-lifestyle. *Alcohol use:* May increase CNS depression. Discourage use together.

EFFECTS ON LAB TEST RESULTS

• May decrease sodium and thyroxine levels.

CONTRAINDICATIONS & CAUTIONS

• Contraindicated in patients hypersensitive to drug or its components.

NURSING CONSIDERATIONS

🛈 **Alert:** Between 25% and 30% of patients with history of hypersensitivity reaction to carbamazepine may develop hypersensitivities to oxcarbazepine. Ask patient about carbamazepine hypersensitivity and stop drug immediately if signs or symptoms of hypersensitivity occur.

🛈 **Alert:** Closely monitor all patients taking or starting antiepileptic drugs for changes in behavior indicating worsening of suicidal thoughts or behavior or depression. Symptoms such as anxiety, agitation, hostility, mania, and hypomania may be precursors to emerging suicidality.

🛈 **Alert:** Withdraw drug gradually to minimize potential for increased seizure frequency.

🛈 **Alert:** Rare serious and sometimes fatal dermatologic reactions can occur. If skin reactions occur, discontinue drug.

• Watch for signs and symptoms of hyponatremia, including nausea, malaise, headache, lethargy, confusion, and decreased sensation.

• Monitor sodium level in patients receiving oxcarbazepine for maintenance treatment, especially patients receiving other therapies that may decrease sodium levels.

• Oxcarbazepine use has been linked to several nervous system–related adverse reactions, including psychomotor slowing, difficulty with concentration, speech or language problems, somnolence, fatigue, and coordination abnormalities, such as ataxia and gait disturbances.

PATIENT TEACHING

• Tell patient to take drug with or without food. For extended-release, tell patient to take on an empty stomach and not to cut, crush, or chew tablets.

• Tell patient to contact prescriber before interrupting or stopping drug.

• Advise patient to report signs and symptoms of low sodium in the blood, such as nausea, malaise, headache, lethargy, and confusion.

🛈 **Alert:** Multiorgan hypersensitivity reactions may occur. Tell patient to report fever and swollen lymph nodes to prescriber.

🛈 **Alert:** Serious skin reactions, including Stevens-Johnson syndrome and toxic epidermal necrolysis, can occur. Advise patient to immediately report rashes to prescriber.

• Caution patient to avoid driving and other potentially hazardous activities that require mental alertness until effects of drug are known.

• Instruct woman using hormonal contraceptives to use alternative form of contraception while taking drug.

• Tell patient to avoid alcohol while taking drug.

• Advise patient to inform prescriber if he has ever experienced hypersensitivity reaction to carbamazepine.

Reactions in bold italics are *life-threatening*. Interactions may have a *rapid onset* or a *delayed onset*.

oxybutynin chloride
ox-i-BYOO-ti-nin

Ditropan, Ditropan XL, Gelnique, Oxytrol

Therapeutic class: Urinary antispasmodics
Pharmacologic class: Antimuscarinics
Pregnancy risk category: B

AVAILABLE FORMS
Syrup: 5 mg/5 mL
Tablets: 5 mg
Tablets (extended-release): 5 mg, 10 mg, 15 mg
Topical gel: 3%, 10%
Transdermal patch: 36-mg patch delivering 3.9 mg/day

INDICATIONS & DOSAGES
➤ **Uninhibited or reflex neurogenic bladder**
Adults: 5 mg P.O. b.i.d. to t.i.d., to maximum of 5 mg q.i.d.
Children age 5 and older: 5 mg P.O. b.i.d., to maximum of 5 mg t.i.d.
Elderly patients: A lower initial starting dose of 2.5 mg P.O. b.i.d. or t.i.d. is recommended.
➤ **Overactive bladder**
Adults: Initially, 5 mg Ditropan XL P.O. once daily. Dosage adjustments may be made weekly in 5-mg increments, as needed, to maximum of 30 mg P.O. daily. Or, apply one patch twice weekly to dry, intact skin on the abdomen, hip, or buttock. Or, 1 g topical gel (10%) or 3 pumps (84 mg) of 3% topical gel once daily applied to dry, intact skin on the abdomen, upper arms or shoulders, or thighs.
Elderly patients: A lower initial starting dose of 2.5 mg P.O. b.i.d. or t.i.d. is recommended.
➤ **Symptoms of detrusor overactivity associated with a neurologic condition (e.g., spina bifida)**
Children age 6 and older: 5 mg Ditropan XL P.O. once daily. May increase in 5-mg increments, as needed, to maximum of 20 mg P.O. daily.

ADMINISTRATION
P.O.
● Don't crush extended-release tablets.
● Give extended-release tablets without regard for food.
Topical
● Use immediately after sachets are opened.
● Apply to dry, intact skin on the abdomen, upper arms or shoulders, or thighs.
● Rotate application sites.
Transdermal
● Apply to dry, intact skin on the abdomen, hip, or buttock.
● Avoid reapplication to the same site within 7 days.
● Don't expose patch to sunlight.

ACTION
Relaxes smooth muscle of bladder by antagonizing muscarinic receptors, relieving symptoms of overactive bladder.

Route	Onset	Peak	Duration
P.O.	30–60 min	3–4 hr	6–10 hr
P.O. (extended-release)	Unknown	4–6 hr	24 hr
Topical	Unknown	Unknown	Unknown
Transdermal	24–48 hr	Varies	96 hr

Half-life: For tablets or oral solution, 2 to 3 hours; for extended-release tablets, 12 to 13 hours; for patch, 7 to 8 hours; for gel, 64 hours.

ADVERSE REACTIONS
CNS: dizziness, insomnia, restlessness, hallucinations, asthenia, fever, headache.
CV: palpitations, tachycardia, vasodilation.
EENT: mydriasis, cycloplegia, decreased lacrimation, amblyopia, blurred vision, dry eyes.
GI: constipation, dry mouth, nausea, vomiting, decreased GI motility, abdominal pain.
GU: urinary hesitancy, urine retention, impotence, UTI.
Skin: rash, decreased diaphoresis.
Other: suppression of lactation.
Transdermal patch
CNS: fatigue, somnolence, headache.
CV: flushing.
EENT: abnormal vision.
GI: dry mouth, diarrhea, abdominal pain, nausea, flatulence.
GU: dysuria.
Musculoskeletal: back pain.

O

Skin: pruritus, erythema, vesicles, macules, rash, burning at application site.

INTERACTIONS
Drug-drug. *Amantadine, anticholinergics:* May increase anticholinergic effects. Use together cautiously.
Beta blockers (such as atenolol), digoxin: May increase levels of these drugs. Monitor drug levels closely.
CNS depressants: May increase CNS effects. Use together cautiously.
CYP3A4 inhibitors (such as ketoconazole): May alter oxybutynin concentration. Use together cautiously.
Haloperidol: May decrease haloperidol level. Monitor drug level closely.
Drug-lifestyle. *Alcohol use:* May increase CNS effects. Discourage use together.
Exercise, hot weather: May cause heatstroke. Advise patient to use with caution in hot weather.

EFFECTS ON LAB TEST RESULTS
None reported.

CONTRAINDICATIONS & CAUTIONS
● Contraindicated in patients hypersensitive to drug or its components and in those with myasthenia gravis, GI obstruction, untreated angle-closure glaucoma, megacolon, adynamic ileus, severe colitis, ulcerative colitis with megacolon, urine or gastric retention, or obstructive uropathy.
● Contraindicated in elderly or debilitated patients with intestinal atony and in hemorrhaging patients with unstable CV status.
● Use cautiously in elderly, pregnant, or breast-feeding patients and in those with autonomic neuropathy, reflux esophagitis, or hepatic or renal disease.
● Extended-release form is not recommended for children who can't swallow the tablet whole without chewing, dividing, or crushing, or children younger than age 6.
● Use extended-release form cautiously in patients with bladder outflow obstruction, gastric obstruction, ulcerative colitis, intestinal atony, myasthenia gravis, or gastroesophageal reflux and in those taking drugs that worsen esophagitis (bisphosphonates).
⚠ **Overdose S&S:** Restlessness, tremors, irritability, seizures, delirium, hallucinations, flushing, fever, dehydration, cardiac arrhythmias, vomiting, urine retention, hypotension or hypertension, respiratory failure, paralysis, coma.

NURSING CONSIDERATIONS
● Before giving drug, get confirmation of neurogenic bladder by cystometry and rule out partial intestinal obstruction in patients with diarrhea, especially those with colostomy or ileostomy.
● If patient has UTI, treat him with antibiotics.
● Drug may aggravate symptoms of hyperthyroidism, coronary artery disease, heart failure, arrhythmias, tachycardia, hypertension, or prostatic hyperplasia.
● Obtain periodic cystometry as directed to evaluate response to therapy.
● Monitor patient for residual urine after voiding.
● Oxytrol for Women has been FDA-approved as an OTC product. The 3.9-mg/day patch should be applied to the skin every 4 days.
● *Look alike–sound alike:* Don't confuse Ditropan with diazepam or Dithranol. Don't confuse oxybutynin with Oxycontin.

PATIENT TEACHING
● Warn patient to avoid hazardous activities, such as operating machinery or driving, until CNS effects of drug are known.
● Caution patient that using drug during very hot weather may cause fever or heatstroke because it suppresses sweating.
● Tell patient to swallow Ditropan XL whole and not to chew or crush it.
● Instruct patient to measure syrup with a teaspoon.
● Advise patient to store drug in tightly closed container at 59° to 86° F (15° to 30° C).
● Instruct patient using transdermal patch to change patch twice a week and to choose a new application site with each new patch to avoid the same site within 7 days. Warn patient to only wear one patch at a time. Tell patient to dispose of old patches carefully in the trash in a manner that prevents accidental application or ingestion by children and pets.

Reactions in bold italics are *life-threatening*. Interactions may have a *rapid onset* or a *delayed onset*.

• Tell patient using transdermal patch to keep patch in sealed pouch until immediately before application, not to expose patch to sunlight, and to wear patch under clothing.

• Tell patient to remove patch before undergoing a magnetic resonance imaging scan.

• Advise patient using topical gel to rotate application sites.

• Advise patient to avoid alcohol while taking drug.

• Tell patient that drug may cause dry mouth.

SAFETY ALERT!

oxycodone hydrochloride
ox-i-KOE-done

OxyContin🖉, Oxecta, Oxy IR†, Roxicodone, Supeudol†

Therapeutic class: Opioid analgesics
Pharmacologic class: Opioids
Pregnancy risk category: B
Controlled substance schedule: II

AVAILABLE FORMS
Capsules: 5 mg
Oral solution: 5 mg/5 mL, 20 mg/mL
Suppository: 10 mg†, 20 mg†
Tablets (controlled-release): 10 mg, 15 mg, 20 mg, 30 mg, 40 mg, 60 mg, 80 mg
Tablets (immediate-release): 5 mg, 7.5 mg, 10 mg, 15 mg, 20 mg, 30 mg

INDICATIONS & DOSAGES
➤ **Moderate to severe pain**
Adults: 5 to 15 mg immediate-release form or oral solution P.O. every 4 to 6 hours. Titrate dosage based on response. Usual dosage is 10 to 30 mg every 4 hours p.r.n. For control of severe, chronic pain, give on a regularly scheduled basis every 4 to 6 hours. Or, one suppository P.R. t.i.d. to q.i.d. p.r.n.
➤ **Moderate to severe pain in patients not currently receiving opioids, who need a continuous, around-the-clock analgesic for an extended period of time**
Adults: 10 mg controlled-release tablets P.O. every 12 hours. May increase dose every 1 to 2 days as needed.

Adjust-a-dose: For elderly patients and patients with hepatic impairment, decrease initial starting dose by one-third to one-half.

ADMINISTRATION
P.O.
• To minimize GI upset, give drug after meals or with milk.
Black Box Warning Patient must swallow extended-release tablets whole. ∎
Black Box Warning The 60- and 80-mg controlled-release tablets, or a single 40-mg dose, or a total daily dose of more than 80 mg is limited to opioid-tolerant patients. ∎
• Don't crush or dissolve controlled-release tablets.
• Patients taking the controlled-release form around-the-clock may need to take the immediate-release form for worsening of pain or prevention of incident pain.
Rectal
• Chill wrapped suppository in refrigerator for 30 minutes or under cold running water if too soft to administer.

ACTION
Unknown. Binds with opioid receptors in the CNS, altering perception of and emotional response to pain.

Route	Onset	Peak	Duration
P.O. (immediate-release)	10–15 min	1 hr	3–6 hr
P.O. (controlled-release)	Unknown	2½ hr	12 hr
P.R.	Unknown	Unknown	Unknown

Half-life: 2 to 3 hours; controlled-release, 4.5 hours.

ADVERSE REACTIONS
CNS: clouded sensorium, dizziness, euphoria, light-headedness, physical dependence, sedation, somnolence, headache, asthenia.
CV: *bradycardia,* hypotension.
GI: constipation, nausea, vomiting, ileus.
GU: urine retention.
Respiratory: *respiratory depression.*
Skin: diaphoresis, pruritus.

INTERACTIONS
Drug-drug. *Anticoagulants:* Oxycodone hydrochloride products containing aspirin may increase anticoagulant effect. Monitor clotting times. Use together cautiously.

CNS depressants, general anesthetics, hypnotics, MAO inhibitors, other opioid analgesics, sedatives, TCAs, tranquilizers: May cause additive effects. Use together with caution. Reduce oxycodone dose and monitor patient response.

Black Box Warning *CYP3A4 inhibitors such as azole antifungals (ketoconazole), macrolide antibiotics (erythromycin), protease inhibitors (ritonavir):* May increase oxycodone level, increase or prolong adverse effects, and cause fatal respiratory depression. Carefully monitor patient over extended period of time and adjust oxycodone dosage as needed. ∎

Drug-lifestyle. *Alcohol use:* May cause additive effects. Discourage use together.

EFFECTS ON LAB TEST RESULTS
● May increase amylase and lipase levels.

CONTRAINDICATIONS & CAUTIONS
● Contraindicated in patients hypersensitive to drug.
● Contraindicated in known or suspected paralytic ileus, significant respiratory depression, and acute or severe bronchial asthma.
● Contraindicated in women immediately before and during labor and delivery, and in breast-feeding women.
● Use with caution in elderly and debilitated patients and in those with head injury, increased intracranial pressure, seizures, asthma, COPD, prostatic hyperplasia, severe hepatic or renal disease, acute abdominal conditions, urethral stricture, hypothyroidism, Addison disease, and arrhythmias.

Black Box Warning Patients must be screened for increased risk of opioid abuse (personal or family history of substance abuse or mental illness) before being prescribed opioids. ∎

Black Box Warning Oxycodone controlled-release tablets are indicated for the management of moderate to severe pain, when a continuous, around-the-clock opioid analgesic is needed for an extended period of time. They aren't intended for use as as-needed analgesics. ∎

⚠ Overdose S&S: CNS depression, respiratory depression, apnea, flaccid skeletal muscles, bradycardia, hypotension, circulatory collapse, cardiac arrest, respiratory arrest, death.

NURSING CONSIDERATIONS
● Reassess patient's level of pain at least 15 and 30 minutes after administration.
● For full analgesic effect, give drug before patient has intense pain.
● Single-drug oxycodone solution or tablets are especially useful for patients who shouldn't take aspirin or acetaminophen.
● Monitor circulatory and respiratory status. Withhold dose and notify prescriber if respirations are shallow or if respiratory rate falls below 12 breaths/minute.
● Monitor patient's bladder and bowel patterns. Patient may need a stimulant laxative because drug has a constipating effect.
● For patients who are taking more than 60 mg daily, stop drug gradually to prevent withdrawal symptoms.
● Drug isn't intended for as-needed use or for immediate postoperative pain. Drug is indicated only for postoperative use if patient was receiving it before surgery or if pain is expected to persist for an extended time.

Black Box Warning Drug is potentially addictive and is abused as much as morphine. Chewing, crushing, snorting, or injecting it can lead to overdose and death. ∎

Black Box Warning All patients on opioids should be routinely monitored for signs and symptoms of misuse, abuse, and addiction. ∎

● OxyContin has been formulated to prevent immediate access to full-dose oxycodone by cutting, chewing, or breaking the tablet. Attempts to dissolve tablets will result in a gummy substance that can't be drawn up into a syringe or injected.

PATIENT TEACHING
● Instruct patient to take drug before pain is intense.
● Tell patient to take drug with milk or after eating.

Black Box Warning Tell patient to swallow controlled-release tablets whole. ∎

● Caution ambulatory patient about getting out of bed or walking. Warn outpatient to avoid driving and other hazardous activities

---

that require mental alertness until drug's CNS effects are known.
• Advise patient to avoid alcohol use during therapy.
• Tell patient not to stop drug abruptly.

SAFETY ALERT!

oxycodone hydrochloride–acetaminophen
ox-i-KOE-done/a-seet-a-MIN-a-fen

Endocet†, Oxycet, Percocet, Primlev, Roxicet, Roxilox, Tylox

Therapeutic class: Opioid analgesics
Pharmacologic class: Opioid agonists–para-aminophenol derivatives
Pregnancy risk category: C
Controlled substance schedule: II

AVAILABLE FORMS
Capsules: 5 mg oxycodone hydrochloride and 500 mg acetaminophen
Oral solution*: 325 mg acetaminophen and 5 mg oxycodone hydrochloride per 5 mL
Tablets: 5 mg oxycodone hydrochloride and 300 mg acetaminophen, 7.5 mg oxycodone hydrochloride and 300 mg acetaminophen, 10 mg oxycodone hydrochloride and 300 mg acetaminophen, 2.5 mg oxycodone hydrochloride and 325 mg acetaminophen, 5 mg oxycodone hydrochloride and 325 mg acetaminophen, 7.5 mg oxycodone hydrochloride and 325 mg acetaminophen, 10 mg oxycodone hydrochloride and 325 mg acetaminophen, 5 mg oxycodone hydrochloride and 400 mg acetaminophen, 7.5 mg oxycodone hydrochloride and 400 mg acetaminophen, 10 mg oxycodone hydrochloride and 400 mg acetaminophen, 5 mg oxycodone hydrochloride and 500 mg acetaminophen, 7.5 mg oxycodone hydrochloride and 500 mg acetaminophen, 10 mg oxycodone hydrochloride and 500 mg acetaminophen, 10 mg oxycodone hydrochloride and 650 mg acetaminophen

INDICATIONS & DOSAGES
➤ **Moderate to moderately severe pain**
Adults: Oxycodone 2.5 to 10 mg and acetaminophen 325 to 650 mg P.O. every 6 hours as needed for pain. Adjust dosage based on pain severity and patient response. Maximum daily doses shouldn't exceed 60 mg oxycodone or 4 g acetaminophen.
Adjust-a-dose: Consider decreased dosage in patients with renal or hepatic impairment, chronic alcoholics, elderly patients, and patients overly sensitive to effects of opioids. Gradually taper dosage if therapy lasts for more than a few weeks.

ADMINISTRATION
P.O.
• Store drug at room temperature.

ACTION
Oxycodone binds with opioid receptors in the CNS, altering perception of and emotional response to pain. Acetaminophen is thought to produce analgesia by inhibiting prostaglandin and other substances that sensitize pain receptors. The combination reduces pain more effectively than acetaminophen alone.

Route	Onset	Peak	Duration
P.O. (acetaminophen)	Unknown	½–2 hr	3–4 hr
P.O. (oxycodone)	10–15 min	1 hr	3–6 hr

Half-life: Acetaminophen, 1 to 4 hours; oxycodone, 3½ hours.

ADVERSE REACTIONS
CNS: stupor, tremor, paresthesia, hypoesthesia, lethargy, *seizures,* anxiety, mental impairment, agitation, cerebral edema, confusion, dizziness, headache, malaise, asthenia, fatigue, euphoria, dysphoria, insomnia, depressed level of consciousness, nervousness, hallucinations, somnolence, depression, *suicide, hypothermia.*
CV: hypotension, hypertension, tachycardia, orthostatic hypotension, *bradycardia,* palpitations, arrhythmias, chest pain.
EENT: miosis, visual disturbances, red eye, hearing loss, tinnitus.
GI: constipation, dyspepsia, taste disturbances, abdominal pain, abdominal distention, diarrhea, dry mouth, flatulence, GI disorder, nausea, vomiting, *pancreatitis,* intestinal obstruction, ileus, anorexia, biliary spasm.

GU: interstitial nephritis, papillary necrosis, proteinuria, renal insufficiency, *renal failure,* renal tubular necrosis, urine retention.
Hematologic: *thrombocytopenia.*
Hepatic: *hepatitis, hepatic failure,* jaundice, *hepatotoxicity.*
Metabolic: dehydration, *hyperkalemia, metabolic acidosis,* respiratory alkalosis, fever, *hypoglycemia,* hyperglycemia.
Musculoskeletal: myalgia, *rhabdomyolysis.*
Respiratory: *asthma, bronchospasm,* dyspnea, hyperpnea, pulmonary edema, tachypnea, aspiration, *hypoventilation, laryngeal edema.*
Skin: pruritus, erythema, urticaria, rash, flushing.
Other: *anaphylactoid reaction,* allergic reaction, thirst, increased sweating, drug dependence, drug abuse, *accidental overdose, nonaccidental overdose.*

INTERACTIONS
Drug-drug. *Anticholinergics (atropine, dicyclomine, scopolamine):* May increase risk of paralytic ileus. Monitor patient closely.
Benzodiazepines, general anesthetics, neuromuscular blockers, opioid analgesics, sedative-hypnotics, other CNS depressants: May increase CNS depression. Use together cautiously, decreasing dosage of one or both agents.
Beta blockers (propranolol): May inhibit acetaminophen metabolism. Use together carefully.
Lamotrigine, loop diuretics, zidovudine: May decrease effects of these drugs when used with acetaminophen. Use together cautiously.
Mixed opioid agonist–antagonist combinations: May decrease effects of oxycodone and precipitate withdrawal. Use together carefully.
Oral contraceptives: May decrease acetaminophen half-life. Use together cautiously.
Probenecid: May increase effectiveness of acetaminophen. Use together cautiously.
Drug-lifestyle. *Alcohol use:* May increase risk of hepatotoxicity. Discourage use together.

EFFECTS ON LAB TEST RESULTS
• May increase potassium, amylase, bilirubin, or liver enzyme levels. May increase or decrease blood glucose level.
• May decrease platelet count.
• Oxycodone may cause cross-reactivity with urinary assays used to detect cocaine and marijuana.

CONTRAINDICATIONS & CAUTIONS
Black Box Warning Acetaminophen may increase risk of acute liver failure, liver transplant, and death. Liver injury is generally associated with use of acetaminophen at doses exceeding 4,000 mg/day and the use of more than one acetaminophen-containing product. ■
⚠ *Alert:* May cause serious, potentially fatal skin reactions including Stevens-Johnson syndrome, toxic epidermal necrolysis, and acute generalized exanthematous pustulosis. Reaction may occur with first or subsequent use when acetaminophen is used as monotherapy or when it is one component of combination drug therapy. Monitor for reddening of the skin, rash, blisters, and detachment of the upper surface of the skin. Stop drug immediately if skin reaction is suspected.
• Contraindicated in patients hypersensitive to components of drug and in those with significant respiratory depression, acute or severe bronchial asthma, hypercarbia, or suspected or known paralytic ileus.
• Use cautiously in patients with increased sensitivity to codeine, head injury, increased intracranial pressure, intracranial lesions, seizures, alcoholism, delirium tremens, biliary disease including pancreatitis, liver disease, COPD, preexisting respiratory impairment, or cor pulmonale.
• Use cautiously in acute abdominal conditions as this drug may obscure diagnostic signs or markedly increase respiratory depression or cerebrospinal fluid pressure.
• Use cautiously in hypotensive patients, elderly or debilitated patients, and in those with severe renal or hepatic impairment, hypothyroidism, urethral stricture, or Addison disease.
• Use in pregnant women only if benefit justifies risk. Dependence in newborns

---

Reactions in bold italics are *life-threatening*. Interactions may have a *rapid onset* or a *delayed onset*.

may occur. Not recommended immediately before or during labor and delivery.

• Both components appear in breast milk. Breast-feeding patient should discontinue drug or discontinue breast-feeding.

⚠ **Overdose S&S:** Oxycodone: Pinpoint pupils, respiratory depression, loss of consciousness, somnolence, stupor, coma, skeletal muscle flaccidity, cold and clammy skin, bradycardia, hypotension, apnea, circulatory collapse, cardiac arrest, death. Acetaminophen: Nausea, vomiting, diaphoresis, general malaise, hepatic necrosis, renal tubular necrosis, hypoglycemic coma, coagulation defects.

NURSING CONSIDERATIONS

• The lowest effective dosage should be prescribed for the shortest period of time. Inform patients of risks and signs and symptoms of morphine toxicity.

• Assess patients identified as potential abusers; drug should be prescribed with extreme care. Drug may cause physical dependence and tolerance with long-term therapy.

• Monitor patients for orthostatic hypotension.

• Monitor patients with head injury carefully. Oxycodone's effects on pupillary response and consciousness may mask worsening of neurologic status.

• Monitor patients with acute abdominal conditions closely. Drug may mask signs and symptoms in these patients.

• Observe for seizures in patients with convulsive disorders.

• Monitor bowel motility postoperatively, especially after intra-abdominal surgery.

PATIENT TEACHING

Black Box Warning Teach patient to look for acetaminophen on labels of all prescriptions and OTC medications he takes and to not use more than one product containing acetaminophen. Warn patient to seek medical attention if acetaminophen intake exceeds 4,000 mg/day even if feeling well. ∎

☼ **Alert:** Warn patient to stop drug and seek medical attention immediately if skin rash or reaction occurs while using acetaminophen.

• Inform patient with severe hepatic or renal disease that serial blood tests will be needed.

• Advise patient not to drive a car or operate heavy machinery while taking this drug.

• Warn patient to avoid alcohol and other CNS depressants.

• Caution patient that oxycodone may be habit-forming and to take drug only as long as prescribed in the amounts prescribed. Advise patient that if drug is taken for more than a few weeks, it should be tapered off gradually.

• Caution breast-feeding patient that drug may cause morphine toxicity (sleepiness, difficulty breast-feeding, breathing difficulties, limpness) in infants and should be avoided.

---

oxymetazoline hydrochloride (intranasal)
ox-i-met-AZ-oh-leen

Afrin ◇, Dristan 12 Hour Nasal ◇, Duration ◇, Genasal ◇, Nasal Relief ◇, Neo-Synephrine 12 Hour Spray ◇, Vicks Sinex 12 Hour ◇

Therapeutic class: Decongestants
Pharmacologic class: Sympathomimetics
Pregnancy risk category: C

0

AVAILABLE FORMS
Nasal solution: 0.05% ◇

INDICATIONS & DOSAGES
➤ **Nasal congestion**
Adults and children age 6 and older: 2 to 3 sprays of 0.05% solution in each nostril b.i.d. Don't use for more than 3 days.

ADMINISTRATION
Intranasal
• Don't exceed two doses in a 24-hour period.
• Have patient sit upright and tilt head back slightly.
• Have patient occlude opposite nostril during administration.
• Wait 1 to 2 minutes between sprays.
• Rinse tip of container with hot water and dry with a clean tissue.

ACTION

Thought to cause local vasoconstriction of dilated arterioles, reducing blood flow and nasal congestion.

Route	Onset	Peak	Duration
Intranasal	5–10 min	6 hr	<12 hr

Half-life: Unknown.

ADVERSE REACTIONS

CNS: anxiety, dizziness, headache, insomnia, restlessness.
CV: *CV collapse,* hypertension, palpitations.
EENT: dryness of nose and throat, increased nasal discharge, rebound nasal congestion or irritation, sneezing, stinging.
Other: systemic effects in children.

INTERACTIONS

None significant.

EFFECTS ON LAB TEST RESULTS

None reported.

CONTRAINDICATIONS & CAUTIONS

• Contraindicated in patients hypersensitive to drug and in children younger than age 6.
• Use cautiously in patients with hyperthyroidism, cardiac disease, hypertension, or diabetes mellitus.
• Use cautiously in those with difficulty urinating because of an enlarged prostate.

NURSING CONSIDERATIONS

• Monitor patient for rebound congestion or systemic effects.
• Don't give to children younger than age 6.

PATIENT TEACHING

• Teach patient how to use drug.
• Caution patient not to share drug because this could spread infection.
• Tell patient not to exceed recommended dosage and to use only when needed.
• Inform patient that prolonged use may result in rebound congestion.
☻ Alert: Warn patient that excessive use may cause slow or rapid heart rate, high blood pressure, dizziness, and weakness.

oxymetazoline hydrochloride (ophthalmic)

ox-i-met-AZ-oh-leen

OcuClear ◇, Visine L.R. ◇

Therapeutic class: Vasoconstrictors
Pharmacologic class: Direct-acting sympathomimetic amines
Pregnancy risk category: C

AVAILABLE FORMS

Ophthalmic solution: 0.025%

INDICATIONS & DOSAGES

➤ **Relief from eye redness caused by minor eye irritation**
Adults and children age 6 and older: Instill 1 to 2 drops in affected eye every 6 hours, as needed.

ADMINISTRATION

Ophthalmic
• Don't use if solution has become cloudy or changed color.
• Apply light finger pressure on lacrimal sac for 1 minute after drug instillation.
• Don't touch tip of dropper to any surface.

ACTION

Acts on alpha-adrenergic receptors in the arterioles of the conjunctiva to produce vasoconstriction, resulting in decreased conjunctival congestion.

Route	Onset	Peak	Duration
Ophthalmic	5 min	Unknown	6 hr

Half-life: Unknown.

ADVERSE REACTIONS

CNS: headache, insomnia, lightheadedness, nervousness.
CV: irregular heartbeat, palpitations, tachycardia.
EENT: transient stinging on first instillation, blurred vision, increased intraocular pressure, keratitis, lacrimation, reactive hyperemia with excessive doses or prolonged use.
Other: trembling.

Reactions in bold italics are *life-threatening*. Interactions may have a *rapid onset* or a *delayed onset*.

INTERACTIONS
Drug-drug. *Anesthetics:* Cyclopropane and halothane may sensitize the myocardium to sympathomimetics; local anesthetics may increase the absorption of topical drugs. Monitor patient for increased adverse effects.
Beta blockers: May cause more systemic adverse effects. Monitor patient for adverse systemic effects.
MAO inhibitors, maprotiline, TCAs: If significant systemic absorption of oxymetazoline occurs, use together may increase pressor effect of oxymetazoline. Avoid using together.

EFFECTS ON LAB TEST RESULTS
None reported.

CONTRAINDICATIONS & CAUTIONS
• Contraindicated in patients hypersensitive to drug or its components and in those with angle-closure glaucoma.
• Use cautiously in patients with hyperthyroidism, cardiac disease, hypertension, eye disease, infection, or injury.

NURSING CONSIDERATIONS
• Rebound congestion and conjunctivitis may occur with frequent or prolonged use.
• *Look alike–sound alike:* Don't confuse Visine with Visken.

PATIENT TEACHING
• Teach patient how to instill drops. Advise him to wash hands before and after instillation, and warn him not to touch tip of dropper to eye or surrounding tissue.
• Instruct patient to apply light finger pressure on lacrimal sac for 1 minute after drug instillation.
• Advise patient to stop drug and consult prescriber if eye pain occurs, if vision changes, or if redness or irritation continues, worsens, or lasts for longer than 72 hours.

SAFETY ALERT!

oxymorphone hydrochloride
ox-i-MOR-fone

Opana, Opana ER, Opana ER (crush-resistant)

Therapeutic class: Opioid analgesics
Pharmacologic class: Opioids
Pregnancy risk category: C; D if used for prolonged periods or at high doses at term
Controlled substance schedule: II

AVAILABLE FORMS
Injection: 1 mg/mL
Tablets: 5 mg, 10 mg
Tablets (extended-release): 5 mg, 7.5 mg, 10 mg, 15 mg, 20 mg, 30 mg, 40 mg

INDICATIONS & DOSAGES
Adjust-a-dose (for all indications): For patients with mild hepatic impairment or CrCl less than 50 mL/minute, start with the lowest possible dose and slowly increase as tolerated.
➤ **Moderate to severe pain**
Adults: 1 to 1.5 mg I.M. or subcutaneously every 4 to 6 hours p.r.n. Or, 0.5 mg I.V. every 4 to 6 hours p.r.n. Or, in opioid-naive patients, 10 to 20 mg P.O. every 4 to 6 hours. If needed, begin dosing at 5 mg P.O. and adjust based on patient response.
➤ **Moderate to severe pain in patients requiring continuous, around-the-clock opioid treatment for an extended period of time**
Opioid-naive adults: Using extended-release (ER) form, give 5 mg P.O. every 12 hours. Increase 5 to 10 mg every 12 hours every 3 to 7 days as needed and tolerated.
Nonopioid-naive adults: Patients taking Opana immediate-release tablets can be switched to Opana ER tablets by giving one-half the patient's total daily dose as Opana ER every 12 hours.
➤ **Analgesia during labor**
Adults: 0.5 to 1 mg I.M.

ADMINISTRATION

P.O.

❸ Alert: Starting doses of more than 20 mg aren't recommended because of potential serious adverse reactions.

• Take tablets 1 hour before or 2 hours after a meal.

Black Box Warning Don't crush, break, allow patient to chew, or dissolve extended-release tablets. ▮

Black Box Warning Extended-release tablets aren't for as-needed use. ▮

I.V.

▼ Assess respiratory status before giving. Withhold dose and notify prescriber if respirations are shallow or rate falls below 12 breaths/minute.

▼ If necessary, dilute drug in normal saline solution.

▼ Give drug by direct I.V. injection.

▼ **Incompatibilities:** None reported.

I.M.

• Rotate administration sites and document.

• Assess respiratory status before giving. Withhold dose and notify prescriber if respirations are shallow or rate falls below 12 breaths/minute.

Subcutaneous

• Rotate administration sites and document.

• Assess respiratory status before giving. Withhold dose and notify prescriber if respirations are shallow or rate falls below 12 breaths/minute.

ACTION

May bind with opioid receptors in the CNS, altering perception of and emotional response to pain.

Route	Onset	Peak	Duration
P.O.	Varies	Varies	Varies
I.V.	5–10 min	15–30 min	3–4 hr
I.M.	10–15 min	30–90 min	3–6 hr
Subcut.	10–20 min	60–90 min	3–6 hr

Half-life: For parenteral, unknown; extended-release tablets, 7 to 12 hours; immediate-release tablets, 3 to 12 hours.

ADVERSE REACTIONS

CNS: clouded sensorium, dizziness, euphoria, headache, sedation, somnolence, *seizures,* dysphoria, light-headedness, hallucinations, physical dependence, fever, restlessness, confusion.

CV: hypotension, *bradycardia,* palpitations, tachycardia.

EENT: blurred vision, diplopia, miosis.

GI: constipation, nausea, vomiting, ileus.

GU: urine retention.

Respiratory: *respiratory depression, laryngeal edema, bronchospasm.*

Skin: increased sweating, pruritus.

INTERACTIONS

Drug-drug. *Agonist or antagonist analgesics:* May reduce analgesic effect or precipitate withdrawal symptoms. Don't use together.

Anticholinergics: May increase risk of urine retention or severe constipation, leading to paralytic ileus. Monitor patient for abdominal pain or distention.

Cimetidine: May increase CNS reactions. Monitor patient closely.

CNS depressants, general anesthetics, phenothiazines, sedative-hypnotics, TCAs: May cause additive effects. Use together with caution and reduce opioid dosage.

MAO inhibitors: May cause severe opioid potentiation. Don't use opioids if patient has received MAO inhibitors within 14 days.

Propofol: May increase bradycardia risk. Monitor ECG closely.

Black Box Warning **Drug-lifestyle.** *Alcohol use:* Alcoholic beverages or medications containing alcohol may cause additive effects and result in a potentially fatal overdose of oxymorphone. Don't use together. ▮

EFFECTS ON LAB TEST RESULTS

• May increase amylase and lipase levels.

CONTRAINDICATIONS & CAUTIONS

• Contraindicated in patients hypersensitive to drug; in those with acute asthma attacks, severe respiratory depression, upper airway obstruction, or paralytic ileus; or in those with moderate to severe hepatic impairment.

• Contraindicated in patients with pulmonary edema caused by a respiratory irritant.

• Use with caution in elderly or debilitated patients and in those with head injury, increased intracranial pressure, seizures, asthma, COPD, acute abdominal conditions, biliary tract disease (including pancreatitis), acute alcoholism, delirium tremens,

---

Reactions in bold italics are *life-threatening*. Interactions may have a *rapid onset* or a *delayed onset*.

prostatic hyperplasia, renal or mild hepatic impairment, urethral stricture, respiratory depression, hypothyroidism, Addison disease, and arrhythmias.

⚠ **Overdose S&S:** Miosis, CNS depression, respiratory depression, apnea, flaccid skeletal muscles, bradycardia, hypotension, circulatory collapse, cardiac arrest, respiratory arrest, death.

NURSING CONSIDERATIONS
• Keep opioid antagonist (naloxone) and resuscitation equipment available.
• Use of this drug may worsen gallbladder pain.
• Drug isn't for mild pain. For better effect, give drug before patient has intense pain.
• Monitor CV and respiratory status. Withhold dose and notify prescriber if respirations decrease or rate is below 12 breaths/minute.
• Monitor bladder and bowel function. Patient may need a stimulant laxative.
Black Box Warning Drug has an abuse liability similar to other opioid analgesics. Consider this when concerned about an increased risk of misuse, abuse, or diversion. ▪
• **Look alike–sound alike:** Don't confuse oxymorphone with oxymetholone or oxycodone.

PATIENT TEACHING
• Instruct patient to ask for drug before pain is intense. Inform patient that extended-release tablets must be taken around the clock.
• When drug is used I.M. or I.V. after surgery, encourage patient to turn, cough, and deep-breathe and to use incentive spirometer to avoid lung problems.
• Caution ambulatory patient about getting out of bed or walking. Warn outpatient to avoid driving and other hazardous activities that require mental alertness until drug's CNS effects are known.
Black Box Warning Caution patient not to consume alcohol or take any prescription or OTC drug containing alcohol with oral form as this can lead to an overdose. ▪
Black Box Warning Warn patient not to crush, break, chew, or dissolve extended-release tablets; doing so may lead to a fatal overdose. ▪

• Tell patient to take tablets 1 hour before or 2 hours after a meal.
Black Box Warning Instruct patient to keep tablets in a child-resistant container in a safe place. Accidental ingestion by a child can result in death. ▪

SAFETY ALERT!

oxytocin (synthetic injection)
ox-i-TOE-sin

Pitocin

Therapeutic class: Oxytocics
Pharmacologic class: Exogenous hormones
Pregnancy risk category: C

AVAILABLE FORMS
Injection: 10 units/mL in 1-mL ampule; 1-mL, 3-mL, and 10-mL vials; or syringe

INDICATIONS & DOSAGES
➤ **To induce or stimulate labor**
Adults: Initially, 10 units in 1,000 mL of D₅W injection, lactated Ringer, or normal saline solution I.V. infused at 0.5 to 2 milliunits/minute. Increase rate by 1 to 2 milliunits/minute at 30- to 60-minute intervals until normal contraction pattern is established. Decrease rate when labor is firmly established. Rates exceeding 9 to 10 milliunits/minute are rarely required.
➤ **To reduce postpartum bleeding after expulsion of placenta**
Adults: 10 to 40 units in 1,000 mL of D₅W injection, lactated Ringer, or normal saline solution I.V. infused at rate needed to control bleeding, which is usually 20 to 40 milliunits/minute. Also, 10 units may be given I.M. after delivery of placenta.
➤ **Incomplete or inevitable abortion**
Adults: 10 units I.V. in 500 mL of normal saline solution, lactated Ringer, or dextrose 5% in normal saline solution. Infuse at 10 to 20 milliunits (20 to 40 drops)/minute. Don't exceed 30 units in 12 hours.

ADMINISTRATION

I.V.

▼ Never give drug simultaneously by more than one route.

▼ To induce or stimulate labor, dilute drug by adding 10 units to 1 L of normal saline, lactated Ringer, or D₅W solution.

▼ To produce intense uterine contractions and reduce postpartum bleeding, dilute drug by adding 10 units to 500 mL of normal saline, lactated Ringer, or D₅W solution.

▼ Don't give bolus injection; use an infusion pump. Give drug only by piggyback infusion so that it may be stopped without interrupting I.V. line.

▼ **Incompatibilities:** Fibrinolysin (human), norepinephrine bitartrate, Normosol-M with dextrose 5%, plasmin, prochlorperazine, sodium bisulfite, warfarin sodium.

I.M.

● Drug isn't recommended for routine I.M. use, but 10 units may be given I.M. after delivery of placenta to control postpartum uterine bleeding.

● Never give drug simultaneously by more than one route.

ACTION

Causes potent and selective stimulation of uterine and mammary gland smooth muscle.

Route	Onset	Peak	Duration
I.V.	Immediate	Unknown	1 hr
I.M.	3–5 min	Unknown	2–3 hr

Half-life: 3 to 5 minutes.

ADVERSE REACTIONS

Maternal

CNS: *subarachnoid hemorrhage, seizures, coma.*

CV: *arrhythmias,* hypertension, PVCs.

GI: nausea, vomiting.

GU: *abruptio placentae,* tetanic uterine contractions, *postpartum hemorrhage, uterine rupture,* impaired uterine blood flow, pelvic hematoma, increased uterine motility.

Hematologic: *afibrinogenemia, possibly related to postpartum bleeding.*

Other: *anaphylaxis, death from oxytocin-induced water intoxication,* hypersensitivity reactions.

Fetal

CNS: *infant brain damage, seizures.*

CV: *bradycardia, arrhythmias,* PVCs.

EENT: neonatal retinal hemorrhage.

Hepatic: neonatal jaundice.

Other: *low Apgar scores at 5 minutes, death.*

INTERACTIONS

Drug-drug. *Cyclopropane anesthetics:* May cause less pronounced bradycardia and hypotension. Use together cautiously.

Drugs that prolong QT interval: May increase risk of life-threatening cardiac arrhythmias, including torsades de pointes. Use together cautiously.

Thiopental anesthetics: May delay induction. Use together cautiously.

Vasoconstrictors: May cause severe hypertension if oxytocin is given within 3 to 4 hours of vasoconstrictor in patient receiving caudal block anesthetic. Avoid using together.

EFFECTS ON LAB TEST RESULTS

None reported.

CONTRAINDICATIONS & CAUTIONS

● Contraindicated in patients hypersensitive to drug.

● Contraindicated when vaginal delivery isn't advised (placenta previa, vasa previa, invasive cervical carcinoma, genital herpes), when cephalopelvic disproportion is present, or when delivery requires conversion, as in transverse lie.

● Contraindicated in fetal distress when delivery isn't imminent, in prematurity, in other obstetric emergencies, and in patients with severe toxemia or hypertonic uterine patterns.

● Use cautiously during first and second stages of labor because cervical laceration, uterine rupture, and maternal and fetal death have been reported.

● Use cautiously, if at all, in patients with invasive cervical cancer and in those with previous cervical or uterine surgery (including cesarean section), grand multiparity, uterine sepsis, traumatic delivery, or overdistended uterus.

⚠ Overdose S&S: Uterine hypersensitivity, tumultuous labor, uterine rupture, cervical and vaginal lacerations, postpartum hemorrhage, uteroplacental hypoperfusion, variable deceleration of fetal heart rate, fetal hypoxia, hypercapnia, perinatal hepatic necrosis, water intoxication, seizures, death.

NURSING CONSIDERATIONS

Black Box Warning Drug is only indicated for the medical, rather than the elective, induction of labor. ∎

☙ Alert: All patients receiving oxytocin I.V. must be under continuous observation by trained personnel who have a thorough knowledge of the drug and are qualified to identify complications.

● Drug is used to induce or reinforce labor only when pelvis is known to be adequate, when vaginal delivery is indicated, when fetal maturity is assured, and when fetal position is favorable. Use drug only in hospital where critical care facilities and prescriber are immediately available.

● Monitor fluid intake and output. Antidiuretic effect may lead to fluid overload, seizures, and coma from water intoxication.

● Monitor and record uterine contractions, heart rate, blood pressure, intrauterine pressure, fetal heart rate, and character of blood loss every 15 minutes.

● Have 20% magnesium sulfate solution available to relax the myometrium.

● If contractions occur less than 2 minutes apart, exceed 50 mm, or last 90 seconds or longer, stop infusion, turn patient on her side, and notify prescriber.

● Drug doesn't cause fetal abnormalities when used as indicated.

● **Look alike–sound alike:** Don't confuse Pitocin with Pitressin.

PATIENT TEACHING

● Explain use and administration of drug to patient and family.

● Instruct patient to report adverse reactions promptly.

SAFETY ALERT!

paclitaxel
pak-leh-TAX-ell

Taxol

Therapeutic class: Antineoplastics
Pharmacologic class: Taxoids
Pregnancy risk category: D

AVAILABLE FORMS
Injection: 6 mg/mL in 5-, 16.7-, 25-, 50-mL vials

INDICATIONS & DOSAGES
➤ **AIDS-related Kaposi sarcoma**
Adults: 135 mg/m^2 I.V. over 3 hours every 3 weeks, or 100 mg/m^2 I.V. over 3 hours every 2 weeks.

Adjust-a-dose: Don't give drug if baseline or subsequent neutrophil counts are less than 1,000/mm^3. Reduce subsequent doses by 20% for patients who experience neutrophil count less than 500/mm^3 for 1 week or longer. Patient also may need reduction in dexamethasone premedication dose (10 mg P.O. instead of 20 mg P.O.) and start of a hematopoietic growth factor. For patients with hepatic impairment, reduce first 3-hour dose based on transaminase and bilirubin levels. If transaminase levels are less than 10 times upper limit of normal (ULN) and bilirubin levels are 1.25 × ULN or less, give 175 mg/m^2. If transaminase levels are less than 10 × ULN and bilirubin levels are 1.26 to 2 × ULN, give 135 mg/m^2. If transaminase levels are less than 10 × ULN and bilirubin levels are 2.01 to 5 × ULN, give 90 mg/m^2. If transaminase levels are 10 × ULN or more or bilirubin levels are more than 5 × ULN, don't use drug. For subsequent courses, base dosage adjustment on individual tolerance.

➤ **First-line and subsequent therapy for advanced ovarian cancer**
Adults (previously untreated): 175 mg/m^2 over 3 hours every 3 weeks, followed by cisplatin 75 mg/m^2; or, 135 mg/m^2 over 24 hours, followed by cisplatin 75 mg/m^2, every 3 weeks.

P

Adults (previously treated): 135 or 175 mg/m² I.V. over 3 hours every 3 weeks.

Adjust-a-dose: For patients with hepatic impairment, reduce first 3-hour dose based on transaminase and bilirubin levels. If transaminase levels are less than 10 × ULN and bilirubin levels are 1.25 × ULN or less, give 175 mg/m². If transaminase levels are less than 10 × ULN and bilirubin levels are 1.26 to 2 × ULN, give 135 mg/m². If transaminase levels are less than 10 × ULN and bilirubin levels are 2.01 to 5 × ULN, give 90 mg/m². If transaminase levels are 10 × ULN or more or bilirubin levels are more than 5 × ULN, don't use drug. For subsequent courses, base dosage adjustment on individual tolerance.

➤ **Breast cancer after failure of combination chemotherapy for metastatic disease or relapse within 6 months of adjuvant chemotherapy (previous therapy should have included an anthracycline unless contraindicated); adjuvant therapy for node-positive breast cancer given sequentially to standard doxorubicin-containing combination chemotherapy**
Adults: 175 mg/m² I.V. over 3 hours every 3 weeks for four cycles.

Adjust-a-dose: For patients with hepatic impairment, reduce first 3-hour dose based on transaminase and bilirubin levels. If transaminase levels are less than 10 × ULN and bilirubin levels are 1.25 × ULN or less, give 175 mg/m². If transaminase levels are less than 10 × ULN and bilirubin levels are 1.26 to 2 × ULN, give 135 mg/m². If transaminase levels are less than 10 × ULN and bilirubin levels are 2.01 to 5 × ULN, give 90 mg/m². If transaminase levels are 10 × ULN or more or bilirubin levels are more than 5 × ULN, don't use drug. For subsequent courses, base dosage adjustment on individual tolerance.

➤ **First treatment of advanced non–small-cell lung cancer for patients who aren't candidates for curative surgery or radiation**
Adults: 135 mg/m² I.V. infusion over 24 hours, followed by cisplatin 75 mg/m². Repeat cycle every 3 weeks.

Adjust-a-dose: Subsequent courses shouldn't be repeated until neutrophil count is at least 1,500/mm³ and platelet count is at least 100,000/mm³. Reduce subsequent doses by 20% for patients who experience neutrophil count less than 500/mm³ for a week or longer or severe peripheral neuropathy. For patients with hepatic impairment, adjust doses for the first courses of therapy as follows: For first 24-hour infusion if transaminase levels are less than 2 × ULN and bilirubin levels are 1.5 mg/dL or less, give 135 mg/m². If transaminase levels are 2 to <10 × ULN and bilirubin levels are 1.5 mg/dL or less, give 100 mg/m². If transaminase levels are <10 × ULN and bilirubin levels are 1.6 to 7.5 mg/dL, give 50 mg/m². If transaminase levels are 10 × ULN or more, or bilirubin levels are more than 7.5 mg/dL, don't use drug.

ADMINISTRATION

I.V.

▼ Preparing and giving drug may be mutagenic, teratogenic, or carcinogenic. Follow institutional policy to reduce risks. Mark all waste materials with CHEMOTHERAPY HAZARD labels.

▼ Prepare and store infusion solutions in glass containers. Undiluted concentrate shouldn't contact polyvinyl chloride I.V. bags or tubing.

▼ Dilute concentrate before infusion. Compatible solutions include normal saline solution for injection, D₅W, 5% dextrose in normal saline solution for injection, and 5% dextrose in Ringer lactate injection. Dilute to yield 0.3 to 1.2 mg/mL. Diluted solutions are stable for 24 hours at room temperature. Prepared solution may appear hazy.

▼ Give through polyethylene-lined administration sets, and use an in-line 0.22-micron filter.

▼ Watch for irritation and infiltration; extravasation can cause tissue damage and necrosis.

▼ Closely monitor patient and vital signs during infusion, especially during the first hour.

▼ Store diluted solution in glass or polypropylene bottles, or use polypropylene or polyolefin bags.

▼ **Incompatibilities:** Amphotericin B, chlorpromazine, cisplatin, doxorubicin liposomal, hydroxyzine hydrochloride,

---

Reactions in bold italics are *life-threatening*. Interactions may have a *rapid onset* or a *delayed onset*.

methylprednisolone sodium succinate, mitoxantrone.

ACTION

Prevents depolymerization of cellular microtubules, inhibiting normal reorganization of microtubule network needed for mitosis and other vital cellular functions.

Route	Onset	Peak	Duration
I.V.	Unknown	Unknown	Unknown

Half-life: After 6- to 12-hour infusion, distribution and elimination half-lives average about 30 minutes and 6 hours, respectively. For 3-hour infusion, distribution and elimination half-lives average about 30 minutes and 2½ hours, respectively.

ADVERSE REACTIONS

CNS: peripheral neuropathy, asthenia.
CV: *bradycardia,* hypotension, abnormal ECG.
GI: nausea, vomiting, diarrhea, mucositis.
Hematologic: *neutropenia, leukopenia, thrombocytopenia,* anemia, *bleeding.*
Musculoskeletal: myalgia, arthralgia.
Skin: alopecia, cellulitis and phlebitis at injection site.
Other: hypersensitivity reactions, *anaphylaxis,* infections.

INTERACTIONS

Drug-drug. *Carbamazeptne, phenobarbital:* May increase metabolism and may decrease paclitaxel levels. Use together cautiously.
Cisplatin: May cause additive myelosuppressive effects. Give paclitaxel before cisplatin.
Doxorubicin, cyclosporine, felodipine, ketoconazole: May increase plasma levels of doxorubicin and its active metabolite, doxorubicinol. Use together cautiously.
Drugs that inhibit CYP450 (cyclosporine, dexamethasone, diazepam, etoposide, **keto-conazole,** *quinidine, retinoic acid, teniposide, testosterone, verapamil, vincristine):* May increase paclitaxel level. Monitor patient for toxicity.

EFFECTS ON LAB TEST RESULTS

• May increase alkaline phosphatase, AST, and triglyceride levels. May decrease hemoglobin level.
• May decrease neutrophil, WBC, and platelet counts.

CONTRAINDICATIONS & CAUTIONS

• Contraindicated in patients hypersensitive to drug or polyoxyethylated castor oil (also known as Cremophor EL, a vehicle used in drug solution).
Black Box Warning Contraindicated in those with baseline neutrophil counts below 1,500/mm^3 and platelet counts below 100,000/mm^3, or in those with AIDS-related Kaposi sarcoma with baseline neutrophil counts below 1,000/mm^3. ■
• Use cautiously in patients with hepatic impairment.
⚠ **Overdose S&S:** Bone marrow suppression, sensory neurotoxicity, mucositis, acute ethanol toxicity (in children), CNS toxicity (in children).

NURSING CONSIDERATIONS

Black Box Warning Administer drug under the supervision of a physician experienced with cancer chemotherapeutic agents. ■
• Patient may experience peripheral neuropathies, which may be cumulative and dose related. Patients with severe symptoms may need dosage reduction.
Black Box Warning To reduce risk or severity of hypersensitivity, patients must receive pretreatment with corticosteroids, such as dexamethasone, and antihistamines. Both H$_1$-receptor antagonists, such as diphenhydramine, and H$_2$-receptor antagonists, such as cimetidine or ranitidine, may be used. Fatal reactions have occurred despite premedication. ■
Black Box Warning Monitor blood counts before therapy is initiated and often during therapy. Bone marrow toxicity is the most common and dose-limiting toxicity. Institute bleeding precautions, as indicated. ■
• Avoid all I.M. injections when platelet count is below 50,000/mm^3.
• If patient develops significant cardiac conduction abnormalities, use indicated therapy and continuous cardiac monitoring during therapy and subsequent infusions.

P

🛈 *Alert:* When indicated, cisplatin dose should follow dose of paclitaxel.

● *Look alike–sound alike:* Don't confuse paclitaxel with paroxetine.

PATIENT TEACHING

● Advise patient to report any pain or burning at site of injection during or after administration.

● Urge patient to watch for fever, sore throat, and fatigue and for easy bruising, nosebleeds, bleeding gums, or tarry stools. Tell patient to take temperature daily.

● Teach patient symptoms of peripheral neuropathy, such as a tingling or burning sensation or numbness in limbs, and to report these symptoms immediately.

● Warn patient that reversible hair loss will probably occur.

● Caution woman of childbearing age to avoid becoming pregnant during therapy. Recommend that she consult prescriber before becoming pregnant.

SAFETY ALERT!

paclitaxel protein-bound particles

pak-leh-TAX-ell

Abraxane

Therapeutic class: Antineoplastics
Pharmacologic class: Taxoids
Pregnancy risk category: D

AVAILABLE FORMS

Lyophilized powder for injection: 100 mg in single-use vials

INDICATIONS & DOSAGES

➤ **Metastatic breast cancer after failure of combination chemotherapy or relapse within 6 months of adjuvant chemotherapy (previous therapy should have included an anthracycline unless clinically contraindicated at the time)**
Adults: 260 mg/m² I.V. over 30 minutes every 3 weeks.

Adjust-a-dose: For patients with severe sensory neuropathy or a neutrophil count less than 500/mm³ for a week or longer, reduce dose to 220 mg/m². For recurring

severe sensory neuropathy or severe neutropenia, reduce dose to 180 mg/m². For grade 3 (severe) sensory neuropathy, stop drug until condition improves to a grade 1 or 2 (mild to moderate); then restart at a reduced dose for the rest of treatment.

For patients with moderate hepatic impairment (serum bilirubin level 1.26 to 2 times upper limit of normal [ULN] and AST level 1 to 10 × ULN), recommended dosage is 200 mg/m²/dose. For patients with severe hepatic impairment (serum bilirubin level 2.01 to 5 × ULN and AST level 1 to 10 × ULN), recommended dosage is 130 mg/m²/dose initially; may be increased to 200 mg/m²/dose as tolerated. Don't give to patients with very severe hepatic impairment (serum bilirubin level more than 5 × ULN or AST level more than 10 × ULN).

➤ **Non-small-cell lung cancer (NSCLC) as first-line treatment in combination with carboplatin in patients who aren't candidates for surgery or radiation therapy**
Adults: 100 mg/m² I.V over 30 minutes on days 1, 8, and 15 of each 21-day cycle. Give carboplatin immediately after paclitaxel protein-bound particles dose on day 1 of each 21-day cycle. Refer to manufacturer's instructions for carboplatin dosage.

Adjust-a-dose: For patients with moderate hepatic impairment (serum bilirubin level 1.26 to 2 × ULN and AST level 1 to 10 × ULN), recommended dosage is 75 mg/m²/dose. For patients with severe hepatic impairment (serum bilirubin level 2.01 to 5 × ULN and AST level 1 to 10 × ULN), recommended dosage is 50 mg/m²/dose; may be increased to 75 mg/m²/dose as tolerated. Don't give to patients with very severe hepatic impairment (serum bilirubin level more than 5 × ULN or AST level more than 10 × ULN). Don't administer paclitaxel on day 1 of a cycle until ANC is at least 1,500 cells/mm³ and platelet count is at least 100,000 cells/mm³. In patients who develop severe neutropenia or thrombocytopenia, withhold treatment until counts recover to an ANC of at least 1,500 cells/mm³ and platelet count of at least 100,000 cells/mm³ on day 1 or to an ANC of at least 500 cells/mm³ and platelet count of at least 50,000 cells/mm^3 on days 8 or 15 of the cycle. Upon resumption of dosing, permanently reduce paclitaxel and carboplatin doses per manufacturer's instructions.

Withhold paclitaxel for grade 3 to 4 peripheral neuropathy. Resume paclitaxel and carboplatin at reduced doses when peripheral neuropathy improves to grade 1 or completely resolves.

➤ **Metastatic pancreatic adenocarcinoma as first-line treatment in combination with gemcitabine**
Adults: 125 mg/m^2 I.V. over 30 to 40 minutes on days 1, 8, and 15 of each 28-day cycle. Give gemcitabine 1,000 mg/m^2 I.V. immediately after each paclitaxel dose.
Adjust-a-dose: For patients with mild hepatic impairment (bilirubin level greater than ULN to 1.25 × ULN and AST less than 10 × ULN), no dosage adjustment is needed. Drug isn't recommended for patients with moderate to severe hepatic impairment.

If necessary, dose level reductions for paclitaxel and gemcitabine are as follows: First dose level reduction consists of paclitaxel 100 mg/m^2 and gemcitabine 800 mg/m^2; second dose level reduction consists of paclitaxel 75 mg/m^2 and gemcitabine to 600 mg/m^2. If further dosage reductions are needed, discontinue both drugs.

On Day 1, if ANC is less than 1,500 cells/mm^3 or platelet count is less than 100,000 cells/mm^3, delay doses until recovery. On Day 8, if ANC is 500 to less than 1,000 cells/mm^3 or platelet count is 50,000 to less than 75,000 cells/mm^3, reduce one dose level. If Day 8 ANC is less than 500 cells/mm^3 or platelet count is less than 50,000 cells/mm^3, withhold doses. On Day 15, if Day 8 doses were given or reduced and ANC is 500 to less than 1,000 cells/mm^3, or platelet count is 50,000 to less than 75,000 cells/mm^3, reduce one dose level from Day 8; if ANC is less than 500 cells/mm^3 or platelet count is less than 50,000 cells/mm^3, withhold doses. On Day 15, if Day 8 doses were withheld and ANC is 1,000 cells/mm^3 or more or platelet count is 75,000 cells/mm^3 or more, reduce one

dose level from Day 1; if ANC is 500 to less than 1,000 cells/mm^3 or platelet count is 50,000 to less than 75,000 cells/mm^3, reduce two dose levels from Day 1; if ANC is less than 500 cells/mm^3 or platelet count is less than 50,000 cells/mm^3, withhold doses.

For grade 3 or 4 febrile neutropenia, withhold paclitaxel and gemcitabine doses until fever resolves and ANC is 1,500 cells/mm^3 or more; then resume at next lower dose level. For grade 3 or 4 peripheral neuropathy, withhold paclitaxel until improvement to grade 1 or better; then resume at next lower dose level, continuing gemcitabine without dosage reduction. For grade 2 or 3 cutaneous toxicity, reduce paclitaxel and gemcitabine doses to next lower dose level; discontinue treatment if toxicity persists. For grade 3 mucositis or diarrhea, withhold both drugs until improvement to grade 1 or better; then resume at next lower dose level.

ADMINISTRATION
I.V.
▼ Because of drug's cytotoxicity, handle it cautiously and wear gloves. If drug contacts skin, wash area thoroughly with soap and water. If drug contacts mucous membranes, flush them thoroughly with water.
▼ Reconstitute the vial with 20 mL of normal saline solution to yield 5 mg/mL of drug. Direct the stream slowly, over at least 1 minute, onto the inside wall of the vial to avoid foaming. Let the vial sit for 5 minutes to ensure proper wetting of the powder. Gently swirl or turn the vial for at least 2 minutes until completely dissolved. If foaming occurs, let the solution stand for 15 minutes for the foam to subside. If particles are visible, gently invert the vial again to ensure complete resuspension. The solution should appear milky and uniform. Inject the correct dose into an empty polyvinyl chloride–type I.V. bag and use immediately.
▼ Give drug over 30 minutes.
▼ The suspension for infusion, when prepared in an infusion bag, is stable at room temperature and normal lighting for up to 8 hours.

P

▼ Store unopened vials at room temperature in the original package. Store reconstituted vials at 36° to 46° F (2° to 8° C) for up to 8 hours, protected from light.
▼ **Incompatibilities:** None known.

ACTION
Prevents depolymerization of cellular microtubules, inhibiting reorganization of the microtubule network and disrupting mitosis and other vital cell functions.

Route	Onset	Peak	Duration
I.V.	Unknown	Unknown	Unknown

Half-life: 27 hours.

ADVERSE REACTIONS
CNS: asthenia, sensory neuropathy.
CV: abnormal ECG, edema, *cardiac arrest,* chest pain, *supraventricular tachycardia, thromboembolism, thrombosis,* hypertension, hypotension.
EENT: visual disturbances.
GI: diarrhea, nausea, oral candidiasis, vomiting, intestinal obstruction, *ischemic colitis, pancreatitis, perforation,* mucositis.
GU: *renal failure.*
Hematologic: anemia, *neutropenia, thrombocytopenia, bleeding.*
Hepatic: *hepatic encephalopathy, hepatic necrosis.*
Musculoskeletal: arthralgia, myalgia.
Respiratory: *pulmonary embolism,* cough, dyspnea, pneumonia, respiratory tract infection.
Skin: alopecia, injection-site reactions.
Other: infections, hypersensitivity reactions.

INTERACTIONS
Drug-drug. *CYP450 inhibitors:* May decrease paclitaxel metabolism. Use together cautiously.

EFFECTS ON LAB TEST RESULTS
● May increase alkaline phosphatase, AST, bilirubin, creatinine, and GGT levels. May decrease hemoglobin level.
● May decrease neutrophil and platelet counts.

CONTRAINDICATIONS & CAUTIONS
Black Box Warning Contraindicated in patients with baseline neutrophil counts of less than 1,500/mm³. ∎
● Don't repeat dose until neutrophil counts recover to more than 1,500/mm³ and platelet count recovers to more than 100,000/mm³.
● In patients with creatinine level over 2 mg/dL or bilirubin level over 1.5 mg/dL, use hasn't been studied.
⚠ *Overdose S&S:* Bone marrow suppression, sensory neurotoxicity, acute ethanol toxicity (in children), CNS toxicity (in children).

NURSING CONSIDERATIONS
Black Box Warning Give only under supervision of practitioner experienced in using chemotherapy in a facility that can manage complications of therapy. ∎
Black Box Warning Don't substitute Abraxane for other forms of paclitaxel. ∎
Black Box Warning Monitor CBC frequently to evaluate for neutropenia, which may be severe and result in infection. ∎
☺ *Alert:* Obtain CBC before dosing on Day 1 for metastatic breast cancer and before Days 1, 8, and 15 for NSCLC or pancreatic cancer.
☺ *Alert:* If patient becomes febrile (regardless of ANC), initiate treatment with broad-spectrum antibiotics.
☺ *Alert:* Watch for pneumonitis in patients receiving drug in combination with gemcitabine. If pneumonitis is suspected, interrupt treatment. If pneumonitis is diagnosed, permanently discontinue treatment with paclitaxel and gemcitabine.
● Because drug contains human albumin, a remote risk exists of transmitting viruses and Creutzfeldt-Jakob disease.
● Assess patient for symptoms of sensory neuropathy and severe neutropenia.
● Monitor LFT and renal function test results.
● Monitor infusion site closely.

PATIENT TEACHING
● Warn patient that alopecia commonly occurs but is reversible after therapy.

Reactions in bold italics are *life-threatening*. Interactions may have a *rapid onset* or a *delayed onset*.

• Teach patient to recognize signs of neuropathy, such as tingling, burning, and numbness in arms and legs.

• Tell patient to report fever or other signs of infection, severe abdominal pain, or severe diarrhea.

• Advise patient to contact prescriber if nausea and vomiting persist or interfere with adequate nutrition. Reassure patient that an antiemetic can be prescribed.

• Explain that many patients experience weakness and fatigue, so it's important to rest. Tiredness, paleness, and shortness of breath may result from low blood counts, and patient may need a transfusion.

• To reduce or prevent mouth sores, remind patient to perform proper oral hygiene.

• Tell women to avoid becoming pregnant or breast-feeding and men to avoid fathering a child during therapy.

paliperidone
pahl-ee-PEHR-ih-dohn

Invega

paliperidone palmitate
Invega Sustenna

Therapeutic class: Antipsychotics
Pharmacologic class: Benzisoxazole derivatives
Pregnancy risk category: C

AVAILABLE FORMS
Injection: 39 mg, 78 mg, 117 mg, 156 mg, 234 mg
Tablets (extended-release): 1.5 mg, 3 mg, 6 mg, 9 mg

INDICATIONS & DOSAGES
Adjust-a-dose (for all indications): In patients with CrCl of 50 to 80 mL/minute, initial dosage is 3 mg P.O. once daily and maximum dosage is 6 mg once daily; for patients with CrCl of 10 to 49 mL/minute, initial dosage is 1.5 mg P.O. once daily and maximum dosage is 3 mg once daily. If using injectable form and CrCl is 50 to 80 mL/minute, give 156 mg I.M. on day 1 and 117 mg I.M. 1 week later, followed by monthly injections of 78 mg.

➤ **Schizophrenia and schizoaffective disorder**
Adults: 6 mg P.O. once daily in the morning; may increase or decrease dose by 3-mg increments to a range of 3 to 12 mg daily; don't exceed 12 mg/day. Or, 234 mg I.M. on treatment day 1 and 156 mg I.M. 1 week later, both administered in deltoid muscle. Recommended maintenance dosage is 117 mg I.M. monthly (range, 39 to 234 mg based on tolerability and efficacy). Adjustments may be made monthly. See manufacturer's instructions for missed dosage schedules.

➤ **Schizophrenia**
Adolescents ages 12 to 17: Initially, 3 mg P.O. daily. Dosage may be increased by 3 mg/day every 5 days based on clinical response. Maximum dose is 12 mg/day for patients weighing 51 kg (112 lb) or more and 6 mg/day for patients weighing less than 51 kg.

ADMINISTRATION
P.O.
• Give with or without food.
• Don't crush or break tablets.
I.M.
• Inspect for particulate matter and discoloration.
• Shake syringe vigorously for at least 10 seconds to ensure a homogeneous suspension before administration.
• Inject slowly and deeply into muscle.
• Don't give I.V. or subcutaneously.
• Administer first two doses into deltoid muscle. After second dose, monthly maintenance doses can be given in deltoid or gluteal muscle.
• Injection is for single use only. Don't administer dose in divided injections.

ACTION
May antagonize both central dopamine (D_2) and serotonin type 2 receptors, as well as $alpha_1$, $alpha_2$, and H_1 receptors. Drug is a major active metabolite of risperidone.

Route	Onset	Peak	Duration
P.O.	Unknown	24 hr	Unknown
I.M.	24 hr	13 days	126 days

Half-life: 23 hours; 25 to 49 days for I.M.

P

ADVERSE REACTIONS

CNS: akathisia, headache, parkinsonism, somnolence, anxiety, asthenia, dizziness, dystonia, extrapyramidal disorder, fatigue, hypertonia, pyrexia, tremor, dyskinesia, hyperkinesia, insomnia, *suicidal ideation.*

CV: abnormal T waves, hypertension, orthostatic hypotension, palpitations, sinus arrhythmia, tachycardia, *AV block,* bundle branch block, *prolonged QTc interval.*

EENT: blurred vision, nasopharyngitis.

GI: abdominal pain, dry mouth, dyspepsia, nausea, salivary hypersecretion, vomiting, diarrhea, constipation, dry mouth.

Metabolic: blood insulin increases, hyperprolactinemia.

Musculoskeletal: back pain, extremity pain, musculoskeletal stiffness, myalgia.

Respiratory: cough, upper respiratory tract infection.

Skin: injection-site reaction.

INTERACTIONS

Drug-drug. *Anticholinergics:* May worsen side effects. Use cautiously together.

Antihypertensives: May worsen orthostatic hypotension. Avoid using together.

Centrally acting drugs: May worsen CNS side effects. Use cautiously together.

Drugs that prolong QTc interval, such as antiarrhythmics (amiodarone, procainamide, quinidine, sotalol), antipsychotics (chlorpromazine, thioridazine), quinolone antibiotics (moxifloxacin): May further prolong QTc interval. Avoid using together.

Levodopa, dopamine agonists: May antagonize effects of these drugs. Use cautiously together.

Drug-lifestyle. *Alcohol use:* May worsen CNS side effects. Discourage use together.

EFFECTS ON LAB TEST RESULTS

• May increase insulin and prolactin levels.

CONTRAINDICATIONS & CAUTIONS

• Contraindicated in patients hypersensitive to paliperidone or risperidone.

Black Box Warning Elderly patients with dementia-related psychosis treated with atypical or conventional antipsychotics are at increased risk for death. Antipsychotics aren't approved for the treatment of dementia-related psychosis. ∎

• Contraindicated in patients with congenital long QT syndrome or history of cardiac arrhythmias.

• Contraindicated in patients with preexisting severe GI narrowing (esophageal motility disorders, small-bowel inflammatory disease, short gut syndrome).

• Use cautiously in patients with a history of seizures or diabetes; those at risk for aspiration pneumonia; and those with bradycardia, hypokalemia, hypomagnesemia, CV disease, cerebrovascular disease, dehydration, or hypovolemia.

• Use cautiously in patients taking antihypertensives and drugs that lower the seizure threshold.

• Use cautiously in patients with history of suicide attempts.

➌ **Alert:** Neonates exposed to antipsychotics during the third trimester of pregnancy are at increased risk for developing extrapyramidal signs and symptoms (repetitive muscle movements of the face and body) and withdrawal signs and symptoms (agitation, abnormally increased or decreased muscle tone, tremors, sleepiness, severe difficulty breathing, difficulty feeding) following delivery. Use in pregnancy only if the potential benefit to the mother justifies the risk to the fetus.

⚠ **Overdose S&S:** Extrapyramidal symptoms, unsteady gait, drowsiness, sedation, tachycardia, hypotension, prolonged QT interval.

NURSING CONSIDERATIONS

• Establish tolerability with oral paliperidone or oral risperidone before initiating treatment with paliperidone injection.

➌ **Alert:** Monitor patient for atypical ventricular tachycardia, such as torsades de pointes, and ECG changes, particularly lengthening of the QT interval.

• Obtain baseline blood pressure before starting therapy and monitor pressure regularly. Watch for orthostatic hypotension.

➌ **Alert:** Watch for evidence of neuroleptic malignant syndrome (extrapyramidal effects, hyperthermia, autonomic disturbance), which is rare but deadly.

Reactions in bold italics are *life-threatening*. Interactions may have a *rapid onset* or a *delayed onset*.

• Monitor patient for tardive dyskinesia; it may disappear spontaneously or persist for life, despite ending drug. Seek smallest dosage and shortest duration of treatment that produce a satisfactory clinical response. Periodically reassess need for continued treatment.

❸ Alert: Drug may cause hyperglycemia. Monitor patient with diabetes regularly. In patient with risk factors for diabetes, obtain fasting blood glucose test results at baseline and periodically.

• Monitor patient for seizure activity, especially if patient has conditions that lower the seizure threshold.

• Monitor patient for dysphagia that can lead to aspiration and aspiration pneumonia.

• Monitor patient for abnormal body temperature regulation, especially if he exercises, is exposed to extreme heat, takes anticholinergics, or is dehydrated.

• Monitor patient for somnolence and sedation. Antipsychotics, including paliperidone, have the potential to impair judgment, thinking, or motor skills.

• Dispense lowest appropriate quantity of drug, to reduce risk of overdose.

PATIENT TEACHING
• Tell patient that remains of the tablet may appear in feces.

• Tell patient to swallow whole with liquids and not to chew, crush, or break tablets.

• Instruct the patient not to perform activities that require mental alertness until effects of drug are known.

• Warn patient to use caution in performing excessively strenuous activities because his body temperature may be disrupted.

• Advise patient that drug may lower blood pressure and to change positions slowly.

• Advise patient to seek medical attention if he experiences an erection lasting more than 4 hours.

• Instruct patient to contact prescriber before taking any other drugs to avoid potential interactions.

• Advise patient to avoid alcohol while taking this medication.

• Advise patient to contact prescriber if she becomes pregnant or wants to breast-feed.

palonosetron hydrochloride
pal-on-OS-e-tron

Aloxi

Therapeutic class: Antiemetics
Pharmacologic class: Selective serotonin (5-HT$_3$) receptor antagonists
Pregnancy risk category: B

AVAILABLE FORMS
Injection: 0.25 mg in 5-mL, single-use vial

INDICATIONS & DOSAGES
➤ **To prevent acute nausea and vomiting from moderately or highly emetogenic chemotherapy or delayed nausea and vomiting from moderately emetogenic chemotherapy**
Adults: 0.25 mg given I.V. over 30 seconds, 30 minutes before chemotherapy starts. Drug is given on the first day of each cycle, no more than every 7 days.

➤ **To prevent postoperative nausea and vomiting for up to 24 hours following surgery**
Adults: 0.075 mg I.V. over 10 seconds immediately before anesthesia induction.

ADMINISTRATION
I.V.
▼ Flush with normal saline solution before and after injection.

▼ Give by rapid I.V. injection through a peripheral or central I.V. line.

▼ **Incompatibilities:** Other I.V. drugs.

ACTION
Antagonizes 5-HT$_3$ receptors in the GI tract and brain, which inhibits emesis caused by chemotherapy.

Route	Onset	Peak	Duration
I.V.	30 min	Unknown	5 days

Half-life: 40 hours I.V.

ADVERSE REACTIONS
CNS: anxiety, dizziness, headache.
CV: *bradycardia, nonsustained ventricular tachycardia,* hypotension, *QT-interval prolongation.*
GI: constipation, diarrhea.

GU: urine retention.
Metabolic: *hyperkalemia.*
Skin: pruritus.

INTERACTIONS

Drug-drug. *Antiarrhythmics or other drugs that prolong the QTc interval, diuretics that induce electrolyte abnormalities, high-dose anthracycline:* May increase risk of prolonged QTc interval. Use together cautiously.
Apomorphine: May cause profound hypotension and loss of consciousness. Use together is contraindicated.

EFFECTS ON LAB TEST RESULTS

● May increase potassium level.

CONTRAINDICATIONS & CAUTIONS

● Contraindicated in patents hypersensitive to palonosetron or its ingredients.
● Use cautiously in patients hypersensitive to other 5-HT$_3$ antagonists, in those taking drugs that affect cardiac conduction, and in those with cardiac conduction abnormalities, hypokalemia, or hypomagnesemia.
● Safety and effectiveness in children haven't been established.

NURSING CONSIDERATIONS

● Before giving this drug, check patient's potassium level.
● Consider adding corticosteroids to the antiemetic regimen, particularly for patients receiving highly emetogenic chemotherapy.
● Make sure patient has additional antiemetics to take for breakthrough nausea or vomiting.
● If patient has cardiac conduction abnormalities, check the ECG before giving drug.

PATIENT TEACHING

● Advise patient to take a different antiemetic for breakthrough nausea or vomiting at the first sign of nausea rather than waiting until symptoms are severe.
● Urge patient with a history of cardiac conduction abnormalities to report any changes in drug regimen, such as adding or stopping an antiarrhythmic.

pamidronate disodium
pah-MIH-dro-nate

Aredia

Therapeutic class: Antiosteoporotics
Pharmacologic class: Bisphosphonates
Pregnancy risk category: D

AVAILABLE FORMS

Powder for injection: 30 mg/vial, 90 mg/vial
Solution for injection: 3 mg/mL, 6 mg/mL, 9 mg/mL in 10-mL vials

INDICATIONS & DOSAGES

➤ **Moderate to severe hypercalcemia from cancer (with or without bone metastases)**
Adults: Dosage depends on severity of hypercalcemia. Correct calcium level for albumin. Corrected calcium (CCa) level is calculated using this formula:

$$\underset{\text{(mg/dL)}}{\text{CCa}} = \underset{\text{(mg/dL)}}{\text{serum calcium}} + \underset{\text{(g/dL)}}{0.8\,(4 - \text{serum albumin})}$$

Patients with CCa levels of 12 to 13.5 mg/dL may receive 60 to 90 mg by I.V. infusion as a single dose over 2 to 24 hours. Patients with CCa levels greater than 13.5 mg/dL may receive 90 mg by I.V. infusion over 2 to 24 hours. Allow at least 7 days before retreatment to permit full response to first dose.
➤ **Moderate to severe Paget disease**
Adults: 30 mg I.V. as a 4-hour infusion on 3 consecutive days for total dose of 90 mg. Repeat cycle as needed.
➤ **Osteolytic bone metastases of breast cancer with standard antineoplastic therapy**
Adults: 90 mg I.V. infusion over 2 hours every 3 to 4 weeks.
➤ **Osteolytic bone lesions of multiple myeloma**
Adults: 90 mg I.V. over 4 hours once monthly.

➤ **Hyperparathyroidism** ◆
Adults: 15 to 90 mg by I.V. infusion. Additional doses may be given when hypercalcemia recurs or on a set schedule of every 1 or 2 months.

➤ **Immobilization-related hypercalcemia** ◆
Adults: 10 to 90 mg as a single I.V. infusion. May be repeated if necessary to maintain normal calcium levels.

➤ **Prevention of glucocorticoid-induced osteoporosis** ◆
Adults: 90 mg I.V. initially, followed by 30 mg I.V. every 3 months.

ADMINISTRATION

I.V.
▼ Reconstitute drug with 10 mL of sterile water for injection. After drug is completely dissolved, add to 250 mL (2-hour infusion), 500 mL (4-hour infusion), or 1,000 mL (up to 24-hour infusion) of half-normal or normal saline solution for injection or D_5W.
▼ Inspect solution for precipitate before use.
▼ Give drug only by I.V. infusion. Injecting a bolus may cause nephropathy.
▼ Infusions longer than 2 hours may reduce the risk of renal toxicity, particularly in patients with preexisting renal insufficiency.
▼ Solution is stable for 24 hours at room temperature.
▼ Store reconstituted drug at 36° to 46° F (2° to 8° C).
▼ **Incompatibilities:** Calcium-containing infusion solutions, such as Ringer injection or lactated Ringer solution.

ACTION

An antihypercalcemic that inhibits resorption of bone but apparently not bone formation. Adsorbs to hydroxyapatite crystals in bone and may directly block calcium phosphate dissolution and mature osteoclast formation.

Route	Onset	Peak	Duration
I.V.	Unknown	Unknown	Unknown

Half-life: Alpha, 1½ hours; beta, 27¼ hours.

ADVERSE REACTIONS

CNS: *seizures,* fatigue, somnolence, syncope, fever.
CV: atrial fibrillation, tachycardia, hypertension, fluid overload.
GI: abdominal pain, anorexia, constipation, nausea, vomiting, *GI hemorrhage.*
GU: renal dysfunction, UTI, *renal failure.*
Hematologic: *leukopenia, thrombocytopenia,* anemia.
Metabolic: hypophosphatemia, *hypokalemia, hypomagnesemia, hypocalcemia.*
Musculoskeletal: arthralgia, back pain, myalgia, osteonecrosis of the jaw.
Skin: infusion-site reaction, pain at infusion site.

INTERACTIONS
None significant.

EFFECTS ON LAB TEST RESULTS
• May increase creatinine level.
• May decrease phosphate, potassium, magnesium, calcium, and hemoglobin levels.
• May decrease WBC and platelet counts.

CONTRAINDICATIONS & CAUTIONS
• Contraindicated in patients hypersensitive to drug or other bisphosphonates such as etidronate.
🔁 *Alert:* There may be an increased risk of atypical fractures of the thigh in patients treated with bisphosphonates.
• Contraindicated in pregnancy.
• Use with caution, considering risks versus benefits, in patients with renal impairment.
• Use cautiously in breast-feeding women; it's unknown if drug appears in breast milk.
⚠ *Overdose S&S:* High fever, hypotension, taste perversion, hypocalcemia.

NURSING CONSIDERATIONS
• Assess hydration before treatment. Use drug only after patient has been vigorously hydrated with normal saline solution. In patients with mild to moderate hypercalcemia, hydration alone may be sufficient.
• Because drug can cause electrolyte disturbances, carefully monitor electrolyte levels, especially calcium, phosphate, and magnesium. Short-term use of calcium may

P

be needed in patients with severe hypocalcemia. Also monitor CBC and differential count, creatinine and hemoglobin levels, and hematocrit.

• Carefully monitor patients with anemia, leukopenia, or thrombocytopenia during first 2 weeks of therapy.

• Monitor patient's temperature. Patient may experience a slight elevation for 24 to 48 hours after therapy.

❸ **Alert:** Because renal dysfunction may lead to renal failure, single doses shouldn't exceed 90 mg.

• Monitor creatinine level before each treatment.

• In patients treated for bone metastases who have renal dysfunction, withhold dose until renal function returns to baseline. Treating bone metastases in patients with severe renal impairment isn't recommended. For other indications, determine whether the potential benefit outweighs the potential risk.

• Severe musculoskeletal pain has been associated with biophosphate use and may occur within days, months, or years of start of therapy. When drug is stopped, symptoms may resolve partially or completely.

• Bisphosphonates can interfere with bone-imaging agents.

❸ **Alert:** Patients should have a dental examination with appropriate preventive dentistry before taking drug, especially those with risk factors, including cancer, chemotherapy, corticosteroid therapy, and poor oral hygiene.

PATIENT TEACHING

• Explain use and administration of drug to patient and family.

• Instruct patient to report adverse reactions promptly.

• Advise women to alert health care provider if pregnant or breast-feeding.

pancrelipase
pan-kre-LYE-pase

Creon, Pancreaze, Pertzye, Ultrase, Ultrase MT12†, Ultrase MT20†, Ultresa, Viokace, Viokase 16†, Viokase Tablets†, Zenpep

Therapeutic class: Digestive enzymes
Pharmacologic class: Pancreatic enzymes
Pregnancy risk category: C

AVAILABLE FORMS
Creon
Capsules (delayed-release): 6,000 units lipase, 19,000 units protease, 30,000 units amylase; 12,000 units lipase, 38,000 units protease, 60,000 units amylase; 24,000 units lipase, 76,000 units protease, 120,000 units amylase
Pancreaze
Capsules (delayed-release): 4,200 units lipase, 10,000 units protease, 17,500 units amylase; 10,500 units lipase, 25,000 units protease, 43,750 units amylase; 16,800 units lipase, 40,000 units protease, 70,000 units amylase; 21,000 units lipase, 37,000 units protease, 61,000 units amylase
Pertzye
Capsules (delayed-release): 8,000 units lipase, 28,750 units protease, 30,250 units amylase; 16,000 units lipase, 57,500 units protease, 60,500 units amylase
Ultresa
Capsules (delayed-release): 13,800 units lipase, 27,600 units protease, 27,600 units amylase; 20,700 units lipase, 41,400 units protease, 41,400 units amylase; 23,000 units lipase, 46,000 units protease, 46,000 units amylase
Viokace
Tablets: 10,440 units lipase, 39,150 units protease, 39,150 units amylase; 20,880 units lipase, 78,300 units protease, 78,300 units amylase
Viokase 16
Tablets: 16,000 units lipase, 60,000 units protease, 60,000 units amylase
Zenpep
Capsules (enteric-coated beads): 3,000 units lipase, 10,000 units protease,

16,000 units amylase; 5,000 units lipase, 17,000 units protease, 27,000 units amylase; 10,000 units lipase, 34,000 units protease, 55,000 units amylase; 15,000 units lipase, 51,000 units protease, 82,000 units amylase; 20,000 units lipase, 68,000 units protease, 109,000 units amylase; 25,000 units lipase, 85,000 units protease, 136,000 units amylase

INDICATIONS & DOSAGES
➤ **Exocrine pancreatic secretion insufficiency; cystic fibrosis in adults and children; steatorrhea and other disorders of fat metabolism caused by insufficient pancreatic enzymes**
Adults and children older than age 4:
500 lipase units/kg P.O. per meal (up to the maximum dose).
Children older than age 12 months to 4 years: 1,000 lipase units/kg per meal up to maximum dose of 2,500 lipase units/kg per meal, 10,000 lipase units/kg daily, or 4,000 lipase units/g of fat ingested daily.
Infants up to age 12 months: 2,000 to 4,000 lipase units per 120 mL of formula or per breast-feeding.
➤ **Exocrine pancreatic insufficiency due to chronic pancreatitis or pancreatectomy (Creon)**
Adults: 72,000 units lipase P.O. while consuming at least 100 g of fat per day. Or, 500 lipase units/kg per meal. Adjust dosage to patient's response.
➤ **Exocrine pancreatic insufficiency due to chronic pancreatitis or pancreatectomy, with a proton pump inhibitor (Viokace)**
Adults: 500 lipase units/kg P.O. per meal to a maximum of 2,500 lipase units/kg of body weight per meal (or 10,000 lipase units/kg of body weight or less per day), or less than 4,000 lipase units/g fat ingested per day.
➤ **Exocrine pancreatic insufficiency due to cystic fibrosis or other conditions**
Adults and children age 4 and older weighing 16 kg (25 lb) or more: Pertzye: 500 lipase units/kg P.O. per meal to a maximum of 2,500 lipase units/kg per meal (or 10,000 lipase units/kg or less per day), or less than 4,000 lipase units/g fat ingested per day.

Adults and children age 4 and older weighing 28 kg (62 lb) or more: Ultresa: 500 lipase units/kg P.O. per meal to a maximum of 2,500 lipase units/kg per meal (or less than or equal to 10,000 lipase units/kg per day), or less than 4,000 lipase units/g fat ingested per day.
Children age 12 months to 4 years weighing 8 kg (18 lb) or more: Pertzye: 1,000 lipase units/kg P.O. per meal to a maximum of 2,500 lipase units/kg per meal (or 10,000 lipase units/kg or less per day), or less than 4,000 lipase units/g fat ingested per day.
Children age 12 months to 4 years weighing 14 kg (31 lb) or more: Ultresa: 1,000 lipase units/kg P.O. per meal to a maximum of 2,500 lipase units/kg per meal (or less than or equal to 10,000 lipase units/kg per day), or less than 4,000 lipase units/g fat ingested per day.

ADMINISTRATION
P.O.
● Give drug before or with meals and snacks.
● Don't crush or allow patient to chew enteric-coated forms. Capsules containing enteric-coated microspheres may be opened and sprinkled on a small quantity of cool, soft food. Have patient swallow immediately, without chewing, and follow dose with glass of water or juice.
● For infants, mix powder with applesauce and give with meals. Avoid contact with or inhalation of powder because it may be highly irritating. Older children may swallow capsules with food.
● Don't mix Zenpep capsule contents directly into formula or breast milk before administration. Capsule contents may be administered directly into the infant's mouth before feeding.

ACTION
Replaces endogenous exocrine pancreatic enzymes and aids digestion of starches, fats, and proteins.

Route	Onset	Peak	Duration
P.O.	Variable	Variable	Variable

Half-life: Unknown.

ADVERSE REACTIONS
CNS: headache.
EENT: pharyngolaryngeal pain, epistaxis.
GI: nausea, cramping, diarrhea with high doses, dyspepsia.
Respiratory: cough.
Other: biliary tract stones, anal pruritus.

INTERACTIONS
Drug-drug. *Antacids:* May destroy enteric coating and enhance degradation of pancrelipase. Avoid using together.
Oral iron supplement: May decrease iron response. Monitor patient for decreased effectiveness.

EFFECTS ON LAB TEST RESULTS
• May increase uric acid level.

CONTRAINDICATIONS & CAUTIONS
• Contraindicated in patients with severe hypersensitivity to pork and in those with acute pancreatitis or acute worsening of chronic pancreatic diseases.
• Use Ultresa, Viokace, and Pertzye cautiously in patients with gout, renal impairment, or hyperuricemia.
⚠ ***Overdose S&S:*** Transient intestinal upset, diarrhea.

NURSING CONSIDERATIONS
🔵 *Alert:* Use drug only for confirmed exocrine pancreatic insufficiency. It isn't effective in GI disorders unrelated to enzyme deficiency.
🔵 *Alert:* Fibrosing colonopathy is associated with high-dose use of pancreatic enzymes. Use cautiously when doses exceed 2,500 lipase units/kg per meal (or are greater than 10,000 lipase units/kg per day).
• Lipase activity is greater than with other pancreatic enzymes.
• Monitor patient's stools. Adequate replacement decreases number of bowel movements and improves stool consistency.
• Individual products aren't bioequivalent and shouldn't be interchanged without prescriber supervision.
• Dosage varies with degree of maldigestion and malabsorption, amount of fat in diet, and enzyme activity of individual preparations.

• Enteric coating on some products may reduce available enzyme in upper portion of jejunum.

PATIENT TEACHING
• Instruct patient to take drug before or with meals and snacks, but always with food.
• Advise patient not to crush or chew enteric-coated forms. Capsules containing enteric-coated microspheres may be opened and sprinkled on a small quantity of cool, soft food. Stress importance of swallowing immediately, without chewing, and following with glass of water or juice.
• Warn patient not to inhale powder form or powder from capsules; it may irritate skin or mucous membranes.
• Tell patient to store drug in airtight container at room temperature.
• Instruct patient not to change brands without consulting prescriber.

SAFETY ALERT!

pancuronium bromide
pan-kyoo-ROW-nee-uhm

Therapeutic class: Skeletal muscle relaxants
Pharmacologic class: Nondepolarizing neuromuscular blockers
Pregnancy risk category: C

AVAILABLE FORMS
Injection: 1 mg/mL, 2 mg/mL

INDICATIONS & DOSAGES
➤ **Adjunct to anesthesia to relax skeletal muscle, facilitate intubation, and assist with mechanical ventilation**
Adults and children age 1 month and older: Initially, 0.04 to 0.1 mg/kg I.V.; then 0.01 mg/kg every 30 to 60 minutes.
Neonates: Individualize dosage.

ADMINISTRATION
I.V.
Black Box Warning This drug should be administered by adequately trained individuals familiar with its actions, characteristics, and hazards. ■

▼ Only staff skilled in airway management should use drug.

▼ Drug has no known effect on consciousness, pain threshold, or cerebration. To avoid patient distress, don't induce neuromuscular blockade before unconsciousness.

▼ Keep endotracheal equipment, ventilator, oxygen, atropine, edrophonium, epinephrine, and neostigmine immediately available.

▼ Store in refrigerator. Don't store in plastic containers or syringes, although plastic syringes may be used for administration.

▼ Compatible in solution with normal saline, dextrose 5%, dextrose 5% and sodium chloride, and Ringer lactate.

▼ **Incompatibilities:** Alkaline solutions, barbiturates, diazepam, thiopental sodium.

ACTION
Prevents acetylcholine from binding to receptors on the motor end plate, blocking neuromuscular transmission.

Route	Onset	Peak	Duration
I.V.	30–45 sec	3–4½ min	35–65 min

Half-life: About 2 hours.

ADVERSE REACTIONS
CV: tachycardia, increased blood pressure.
EENT: excessive salivation.
Musculoskeletal: residual muscle weakness.
Respiratory: *prolonged respiratory insufficiency or apnea.*
Skin: transient rashes.
Other: allergic or idiosyncratic hypersensitivity reactions.

INTERACTIONS
Drug-drug. *Aminoglycosides (amikacin, gentamicin, neomycin, streptomycin, tobramycin), magnesium salts:* May increase the effects of pancuronium, including prolonged respiratory depression. Use together only when necessary. Dose of pancuronium may need to be reduced.
Azathioprine: May reverse neuromuscular blockade induced by pancuronium. Monitor patient.

Beta blockers, clindamycin, general anesthetics (such as enflurane, halothane, isoflurane), ketamine, lincomycin, magnesium sulfate, polymyxin antibiotics (colistin, polymyxin B sulfate), quinidine, quinine, verapamil: May enhance neuromuscular blockade, increasing skeletal muscle relaxation and prolonging effect of pancuronium. Use together cautiously during and after surgery.
Carbamazepine, phenytoin: May decrease effects of pancuronium. May need to increase pancuronium dose.
Diuretics: May cause electrolyte imbalance or alter neuromuscular blockade. Monitor electrolytes before giving drug.
Lithium, opioid analgesics: May enhance neuromuscular blockade, increasing skeletal muscle relaxation and possibly causing respiratory paralysis. Use cautiously, and reduce dose of pancuronium.
Succinylcholine: May increase intensity and duration of neuromuscular blockade. Allow effects of succinylcholine to subside before giving pancuronium.
Theophylline: May produce a dose-dependent reversal of neuromuscular blocking effects. Monitor patient for clinical effect.
TCAs: May increase risk of ventricular arrhythmias in patients anesthetized with both halothane and pancuronium. Monitor ECG closely in patients taking TCAs before surgery.

EFFECTS ON LAB TEST RESULTS
None reported.

CONTRAINDICATIONS & CAUTIONS
● Contraindicated in patients hypersensitive to bromides, those with tachycardia, and those for whom even a minor increase in heart rate is undesirable.
● Use cautiously in elderly or debilitated patients; in patients with renal, hepatic, or pulmonary impairment; and in those with respiratory depression, myasthenia gravis, myasthenic syndrome related to lung cancer, dehydration, thyroid disorders, CV disease, collagen diseases, porphyria, electrolyte disturbances, hyperthermia, and toxemic states. Also, use large doses cautiously in patients undergoing cesarean section.

P

⚠ *Overdose S&S:* Residual neuromuscular blockade (skeletal muscle weakness, decreased respiratory reserve, low tidal volume, apnea).

NURSING CONSIDERATIONS
● Dosage depends on anesthetic used, individual needs, and response. Dosages are representative and must be adjusted.
● Allow succinylcholine effects to subside before giving this drug.
● Monitor baseline electrolyte determinations (electrolyte imbalance can potentiate neuromuscular effects) and vital signs, especially respirations and heart rate.
● Measure fluid intake and output; renal dysfunction may prolong duration of action because 25% of drug is excreted unchanged in the urine.
● A nerve stimulator and train-of-four monitoring are recommended to confirm antagonism of neuromuscular blockade and recovery of muscle strength. Make sure there's some evidence of spontaneous recovery before attempting pharmacologic reversal with neostigmine.
● Monitor respirations closely until patient recovers fully from neuromuscular blockade, as indicated by tests of muscle strength (hand grip, head lift, and ability to cough).
● After spontaneous recovery starts, neuromuscular blockade may be reversed with an anticholinesterase (such as neostigmine or edrophonium), which is usually given with an anticholinergic (such as atropine).
● Drug doesn't cause histamine release or hypotension, but it may raise heart rate and blood pressure.
● Give analgesics for pain.
⟳ *Alert:* Careful dosage calculation is essential. Always verify dosage with another health care professional.

PATIENT TEACHING
● Explain all events and procedures to patient because he can still hear.

pantoprazole sodium
pan-TOE-pray-zol

Pantoloc†, Panto IV†, Protonix◆, Protonix I.V.

Therapeutic class: Antiulcer drugs
Pharmacologic class: Proton pump inhibitors
Pregnancy risk category: B

AVAILABLE FORMS
Injection: 40 mg/vial
Suspension (delayed-release): 40 mg
Tablets (delayed-release): 20 mg, 40 mg
Tablets (enteric-coated): 20 mg, 40 mg

INDICATIONS & DOSAGES
➤ **Maintenance of healing of erosive esophagitis**
Adults: 40 mg P.O. once daily.
➤ **Short-term treatment of erosive esophagitis associated with GERD**
Adults: 40 mg P.O. once daily for up to 8 weeks. For patients who haven't healed after 8 weeks of treatment, another 8-week course may be considered. Or, 40 mg I.V. once daily for 7 to 10 days. Switch to P.O. form as soon as patient is able to take orally.
➤ **Long-term maintenance of healing erosive esophagitis and reduction in relapse rates of daytime and nighttime heartburn symptoms in patients with GERD**
Adults: 40 mg P.O. once daily.
➤ **Treatment of pathologic hypersecretion caused by Zollinger-Ellison syndrome**
Adults: Individualize dosage. Usual dosage is 40 mg P.O. b.i.d. Usual I.V. dose is 80 mg I.V. every 12 hours for no more than 6 days. For those needing a higher dose, 80 mg every 8 hours is expected to maintain acid output below 10 mEq/hour. Maximum daily dose is 240 mg/day. When converting from I.V. to P.O. form, ensure continuity of suppression of acid secretion.
➤ **Stress ulcer prophylaxis ◆**
Adults: 40 mg P.O. or I.V. every 12 to 24 hours.

Reactions in bold italics are *life-threatening*. Interactions may have a *rapid onset* or a *delayed onset*.

ADMINISTRATION

P.O.
● Give tablets without regard for food and make sure patient swallows them whole.
● May give with antacids.
● Don't crush or split tablets.
● Give delayed-release suspension in apple sauce or apple juice 30 minutes prior to a meal. Don't give in water or other liquids or foods.
● Don't split, crush, or allow patient to chew granules for delayed-release oral suspension.

I.V.
▼ Safety and effectiveness of the I.V. form to start therapy for GERD are unknown.
▼ Reconstitute each vial with 10 mL of normal saline solution.
▼ Compatible diluents for infusion include normal saline solution, D₅W, or lactated Ringer solution for injection.
▼ For patients with GERD, further dilute with 100 mL of diluent to yield 0.4 mg/mL.
▼ For patients with hypersecretion, combine two reconstituted vials and further dilute with 80 mL of diluent to a total volume of 100 mL, to yield 0.8 mg/mL.
▼ Infuse diluted solutions over 15 minutes at a rate of about 7 mL/minute.
▼ For a 2-minute infusion, give the reconstituted vials (final yield of about 4 mg/mL) over at least 2 minutes.
▼ The reconstituted solution may be stored for up to 2 hours and the diluted solutions for up to 22 hours at room temperature.
▼ **Incompatibilities:** Midazolam, zinc-containing products or solutions. Don't give another infusion simultaneously through the same line.

ACTION

Inhibits proton pump activity by binding to hydrogen–potassium adenosine triphosphatase, located at secretory surface of gastric parietal cells, to suppress gastric acid secretion.

Route	Onset	Peak	Duration
P.O.	Unknown	2½ hr	>24 hr
I.V.	15–30 min	Unknown	24 hr

Half-life: 1 hour.

ADVERSE REACTIONS

CNS: anxiety, asthenia, dizziness, headache, insomnia, migraine, pain.
CV: chest pain.
EENT: pharyngitis, rhinitis, sinusitis.
GI: abdominal pain, constipation, diarrhea, dyspepsia, eructation, flatulence, gastroenteritis, GI disorder, nausea, rectal disorder, vomiting.
GU: urinary frequency, UTI.
Metabolic: hyperglycemia, hyperlipidemia.
Musculoskeletal: arthralgia, back pain, hypertonia, neck pain.
Respiratory: bronchitis, dyspnea, increased cough, upper respiratory tract infection.
Skin: rash.
Other: flulike syndrome, infection, injection-site reaction.

INTERACTIONS

Drug-drug. *Ampicillin esters, iron salts, ketoconazole:* May decrease absorption of these drugs. Monitor patient closely and separate doses.
Azole antifungals (itraconazole, ketoconazole): May decrease plasma levels of these drugs. Avoid this combination if possible.
Protease inhibitors (atazanavir, indinavir, nelfinavir): May reduce antiviral activity of these drugs. Adjust dosage as needed; administration of atazanavir with pantoprazole isn't recommended.
Salicylates: Enteric-coated salicylates may dissolve more rapidly, increasing gastric adverse reactions. Monitor patient.
Warfarin: May increase INR and PT. Monitor patient and laboratory values.
Drug-herb. *Ginkgo biloba:* May reduce pantoprazole's therapeutic effect. Avoid this combination.
St. John's wort: May increase risk of sunburn. Advise patient to avoid excessive sunlight exposure.
Drug-lifestyle. *Sunlight:* May increase risk of sunburn. Advise patient to avoid excessive sunlight exposure.

EFFECTS ON LAB TEST RESULTS

● May increase glucose and lipid levels.
● May increase liver function test result values.

• May cause false-positive urine screen test for tetrahydrocannabinol.

CONTRAINDICATIONS & CAUTIONS
• Contraindicated in patients hypersensitive to any component of the formulation.

NURSING CONSIDERATIONS
• Symptomatic response to therapy doesn't preclude the presence of gastric malignancy.
❸ *Alert:* Prolonged use of proton pump inhibitors may cause low magnesium levels. Monitor magnesium levels before start of treatment and periodically thereafter.
❸ *Alert:* Monitor patient for signs and symptoms of low magnesium level, such as abnormal heart rate or rhythm, palpitations, muscle spasms, tremor, or seizures. In children, abnormal heart rate may present as fatigue, upset stomach, dizziness, and lightheadedness. Magnesium supplementation or drug discontinuation may be required.
❸ *Alert:* May increase risk for *Clostridium difficile*–associated diarrhea (CDAD). Evaluate for CDAD in patients who develop diarrhea that doesn't improve.
• *Look alike–sound alike:* Don't confuse Protonix with Prilosec, Prozac, or Prevacid. Don't confuse pantoprazole with aripiprazole.

PATIENT TEACHING
• Instruct patient to take exactly as prescribed and at about the same time every day.
• Advise patient that drug can be taken without regard to meals.
• Tell patient to swallow tablet whole and not to crush, split, or chew it.
• Tell patient that antacids don't affect drug absorption.
• Teach patient to recognize and report signs and symptoms of low magnesium levels.

paroxetine hydrochloride
pah-ROX-a-teen

Paxil, Paxil CR

paroxetine mesylate
Brisdelle, Pexeva

Therapeutic class: Antidepressants
Pharmacologic class: SSRIs
Pregnancy risk category: D

AVAILABLE FORMS
Suspension: 10 mg/5 mL
Tablets: 7.5 mg, 10 mg, 20 mg, 30 mg, 40 mg
Tablets (controlled-release): 12.5 mg, 25 mg, 37.5 mg

INDICATIONS & DOSAGES
Adjust-a-dose (for all indications): For debilitated patients or those with renal or hepatic impairment taking immediate-release form, initially, 10 mg P.O. daily, preferably in morning. If patient doesn't respond after full antidepressant effect has occurred, increase dose by 10 mg daily at weekly intervals to a maximum of 40 mg daily. If using controlled-release form, start therapy at 12.5 mg daily. Don't exceed 50 mg daily.
➤ **Depression**
Adults: Initially, 20 mg P.O. daily, preferably in morning, as indicated. If patient doesn't improve, increase dose by 10 mg daily at intervals of at least 1 week to a maximum of 50 mg daily. If using controlled-release form, initially, 25 mg P.O. daily. Increase dose by 12.5 mg daily at weekly intervals to a maximum of 62.5 mg daily.
Elderly patients: Initially, 10 mg P.O. daily, preferably in morning, as indicated. If patient doesn't improve, increase dose by 10 mg daily at weekly intervals, to a maximum of 40 mg daily. If using controlled-release form, start therapy at 12.5 mg P.O. daily. Don't exceed 50 mg daily.
➤ **Obsessive-compulsive disorder (OCD)**
Adults: Initially, 20 mg P.O. daily, preferably in morning. Increase dose by 10 mg daily at weekly intervals. Recommended daily dose is 40 mg. Maximum daily dose is 60 mg.

Reactions in bold italics are *life-threatening*. Interactions may have a *rapid onset* or a *delayed onset*.

> **Panic disorder**
Adults: Initially, 10 mg P.O. daily. Increase dose by 10 mg at no less than weekly intervals to maximum of 60 mg daily. Or, 12.5 mg Paxil CR P.O. as a single daily dose, usually in the morning, with or without food; increase dose at intervals of at least 1 week by 12.5 mg daily, up to a maximum of 75 mg daily.

> **Social anxiety disorder (excluding Pexeva)**
Adults: Initially, 20 mg P.O. daily, preferably in morning. Dosage range is 20 to 60 mg daily. Adjust dosage to maintain patient on lowest effective dose. Or, 12.5 mg Paxil CR P.O. as a single daily dose, usually in the morning, with or without food. Increase dosage at weekly intervals in increments of 12.5 mg daily, up to a maximum of 37.5 mg daily.

> **Generalized anxiety disorder (excluding Pexeva)**
Adults: 20 mg P.O. daily initially, increasing by 10 mg per day weekly up to 50 mg daily.

> **Posttraumatic stress disorder (excluding Pexeva)**
Adults: Initially, 20 mg P.O. daily. Increase dose by 10 mg daily at intervals of at least 1 week. Maximum daily dose is 50 mg P.O.

> **Premenstrual dysphoric disorder (PMDD)**
Adults: Initially, 12.5 mg Paxil CR P.O. as a single daily dose, usually in the morning, with or without food, daily or during the luteal phase of the menstrual cycle. Dose changes should occur at intervals of at least 1 week. Maximum dose is 25 mg P.O. daily.

✷ *NEW INDICATION:* **Moderate to severe vasomotor symptoms associated with menopause (Brisdelle only)**
Adults: 7.5 mg P.O. daily.

> **Hot flashes (breast cancer)** ◆
Adults: 20 mg P.O. daily or nightly.

> **Hot flashes (menopausal)** ◆
Adults: 10 or 20 mg P.O. daily (immediate release) or 12.5 or 25 mg P.O. daily (controlled-release).

> **Diabetic neuropathy** ◆
Adults: Initially, 10 mg P.O. daily. Titrate dosage to 20 to 60 mg/day.

> **Irritable bowel syndrome** ◆
Adults: 20 to 40 mg P.O. daily for 6 to 12 months.

> **Premenstrual disorders** ◆
Adults: 10 to 30 mg P.O. daily.

ADMINISTRATION
P.O.
● Give drug without regard for food.
● Don't split or crush controlled-release tablets.

ACTION
Thought to be linked to drug's inhibition of CNS neuronal uptake of serotonin.

Route	Onset	Peak	Duration
P.O.	Unknown	2–8 hr	Unknown
P.O. (controlled-release)	Unknown	6–10 hr	Unknown

Half-life: About 24 hours.

ADVERSE REACTIONS
CNS: asthenia, dizziness, headache, insomnia, somnolence, tremor, nervousness, *suicidal behavior,* anxiety, paresthesia, confusion, agitation.
CV: palpitations, vasodilation, hypertension, tachycardia.
EENT: lump or tightness in throat, blurred vision.
GI: dry mouth, nausea, constipation, diarrhea, flatulence, vomiting, dyspepsia, dysgeusia, increased or decreased appetite, abdominal pain.
GU: ejaculatory disturbances, sexual dysfunction, urinary frequency, other urinary disorders.
Musculoskeletal: myopathy, myalgia, myasthenia.
Skin: diaphoresis, rash, pruritus.
Other: decreased libido, yawning.

INTERACTIONS
Drug-drug. *Atomoxetine:* May alter atomoxetine level. Initiate atomoxetine at a reduced dosage.
Barbiturates (phenobarbital), phenytoin: May alter pharmacokinetics of both drugs. Dosage adjustments may be needed.
Cimetidine: May decrease hepatic metabolism of paroxetine, leading to risk of adverse reactions. Dosage adjustments may be needed.
Cyclosporine: May increase cyclosporine level and toxicity. Monitor cyclosporine

P

level when adding or discontinuing paroxetine; adjust cyclosporine dosage as needed.

Digoxin: May decrease digoxin level. Use together cautiously.

Drugs that prolong QT interval (antiarrhythmics [amiodarone, bretylium, disopyramide, dofetilide, procainamide, quinidine, sotalol], arsenic trioxide, chlorpromazine, cisapride, dolasetron, droperidol, mefloquine, mesoridazine, moxifloxacin, pentamidine, pimozide, tacrolimus, thioridazine, ziprasidone): May increase risk of life-threatening cardiac arrhythmias, including torsades de pointes. Monitor patient closely.

Fosamprenavir, ritonavir: May decrease paroxetine plasma level. Adjust dosage as needed.

Galantamine: May alter oral bioavailability of galantamine. Use together cautiously.

Linezolid: May cause serotonin syndrome. Allow at least 2 weeks after stopping linezolid before giving paroxetine.

Lithium: May enhance serotonergic effects of paroxetine. Use with caution.

MAO inhibitors (such as phenelzine, selegiline, tranylcypromine): May cause serotonin syndrome and signs and symptoms resembling neuroleptic malignant syndrome. Avoid using within 14 days of MAO inhibitor therapy.

Metoclopramide, sibutramine, L-tryptophan, sympathomimetics: May increase risk of serotonin syndrome. Monitor patient closely.

NSAIDs: May increase risk of GI bleeding. If possible, avoid concurrent use. If coadministration can't be avoided, consider shortening NSAID treatment duration, decreasing dosage, or switching to acetaminophen or a TCA.

Phenothiazines (thioridazine): May increase phenothiazine plasma level, increasing pharmacologic and adverse reactions of phenothiazine. Use together is contraindicated.

Pimozide: May increase pimozide level. Use together is contraindicated.

Procyclidine: May increase procyclidine level. Reduce procyclidine dosage if anticholinergic effects occur.

Risperidone: May increase risperidone level, increasing risk of adverse reactions;

serotonin syndrome may occur. Use together cautiously.

Sympathomimetics: May increase sensitivity to the effect of sympathomimetics and increase risk of serotonin syndrome. Monitor patient.

Drug-herb. *SAMe:* May increase risk of serotonin syndrome. Avoid use together.

St. John's wort: May increase sedative-hypnotic effects. Discourage use together.

Drug-lifestyle. *Alcohol use:* May alter psychomotor function. Discourage use together.

EFFECTS ON LAB TEST RESULTS
None reported.

CONTRAINDICATIONS & CAUTIONS
• Contraindicated in patients hypersensitive to drug, within 14 days of MAO inhibitor therapy, and in those taking thioridazine.

Black Box Warning Contraindicated in children and adolescents younger than age 18. ▮

❸ *Alert:* Use with linezolid or methylene blue can cause serotonin syndrome (fever, mental status changes, muscle twitching, excessive sweating, shivering or shaking, diarrhea, loss of coordination). Use drug with linezolid or methylene blue only for life-threatening or urgent conditions when the potential benefits outweigh the risks of toxicity.

• Use cautiously in patients with history of seizure disorders or mania and in those with other severe, systemic illness.

• Use cautiously in patients at risk for volume depletion and monitor them appropriately.

• Using drug in the first trimester may increase the risk of congenital fetal malformations; using drug in the third trimester may cause neonatal complications at birth. Consider the risk versus benefit of therapy.

⚠ *Overdose S&S:* Coma, confusion, dizziness, nausea, somnolence, tachycardia, tremor, vomiting, acute renal failure, aggressive reactions, bradycardia, dystonia, hepatic necrosis, hypertension, hypotension, jaundice, manic reactions, mydriasis, myoclonus, rhabdomyolysis, seizures,

---

serotonin syndrome, stupor, hepatic impairment, syncope, urine retention, ventricular arrhythmias.

NURSING CONSIDERATIONS
• Patients taking Paxil CR for PMDD should be periodically reassessed to determine the need for continued treatment.
• If signs or symptoms of psychosis occur or increase, expect prescriber to reduce dosage. Record mood changes. Monitor patient for suicidal tendencies, and allow only a minimum supply of drug.
Black Box Warning Drug may increase the risk of suicidal thinking and behavior in children, adolescents, and young adults ages 18 to 24 during the first 2 months of treatment, especially in those with major depressive disorder or other psychiatric disorder. ∎

❸ *Alert:* If linezolid or methylene blue must be given, stop paroxetine and monitor patient for serotonin toxicity for 2 weeks or until 24 hours after the last dose of methylene blue or linezolid, whichever comes first. Treatment with paroxetine may be resumed 24 hours after the last dose of methylene blue or linezolid.
• Monitor patient for complaints of sexual dysfunction. In men, they include anorgasmia, erectile difficulties, delayed ejaculation or orgasm; in women, they include anorgasmia or difficulty with orgasm.

❸ *Alert:* Don't stop drug abruptly. Withdrawal or discontinuation syndrome may occur if drug is stopped abruptly. Symptoms include headache, myalgia, lethargy, and general flulike symptoms. Taper drug slowly over 1 to 2 weeks.

❸ *Alert:* Combining triptans with an SSRI or an SSNRI may cause serotonin syndrome or neuroleptic malignant syndrome–like reactions. Signs and symptoms of serotonin syndrome may include restlessness, hallucinations, loss of coordination, fast heartbeat, rapid changes in blood pressure, increased body temperature, overactive reflexes, nausea, vomiting, and diarrhea. Serotonin syndrome may be more likely to occur when starting or increasing the dose of triptan, SSRI, or SSNRI.
• *Look alike–sound alike:* Don't confuse paroxetine with fluoxetine or paclitaxel.

Don't confuse Paxil with Doxil, paclitaxel, Plavix, or Taxol.

PATIENT TEACHING
Black Box Warning Advise families and caregivers to closely observe patient for increased suicidal thinking and behavior. ∎
❸ *Alert:* Teach patient to recognize and immediately report signs and symptoms of serotonin toxicity.
• Tell patient that drug may be taken with or without food, usually in morning.
• Tell patient not to break, crush, or chew controlled-release tablets.
• Warn patient to avoid activities that require alertness and good coordination until effects of drug are known.
• Advise woman of childbearing age to contact prescriber if she becomes pregnant or plans to become pregnant during therapy or if she's currently breast-feeding.
• Tell patient to avoid alcohol and to consult prescriber before taking other prescription or OTC drugs or herbal medicines.
• Instruct patient not to stop taking drug abruptly.

SAFETY ALERT!

pegaspargase (PEG-L-asparaginase)
peg-AHS-per-jays

Oncaspar

Therapeutic class: Antineoplastics
Pharmacologic class: Modified L-asparaginases
Pregnancy risk category: C

AVAILABLE FORMS
Injection: 750 international units/mL

INDICATIONS & DOSAGES
➤ **As part of a multidrug chemotherapy regimen in the treatment of acute lymphoblastic leukemia, and acute lymphoblastic leukemia with hypersensitivity to asparaginase**
Adults and children older than age 1: 2,500 international units/m^2 I.V. or I.M. every 14 days.

ADMINISTRATION

I.V.

▼ Give I.V. only if I.M. route is contraindicated.

▼ Give I.V. over 1 to 2 hours in 100 mL of normal saline solution or D_5W injection through an infusion that's already running.

▼ Drug may be a contact irritant, and solution must be handled and given with care. Wear gloves. Avoid inhalation of vapors and contact with skin or mucous membranes, especially in the eyes. If contact occurs, wash with generous amounts of water for at least 15 minutes.

▼ Don't use if cloudy or contains precipitate. Avoid excessive agitation of drug; don't shake.

▼ Don't freeze or use drug that has been frozen because freezing destroys drug's effectiveness.

▼ Discard unused portions. Use only one dose per vial; don't reenter vial.

▼ Don't use if stored at room temperature for longer than 48 hours. Keep refrigerated at 36° to 46° F (2° to 8° C).

▼ **Incompatibilities:** None reported, but don't mix with other I.V. drugs.

I.M.

● I.M. is the preferred route and is associated with lower incidence of adverse effects.

● When giving I.M., limit volume given at a single injection site to 2 mL. If volume to be given exceeds 2 mL, use multiple injection sites.

ACTION

A modified version of the enzyme L-asparaginase that exerts cytotoxic effects by inactivating the amino acid asparagine, which tumor cells need to synthesize proteins.

Route	Onset	Peak	Duration
I.V., I.M.	Unknown	Unknown	Unknown

Half-life: Unknown.

ADVERSE REACTIONS

CNS: *coma, seizures, status epilepticus,* confusion, dizziness, emotional lability, fatigue, headache, malaise, paresthesia, parkinsonism, peripheral neuritis, somnolence, *stroke.*

CV: hypertension, hypotension, peripheral edema, tachycardia.

EENT: epistaxis.

GI: *pancreatitis,* abdominal pain, anorexia, constipation, diarrhea, flatulence, mouth tenderness, mucositis, nausea, severe colitis, vomiting.

GU: *renal failure,* hematuria, increased urinary frequency, proteinuria, renal dysfunction, severe hemorrhagic cystitis.

Hematologic: *agranulocytosis, disseminated intravascular coagulation, hemorrhage, leukopenia, pancytopenia, thrombocytopenia, thrombosis,* easy bruising, hemolytic anemia.

Hepatic: *liver failure,* ascites, fatty changes in liver, hypoalbuminemia, jaundice.

Metabolic: *hypoglycemia,* hyperglycemia, hyperuricemia, hypoproteinemia, *metabolic acidosis,* uric acid nephropathy.

Musculoskeletal: arthralgia, cramps, joint stiffness, myalgia, musculoskeletal pain.

Respiratory: *bronchospasm,* cough, upper respiratory tract infection.

Skin: ecchymoses, erythema, erythema simplex, fungal changes, hand whiteness, injection pain or reaction, itching, localized edema, nail whiteness and ridging, petechial rash, purpura, rash, urticaria.

Other: *anaphylaxis, sepsis, septic shock,* hypersensitivity reactions, infection, night sweats.

INTERACTIONS

Drug-drug. *Aspirin, dipyridamole, heparin, NSAIDs, warfarin:* May cause imbalances in coagulation factors, predisposing patient to bleeding or thrombosis. Use together cautiously.

Protein-bound drugs: May increase toxicity of other drugs that bind to proteins and may interfere with enzymatic detoxification of other drugs, especially in the liver. Check for toxicity, and use together cautiously.

EFFECTS ON LAB TEST RESULTS

● May increase BUN, creatinine, amylase, lipase, bilirubin, ALT, AST, uric acid, and ammonia levels. May decrease sodium and protein levels. May increase or decrease glucose level.

● May increase PT, INR, activated PTT, and thromboplastin. May decrease hemoglobin

---

level and antithrombin III, WBC, RBC, platelet, and granulocyte counts.

CONTRAINDICATIONS & CAUTIONS
• Contraindicated in patients with pancreatitis or history of pancreatitis, in those who have had significant hemorrhagic events related to previous treatment with L-asparaginase, and in those with history of serious allergic reactions to drug, such as generalized urticaria, bronchospasm, laryngeal edema, hypotension, or other unacceptable adverse reactions.
• Discontinue drug in patients with serious thrombotic events.
• Use cautiously in patients with liver dysfunction.
• Use only when clearly indicated in pregnant women.
⚠ **Overdose S&S:** Elevated liver enzyme levels, rash.

NURSING CONSIDERATIONS
• Take preventive measures (including adequate hydration) before starting treatment. Hyperuricemia may result from rapid lysis of leukemic cells.
🟊 **Alert:** Monitor patients closely for hypersensitivity (including life-threatening anaphylaxis), especially those hypersensitive to other forms of L-asparaginase. Observe patient for 1 hour after giving drug and have emergency equipment and other drugs needed to treat anaphylaxis readily available. Moderate to life-threatening hypersensitivity requires stopping L-asparaginase.
• To assess effects of therapy, monitor patient's peripheral blood count and bone marrow. A drop in circulating lymphoblasts is often noted after therapy starts, sometimes accompanied by a marked rise in uric acid level.
• Obtain frequent amylase and lipase determinations to detect pancreatitis. Monitor patient's glucose level during therapy to detect hyperglycemia.
• Monitor patient for liver dysfunction when drug is used with hepatotoxic chemotherapeutic drugs.
• Drug may affect several plasma proteins; monitor fibrinogen, PT, INR, and PTT at baseline and periodically during and after treatment.

• **Look alike–sound alike:** Don't confuse pegaspargase with asparaginase.

PATIENT TEACHING
• Inform patient of risk of hypersensitivity reactions and importance of reporting them immediately.
• Tell patient not to take other drugs, including OTC preparations, until approved by prescriber because risk of bleeding is higher when pegaspargase is given with drugs such as aspirin. Drug may also increase toxicity of other drugs.
• Urge patient to report signs and symptoms of infection (fever, chills, and malaise); drug may suppress the immune system.
• Caution woman of childbearing age to avoid pregnancy and breast-feeding during therapy.

SAFETY ALERT!

pegfilgrastim
peg-fill-GRASS-tim

Neulasta

Therapeutic class: Colony stimulating factors
Pharmacologic class: Hematopoietics
Pregnancy risk category: C

AVAILABLE FORMS
Injection: 6 mg/0.6-mL syringe

INDICATIONS & DOSAGES
➤ **To reduce frequency of infection in patients with nonmyeloid malignancies receiving myelosuppressive chemotherapy that may cause febrile neutropenia**
Adults weighing more than 45 kg (99 lb): 6 mg subcutaneously once per chemotherapy cycle. Don't give in period between 14 days before and 24 hours after administration of cytotoxic chemotherapy.

ADMINISTRATION
Subcutaneous
• Allow drug to come to room temperature before giving; protect from light.
• Don't shake.
• Don't use if discoloration or particulate matter is seen.

P

• Discard drug if left at room temperature for more than 48 hours.

ACTION

Binds cell receptors to stimulate proliferation, differentiation, commitment, and end-cell function of neutrophils.

Route	Onset	Peak	Duration
Subcut.	Unknown	Unknown	Unknown

Half-life: 15 to 80 hours.

ADVERSE REACTIONS

CNS: dizziness, fatigue, fever, headache, insomnia, asthenia.
GI: abdominal pain, anorexia, constipation, diarrhea, dyspepsia, mucositis, nausea, stomatitis, taste perversion, vomiting.
Hematologic: *granulocytopenia, neutropenic fever.*
Musculoskeletal: arthralgia, bone pain, generalized weakness, myalgia, skeletal pain.
Skin: alopecia.
Other: peripheral edema.

INTERACTIONS

Drug-drug. *Lithium:* May increase the release of neutrophils. Monitor neutrophil counts closely.

EFFECTS ON LAB TEST RESULTS

• May increase LDH, alkaline phosphatase, and uric acid levels.
• May decrease granulocyte, platelet, and RBC counts.

CONTRAINDICATIONS & CAUTIONS

• Contraindicated in patients hypersensitive to *Escherichia coli*–derived proteins, filgrastim, or any component of the drug. Don't use for peripheral blood progenitor cell mobilization.
• Use cautiously in patients with sickle cell disease, those receiving chemotherapy causing delayed myelosuppression, or those receiving radiation therapy.
• Infants, children, and adolescents who weigh less than 45 kg (99 lb) shouldn't receive the 6-mg single-use syringe dose. Safety and effectiveness in children haven't been established.
⚠ *Overdose S&S:* Leukocytosis.

NURSING CONSIDERATIONS

⊙ *Alert:* Splenic rupture may occur rarely. Assess patient who experiences signs or symptoms of left upper abdominal or shoulder pain for an enlarged spleen or splenic rupture.
• Obtain CBC and platelet count before therapy.
• Monitor patient's hemoglobin level, hematocrit, CBC, and platelet count, as well as LDH, alkaline phosphatase, and uric acid levels during therapy.
• Monitor patient for allergic-type reactions, including anaphylaxis, skin rash, and urticaria, which can occur with first or subsequent treatment.
• Evaluate patient with fever, lung infiltrates, or respiratory distress for adult respiratory distress syndrome. Notify prescriber if respiratory status worsens.
• Keep patient with sickle cell disease well hydrated, and monitor him for symptoms of sickle cell crisis.
• Pegfilgrastim may act as a growth factor for tumors.
• *Look alike–sound alike:* Don't confuse Neulasta with Neumega, Neupogen, or Lunesta.

PATIENT TEACHING

• Inform patient of the potential side effects of the drug.
• Tell patient to report signs and symptoms of allergic reactions, fever, or breathing problems.
⊙ *Alert:* Rarely, splenic rupture may occur. Advise patient to immediately report upper left abdominal or shoulder tip pain.
• Tell patient with sickle cell disease to keep drinking fluids and report signs or symptoms of sickle cell crisis.
• Instruct patient or caregiver how to give drug if it's to be given at home.

Reactions in bold italics are *life-threatening*. Interactions may have a *rapid onset* or a *delayed onset*.

peginterferon alfa-2a
peg-in-ter-FEER-on

Pegasys, Pegasys ProClick

Therapeutic class: Antivirals
Pharmacologic class: Biological
response modifiers
Pregnancy risk category: C

AVAILABLE FORMS
Injection: 180 mcg/1 mL single-dose vials;
135 mcg/0.5 mL, 180 mcg/0.5 mL prefilled
syringes

INDICATIONS & DOSAGES
Adjust-a-dose (for all indications): For patients who experience moderate adverse
reactions, decrease dose to 135 mcg subcutaneously once a week; for severe adverse
reactions, decrease to 90 mcg subcutaneously once a week. For patients who
experience hematologic reactions, if the
ANC is less than $750/mm^3$, reduce dose to
135 mcg subcutaneously once a week; if
the ANC is less than $500/mm^3$, stop drug
until ANC exceeds $1,000/mm^3$ and restart
at 90 mcg subcutaneously once a week. If
platelet count is less than $50,000/mm^3$, reduce dose to 90 mcg subcutaneously once
a week; stop drug if platelet count drops
below $25,000/mm^3$. In patients with ESRD
requiring hemodialysis, decrease dose to
135 mcg subcutaneously once a week. In
chronic hepatitis C patients with ALT increases above baseline, decrease dose to
135 mcg subcutaneously once a week. For
chronic hepatitis B patients with elevations
in ALT more than 5 times the upper limit
of normal (ULN), reduce dose to 135 mcg
subcutaneously once a week or temporarily stop treatment; if less than $10 \times$ ULN,
consider stopping treatment. For patients
also taking ribavirin therapy, if hemoglobin
level is less than 10 g/dL in patients with
no cardiac disease, reduce ribavirin dose to
600 mg/day. If less than 8.5 g/dL in this
population, stop ribavirin. If hemoglobin
level decreases by 2 g/dL or more during
any 4-week period in patients with history
of stable cardiac disease, reduce ribavirin
dose to 600 mg daily. If less than 12 g/dL
despite 4 weeks at reduced dose, stop ribavirin. Don't use ribavirin in patients with
a CrCl less than 50 mL/minute.
➤ **Chronic hepatitis C with compensated
hepatic disease in patients not previously
treated with interferon alfa**
Adults: 180 mcg subcutaneously in abdomen or thigh, once weekly for 48 weeks.
May be used with 800 to 1,200 mg ribavirin
daily, in two divided doses, depending on
viral genotype.
Children age 5 and older: 180 mcg/1.73 m^2
times body surface area subcutaneously
once weekly in combination with ribavirin.
Treat patients with genotype 2 or 3 for
24 weeks; other genotypes for 48 weeks.
➤ **Chronic hepatitis C (regardless of
genotype) in HIV-infected patients who
have not previously been treated with
interferon**
Adults: 180 mcg subcutaneously in abdomen or thigh, once weekly for 48 weeks.
May be used with 800 mg ribavirin P.O.
daily in two divided doses.
➤ **Chronic hepatitis B who have compensated liver disease and evidence of viral
replication and liver inflammation**
Adults: 180 mcg subcutaneously in abdomen or thigh, once weekly for 48 weeks.

ADMINISTRATION
Subcutaneous
● Vials and prefilled syringes are for single
use only. Discard unused portion.
● Do not shake. Allow to reach room temperature before use, but don't leave out of
refrigerator for more than 24 hours.
● Protect from light.
● Visually inspect drug for particulate
matter and discoloration before administration; don't use if particulate matter is
visible or product is discolored.

ACTION
Causes reversible decreases in leukocyte
and platelet counts, partially through stimulation of production of effector proteins in
vitro.

Route	Onset	Peak	Duration
Subcut.	Unknown	3–4 days	<1 wk

Half-life: 80 hours.

ADVERSE REACTIONS

CNS: depression, dizziness, fatigue, headache, insomnia, irritability, pain, pyrexia, anxiety, asthenia, concentration impairment, memory impairment, mood alteration.
GI: abdominal pain, anorexia, diarrhea, nausea, dry mouth, vomiting.
Hematologic: *neutropenia, thrombocytopenia,* anemia, *lymphopenia.*
Musculoskeletal: arthralgia, myalgia, back pain.
Respiratory: cough, dyspnea.
Skin: alopecia, pruritus, dermatitis, increased sweating, rash, dry skin, eczema.
Other: injection-site reaction, rigors.

INTERACTIONS

Drug-drug. *Methadone:* May increase methadone level. Monitor patient closely and decrease methadone dosage as needed.
Nucleoside reverse transcriptase inhibitors (NRTIs): May cause severe and potentially fatal hepatic decompensation. If used together in patients coinfected with HIV who are taking NRTIs, monitor for toxicities.
Ribavirin: May cause additive hematologic toxicity. Monitor hematologic function.
Telbivudine: May increase risk of peripheral neuropathy. Avoid use together.
Theophylline, other drugs metabolized by CYP1A2: May increase theophylline level and may interact with other drugs metabolized by this enzyme system. Monitor theophylline level and adjust dosage as needed.

EFFECTS ON LAB TEST RESULTS

• May increase triglyceride and ALT levels. May decrease hemoglobin level and hematocrit.

• May decrease ANC, WBC, and platelet counts. May increase or decrease thyroid function test values.

CONTRAINDICATIONS & CAUTIONS

• Contraindicated in patients hypersensitive to interferon alfa-2a or any components of formulation.
• Contraindicated in patients with autoimmune hepatitis or decompensated liver disease (with monoinfection or coinfection with HIV) before or during treatment with drug and in neonates and infants.
• Use cautiously in patients with a history of depression.
• Use cautiously in patients with baseline neutrophil counts less than 1,500/mm^3, baseline platelet counts less than 90,000/mm^3, or baseline hemoglobin level less than 10 g/dL.
• Use cautiously in patients with CrCl less than 50 mL/minute.
• Use cautiously in patients with cardiac disease or hypertension, thyroid disease, autoimmune disorders, pulmonary disorders, colitis, pancreatitis, and ophthalmologic disorders.
• Use cautiously in elderly patients because they may be at increased risk for adverse reactions.
Black Box Warning Use cautiously in patients also taking ribavirin. Ribavirin may cause birth defects or fetal demise. Ribavirin is also known to cause hemolytic anemia, which may worsen cardiac disease. ∎
• It isn't known if drug appears in breast milk. Either discontinue drug or discontinue breast-feeding.
• Safety and effectiveness haven't been established in patients who have failed to respond to other interferon alfa treatments, in organ transplant recipients, and in patients who are also infected with hepatitis B.
⚠ **Overdose S&S:** Fatigue, elevated liver enzyme levels, neutropenia, thrombocytopenia.

NURSING CONSIDERATIONS

Black Box Warning Alpha interferons cause or aggravate fatal or life-threatening neuropsychiatric, autoimmune, ischemic, and infectious disorders. Monitor patients closely with periodic clinical and laboratory evaluations. Withdraw patients with persistently severe or worsening signs or symptoms of these conditions from therapy. ∎

Reactions in bold italics are *life-threatening*. Interactions may have a *rapid onset* or a *delayed onset*.

- Obtain CBC before treatment and monitor counts routinely during therapy. Stop drug in patients who develop severe decrease in neutrophil or platelet counts.
- Stop drug if uncontrollable thyroid disease, hyperglycemia, hypoglycemia, or diabetes mellitus occurs during treatment.
- If persistent or unexplained pulmonary infiltrates or pulmonary dysfunction occur, stop drug.
- Stop drug if signs and symptoms of colitis occur, such as abdominal pain, bloody diarrhea, and fever. Symptoms should resolve within 1 to 3 weeks.
- Stop drug if signs and symptoms of pancreatitis occur, including fever, malaise, and abdominal pain.
- Obtain baseline eye examination and periodically monitor eye examinations during treatment. Stop drug if new or worsening eye disorders occur.
- Monitor patient with impaired renal function for interferon toxicity.
- Use in women of childbearing age only when effective contraception is being used.

PATIENT TEACHING
- Advise patient to read medication guide that comes with drug.
- Teach patient proper way to give drug and dispose of needles and syringes.
- Tell patient to immediately report depression or suicidal ideation.
- Tell patient to report signs and symptoms of pancreatitis, colitis, eye disorders, or respiratory disorders.
- Advise patient to avoid driving or operating machinery if he feels dizzy, tired, confused, or sleepy.
- Advise patient not to switch to another brand of interferon without consulting health care provider.
- Advise female patient that drug may alter menstrual cycles and impaired fertility is possible.

Black Box Warning Tell male and female patients and their partners to take extreme care to avoid pregnancy during treatment and for 6 months after treatment stops. ∎

SAFETY ALERT!

peginterferon alfa-2b
peg-in-ter-FEER-on

PEG-Intron, PEG-Intron Redipen, Sylatron

Therapeutic class: Antivirals
Pharmacologic class: Biological response modifiers
Pregnancy risk category: C

AVAILABLE FORMS
Injection: 50 mcg/0.5 mL, 80 mcg/0.5 mL, 120 mcg/0.5 mL, 150 mcg/0.5 mL
Powder for injection: 296 mcg, 444 mcg, 888 mcg

INDICATIONS & DOSAGES
➤ **Chronic hepatitis C in patients with compensated liver disease not previously treated with interferon alfa (PEG-Intron)**
Adults: 1 mcg/kg subcutaneously once weekly for up to 1 year, on same day each week. The volume of PEG-Intron to be injected depends on the patient's weight and the vial strength used.
Adults weighing 137 to 160 kg (301 to 353 lb): 150 mcg (0.5 mL) of 300-mcg/mL strength.
Adults weighing 107 to 136 kg (235 to 300 lb): 120 mcg (0.5 mL) of 240-mcg/mL strength.
Adults weighing 89 to 106 kg (196 to 234 lb): 96 mcg (0.4 mL) of 240-mcg/mL strength.
Adults weighing 73 to 88 kg (160 to 195 lb): 80 mcg (0.5 mL) of 160-mcg/mL strength.
Adults weighing 57 to 72 kg (125 to 159 lb): 64 mcg (0.4 mL) of 160-mcg/mL strength.
Adults weighing 46 to 56 kg (101 to 124 lb): 50 mcg (0.5 mL) of 100-mcg/mL strength.
Adults weighing 45 kg (100 lb) or less: 40 mcg (0.4 mL) of 100-mcg/mL strength.
Adjust-a-dose: Decrease peginterferon alfa-2b dose by 50% in patients with WBC count less than 1,500/mm³, neutrophil count less than 750/mm³, or platelet count less than 80,000/mm³. Oral ribavirin dose can be continued. If hemoglobin level is less

P

---

than 10 g/dL, reduce oral ribavirin dose by 200 mg. Stop both drugs if hemoglobin level is less than 8.5 g/dL, WBC count less than 1,000/mm³, neutrophil count less than 500/mm³, or platelet count less than 50,000/mm³. If symptoms improve and remain stable for 4 weeks, continue at present dose or resume previous dose.

If patient develops mild depression, continue peginterferon alfa-2b, but evaluate patient once weekly. In adults with moderate depression, reduce peginterferon alfa-2b dose by 50% for 4 to 8 weeks and evaluate patient every week. In severe depression, stop peginterferon alfa-2b.

For patients with stable CV disease, decrease peginterferon alfa-2b dose by 50% and ribavirin dosage by 200 mg daily if hemoglobin level drops more than 2 g/dL in any 4-week period. Stop both drugs if hemoglobin level goes below 12 g/dL after 4 weeks of reduced dosages.

Decrease dosage by 25% for CrCl of 30 to 50 mL/minute and by 50% for CrCl of 10 to 29 mL/minute. Discontinue for CrCl of less than 10 mL/minute. Don't use with ribavirin if CrCl is less than 50 mL/minute.

➤ **Chronic hepatitis C in patients with compensated liver disease not previously treated with interferon alfa, combined with ribavirin (PEG-Intron)**
Adults: 1.5 mcg/kg subcutaneously once weekly for 24 to 48 weeks on same day every week. The volume of PEG-Intron to be injected depends on the patient's weight and the vial strength used.
Adults weighing more than 85 kg (187 lb): 150 mcg (0.5 mL) of 300-mcg/mL strength.
Adults weighing 76 to 85 kg (167 to 187 lb): 120 mcg (0.5 mL) of 240-mcg/mL strength.
Adults weighing 61 to 75 kg (134 to 165 lb): 96 mcg (0.4 mL) of 240-mcg/mL strength.
Adults weighing 51 to 60 kg (112 to 132 lb): 80 mcg (0.5 mL) of 160-mcg/mL strength.
Adults weighing 40 to 50 kg (88 to 110 lb): 64 mcg (0.4 mL) of 160-mcg/mL strength.
Adults weighing less than 40 kg (88 lb): 50 mcg (0.5 mL) of 100-mcg/mL strength.
Children ages 3 to 17: 60 mcg/m² subcutaneously on same day every week.
Adjust-a-dose: See the preceding indication on chronic hepatitis C for specific guidelines.

➤ **Chronic hepatitis C genotype 1 infection in combination with ribavirin and an approved hepatitis C virus (HCV) NS3/4A protease inhibitor (PEG-Intron)**
Adults: 1.5 mcg/kg subcutaneously once weekly for 24 to 48 weeks on same day each week. Volume of PEG-Intron to be injected depends on patient's weight and vial strength used.
Adults weighing more than 85 kg (187 lb): 150 mcg (0.5 mL) of 300-mcg/mL strength.
Adults weighing 76 to 85 kg (167 to 187 lb): 120 mcg (0.5 mL) of 240-mcg/mL strength.
Adults weighing 61 to 75 kg (134 to 165 lb): 96 mcg (0.4 mL) of 240-mcg/mL strength.
Adults weighing 51 to 60 kg (112 to 132 lb): 80 mcg (0.5 mL) of 160-mcg/mL strength.
Adults weighing 40 to 50 kg (88 to 110 lb): 64 mcg (0.4 mL) of 160-mcg/mL strength.
Adults weighing less than 40 kg (88 lb): 50 mcg (0.5 mL) of 100-mcg/mL strength.
Adjust-a-dose: Base dosage modification on patient response. Refer to package insert for manufacturer's instructions.

➤ **For adjuvant treatment of melanoma with microscopic or gross nodal involvement within 84 days of definitive surgical resection including complete lymphadenectomy (Sylatron)**
Adults: 6 mcg/kg/week subcutaneously for 8 doses, followed by 3 mcg/kg/week subcutaneously for up to 5 years. Premedicate with acetaminophen 500 to 1,000 mg P.O. 30 minutes before the first dose and as needed for subsequent doses.
Adjust-a-dose: Dosage modification is based on patient response to treatment. Refer to the package insert for manufacturer's instructions.

ADMINISTRATION
Subcutaneous
● To reconstitute the lyophilized peginterferon alfa-2b in the Redipen, hold the Redipen upright (dose button down) and press the two halves of the pen together until there is an audible click.
● Gently invert the pen to mix the solution. Don't shake.
● Keeping the pen upright, attach the supplied needle, and select the appropriate peginterferon alfa-2b dose by pulling back on the dosing button until the dark bands are

---

visible and turning the button until the dark band is aligned with the correct dose.

• The Redipen is for single use only.

• Reconstitute the peginterferon alfa-2b lyophilized product with only 0.7 mL of supplied diluent (sterile water for injection). Discard the remaining diluent.

• Swirl gently to dissolve completely.

• Use immediately after reconstitution or store for up to 24 hours at 36° to 46° F (2° to 8° C).

• **Incompatibilities:** Don't add any other medication to solutions containing peginterferon alfa-2b.

ACTION

Binds to specific membrane receptors on the cell surface, inducing certain enzymes, suppressing cell proliferation and immunomodulating activities, and inhibiting virus replication in virus-infected cells. Increases levels of effector proteins and body temperature, and decreases leukocyte and platelet counts.

Route	Onset	Peak	Duration
Subcut.	Unknown	15–44 hr	Unknown

Half-life: 40 hours.

ADVERSE REACTIONS

CNS: anxiety, depression, dizziness, emotional lability, fatigue, fever, headache, insomnia, irritability, *suicidal behavior,* hypertonia, malaise, agitation, nervousness.

CV: flushing, chest pain.

EENT: pharyngitis, sinusitis, rhinitis, conjunctivitis, blurred vision, dry mouth, taste perversion.

GI: abdominal pain, anorexia, diarrhea, nausea, dyspepsia, right upper quadrant pain, vomiting.

GU: menstrual disorder.

Hematologic: *neutropenia, thrombocytopenia.*

Hepatic: hepatomegaly.

Metabolic: weight loss, hypothyroidism.

Musculoskeletal: musculoskeletal pain, myalgia, arthralgia.

Respiratory: cough, dyspnea.

Skin: alopecia, dry skin, increased sweating, injection-site inflammation or reaction, pruritus, rash, injection-site pain.

Other: flulike symptoms, rigors, viral infection.

INTERACTIONS

Drugs metabolized by CYP2C8, CYP2C9 (phenytoin, warfarin), or CYP2D6 (flecainide): May decrease serum levels of these drugs. Monitor patient response and drug levels; adjust dosage as needed.

Methadone: May increase methadone level. Monitor patient closely and decrease methadone dosage as needed.

Nucleoside reverse transcriptase inhibitors (NRTIs): May cause severe and potentially fatal hepatic decompensation. If used together in patient coinfected with HIV, monitor patient for toxicities.

Telbivudine: May increase risk of peripheral neuropathy. Avoid use together.

EFFECTS ON LAB TEST RESULTS

• May increase serum bilirubin, uric acid, triglyceride, and ALT levels. May increase or decrease thyroid-stimulating hormone (TSH) level.

• May decrease hemoglobin.

• May decrease neutrophil and platelet counts.

CONTRAINDICATIONS & CAUTIONS

• Contraindicated in patients hypersensitive to drug or any of its components, in patients with autoimmune hepatitis or decompensated liver disease, in those with diabetes or thyroid disorders that can't be controlled with medication, in patients who have failed to respond to other alpha interferon treatment or have had an organ transplant, and in those with HIV or hepatitis B virus.

• Use cautiously in patients with psychiatric disorders, diabetes mellitus, CV disease, CrCl less than 50 mL/minute, pulmonary infiltrates, pulmonary function impairment, or autoimmune, ischemic, or infectious disorders.

NURSING CONSIDERATIONS

• Obtain eye examination in patient with diabetes or hypertension before starting drug. Retinal hemorrhages, cotton-wool spots, and retinal artery or vein obstruction may occur.

P

Black Box Warning Drug may cause or aggravate fatal or life-threatening neuro-psychiatric, autoimmune, ischemic, and infectious disorders. Monitor patients closely with periodic clinical and labora-tory evaluations. In patient with persistently severe or worsening signs or symptoms of these conditions from therapy, withhold drug. In many but not all cases, these dis-orders resolve after stopping PEG-Intron therapy. ∎

Black Box Warning The risk of serious de-pression with suicidal ideation, completed suicides, and other neuropsychiatric disor-ders increases with use of alpha interferons, including Sylatron. Permanently discon-tinue Sylatron in patients with persistently severe or worsening signs or symptoms of depression, psychosis, or encephalop-athy. These disorders may not resolve after stopping Sylatron. ∎

• Combination therapy with ribavirin is preferred over monotherapy because of better response rates, unless contraindica-tion or intolerance exists.

Black Box Warning If used in combination therapy with ribavirin, ensure extreme care to avoid pregnancy. Also, monitor patient for worsening cardiac disease secondary to anemia. ∎

• Drug may cause or aggravate hypothy-roidism, hyperthyroidism, or diabetes.

• Perform ECG on patient with history of MI or arrhythmias before starting drug.

• Start treatment in patient who is well hydrated.

• Monitor patient with history of MI or arrhythmias closely for hypotension, arrhythmias, tachycardia, cardiomyopathy, and signs and symptoms of MI.

• Monitor patient for depression and other mental health disorders. If symptoms are severe, stop drug and refer patient for psychiatric care.

• Monitor patient for signs and symp-toms of colitis, such as abdominal pain, bloody diarrhea, and fever. Stop drug if colitis occurs. Symptoms should resolve 1 to 3 weeks after stopping drug.

• Monitor patient for signs and symptoms of pancreatitis (due to elevated triglyceride levels) or hypersensitivity reactions, and stop drug if these occur.

• Monitor patient with pulmonary disease for dyspnea, pulmonary infiltrates, pneu-monitis, and pneumonia.

• Monitor patient with renal disease for signs and symptoms of toxicity.

• Monitor CBC count, platelet count, and AST, ALT, bilirubin, and TSH levels be-fore starting drug and periodically during treatment.

• Notify prescriber if severe neutropenia or thrombocytopenia occurs.

• Children may experience growth delays in height and weight.

• *Look alike–sound alike:* Don't confuse peginterferon alfa-2b with interferon alfa-2a, interferon alfa-2b, interferon alfa-n3, or peginterferon alfa-2a. Don't confuse PEG-Intron with Intron A.

PATIENT TEACHING

• Teach patient the appropriate use of the drug and the benefits and risks of treatment. Tell patient that adverse reactions may continue for several months after treatment is stopped.

• Tell patient to immediately report symp-toms of depression or suicidal thoughts.

• Instruct patient on importance of proper disposal of needles and syringes, and cau-tion him against reuse of old needles and syringes.

• Tell patient that drug won't prevent trans-mission of HCV to others and may not cure hepatitis C or prevent cirrhosis, liver failure, or liver cancer that may result from HCV infection.

• Advise patient that laboratory tests are needed before starting therapy and period-ically thereafter.

• Tell patient to take drug at bedtime and to use fever-reducing drugs to decrease risk of flulike signs and symptoms.

• Inform breast-feeding patient of the potential for adverse reactions in infants. Tell her to either stop using drug or stop breast-feeding.

• Advise patient to brush teeth thoroughly at least twice a day, have regular dental exam-inations, and rinse mouth thoroughly after emesis.

Black Box Warning Tell patient to avoid pregnancy. ∎

---

pegloticase

peg-LOE-tih-kase

Krystexxa

Therapeutic class: Antigout agents
Pharmacologic class: Uric acid–specific enzymes
Pregnancy risk category: C

AVAILABLE FORMS

Injection: 8 mg/mL in 2-mL single-use vial

INDICATIONS & DOSAGES

➤ **Treatment of chronic gout in patients refractory to conventional therapy**
Adults: 8 mg by I.V. infusion every 2 weeks over at least 120 minutes.

ADMINISTRATION

I.V.
▼ Keep drug refrigerated until ready to use.
▼ Inspect vial for particulate matter and discoloration. Don't use unless solution is clear and colorless.
▼ Withdraw 8 mg (1 mL) and place into 250 mL normal saline or half-normal saline solution. Invert bag several times to ensure mixing; don't shake. After mixing, drug is stable for 4 hours at room temperature or refrigerated. Use within 4 hours of dilution.
▼ Protect from light.
▼ Don't administer diluted drug until it's at room temperature.
▼ Don't administer as I.V. push or bolus.
▼ **Black Box Warning** Premedicate with antihistamine and corticosteroid. ■
▼ **Incompatibilities:** Solutions other than normal saline or half-normal saline.

ACTION

Enables oxidation of uric acid to allantoin, thereby lowering serum uric acid level.

Route	Onset	Peak	Duration
I.V.	Unknown	Unknown	Unknown

Half-life: Unknown.

ADVERSE REACTIONS

CV: chest pain.
EENT: nasopharyngitis.
GI: nausea, constipation, vomiting.
Musculoskeletal: gout flare.
Skin: contusion, ecchymosis, urticaria.
Other: *infusion reaction, anaphylaxis.*

INTERACTIONS

Drug-drug. *Other pegylated drugs (pegylated interferon, pegylated liposomal doxorubicin):* May cause excessive binding. Avoid use together.

EFFECTS ON LAB TEST RESULTS

● May increase or decrease uric acid levels.

CONTRAINDICATIONS & CAUTIONS

● Contraindicated in patients with G6PD deficiency because of risk of hemolysis and methemoglobinemia and possible hypersensitivity to pegloticase.
● Use cautiously in patients with heart failure and in those with history of anaphylactic or infusion reactions.
● Drug isn't recommended for treatment of asymptomatic hyperuricemia.
● Use cautiously in pregnant women and only if clearly needed.
● It isn't known if drug appears in breast milk. Don't use in breast-feeding women.
● Safety and effectiveness in children haven't been established.

NURSING CONSIDERATIONS

● Screen high-risk patients, such as those with African or Mediterranean ancestry, for G6PD deficiency because of increased risk of hemolysis and methemoglobinemia.
Black Box Warning Administer drug in health care setting. Monitor patient for anaphylactic and infusion reactions. Anaphylaxis may occur with any infusion (including the first one) and at any time, although most reactions have occurred within 2 hours of initiation. Premedicate with antihistamine and corticosteroid. If reaction occurs, slow or stop infusion at physician discretion. ■
Black Box Warning Monitor patient for anaphylactic and infusion reactions for at least 1 hour after administration; realize that hypersensitivity reaction may be delayed. ■

P

Black Box Warning Monitor uric acid levels and discontinue drug if levels are greater than 6 mg/dL, especially after two successive readings, because risk of anaphylaxis rises with increases in uric acid levels and loss of therapeutic response. ■

• Monitor patient for gout flares and treat with an NSAID or colchicine for at least 1 week before initiation of infusion. Gout flare prophylaxis is recommended for at least the first 6 months of therapy unless medically contraindicated or not tolerated. Drug may still be given during gout flare.

• Carefully monitor patient who requires retreatment after 4-week drug-free interval because he may be at higher risk for infusion reaction or anaphylaxis.

• Monitor patient for signs and symptoms of heart failure (peripheral edema, shortness of breath, chest pain).

PATIENT TEACHING

• Tell patient to immediately report signs and symptoms of allergic reaction (wheezing, shortness of breath, cough, chest tightness, trouble breathing, reddening of skin or face, tongue swelling, trouble swallowing).

• Caution patient that he shouldn't take drug if he has G6PD deficiency and to inform prescriber if he does.

• Tell patient that drug shouldn't be given for high uric acid levels with no symptoms.

• Instruct patient to notify prescriber if he has heart failure.

• Before treatment begins, tell female patient to inform prescriber if she is pregnant, plans to become pregnant, or is breast-feeding.

• Teach patient to report gout flares during treatment.

• Instruct patient that periodic monitoring of serum uric acid levels will be needed during and after treatment.

SAFETY ALERT!

pemetrexed disodium
peh-meh-TREX-ed

Alimta

Therapeutic class: Antineoplastics
Pharmacologic class: Folate antagonists
Pregnancy risk category: D

AVAILABLE FORMS
Injection: 100 mg, 500 mg in single-use vials

INDICATIONS & DOSAGES
Adjust-a-dose (for all indications): In patients who develop toxic reactions, adjust dosage according to the table.

Toxic reaction	Dosage change
– Grade 3 (severe or undesirable) or grade 4 (life-threatening or disabling) diarrhea – Diarrhea that warrants hospitalization – Any grade 3 toxicity (except mucositis and increased transaminase levels) – Any grade 4 toxicity (except mucositis) – Platelet count $\geq$ 50,000/mm^3 and absolute neutrophil count < 500/mm^3	Give 75% of previous pemetrexed and cisplatin doses.
– Platelet count < 50,000/mm^3	Give 50% of previous pemetrexed and cisplatin doses.
Grade 3 or 4 mucositis	Give 50% of previous pemetrexed dose and 100% of previous cisplatin dose.
Grade 2 (moderate) neurotoxicity	Give 100% of previous pemetrexed dose and 50% of previous cisplatin dose.
– Grade 3 or 4 neurotoxicity – Any grade 3 or 4 toxicity (except increased transaminase levels) present after two dose reductions	Stop therapy.

Reactions in bold italics are *life-threatening*. Interactions may have a *rapid onset* or a *delayed onset*.

➤ **Malignant pleural mesothelioma or non–small-cell (nonsquamous) lung cancer (NSCLC) with cisplatin, in patients whose disease is unresectable or who aren't candidates for surgery**

Adults: 500 mg/m^2 I.V. over 10 minutes on day 1 of each 21-day cycle. Starting 30 minutes after pemetrexed infusion ends, give cisplatin 75 mg/m^2 I.V. over 2 hours.

➤ **Locally advanced or metastatic NSCLC after chemotherapy**

Adults: 500 mg/m^2 I.V. over 10 minutes on day 1 of each 21-day cycle.

ADMINISTRATION

I.V.

▼ Premedicate with folic acid 400 to 1,000 mcg P.O. once daily beginning 7 days before first dose of drug and continued during therapy and for 21 days after last dose. Administer vitamin B$_{12}$ 1 mg I.M. 1 week before first dose of pemetrexed and every three cycles thereafter. Administer dexamethasone 4 mg P.O. b.i.d. the day before, the day of, and the day after pemetrexed administration.

▼ Reconstitute 100-mg vial with 4.2 mL or 500-mg vial with 20 mL of preservative-free normal saline solution to yield 25 mg/mL.

▼ Swirl vial gently until powder is completely dissolved. Solution should be clear and colorless to yellow or yellow-green.

▼ Calculate appropriate dose, and further dilute with normal saline solution so total volume of solution is 100 mL.

▼ Give over 10 minutes.

▼ Reconstituted solution and dilution are stable for 24 hours refrigerated or at room temperature.

▼ **Incompatibilities:** Calcium-containing diluents, including Ringer's or lactated Ringer's for injection; other drugs or diluents.

ACTION

Disturbs cell replication by inhibiting several folate-dependent enzymes involved in nucleotide synthesis. When given with other antineoplastics, drug inhibits growth of mesothelioma cell lines.

Route	Onset	Peak	Duration
I.V.	Unknown	Unknown	Unknown

Half-life: 3½ hours.

ADVERSE REACTIONS

CNS: depression, fatigue, fever, neuropathy.

CV: *cardiac ischemia,* chest pain, edema, *emboli,* thrombosis.

EENT: pharyngitis, conjunctivitis.

GI: anorexia, constipation, diarrhea, nausea, stomatitis, vomiting, esophagitis, painful, difficult swallowing, taste disturbance.

GU: *renal failure.*

Hematologic: anemia, *leukopenia, neutropenia, thrombocytopenia.*

Metabolic: dehydration.

Musculoskeletal: arthralgia, myalgia.

Respiratory: dyspnea.

Skin: alopecia, rash.

Other: allergic reaction, infection.

INTERACTIONS

Drug-drug. *Nephrotoxic drugs, probenecid:* May delay pemetrexed clearance. Monitor patient.

NSAIDs: May decrease pemetrexed clearance in patients with mild to moderate renal insufficiency. For NSAIDs with short half-lives, avoid use for 2 days before, during, and 2 days after pemetrexed therapy. For NSAIDs with long half-lives, avoid use for 5 days before, during, and 2 days after pemetrexed therapy.

EFFECTS ON LAB TEST RESULTS

● May increase ALT, AST, and creatinine levels. May decrease hemoglobin level and hematocrit.

● May decrease absolute neutrophil, platelet, and WBC counts.

CONTRAINDICATIONS & CAUTIONS

● Contraindicated in patients with a history of severe hypersensitivity reaction to drug or its ingredients. Don't use in patients with CrCl less than 45 mL/minute.

⚠ *Overdose S&S:* Neutropenia, anemia, thrombocytopenia, mucositis, rash, infection with or without fever, diarrhea.

P

NURSING CONSIDERATIONS

• Patient shouldn't start a new cycle of treatment unless ANC is 1,500 cells/mm^3 or more, platelet count is 100,000 cells/mm^3 or more, and CrCl is 45 mL/minute or more.

• Patients with pleural effusion and ascites may need to have effusion drained before therapy.

• Monitor renal function, CBC, platelet count, hemoglobin level, hematocrit, and LFT values.

• Assess patient for neurotoxicity, mucositis, and diarrhea. Severe symptoms may warrant dosage adjustment.

🜂 **Alert:** To reduce the occurrence and severity of cutaneous reactions, give a corticosteroid, such as dexamethasone 4 mg P.O. b.i.d., the day before, the day of, and the day after giving this drug.

🜂 **Alert:** To reduce toxicity, patient should take 350 to 1,000 mcg of folic acid daily, 5 days before therapy until 21 days after therapy.

🜂 **Alert:** Give vitamin B$_{12}$ 1,000 mcg I.M. once during the week before the first dose and every three cycles thereafter. After the first cycle, vitamin injections may be given on the first day of the cycle.

• **Look alike–sound alike:** Don't confuse pemetrexed with methotrexate or pralatrexate.

PATIENT TEACHING

• Inform patient that he may receive corticosteroids and vitamins before pemetrexed to help minimize its adverse effects.

• Tell patient to avoid NSAIDs for several days before, during, and after treatment.

• Urge patient to report adverse effects, especially fever, sore throat, infection, diarrhea, fatigue, and limb pain.

• It's unknown if drug appears in breast milk. Advise patient to stop breast-feeding during treatment.

penicillin G benzathine (benzathine benzylpenicillin)
pen-i-SILL-in

Bicillin L-A

Therapeutic class: Antibiotics
Pharmacologic class: Natural penicillins
Pregnancy risk category: B

AVAILABLE FORMS
Injection: 300,000 units/mL, 600,000 units/mL, 1.2 million units/2 mL, 2.4 million units/4 mL

INDICATIONS & DOSAGES
➤ **Congenital syphilis**
Children younger than age 2: 50,000 units/kg (up to 2.4 million units) I.M. as a single dose.
➤ **Group A streptococcal upper respiratory tract infections**
Adults: 1.2 million units I.M. as a single injection.
Children weighing 27 kg (59.5 lb) or more: 900,000 units I.M. as a single injection.
Infants and children weighing less than 27 kg: 300,000 to 600,000 units I.M. as a single injection.
➤ **To prevent poststreptococcal rheumatic fever and glomerulonephritis**
Adults and children: 1.2 million units I.M. once monthly or 600,000 units I.M. every 2 weeks.
➤ **Syphilis (primary, secondary, and latent)**
Adults: 2.4 million units I.M. as a single dose.
➤ **Syphilis (tertiary and neurosyphilis)**
Adults: 2.4 million units I.M. weekly for 3 weeks.
➤ **Yaws, bejel, and pinta**
Adults: 1.2 million units I.M. as a single injection.

ADMINISTRATION
I.M.
Black Box Warning Inadvertent I.V. use may cause cardiac arrest and death. Never give I.V., intra-arterially, or subcutaneously. ∎

Reactions in bold italics are *life-threatening*. Interactions may have a *rapid onset* or a *delayed onset*.

• Before giving drug, ask patient about allergic reactions to penicillin.
• Obtain specimen for culture and sensitivity tests before giving first dose. Begin therapy while awaiting results.
• Shake well before injecting.
• Inject deep into upper outer quadrant of buttocks in adults and in midlateral thigh in infants and small children. Rotate injection sites. Avoid injection into or near major nerves or blood vessels to prevent permanent neurovascular damage.
• Injection may be painful, but ice applied to the site may ease discomfort.

ACTION
Inhibits cell-wall synthesis during bacterial multiplication.

Route	Onset	Peak	Duration
I.M.	Unknown	13–24 hr	1–4 wk

Half-life: 30 to 60 minutes.

ADVERSE REACTIONS
CNS: neuropathy.
GI: *pseudomembranous colitis,* enterocolitis, nausea, vomiting.
GU: nephropathy.
Hematologic: *agranulocytosis, leukopenia, thrombocytopenia,* eosinophilia, hemolytic anemia.
Skin: exfoliative dermatitis, maculopapular rash.
Other: *anaphylaxis,* hypersensitivity reactions, sterile abscess at injection site.

INTERACTIONS
Drug-drug. *Aminoglycosides:* Physical and chemical incompatibility. Give separately.
Anticogulants (warfarin): May increase or decrease anticoagulant effects of warfarin. Monitor coagulation studies and adjust warfarin dosages as needed.
Hormonal contraceptives: May decrease hormonal contraceptive effectiveness. Advise use of additional form of contraception during therapy.
Live-virus vaccines: May decrease effectiveness of live-virus vaccines. Avoid concurrent use.
Methotrexate: May increase risk of methotrexate toxicity. Monitor patient closely.

Probenecid: May increase penicillin level. Probenecid may be used for this purpose.
Tetracycline: May antagonize penicillin G benzathine effects. Avoid using together.

EFFECTS ON LAB TEST RESULTS
• May decrease hemoglobin level.
• May increase eosinophil count. May decrease platelet, WBC, and granulocyte counts. May cause positive Coombs test results.
• May falsely decrease aminoglycoside level. May cause false-positive CSF protein test results. May alter urine glucose testing using cupric sulfate (Benedict reagent).

CONTRAINDICATIONS & CAUTIONS
• Contraindicated in patients hypersensitive to drug or other penicillins.
• Inadvertent intravascular administration has resulted in severe neurovascular damage, including transverse myelitis with permanent paralysis and gangrene.
• Use cautiously in patients allergic to other drugs, especially to cephalosporins, because of possible cross-sensitivity.
• Use cautiously in patients with a history of significant allergies or asthma.
⚠ *Overdose S&S:* Neuromuscular hyperexcitability, seizures.

NURSING CONSIDERATIONS
🕐 *Alert:* Bicillin L-A is the only penicillin G benzathine product indicated for sexually transmitted infections. Don't substitute Bicillin C-R because it may not be effective.
• Drug may alter colon flora. Monitor patient for diarrhea. Drug may need to be stopped.
• Drug's extremely slow absorption time makes allergic reactions difficult to treat.
• If large doses are given or if therapy is prolonged, bacterial or fungal superinfection may occur, especially in elderly, debilitated, or immunosuppressed patients.
• *Look alike–sound alike:* Don't confuse penicillin G benzathine with Polycillin, penicillamine, or the various other types of penicillin.

PATIENT TEACHING
• Tell patient to report adverse reactions promptly.

P

- Inform patient that fever and increased WBC count are the most common reactions.
- Warn patient that I.M. injection may be painful but that ice applied to the site may ease discomfort.

penicillin G potassium (benzylpenicillin potassium)
pen-i-SILL-in

Pfizerpen

Therapeutic class: Antibiotics
Pharmacologic class: Natural penicillins
Pregnancy risk category: B

AVAILABLE FORMS
Injection: 5 million units, 20 million units
Premixed injection: 1 million units/50 mL, 2 million units/50 mL, 3 million units/ 50 mL

INDICATIONS & DOSAGES
Adjust-a-dose (for all indications): If CrCl is 10 to 50 mL/minute, give the usual dose every 8 to 12 hours. If CrCl is less than 10 mL/minute, give 50% of usual dose every 8 to 10 hours or the usual dose every 12 to 18 hours. If patient is uremic and CrCl is more than 10 mL/minute, give full loading dose; then give half the loading dose every 4 to 5 hours for additional doses.
➤ **Actinomycosis**
Adults: For cervicofacial infections, 1 to 6 million units/day in divided doses I.M. or I.V. every 4 to 6 hours. For thoracic or abdominal infections, 10 to 20 million units/day in divided doses I.M. or I.V. every 4 to 6 hours or by continuous I.V. infusion.
➤ **Anthrax**
Adults: 8 million units/day in divided doses I.M. or I.V. every 6 hours; higher doses may be required depending on susceptibility of the organism.
➤ **Clostridial infections**
Adults: 20 million units/day in divided doses I.M. or I.V. every 4 to 6 hours.
➤ **Diphtheria**
Adults: 2 to 3 million units/day in divided doses I.M. or I.V. every 4 to 6 hours for 10 to 12 days.

Children: 150,000 to 250,000 units/kg/day in equal doses I.M. or I.V. every 6 hours for 7 to 10 days.
➤ **Disseminated gonococcal infections**
Adults: 10 million units/day in divided doses I.M. or I.V. every 4 to 6 hours.
Children weighing 45 kg (99 lb) or more with arthritis, endocarditis, or meningitis: 10 million units/day in four equally divided doses I.M. or I.V., with duration of therapy depending on type of infection.
Children weighing less than 45 kg with arthritis: 100,000 units/kg/day in four equally divided doses I.M. or I.V. for 7 to 10 days.
Children weighing less than 45 kg with endocarditis: 250,000 units/kg/day in equal doses I.M. or I.V. every 4 hours for 4 weeks.
Children weighing less than 45 kg with meningitis: 250,000 units/kg/day in equal doses I.M. or I.V. every 4 hours for 10 to 14 days.
➤ *Erysipelothrix* **endocarditis**
Adults: 12 to 20 million units/day in divided doses I.M. or I.V. every 4 to 6 hours for 4 to 6 weeks.
➤ **Fusospirochetosis**
Adults: 5 to 10 million units/day in divided doses I.M. or I.V. every 4 to 6 hours.
➤ **Gram-negative bacillary bacteremia**
Adults: 20 to 80 million units/day by continuous I.V. infusion. Penicillin G isn't drug of choice for treatment of gram-negative bacillary infections.
➤ **Haverhill fever**
Adults: 12 to 20 million units/day in divided doses I.M. or I.V. every 4 to 6 hours for 3 to 4 weeks.
➤ *Listeria monocytogenes* **endocarditis or meningitis**
Adults: 15 to 20 million units/day in divided doses I.M. or I.V. every 4 to 6 hours. Treat for 2 weeks for meningitis and 4 weeks for endocarditis.
Neonates: 500,000 to 1 million units daily in divided doses.
➤ **Meningococcal meningitis or septicemia**
Adults: 24 million units/day as 2 million units I.M. or I.V. every 2 hours. Or, a continuous I.V. infusion of 20 to 30 million units/day.

➤ **Neurosyphilis**
Adults: 12 to 24 million units/day (2 to 4 million units every 4 hours) I.M. or I.V. for 10 to 14 days. Many experts recommend benzathine penicillin G 2.4 million units I.M. weekly for 3 weeks following completion of this regimen.

➤ *Pasteurella multocida* **bacteremia or meningitis**
Adults: 4 to 6 million units/day in divided doses I.M. or I.V. every 4 to 6 hours for 2 weeks.

➤ **Rat bite fever**
Adults: 12 to 20 million units/day in divided doses I.M. or I.V. every 4 to 6 hours for 3 to 4 weeks.

➤ **Serious staphylococcal infections**
Adults: 5 to 24 million units/day in equally divided doses I.M. or I.V. every 4 to 6 hours.

➤ **Serious streptococcal infections**
Adults: 12 to 24 million units/day in equally divided doses I.M. or I.V. every 4 to 6 hours.

➤ **Haverhill fever (with endocarditis caused by** *Streptobacillus moniliformis***)**
Children: 150,000 to 250,000 units/kg/day in equal doses I.M. or I.V. every 4 hours for 4 weeks.

➤ **Meningitis caused by susceptible strains of pneumococcus and meningococcus**
Children: 250,000 units/kg/day in equal doses every 4 hours for 7 to 14 days, depending on infecting organism. Maximum dosage is 12 to 20 million units/day.

➤ **Rat bite fever (with endocarditis caused by** *S. moniliformis***)**
Children: 150,000 to 250,000 units/kg/day in equal doses every 4 hours for 4 weeks.

➤ **Serious streptococcal infections, such as pneumonia and endocarditis (***Streptococcus pneumoniae***), and meningococcal infections**
Children: 150,000 to 300,000 units/kg/day in equal doses every 4 to 6 hours. Duration of therapy depends on infecting organism and type of infection.

➤ **Syphilis (congenital and neurosyphilis) after newborn period**
Children: 200,000 to 300,000 units/kg/day (administered as 50,000 units/kg I.V. every 4 to 6 hours) for 10 to 14 days.

➤ **Lyme neuroborreliosis** ◆
Adults: 18 to 24 million units/day in divided doses I.V. every 4 hours for 14 days.

ADMINISTRATION
I.V.
▼ Before giving drug, ask patient about allergic reactions to penicillin.
▼ Obtain specimen for culture and sensitivity tests before giving first dose. Begin therapy while awaiting results.
▼ Reconstitute drug with sterile water for injection, D_5W, or normal saline solution for injection. Volume of diluent varies with manufacturer.
▼ Reconstituted solution may be stored in refrigerator for up to 7 days.
▼ For intermittent infusion in adults, give drug over 1 to 2 hours. For intermittent infusion in infants, give drug over 15 to 30 minutes.
⊕ *Alert:* Don't use in children requiring less than 1 million units/dose.
▼ For continuous infusion, add reconstituted drug to 1 to 2 L of compatible solution. Determine how much fluid is needed and what the rate should be for a 24-hour period; then, add the drug to this fluid.
▼ Don't administer premixed solutions to patients requiring less than 1 million units per dose.
▼ **Incompatibilities:** Alcohol 5%, amikacin, aminoglycosides, aminophylline, amphotericin B sodium, chlorpromazine, dextran, dopamine, heparin sodium, hydroxyzine hydrochloride, lincomycin, metoclopramide, pentobarbital sodium, phenytoin sodium, prochlorperazine mesylate, promethazine hydrochloride, sodium bicarbonate, thiopental, vancomycin, vitamin B complex with C.
I.M.
● Before giving drug, ask patient about allergic reactions to penicillin.
● Obtain specimen for culture and sensitivity tests before giving first dose. Begin therapy while awaiting results.
⊕ *Alert:* Don't use in children requiring less than 1 million units/dose.
● I.M. is the preferred route. Keep total volume of injection small.

P

● Give deep into large muscle; injection may be extremely painful.
● I.M. injection may be painful, but ice applied to the site may help alleviate discomfort.

ACTION
Inhibits cell-wall synthesis during bacterial multiplication.

Route	Onset	Peak	Duration
I.V.	Immediate	Immediate	Unknown
I.M.	Unknown	15–30 min	Unknown

Half-life: 30 to 60 minutes.

ADVERSE REACTIONS
CNS: *seizures,* agitation, anxiety, confusion, depression, dizziness, fatigue, hallucinations, lethargy, neuropathy.
CV: thrombophlebitis, *cardiac arrest, arrhythmias.*
GI: *pseudomembranous colitis,* enterocolitis, nausea, vomiting.
GU: interstitial nephritis, nephropathy.
Hematologic: *agranulocytosis, leukopenia, thrombocytopenia,* anemia, eosinophilia, hemolytic anemia.
Metabolic: *severe potassium poisoning.*
Skin: exfoliative dermatitis, maculopapular eruptions, pain at injection site.
Other: *anaphylaxis,* hypersensitivity reactions, overgrowth of nonsusceptible organisms.

INTERACTIONS
Drug-drug. *Bacteriostatic antibacterial agents (chloramphenicol, macrolide antibiotics, sulfonamides, tetracyclines):* Physically and chemically incompatible. Give separately.
Colestipol: May decrease penicillin G potassium level. Give penicillin G potassium 1 hour before or 4 hours after colestipol.
Heparin: May increase risk of bleeding. Closely monitor patient and adjust heparin dose as needed.
Hormonal contraceptives: May decrease hormonal contraceptive effectiveness. Advise use of additional form of contraception during therapy.

Live-virus vaccines: May decrease effectiveness of live-virus vaccines. Don't use together.
Methotrexate: May increase risk of methotrexate toxicity. Monitor patient closely.
Oral anticoagulants: May increase or decrease anticoagulant effects. Monitor PT and INR.
Potassium-sparing diuretics: May increase risk of hyperkalemia. Avoid using together.
Probenecid: May increase penicillin level. Probenecid may be used for this purpose.

EFFECTS ON LAB TEST RESULTS
● May increase potassium level. May decrease hemoglobin level.
● May increase eosinophil count. May decrease platelet, WBC, and granulocyte counts. May cause positive Coombs test result.
● May falsely decrease aminoglycoside levels. May cause false-positive CSF protein test result. May alter urine glucose testing using cupric sulfate (Benedict reagent).

CONTRAINDICATIONS & CAUTIONS
● Contraindicated in patients hypersensitive to drug or other penicillins.
● Use cautiously in patients with other drug allergies, especially to cephalosporins, because of possible cross-sensitivity.
● Use cautiously in patients with renal impairment.
⚠ *Overdose S&S:* Agitation, confusion, asterixis, hallucinations, stupor, coma, multifocal myoclonus, seizures, encephalopathy, hyperkalemia.

NURSING CONSIDERATIONS
● Monitor renal function closely. Patients with poor renal function are predisposed to high levels.
● Due to increased risk of electrolyte imbalances, monitor potassium and sodium levels closely in patients receiving more than 10 million units I.V. daily.
● Observe patient closely. With large doses and prolonged therapy, bacterial or fungal superinfection may occur, especially in elderly, debilitated, or immunosuppressed patients.

Reactions in bold italics are *life-threatening.* Interactions may have a *rapid onset* or a *delayed onset.*

• **Look alike–sound alike:** Don't confuse penicillin G potassium with Polycillin, penicillamine, or the various other types of penicillin.

PATIENT TEACHING

• Tell patient to notify prescriber if rash, fever, or chills develop. A rash is the most common allergic reaction.

• Warn patient that I.M. injection may be painful but that ice applied to the site may help alleviate discomfort.

penicillin G procaine (benzylpenicillin procaine)
pen-i-SILL-in

Therapeutic class: Antibiotics
Pharmacologic class: Natural penicillins
Pregnancy risk category: B

AVAILABLE FORMS
Injection: 300,000 units/mL, 600,000 units/mL

INDICATIONS & DOSAGES
➤ **Cutaneous anthrax**
Adults: 600,000 to 1 million units/day I.M.
➤ **Inhalational anthrax (postexposure)**
Adults: 1.2 million units I.M. every 12 hours. Available safety data for penicillin G procaine at this dose would best support a duration of therapy of 2 weeks or less.
Children: 25,000 units/kg (maximum, 1.2 million units) I.M. every 12 hours.
Note: Treatment of inhalational anthrax (postexposure) must be continued for a total of 60 days. Consider risks and benefits of continuing administration of penicillin G procaine for more than 2 weeks or switching to an effective alternative treatment.
➤ **Bacterial endocarditis (group A streptococci), only in extremely sensitive infections**
Adults: 600,000 to 1 million units/day I.M.
➤ **Adjunctive therapy for diphtheria with antitoxin**
Adults: 300,000 to 600,000 units/day I.M.
➤ **Diphtheria carrier state**
Adults: 300,000 units/day I.M. for 10 days.
➤ **Erysipeloid**
Adults: 600,000 to 1 million units/day I.M.

➤ **Fusospirochetosis (Vincent infection)**
Adults: 600,000 to 1 million units/day I.M.
➤ **Pneumonia (pneumococcal), moderately severe (uncomplicated)**
Adults and children weighing 27.3 kg (60 lb) or more: 600,000 to 1 million units/day I.M.
Children weighing less than 27.3 kg: 300,000 units/day I.M.
➤ **Rat bite fever (*Streptobacillus moniliformis and Spirillum minus*)**
Adults: 600,000 to 1 million units/day I.M.
➤ **Staphylococcal infections, moderately severe to severe**
Adults and children weighing 27.3 kg (60 lb) or more: 600,000 to 1 million units/day I.M.
Children weighing less than 27.3 kg: 300,000 units/day I.M.
➤ **Streptococcal infections (group A), including moderately severe to severe tonsillitis, erysipelas, scarlet fever, and upper respiratory tract, skin, and soft-tissue infections**
Adults and children weighing 27.3 kg (60 lb) or more: 600,000 to 1 million units/day I.M. for minimum of 10 days.
Children weighing less than 27.3 kg: 300,000 units/day I.M.
➤ **Syphilis (primary, secondary, and latent syphilis with negative spinal fluid)**
Adults and children older than age 12: 600,000 units/day I.M. for 8 days; total, 4.8 million units.
➤ **Late syphilis (tertiary syphilis, neurosyphilis, and latent syphilis with positive spinal fluid examination or no spinal fluid examination)**
Adults: 600,000 units/day I.M. for 10 to 15 days; total, 6 to 9 million units.
➤ **Yaws, bejel, pinta**
Adults: Treatment as for syphilis in the corresponding stage of disease.

ADMINISTRATION
I.M.
• Before giving drug, ask patient about allergic reactions to penicillin.
• Obtain specimen for culture and sensitivity tests before giving first dose. Begin therapy while awaiting results.
• Give deep in upper outer quadrant of buttocks in adults and in midlateral thigh in

P

small children. Rotate injection sites. Don't give subcutaneously. Don't massage injection site. Avoid injection near major nerves or blood vessels to prevent permanent neurovascular damage and tissue necrosis.

❸ **Alert:** Inadvertent I.V. use may cause CNS toxicity and death. Toxic reaction may occur after one dose. Never give I.V.

● I.M. injection may be painful, but ice applied to the site may help alleviate discomfort.

ACTION

Inhibits cell-wall synthesis during bacterial multiplication.

Route	Onset	Peak	Duration
I.M.	Unknown	1–4 hr	1–5 days

Half-life: 30 to 60 minutes.

ADVERSE REACTIONS

CNS: *seizures,* agitation, anxiety, confusion, depression, dizziness, fatigue, hallucinations, lethargy.
GI: *pseudomembranous colitis,* enterocolitis, nausea, vomiting.
GU: interstitial nephritis, nephropathy.
Hematologic: *agranulocytosis, thrombocytopenia,* hemolytic anemia, *leukopenia,* anemia, eosinophilia.
Musculoskeletal: arthralgia.
Other: *anaphylaxis,* hypersensitivity reactions, overgrowth of nonsusceptible organisms.

INTERACTIONS

Drug-drug. *Aminoglycosides:* Physically and chemically incompatible. Give separately.
Hormonal contraceptives: May decrease hormonal contraceptive effectiveness. Advise use of additional form of contraception during therapy.
Live-virus vaccines: May decrease vaccine effectiveness. Avoid concurrent use.
Methotrexate: May increase risk of methotrexate toxicity. Monitor patient closely.
Oral anticoagulants (warfarin): May increase or decrease effects of warfarin. Monitor coagulation status and adjust warfarin dosage as needed.

Probenecid: May increase penicillin level. Probenecid may be used for this purpose.

EFFECTS ON LAB TEST RESULTS

● May decrease hemoglobin level.
● May increase eosinophil count. May decrease platelet, WBC, and granulocyte counts.

CONTRAINDICATIONS & CAUTIONS

● Contraindicated in patients hypersensitive to drug or other penicillins.
● Use cautiously in patients with other drug allergies, especially to cephalosporins, because of possible cross-sensitivity. Some formulations contain sulfites, which may cause allergic reactions in sensitive people.

⚠ **Overdose S&S:** Neuromuscular hyperexcitability, seizures.

NURSING CONSIDERATIONS

❸ **Alert:** Continue postexposure treatment for inhalation anthrax for 60 days. Prescriber should consider the risk-benefit ratio of continuing penicillin longer than 2 weeks, compared with switching to another drug.
● Drug may alter normal colon flora. Monitor patient for diarrhea and initiate therapeutic measures as needed. Drug may need to be stopped.
● Allergic reactions are hard to treat because of drug's slow absorption rate.
● Monitor renal and hematopoietic function periodically.
● If large doses are given or if therapy is prolonged, bacterial or fungal superinfection may occur, especially in elderly, debilitated, or immunosuppressed patients.
● Treatment duration depends on site and cause of infection.
● **Look alike–sound alike:** Don't confuse penicillin G procaine with Polycillin, penicillamine, or the various other types of penicillin.

PATIENT TEACHING

● Tell patient to report adverse reactions promptly. A rash is the most common allergic reaction.
● Warn patient that I.M. injection may be painful but that ice applied to the site may help alleviate discomfort.

Reactions in bold italics are *life-threatening*. Interactions may have a *rapid onset* or a *delayed onset*.

penicillin G sodium (benzylpenicillin sodium)

pen-i-SILL-in

Crystapen†

Therapeutic class: Antibiotics
Pharmacologic class: Natural penicillins
Pregnancy risk category: B

AVAILABLE FORMS

Injection: 5 million-unit vial

INDICATIONS & DOSAGES

Adjust-a-dose (for all indications): If CrCl is 10 to 50 mL/minute, give the usual dose every 8 to 12 hours. If CrCl is less than 10 mL/minute, give the full loading dose followed by 50% of the loading dose every 8 to 10 hours. If patient is uremic and CrCl is more than 10 mL/minute, give full loading dose; then give half the loading dose every 4 to 5 hours for additional doses.

➤ **Actinomycosis**
Adults: For cervicofacial infections, 1 to 6 million units/day in divided doses I.M. or I.V. every 4 to 6 hours. For thoracic or abdominal infections, 10 to 20 million units/day in divided doses every 4 to 6 hours.

➤ **Anthrax**
Adults: 8 million units/day in divided doses I.M. or I.V. every 6 hours; higher dosages may be required depending on susceptibility of the organism.

➤ **Clostridial infections**
Adults: 20 million units/day in divided doses I.M. or I.V. every 4 to 6 hours.

➤ **Diphtheria**
Adults: 2 to 3 million units/day in divided doses I.M. or I.V. every 4 to 6 hours for 10 to 12 days.

➤ **Disseminated gonococcal infection**
Adults: 10 million units/day in divided doses I.M. or I.V. every 4 to 6 hours.

➤ ***Erysipelothrix* endocarditis**
Adults: 12 to 20 million units/day in divided doses I.M. or I.V. every 4 to 6 hours for 4 to 6 weeks.

➤ **Fusospirochetosis**
Adults: 5 to 10 million units/day in divided doses I.M. or I.V. every 4 to 6 hours.

➤ **Haverhill fever**
Adults: 12 to 20 million units/day in divided doses I.M. or I.V. every 4 to 6 hours for 3 to 4 weeks.

➤ ***Listeria monocytogenes* endocarditis or meningitis**
Adults: 15 to 20 million units/day in divided doses I.M. or I.V. every 4 to 6 hours. Treat for 2 weeks for meningitis and 4 weeks for endocarditis.

➤ **Meningococcal meningitis or septicemia**
Adults: 24 million units/day as 2 million units I.M. or I.V. every 2 hours.

➤ **Neurosyphilis**
Adults: 12 to 24 million units/day (2 to 4 million units I.M. or I.V. every 4 hours) for 10 to 14 days. Many experts recommend benzathine penicillin G 2.4 million units I.M. weekly for 3 weeks following completion of this regimen.

➤ ***Pasteurella multocida* bacteremia or meningitis**
Adults: 4 to 6 million units/day in divided doses I.M. or I.V. every 4 to 6 hours for 2 weeks.

➤ **Rat bite fever**
Adults: 12 to 20 million units/day in divided doses I.M. or I.V. every 4 to 6 hours for 3 to 4 weeks.
Children: 150,000 to 250,000 units/kg/day in equal doses I.M. or I.V. every 4 to 6 hours for 4 weeks.

➤ **Serious staphylococcal and streptococcal infections**
Adults: 5 to 24 million units/day in equally divided doses I.M. or I.V. every 4 to 6 hours.

➤ **Diphtheria (adjunctive therapy to antitoxin and for prevention of carrier state)**
Children: 150,000 to 250,000 units/kg/day in equal doses I.M. or I.V. every 6 hours for 7 to 10 days.

➤ **Disseminated gonococcal infections (penicillin-susceptible strains)**
Children weighing 45 kg (99 lb) or more with arthritis, endocarditis, or meningitis: 10 million units/day in four equally divided doses I.M. or I.V., with duration of therapy depending on type of infection.

P

Children weighing less than 45 kg with arthritis: 100,000 units/kg/day in four equally divided doses I.M. or I.V. for 7 to 10 days.

Children weighing less than 45 kg with endocarditis: 250,000 units/kg/day in equal doses I.M. or I.V. every 4 hours for 4 weeks.

Children weighing less than 45 kg with meningitis: 250,000 units/kg/day in equal doses I.M. or I.V. every 4 hours for 10 to 14 days.

➤ **Haverhill fever (with endocarditis caused by *Streptobacillus moniliformis*)**
Children: 150,000 to 250,000 units/kg/day in equal doses I.M. or I.V. every 4 hours for 4 weeks.

➤ **Meningitis caused by susceptible strains of pneumococcus and meningococcus**
Children: 250,000 units/kg/day in equal doses I.M. or I.V. every 4 hours for 7 to 14 days, depending on infecting organism. Maximum dosage is 12 to 20 million units/day.

➤ **Serious streptococcal infections, such as pneumonia and endocarditis (*Streptococcus pneumoniae*), and meningococcal infections**
Children: 150,000 units/kg/day in equal doses I.M. or I.V. every 4 to 6 hours. Duration of therapy depends on infecting organism and type of infection.

➤ **Syphilis (congenital and neurosyphilis) after newborn period**
Children: 200,000 to 300,000 units/kg/day (administered as 50,000 units/kg I.M. or I.V. every 4 to 6 hours) for 10 to 14 days.

ADMINISTRATION

I.V.
▼ Before giving drug, ask patient about allergic reactions to penicillin.
▼ Obtain specimen for culture and sensitivity tests before giving first dose. Begin therapy while awaiting results.
▼ Reconstitute drug with sterile water for injection, normal saline solution for injection, or D_5W. Check manufacturer's instructions for volume of diluent necessary to produce desired drug level.
▼ Give by intermittent infusion: Dilute drug in 50 to 100 mL, and give over 30 minutes to 2 hours every 4 to 6 hours.

⊘ *Alert:* Don't use in children requiring less than 1 million units/dose.
▼ In infants and children, give divided doses over 15 to 30 minutes.
▼ **Incompatibilities:** Aminoglycosides, amphotericin B, bleomycin, carbohydrate solutions at alkaline pH, chlorpromazine, cytarabine, fat emulsions 10%, heparin sodium, hydroxyzine hydrochloride, invert sugar 10%, lincomycin, methylprednisolone sodium succinate, potassium chloride, prochlorperazine mesylate, promethazine hydrochloride.

I.M.
● Before giving drug, ask patient about allergic reactions to penicillin.
● I.M. is the preferred route.
● Obtain specimen for culture and sensitivity tests before giving first dose. Begin therapy while awaiting results.
⊘ *Alert:* Don't use in children requiring less than 1 million units/dose.
● Injection may be painful, but ice applied to site may help alleviate discomfort.

ACTION

Inhibits cell-wall synthesis during bacterial multiplication.

Route	Onset	Peak	Duration
I.V.	Immediate	Immediate	Unknown
I.M.	Unknown	15–30 min	Unknown

Half-life: 30 to 60 minutes.

ADVERSE REACTIONS

CNS: neuropathy, *seizures,* agitation, anxiety, confusion, depression, dizziness, fatigue, hallucinations, lethargy.
CV: *heart failure,* thrombophlebitis.
GI: enterocolitis, ischemic colitis, nausea, vomiting, *pseudomembranous colitis.*
GU: nephropathy, interstitial nephritis.
Hematologic: hemolytic anemia, *agranulocytosis, leukopenia, thrombocytopenia, anemia,* eosinophilia.
Musculoskeletal: arthralgia.
Other: hypersensitivity reactions, *anaphylaxis,* overgrowth of nonsusceptible organisms, injection-site pain, vein irritation.

Reactions in bold italics are *life-threatening*. Interactions may have a *rapid onset* or a *delayed onset*.

INTERACTIONS

Drug-drug. *Aminoglycosides:* Physically and chemically incompatible. Give separately.
Aspirin, furosemide, indomethacin, sulfonamides, thiazide diuretics: May compete with penicillin for renal tubular secretion, prolonging the half-life of penicillin. Monitor patient.
Bacteriostatic antibacterial agents (chloramphenicol, macrolide antibiotics, sulfonamides, tetracyclines): May antagonize bactericidal effect of penicillin. Avoid concomitant use.
Colestipol: May decrease penicillin G sodium level. Give penicillin G sodium 1 hour before or 4 hours after colestipol.
Heparin: May increase risk of bleeding. Closely monitor coagulation status. Adjust heparin dose as needed.
Hormonal contraceptives: May decrease hormonal contraceptive effectiveness. Advise use of additional form of contraception during penicillin therapy.
Live-virus vaccines: May decrease effectiveness of live-virus vaccines. Avoid concurrent use.
Oral anticoagulants: May increase or decrease anticoagulant effects. Monitor PT and INR.
Probenecid: May increase penicillin level. Probenecid may be used for this purpose.

EFFECTS ON LAB TEST RESULTS

● May decrease hemoglobin level.
● May cause positive Coombs test result. May increase eosinophil count. May decrease platelet, WBC, granulocyte, and RBC counts.
● May cause false-positive CSF protein test result. May falsely decrease aminoglycoside level. May alter urine glucose testing using cupric sulfate (Benedict reagent).

CONTRAINDICATIONS & CAUTIONS

● Contraindicated in patients hypersensitive to drug or other penicillins and in those on sodium-restricted diets.
● Use cautiously in patients with other drug allergies, especially to cephalosporins, because of possible cross-sensitivity.
⚠ Overdose S&S: Neuromuscular hyperexcitability, seizures.

NURSING CONSIDERATIONS

● Drug may alter normal colon flora. Monitor patient for diarrhea, and initiate therapeutic measures as needed. Drug may need to be stopped.
● Observe patient closely. With large doses and prolonged therapy, bacterial or fungal superinfection may occur, especially in elderly, debilitated, or immunosuppressed patients.
● **Look alike–sound alike:** Don't confuse penicillin G sodium with Polycillin, penicillamine, or the various other types of penicillin.

PATIENT TEACHING

● Tell patient to report adverse reactions promptly.
● Instruct patient to report discomfort at I.V. site.
● Warn patient receiving I.M. injection that the injection may be painful but that ice applied to site may help alleviate discomfort.

penicillin V potassium (phenoxymethyl penicillin potassium)

pen-i-SILL-in

Apo-Pen VK†, Novo-Pen-VK†, Nu-Pen-VK†, Penicillin-VK

Therapeutic class: Antibiotics
Pharmacologic class: Natural penicillins
Pregnancy risk category: B

AVAILABLE FORMS

Oral suspension: 125 mg/5 mL, 250 mg/ 5 mL (after reconstitution)
Tablets: 250 mg, 500 mg

INDICATIONS & DOSAGES

➤ **Fusospirochetosis (Vincent infection) and staphylococcal infections**
Adults and children age 12 and older: 250 to 500 mg P.O. every 6 to 8 hours.
➤ **Pneumococcal infections**
Adults and children age 12 and older: 250 to 500 mg P.O. every 6 hours until patient has been afebrile for at least 2 days.

➤ **Streptococcal infections**
Adults and children age 12 and older: 125 to 250 mg P.O. every 6 to 8 hours for 10 days.
➤ **To prevent recurrent rheumatic fever**
Adults and children age 12 and older: 125 to 250 mg P.O. b.i.d.

ADMINISTRATION
P.O.
● Before giving drug, ask patient about allergic reactions to penicillins.
● Obtain specimen for culture and sensitivity tests before giving first dose. Begin therapy while awaiting results.
● Give drug with food if patient has stomach upset.
● Store oral solution in refrigerator.

ACTION
Inhibits cell-wall synthesis during bacterial multiplication.

Route	Onset	Peak	Duration
P.O.	Unknown	30–60 min	Unknown

Half-life: 30 minutes.

ADVERSE REACTIONS
GI: epigastric distress, nausea, diarrhea, black hairy tongue, vomiting.
Hematologic: *leukopenia, thrombocytopenia,* eosinophilia, hemolytic anemia.
Other: *anaphylaxis,* hypersensitivity reactions, overgrowth of nonsusceptible organisms.

INTERACTIONS
Drug-drug. *Hormonal contraceptives:* May decrease hormonal contraceptive effectiveness. Advise use of another form of contraception during therapy.
Methotrexate: May increase risk of methotrexate toxicity. Monitor patient closely.
Probenecid: May increase penicillin level. Probenecid may be used for this purpose.
Tetracyclines: May impair bactericidal effects of penicillin V. Avoid use together.

EFFECTS ON LAB TEST RESULTS
● May decrease hemoglobin level.
● May increase eosinophil count. May decrease platelet, WBC, and granulocyte counts.

● May alter results of turbidimetric test methods using sulfosalicylic acid, acetic acid, trichloroacetic acid, and nitric acid.

CONTRAINDICATIONS & CAUTIONS
● Contraindicated in patients hypersensitive to drug or other penicillins.
● Use cautiously in patients with GI disturbances and in those with other drug allergies, especially to cephalosporins, because of possible cross-sensitivity.
⚠ *Overdose S&S:* Neuromuscular hyperexcitability, seizures.

NURSING CONSIDERATIONS
● Drug may alter normal colon flora. Monitor patient for diarrhea, and initiate therapeutic measures as needed. Drug may need to be stopped.
● Periodically assess renal and hematopoietic function in patients receiving long-term therapy.
● If large doses are given or if therapy is prolonged, bacterial or fungal superinfection may occur, especially in elderly, debilitated, or immunosuppressed patients.
● Amoxicillin is the preferred drug to prevent endocarditis because GI absorption is better and drug levels are sustained longer. Penicillin V is considered an alternative drug.
● *Look alike–sound alike:* Don't confuse penicillin V potassium with Polycillin, penicillamine, or the various other types of penicillin.

PATIENT TEACHING
● Instruct patient to take entire quantity of drug exactly as prescribed, even after he feels better.
● Tell patient to take drug with food if stomach upset occurs.
● Advise patient to notify prescriber if rash, fever, or chills develop. A rash is the most common allergic reaction.

---

pentamidine isethionate
pen-TA-ma-deen

NebuPent, Pentam

Therapeutic class: Antiprotozoals
Pharmacologic class: Diamidine
derivatives
Pregnancy risk category: C

AVAILABLE FORMS
Aerosol, injection, powder for injection:
300-mg vial

INDICATIONS & DOSAGES
➤ *Pneumocystis jiroveci (carinii)*
pneumonia
Adults and children age 4 months and older:
4 mg/kg I.V. or I.M. once daily for 14 to
21 days.
➤ **To prevent** *P. jiroveci (carinii)* **pneu-**
monia in high-risk patients
Adults and children capable of using a
nebulizer effectively: 300 mg by inhalation
using a Respirgard II nebulizer once every
4 weeks.

ADMINISTRATION
I.V.
▼ Reconstitute drug with 3 to 5 mL sterile
water for injection.
▼ Dilute reconstituted drug in 50 to
250 mL D₅W.
▼ Infuse over 60 to 120 minutes.
▼ To minimize risk of hypotension,
infuse drug slowly with patient lying down.
Closely monitor blood pressure.
▼ **Incompatibilities:** Aldesleukin,
cephalosporins, fluconazole, foscarnet,
linezolid.
I.M.
● Reconstitute drug with 3 mL sterile water
for a solution containing 100 mg/mL.
● Give deep into muscle.
● Patient may have pain and induration at
injection site.
● Rotate injection sites.
Inhalational
● Drug is considered a biohazardous agent.
Follow safe-handling procedures.
● Give aerosol form only by Respirgard II
nebulizer. Dosage recommendations are

based on particle size and delivery rate of
this device. To give aerosol, mix contents of
one vial in 6 mL sterile water for injection.
Don't use normal saline solution. Don't mix
with other drugs.
● Don't use the Respirgard II to administer a
bronchodilator.
● Don't use low-pressure (less than
20 pounds per square inch [psi]) com-
pressors. The flow rate should be 5 to
7 L/minute from 40- to 50-psi air or
oxygen source.

ACTION
May interfere with biosynthesis of DNA,
RNA, phospholipids, and proteins in sus-
ceptible organisms.

Route	Onset	Peak	Duration
I.V.	Unknown	1 hr	Unknown
I.M.	Unknown	30 min	Unknown
Inhalation	Unknown	Unknown	Unknown

Half-life: I.M., 9 to 13 hours; I.V., about 6½ hours;
inhalation, unknown.

ADVERSE REACTIONS
CNS: confusion, hallucinations, headache.
CV: chest pain, hypotension.
GI: nausea, metallic taste, diarrhea,
anorexia.
Hematologic: *leukopenia, thrombocyto-*
penia, anemia.
Metabolic: *hypoglycemia.*
Respiratory: cough, wheezing.
Skin: rash; sterile abscess or necrosis, pain,
or induration at site of I.M. injection.
Other: night sweats, infection.

INTERACTIONS
Drug-drug. *Aminoglycosides, ampho-*
tericin B, capreomycin, cisplatin, methoxy-
flurane, polymyxin B, vancomycin: May
increase risk of nephrotoxicity. Monitor
renal function test results closely.
Antineoplastics: May cause additive bone
marrow suppression. Use together cautiously; monitor hematologic study results.
Drugs that prolong the QT interval (anti-
psychotics; antiarrhythmics, such as amio-
darone, disopyramide, procainamide,
quinidine, and sotalol; fluoroquinolones;
macrolides; TCAs): May cause additive

P

effect. Use together cautiously; monitor patient for adverse cardiac effects.

EFFECTS ON LAB TEST RESULTS
• May increase BUN, creatinine, and potassium levels and LFT values. May decrease hemoglobin level and hematocrit. May increase or decrease glucose level.
• May decrease WBC and platelet counts.

CONTRAINDICATIONS & CAUTIONS
• Contraindicated in patients with history of anaphylactic reaction to drug.
• Use cautiously in patients with hypertension, hypotension, hypoglycemia, hypocalcemia, leukopenia, thrombocytopenia, anemia, diabetes, pancreatitis, Stevens-Johnson syndrome, or hepatic or renal dysfunction.
• Use cautiously in breast-feeding women; it's unknown if drug appears in breast milk.
⚠ *Overdose S&S:* Renal and hepatic impairment, hypotension, cardiopulmonary arrest.

NURSING CONSIDERATIONS
۞ *Alert:* Monitor glucose, creatinine, and BUN levels daily. After parenteral administration, glucose level may decrease initially; hypoglycemia may be severe in 5% to 10% of patients. After several months of therapy, this may be followed by hyperglycemia and type 1 diabetes mellitus, which may be permanent.
• Monitor CBC, platelet count, LFT, calcium level, and ECG before, during, and after therapy.
۞ *Alert:* Monitor blood pressure during and after infusion because of increased risk of severe hypotension with I.V. or I.M. administration.
• Extravasation can lead to ulceration, tissue necrosis, or sloughing at injection site. Monitor I.V. site closely.
• Use of aerosolized drug has been associated with acute pancreatitis. Discontinue drug if signs or symptoms of acute pancreatitis occur.
• Obtain the following tests before, during, and after therapy: CBC, platelet count, LFT, serum calcium, and ECG.

• In patients with AIDS, drug may produce less severe adverse reactions than sulfamethoxazole–trimethoprim.

PATIENT TEACHING
• Instruct patient to use the aerosol device until the chamber is empty, which may take up to 45 minutes.
• Warn patient that I.M. injection is painful.
• Instruct patient to complete the full course, even if he's feeling better.
• Tell patient to report signs and symptoms of pulmonary infection, such as shortness of breath, fever, or cough.

SAFETY ALERT!

pentazocine hydrochloride†
pen-TAZ-oh-seen

Talwin†

pentazocine lactate
Talwin

Therapeutic class: Analgesics
Pharmacologic class: Opioid agonist-antagonists–opioid partial agonists
Pregnancy risk category: C
Controlled substance schedule: IV

AVAILABLE FORMS
pentazocine hydrochloride
Tablets: 50 mg†
pentazocine lactate
Injection: 30 mg/mL

INDICATIONS & DOSAGES
➤ **Moderate to severe pain; preoperative or preanesthetic supplement to surgical anesthesia**
Adults and children older than age 12:
30 mg I.M., I.V., or subcutaneously every 3 to 4 hours p.r.n. Maximum parenteral dose is 360 mg/day. Single doses above 30 mg I.V. or 60 mg I.M. or subcutaneously aren't recommended.
➤ **Labor**
Adults and children older than age 12:
30 mg I.M. as a single dose or 20 mg I.V. every 2 to 3 hours when contractions become regular for two to three doses.

ADMINISTRATION
P.O.
● Give drug with aspirin or acetaminophen for additive analgesic effect.
I.V.
▼ Give drug slowly by direct I.V. injection.
▼ **Incompatibilities:** Alkaline solutions, aminophylline, amobarbital, glycopyrrolate, heparin sodium, nafcillin sodium, pentobarbital sodium, phenobarbital sodium, sodium bicarbonate.
I.M.
● Rotate injection sites to minimize tissue irritation.
Subcutaneous
● Rotate injection sites to minimize tissue irritation. If possible, avoid giving subcutaneously.

ACTION
Unknown. Binds with opioid receptors in the CNS, altering perception of and emotional response to pain.

Route	Onset	Peak	Duration
P.O.	15–30 min	1–3 hr	2–3 hr
I.V.	2–3 min	15–30 min	2–3 hr
I.M., subcut.	15–20 min	30–60 min	2–3 hr

Half-life: 2 to 3 hours.

ADVERSE REACTIONS
CNS: dizziness, euphoria, lightheadedness, sedation, confusion, drowsiness, hallucinations, headache, psychotomimetic effects, visual disturbances.
CV: *shock, circulatory depression,* hypertension, hypotension.
EENT: dry mouth.
GI: nausea, vomiting, constipation.
GU: urine retention.
Respiratory: *apnea, respiratory depression,* dyspnea.
Skin: diaphoresis, induration, nodules, sclerosis at injection site, pruritus, sloughing.
Other: *anaphylaxis,* hypersensitivity reactions, physical and psychological dependence.

INTERACTIONS
Drug-drug. *CNS depressants:* May cause additive effects. Use together cautiously.

Fluoxetine: May cause additive effects resulting in serotonin syndrome. Use together cautiously.
Opioid analgesics: May decrease analgesic effect. Avoid using together.
Drug-lifestyle. *Alcohol use:* May cause additive effects. Discourage use together.
Smoking: May increase requirements for pentazocine. Monitor drug's effectiveness.

EFFECTS ON LAB TEST RESULTS
● May interfere with laboratory tests for urinary 17-hydroxycorticosteroids.

CONTRAINDICATIONS & CAUTIONS
● Contraindicated in patients hypersensitive to drug or its components and in children younger than age 12.
● Use cautiously in patients with hepatic or renal disease, acute MI, head injury, increased intracranial pressure, and respiratory depression.

NURSING CONSIDERATIONS
● Reassess patient's level of pain at least 15 and 30 minutes after parenteral administration and 30 minutes after oral administration.
● Drug may cause constipation. Assess bowel function and need for stool softeners or stimulant laxatives. Encourage fluids.
● Have naloxone readily available. Respiratory depression can be reversed with naloxone.
● Drug has opioid antagonist properties. May cause withdrawal syndrome in opioid-dependent patients.
● Psychological and physical dependence may occur with prolonged use.

PATIENT TEACHING
● Instruct patient to ask for drug before pain is intense.
● Caution ambulatory patient about getting out of bed or walking. Warn outpatient to avoid driving and other hazardous activities that require mental alertness until drug's CNS effects are known.
● Advise patient to avoid alcohol during therapy.
● Instruct patient or family to report rash, disorientation, or confusion to prescriber.

perindopril erbumine
pur-IN-doh-pril

Aceon, Coversyl†

Therapeutic class: Antihypertensives
Pharmacologic class: ACE inhibitors
Pregnancy risk category: D

AVAILABLE FORMS
Tablets: 2 mg, 4 mg, 8 mg

INDICATIONS & DOSAGES
Adjust-a-dose (for all indications): For patients with renal insufficiency and CrCl of 30 mL/minute or greater, initially 2 mg P.O. daily. Maximum daily maintenance dose is 8 mg. Not recommended for patients with CrCl of less than 30 mL/minute. In patients taking diuretics, initially 2 to 4 mg P.O. daily as single dose or in two divided doses, with close medical supervision for several hours and until blood pressure has stabilized. Adjust dosage based on patient's blood pressure response.
➤ **To reduce the risk of CV death or nonfatal MI in patients with stable coronary artery disease**
Adults age 70 or younger: 4 mg P.O. once daily for 2 weeks; then, increase as tolerated to 8 mg once daily.
Elderly adults older than age 70: Initially, 2 mg P.O. once daily for the first week; then, 4 mg once daily for the second week and 8 mg once daily after that, if tolerated.
➤ **Essential hypertension**
Adults: Initially, 4 mg P.O. once daily. Increase dosage until blood pressure is controlled or to maximum of 16 mg/day; usual maintenance dosage is 4 to 8 mg once daily; may be given in two divided doses.
Adults older than age 65: Initially, 4 mg P.O. daily as one dose or in two divided doses. Dosage may be increased by more than 8 mg/day only under close medical supervision.
➤ **Heart failure ♦**
Adults: 2 mg P.O. once daily, to maximum of 8 to 16 mg daily.

ADMINISTRATION
P.O.
● Give drug without regard for food.

ACTION
Prevents conversion of angiotensin I to angiotensin II, a potent vasoconstrictor. Less angiotensin II decreases peripheral arterial resistance, decreasing aldosterone secretion, which reduces sodium and water retention and lowers blood pressure.

Route	Onset	Peak	Duration
P.O.	Unknown	1 hr	Unknown

Half-life: About 1 hour for perindopril; mean half-life, 3 to 10 hours, and terminal elimination half-life, 30 to 120 hours for perindoprilat.

ADVERSE REACTIONS
CNS: headache, dizziness, asthenia, sleep disorder, paresthesia, depression, somnolence, nervousness, fever.
CV: palpitations, edema, chest pain, hypotension, abnormal ECG.
EENT: rhinitis, sinusitis, ear infection, pharyngitis, tinnitus.
GI: dyspepsia, diarrhea, abdominal pain, nausea, vomiting, flatulence.
GU: *acute renal failure,* proteinuria, UTI, male sexual dysfunction, menstrual disorder.
Metabolic: *hyperkalemia.*
Musculoskeletal: back pain, hypertonia, neck pain, joint pain, myalgia, arthritis, arm or leg pain.
Respiratory: cough, upper respiratory tract infection.
Skin: rash.
Other: viral infection, injury, seasonal allergy.

INTERACTIONS
Drug-drug. ❸ *Alert: Aliskiren:* May increase risk of renal impairment, hypotension, and hyperkalemia in diabetic patients and those with moderate to severe renal impairment (GFR less than 60 mL/minute). Concomitant use is contraindicated in diabetic patients. Avoid concomitant use in those with moderate to severe renal impairment.
Diuretics: May increase hypotensive effect. Monitor patient closely.

Reactions in bold italics are *life-threatening*. Interactions may have a *rapid onset* or a *delayed onset*.

Lithium: May increase lithium level and risk of lithium toxicity. Use together cautiously; monitor lithium level.

NSAIDs: May decrease antihypertensive effects. Monitor blood pressure.

Potassium-sparing diuretics (amiloride, spironolactone, triamterene), potassium supplements, other drugs capable of increasing potassium level (cyclosporine, heparin, indomethacin): May increase hyperkalemic effect. Use together cautiously; monitor potassium level.

Drug-herb. *Capsaicin:* May cause cough. Discourage use together.

Drug-food. *Salt substitutes containing potassium:* May cause hyperkalemia. Discourage use together.

EFFECTS ON LAB TEST RESULTS

• May increase ALT, alkaline phosphatase, uric acid, cholesterol, and creatinine levels. May increase potassium level.

• May decrease hemoglobin level and hematocrit.

CONTRAINDICATIONS & CAUTIONS

• Contraindicated in patients hypersensitive to drug or other ACE inhibitors and in those with a history of angioedema caused by ACE inhibitor use.

Black Box Warning Use during pregnancy can cause injury and death to the developing fetus. When pregnancy is detected, stop drug as soon as possible. ∎

• Use cautiously in patients with a history of angioedema unrelated to ACE inhibitor use.

• Use cautiously in patients with renal impairment, heart failure, ischemic heart disease, cerebrovascular disease, or renal artery stenosis and in those with collagen vascular disease, such as systemic lupus erythematosus or scleroderma.

⚠ *Overdose S&S:* Hypotension.

NURSING CONSIDERATIONS

• When used alone in black patients, drug affects blood pressure less than in other patients. Monitor blood pressure closely.

• Patients with a history of angioedema unrelated to ACE inhibitor use may be at increased risk for angioedema during therapy. Black patients are at a higher risk

for angioedema regardless of prior ACE inhibitor use.

⊙ *Alert:* If angioedema occurs, stop drug and observe patient until swelling disappears. Antihistamines may relieve swelling of the face and lips. Swelling of the tongue, glottis, or throat may cause life-threatening airway obstruction. Give prompt treatment, such as epinephrine.

• Monitor CBC with differential for agranulocytosis and neutropenia before therapy, especially in renally impaired patients with lupus or scleroderma.

• Monitor patient for hypotension when starting therapy and when adjusting dosage. If severe hypotension occurs, place patient in supine position and treat symptomatically.

• Severe hypotension can occur when drug is given with diuretics. If possible, stop diuretic 2 to 3 days before starting this drug. If impossible, use lower doses of either drug.

• In patient who is volume- or sodium-depleted from prolonged diuretic therapy, dietary sodium restriction, dialysis, diarrhea, or vomiting, correct fluid and sodium deficits before starting drug.

• Monitor renal function before and periodically throughout therapy.

• Monitor potassium level closely.

PATIENT TEACHING

• Inform patient that throat and facial swelling, including swelling of the throat, can occur during therapy, especially with the first dose. Advise patient to stop taking drug and immediately report any signs or symptoms of swelling of face, extremities, eyes, lips, or tongue; hoarseness; or difficulty in swallowing or breathing.

• Advise patient to report promptly any sign or symptom of infection (sore throat, fever) or jaundice (yellowing of eyes or skin).

• Advise patient to avoid salt substitutes containing potassium unless instructed otherwise by prescriber.

• Caution patient that light-headedness may occur, especially during first few days of therapy. Advise patient to report light-headedness and, if fainting occurs, to stop drug and consult prescriber promptly.

P

• Caution patient that inadequate fluid intake or excessive perspiration, diarrhea, or vomiting can lead to an excessive drop in blood pressure.

• Advise woman of childbearing age of the consequences of second- and third-trimester exposure to drug. Advise her to notify prescriber immediately if she suspects pregnancy.

permethrin
per-METH-rin

Elimite, Kwellada-P†, Nix ◊

Therapeutic class: Scabicides–pediculicides
Pharmacologic class: Pyrethroids
Pregnancy risk category: B

AVAILABLE FORMS
Cream: 5%
Lotion: 1%
Topical liquid (cream rinse): 1%

INDICATIONS & DOSAGES
➤ **Infestation with *Pediculus humanus capitis* (head louse) and its nits**
Adults and children age 2 and older: Use after hair has been washed with shampoo, rinsed with water, and towel dried. Apply 25 to 50 mL of liquid to saturate hair and scalp. Allow drug to remain on hair for 10 minutes before rinsing off with water. Remove remaining nits with comb. Usually only one application is needed.
➤ **Infestation with *Sarcoptes scabiei***
Adults and children age 2 months and older: Thoroughly massage into the skin from the head to the soles. Treat infants on hairline, neck, scalp, temple, and forehead. Wash cream off after 8 to 14 hours.

ADMINISTRATION
Topical
• Usually only one application is needed.
• Don't use drug on eyes, eyelashes, eyebrows, nose, mouth, or mucous membranes.

ACTION
Acts on parasite nerve cells to disrupt the sodium channel current, causing parasitic paralysis.

Route	Onset	Peak	Duration
Topical	10–15 min	Unknown	10 days

Half-life: Unknown.

ADVERSE REACTIONS
Skin: burning, stinging, edema, mild erythema, pruritus, scalp numbness or discomfort, scalp rash, tingling.

INTERACTIONS
None significant.

EFFECTS ON LAB TEST RESULTS
None reported.

CONTRAINDICATIONS & CAUTIONS
• Contraindicated in patients hypersensitive to pyrethrins, chrysanthemums, or components of drug.
⚠ Overdose S&S: Increased skin irritation and erythema.

NURSING CONSIDERATIONS
• Combing of nits isn't needed for effectiveness, but drug package supplies a fine-tooth comb for cosmetic use and to decrease diagnostic confusion that may lead to retreatment.
• Retreat for lice if they are seen 7 days after first application.
• Treat sexual partners simultaneously.

PATIENT TEACHING
• Explain that treatment may temporarily worsen signs and symptoms of head lice infestation, such as itching, redness, and swelling.
• Tell patient to disinfect headgear, combs and brushes, scarves, coats, and bed linens by machine washing with hot water and machine drying for at least 20 minutes, using hot cycle. Tell him to seal nonwashable items in plastic bag for 2 weeks or spray with product designed to eliminate lice and their nits.
• Warn patient not to use drug on eyes, eyelashes, eyebrows, nose, mouth, or mucous membranes.

Reactions in bold italics are *life-threatening*. Interactions may have a *rapid onset* or a *delayed onset*.

• Tell patient to warn other family members and sexual contacts about infestation.

SAFETY ALERT!

pertuzumab
per-TOO-zoo-mab

Perjeta

Therapeutic class: Antineoplastics
Pharmacologic class: Monoclonal antibodies
Pregnancy risk category: D

AVAILABLE FORMS
Injection: 420 mg/14 mL (30 mg/mL) in single-use vials

INDICATIONS & DOSAGES
Adjust-a-dose (for all indications): If a dose is missed or delayed and the time between infusions is less than 6 weeks, give 420-mg dose when possible; don't wait until the next planned dose. If the time between the two infusions is 6 weeks or more, give 840 mg loading dose followed by maintenance dose 3 weeks later. Withhold drug for at least 3 weeks if LVEF is less than 40% or is 40% to 45% with a 10% or more decrease below pretreatment values. Repeat LVEF assessment in 3 weeks. Discontinue both pertuzumab and trastuzumab if LVEF isn't improved or is worse, unless benefit outweighs risk. Dosage reductions aren't recommended for pertuzumab.
➤ **HER2-positive metastatic breast cancer with trastuzumab and docetaxel in patients who haven't received prior anti-*HER2* therapy or chemotherapy for metastatic disease**
Adults: Initial loading dose of 840 mg I.V. as a 60-minute infusion in combination with trastuzumab 8 mg/kg and docetaxel 75 mg/m². Administer a maintenance regimen every 3 weeks with pertuzumab 420 mg I.V. as a 30- to 60-minute infusion in combination with trastuzumab 6 mg/kg and docetaxel (may increase docetaxel dose to 100 mg/m² if tolerated).
✳ *NEW INDICATION:* **Neoadjuvant treatment of HER-2 positive, locally advanced, inflammatory, or early stage breast**
cancer (either greater than 2 cm in diameter or node positive) in combination with other drugs
Adults: Initial loading dose of 840 mg I.V. as a 60-minute infusion, then a maintenance regimen every 3 weeks with pertuzumab 420 mg I.V. as a 30- to 60-minute infusion in combination with either 4 preoperative cycles with trastuzumab and docetaxel followed by 3 postoperative cycles of fluorouracil, epirubicin, and cyclophosphamide (FEC); or 3 preoperative cycles of FEC alone followed by 3 postoperative cycles of pertuzumab in combination with docetaxel and trastuzumab; or 6 preoperative cycles of pertuzumab in combination with docetaxel, carboplatin, and trastuzumab (TCH). Following surgery, continue trastuzumab to complete 1 year of treatment regardless of regimen used.

ADMINISTRATION
I.V.
▼ Don't administer as I.V. push or bolus.
▼ Refrigerate vials. Store in outer carton to protect from light.
▼ Inspect solution for particulates and discoloration. Solution should be clear to slightly opalescent and colorless to pale brown.
▼ Withdraw appropriate amount of pertuzumab and dilute in 250 mL normal saline solution in a PVC or non-PVC polyolefin infusion bag.
▼ Invert bag gently to mix solution; don't shake. Administer immediately.
▼ May store diluted solution, refrigerated, for up to 24 hours.
▼ **Incompatibilities:** Other drugs. Only mix with normal saline solution.

ACTION
Binds to HER2 protein receptor, causing inhibition of signaling pathways, which results in cell growth arrest and apoptosis. The combination of pertuzumab and trastuzumab synergistically increases their antitumor activity.

Route	Onset	Peak	Duration
I.V.	Unknown	Unknown	Unknown

Half-life: 18 days.

P

ADVERSE REACTIONS

CNS: fatigue, asthenia, pyrexia, peripheral neuropathy, headache, dizziness, insomnia.
CV: peripheral edema, *left ventricular dysfunction.*
EENT: nasopharyngitis, increased tearing.
GI: diarrhea, nausea, vomiting, constipation, stomatitis, dysgeusia, decreased appetite.
Hematologic: *neutropenia,* anemia, *leukopenia, febrile neutropenia.*
Musculoskeletal: myalgia, arthralgia.
Respiratory: upper respiratory tract infection, dyspnea, pleural effusion.
Skin: alopecia, rash, pruritus, dry skin, paronychia, nail disorder.
Other: mucosal inflammation, infusion-related hypersensitivity, immunogenicity.

INTERACTIONS

Drug-drug. *Anthracyclines:* Prior exposure to anthracyclines may increase risk of left ventricular dysfunction. Use pertuzumab cautiously.

EFFECTS ON LAB TEST RESULTS

• May decrease WBC and RBC counts.

CONTRAINDICATIONS & CAUTIONS

Black Box Warning Pertuzumab can result in subclinical and clinical cardiac failure. Evaluate LVEF in all patients prior to and during treatment. Discontinue drug treatment for a confirmed clinically significant decrease in left ventricular function. ▮
۞ Alert: The safe use of pertuzumab with a doxorubicin-containing regimen or administration of more than 6 cycles for early breast cancer has not been established.
• Contraindicated in patients hypersensitive to drug or its components and in pregnant and breast-feeding women.
• Use cautiously in patients with a history of congestive heart failure or reduced LVEF and in those with severe renal impairment. Prior exposure to radiotherapy may increase risk of left ventricular dysfunction.
Black Box Warning Exposure to drug during pregnancy can result in embryo death or fetal death, delayed renal development, and other birth defects. Verify pregnancy status before initiating drug. ▮

NURSING CONSIDERATIONS

• If patient becomes pregnant during treatment, monitor closely. If oligohydramnios (low amniotic fluid level) occurs, perform fetal testing appropriate for gestational age and consistent with community standards of care.
• Verify HER2 status with reputable laboratory. Drug is only useful in patients with HER2 protein overexpression.
• Assess LVEF before starting treatment and every 3 months during treatment for metastatic disease or every 6 weeks during neoadjuvant treatment.
• Withhold or discontinue pertuzumab if trastuzumab is withheld or discontinued. If docetaxel is discontinued, treatment with pertuzumab and trastuzumab may continue.
• Monitor patient for hypersensitivity or infusion reactions for 60 minutes after first infusion and for 30 minutes after subsequent infusions. For significant infusion-related reactions, slow or interrupt infusion and treat symptoms. If severe reactions occur, consider permanently discontinuing drug.
• Monitor CBC regularly.
• Monitor patients for fever or infection.
• An increased incidence of febrile neutropenia has occurred in Asian patients.
• Assess LVEF before starting treatment and every 3 months during treatment.

PATIENT TEACHING

Black Box Warning Inform women of childbearing potential that drug may cause fetal harm. Counsel patient to use reliable birth control methods while taking this drug and for 6 months after therapy ends. ▮
• Teach patient that hair loss (alopecia) and skin and nail adverse reactions are common during treatment.
• Instruct patient to immediately report fever or other signs and symptoms of infection.
• Caution patient to immediately report shortness of breath, unusual edema, weight gain, or excessive fatigue.
• Advise women who are exposed to pertuzumab during pregnancy to enroll in the MotHER Pregnancy Registry by calling 1-800-690-6720.

Reactions in bold italics are *life-threatening*. Interactions may have a *rapid onset* or a *delayed onset*.

phentermine hydrochloride
FEN-ter-meen

Adipex-P, Suprenza

Therapeutic class: Anorexiants
Pharmacologic class: Sympathomimetic amines
Pregnancy risk category: X
Controlled substance schedule: IV

AVAILABLE FORMS
Capsules: 30 mg, 37.5 mg
Capsules (resin complex, sustained-release): 15 mg, 30 mg
Tablets: 37.5 mg
Tablets (dispersible): 15 mg, 30 mg, 37.5 mg

INDICATIONS & DOSAGES
➤ **Short-term adjunct in exogenous obesity**
Adults: 15 to 37.5 mg or 15 to 30 mg (as resin complex) P.O. daily as a single dose in the morning. Or 1 tablet Suprenza in the morning with or without food.

ADMINISTRATION
P.O.
● Give sustained-release capsule whole before breakfast or at least 10 to 14 hours before bedtime.
● For dispersible tablets, use dry hands to immediately place the tablet on the tongue, where it will dissolve; then have patient swallow with or without water.

ACTION
Unknown. Probably promotes nerve impulse transmission by releasing stored norepinephrine from nerve terminals in the brain, especially in the cerebral cortex and reticular activating system.

Route	Onset	Peak	Duration
P.O.	Unknown	Unknown	12–14 hr

Half-life: 19 to 24 hours.

ADVERSE REACTIONS
CNS: insomnia, overstimulation, headache, euphoria, dysphoria, dizziness.
CV: palpitations, tachycardia, increased blood pressure, *primary pulmonary hypertension.*
GI: dry mouth, dysgeusia, constipation, diarrhea, unpleasant taste, other GI disturbances.
GU: erectile dysfunction.
Skin: urticaria.
Other: altered libido.

INTERACTIONS
Drug-drug. *Acetazolamide, antacids, sodium bicarbonate:* May increase renal reabsorption. Monitor patient for enhanced effects.
Ammonium chloride, ascorbic acid: May decrease level and increase renal excretion of phentermine. Monitor patient for decreased phentermine effects.
Hormonal contraceptives: May reduce effectiveness of hormonal contraceptives. Advise patient to use alternative methods of contraception during treatment and for 1 month after discontinuation of therapy.
Insulin, oral antidiabetics: May alter antidiabetic requirements. Monitor glucose level.
MAO inhibitors: May cause severe hypertension or hypertensive crisis. Avoid using within 14 days of MAO inhibitor therapy.
Drug-food. *Alcohol use:* May increase risk of adverse drug reactions. Monitor patient.
Caffeine: May increase CNS stimulation. Discourage use together.

EFFECTS ON LAB TEST RESULTS
None reported.

CONTRAINDICATIONS & CAUTIONS
● Contraindicated in patients hypersensitive to sympathomimetic amines, in those with idiosyncratic reactions to them, in agitated patients, and in those with hyperthyroidism, moderate-to-severe hypertension, advanced arteriosclerosis, symptomatic CV disease, or glaucoma.
● Contraindicated within 14 days of MAO inhibitor therapy.
● Use cautiously in patients with mild hypertension.

P

⚠ **Overdose S&S:** Restlessness, tremor, hyperreflexia, rapid respiration, confusion, assaultiveness, hallucinations, panic states, fatigue, depression, arrhythmias, hypertension, hypotension, circulatory collapse, nausea, vomiting, diarrhea, abdominal cramps, seizures, coma.

NURSING CONSIDERATIONS
● Use drug with a weight-reduction program.
● Monitor patient for tolerance or dependence.
● **Look alike–sound alike:** Don't confuse phentermine with phentolamine or phenytoin.

PATIENT TEACHING
● Tell patient to take sustained-release drug at least 10 to 14 hours before bedtime to avoid sleep interference.
● Advise patient to avoid products that contain caffeine. Tell him to report evidence of excessive stimulation.
● Warn patient that fatigue may result as drug effects wear off and that he'll need more rest.
● Warn patient that drug may lose its effectiveness over time.
● Tell patient to take sustained-release capsule whole and not to chew, crush, or open it.
● Instruct patient on proper administration of dispersible tablet.

---

phentermine hydrochloride–topiramate
FEN-ter-meen/toe-PIE-rah-mate

Qsymia

Therapeutic class: Anorexiants–anticonvulsants
Pharmacologic class: Sympathomimetic amines–sulfamate-substituted monosaccharides
Pregnancy risk category: X
Controlled substance schedule: IV

AVAILABLE FORMS
Capsules: 3.75 mg phentermine and 23 mg topiramate extended-release, 7.5 mg phen-termine and 46 mg topiramate extended-release, 11.25 mg phentermine and 69 mg topiramate extended-release, 15 mg phentermine and 92 mg topiramate extended-release

INDICATIONS & DOSAGES
➤ **Chronic weight management, as an adjunct to diet and increased physical activity in patients with initial body mass index (BMI) of 30 kg/m² or greater (obese) or 27 kg/m² or greater (overweight) and at least one weight-related comorbidity, such as hypertension, type 2 diabetes mellitus, or dyslipidemia**
Adults: Initially, 3.75 mg phentermine/ 23 mg topiramate extended-release P.O. every morning for 14 days; then increase to 7.5 mg phentermine/46 mg topiramate extended-release every morning. Evaluate weight loss after 12 weeks of treatment. If patient hasn't lost at least 3% of baseline body weight, discontinue drug or escalate dosage to 11.25 mg phentermine/69 mg topiramate extended-release every morning for 14 days, followed by 15 mg phentermine/ 92 mg topiramate extended-release every morning. Evaluate weight loss 12 weeks after dosage escalation. If patient hasn't lost at least 5% of baseline body weight, discontinue drug by decreasing dosage to every other day for at least 1 week before stopping treatment altogether.
Adjust-a-dose: For patients with moderate renal impairment (CrCl of 30 to less than 50 mL/minute), severe renal impairment (CrCl less than 30 mL/minute), or moderate hepatic impairment (Child-Pugh class B), don't exceed 7.5 mg phentermine/ 46 mg topiramate once daily. Drug isn't for use in patients with ESRD on dialysis or those with severe hepatic impairment.

ADMINISTRATION
P.O.
● Give drug in morning with or without food. Don't give in evening due to risk of insomnia.

ACTION
Phentermine: Unknown. May be mediated by release of catecholamines in hypothalamus, resulting in decreased appetite and

decreased food consumption. Topiramate: Unknown in weight management. May involve appetite suppression and satiety enhancement via a variety of neurotransmitter or enzymatic effects.

Route	Onset	Peak	Duration
P.O.	Unknown	6 hr (phentermine); 9 hr (topiramate)	Unknown

Half-life: Phentermine, 20 hours; topiramate, 65 hours.

ADVERSE REACTIONS

CNS: paresthesia, headache, dizziness, dysgeusia, hypoesthesia, disturbance in attention or memory, cognitive disorder, insomnia, depression, anxiety, fatigue, irritability.
CV: palpitations, chest discomfort.
EENT: blurred vision, eye pain, dry eye, dry mouth, nasopharyngitis, sinusitis, sinus congestion, pharyngolaryngeal pain, nasal congestion.
GI: constipation, nausea, diarrhea, dyspepsia, GERD, oral paresthesia, gastroenteritis, decreased appetite, thirst.
GU: UTI, kidney stones, dysmenorrhea.
Metabolic: *hypokalemia, metabolic acidosis.*
Musculoskeletal: back pain, extremity pain, muscle spasms, musculoskeletal pain, neck pain.
Respiratory: cough, bronchitis, upper respiratory tract infection.
Skin: alopecia, rash.
Other: procedural pain, flulike symptoms.

INTERACTIONS

Drug-drug. *Amitriptyline:* May increase amitriptyline level. Adjust amitriptyline dosage based on patient clinical response.
Anticholinergics (atropine, benztropine): May increase risk of heat-related disorders. Use together cautiously.
Carbamazepine, phenytoin: May decrease topiramate plasma concentration. Use together cautiously.
Carbonic anhydrase inhibitors (acetazolamide, methazolamide, zonisamide): May increase risk of metabolic acidosis and kidney stones. Avoid concurrent use.

CNS depressants (barbiturates, benzodiazepines, sleep medications): May increase CNS depressant effects. Avoid use together.
Lithium: High topiramate dosage may increase lithium level. Monitor lithium level.
MAO inhibitors: May increase risk of hypertensive crisis. Use is contraindicated during or within 14 days of MAO inhibitor administration.
Nonpotassium-sparing diuretics: May increase risk of hypokalemia. Monitor potassium level.
Oral antidiabetics, insulin: May increase risk of hypoglycemia. Monitor glucose level closely.
Oral contraceptives: May cause irregular bleeding but not increased risk of pregnancy. Advise patients not to discontinue oral contraceptives if spotting occurs.
Other weight-loss drugs: Use with other weight-loss drugs hasn't been studied. Avoid use together.
Valproic acid: May increase risk of hyperammonemia and encephalopathy. Monitor patient and measure blood ammonia level if symptoms develop.
Drug-herb. *Weight-loss supplements:* Use with other weight-loss products hasn't been studied. Avoid use together.
Drug-food. *Ketogenic diet (high-protein, low-carbohydrate):* May increase risk of kidney stones. Use together cautiously.
Drug-lifestyle. *Alcohol use:* May increase CNS depressant effects. Discourage use together.

EFFECTS ON LAB TEST RESULTS

● May increase creatinine level. May decrease sodium bicarbonate, potassium, and glucose levels.

CONTRAINDICATIONS & CAUTIONS

● Contraindicated in patients hypersensitive to drug or its components; in those with glaucoma, hyperthyroidism, severe hepatic dysfunction, or ESRD; in patients with a history of or active suicidal ideation or attempts; during or within 14 days of MAO inhibitor; and in pregnant or breast-feeding women.

P

• Use cautiously in patients with increased resting heart rate, especially those with cardiac or cerebrovascular disease (history of MI or stroke in the past 6 months, life-threatening arrhythmias, congestive heart failure); in patients with depression or suicidal thoughts; in elderly patients; and in those at risk for development of metabolic acidosis or kidney stones.

• The safety and effectiveness of this drug in combination with other products intended for weight loss, including prescription and OTC drugs and herbal preparations, haven't been established.

• Drug is only available through certified pharmacies that are enrolled in the Qsymia certified pharmacy network; see www.qsymiarems.com or call 1-888-998-4887.

⚠ **Overdose S&S:** Phentermine: Restlessness, tremor, rapid respiration, confusion, hallucinations, arrhythmias, changes in blood pressure, nausea, vomiting, diarrhea. Topiramate: Metabolic acidosis, seizures, drowsiness, speech disturbance, blurred vision, hypotension, abdominal pain, agitation, dizziness, depression.

NURSING CONSIDERATIONS

• Gradually decrease dosage when discontinuing drug to lower risk of seizures. If it's necessary to stop drug immediately, monitor patient closely.

• Monitor patient for mood disorders and insomnia; if present, decrease dosage or discontinue drug.

• Monitor patient for emergence or worsening of depression, suicidal thoughts or behavior, or unusual changes in mood or behavior. Discontinue drug in patients who experience suicidal thoughts or behaviors.

• Monitor resting heart rate. If sustained tachycardia occurs, decrease dosage or stop drug.

• Assess electrolyte, glucose, and bicarbonate levels before and periodically during treatment.

• Drug causes decreased sweating, which can predispose patients to heat-related disorders. Monitor fluid loss, especially in hot weather.

• Monitor blood pressure regularly, especially in patients with history of hypertension.

• Monitor patient for ocular changes (acute myopia, severe and persistent eye pain, vision changes, anterior chamber shallowing, redness, increased intraocular pressure, mydriasis). Discontinue drug immediately if any of these symptoms occur.

• Monitor patient for potential abuse of drug. Phentermine has a known potential for abuse.

• Phentermine is related chemically and pharmacologically to amphetamines.

• Assess for pregnancy before and monthly during treatment.

PATIENT TEACHING

• Advise patient to take drug once daily in the morning and to avoid nighttime dosing because of insomnia.

• Inform patient that drug is only available through certified pharmacies that are enrolled in the Qsymia certified pharmacy network. Pharmacies can be found at www.qsymiarems.com or by calling 1-888-998-4887.

• Warn patient not to increase dosage without first discussing with prescriber.

• Advise woman of childbearing potential that pregnancy testing will be done before start of therapy and monthly during therapy.

• Counsel patient in use of effective contraception. Advise her to inform prescriber immediately if pregnancy occurs.

• Instruct patient to tell all health care providers about all medications, nutritional supplements, and vitamins (including weight-loss products) that are being taken or may be taken during therapy.

• Caution patient to report sustained periods of heart pounding or racing while at rest; mood changes, depression, or suicidal ideation; prolonged diarrhea; scheduled surgery; occurrence or history of seizures; or use of a high-protein, low-carbohydrate diet.

• Teach patient to immediately report severe and persistent eye pain or significant vision changes.

• Instruct patient to report changes in attention, concentration, memory, or difficulty finding words.

• Tell patient to avoid operating hazardous machinery, including automobiles, until effects of drug are known.

• Advise diabetic patient to monitor glucose level closely and to report episodes of hypoglycemia. Medication regimen may need adjustment.
• Caution patient to watch for decreased sweating or increased body temperature during physical activity, especially during hot weather.
• Warn patient not to stop drug abruptly as seizures may result.
• Advise patient to increase fluid intake to avoid kidney stones and to report severe side or back pain or blood in urine.

phenylephrine hydrochloride (intranasal)
fen-ill-EF-rin

4-Way Fast Acting ◊, Contac-D ◊, Little Noses Gentle Formula ◊, Neo-Synephrine ◊, Rhinall ◊, Sudafed RE Children's ◊, Sudafed PE Maximum Strength ◊

Therapeutic class: Vasoconstrictors
Pharmacologic class: Adrenergics
Pregnancy risk category: C

AVAILABLE FORMS
Nasal solution: 0.125%, 0.25%, 0.5%, 1%

INDICATIONS & DOSAGES
➤ **Nasal congestion**
Adults and children age 12 and older: 2 to 3 drops or 2 to 3 sprays of 0.25% or 0.5% solution in each nostril every 4 hours, p.r.n. Don't use for longer than 3 to 5 days.
Children ages 6 to 12: 2 to 3 drops or 2 to 3 sprays of 0.25% solution in each nostril every 4 hours, p.r.n.
Children ages 2 to 6: 2 to 3 drops of 0.125% solution every 4 hours, p.r.n.

ADMINISTRATION
Intranasal
• Give 1% solution no more often than every 4 hours. Don't give the 1% solution to children younger than age 12 unless directed by prescriber.
• To instill nose drops, have patient lie down and tilt his head back. Insert dropper no more than ⅓ inch into nostril. Don't touch

side of nose. Patient should remain supine with head back for 2 minutes after dose.
• Tilt patient's head back slightly to give nasal spray. Gently occlude opposite nostril.
• When giving more than one spray, wait 1 to 2 minutes between sprays.
• Rinse tip of spray under hot water and dry with a clean tissue.

ACTION
Causes local vasoconstriction of dilated arterioles, reducing blood flow and nasal congestion.

Route	Onset	Peak	Duration
Intranasal	Rapid	Unknown	30 min–4 hr

Half-life: Unknown.

ADVERSE REACTIONS
CNS: dizziness, headache, nervousness, psychological disturbances, restlessness, tremor.
CV: palpitations, tachycardia, hypertension, pallor, PVCs.
EENT: dryness of nasal mucosa, rebound nasal congestion, transient burning or stinging.
GI: nausea.
Other: hypersensitivity reactions, sweating.

INTERACTIONS
Drug-drug. *Beta blockers:* May cause hypertension, then bradycardia. Avoid using together.
MAO inhibitors, methyldopa, TCAs: May potentiate the pressor response of phenylephrine. Avoid using within 14 days of an MAO inhibitor.

EFFECTS ON LAB TEST RESULTS
None reported.

CONTRAINDICATIONS & CAUTIONS
• Contraindicated in patients hypersensitive to drug.
• Use cautiously in patients with hyperthyroidism, marked hypertension, type 1 diabetes mellitus, cardiac disease, or advanced arteriosclerotic changes; in children with low body weight; and in elderly patients.

P

NURSING CONSIDERATIONS

• Monitor patient for systemic adverse effects.

• Don't use in children who are younger than age 2.

• *Look alike–sound alike:* Don't confuse Neo-Synephrine (phenylephrine) with Neo-Synephrine 12 Hour (oxymetazoline).

PATIENT TEACHING

• Teach patient how to use drug.

• Caution patient not to share drug because this could spread infection.

• Tell patient not to exceed recommended dosage and to use only when needed.

• Advise patient to contact prescriber if signs and symptoms persist longer than 3 days.

• Inform patient that prolonged use may result in rebound congestion.

phenylephrine hydrochloride (ophthalmic)

fen-ill-EF-rin

AK-Dilate, Altafrin ◇, Mydfrin, Neofrin, OcuNefrin ◇, Refresh Redness Relief ◇

Therapeutic class: Mydriatics
Pharmacologic class: Sympathomimetic amines–adrenergics
Pregnancy risk category: C

AVAILABLE FORMS

Ophthalmic solution: 0.12%, 2.5%, 10%

INDICATIONS & DOSAGES

➤ **Mydriasis without cycloplegia**
Adults and children: Instill 1 drop of 2.5% or 10% solution before examination. May repeat in 1 hour, as needed. May need to apply topical anesthetic before use to prevent stinging and dilution from lacrimation.

➤ **Mydriasis and vasoconstriction**
Adults and adolescents: Instill 1 drop of 2.5% or 10% solution.
Children: Instill 1 drop of 2.5% solution.

➤ **Chronic mydriasis**
Adults and adolescents: Instill 1 drop of 2.5% or 10% solution b.i.d. or t.i.d.
Children: Instill 1 drop of 2.5% solution b.i.d. or t.i.d.

➤ **Posterior synechiae (adhesion of iris)**
Adults and children: To prevent or break posterior synechiae in patients with anterior uveitis, instill 1 drop of 2.5% or 10% solution t.i.d. or more often in combination with atropine sulfate ophthalmic solution or ointment. To prevent posterior synechiae after iridectomy, instill 1 drop of 10% solution once daily to b.i.d.; give in combination with atropine sulfate ophthalmic solution or ointment if inflammation is severe. Don't use 10% concentration in children younger than 1.

➤ **Minor eye irritations**
Adults and children: Instill 1 or 2 drops of the 0.12% solution in affected eye up to q.i.d., as needed.

ADMINISTRATION

Ophthalmic

• Don't touch tip of dropper to eye or surrounding tissue.

• Apply light finger pressure on lacrimal sac for 1 minute after instilling drug to minimize systemic absorption.

• Don't use brown solution or solution that contains precipitate.

ACTION

Dilates the pupil by contracting the dilator muscle.

Route	Onset	Peak	Duration
Ophthalmic	Rapid	10–90 min	3–7 hr

Half-life: Unknown.

ADVERSE REACTIONS

CNS: brow ache, headache.
CV: hypertension with 10% solution, *MI,* palpitations, PVCs, tachycardia.
EENT: allergic conjunctivitis, blurred vision, increased intraocular pressure (IOP), keratitis, lacrimation, reactive hyperemia of eye, rebound miosis, transient eye burning or stinging on instillation.
Skin: dermatitis, diaphoresis, pallor.
Other: trembling.

INTERACTIONS

Drug-drug. *Atropine (topical), cyclopentolate, homatropine, scopolamine:* May increase pupil dilation. Use together cautiously.

Reactions in bold italics are *life-threatening*. Interactions may have a *rapid onset* or a *delayed onset*.

Beta blockers, MAO inhibitors: May cause arrhythmias because of increased pressor effect. Use together cautiously.

Levodopa: May reduce mydriatic effect of phenylephrine. Use together cautiously.

TCAs: May increase cardiac effects of epinephrine. Use together cautiously.

Drug-lifestyle. *Sun exposure:* May cause photophobia. Advise patient to wear sunglasses.

EFFECTS ON LAB TEST RESULTS
• May lower IOP in normal eyes or in angle-closure glaucoma.
• May cause false-normal tonometry readings.

CONTRAINDICATIONS & CAUTIONS
• Contraindicated in patients hypersensitive to drug, in those with angle-closure glaucoma, and in those who wear soft contact lenses.
• Use cautiously in patients with marked hypertension, cardiac disorders, advanced arteriosclerotic changes, type 1 diabetes, or hyperthyroidism; in children with low body weight; and in elderly patients.

NURSING CONSIDERATIONS
• Systemic adverse reactions are least likely with 0.12% and 2.5% solutions and most likely with 10% solution.
• *Look alike–sound alike:* Don't confuse Mydfrin with Midrin.

PATIENT TEACHING
• Teach patient how to instill drug. Advise him to wash hands before and after instillation and to apply light finger pressure on lacrimal sac for 1 minute after drops are instilled. Warn him not to touch tip of dropper to eye or surrounding tissue.
• Warn patient not to exceed recommended dosage because systemic effects can result. Monitor blood pressure and pulse rate.
• Tell patient not to use brown solution or solution that contains precipitate.
• Warn patient to avoid hazardous activities, such as operating machinery or driving, until temporary blurring subsides.
• Advise patient to contact prescriber if condition persists longer than 12 hours after stopping drug.

• Advise patient to ease photophobia by wearing dark glasses.

phenytoin (diphenylhydantoin)
FEN-i-toe-in

Dilantin 125, Dilantin Infatabs

phenytoin sodium

phenytoin sodium (extended)
Dilantin, Phenytek

Therapeutic class: Anticonvulsants
Pharmacologic class: Hydantoin derivatives
Pregnancy risk category: D

AVAILABLE FORMS
phenytoin
Oral suspension: 125 mg/5 mL*
Tablets (chewable): 50 mg
phenytoin sodium
Injection: 50 mg/mL (46 mg base)
phenytoin sodium (extended)
Capsules: 30 mg (27.6 mg base), 100 mg (92 mg base), 200 mg (184 mg base), 300 mg (276 mg base)

INDICATIONS & DOSAGES
➤ **To control tonic-clonic (grand mal) and complex partial (temporal lobe) seizures**
Adults: Highly individualized. Initially, 100 mg P.O. t.i.d., increasing by 100 mg P.O. every 2 to 4 weeks until desired response is obtained. Usual range is 300 to 600 mg daily. If patient is stabilized with extended-release capsules, once-daily dosing with 300-mg extended-release capsules is possible as an alternative.

Children: 5 mg/kg or 250 mg/m^2 P.O. divided in two or three doses. Usual dose range is 4 to 8 mg/kg daily. Maximum daily dose is 300 mg.

➤ **For patients requiring a loading dose**
Adults: Initially, 1 g P.O. daily divided into three doses and given at 2-hour intervals. Or, 10 to 15 mg/kg I.V. at a rate not exceeding 50 mg/minute. Normal maintenance

P

dosage is started 24 hours after loading dose.

Children: 500 to 600 mg P.O. in divided doses, followed by maintenance dosage 24 hours after loading dose. Or, 15 to 20 mg/kg I.V.

➤ **To prevent and treat seizures occurring during neurosurgery**

Adults: 100 to 200 mg I.M. every 4 hours during and after surgery.

➤ **Status epilepticus**

Adults: Loading dose of 10 to 15 mg/kg I.V. (1 to 1.5 g may be needed) at a rate not exceeding 50 mg/minute; then maintenance dosage of 100 mg P.O. or I.V. every 6 to 8 hours.

Children: Loading dose of 15 to 20 mg/kg I.V., at a rate not exceeding 1 to 3 mg/kg/minute; then highly individualized maintenance dosages.

Elderly patients: May need lower dosages.

ADMINISTRATION
P.O.
● Give divided doses with or after meals to decrease adverse GI reactions.

I.V.
▼ Clear tubing with normal saline solution. Use only clear solution for injection. A slight yellow color is acceptable.

▼ Mix with normal saline solution, if needed, and give as an infusion over 30 minutes to 1 hour, when possible.

▼ Infusion must begin within 1 hour after preparation and should run through an in-line filter.

▼ Check patency of catheter before giving. Monitor site for extravasation because it can cause severe tissue damage.

Black Box Warning Drug must be administered slowly. In adults, don't exceed 50 mg/minute I.V. In neonates, administer drug at a rate not exceeding 1 to 3 mg/kg/minute. ∎

▼ Follow each injection with injection of sterile saline through the same needle or catheter.

▼ If possible, don't give by I.V. push into veins on back of hand to avoid purple glove syndrome. Inject into larger veins or central venous catheter, if available.

▼ Check vital signs, blood pressure, and ECG during I.V. administration.

▼ Discard 4 hours after preparation. Don't refrigerate.

▼ **Incompatibilities:** Amikacin, aminophylline, amphotericin B, bretylium, cephapirin, ciprofloxacin, D_5W, diltiazem, dobutamine, enalaprilat, fat emulsions, hydromorphone, insulin (regular), levorphanol, lidocaine, lincomycin, meperidine, morphine sulfate, nitroglycerin, norepinephrine, other I.V. drugs or infusion solutions, pentobarbital sodium, potassium chloride, procaine, propofol, streptomycin, sufentanil citrate, theophylline, vitamin B complex with C. If giving as an infusion, don't mix drug with D_5W because it will precipitate.

I.M.
● Give I.M. only if dosage adjustments are made; I.M. dose is 50% greater than oral dose.

● Be aware that drug may precipitate at injection site, cause pain, and be absorbed erratically.

ACTION
May stabilize neuronal membranes and limit seizure activity either by increasing efflux or decreasing influx of sodium ions across cell membranes in the motor cortex during generation of nerve impulses.

Route	Onset	Peak	Duration
P.O.	Unknown	1½–12 hr	Unknown
P.O. (Phenytek)	Unknown	4–12 hr	Unknown
I.V.	Immediate	1–2 hr	Unknown
I.M.	Unknown	Unknown	Unknown

Half-life: Varies with dose and concentration changes.

ADVERSE REACTIONS
CNS: ataxia, decreased coordination, mental confusion, slurred speech, dizziness, headache, insomnia, nervousness, twitching, peripheral neuropathy.
CV: bradycardia, periarteritis nodosa, hypotension.
EENT: diplopia, nystagmus, blurred vision, thickening of facial features.
GI: gingival hyperplasia, nausea, vomiting, constipation.

Reactions in bold italics are *life-threatening*. Interactions may have a *rapid onset* or a *delayed onset*.

Hematologic: *agranulocytosis, leuko-penia, pancytopenia, thrombocytopenia,* macrocythemia, megaloblastic anemia.
Hepatic: *toxic hepatitis.*
Metabolic: hyperglycemia.
Musculoskeletal: osteomalacia.
Skin: *Stevens-Johnson syndrome, toxic epidermal necrolysis,* bullous or purpuric dermatitis, discoloration of skin if given by I.V. push in back of hand, exfoliative dermatitis, hypertrichosis, inflammation at injection site, necrosis, pain, photosensitivity reactions, scarlatiniform or morbilliform rash.
Other: lymphadenopathy, systemic lupus erythematosus.

INTERACTIONS
Drug-drug. *Acetaminophen:* May decrease the therapeutic effects of acetaminophen and increase the incidence of hepatotoxicity. Monitor for toxicity.
Amiodarone, antihistamines, chloramphenicol, **cimetidine,** *cycloserine, diazepam,* **fluconazole, isoniazid,** *metronidazole, omeprazole, phenylbutazone, salicylates,* **sulfonamides, ticlodipine,** *valproate:* May increase phenytoin activity and toxicity. Monitor patient for toxicity and adjust dose as needed.
Atracurium, cisatracurium, pancuronium, rocuronium, vecuronium: May decrease the effects of nondepolarizing muscle relaxant. May need to increase the nondepolarizing muscle relaxant dose.
Barbiturates, carbamazepine, dexa-methasone, diazoxide, folic acid, rifampin: May decrease phenytoin activity. Monitor phenytoin level.
Carbamazepine, cardiac glycosides, doxycycline, hormonal contraceptives, quinidine, theophylline, valproic acid: May decrease effects of these drugs. Monitor patient.
Colesevelam: May impair phenytoin absorption. Administer phenytoin 4 hours prior to colesevelam.
Corticosteroids: May decrease phenytoin level and corticosteroid effects. Measure phenytoin level and adjust phenytoin and corticosteroid dosages as needed.
Cyclosporine: May decrease cyclosporine levels, risking organ rejection. Monitor

cyclosporine levels closely and adjust dose as needed.
Delavirdine: May cause loss of virologie response. Use together is contraindicated.
Disulfiram: May increase toxic effects of phenytoin. Monitor phenytoin level closely and adjust dose as needed.
Efavirenz: May increase phenytoin level and decrease efavirenz level. Monitor patient and adjust dosages of either or both drugs if needed.
Erlotinib: May increase phenytoin level and decrease erlotinib level. Monitor patient response.
Hormonal contraceptives: May increase phenytoin level and decrease contraceptive effectiveness. Monitor phenytoin level and adjust dosage if needed. Alternative form of contraception is recommended during therapy.
Isoniazid: May increase phenytoin level. Monitor phenytoin level and patient for toxicity.
Lithium: May increase toxicity of lithium, despite normal lithium levels. Monitor patient for adverse effects.
Methylphenidate: May increase phenytoin level. Monitor phenytoin level and adjust phenytoin dosage as needed.
Protease inhibitors (fosamprenavir, lopinavir–ritonavir): May decrease levels of both drugs. Measure phenytoin level and adjust dosage of phenytoin or protease inhibitor as needed.
Warfarin: May increase effects of warfarin. Monitor patient for bleeding.
Drug-food. *Enteral tube feedings:* May interfere with absorption of oral drug. Stop enteral feedings for 2 hours before and 2 hours after drug use.
Drug-lifestyle. *Long-term alcohol use:* May decrease drug's activity. Strongly discourage use together.

EFFECTS ON LAB TEST RESULTS
• May increase alkaline phosphatase, GGT, and glucose levels. May decrease urinary 17-hydroxysteroid, 17-ketosteroid, and hemoglobin levels and hematocrit.
• May decrease platelet, WBC, RBC, and granulocyte counts.

P

• May increase urine 6-hydroxycortisol excretion. May decrease dexamethasone suppression and metyrapone test results.
• May falsely reduce protein-bound iodine or free T_4 level test results.

CONTRAINDICATIONS & CAUTIONS
• Contraindicated in patients hypersensitive to hydantoin, in those taking delavirdine, and in those with sinus bradycardia, SA block, second- or third-degree AV block, or Adams-Stokes syndrome.
• Use cautiously in patients with hepatic dysfunction, hypotension, myocardial insufficiency, diabetes, or respiratory depression; in elderly or debilitated patients; and in those receiving other hydantoin derivatives.
• Elderly patients tend to metabolize drug slowly and may need reduced dosages.
⚠ **Overdose S&S:** Ataxia, dysarthria, nystagmus, hyperreflexia, lethargy, nausea, slurred speech, tremor, vomiting, coma, hypotension, circulatory and respiratory depression.

NURSING CONSIDERATIONS
• Therapeutic dose usually increases during pregnancy.
• Asian patients who have tested positive for the allele HLA-B*1502 have a potentially increased risk of serious skin reactions, including Stevens-Johnson syndrome and toxic epidermal necrolysis. Monitor these patients carefully.
• If rash appears, stop drug. If rash is scarlatiniform or morbilliform, resume drug after rash clears. If rash reappears, stop drug. If rash is exfoliative, purpuric, or bullous, don't resume drug.
• Don't stop drug suddenly because this may worsen seizures. Call prescriber immediately if adverse reactions develop.
• Monitor drug level. Therapeutic level of total phenytoin is 10 to 20 mcg/mL. The therapeutic range of free phenytoin is 1 to 2 mcg/mL.
• Allow at least 7 to 10 days to elapse between dosage changes.
• Because of the risks of cardiac and local toxicity with parenteral phenytoin, use oral form when possible.

• Monitor CBC and calcium level every 6 months, and periodically monitor hepatic function. If megaloblastic anemia is evident, prescriber may order folic acid and vitamin B_{12}.
• Maintain seizure precautions, as needed.
• Mononucleosis may decrease level. Watch for increased seizures.
❸ **Alert:** Closely monitor all patients for changes in behavior that may indicate worsening of suicidal thoughts or behavior or depression.
• Watch for gingival hyperplasia, especially in children.
❸ **Alert:** Doubling the dose doesn't double the level but may cause toxicity. Consult pharmacist for specific dosing recommendations.
• If seizure control is established with divided doses, once-daily dosing may be considered.
• **Look alike–sound alike:** Don't confuse phenytoin with mephenytoin, fosphenytoin, phenelzine, phentermine, or phenobarbital. Don't confuse Dilantin with Dilaudid, diltiazem, or Dipentum.

PATIENT TEACHING
• Tell patient to notify prescriber if skin rash develops.
• Advise patient to avoid driving and other potentially hazardous activities that require mental alertness until drug's CNS effects are known.
• Advise patient not to change brands or dosage forms once he's stabilized on therapy.
• Dilantin capsules are the only oral form that can be given once daily. Toxic levels may result if any other brand or form is given once daily. Dilantin tablets and oral suspension should never be taken once daily.
• Tell patient not to use capsules that are discolored.
• Advise patient to avoid alcohol.
• Warn patient and parents not to stop drug abruptly.
• Stress importance of good oral hygiene and regular dental examinations. Surgical removal of excess gum tissue may be needed periodically if dental hygiene is poor.
• Caution patient that drug may color urine pink, red, or reddish brown.

Reactions in bold italics are *life-threatening*. Interactions may have a *rapid onset* or a *delayed onset*.

pilocarpine hydrochloride (ophthalmic)
pie-low-KAR-peen

Akarpine†, Diocarpine†, Isopto Carpine, Pilopine HS

pilocarpine nitrate†

Therapeutic class: Miotics
Pharmacologic class: Direct-acting parasympathomimetics
Pregnancy risk category: C

AVAILABLE FORMS
pilocarpine hydrochloride
Ophthalmic gel: 4%
Ophthalmic solution: 1%, 2%, 4%
pilocarpine nitrate
Ophthalmic solution: 2%

INDICATIONS & DOSAGES
➤ **Primary open-angle glaucoma**
Adults and children: Instill 1 or 2 drops every 6 to 8 hours; adjust concentration and frequency to control intraocular pressure (IOP). Or apply 1.3-cm (½-inch) ribbon of 4% gel into the lower conjunctival sac once daily at bedtime.
➤ **Mydriasis caused by mydriatic or cycloplegic drugs**
Adults and children: Instill 1 drop of 1% solution.

ADMINISTRATION
Ophthalmic
• Don't touch tip of dropper to eye or surrounding tissue.
• Apply light finger pressure on lacrimal sac for 1 minute after instilling to minimize systemic absorption.
• If both solution and gel are used, the solution should be applied first; wait at least 5 minutes before applying the gel.

ACTION
A cholinergic that causes contraction of iris sphincter muscles, resulting in miosis, and that produces ciliary spasm, deepening of the anterior chamber, and vasodilation of conjunctival vessels of the outflow tract.

Route	Onset	Peak	Duration
Ophthalmic	10–30 min	30–85 min	4–8 hr

Half-life: Unknown.

ADVERSE REACTIONS
EENT: blurred vision, brow pain, myopia, changes in visual field, ciliary spasm, conjunctival irritation, keratitis, lacrimation, lens opacity, periorbital or supraorbital headache, retinal detachment, transient stinging and burning.
GI: diarrhea, nausea, vomiting.
Other: diaphoresis.

INTERACTIONS
Drug-drug. *Carbachol, echothiophate:* May cause additive effects. Avoid using together.
Cyclopentolate, ophthalmic belladonna alkaloids such as atropine, scopolamine: May decrease pilocarpine's antiglaucoma effect and block mydriatic effects of these drugs. Avoid using together.
Phenylephrine: May decrease dilation by phenylephrine. Avoid using together.

EFFECTS ON LAB TEST RESULTS
None reported.

CONTRAINDICATIONS & CAUTIONS
• Contraindicated in patients hypersensitive to drug and in conditions in which cholinergic effects, such as constriction, are undesirable (acute iritis, some forms of secondary glaucoma, pupillary block glaucoma, or acute inflammatory disease of the anterior chamber).
• Use cautiously in patients with acute cardiac failure, bronchial asthma, peptic ulcer, hyperthyroidism, GI spasm, urinary tract obstruction, and Parkinson disease.
⚠ *Overdose S&S:* Excess salivation, tearing, sweating, nausea, vomiting, diarrhea, bronchial constriction, tremors, bradycardia, hypotension.

NURSING CONSIDERATIONS
• Monitor vital signs.
☞ *Alert:* Patients with hazel or brown irises may need stronger solutions or more frequent instillation because eye pigment may absorb drug.

• *Look alike–sound alike:* Don't confuse Isopto Carpine with Isopto Carbachol.

PATIENT TEACHING
• Instruct patient to apply gel at bedtime because it will blur vision. Warn him to avoid hazardous activities, such as operating machinery or driving, until temporary blurring subsides.
• Teach patient how to instill drug. Advise him to wash hands before and after instillation and to apply light finger pressure on lacrimal sac for 1 minute after drops are instilled. Warn patient not to touch applicator tip to eye or surrounding tissue.
• Tell patient that if other glaucoma medications and gel are used at bedtime, to apply the drops first and to wait at least 5 minutes before applying the gel.
• Warn patient that transient brow pain and nearsightedness are common at first but usually disappear in 10 to 14 days.
• Advise patient to carry medical identification at all times during therapy.

pilocarpine hydrochloride (oral)
pye-loe-CAR-peen

Salagen

Therapeutic class: Cholinergic agonists
Pharmacologic class: Cholinergic agonists
Pregnancy risk category: C

AVAILABLE FORMS
Tablets: 5 mg, 7.5 mg

INDICATIONS & DOSAGES
Adjust-a-dose (for all indications): For patients with moderate hepatic impairment, initial dose is 5 mg P.O. b.i.d. Adjust dose based on tolerance.
➤ **Xerostomia from salivary gland hypofunction caused by radiotherapy for cancer of head and neck**
Adults: 5 mg P.O. t.i.d.; may increase to 10 mg P.O. t.i.d., as needed.
➤ **Dry mouth in patients with Sjögren syndrome**
Adults: 5 mg P.O. q.i.d.

➤ **Keratoconjunctivitis sicca (dry eye syndrome)** ◆
Adult: 5 mg P.O. q.i.d. to maximum of 30 mg/day.

ADMINISTRATION
P.O.
• Don't give drug with a high-fat meal.

ACTION
Cholinergic parasympathomimetic that increases secretion of salivary glands, eliminating dryness.

Route	Onset	Peak	Duration
P.O.	20 min	1 hr	3–5 hr

Half-life: 45 minutes to 1½ hours.

ADVERSE REACTIONS
CNS: asthenia, dizziness, headache, tremor.
CV: flushing, hypertension, tachycardia, edema.
EENT: abnormal vision, rhinitis, sinusitis, lacrimation, amblyopia, pharyngitis, voice alteration, conjunctivitis, epistaxis.
GI: nausea, dyspepsia, diarrhea, abdominal pain, vomiting, dysphagia, taste perversion.
GU: urinary frequency.
Musculoskeletal: myalgia.
Skin: sweating, rash, pruritus.
Other: chills.

INTERACTIONS
Drug-drug. *Beta blockers:* May increase risk of conduction disturbances. Use together cautiously.
Drugs with anticholinergic effects: May antagonize anticholinergic effects. Use together cautiously.
Drugs with parasympathomimetic effects: May result in additive pharmacologic effects. Monitor patient closely.
Drug-food. *High-fat meals:* May reduce drug absorption. Discourage patient from eating high-fat meals.

EFFECTS ON LAB TEST RESULTS
None reported.

CONTRAINDICATIONS & CAUTIONS
• Contraindicated in patients hypersensitive to pilocarpine, in breast-feeding women, in those with uncontrolled asthma, and in those

---

Reactions in bold italics are *life-threatening*. Interactions may have a *rapid onset* or a *delayed onset*.

for whom miosis is undesirable, as in acute iritis or angle-closure glaucoma.
• Use in severe hepatic insufficiency isn't recommended.
• Use cautiously in patients with CV disease, controlled asthma, chronic bronchitis, COPD, cholelithiasis, biliary tract disease, nephrolithiasis, cognitive or psychiatric disturbances, or in pregnant women.
• Safety and effectiveness of drug in children haven't been established.
⚠ **Overdose S&S:** CV depression, bronchoconstriction, death.

NURSING CONSIDERATIONS
• Examine patient's fundus carefully before beginning therapy because retinal detachment may occur in patients with retinal disease.
• Monitor patient for signs and symptoms of toxicity: headache, visual disturbance, lacrimation, sweating, respiratory distress, GI spasm, nausea, vomiting, diarrhea, AV block, tachycardia, bradycardia, hypotension, hypertension, shock, mental confusion, arrhythmia, and tremors. Immediately notify prescriber of suspected toxicity.
• **Look alike–sound alike:** Don't confuse Salagen with selegiline.

PATIENT TEACHING
• Warn patient that driving ability may be impaired, especially at night, by drug-induced visual disturbances.
• Advise patient to drink plenty of fluids to prevent dehydration.
• Tell elderly patient with Sjögren syndrome that he may be especially prone to urinary frequency, diarrhea, and dizziness.
• Advise patient not to take drug with a high-fat meal.

pimecrolimus
py-meck-roh-LY-mus

Elidel

Therapeutic class: Immunosuppressants (topical)
Pharmacologic class: Topical immunomodulators
Pregnancy risk category: C

AVAILABLE FORMS
Cream: 1%. Base contains benzyl alcohol, cetyl alcohol, oleyl alcohol, and stearyl alcohol.

INDICATIONS & DOSAGES
➤ **Short- and intermittent long-term treatment of mild to moderate atopic dermatitis in nonimmunocompromised patients in whom the use of other conventional therapies is deemed inadvisable, or in patients with inadequate response to or intolerance of conventional therapies**
Adults and children age 2 and older: Apply a thin layer to the affected skin b.i.d. and rub in gently and completely. Discontinue therapy when signs and symptoms (itch, rash, redness) resolve.

ADMINISTRATION
Topical
• Drug may be used on all skin surfaces, including the head, neck, and intertriginous areas.
• Clear infections at treatment sites before using.
• Don't use with occlusive dressing.

ACTION
Unknown. Inhibits T-cell activation and prevents the release of inflammatory cytokines and mediators from mast cells.

Route	Onset	Peak	Duration
Topical	Unknown	Unknown	Unknown

Half-life: Unknown.

ADVERSE REACTIONS
CNS: headache, fever.
EENT: nasopharyngitis, otitis media, sinusitis, pharyngitis, tonsillitis, eye

P

infection, nasal congestion, rhinorrhea, sinus congestion, rhinitis, epistaxis, conjunctivitis, earache.

GI: gastroenteritis, abdominal pain, vomiting, diarrhea, nausea, constipation, loose stools.

GU: dysmenorrhea.

Musculoskeletal: back pain, arthralgias.

Respiratory: upper respiratory tract infections, bronchitis, cough, *asthma,* pneumonia, wheezing, dyspnea.

Skin: application-site reaction (burning, irritation, erythema, pruritus), skin infections, impetigo, folliculitis, molluscum contagiosum, herpes simplex, varicella, papilloma, urticaria, acne.

Other: influenza, flulike illness, hypersensitivity, toothache, bacterial infection, staphylococcal infection, viral infection.

INTERACTIONS

Drug-drug. *CYP450 inhibitors (such as calcium channel blockers, erythromycin, fluconazole, itraconazole, ketoconazole):* May affect metabolism of pimecrolimus. Use together cautiously.

Drug-lifestyle. *Natural or artificial sunlight exposure:* May worsen atopic dermatitis. Advise patient to avoid or minimize sunlight exposure.

EFFECTS ON LAB TEST RESULTS

None reported.

CONTRAINDICATIONS & CAUTIONS

• Contraindicated in patients hypersensitive to drug or its components, in patients with Netherton syndrome, and in immunocompromised patients.

• Contraindicated in patients with active cutaneous viral infections or infected atopic dermatitis.

Black Box Warning Contraindicated in children younger than age 2. ∎

• Use cautiously in patients with varicella zoster virus infection, herpes simplex virus infection, or eczema herpeticum.

• Safety of use in pregnant women hasn't been established.

NURSING CONSIDERATIONS

❸ *Alert:* Use drug only after other therapies have failed because of the risk of cancer.

Black Box Warning Long-term safety hasn't been established. Avoid continuous long-term use of drug and limit application to areas of involvement of atopic dermatitis. ∎

• If symptoms persist longer than 6 weeks, reevaluate the patient.

• May cause local symptoms such as skin burning. Most local reactions start within 1 to 5 days after treatment, are mild to moderately severe, and last no longer than 5 days.

• Monitor patient for lymphadenopathy. If lymphadenopathy occurs and its cause is unknown, or if the patient develops acute infectious mononucleosis, consider stopping drug.

• Drug use may cause papillomas or warts. Consider stopping drug if papillomas worsen or don't respond to conventional treatment.

• It's unknown if drug appears in breast milk. Serious adverse reactions may occur in breast-feeding infants exposed to drug. Patient should either stop breast-feeding or stop treatment.

• *Look alike–sound alike:* Don't confuse pimecrolimus with tacrolimus.

PATIENT TEACHING

• Inform patient that this drug is for external use only and that he should use it as directed.

• Tell patient to report adverse reactions.

• Tell patient not to use with an occlusive dressing.

• Instruct patient to wash hands after application if hands are not treated.

• Tell patient to stop therapy after signs and symptoms have resolved. If symptoms persist longer than 6 weeks, tell him to contact his prescriber.

• Tell patient to resume treatment at first signs of recurrence.

• Stress that patient should minimize or avoid exposure to natural or artificial sunlight (including tanning beds and UVA-UVB treatment) while using this drug.

• Tell patient to expect application-site reactions but to notify his prescriber if reaction is severe or persists for longer than 1 week.

Reactions in bold italics are *life-threatening*. Interactions may have a *rapid onset* or a *delayed onset*.

pioglitazone hydrochloride
pie-oh-GLIT-ah-zohn

Actos⌾

Therapeutic class: Antidiabetics
Pharmacologic class: Thiazolidinediones
Pregnancy risk category: C

AVAILABLE FORMS
Tablets: 15 mg, 30 mg, 45 mg

INDICATIONS & DOSAGES
➤ **Type 2 diabetes mellitus, alone or with a sulfonylurea, metformin, or insulin**
Adults: Initially, 15 or 30 mg P.O. once daily. Maximum daily dose, if used alone or in combination therapy, is 45 mg.
Adjust-a-dose: For patients taking pioglitazone with insulin, reduce insulin by 10% to 25% if patient reports hypoglycemia or if glucose level is less than 100 mg/dL. Maximum recommended dose of pioglitazone is 15 mg when used with gemfibrozil or other strong CYP2C8 inhibitors. Start with 15 mg in patients with New York Heart Association (NYHA) class I or II heart failure.
➤ **Polycystic ovary syndrome ◆**
Adults: 15 to 30 mg P.O. once daily.

ADMINISTRATION
P.O.
● Give drug without regard for meals.

ACTION
Lowers glucose level by decreasing insulin resistance and hepatic glucose production. Improves sensitivity of insulin in muscle and adipose tissue.

Route	Onset	Peak	Duration
P.O.	30 min	≤2 hr	Unknown

Half-life: 3 to 7 hours.

ADVERSE REACTIONS
CNS: headache.
CV: edema, *heart failure.*
EENT: sinusitis, pharyngitis, macular edema.
Hematologic: anemia.

Metabolic: *hypoglycemia with combination therapy, aggravated diabetes,* weight gain.
Musculoskeletal: myalgia, fractures.
Respiratory: upper respiratory tract infection.
Other: tooth disorder.

INTERACTIONS
Drug-drug. *Atorvastatin:* May decrease atorvastatin and pioglitazone levels. Monitor patient and glucose level.
Gemfibrozil: May increase pioglitazone level. Monitor patient and glucose level. Maximum pioglitazone dose is 15 mg.
Hormonal contraceptives: May decrease level of hormonal contraceptives, reducing contraceptive effectiveness. Advise patient taking drug and hormonal contraceptives to consider additional birth control measures.
Ketoconazole: May inhibit pioglitazone metabolism. Monitor glucose level more frequently.
Rifampin: May decrease pioglitazone concentration. Don't exceed maximum recommended pioglitazone dose.
Drug-herb. *Burdock, dandelion, eucalyptus, marshmallow:* May increase hypoglycemic effects. Discourage use together.
Drug-lifestyle. *Alcohol use:* May alter glycemic control and increase risk of hypoglycemia. Discourage use together.

EFFECTS ON LAB TEST RESULTS
● May increase CK, ALT, HDL, LDL, and total cholesterol levels.
● May decrease glucose, triglyceride, hematocrit, and hemoglobin levels.

CONTRAINDICATIONS & CAUTIONS
Black Box Warning Contraindicated in patients with symptomatic heart failure and in those with NYHA class III or IV heart failure. ∎
● Contraindicated in patients hypersensitive to drug or its components and in those with active bladder disease, type 1 diabetes mellitus, diabetic ketoacidosis, active liver disease, ALT level greater than 2½ times the upper limit of normal (ULN), and in those who experienced jaundice while taking troglitazone.

Black Box Warning Use cautiously in patients with edema or heart failure or patients at risk for heart failure. ∎

• Use cautiously in patients with a history of bladder cancer.

• Use during pregnancy only if the benefit justifies risk to fetus; insulin is the preferred antidiabetic during pregnancy.

• Safety and effectiveness in children haven't been established.

NURSING CONSIDERATIONS

❸ *Alert:* Measure liver enzyme levels at start of therapy, every 2 months for first year of therapy, and periodically thereafter. Obtain LFT results in patients who develop signs and symptoms of liver dysfunction, such as nausea, vomiting, abdominal pain, fatigue, anorexia, or dark urine. Stop drug if patient develops jaundice or if LFT results show ALT level greater than $3 \times$ ULN.

Black Box Warning Drug can cause fluid retention, leading to or worsening heart failure. Observe patients carefully for signs and symptoms of heart failure (including excessive, rapid weight gain; dyspnea; and edema). If these signs and symptoms develop, the heart failure should be managed according to the current standards of care. Also, stopping or reducing dose of pioglitazone must be considered. ∎

• Hemoglobin level and hematocrit may drop, usually during first 4 to 12 weeks of therapy.

• Management of type 2 diabetes should include diet control. Because caloric restrictions, weight loss, and exercise help improve insulin sensitivity and help make drug therapy effective, these measures are essential for proper diabetes management.

• Watch for hypoglycemia, especially in patients receiving combination therapy. Dosage adjustments of these drugs may be needed.

• Monitor glucose level regularly, especially during situations of increased stress, such as infection, fever, surgery, and trauma.

❸ *Alert:* Drug may be associated with an increased risk of bladder cancer when used for more than 1 year. Monitor patients for signs and symptoms of bladder cancer (such as blood in urine or abdominal pain). If considering use in patients with a history of bladder cancer, weigh benefits of blood

glucose control with drug against unknown risks of cancer recurrence.

• Risk of fractures (forearm, hand, wrist, foot, ankle, fibula, and tibia) in female patients receiving long-term treatment is increased. Give only if risk outweighs benefits.

• *Look alike–sound alike:* Don't confuse pioglitazone with rosiglitazone. Don't confuse Actos with Actidose or Actonel.

PATIENT TEACHING

• Instruct patient to adhere to dietary instructions and to have glucose and glycosylated hemoglobin levels tested regularly.

• Teach patient taking pioglitazone with insulin or oral antidiabetics the signs and symptoms of hypoglycemia.

• Advise patient to notify prescriber during periods of stress, such as fever, trauma, infection, or surgery, because dosage may need adjustment.

• Instruct patient how and when to monitor glucose level.

• Notify patient that blood tests of liver function will be performed before therapy starts, every 2 months for the first year, and periodically thereafter.

• Tell patient to report unexplained nausea, vomiting, abdominal pain, fatigue, anorexia, and dark urine immediately because these symptoms may indicate liver problems.

• Warn patient to contact his health care provider if he has signs or symptoms of heart failure (unusually rapid increase in weight, swelling, or shortness of breath).

• Advise anovulatory, premenopausal women with insulin resistance that therapy may cause resumption of ovulation; recommend using contraception.

• Tell patient to have regular eye examinations and to report any visual changes immediately.

piperacillin sodium–tazobactam sodium

pie-PER-us-sil-in–taz-oh-BAK-tem

Tazocin†, Zosyn

Therapeutic class: Antibiotics
Pharmacologic class: Extended-spectrum penicillins–beta-lactamase inhibitors
Pregnancy risk category: B

AVAILABLE FORMS

Powder for injection: 2 g piperacillin and 0.25 g tazobactam per vial, 3 g piperacillin and 0.375 g tazobactam per vial, 4 g piperacillin and 0.5 g tazobactam per vial

INDICATIONS & DOSAGES

➤ **Moderate to severe infections from piperacillin-resistant, piperacillin–tazobactam-susceptible, beta-lactamase–producing strains of microorganisms in appendicitis (complicated by rupture or abscess) and peritonitis caused by *Escherichia coli, Bacteroides fragilis, B. ovatus, B. thetaiotaomicron,* and *B. vulgatus;* skin and skin-structure infections caused by *Staphylococcus aureus;* postpartum endometritis or pelvic inflammatory disease caused by *E. coli;* moderately severe community-acquired pneumonia caused by *Haemophilus influenzae***

Adults: 3.375 g (3 g piperacillin/0.375 g tazobactam) every 6 hours by I.V. infusion for 7 to 10 days.

Adjust-a-dose: If CrCl is 20 to 40 mL/minute, give 2.25 g (2 g piperacillin/0.25 g tazobactam) every 6 hours; if CrCl is less than 20 mL/minute, give 2.25 g (2 g piperacillin/0.25 g tazobactam) every 8 hours. In continuous ambulatory peritoneal dialysis (CAPD) patients, give 2.25 g (2 g piperacillin/0.25 g tazobactam) every 12 hours. In hemodialysis patients, give 2.25 g (2 g piperacillin/0.25 g tazobactam) every 12 hours with a supplemental dose of 0.75 g (0.67 g piperacillin/0.08 g tazobactam) after each dialysis period.

➤ **Appendicitis, peritonitis**
Children weighing more than 40 kg (88 lb) with normal renal function: 3.375 g (3 g piperacillin/0.375 g tazobactam) every 6 hours by I.V. infusion for 7 to 10 days.
Children age 9 months and older weighing 40 kg or less with normal renal function: 100 mg piperacillin/12.5 mg tazobactam per kg of body weight every 8 hours by I.V. infusion.
Children age 2 to 9 months: 80 mg piperacillin/10 mg tazobactam per kg of body weight every 8 hours by I.V. infusion.

➤ **Moderate to severe nosocomial pneumonia caused by piperacillin-resistant, beta-lactamase–producing strains of *S. aureus* and by piperacillin–tazobactam-susceptible *Acinetobacter baumannii, H. influenzae, Klebsiella pneumoniae,* and *Pseudomonas aeruginosa***

Adults: 4.5 g (4 g piperacillin/0.5 g tazobactam) every 6 hours with aminoglycoside. Patients with *P. aeruginosa* should continue aminoglycoside treatment; if *P. aeruginosa* isn't isolated, aminoglycoside treatment may be stopped. Duration of treatment is usually 7 to 14 days.

Adjust-a-dose: If CrCl is 20 to 40 mL/minute, give 3.375 g (3 g piperacillin/0.375 g tazobactam) every 6 hours; if CrCl is less than 20 mL/minute, give 2.25 g (2 g piperacillin/0.25 g tazobactam) every 6 hours. In CAPD patients, give 2.25 g (2 g piperacillin/0.25 g tazobactam) every 8 hours. In hemodialysis patients, give 2.25 g (2 g piperacillin/0.25 g tazobactam) every 8 hours with a supplemental dose of 0.75 g (0.67 g piperacillin/0.08 g tazobactam) after each dialysis period.

➤ **Catheter-related bloodstream infection ◆**
Adults: 4.5 g I.V. every 6 hours for 7 to 14 days. Refer to the package insert for dosing in renal insufficiency.

ADMINISTRATION

I.V.
▼ Before giving drug, ask patient about allergic reactions to penicillins.
▼ Obtain specimen for culture and sensitivity tests before giving first dose. Therapy may begin while awaiting results.

P

▼ Reconstitute each gram with 5 mL of diluent, such as sterile or bacteriostatic water for injection, normal saline solution for injection, bacteriostatic normal saline solution for injection, D_5W, dextrose 5% in normal saline solution for injection, or dextran 6% in normal saline solution for injection.

▼ Shake until dissolved.

▼ Further dilute to 50 to 150 mL before infusion.

▼ Use drug immediately after reconstitution.

▼ Stop any primary infusion during administration, if possible.

▼ Infuse over at least 30 minutes.

▼ Discard unused drug in single-dose vials after 24 hours if stored at room temperature or 48 hours if refrigerated.

▼ Change I.V. site every 48 hours.

▼ Diluted drug is stable in I.V. bags for 24 hours at room temperature or for 1 week refrigerated.

▼ **Incompatibilities:** Acyclovir sodium, aminoglycosides, amphotericin B, chlorpromazine, cisatracurium, cisplatin, dacarbazine, daunorubicin, dobutamine, doxorubicin, doxycycline hyclate, droperidol, famotidine, ganciclovir, gemcitabine, haloperidol lactate, hydroxyzine hydrochloride, idarubicin, lactated Ringer's solution, minocycline, mitomycin, mitoxantrone, nalbuphine, prochlorperazine edisylate, promethazine hydrochloride, streptozocin, vancomycin.

ACTION

Inhibits cell-wall synthesis during bacterial multiplication.

Route	Onset	Peak	Duration
I.V.	Immediate	Immediate	Unknown

Half-life: About 1 hour.

ADVERSE REACTIONS

CNS: headache, insomnia, fever, *seizures,* agitation, anxiety, dizziness, pain.
CV: *arrhythmia,* chest pain, edema, hypertension, tachycardia.
EENT: rhinitis.
GI: diarrhea, constipation, nausea, *pseudomembranous colitis,* abdominal pain, dyspepsia, stool changes, vomiting.

GU: candidiasis, interstitial nephritis.
Hematologic: *leukopenia, neutropenia, thrombocytopenia,* anemia, eosinophilia.
Respiratory: dyspnea.
Skin: pruritus, rash.
Other: *anaphylaxis,* hypersensitivity reactions, inflammation, phlebitis at I.V. site.

INTERACTIONS

Drug-drug. *Anticoagulants, heparin:* May prolong effectiveness and increase risk of bleeding. Monitor PT and INR closely.
Hormonal contraceptives: May decrease contraceptive effectiveness. Advise use of another form of contraception during therapy.
Live-virus vaccines: May decrease vaccine effectiveness. Don't use together.
Methotrexate: May increase risk of methotrexate toxicity. Monitor patient closely.
Probenecid: May increase piperacillin level. Probenecid may be used for this purpose.
Vecuronium: May prolong neuromuscular blockade. Monitor patient closely.

EFFECTS ON LAB TEST RESULTS

● May decrease hemoglobin level.
● May increase eosinophil count. May decrease neutrophil, platelet, and WBC counts.
● May cause false-positive result for urine glucose tests using copper reduction method such as Clinitest. May cause false-positive test for *Aspergillus.*

CONTRAINDICATIONS & CAUTIONS

● Contraindicated in patients hypersensitive to drug or other penicillins.
● Use cautiously in patients with bleeding tendencies, uremia, hypokalemia, and allergies to other drugs, especially cephalosporins, because of possible cross-sensitivity.
⚠ *Overdose S&S:* Neuromuscular hyperexcitability, seizures.

NURSING CONSIDERATIONS

● Drug may alter normal colon flora. Monitor patient for diarrhea and initiate therapeutic measures as needed. Drug may need to be stopped.

Reactions in bold italics are *life-threatening*. Interactions may have a *rapid onset* or a *delayed onset*.

• Because peritoneal dialysis removes 6% of the piperacillin dose and 21% of the tazobactam dose, and hemodialysis removes 30% to 40% of a dose in 4 hours, additional doses may be needed after each dialysis period.

• If large doses are given or if therapy is prolonged, bacterial or fungal superinfection may occur, especially in elderly, debilitated, or immunosuppressed patients.

• Drug contains 2.35 mEq sodium/g of piperacillin. Monitor patient's sodium intake and electrolyte levels.

• Monitor hematologic and coagulation parameters.

• Patients with cystic fibrosis may have a higher rate of fever and rash. Monitor these patients closely.

• *Look alike–sound alike:* Don't confuse Zosyn with Zofran or Zyvox.

PATIENT TEACHING

• Tell patient to report adverse reactions promptly.

• Tell patient to alert a health care professional about discomfort at the I.V. site.

pirbuterol acetate
peer-BYOO-ter-ole

Maxair Autohaler

Therapeutic class: Bronchodilators
Pharmacologic class: Beta₂ agonists
Pregnancy risk category: C

AVAILABLE FORMS
Inhaler: 0.2 mg/metered dose

INDICATIONS & DOSAGES
➤ **To prevent and reverse bronchospasm; asthma**
Adults and children age 12 and older: 1 or 2 inhalations (0.2 to 0.4 mg), repeated every 4 to 6 hours. Don't exceed 12 inhalations daily.

ADMINISTRATION
Inhalational
• Shake well before using. "Test spray" pirbuterol inhaler into the air before using

for the first time and when the aerosol hasn't been used for a prolonged period.

• If more than 1 inhalation is ordered, wait 1 minute between inhalations.

• Have patient hold his breath for 10 seconds after inhalation, then exhale slowly.

• Give corticosteroid inhaler 5 minutes after bronchodilator.

ACTION
Relaxes bronchial smooth muscle by stimulating beta₂ receptors.

Route	Onset	Peak	Duration
Inhalation	5 min	30–60 min	5 hr

Half-life: About 2 hours.

ADVERSE REACTIONS
CNS: tremor, nervousness, dizziness, insomnia, headache, vertigo.
CV: tachycardia, palpitations, chest tightness.
EENT: dry or irritated throat.
GI: nausea, vomiting, diarrhea, dry mouth.
Respiratory: cough.

INTERACTIONS
Drug-drug. *Beta blockers, propranolol:* May decrease bronchodilating effects. Avoid using together.
MAO inhibitors, TCAs: May potentiate action of beta agonist on vascular system. Use together cautiously.
Non-potassium-sparing diuretics: May cause ECG changes or hypokalemia. Use together cautiously.

EFFECTS ON LAB TEST RESULTS
None reported.

CONTRAINDICATIONS & CAUTIONS
• Contraindicated in patients hypersensitive to drug.
✪ Alert: Drug can cause paradoxical bronchospasm, which may be life-threatening. Bronchospasm frequently occurs with the first use of a new canister. If bronchospasm occurs, immediately discontinue drug and institute alternative therapy.

• Use cautiously in patients unusually responsive to sympathomimetic amines and patients with CV disorders, hyperthyroidism, diabetes, and seizure disorders.

P

⚠ Overdose S&S: Exaggeration of adverse reactions, hypokalemia, seizures, angina, hypertension, hypotension, arrhythmias, fatigue, malaise, insomnia, cardiac arrest, sudden death.

NURSING CONSIDERATIONS
• Monitor patient for increased pulse or blood pressure during therapy.
• Stop drug immediately and notify prescriber if paradoxical bronchospasm occurs.
• Notify prescriber of decreasing effectiveness of the drug.

PATIENT TEACHING
• Tell patient to prime inhaler before first use and if it hasn't been used in 48 hours.
• Give the following instructions for using Autohaler:
– Remove mouthpiece cover by pulling down lip on back cover. Inspect mouthpiece for foreign objects. Locate "Up" arrows and air vents.
– Hold Autohaler upright so that arrows point up; raise lever until it snaps into place.
– Hold Autohaler around the middle, and shake gently several times.
– Continue to hold upright, and be careful not to block air vents at bottom. Exhale normally before use.
– Seal lips around mouthpiece. Inhale deeply through mouthpiece with steady, moderate force to trigger release of the drug. You'll hear a click and feel a soft puff when drug is released. Continue to take a full, deep breath.
– Take Autohaler away from mouth when done inhaling. Hold breath for 10 seconds; then exhale slowly.
– Continue to hold Autohaler upright while lowering lever. Lower lever after each puff. If additional puffs are ordered, wait 1 minute before repeating process to obtain the next puff.
• Have patient clean inhaler per manufacturer's instructions.
• If patient also uses a corticosteroid inhaler, tell him to use the bronchodilator first, and then wait about 5 minutes before using the corticosteroid. This allows the bronchodilator to open air passages for maximal effectiveness of the corticosteroid.

• Instruct patient to call prescriber if bronchospasm increases after using drug.
• Advise patient to seek medical attention if a previously effective dosage doesn't control symptoms; this may signal worsening of disease.

pitavastatin
pih-tav-a-STAT-in

Livalo

Therapeutic class: Antilipemics
Pharmacologic class: HMG-CoA reductase inhibitors
Pregnancy risk category: X

AVAILABLE FORMS
Tablets: 1 mg, 2 mg, 4 mg

INDICATIONS & DOSAGES
➤ **Adjunctive therapy with diet to reduce total and LDL cholesterol and apolipoprotein B triglyceride levels, and to increase HDL cholesterol level in patients with primary hyperlipidemia and mixed dyslipidemia**
Adults: Initially, 2 mg P.O. daily. May increase dosage as needed, to maximum of 4 mg P.O. daily.
Adjust-a-dose: For patients with CrCl of 30 to 60 mL/minute, start with 1 mg P.O. daily; maximum dosage is 2 mg daily. If CrCl is less than 30 mL/minute, avoid use if patient isn't receiving dialysis. If ALT or AST level rises to more than 3 times the upper limit of normal and persists, reduce dosage or discontinue drug.

ADMINISTRATION
P.O.
• May be given without regard to food.

ACTION
Inhibits HMG-CoA reductase, a hepatic enzyme that's needed for cholesterol biosynthesis.

Route	Onset	Peak	Duration
P.O.	Unknown	1 hr	Unknown

Half-life: 12 hours.

ADVERSE REACTIONS
GI: constipation, diarrhea.
Musculoskeletal: back pain, myalgia, extremity pain, *rhabdomyolysis.*

INTERACTIONS
Drug-drug. ☻ *Alert: Atazanavir, atazanavir and ritonavir, darunavir and ritonavir, lopinavir–ritonavir:* May increase statin level and risk of myopathy and rhabdomyolysis. Avoid concurrent use with lopinavir–ritonavir combination; use together cautiously with other agents.
Cyclosporine: May increase pitavastatin level. Use together is contraindicated.
Erythromycin: May increase pitavastatin levels. Don't exceed 1 mg pitavastatin daily.
Fibrates (such as gemfibrozil, niacin): May increase risk of myopathy. Use together cautiously; consider reducing pitavastatin dosage when combined with niacin.
Rifampin: May increase pitavastatin levels. Don't exceed 2 mg pitavastatin daily.
Drug-herb. *Herbal cholesterol-lowering products:* May increase pitavastatin levels. Discourage using together.
Drug-food. *Grapefruit juice:* May increase pitavastatin levels and increase risk of adverse effects, including rhabdomyolysis and myopathy. Avoid using together.

EFFECTS ON LAB TEST RESULTS
● May increase AST, ALT, CK, bilirubin, and glucose levels.

CONTRAINDICATIONS & CAUTIONS
● Contraindicated in patients hypersensitive to drug or its components and in those with active liver disease.
● Contraindicated in pregnant and breast-feeding women.
● Avoid use in patients taking cyclosporine.
● Use cautiously in elderly patients and in those with renal impairment, inadequately treated hypothyroidism, or a history of myopathy or rhabdomyolysis.
● Statin therapy should be interrupted if the patient shows signs of serious liver injury, hyperbilirubinemia, or jaundice. The drug shouldn't be restarted if another cause can't be found.
● Safety and effectiveness in children haven't been established.

NURSING CONSIDERATIONS
● Start pitavastatin only after diet and other nondrug therapies have proved ineffective.
● Monitor PT and INR in patients taking warfarin when pitavastatin is added.
● Monitor LFT results and CK levels before therapy is started, 12 weeks after therapy is initiated, after a dosage change, and periodically thereafter.
● Discontinue drug if myopathy develops or if CK level markedly increases.
● Temporarily withhold drug if patient develops sepsis; hypotension; dehydration; severe metabolic, endocrine, or electrolyte disorders; uncontrolled seizures; or trauma or if patient requires major surgery. These conditions may predispose patient to myopathy or rhabdomyolysis.
● Adjust dosage about every 4 weeks.
● *Look alike–sound alike:* Don't confuse pitavastatin with atorvastatin, fluvastatin, lovastatin, nystatin, pravastatin, rosuvastatin, or simvastatin.

PATIENT TEACHING
● Tell patient that drug may be taken without regard to meals.
● Explain the importance of controlling serum lipid levels. Teach appropriate dietary management (restricting total fat and cholesterol intake), weight control, and exercise.
● Advise women of childbearing age to use birth control while taking pitavastatin and to discuss future pregnancy and breast-feeding plans with their health care provider.
● Advise patient to report unexplained muscle pain, tenderness, or weakness, especially if accompanied by fever or malaise.
● Advise patient that blood tests to check liver enzyme levels will be needed at 12 weeks after the start of therapy, after a dosage increase, and periodically thereafter.
● Tell patient that the drug may increase blood sugar levels; however, the CV benefits are thought to outweigh the slight increase in risk.

P

polyethylene glycol (PEG)
pol-ee-ETH-ih-leen

Clearlax† ◇, GlycoLax, Lax-A-Day† ◇, MiraLax ◇, PEG 3350†, Pegalax† ◇, Polylax†, Relaxa† ◇, Restoralax† ◇

Therapeutic class: Laxatives
Pharmacologic class: Osmotic drugs
Pregnancy risk category: C

AVAILABLE FORMS
Powder: single-dose 17-g packets; 16-ounce (255-g), 24-ounce (527-g) containers

INDICATIONS & DOSAGES
➤ **Short-term treatment of occasional constipation**
Adults: 17 g (about 1 heaping tablespoon) powder P.O. daily.

ADMINISTRATION
P.O.
● Before giving, rule out bowel obstruction in patients who have nausea, vomiting, abdominal pain, or distention.
● Dissolve powder in 8 ounces (240 mL) of water, juice, soda, coffee, or tea.

ACTION
Causes water to be retained in stool.

Route	Onset	Peak	Duration
P.O.	48–96 hr	Unknown	Unknown

Half-life: Unknown.

ADVERSE REACTIONS
GI: abdominal bloating, cramping, diarrhea, excess stool frequency, flatulence, nausea.

INTERACTIONS
Drug-drug. *Drugs containing polyethylene glycol:* May cause urticaria. Monitor patient.

EFFECTS ON LAB TEST RESULTS
None reported.

CONTRAINDICATIONS & CAUTIONS
● Contraindicated in patients allergic to drug and those with known or suspected bowel obstruction.
⚠ *Overdose S&S:* Diarrhea.

NURSING CONSIDERATIONS
● It may take 2 to 4 days before a bowel movement occurs.
● Drug should be taken for 2 weeks or less to avoid risk of laxative dependence.
● Occasional use as directed doesn't affect absorption or secretion of glucose or electrolytes.
● Prolonged, frequent, or excessive use may cause electrolyte imbalance and laxative dependence.
● Drug may be more likely to cause diarrhea in older patients.

PATIENT TEACHING
● Explain that proper eating habits and lifestyle changes may produce more regular bowel movements. Tell patient to eat adequate amounts of dietary fiber, drink ample fluids, and get appropriate exercise.
● If patient uses bottled form of drug, urge him to measure each 17-g dose using the measuring cup provided in the package. If patient uses drug packets, each one contains 17 g.
● Instruct patient to dissolve dose in 8 ounces of water, juice, soda, coffee, or tea.
● Inform patient that it may take 2 to 4 days to produce a bowel movement.
● Warn patient that taking more than the recommended dose can cause dehydration and severe diarrhea.
● Tell patient that drug should be used for 2 weeks or less to avoid risk of laxative dependence.
● Urge patient to report unusual cramping, bloating, or diarrhea.

Reactions in bold italics are *life-threatening*. Interactions may have a *rapid onset* or a *delayed onset*.

polyethylene glycol (PEG)–electrolyte solution
pol-ee-ETH-ih-leen

Colyte, GoLYTELY, MoviPrep, NuLYTELY, TriLyte

Therapeutic class: Laxatives
Pharmacologic class: Osmotic laxatives
Pregnancy risk category: C

AVAILABLE FORMS
Oral solution: PEG 3350 (6 g), sodium sulfate decahydrate (1.29 g), sodium chloride (146 mg), potassium chloride (75 mg), sodium bicarbonate (168 mg), polysorbate-80 (30 mg) per 100 mL (OCL)
Powder for oral solution: 4-L dose of solution contains PEG 3350 (17.6 mmol/L), sodium (125 mmol/L), sulfate (40 mmol/L; Colyte 80 mmol/L), chloride (35 mmol/L), bicarbonate (20 mmol/L), and potassium (10 mmol/L)

INDICATIONS & DOSAGES
➤ **Bowel preparation before GI examination**
Adults: 240 mL P.O. every 10 minutes until 4 L are consumed or until watery stool is clear. Typically, give 4 hours before examination, allowing 3 hours for drinking and 1 hour for bowel evacuation. Or, for MoviPrep, refer to package instructions for split-dose or full-dose regimen.

ADMINISTRATION
P.O.
• Use tap water to reconstitute powder according to package instructions. Shake vigorously to dissolve all powder. Refrigerate reconstituted solution, but use within 48 hours.
• Chilling solution improves palatability.
• Give solution early in the morning if patient is scheduled for a midmorning examination. Oral solution induces diarrhea (onset 30 to 60 minutes) that rapidly cleans the bowel, usually within 4 hours.
• When using to prepare for barium enema, give solution the evening before the examination to avoid interfering with barium coating of the colonic mucosa.

• If given to semiconscious patient or to patient with impaired gag reflex, take care to prevent aspiration.
• Give drug at least 2 hours after solid food.

ACTION
PEG 3350, a nonabsorbable solution, acts as an osmotic. Sodium sulfate greatly reduces sodium absorption. The electrolyte level causes virtually no net absorption or secretion of ions.

Route	Onset	Peak	Duration
P.O.	1 hr	Variable	Variable

Half-life: None.

ADVERSE REACTIONS
EENT: rhinorrhea.
GI: abdominal fullness, bloating, cramps, nausea, vomiting.
Skin: allergic reaction, anal irritation, dermatitis, urticaria.

INTERACTIONS
Drug-drug. *Oral drugs:* May decrease absorption if given within 1 hour of starting therapy. Give at least 2 to 3 hours before starting therapy.

EFFECTS ON LAB TEST RESULTS
None reported.

CONTRAINDICATIONS & CAUTIONS
• Contraindicated in patients with GI obstruction or perforation, gastric retention, toxic colitis, or megacolon.
⚠ *Overdose S&S:* Diarrhea.

NURSING CONSIDERATIONS
• No major shifts in fluid or electrolyte balance have been reported.
• Patient preparation for barium enema may be less satisfactory with this solution because it may interfere with the barium coating of the colonic mucosa using the double-contrast technique.
• *Look alike–sound alike:* Don't confuse GoLYTELY with NuLYTELY. Don't confuse TriLyte with TriLipix.

P

PATIENT TEACHING
● Tell patient to fast for 3 to 4 hours before taking solution, and thereafter to drink only clear fluids until examination is complete.
● Tell patient to improve drug's taste by chilling.
● Warn patient about adverse reactions.

posaconazole
pahs-ah-KON-ah-zall

Noxafil, Posanol†

Therapeutic class: Antifungals
Pharmacologic class: Triazole antifungals
Pregnancy risk category: C

AVAILABLE FORMS
Oral suspension: 40 mg/mL

INDICATIONS & DOSAGES
➤ **Prevention of invasive *Aspergillus* and *Candida* infections in high-risk immuno-compromised patients**
Adults and children age 13 and older:
200 mg (5 mL) P.O. t.i.d. with a full meal or a liquid nutritional supplement; duration of therapy is based on recovery from neutropenia or immunosuppression.
➤ **Oropharyngeal candidiasis**
Adults and children age 13 and older:
100 mg (2.5 mL) P.O. b.i.d. on first day, then 100 mg (2.5 mL) once daily for 13 days with a full meal or a liquid nutritional supplement.
➤ **Oropharyngeal candidiasis resistant to itraconazole or fluconazole treatment**
Adults and children age 13 and older:
400 mg (10 mL) P.O. b.i.d. with a full meal or a liquid nutritional supplement; duration of treatment is based on severity of underlying disease and patient response.

ADMINISTRATION
P.O.
● Give drug with a full meal or a liquid nutritional supplement.
● Shake the suspension well before giving it.
● Measure doses using calibrated spoon provided with the drug, which has two markings, one for 2.5 mL and one for 5 mL.

After patient takes dose, fill spoon with water and have him drink it to ensure a full dose.
● Store oral suspension at room temperature.

ACTION
Blocks the synthesis of ergosterol, a vital component of the fungal cell membrane.

Route	Onset	Peak	Duration
P.O.	Unknown	3–5 hr	Unknown

Half-life: 35 hours.

ADVERSE REACTIONS
CNS: anxiety, dizziness, fatigue, fever, headache, insomnia, weakness.
CV: edema, hypertension, hypotension, tachycardia.
EENT: epistaxis, pharyngitis, altered taste, blurred vision.
GI: abdominal pain, constipation, diarrhea, dyspepsia, mucositis, nausea, vomiting.
GU: *vaginal hemorrhage.*
Hematologic: anemia, petechiae, *febrile neutropenia, neutropenia, thrombocytopenia.*
Hepatic: bilirubinemia.
Metabolic: anorexia, hyperglycemia, *hypokalemia, hypomagnesemia, hypocalcemia.*
Musculoskeletal: arthralgia, back pain, musculoskeletal pain.
Respiratory: cough, dyspnea, upper respiratory tract infection.
Skin: pruritus, rash, diaphoresis.
Other: bacteremia, CMV infection, herpes simplex, rigors.

INTERACTIONS
Drug-drug. *Calcium channel blockers, cyclosporine, HMG-CoA reductase inhibitors, midazolam, phenytoin, sirolimus, tacrolimus, vinca alkaloids:* May increase levels of these drugs. Reduce dosages, increase monitoring of levels, and observe patient for adverse effects.
Cimetidine, phenytoin: May decrease level and effectiveness of posaconazole. Avoid using together.
CYP3A4 substrates (astemizole, cisapride, halofantrine, pimozide, quinidine, terfenadine): May lead to QT-interval prolongation

---

Reactions in bold italics are *life-threatening*. Interactions may have a *rapid onset* or a *delayed onset*.

and torsades de pointes. Use together is contraindicated.

Ergot alkaloids (dihydroergotamine, ergotamine): May increase ergot level. Use together is contraindicated.

Rifabutin: May decrease level and effectiveness of posaconazole while increasing rifabutin level and risk of toxicity. Avoid using together. If unavoidable, monitor patient for uveitis, leukopenia, and other adverse effects.

Drug-food. *Any food, liquid nutritional supplements:* May greatly enhance absorption of drug. Always give drug with liquid supplement or food.

EFFECTS ON LAB TEST RESULTS
● May increase AST, ALT, bilirubin, creatinine, alkaline phosphatase, and glucose levels.
● May decrease potassium, magnesium, and calcium levels.
● May decrease WBC, RBC, and platelet counts.

CONTRAINDICATIONS & CAUTIONS
● Contraindicated in patients hypersensitive to drug or its components and in patients taking sirolimus, HMG-CoA reductase inhibitors that are primarily metabolized through CYP3A4 (atorvastatin, lovastatin, simvastatin), CYP3A4 substrates that prolong the QT interval (pimozide, quinidine), other antifungal agents, or ergot derivatives.
● Use cautiously in patients hypersensitive to other azole antifungals, patients with potentially proarrhythmic conditions, and patients with hepatic or renal insufficiency.
● Safe use in children younger than age 13 hasn't been established.
🛈 *Alert:* Drug may prolong QT interval and increase risk of torsades de pointes.

NURSING CONSIDERATIONS
● Correct electrolyte imbalances, especially potassium, magnesium, and calcium imbalances, before therapy.
● Monitor patient for signs and symptoms of electrolyte imbalance, including a slow, weak, or irregular pulse; ECG change; nausea; neuromuscular irritability; and tetany.

● Obtain baseline LFTs, including bilirubin level, before therapy and periodically during treatment. Notify prescriber if patient develops signs or symptoms of hepatic dysfunction.
● Monitor patient who has severe vomiting or diarrhea for breakthrough fungal infection.
● *Look alike–sound alike:* Don't confuse Noxafil with minoxidil.

PATIENT TEACHING
● If patient can't take a liquid supplement or eat a full meal, instruct him to notify prescriber. A different anti-infective may be needed, or monitoring may need to be increased.
● Tell patient to notify prescriber about an irregular heartbeat, fainting, or severe diarrhea or vomiting.
● Explain the signs and symptoms of liver dysfunction, including abdominal pain, yellowing skin or eyes, pale stools, and dark urine.
● Urge patient to contact the prescriber or pharmacist before taking other prescription or OTC drugs, herbal supplements, or dietary supplements.
● Tell patient to shake the suspension well before taking it.
● Instruct patient to measure doses using the spoon provided with the drug. Household spoons vary in size and may yield an incorrect dose.
● Point out that the calibrated spoon has two markings: one for 2.5 mL and one for 5 mL. Make sure patient understands which mark to use for his prescribed dose.
● After patient takes dose, tell him to fill the spoon with water and drink it, to ensure a full dose. Tell him to clean the spoon with water before putting it away.

P

potassium acetate

Therapeutic class: Potassium supplements
Pharmacologic class: Potassium salts
Pregnancy risk category: C

AVAILABLE FORMS
Injection: 2 mEq/mL in 20-, 50-, and 100-mL vials; 4 mEq/mL in 50-mL vial

INDICATIONS & DOSAGES
➤ **Hypokalemia**
Adults: Individualize dosage. 40 to 80 mEq/24 hours by I.V. infusion.
Children: Individualize dosage. 2 to 3 mEq/kg/24 hours by I.V. infusion. For newborns, normal daily requirement is 2 to 6 mEq/kg/hour.

ADMINISTRATION
I.V.
▼ Use only in life-threatening hypokalemia or when oral replacement isn't feasible.
▼ Don't give undiluted potassium. Maximum infusion rate is 1 mEq/kg/hour.
▼ Don't add potassium to a hanging bag. Mix well to avoid layering.
▼ To prevent pain, use largest peripheral vein and a well-placed small-bore needle.
▼ Give only by infusion, never I.V. push or I.M. Watch for pain and redness at infusion site.
▼ Give slowly as diluted solution; rapid infusion may cause fatal hyperkalemia.
▼ **Incompatibilities:** None reported.

ACTION
Replaces potassium and maintains potassium level.

Route	Onset	Peak	Duration
I.V.	Immediate	Immediate	Unknown

Half-life: Unknown.

ADVERSE REACTIONS
CNS: paresthesia of limbs, listlessness, mental confusion, weakness or heaviness of legs, flaccid paralysis, pain, fever.
CV: *arrhythmias, cardiac arrest, heart block,* ECG changes, hypotension.
GI: nausea, vomiting, abdominal pain, diarrhea.
Metabolic: *hyperkalemia.*
Respiratory: *respiratory paralysis.*
Skin: redness at infusion site.

INTERACTIONS
Drug-drug. *ACE inhibitors, aldosterone blockers, potassium-sparing diuretics:* May increase risk of hyperkalemia. Use together with caution.
Digoxin: May cause digoxin toxicity from hypokalemia if drug is stopped. Stop potassium cautiously if patient is taking digoxin.
Drug-food. *Potassium-containing salt substitutes:* May increase risk of hyperkalemia. Use together cautiously.

EFFECTS ON LAB TEST RESULTS
● May increase potassium level.

CONTRAINDICATIONS & CAUTIONS
● Contraindicated in patients with severe renal impairment with oliguria, anuria, or azotemia.
● Contraindicated in those with untreated Addison disease, acute dehydration, heat cramps, hyperkalemia, hyperkalemic form of familial periodic paralysis, or conditions linked to extensive tissue breakdown.
● Use cautiously in patients with cardiac disease or renal impairment.
⚠ *Overdose S&S:* Paresthesia, flaccid paralysis, listlessness, confusion, weakness and heaviness of legs, hypotension, cardiac arrhythmias, heart block, ECG changes, cardiac arrest.

NURSING CONSIDERATIONS
● During therapy, monitor ECG, renal function, fluid intake and output, and potassium, creatinine, and BUN levels. Never give potassium postoperatively until urine flow is established.
● Many adverse reactions may reflect hyperkalemia.
🛑 *Alert:* Consider a separate storage area for concentrated I.V. potassium. Fatal outcomes are possible if concentrated potassium is administered by I.V. push.
● *Look alike–sound alike:* Potassium preparations aren't interchangeable; verify preparation before use.

PATIENT TEACHING
● Explain use and administration to patient and family.
● Tell patient to report adverse effects, especially pain at insertion site.

Reactions in bold italics are *life-threatening*. Interactions may have a *rapid onset* or a *delayed onset*.

SAFETY ALERT!

potassium chloride

K 10†, K-Dur 10, K-Dur 20, K-Lor,
Klor-Con, Klor-Con 8, Klor-Con 10,
Klor-Con/25, Klor-Con M10, Klor-Con
M15, Klor-Con M20, K-Lyte/Cl, K-
Tab, K-Vescent, Micro-K, Micro-K 10,
Pro-600 K SRT†, Slow K†, Slow Pot†

Therapeutic class: Potassium
supplements
Pharmacologic class: Potassium salts
Pregnancy risk category: C

AVAILABLE FORMS
Capsules (controlled-release): 8 mEq,
10 mEq
Injection concentrate: 1.5 mEq/mL,
2 mEq/mL
Injection for I.V. infusion: 0.1 mEq/mL,
0.2 mEq/mL, 0.3 mEq/mL, 0.4 mEq/mL
Oral liquid: 20 mEq/15 mL, 40 mEq/15 mL
Powder for oral administration: 20 mEq/
packet, 25 mEq/packet
Tablets (controlled-release): 8 mEq,
10 mEq, 20 mEq
Tablets (extended-release): 8 mEq, 10 mEq,
15 mEq, 20 mEq

INDICATIONS & DOSAGES
➤ **To prevent hypokalemia**
Adults: Initially, 16 to 24 mEq of potassium
supplement P.O. daily, in divided doses. Adjust dosage, as needed, based on potassium
levels.
➤ **Hypokalemia**
Adults: 40 to 100 mEq P.O. in two to four
divided doses daily. Maximum dose of
diluted I.V. potassium chloride is 40 mEq/L
at 10 mEq/hour. Don't exceed 200 mEq
daily. Further doses are based on potassium
levels and blood pH. Give I.V. potassium
replacement only with monitoring of ECG
and potassium level.
➤ **Severe hypokalemia**
Adults: Dilute potassium chloride in a suitable I.V. solution of less than 80 mEq/L, and
give at no more than 40 mEq/hour.

Further doses are based on potassium
level. Don't exceed 400 mEq I.V. daily.
Give I.V. potassium replacement only with
monitoring of ECG and potassium level.

ADMINISTRATION
P.O.
● Make sure powders are completely
dissolved before giving.
● Enteric-coated tablets are not recommended because of increased risk of GI
bleeding and small-bowel ulcerations.
● Tablets in wax matrix may lodge in the
esophagus and cause ulceration in cardiac
patients with esophageal compression from
an enlarged left atrium. Use sugar-free
liquid form in these patients and in those
with esophageal stasis or obstruction. Have
patient sip slowly to minimize GI irritation.
● Don't crush controlled-release or
extended-release forms.

I.V.
▼ Use only when oral replacement isn't
feasible or when hypokalemia is life-
threatening.
▼ Give by infusion only, never I.V. push or
I.M. Give slowly as dilute solution; rapid
infusion may cause fatal hyperkalemia.
▼ If burning occurs during infusion,
decrease rate.
▼ **Incompatibilities:** Amikacin, amoxicillin, amphotericin B, azithromycin,
diazepam, dobutamine, ergotamine,
etoposide with cisplatin and mannitol,
fat emulsion 10%, methylprednisolone,
penicillin G, phenytoin, promethazine.

ACTION
Replaces potassium and maintains potassium level.

Route	Onset	Peak	Duration
P.O.	Unknown	Unknown	Unknown
I.V.	Immediate	Immediate	Unknown

Half-life: Unknown.

ADVERSE REACTIONS
CNS: paresthesia of limbs, listlessness,
confusion, weakness or heaviness of limbs,
flaccid paralysis.
CV: postinfusion phlebitis, *arrhythmias,
heart block, cardiac arrest,* ECG changes,
hypotension.
GI: nausea, vomiting, abdominal pain,
diarrhea.
Metabolic: *hyperkalemia.*
Respiratory: *respiratory paralysis.*

P

INTERACTIONS
Drug-drug. *ACE inhibitors, digoxin, potassium-sparing diuretics:* May cause hyperkalemia. Use together with extreme caution. Monitor potassium level.

EFFECTS ON LAB TEST RESULTS
● May increase potassium level.

CONTRAINDICATIONS & CAUTIONS
● Contraindicated in patients with severe renal impairment with oliguria, anuria, or azotemia; with untreated Addison disease; or with acute dehydration, heat cramps, hyperkalemia, hyperkalemic form of familial periodic paralysis, or other conditions linked to extensive tissue breakdown.
● Use cautiously in patients with cardiac disease or renal impairment.
⚠ **Overdose S&S:** ECG changes, weakness, flaccidity, respiratory paralysis, cardiac arrhythmias, death.

NURSING CONSIDERATIONS
● Patients at an increased risk of GI lesions include those with scleroderma, diabetes, mitral valve replacement, cardiomegaly, or esophageal strictures, and elderly or immobile patients.
● Drug is commonly used orally with potassium-wasting diuretics to maintain potassium levels.
● Monitor continuous ECG and electrolyte levels during therapy.
● Monitor renal function. After surgery, don't give drug until urine flow is established.
● Many adverse reactions may reflect hyperkalemia.
● Patient may be sensitive to tartrazine in some of these products.
🔱 **Alert:** Consider a separate storage area for concentrated I.V. potassium. Fatal outcomes are possible if concentrated potassium is administered by I.V. push.
● **Look alike–sound alike:** Potassium preparations aren't interchangeable; verify preparation before use and don't switch products. Don't confuse Kaon-Cl-10 with Kaolin, KCl with HCl, KlorCon with Klaron, or Micro-K with Macrobid or Micronase.

PATIENT TEACHING
● Teach patient how to prepare powders and how to take drug. Tell patient to take with or after meals with full glass of water or fruit juice to lessen GI distress.
● Teach patient signs and symptoms of hyperkalemia, and tell patient to notify prescriber if they occur.
● Tell patient to report discomfort at I.V. insertion site.
● Warn patient not to use salt substitutes concurrently, except with prescriber's permission.
● Tell patient not to be concerned if wax matrix appears in stool because the drug has already been absorbed.

---

potassium iodide
po-TASS-ee-um

Iosat ◊, Pima, saturated solution (SSKI), strong iodine solution (Lugol solution), ThyroSafe ◊, ThyroShield ◊

Therapeutic class: Antihyperthyroid drugs
Pharmacologic class: Salts of stable iodine
Pregnancy risk category: D

AVAILABLE FORMS
Oral solution (Lugol solution): iodine 5% and potassium iodide 10%
Oral solution (SSKI): 1 g/mL
Oral solution (ThyroShield): 65 mg/mL
Syrup (Pima): 325 mg/5 mL
Tablets: 65 mg, 130 mg

INDICATIONS & DOSAGES
➤ **To prepare for thyroidectomy**
Adults and children: 0.3 mL P.O. t.i.d. (range, 0.1 to 0.9 mL daily). Administer for 10 days before surgery.
➤ **Radiation protectant for thyroid gland (Iosat, ThyroSafe, ThyroShield)**
Adults and children ages 12 to 18 weighing at least 68 kg (150 lb): 130 mg (2 mL) P.O. every 24 hours for 10 to 14 days as directed by public health authorities. Start no later than 3 to 4 hours after exposure. Avoid

---

repeat dosing in pregnant or breast-feeding women.

Children ages 3 to 12 or children ages 12 to 18 weighing less than 68 kg (150 lb): 65 mg (1 mL) P.O. every 24 hours as directed by public health authorities. Start no later than 3 to 4 hours after exposure.

Children ages 1 month to 3 years: 32.5 mg (0.5 mL) P.O. every 24 hours as directed by public health authorities. Start no later than 3 to 4 hours after exposure.

Neonates from birth to 1 month: 16.25 mg (0.25 mL) P.O. every 24 hours as directed by public health authorities. Start no later than 3 to 4 hours after exposure. Avoid repeat dosing, if possible.

➤ **Expectorant**

Adults: 5 to 10 mL (325 to 650 mg) Pima P.O. t.i.d. Or, 300 to 600 mg SSKI P.O. t.i.d. to q.i.d.

Children older than age 3: 5 mL (325 mg) Pima P.O. t.i.d.

Children younger than age 3: 2.5 mL (162.5 mg) Pima P.O. t.i.d.

ADMINISTRATION

P.O.
● Dilute oral solution in 120 to 240 mL water, milk, or fruit juice, and give after meals to prevent gastric irritation, hydrate patient, and mask salty taste.
● Give iodides through straw to avoid tooth discoloration.
● Preparations aren't interchangeable. Verify preparation before use and don't switch products.
● Store in light-resistant container.

ACTION

Inhibits thyroid hormone formation, limits iodide transport into the thyroid gland, and blocks thyroid hormone release. Also decreases mucus viscosity by enhancing the secretion of respiratory fluids.

Route	Onset	Peak	Duration
P.O.	<24 hr	10–15 days	Unknown

Half-life: Unknown.

ADVERSE REACTIONS

CNS: fever.
EENT: periorbital edema.

GI: nausea, vomiting, diarrhea, inflammation of salivary glands, burning mouth and throat, sore teeth and gums, metallic taste.
Metabolic: *potassium toxicity.*
Skin: acneiform rash.
Other: hypersensitivity reactions (including *angioedema*).

INTERACTIONS

Drug-drug. *ACE inhibitors, potassium-sparing diuretics:* May cause hyperkalemia. Avoid using together.
Antithyroid drugs: May increase hypothyroid or goitrogenic effects. Monitor patient closely.
Lithium carbonate: May cause hypothyroidism. Use together cautiously.
Drug-food. *Iodized salt, shellfish:* May alter drug's effectiveness. Urge caution.

EFFECTS ON LAB TEST RESULTS

● May increase potassium level.
● May alter thyroid function test results.

CONTRAINDICATIONS & CAUTIONS

● Contraindicated in patients allergic to iodine.
● Contraindicated in patients with tuberculosis, acute bronchitis, iodide hypersensitivity, or hyperkalemia. Some formulations contain sulfites, which may cause allergic reactions in hypersensitive patients.
● Use cautiously in patients with hypocomplementemic vasculitis, goiter, or autoimmune thyroid disease.
⚠ *Overdose S&S:* Gastroenteritis, abdominal pain, diarrhea (sometimes bloody), death from circulatory collapse caused by shock, corrosive gastritis, or asphyxiation from swelling of the glottis or larynx.

NURSING CONSIDERATIONS

● Potassium iodide should be used during a nuclear radiation emergency only when recommended by public health officials. It should not be taken more than once every 24 hours.
● The FDA doesn't recommend prophylaxis with potassium iodide for a radiation emergency in adults over age 40 unless a large internal radiation dose is anticipated.
● For thyrotoxicosis, first iodine dose is given at least 1 hour after first dose of propylthiouracil and methimazole.

P

❸ *Alert:* Earliest signs of delayed hypersensitivity reactions caused by iodides are irritation and swollen eyelids.

● Signs of an iodide hypersensitivity reaction include angioedema, cutaneous and mucosal hemorrhage, fever, arthralgia, lymph node enlargement, and eosinophilia.

● Monitor patient for iodism, which can cause metallic taste, burning in mouth and throat, sore teeth and gums, increased salivation, coryza, sneezing, eye irritation with swelling of eyelids, severe headache, productive cough, GI irritation, diarrhea, rash, or soreness of the pharynx, larynx, and tonsils.

PATIENT TEACHING

● Show patient how to mask salty taste of oral solution. Tell him to take all forms of drug after meals.

❸ *Alert:* Warn patient that sudden withdrawal may precipitate thyroid crisis.

❸ *Alert:* Teach patient signs and symptoms of potassium toxicity, including confusion, irregular heartbeat, numbness, tingling, pain or weakness of hands or feet, and tiredness.

● Tell patient to ask prescriber about using iodized salt and eating shellfish. These foods contain iodine and may alter drug's effectiveness.

● Tell patient not to increase the amount of potassium through diet.

● Tell patient to stop drug and notify prescriber if epigastric pain, rash, metallic taste, nausea, or vomiting occurs.

---

pralidoxime chloride (2-PAM chloride, 2-pyridine-aldoxime methochloride)
pra-li-DOX-eem

Protopam Chloride

Therapeutic class: Antidotes
Pharmacologic class: Quaternary ammonium oximes
Pregnancy risk category: C

AVAILABLE FORMS

Injection: 1 g/20 mL in 20-mL vial
Injection (for I.M. use): 300 mg/mL

INDICATIONS & DOSAGES
➤ **Antidote for organophosphate poisoning**

Adults: 1 to 2 g in 100 mL of normal saline solution by I.V. infusion over 15 to 30 minutes. If not practical or pulmonary edema is present, give dose as a 5% solution in sterile water by slow I.V. push over at least 5 minutes. Repeat in 1 hour if muscle weakness persists. Additional doses may be given cautiously. I.M. or subcutaneous injection may be used if I.V. isn't feasible.

For I.M. dosing: *For mild symptoms,* give 600 mg I.M. Wait 15 minutes; if symptoms persist, give a second dose. A third dose may be given after an additional 15 minutes. If at any time after the first dose patient develops severe symptoms, give two additional 600-mg doses in rapid succession for a total cumulative dose of 1,800 mg. *For severe symptoms,* give three 600-mg doses in rapid succession. If symptoms persist after the complete 1,800-mg regimen (three injections of 600 mg each), the series may be repeated beginning approximately 1 hour after the last injection.

Children age 16 and younger (I.V. dosing): Give loading dose of 20 to 50 mg/kg (maximum 2 g) I.V. over 15 to 30 minutes, followed by 10 to 20 mg/kg/hour by continuous I.V. infusion. Or, give initial dose of 20 to 50 mg/kg I.V. over 15 to 30 minutes. May give second dose of 20 to 50 mg/kg I.V. in 1 hour if muscle weakness persists. May repeat dose every 10 to 12 hours p.r.n. Maximum is 2 g/dose. Or, if pulmonary edema is present or it isn't practical to give intermittent or continuous I.V. infusions, give dose of 20 to 50 mg/kg as 50-mg/mL solution in water by I.V. push slowly over 5 minutes. If muscle weakness persists, additional doses may be given every 10 to 12 hours.

Children age 16 and younger with mild symptoms who weigh 40 kg (88 lb) or more (I.M. dosing): Give 600 mg I.M. If symptoms persist after 15 minutes, give second dose of 600 mg I.M. If symptoms persist 15 minutes after second dose, give third dose of 600 mg I.M. Maximum combined dose for three injections is 1,800 mg. If patient develops severe symptoms at any time after first dose, administer second and third

---

doses in rapid succession. For severe symptoms, give all three doses of 600 mg I.M. each in rapid succession for total combined dose of 1,800 mg.

Children age 16 and younger with mild symptoms who weigh less than 40 kg (I.M. dosing): Give 15 mg/kg I.M. in anterolateral thigh. If symptoms persist after 15 minutes, give second dose of 15 mg/kg I.M. If symptoms persist after second dose, give third dose of 15 mg/kg I.M. If patient develops severe symptoms at any time after first dose, give second and third doses in rapid succession. For severe symptoms, give all three doses of 15 mg/kg I.M. each in rapid succession. Maximum combined dose for three injections is 45 mg/kg.

➤ **Cholinergic crisis in myasthenia gravis**
Adults: 1 to 2 g I.V.; then 250 mg I.V. every 5 minutes, p.r.n.

ADMINISTRATION
I.V.
▼ Reconstitute by adding 20 mL of sterile water for injection to vial containing 1 g of drug.
▼ Dilute by adding 100 mL of normal saline solution.
▼ Infuse over 15 to 30 minutes. Too-rapid infusion may cause tachycardia, laryngospasm, and muscle rigidity.
▼ **Incompatibilities:** None reported.
I.M.
● Visually inspect parenteral drug products for particulate matter and discoloration before administration, whenever solution and container permit.

ACTION
Reactivates cholinesterase inactivated by organophosphorus pesticides and related compounds, permitting degradation of accumulated acetylcholine and facilitating normal functioning of neuromuscular junctions.

Route	Onset	Peak	Duration
I.V.	Unknown	5–15 min	Unknown
I.M.	Unknown	10–20 min	Unknown

Half-life: 1½ hours.

ADVERSE REACTIONS
CNS: dizziness, headache, drowsiness.
CV: tachycardia, increased systolic and diastolic blood pressure.
EENT: blurred vision, diplopia, impaired accommodation.
GI: nausea.
Musculoskeletal: muscle weakness.
Respiratory: hyperventilation.
Other: mild to moderate pain at injection site.

INTERACTIONS
Drug-drug. *Atropine:* May cause atropinization (flushing, mydriasis, tachycardia, dryness of the mouth and nose) earlier than might be expected when atropine is used alone. Closely monitor clinical response.
Barbiturates: May increase anticholinesterase level. Use together cautiously to treat seizures.

EFFECTS ON LAB TEST RESULTS
● May increase liver enzyme levels.

CONTRAINDICATIONS & CAUTIONS
● Contraindicated in patients hypersensitive to drug.
● Use cautiously in patients with myasthenia gravis (overdose may trigger myasthenic crisis) and in those with impaired renal function.
⚠ *Overdose S&S:* Dizziness, blurred vision, diplopia, headache, impaired accommodation, nausea, tachycardia.

NURSING CONSIDERATIONS
● Initially, remove secretions, maintain patent airway, and institute mechanical ventilation, if needed. After dermal exposure to organophosphate, remove patient's clothing and wash his skin and hair with sodium bicarbonate, soap, water, and alcohol as soon as possible. A second washing may be needed. When washing patient, wear protective gloves and clothes to avoid exposure.
● Draw blood for cholinesterase level before giving drug.

P

• Use drug only in hospitalized patients; have respiratory and other supportive measures available. If possible, obtain accurate medical history and chronology of poisoning. Give drug as soon as possible after poisoning; drug is most effective if started within 24 hours after exposure.

• To improve muscarinic effects and block accumulation of acetylcholine from organophosphate poisoning in adults, give atropine 2 to 4 mg I.V. with pralidoxime if cyanosis isn't present; if cyanosis is present, give atropine I.M. Give atropine every 5 to 10 minutes until signs of atropine toxicity (flushing, tachycardia, dry mouth, blurred vision, excitement, delirium, and hallucinations) appear; maintain atropinization for at least 48 hours.

• Observe patient for 48 to 72 hours if he ingested poison. Delayed absorption may occur from lower bowel. It's difficult to distinguish between toxic effects produced by atropine or organophosphate compounds and those resulting from pralidoxime.

• In a patient with myasthenia gravis being treated for overdose of cholinergics, watch for signs of rapid weakening. He can pass quickly from cholinergic crisis to myasthenic crisis and need more cholinergics to treat myasthenia. Keep edrophonium available for differentiating diagnoses.

• Avoid use of aminophylline, morphine, phenothiazine-like tranquilizers, reserpine, succinylcholine, and theophylline in patients with organophosphate poisoning.

• Drug isn't effective against poisoning caused by phosphorus, inorganic phosphates, or organophosphates with no anticholinesterase activity.

• *Look alike–sound alike:* Don't confuse pralidoxime with pramoxine or pyridoxine. Don't confuse Protopam with protamine.

PATIENT TEACHING

• Explain use and administration of drug to patient and family.

• Tell patient to report adverse effects.

• Caution patient treated for organophosphate poisoning to avoid contact with insecticides for several weeks.

pramipexole dihydrochloride
pram-ah-PEX-ole

Mirapex, Mirapex ER

Therapeutic class: Antiparkinsonians
Pharmacologic class: Nonergot dopamine agonists
Pregnancy risk category: C

AVAILABLE FORMS
Tablets: 0.125 mg, 0.25 mg, 0.5 mg, 0.75 mg, 1 mg, 1.5 mg
Tablets (extended-release): 0.375 mg, 0.75 mg, 1.5 mg, 2.25 mg, 3 mg, 3.75 mg, 4.5 mg

INDICATIONS & DOSAGES
➤ **Signs and symptoms of idiopathic Parkinson disease**
Adults: Initially, 0.375 mg P.O. daily in three divided doses. Adjust doses slowly (not more often than every 5 to 7 days) over several weeks until desired therapeutic effect is achieved. Maintenance dosage is 1.5 to 4.5 mg daily in three divided doses. Or, 0.375 mg (extended-release form) P.O. once daily. May titrate dosage gradually (not more often than every 5 to 7 days), first to 0.75 mg P.O. daily, then by 0.75-mg increments to maximum recommended dosage of 4.5 mg/day.

Adjust-a-dose: For patients with CrCl over 50 mL/minute, first dosage of immediate-release tablets is 0.125 mg P.O. t.i.d., up to 1.5 mg t.i.d. For those with CrCl of 30 to 50 mL/minute, first dosage is 0.125 mg P.O. b.i.d., up to 0.75 mg t.i.d. For those with CrCl of 15 to less than 30 mL/minute, first dosage is 0.125 mg P.O. daily, up to 1.5 mg daily. If using extended-release tablets, in patients with CrCl of 30 to 50 mL/minute, initially give dose every other day. Use caution and assess response and tolerability before increasing to daily dosing after 1 week and before titration. Titrate dosage in 0.375-mg increments up to 2.25 mg/day, no more frequently than at weekly intervals. Don't use extended-release tablets in patients with CrCl of less than 30 mL/minute or in hemodialysis patients.

➤ **Moderate to severe primary restless leg syndrome (immediate-release only)**
Adults: 0.125 mg P.O. daily, 2 to 3 hours before bedtime. May increase after 4 to 7 days to 0.25 mg P.O. daily, as needed. May increase again after 4 to 7 days to 0.5 mg P.O. daily, if needed.
Adjust-a-dose: For patients with CrCl of 20 to 60 mL/minute, increase the duration between titration steps to 14 days.

ADMINISTRATION
P.O.
● Give drug with or without food; giving with food may reduce nausea.

ACTION
Thought to stimulate dopamine receptors.

Route	Onset	Peak	Duration
P.O.	Rapid	2 hr	8–12 hr

Half-life: Approximately 8 hours.

ADVERSE REACTIONS
CNS: asthenia, confusion, dizziness, dream abnormalities, dyskinesia, extrapyramidal syndrome, hallucinations, insomnia, somnolence, amnesia, akathisia, drowsiness, delusions, dystonia, gait abnormalities, hypoesthesia, hypertonia, myoclonus, paranoid reaction, malaise, sleep disorders, thought abnormalities, fever.
CV: orthostatic hypotension, chest pain, peripheral edema.
EENT: accommodation abnormalities, diplopia, rhinitis, vision abnormalities.
GI: constipation, nausea, dry mouth, anorexia, dysphagia.
GU: erectile dysfunction, urinary frequency, UTI, urinary incontinence.
Metabolic: weight loss.
Musculoskeletal: arthritis, bursitis, myasthenia, twitching.
Respiratory: dyspnea, pneumonia.
Skin: skin disorders.
Other: accidental injury, decreased libido, general edema.

INTERACTIONS
Drug-drug. *Cimetidine, diltiazem, quinidine, quinine, ranitidine, triamterene, verapamil:* May decrease pramipexole clearance. Adjust dosage as needed.

Dopamine antagonists: May reduce pramipexole effectiveness. Monitor patient closely.
Drug-lifestyle. *Alcohol use:* May increase risk of falling asleep. Tell patient to avoid alcohol.

EFFECTS ON LAB TEST RESULTS
● May increase CK level.

CONTRAINDICATIONS & CAUTIONS
● Contraindicated in patients hypersensitive to drug or its components.
● Use cautiously in renally impaired patients.
● Use cautiously in breast-feeding women. It's unknown if drug appears in breast milk.

NURSING CONSIDERATIONS
● If drug must be stopped, withdraw over 1 week.
● Drug may cause orthostatic hypotension, especially during dosage increases. Monitor patient carefully.
● Drug may cause intense impulse control and compulsive behaviors. Monitor patient for problems with impulse control (such as gambling urges, intense sexual urges, binge eating).
● Adjust dosage gradually to achieve maximal therapeutic effect, balanced against the main adverse effects of dyskinesia, hallucinations, somnolence, and dry mouth.
● *Look alike–sound alike:* Don't confuse Mirapex with Hiprex, Mifeprex, or MiraLax.

PATIENT TEACHING
● Instruct patient not to rise rapidly after sitting or lying down because of risk of dizziness.
● Caution patient to avoid hazardous activities until CNS response to drug is known.
● Tell patient to use caution before taking drug with other CNS depressants.
● Tell patient (especially elderly patient) that hallucinations may occur.
● Advise patient to take drug with food if nausea develops.
● Tell woman to notify prescriber if she is or will be breast-feeding.

P

• Advise patient that it may take 4 weeks for effects of drug to be noticed because of slow adjustment schedule.

SAFETY ALERT!

pramlintide acetate
PRAM-lin-tyde

Symlin, SymlinPen 60,
SymlinPen 120

Therapeutic class: Antidiabetics
Pharmacologic class: Human amylin analogues
Pregnancy risk category: C

AVAILABLE FORMS
Injection: 0.6 mg/mL in 5-mL vials, 1 mg/mL in 1.5-mL and 2.7-mL multidose pen injectors

INDICATIONS & DOSAGES
➤ **Adjunct to insulin in patients with type 1 diabetes mellitus**
Adults: Initially, 15 mcg subcutaneously before major meals (more than 250 calories or 30 g of carbohydrates). Reduce preprandial rapid-acting or short-acting insulin dose, including fixed-mix insulin such as 70/30, by 50%. Increase pramlintide dose by 15-mcg increments every 3 days if no nausea occurs, to a maintenance dose of 30 to 60 mcg. Adjust insulin dose as needed.
Adjust-a-dose: If significant nausea at 45 or 60 mcg persists, decrease to 30 mcg. If nausea persists at 30 mcg, consider stopping.
➤ **Adjunct to insulin in patients with type 2 diabetes mellitus, with or without a sulfonylurea or metformin**
Adults: Initially, 60 mcg subcutaneously immediately before major meals. Reduce preprandial rapid-acting or short-acting insulin dose, including fixed-mix insulin, by 50%. Increase pramlintide dose to 120 mcg if no significant nausea occurs for 3 to 7 days. Adjust insulin dose as needed.
Adjust-a-dose: If significant nausea persists at 120 mcg, decrease to 60 mcg.

ADMINISTRATION
Subcutaneous
• Before starting drug, review patient's glycosylated hemoglobin (HbA$_{1c}$) level, recent blood glucose monitoring data, hypoglycemic episodes, current insulin regimen, and body weight. Reduce preprandial, rapid-acting or short-acting insulin dosages, including fixed-mix insulins, by 50%.
• To give drug, use a U-100 insulin syringe, preferably a 0.3-mL size.
• Give each dose subcutaneously into abdomen or thigh. Rotate injection sites.
• Always administer pramlintide and insulin as separate injections. The injection site for pramlintide should be distinct from the site for concomitant insulin injection.
• Drug concentration in pen injector is higher than in vials. Don't transfer drug to syringe for administration.
• Refrigerate pen injectors and unopened and opened vials. Contents of opened vials should be used within 28 days and those of unopened vials before their expiration date.

ACTION
Slows rate at which food leaves the stomach, reducing the initial postprandial increase in glucose level. Decreases hyperglycemia by reducing postprandial glucagon level and reduces total caloric intake by reducing appetite.

Route	Onset	Peak	Duration
Subcut.	Unknown	19–21 min	Unknown

Half-life: About 48 minutes each (parent drug and active metabolite).

ADVERSE REACTIONS
CNS: dizziness, fatigue, headache.
EENT: pharyngitis.
GI: abdominal pain, anorexia, nausea, vomiting.
Metabolic: *hypoglycemia.*
Musculoskeletal: arthralgia.
Respiratory: cough.
Skin: injection-site reaction.
Other: allergic reaction, accidental injury.

Reactions in bold italics are *life-threatening*. Interactions may have a *rapid onset* or a *delayed onset*.

INTERACTIONS
Drug-drug. *ACE inhibitors, disopyramide, fibrates, fluoxetine, MAO inhibitors, oral antidiabetics, pentoxifylline, propoxyphene, salicylates, sulfonamide antibiotics:* May increase risk of hypoglycemia. Monitor glucose level closely.
Alpha glucosidase inhibitors (such as acarbose), anticholinergics (such as atropine, benztropine, TCAs): May alter GI motility and slow intestinal absorption. Avoid using together.
Beta blockers, clonidine, guanethidine, reserpine: May mask signs of hypoglycemia. Monitor glucose level closely.
Oral drugs dependent on rapid onset of action (such as analgesics): May delay absorption because of slowed gastric emptying. If rapid effect is needed, give oral drug 1 hour before or 2 hours after pramlintide.

EFFECTS ON LAB TEST RESULTS
None reported.

CONTRAINDICATIONS & CAUTIONS
• Contraindicated in patients hypersensitive to drug or its components, including metacresol, and in patients with gastroparesis or hypoglycemia unawareness.
• Don't use in patients noncompliant with current insulin and glucose monitoring regimen, patients with a HbA$_{1c}$ level greater than 9%, patients with severe hypoglycemia during the previous 6 months, and patients who take drugs that stimulate GI motility.
• Use cautiously in pregnant or breastfeeding women and in elderly patients.
⚠ **Overdose S&S:** Severe nausea, vomiting, diarrhea, vasodilation, dizziness.

NURSING CONSIDERATIONS
Black Box Warning Drug may increase the risk of insulin-induced severe hypoglycemia, particularly in patients with type 1 diabetes. The risk of severe hypoglycemia is highest within the first 3 hours after an injection. ∎
• Symptoms of hypoglycemia may be masked in patients with a long history of diabetes, diabetic nerve disease, or intensified diabetes control.

• Notify prescriber of severe nausea and vomiting. A reduced dose may be needed.
• If patient has persistent nausea or recurrent, unexplained hypoglycemia that requires medical assistance, stop drug.
• If patient doesn't comply with glucose monitoring or drug dosage adjustments, stop drug.

PATIENT TEACHING
• Teach patient how to take drug exactly as prescribed, at mealtimes. Explain that it doesn't replace daily insulin but may lower the amount of insulin needed.
• Explain that a meal is considered more than 250 calories or 30 g of carbohydrates.
• Caution patient not to mix drug with insulin; instruct him to give the injections at separate sites.
• Instruct patient not to change doses of pramlintide or insulin without consulting prescriber.
• Instruct patient not to transfer drug from pen injector to syringe. Drug in pen injector is a higher concentration than in vial.
• Tell patient to refrain from driving, operating heavy machinery, or performing other risky activities where he could hurt himself or others until it's known how drug affects his glucose level.
• Caution patient about possibility of severe hypoglycemia, particularly within 3 hours after injection.
• Teach patient and family members the signs and symptoms of hypoglycemia, including hunger, headache, sweating, tremor, irritability, and difficulty concentrating.
• Instruct patient and family members what to do if patient develops hypoglycemia.
• Tell patient to report severe nausea and vomiting to prescriber.
• Advise women of childbearing age to tell the prescriber if they are, could be, or are planning to become pregnant.
• Teach patient how to handle unplanned situations, such as illness or stress, low or forgotten insulin dose, accidental use of too much insulin or drug, not enough food, or missed meals.

P

• Tell patient to refrigerate pen injectors and unopened and opened vials. Contents of opened vials should be used within 28 days and those of unopened vials before expiration date.

SAFETY ALERT!

prasugrel
PRAH-soo-grel

Effient◆

Therapeutic class: Antiplatelet drugs
Pharmacologic class: Adenosine diphosphate–induced platelet aggregation inhibitors
Pregnancy risk category: B

AVAILABLE FORMS
Tablets: 5 mg, 10 mg

INDICATIONS & DOSAGES
➤ **To reduce thrombotic events in patients with acute coronary syndrome (ACS) (unstable angina and non-ST-elevation MI) managed with percutaneous coronary intervention [PCI]); to reduce thrombotic events in patients with ACS (ST-elevation MI) managed with primary or delayed PCI**
Adults: Initially, single 60-mg loading dose; then 10 mg P.O. once daily. Patient should also take aspirin 75 to 325 mg P.O. daily.
Adjust-a-dose: For adults weighing less than 60 kg (132 lb), consider reducing dosage to 5 mg P.O. once daily.

ADMINISTRATION
P.O.
• May give drug with or without food.
• Don't break tablets.

ACTION
Inhibits platelet activation and aggregation through irreversible binding of its active metabolite to the P2Y12 class of adenosine diphosphate receptors on platelets.

Route	Onset	Peak	Duration
P.O.	Rapid	30 min	5–9 days

Half-life: 7 hours.

ADVERSE REACTIONS
CNS: dizziness, fatigue, headache, fever.
CV: atrial fibrillation, bradycardia, hypertension or hypotension, peripheral edema.
GI: *GI bleeding,* nausea, diarrhea.
EENT: epistaxis.
Hematologic: *bleeding,* leukopenia, *thrombotic thrombocytopenic purpura.*
Metabolic: hypercholesterolemia, hyperlipidemia.
Musculoskeletal: back pain, extremity pain.
Respiratory: cough, dyspnea.
Skin: rash.
Other: noncardiac chest pain.

INTERACTIONS
Drug-drug. *Direct factor Xa inhibitors (rivaroxaban), direct thrombin inhibitors (dabigatran, desirudin), fibrinolytics (tenecteplase), heparin, NSAIDs (long-term use), warfarin:* May increase the risk of bleeding. Use together cautiously.

EFFECTS ON LAB TEST RESULTS
• May increase cholesterol and lipid levels.
• May decrease WBC and platelet counts.

CONTRAINDICATIONS & CAUTIONS
Black Box Warning Contraindicated in patients with pathologic bleeding (such as peptic ulcer or intracranial hemorrhage) and in those with a history of transient ischemic attack or stroke. ∎
Black Box Warning Prasugrel is generally not recommended in patients age 75 and older because of the increased risk of intracranial and fatal bleeding and uncertain benefit, except in high-risk situations (patients with diabetes or a history of prior MI). In these situations, drug's effect appears to be greater and its use may be considered. ∎
Black Box Warning Use cautiously in patients who weigh less than 60 kg because of the increased risk of bleeding. ∎
• Use cautiously in patients at risk for increased bleeding from trauma, surgery, or other pathologic conditions and in those with severe hepatic impairment.
⚠ *Overdose S&S:* Bleeding due to impaired clotting ability.

Reactions in bold italics are *life-threatening*. Interactions may have a *rapid onset* or a *delayed onset*.

NURSING CONSIDERATIONS

Black Box Warning Drug may cause significant, sometimes fatal, bleeding. Suspect bleeding in patient who is hypotensive and has recently undergone PCI, CABG, or other surgical procedure. Manage bleeding without stopping drug, if possible. Stopping drug within first few weeks after ACS occurrence increases the risk of further CV events. ∎

• Monitor patient for unusual bleeding or bruising.

• Drug should be taken with aspirin (75 to 325 mg daily).

Black Box Warning Discontinue drug 7 days before CABG. Don't start drug if patient is likely to undergo urgent CABG. ∎

• Bleeding associated with CABG may be treated with transfusion of blood products, such as RBCs and platelets; however, platelets may be ineffective if given within 6 hours of loading dose or within 4 hours of maintenance dose.

❂ **Alert:** Drug may cause fatal thrombotic thrombocytopenic purpura (thrombocytopenia, hemolytic anemia, neurologic signs and symptoms, renal dysfunction, and fever) that requires urgent treatment, including plasmapheresis.

• **Look alike–sound alike:** Don't confuse prasugrel with pravastatin or propranolol.

PATIENT TEACHING

• Advise patient that drug can be taken without regard to food.

• Inform patient that he will bruise more easily and that it may take longer than usual to stop bleeding.

• Instruct patient to report prolonged or excessive bleeding or blood in his stool or urine.

• Advise patient to inform health care providers that he's taking prasugrel before scheduling surgery or taking new drugs.

pravastatin sodium (eptastatin)
prah-va-STA-tin

Pravachol🖋

Therapeutic class: Antilipemics
Pharmacologic class: HMG-CoA reductase inhibitors
Pregnancy risk category: X

AVAILABLE FORMS
Tablets: 10 mg, 20 mg, 40 mg, 80 mg

INDICATIONS & DOSAGES
Adjust-a-dose (for all indications): In patients with renal or hepatic dysfunction, start with 10 mg P.O. daily. In patients taking immunosuppressants, begin with 10 mg P.O. at bedtime and adjust to higher dosages with caution. Most patients treated with the combination of immunosuppressants and pravastatin receive up to 20 mg pravastatin daily.

➤ **Primary and secondary prevention of coronary events; hyperlipidemia**
Adults: Initially, 40 mg P.O. once daily at the same time each day, with or without food. Adjust dosage every 4 weeks, based on patient tolerance and response; maximum daily dose is 80 mg.

➤ **Heterozygous familial hypercholesterolemia**
Adolescents ages 14 to 18: Give 40 mg P.O. once daily. Maximum dose is 40 mg daily.
Children ages 8 to 13: Give 20 mg P.O. once daily. Maximum dose is 20 mg daily.

ADMINISTRATION
P.O.
• Give drug without regard for meals.
• If patient is also taking a bile acid resin (cholestyramine), administer pravastatin 1 hour before or 4 hours after the resin.

ACTION
Inhibits HMG-CoA reductase, an early (and rate-limiting) step in cholesterol biosynthesis.

Route	Onset	Peak	Duration
P.O.	Unknown	60–90 min	Unknown

Half-life: 1¼ to 2¼ hours.

P

ADVERSE REACTIONS
CNS: dizziness, fatigue, headache.
CV: chest pain.
EENT: rhinitis.
GI: nausea, abdominal pain, constipation, diarrhea, flatulence, heartburn, vomiting.
GU: *renal failure caused by myoglobinuria,* urinary abnormality.
Musculoskeletal: localized muscle pain, *rhabdomyolysis,* myalgia, myopathy, myositis.
Respiratory: common cold, cough.
Skin: rash.
Other: flulike symptoms, influenza.

INTERACTIONS
Drug-drug. *Azole antifungals (such as fluconazole, ketoconazole), erythromycin, fibric acid derivatives (such as gemfibrozil), niacin:* May increase risk of severe myopathy or rhabdomyolysis. Avoid using together.
Cholestyramine, colestipol: May decrease pravastatin level. Give pravastatin 1 hour before or 4 hours after these drugs.
Clarithromycin: May increase pravastatin level. Limit pravastatin to 40 mg once daily.
Cyclosporine: May increase pravastatin level and pravastatin-related adverse reactions. If concomitant use can't be avoided, begin therapy with pravastatin 10 mg once daily at bedtime and titrate to higher doses with caution. Most patients received a maximum dose of pravastatin 20 mg daily.
❸ Alert: *Darunavir and ritonavir, lopinavir–ritonavir:* May increase pravastatin level and risk of myopathy and rhabdomyolysis. Use together cautiously.
Hepatotoxic drugs: May increase risk of hepatotoxicity. Avoid using together.
Protease inhibitors (ritonavir, saquinavir): May reduce pravastatin level. Monitor clinical response.
Rifamycins: May increase or decrease pravastatin levels. Carefully monitor clinical response.
Drug-herb. *Eucalyptus, jin bu huan, kava:* May increase the risk of hepatotoxicity. Discourage use together.
Red yeast rice: May increase risk of adverse reactions because herb contains compounds similar to those in drug. Discourage use together.

Drug-food. *Oat bran:* May decrease effectiveness of pravastatin. Separate administration times as much as possible.
Drug-lifestyle. *Alcohol use:* May increase risk of hepatotoxicity. Discourage use together.

EFFECTS ON LAB TEST RESULTS
● May increase ALT, AST, CK, alkaline phosphatase, HbA_{1c}, fasting glucose, and bilirubin levels.
● May alter thyroid function test values.

CONTRAINDICATIONS & CAUTIONS
● Contraindicated in patients hypersensitive to drug and in those with active liver disease or conditions that cause unexplained, persistent elevations of transaminase levels.
● Contraindicated in pregnant and breast-feeding women and in women of childbearing age.
● Use cautiously in patients who consume large quantities of alcohol or have history of liver disease.
● Statin therapy should be interrupted if the patient shows signs of serious liver injury, hyperbilirubinemia, or jaundice. The drug shouldn't be restarted if another cause can't be found.
● Safety and effectiveness in children younger than age 8 haven't been established.

NURSING CONSIDERATIONS
● Patient should follow a diet restricted in saturated fat and cholesterol during therapy.
● Use in children with heterozygous familial hypercholesterolemia if LDL cholesterol level is at least 190 mg/dL, or if LDL cholesterol is at least 160 mg/dL and patient has either a positive family history of premature CV disease or two or more other CV disease risk factors.
● Obtain LFT results at start of therapy and then periodically. A liver biopsy may be performed if elevated liver enzyme levels persist.
● **Look alike–sound alike:** Don't confuse Pravachol with Prevacid, Prinivil, or propranolol. Don't confuse pravastatin with nystatin, pitavastatin, or prasugrel.

Reactions in bold italics are *life-threatening*. Interactions may have a *rapid onset* or a *delayed onset*.

PATIENT TEACHING
• Advise patient who is also taking a bile acid resin such as cholestyramine to take pravastatin at least 1 hour before or 4 hours after taking resin.
• Tell patient to notify prescriber of adverse reactions, particularly muscle aches and pains.
• Inform patient that LFTs will be performed before and periodically throughout treatment.
• Tell patient to promptly report signs and symptoms of liver injury, including fatigue, anorexia, right upper quadrant discomfort, dark urine, or jaundice.
• Tell patient that the drug may increase blood sugar levels; however, the CV benefits are thought to outweigh the slight increase in risk.
• Teach patient about proper dietary management of cholesterol and triglycerides. When appropriate, recommend weight control, exercise, and smoking cessation programs.
• Inform patient that it will take up to 4 weeks to achieve full therapeutic effect.
⊙ **Alert:** Tell woman of childbearing age to stop drug and notify prescriber immediately if she is or may be pregnant or if she's breast-feeding.

---

prazosin hydrochloride
PRA-zo-sin

Minipress

Therapeutic class: Antihypertensives
Pharmacologic class: Alpha blockers
Pregnancy risk category: C

AVAILABLE FORMS
Capsules: 1 mg, 2 mg, 5 mg

INDICATIONS & DOSAGES
➤ **Mild to moderate hypertension**
Adults: Test dose is 1 mg P.O. at bedtime to prevent first-dose syncope (severe syncope with loss of consciousness). First dosage is 1 mg P.O. b.i.d. or t.i.d. Dosage may be increased slowly. Maximum daily dose is 20 mg. Maintenance dosage is 6 to 15 mg

daily in divided doses. Some patients need larger dosages (up to 40 mg daily).
   If other antihypertensives or diuretics are added to therapy, decrease prazosin dosage to 1 to 2 mg t.i.d. and readjust to maintenance dosage.
➤ **Pediatric hypertension** ◆
Children ages 1 to 17: Initially, 0.05 to 0.1 mg/kg P.O. t.i.d. Maximum dosage is 0.5 mg/kg P.O. t.i.d.

ADMINISTRATION
P.O.
• Give drug without regard for meals.

ACTION
Unknown. Thought to act by blocking alpha-adrenergic receptors.

Route	Onset	Peak	Duration
P.O.	30–90 min	2–4 hr	7–10 hr

Half-life: 2 to 3 hours.

ADVERSE REACTIONS
CNS: dizziness, first-dose syncope, headache, drowsiness, nervousness, paresthesia, weakness, depression, vertigo, lack of energy.
CV: orthostatic hypotension, palpitations, edema.
EENT: blurred vision, conjunctivitis, epistaxis, nasal congestion.
GI: vomiting, diarrhea, abdominal cramps, nausea, constipation.
GU: urinary frequency.
Musculoskeletal: arthralgia, myalgia.
Respiratory: dyspnea.
Skin: rash.

INTERACTIONS
Drug-drug. *Acebutolol, atenolol, betaxolol, carteolol, esmolol, metoprolol, nadolol, pindolol, propranolol, sotalol, timolol:* May increase the risk of orthostatic hypotension in the early phases of use together. Help patient stand slowly until effects are known. *Diuretics:* May increase frequency of syncope with loss of consciousness. Advise patient to sit or lie down if dizziness occurs. *Verapamil:* May increase prazosin level. Monitor patient closely.

P

Drug-herb. *Butcher's broom:* May reduce effect. Discourage use together.
Ma huang: May decrease antihypertensive effects. Discourage use together.

EFFECTS ON LAB TEST RESULTS
• May increase levels of BUN, uric acid, and urinary metabolite of norepinephrine and vanillylmandelic acid.
• May increase LFT values. May alter results of screening tests for pheochromocytoma.
• May cause positive ANA titer.

CONTRAINDICATIONS & CAUTIONS
• Contraindicated in patients hypersensitive to drug or other alpha blockers.
• Use cautiously in patients receiving other antihypertensives.
⚠ Overdose S&S: Profound drowsiness, depressed reflexes, hypotension.

NURSING CONSIDERATIONS
• Monitor patient's blood pressure and pulse rate frequently.
• Elderly patients may be more sensitive to drug's hypotensive effects.
• Compliance might be improved with twice-daily dosing. Discuss dosing change with prescriber if compliance problems are suspected.
☹ Alert: If first dose is more than 1 mg, first-dose syncope may occur.
• **Look alike–sound alike:** Don't confuse prazosin with prednisone.

PATIENT TEACHING
• Warn patient that dizziness may occur with first dose. If he experiences dizziness, tell him to sit or lie down. Reassure him that this effect disappears with continued dosing.
• Caution patient to avoid driving or performing hazardous tasks for the first 24 hours after starting this drug or increasing the dose.
• Tell patient not to suddenly stop taking drug, but to notify prescriber if unpleasant adverse reactions occur.
• Advise patient to minimize low blood pressure and dizziness upon standing by rising slowly and avoiding sudden position changes. Dry mouth can be relieved by chewing gum or sucking on hard candy or ice chips.

prednisoLONE
pred-NISS-oh-lone

Prelone

prednisoLONE acetate
Flo-Pred

prednisoLONE sodium phosphate
Orapred, Orapred ODT, Pediapred

Therapeutic class: Corticosteroids
Pharmacologic class: Glucocorticoids–mineralocorticoids
Pregnancy risk category: C

AVAILABLE FORMS
prednisolone
Syrup: 5 mg/5 mL, 15 mg/5 mL*
Tablets: 5 mg
prednisolone acetate
Oral suspension: 5 mg/5 mL, 15 mg/5 mL
prednisolone sodium phosphate
Orally disintegrating tablets (ODTs): 10 mg, 15 mg, 30 mg
Oral solution: 5 mg/5 mL, 10 mg/5 mL, 15 mg/5 mL

INDICATIONS & DOSAGES
➤ **Severe inflammation, immunosuppression**
Adults: 5 to 60 mg P.O. daily.
Children: 0.14 to 2 mg/kg/day P.O. in three or four divided doses (4 to 60 mg/m^2/day).
➤ **Uncontrolled asthma in those taking inhaled corticosteroids and long-acting bronchodilators**
Children: 1 to 2 mg/kg/day prednisolone sodium phosphate or prednisolone acetate P.O. in single or divided doses. Continue short course (or "burst" therapy) until child achieves a peak expiratory flow rate of 80% of his personal best, or until symptoms resolve. This usually requires 3 to 10 days of treatment but can take longer. Tapering the dose after improvement doesn't necessarily prevent relapse.

➤ **Acute exacerbations of MS**
Adults and children: 200 mg/day prednisolone sodium phosphate P.O. as single or divided dose for 7 days; then 80 mg every other day for 1 month.

➤ **Nephrotic syndrome**
Children: 60 mg/m² prednisolone sodium phosphate or prednisolone acetate P.O. in three divided doses daily for 4 weeks, followed by 4 weeks of single-dose alternate-day therapy at 40 mg/m²/day.

ADMINISTRATION

P.O.
● Give drug with food to reduce GI irritation. Patient may need another drug to prevent GI irritation.
● Don't cut or crush ODTs.

ACTION

Not clearly defined. Decreases inflammation, mainly by stabilizing leukocyte lysosomal membranes; suppresses immune response; stimulates bone marrow; and influences protein, fat, and carbohydrate metabolism.

Route	Onset	Peak	Duration
P.O.	Rapid	1–2 hr	3–36 hr

Half-life: 2 to 4 hours.

ADVERSE REACTIONS

CNS: euphoria, insomnia, *pseudotumor cerebri, seizures,* psychotic behavior, vertigo, headache, paresthesia.
CV: *arrhythmias, heart failure, thromboembolism,* hypertension, edema, thrombophlebitis.
EENT: cataracts, glaucoma.
GI: peptic ulceration, *pancreatitis,* GI irritation, increased appetite, nausea, vomiting.
GU: menstrual irregularities, increased urine calcium levels.
Metabolic: *hypokalemia,* hyperglycemia, carbohydrate intolerance, hypercholesterolemia, *hypocalcemia.*
Musculoskeletal: growth suppression in children, muscle weakness, osteoporosis.
Skin: hirsutism, delayed wound healing, acne, various skin eruptions.

Other: (after increased stress) *acute adrenal insufficiency,* susceptibility to infections, cushingoid state; (after abrupt withdrawal) rebound inflammation, fatigue, weakness, arthralgia, fever, dizziness, lethargy, depression, fainting, orthostatic hypotension, dyspnea, anorexia, *hypoglycemia;* (after prolonged use followed by sudden withdrawal) *possible death.*

INTERACTIONS

Drug-drug. *Aspirin, indomethacin, other NSAIDs:* May increase risk of GI distress and bleeding. Use together cautiously.
Azole antifungals (fluconazole, ketoconazole): May increase antifungal toxicity. Reduce steroid dosage as needed.
Barbiturates, carbamazepine, fosphenytoin, phenytoin, rifampin: May decrease corticosteroid effect. Increase corticosteroid dosage.
Cyclosporine: May increase toxicity and risk of seizures. Monitor patient closely.
Drugs that deplete potassium, such as thiazide diuretics and amphotericin B: May enhance potassium-wasting effects of prednisolone. Monitor potassium level.
Estrogens: May increase pharmacologic and toxic effects of prednisolone. Monitor patient closely.
Oral anticoagulants: May alter dosage requirements. Monitor PT and INR closely.
Salicylates: May decrease salicylate level. Monitor patient for lack of salicylate effectiveness.
Skin-test antigens: May decrease response. Postpone skin testing until therapy is completed.
Toxoids, vaccines: May decrease antibody response and may increase risk of neurologic complications. Avoid using together.

EFFECTS ON LAB TEST RESULTS

● May increase glucose and cholesterol levels. May decrease T₃, T₄, potassium, and calcium levels.
● May decrease ¹³¹I uptake and protein-bound iodine levels in thyroid function tests. May alter skin-test results. May cause false-negative results in nitroblue tetrazolium test for systemic bacterial infections.

P

CONTRAINDICATIONS & CAUTIONS

● Contraindicated in patients hypersensitive to drug or its ingredients, in those with systemic fungal infections, and in those receiving immunosuppressive doses together with live-virus vaccines.

● Use with caution in patients with recent MI.

● Use cautiously in patients with GI ulcer, renal disease, hypertension, osteoporosis, diabetes mellitus, hypothyroidism, cirrhosis, active hepatitis, diverticulitis, nonspecific ulcerative colitis, recent intestinal anastomoses, thromboembolic disorders, seizures, myasthenia gravis, heart failure, tuberculosis, ocular herpes simplex, emotional instability, and psychotic tendencies or in breast-feeding women.

⚠ *Overdose S&S:* Abnormal fat deposits, accentuated menopausal symptoms, acne, adrenal insufficiency, decreased glucose tolerance, decreased resistance to infection, dry scaly skin, ecchymosis, excessive appetite, fluid retention, fractures, headache, hypertrichosis, hypokalemia, increased blood pressure, increased sweating, menstrual disorder, mental symptoms, moon face, negative nitrogen balance with delayed bone and wound healing, neuropathy, osteoporosis, peptic ulcer, pigmentation, striae, tachycardia, thinning scalp hair, thrombophlebitis, weakness, weight gain; hepatomegaly, abdominal distention (in children).

NURSING CONSIDERATIONS

● Determine whether patient is sensitive to other corticosteroids.

● Always adjust to lowest effective dose.

● Drug may be used for alternate-day therapy.

● Most adverse reactions to corticosteroids are dose- or duration-dependent.

● Monitor patient's weight, blood pressure, and electrolyte level.

● Monitor patient for cushingoid effects, including moon face, buffalo hump, central obesity, thinning hair, hypertension, and increased susceptibility to infection.

● Watch for depression or psychotic episodes, especially during high-dose therapy.

● Diabetic patient may need increased insulin; monitor glucose level.

● Give patient low-sodium diet that's high in potassium and protein. Give potassium supplements as needed.

● Drug may mask or worsen infections, including latent amebiasis.

● Elderly patients may be more susceptible to osteoporosis with long-term use.

● Gradually reduce dosage after long-term therapy.

● *Look alike–sound alike:* Don't confuse prednisolone with prednisone. Don't confuse Pediapred with Pediazole or Prelone with Prozac.

PATIENT TEACHING

● Tell patient not to stop drug abruptly or without prescriber's consent.

● Instruct patient to take oral form of drug with food or milk.

● Teach patient signs and symptoms of early adrenal insufficiency: fatigue, muscle weakness, joint pain, fever, anorexia, nausea, shortness of breath, dizziness, and fainting.

● Instruct patient to carry medical identification that includes prescriber's name and name and dosage of drug and indicates his need for supplemental systemic glucocorticoids during stress.

● Warn patient on long-term therapy about cushingoid effects and the need to notify prescriber about sudden weight gain or swelling.

● Tell patient to report slow healing.

● Advise patient receiving long-term therapy to consider exercise or physical therapy. Also, tell him to ask prescriber about vitamin D or calcium supplement.

● Instruct patient to avoid exposure to infections and to notify prescriber if exposure occurs.

● Tell patient to avoid immunizations while taking drug.

● *Alert:* Tell patient not to cut, crush, or chew ODTs.

● Instruct patient not to remove the ODT from the blister pack until he's ready to take it. The tablet can be swallowed whole or allowed to dissolve on the tongue with or without water.

Reactions in bold italics are *life-threatening*. Interactions may have a *rapid onset* or a *delayed onset*.

prednisoLONE acetate (ophthalmic suspension)
pred-NISS-oh-lone

Omnipred, Pred Forte, Pred Mild

prednisoLONE sodium phosphate (solution)

Therapeutic class: Anti-inflammatory drugs (ophthalmic)
Pharmacologic class: Corticosteroids
Pregnancy risk category: C

AVAILABLE FORMS
prednisolone acetate
Ophthalmic suspension: 0.12%, 1%
prednisolone sodium phosphate
Ophthalmic solution: 1%

INDICATIONS & DOSAGES
➤ **Inflammation of palpebral and bulbar conjunctiva, cornea, and anterior segment of globe**
Adults: 1 or 2 drops into eye. In severe conditions, may be used hourly, tapering as inflammation subsides. In mild or moderate inflammation or when a favorable response is attained in severe conditions, dosage may be reduced to 1 or 2 drops every 3 to 12 hours.

ADMINISTRATION
Ophthalmic
• Shake suspension and check dosage before giving to ensure correct strength. Store in tightly covered container.
• Apply light finger pressure on lacrimal sac for 1 minute after instillation.

ACTION
Suppresses edema, fibrin deposition, capillary dilation, leukocyte migration, capillary proliferation, and collagen deposition.

Route	Onset	Peak	Duration
Ophthalmic	Unknown	Unknown	Unknown

Half-life: Unknown.

ADVERSE REACTIONS
EENT: cataracts, corneal ulceration, discharge, discomfort, foreign body sensation, glaucoma worsening, increased intraocular pressure (IOP), increased susceptibility to viral or fungal corneal infection, interference with corneal wound healing, optic nerve damage with excessive or long-term use, visual acuity and visual field defects.
Other: adrenal suppression with excessive or long-term use, systemic effects.

INTERACTIONS
None significant.

EFFECTS ON LAB TEST RESULTS
None reported.

CONTRAINDICATIONS & CAUTIONS
• Contraindicated in patients with acute, untreated, purulent ocular infections; acute superficial herpes simplex (dendritic keratitis); vaccinia, varicella, or other viral or fungal eye diseases; or ocular tuberculosis.
• Use cautiously in patients with corneal abrasions that may be contaminated (especially with herpes).

NURSING CONSIDERATIONS
• *Look alike–sound alike:* Don't confuse prednisolone with prednisone.

PATIENT TEACHING
• Teach patient how to instill drops. Advise him to wash hands before and after instillation, and warn him not to touch tip of dropper to eye or surrounding area.
• Advise patient to apply light finger pressure on lacrimal sac for 1 minute after instillation.
• Tell patient on long-term therapy to have IOP tested frequently.
• Tell patient not to share drug, washcloths, or towels with family members and to notify prescriber if anyone develops the same signs or symptoms.
• Stress importance of compliance with recommended therapy.
• Tell patient to notify prescriber if improvement doesn't occur within several days or if pain, itching, or swelling of eye occurs.

P

• Warn patient not to use leftover drug for new eye inflammation because serious problems may occur.

predniSONE
PRED-ni-sone

Prednisone Intensol*, Winpred†

Therapeutic class: Corticosteroids
Pharmacologic class: Adrenocorticoids
Pregnancy risk category: C

AVAILABLE FORMS
Oral solution: 5 mg/5 mL*, 5 mg/mL (concentrate)*
Tablets: 1 mg, 2.5 mg, 5 mg, 10 mg, 20 mg, 50 mg

INDICATIONS & DOSAGES
➤ **Severe inflammation, immuno-suppression, endocrine disorders**
Adults and children: 5 to 60 mg P.O. daily in single dose or as two to four divided doses. Maintenance dose given daily or every other day. Dosage must be individualized, and constant monitoring is needed.
➤ **Acute exacerbations of MS**
Adults and children: 200 mg P.O. daily for 7 days; then 80 mg P.O. every other day for 1 month.

ADMINISTRATION
P.O.
• Unless contraindicated, give drug with food to reduce GI irritation. Patient may need another drug to prevent GI irritation.
• Solution may be diluted in juice or other flavored diluent or semisolid food such as applesauce before using.

ACTION
Not clearly defined. Decreases inflammation, mainly by stabilizing leukocyte lysosomal membranes; suppresses immune response; stimulates bone marrow; and influences protein, fat, and carbohydrate metabolism.

Route	Onset	Peak	Duration
P.O.	Variable	Variable	Variable

Half-life: 18 to 36 hours.

ADVERSE REACTIONS
CNS: euphoria, insomnia, psychotic behavior, *pseudotumor cerebri,* vertigo, headache, paresthesia, *seizures.*
CV: *heart failure,* hypertension, edema, *arrhythmias,* thrombophlebitis, *thromboembolism.*
EENT: cataracts, glaucoma.
GI: peptic ulceration, *pancreatitis,* GI irritation, increased appetite, nausea, vomiting.
GU: menstrual irregularities, increased urine calcium level.
Metabolic: *hypokalemia,* hyperglycemia, carbohydrate intolerance, hypercholesterolemia, *hypocalcemia.*
Musculoskeletal: growth suppression in children, muscle weakness, osteoporosis.
Skin: hirsutism, delayed wound healing, acne, various skin eruptions.
Other: cushingoid state, susceptibility to infections, *acute adrenal insufficiency* after increased stress or abrupt withdrawal after long-term therapy.
After abrupt withdrawal: rebound inflammation, fatigue, weakness, arthralgia, fever, dizziness, lethargy, depression, fainting, orthostatic hypotension, dyspnea, anorexia, *hypoglycemia. After prolonged use, sudden withdrawal may be fatal.*

INTERACTIONS
Drug-drug. *Aspirin, indomethacin, other NSAIDs:* May increase risk of GI distress and bleeding. Use together cautiously.
Barbiturates, carbamazepine, fosphenytoin, phenobarbital, phenytoin, rifampin: May decrease corticosteroid effect. Increase corticosteroid dosage.
Cyclosporine: May increase toxicity and cause seizures. Monitor patient closely.
Ketoconazole, troleandomycin: May inhibit the metabolism of corticosteroids and decrease their clearance. Titrate the dose of corticosteroid to avoid toxicity.
Oral anticoagulants: May alter dosage requirements. Monitor PT and INR closely.
Potassium-depleting drugs, such as thiazide diuretics and amphotericin B: May enhance potassium-wasting effects of prednisone. Monitor potassium level.

Reactions in bold italics are *life-threatening*. Interactions may have a *rapid onset* or a *delayed onset*.

Salicylates: May decrease salicylate level. Monitor patient for lack of salicylate effectiveness.

Skin-test antigens: May decrease response. Postpone skin testing until therapy is completed.

Toxoids, vaccines: May decrease antibody response and may increase risk of neurologic complications. Avoid using together.

EFFECTS ON LAB TEST RESULTS

• May increase glucose and cholesterol levels. May decrease T_3, T_4, potassium, and calcium levels.

• May decrease ^{131}I uptake and protein-bound iodine values in thyroid function tests. May cause false-negative results in nitroblue tetrazolium test for systemic bacterial infections. May alter reactions to skin tests.

CONTRAINDICATIONS & CAUTIONS

• Contraindicated in patients hypersensitive to drug or its ingredients, in those with systemic fungal infections, and in those receiving immunosuppressive doses together with live-virus vaccines.

• Use cautiously in patients with recent MI, GI ulcer, renal disease, hypertension, osteoporosis, diabetes mellitus, hypothyroidism, cirrhosis, active hepatitis, diverticulitis, nonspecific ulcerative colitis, recent intestinal anastomoses, thromboembolic disorders, seizures, myasthenia gravis, heart failure, tuberculosis, ocular herpes simplex, emotional instability, and psychotic tendencies or in breast-feeding women.

NURSING CONSIDERATIONS

• Determine whether patient is sensitive to other corticosteroids.

• Drug may be used for alternate-day therapy.

• Always adjust to lowest effective dose.

• Most adverse reactions to corticosteroids are dose- or duration-dependent.

• For better results and less toxicity, give a once-daily dose in the morning.

• Drug may be used in conjunction with mineralocorticoids when needed.

• Monitor patient's blood pressure, sleep patterns, and potassium level.

• Weigh patient daily; report sudden weight gain to prescriber.

• Monitor patient for cushingoid effects, including moon face, buffalo hump, central obesity, thinning hair, hypertension, and increased susceptibility to infection.

• Watch for depression or psychotic episodes, especially during high-dose therapy.

• Diabetic patient may need increased insulin; monitor glucose level.

• Elderly patients may be more susceptible to osteoporosis with long-term use.

• Drug may mask or worsen infections, including latent amebiasis.

• Unless contraindicated, give low-sodium diet that's high in potassium and protein. Give potassium supplements as needed.

• Gradually reduce dosage after long-term therapy.

• *Look alike–sound alike:* Don't confuse prednisone with prednisolone or primidone.

PATIENT TEACHING

• Tell patient not to stop drug abruptly or without prescriber's consent.

• Instruct patient to take drug with food or milk.

• Teach patient signs and symptoms of early adrenal insufficiency: fatigue, muscle weakness, joint pain, fever, anorexia, nausea, shortness of breath, dizziness, and fainting.

• Instruct patient to carry or wear medical identification indicating his need for supplemental systemic glucocorticoids during stress. It should include prescriber's name and name and dosage of drug.

• Warn patient on long-term therapy about cushingoid effects (moon face, buffalo hump) and the need to notify prescriber about sudden weight gain or swelling.

• Advise patient receiving long-term therapy to consider exercise or physical therapy. Also, tell patient to ask prescriber about vitamin D or calcium supplement.

• Tell patient to report slow healing.

• Advise patient receiving long-term therapy to have periodic eye examinations.

• Instruct patient to avoid exposure to infections and to contact prescriber if exposure occurs.

P

pregabalin
pray-GAB-ah-lin

Lyrica◆

Therapeutic class: Anticonvulsants
Pharmacologic class: CNS drugs
Pregnancy risk category: C
Controlled substance schedule: V

AVAILABLE FORMS
Capsules: 25 mg, 50 mg, 75 mg, 100 mg,
150 mg, 200 mg, 225 mg, 300 mg
Oral solution: 20 mg/mL

INDICATIONS & DOSAGES
Adjust-a-dose (for all indications): If CrCl is
30 to 60 mL/minute, give 75 to 300 mg/day
in two or three divided doses. If CrCl is 15
to 30 mL/minute, give 25 to 150 mg/day in
one dose or divided into two doses. If CrCl
is less than 15 mL/minute, give 25 to 75 mg/
day in one dose. If patient undergoes hemodialysis, give one supplemental dose according to these guidelines. If patient
takes 25 mg daily, give 25 or 50 mg. If
patient takes 25 to 50 mg daily, give 50 or
75 mg. If patient takes 75 mg daily, give
100 or 150 mg.
➤ **Fibromyalgia**
Adults: 75 mg P.O. b.i.d. (150 mg/day).
May increase to 150 mg b.i.d. (300 mg/day)
within 1 week, based on patient response.
If pain relief insufficient with 300 mg/day,
increase to 225 mg b.i.d. (450 mg/day).
➤ **Diabetic peripheral neuropathy**
Adults: Initially, 50 mg P.O. t.i.d. May
increase to 100 mg P.O. t.i.d. within 1 week.
➤ **Neuropathic pain associated with
spinal cord injury**
Adults: Initially, 75 mg P.O. b.i.d. (150 mg/
day). May increase to 150 mg b.i.d.
(300 mg/day) within 1 week based on patient response. If pain relief is insufficient
after 2 to 3 weeks, increase to 300 mg b.i.d.
Maximum dose is 600 mg/day.
➤ **Postherpetic neuralgia**
Adults: Initially, 75 mg P.O. b.i.d. or 50 mg
P.O. t.i.d. May increase to 300 mg/day in
two or three equally divided doses within
1 week. If pain relief insufficient after 2 to

4 weeks, may increase to 300 mg b.i.d. or
200 mg t.i.d.
➤ **Partial onset seizures**
Adults: Initially, 75 mg P.O. b.i.d. or 50 mg
P.O. t.i.d. Range, 150 to 600 mg/day. Dosage
may be increased to maximum 600 mg/day.

ADMINISTRATION
P.O.
● Give drug without regard for food.
● Don't stop drug abruptly. Instead, taper
gradually over at least 1 week.

ACTION
May contribute to analgesic and anticonvulsant effects by binding to sites in CNS.

Route	Onset	Peak	Duration
P.O.	Unknown	1½–3 hr	Unknown

Half-life: 6 hours.

ADVERSE REACTIONS
CNS: ataxia, dizziness, somnolence,
tremor, abnormal gait, abnormal thinking,
amnesia, anxiety, asthenia, confusion,
depersonalization, euphoria, headache,
hypesthesia, hypertonia, incoordination,
myoclonus, nervousness, nystagmus, pain,
paresthesia, stupor, twitching, vertigo.
CV: edema, PR-interval prolongation.
EENT: blurred or abnormal vision,
conjunctivitis, diplopia, eye disorder,
otitis media, tinnitus.
GI: dry mouth, abdominal pain, constipation, flatulence, gastroenteritis, vomiting.
GU: anorgasmia, impotence, urinary incontinence, urinary frequency.
Metabolic: *hypoglycemia,* weight gain,
increased or decreased appetite.
Musculoskeletal: arthralgia, back and chest
pain, leg cramps, myalgia, myasthenia,
neuropathy, tremor.
Respiratory: bronchitis, dyspnea.
Skin: ecchymosis, pruritus.
Other: accidental injury, infection, allergic
reaction, decreased libido, flu syndrome.

INTERACTIONS
Drug-drug. *ACE inhibitors:* May increase
risk of swelling and hives with concomitant
use. Monitor patient.

Reactions in bold italics are *life-threatening*. Interactions may have a *rapid onset* or a *delayed onset*.

CNS depressants: May have additive effects on cognitive and gross motor function. Monitor patient for increased dizziness and somnolence.

Pioglitazone, rosiglitazone: May cause additive fluid retention and weight gain. Monitor patient closely.

Drug-lifestyle. *Alcohol use:* May have additive depressant effects on cognitive and gross motor function. Discourage alcohol use.

EFFECTS ON LAB TEST RESULTS
● May increase CK level.
● May decrease platelet count.

CONTRAINDICATIONS & CAUTIONS
● Contraindicated in patients hypersensitive to drug or its components.
● Use cautiously in patients with New York Heart Association class III or IV heart failure.
⚠ Overdose S&S: Exaggerated adverse effects.

NURSING CONSIDERATIONS
🕔 **Alert:** Monitor patient for signs and symptoms of angioedema (including swelling of face, mouth, and neck), which may compromise breathing. Discontinue drug immediately if angioedema occurs.
● Monitor patient's weight and fluid status, especially if he has heart failure.
● Monitor patient for depression, suicidal thoughts or behavior, and unusual mood changes.
● Check for changes in vision.
🕔 **Alert:** Watch for signs of rhabdomyolysis, such as dark, red, or cola-colored urine; muscle tenderness; generalized weakness; or muscle stiffness or aching.
● **Look alike–sound alike:** Don't confuse Lyrica with Lopressor.

PATIENT TEACHING
● Explain that drug may be taken without regard to food.
● Warn patient not to stop drug abruptly.
● Caution patient to avoid hazardous activities until drug's effects are known.
● Instruct patient to watch for weight changes and water retention.

● Advise patient to report vision changes and malaise or fever accompanied by muscle pain, tenderness, or weakness.
● Tell women to immediately report planned or suspected pregnancy.
● Tell a man who plans to father a child that he should consult prescriber about possible risks to fetus.
● If patient has diabetes, urge him to inspect his skin closely for ulcer formation.
● Advise patient to avoid alcohol.

primaquine phosphate
PRIM-uh-kween

Therapeutic class: Antimalarials
Pharmacologic class: Aminoquinolines
Pregnancy risk category: C

AVAILABLE FORMS
Tablets: 26.3 mg (equivalent to 15-mg base)

INDICATIONS & DOSAGES
Black Box Warning Prescribers should be completely familiar with this drug before prescribing. ∎
➤ **Relapsing** *Plasmodium vivax* **malaria, eliminating symptoms and infection completely; to prevent relapse**
Adults: 15 mg base P.O. daily for 14 days. Begin therapy during the last 2 weeks of, or after, a course of suppression with chloroquine or comparable drug.

ADMINISTRATION
P.O.
🕔 **Alert:** Drug dosage may be discussed in "mg" or "mg base"; be aware of the difference.
● Give drug with or without food. Give with a meal if stomach irritation occurs.

ACTION
May bind to and alter the properties of DNA in susceptible parasites.

Route	Onset	Peak	Duration
P.O.	Unknown	1–3 hr	Unknown

Half-life: 4 to 10 hours.

ADVERSE REACTIONS
GI: nausea, vomiting, epigastric distress, abdominal cramps.
Hematologic: *hemolytic anemia, leukopenia, methemoglobinemia.*

INTERACTIONS
Drug-drug. *Aluminum salts, magnesium:* Decreases GI absorption. Separate dose times.
Quinacrine: May increase risk of toxicity. Avoid concomitant use.
Drug-food. *Grapefruit juice:* May increase drug plasma concentration and toxic effects. Advise patient to avoid grapefruit products.

EFFECTS ON LAB TEST RESULTS
● May decrease hemoglobin level.
● May decrease RBC count. May increase or decrease WBC count.

CONTRAINDICATIONS & CAUTIONS
● Contraindicated in patients with systemic diseases in which agranulocytosis may develop, such as lupus erythematosus or rheumatoid arthritis, and in those taking a bone marrow suppressant, quinacrine, or hemolytic drugs.
● Use cautiously in patients with previous idiosyncratic reaction involving hemolytic anemia, methemoglobinemia, or leukopenia; in those with a family or personal history of favism; and in those with erythrocytic G6PD or nicotinamide-adenine-dinucleotide (NADH) methemoglobin reductase deficiency.
⚠ *Overdose S&S:* Abdominal cramps, anemia, burning epigastric distress, CNS and CV disturbances, cyanosis, methemoglobinemia, moderate leukocytosis or leukopenia, vomiting, granulocytopenia, acute hemolytic anemia, acute hemolysis.

NURSING CONSIDERATIONS
● Use drug with a fast-acting antimalarial such as chloroquine to reduce possibility of drug-resistant strains.
● Obtain frequent blood studies and urinalysis in light-skinned patients taking more than 30 mg base daily, dark-skinned patients taking more than 15 mg base daily, and patients with severe anemia or suspected sensitivity.

● Monitor patient for markedly darkened urine and for suddenly reduced hemoglobin level or RBC or WBC count, which suggest impending hemolytic reactions. Stop drug immediately and notify prescriber.
● Safe use during pregnancy hasn't been established.
● *Look alike–sound alike:* Don't confuse primaquine with primidone.

PATIENT TEACHING
● Instruct patient to take drug with meals to minimize stomach upset. If nausea, vomiting, or stomach pain persists, tell patient to notify prescriber.
● Tell patient to report to prescriber chills, fever, chest pain, and bluish skin discoloration; these signs and symptoms may suggest a hemolytic reaction.
● Tell patient to stop drug and notify prescriber immediately if urine darkens markedly.
● Stress importance of completing full course of therapy.

probenecid
proe-BEN-e-sid

Probalan

Therapeutic class: Uricosurics
Pharmacologic class: Sulfonamide derivatives
Pregnancy risk category: C

AVAILABLE FORMS
Tablets: 500 mg

INDICATIONS & DOSAGES
➤ **Adjunct to penicillin therapy**
Adults and children age 15 and older weighing more than 50 kg (110 lb): 500 mg P.O. q.i.d.
Children ages 2 to 14 or weighing 50 kg or less: Initially, 25 mg/kg P.O.; then 40 mg/kg/day in four divided doses daily.
➤ **Alternative therapy for uncomplicated gonorrhea**
Adults: 4.8 million units aqueous procaine penicillin G I.M. (divided into two injected doses at one visit) or 3.5 g ampicillin P.O. plus probenecid 1 g P.O.

➤ **Hyperuricemia of gout, gouty arthritis**
Adults: 250 mg P.O. b.i.d. for first week;
then 500 mg b.i.d., to maximum of 2 to
3 g daily. Review maintenance dose every 6 months and reduce by increments of
500 mg, if indicated.

ADMINISTRATION
P.O.
● To minimize GI distress, give drug with
milk, food, or antacids. If unrelieved,
consider reducing dosage.

ACTION
Blocks renal tubular reabsorption of uric
acid, increasing excretion, and inhibits
active renal tubular secretion of many
weak organic acids, such as penicillins
and cephalosporins.

Route	Onset	Peak	Duration
P.O.	Unknown	2–4 hr	Unknown

Half-life: 3 to 8 hours after 500-mg dose; 4 to
17 hours after larger doses.

ADVERSE REACTIONS
CNS: fever, headache, dizziness.
CV: flushing.
GI: anorexia, nausea, vomiting, sore gums.
GU: urinary frequency, renal colic,
nephrotic syndrome, costovertebral pain.
Hematologic: *aplastic anemia,* hemolytic
anemia, anemia.
Hepatic: *hepatic necrosis.*
Skin: dermatitis, pruritus.
Other: worsening of gout, hypersensitivity
reactions including *anaphylaxis.*

INTERACTIONS
Drug-drug. *Acyclovir, cephalosporins,
clofibrate, dapsone, indomethacin, ketamine, lorazepam, meclofenamate, penicillin, rifampin, sulfonamides, thiopental:*
May increase levels of these drugs. Use
together cautiously.
Allopurinol: May increase uric acid–
lowering effects. May be used to therapeutic
advantage.
Methotrexate: May impair excretion of
methotrexate, causing increased level,
effects, and toxicity of methotrexate.
Don't use together.

Nitrofurantoin: May increase toxicity and
reduce effectiveness of nitrofurantoin.
Reduce probenecid dose.
NSAIDs: May increase NSAID toxicity.
Avoid using together.
Salicylates: May inhibit uricosuric effect of
probenecid, causing urate retention. Don't
use together.
Sulfonylureas: May increase hypoglycemic
effect. Monitor glucose level closely.
Dosage may need to be adjusted.
Zidovudine: May increase zidovudine level
and toxicity symptoms. Monitor patient.
Drug-lifestyle. *Alcohol use:* May increase
urate level. Discourage use together.

EFFECTS ON LAB TEST RESULTS
● May decrease hemoglobin level and
hematocrit.
● May falsely elevate theophylline level.

CONTRAINDICATIONS & CAUTIONS
● Contraindicated in patients hypersensitive to drug and in those with uric acid
kidney stones or blood dyscrasias; also
contraindicated in patients with an acute
gout attack and in children younger than
age 2.
● Use cautiously in patients with peptic
ulcer or renal impairment.
● Use cautiously in patients with sulfa
allergy because probenecid is a sulfonamide
derivative.

NURSING CONSIDERATIONS
● Force fluids to maintain minimum daily
output of 2 to 3 L. Alkalinize urine with
sodium bicarbonate or potassium citrate.
These measures prevent hematuria, renal
colic, urate stone development, and costovertebral pain.
● Don't use to treat gout until acute attack
subsides. Drug has no analgesic or antiinflammatory effects and is of no value
during acute gout attacks.
● Monitor BUN and renal function test
results periodically in long-term therapy.
● Drug is suitable for long-term use; no
cumulative effects or tolerance have been
reported.
● Drug is ineffective in patients with GFR
below 30 mL/minute.

P

• Drug may increase frequency, severity, and length of acute gout attacks during first 6 to 12 months of therapy. Appropriate therapy may be used preventively during first 3 to 6 months.
• *Look alike–sound alike:* Don't confuse probenecid with Procanbid.

PATIENT TEACHING
• Instruct patient with gout to take drug regularly to prevent recurrence.
• Tell patient to visit prescriber regularly so that uric acid can be monitored and dosage adjusted, if needed. Lifelong therapy may be needed in patients with hyperuricemia.
• Advise patient with gout to avoid all drugs that contain aspirin, which may precipitate gout. Acetaminophen may be used for pain.
• Instruct patient to drink at least 6 to 8 glasses of water per day.
• Urge patient with gout to avoid alcohol; it increases urate level.
• Tell patient with gout to limit intake of foods high in purine, such as anchovies, liver, sardines, kidneys, sweetbreads, peas, and lentils. Also tell him to identify and avoid other foods that may trigger gout attacks.
• Because drug may be prescribed with an antibiotic, instruct patient to take all medicine as prescribed.

SAFETY ALERT!

procainamide hydrochloride
proe-KANE-a-myed

Apo-Procainamide†, Procan SR†

Therapeutic class: Antiarrhythmics
Pharmacologic class: Procaine derivatives
Pregnancy risk category: C

AVAILABLE FORMS
Capsules†: 250 mg, 375 mg, 500 mg
Injection: 100 mg/mL, 500 mg/mL
Tablets (extended-release)†: 250 mg, 500 mg, 750 mg

INDICATIONS & DOSAGES
➤ **Symptomatic PVCs, life-threatening ventricular tachycardia**
Adults: For oral therapy, start at 50 mg/kg/day P.O. of conventional capsules in divided doses every 3 hours until therapeutic level is reached. For maintenance, substitute extended-release form to deliver the total daily dose divided every 6 hours or extended-release form at a dose of 50 mg/kg P.O. in two divided doses every 12 hours.

For I.V. administration, 100 mg every 5 minutes by slow I.V. push, no faster than 25 to 50 mg/minute, until arrhythmias disappear, adverse effects develop, or 500 mg has been given. Usual effective loading dose is 500 to 600 mg. Or, give a loading dose of 500 to 600 mg I.V. infusion over 25 to 30 minutes. Maximum total dose is 1 g. When arrhythmias disappear, give continuous infusion of 2 to 6 mg/minute. If arrhythmias recur, repeat bolus as above and increase infusion rate.

For I.M. administration, give 50 mg/kg divided into fractional doses of ⅛ to ¼ every 3 to 6 hours until oral therapy is possible; if arrhythmias occur during surgery, give 100 to 500 mg I.M.
Adjust-a-dose: For patients with renal or hepatic dysfunction, decrease dose or increase dosing interval, as needed.

ADMINISTRATION
P.O.
☻ *Alert:* Don't crush the extended-release tablets.
I.V.
▼ Vials for I.V. injection contain 1 g of drug: 100 mg/mL (10 mL) or 500 mg/mL (2 mL).
▼ Dilute with compatible I.V. solution, such as D_5W injection (1 g diluted to 50 mL), and give with the patient supine at a rate not exceeding 25 to 50 mg/minute. Keep patient supine during I.V. administration.
▼ Attend patient receiving infusion at all times. Use an infusion-control device to give infusion precisely.
▼ Monitor blood pressure and ECG continuously during I.V. administration. Watch for prolonged QTc intervals and QRS

complexes, heart block, or increased arrhythmias. If such reactions occur, withhold drug, obtain rhythm strip, and notify prescriber immediately. If drug is given too rapidly, hypotension can occur. Watch closely for adverse reactions during infusion, and notify prescriber if they occur.

▼ **Incompatibilities:** Bretylium, esmolol, ethacrynate, milrinone, phenytoin sodium.

I.M.

● I.M. injections are a substitute for oral administration in patients who are not allowed anything by mouth. Oral dosing should be resumed as soon as possible.

ACTION

Decreases excitability, conduction velocity, automaticity, and membrane responsiveness with prolonged refractory period. Larger than usual doses may induce AV block.

Route	Onset	Peak	Duration
P.O.	Unknown	90–120 min	Unknown
I.V.	Immediate	Immediate	Unknown
I.M.	10–30 min	15–60 min	Unknown

Half-life: About 2½ to 4¾ hours.

ADVERSE REACTIONS

CNS: fever, *seizures,* hallucinations, psychosis, giddiness, confusion, depression, dizziness.
CV: hypotension, *bradycardia, AV block, ventricular fibrillation, ventricular asystole.*
GI: abdominal pain, nausea, vomiting, anorexia, diarrhea, bitter taste.
Skin: maculopapular rash, urticaria, pruritus, flushing.
Other: lupuslike syndrome, *angioneurotic edema.*

INTERACTIONS

Drug-drug. *Amiodarone:* May increase procainamide level and toxicity and have additive effects on QTc interval and QRS complex. Avoid using together.
Antiarrhythmics: May enhance antiarrhythmic and hypotensive effects. Avoid using together.
Anticholinergics: May increase antivagal effects. Monitor patient closely.

Beta blockers, ranitidine, trimethoprim: May increase procainamide level. Watch for toxicity.
Cimetidine, ranitidine: May increase procainamide level. Avoid using together if possible. Monitor procainamide level closely and adjust the dosage as necessary.
Macrolides and related antibiotics (azithromycin, clarithromycin, erythromycin, telithromycin): May prolong the QT interval. Use with caution. Avoid use with telithromycin.
Neuromuscular blockers: May increase skeletal muscle relaxant effect. May need to decrease dosage of neuromuscular blocker.
Quinolones: Life-threatening arrhythmias, including torsades de pointes, can occur. Avoid using together; sparfloxacin is contraindicated.
Thioridazine, ziprasidone: May prolong QTc interval. Avoid using together.
Drug-herb. *Jimsonweed:* May adversely affect CV function. Discourage use together.
Licorice: May prolong QTc interval. Urge caution.
Drug-lifestyle. *Alcohol use:* May reduce drug level. Discourage use together.

EFFECTS ON LAB TEST RESULTS

● May increase ALT, AST, alkaline phosphatase, LDH, and bilirubin levels.
● May decrease hemoglobin level, hematocrit, and WBC and platelet counts.
● May cause positive ANA titers and positive direct antiglobulin (Coombs) tests.

CONTRAINDICATIONS & CAUTIONS

● Contraindicated in patients hypersensitive to this drug and related drugs.
● Contraindicated in those with complete second- or third-degree heart block in the absence of an artificial pacemaker. Also contraindicated in those with myasthenia gravis, systemic lupus erythematosus, or atypical ventricular tachycardia (torsades de pointes).
● Use with extreme caution in patients with ventricular tachycardia during coronary occlusion.

P

• Use cautiously in patients with heart failure or other conduction disturbances, such as bundle-branch heart block, sinus bradycardia, or digoxin intoxication, and in those with hepatic or renal insufficiency.

Black Box Warning Use cautiously in patients with blood dyscrasias or bone marrow suppression. ∎

⚠ **Overdose S&S:** Progressive widening of QRS complex, prolonged QT and PR intervals, lowered R and T waves, increasing AV block, ventricular ectopy, ventricular tachycardia, hypotension, CNS depression, tremor, respiratory depression.

NURSING CONSIDERATIONS

Black Box Warning Because of its proarrhythmic effects, procainamide should be reserved for patients with life-threatening ventricular arrhythmias. ∎

• Digitalize or cardiovert patients with atrial flutter or fibrillation before therapy with procainamide to prevent ventricular rate acceleration in patient.

• Monitor level of drug and its active metabolite N-acetylprocainamide (NAPA). To suppress ventricular arrhythmias, therapeutic levels of procainamide are 4 to 8 mcg/mL; therapeutic levels of NAPA are 10 to 30 mcg/mL.

• Monitor ECG closely. If QRS widens more than 25% or marked prolongation of the QTc interval occurs, check for overdosage.

• Hypokalemia predisposes patient to arrhythmias. Monitor electrolytes, especially potassium level.

• Elderly patients may be more likely to develop hypotension. Monitor blood pressure carefully.

Black Box Warning Agranulocytosis, bone marrow depression, neutropenia, hypoplastic anemia, and thrombocytopenia have been noted in patients during the first 12 weeks of therapy. It is recommended that CBCs be performed at weekly intervals for the first 3 months of therapy and periodically thereafter. ∎

Black Box Warning Perform CBCs promptly if patient develops signs of infection, bruising, or bleeding. If hematologic disorder is identified, discontinue drug. Blood counts usually return to normal within 1 month of discontinuation. ∎

Black Box Warning Positive ANA titer is common in about 60% of patients who don't have symptoms of lupuslike syndrome. This response seems to be related to prolonged use, not dosage. If positive ANA titer develops, assess the benefits and risks of continued therapy. ∎

• Discontinue I.V. therapy if persistent conduction disturbances or hypotension develops. As soon as cardiac rhythm is stabilized, oral antiarrhythmic maintenance therapy is preferable.

PATIENT TEACHING

• Stress importance of taking drug exactly as prescribed. This may require use of an alarm clock for nighttime doses.

• Instruct patient to report fever, rash, muscle pain, diarrhea, bleeding, bruises, or pleuritic chest pain.

• Tell patient not to crush or break extended-release tablets.

• Reassure patient who is taking extended-release form that a wax-matrix "ghost" from the tablet may be passed in stools. Drug is completely absorbed before this occurs.

SAFETY ALERT!

procarbazine hydrochloride
proe-KAR-buh-zeen

Matulane

Therapeutic class: Antineoplastics
Pharmacologic class: Methylhydrazine derivatives
Pregnancy risk category: D

AVAILABLE FORMS
Capsules: 50 mg

INDICATIONS & DOSAGES
➤ **Adjunctive treatment of Hodgkin lymphoma (stages III and IV) and other cancers using nitrogen mustard, vincristine, procarbazine, prednisone (known as MOPP) regimen**
Adults: 2 to 4 mg/kg P.O. daily in single dose or divided doses for first week. Then, 4 to 6 mg/kg daily until WBC count falls below 4,000/mm³, platelet count falls below 100,000/mm³, or maximum response

is obtained. Maintenance dose is 1 to 2 mg/kg daily after bone marrow recovery. For MOPP regimen, 100 mg/m^2 daily P.O. for first 14 days of 28-day cycle. Treat with minimum of six cycles of MOPP plus two to three cycles of consolidation chemotherapy.

Children: 50 mg/m^2 P.O. daily for first week; then 100 mg/m^2 until response or toxicity occurs. Maintenance dose is 50 mg/m^2 P.O. daily after bone marrow recovery.

Adjust-a-dose: If serum bilirubin level is 5 mg/dL or less and AST or ALT level is 1.6 to 6 times the upper limit of normal (ULN), give 75% of usual dose. If serum bilirubin level is 5 mg/dL or less and AST or ALT level is more than 6 × ULN, use clinical judgment to determine dose. Don't give if serum bilirubin level is greater than 5 mg/dL.

ADMINISTRATION
P.O.
• Give drug with or after meals. May give once daily or in two to three divided doses.
• For patient unable to swallow capsules whole, empty capsule contents into sterile water for injection. Stir until dissolved; then have patient drink the mixture immediately. Rinse the container with additional water and have patient drink.

ACTION
Unknown. Thought to inhibit DNA, RNA, and protein synthesis.

Route	Onset	Peak	Duration
P.O.	Unknown	Unknown	Unknown

Half-life: 10 minutes.

ADVERSE REACTIONS
CNS: ataxia, hallucinations, *coma,* confusion, depression, dizziness, headache, insomnia, nervousness, neuropathy, nightmares, paresthesia, syncope, *seizures.*
CV: flushing, hypotension, tachycardia.
EENT: nystagmus, photophobia, retinal hemorrhage, diplopia, hearing loss.
GI: nausea, vomiting, abdominal pain, anorexia, constipation, diarrhea, dry mouth, dysphagia, *hematemesis, melena,* stomatitis.
GU: hematuria, nocturia, urinary frequency.

Hematologic: *anemia, bleeding tendency, leukopenia, thrombocytopenia,* eosinophilia, hemolytic anemia.
Hepatic: *hepatotoxicity,* jaundice.
Respiratory: pleural effusion, cough, pneumonitis.
Skin: dermatitis, hyperpigmentation, pruritus, rash, reversible alopecia.
Other: *secondary malignancies,* allergic reaction, gynecomastia, herpes outbreak.

INTERACTIONS
Drug-drug. *CNS depressants:* May cause additive depressant effects. Avoid using together.
Digoxin: May decrease digoxin level. Monitor digoxin level closely.
Drugs high in tyramine, local anesthetics, MAO inhibitors, sympathomimetics, TCAs: May cause tremor, palpitations, and increased blood pressure. Monitor patient closely.
Methotrexate: The nephrotoxicity of methotrexate may be increased. Wait 72 hours or longer between giving the final dose of procarbazine and starting a high-dose methotrexate infusion.
Drug-food. *Caffeine:* May result in arrhythmias and severe hypertension. Discourage caffeine intake.
Foods high in tyramine (cheese, Chianti): May cause tremor, palpitations, and increased blood pressure. Monitor patient closely; advise him to avoid or limit intake.
Drug-lifestyle. *Alcohol use:* Mild disulfiram-like reaction may cause flushing, headache, nausea, and hypotension. Warn patient to avoid alcoholic beverages.

EFFECTS ON LAB TEST RESULTS
• May decrease hemoglobin level.
• May increase eosinophil count. May decrease platelet, RBC, and WBC counts.

CONTRAINDICATIONS & CAUTIONS
• Contraindicated in patients hypersensitive to drug and in those with inadequate bone marrow reserve as shown by bone marrow aspiration.
• Use cautiously in patients with impaired hepatic or renal function.

⚠ *Overdose S&S:* Nausea, vomiting, diarrhea, enteritis, hypotension, tremors, seizures, coma.

NURSING CONSIDERATIONS

Black Box Warning Give drug only under the supervision of a physician experienced with potent antineoplastic drugs. Adequate clinical and laboratory facilities should be available. ∎

• Monitor CBC and platelet counts.

۞ *Alert:* Prompt discontinuation of therapy is recommended if patient develops CNS signs or symptoms, such as paresthesia, neuropathies, or confusion; leukopenia (WBC count less than 4,000 cell/mm^3); thrombocytopenia (platelet count less than 100,000 cells/mm^3); hypersensitivity reaction; stomatitis; diarrhea; or hemorrhage or bleeding tendencies.

• Bone marrow depression begins 2 to 8 weeks after the start of treatment.

• Avoid all I.M. injections when platelet count is below 50,000/mm^3.

• The manufacturer recommends that if radiation or chemotherapeutic agents with bone marrow depressant activity have been used, give patient a 1-month interval without such therapy before beginning procarbazine therapy.

• *Look alike–sound alike:* Don't confuse procarbazine with dacarbazine.

PATIENT TEACHING

• To decrease nausea and vomiting, advise patient to take drug at bedtime and in divided doses.

• Tell patient to watch for fever, sore throat, fatigue, easy bruising, nosebleeds, bleeding gums, or tarry stools. Tell patient to take temperature daily.

• Advise patient to discontinue alcohol during therapy.

• Instruct patient to avoid OTC medications that contain antihistamines and sympathomimetics and to avoid foods and drinks high in tyramine, such as wine, tea, coffee, cola, cheese, and bananas.

• Warn patient to avoid hazardous activities that require alertness and good motor coordination until CNS effects of drug are known.

• Caution women of childbearing age to avoid becoming pregnant during therapy and to consult prescriber before becoming pregnant.

prochlorperazine
proe-klor-PER-a-zeen

Compro

prochlorperazine edisylate

prochlorperazine maleate
Nu-Prochlor†, Procomp

Therapeutic class: Antiemetics
Pharmacologic class: Dopamine antagonists
Pregnancy risk category: C

AVAILABLE FORMS
prochlorperazine
Suppositories: 10 mg†, 25 mg
prochlorperazine edisylate
Injection: 5 mg/mL
Suppositories: 25 mg
prochlorperazine maleate
Tablets: 5 mg, 10 mg, 25 mg

INDICATIONS & DOSAGES
➤ **To control preoperative nausea**
Adults: 5 to 10 mg I.M. 1 to 2 hours before induction of anesthesia; repeat once in 30 minutes, if needed. Or, 5 to 10 mg I.V. 15 to 30 minutes before induction of anesthesia; repeat once, if needed.

➤ **Severe nausea and vomiting**
Adults: 5 to 10 mg P.O. t.i.d. or q.i.d.; 25 mg P.R. b.i.d.; or 5 to 10 mg I.M., repeated every 3 to 4 hours, as needed. Maximum I.M. dose is 40 mg daily. Or, 2.5 to 10 mg I.V. at no more than 5 mg/minute. Maximum I.V. dose is 40 mg daily.
Children weighing 18 to 39 kg (39 to 86 lb): 2.5 mg P.O. or P.R. t.i.d.; or 5 mg P.O. or P.R. b.i.d. Maximum, 15 mg daily. Or, 0.132 mg/kg by deep I.M. injection. Control is usually achieved with one dose.
Children weighing 14 to 17 kg (30 to 38 lb): 2.5 mg P.O. or P.R. b.i.d. or t.i.d. Maximum, 10 mg daily. Or, 0.132 mg/kg by deep I.M.

---

injection. Control is usually achieved with one dose.

Children weighing 9 to 13 kg (20 to 29 lb): 2.5 mg P.O. or P.R. once daily or b.i.d. Maximum, 7.5 mg daily. Or, 0.132 mg/kg by deep I.M. injection. Control is usually achieved with one dose.

➤ **Schizophrenia**

Adults: For mild conditions, 5 or 10 mg P.O. t.i.d. or q.i.d. For moderate to severe conditions, start with 10 mg P.O. t.i.d. or q.i.d.; increase by small increments every 2 or 3 days until symptoms are controlled or adverse reactions become bothersome. For severe conditions, 100 to 150 mg P.O. daily. Or, for severe symptoms, 10 to 20 mg by deep I.M. injection. Repeat the initial I.M. dose every 2 to 4 hours (or, in resistant cases, every hour) to gain control of patient, as necessary. More than three or four I.M. doses is seldom necessary. If, in rare cases, parenteral therapy is needed for a prolonged period, give 10 to 20 mg I.M. every 4 to 6 hours. After control is achieved, switch patient to an oral form of drug at same dosage level or higher.

Children ages 2 to 12: Initially, 2.5 mg P.O. b.i.d. or t.i.d., not to exceed 10 mg on the first day. Increase dosage according to patient's response. Maximum dose is 20 mg/day (ages 2 to 5) or 25 mg/day (ages 6 to 12). Or, give 0.132 mg/kg (0.06 mg/lb) by deep I.M. injection. Control is usually achieved with one I.M. dose. After control is achieved, switch patient to an oral form of drug at same dosage level or higher.

➤ **Nonpsychotic anxiety**

Adults: 5 mg P.O. t.i.d. or q.i.d. Maximum dose is 20 mg/dL for no longer than 12 weeks.

ADMINISTRATION
P.O.
● Protect from light.
I.V.
▼ Add 20 mg of drug per liter of D_5W and normal saline solution, 15 to 30 minutes before induction of anesthesia.
▼ Infuse slowly; rate shouldn't exceed 5 mg/minute. Maximum parenteral dose is 40 mg daily.

▼ To prevent contact dermatitis, avoid getting injection solution on hands or clothing.
▼ **Incompatibilities:** Aldesleukin, allopurinol, amifostine, aminophylline, amphotericin B, ampicillin sodium, aztreonam, calcium gluconate, chloramphenicol sodium succinate, chlorothiazide, dexamethasone sodium phosphate, dimenhydrinate, etoposide, filgrastim, fludarabine, foscarnet, furosemide, gemcitabine, heparin sodium, hydrocortisone sodium succinate, hydromorphone, ketorolac, solutions containing methylparabens, midazolam hydrochloride, morphine, penicillin G potassium, penicillin G sodium, pentobarbital, phenobarbital sodium, phenytoin sodium, piperacillin sodium–tazobactam sodium, solutions containing propylparabens, thiopental, vitamin B complex with C.
I.M.
● For I.M. use, inject deeply into upper outer quadrant of gluteal region.
● Don't give by subcutaneous route or mix in syringe with another drug.
● To prevent contact dermatitis, avoid getting injection solution on hands or clothing.
● Store in light-resistant container. Slight yellowing doesn't affect potency; discard extremely discolored solutions.
Rectal
● Protect from light.

ACTION
Acts on the chemoreceptor trigger zone to inhibit nausea and vomiting; in larger doses, it partially depresses vomiting center.

Route	Onset	Peak	Duration
P.O.	30–40 min	Unknown	3–12 hr
I.V.	Unknown	Unknown	Unknown
I.M.	10–20 min	Unknown	3–4 hr
P.R.	1 hr	Unknown	3–4 hr

Half-life: Unknown.

ADVERSE REACTIONS
CNS: extrapyramidal reactions, dizziness, EEG changes, pseudoparkinsonism, sedation, drowsiness, motor restlessness, dystonia, tardive dyskinesia.

CV: orthostatic hypotension, ECG changes, tachycardia.
EENT: blurred vision, ocular changes.
GI: constipation, dry mouth, increased appetite.
GU: urine retention, dark urine, inhibited ejaculation, menstrual irregularities.
Hematologic: *agranulocytosis, transient leukopenia.*
Hepatic: cholestatic jaundice.
Metabolic: weight gain.
Skin: mild photosensitivity reactions, allergic reactions, exfoliative dermatitis.
Other: gynecomastia, hyperprolactinemia.

INTERACTIONS
Drug-drug. *Antacids:* May inhibit absorption of oral phenothiazines. Separate antacid and phenothiazine doses by at least 2 hours.
Anticholinergics, including antidepressants and antiparkinsonians: May increase anticholinergic activity and may aggravate parkinsonian symptoms. Use together cautiously.
Barbiturates: May decrease phenothiazine effect. Monitor patient for decreased antiemetic effect.
CNS depressants (anesthetics, opioids): May intensify or prolong action of these drugs. Monitor patient.
Drug-herb. *Dong quai, St. John's wort:* May increase risk of photosensitivity. Advise patient to avoid excessive sun exposure.
Kava: May increase risk of dystonic reactions. Discourage use together.
Drug-lifestyle. *Alcohol use:* May increase CNS depression, particularly psychomotor skills. Strongly discourage use together.

EFFECTS ON LAB TEST RESULTS
• May decrease WBC and granulocyte counts.
• May cause false-positive results for phenylketonuria tests. May cause abnormal LFT results.

CONTRAINDICATIONS & CAUTIONS
• Contraindicated in patients hypersensitive to phenothiazines and in patients with CNS depression, including those in a coma.

• Contraindicated during pediatric surgery, when using spinal or epidural anesthetic or adrenergic blockers, and in children younger than age 2.
Black Box Warning Drug isn't approved for the treatment of patients with dementia-related psychosis. ∎
• Use cautiously in patients with impaired CV function, glaucoma, seizure disorders, and Parkinson disease; in those who have been exposed to extreme heat; and in children with acute illness.
❸ Alert: Neonates exposed to antipsychotics during the third trimester of pregnancy are at risk for developing extrapyramidal signs and symptoms (repetitive muscle movements of the face and body) and withdrawal signs and symptoms (agitation, abnormally increased or decreased muscle tone, tremors, sleepiness, severe difficulty breathing, difficulty feeding) following delivery. Use in pregnancy only if the potential benefit to the mother justifies the risk to the fetus. ∎
⚠ Overdose S&S: Dystonic reactions, CNS depression, agitation, restlessness, seizures, ECG changes, cardiac arrhythmias, fever, hypotension, dry mouth, ileus.

NURSING CONSIDERATIONS
Black Box Warning Elderly patients with dementia-related psychosis treated with antipsychotics are at an increased risk for death. ∎
• Watch for orthostatic hypotension, especially when giving drug I.V.
• Monitor CBC and LFTs during long-term therapy.
❸ Alert: Use drug only when vomiting can't be controlled by other measures or when only a few doses are needed. If more than four doses are needed in 24 hours, notify prescriber.
• **Look alike–sound alike:** Don't confuse prochlorperazine with chlorpromazine.

PATIENT TEACHING
• Advise patient to wear protective clothing when exposed to sunlight.
• Tell patient to call prescriber if more than four doses are needed within 24 hours.

Reactions in bold italics are *life-threatening*. Interactions may have a *rapid onset* or a *delayed onset*.

promethazine hydrochloride
proe-METH-a-zeen

Promethegan

Therapeutic class: Antiemetics
Pharmacologic class: Phenothiazines
Pregnancy risk category: C

AVAILABLE FORMS
Injection: 25 mg/mL, 50 mg/mL
Suppositories: 12.5 mg, 25 mg, 50 mg
Syrup: 6.25 mg/5 mL*
Tablets: 12.5 mg, 25 mg, 50 mg

INDICATIONS & DOSAGES
➤ **Motion sickness**
Adults: 25 mg P.O. or P.R. taken 30 minutes to 1 hour before departure. May repeat dose 8 to 12 hours later p.r.n. Then, 25 mg P.O. b.i.d. on successive travel days.
Children older than age 2: 12.5 to 25 mg P.O. or P.R. 30 minutes to 1 hour before departure. May repeat dose 8 to 12 hours later p.r.n.
➤ **Nausea and vomiting**
Adults: 12.5 to 25 mg P.O., I.M., or P.R. every 4 to 6 hours p.r.n.
Children older than age 2: 12.5 to 25 mg P.O. or P.R. every 4 to 6 hours p.r.n. Or, 6.25 to 12.5 mg I.M. every 4 to 6 hours p.r.n.
➤ **Rhinitis, allergy symptoms**
Adults: 25 mg P.O. or P.R. at bedtime; or, 12.5 mg P.O. or P.R. t.i.d. and at bedtime. Or, 25 mg deep I.M. or I.V. May repeat dose within 2 hours if needed. Resume oral dosing as soon as possible.
Children older than age 2: 25 mg P.O. or P.R. at bedtime; or, 6.25 to 12.5 mg P.O. or P.R. t.i.d.
➤ **Nighttime sedation**
Adults: 25 to 50 mg P.O., I.M., or P.R. at bedtime. Or, 25 mg I.V. at bedtime.
Children older than age 2: 12.5 to 25 mg P.O., I.M., or P.R. at bedtime.
➤ **Adjunct to analgesics for routine preoperative or postoperative sedation**
Adults: 25 to 50 mg I.M., P.O. or P.R. Or, 25 mg I.V.
Children older than age 2: 0.5 to 1.1 mg/kg P.O., I.M., or P.R.

➤ **Obstetric sedation**
Adults: 50 mg deep I.M. or I.V. in the early stages of labor. When labor is definitely established, give 25 to 75 mg I.M. or I.V. with an appropriately reduced dose of desired opioid. If necessary, may repeat once or twice at 4-hour intervals. Maximum dose is 100 mg/24 hours.
➤ **Nausea and vomiting of pregnancy** ◆
Adults: 12.5 to 25 mg P.O., I.V., or P.R. every 4 hours.

ADMINISTRATION
P.O.
● Reduce GI distress by giving drug with food or milk.
I.V.
▼ If solution is discolored or contains a precipitate, discard.
▼ Give injection through a free-flowing I.V. line.
Black Box Warning Be alert for extravasation. Severe chemical irritation and damage can result. ■
✪ *Alert:* Don't give at a concentration above 25 mg/mL or a rate above 25 mg/minute.
Black Box Warning Don't give I.V. solution subcutaneously or intra-arterially. ■
▼ **Incompatibilities:** Aldesleukin, allopurinol, aminophylline, amphotericin B, cephalosporins, chloramphenicol sodium succinate, chloroquine phosphate, chlorothiazide, diatrizoate, dimenhydrinate, doxorubicin liposomal, foscarnet, furosemide, heparin sodium, hydrocortisone sodium succinate, iodipamide meglumine (52%), iothalamate, ketorolac, methohexital, morphine, nalbuphine, penicillin G potassium, penicillin G sodium, pentobarbital sodium, phenobarbital sodium, phenytoin sodium, thiopental, vitamin B complex.
I.M.
Black Box Warning I.M. injection is the preferred parenteral route. Inject deep I.M. into large muscle mass. ■
● Rotate injection sites.
Rectal
● If suppository is too soft, place wrapped in refrigerator for 15 minutes or run under cold water.

P

ACTION

Phenothiazine derivative that competes with histamine for H_1-receptor sites on effector cells. Prevents, but doesn't reverse, histamine-mediated responses. At high doses, drug also has local anesthetic effects.

Route	Onset	Peak	Duration
P.O.	15–60 min	Unknown	<12 hr
I.V.	3–5 min	Unknown	<12 hr
I.M., P.R.	20 min	Unknown	<12 hr

Half-life: Unknown.

ADVERSE REACTIONS

CNS: drowsiness, sedation, confusion, sleepiness, dizziness, disorientation, extrapyramidal symptoms.
CV: hypotension, hypertension.
EENT: dry mouth, blurred vision.
GI: nausea, vomiting.
GU: urine retention.
Hematologic: *leukopenia, agranulocytosis, thrombocytopenia.*
Metabolic: hyperglycemia.
Respiratory: *respiratory depression, apnea.*
Skin: photosensitivity, rash.

INTERACTIONS

Drug-drug. *Anticholinergics, TCAs:* May increase anticholinergic effects. Avoid using together.
Antipsychotics: May increase risk of neuroleptic malignant syndrome. Monitor patient; discontinue promethazine if interaction is suspected.
CNS depressants: May increase sedation. Use together cautiously. If used together, reduce opiate dose by at least 25% to 50%, and reduce barbiturate dose by at least 50%.
Epinephrine: May block or reverse effects of epinephrine. Use other pressor drugs instead.
Levodopa: May decrease antiparkinsonian action of levodopa. Avoid using together.
Lithium: May reduce GI absorption or enhance renal elimination of lithium. Avoid using together.
MAO inhibitors: May increase extrapyramidal effects. Avoid using together.

Drug-herb. *Yohimbe:* May increase risk of herb toxicity. Ask patient about use of herbal remedies, and recommend caution.
Drug-lifestyle. *Alcohol use:* May increase sedation. Discourage use together.
Sun exposure: May cause photosensitivity reactions. Advise patient to avoid extensive sunlight exposure and to use sunblock.

EFFECTS ON LAB TEST RESULTS

• May increase hemoglobin level and hematocrit and blood glucose level.
• May decrease WBC, platelet, and granulocyte counts.
• May prevent, reduce, or mask positive result in diagnostic skin test. May cause false-positive or false-negative pregnancy test result. May interfere with blood grouping in the ABO system.

CONTRAINDICATIONS & CAUTIONS

• Contraindicated in patients hypersensitive to drug, those who have experienced adverse reactions to phenothiazines, breast-feeding women, comatose patients, and acutely ill or dehydrated children.
Black Box Warning Contraindicated in children younger than age 2 because of the potential for fatal respiratory depression. Use the lowest effective dose in children older than age 2 and avoid administering with drugs that can cause respiratory depression. ▌
• Use cautiously in patients with asthma or pulmonary, hepatic, or CV disease and in those with intestinal obstruction, prostatic hyperplasia, bladder-neck obstruction, angle-closure glaucoma, seizure disorders, CNS depression, and stenosing or peptic ulcerations.

⚠ Overdose S&S: Hypotension, respiratory depression, ataxia, athetosis, positive Babinski reflex, unconsciousness, hyperreflexia, hypertonia, dry mouth, fixed dilated pupils, flushing, GI symptoms, seizures, sudden death; hyperexcitability, nightmares (in children).

NURSING CONSIDERATIONS

Black Box Warning Perivascular extravasation, unintentional intra-arterial injection, or intraneuronal or perineuronal infiltration

---

Reactions in bold italics are *life-threatening*. Interactions may have a *rapid onset* or a *delayed onset*.

of the drug may result in irritation and tissue damage. Adverse reactions include burning, pain, thrombophlebitis, tissue necrosis, and gangrene. ∎

• Monitor patient for neuroleptic malignant syndrome: altered mental status, autonomic instability, muscle rigidity, and hyperpyrexia.

• Stop drug 4 days before diagnostic skin testing because antihistamines can prevent, reduce, or mask positive skin test response.

• Drug is used as an adjunct to analgesics, usually to increase sedation; it has no analgesic activity.

• Drug may be mixed with meperidine in same syringe.

• In patients scheduled for a myelogram, stop drug 48 hours before procedure. Don't resume drug until 24 hours after procedure because of the risk of seizures.

• *Look alike–sound alike:* Don't confuse promethazine with chlorpromazine or prednisone.

PATIENT TEACHING

• Tell patient to take oral form with food or milk.

• When treating motion sickness, tell patient to take first dose 30 to 60 minutes before travel; dose may be repeated in 8 to 12 hours, if necessary. On succeeding days of travel, patient should take dose upon arising and with evening meal.

• Warn patient to avoid alcohol and hazardous activities that require alertness until CNS effects of drug are known.

• Inform patient that sugarless gum, hard candy, or ice chips may relieve dry mouth.

• Warn patient about possible photosensitivity reactions. Advise use of a sunblock.

• Advise patient to report discomfort at I.V. site immediately.

propafenone hydrochloride
proe-PAF-a-non

Rythmol, Rythmol SR

Therapeutic class: Antiarrhythmics
Pharmacologic class: Sodium channel antagonists
Pregnancy risk category: C

AVAILABLE FORMS
Capsules (extended-release): 225 mg, 325 mg, 425 mg
Tablets (immediate-release): 150 mg, 225 mg, 300 mg

INDICATIONS & DOSAGES
Adjust-a-dose (for all indications): For patients with hepatic impairment, reduce initial dose of immediate-release tablets by 70% to 80%.

➤ **To suppress life-threatening ventricular arrhythmias such as sustained ventricular tachycardia; to prevent paroxysmal supraventricular tachycardia (PSVT) and paroxysmal atrial fibrillation or flutter**

Adults: Initially, 150 mg immediate-release tablet P.O. every 8 hours. May increase dosage every 3 or 4 days to 225 mg every 8 hours. If needed, increase dosage to 300 mg every 8 hours. Maximum daily dose, 900 mg.

➤ **To prolong time until recurrence of symptomatic atrial fibrillation**

Adults: Initially, 150-mg immediate-release tablet P.O. every 8 hours. May increase dosage after 3 days to 225- to 300-mg immediate-release tablet P.O. every 8 hours. Maximum dosage is 900 mg/day. Or, 225 mg extended-release capsule P.O. every 12 hours. May increase dose after 5 days to 325 mg P.O. every 12 hours. May increase dose to 425 mg every 12 hours.

Adjust-a-dose: Reduce dose in patients with hepatic impairment, significant QRS complex widening, or second- or third-degree AV block.

P

ADMINISTRATION
P.O.
- Give without regard to food.
- Don't crush or open the extended-release capsules.

ACTION
Reduces inward sodium current in cardiac cells, prolongs refractory period in AV node, and decreases excitability, conduction velocity, and automaticity in cardiac tissue.

Route	Onset	Peak	Duration
P.O. (immediate-release)	Unknown	3½ hr	Unknown
P.O. (extended-release)	Unknown	3–8 hr	Unknown

Half-life: Estimated at 10 to 32 hours.

ADVERSE REACTIONS
CNS: dizziness, anxiety, ataxia, drowsiness, fatigue, headache, insomnia, syncope, tremor, weakness.
CV: *heart failure, bradycardia, arrhythmias, ventricular tachycardia, PVCs, ventricular fibrillation,* atrial fibrillation, bundle-branch block, angina, chest pain, edema, first-degree AV block, hypotension, prolonged QRS complex, intraventricular conduction delay, palpitations.
EENT: blurred vision.
GI: nausea, vomiting, abdominal pain or cramps, constipation, diarrhea, dyspepsia, anorexia, flatulence, dry mouth, unusual taste.
Musculoskeletal: arthralgia.
Respiratory: dyspnea.
Skin: rash, diaphoresis.

INTERACTIONS
Drug-drug. *Antiarrhythmics, paroxetine, sertraline:* May increase risk of prolonged QTc interval. Monitor patient closely.
Beta blockers (metoprolol, propranolol): May decrease metabolism of these drugs. Adjust dosage of beta blocker as needed.
Cimetidine: May increase propafenone levels. Monitor patient for adverse effects and toxicity.
*Cyclosporine, **digoxin:*** May increase levels of these drugs, causing toxicity. Monitor patient closely; dosage adjustment may be necessary.

Desipramine, haloperidol, imipramine, venlafaxine: May decrease metabolism of these drugs. Monitor patient closely.
Lidocaine: May decrease lidocaine metabolism. Monitor patient for increased CNS adverse effects and lidocaine toxicity.
Local anesthetics: May increase risk of CNS toxicity. Monitor patient closely.
Mexiletine: May decrease mexiletine metabolism, increasing level and adverse reactions. Monitor mexiletine level and patient closely.
Orlistat: May reduce fraction of propafenone available for absorption. Abrupt discontinuation of orlistat can result in severe adverse events. Use together with caution.
Phenobarbital, rifampin: May increase propafenone clearance. Watch for decreased antiarrhythmic effect.
Quinidine: May decrease propafenone metabolism; may be useful in certain patients refractory to propafenone and quinidine monotherapy. Monitor patient closely.
Ritonavir: May increase propafenone level, causing life-threatening arrhythmias. Avoid using together.
SSRIs, TCAs: May increase risk of cardiac arrhythmias. Avoid use together.
Theophylline: May decrease theophylline metabolism. Monitor theophylline level and ECG closely.
Warfarin: May increase warfarin level. Monitor PT and INR closely, and adjust warfarin dose as needed.
Drug-food. *Grapefruit juice:* May increase drug level. Discourage use together.

EFFECTS ON LAB TEST RESULTS
- May increase alkaline phosphatase, ALT, and AST levels.
- May cause positive ANA titers.

CONTRAINDICATIONS & CAUTIONS
- Contraindicated in patients hypersensitive to drug and in those with severe or uncontrolled heart failure; cardiogenic shock; SA, AV, or intraventricular disorders of impulse conduction without a pacemaker; bradycardia; Brugada syndrome; marked hypotension; bronchospastic disorders; or electrolyte imbalances.

Reactions in bold italics are *life-threatening*. Interactions may have a *rapid onset* or a *delayed onset*.

- Use cautiously in patients with a history of heart failure because drug may weaken the contraction of the heart.
- Use cautiously in patients taking other cardiac depressants and in those with hepatic or renal impairment.
- Use cautiously in patients with myasthenia gravis; may cause exacerbation.

⚠ **Overdose S&S:** Hypotension, somnolence, bradycardia, intra-atrial and intraventricular conduction disturbance.

NURSING CONSIDERATIONS
Black Box Warning Because of its proar-rhythmic effects, propafenone should be reserved for patients with life-threatening ventricular arrhythmias. ∎

☺ **Alert:** Perform continuous cardiac moni-toring at start of therapy and during dosage adjustments. If PR interval or QRS complex increases by more than 25%, reduce dosage.
- If using with digoxin, frequently monitor ECG and digoxin level.
- Pacing and sensing thresholds of arti-ficial pacemakers may change; monitor pacemaker function.
- Agranulocytosis may develop during the first 2 to 3 months of therapy. If patient has an unexplained fever, monitor leukocyte count.

PATIENT TEACHING
- Stress importance of taking drug exactly as prescribed.
- Tell patient not to double the dose if he misses one, but to take the next dose at the usual time.
- Tell patient to report adverse reactions promptly, including fever, sore throat, chills, and other signs and symptoms of infection.
- Tell patient to report swelling in arms or legs, trouble breathing, or sudden weight gain.
- Instruct patient to notify prescriber if prolonged diarrhea, sweating, vomiting, or loss of appetite or thirst occurs; these may cause an electrolyte imbalance.
- Tell patient not to crush, chew, or open the extended-release capsules.
- Tell patient to avoid grapefruit juice.

SAFETY ALERT!

propofol
PRO-puh-fole

Diprivan

Therapeutic class: Hypnotics
Pharmacologic class: Phenol derivatives
Pregnancy risk category: B

AVAILABLE FORMS
Injection: 10 mg/mL in ampules, vials, and prefilled syringes

INDICATIONS & DOSAGES
➤ **To induce anesthesia**
Adults younger than age 55 classified as American Society of Anesthesiologists (ASA) Physical Status (PS) category I or II: 2 to 2.5 mg/kg I.V. Give in 40-mg boluses every 10 seconds until desired response is achieved.
Children ages 3 to 16 classified as ASA PS I or II: 2.5 to 3.5 mg/kg I.V. over 20 to 30 seconds.
Adjust-a-dose: In geriatric, debilitated, hypovolemic, or ASA PS III or IV patients, give half the usual induction dose, in 20-mg boluses, every 10 seconds. For cardiac anesthesia, give 20 mg (0.5 to 1.5 mg/kg) every 10 seconds until desired response is achieved. For neurosurgical patients, give 20 mg (1 to 2 mg/kg) every 10 seconds until desired response is achieved.
➤ **To maintain anesthesia**
Healthy adults younger than age 55: 0.1 to 0.2 mg/kg/minute (6 to 12 mg/kg/hour) I.V. Or, 20- to 50-mg intermittent boluses, p.r.n.
Healthy children ages 3 to 16: 125 to 300 mcg/kg/minute (7.5 to 18 mg/kg/hour) I.V.
Adjust-a-dose: In geriatric, debilitated, hypovolemic, or ASA PS III or IV patients, give half the usual maintenance dose (0.05 to 0.1 mg/kg/minute or 3 to 6 mg/kg/hour). For cardiac anesthesia with sec-ondary opioid, 100 to 150 mcg/kg/minute; low dose with primary opioid, 50 to 100 mcg/kg/minute. For neurosurgical patients, 100 to 200 mcg/kg/minute (6 to 12 mg/kg/hour).

➤ **Monitored anesthesia care**
Healthy adults younger than age 55:
Initially, 100 to 150 mcg/kg/minute (6 to 9 mg/kg/hour) I.V. for 3 to 5 minutes or a slow injection of 0.5 mg/kg over 3 to 5 minutes. For maintenance dose, give infusion of 25 to 75 mcg/kg/minute (1.5 to 4.5 mg/kg/hour), or incremental 10- or 20-mg boluses.
Adjust-a-dose: In geriatric, debilitated, or ASA PS III or IV patients, give 80% of usual adult maintenance dose. Don't use rapid bolus.
➤ **To sedate intubated intensive care unit (ICU) patients**
Adults: Initially, 5 mcg/kg/minute (0.3 mg/kg/hour) I.V. for 5 minutes. Increments of 5 to 10 mcg/kg/minute (0.3 to 0.6 mg/kg/hour) over 5 to 10 minutes may be used until desired sedation is achieved. Maintenance rate, 5 to 50 mcg/kg/minute (0.3 to 3 mg/kg/hour).

ADMINISTRATION
I.V.
▼ Maintain aseptic technique when handling the solution. Drug can support the growth of microorganisms; don't use if solution might be contaminated.
▼ Protect drug from light. Shake well.
▼ Dilute only with D₅W. Don't dilute to less than 2 mg/mL.
▼ Don't use if emulsion shows evidence of separation.
▼ Don't infuse through a filter with a pore size smaller than 5 microns. Give via larger veins in arms to decrease injection-site pain.
▼ Titrate drug daily to maintain minimum effective level. Allow 3 to 5 minutes between dosage adjustments to assess effects.
▼ Discard tubing and unused portions of drug after 12 hours.
▼ **Incompatibilities:** Other I.V. drugs, blood and plasma.

ACTION
Unknown. Rapid-acting I.V. sedative-hypnotic.

Route	Onset	Peak	Duration
I.V.	<40 sec	Unknown	10–15 min

Half-life: Initial (distribution) phase, about 2 to 10 minutes; second (redistribution) phase, 21 to 70 minutes; terminal (elimination) phase, 1½ to 31 hours.

ADVERSE REACTIONS
CNS: dystonic or choreiform movement.
CV: *bradycardia,* hypotension, hypertension, decreased cardiac output.
Metabolic: hyperlipidemia.
Respiratory: *apnea, respiratory acidosis.*
Skin: rash, pruritus.
Other: burning or stinging at injection site.

INTERACTIONS
Drug-drug. *Inhaled anesthetics (such as enflurane, halothane, isoflurane), opioids (alfentanil, fentanyl, meperidine, morphine), sedatives (such as barbiturates, benzodiazepines, chloral hydrate, droperidol):* May increase anesthetic and sedative effects and further decrease blood pressure and cardiac output. Monitor patient closely.
Drug-herb. *St. John's wort:* May prolong anesthetic effects. Advise patient to stop using herb 5 days before surgery.

EFFECTS ON LAB TEST RESULTS
● May increase serum triglyceride levels.

CONTRAINDICATIONS & CAUTIONS
● Contraindicated in patients hypersensitive to drug or its components (including egg lecithin, soybean oil, and glycerol), in pregnant women (because it may cause fetal depression), and in those unable to undergo general anesthesia or sedation.
● Use cautiously in patients who are hemodynamically unstable or who have seizures, disorders of lipid metabolism, or increased intracranial pressure.
● Because drug appears in breast milk, avoid using in breast-feeding women.
⚠ *Overdose S&S:* Cardiorespiratory depression.

NURSING CONSIDERATIONS
● If drug is used for prolonged sedation in ICU, urine may turn green.
● For general anesthesia or monitored anesthesia care sedation, trained staff not

involved in the surgical or diagnostic procedure should give drug. For ICU sedation, persons skilled in managing critically ill patients and trained in cardiopulmonary resuscitation and airway management should give drug.

• Continuously monitor vital signs.

❸ **Alert:** The FDA issued an alert after receiving reports of chills, fever, and body aches in several clusters of patients shortly after patients received propofol for sedation or general anesthesia. Various lots of the drug were tested, but no toxins, bacteria, or other signs of contamination were found. The FDA advises all health care providers to carefully follow the handling and use sections of the prescribing information for this drug. They recommend that all patients be evaluated for possible reactions following use of the drug, and that anyone experiencing signs of acute febrile reactions be evaluated for possible bacterial sepsis. They ask that any adverse events following the use of propofol be reported to MedWatch.

• Monitor patient at risk for hyperlipidemia for elevated triglyceride levels.

• Drug contains 0.1 g of fat (1.1 kcal)/mL. Reduce other lipid products if given together.

• Drug contains ethylenediaminetetraacetic acid (EDTA), a strong metal chelator. Consider supplemental zinc during prolonged therapy.

• When giving drug in the ICU, assess patient's CNS function daily to determine minimum dose needed.

• Stop drug gradually to prevent abrupt awakening and increased agitation.

• **Look alike–sound alike:** Don't confuse Diprivan with Ditropan, Diflucan, or Dipivefrin.

PATIENT TEACHING
• Advise patient that performance of activities requiring mental alertness may be impaired for some time after drug use.

• Tell patient that abnormal dreams or anesthesia awareness may occur.

propranolol hydrochloride
proe-PRAN-oh-lol

Inderal⬦, Inderal LA⬦, InnoPran XL

Therapeutic class: Antihypertensives
Pharmacologic class: Nonselective beta blockers
Pregnancy risk category: C (first trimester); D (second and third trimesters)

AVAILABLE FORMS
Capsules (extended-release): 60 mg, 80 mg, 120 mg, 160 mg
Injection: 1 mg/mL
Oral solution: 4 mg/mL, 8 mg/mL
Tablets: 10 mg, 20 mg, 40 mg, 60 mg, 80 mg

INDICATIONS & DOSAGES
➤ **Angina pectoris**
Adults: Total daily doses of 80 to 320 mg P.O. given in two to four divided doses. Or, one 80-mg extended-release capsule daily. Dosage increased at 3- to 7-day intervals.

➤ **To decrease risk of death after MI**
Adults: Initially, 40 mg P.O. t.i.d. After 1 month, titrate to 60 to 80 mg t.i.d. as tolerated.

➤ **Supraventricular, ventricular, and atrial arrhythmias; tachyarrhythmias caused by excessive catecholamine action during anesthesia, hyperthyroidism, or pheochromocytoma**
Adults: 1 to 3 mg by slow I.V. push, not to exceed 1 mg/minute. After 3 mg have been given, another dose may be given in 2 minutes; subsequent doses, no sooner than every 4 hours. Usual maintenance dose is 10 to 30 mg P.O. t.i.d. or q.i.d.

➤ **Hypertension**
Adults: Initially, 80 mg P.O. daily in two divided doses or extended-release form once daily. Increase at 3- to 7-day intervals to maximum daily dose of 640 mg. Usual maintenance dose is 120 to 240 mg daily or 120 to 160 mg daily as extended-release. For InnoPran XL, dose is 80 mg P.O. once daily at bedtime. Give consistently with or without food. Adjust to maximum of

P

120 mg daily if needed. Full effects are seen in about 2 to 3 weeks.

➤ **Essential tremor**
Adults: 40 mg (tablets or oral solution) P.O. b.i.d. Usual maintenance dose is 120 to 320 mg daily in three divided doses.

➤ **Hypertrophic subaortic stenosis**
Adults: 20 to 40 mg P.O. t.i.d. or q.i.d., or 80 to 160 mg extended-release capsules once daily.

➤ **Adjunctive therapy in pheochromocytoma**
Adults: 60 mg P.O. daily in divided doses with an alpha blocker 3 days before surgery.

➤ **Prevention of migraine**
Adults: Initially, 80 mg P.O. daily in divided doses. May increase to 160 to 240 mg/day.

➤ **Traumatic brain injury ◆**
Adults: 60 mg P.O. daily. Increase in 60-mg/day increments every third day until agitation ceases, adverse reactions occur, or the maximum dosage of 520 mg/day is reached.

ADMINISTRATION
P.O.
● Give drug consistently with meals. Food may increase absorption of propranolol.
● Compliance may be improved by giving drug twice daily or as extended-release capsules. Check with prescriber.
● Check blood pressure and apical pulse before giving drug. If hypotension or extremes in pulse rate occur, withhold drug and notify prescriber.
● Don't substitute extended-release form for immediate-release on a mg-for-mg basis. Retitration may be necessary.

I.V.
▼ For direct injection, give into a large vessel or into the tubing of a free-flowing, compatible I.V. solution; don't give by continuous I.V. infusion.
▼ Drug is compatible with D₅W, half-normal saline solution, normal saline solution, and lactated Ringer solution.
▼ Infusion rate shouldn't exceed 1 mg/minute.
▼ Double-check dose and route. I.V. doses are much smaller than oral doses.
▼ Monitor blood pressure, ECG, central venous pressure, and heart rate and

rhythm frequently, especially during I.V. administration. If patient develops severe hypotension, notify prescriber; a vasopressor may be prescribed.
▼ For overdose, give I.V. isoproterenol, I.V. atropine, or glucagon; refractory cases may require a pacemaker.
▼ **Incompatibilities:** Amphotericin B, diazoxide.

ACTION
Reduces cardiac oxygen demand by blocking catecholamine-induced increases in heart rate, blood pressure, and force of myocardial contraction. Drug depresses renin secretion and prevents vasodilation of cerebral arteries.

Route	Onset	Peak	Duration
P.O.	30 min	60–90 min	12 hr
P.O. (extended-release)	Unknown	6–14 hr	24 hr
I.V.	Immediate	1 min	5 min

Half-life: About 4 hours; 8 hours for InnoPran XL.

ADVERSE REACTIONS
CNS: fatigue, lethargy, fever, vivid dreams, hallucinations, mental depression, lightheadedness, dizziness, insomnia.
CV: hypotension, *bradycardia, heart failure, intensification of AV block,* intermittent claudication.
GI: abdominal cramping, constipation, diarrhea, nausea, vomiting.
Hematologic: *agranulocytosis.*
Respiratory: *bronchospasm.*
Skin: rash.

INTERACTIONS
Drug-drug. *Aminophylline:* May antagonize beta-blocking effects of propranolol. Use together cautiously.
Amiodarone, diltiazem, verapamil: May cause hypotension, bradycardia, and increased depressant effect on myocardium. Use together cautiously.
Cardiac glycosides: May reduce the positive inotrope effect of the glycoside. Monitor patient for clinical effect.

Cimetidine, ciprofloxacin, fluconazole, fluoxetine, paroxetine: May inhibit metabolism of propranolol. Watch for increased beta-blocking effect.

Epinephrine: May cause severe vaso-constriction. Monitor blood pressure and observe patient carefully.

Glucagon, isoproterenol: May antagonize propranolol effect. May be used therapeutically and in emergencies.

Haloperidol: May cause cardiac arrest. Avoid using together.

Insulin, oral antidiabetics: May alter requirements for these drugs in previously stabilized diabetics. Monitor patient for hypoglycemia.

Lidocaine: May reduce clearance of lidocaine. Monitor lidocaine level closely.

Phenothiazines (chlorpromazine, thioridazine): May increase risk of serious adverse reactions to either drug. Use with thioridazine is contraindicated. If chlorpromazine must be used, monitor patient's pulse and blood pressure; decrease propranolol dose as needed.

Propafenone, quinidine: May increase propranolol level. Monitor cardiac function, and adjust propranolol dose as needed.

Drug-herb. *Betel palm:* May decrease temperature-elevating effects and enhanced CNS effects. Discourage use together.

Ma huang: May decrease antihypertensive effects. Discourage use together.

Drug-lifestyle. *Alcohol use:* May increase propranolol level. Discourage alcohol use.

Cocaine use: May increase angina-inducing potential of cocaine. Inform patient of this interaction.

Smoking: May decrease propranolol level. Monitor clinical response and adjust dosage as needed.

EFFECTS ON LAB TEST RESULTS

● May increase T_4, BUN, transaminase, alkaline phosphatase, potassium, and LDH levels. May decrease T_3 level.

● May decrease granulocyte count.

CONTRAINDICATIONS & CAUTIONS

Black Box Warning Abrupt withdrawal of drug may cause exacerbation of angina or MI. To discontinue drug, gradually reduce dosage over a few weeks. Because coronary artery disease may be unrecognized, don't discontinue drug abruptly, even when taken for other indications. ■

● Contraindicated in patients with known hypersensitivity to drug, bronchial asthma, sinus bradycardia and heart block greater than first-degree, cardiogenic shock, and overt and decompensated heart failure (unless failure is secondary to a tachyarrhythmia that can be treated with propranolol).

● Use cautiously in patients with hepatic or renal impairment, Wolff-Parkinson-White syndrome, nonallergic bronchospastic diseases, or hepatic disease and in those taking other antihypertensives.

● Use cautiously in patients who have diabetes mellitus because drug masks some symptoms of hypoglycemia.

● In patients with thyrotoxicosis, use drug cautiously because it may mask the signs and symptoms. Abrupt withdrawal may exacerbate symptoms of hyperthyroidism, including thyroid storm.

● Elderly patients may experience enhanced adverse reactions and may need dosage adjustment.

● Use cautiously in pregnant women because drug may be associated with small placenta and congenital anomalies.

⚠ Overdose S&S: Bradycardia, cardiac failure, hypotension, bronchospasm.

NURSING CONSIDERATIONS

● Drug masks common signs and symptoms of shock and hypoglycemia.

● Monitor black patients for expected therapeutic effects; dosage adjustments may be necessary.

⊙ Alert: Don't stop drug before surgery for pheochromocytoma. Before any surgical procedure, tell anesthesiologist that patient is receiving propranolol.

● **Look alike–sound alike:** Don't confuse propranolol with prasugrel or Pravachol. Don't confuse Inderal with Inderide, Isordil, Adderall, or Imuran.

PATIENT TEACHING

● Caution patient to continue taking this drug as prescribed, even when he's feeling well.

● Instruct patient to take drug with food.

• Advise patient that propranolol may interfere with glaucoma screening because it can reduce intraocular pressure.

۞ Alert: Tell patient not to stop drug suddenly because this can worsen chest pain and trigger a heart attack.

• Advise patient to avoid smoking, alcohol, and illicit drug use.

propylthiouracil (PTU)
proe-pill-thye-oh-YOOR-a-sill

PTU Propyl-Thyracil†

Therapeutic class: Antihyperthyroids
Pharmacologic class: Thyroid hormone antagonists
Pregnancy risk category: D

AVAILABLE FORMS
Tablets: 50 mg, 100 mg†

INDICATIONS & DOSAGES
Black Box Warning Reserve drug for patients who can't tolerate methimazole and in whom radioactive iodine therapy or surgery isn't appropriate. ▮

➤ **Hyperthyroidism**
Adults: 300 to 400 mg P.O. daily in three divided doses at 8-hour intervals. Patients with severe hyperthyroidism or very large goiters may need initial dose of 600 to 900 mg daily. Continue until patient is euthyroid; then start maintenance dose of 100 to 150 mg P.O. daily in three divided doses every 8 hours.
Children age 6 and older: Initially, 50 mg P.O. daily in divided doses every 8 hours. Carefully titrate upward.

➤ **Hyperthyroidism ◆**
Children older than age 10: Initially, 150 to 300 mg or 150 mg/m² P.O. daily in divided doses. Continue until patient is euthyroid. Individualize maintenance dose.
Children ages 6 to 10: Initially, 50 to 150 mg P.O. daily in divided doses every 8 hours. Continue until patient is euthyroid. Individualize maintenance dose. Or, 5 to 7 mg/kg/day P.O. or 150 to 200 mg/m²/day P.O. in divided doses every 8 hours. Maintenance dose is one-third to two-thirds

the initial dose beginning when patient is euthyroid.
Infants and children younger than age 6: 5 to 7 mg/kg/day P.O. daily divided every 8 hours. Maintenance dose is one-third to two-thirds the initial dose divided every 8 to 12 hours when patient is euthyroid.
Neonates: 5 to 10 mg/kg P.O. daily in three divided doses.

➤ **Thyrotoxic crisis**
Adults: 200 mg P.O. every 4 to 6 hours on first day; after symptoms are fully controlled, gradually reduce dosage to usual maintenance levels.

ADMINISTRATION
P.O.
• Give in three equally divided doses about 8 hours apart.
• Give drug with meals to reduce adverse GI reactions.
• Store drug in light-resistant container.

ACTION
Inhibits oxidation of iodine in thyroid gland, blocking ability of iodine to combine with tyrosine to form T_4, and may prevent coupling of monoiodotyrosine and diiodotyrosine to form T_4 and T_3.

Route	Onset	Peak	Duration
P.O.	Unknown	60–90 min	Unknown

Half-life: 1 to 2 hours.

ADVERSE REACTIONS
CNS: headache, drowsiness, vertigo, paresthesia, neuritis, neuropathies, CNS stimulation, depression, fever.
CV: vasculitis.
EENT: visual disturbances, loss of taste.
GI: diarrhea, nausea, vomiting, epigastric distress, salivary gland enlargement.
GU: nephritis.
Hematologic: *agranulocytosis, leukopenia, thrombocytopenia, aplastic anemia.*
Hepatic: jaundice, *hepatotoxicity.*
Metabolic: dose-related hypothyroidism.
Musculoskeletal: arthralgia, myalgia.
Skin: rash, urticaria, skin discoloration, pruritus, erythema nodosum, exfoliative dermatitis, lupuslike syndrome.
Other: lymphadenopathy.

Reactions in bold italics are *life-threatening*. Interactions may have a *rapid onset* or a *delayed onset*.

INTERACTIONS

Drug-drug. *Aminophylline, oxtriphylline, theophylline:* May decrease clearance of these drugs. Dosage may need to be adjusted.

Beta blockers: Hyperthyroidism may increase clearance of beta blockers. Monitor thyroid status; beta blocker dosage reduction may be necessary when hyperthyroid patient becomes euthyroid.

Cardiac glycosides: May increase glycoside level. Dosage may need to be reduced.

Potassium iodide: May decrease response to drug. Dosage of antithyroid drug may need to be increased.

Warfarin: May increase anticoagulation. Monitor PT and INR.

Drug-food. *Iodized salt, shellfish:* May alter drug's effectiveness. Urge caution.

EFFECTS ON LAB TEST RESULTS

• May increase PT. May decrease hemoglobin level.

• May decrease granulocyte, WBC, and platelet counts and liothyronine uptake.

CONTRAINDICATIONS & CAUTIONS

• Contraindicated in patients hypersensitive to drug and in breast-feeding women.

Black Box Warning Not recommended for use in children except in rare instances in which methimazole isn't well tolerated and surgery or radioactive iodine therapy isn't appropriate. ∎

• Use cautiously in pregnant patients.

⚠ Overdose S&S: Nausea, vomiting, epigastric distress, headache, fever, arthralgia, pruritus, edema, pancytopenia, agranulocytosis, exfoliative dermatitis, hepatitis, neuropathies, CNS stimulation or depression.

NURSING CONSIDERATIONS

Black Box Warning Because of risk of fetal abnormalities associated with methimazole, propylthiouracil may be treatment of choice when an antithyroid drug is indicated during or just before first trimester. ∎

• Pregnant women may need less drug as pregnancy progresses. Monitor thyroid function studies closely. Thyroid hormone may be added to regimen. Drug may be stopped during last few weeks of pregnancy.

⊙ Alert: Patients older than age 40 may have an increased risk of agranulocytosis.

• Watch for hypothyroidism (mental depression, cold intolerance, and hard, nonpitting edema); adjust dosage.

• Monitor CBC periodically to detect impending leukopenia, thrombocytopenia, and agranulocytosis.

⊙ Alert: Stop drug and notify prescriber if severe rash develops or cervical lymph nodes enlarge.

Black Box Warning Severe liver injury or acute liver failure requiring transplantation or causing death may occur in patients taking drug; monitor patient closely. ∎

• Monitor hepatic function. Stop drug if transaminase levels are greater than 3 times the upper limit of normal.

• **Look alike–sound alike:** Don't confuse propylthiouracil with Purinethol.

PATIENT TEACHING

• Instruct patient to take drug with meals.

• Warn patient to report fever, sore throat, mouth sores, and skin eruptions.

• Tell patient to report unusual bleeding or bruising.

• Tell patient to ask prescriber about using iodized salt and eating shellfish. These foods contain iodine and may alter effectiveness of drug.

• Teach patient to watch for signs and symptoms of hypothyroidism (unexplained weight gain, fatigue, cold intolerance) and to notify prescriber if they occur.

• Tell female patient to contact prescriber if she becomes pregnant or intends to become pregnant.

P

pseudoephedrine hydrochloride

soo-dow-e-FED-rin

CongestAid ◊, ElixSure Children's Congestion ◊, Genaphed ◊, Silfedrine ◊, Simply Stuffy ◊, Sudafed ◊, SudoGest ◊, Unified ◊

Therapeutic class: Decongestants
Pharmacologic class: Adrenergics
Pregnancy risk category: C

AVAILABLE FORMS

Oral solution: 15 mg/5 mL ◊,
30 mg/5 mL ◊
Syrup: 15 mg/5 mL ◊, 30 mg/5 mL ◊
Tablets: 30 mg ◊, 60 mg ◊
Tablets (chewable): 15 mg ◊
Tablets (extended-release): 120 mg ◊,
240 mg ◊

INDICATIONS & DOSAGES

➤ **To decongest nose and eustachian tubes**

Adults and children older than age 12:
60 mg P.O. every 4 to 6 hours; or 120 mg P.O. extended-release tablet every 12 hours; or 240 mg P.O. extended-release tablet once daily. Maximum dosage is 240 mg daily.
Children ages 6 to 12: 30 mg P.O. every 4 to 6 hours. Maximum dosage is 120 mg daily.
Children ages 2 to 5: 15 mg P.O. every 4 to 6 hours. Maximum dosage is 60 mg daily.

ADMINISTRATION

P.O.

● Don't crush or break extended-release tablets.

ACTION

Stimulates alpha receptors in the respiratory tract, constricting blood vessels, shrinking swollen nasal mucous membranes, increasing airway patency, and reducing tissue hyperemia, edema, and nasal congestion.

Route	Onset	Peak	Duration
P.O.	30 min	30–60 min	4–12 hr

Half-life: Unknown.

ADVERSE REACTIONS

CNS: anxiety, nervousness, dizziness, headache, insomnia, tremor.
CV: palpitations, *arrhythmias, CV collapse,* tachycardia.
GI: anorexia, dry mouth, nausea, vomiting.
GU: urine retention.
Skin: pallor.
Other: diaphoresis, rash.

INTERACTIONS

Drug-drug. *Antihypertensives:* May inhibit hypotensive effect. Monitor blood pressure closely.
Linezolid, methyldopa, reserpine: May increase pressor response. Monitor patient closely.
MAO inhibitors (phenelzine, tranylcypromine): May cause severe headache, hypertension, fever, and hypertensive crisis. Avoid using together and within 14 days of MAO inhibitor use.

EFFECTS ON LAB TEST RESULTS

None reported.

CONTRAINDICATIONS & CAUTIONS

● Contraindicated in patients with severe hypertension or severe coronary artery disease, in those receiving MAO inhibitors, and in breast-feeding women. Extended-release forms are contraindicated in children younger than age 12.
● Use cautiously in patients with hypertension, cardiac disease, diabetes, glaucoma, hyperthyroidism, bowel narrowing, and prostatic hyperplasia.
⚠ *Overdose S&S:* Hypertension, bradycardia, drowsiness, rebound hypotension.

NURSING CONSIDERATIONS

● Elderly patients are more sensitive to drug's effects. Extended-release tablets shouldn't be given to elderly patients until safety with short-acting preparations has been established.

PATIENT TEACHING

● Tell patient not to crush or break extended-release tablets.
● Warn against using OTC products containing other sympathomimetics.

Reactions in bold italics are *life-threatening*. Interactions may have a *rapid onset* or a *delayed onset*.

• Instruct patient not to take drug within 2 hours of bedtime because it can cause insomnia.

• Tell patient to stop drug and notify prescriber if he becomes unusually restless.

pyrethrins–piperonyl butoxide
pi-RETH-rinz and PI-per-oh-nel

A-200 ◊, Licide ◊, Pronto ◊, Pyrinyl Plus ◊, R & C† ◊, RID ◊, Tisit ◊

Therapeutic class: Pediculicides
Pharmacologic class: Pyrethrins
Pregnancy risk category: C

AVAILABLE FORMS
Lotion: pyrethrins 0.3% and piperonyl butoxide 2%
Mousse: pyrethrins 0.33% and piperonyl butoxide 4%
Shampoo: pyrethrins 0.33% and piperonyl butoxide 4%
Topical gel: pyrethrins 0.3% and piperonyl butoxide 3%

INDICATIONS & DOSAGES
➤ **Infestations of head, body, and pubic (crab) lice and their eggs**
Adults and children: Apply to hair, scalp, or other infested areas until entirely wet. Allow to remain for 10 minutes but no longer. Wash thoroughly with warm water and soap or shampoo. Remove dead lice and eggs with fine-tooth comb. Repeat treatment in 7 to 10 days to kill newly hatched lice; don't use more than two applications within 24 hours.

ADMINISTRATION
Topical
• Don't apply to open areas, acutely inflamed skin, eyebrows, eyelashes, face, eyes, mucous membranes, or urethral opening. If accidental contact with eyes occurs, flush with water and notify prescriber.

• Stop using drug, wash it off skin, and notify prescriber immediately if skin irritation develops.

• All preparations contain petroleum distillates.

ACTION
Acts as contact poison that disrupts parasite's nervous system, causing parasite's paralysis and death.

Route	Onset	Peak	Duration
Topical	Unknown	Unknown	Unknown

Half-life: Unknown.

ADVERSE REACTIONS
Skin: irritation with repeated use, edema, erythema, eczema, pruritus, urticaria.

INTERACTIONS
None significant.

EFFECTS ON LAB TEST RESULTS
None reported.

CONTRAINDICATIONS & CAUTIONS
• Contraindicated in patients hypersensitive to drug, ragweed, or chrysanthemums.
• Use cautiously in infants and small children.

NURSING CONSIDERATIONS
• Apply topical corticosteroids or give oral antihistamines if dermatitis develops from scratching.
• Discard container by wrapping in several layers of newspaper.
• Inspect all family members daily for at least 2 weeks for infestation.
• Drug isn't effective against scabies.
• Treat sexual contacts simultaneously.

PATIENT TEACHING
• Instruct patient not to apply to open areas, acutely inflamed skin, eyebrows, eyelashes, face, eyes, mucous membranes, or urethral opening. If accidental contact with eyes occurs, advise patient to flush with water and notify prescriber.
• Warn patient not to swallow or inhale vapors from the drug.
• Tell patient to stop using drug, wash it off skin, and notify prescriber immediately if skin irritation develops. All preparations contain petroleum distillates.
• Instruct patient to change all clothing and bed linens after drug is washed off body. Tell him to disinfect washable items by machine washing in hot water and drying on

P

hot cycle for at least 20 minutes. Other items can be dry-cleaned and sealed in plastic bags for 2 weeks, or treated with products made for this purpose.

• Teach patient to remove dead parasites with a fine-tooth comb.

• Tell patient to repeat treatment in 7 to 10 days to kill any newly hatched eggs.

• Urge patient to warn other family members and sexual partners so that they can be examined for the presence of lice.

pyridostigmine bromide
peer-id-oh-STIG-meen

Mestinon*, Mestinon-SR†, Regonol*

Therapeutic class: Muscle stimulants
Pharmacologic class: Cholinesterase inhibitors
Pregnancy risk category: C

AVAILABLE FORMS
Injection: 5 mg/mL
Syrup: 60 mg/5 mL*
Tablets: 60 mg
Tablets (extended-release): 180 mg

INDICATIONS & DOSAGES
Adjust-a-dose (for all indications): Smaller doses may be required in patients with renal disease. Adjust dosage to achieve desired effect.

➤ **Antidote for nondepolarizing neuro-muscular blockers**
Adults: 0.1 to 0.25 mg/kg I.V., preceded by atropine sulfate 0.6 to 1.2 mg I.V.
➤ **Myasthenia gravis**
Adults: 60 to 120 mg P.O. every 3 or 4 hours. Average dosage is 600 mg daily, but dosages up to 1,500 mg daily may be needed. For I.M. or I.V. use, give ⅓₀ of oral dose. Dosage must be adjusted for each patient, based on response and tolerance. Or, 180 to 540 mg extended-release tablets P.O. daily or b.i.d., with at least 6 hours between doses.

ADMINISTRATION
P.O.
• Don't crush extended-release tablets.

• If patient has trouble swallowing, give syrup form. If patient can't tolerate sweet flavor, give over ice chips.
I.V.
▼ **Black Box Warning** Drug should only be administered by individuals familiar with its actions, characteristics, and hazards. ▮
▼ Don't use solution if it contains particulate matter or is discolored.
▼ Position patient to ease breathing. Keep atropine injection available, and be prepared to give it immediately.
▼ Monitor vital signs frequently, especially respirations. Provide respiratory support as needed.
▼ Give injection no faster than 1 mg/minute. Rapid infusion may cause bradycardia and seizures.
▼ If patient's muscle weakness is severe, prescriber will determine if it results from drug toxicity or worsening myasthenia gravis. Test dose of edrophonium I.V. will aggravate drug-induced weakness but will temporarily relieve disease-induced weakness.
▼ **Incompatibilities:** Alkaline solutions.
I.M.
• Don't use solution if it contains particulate matter or is discolored.

ACTION
Inhibits acetylcholinesterase, blocking destruction of acetylcholine from the parasympathetic and somatic efferent nerves. Acetylcholine accumulates, promoting increased stimulation of the receptors.

Route	Onset	Peak	Duration
P.O.	20–30 min	2 hr	3–6 hr
P.O. (extended-release)	30–60 min	1–2 hr	6–12 hr
I.V.	2–5 min	Unknown	2–4 hr
I.M.	15 min	Unknown	2–4 hr

Half-life: 1 to 3 hours, depending on route.

ADVERSE REACTIONS
CNS: headache with high doses, weakness, syncope.
CV: ***bradycardia, cardiac arrest,*** hypotension, thrombophlebitis.
EENT: miosis, rhinorrhea.

GI: nausea, vomiting, abdominal cramps, diarrhea, excessive salivation, increased peristalsis.
GU: urinary frequency, urinary urgency.
Musculoskeletal: muscle cramps, muscle fasciculations, muscle weakness, tingling in extremities.
Respiratory: *bronchospasm, bronchoconstriction,* increased bronchial secretions.
Skin: rash, diaphoresis.

INTERACTIONS
Drug-drug. *Anticholinergics, atropine, corticosteroids, general or local anesthetics, magnesium, procainamide, quinidine:* May antagonize cholinergic effects. Observe patient for lack of drug effect.
Ganglionic blockers: May increase risk of hypotension. Monitor patient closely.
Succinylcholine: May prolong the phase I block of the depolarizing muscle relaxant. Avoid using together.

EFFECTS ON LAB TEST RESULTS
None reported.

CONTRAINDICATIONS & CAUTIONS
• Contraindicated in patients hypersensitive to anticholinesterases or bromides and in those with mechanical obstruction of the intestinal or urinary tract.
• Use cautiously in patients with bronchial asthma, bradycardia, arrhythmias, epilepsy, recent coronary occlusion, vagotonia, renal impairment, hyperthyroidism, or peptic ulcer.
• Use cautiously in patients taking beta blockers for hypertension or glaucoma.
• Use cautiously in pregnant and breast-feeding women; drug appears in breast milk.

NURSING CONSIDERATIONS
• Stop all other cholinergics before giving this drug.
• Monitor and document patient's response after each dose. Optimum dosage is difficult to judge.
• **Alert:** Regonol contains benzyl ethanol preservative, which may cause toxicity in neonates if given in high doses.
• *Look alike–sound alike:* Don't confuse pyridostigmine with physostigmine. Don't confuse Regonol with Reglan or Renagel.

PATIENT TEACHING
• When giving drug for myasthenia gravis, stress importance of taking exactly as prescribed, on time, in evenly spaced doses. For extended-release tablets, tell patient to take at same time each day, at least 6 hours apart.
• Advise patient not to crush or chew extended-release tablets.
• Explain that patient may have to take drug for life.
• Advise patient to wear or carry medical identification that identifies his myasthenia gravis.

pyrimethamine
pihr-ih-METH-ah-meen

Daraprim

Therapeutic class: Antimalarials
Pharmacologic class: Folate antagonists
Pregnancy risk category: C

AVAILABLE FORMS
Tablets: 25 mg

INDICATIONS & DOSAGES
➤ **To prevent and control transmission of malaria**
Adults and children older than age 10: 25 mg P.O. weekly for 6 to 10 weeks or longer after leaving malaria-endemic areas.
Children ages 4 to 10: Give 12.5 mg P.O. weekly, continued for 6 to 10 weeks or longer after leaving malaria-endemic areas.
Infants and children younger than age 4: Give 6.25 mg P.O. weekly, continued for 6 to 10 weeks or longer after leaving malaria-endemic areas.
➤ **Acute attacks of malaria**
Adults and children age 10 and older: 25 mg P.O. daily for 2 days with a sulfonamide. Clinical cure should be followed with 25 mg P.O. once weekly for at least 10 weeks. Or, 50 mg P.O. daily for 2 days; then 25 mg once weekly for at least 10 weeks.
Children ages 4 to 10: Give 25 mg P.O. once daily for 2 days; then 12.5 mg once weekly for at least 10 weeks.
➤ **Toxoplasmosis**
Adults: Initially, 50 to 75 mg P.O. with 1 to 4 g of a sulfonamide of the sulfapyrimidine

P

type; continue for 1 to 3 weeks. After 3 weeks, reduce dosage by half and continue for 4 to 5 weeks.
Children: Initially, 1 mg/kg/day P.O. in two equally divided doses for 2 to 4 days; then 0.5 mg/kg daily divided into two equal doses for 4 weeks, along with a sulfonamide at a pediatric dosage.

ADMINISTRATION
P.O.
● Patient should take first preventive dose 1 to 2 days before traveling.
● Give drug with meals.

ACTION
Blocks creation of folic acid, which is required for the reproduction of the infecting organism. Sulfadoxine competitively inhibits use of PABA.

Route	Onset	Peak	Duration
P.O.	Unknown	1½–8 hr	2 wk

Half-life: 4 days.

ADVERSE REACTIONS
CV: *arrhythmias.*
GI: anorexia, vomiting, atrophic glossitis.
Hematologic: *agranulocytosis, aplastic anemia, leukopenia, thrombocytopenia, pancytopenia,* megaloblastic anemia.
Skin: *Stevens-Johnson syndrome.*
Other: *hypersensitivity reactions,* hyperphenylalaninemia.

INTERACTIONS
Drug-drug. *Lorazepam:* May increase risk of hepatotoxicity. Avoid using together.
Methotrexate, sulfamethoxazole–trimethoprim, sulfonamides: May increase risk of bone marrow suppression. Avoid using together.
PABA: May decrease action against toxoplasmosis. May need to adjust dosage.

EFFECTS ON LAB TEST RESULTS
● May decrease hemoglobin level.
● May decrease granulocyte, WBC, platelet, and RBC counts.

CONTRAINDICATIONS & CAUTIONS
● Pyrimethamine is contraindicated in patients hypersensitive to drug and in those

with megaloblastic anemia from folic acid deficiency.
● Contraindicated in infants younger than age 2 months and in pregnant (at term) and breast-feeding women.
● Use cautiously after treatment with chloroquine and in patients with impaired hepatic or renal function, severe allergy or bronchial asthma, G6PD deficiency, or seizure disorders (smaller doses may be needed).
⚠ *Overdose S&S:* Abdominal pain, nausea, vomiting, hematemesis, excitability, respiratory depression, circulatory collapse.

NURSING CONSIDERATIONS
● Pyrimethamine alone isn't recommended for malaria. Use drug with faster-acting antimalarials, such as chloroquine, for 2 days to start transmission control and suppressive cure.
● For toxoplasmosis, obtain twice-weekly blood counts, including platelets, because usual dosages approach toxic levels. If signs of folic acid or folinic acid deficiency develop, reduce dosage or stop drug and give parenteral folinic acid (leucovorin) until blood counts return to normal.
● Adverse drug reactions related to sulfadiazine are similar to those related to sulfonamides.
● When used for toxoplasmosis in patients with AIDS, therapy may be lifelong.

PATIENT TEACHING
● Instruct patient to take drug with meals.
● Inform patient with toxoplasmosis of importance of frequent laboratory studies and compliance with therapy. Tell patient he may need long-term therapy.
● Tell patient to take first preventive dose 1 to 2 days before traveling.
● Tell patient to discontinue drug at first sign of rash and to immediately seek medical attention.
● Advise female patient against becoming pregnant.
● Tell patient that sore throat, pallor, purpura, or inflammation of the tongue may be early signs of serious disorders that require medical attention.

---

quetiapine fumarate
kwe-TIE-ah-peen

Seroquel◆, Seroquel XR

Therapeutic class: Antipsychotics
Pharmacologic class: Dibenzothiazepine
derivatives
Pregnancy risk category: C

AVAILABLE FORMS
Tablets: 25 mg, 50 mg, 100 mg, 200 mg,
300 mg, 400 mg
Tablets (extended-release): 50 mg, 150 mg,
200 mg, 300 mg, 400 mg

INDICATIONS & DOSAGES
➤ Schizophrenia
Adults: Initially, 25 mg P.O. b.i.d., with increases in increments of 25 to 50 mg b.i.d.
or t.i.d. on days 2 and 3, as tolerated. Target
range is 300 to 400 mg daily divided into
two or three doses by day 4. Further dosage
adjustments, if indicated, should occur at
intervals of not less than 2 days. Dosage can
be increased or decreased by 25 to 50 mg
b.i.d. Effect generally occurs at 150 to
750 mg daily. Safety of dosages over
800 mg daily hasn't been evaluated.

Or, 300 mg/day extended-release tablets
P.O. once daily, preferably in the evening.
Titrate within a dose range of 400 to
800 mg/day, depending on the response
and tolerance of the individual. Increase at
intervals as short as 1 day and in increments
of 300 mg/day.
Adolescents ages 13 to 17: Total daily
dosage for initial 5 days of therapy is 50 mg
P.O. on day 1, then 100 mg on day 2, then
200 mg on day 3, then 300 mg on day 4, and
400 mg on day 5. Then adjust dosage within
the recommended range of 400 to 800 mg
daily. Make adjustments in increments of no
greater than 100 mg/day. Effectiveness of
therapy for longer than 6 weeks hasn't been
evaluated.
Adjust-a-dose: Elderly patients: For
immediate-release formula, use slow titration and regular monitoring. Or, begin
extended-release formula at 50 mg/day;
may increase dosage in increments of
50 mg/day depending on clinical response

and tolerance. In patients with hepatic impairment, initial dose (immediate-release) is
25 mg daily. Increase daily in increments
of 25 to 50 mg daily to an effective dose.
Or, begin extended-release formula at
50 mg/day; may increase dosage in increments of 50 mg/day depending on clinical
response and tolerance. For debilitated patients and those with hypotension, consider
lower dosages and slower adjustment.
➤ **Monotherapy and adjunctive therapy
with lithium or divalproex for the short-
term treatment of acute manic episodes
associated with bipolar I disorder;
adjunctive maintenance therapy with
lithium or divalproex**
Adults: Initially, 50 mg P.O. b.i.d. Increase
dosage in increments of 100 mg daily in two
divided doses up to 400 mg P.O. b.i.d. on
day 4. May increase dosage in increments
no greater than 200 mg daily up to 800 mg
daily by day 6. Usual dose is 400 to 800 mg
daily. For maintenance therapy with lithium
or divalproex, continue treatment at the
dosage required to maintain symptom
remission.

Or, start with 300 mg (extended-release)
P.O. on day 1 and 600 mg P.O. on day
2 once daily in the evening. Dosage may
be adjusted between 400 and 800 mg beginning on day 3.
Adjust-a-dose: Elderly patients: For
immediate-release formula, use slow
titration and regular monitoring. Or, begin
extended-release formula at 50 mg/day; may
increase dosage in increments of 50 mg/day
depending on clinical response and tolerance. In patients with hepatic impairment,
initial dose (immediate-release) is 25 mg
daily. Increase daily in increments of 25 to
50 mg daily to an effective dose. Or, begin
extended-release formula at 50 mg/day;
may increase dosage in increments of
50 mg/day depending on clinical response
and tolerance. For debilitated patients and
those with hypotension, consider lower
dosages and slower adjustment.
➤ **Bipolar I disorder, acute manic
episodes (immediate-release)**
Children ages 10 to 17: Total daily dosage
for initial 5 days of therapy is 50 mg P.O. on
day 1, then 100 mg on day 2, then 200 mg
on day 3, then 300 mg on day 4, and 400 mg

Q

on day 5. After day 5, adjust dosage within recommended range of 400 to 600 mg/day. Effectiveness of therapy for longer than 3 weeks hasn't been evaluated.

➤ **Depression associated with bipolar disorder**

Adults: Initially, 50 mg P.O. once daily at bedtime; increase on day 2 to 100 mg; increase on day 3 to 200 mg; increase on day 4 to maintenance dose of 300 mg.

Adjust-a-dose: Elderly patients: For immediate-release formula, use slow titration and regular monitoring. Or, begin extended-release formula at 50 mg/day; may increase dosage in increments of 50 mg/day depending on clinical response and tolerance. In patients with hepatic impairment, initial dose (immediate-release) is 25 mg daily. Increase daily in increments of 25 to 50 mg daily to an effective dose. Or, begin extended-release formula at 50 mg/day; may increase dosage in increments of 50 mg/day depending on clinical response and tolerance. For debilitated patients and those with hypotension, consider lower dosages and slower adjustment.

➤ **Major depressive disorder, adjunctive therapy**

Adults: 50 mg P.O. (extended-release) once daily in the evening. On day 3, may increase dosage to 150 mg P.O. once daily in the evening. Dosages ranging from 150 to 300 mg/day have proved effective.

➤ **Obsessive-compulsive disorder ◆**

Adults: 50 mg P.O. daily; increase dosage based on therapeutic effect and tolerance. Continue for 1 to 2 years before tapering; then reduce dosage by 10% to 25% every 1 to 2 months.

ADMINISTRATION

P.O.

● Don't break or crush extended-release tablets.

● Give drug without regard for food; give extended-release tablets without food or with a light meal (about 300 calories).

● Schizophrenic patients who are currently being treated with divided doses of the immediate-release form may be switched to extended-release tablets at the equivalent total daily dose taken once daily. Individual dosage adjustments may be necessary. Those requiring less than 200 mg/dose should remain on the immediate-release form.

ACTION

Blocks dopamine and serotonin 5-HT$_2$ receptors. Its action may be mediated through this antagonism.

Route	Onset	Peak	Duration
P.O.	Unknown	1½ hr	Unknown
P.O. (extended-release)	Unknown	6 hr	Unknown

Half-life: 6 hours; extended-release, 7 to 12 hours.

ADVERSE REACTIONS

CNS: dizziness, headache, somnolence, ***neuroleptic malignant syndrome, seizures,*** hypertonia, dysarthria, asthenia, agitation.

CV: orthostatic hypotension, tachycardia, palpitations, peripheral edema.

EENT: ear pain, pharyngitis, rhinitis.

GI: dry mouth, dyspepsia, abdominal pain, constipation, anorexia, vomiting.

Hematologic: *leukopenia.*

Metabolic: weight gain, hyperglycemia.

Musculoskeletal: back pain.

Respiratory: increased cough, dyspnea.

Skin: rash, diaphoresis.

Other: flulike syndrome.

INTERACTIONS

Drug-drug. *Antihypertensives:* May increase effects of antihypertensives. Monitor blood pressure.

Carbamazepine, glucocorticoids, phenobarbital, phenytoin, rifampin, thioridazine: May increase quetiapine clearance. May need to adjust quetiapine dosage.

CNS depressants: May increase CNS effects. Use together cautiously.

Dopamine agonists, levodopa: May antagonize the effects of these drugs. Monitor patient.

Erythromycin, fluconazole, itraconazole, ketoconazole: May decrease quetiapine clearance. Use together cautiously.

Lorazepam: May decrease lorazepam clearance. Monitor patient for increased CNS effects.

Drug-lifestyle. *Alcohol use:* May increase CNS effects. Discourage use together.

Reactions in bold italics are *life-threatening*. Interactions may have a *rapid onset* or a *delayed onset*.

EFFECTS ON LAB TEST RESULTS

- May increase liver enzyme, cholesterol, triglyceride, and glucose levels. May decrease T_4 and thyroid-stimulating hormone levels.
- May decrease WBC count.
- May cause false-positive results in urine enzyme immunoassays for methadone and TCAs.

CONTRAINDICATIONS & CAUTIONS

- Contraindicated in patients hypersensitive to drug or its ingredients.
- Use cautiously in patients with CV disease, cerebrovascular disease, conditions that predispose to hypotension, a history of seizures or conditions that lower the seizure threshold, and conditions in which core body temperature may be elevated.
- Use cautiously in patients at risk for aspiration pneumonia.

Black Box Warning Drug isn't approved for use in children younger than age 10 (immediate-release) or younger than age 18 (extended-release). ∎

⚠ **Overdose S&S:** Drowsiness, hypotension, sedation, tachycardia, hypokalemia, first-degree heart block.

NURSING CONSIDERATIONS

- Dispense lowest appropriate quantity of drug to reduce risk of overdose.

Black Box Warning Drug isn't indicated for use in elderly patients with dementia-related psychosis because of increased risk of death from CV disease or infection. ∎

🔵 **Alert:** Watch for evidence of neuroleptic malignant syndrome (extrapyramidal effects, hyperthermia, autonomic disturbance), which is rare but deadly.

- Monitor patient for tardive dyskinesia, which may occur after prolonged use. It may not appear until months or years later and may disappear spontaneously or persist for life, despite ending drug.
- Hyperglycemia may occur in patients taking drug. Monitor patients with diabetes regularly.
- Monitor patient for weight gain.

🔵 **Alert:** Monitor patient for symptoms of metabolic syndrome (significant weight gain and increased body mass index, hypertension, hyperglycemia, hypercholesterolemia, and hypertriglyceridemia).

- Drug use may cause cataract formation. Obtain baseline ophthalmologic examination and reassess every 6 months.

Black Box Warning Drug may increase the risk of suicidal thinking and behavior in children, adolescents, and young adults ages 18 to 24, especially during the first few months of treatment, especially in those with major depressive or other psychiatric disorder. ∎

🔵 **Alert:** Neonates exposed to antipsychotics during the third trimester of pregnancy are at risk for developing extrapyramidal signs and symptoms (repetitive muscle movements of the face and body) and withdrawal signs and symptoms (agitation, abnormally increased or decreased muscle tone, tremors, sleepiness, severe difficulty breathing, difficulty feeding) following delivery. Use in pregnancy only if the potential benefit to the mother justifies the risk to the fetus.

PATIENT TEACHING

- Warn patient about risk of dizziness when standing up quickly. The risk is greatest during the 3- to 5-day period of first dosage adjustment, when resuming treatment, and when increasing dosages.
- Tell patient to avoid becoming overheated or dehydrated.
- Warn patient to avoid activities that require mental alertness until effects of drug are known, especially during first dosage adjustment or dosage increases.
- Remind patient to have an eye examination at start of therapy and every 6 months during therapy to check for cataracts.
- Tell patient to notify prescriber about other prescription or OTC drugs he's taking or plans to take.
- Tell women of childbearing age to notify prescriber about planned, suspected, or known pregnancy.
- Advise women not to breast-feed during therapy.
- Advise patient to avoid alcohol while taking drug.
- Tell patient to take drug with or without food.
- Tell patient not to crush, chew, or break extended-release tablets.
- Tell patient to take extended-release tablets without food or with a light meal.

Q

• Tell patient and caregivers to be alert for anxiety, agitation, panic attacks, insomnia, irritability, hostility, aggressiveness, impulsivity, motor restlessness, hypomania, mania, other unusual changes in behavior, worsening of depression, and suicidal thoughts.

• Tell patient not to stop medication abruptly.

quinapril hydrochloride
KWIN-ah-pril

Accupril

Therapeutic class: Antihypertensives
Pharmacologic class: ACE inhibitors
Pregnancy risk category: C; D in 2nd and 3rd trimesters

AVAILABLE FORMS
Tablets: 5 mg, 10 mg, 20 mg, 40 mg

INDICATIONS & DOSAGES
➤ **Hypertension**
Adults: Initially, 10 to 20 mg P.O. daily. Dosage may be adjusted based on patient response at intervals of about 2 weeks. Most patients are controlled at 20, 40, or 80 mg daily as a single dose or in two divided doses. If patient is taking a diuretic, start therapy with 5 mg daily.
Elderly patients: For patients older than age 65, start therapy at 10 mg P.O. daily.
Adjust-a-dose: For adults with CrCl over 60 mL/minute, initially, 10 mg maximum daily; for CrCl of 30 to 60 mL/minute, 5 mg; for CrCl of 10 to 30 mL/minute, 2.5 mg.
➤ **Heart failure**
Adults: 5 mg P.O. b.i.d. initially. Dosage may be increased at weekly intervals. Usual effective dose is 20 to 40 mg daily in two equally divided doses.
Adjust-a-dose: For patients with CrCl over 30 mL/minute, first dose is 5 mg daily; if CrCl is 10 to 30 mL/minute, 2.5 mg.

ADMINISTRATION
P.O.
• Don't give drug with a high-fat meal because this may decrease absorption of drug.

ACTION
Prevents conversion of angiotensin I to angiotensin II, a potent vasoconstrictor. Less angiotensin II decreases peripheral arterial resistance, decreasing aldosterone secretion, which reduces sodium and water retention and lowers blood pressure.

Route	Onset	Peak	Duration
P.O.	1 hr	2–6 hr	24 hr

Half-life: 25 hours.

ADVERSE REACTIONS
CNS: headache, dizziness, fatigue, depression.
CV: *hypertensive crisis,* hypotension, chest pain.
GI: abdominal pain, vomiting, nausea, diarrhea.
Metabolic: *hyperkalemia.*
Musculoskeletal: back pain, myalgia.
Respiratory: dry, persistent, tickling, nonproductive cough; dyspnea.
Skin: rash.

INTERACTIONS
Drug-drug. ❸ Alert: *Aliskiren:* May increase risk of renal impairment, hypotension, and hyperkalemia in diabetic patients and those with moderate to severe renal impairment (GFR less than 60 mL/minute). Concomitant use is contraindicated in diabetic patients. Avoid concomitant use in those with moderate to severe renal impairment.
Diuretics, other antihypertensives: May cause excessive hypotension. Stop diuretic or reduce dose of quinapril, as needed.
Lithium: May increase lithium level and lithium toxicity. Monitor lithium level.
NSAIDs: May decrease antihypertensive effects. Monitor blood pressure.
Potassium-sparing diuretics, potassium supplements: May cause hyperkalemia. Monitor patient closely.
Tetracycline: May decrease absorption if taken with quinapril. Avoid using together.

Reactions in bold italics are *life-threatening*. Interactions may have a *rapid onset* or a *delayed onset*.

Drug-herb. *Capsaicin:* May cause cough. Discourage use together.
Ma huang: May decrease antihypertensive effects. Discourage use together.
Drug-food. *Salt substitutes containing potassium:* May cause hyperkalemia. Discourage use together.

EFFECTS ON LAB TEST RESULTS
• May increase potassium, BUN, and creatinine levels.
• May increase LFT values.

CONTRAINDICATIONS & CAUTIONS
• Contraindicated in patients hypersensitive to ACE inhibitors and in those with a history of angioedema related to treatment with an ACE inhibitor.
Black Box Warning Use during pregnancy can cause injury and death to the developing fetus. When pregnancy is detected, stop drug as soon as possible. ∎
• Use cautiously in patients with impaired renal function.
⚠ Overdose S&S: Hypotension.

NURSING CONSIDERATIONS
• Assess renal and hepatic function before and periodically throughout therapy.
• Monitor blood pressure for effectiveness of therapy. When adjusting dosage, measure blood pressure before giving dose (trough) and 2 to 6 hours after dosing (peak).
• Monitor potassium level. Risk factors for the development of hyperkalemia include renal insufficiency, diabetes, and concomitant use of drugs that raise potassium level.
• Although ACE inhibitors reduce blood pressure in all races, they reduce it less in blacks taking an ACE inhibitor alone. Black patients should take drug with a thiazide diuretic for a better response.
• ACE inhibitors appear to increase risk of angioedema in black patients.
• Other ACE inhibitors have caused agranulocytosis and neutropenia. Monitor CBC with differential counts before therapy and periodically thereafter.

PATIENT TEACHING
• Advise patient to report signs of infection, such as fever and sore throat.

⚠ Alert: Facial and throat swelling (including swelling of the tongue and larynx) may occur, especially after first dose. Advise patient to report signs or symptoms of breathing difficulty or swelling of face, eyes, lips, or tongue.
• Light-headedness can occur, especially during first few days of therapy. Tell patient to rise slowly to minimize effect and to report signs and symptoms to prescriber. If he faints, patient should stop taking drug and call prescriber immediately.
• Inform patient that inadequate fluid intake, vomiting, diarrhea, and excessive perspiration can lead to light-headedness and fainting. Tell him to use caution in hot weather and during exercise.
• Tell patient to avoid salt substitutes. These products may contain potassium, which can cause high potassium level in patients taking quinapril.
• Advise women of childbearing age to notify prescriber if pregnancy occurs. Drug will need to be stopped.
• Tell patient to avoid taking with a high-fat meal because this may decrease absorption of drug.

SAFETY ALERT!

quinidine gluconate
KWIN-i-deen

quinidine sulfate
Therapeutic class: Antiarrhythmics
Pharmacologic class: Cinchona alkaloids
Pregnancy risk category: C

Q

AVAILABLE FORMS
quinidine gluconate (62% quinidine base)
Injection: 80 mg/mL
Tablets (extended-release): 324 mg
quinidine sulfate (83% quinidine base)
Injection: 190 mg/mL†
Tablets: 200 mg, 300 mg
Tablets (extended-release): 300 mg

INDICATIONS & DOSAGES
Adjust-a-dose (for all indications): In patients with hepatic impairment or heart failure, reduce dosage.

➤ **Atrial flutter or fibrillation**
Adults: 400 mg quinidine sulfate
(immediate-release) or equivalent base
P.O. every 6 hours. Or, 300 mg quinidine
sulfate (extended-release) P.O. every 8 to
12 hours. Or, quinidine gluconate 648 mg
(2 tablets) P.O. every 8 hours. Or, begin
quinidine gluconate I.V. infusion no faster
than 0.25 mg/kg/minute (1 mg/kg/hour).
Discontinue infusion if patient hasn't
converted to sinus rhythm after receiving
10 mg/kg. Discontinue drug if QRS complex widens to 130% of pretreatment duration, QTc interval widens to 130% of
pretreatment duration and is longer than
50 msec, P waves disappear, or patient develops significant tachycardia, symptomatic
bradycardia, or hypotension.
➤ **Severe *Plasmodium falciparum* malaria**
Adults: 10 mg/kg quinidine gluconate I.V.
diluted in 250 mL normal saline solution
and infused over 1 to 2 hours; then begin a
continuous infusion of 0.02 mg/kg/minute.
In patients able to swallow, discontinue
infusion and give oral quinine sulfate every
8 hours. Continue quinidine/quinine therapy
for 72 hours or until parasitemia is reduced
to less than 1%, whichever occurs first. Or,
give a loading dose of 24 mg/kg of quinidine
gluconate I.V. diluted in 250 mL of normal
saline solution and infused over 4 hours;
4 hours later, give maintenance dose of
12 mg/kg of quinidine gluconate by I.V.
infusion over 4 hours at 8-hour intervals
until three maintenance doses have been
given and parasitemia is reduced to less
than 1% and oral quinidine sulfate can be
initiated.
Children: 10 mg/kg gluconate I.V. over
1 to 2 hours; then continuous infusion of
0.02 mg/kg/minute for up to 72 hours or
until parasitemia is reduced to 1% or less,
whichever comes first. For patients able to
swallow pills, maintenance therapy may
be given P.O. with quinine sulfate every
8 hours in divided doses of same quinine
base amount.

ADMINISTRATION
P.O.
● Give drug with food to avoid adverse GI
reactions.

● Don't crush extended-release tablets. If
necessary, scored tablets may be broken in
half to adjust quinidine dose.
● Don't give drug with grapefruit juice.
I.V.
▼ For quinidine gluconate infusion to
treat atrial fibrillation or flutter in adults,
dilute 800 mg (10 mL of injection)
with 40 mL D_5W and infuse at up to
0.25 mg/kg/minute.
▼ For quinidine gluconate infusion to
treat malaria, dilute in 5 mL/kg (usually
250 mL) normal saline solution and infuse
over 1 to 2 hours, followed by a continuous
maintenance infusion.
▼ During infusion, continuously monitor
patient's blood pressure and ECG.
▼ Adjust rate so that the arrhythmia is
corrected without disturbing the normal
mechanism of the heartbeat.
▼ Never use discolored (brownish)
quinidine solution.
▼ Store drug away from heat and direct
light.
▼ **Incompatibilities:** Alkalies, amiodarone, atracurium besylate, furosemide,
heparin sodium, iodides.

ACTION
A class IA antiarrhythmic with direct and
indirect (anticholinergic) effects on cardiac
tissue. Decreases automaticity, conduction
velocity, and membrane responsiveness;
prolongs effective refractory period; and
reduces vagal tone.

Route	Onset	Peak	Duration
P.O.	1–3 hr	1–6 hr	6–8 hr
I.V.	Immediate	Immediate	Unknown

Half-life: 5 to 12 hours.

ADVERSE REACTIONS
CNS: vertigo, fever, headache, light-
headedness, ataxia, confusion, depression,
dementia.
CV: ECG changes, tachycardia, *PVCs,
ventricular tachycardia, atypical ventricular tachycardia, complete AV block,
aggravated heart failure,* hypotension.
EENT: tinnitus, blurred vision, diplopia,
photophobia.
GI: diarrhea, nausea, vomiting, anorexia,
excessive salivation, abdominal pain.

Reactions in bold italics are *life-threatening*. Interactions may have a *rapid onset* or a *delayed onset*.

Hematologic: *thrombocytopenia, agranulocytosis,* hemolytic anemia.
Hepatic: *hepatotoxicity.*
Respiratory: *acute asthmatic attack, respiratory arrest.*
Skin: rash, petechial hemorrhage of buccal mucosa, pruritus, urticaria, photosensitivity reactions.
Other: cinchonism, *angioedema,* lupus erythematosus.

INTERACTIONS
Drug-drug. *Amiloride:* May increase the risk of arrhythmias. If use together can't be avoided, monitor ECG closely.
Amiodarone: May increase quinidine level, producing life-threatening cardiac arrhythmias. Monitor quinidine level closely if use together can't be avoided. Adjust quinidine as needed.
Antacids, sodium bicarbonate: May increase quinidine level. Monitor patient for increased effect.
Azole antifungals: May increase the risk of CV events. Use together is contraindicated.
Barbiturates, phenytoin, rifampin: May decrease quinidine level. Monitor patient for decreased effect.
Cimetidine: May increase quinidine level. Monitor patient for increased arrhythmias.
Digoxin: May increase digoxin level after starting quinidine therapy. Monitor digoxin level.
Drugs that prolong the QT interval (antipsychotics, disopyramide, procainamide, sotalol, TCAs): May have additive effect with quinidine and cause life-threatening cardiac arrhythmias. Avoid using together when possible.
Fluvoxamine, nefazodone, TCAs: May increase antidepressant level, thus increasing its effect. Monitor patient for adverse reactions.
Macrolides and related antibiotics (azithromycin, clarithromycin, erythromycin, telithromycin): May cause additive effects or prolongation of the QT interval. Use with caution. Avoid use with telithromycin.
Neuromuscular blockers: May potentiate effects of these drugs. Avoid use of quinidine immediately after surgery.

Nifedipine: May decrease quinidine level. May need to adjust dosage.
Other antiarrhythmics (such as lidocaine, procainamide, propranolol): May increase risk of toxicity. Use together cautiously.
Protease inhibitors (nelfinavir, ritonavir): May significantly increase quinidine levels and toxicity. Use together is contraindicated.
Quinolones: May cause life-threatening arrhythmias, including torsades de pointes. Avoid using together.
Verapamil: May decrease quinidine clearance and cause hypotension, bradycardia, AV block, or pulmonary edema. Monitor blood pressure and heart rate.
Warfarin: May increase anticoagulant effect. Monitor patient closely.
Drug-herb. *Jimsonweed:* May adversely affect CV function. Discourage use together.
Licorice: May have additive effect and prolong QT interval. Urge caution.
Drug-food. *Grapefruit:* May delay absorption and onset of action of drug. Discourage use together.

EFFECTS ON LAB TEST RESULTS
• May decrease hemoglobin level.
• May decrease platelet and granulocyte counts.

CONTRAINDICATIONS & CAUTIONS
• Contraindicated in patients with idiosyncrasy or hypersensitivity to quinidine or related cinchona derivatives.
• Contraindicated in those with myasthenia gravis, intraventricular conduction defects, digoxin toxicity when AV conduction is grossly impaired, abnormal rhythms caused by escape mechanisms, complete AV block, history of drug-induced torsades de pointes, and history of prolonged QT interval syndrome.
• Contraindicated in patients who developed thrombocytopenia after exposure to quinidine or quinine.
• Use cautiously in patients with asthma, muscle weakness, or infection accompanied by fever because hypersensitivity reactions to drug may be masked.
• Use cautiously in patients with hepatic or renal impairment because systemic accumulation may occur.

Q

⚠ Overdose S&S: Depressed mental function, headache, nausea, vomiting, diarrhea, abdominal pain, tachyarrhythmias, depressed cardiac automaticity and conduction, hypotension, heart failure, hypokalemia, acidosis.

NURSING CONSIDERATIONS

• Check apical pulse rate and blood pressure before therapy. If extremes in pulse rate are detected, withhold drug and notify prescriber at once.

• Anticoagulant therapy is commonly advised before quinidine therapy in long-standing atrial fibrillation because restoration of normal sinus rhythm may result in thromboembolism caused by dislodgment of thrombi from atrial wall.

• Monitor patient for atypical ventricular tachycardia, such as torsades de pointes and ECG changes, particularly widening of QRS complex and widened QT and PR intervals.

❸ Alert: When changing route of administration or oral salt form, prescriber should alter dosage to compensate for variations in quinidine base content.

❸ Alert: Hospitalize patients with severe malaria in an intensive care setting, with continuous monitoring. Decrease infusion rate if quinidine level exceeds 6 mcg/mL, uncorrected QT interval exceeds 0.6 seconds, or QRS complex widening exceeds 25% of baseline.

• Monitor LFT results during first 4 to 8 weeks of therapy.

• Monitor quinidine level. Therapeutic levels for antiarrhythmic effects are 4 to 8 mcg/mL.

• Monitor patient response carefully. If adverse GI reactions occur, especially diarrhea, notify prescriber. Check quinidine level, which is increasingly toxic when greater than 10 mcg/mL. GI symptoms may be decreased by giving drug with meals or aluminum hydroxide antacids.

• **Look alike–sound alike:** Don't confuse quinidine with quinine or clonidine.

PATIENT TEACHING

• Stress importance of taking drug exactly as prescribed and taking it with food if adverse GI reactions occur.

❸ Alert: Instruct patient not to crush or chew extended-release tablets. If necessary, he may break scored tablets in half to adjust quinidine dose.

• Tell patient to avoid grapefruit juice because it may delay drug absorption and inhibit drug metabolism.

• Advise patient to report persistent or serious adverse reactions promptly, especially signs and symptoms of quinidine toxicity (ringing in the ears, visual disturbances, dizziness, headache, nausea).

quinupristin–dalfopristin
QUIN-uh-pris-tin/DALF-oh-pris-tin

Synercid

Therapeutic class: Antibiotics
Pharmacologic class: Streptogramins
Pregnancy risk category: B

AVAILABLE FORMS
Injection: 500-mg vial (150 mg quinupristin and 350 mg dalfopristin)

INDICATIONS & DOSAGES
➤ **Complicated skin and skin-structure infections caused by methicillin-susceptible *Staphylococcus aureus* or *Streptococcus pyogenes***
Adults and adolescents age 12 and older: 7.5 mg/kg I.V. over 1 hour every 12 hours for at least 7 days.
➤ **Infective endocarditis ◆**
Adults and children: 22.5 mg/kg I.V. in three divided doses daily for at least 8 weeks.

ADMINISTRATION
I.V.
▼ Reconstitute powder for injection by adding 5 mL of either sterile water for injection or D₅W and gently swirling vial by manual rotation to ensure dissolution; avoid shaking to limit foaming. Reconstituted solutions must be further diluted within 30 minutes.
▼ Add appropriate dose of reconstituted solution to 250 mL of D₅W, according to patient's weight, to yield no more than

2 mg/mL. This diluted solution is stable for 5 hours at room temperature or 54 hours if refrigerated.

▼ Flush line with D_5W before and after each dose.

▼ Fluid-restricted patients with a central venous catheter may receive dose in 100 mL of D_5W. This concentration isn't recommended for peripheral venous administration.

▼ If moderate to severe peripheral venous irritation occurs, consider increasing infusion volume to 500 or 750 mL, changing injection site, or infusing by a central venous catheter.

▼ Give all doses by I.V. infusion over 1 hour. An infusion pump or device may be used to control infusion rate.

▼ **Incompatibilities:** Saline and heparin solutions.

ACTION

The two antibiotics work synergistically to inhibit or destroy susceptible bacteria through combined inhibition of protein synthesis in bacterial cells. Without the ability to manufacture new proteins, the bacterial cells are inactivated or die.

Route	Onset	Peak	Duration
I.V.	Unknown	Unknown	Unknown

Half-life: Quinupristin, 1 hour; dalfopristin, ¾ hour.

ADVERSE REACTIONS

CNS: headache, pain.
CV: thrombophlebitis.
GI: diarrhea, nausea, vomiting.
Musculoskeletal: arthralgia, myalgia.
Skin: edema at infusion site, inflammation, infusion-site reaction, pain at infusion site, pruritus, rash.

INTERACTIONS

Drug-drug. *Cyclosporine:* May lower metabolism; may increase drug level. Monitor cyclosporine level.

Drugs metabolized by CYP3A4 (such as carbamazepine, delavirdine, diazepam, diltiazem, disopyramide, docetaxel, indinavir, lidocaine, lovastatin, methylprednisolone, midazolam, nevirapine, nifedipine, paclitaxel, ritonavir, tacrolimus, verapamil, vinblastine): May increase

levels of these drugs, which could increase both their therapeutic effects and adverse reactions. Use together cautiously.

Drugs metabolized by CYP3A4 that may prolong the QTc interval, such as quinidine: May decrease metabolism of these drugs, prolonging QTc interval. Avoid using together.

EFFECTS ON LAB TEST RESULTS

● May increase AST, ALT, and bilirubin levels.

CONTRAINDICATIONS & CAUTIONS

● Contraindicated in patients hypersensitive to drug or other streptogramin antibiotics.
● Safety and effectiveness haven't been established in patients younger than age 16.
● Use during pregnancy only if clearly needed. Use cautiously in breast-feeding women.

NURSING CONSIDERATIONS

● Drug isn't active against *Enterococcus faecalis.* Blood cultures are needed to avoid misidentifying *E. faecalis* as *E. faecium.*
● Because drug may cause mild to life-threatening pseudomembranous colitis, consider this diagnosis in patient who develops diarrhea during or after therapy.
● Adverse reactions, such as arthralgia and myalgia, may be reduced by decreasing dosage interval to every 12 hours.
● Because overgrowth of nonsusceptible organisms may occur, monitor patient closely for signs and symptoms of super-infection.
● Monitor LFT results during therapy.

PATIENT TEACHING

● Advise patient to immediately report irritation at I.V. site, pain in joints or muscles, and diarrhea.
● Tell patient about importance of reporting persistent or worsening signs and symptoms of infection, such as pain or redness.
● Tell patient to report watery and bloody stools, even as late as 2 or more months after the last antibiotic dose.

Q

rabeprazole sodium
rah-BEH-pray-zol

Aciphex◆, Aciphex Sprinkle

Therapeutic class: Antiulcer drugs
Pharmacologic class: Proton pump inhibitors
Pregnancy risk category: B

AVAILABLE FORMS
Capsules (delayed-release): 5 mg, 10 mg
Tablets (delayed-release): 20 mg

INDICATIONS & DOSAGES
➤ **Healing of erosive or ulcerative GERD**
Adults: 20 mg P.O. daily for 4 to 8 weeks. Additional 8-week course may be considered, if needed.
➤ **Maintenance of healing of erosive or ulcerative GERD**
Adults: 20 mg P.O. daily.
➤ **Healing of duodenal ulcers**
Adults: 20 mg P.O. daily after morning meal for up to 4 weeks.
➤ **Pathologic hypersecretory conditions, including Zollinger-Ellison syndrome**
Adults: 60 mg P.O. daily; may be increased, as needed, to 100 mg P.O. daily or 60 mg P.O. b.i.d.
➤ **Symptomatic GERD, including daytime and nighttime heartburn**
Adults: 20 mg P.O. daily for 4 weeks. Additional 4-week course may be considered, if needed.
Children age 12 and older: 20 mg P.O. daily for up to 8 weeks.
✱ *NEW INDICATION:* **GERD (Aciphex Sprinkle)**
Children ages 1 to 11 weighing 15 kg (33 lb) or more: 10 mg P.O. once daily for up to 12 weeks.
Children ages 1 to 11 weighing less than 15 kg: 5 mg P.O. once daily for up to 12 weeks. May increase to 10 mg once daily if inadequate response.
➤ *Helicobacter pylori* **eradication, to reduce the risk of duodenal ulcer recurrence**
Adults: 20 mg P.O. b.i.d., combined with amoxicillin 1,000 mg P.O. b.i.d. and clarithromycin 500 mg P.O. b.i.d., for 7 days.

ADMINISTRATION
P.O.
● Don't crush or split tablets.
● Give drug without regard for food.
● Open Sprinkle delayed-release capsules and empty onto a spoonful of soft food (applesauce) or liquid that's at or below room temperature.
● Give whole dose within 15 minutes of sprinkling and 30 minutes before a meal.
● Sprinkle granules shouldn't be chewed or crushed.

ACTION
Blocks proton pump activity and gastric acid secretion by inhibiting gastric hydrogen–potassium adenosine triphosphatase (an enzyme) at secretory surface of gastric parietal cells.

Route	Onset	Peak	Duration
P.O.	<1 hr	2–5 hr	>24 hr

Half-life: 1 to 2 hours.

ADVERSE REACTIONS
CNS: headache, pain, dizziness.
CV: edema.
EENT: pharyngitis, dry mouth.
GI: abdominal pain, constipation, diarrhea, flatulence.
Hepatic: elevated liver enzyme levels, hepatitis, hepatic encephalopathy.
Musculoskeletal: arthralgia, myalgia.
Other: infection.

INTERACTIONS
Drug-drug. *Clarithromycin:* May increase rabeprazole level. Monitor patient closely.
Cyclosporine: May inhibit cyclosporine metabolism. Use together cautiously.
Digoxin, ketoconazole, other gastric pH-dependent drugs: May decrease or increase drug absorption at increased pH values. Monitor patient closely.
Methotrexate: May increase methotrexate concentration and risk of toxicity. Closely monitor methotrexate concentration and watch for signs and symptoms of methotrexate toxicity. Rabeprazole may need to be suspended or stopped.
Protease inhibitors (atazanavir, indinavir, nelfinavir, saquinavir): May decrease levels

---

Reactions in bold italics are *life-threatening*. Interactions may have a *rapid onset* or a *delayed onset*.

of these drugs. Monitor clinical response. Contraindicated with atazanavir.

Salicylates (aspirin): May increase release of salicylate from enteric coating, increasing gastric side effects. Use together cautiously.

Warfarin: May inhibit warfarin metabolism. Monitor PT and INR.

EFFECTS ON LAB TEST RESULTS
• May decrease magnesium level.

CONTRAINDICATIONS & CAUTIONS
• Contraindicated in patients hypersensitive to drug, other benzimidazoles (lansoprazole, omeprazole), or components of these formulations.

• In *H. pylori* eradication, clarithromycin is contraindicated in pregnant women, patients hypersensitive to macrolides, and those taking pimozide; amoxicillin is contraindicated in patients hypersensitive to penicillin.

• Use cautiously in patients with severe hepatic impairment.

• Long-term (1 year or more) and multiple daily-dose rabeprazole therapy may be associated with an increased risk of osteoporosis-related fractures of the hip, wrist, or spine. Use lowest dosage and shortest duration of therapy appropriate to the condition being treated.

NURSING CONSIDERATIONS
• Consider additional courses of therapy if duodenal ulcer or GERD isn't healed after first course of therapy.

• If *H. pylori* eradication is unsuccessful, do susceptibility testing. If patient is resistant to clarithromycin or susceptibility testing isn't possible, expect to start therapy using a different antimicrobial.

⚠ *Alert:* Prolonged use of proton pump inhibitors may cause low magnesium levels. Monitor magnesium levels before starting treatment and periodically thereafter.

⚠ *Alert:* Monitor patients for signs and symptoms of low magnesium level, such as abnormal heart rate or rhythm, palpitations, muscle spasms, tremor, or seizures. In children, abnormal heart rate may present as fatigue, upset stomach, dizziness, and lightheadedness. Magnesium supplementation or drug discontinuation may be needed.

• Symptomatic response to therapy doesn't preclude presence of gastric malignancy.

⚠ *Alert:* Patients treated for *H. pylori* eradication have developed pseudomembranous colitis with nearly all antibiotics, including clarithromycin and amoxicillin. Monitor patient closely.

⚠ *Alert:* May increase *Clostridium difficile*–associated diarrhea (CDAD). Evaluate for CDAD in patients who develop diarrhea that doesn't improve.

• *Look alike–sound alike:* Don't confuse Aciphex with Accupril or Aricept. Don't confuse rabeprazole with aripiprazole.

PATIENT TEACHING
• Explain importance of taking drug exactly as prescribed.

• Advise patient to swallow delayed-release tablet whole and not to crush, chew, or split.

• Inform patient that delayed-release tablet may be taken without regard to meals.

• Tell patient or caregiver to open Sprinkle delayed-release capsules and empty onto a spoonful of soft food (applesauce) or liquid that's at or below room temperature, and to take the whole dose within 15 minutes of sprinkling and 30 minutes before a meal.

• Advise patient or caregiver that Sprinkle granules shouldn't be chewed or crushed.

• Inform patient that drug may increase the risk of osteoporosis-related fractures of the hip, wrist, or spine with multiple daily doses that are continued for longer than 1 year.

• Teach patient to recognize and report signs and symptoms of low magnesium levels.

raloxifene hydrochloride
rah-LOX-i-feen

Evista⌀

Therapeutic class: Antiosteoporotics
Pharmacologic class: Selective estrogen receptor modulators
Pregnancy risk category: X

AVAILABLE FORMS
Tablets: 60 mg

INDICATIONS & DOSAGES

➤ **To prevent or treat osteoporosis; to reduce the risk of invasive breast cancer in postmenopausal women with osteoporosis and postmenopausal women at high risk for invasive breast cancer**
Postmenopausal women: 60 mg P.O. once daily.

ADMINISTRATION

P.O.
● Give drug without regard for food.
● Stop drug at least 72 hours before prolonged immobilization and resume only after patient is fully mobilized.

ACTION

Reduces resorption of bone and decreases overall bone turnover. These effects on bone are manifested as reductions in serum and urine levels of bone turnover markers and increases in bone mineral density.

Route	Onset	Peak	Duration
P.O.	Unknown	Unknown	24 hr

Half-life: 27½ hours.

ADVERSE REACTIONS

CNS: depression, insomnia, fever, migraine.
CV: chest pain.
EENT: sinusitis, pharyngitis, laryngitis.
GI: nausea, dyspepsia, vomiting, flatulence, gastroenteritis, abdominal pain.
GU: vaginitis, UTI, cystitis, leukorrhea, endometrial disorder, vaginal bleeding.
Metabolic: weight gain.
Musculoskeletal: arthralgia, myalgia, arthritis, leg cramps.
Respiratory: increased cough, pneumonia.
Skin: rash, diaphoresis.
Other: infection, flulike syndrome, hot flashes, breast pain, peripheral edema.

INTERACTIONS

Drug-drug. *Cholestyramine:* May cause significant reduction in absorption of raloxifene. Avoid using together.
Highly protein-bound drugs (such as clofibrate, diazepam, diazoxide, ibuprofen, indomethacin, naproxen): May interfere with binding sites. Use together cautiously.

Warfarin: May cause a decrease in PT. Monitor PT and INR closely.

EFFECTS ON LAB TEST RESULTS

● May increase triglyceride level.

CONTRAINDICATIONS & CAUTIONS

● Contraindicated in women hypersensitive to drug or its components; in women who are pregnant, planning to get pregnant, or breast-feeding; and in children.
Black Box Warning Increased risk of venous thromboembolism and death from stroke. Contraindicated in women with a history of, or active, venous thromboembolism. Consider the risk-benefit balance in women at risk for stroke. ∎
● Use cautiously in patients with severe hepatic or renal impairment.
● Safety and effectiveness of drug haven't been evaluated in men.
⚠ Overdose S&S: Leg cramps, dizziness, ataxia, flushing, rash, tremors, vomiting, elevated alkaline phosphatase level.

NURSING CONSIDERATIONS

● Watch for signs of blood clots. Greatest risk of thromboembolic events occurs during first 4 months of treatment.
● Watch for breast abnormalities; drug doesn't eliminate risk of breast cancer.
● Effect on bone mineral density beyond 2 years of drug treatment isn't known.
● Use with hormone replacement therapy or systemic estrogen hasn't been evaluated and isn't recommended.
● Monitor triglyceride level if previous treatment with estrogen caused elevation.

PATIENT TEACHING

● Advise patient to avoid long periods of restricted movement (such as during traveling) because of increased risk of venous thromboembolic events.
● Inform patient that hot flashes or flushing may occur and that drug doesn't aid in reducing them.
● Instruct patient to practice other bone loss-prevention measures, including taking supplemental calcium and vitamin D if dietary intake is inadequate, performing weight-bearing exercises, and stopping alcohol consumption and smoking.

Reactions in bold italics are *life-threatening*. Interactions may have a *rapid onset* or a *delayed onset*.

• Tell patient that drug may be taken without regard for food.
• Advise patient to report unexplained uterine bleeding or breast abnormalities during therapy.
• Explain adverse reactions and instruct patient to read patient package insert before starting therapy and each time prescription is renewed.

raltegravir potassium
ral-TEG-rah-veer

Isentress

Therapeutic class: Antiretrovirals
Pharmacologic class: HIV integrase strand transfer inhibitors
Pregnancy risk category: C

AVAILABLE FORMS
Tablets: 400 mg
Tablets (chewable): 25 mg, 100 mg

INDICATIONS & DOSAGES
➤ **HIV-1 infection, with other antiretrovirals, in treatment-experienced and treatment-naive patients who have continued HIV-1 replication despite antiretroviral therapy**
Adults and children age 16 and older:
400 mg P.O. b.i.d. When administered concomitantly with rifampin, give 800 mg P.O. b.i.d.
➤ **HIV-1 infection, with other antiretrovirals, in children and adolescents age 2 and older weighing at least 10 kg**
Children ages 12 to 15 and children ages 6 to 11 weighing at least 25 kg (55 lb):
400 mg P.O. b.i.d.
Children ages 2 to 11 weighing at least 40 kg (88 lb): 300 mg (chewable tablets) P.O. b.i.d.
Children ages 2 to 11 weighing 28 kg (62 lb) to less than 40 kg: 200 mg (chewable tablets) P.O. b.i.d.
Children ages 2 to 11 weighing 20 kg (44 lb) to less than 28 kg: 150 mg (chewable tablets) P.O. b.i.d.
Children ages 2 to 11 weighing 14 kg (31 lb) to less than 20 kg: 100 mg (chewable tablets) P.O. b.i.d.

Children ages 2 to 11 weighing 10 kg (22 lb) to less than 14 kg: 75 mg (chewable tablets) P.O. b.i.d.

ADMINISTRATION
P.O.
• Give drug without regard for meals.

ACTION
Inhibits HIV-1 integrase, an enzyme required for HIV-1 replication.

Route	Onset	Peak	Duration
P.O.	Rapid	3 hr	Unknown

Half-life: About 9 hours.

ADVERSE REACTIONS
CNS: headache, fever, fatigue, dizziness, insomnia.
GI: nausea, abdominal pain, vomiting.
Hematologic: anemia, *neutropenia, thrombocytopenia.*
Metabolic: hyperglycemia.
Musculoskeletal: asthenia, myopathy, *rhabdomyolysis.*
Skin: lipodystrophy.
Other: immune reconstitution syndrome.

INTERACTIONS
Drug-drug. *Atazanavir:* May increase raltegravir level. Use together cautiously.
UGT1A1 inhibitors, such as rifampin: May decrease raltegravir level. Use together cautiously.

EFFECTS ON LAB TEST RESULTS
• May increase bilirubin, AST, ALT, alkaline phosphatase, amylase, lipase, glucose, and CK levels. May decrease hemoglobin level.
• May decrease neutrophil and platelet counts.

CONTRAINDICATIONS & CAUTIONS
• Contraindicated in patients hypersensitive to drug or its components.
⊗ **Alert:** Severe, potentially life-threatening and fatal skin reactions have been reported. Discontinue drug immediately if signs or symptoms of severe skin reactions occur.
• Use cautiously in patients taking drugs known to cause myopathy or rhabdomyolysis, such as statins.

R

• Use cautiously in elderly patients, especially those with hepatic, renal, and cardiac insufficiency.

NURSING CONSIDERATIONS
• Perform laboratory tests, including CBC, platelet count, and LFTs, before therapy and regularly throughout therapy.
• Use drug with at least one other antiretroviral.
• Drug should be reserved for patients who demonstrate resistance to other regimens.
• Watch for signs of myopathy or rash.
• Give drug to pregnant women only if the potential benefit justifies the risk to the fetus.
• Register pregnant women for monitoring of maternal-fetal outcomes by calling the Antiretroviral Pregnancy Registry at 1-800-258-4263.
• Safety and effectiveness haven't been established in children younger than age 2.
• Breast-feeding isn't recommended during therapy.
• Monitor patient for immune reconstitution syndrome. During initial phase of treatment, patients responding to antiretroviral therapy may develop an inflammatory response to indolent or residual opportunistic infections (CMV, *Mycobacterium avium* complex, *Pneumocystis jiroveci* pneumonia, tuberculosis), which may necessitate further evaluation and treatment. Autoimmune disorders (such as Graves disease, polymyositis, and Guillain-Barré syndrome) have also been reported in the setting of immune reconstitution; however, time to onset is more variable, and can occur many months after initiation of antiretroviral treatment.

PATIENT TEACHING
• Inform patient that drug doesn't cure HIV infection. He may continue to develop opportunistic infections and other complications of HIV infection, and transmission of HIV to others through sexual contact or blood contamination is still possible.
• Advise patient to use barrier protection during sexual intercourse.
• Tell women that breast-feeding isn't recommended during therapy.

• Advise patient to immediately report worsening symptoms or unexplained muscle pain, tenderness, or weakness while taking the drug.
• Instruct patient to avoid missing any doses to decrease the risk of developing HIV resistance.
• Inform patient that severe and potentially life-threatening rash has been reported and to immediately contact the health care provider if a rash develops. Instruct patient to immediately stop taking raltegravir and seek medical attention if the rash is associated with any of the following signs or symptoms: fever; generally ill feeling; extreme tiredness; muscle or joint aches; blisters; oral lesions; eye inflammation; facial swelling; swelling of the eyes, lips, or mouth; breathing difficulty; or signs and symptoms of liver problems (such as yellowing of the skin or whites of the eyes, dark or tea colored urine, pale-colored stools or bowel movements, nausea, vomiting, loss of appetite, pain, aching or sensitivity on the right side below the ribs).
• Advise patient with phenylketonuria that the 25-mg and 100-mg chewable tablets contain phenylalanine.
• Tell patient if a dose is missed to take the next dose as soon as possible and not to double the next dose.
• Advise patient to report use of other drugs, including OTC drugs; this drug interacts with other drugs.
• Tell patient that drug may be taken without regard for meals.

ramelteon
rah-MELL-tee-on

Rozerem

Therapeutic class: Hypnotics
Pharmacologic class: Melatonin receptor agonists
Pregnancy risk category: C

AVAILABLE FORMS
Tablets: 8 mg

INDICATIONS & DOSAGES
➤ **Insomnia characterized by trouble falling asleep**
Adults: 8 mg P.O. within 30 minutes of bedtime.

ADMINISTRATION
P.O.
● Don't give drug with or immediately after a high-fat meal.
● Give drug within 30 minutes of bedtime.

ACTION
Acts on receptors believed to maintain the circadian rhythm underlying the normal sleep-wake cycle.

Route	Onset	Peak	Duration
P.O.	Rapid	½–1½ hr	Unknown

Half-life: Parent compound, 1 to 2½ hours; metabolite M-II, 2 to 5 hours.

ADVERSE REACTIONS
CNS: complex sleep-related behaviors, depression, dizziness, fatigue, headache, somnolence, worsened insomnia.
GI: diarrhea, impaired taste, nausea.
Musculoskeletal: arthralgia, myalgia.
Respiratory: upper respiratory tract infection.
Other: *anaphylaxis, angioedema,* flulike symptoms.

INTERACTIONS
Drug-drug. *CNS depressants:* May cause excessive CNS depression. Use together cautiously.
Fluconazole (strong CYP2C9 inhibitor), ketoconazole (strong CYP3A4 inhibitor), weak CYP1A2 inhibitors: May increase ramelteon level. Use together cautiously.
Fluvoxamine (strong CYP1A2 inhibitor): May increase ramelteon level. Don't use together.
Rifampin (strong CYP enzyme inducer): May decrease ramelteon level. Monitor patient for lack of effect.
Drug-food. *Food (especially high-fat meals):* May delay time to peak drug effect. Tell patient to take drug on an empty stomach.

Drug-lifestyle. *Alcohol use:* May cause excessive CNS depression. Discourage alcohol use.

EFFECTS ON LAB TEST RESULTS
● May increase prolactin level.
● May decrease testosterone level.

CONTRAINDICATIONS & CAUTIONS
● Contraindicated in those hypersensitive to drug or its components. Don't use in patients taking fluvoxamine or in those with severe hepatic impairment, severe sleep apnea, or severe COPD.
● Use cautiously in patients with depression or moderate hepatic impairment.

NURSING CONSIDERATIONS
⊙ *Alert:* Anaphylaxis and angioedema may occur as early as the first dose. Monitor patient closely.
● Thoroughly evaluate the cause of insomnia before starting drug.
● Assess patient for behavioral or cognitive disorders.
● Drug doesn't cause physical dependence.
● *Look alike–sound alike:* Don't confuse Rozerem with Razadyne. Don't confuse ramelteon with Remeron.

PATIENT TEACHING
⊙ *Alert:* Warn patient that drug may cause allergic reactions, facial swelling, and complex sleep-related behaviors, such as driving, eating, and making phone calls while asleep. Advise patient to report these adverse effects.
● Instruct patient to take dose within 30 minutes of bedtime.
● Tell patient not to take drug with or after a heavy meal.
● Caution against performing activities that require mental alertness or physical coordination after taking drug.
● Caution patient to avoid alcohol while taking drug.
● Tell patient to consult prescriber if insomnia worsens or behavior changes.
● Urge women to consult prescriber if menses stops, libido decreases, or galactorrhea or fertility problems develop.

R

ramipril
ra-MI-pril

Altace

Therapeutic class: Antihypertensives
Pharmacologic class: ACE inhibitors
Pregnancy risk category: C; D in 2nd and 3rd trimesters

AVAILABLE FORMS
Capsules: 1.25 mg, 2.5 mg, 5 mg, 10 mg
Tablets: 1.25 mg, 2.5 mg, 5 mg, 10 mg

INDICATIONS & DOSAGES
➤ **Hypertension**
Adults: Initially, 2.5 mg P.O. once daily for patients not taking a diuretic, and 1.25 mg P.O. once daily for patients taking a diuretic. Increase dosage, if needed, based on patient response. Maintenance dose is 2.5 to 20 mg daily as a single dose or in divided doses.
Adjust-a-dose: For patients with CrCl less than 40 mL/minute, give 1.25 mg P.O. daily. Adjust dosage gradually based on response. Maximum daily dose is 5 mg.
➤ **Heart failure after an MI**
Adults: Initially, 2.5 mg P.O. b.i.d. If hypotension occurs, decrease dosage to 1.25 mg P.O. b.i.d. Adjust as tolerated, with dosage increases about 3 weeks apart, to target dosage of 5 mg P.O. b.i.d.
Adjust-a-dose: For patients with CrCl less than 40 mL/minute, give 1.25 mg P.O. daily. Adjust dosage gradually based on response. Maximum dosage is 2.5 mg b.i.d.
➤ **To reduce risk of MI, stroke, and death from CV causes**
Adults age 55 and older: 2.5 mg P.O. once daily for 1 week, then 5 mg P.O. once daily for 3 weeks. Increase as tolerated to a maintenance dose of 10 mg P.O. once daily.
Adjust-a-dose: In patients who are hypertensive or who have recently had an MI, daily dose may be divided.
➤ **Heart failure due to left ventricular systolic dysfunction with reduced LVEF** ◆
Adults: Initially, 1.25 to 2.5 mg P.O. once daily, titrated to a maximum dosage of 10 mg once daily.

Adjust-a-dose: In patients with CrCl of less than 40 mL/minute, 25% of normal dose will usually induce full therapeutic levels. Adjust dosage accordingly.

ADMINISTRATION
P.O.
● Give drug without regard for meals.
● Open capsule and sprinkle contents on a small amount of applesauce or mix with 4 oz of water or apple juice. Give to patient immediately.

ACTION
Prevents conversion of angiotensin I to angiotensin II, a potent vasoconstrictor. Less angiotensin II decreases peripheral arterial resistance, decreasing aldosterone secretion, which reduces sodium and water retention and lowers blood pressure.

Route	Onset	Peak	Duration
P.O.	1–2 hr	1–3 hr	24 hr

Half-life: 13 to 17 hours.

ADVERSE REACTIONS
CNS: headache, dizziness, fatigue, asthenia, malaise, light-headedness, vertigo, syncope.
CV: hypotension, *heart failure, MI,* postural hypotension, angina pectoris, chest pain, edema.
GI: nausea, vomiting, diarrhea.
Metabolic: *hyperkalemia,* hyperglycemia, weight gain.
Musculoskeletal: arthralgia, arthritis, myalgia.
Respiratory: dyspnea; dry, persistent, tickling, nonproductive cough.
Other: hypersensitivity reactions.

INTERACTIONS
Drug-drug. ● *Alert: Aliskiren:* May increase risk of renal impairment, hypotension, and hyperkalemia in diabetic patients and those with moderate to severe renal impairment (GFR less than 60 mL/minute). Concomitant use is contraindicated in diabetic patients. Avoid concomitant use in those with moderate to severe renal impairment.

Reactions in bold italics are *life-threatening*. Interactions may have a *rapid onset* or a *delayed onset*.

Diuretics: May cause excessive hypotension, especially at start of therapy. Stop diuretic at least 3 days before therapy begins, increase sodium intake, or reduce starting dose of ramipril.

Insulin, oral antidiabetics: May cause hypoglycemia, especially at start of ramipril therapy. Monitor glucose level closely.

Lithium: May increase lithium level. Use together cautiously and monitor lithium level.

NSAIDs: May decrease antihypertensive effects. Monitor blood pressure.

Potassium-sparing diuretics, potassium supplements: May cause hyperkalemia; ramipril attenuates potassium loss. Monitor potassium level closely.

Salicylates (aspirin): May decrease antihypertensive effects of ramipril. Ramipril dosage increase or aspirin dosage decrease may be needed.

Telmisartan: May increase risk of renal dysfunction. Avoid use together.

Tizanidine: May cause severe hypotension. Use cautiously and monitor blood pressure closely.

Drug-herb. *Capsaicin:* May cause cough. Discourage use together.

Ma huang: May decrease antihypertensive effects. Discourage use together.

Drug-food. *Salt substitutes containing potassium:* May cause hyperkalemia; ramipril attenuates potassium loss. Discourage use of salt substitutes during therapy.

EFFECTS ON LAB TEST RESULTS
● May increase BUN, creatinine, bilirubin, liver enzymes, glucose, and potassium levels. May decrease hemoglobin level and hematocrit.
● May decrease RBC and platelet counts.

CONTRAINDICATIONS & CAUTIONS
● Contraindicated in patients hypersensitive to ACE inhibitors, in those with a history of angioedema related to treatment with an ACE inhibitor, and in breast-feeding women.

Black Box Warning Use during pregnancy can cause injury and death to the developing fetus. When pregnancy is detected, stop drug as soon as possible. ∎

● Use cautiously in patients with renal impairment.
⚠ Overdose S&S: Hypotension.

NURSING CONSIDERATIONS
● Monitor blood pressure regularly for drug effectiveness.
● Correct fluid and electrolyte imbalances before starting therapy.
● Closely assess renal function in patients during first few weeks of therapy. Regular assessment of renal function is advisable. Patients with severe heart failure whose renal function depends on the renin-angiotensin-aldosterone system have experienced acute renal failure during ACE inhibitor therapy. Hypertensive patients with unilateral or bilateral renal artery stenosis also may show signs of worsening renal function during first few days of therapy. Dose reduction or drug stoppage may be necessary.
● Although ACE inhibitors reduce blood pressure in all races, they reduce it less in blacks taking the ACE inhibitor alone. Black patients should take drug with a thiazide diuretic for a more favorable response.
● ACE inhibitors appear to increase risk of angioedema in black patients.
● Discontinue drug if patient develops jaundice or significant hepatic enzyme elevation.
● Monitor CBC with differential counts before therapy and periodically thereafter.
● Drug may reduce hemoglobin and WBC, RBC, and platelet counts, especially in patients with impaired renal function or collagen vascular diseases (systemic lupus erythematosus or scleroderma).
● Monitor potassium level. Risk factors for the development of hyperkalemia include renal insufficiency, diabetes, and concomitant use of drugs that raise potassium level.

PATIENT TEACHING
● Tell patient to notify prescriber if any adverse reactions occur. Dosage adjustment or stoppage of drug may be needed.
❸ Alert: Rarely, swelling of the face and throat (including swelling of the larynx) may occur, especially after first dose. Advise patient to report signs or symptoms

R

of breathing difficulty or swelling of face, eyes, lips, or tongue.
• Inform patient that light-headedness can occur, especially during the first few days of therapy. Tell him to rise slowly to minimize this effect and to report signs and symptoms to prescriber. If he faints, patient should stop taking drug and call prescriber immediately.
• Tell patient that if he has difficulty swallowing capsules, he can open drug and sprinkle contents on a small amount of applesauce.
• Advise patient to report signs and symptoms of infection, such as fever and sore throat.
• Tell patient to avoid salt substitutes. These products may contain potassium, which can cause high potassium level in patients taking ramipril.
• Tell women of childbearing age to notify prescriber if pregnancy occurs. Drug will need to be stopped.

ranibizumab
RA-ni-BIZ-oo-mab

Lucentis

Therapeutic class: Vascular endothelial growth factor A inhibitors
Pharmacologic class: Monoclonal antibodies
Pregnancy risk category: C

AVAILABLE FORMS
Intravitreal injection: 6 mg/mL, 10 mg/mL

INDICATIONS & DOSAGES
➤ **Neovascular (wet) age-related macular degeneration or macular edema after retinal vein occlusion**
Adults: 0.5 mg (0.05 mL of 10-mg/mL solution) by intravitreal injection once a month (approximately 28 days between doses), or 0.5 mg administered by intravitreal injection once a month for 4 months followed by 0.5 mg every 3 months thereafter.
➤ **Diabetic macular edema**
Adults: 0.3 mg (0.05 mL of 6-mg/mL solution) by intravitreal injection once a month (approximately 28 days between doses).

ADMINISTRATION
Ophthalmic intravitreal injection
• Store vials in original carton under refrigeration until use. Don't freeze.
• Protect from light.
• Withdraw vial contents through a 5-micron, 19G filter needle attached to a 1-mL tuberculin syringe; discard filter needle after withdrawal of vial contents.
• Replace filter needle with a sterile 30G × ½-inch needle for the intravitreal injection. Expel contents until 0.05 mL remains in syringe.

ACTION
Binds to the receptor-binding site of active forms of vascular endothelial growth factor A, reducing endothelial cell proliferation, vascular leakage, and new blood vessel formation.

Route	Onset	Peak	Duration
Intravitreal injection	Unknown	1 day	Unknown

Half-life: 9 days.

ADVERSE REACTIONS
CNS: headache, peripheral neuropathy.
CV: atrial fibrillation, peripheral edema, *arterial thromboembolic events.*
EENT: conjunctival hemorrhage, eye pain, vitreous floaters, increased intraocular pressure (IOP), vitreous detachment, intraocular inflammation, cataract, foreign body sensation in eyes, eye irritation, increased lacrimation, blepharitis, dry eye, visual disturbance or blurred vision, eye pruritus, ocular hyperemia, retinal disorder, maculopathy, retinal degeneration, ocular discomfort, conjunctival hyperemia, posterior capsule opacification, injection-site hemorrhage, nasopharyngitis, sinusitis.
GI: nausea, constipation, GERD.
GU: renal failure, chronic renal failure.
Hematologic: anemia.
Metabolic: hypercholesterolemia.
Musculoskeletal: arthralgia.
Respiratory: upper respiratory tract infection, bronchitis, COPD, cough.
Skin: wound healing complications.
Other: seasonal allergy, flulike symptoms, antibody formation.

Reactions in bold italics are *life-threatening*. Interactions may have a *rapid onset* or a *delayed onset*.

INTERACTIONS
Drug-lifestyle. *Increased light exposure , photodynamic therapy:* May increase risk of photosensitivity. Avoid increased light exposure.

EFFECTS ON LAB TEST RESULTS
● None reported.

CONTRAINDICATIONS & CAUTIONS
● Contraindicated in patients with known hypersensitivity to drug or its components and in patients with ocular or periocular infections.
● Use cautiously in pregnant or breast-feeding women. Use only if clearly needed because effects of drug are unknown.
● May increase risk of arterial thromboem-bolic events (nonfatal stroke, nonfatal MI, vascular death, or death of unknown cause), especially in diabetic patients.

NURSING CONSIDERATIONS
● Carry out intravitreal injection procedure under aseptic conditions with adequate anesthesia and a broad-spectrum microbi-cide given before injection.
● Before and 30 minutes after intravitreal injection, monitor patient for elevated IOP using tonometry.
● Check for perfusion of the optic nerve head immediately after injection.
● Use one vial per treatment of a single eye. If second eye treatment is necessary, use new vial and reestablish sterile field.
● Monitor patient for hypersensitivity reac-tions, which may present as severe intraocu-lar inflammation.
● Monitor patient for signs and symptoms suggestive of endophthalmitis (eye red-ness, sensitivity to light, eye pain, vision changes).
● Monitor patient for arterial thromboem-bolic events.

PATIENT TEACHING
● Instruct patient to seek immediate care from the ophthalmologist for eye redness, sensitivity to light, eye pain, or vision changes.

ranitidine hydrochloride
ra-NYE-te-deen

Acid Reducer† ◇, Zantac✐*, Zantac 75 ◇, Zantac 150 ◇, Zantac 300, Zantac EFFERdose

Therapeutic class: Antiulcer drugs
Pharmacologic class: H_2-receptor antagonists
Pregnancy risk category: B

AVAILABLE FORMS
Capsules: 150 mg, 300 mg
Injection: 25 mg/mL
Syrup: 15 mg/mL*
Tablets: 75 mg ◇, 150 mg ◇, 300 mg
Tablets (effervescent): 25 mg

INDICATIONS & DOSAGES
Adjust-a-dose (for all indications): For patients with CrCl below 50 mL/minute, 150 mg P.O. every 24 hours or 50 mg I.V. every 18 to 24 hours.
➤ **Active duodenal and gastric ulcer**
Adults: 150 mg P.O. b.i.d. or 300 mg daily at bedtime. Or, 50 mg I.V. or I.M. every 6 to 8 hours. Maximum daily I.V. dose, 400 mg. Or, 150 mg by continuous infusion at 6.25 mg/hour over 24 hours.
Children ages 1 month to 16 years: For duodenal and gastric ulcers only, 2 to 4 mg/kg P.O. b.i.d., up to 300 mg/day.
➤ **Maintenance therapy for duodenal or gastric ulcer**
Adults: 150 mg P.O. at bedtime.
Children ages 1 month to 16 years: 2 to 4 mg/kg P.O. daily, up to 150 mg daily.
➤ **Pathologic hypersecretory conditions, such as Zollinger-Ellison syndrome**
Adults: 150 mg P.O. b.i.d.; doses up to 6 g or more frequent intervals may be needed in patients with severe disease. Or, infuse continuously at 1 mg/kg/hour. After 4 hours, if patient remains symptomatic or gastric acid output is greater than 10 mEq/hour, in-crease dose in increments of 0.5 mg/kg/hour and recheck gastric acid output. Doses up to 2.5 mg/kg/hour and infusion rates up to 220 mg/hour have been used.

R

➤ **GERD**
Adults: 150 mg P.O. b.i.d.
Children ages 1 month to 16 years: 5 to 10 mg/kg P.O. daily given as two divided doses.

➤ **Erosive esophagitis**
Adults: 150 mg P.O. q.i.d. Maintenance dosage is 150 mg P.O. b.i.d.
Children ages 1 month to 16 years: 5 to 10 mg/kg P.O. daily given as two divided doses.

➤ **Heartburn**
Adults and children age 12 and older: 75 mg of Zantac 75 P.O. as symptoms occur, up to 150 mg daily, not to exceed 2 weeks of continuous treatment.

➤ **To prevent stress ulcer development ◆**
Adults with normal renal function:
150 mg P.O. or via nasogastric (NG) tube b.i.d. Or, 50 mg I.V. every 6 to 8 hours. Or, 6.25 mg/hour via I.V. continuous infusion.
Adults with CrCl of less than 50 mL/ minute: 150 mg P.O. or via NG tube once daily or b.i.d. Or, 50 mg I.V. every 12 to 24 hours. Or, 2 to 4 mg/hour I.V. continuous infusion.

➤ **To prevent aspiration pneumonia in patients undergoing elective surgery ◆**
Adults: 150 mg P.O. the evening before and again 2 to 3 hours before surgery, or a single 50-mg I.V. dose 1 hour before surgery.

ADMINISTRATION
P.O.
● Give once-daily dose at bedtime.
● For effervescent tablets, make sure patient doesn't chew, swallow whole, or dissolve them on the tongue. Dissolve each dose in 6 to 8 ounces of water, then have patient drink the liquid.

I.V.
▼ To prepare I.V. injection, dilute 2 mL (50 mg) ranitidine with compatible I.V. solution to a total volume of 20 mL, and inject over at least 5 minutes. Compatible solutions include sterile water for injection, normal saline solution for injection, D_5W, or lactated Ringer injection.
▼ To give drug by intermittent I.V. infusion, dilute 50 mg (2 mL) in 100 mL compatible solution and infuse at a rate of 5 to 7 mL/minute. Infuse over 15 to 20 minutes.

▼ For continuous infusion to treat active duodenal or gastric ulcer, dilute 150 mg in 250 mL of D_5W. For hypersecretory conditions such as Zollinger-Ellison syndrome, dilute with D_5W or other compatible solution to no more than 2.5 mg/mL.
▼ After dilution, solution is stable for 48 hours at room temperature.
▼ Store I.V. injection at 39° to 86° F (4° to 30° C). Store premixed containers at 36° to 77° F (2° to 25° C).
▼ **Incompatibilities:** Amphotericin B, atracurium, cefazolin, cefoxitin, ceftazidime, cefuroxime, chlorpromazine, clindamycin phosphate, diazepam, ethacrynate sodium, hetastarch, hydroxyzine, insulin, methotrimeprazine, midazolam, norepinephrine, pentobarbital sodium, phenobarbital, phytonadione.

ACTION
Competitively inhibits action of histamine at H_2-receptor sites of parietal cells, decreasing gastric acid secretion.

Route	Onset	Peak	Duration
P.O.	1 hr	1–3 hr	13 hr
I.V.	Unknown	Unknown	Unknown

Half-life: 2 to 3 hours.

ADVERSE REACTIONS
CNS: headache, malaise, vertigo.
EENT: blurred vision.
Hepatic: jaundice.
Other: *anaphylaxis, angioedema,* burning and itching at injection site.

INTERACTIONS
Drug-drug. *Glipizide:* May increase hypoglycemic effect. Adjust glipizide dosage, as directed.
Procainamide: May decrease renal clearance of procainamide. Monitor patient closely for toxicity.
Warfarin: May interfere with warfarin clearance. Monitor patient closely.

EFFECTS ON LAB TEST RESULTS
● May increase creatinine and ALT levels.
● May cause false-positive results in urine protein tests using Multistix.

Reactions in bold italics are *life-threatening*. Interactions may have a *rapid onset* or a *delayed onset*.

CONTRAINDICATIONS & CAUTIONS
• Contraindicated in patients hypersensitive to drug and in those with acute porphyria.
• Use cautiously in patients with hepatic dysfunction. Adjust dosage in patients with impaired renal function.
⚠ **Overdose S&S:** Exaggeration of adverse reactions, abnormal gait, hypotension.

NURSING CONSIDERATIONS
• Assess patient for abdominal pain. Note presence of blood in emesis, stool, or gastric aspirate.
• Drug may be added to total parenteral nutrition solutions.
• **Look alike–sound alike:** Don't confuse ranitidine with rimantadine. Don't confuse Zantac with Xanax or Zyrtec.

PATIENT TEACHING
• Instruct patient on proper use of OTC preparation, as indicated.
• Remind patient to take once-daily prescription drug at bedtime for best results.
• Instruct patient to take without regard to meals because absorption isn't affected by food.
• Urge patient to avoid cigarette smoking because this may increase gastric acid secretion and worsen disease.
• Advise patient to report abdominal pain, blood in stool or emesis, black, tarry stools, or coffee-ground emesis.

ranolazine
ran-OH-lah-zeen

Ranexa✐

Therapeutic class: Antianginals
Pharmacologic class: Cardiovascular drugs
Pregnancy risk category: C

AVAILABLE FORMS
Tablets (extended-release): 500 mg, 1,000 mg

INDICATIONS & DOSAGES
➤ **Chronic angina**
Adults: Initially, 500 mg P.O. b.i.d. Increase, if needed, to maximum of 1,000 mg b.i.d.

ADMINISTRATION
P.O.
• Give drug without regard for meals.
• Give drug whole; don't crush or cut tablets.
• Don't give drug with grapefruit juice.

ACTION
May result from increased efficiency of myocardial oxygen use when myocardial metabolism is shifted away from fatty acid oxidation toward glucose oxidation. Antianginal and anti-ischemic properties don't decrease heart rate or blood pressure and don't increase myocardial work.

Route	Onset	Peak	Duration
P.O.	Rapid	2–5 hr	Unknown

Half-life: 7 hours.

ADVERSE REACTIONS
CNS: dizziness, headache.
CV: palpitations, peripheral edema, syncope.
EENT: tinnitus, vertigo.
GI: abdominal pain, constipation, dry mouth, nausea, vomiting.
Respiratory: dyspnea.

INTERACTIONS
Drug-drug. *Antipsychotics or TCAs metabolized by CYP2D6:* May increase levels of these drugs. Dosage reduction may be needed.
Clarithromycin, nefazodone, protease inhibitors: May cause QTc prolongation. Use together is contraindicated.
Cyclosporine, paroxetine, ritonavir: May increase ranolazine level. Use cautiously together, and monitor patient for increased adverse effects.
Digoxin: May increase digoxin level. Monitor digoxin level periodically; digoxin dosage may need to be reduced.
Diltiazem, ketoconazole and other azole antifungals, macrolide antibiotics (azithromycin, erythromycin), verapamil, other CYP3A inhibitors: May increase ranolazine level and prolong QT interval. Avoid using together.
Drugs that prolong the QT interval (antiarrhythmics, such as dofetilide, quinidine, and sotalol), antipsychotics (such as chlorpromazine and ziprasidone): May increase

R

the risk of prolonged QT interval. Use cautiously together.

Rifabutin, rifampin, rifapentine, other CYP3A inducers (carbamazepine, phenobarbital, phenytoin): May reduce plasma concentration of ranolazine to subtherapeutic levels. Don't use together.

Simvastatin: May increase simvastatin level. Limit simvastatin dosage to 20 mg once daily, and monitor patient for adverse effects.

Drug-herb. *St. John's wort:* May reduce plasma concentration of ranolazine to subtherapeutic levels. Don't use together.

Drug-food. *Grapefruit:* May increase drug level and prolong QT interval. Discourage use together.

EFFECTS ON LAB TEST RESULTS
● May increase creatinine and BUN levels. May decrease hemoglobin and glycosylated hemoglobin levels and hematocrit.
● May decrease eosinophil count.

CONTRAINDICATIONS & CAUTIONS
● Contraindicated in patients taking QT interval-prolonging drugs, CYP3A inducers (including rifampin, phenobarbital), or CYP3A inhibitors (including clarithromycin, ketoconazole and nelfinavir), and in patients with ventricular tachycardia, hepatic impairment, or prolonged QT interval.
● Use cautiously in patients with renal impairment.
● It isn't known whether drug appears in breast milk. Patient should either stop breast-feeding or stop the drug.

NURSING CONSIDERATIONS
🚯 **Alert:** Drug prolongs the QT interval according to the dose. If drug is given with other drugs that prolong the QTc interval, torsades de pointes or sudden death may occur. Don't exceed maximum dosage.
● Obtain baseline ECG and monitor subsequent ECG for prolonged QT interval. Measure the QTc interval regularly.
● If patient has renal insufficiency, monitor blood pressure closely.

PATIENT TEACHING
● Teach patient about this drug's potential to affect the heart's rhythm. Advise patient to immediately report palpitations or fainting.
● Urge patient to tell prescriber about all other prescription or OTC drugs or herbal supplements he takes.
● Tell patient that he should keep taking other drugs prescribed for angina.
● Tell patient that drug may be taken with or without food.
● Advise patient to avoid grapefruit juice while taking this drug.
🚯 **Alert:** Warn patient that tablets must be swallowed whole and not crushed, broken, or chewed.
● Explain that drug won't stop a sudden anginal attack; advise him to keep other treatments, such as S.L. nitroglycerin, readily available.
● Tell patient to avoid activities that require mental alertness until effects of the drug are known.

rasagiline mesylate
reh-SAH-jih-leen

Azilect◆

Therapeutic class: Antiparkinsonians
Pharmacologic class: Irreversible, selective MAO inhibitors type B
Pregnancy risk category: C

AVAILABLE FORMS
Tablets: 0.5 mg, 1 mg

INDICATIONS & DOSAGES
➤ **Idiopathic Parkinson disease, as monotherapy or with levodopa**
Adults: As monotherapy, 1 mg P.O. once daily. As adjunctive therapy, initial dose is 0.5 mg P.O. once daily. May increase to 1 mg P.O. once daily.
Adjust-a-dose: If patient has mild hepatic impairment or takes a CYP1A2 inhibitor such as ciprofloxacin, give 0.5 mg once daily.

ADMINISTRATION
P.O.
● Give drug without regard for food.

ACTION
Unknown. May increase extracellular dopamine level in the CNS, improving neurotransmission and relieving signs and symptoms of Parkinson disease.

Route	Onset	Peak	Duration
P.O.	Variable	1 hr	1 wk

Half-life: 3 hours.

ADVERSE REACTIONS
Monotherapy
CNS: dizziness, falls, headache, depression, fever, hallucinations, malaise, paresthesia, syncope, vertigo.
CV: chest pain, angina pectoris, postural hypotension.
EENT: gingivitis.
GI: anorexia, diarrhea, dyspepsia, gastroenteritis, vomiting.
GU: albuminuria, impotence.
Hematologic: *leukopenia.*
Musculoskeletal: arthralgia, arthritis, neck pain.
Respiratory: asthma, flu syndrome, rhinitis.
Skin: alopecia, *carcinoma,* ecchymosis, vesiculobullous rash.
Other: allergic reaction, decreased libido.
Combined with levodopa
CNS: confusion, falls, headache, abnormal dreams, amnesia, ataxia, dyskinesia, dystonia, hallucinations, paresthesia, somnolence, sweating.
EENT: epistaxis, gingivitis.
GI: nausea, abdominal pain, anorexia, constipation, diarrhea, dry mouth, dyspepsia, dysphagia, vomiting, weight loss.
GU: albuminuria.
Hematologic: *hemorrhage,* anemia.
Musculoskeletal: arthralgia, arthritis, bursitis, hernia, leg cramps, myasthenia, neck pain, tenosynovitis.
Respiratory: dyspnea.
Skin: *carcinoma,* ecchymosis, pruritus, rash, ulcer.
Other: infection.

INTERACTIONS
Drug-drug. *Ciprofloxacin and other CYP1A2 inhibitors:* May double rasagiline level. Decrease rasagiline dosage to 0.5 mg daily.

Levodopa: May increase rasagiline level. Watch for dyskinesia, dystonia, hallucinations, and hypotension, and reduce levodopa dosage if needed.
SSRIs, SNRIs, TCAs: May cause severe or fatal CNS toxicity. Stop rasagiline for at least 14 days before starting an antidepressant. Stop fluoxetine for 5 weeks before starting rasagiline.
Drug-herb. *St. John's wort:* May cause severe reaction. Use together is contraindicated.
Drug-food. *Foods with very high levels of tyramine (more than 150 mg), such as aged cheeses:* May cause hypertensive reaction. Urge patient to avoid aged cheeses such as Stilton.

EFFECTS ON LAB TEST RESULTS
● May increase liver enzyme levels.
● May decrease WBC count.

CONTRAINDICATIONS & CAUTIONS
● Contraindicated in patients with pheochromocytoma, those with moderate to severe hepatic impairment, and those taking amphetamines, cold products, dextromethorphan, ephedrine, MAO inhibitors, meperidine, methadone, phenylephrine, propoxyphene, pseudoephedrine, St. John's wort, sympathomimetic amines, or tramadol.
● Use cautiously in patients with mild hepatic impairment and in pregnant or breastfeeding women.
⚠ *Overdose S&S:* Drowsiness, dizziness, faintness, irritability, hyperactivity, agitation, severe headache, hallucinations, trismus, opisthotonos, seizures, coma, rapid and irregular pulse, hypertension, hypotension and vascular collapse, precordial pain, respiratory depression and failure, hyperpyrexia, diaphoresis, cool and clammy skin.

NURSING CONSIDERATIONS
● Orthostatic hypotension may occur during first 2 months of therapy; help patient to rise from a reclining position.
● Notify prescriber if patient experiences adverse effects; levodopa dose may need to be reduced.

R

• Examine the patient's skin periodically for possible melanoma because of drug's associated risk of skin cancer.
• Notify prescriber if patient is having elective surgery; drug should be stopped at least 2 weeks before.
• *Look alike–sound alike:* Don't confuse Azilect with Aricept.

PATIENT TEACHING
• Explain the risk of hypertensive crisis if patient ingests foods containing very high levels of tyramine while taking rasagiline. Give patient a list of these foods and products.
• Tell patient to contact prescriber if hallucinations occur.
• Urge patient to watch for skin changes that could suggest melanoma and to have periodic skin examinations by a health professional.
• Instruct patient to maintain his usual dosage schedule if he misses a dose and not to double the next dose to make up for a missed one.
• Advise patient to contact health care provider before discontinuing rasagiline.

SAFETY ALERT!

repaglinide
re-PAG-lah-nyde

Prandin

Therapeutic class: Antidiabetics
Pharmacologic class: Meglitinides
Pregnancy risk category: C

AVAILABLE FORMS
Tablets: 0.5 mg, 1 mg, 2 mg

INDICATIONS & DOSAGES
➤ **Type 2 diabetes alone or with metformin or a thiazolidinedione**
Adults: For patients not previously treated or whose glycosylated hemoglobin (HbA_{1c}) level is below 8%, starting dose is 0.5 mg P.O. taken about 15 minutes before each meal. For patients previously treated with glucose-lowering drugs and whose HbA_{1c} is 8% or more, first dose is 1 to 2 mg P.O. with each meal. Recommended dosage range is

0.5 to 4 mg with meals b.i.d., t.i.d., or q.i.d. Maximum daily dose is 16 mg.
  Determine dosage by glucose response. May double dosage up to 4 mg with each meal until satisfactory glucose response is achieved. At least 1 week should elapse between dosage adjustments to assess response to each dose.
  Metformin or a thiazolidinedione may be added if repaglinide monotherapy is inadequate; no repaglinide dosage adjustment is necessary.
Adjust-a-dose: In patients with severe renal impairment, starting dose is 0.5 mg P.O. with meals.

ADMINISTRATION
P.O.
• Give drug before meals, usually 15 minutes before start of meal; however, time can vary from immediately preceding meal to up to 30 minutes before meal.

ACTION
Stimulates insulin release from beta cells in the pancreas by closing adenosine triphosphate (ATP)-dependent potassium channels in beta cell membranes, which causes calcium channels to open. Increased calcium influx induces insulin secretion; the overall effect is to lower glucose level.

Route	Onset	Peak	Duration
P.O.	30 min	1 hr	Unknown

Half-life: 1 hour.

ADVERSE REACTIONS
CNS: headache, paresthesia.
CV: angina.
EENT: rhinitis, sinusitis.
GI: constipation, diarrhea, dyspepsia, nausea, vomiting.
GU: UTI.
Metabolic: *hypoglycemia,* hyperglycemia.
Musculoskeletal: arthralgia, back pain.
Respiratory: bronchitis, upper respiratory tract infection.
Other: tooth disorder.

INTERACTIONS
Drug-drug. *Barbiturates, carbamazepine, rifampin:* May increase repaglinide metabolism. Monitor glucose level.

Reactions in bold italics are *life-threatening*. Interactions may have a *rapid onset* or a *delayed onset*.

Beta blockers, chloramphenicol, coumarin derivatives, MAO inhibitors, NSAIDs, other drugs that are highly protein bound, probenecid, salicylates, sulfonamides: May increase hypoglycemic action of repaglinide. Monitor glucose level.

Calcium channel blockers, corticosteroids, estrogens, fosphenytoin, hormonal contraceptives, isoniazid, nicotinic acid, phenothiazines, phenytoin, sympathomimetics, thiazides and other diuretics, thyroid products: May produce hyperglycemia, resulting in a loss of glycemic control. Monitor glucose level.

Clarithromycin: May increase repaglinide levels. Adjust repaglinide dosage.

Erythromycin, itraconazole, ketoconazole, miconazole, similar inhibitors of CYP3A4: May inhibit repaglinide metabolism. Monitor glucose level.

Gemfibrozil: May increase repaglinide levels. Avoid using together, if possible. Monitor glucose level and adjust repaglinide dosage, if indicated.

Drug-herb. *Burdock, dandelion, eucalyptus, marshmallow:* May increase hypoglycemic effects. Discourage use together.

Drug-food. *Grapefruit juice:* May inhibit metabolism of drug. Discourage use together.

Drug-lifestyle. *Alcohol use:* May alter glycemic control, most commonly causing hypoglycemia. Discourage use together.

EFFECTS ON LAB TEST RESULTS
● May increase or decrease glucose level.

CONTRAINDICATIONS & CAUTIONS
● Contraindicated in patients hypersensitive to drug or its inactive ingredients and in those with type 1 diabetes or diabetic ketoacidosis.
● Drug isn't indicated for use in combination with NPH insulin.
● Use cautiously in elderly, debilitated, or malnourished patients and in those with hepatic, adrenal, or pituitary insufficiency.

⚠ Overdose S&S: Hypoglycemia, severe hypoglycemic reactions (coma, seizures, neurologic impairment).

NURSING CONSIDERATIONS
● Increase dosage carefully in patients with impaired renal function or renal failure requiring dialysis.
● Metformin may be added if repaglinide alone is inadequate.
● Drug may increase CV mortality compared with diet alone or diet plus insulin.
● Monitor patient for loss of glycemic control, especially during stress, such as fever, trauma, infection, or surgery.
● Hypoglycemia may be difficult to recognize in elderly patients and in patients taking beta blockers.
● When switching to a different oral antidiabetic, begin new drug on day after last dose of repaglinide.
● *Look alike–sound alike:* Don't confuse Prandin with Avandia.

PATIENT TEACHING
● Stress importance of diet and exercise with drug therapy.
● Discuss symptoms of hypoglycemia with patient and family.
● Encourage patient to keep regular appointments and have his HbA_{1c} level checked every 3 months to determine long-term glucose control.
● Tell patient to take drug before meals, usually 15 minutes before start of meal; however, time can vary from immediately preceding meal to up to 30 minutes before meal.
● Tell patient that, if a meal is skipped or added, he should skip dose or add an extra dose of drug for that meal, respectively.
● Instruct patient to monitor glucose level carefully and tell him what to do when he's ill, undergoing surgery, or under added stress.
● Advise women planning pregnancy to first consult prescriber. Insulin may be needed during pregnancy and breast-feeding.
● Teach patient to carry candy or other simple sugars to treat mild hypoglycemia episodes. Patient experiencing severe episode may need emergency treatment.
● Advise patient to avoid alcohol, which lowers glucose level.

R

retapamulin
re-te-PAM-ue-lin

Altabax

Therapeutic class: Antibiotics
Pharmacologic class: Pleuromutilins
Pregnancy risk category: B

AVAILABLE FORMS
Topical ointment: 1%

INDICATIONS & DOSAGES
➤ **Impetigo**
Adults and children age 9 months and older:
Apply a thin layer to affected area b.i.d. for 5 days.

ADMINISTRATION
Topical
- Wash hands before and after application, and use glove if available.
- Affected area may be covered with sterile bandage or gauze if needed.

ACTION
Inhibits bacterial protein synthesis in methicillin-susceptible *Staphylococcus aureus* or *Streptococcus pyogenes*.

Route	Onset	Peak	Duration
Topical	Within 24 hr	Unknown	Unknown

Half-life: Unknown.

ADVERSE REACTIONS
CNS: headache, pyrexia.
GI: diarrhea, nausea.
Respiratory: nasopharyngitis.
Skin: application-site irritation, eczema, pruritus.

INTERACTIONS
None significant.

EFFECTS ON LAB TEST RESULTS
- May increase CK levels.

CONTRAINDICATIONS & CAUTIONS
- Contraindicated in patients hypersensitive to drug or its components.
- Safety and effectiveness in children under age 9 months haven't been established.

- Safety and effectiveness in pregnant and breast-feeding women haven't been established.

NURSING CONSIDERATIONS
- To reduce drug resistance or superinfection, treat infection only from organisms proven to be susceptible to this drug.
- Monitor the site for local irritation; if the reaction is severe, wipe the drug off the skin and don't reapply.
- Drug is for topical use only. Don't apply to nasal mucosa because epistaxis may occur.
- Treatment area shouldn't exceed 100 cm² BSA in adults or 2% of total BSA in children.

PATIENT TEACHING
- Tell patient to wash his hands before and after application, and to use a glove if available.
- Tell patient to notify prescriber if his condition doesn't improve in 3 to 4 days, or if a local reaction develops.
- Advise patient to continue using drug for entire prescribed course of therapy.
- Warn patient that drug is for external use only.

SAFETY ALERT!

reteplase (recombinant)
RET-ah-place

Retavase

Therapeutic class: Thrombolytics
Pharmacologic class: Tissue plasminogen activators
Pregnancy risk category: C

AVAILABLE FORMS
Injection: 10.4 units (18.1 mg)/vial, supplied in a kit with components for reconstitution for two single-use vials

INDICATIONS & DOSAGES
➤ **To manage acute MI**
Adults: Double-bolus injection of 10 + 10 units. Give each bolus I.V. over 2 minutes. If complications, such as serious bleeding or anaphylactoid reaction, don't

---

Reactions in bold italics are ***life-threatening***. Interactions may have a *rapid onset* or a ***delayed onset***.

occur after first bolus, give second bolus 30 minutes after start of first.

▶ **Catheter occlusion ◆**
Adults: 0.4 units/lumen with a dwell time of 20 to 30 minutes.

ADMINISTRATION
I.V.

▼ Reconstitute drug according to manufacturer's instructions using items provided in kit and sterile water for injection, without preservatives. Make sure reconstituted solution is colorless; resulting concentration is 1 unit/mL. If foaming occurs, let vial stand for several minutes. Inspect for precipitation. Use within 4 hours of reconstitution; discard unused portions.

▼ Give as a double-bolus injection. If bleeding or anaphylactoid reaction occurs after first bolus, notify prescriber; second bolus may be withheld.

▼ **Incompatibilities:** Other I.V. drugs.

ACTION
Enhances cleavage of plasminogen to generate plasmin, which leads to fibrinolysis.

Route	Onset	Peak	Duration
I.V.	Unknown	Unknown	Unknown

Half-life: 13 to 16 minutes.

ADVERSE REACTIONS
CNS: *intracranial hemorrhage.*
CV: *arrhythmias, cholesterol embolization, hemorrhage.*
GI: *hemorrhage.*
GU: hematuria.
Hematologic: *bleeding tendency,* anemia.
Other: bleeding at puncture sites, hypersensitivity reactions.

INTERACTIONS
Drug-drug. *Heparin, oral anticoagulants, platelet inhibitors (abciximab, aspirin, dipyridamole, eptifibatide, tirofiban):* May increase risk of bleeding. Use together cautiously.

EFFECTS ON LAB TEST RESULTS
● May increase PT, PTT, and INR.
● May decrease plasminogen and fibrinogen levels.
● May alter coagulation study results.

CONTRAINDICATIONS & CAUTIONS
● Contraindicated in patients with active internal bleeding, known bleeding diathesis, history of stroke, recent intracranial or intraspinal surgery or trauma, severe uncontrolled hypertension, intracranial neoplasm, arteriovenous malformation, or aneurysm.
● Use cautiously in patients with previous puncture of noncompressible vessels; in those with recent (within 10 days) major surgery, obstetric delivery, organ biopsy, GI or GU bleeding, or trauma; in those with cerebrovascular disease, systolic blood pressure 180 mm Hg or higher or diastolic pressure 110 mm Hg or higher, and conditions that may lead to left heart thrombus, including mitral stenosis, acute pericarditis, subacute bacterial endocarditis, severe renal or hepatic dysfunction, and hemostatic defects.
● Use cautiously in patients taking oral anticoagulants and in those with diabetic hemorrhagic retinopathy, septic thrombophlebitis, and other conditions in which bleeding would be difficult to manage.
● Use cautiously in patients age 75 and older and in breast-feeding women.

NURSING CONSIDERATIONS
● Drug remains active in vitro and can lead to degradation of fibrinogen in sample, changing coagulation study results. Collect blood samples with chloromethylketone at 2-micromolar concentrations.
● Drug may be given to menstruating women.
● Carefully monitor ECG during treatment. Coronary thrombolysis may cause arrhythmias linked with reperfusion. Be prepared to treat bradycardia or ventricular irritability.
● Closely monitor patient for bleeding. Avoid I.M. injections, invasive procedures, and nonessential handling of patient. Bleeding is the most common adverse reaction and may occur internally or at external puncture sites. If local measures don't control serious bleeding, stop anticoagulant and notify prescriber. Withhold second bolus of reteplase.
● Monitor patient for cholesterol embolization.

R

• Potency is expressed in units specific to reteplase and isn't comparable with other thrombolytics.

• Avoid use of noncompressible puncture sites during therapy. If an arterial puncture is needed, use an arm vessel that can be compressed manually. Apply pressure for at least 30 minutes; then apply a pressure dressing. Check site frequently.

PATIENT TEACHING

• Explain use and administration of drug to patient and family.

• Tell patient to report adverse reactions immediately.

ribavirin
rye-ba-VYE-rin

Copegus, Rebetol, RibaPak, Ribasphere, Virazole

Therapeutic class: Antivirals
Pharmacologic class: Nucleosides–nucleotides
Pregnancy risk category: X

AVAILABLE FORMS
Capsules: 200 mg
Oral solution: 40 mg/mL
Powder to be reconstituted for inhalation: 6 g in 100-mL glass vial
Tablets: 200 mg, 400 mg, 500 mg, 600 mg

INDICATIONS & DOSAGES
➤ **Hospitalized infants and young children infected by respiratory syncytial virus (RSV)**
Infants and young children: Solution in concentration of 20 mg/mL delivered via the Viratek Small Particle Aerosol Generator (SPAG-2) and mechanical ventilator or oxygen hood, face mask, or oxygen tent at a rate of about 12.5 L of mist/minute. Treatment is given for 12 to 18 hours/day for at least 3 days, and no longer than 7 days.
➤ **Chronic hepatitis C in patients with compensated liver disease previously untreated with interferon alfa or who have relapsed following interferon alfa therapy**

Black Box Warning Ribavirin alone isn't effective for treatment of chronic hepatitis C. ■
Adults weighing more than 75 kg (165 lb): 1,200 mg P.O. (Rebetol) in two divided doses (600 in morning, 600 mg in evening) with interferon alfa-2b, 3 million units subcutaneously three times weekly. Or, 1,200 mg (Copegus) with 180 mcg of peginterferon alfa-2a.
Adults weighing 75 kg or less: 1,000 mg P.O. (Rebetol) daily in divided dose (400 mg in morning, 600 mg in evening) with interferon alfa-2b, 3 million units subcutaneously three times weekly. Or, 1,000 mg (Copegus) with 180 mcg of peginterferon alfa-2a.
Children age 3 and older weighing 50 to 61 kg (110 to 134 lb): 400 mg P.O. (Rebetol) every morning and 400 mg P.O. every evening with interferon alfa-2b, 3 million units/m^2 subcutaneously three times weekly.
Children age 3 and older weighing 37 to 49 kg (81 to 108 lb): 200 mg P.O. (Rebetol) every morning and 400 mg P.O. every evening with interferon alfa-2b, 3 million units/m^2 subcutaneously three times weekly.
Children age 3 and older weighing 25 to 36 kg (55 to 79 lb): 200 mg P.O. (Rebetol) every morning and 200 mg P.O. every evening with interferon alfa-2b, 3 million units/m^2 subcutaneously three times weekly.
➤ **Chronic hepatitis C in patients with compensated liver disease not previously treated with interferon alfa**
Black Box Warning Ribavirin alone isn't effective for treatment of chronic hepatitis C. ■
Adults with viral genotypes 1 or 4 weighing 75 kg (165 lb) or more: 1,200 mg P.O. (Copegus) daily in two divided doses with 180 mcg peginterferon alfa-2a for 48 weeks.
Adults with viral genotypes 1 or 4 weighing less than 75 kg: 1,000 mg P.O. (Copegus) daily in two divided doses with 180 mcg peginterferon alfa-2a for 48 weeks.
Adults with viral genotypes 2 or 3: 800 mg P.O. (Copegus) daily in two divided doses with 180 mcg peginterferon alfa-2a for 24 weeks.
Adjust-a-dose: In patient with no cardiac disease history and hemoglobin level less

---

Reactions in bold italics are *life-threatening*. Interactions may have a *rapid onset* or a *delayed onset*.

than 10 g/dL, reduce dosage to 600 mg daily (200 mg in morning, 400 mg in evening). If hemoglobin level is less than 8.5 g/dL, stop drug. In patient with history of stable cardiac disease and whose hemoglobin level falls 2 g/dL or more during any 4-week period, reduce dosage to 600 mg daily (200 mg in morning, 400 mg in evening). If hemoglobin level is less than 12 g/dL after 4 weeks of reduced dosage, stop drug.

➤ **Chronic hepatitis C (regardless of genotype) in HIV-infected patients who haven't previously been treated with interferon**

Adults: 800 mg P.O. (Copegus) daily in two divided doses with peginterferon alfa-2a, 180 mcg subcutaneously weekly for 48 weeks.

Adjust-a-dose: In patient with no cardiac history and hemoglobin level less than 10 g/dL, reduce dosage to 600 mg daily (200 mg in morning, 400 mg in evening) for adults and 7.5 mg/kg daily for children. If hemoglobin level is less than 8.5 g/dL, stop drug. In patient with cardiac history and whose hemoglobin level falls 2 g/dL or more during any 4-week period, reduce dosage to 600 mg daily (200 mg in morning, 400 mg in evening) for adults and 7.5 mg/kg daily for children. If hemoglobin level is less than 12 g/dL after 4 weeks of reduced dosage, stop drug.

ADMINISTRATION
Inhalational
● Give by the Viratek SPAG-2 only. Don't use any other aerosol-generating device.
● Use sterile USP water for injection, not bacteriostatic water. Water used to reconstitute this drug must not contain any antimicrobial product.
● Discard solutions placed in the SPAG-2 unit at least every 24 hours before adding newly reconstituted solution.
● Store reconstituted solutions at room temperature for 24 hours.
P.O.
● Give drug with food and at the same time every day.
● **⚠ Alert:** Capsules should never be opened, crushed, or broken.

ACTION
Inhibits viral activity by an unknown mechanism, possibly by inhibiting RNA and DNA synthesis by depleting intracellular nucleotide pools.

Route	Onset	Peak	Duration
Inhalation	Unknown	Unknown	Unknown
P.O.	Unknown	2 hr	Unknown

Half-life: First phase, 9¼ hours; second phase, 40 hours.

ADVERSE REACTIONS
CNS: fatigue, anxiety, depression, dizziness, headache, insomnia.
CV: *bradycardia, cardiac arrest.*
EENT: conjunctivitis.
GI: anorexia, diarrhea, nausea, vomiting, weight loss.
Hematologic: anemia, reticulocytosis.
Respiratory: *apnea, bronchospasm,* bacterial pneumonia, *pneumothorax, pulmonary edema,* worsening respiratory state.
Skin: flushing, alopecia, pruritus, rash, dry skin, injection-site reaction.
Other: chills, pyrexia, flulike illness, pain.

INTERACTIONS
Drug-drug. *Acetaminophen; antacids that contain magnesium, aluminum, or simethicone; aspirin; cimetidine:* May affect drug level. Monitor patient.
Didanosine: May increase toxicity. Avoid using together.
Lamivudine, stavudine, zidovudine: May decrease antiretroviral activity. Use together cautiously.

EFFECTS ON LAB TEST RESULTS
● May increase ALT, AST, and bilirubin levels. May decrease hemoglobin level.
● May increase reticulocyte count. May decrease WBC and platelet counts.

CONTRAINDICATIONS & CAUTIONS
Black Box Warning Monotherapy is ineffective for treatment of chronic hepatitis C infection. ■
Black Box Warning Aerosol form contraindicated in patients hypersensitive to drug, and isn't indicated for use in adults. ■

R

Black Box Warning Ribavirin may cause hemolytic anemia and worsen cardiac disease, leading to potentially fatal MI. Contraindicated for use in patients with a history of significant or unstable cardiac disease. ∎

• Oral form is contraindicated in patients hypersensitive to drug and in those with thalassemia major or sickle cell anemia.

Black Box Warning Contraindicated for use in pregnant women and men whose partners are pregnant or may become pregnant within 6 months. ∎

Black Box Warning In infants, aerosolized ribavirin has been associated with sudden deterioration of respiratory function. Monitor respiratory function carefully and stop treatment if sudden respiratory deterioration occurs. ∎

• Use cautiously in elderly patients and patients with hepatic or renal insufficiency.

⚠ **Overdose S&S:** Increased severity of adverse reactions.

NURSING CONSIDERATIONS
Aerosol form
❸ **Alert:** The long-term and cumulative effects in health care personnel exposed to this form aren't known. Eye irritation and headache may occur. Advise pregnant women to avoid unnecessary exposure.

Black Box Warning Monitor ventilator function frequently. Drug may precipitate in ventilator, causing equipment to malfunction with serious consequences. ∎

• This form is indicated only for severe lower respiratory tract infection caused by RSV. Although you should begin treatment while awaiting test results, an RSV infection must be documented eventually.

• Most infants and children with RSV infection don't require treatment with antivirals because the disease is commonly mild and self-limiting. Premature infants or those with cardiopulmonary disease experience RSV in its severest form and benefit most from treatment with ribavirin aerosol.

Oral form
• Don't start therapy until a negative pregnancy test is confirmed in patient or partner of patient; they should take a pregnancy test every month during therapy and for 6 months afterward.

• Women or female partner of patient should use two reliable forms of contraception before and during treatment and for 6 months afterward.

• Report pregnancies that occur during treatment by calling the Ribavirin Pregnancy Registry at 800-593-2214.

• Monitor hematologic status, liver and renal function, and thyroid-stimulating hormone level at baseline and throughout therapy.

❸ **Alert:** Monitor patient for suicidal ideation, severe depression, hemolytic anemia, bone marrow suppression, autoimmune and infective disorders, pulmonary dysfunction, pancreatitis, and diabetes.

• Stop drug if pulmonary infiltrates or severe pulmonary impairment or pancreatitis occurs.

PATIENT TEACHING
• Inform parents of need for drug, and answer any questions.

• Encourage parents to immediately report any subtle change in child.

• Inform patient that oral form may be taken without regard to meals but should be taken in a consistent manner.

• Warn patient of childbearing age that drug is a teratogen, and provide contraception counseling. Advise patient that extreme care must be taken to avoid pregnancy during therapy and for 6 months after completion of treatment.

rifabutin
rif-ah-BYOO-tin

Mycobutin

Therapeutic class: Antituberculotics
Pharmacologic class: Semisynthetic ansamycins
Pregnancy risk category: B

AVAILABLE FORMS
Capsules: 150 mg

INDICATIONS & DOSAGES
Adjust-a-dose (for all indications): For patients with CrCl of less than 30 mL/minute, reduce rifabutin dosage by 50%.

➤ To prevent disseminated *Mycobacterium avium* complex in patients with advanced HIV infection
Adults: 300 mg P.O. daily as a single dose or in two divided doses.
➤ Substitute for rifampin in patients with tuberculosis (TB) concurrently receiving medications that have unacceptable interactions with rifampin or who have intolerance to rifampin ♦
Adults: 5 mg/kg P.O. two or three times weekly, not to exceed 300 mg/day.

ADMINISTRATION
P.O.
• For patient who has difficulty swallowing, mix drug with soft foods such as applesauce.
• Patient experiencing GI adverse effects, such as nausea or vomiting, may divide total daily dose into two doses and take with food.

ACTION
Inhibits DNA-dependent RNA polymerase in susceptible bacteria, blocking bacterial protein synthesis.

Route	Onset	Peak	Duration
P.O.	Unknown	2–4 hr	Unknown

Half-life: About 2 days.

ADVERSE REACTIONS
CNS: headache, fever, insomnia.
EENT: eye inflammation.
GI: dyspepsia, eructation, flatulence, diarrhea, nausea, vomiting, abdominal pain, anorexia, taste perversion.
GU: discolored urine.
Hematologic: *neutropenia, leukopenia, thrombocytopenia,* eosinophilia.
Musculoskeletal: myalgia.
Skin: rash.

INTERACTIONS
Drug-drug. *Benzodiazepines, beta blockers, buspirone,* **corticosteroids**, **cyclosporine**, *delavirdine, doxycycline, fluconazole, hydantoins, indinavir, itraconazole, ketoconazole, losartan, macrolides, methadone, morphine, nelfinavir, quinidine, quinine,* **tacrolimus**, *TCAs, theophylline,*

zolpidem: May decrease effectiveness of these drugs. Monitor patient for drug effects.
Hormonal contraceptives: May decrease contraceptive effectiveness. Tell patient to use another form of birth control.
Indinavir: May increase rifabutin level. Decrease rifabutin dosage by 50%.
Lurasidone, praziquantel, ranolazine: May decrease plasma concentrations and pharmacologic effects of lurasidone, praziquantel, and ranolazine. Using together is contraindicated.
Ritonavir: May increase the risk of rifabutin hematologic toxicity. Use together is contraindicated.
Rivaroxaban: May decrease effects of rivaroxaban. Avoid use together.
Voriconazole: May decrease therapeutic effects of voriconazole while increasing the risk of rifabutin adverse effects. Use together is contraindicated.
Warfarin: May decrease effectiveness of warfarin. May require higher dosages of anticoagulants. Monitor PT and INR.
Drug-food. *High-fat foods:* May reduce rate but not extent of absorption. Discourage use together.

EFFECTS ON LAB TEST RESULTS
• May increase aminotransferase level.
• May decrease neutrophil, WBC, and platelet counts.

CONTRAINDICATIONS & CAUTIONS
• Contraindicated in patients hypersensitive to drug or other rifamycin derivatives, such as rifampin, and in patients with active TB because single-drug therapy with rifabutin increases risk of inducing bacterial resistance to both rifabutin and rifampin.
• Use cautiously in patients with neutropenia and thrombocytopenia.

NURSING CONSIDERATIONS
• In patients with neutropenia or thrombocytopenia, obtain baseline hematologic studies and repeat periodically.
• **Look alike–sound alike:** Don't confuse rifabutin with rifampin or rifapentine.

R

PATIENT TEACHING
● Instruct patient to take drug for as long as prescribed, exactly as directed, even after feeling better.
● Tell patient experiencing GI adverse effects, such as nausea or vomiting, to divide total daily dose into two doses and to take with food.
● Tell patient that drug may cause brownish orange staining of urine, feces, sputum, saliva, tears, and skin. Tell him to avoid wearing soft contact lenses because they may be permanently stained.
● Instruct patient to report sensitivity to light, excessive tears, or eye pain immediately.
● Advise patient to report tingling and joint stiffness, swelling, or tenderness.
● Advise patients using hormonal contraceptives to change to nonhormonal birth control because rifabutin may decrease hormonal contraceptive effectiveness.

rifampin (rifampicin)
rif-AM-pin

Rifadin, Rimactane, Rofact†

Therapeutic class: Antituberculotics
Pharmacologic class: Semisynthetic rifamycins
Pregnancy risk category: C

AVAILABLE FORMS
Capsules: 150 mg, 300 mg
Powder for injection: 600 mg

INDICATIONS & DOSAGES
Adjust-a-dose (for all indications): For patients with CrCl of less than 50 mL/minute or for patients receiving hemodialysis or continuous ambulatory peritoneal dialysis, give 50% to 100% of the usual dose.
➤ **Pulmonary tuberculosis (TB), with other antituberculotics**
Adults: 10 mg/kg P.O. or I.V. daily in single dose. Give oral doses 1 hour before or 2 hours after meals with a full glass of water. Maximum daily dose is 600 mg.
Children age 5 and older: 10 to 20 mg/kg P.O. or I.V. daily in single dose. Give oral doses 1 hour before or 2 hours after meals

with a full glass of water. Maximum daily dose is 600 mg. Give with other antituberculotics.
➤ **Meningococcal carriers**
Adults: 600 mg P.O. or I.V. every 12 hours for 2 days; or 600 mg P.O. or I.V. once daily for 4 days.
Children ages 1 month to 12 years: 10 mg/kg P.O. or I.V. every 12 hours for 2 days, not to exceed 600 mg/day; or 20 mg/kg once daily for 4 days.
Neonates: 5 mg/kg P.O. or I.V. every 12 hours for 2 days.
➤ **Catheter-related bloodstream infection ♦**
Adults: 10 mg/kg P.O. or I.V. as a single daily dose, not to exceed 600 mg.
➤ **Cholestatic pruritus ♦**
Adults: 150 mg/day P.O. if bilirubin level is less than 3 mg/dL or 150 mg P.O. b.i.d. if bilirubin level is 3 mg/dL or higher.
➤ **Methicillin-resistant *Staphylococcus aureus* brain abscess, empyema, epidural abscess ♦**
Adults: 600 mg P.O. or I.V. once daily or 300 to 450 mg I.V. b.i.d. in addition to I.V. vancomycin for 4 to 6 weeks.
➤ **Methicillin-resistant *S. aureus* osteomyelitis ♦**
Adults: 600 mg P.O. or I.V. once daily for at least 8 weeks in combination with sulfamethoxazole–trimethoprim. Or, 600 mg P.O. or I.V. once daily or 300 to 450 mg P.O. or I.V. b.i.d. with linezolid or clindamycin.
➤ **Methicillin-resistant *S. aureus* septic thrombosis of cavernous or dural venous sinus ♦**
Adults: 600 mg P.O. or I.V. once daily or 300 to 450 mg P.O. or I.V. b.i.d. in addition to I.V. vancomycin for 4 to 6 weeks.
➤ **Device-related osteoarticular infections (methicillin-resistant *S. aureus*) ♦**
Adults: 600 mg P.O. daily or 300 to 450 mg P.O. b.i.d.
➤ **Methicillin-resistant *S. aureus* septic arthritis ♦**
Adults: 600 mg P.O. or I.V. daily for 3 to 4 weeks in combination with sulfamethoxazole–trimethoprim. Or, rifampin 600 mg daily or 300 to 450 mg b.i.d. with linezolid or clindamycin.

Reactions in bold italics are *life-threatening*. Interactions may have a *rapid onset* or a *delayed onset*.

➤ **TB (intermittent dosing)** ◆
Adults: 10 mg/kg P.O. or I.V. two or three
times weekly, not to exceed 600 mg/dose.

ADMINISTRATION
P.O.
● Give drug with at least one other antituberculotic.
● For best absorption, give capsules 1 hour
before or 2 hours after a meal with a full
glass of water.
● For patients who can't tolerate capsules
on an empty stomach or those who have
difficulty swallowing capsules or when
lower doses are needed, consult pharmacist
for preparation of an oral suspension.
I.V.
▼ Reconstitute drug with 10 mL of sterile
water for injection to yield 60 mg/mL.
▼ Add to 100 mL of D₅W and infuse over
30 minutes, or add to 500 mL of D₅W and
infuse over 3 hours.
▼ When dextrose is contraindicated, dilute
with normal saline solution for injection.
▼ Once prepared, dilutions in D₅W are
stable for up to 4 hours and dilutions in
normal saline solution are stable for up to
24 hours at room temperature.
▼ **Incompatibilities:** Diltiazem, minocycline, other I.V. solutions.

ACTION
Inhibits DNA-dependent RNA polymerase,
which impairs RNA synthesis; bactericidal.

Route	Onset	Peak	Duration
P.O.	Unknown	2–4 hr	Unknown
I.V.	Unknown	Unknown	Unknown

Half-life: 1¼ to 5 hours.

ADVERSE REACTIONS
CNS: headache, fatigue, drowsiness, behavioral changes, dizziness, mental confusion,
generalized numbness, ataxia.
CV: *shock.*
EENT: visual disturbances, exudative
conjunctivitis.
GI: *pancreatitis, pseudomembranous colitis,* epigastric distress, anorexia, nausea,
vomiting, abdominal pain, diarrhea, flatulence, sore mouth and tongue.
GU: *acute renal failure,* hemoglobinuria,
hematuria, menstrual disturbances.

Hematologic: *thrombocytopenia, tran-
sient leukopenia,* eosinophilia, hemolytic
anemia.
Hepatic: *hepatotoxicity.*
Metabolic: hyperuricemia.
Musculoskeletal: osteomalacia.
Respiratory: shortness of breath, wheezing.
Skin: pruritus, urticaria, rash.
Other: flulike syndrome, discoloration of
body fluids, porphyria exacerbation.

INTERACTIONS
Drug-drug. *Acetaminophen, amiodarone,
analgesics, anticonvulsants, barbiturates,
beta blockers, cardiac glycosides, chloramphenicol, clofibrate,* **corticosteroids,
cyclosporine,** *dapsone, delavirdine, diazepam, digoxin, disopyramide, doxycycline, enalapril, fluoroquinolones,
hormonal contraceptives, hydantoins,
losartan, methadone, mexiletine, midazolam, nifedipine, ondansetron, opioids,
progestins, propafenone, quinidine,* **ritonavir,** *sulfonylureas,* **tacrolimus,** *TCAs,
theophylline, tocainide, triazolam, verapamil, zidovudine, zolpidem:* May decrease
effectiveness of these drugs. Monitor effectiveness.
Anticoagulants: May increase requirements
for anticoagulant. Monitor PT and INR
closely, and adjust dosage of anticoagulants.
Halothane: May increase risk of hepatotoxicity. Monitor LFT results.
Isoniazid: May increase risk of hepatotoxicity. Monitor LFT results.
*Ketoconazole, para-aminosalicylate
sodium:* May interfere with absorption of
rifampin. Separate doses by 8 to 12 hours.
Macrolide antibiotics, protease inhibitors:
May inhibit rifampin metabolism but increase metabolism of other drug. Monitor
patient for clinical and adverse effects.
Probenecid: May increase rifampin levels.
Use together cautiously.
Voriconazole: May decrease voriconazole's
therapeutic effects while increasing the risk
of rifampin adverse effects. Use together is
contraindicated.
Drug-lifestyle. *Alcohol use:* May increase
risk of hepatotoxicity. Discourage use
together.

R

EFFECTS ON LAB TEST RESULTS
● May increase ALT, AST, alkaline phosphatase, bilirubin, and uric acid levels. May decrease hemoglobin level.
● May increase eosinophil counts. May decrease platelet and WBC counts.
● May alter standard folate and vitamin B_{12} assay results.

CONTRAINDICATIONS & CAUTIONS
● Contraindicated in patients hypersensitive to rifampin or related drugs.
● Use cautiously in patients with liver disease or diabetes.
● Use in pregnant women only if potential benefit justifies potential risk to fetus.
⚠ *Overdose S&S:* Nausea; vomiting; abdominal pain; pruritus; headache; increasing lethargy; unconsciousness; transient increases in liver enzyme or bilirubin levels; brownish red or orange discoloration of skin, urine, sweat, saliva, tears, and feces; facial or periorbital edema; hypotension; tachycardia; ventricular arrhythmias; seizures; cardiac arrest; liver enlargement; jaundice.

NURSING CONSIDERATIONS
● Monitor hepatic function, hematopoietic studies, and uric acid levels. Drug's systemic effects may asymptomatically raise LFT results and uric acid level.
● Watch for and report to prescriber signs and symptoms of hepatic impairment.
● Drug may cause hemorrhage in neonates and mother when drug is given during last few weeks of pregnancy. Monitor clotting parameters closely, and treat with vitamin K as needed.
● *Look alike–sound alike:* Don't confuse rifampin with rifabutin, rifaximin, rifapentine, or Rifamate.

PATIENT TEACHING
● Advise patient who is unable to swallow capsules whole or can't tolerate capsules on an empty stomach that an oral suspension can be prepared by the pharmacist.
● Warn patient that he may feel drowsy and that drug can turn body fluids red-orange and permanently stain contact lenses.

● Advise women using hormonal contraceptives to consider another form of birth control.
● Advise patient to contact prescriber if he experiences fever, loss of appetite, malaise, nausea, vomiting, dark urine, or yellow discoloration of the eyes or skin.
● Advise patient to avoid alcohol during drug therapy.

rifapentine
RIF-a-PEN-teen

Priftin

Therapeutic class: Antituberculotics
Pharmacologic class: Synthetic rifamycins
Pregnancy risk category: C

AVAILABLE FORMS
Tablets (film-coated): 150 mg

INDICATIONS & DOSAGES
➤ **Pulmonary tuberculosis (TB), with at least one other antituberculotic to which the isolate is susceptible**
Adults and children age 12 and older: During intensive phase of short-course therapy, 600 mg P.O. twice weekly for 2 months, with an interval between doses of at least 3 days (72 hours). During continuation phase of short-course therapy, 600 mg P.O. once weekly for 4 months, combined with isoniazid or another drug to which the isolate is susceptible.
Elderly patients: Begin therapy at low end of dosing range.

ADMINISTRATION
P.O.
● Give drug with pyridoxine (vitamin B_6) in malnourished patients; in those predisposed to neuropathy, such as alcoholics and diabetics; and in adolescents.
⚠ *Alert:* Give drug with appropriate daily companion drugs. Compliance with all drug regimens, especially with daily companion drugs on the days when rifapentine isn't given, is crucial for early sputum conversion and protection from relapse of TB.

ACTION

Inhibits DNA-dependent RNA polymerase in susceptible strains of *Mycobacterium tuberculosis*. Demonstrates bactericidal activity against the organism both intracellularly and extracellularly.

Route	Onset	Peak	Duration
P.O.	Unknown	5–6 hr	Unknown

Half-life: 13 hours.

ADVERSE REACTIONS

CNS: headache, dizziness, pain.
CV: hypertension.
GI: anorexia, nausea, vomiting, dyspepsia, diarrhea.
GU: hyperuricemia, pyuria, proteinuria, hematuria, urinary casts.
Hematologic: *leukopenia, neutropenia,* anemia, *thrombocytosis.*
Metabolic: hyperuricemia.
Musculoskeletal: arthralgia.
Respiratory: hemoptysis.
Skin: rash, pruritus, acne, maculopapular rash.

INTERACTIONS

Drug-drug. *Antiarrhythmics (disopyramide, mexiletine, quinidine, tocainide), antibiotics (chloramphenicol, clarithromycin, dapsone, doxycycline, fluoroquinolones), anticonvulsants (phenytoin), antifungals (fluconazole, itraconazole, ketoconazole), barbiturates, benzodiazepines (diazepam), beta blockers, calcium channel blockers (diltiazem, nifedipine, verapamil), cardiac glycosides, clofibrate,* **corticosteroids***, haloperidol, HIV protease inhibitors (indinavir, nelfinavir, ritonavir, saquinavir), hormonal contraceptives,* **immunosuppressants (cyclosporine, tacrolimus)***, levothyroxine, opioid analgesics (methadone), oral anticoagulants (warfarin), oral antidiabetics (sulfonylureas), progestins, quinine, reverse transcriptase inhibitors (delavirdine, zidovudine), sildenafil, TCAs (amitriptyline, nortriptyline), theophylline:* May decrease activity of these drugs because of cytochrome P-450 enzyme metabolism. May need to adjust dosage.
Ritonavir: May decrease ritonavir levels. Carefully monitor patient's response.

EFFECTS ON LAB TEST RESULTS

● May increase uric acid, ALT, and AST levels. May decrease hemoglobin level.
● May increase platelet count. May decrease neutrophil and WBC counts.
● May alter folate and vitamin B_{12} assay results.

CONTRAINDICATIONS & CAUTIONS

● Contraindicated in patients hypersensitive to rifamycins (rifapentine, rifampin, or rifabutin).
● Use drug cautiously and with frequent monitoring in patients with liver disease.
⚠ *Overdose S&S:* Heartburn, headache, increased urinary frequency, transient increase in AST, pruritus.

NURSING CONSIDERATIONS

● Rifamycin antibiotics may cause hepatotoxicity. Obtain baseline LFT results before therapy.
● If used during the last 2 weeks of pregnancy, drug may lead to postnatal hemorrhage in mother or infant. Monitor clotting parameters closely if drug is used at that time.
● *Look alike–sound alike:* Don't confuse rifapentine with rifabutin or rifampin.

PATIENT TEACHING

● Stress importance of strict compliance with this drug regimen and that of daily companion drugs, as well as needed follow-up visits and laboratory tests.
● Advise women to use nonhormonal birth control methods.
● Tell patient to take drug with food if nausea, vomiting, or GI upset occurs.
● Instruct patient to report to prescriber fever, appetite loss, malaise, nausea, vomiting, darkened urine, yellowish skin and eyes, joint pain or swelling, or excessive loose stools or diarrhea.
● Instruct patient to protect pills from excessive heat.
● Tell patient that drug may turn body fluids red-orange and permanently stain contact lenses.

R

rifaximin
reh-FACKS-ah-men

Xifaxan

Therapeutic class: Antibiotics
Pharmacologic class: Rifamycin
antibacterials
Pregnancy risk category: C

AVAILABLE FORMS
Tablets: 200 mg, 550 mg

INDICATIONS & DOSAGES
➤ **Traveler's diarrhea from noninvasive strains of *Escherichia coli***
Adults and children age 12 and older:
200 mg P.O. t.i.d. for 3 days.
➤ **Hepatic encephalopathy**
Adults: 550 mg P.O. b.i.d.
➤ **Irritable bowel syndrome** ♦
Adults: 400 mg P.O. b.i.d. or t.i.d. for 10 days.

ADMINISTRATION
P.O.
● Give drug without regard for food.

ACTION
Binds to the beta-subunit of bacterial DNA-dependent RNA polymerase, which inhibits bacterial RNA synthesis and kills *E. coli.*

Route	Onset	Peak	Duration
P.O.	Unknown	½–4 hr	Unknown

Half-life: 1.8 to 4.8 hours.

ADVERSE REACTIONS
CNS: depression, dizziness, fatigue, fever, headache, insomnia.
CV: peripheral edema.
EENT: nasopharyngitis.
GI: ascites, abdominal pain, constipation, defecation urgency, flatulence, nausea, rectal tenesmus, vomiting.
Hematologic: anemia.
Musculoskeletal: arthralgia, muscle spasms.
Respiratory: dyspnea.
Skin: rash, pruritus.

INTERACTIONS
None significant.

EFFECTS ON LAB TEST RESULTS
None reported.

CONTRAINDICATIONS & CAUTIONS
● Contraindicated in patients hypersensitive to rifaximin or any rifamycin antibacterial.
● Use with caution in patients with severe hepatic impairment.

NURSING CONSIDERATIONS
● Don't use drug in patients whose illness may be caused by *Campylobacter jejuni, Shigella,* or *Salmonella.*
🟡 *Alert:* Don't use drug in patients with blood in the stool, diarrhea with fever, or diarrhea from pathogens other than *E. coli.*
● Stop drug if diarrhea worsens or lasts longer than 24 to 48 hours. The patient may need a different antibiotic.
● Patients who have diarrhea after antibiotic therapy may have *Clostridium difficile–*associated diarrhea, which may range from mild to life-threatening.
● Monitor patient for overgrowth of nonsusceptible organisms.

PATIENT TEACHING
● Explain that drug may be taken with or without food.
● Tell patient to take all the prescribed drug, even if he feels better before the drug is finished.
● Advise patient to notify his prescriber if diarrhea worsens or lasts longer than 1 or 2 days after starting treatment. A different treatment may be needed.
● Tell patient to call the prescriber if he develops a fever or has blood in his stool.
● Explain that this drug is only for treating diarrhea caused by contaminated foods or beverages while traveling and not for any other type of infection.
● Caution patient not to share this drug with others.

Reactions in bold italics are ***life-threatening***. Interactions may have a *rapid onset* or a ***delayed onset***.

rilpivirine
ril-pi-VIR-een

Edurant

Therapeutic class: Antiretrovirals
Pharmacologic class: Nonnucleoside
reverse transcriptase inhibitors
Pregnancy risk category: B

AVAILABLE FORMS
Tablets: 25 mg

INDICATIONS & DOSAGES
➤ **Treatment of HIV-1 infection in antiretroviral-naive patients in combination with other antiretrovirals**
Adults: 25 mg P.O. once daily.

ADMINISTRATION
P.O.
- Give drug with a full meal.
- Store tablets at room temperature and in the original bottle to protect from light.

ACTION
Inhibits HIV-1 replication by noncompetitive inhibition of HIV-1 reverse transcriptase but doesn't inhibit the human cellular DNA polymerases alpha, beta, and gamma.

Route	Onset	Peak	Duration
P.O.	Rapid	4–5 hr	Unknown

Half-life: 50 hours.

ADVERSE REACTIONS
CNS: abnormal dreams, dizziness, fatigue, headache, insomnia, depression.
GI: nausea, vomiting, abdominal pain.
Skin: rash.

INTERACTIONS
Drug-drug. *Antacids (aluminum or magnesium hydroxide, calcium carbonate):* May significantly decrease rilpivirine level. Give antacids either 2 hours before or at least 4 hours after rilpivirine.
Anticonvulsants (carbamazepine, oxcarbazepine, phenobarbital, phenytoin): May decrease rilpivirine level, decrease response, and increase risk of resistance to nonnucleoside reverse transcriptase inhibitors (NNRTIs). Use together is contraindicated.
Azole antifungals (fluconazole, itraconazole, ketoconazole, posaconazole, voriconazole): May increase rilpivirine level and decrease antifungal level. Monitor effectiveness of antifungal.
Delavirdine: May increase rilpivirine level. Don't use together.
Didanosine (buffered): May decrease rilpivirine level. Administer didanosine at least 2 hours before or 4 hours after rilpivirine.
Drugs that prolong QT interval: May increase levels of both drugs, increasing risk of torsades de pointes. Use together cautiously.
H_2-receptor antagonists (cimetidine, famotidine, nizatidine, ranitidine): May significantly decrease rilpivirine level. Give H_2-receptor antagonists at least 12 hours before or 4 hours after rilpivirine.
Macrolide antibiotics (clarithromycin, erythromycin, troleandomycin): May increase rilpivirine level. When possible, consider an alternative such as azithromycin.
Methadone: May decrease levels of both drugs. Monitor effectiveness of methadone and adjust methadone dosage as needed.
Other NNRTIs (efavirenz, etravirine, nevirapine): May decrease rilpivirine level. Don't use together.
Proton pump inhibitors (esomeprazole, lansoprazole, pantoprazole, rabeprazole): May decrease rilpivirine level, decrease virologic response, and increase risk of resistance to NNRTIs. Use together is contraindicated.
Rifamycins (rifabutin, rifampin, rifapentine): May decrease rilpivirine level, decrease virologic response, and increase risk of resistance to NNRTIs. Use together is contraindicated.
Systemic glucocorticoids (dexamethasone): May decrease rilpivirine level. Use together is contraindicated.
Drug-herb. *St. John's wort:* May decrease rilpivirine level, decrease virologic response, and increase risk of resistance to NNRTIs. Use together is contraindicated.

R

EFFECTS ON LAB TEST RESULTS

• May increase AST, ALT, bilirubin, creatinine, total cholesterol, and LDL and triglyceride levels.

CONTRAINDICATIONS & CAUTIONS

• Contraindicated in patients hypersensitive to drug or its components.

• Use cautiously when administering with drugs known to prolong QT interval, in elderly patients, and in those with severe renal impairment, ESRD, or severe hepatic impairment.

• Redistribution or accumulation of body fat, including central obesity, dorsocervical fat enlargement (buffalo hump), peripheral wasting, facial wasting, breast enlargement, and "cushingoid appearance," has occurred in patients receiving antiretroviral therapy. The mechanism and long-term consequences of these events are currently unknown. A causal relationship hasn't been established.

• Hepatic adverse events have been reported. Patients with underlying hepatitis B or C or marked elevations in transaminase levels before treatment may be at increased risk for worsening or development of transaminase elevations. A few cases of hepatotoxicity have been reported in patients who had no preexisting hepatic disease or other identifiable risk factors.

• Use during pregnancy only if the potential benefit to the mother justifies the potential risk to the fetus.

• The Centers for Disease Control and Prevention recommends that an HIV-infected mother not breast-feed to avoid risking postnatal transmission of HIV.

NURSING CONSIDERATIONS

• Patients should take drug with a regular meal and not with a protein drink; taking drug with a protein-rich nutritional drink alone may lower the exposure of rilpivirine by 50%.

• Always use rilpivirine in combination with other antiretrovirals.

• Drug isn't a cure for HIV infection. Patients must stay on continuous HIV therapy to control HIV infection and decrease HIV-related illnesses.

• Assess patient for redistribution or accumulation of body fat.

• Monitor patients for reemergence of infections, such as *Mycobacterium avium,* cytomegalovirus, *Pneumocystis jiroveci* pneumonia, and tuberculosis, during initial phase of combination treatment. Treat infections appropriately.

• Monitor patients for depressive disorders (depressed mood, dysphoria, negative thoughts, suicidal ideation or attempt). Weigh risks of continued therapy against benefits of treatment.

• Monitor liver enzyme levels before and during treatment for patients with underlying hepatic disease, including hepatitis B or C infection, and for patients with marked transaminase elevations. Consider monitoring liver enzyme levels for patients without preexisting hepatic dysfunction or other risk factors. Monitor patients with severe renal impairment or ESRD for adverse reactions during treatment.

• Enroll pregnant women exposed to rilpivirine in the Antiretroviral Pregnancy Registry for monitoring maternal-fetal outcomes at 1-800-258-4263.

PATIENT TEACHING

• Advise patient that rilpivirine isn't a cure for HIV infection or AIDS and that he must stay on continuous antiretroviral therapy so that the HIV infection can be controlled.

• Tell patient to report all medications and supplements he is taking because many drugs interact with rilpivirine.

• Instruct patient to take rilpivirine once daily with a full meal and to keep the tablets in the original container to protect them from light.

• Inform patient that, if he misses a dose, not to take the missed dose if the next scheduled dose is within 12 hours.

• Warn patient that rilpivirine may cause depressed or altered mood and to report mood changes or symptoms of depression immediately.

• Tell female patient to report pregnancy immediately.

Reactions in bold italics are *life-threatening*. Interactions may have a *rapid onset* or a *delayed onset*.

risedronate sodium
rah-SED-dro-nate

Actonel✒, Atelvia

Therapeutic class: Antiosteoporotics
Pharmacologic class: Bisphosphonates
Pregnancy risk category: C

AVAILABLE FORMS
Tablets: 5 mg, 30 mg, 35 mg, 150 mg
Tablets (delayed-release): 35 mg

INDICATIONS & DOSAGES
Adjust-a-dose (for all indications): Don't use if CrCl is less than 30 mL/minute.
➤ **To prevent and treat postmenopausal osteoporosis**
Women: 5-mg immediate-release tablet P.O. once daily, or 35-mg immediate-release tablet P.O. once weekly.
➤ **To treat postmenopausal osteoporosis**
Women: 35-mg delayed-release tablet P.O. once weekly.
➤ **To prevent or treat postmenopausal osteoporosis when fewer dosing days are desirable**
Adults: 75 mg P.O. on 2 consecutive days for a total of 2 immediate-release tablets each month. Or, one 150-mg immediate-release tablet P.O. once each month.
➤ **To increase bone mass in men with osteoporosis**
Men: One 35-mg immediate-release tablet P.O. once weekly.
➤ **Glucocorticoid-induced osteoporosis in patients taking 7.5 mg or more of prednisone or equivalent glucocorticoid daily**
Adults: 5 mg immediate-release tablet P.O. daily.
➤ **Paget disease (Actonel)**
Adults: 30 mg P.O. daily for 2 months. If relapse occurs or alkaline phosphatase level doesn't normalize, may repeat treatment course 2 months or more after completing first treatment course.

ADMINISTRATION
P.O.
● Give immediate-release tablets (Actonel) at least 30 minutes before the first food, drink, or medication of the day, other than water. Give with 6 to 8 ounces of plain water while patient is sitting or standing.
● Give delayed-release tablet in the morning immediately after breakfast and not under fasting conditions because of a higher risk of abdominal pain if taken when fasting. Give with at least 4 ounces of plain water while patient is sitting or standing.
● Warn patient against lying down for 30 minutes after taking drug.
● Make sure patient doesn't chew, crush, cut, or suck tablets.

ACTION
Reverses the loss of bone mineral density by reducing bone turnover and bone resorption. In patients with Paget disease, drug causes bone turnover to return to normal.

Route	Onset	Peak	Duration
P.O.	1 hr	Unknown	Unknown
P.O. (delayed-release)	Unknown	3 hr	Unknown

Half-life: 23 hours immediate-release; 561 hours delayed-release.

ADVERSE REACTIONS
CNS: asthenia, headache, depression, dizziness, insomnia, anxiety, neuralgia, vertigo, hypertonia, paresthesia, pain.
CV: hypertension, CV disorder, angina pectoris, chest pain, peripheral edema.
EENT: pharyngitis, rhinitis, sinusitis, cataract, conjunctivitis, otitis media, amblyopia, tinnitus.
GI: nausea, diarrhea, abdominal pain, flatulence, gastritis, rectal disorder, constipation.
GU: UTI, cystitis.
Hematologic: ecchymosis, anemia.
Musculoskeletal: arthralgia, neck pain, back pain, myalgia, bone pain, leg cramps, bursitis, tendon disorder.
Respiratory: dyspnea, pneumonia, bronchitis.
Skin: rash, pruritus.
Other: infection, tooth disorder.

INTERACTIONS
Drug-drug. *Aspirin, NSAIDs:* May increase risk of gastric ulcers. Use cautiously together.
Calcium supplements, antacids that contain calcium, magnesium, or aluminum: May interfere with risedronate absorption. Advise patient to separate dosing times.

R

H₂ antagonists, proton pump inhibitors:
May affect enteric coating on delayed-release tablets, decreasing bioavailability. Use together isn't recommended.

Drug-food. *Any food:* May interfere with absorption of drug. Advise patient to take immediate-release tablets at least 30 minutes before first food or drink of the day (other than water).

EFFECTS ON LAB TEST RESULTS
● May decrease calcium and phosphorus levels.

CONTRAINDICATIONS & CAUTIONS
● Contraindicated in patients hypersensitive to any component of the product, in hypocalcemic patients, in patients with conditions that delay esophageal emptying, in patients with CrCl less than 30 mL/minute, and in those who can't stand or sit upright for 30 minutes after administration.
❸ **Alert:** There may be an increased risk of fractures of the thigh in patients treated with bisphosphonates.
● Drug increases risk of osteonecrosis of the jaw, which can occur spontaneously. For patients requiring invasive dental procedures, discontinuing bisphosphonate treatment may reduce the risk.
● Use cautiously in patients with upper GI disorders, such as dysphagia, esophagitis, and esophageal or gastric ulcers.
● Treat hypocalcemia and other disturbances of bone and mineral metabolism before starting treatment.
● Actonel and Atelvia contain the same active ingredient and must not be given together.
⚠ **Overdose S&S:** Hypocalcemia, hypophosphatemia.

NURSING CONSIDERATIONS
● Risk factors for the development of osteoporosis include family history, previous fracture, smoking, a decrease in bone mineral density below the premenopausal mean, a thin body frame, White or Asian race, and early menopause.
● Monitor patient for osteonecrosis of the jaw. Associated risk factors include invasive dental procedures, cancer diagnosis, concomitant treatment such as chemotherapy

and steroids, poor oral hygiene, and preexisting dental disease. If signs or symptoms occur, stop drug and refer patient to oral surgeon.
❸ **Alert:** Drug may cause dysphagia, esophagitis, and esophageal or gastric ulcers. Monitor patient for symptoms of esophageal disease.
● Severe musculoskeletal pain has been associated with biophosphate use and may occur within days, months, or years of start of therapy. When drug is stopped, symptoms may resolve partially or completely.
● Give supplemental calcium and vitamin D if dietary intake is inadequate. Because calcium supplements and drugs containing calcium, aluminum, or magnesium may interfere with risedronate absorption, separate dosing times.
● Bisphosphonates can interfere with bone-imaging agents.
● **Look alike–sound alike:** Don't confuse Actonel with Actos.

PATIENT TEACHING
● Explain that drug may reverse bone loss by stopping more bone loss and increasing bone strength.
● Caution patient about the importance of adhering to special dosing instructions.
● Tell patient not to chew, cut, crush, or suck the tablet because doing so may irritate his mouth.
● Advise patient to contact prescriber immediately if he develops GI discomfort (such as difficulty or pain when swallowing, retrosternal pain, or severe heartburn).
● Tell patient that Actonel and Atelvia contain the same active ingredient and must not be taken together.
● Advise patient to take calcium and vitamin D if dietary intake is inadequate, but to take them at a different time than risedronate.
● Advise patient to stop smoking and drinking alcohol, as appropriate. Also, advise patient to perform weight-bearing exercise.
● Tell patient to store drug in a cool, dry place, at room temperature, and away from children.
● Urge patient to read the Patient Information Guide before starting therapy.

• Tell patient if he misses a dose of the 35-mg delayed-release tablet, he should take 1 tablet on the morning after he remembers and return to taking 1 tablet once a week, as originally scheduled on his chosen day. Patient shouldn't take two tablets on the same day.

risperiDONE
ris-PEER-i-dohn

Risperdal◈, Risperdal Consta, Risperdal M-TAB

Therapeutic class: Antipsychotics
Pharmacologic class: Benzisoxazole derivatives
Pregnancy risk category: C

AVAILABLE FORMS
Injection: 12.5 mg, 25 mg, 37.5 mg, 50 mg
Solution: 1 mg/mL
Tablets: 0.25 mg, 0.5 mg, 1 mg, 2 mg, 3 mg, 4 mg
Tablets (orally disintegrating): 0.25 mg, 0.5 mg, 1 mg, 2 mg, 3 mg, 4 mg

INDICATIONS & DOSAGES
➤ **Schizophrenia**
Adults: Drug may be given once daily or b.i.d. Initial dosing is generally 2 mg P.O. daily. Increase dosage at intervals not less than 24 hours, in increments of 1 to 2 mg/day, as tolerated, to a recommended dose of 4 to 8 mg/day. Periodically reassess to determine the need for maintenance treatment with an appropriate dose. Maximum dose is 16 mg/day.
Adolescents ages 13 to 17: Start treatment with 0.5 mg P.O. once daily, given as a single daily dose in either the morning or evening. Adjust dose, if indicated, at intervals of not less than 24 hours, in increments of 0.5 or 1 mg/day, as tolerated, to a recommended dose of 3 mg/day. There are no data to support use beyond 8 weeks.
➤ **12-week parenteral therapy for schizophrenia**
Adults: Establish tolerance to oral risperidone before giving I.M. Give 25 mg deep I.M. into the buttock every 2 weeks, alternating injections between the two buttocks.

Adjust dose no sooner than every 4 weeks. Maximum, 50 mg I.M. every 2 weeks. Continue oral antipsychotic for 3 weeks after first I.M. injection, then stop oral therapy.
Adjust-a-dose: In patients with hepatic or renal impairment, titrate slowly to 2 mg P.O. if tolerated, give 25 mg I.M. every 2 weeks, or give initial dose of 12.5 mg I.M. Continue oral form of risperidone (or another antipsychotic drug) with the first injection and for 3 subsequent weeks to maintain therapeutic drug levels.
➤ **Monotherapy or combination therapy with lithium or valproate for 3-week treatment of acute manic or mixed episodes from bipolar I disorder**
Adults: 2 to 3 mg P.O. once daily. Adjust dose by 1 mg daily. Dosage range is 1 to 6 mg daily. Or, 25 mg I.M. every 2 weeks. Some patients may benefit from a higher dose of 37.5 or 50 mg.
Adjust-a-dose: In elderly or debilitated patients, hypotensive patients, or those with severe renal or hepatic impairment, start with 0.5 mg P.O. b.i.d. Increase dosage by 0.5 mg b.i.d. Increase in dosages above 1.5 mg b.i.d. should occur at least 1 week apart. Subsequent switches to once-daily dosing may be made after patient is on a twice-daily regimen for 2 to 3 days at the target dose.
Children and adolescents ages 10 to 17: 0.5 mg P.O. as a single daily dose in either the morning or evening. Adjust dose, if indicated, at intervals not less than 24 hours, in increments of 0.5 or 1 mg/day, as tolerated, to a recommended dose of 2.5 mg/day.
➤ **Irritability, including aggression, self-injury, and temper tantrums, associated with an autistic disorder**
Adolescents and children ages 5 to 16 weighing 20 kg (44 lb) or more: Initially, 0.5 mg P.O. once daily or in two divided doses. After 4 days, increase dose to 1 mg. Increase dosage further in 0.5-mg increments at intervals of at least 2 weeks.
Children ages 5 to 16 weighing more than 15 kg (33 lb) and less than 20 kg: Initially, 0.25 mg P.O. once daily or in two divided doses. After 4 days, increase dose to 0.5 mg. Increase dosage further in

R

0.25-mg increments at intervals of at least 2 weeks. Increase cautiously in children who weigh less than 15 kg (33 lb).

➤ **Tourette syndrome ◆**
Adults and children: Initially, 0.5 to 1 mg P.O. daily. Titrate by 0.5 or 1 mg every 5 days. Average dose is less than 4 mg daily; maximum dose, 6 to 9 mg daily.

➤ **Obsessive-compulsive disorder ◆**
Adults: 0.5 or 1 mg P.O. daily, increased by 0.5 to 1 mg weekly. Continue for 1 to 2 years before tapering; then may reduce dosage by 10% to 25% every 1 to 2 months.

ADMINISTRATION

P.O.
● Give drug without regard for meals.
● Open package for orally disintegrating tablets (ODTs) immediately before giving by peeling off foil backing with dry hands. Don't push tablets through the foil.
● Phenylalanine contents of ODTs are as follows: 0.5-mg tablet contains 0.14 mg phenylalanine; 1-mg tablet contains 0.28 mg phenylalanine; 2-mg tablet contains 0.56 mg phenylalanine; 3-mg tablet contains 0.63 mg phenylalanine; 4-mg tablet contains 0.84 mg phenylalanine.

I.M.
● Continue oral therapy for the first 3 weeks of I.M. injection therapy until injections take effect, then stop oral therapy.
● To reconstitute I.M. injection, inject premeasured diluent into vial and shake vigorously for at least 10 seconds. Suspension appears uniform, thick, and milky; particles are visible, but no dry particles remain. Use drug immediately, or refrigerate for up to 6 hours after reconstitution. If more than 2 minutes pass before injection, shake vigorously again. See manufacturer's package insert for more detailed instructions.
● Refrigerate I.M. injection kit and protect it from light. Drug can be stored at temperature less than 77° F (25° C) for no more than 7 days before administration.

ACTION

Blocks dopamine and 5-HT₂ receptors in the brain.

Route	Onset	Peak	Duration
P.O.	Unknown	1 hr	Unknown
I.M.	3 wk	4–6 wk	7 wk

Half-life: 3 to 20 hours.

ADVERSE REACTIONS

CNS: akathisia, somnolence, dystonia, headache, insomnia, agitation, anxiety, pain, parkinsonism, *neuroleptic malignant syndrome, suicide attempt,* dizziness, fever, hallucination, mania, impaired concentration, abnormal thinking and dreaming, tremor, hypoesthesia, fatigue, depression, nervousness, parkinsonism.
CV: tachycardia, chest pain, orthostatic hypotension, peripheral edema, syncope, hypertension.
EENT: rhinitis, sinusitis, pharyngitis, abnormal vision, ear disorder (I.M.).
GI: constipation, nausea, vomiting, dyspepsia, abdominal pain, anorexia, dry mouth, increased saliva, diarrhea.
GU: urinary incontinence, increased urination, abnormal orgasm, vaginal dryness.
Metabolic: weight gain, hyperglycemia, weight loss.
Musculoskeletal: arthralgia, back pain, leg pain, myalgia.
Respiratory: coughing, dyspnea, upper respiratory tract infection.
Skin: rash, dry skin, photosensitivity reactions, acne, injection-site pain (I.M.).
Other: tooth disorder, toothache, injury, decreased libido.

INTERACTIONS

Drug-drug. *Antihypertensives:* May enhance hypotensive effects. Monitor blood pressure.
Azole antifungal (such as fluconazole, itraconazole, ketoconazole): May increase risperidone plasma level. Monitor clinical response and adjust risperidone dosage.
Carbamazepine: May increase risperidone clearance and decrease effectiveness. Monitor patient closely.
Clozapine: May decrease risperidone clearance, increasing toxicity. Monitor patient closely.
CNS depressants: May cause additive CNS depression. Use together cautiously.

Reactions in bold italics are *life-threatening*. Interactions may have a *rapid onset* or a *delayed onset*.

Dopamine agonists, levodopa: May antagonize effects of these drugs. Use together cautiously and monitor patient.

Fluoxetine, paroxetine: May increase the risk of risperidone's adverse effects, including serotonin syndrome. Monitor patient closely and adjust risperidone dose, as needed.

Drug-lifestyle. *Alcohol use:* May cause additive CNS depression. Discourage use together.

Sun exposure: May increase risk of photosensitivity reactions. Advise patient to avoid excessive sunlight exposure.

EFFECTS ON LAB TEST RESULTS
• May increase prolactin level.
• May decrease hemoglobin level and hematocrit.

CONTRAINDICATIONS & CAUTIONS
• Contraindicated in patients hypersensitive to drug and in breast-feeding women.
◑ **Alert:** Neonates exposed to antipsychotics during the third trimester of pregnancy are at risk for developing extrapyramidal signs and symptoms (repetitive muscle movements of the face and body) and withdrawal symptoms (agitation, abnormally increased or decreased muscle tone, tremors, sleepiness, severe difficulty breathing, difficulty feeding) following delivery. Use in pregnancy only if the potential benefit to the mother justifies the risk to the fetus.
• Use cautiously in patients with prolonged QT interval, CV disease, cerebrovascular disease, dehydration, hypovolemia, history of seizures, or conditions that could affect metabolism or hemodynamic responses.
• Use cautiously in patients exposed to extreme heat.
• Use caution in patients at risk for aspiration pneumonia.
• Use I.M. injection cautiously in those with hepatic or renal impairment.
⚠ **Overdose S&S:** Drowsiness, sedation, tachycardia, hypotension, extrapyramidal symptoms, QT-interval prolongation, seizures, torsades de pointes.

NURSING CONSIDERATIONS
◑ **Alert:** Obtain baseline blood pressure measurements before starting therapy, and monitor pressure regularly. Watch for orthostatic hypotension, especially during first dosage adjustment.

Black Box Warning Elderly patients with dementia-related psychosis treated with antipsychotics are at increased risk for death. Drug isn't approved to treat elderly patients with dementia-related psychosis. ∎
• Monitor patient for tardive dyskinesia, which may occur after prolonged use. It may not appear until months or years later and may disappear spontaneously or persist for life, despite stopping drug.
◑ **Alert:** Watch for evidence of neuroleptic malignant syndrome (extrapyramidal effects, hyperthermia, autonomic disturbance), which is rare but can be fatal.
• Life-threatening hyperglycemia may occur in patients taking atypical antipsychotics. Monitor patients with diabetes regularly.
◑ **Alert:** Monitor patient for symptoms of metabolic syndrome (significant weight gain and increased body mass index, hypertension, hyperglycemia, hypercholesterolemia, and hypertriglyceridemia).
• Periodically reevaluate drug's risks and benefits, especially during prolonged use.
• Monitor patient for weight gain.
• *Look alike–sound alike:* Don't confuse risperidone with reserpine or ropinirole. Don't confuse Risperdal with Restoril.

PATIENT TEACHING
• Warn patient to avoid activities that require alertness until effects of drug are known.
• Warn patient to rise slowly, avoid hot showers, and use other precautions to avoid fainting when starting therapy.
• Advise patient to use caution in hot weather to prevent heatstroke.
• Tell patient to take drug with or without food.
• Instruct patient to keep the ODT in the blister pack until just before taking it. After opening the pack, he should dissolve the tablet on tongue without cutting or chewing. Tell the patient to use dry hands to peel apart the foil to expose the tablet; he shouldn't attempt to push it through the foil.
• Tell patient to use sunblock and wear protective clothing outdoors.

R

- Advise women not to become pregnant or to breast-feed for 12 weeks after the last I.M. injection.
- Advise patient to avoid alcohol during therapy.

ritonavir
ri-TON-ah-veer

Norvir

Therapeutic class: Antiretrovirals
Pharmacologic class: Protease inhibitors
Pregnancy risk category: B

AVAILABLE FORMS
Capsules: 100 mg
Oral solution: 80 mg/mL*
Tablets: 100 mg

INDICATIONS & DOSAGES
➤ **HIV infection, with other antiretrovirals**
Adults: 600 mg P.O. b.i.d. with meals. To reduce adverse GI effects, begin with 300 mg P.O. b.i.d. and increase by 100 mg b.i.d. at 2- to 3-day intervals.
Children older than age 1 month: 350 to 400 mg/m^2 P.O. b.i.d.; don't exceed 600 mg P.O. b.i.d. Initially, start with 250 mg/m^2 b.i.d. and increase by 50 mg/m^2 P.O. every 12 hours at 2- to 3-day intervals. If children can't reach b.i.d. doses of 400 mg/m^2 because of adverse effects, consider alternative therapy.

ADMINISTRATION
P.O.
- Give drug with meals.
- Oral solution may be mixed with chocolate milk or enteral nutrition therapy liquids within 1 hour of dosing. Shake well.
- When giving oral solution to children, use a calibrated dosing syringe, if possible.
- Make sure patient swallows tablets whole and doesn't break, crush, or chew them.

ACTION
An HIV-1 and HIV-2 protease inhibitor. Drug binds to the protease-active site and inhibits activity of the enzyme, preventing cleavage of the viral polyproteins and causing formation of immature, noninfectious viral particles.

Route	Onset	Peak	Duration
P.O.	Unknown	2–4 hr	Unknown

Half-life: 3 to 5 hours.

ADVERSE REACTIONS
CNS: asthenia, *generalized tonic-clonic seizure,* anxiety, circumoral paresthesia, confusion, depression, dizziness, fever, headache, insomnia, malaise, pain, paresthesia, peripheral paresthesia, somnolence, thinking abnormality.
CV: syncope, vasodilation.
EENT: pharyngitis.
GI: diarrhea, nausea, taste perversion, vomiting, *pancreatitis, pseudomembranous colitis,* abdominal pain, anorexia, constipation, dyspepsia, flatulence.
Hematologic: *leukopenia, thrombocytopenia.*
Hepatic: *hepatitis.*
Metabolic: *diabetes mellitus,* weight loss.
Musculoskeletal: arthralgia, myalgia.
Skin: sweating.
Other: hypersensitivity reactions, fat redistribution or accumulation, immune reconstitution syndrome.

INTERACTIONS
Drug-drug. Black Box Warning *Alfuzosin, amiodarone, bepridil, ergot derivatives, flecainide, oral midazolam, pimozide, propafenone, quinidine, sildenafil (Revatio when used to treat pulmonary arterial hypertension), simvastatin, triazolam, voriconazole:* May cause life-threatening adverse reactions due to possible effects of ritonavir on the hepatic metabolism of these drugs. Use together is contraindicated. ■
✪ *Alert: Atorvastatin, pitavastatin, pravastatin, rosuvastatin:* May increase statin level and risk of myopathy and rhabdomyolysis. Use together cautiously at the recommended dosage for the statin given in combination with ritonavir. Refer to prescribing information for statin drug dosage limitations.

---

*Reactions in bold italics are **life-threatening**. Interactions may have a **rapid onset** or a **delayed onset**.*

Atovaquone, divalproex, lamotrigine, phenytoin, warfarin: May decrease levels of these drugs. Use together cautiously and monitor drug levels closely.

Beta blockers, disopyramide, fluoxetine, mexiletine, nefazodone: May increase levels of these drugs, causing cardiac and neurologic events. Use together cautiously.

Bupropion, buspirone, calcium channel blockers, carbamazepine, clonazepam, clorazepate, cyclosporine, desipramine, dexamethasone, diazepam, **digoxin,** *dronabinol, estazolam, ethosuximide, flurazepam, lidocaine, methamphetamine, metoprolol, perphenazine, prednisone, propoxyphene, quinine, risperidone, sirolimus, SSRIs, tacrolimus, TCAs, thioridazine, timolol, tramadol, zolpidem:* May increase levels of these drugs. Use cautiously together and consider decreasing the dosage of these drugs by almost 50%. Monitor therapeutic levels.

Clarithromycin: May increase clarithromycin level. If CrCl is 30 to 60 mL/minute, reduce clarithromycin dosage by 50%. If CrCl is less than 30 mL/minute, reduce clarithromycin dosage by 75%.

Clozapine, piroxicam: May increase levels and toxicity of these drugs. Avoid using together.

Delavirdine: May increase ritonavir level. Adjusted dose recommendations aren't established. Use together cautiously.

Didanosine: May decrease didanosine absorption. Separate doses by 2½ hours.

Disulfiram, metronidazole: May increase risk of disulfiram-like reactions because ritonavir formulations contain alcohol. Monitor patient.

Ethinyl estradiol: May decrease ethinyl estradiol level. Use an alternative or additional method of birth control.

Fluticasone: May significantly increase fluticasone exposure, significantly decreasing cortisol concentrations and causing systemic corticosteroid effects (including Cushing syndrome). Don't use together, if possible.

HMG-CoA reductase inhibitors: May cause large increase in statin levels, resulting in myopathy. Use cautiously with atorvastatin. Consider using fluvastatin or pravastatin.

Indinavir: May increase indinavir levels. Use together cautiously.

Itraconazole, ketoconazole: May increase levels of these drugs. Don't exceed 200 mg/day of these drugs.

❸ Alert: *Lovastatin, simvastatin:* May increase statin level and risk of myopathy and rhabdomyolysis. Use together is contraindicated.

Meperidine: May decrease levels of meperidine and its metabolite. Dosage increases and long-term use together aren't recommended because of CNS effects. Use cautiously together.

Methadone: May decrease methadone levels. Consider increasing methadone dosage.

PDE5 inhibitors (sildenafil, tadalafil, vardenafil): May increase levels of PDE5 inhibitor, causing hypotension, syncope, visual changes, or prolonged erection. Use together cautiously and increase monitoring for adverse reactions. Tell patient not to exceed 25 mg of sildenafil in a 48-hour period, 10 mg of tadalafil in a 72-hour period, or 2.5 mg of vardenafil in a 72-hour period.

Rifabutin: May increase rifabutin levels. Monitor patient and reduce rifabutin daily dosage by at least 75% of usual dose.

Rifampin, rifapentine: May decrease ritonavir levels. Consider using rifabutin.

Saquinavir: May increase saquinavir plasma levels. Adjust dose by taking saquinavir 400 mg b.i.d. and ritonavir 400 mg b.i.d.

Saquinavir: May prolong QT and PR intervals. Avoid concomitant use in patients with history of prolonged QT interval and in those already receiving drugs known to prolong QT interval (class I or class III antiarrythmics).

Theophylline: May decrease theophylline levels. Increase dose based on blood levels.

Trazodone: May increase trazodone level, causing nausea, dizziness, hypotension, and syncope. Avoid using together. If unavoidable, use cautiously and lower trazodone dose.

Drug-herb. *St. John's wort:* May substantially reduce drug levels. Use together is contraindicated.

R

Drug-food. *Any food:* May increase absorption. Advise patient to take drug with food.

Drug-lifestyle. *Smoking:* May decrease drug levels. Discourage smoking.

EFFECTS ON LAB TEST RESULTS

• May increase ALT, AST, GGT, glucose, triglyceride, lipid, CK, and uric acid levels. May decrease hemoglobin level and hematocrit.

• May decrease WBC, RBC, platelet, and neutrophil counts.

CONTRAINDICATIONS & CAUTIONS

• Contraindicated in patients hypersensitive to drug or its components.

• Use cautiously in patients with hepatic disease, liver enzyme abnormalities, or hepatitis.

◐ Alert: Patients with advanced HIV infection may have increased risk of elevated triglyceride levels and in some cases fatal pancreatitis.

• In postmarketing surveillance, hyperglycemia requiring treatment has been reported. A causal relationship with ritonavir hasn't been established.

• Safety and effectiveness in children younger than 1 month haven't been established.

• May cause toxicity in preterm neonates. Don't use oral solution in preterm neonates in the immediate postnatal period. A safe and effective dose in this patient population hasn't been established.

• It's unknown if ritonavir appears in breast milk. Use cautiously in breast-feeding women.

⚠ Overdose S&S: Paresthesia, renal failure with eosinophilia, alcohol-related toxicity with oral solution.

NURSING CONSIDERATIONS

Black Box Warning Coadministration with sedative-hypnotics, antiarrhythmics, or ergot alkaloid preparations may result in potentially serious or life-threatening adverse events because of possible effects on the hepatic metabolism of certain drugs. Review medications taken by patients before administering ritonavir or when adminis-

tering other medications to patients already taking ritonavir. ▮

• Monitor patient for immune reconstitution syndrome. During initial phase of treatment, patients responding to antiretroviral therapy may develop an inflammatory response to indolent or residual opportunistic infections (CMV, *Mycobacterium avium* complex, *Pneumocystis jiroveci* pneumonia, tuberculosis), which may necessitate further evaluation and treatment. Autoimmune disorders (such as Graves disease, polymyositis, and Guillain-Barré syndrome) have also been reported in the setting of immune reconstitution; however, time to onset is more variable, and can occur many months after initiation of antiretroviral treatment.

• Patients beginning regimens with ritonavir and nucleosides may improve GI tolerance by starting ritonavir alone and then adding nucleosides before completing 2 weeks of ritonavir.

• In patients with liver disease, monitor liver enzyme and triglyceride levels frequently, especially during the first 3 months of treatment.

• Monitor patient for redistribution or accumulation of body fat, which has been observed with antiretroviral therapy.

• **Look alike–sound alike:** Don't confuse Norvir with Norvasc.

PATIENT TEACHING

• Inform patient that drug doesn't cure HIV infection. He may continue to develop opportunistic infections and other complications of HIV infection. Drug hasn't been shown to reduce the risk of transmitting HIV to others through sexual contact or blood contamination.

• Caution patient to take drug as prescribed and not to adjust dosage or stop therapy without first consulting prescriber.

• Tell patient that taste of oral solution may be improved by mixing it with chocolate milk, Ensure, or Advera within 1 hour of the scheduled dose.

• Advise patient not to chew, crush, or break tablets.

• Instruct patient to take drug with a meal to improve absorption.

• Tell patient that if a dose is missed, he should take the next dose as soon as possible. If a dose is skipped, he shouldn't double the next dose.

• Advise patients taking a PDE5 inhibitor for erectile dysfunction to promptly report hypotension, dizziness, visual changes, and prolonged erection to their prescriber. Caution against exceeding the recommended reduced dosage.

• Advise patient using estrogen-based contraceptives to use an alternative method during therapy.

• Caution patient to report signs and symptoms of pancreatitis (nausea, vomiting, and abdominal pain) immediately.

• Counsel patient that ritonavir must always be taken in combination with other antiretrovirals.

• Advise patient to report use of other drugs, including OTC drugs; this drug interacts with many drugs.

SAFETY ALERT!

rituximab
ri-TUX-i-mab

Rituxan

Therapeutic class: Antineoplastics
Pharmacologic class: Monoclonal antibodies
Pregnancy risk category: C

AVAILABLE FORMS
Injection: 10 mg/mL in 10-mL and 50-mL single-use, sterile vials

INDICATIONS & DOSAGES
➤ **Maintenance therapy for patients with previously untreated follicular, CD20-positive, B-cell non-Hodgkin lymphoma (NHL) who achieve response to rituximab in combination with chemotherapy**
Adults: 375 mg/m² I.V. as single agent every 8 weeks for 12 doses beginning 8 weeks after completion of combination therapy.
➤ **Wegener granulomatosis (WG); microscopic polyangiitis (MPA) in combination with glucocorticoids**
Adults: 375 mg/m² I.V. once weekly for 4 weeks. Give methylprednisolone 1,000

mg/day I.V. for 1 to 3 days followed by oral prednisone 1 mg/kg/day (not to exceed 80 mg/day and tapered per clinical need) to treat severe vasculitis symptoms. This regimen should begin within 14 days before or with the initiation of rituximab and may continue during and after the 4-week course of rituximab treatment.
➤ **Previously untreated, follicular CD20-positive, B-cell NHL with cyclophosphamide-vincristine-prednisolone (CVP) chemotherapy regimen**
Adults: 375 mg/m² I.V. given on day 1 of each CVP cycle, for up to eight doses.
➤ **Previously untreated low-grade, CD20-positive, B-cell NHL following first-line treatment with CVP chemotherapy**
Adults: For patients who fail to progress after six to eight cycles of CVP chemotherapy, give 375 mg/m² I.V. once weekly for 4 doses every 6 months for up to 16 doses.
➤ **CD20-positive chronic lymphocytic leukemia (CLL) in combination with fludarabine and cyclophosphamide**
Adults: 375 mg/m² I.V. given day before combination treatment. Then give 500 mg/m² I.V. on day 1 of cycles two through six in combination with fludarabine and cyclophosphamide (every 28 days).
➤ **Relapsed or refractory low-grade or follicular, CD20-positive, B-cell NHL**
Adults: Initially, 375 mg/m² I.V. once weekly for four or eight doses. Retreatment for patients with progressive disease, 375 mg/m² I.V. infusion once weekly for four doses.
➤ **With ibritumomab tiuxetan (Zevalin) for relapsed or refractory low-grade, follicular or transformed B-cell NHL**
Adults: 250 mg/m² I.V. 4 hours before indium-111 Zevalin infusion. Repeat in 7 to 9 days, 4 hours before yttrium-90 Zevalin infusion.
➤ **With methotrexate to reduce the signs and symptoms of moderate to severely active rheumatoid arthritis in patients who have had an inadequate response to one or more TNF antagonists**

R

Adults: Two 1,000-mg I.V. infusions 2 weeks apart. To reduce the incidence and severity of infusion reactions, give methylprednisolone 100 mg I.V., or its equivalent, 30 minutes before each infusion.

➤ **Diffuse large B-cell, CD20-positive NHL, given with cyclophosphamide-Adriamycin (doxorubicin)-Oncovin (vincristine)-prednisone (CHOP) chemotherapy regimen or other anthracycline-based chemotherapy regimens**
Adults: 375 mg/m^2 I.V. given on day 1 of each chemotherapy cycle for up to eight infusions.

ADMINISTRATION
I.V.
▼ Give acetaminophen and diphenhydramine before each infusion.
▼ Protect vials from direct sunlight.
▼ Give as an infusion; don't give as I.V. push or bolus.
▼ Begin infusion at rate of 50 mg/hour. If no hypersensitivity or infusion-related events occur, increase rate by 50 mg/hour every 30 minutes, to maximum of 400 mg/hour. Start subsequent infusions at 100 mg/hour and increase by 100 mg/hour every 30 minutes, to maximum of 400 mg/hour as tolerated.
▼ Dilute to yield 1 to 4 mg/mL in bag of D$_5$W or normal saline solution. Gently invert bag to mix solution.
▼ Discard unused portion left in vial.
▼ Diluted solutions are stable for 24 hours if refrigerated and for 12 hours at room temperature.
▼ **Incompatibilities:** Other I.V. drugs.

ACTION
A murine and human monoclonal antibody directed against CD20 antigen found on the surface of normal and malignant B lymphocytes. Binding to this antigen mediates the lysis of the B cells.

Route	Onset	Peak	Duration
I.V.	Variable	Variable	6–12 mo

Half-life: Varies widely, possibly because of differences in tumor burden among patients and changes in CD-positive B-cell populations on repeated therapy.

ADVERSE REACTIONS
CNS: asthenia, fever, headache, agitation, dizziness, fatigue, hypesthesia, hypertonia, insomnia, malaise, nervousness, pain, paresthesia, somnolence, vertigo.
CV: hypotension, *arrhythmias, bradycardia,* chest pain, edema, flushing, hypertension, peripheral edema, tachycardia, *heart failure.*
EENT: conjunctivitis, lacrimation disorder, rhinitis, sinusitis, sore throat.
GI: nausea, abdominal pain or enlargement, anorexia, diarrhea, dyspepsia, taste perversion, vomiting, *bowel perforation.*
GU: *acute renal failure.*
Hematologic: *leukopenia, neutropenia, thrombocytopenia,* anemia.
Metabolic: hyperglycemia, hypocalcemia, weight decrease.
Musculoskeletal: arthritis, back pain, myalgia.
Respiratory: *bronchospasm,* bronchitis, cough increase, dyspnea.
Skin: pruritus, rash, *severe mucocutaneous reactions,* pain at injection site, urticaria.
Other: chills, rigors, *angioedema, infusion reaction,* infection, *tumor lysis syndrome,* tumor pain.

INTERACTIONS
Drug-drug. *Cisplatin:* May cause renal toxicity. Monitor renal function tests.
Live-virus vaccines: Virus replication may occur. Avoid vaccination with live-virus vaccines.
Tocilizumab: May increase risk of serious infection. Avoid use together.

EFFECTS ON LAB TEST RESULTS
● May increase glucose and LDH levels. May decrease calcium and hemoglobin levels.
● May decrease WBC, platelet, and neutrophil counts.

CONTRAINDICATIONS & CAUTIONS
● Contraindicated in patients with type I hypersensitivity or anaphylactic reactions to murine proteins or components of drug.
Black Box Warning Hepatitis B virus (HBV) reactivation, including fulminant hepatitis, hepatic failure, and death, may occur in patients treated with rituximab. Screen all patients for HBV infection

before treatment by measuring hepatitis B surface antigen and hepatitis B core antibody. Monitor patients with evidence of current or prior HBV infection during and for several months after therapy. If HBV reactivation occurs, discontinue rituximab and concomitant chemotherapy and begin appropriate treatment. ■

🛈 *Alert:* Consult hepatitis expert when screening identifies patients at risk for HBV reactivation due to prior HBV infection.

NURSING CONSIDERATIONS

Black Box Warning Deaths from infusion reactions have occurred. Eighty percent of fatal reactions are associated with the first infusion. Monitor patient for infusion reaction complex, including hypoxia, pulmonary infiltrates, acute respiratory distress syndrome, MI, or cardiogenic shock. ■

• Monitor patient closely for signs and symptoms of hypersensitivity. Have drugs, such as epinephrine, antihistamines, and corticosteroids, available to immediately treat such a reaction.

• Monitor patient's blood pressure closely during infusion. If hypotension, bronchospasm, or angioedema occurs, stop infusion and restart at half the rate when symptoms resolve.

• Withhold antihypertensives 12 hours before infusion because transient hypotension may occur.

• If serious or life-threatening arrhythmias occur, stop infusion. If patient develops significant arrhythmias, monitor cardiac function during and after subsequent infusions.

• *Pneumocystis jiroveci* pneumonia and antiherpetic viral prophylaxis is recommended for patients with CLL during and for up to 12 months after treatment ends.

• HBV reactivation, including fulminant hepatitis, hepatic failure, and death, may occur in patients treated with rituximab. Screen patients at high risk for HBV before start of therapy and monitor carriers for active HBV infection for several months after therapy.

• Monitor patients with WG and MPA carefully for signs and symptoms of infection (fever, pain, cold or flu symptoms, erythema) if biological agents or disease-modifying antirheumatic drugs are used concomitantly.

🛈 *Alert:* Prophylaxis for *P. jiroveci* pneumonia is recommended for patients with WG and MPA during treatment with rituximab and for at least 6 months after the last infusion.

Black Box Warning Severe mucocutaneous reactions (including toxic epidermal necrolysis, Stevens-Johnson syndrome, paraneoplastic pemphigus, and lichenoid or vesiculobullous dermatitis) may occur 1 to 13 weeks after administration. Avoid further infusions and promptly start treatment of the skin reaction. ■

• Infusion-related reactions are most severe with the first infusion. Subsequent infusions are generally well tolerated.

Black Box Warning Acute renal failure requiring dialysis has been reported in the setting of tumor lysis syndrome (TLS) following treatment of patients with NHL. ■

• Patients at high risk for TLS may receive prophylactic allopurinol and hydration to correct hyperuricemia. Monitor renal function and fluid balance, and correct electrolyte abnormalities.

Black Box Warning JC virus infection resulting in progressive multifocal leukoencephalopathy has been reported in patients within 12 months of their last rituximab infusion. Monitor patient for new-onset neurologic manifestations. ■

• Obtain CBC at regular intervals and more frequently in patients in whom cytopenias develop.

• Monitor patients at risk for hepatitis B closely. Discontinue drug at first sign of hepatitis B infection.

• Monitor patient for abdominal pain. Bowel obstruction and perforation have occurred with chemotherapy.

PATIENT TEACHING

• Tell patient to report symptoms of hypersensitivity, such as itching, rash, chills, or rigor, during and after infusion.

• Urge patient to watch for fever, sore throat, fatigue, easy bruising, nosebleeds, bleeding gums, abdominal pain, or tarry stools. Tell him to take temperature daily.

R

• Advise breast-feeding women to stop breast-feeding until drug levels are undetectable.

SAFETY ALERT!

rivaroxaban
ri-va-ROX-a-ban

Xarelto

Therapeutic class: Anticoagulants
Pharmacologic class: Factor Xa inhibitors
Pregnancy risk category: C

AVAILABLE FORMS
Tablets: 10 mg, 15 mg, 20 mg

INDICATIONS & DOSAGES
➤ **Prophylaxis of DVT that may lead to PE in patients undergoing knee or hip replacement surgery**
Adults: 10 mg P.O. once daily, 6 to 10 hours after surgery once hemostasis has been established. Treat for 35 days after hip replacement surgery and 12 days after knee replacement surgery.
Adjust-a-dose: Use with caution in patients with moderate renal impairment (CrCl ranging from 30 to less than 50 mL/minute).
✴ **NEW INDICATION: Treatment of DVT or PE**
Adults: 15 mg P.O. b.i.d. with food for 21 days; then 20 mg P.O. once daily for remainder of treatment.
Adjust-a-dose: If CrCl is less than 30 mL/minute, avoid use.
✴ **NEW INDICATION: To decrease risk of recurrent DVT or PE**
Adults: 20 mg P.O. once daily with food.
Adjust-a-dose: If CrCl is less than 30 mL/minute, avoid use.
➤ **Stroke and systemic embolism risk reduction in patients with nonvalvular atrial fibrillation**
Adults: 20 mg once daily with evening meal.
Adjust-a-dose: In patients with CrCl of 15 to 50 mL/minute, reduce dosage to 15 mg once daily with evening meal. Avoid use in patients with CrCl less than 15 mL/minute.

ADMINISTRATION
P.O.
• For prophylaxis of DVT, give without regard for food. For nonvalvular atrial fibrillation, give with evening meal.
• May crush drug and give through a feeding tube that has confirmed gastric placement. Delivery of drug into the small intestine results in reduced absorption.

ACTION
Selectively blocks the active site of factor Xa, which is necessary for coagulation.

Route	Onset	Peak	Duration
P.O.	Unknown	2–4 hr	Unknown

Half-life: 5 to 9 hours.

ADVERSE REACTIONS
CNS: syncope.
Hematologic: *bleeding events (including hemorrhage).*
Musculoskeletal: extremity pain, muscle spasm.
Skin: wound secretion, pruritus, blister.

INTERACTIONS
Drug-drug. *Anticoagulants (warfarin), aspirin, clopidogrel, NSAIDs:* May increase bleeding risk. Avoid use together. Monitor patient carefully for bleeding if drugs must be given together.
Combined P-glycoprotein (P-gp) and strong CYP3A4 inducers (carbamazepine, phenytoin, rifampin): May significantly decrease rivaroxaban level. Avoid use together.
Combined P-gp and strong CYP3A4 inhibitors (clarithromycin, conivaptan, indinavir–ritonavir, itraconazole, ketoconazole, lopinavir–ritonavir, ritonavir): May significantly increase rivaroxaban level. Avoid use together.
Combined P-gp and weak or moderate CYP3A4 inhibitors (amiodarone, azithromycin, diltiazem, dronedarone, erythromycin, felodipine, quinidine, ranolazine, verapamil): May increase rivaroxaban level. Use together only if benefit outweighs risk.
Drug-herb. *St. John's wort:* May significantly decrease rivaroxaban level. Avoid use together.

EFFECTS ON LAB TEST RESULTS
● May increase AST, ALT, total bilirubin, and GGT levels.
● May decrease platelet count.

CONTRAINDICATIONS & CAUTIONS
Black Box Warning There is an increased risk of epidural or spinal hematomas, possibly resulting in long-term or permanent paralysis, in patients who have received anticoagulants and are receiving neuraxial anesthesia or undergoing spinal puncture. Factors that can increase the risk of epidural or spinal hematomas in these patients include use of indwelling epidural catheters; concomitant use of other drugs that affect hemostasis, such as NSAIDs, platelet inhibitors, and other anticoagulants; history of traumatic or repeated epidural or spinal punctures; and history of spinal deformity or spinal surgery. Monitor patients frequently for neurologic impairment. If neurologic compromise is noted, urgent treatment is necessary. Consider risks and benefits before neuraxial procedures in patients who have received anticoagulants for thromboprophylaxis. ■

Black Box Warning Discontinuing rivaroxaban places patients with nonvalvular atrial fibrillation at increased risk for thrombotic events. An increased rate of stroke was observed after rivaroxaban discontinuation in clinical trials in patients with atrial fibrillation. If anticoagulation with rivaroxaban must be discontinued for a reason other than pathological bleeding, consider using another anticoagulant. ■

● Contraindicated in patients hypersensitive to drug and in those with active major bleeding.
● Use isn't recommended in patients with prosthetic heart valves.
● Use cautiously in conditions associated with increased risk of hemorrhage, with concurrent use of drugs affecting hemostasis (platelet aggregation inhibitors, other antithrombotic agents, fibrinolytics, thienopyridines, long-term NSAIDs), and in elderly patients.
● Use cautiously in pregnant and breast-feeding women; use only if benefits outweigh risks.

● Avoid use in patients with CrCl of less than 50 mL/minute who are taking drug for DVT prophylaxis. Discontinue drug if acute renal failure occurs.
● Avoid use in patients with moderate or severe hepatic impairment (Child-Pugh class B or C) and in those with hepatic disease associated with coagulopathy.
● Consider alternative therapy in patients with renal impairment and in those receiving drugs that are concurrent P-gp and weak to moderate CYP3A4 inhibitors; bleeding risk may increase.
● Use cautiously in Japanese patients because drug exposure in these patients may be increased up to 50% when compared to other ethnicities.
⚠ Overdose S&S: Hemorrhage.

NURSING CONSIDERATIONS
Black Box Warning Monitor patient frequently for signs and symptoms of neurologic impairment. If neurologic compromise is noted, urgent treatment is necessary. ■
Black Box Warning Consider the benefits and risks before neuraxial intervention in patients anticoagulated or to be anticoagulated for thromboprophylaxis. ■
● Don't remove an epidural catheter earlier than 18 hours after last administration of drug, and don't give next dose until 6 hours after catheter removal unless traumatic puncture occurred; if puncture has occurred, wait 24 hours before giving next dose.
● Monitor patient carefully for bleeding, which can occur at any site during therapy.
� Alert: Watch for signs and symptoms of blood loss. Search for a bleeding site if an unexplained fall in hematocrit or blood pressure occurs. Patients with moderate renal failure (CrCl ranging from 30 to less than 50 mL/minute) are at increased risk.

PATIENT TEACHING
● Instruct patient to take drug only as directed and not to discontinue drug without consulting prescriber.
● Tell patient if a dose is missed, to take dose as soon as he remembers and to resume the normal regimen the following day.
� Alert: If patient has had neuraxial anesthesia or spinal puncture, especially if he is taking concomitant NSAIDs or platelet

R

inhibitors, advise him to watch for signs and symptoms of spinal or epidural hematoma (tingling, numbness of the limbs, muscular weakness). If any of these symptoms occur, advise him to contact his physician immediately.

• Advise patient to watch for bleeding risks, especially if he had a spinal catheter or is currently taking drugs or supplements that increase bleeding risk.

• Instruct female patient to consult prescriber if she is pregnant, plans to become pregnant, or intends to breast-feed.

• Caution patient to report changes in medications or herbal supplements or unusual bleeding or bruising.

• Advise patient who can't swallow the tablet whole to crush tablet and combine with a small amount of applesauce followed by food.

• Instruct patient with a nasogastric or gastric feeding tube to crush the tablet and mix it with a small amount of water before administering via the tube.

• Instruct patient to inform all health care providers that he or she is taking rivaroxaban before any invasive procedure (including dental procedures) is scheduled.

rivastigmine
riv-ah-STIG-meen

Exelon Patch

rivastigmine tartrate✦
Exelon

Therapeutic class: Anti-Alzheimer drugs
Pharmacologic class: Cholinesterase inhibitors
Pregnancy risk category: B

AVAILABLE FORMS
Capsules: 1.5 mg, 3 mg, 4.5 mg, 6 mg
Solution: 2 mg/mL
Transdermal patch: 4.6 mg/24 hours, 9.5 mg/24 hours, 13.3 mg/24 hours

INDICATIONS & DOSAGES
Adjust-a-dose (for all indications): For patients with mild to moderate hepatic impairment (Child-Pugh score 5 to 9), consider using 4.6 mg/24 hours transdermal patch for both initial and maintenance dose. For patients with low body weight (less than 50 kg [110 lb]), watch for toxicities (nausea, vomiting) and, if they occur, consider reducing maintenance dosage to 4.6 mg/24 hours transdermal patch.

➤ **Mild to moderate Alzheimer dementia**
Adults: Initially, 1.5 mg P.O. b.i.d. with food. If tolerated, may increase to 3 mg b.i.d. after 2 weeks. After 2 weeks at this dose, may increase to 4.5 mg b.i.d. and 6 mg b.i.d., as tolerated. Effective dosage range is 6 to 12 mg daily; maximum, 12 mg daily. Or, 4.6 mg/24 hours transdermal patch. After 4 weeks, if tolerated, increase to 9.5 mg/24 hours transdermal patch, then to 13.3 mg/24 hours transdermal patch. Maximum dose is 13.3 mg/24 hours.

✴ *NEW INDICATION:* **Severe Alzheimer dementia (transdermal patch only)**
Adults: Initially, 4.6 mg/24 hours transdermal patch once daily. After 4 weeks, if tolerated, increase to 9.5 mg/24 hours transdermal patch; then, if tolerated after an additional 4 weeks, may increase to 13.3 mg/24 hours transdermal patch.

➤ **Mild to moderate dementia associated with Parkinson disease**
Adults: Initially, 1.5 mg P.O. b.i.d. May increase, as tolerated, to 3 mg b.i.d., then 4.5 mg b.i.d., and finally to 6 mg b.i.d. after a minimum of 4 weeks at each dose. Or, 4.6 mg/24 hours transdermal patch. After 4 weeks, if tolerated, increase to 9.5 mg/ 24 hours transdermal patch, then to 13.3 mg/24 hours transdermal patch. Maximum dose is 13.3 mg/24 hours.

➤ **Treatment of neuropsychiatric symptoms associated with Lewy body dementia ◆**
Adults: Initially, 1.5 P.O. b.i.d.; increase as tolerated by 1.5 mg b.i.d. every 2 weeks to a maximum of 6 mg b.i.d. Ongoing therapy is required.

ADMINISTRATION
P.O.
• Give drug with food in the morning and evening.
• Solution may be taken directly or mixed with small glass of water, cold fruit juice, or soda.

• Capsule and solution doses are interchangeable.

Transdermal

• Apply patch once daily to clean, dry, hairless skin on the upper or lower back, upper arm, or chest, in a place not rubbed by tight clothing.

• Change the site daily, and don't use the same site within 14 days.

• Press patch firmly into place until the edges stick well.

ACTION

Thought to increase acetylcholine level by inhibiting cholinesterase enzyme, which causes acetylcholine hydrolysis.

Route	Onset	Peak	Duration
P.O.	Unknown	1 hr	12 hr
Transdermal	Unknown	8 hr	24 hr

Half-life: 1½ hours (oral); 3 hours (transdermal).

ADVERSE REACTIONS

CNS: headache, dizziness, syncope, fatigue, asthenia, malaise, somnolence, tremor, insomnia, confusion, depression, anxiety, hallucinations, aggressive reaction, vertigo, agitation, nervousness, delusion, paranoid reaction, pain.

CV: hypertension, chest pain, peripheral edema, *bradycardia.*

EENT: rhinitis, pharyngitis.

GI: nausea, vomiting, diarrhea, anorexia, abdominal pain, dyspepsia, constipation, flatulence, eructation.

GU: UTI, incontinence.

Metabolic: weight loss.

Musculoskeletal: back pain, arthralgia, bone fracture.

Respiratory: upper respiratory tract infection, cough, bronchitis.

Skin: increased sweating, rash.

Other: accidental trauma, flulike symptoms.

INTERACTIONS

Drug-drug. *Anticholinergics:* May decrease effectiveness of anticholinergic. Monitor patient for expected therapeutic effects.

Bethanechol, succinylcholine, other neuromuscular-blocking drugs or cholinergic antagonists: May have synergistic effect. Monitor patient closely.

NSAIDs: May increase gastric acid secretions. Monitor patient for symptoms of active or occult GI bleeding.

Drug-lifestyle. *Smoking:* May increase drug clearance. Discourage smoking.

EFFECTS ON LAB TEST RESULTS

None reported.

CONTRAINDICATIONS & CAUTIONS

• Contraindicated in patients hypersensitive to drug, other carbamate derivatives, or other components of the drug.

• Use cautiously in patients with history of CV disease, GI bleeding, seizure disorder, genitourinary conditions, asthma, or obstructive pulmonary disease.

⚠ *Overdose S&S:* Nausea, vomiting, excessive salivation, sweating, bradycardia, hypotension, respiratory depression, syncope, seizures, muscle weakness.

NURSING CONSIDERATIONS

• Expect significant GI adverse effects (such as nausea, vomiting, anorexia, and weight loss). These effects are less common during maintenance doses.

• Monitor patient for evidence of active or occult GI bleeding.

• Dramatic memory improvement is unlikely. As disease progresses, the benefits of drug may decline.

• Monitor patient for severe nausea, vomiting, and diarrhea, which may lead to dehydration and weight loss.

• Carefully monitor patient with a history of GI bleeding, NSAID use, arrhythmias, seizures, or pulmonary conditions for adverse effects.

• If adverse reactions, such as diarrhea, loss of appetite, nausea, or vomiting, occur with transdermal patch, stop use for several days, then restart at the same or lower dose. If treatment is interrupted for more than several days, restart patch at the lowest dose and retitrate.

• Patients weighing less than 50 kg (110 lb) may experience more adverse reactions when using the transdermal patch.

• Application-site reactions may occur with the transdermal patch. Discontinue treatment if application-site reaction spreads

R

beyond the patch size, if there's evidence of a more intense local reaction (increasing erythema, edema, papules, vesicles), and if symptoms don't significantly improve within 48 hours after patch removal.

• When switching from an oral form to the transdermal patch, patients on a total daily dose of less than 6 mg can be switched to 4.6 mg/24 hours. Patients taking 6 to 12 mg orally can switch to the 9.5 mg/24 hour patch. The patch should be applied on the day after the last oral dose.

PATIENT TEACHING

• Tell caregiver to give drug with food in the morning and evening.

• Advise patient that memory improvement may be subtle and that drug more likely slows future memory loss.

• Tell patient to report nausea, vomiting, or diarrhea.

• Tell patient to consult prescriber before using OTC drugs.

• Tell patient to apply patch once daily to clean, dry, hairless skin in a place not rubbed by tight clothing.

• Teach patient that the recommended sites for patch placement include the upper or lower back, upper arm, or chest.

• Tell patient to change the site daily and not to use the same site within 14 days.

• Tell patient to press the patch firmly into place until the edges stick well.

rizatriptan benzoate
rih-zah-TRIP-tan

Maxalt, Maxalt-MLT

Therapeutic class: Antimigraine drugs
Pharmacologic class: Serotonin 5-HT$_1$ receptor agonists
Pregnancy risk category: C

AVAILABLE FORMS
Tablets: 5 mg, 10 mg
Tablets (orally disintegrating): 5 mg, 10 mg

INDICATIONS & DOSAGES
➤ **Acute migraine headaches with or without aura**
Adults: Initially, 5 or 10 mg P.O. If first dose is ineffective, may give another dose at least

2 hours after first dose; maximum, 30 mg in 24 hours. For patients receiving propranolol, 5 mg P.O.; maximum, 15 mg in 24 hours.
Children ages 6 to 17 weighing less than 40 kg (88 lb): 5 mg P.O. daily; maximum of 5 mg in 24 hours. Don't administer concomitantly with propranolol.
Children ages 6 to 17 weighing 40 kg or more: 10 mg P.O. daily; maximum, 10 mg in 24 hours.
Adjust-a-dose: For children weighing 40 kg or more taking propranolol, only a single 5-mg dose of rizatriptan is recommended; maximum of 5 mg in a 24 hours.

ADMINISTRATION
P.O.
• Give drug with or without food, although food may delay onset of drug action.

• Give tablet with plenty of fluid.

• Give orally disintegrating tablet (ODT) with or without fluid.

• For Maxalt-MLT, remove blister pack from pouch and remove drug from blister pack immediately before use. Tablet shouldn't be popped out of blister pack; carefully peel away package with dry hands, place tablet on patient's tongue, and let tablet dissolve until it can be swallowed with saliva.

ACTION
May act as an agonist at serotonin receptors on extracerebral intracranial blood vessels, which constricts the affected vessels, inhibits neuropeptide release, and reduces pain transmission in the trigeminal pathways.

Route	Onset	Peak	Duration
P.O.	Unknown	60–90 min	Unknown

Half-life: 2 to 3 hours.

ADVERSE REACTIONS
CNS: dizziness, headache, somnolence, paresthesia, asthenia, fatigue, decreased mental acuity, euphoria, tremor, pain.
CV: *coronary artery vasospasm; transient myocardial ischemia; MI; ventricular tachycardia; ventricular fibrillation;* chest pain, pressure, or heaviness; palpitations; flushing.
EENT: neck, throat, and jaw pain.
GI: dry mouth, nausea, diarrhea, vomiting.

Reactions in bold italics are *life-threatening*. Interactions may have a *rapid onset* or a *delayed onset*.

Respiratory: dyspnea.
Other: hot flashes, warm or cold feelings.

INTERACTIONS
Drug-drug. *Ergot-containing or ergot-type drugs (dihydroergotamine, methysergide), other 5-HT₁ agonists:* May prolong vasospastic reactions. Avoid using within 24 hours of rizatriptan.
MAO inhibitors: May increase rizatriptan level. Avoid using within 2 weeks of MAO inhibitor.
Propranolol: May increase rizatriptan level. Reduce rizatriptan dose to 5 mg.
SSRIs (fluoxetine, fluvoxamine, paroxetine, sertraline): May cause weakness, hyperreflexia, and incoordination. Monitor patient.

EFFECTS ON LAB TEST RESULTS
None reported.

CONTRAINDICATIONS & CAUTIONS
• Contraindicated in patients hypersensitive to drug or its components and in those with a history or symptoms of ischemic heart disease, coronary artery vasospasm (Prinzmetal variant angina), or other significant underlying CV disease.
• Contraindicated in patients with uncontrolled hypertension; within 24 hours of another 5-HT₁ agonist, drug containing ergotamine, or ergot-type drug, such as dihydroergotamine or methysergide; or within 2 weeks of MAO inhibitor.
• Contraindicated in patients with hemiplegic or basilar migraine.
• Use cautiously in patients with risk factors for coronary artery disease (CAD), such as hypertension, hypercholesterolemia, smoking, obesity, diabetes, strong family history of CAD, postmenopausal women, or men older than age 40, unless patient is free from cardiac disease. Monitor patient closely after first dose.
• Use cautiously in patients with hepatic or renal impairment.
• Safety and effectiveness in children younger than age 6 are unknown.
• Safety of treating more than four headaches in 30 days hasn't been established.

⚠ *Overdose S&S:* Dizziness, somnolence, syncope, bradycardia, vomiting, third-degree AV block, hypertension, other more serious CV symptoms.

NURSING CONSIDERATIONS
• Assess CV status in patients who develop risk factors for CAD during treatment.
• Use drug only when patient has a clear diagnosis of migraine.
• Don't use drug to prevent migraines or to treat hemiplegic or basilar migraine or cluster headaches.
ℹ Alert: Combining drug with an SSRI or an SSNRI may cause serotonin syndrome. Symptoms include restlessness, hallucinations, loss of coordination, fast heartbeat, rapid changes in blood pressure, increased body temperature, hyperreflexia, nausea, vomiting, and diarrhea. Serotonin syndrome is more likely to occur when starting or increasing the dose of this drug, the SSRI, or the SSNRI.
• The ODTs contain phenylalanine.

PATIENT TEACHING
• Inform patient that drug doesn't prevent migraine headache.
• For Maxalt-MLT, tell patient to remove blister pack from pouch and remove drug from blister pack immediately before use. Tablet shouldn't be popped out of blister pack; tell patient to carefully peel away package with dry hands, place tablet on tongue, and allow tablet to dissolve. Tablet is then swallowed with saliva. No water is needed or recommended. Tell patient that ODT doesn't relieve headache more quickly.
• Instruct patient to take regular tablets with plenty of fluid.
• Advise patient that, if headache returns after first dose, he may take a second dose at least 2 hours after the first dose. Warn against taking more than 30 mg in a 24-hour period.
• Inform patient that drug may cause sleepiness and dizziness, and warn him to avoid hazardous activities until effects are known.
• Tell patient that food may delay onset of drug action.
• Advise patient to notify prescriber about suspected or known pregnancy.

R

● Instruct patient not to breast-feed during therapy because effects on the infant are unknown.
● Warn patients with phenylketonuria that ODTs contain phenylalanine.

roflumilast
roe-FLUE-mi-last

Daliresp

Therapeutic class: Miscellaneous respiratory drugs
Pharmacologic class: Selective phosphodiesterase inhibitors
Pregnancy risk category: C

AVAILABLE FORMS
Tablets: 500 mcg

INDICATIONS & DOSAGES
➤ To reduce risk of COPD exacerbations in patients with severe COPD associated with chronic bronchitis and a history of exacerbations
Adults: 500 mcg P.O. daily.

ADMINISTRATION
P.O.
● Give drug without regard to food.

ACTION
Selectively inhibits phosphodiesterase-4 (PDE$_4$), which is a cAMP-metabolizing enzyme in the lung tissue. Inhibition of PDE$_4$ leads to accumulation of intracellular cAMP. Effects of drug are thought to be related to the increased intracellular cAMP in lung cells.

Route	Onset	Peak	Duration
P.O.	Unknown	1–2 hr	Unknown

Half-life: 17 hours.

ADVERSE REACTIONS
CNS: headache, insomnia, dizziness, tremor, anxiety, depression.
EENT: rhinitis, sinusitis.
GI: diarrhea, nausea, decreased appetite, abdominal pain, dyspepsia, gastritis, vomiting.
GU: UTI.

Metabolic: weight loss.
Musculoskeletal: back pain, muscle spasms.
Other: influenza.

INTERACTIONS
Drugs that induce CYP450 enzymes (carbamazepine, phenobarbital, phenytoin, rifampin): May decrease the effectiveness of roflumilast. Avoid use together.
Drugs that inhibit CYP450 enzymes (cimetidine, enoxacin, erythromycin, fluvoxamine, ketoconazole), hormonal contraceptives containing gestodene and ethinyl estradiol: May increase roflumilast concentration and risk of adverse reactions. Use together cautiously.

EFFECTS ON LAB TEST RESULTS
None reported.

CONTRAINDICATIONS & CAUTIONS
● Contraindicated in patients hypersensitive to drug or its components, in those with moderate to severe hepatic impairment (Child-Pugh class B or C), and in breast-feeding women.
● Use cautiously in patients with history of depression or suicidal thoughts and behaviors.
● Use drug in pregnant women only if the potential benefit to the mother outweighs the potential risk to the fetus.

NURSING CONSIDERATIONS
● Drug isn't a bronchodilator and isn't indicated for the relief of acute bronchospasm.
● Monitor patients for signs and symptoms of psychiatric adverse events, including insomnia, anxiety, depression, suicidal ideation, and suicide attempts. If events occur, evaluate the risks versus benefits of continuing drug.
● Monitor weight regularly; if unexplained or significant weight loss occurs, evaluate cause and consider stopping drug.

PATIENT TEACHING
● Educate patient that drug isn't a bronchodilator and isn't to be used for the relief of acute bronchospasm.

• Advise patient, family, and caregivers to watch for signs and symptoms of psychiatric adverse events, including insomnia, anxiety, depression, suicidal ideation, and suicide attempts, and to report any occurrences to the health care provider.

• Tell patient to report unexplained or significant weight loss.

rOPINIRole hydrochloride
row-PIN-ah-roll

Requip, Requip XL

Therapeutic class: Antiparkinsonians
Pharmacologic class: Nonergot dopamine agonists
Pregnancy risk category: C

AVAILABLE FORMS
Tablets: 0.25 mg, 0.5 mg, 1 mg, 2 mg, 3 mg, 4 mg, 5 mg
Tablets (extended-release): 2 mg, 4 mg, 6 mg, 8 mg, 12 mg

INDICATIONS & DOSAGES
➤ **Idiopathic Parkinson disease**
Adults: Initially, 0.25 mg P.O., t.i.d. Increase dose by 0.25 mg t.i.d. at weekly intervals for 4 weeks. After week 4, daily dosage may be increased by 1.5 mg/day on a weekly basis up to a dose of 9 mg/day, and then by up to 3 mg/day weekly to a total dose of 24 mg/day. For extended-release form, starting dosage is 2 mg P.O. once daily for 1 to 2 weeks. May increase by 2 mg/day at 1-week or longer intervals. Maximum dosage is 24 mg/day. To switch from immediate-release to extended-release tablets, use the following table:

Immediate-release total daily dosage	Extended-release total daily dosage
0.75 to 2.25 mg	2 mg
3 to 4.5 mg	4 mg
6 mg	6 mg
7.5 to 9 mg	8 mg
12 mg	12 mg
15 to 18 mg	16 mg
21 mg	20 mg
24 mg	24 mg

Elderly patients: Adjust dosages individually, according to patient response; clearance may be reduced in these patients.
➤ **Moderate to severe restless legs syndrome (immediate-release)**
Adults: Initially, 0.25 mg P.O. 1 to 3 hours before bedtime. May increase dose as needed and tolerated after 2 days to 0.5 mg, then to 1 mg by the end of the first week. May further increase dose as needed and tolerated as follows: week 2, give 1 mg once daily. Week 3, give 1.5 mg once daily. Week 4, give 2 mg once daily. Week 5, give 2.5 mg once daily. Week 6, give 3 mg once daily. And week 7, give 4 mg once daily. All doses should be taken 1 to 2 hours before bedtime.

ADMINISTRATION
P.O.
• Give drug with food if nausea occurs.

ACTION
Thought to stimulate dopamine (D2) receptors.

Route	Onset	Peak	Duration
P.O.	Unknown	1–2 hr	6 hr

Half-life: 6 hours.

ADVERSE REACTIONS
Early Parkinson disease (without levodopa)
CNS: dizziness, fatigue, somnolence, syncope, hallucinations, aggravated Parkinson disease, headache, confusion, hyperkinesia, hypoesthesia, vertigo, amnesia, impaired concentration, malaise, asthenia, pain.
CV: orthostatic hypotension, orthostatic symptoms, hypertension, edema, chest pain, extrasystoles, atrial fibrillation, palpitations, tachycardia, flushing.
EENT: pharyngitis, abnormal vision, eye abnormality, xerophthalmia, rhinitis, sinusitis.
GI: nausea, vomiting, dyspepsia, dry mouth, flatulence, abdominal pain, anorexia, constipation.
GU: UTI, impotence.
Respiratory: bronchitis, dyspnea, yawning.
Other: viral infection, increased sweating, peripheral ischemia.

R

Advanced Parkinson disease (with levodopa)
CNS: dizziness, somnolence, headache, hallucinations, aggravated parkinsonism, insomnia, abnormal dreaming, confusion, tremor, anxiety, nervousness, amnesia, paresis, paresthesia, syncope, pain.
CV: hypotension.
EENT: diplopia.
GI: nausea, abdominal pain, dry mouth, vomiting, constipation, diarrhea, dysphagia, flatulence, increased saliva.
GU: UTI, pyuria, urinary incontinence.
Hematologic: anemia.
Metabolic: weight decrease, suppressed prolactin.
Musculoskeletal: dyskinesia, arthralgia, arthritis, hypokinesia.
Respiratory: upper respiratory tract infection, dyspnea.
Skin: increased sweating.
Other: falls, injury, viral infection.
Restless legs syndrome
CNS: fatigue, somnolence, dizziness, vertigo, paresthesia.
CV: peripheral edema.
EENT: nasopharyngitis, nasal congestion.
GI: nausea, vomiting, diarrhea, dyspepsia, dry mouth.
Musculoskeletal: arthralgia, muscle cramps, extremity pain.
Respiratory: cough.
Skin: increased sweating.
Other: influenza.

INTERACTIONS
Drug-drug. *Cimetidine, ciprofloxacin, fluvoxamine, inhibitors or substrates of CYP1A2, ritonavir:* May alter ropinirole clearance. Adjust ropinirole dose if other drugs are started or stopped during treatment.
CNS depressants: May increase CNS effects. Use together cautiously.
Dopamine antagonists (neuroleptics), metoclopramide: May decrease ropinirole effects. Avoid using together.
Estrogens: May decrease ropinirole clearance. Adjust ropinirole dosage if estrogen therapy is started or stopped during treatment.

Warfarin: May increase anticoagulation. Monitor coagulation parameters and adjust warfarin dosage as needed.
Drug-lifestyle. *Alcohol use:* May increase sedative effect. Discourage use together.
Smoking: May increase drug clearance. Discourage use together.

EFFECTS ON LAB TEST RESULTS
● May increase BUN and alkaline phosphatase levels. May decrease hemoglobin level.

CONTRAINDICATIONS & CAUTIONS
● Contraindicated in patients hypersensitive to drug.
● Use cautiously in patients with severe hepatic or renal impairment.
⚠ **Overdose S&S:** Nausea, dizziness, visual hallucinations, hyperhidrosis, claustrophobia, chorea, palpitations, asthenia, nightmares, vomiting, increased coughing, fatigue, syncope, vasovagal syncope, dyskinesia, agitation, chest pain, orthostatic hypotension, somnolence, confusion.

NURSING CONSIDERATIONS
◑ **Alert:** Monitor patient carefully for orthostatic hypotension, especially during dosage increases.
● Drug may potentiate the adverse effects of levodopa and may cause or worsen dyskinesia. Dosage may be decreased.
● Although not reported with ropinirole, other adverse reactions reported with dopaminergic therapy include hyperpyrexia, fibrotic complications, and confusion, which may occur with rapid dosage reduction or withdrawal of drug.
● Patient may have syncope, with or without bradycardia. Monitor patient carefully, especially for 4 weeks after start of therapy and with dosage increases.
● When used for Parkinson disease, withdraw drug gradually over 7 days.
● When used for restless legs syndrome, stop drug without tapering.
● Drug can cause somnolence and sudden episodes of falling asleep. Continually reassess patient for drowsiness or sleepiness and for factors that could contribute to sleepiness.

Reactions in bold italics are *life-threatening*. Interactions may have a *rapid onset* or a *delayed onset*.

● **Look alike–sound alike:** Don't confuse ropinirole with risperidone.

PATIENT TEACHING

● Advise patient to take drug with food if nausea occurs.

● Inform patient (especially elderly patient) that hallucinations can occur.

● Instruct patient not to rise rapidly after sitting or lying down because of risk of dizziness, which may occur more frequently early in therapy or when dosage increases.

● Sleepiness and sudden episodes of falling asleep can occur, sometimes without warning. Warn patient to minimize hazardous activities until CNS effects of drug are known.

● Advise patient to avoid alcohol.

● Tell woman to notify prescriber about planned, suspected, or known pregnancy; also tell her to inform prescriber if she's breast-feeding.

SAFETY ALERT!

rosiglitazone maleate
roh-zee-GLIT-ah-zohn

Avandia⚘

Therapeutic class: Antidiabetics
Pharmacologic class: Thiazolidinediones
Pregnancy risk category: C

AVAILABLE FORMS
Tablets: 2 mg, 4 mg, 8 mg

INDICATIONS & DOSAGES

➤ **Type 2 diabetes mellitus, alone or with a sulfonylurea or metformin, in patients currently benefiting from therapy or in patients unable to achieve glucose control with other medications**
Adults: Initially, 4 mg P.O. daily in the morning or in two divided doses (morning and evening). Increase to 8 mg P.O. daily or in two divided doses if fasting glucose level doesn't improve after 8 to 12 weeks of treatment.

➤ **Polycystic ovary syndrome ◆**
Adults: 2 to 8 mg P.O. daily in one to two divided doses as monotherapy or in combination therapy.

ADMINISTRATION
P.O.
❂ *Alert:* Check liver enzyme levels before therapy starts. Don't use drug in patients with increased baseline liver enzyme levels.
● Give drug without regard for food.

ACTION
Lowers glucose level by improving insulin sensitivity.

Route	Onset	Peak	Duration
P.O.	Unknown	1 hr	Unknown

Half-life: 3 to 4 hours.

ADVERSE REACTIONS
CNS: headache, fatigue.
CV: edema, *worsening heart failure.*
EENT: sinusitis.
GI: diarrhea.
Hematologic: anemia.
Metabolic: hyperglycemia, weight gain.
Musculoskeletal: back pain, fractures.
Respiratory: upper respiratory tract infection.
Other: accidental injury.

INTERACTIONS
Drug-drug. *Fluvoxamine, gemfibrozil, ketoconazole, trimethoprim:* May increase rosiglitazone levels, increasing hypoglycemic effects and adverse reactions. Monitor glucose; dosage adjustment may be necessary.
Insulin: May increase incidence of edema and risk of MI. Use together isn't recommended.
Rifampin: May decrease rosiglitazone levels. Monitor glucose; dosage adjustment may be necessary.

EFFECTS ON LAB TEST RESULTS
● May increase glucose, HDL, LDL, total cholesterol, and ALT levels.
● May decrease hemoglobin level and hematocrit.

R

CONTRAINDICATIONS & CAUTIONS

• Don't use for treatment of diabetic ke-toacidosis or type 1 diabetes mellitus.
• Administration with insulin isn't recommended.
• Contraindicated in patients hypersensitive to drug or its components.

Black Box Warning Contraindicated in patients with symptomatic heart failure or those with established New York Heart Association class III or IV heart failure. ■

• Contraindicated in patients with active liver disease, increased baseline liver enzyme levels (ALT level greater than 2½ times upper limit of normal), type 1 diabetes, or diabetic ketoacidosis and in those who experienced jaundice while taking troglitazone.
• Don't start drug in patients experiencing acute coronary syndrome.
• Use cautiously in patients with edema or heart failure.

NURSING CONSIDERATIONS

◐ **Alert:** Monitor liver enzyme levels every 2 months for first 12 months and periodically thereafter. If ALT level becomes elevated, recheck as soon as possible. Stop drug if levels remain elevated.

◐ **Alert:** Drug can cause fluid retention leading to or worsening heart failure. Monitor patients for signs and symptoms of heart failure. Notify prescriber if any deterioration in cardiac status occurs.

• Management of type 2 diabetes should include diet control. Because caloric restriction, weight loss, and exercise help improve insulin sensitivity and effectiveness of drug therapy, these measures are essential to proper diabetes treatment.
• Check glucose and glycosylated hemoglobin levels periodically to monitor therapeutic response to drug.
• Hemoglobin level and hematocrit may drop during therapy, usually during first 4 to 8 weeks. Increases in total cholesterol, LDL, and HDL levels and decreases in free fatty acid level also may occur.
• For patients inadequately controlled with a maximum dose of a sulfonylurea or met-formin, add rosiglitazone to, rather than

substituting it for, the sulfonylurea or met-formin.
• Drug may increase the incidence of bone fractures (most common in the arm, hand, and foot) in women.
• **Look alike–sound alike:** Don't confuse rosiglitazone with pioglitazone. Don't confuse Avandia with Prandin.

PATIENT TEACHING

• Advise patient that drug can be taken with or without food.
• Notify patient that blood will be tested to check liver function before therapy starts, every 2 months for first 12 months, and then periodically thereafter.
• Tell patient to immediately notify pre-scriber about unexplained signs and symptoms, such as nausea, vomiting, abdominal pain, fatigue, anorexia, or dark urine; these may indicate liver problems.
• Tell patient to immediately notify pre-scriber of changes in vision as this may indicate macular edema.
• Warn patient to contact his health care provider about signs or symptoms of heart failure (unusually rapid increase in weight or swelling, shortness of breath).
• Recommend use of contraceptives to premenopausal, anovulatory women with insulin resistance because ovulation may resume with therapy.
• Advise patient that management of diabetes includes diet control, calorie re-striction, weight loss, and exercise, and that these measures improve effectiveness of drug therapy.
• Instruct patient to monitor glucose level carefully and tell him what to do when he's ill, undergoing surgery, or under added stress.

Reactions in bold italics are *life-threatening*. Interactions may have a *rapid onset* or a *delayed onset*.

rosuvastatin calcium
row-SUE-va-sta-tin

Crestor⟋

Therapeutic class: Antilipemics
Pharmacologic class: HMG-CoA
reductase inhibitors
Pregnancy risk category: X

AVAILABLE FORMS
Tablets: 5 mg, 10 mg, 20 mg, 40 mg

INDICATIONS & DOSAGES
Adjust-a-dose (for all indications): If CrCl
is less than 30 mL/minute, initially, 5 mg
once daily; don't exceed 10 mg once daily.
For Asian patients, initial dose is 5 mg.
For patients also taking cyclosporine, limit
rosuvastatin dose to 5 mg once daily. For
patients taking combination of lopinavir or
gemfibrozil and ritonavir, limit rosuvastatin
dose to 10 mg once daily.
➤ **Risk reduction in patients without
clinical evidence of coronary artery
disease (CAD) but with multiple risk
factors**
Adults: Initially, 10 mg P.O. once daily;
5 mg P.O. once daily in patients needing
less aggressive LDL cholesterol reduction.
For aggressive lipid reduction (LDL greater
than 190 mg/dL) initially, 20 mg P.O. once
daily. Increase as needed to maximum of
40 mg P.O. daily. Dosage may be titrated
every 2 to 4 weeks, based on lipid
levels.
➤ **Children with heterozygous familial
hypercholesterolemia after failing an
adequate trial of diet therapy**
Children ages 10 to 17: 5 to 20 mg P.O.
daily. Dosage may be titrated every 4 weeks
or more, based on lipid levels.
➤ **Adjunct to diet to reduce LDL cholesterol, total cholesterol, apolipoprotein B,
non-HDL cholesterol, and triglyceride
(TG) levels and to increase HDL cholesterol level in patients with primary hypercholesterolemia (heterozygous familial
and nonfamilial) and mixed dyslipidemia (Fredrickson types IIa and IIb);
adjunct to diet to treat elevated TG level**

**(Fredrickson type IV); adjunct to diet to
treat primary dysbetalipoproteinemia**
Adults: Initially, 10 mg P.O. once daily;
5 mg P.O. once daily in patients needing
less aggressive LDL cholesterol reduction or those predisposed to myopathy. For
aggressive lipid lowering when LDL is
greater than 190 mg/dL, initially, 20 mg
P.O. once daily. Increase as needed to maximum of 40 mg P.O. daily. Dosage may be
titrated every 2 to 4 weeks, based on lipid
levels.
➤ **Adjunct to diet to slow atherosclerosis
progression in patients with elevated
cholesterol**
Adults: Initially, 10 mg P.O. daily. Increase
as needed every 2 to 4 weeks based on lipid
levels, to maximum of 40 mg daily.
➤ **Adjunct to lipid-lowering therapies; to
reduce LDL cholesterol, apolipoprotein
B, and total cholesterol levels in homozygous familial hypercholesterolemia**
Adults: Initially, 20 mg P.O. once daily.
Maximum, 40 mg once daily.

ADMINISTRATION
P.O.
● Give drug without regard for meals.
● Wait 2 hours after giving dose to give
aluminum- or magnesium-containing
antacid.

ACTION
Inhibits HMG-CoA reductase, increases
LDL receptors on liver cells, and inhibits
hepatic synthesis of very–low-density
lipoprotein.

Route	Onset	Peak	Duration
P.O.	Unknown	3–5 hr	Unknown

Half-life: About 19 hours.

ADVERSE REACTIONS
CNS: asthenia, dizziness, headache,
insomnia.
EENT: pharyngitis, rhinitis, sinusitis.
GI: abdominal pain, constipation, diarrhea,
dyspepsia, nausea, vomiting.
Hematologic: anemia, ecchymosis.
Metabolic: diabetes mellitus.
Musculoskeletal: arthralgia, myalgia, neck
pain.

R

Skin: pruritus, rash.
Other: accidental injury, flulike syndrome, infection.

INTERACTIONS

Drug-drug. *Antacids:* May decrease rosuvastatin level. Give antacids at least 2 hours after rosuvastatin.
Atazanavir, atazanavir–ritonavir, lopinavir–ritonavir: May increase rosuvastatin level and risk of myopathy and rhabdomyolysis. Rosuvastatin dosage shouldn't exceed 10 mg daily.
Bile acid sequestrants (cholestyramine, colestipol): May decrease GI absorption of rosuvastatin. Separate doses by at least 4 hours.
Colchicine: May increase risk of myopathy and rhabdomyolysis. Avoid use together. If use together is necessary, monitor patient for signs and symptoms of myopathy and elevated CK level during use and after dosage increases.
Cyclosporine: May increase rosuvastatin level and risk of myopathy or rhabdomyolysis. Don't exceed 5 mg of rosuvastatin daily. Watch for evidence of toxicity.
Daptomycin: May increase risk of rhabdomyolysis. Withhold rosuvastatin temporarily or monitor patient and CK level closely during coadministration.
Eltrombopag: May increase rosuvastatin level and risk of toxicity. Consider reducing rosuvastatin dosage.
Fenofibrate, gemfibrozil: May increase rosuvastatin level and risk of myopathy or rhabdomyolysis. Don't exceed 10 mg of rosuvastatin once daily. Watch for evidence of toxicity.
Hormonal contraceptives: May increase ethinyl estradiol and norgestrel levels. Watch for adverse effects.
Niacin: May increase risk of myopathy or rhabdomyolysis. Decrease rosuvastatin dosage and monitor patient closely.
Warfarin: May increase INR and risk of bleeding. Monitor INR, and watch for evidence of increased bleeding.
Drug-lifestyle. *Alcohol use:* May increase risk of hepatotoxicity. Discourage use together.

EFFECTS ON LAB TEST RESULTS
● May increase glycosylated hemoglobin (HbA_{1c}), fasting blood sugar, CK, transaminase, glucose, glutamyl transpeptidase, alkaline phosphatase, and bilirubin levels.
● May decrease hemoglobin level and hematocrit.
● May cause thyroid function abnormalities, dipstick-positive proteinuria, and microscopic hematuria.

CONTRAINDICATIONS & CAUTIONS
● Contraindicated in patients hypersensitive to rosuvastatin or its components, pregnant or breast-feeding patients, patients with active liver disease, and those with unexplained persistently increased transaminase levels.
● Use cautiously in patients who drink substantial amounts of alcohol or have a history of liver disease and in those at increased risk for myopathies, such as those with renal impairment, advanced age, or hypothyroidism.
● Use cautiously in Asian patients because they have a greater risk of elevated drug levels.
● Rare reports of cognitive impairment (memory loss, forgetfulness, amnesia, memory impairment, confusion) have been associated with statin use. These reported symptoms are generally not serious and are reversible upon statin discontinuation, with variable times to symptom onset (1 day to years) and symptom resolution (median of 3 weeks).
⚠ *Overdose S&S:* Unexplained muscle pain, tenderness, or weakness, especially with malaise or fever.

NURSING CONSIDERATIONS
● Before therapy starts, assess patient for underlying causes of hypercholesterolemia, including poorly controlled diabetes, hypothyroidism, nephrotic syndrome, dyslipoproteinemias, obstructive liver disease, drug interaction, and alcoholism.
● Before therapy starts, advise patient to control hypercholesterolemia with diet, exercise, and weight reduction.
● Interrupt statin therapy if patient shows signs or symptoms of serious liver injury,

---

Reactions in bold italics are *life-threatening*. Interactions may have a *rapid onset* or a *delayed onset*.

hyperbilirubinemia, or jaundice. Don't restart drug if another cause can't be found.

◑ Alert: Rarely, rhabdomyolysis with acute renal failure has developed in patients taking drugs in this class, including rosuvastatin.

• Patients who are age 65 or older, have hypothyroidism, or have renal insufficiency may be at a greater risk for developing myopathy while receiving a statin.

• Notify prescriber if CK level becomes markedly elevated or myopathy is suspected, or if routine urinalysis shows persistent proteinuria and patient is taking 40 mg daily.

• Withhold drug temporarily if patient becomes predisposed to myopathy or rhabdomyolysis because of sepsis, hypotension, major surgery, trauma, uncontrolled seizures, or severe metabolic, endocrine, or electrolyte disorders.

PATIENT TEACHING

• Instruct patient to take drug exactly as prescribed.

• Teach patient about diet, exercise, and weight control.

• Inform patient that rare instances of memory loss and confusion have occurred with statin use. These reported events were generally not serious and resolved when drug was discontinued.

• Tell patient that drug may increase blood sugar level but that the CV benefits are thought to outweigh the slight increase in risk.

• Tell patient to immediately report unexplained muscle pain, tenderness, or weakness (especially if accompanied by malaise or fever) and loss of appetite, upper abdominal pain, dark-colored urine, or yellowing of skin or eyes.

• Instruct patient to take drug at least 2 hours before taking aluminum- or magnesium-containing antacids.

◑ Alert: Tell female patient to stop drug and notify prescriber immediately if she is or may be pregnant or if she's breast-feeding.

SAFETY ALERT!

ruxolitinib phosphate
RUX-oh-LI-ti-nib

Jakafi

Therapeutic class: Antineoplastics
Pharmacologic class: Janus-associated kinase inhibitors
Pregnancy risk category: C

AVAILABLE FORMS
Tablets: 5 mg, 10 mg, 15 mg, 20 mg, 25 mg

INDICATIONS & DOSAGES
➤ **Treatment of patients with intermediate or high-risk myelofibrosis, including primary myelofibrosis, post–polycythemia vera myelofibrosis, and post–essential thrombocythemia myelofibrosis**
Adults: Initially, 20 mg P.O. b.i.d. if platelet count is greater than 200×10^9/L, 15 mg P.O. b.i.d. if platelet count is 100 to 200×10^9/L, or 5 mg P.O. b.i.d. if platelet count is 50 to less than 100×10^9/L. May increase in 5-mg increments b.i.d. to a maximum of 25 mg b.i.d. Don't increase during the first 4 weeks of therapy and not more frequently than every 2 weeks. Consider dosage increases in patients who meet all of the following conditions: failure to achieve either a 50% reduction from pretreatment baseline in palpable spleen length or a 35% reduction in spleen volume as measured by computed tomography or magnetic resonance imaging; platelet count greater than 125×10^9/L at 4 weeks and platelet count never below 100×10^9/L; and ANC greater than 0.75 $\times 10^9$/L. Long-term maintenance at a 5-mg b.i.d. dosage hasn't shown response; limit continued use at this dosage to patients in whom benefits outweigh risks. Discontinue drug after 6 months if there is no spleen reduction or symptom improvement. If drug needs to be stopped for any reason except thrombocytopenia, taper gradually by 5 mg b.i.d. each week.

Adjust-a-dose: To avoid thrombocytopenia, reduce dosage if platelet count begins to fall. If platelet count is 100 to less than

---

125×10^9/L and current dosage is 25 mg b.i.d., decrease to 20 mg b.i.d.; if current dosage is 20 mg b.i.d., decrease to 15 mg b.i.d. If platelet count is 75 to less than 100 $\times 10^9$/L and current dosage is 15 to 25 mg b.i.d., decrease to 10 mg b.i.d. If platelet count is 50 to less than 75×10^9/L and current dosage is 10 to 25 mg b.i.d., decrease to 5 mg b.i.d. If platelet count is less than 50×10^9/L, withhold drug. When platelet count begins to recover, refer to manufacturer's dosing instructions to restart drug. For moderate to severe renal impairment (CrCl of 15 to 59 mL/minute) and platelet count between 100 and 150×10^9/L, initial dose is 10 mg b.i.d. For patients with ESRD on dialysis and with platelet count between 100 and 200×10^9/L, initial dose is 15 mg b.i.d. For patients with ESRD on dialysis and with platelet count greater than 200×10^9/L, initial dose is 20 mg b.i.d. Give subsequent doses on dialysis days after each dialysis session. For patients with hepatic impairment and platelet count between 100 and 150×10^9/L, initial dose is 10 mg b.i.d.

ADMINISTRATION
P.O.
● May give without regard to food.
● To give through a nasogastric (NG) tube (8 French or greater), place one tablet in approximately 40 mL water and stir for 10 minutes to dissolve. Give within 6 hours of preparing the suspension, using an appropriate syringe. Rinse NG tube with 75 mL water.

ACTION
Inhibits signaling of cytokines and growth factors important for hematopoiesis and immune functions. Prevents splenomegaly by decreasing circulating inflammatory cytokines.

Route	Onset	Peak	Duration
P.O.	Rapid	1–2 hr	10 hr

Half-life: 3 hours.

ADVERSE REACTIONS
CNS: dizziness, headache.
GU: UTI.

GI: flatulence.
Hematologic: neutropenia, thrombocytopenia, anemia.
Metabolic: hypercholesterolemia, weight gain.
Skin: bruising.
Other: serious bacterial, mycobacterial, fungal, or viral infections.

INTERACTIONS
Drug-drug. *CYP3A4 inducers (such as rifampin):* May decrease ruxolitinib level. No initial dosage adjustment is necessary. Monitor patients closely and titrate dosage if necessary.
Strong CYP3A4 inhibitors (boceprevir, clarithromycin, conivaptan, infinavir, itraconazole, ketoconazole, lopinavir– ritonavir, mibefradil, nefazodone, nelfinavir, posaconazole, ritonavir, saquinavir, telaprevir, telithromycin, voriconazole): May increase ruxolitinib level. If patient is taking a strong CYP3A4 inhibitor and platelet count is 100×10^9/L or more, start ruxolitinib at 10 mg b.i.d. If patient is taking a strong CYP3A4 inhibitor and platelet count is less than 100×10^9/L, don't give drug.
Drug-food. *Grapefruit juice:* May increase ruxolitinib level. Discourage use together.

EFFECTS ON LAB TEST RESULTS
● May increase cholesterol, AST, and ALT levels.
● May decrease platelet and neutrophil counts.
● May decrease hemoglobin level.

CONTRAINDICATIONS & CAUTIONS
● Contraindicated in patients hypersensitive to drug and in those with ESRD not requiring dialysis, moderate to severe renal failure and platelet count less than 100×10^9/L, or hepatic impairment with platelet count less than 100×10^9/L.
● Use cautiously in patients with thrombocytopenia, anemia, or neutropenia, and in those at risk for developing serious bacterial, mycobacterial, fungal, or viral infections (such as herpes zoster).
● Use in pregnant women only if benefit outweighs risk to fetus.

Reactions in bold italics are *life-threatening*. Interactions may have a *rapid onset* or a *delayed onset*.

• It's unknown if drug appears in breast milk. A decision should be made whether patient should discontinue drug or discontinue breast-feeding, taking into account importance of drug to the mother.

NURSING CONSIDERATIONS
• Obtain platelet, RBC, and WBC counts before starting drug, every 2 to 4 weeks until dosage is stabilized, then as needed.
• Resolve active infections before starting therapy.
• Blood transfusions may be necessary to manage anemia.
• Monitor patient for signs and symptoms of serious bacterial, mycobacterial, fungal, or viral infections (such as herpes zoster) during therapy; begin treatment for infection, if necessary, as soon as possible.

PATIENT TEACHING
• Inform patient that drug must be taken daily and not to change dosage or stop drug without consulting health care provider. Myelofibrosis and related signs and symptoms will return if drug is discontinued.
• Instruct patient that if a dose is missed, not to take an additional dose but to take the next usual prescribed dose.
• Inform patient on dialysis to not take a dose before dialysis, but to wait and take it after dialysis.
• Inform patient that blood tests will be needed to monitor for adverse effects and that dosage may be adjusted based on test results.
• Inform patient of increased risk of infection. Advise patient to immediately report signs and symptoms of illness (fever, cough, malaise, skin eruptions).

salmeterol xinafoate
sal-MEE-ter-ol

Serevent Diskus

Therapeutic class: Bronchodilators
Pharmacologic class: Long-acting selective beta$_2$ agonists
Pregnancy risk category: C

AVAILABLE FORMS
Inhalation powder: 50 mcg/blister

INDICATIONS & DOSAGES
➤ **Long-term maintenance of asthma; to prevent bronchospasm in patients with nocturnal asthma or reversible obstructive airway disease who need regular treatment with short-acting beta agonists**
Adults and children age 4 and older:
1 inhalation (50 mcg) b.i.d. in the morning and evening, about 12 hours apart.
➤ **To prevent exercise-induced bronchospasm**
Adults and children age 4 and older:
1 inhalation (50 mcg) at least 30 minutes before exercise. Additional doses shouldn't be taken for at least 12 hours.
➤ **COPD or emphysema**
Adults: 1 inhalation (50 mcg) b.i.d. in the morning and evening, about 12 hours apart.

ADMINISTRATION
Inhalational
• Give drug 30 to 60 minutes before exercise to prevent exercise-induced bronchospasm.
• Don't use a spacer device with this drug.

ACTION
Unclear. Selectively activates beta$_2$ receptors, which results in bronchodilation; also, blocks the release of allergic mediators from mast cells lining the respiratory tract.

Route	Onset	Peak	Duration
Inhalation	30–48 min	3 hr	12 hr

Half-life: 5½ hours; xinafoate salt, 11 days.

S

ADVERSE REACTIONS

CNS: headache, sinus headache, tremor, nervousness, giddiness, paresthesia, sleep disturbance, fever.
CV: *ventricular arrhythmias,* tachycardia, palpitations.
EENT: nasopharyngitis, pharyngitis, hoarseness, nasal cavity or sinus disorder.
GI: nausea, vomiting, diarrhea, heartburn.
Musculoskeletal: joint and back pain, myalgia.
Respiratory: upper respiratory tract infection, *bronchospasm,* cough, lower respiratory tract infection.
Other: hypersensitivity reactions, rash, urticaria, flulike symptoms.

INTERACTIONS

Drug-drug. *Antiarrhythmics (such as amiodarone, disopyramide, sotalol), chlorpromazine, dolasetron, droperidol, moxifloxacin, pentamidine, pimozide, tacrolimus, thioridazine, ziprasidone:* May prolong QT interval and increase risk of life-threatening cardiac arrhythmias. Monitor QT interval closely.
Beta agonists, other methylxanthines, theophylline: May cause adverse cardiac effects with excessive use. Monitor patient.
CYP3A4 inhibitors (ketoconazole, ritonavir): May increase cardiac effects. Avoid use together.
Diuretics: May worsen hypokalemia and ECG changes. Use cautiously together.
MAO inhibitors: May cause risk of severe adverse CV effects. Avoid use within 14 days of MAO inhibitor therapy.
TCAs: May cause risk of moderate to severe adverse CV effects. Use together with caution.

EFFECTS ON LAB TEST RESULTS

None reported.

CONTRAINDICATIONS & CAUTIONS

• Contraindicated in patients hypersensitive to drug or its ingredients.
❸ **Alert:** Don't use drug with other medications containing long-acting beta$_2$ agonists.
• Use cautiously in patients unusually responsive to sympathomimetics and those

with coronary insufficiency, arrhythmias, hypertension, other CV disorders, thyrotoxicosis, hepatic impairment, or seizure disorders.
⚠ *Overdose S&S:* Exaggeration of adverse reactions, hypokalemia, seizures, angina, hypertension, hypotension, dry mouth, muscle cramps, dizziness, fatigue, insomnia, tachycardia, ventricular arrhythmias, cardiac arrest, sudden death.

NURSING CONSIDERATIONS

Black Box Warning Drug may increase the risk of asthma-related death. Only use salmeterol as additional therapy for patients whose condition is not adequately controlled on other medications or patients whose disease severity warrants initiation of treatment with two maintenance therapies. ▌

Black Box Warning Long-acting beta$_2$-adrenergic agonists may increase risk of asthma-related hospitalization in children and adolescents. For children and adolescents with asthma who require addition of a long-acting beta$_2$-adrenergic agonist to an inhaled corticosteroid, a fixed-dose combination product containing both an inhaled corticosteroid and a long-acting beta$_2$-adrenergic agonist should ordinarily be used to ensure adherence with both drugs. In cases in which use of a separate long-term asthma-control medication (such as an inhaled corticosteroid) and a long-acting beta$_2$-adrenergic agonist is clinically indicated, appropriate steps must be taken to ensure adherence with both treatment components. If adherence can't be ensured, a fixed-dose combination product containing both an inhaled corticosteroid and a long-acting beta$_2$-adrenergic agonist is recommended. ▌
• Drug isn't indicated for acute bronchospasm.
❸ *Alert:* Monitor patient for rash and urticaria, which may signal a hypersensitivity reaction.
• *Look alike–sound alike:* Don't confuse Serevent with Serentil.

PATIENT TEACHING

Black Box Warning Teach parents of child or adolescent who requires the use of a separate long-term asthma-control medication (such as an inhaled corticosteroid) and a long-acting beta$_2$-adrenergic agonist that appropriate steps must be taken to ensure adherence with both treatment components. If adherence can't be ensured, a fixed-dose combination product containing both an inhaled corticosteroid and a long-acting beta$_2$-adrenergic agonist is recommended. ∎

• Remind patient to take drug at about 12-hour intervals for optimal effect and to take drug even when feeling better.

• If patient is taking drug to prevent exercise-induced bronchospasm, tell him to take it 30 to 60 minutes before exercise.

☉ Alert: Tell patient drug shouldn't be used to treat acute bronchospasm. He must use a short-acting beta agonist, such as albuterol, to treat worsening symptoms.

☉ Alert: Rare serious asthma episodes or asthma-related deaths may occur in patients using salmeterol. Black patients may be at greater risk.

• Tell patient to contact prescriber if the short-acting agonist no longer provides sufficient relief or if he needs more than 4 inhalations daily. This may be a sign that the asthma symptoms are worsening. Tell him not to increase the dosage of salmeterol.

• If patient takes an inhaled corticosteroid, he should continue to use it regularly. Warn patient not to take other drugs without prescriber's consent.

• If patient takes the inhalation powder (in a multidose inhaler), instruct him not to exhale into the device. He should activate and use it only in a level, horizontal position.

• Tell patient not to use the dry-powder multidose inhaler with a spacer.

• Instruct patient never to wash the mouthpiece or any part of the dry-powder multidose inhaler; it must be kept dry.

SAFETY ALERT!

sargramostim (GM-CSF; granulocyte-macrophage colony-stimulating factor)
sar-GRAM-oh-stim

Leukine

Therapeutic class: Hematopoietics
Pharmacologic class: Colony-stimulating factors
Pregnancy risk category: C

AVAILABLE FORMS
Powder for injection: 250 mcg
Solution for injection: 500 mcg/mL*

INDICATIONS & DOSAGES
➤ **To accelerate hematopoietic reconstitution after autologous or allogenic bone marrow transplantation in patients with malignant lymphoma or acute lymphoblastic leukemia or in patients with Hodgkin lymphoma**
Adults: 250 mcg/m^2 daily given as 2-hour I.V. infusion beginning 2 to 4 hours after bone marrow transplantation. Continue until ANC is more than 1,500/mm^3 for 3 consecutive days.

➤ **Neutrophil recovery following chemotherapy in acute myelogenous leukemia**
Adults age 55 and older: Initially, 250 mcg/m^2 I.V. once daily over 4 hours beginning day 11 or 4 days after completion of induction therapy; initiate only if bone marrow is hypoplastic with less than 5% blasts on day 10. If a second induction cycle is needed, begin sargramostim 4 days after completing chemotherapy and only if bone marrow is hypoplastic with less than 5% blasts. Continue until the ANC is more than 1,500/mm^3 for 3 consecutive days or for a maximum of 42 days.

➤ **Mobilization of peripheral blood progenitor cells (PBPC)**
Adults: 250 mcg/m^2 by continuous I.V. infusion over 24 hours or by subcutaneous injection once daily. Continue through PBPC collection.

S

➤ **Post-PBPC transplantation**
Adults: 250 mcg/m^2 by continuous I.V. infusion over 24 hours or by subcutaneous injection once daily beginning immediately following PBPC infusion; continue until ANC is more than 1,500/mm^3 for 3 consecutive days.

➤ **Bone marrow transplantation failure or engraftment delay**
Adults: 250 mcg/m^2 as a 2-hour I.V. infusion daily for 14 days. This course of therapy may be repeated after 7 days of no therapy. If engraftment still hasn't occurred, a third course of 500 mcg/m^2 daily I.V. for 14 days may be attempted after another therapy-free 7 days.

Adjust-a-dose: Stimulation of marrow precursors may result in rapid rise of WBC count. If blast cells appear or increase to 10% or more of WBC count or if the underlying disease progresses, stop therapy. If ANC is above 20,000/mm^3 or if platelet count is above 500,000/mm^3, temporarily stop drug or reduce dose by 50%.

➤ **Moderate to severe Crohn disease ◆**
Adults: 4 to 6 mcg/kg daily as a subcutaneous injection.

ADMINISTRATION

I.V.

▼ Reconstitute with 1 mL of sterile or bacteriostatic water for injection. Direct stream of sterile water against side of vial and gently swirl contents to minimize foaming. Avoid excessive or vigorous agitation or shaking.

▼ Dilute in normal saline solution. If drug yield is below 10 mcg/mL, add human albumin at final concentration of 0.1% to saline solution before adding sargramostim to prevent adsorption to components of the delivery system. To yield 0.1% human albumin, add 1 mg human albumin to each milliliter of saline solution (dilute 1 mL of 5% human albumin in 50 mL of saline solution).

▼ Don't use in-line filter.

▼ Give as soon as possible after mixing and no later than 6 hours after reconstituting.

▼ **Incompatibilities:** Other I.V. drugs, unless specific compatibility data are available.

Subcutaneous

● Further dilution of injection or reconstituted solution isn't needed.

ACTION

Induces cellular responses by binding to specific receptors on surfaces of target cells.

Route	Onset	Peak	Duration
I.V.	15 min	1–3 hr	Unknown
Subcut.	15 min	2–4 hr	Unknown

Half-life: About 1 hour (I.V.); about 3 hours (subcutaneous).

ADVERSE REACTIONS

CNS: asthenia, CNS disorders, fever, headache, malaise.
CV: *hemorrhage,* edema, peripheral edema, hypertension, *supraventricular arrhythmias,* pericardial effusion.
GI: anorexia, diarrhea, GI disorders, nausea, stomatitis, vomiting, *GI hemorrhage.*
GU: urinary tract disorder, abnormal kidney function.
Hematologic: blood dyscrasias.
Hepatic: liver damage.
Musculoskeletal: arthralgias.
Respiratory: dyspnea, lung disorders, pleural effusion.
Skin: alopecia, pruritus, rash.
Other: *sepsis,* mucous membrane disorder.

INTERACTIONS

Drug-drug. *Corticosteroids, lithium:* May increase myeloproliferative effects of sargramostim. Use cautiously together.

EFFECTS ON LAB TEST RESULTS

● May increase BUN, creatinine, AST, ALT, alkaline phosphatase, bilirubin, glucose, and cholesterol levels.
● May decrease calcium and albumin levels.

CONTRAINDICATIONS & CAUTIONS

● Contraindicated in patients hypersensitive to drug or its components or to yeast-derived products and in those with excessive leukemic myeloid blasts in bone marrow or peripheral blood.
● Giving within 24 hours of chemotherapy or radiation is contraindicated.

Reactions in bold italics are *life-threatening*. Interactions may have a *rapid onset* or a *delayed onset*.

• Use cautiously in patients with cardiac disease, hypoxia, fluid retention, pulmonary infiltrates, heart failure, or impaired renal or hepatic function because these conditions may be worsened.

• Safety and effectiveness haven't been established in children.

⚠ **Overdose S&S:** Dyspnea, malaise, nausea, fever, rash, sinus tachycardia, headache, chills.

NURSING CONSIDERATIONS

• If severe adverse reactions occur, reduce dose by 50% or temporarily stop drug and notify prescriber. Resume therapy when reactions decrease. Transient rash and local reactions at injection site may occur.

• Solution for injection contains benzyl alcohol, which has been associated with fatal "gasping syndrome" in neonates. Don't administer to neonates.

• Rapidly dividing progenitor cells may be sensitive to cytotoxic therapies, making the drug ineffective; don't give within 24 hours of last dose of chemotherapy or within 12 hours of last dose of radiotherapy.

• Monitor CBC with differential, including examination for presence of blast cells, biweekly.

• Drug accelerates myeloid recovery in patients receiving bone marrow that is either unpurged or purged by anti-B cell monoclonal antibodies more than in those who receive bone marrow that is chemically purged.

• Drug may produce a limited response in transplant patients who have received extensive radiotherapy or who have received other myelotoxic drugs.

• Drug can act as a growth factor for any tumor type, particularly myeloid malignant disease.

PATIENT TEACHING

• Review administration schedule with patient and caregivers, and address their concerns.

• Urge patient to report adverse reactions promptly.

SAFETY ALERT!

saxagliptin
sax-ah-GLIP-ten

Onglyza⚬

Therapeutic class: Antidiabetics
Pharmacologic class: DPP-4 enzyme inhibitors
Pregnancy risk category: B

AVAILABLE FORMS
Tablets: 2.5 mg, 5 mg

INDICATIONS & DOSAGES
➤ **Adjunct to diet and exercise to improve glycemic control in type 2 diabetes**
Adults: 2.5 or 5 mg P.O. once daily.
Adjust-a-dose: For patient with CrCl of 50 mL/minute or less, give 2.5 mg P.O. once daily; if patient requires dialysis, give drug after treatment.

ADMINISTRATION
P.O.
• Give drug with or without food.
• Don't split or cut tablets.

ACTION
Inhibits DPP-4, an enzyme that rapidly inactivates incretin hormones, which play a part in the body's regulation of glucose. By increasing active incretin levels, drug helps to increase insulin release and decrease circulating glucose.

Route	Onset	Peak	Duration
P.O.	Unknown	2 hr	Unknown

Half-life: 2½ hours.

ADVERSE REACTIONS
CNS: headache.
CV: facial edema, peripheral edema.
EENT: sinusitis.
GI: abdominal pain, gastroenteritis, vomiting.
GU: UTI.
Metabolic: hypoglycemia.
Respiratory: upper respiratory tract infection.
Skin: urticaria.

S

INTERACTIONS
Drug-drug. *Strong CYP3A4/5 inhibitors (atazanavir, clarithromycin, indinavir, itraconazole, ketoconazole, nefazodone, nelfinavir, ritonavir, saquinavir, telithromycin):* May increase saxagliptin level. Reduce dosage to 2.5 mg P.O. daily.

EFFECTS ON LAB TEST RESULTS
• May decrease lymphocyte count.

CONTRAINDICATIONS & CAUTIONS
• Use cautiously in patients taking secretagogues (such as sulfonylureas) because of increased risk of hypoglycemia.
• Use cautiously in pregnant and breast-feeding women.
• Discontinue drug if pancreatitis is suspected.
• Safety and effectiveness in children haven't been established.

NURSING CONSIDERATIONS
• Monitor blood glucose level and watch for signs and symptoms of hypoglycemia.
• Monitor glycosylated hemoglobin level periodically to assess long-term glycemic control.
• Monitor patient for signs and symptoms of pancreatitis. If pancreatitis is suspected, discontinue drug and initiate appropriate management.
• Assess renal function before starting drug and periodically thereafter.
• Management of type 2 diabetes should also include diet control and exercise. Because calorie restriction, weight loss, and exercise help improve insulin sensitivity and help make drug therapy effective, these measures are essential for proper diabetes management.
• *Look alike–sound alike:* Don't confuse saxagliptin with sitagliptin.

PATIENT TEACHING
• Tell patient drug may be taken with or without food.
• Advise patient that drug isn't a substitute for diet and exercise and that it's important to follow a prescribed dietary and physical activity routine and to monitor glucose levels.

• Inform patient and family members of the signs and symptoms of hypoglycemia and hyperglycemia and the steps to take should these occur, including notifying the prescriber.
• Tell patient to notify prescriber during periods of stress, such as fever, infection, or surgery, because dosage may need adjustment.
• Tell patient to stop drug if signs and symptoms of pancreatitis (persistent severe abdominal pain, sometimes radiating to the back, vomiting) occur.

selegiline
se-LEH-ge-leen

Emsam

selegiline hydrochloride (L-deprenyl hydrochloride)
Eldepryl, Zelapar

Therapeutic class: Antiparkinsonians
Pharmacologic class: MAO inhibitors
Pregnancy risk category: C

AVAILABLE FORMS
selegiline
Transdermal system: 6 mg/24 hours, 9 mg/24 hours, 12 mg/24 hours
selegiline hydrochloride
Capsules: 5 mg
Tablets: 5 mg
Tablets (orally disintegrating): 1.25 mg

INDICATIONS & DOSAGES
➤ **Adjunctive treatment with levodopa–carbidopa in managing signs and symptoms of Parkinson disease**
Adults: For capsules and tablets, 10 mg P.O. daily divided as 5 mg at breakfast and 5 mg at lunch. After 2 or 3 days, gradual decrease of levodopa–carbidopa dosage may be needed. Or, if using orally disintegrating tablets (ODTs), start with 1.25 mg P.O. once daily before breakfast and without liquid. Increase to 2.5 mg daily after at least 6 weeks, if tolerated and needed.
➤ **Major depressive disorder**
Adults: Apply one patch daily to dry intact skin on the upper torso, upper thigh, or upper arm. Initially, use 6 mg/day. Increase,

if needed, in increments of 3 mg/day at intervals of 2 or more weeks. Maximum daily dose, 12 mg.

Elderly patients: 6 mg transdermal patch daily.

ADMINISTRATION

P.O.

• Don't give food or liquids for 5 minutes before and after giving ODTs.

• Don't push ODTs through the foil backing; peel the backing off and gently remove the tablet.

Transdermal

• Apply patch to dry, intact skin on the upper torso, upper thigh, or outer surface of the upper arm once every 24 hours.

• Don't cut the transdermal patch into smaller pieces.

ACTION

May inhibit MAO type B (mainly found in the brain) and dopamine metabolism. At higher-than-recommended doses, drug non-selectively inhibits MAO, including MAO type A (mainly found in the intestine). May also directly increase dopaminergic activity by decreasing the reuptake of dopamine into nerve cells.

Route	Onset	Peak	Duration
P.O. (tablet, capsule)	Unknown	30–120 min	Unknown
P.O. (ODT)	5 min	10–15 min	Unknown
Transdermal	Unknown	Unknown	24 hr

Half-life: Selegiline, 2 to 10 hours; N-desmethyl-deprenyl, 2 hours; L-amphetamine, 17¾ hours; L-methamphetamine, 20½ hours.

ADVERSE REACTIONS

Transdermal form

CNS: headache, insomnia.

CV: chest pain, hypotension, orthostatic blood pressure.

GI: diarrhea, dry mouth, dyspepsia.

Metabolic: weight gain, weight loss.

Respiratory: pharyngitis, sinusitis.

Skin: application-site reaction, rash.

Oral form

CNS: dizziness, agitation, delusions, loss of balance, depression, increased bradykinesia, involuntary movements, headache,

confusion, hallucinations, vivid dreams, insomnia, syncope, pain.

CV: *arrhythmias,* orthostatic hypotension, hypertension, new or increased angina.

EENT: pharyngitis, rhinitis.

GI: nausea, dry mouth, abdominal pain, diarrhea.

Musculoskeletal: leg cramps, myalgia, back pain.

Respiratory: dyspnea.

Skin: rash, ecchymosis.

INTERACTIONS

Drug-drug. *Bupropion; cyclobenzaprine; dextromethorphan; meperidine; methadone; mirtazapine; MAO inhibitors; sympath-omimetic amines, including amphetamines, cold products, and weight-loss preparations containing vasoconstrictors; TCAs; tramadol:* May cause hypertensive crisis. Separate use by at least 2 weeks.

Carbamazepine, oxcarbazepine: May increase selegiline levels. Use together is contraindicated.

Citalopram, duloxetine, fluoxetine, fluvoxamine, nefazodone, paroxetine, sertraline, venlafaxine: May cause serotonin syndrome (CNS irritability, shivering, and altered consciousness). Separate use by at least 2 weeks (5 weeks if switching to or from fluoxetine).

Hormonal contraceptives: May increase plasma selegiline level and increase adverse reactions. Monitor patient closely.

Linezolid, methylene blue: May cause serotonin syndrome. Use extreme caution and monitor patient closely.

Drug-herb. *Ginseng:* May cause headache, tremors, or mania. Discourage use together.

St. John's wort: May cause increased serotonergic effects. Warn patient against use together.

Drug-food. *Foods high in tyramine:* May cause hypertensive crisis, especially at increased doses. Provide patient with a list of foods to avoid.

EFFECTS ON LAB TEST RESULTS

• May cause positive result for amphetamine on urine drug screen.

S

CONTRAINDICATIONS & CAUTIONS

● Contraindicated in patients hypersensitive to drug, in patients with pheochromocytoma, and in those taking bupropion, carbamazepine, cyclobenzaprine, dextromethorphan, duloxetine, methadone, meperidine, mirtazapine, MAO inhibitors, oxcarbazepine, SSRIs, sympathomimetics, tramadol, TCAs, or venlafaxine.

◐ *Alert:* Concomitant use with linezolid or methylene blue can cause serotonin syndrome (fever, mental status changes, muscle twitching, excessive sweating, shivering or shaking, diarrhea, loss of coordination). Use drug with linezolid or methylene blue only for life-threatening or urgent conditions when the potential benefits outweigh the risks of toxicity.

● Don't use oral drug with the transdermal system.

Black Box Warning Selegiline isn't approved for use in children. Emsam shouldn't be used in children under age 12, even when administered with dietary modifications. ■

⚠ *Overdose S&S:* Drowsiness, dizziness, faintness, irritability, hyperactivity, agitation, severe headache, hallucinations, trismus, opisthotonos, seizures, coma, rapid and irregular pulse, hypertension, hypotension and vascular collapse, precordial pain, respiratory depression and failure, hyperpyrexia, diaphoresis, cool and clammy skin.

NURSING CONSIDERATIONS

◐ *Alert:* Some patients experience increased adverse reactions to levodopa when it's used with selegiline and need a 10% to 30% reduction of levodopa–carbidopa dosage.

Black Box Warning Drug may increase the risk of suicidal thinking and behavior in children, adolescents, and young adults ages 18 to 24, especially during the first few months of treatment, especially in those with major depressive or other psychiatric disorder. ■

◐ *Alert:* If linezolid or methylene blue must be given, stop selegiline and monitor patient for serotonin toxicity for 2 weeks, or until 24 hours after the last dose of methylene blue or linezolid, whichever comes first. May resume selegiline 24 hours after last dose of methylene blue or linezolid.

● Monitor patients with major depressive disorder for worsening of symptoms and of suicidal behavior, especially during the first few weeks of treatment and during dosage changes.

● *Look alike–sound alike:* Don't confuse selegiline with Stelazine. Don't confuse Eldepryl with enalapril.

PATIENT TEACHING

◐ *Alert:* Teach patient to recognize and immediately report signs and symptoms of serotonin toxicity (fever, mental status changes, muscle twitching, excessive sweating, shivering or shaking, diarrhea, loss of coordination).

● Warn patient to move cautiously or change positions slowly at start of therapy because he may become dizzy or lightheaded.

● Caution patient to avoid driving and other hazardous activities that require mental alertness until the drug's effects are known.

● Advise patient not to take drug in the evening because doing so may cause insomnia.

● Advise patient not to overindulge in tyramine-rich foods or beverages. If using a 9 mg/day or higher transdermal system, avoid these products altogether.

● Advise patient to avoid liquids for 5 minutes before and after taking ODTs.

◐ *Alert:* Warn patient about the many drugs, including OTC drugs, that may interact with this drug and about the need to consult a pharmacist or his prescriber before using them.

● Teach patient and family the signs and symptoms of hypertensive crisis, including severe headache, sore or stiff neck, nausea, vomiting, sweating, rapid heartbeat, dilated pupils, and photophobia.

Black Box Warning Advise family members to watch patient for anxiety, agitation, insomnia, irritability, hostility, and aggressiveness and to report these immediately to prescriber. ■

● Tell patient to avoid exposing transdermal system to direct external heat sources, such as heating pads, electric blankets, hot tubs, heated water beds, and prolonged sunlight.

• Tell patient to stop using the transdermal system 10 days before having surgery requiring general anesthesia.
• Tell patient not to cut the transdermal system into smaller pieces.
• Advise women planning pregnancy or breast-feeding to first contact prescriber.

sertraline hydrochloride
SIR-trah-leen

Apo-Sertraline†, Zoloft⌀

Therapeutic class: Antidepressants
Pharmacologic class: SSRIs
Pregnancy risk category: C

AVAILABLE FORMS
Capsules †: 25 mg, 50 mg, 100 mg
Oral concentrate*: 20 mg/mL
Tablets: 25 mg, 50 mg, 100 mg

INDICATIONS & DOSAGES
Adjust-a-dose (for all indications): Dosage changes shouldn't occur at intervals of less than 1 week. For patients with hepatic disease, use lower or less-frequent dosages.
➤ **Depression**
Adults: 50 mg P.O. daily. Adjust dosage as needed and tolerated; dosage range is 50 to 200 mg daily.
➤ **Obsessive-compulsive disorder**
Adults: 50 mg P.O. once daily. If patient doesn't improve, increase dosage, up to 200 mg daily.
Children ages 6 to 17: Initially, 25 mg P.O. daily in children ages 6 to 12, or 50 mg P.O. daily in adolescents ages 13 to 17. Increase dosage, as needed, up to 200 mg daily at intervals of no less than 1 week.
➤ **Panic disorder**
Adults: Initially, 25 mg P.O. daily. After 1 week, increase dose to 50 mg P.O. daily. If patient doesn't improve, increase dose to maximum of 200 mg daily.
➤ **Posttraumatic stress disorder**
Adults: Initially, 25 mg P.O. once daily. Increase dosage to 50 mg P.O. once daily after 1 week. Increase at weekly intervals to a maximum of 200 mg daily. Maintain patient on lowest effective dose.

➤ **Premenstrual dysphoric disorder**
Adults: Initially, 50 mg P.O. daily either continuously or only during the luteal phase of the menstrual cycle. If patient doesn't respond, dose may be increased 50 mg per menstrual cycle, up to 150 mg daily for use throughout the menstrual cycle or 100 mg daily for luteal-phase doses. If a 100-mg daily dose has been established with luteal-phase dose, use a 50-mg daily adjustment for 3 days at the beginning of each luteal phase.
➤ **Social anxiety disorder**
Adults: Initially, 25 mg P.O. once daily. Increase dosage to 50 mg P.O. once daily after 1 week of therapy. Dose range is 50 to 200 mg daily. Adjust to the lowest effective dosage and periodically reassess patient to determine the need for long-term treatment.

ADMINISTRATION
P.O.
• Give drug without regard for food.
• Don't use oral concentrate dropper, which is made of rubber, for a patient with latex allergy.
• Mix oral concentrate with 4 oz (118 mL) of water, ginger ale, lemon-lime soda, lemonade, or orange juice only, and give immediately.

ACTION
Thought to be linked to drug's inhibition of CNS neuronal uptake of serotonin.

Route	Onset	Peak	Duration
P.O.	1 wk	4–8 hr	Unknown

Half-life: 26 hours.

ADVERSE REACTIONS
CNS: fatigue, headache, tremor, dizziness, insomnia, somnolence, *suicidal behavior,* paresthesia, hypesthesia, nervousness, anxiety, agitation, hypertonia, pain.
CV: palpitations, chest pain, hot flashes.
GI: dry mouth, nausea, diarrhea, loose stools, dyspepsia, vomiting, constipation, thirst, flatulence, anorexia, abdominal pain, increased appetite.
GU: male sexual dysfunction.
Musculoskeletal: myalgia.
Skin: rash, pruritus, diaphoresis.

S

INTERACTIONS

Drug-drug. *Amphetamines, buspirone, dextromethorphan, dihydroergotamine, lithium salts, meperidine, other SSRIs or SSNRIs (duloxetine, venlafaxine), sumatriptan, TCAs,* **tramadol,** *trazodone, tryptophan:* May increase the risk of serotonin syndrome. Avoid combinations of drugs that increase the availability of serotonin in the CNS; monitor patient closely if used together.

Benzodiazepines, tolbutamide: May decrease clearance of these drugs. Significance unknown; monitor patient for increased drug effects.

Cimetidine: May decrease clearance of sertraline. Monitor patient closely.

Disulfiram: Oral concentrate contains alcohol, which may react with drug. Avoid using together.

Linezolid, methylene blue: May cause serotonin syndrome. Use extreme caution and monitor patient closely.

MAO inhibitors, such as phenelzine, selegiline, tranylcypromine: May cause serotonin syndrome or signs and symptoms resembling neuroleptic malignant syndrome. Avoid using within 14 days of MAO inhibitor therapy.

Pimozide: May increase pimozide level. Avoid using together.

Triptans: May cause serotonin syndrome (restlessness, hallucinations, loss of coordination, fast heartbeat, rapid changes in blood pressure, increased body temperature, hyperreflexia, nausea, vomiting, and diarrhea) or neuroleptic malignant syndrome–like reactions. Use cautiously, with close monitoring, especially at the start of treatment and during dosage adjustments.

Warfarin, other highly protein-bound drugs: May increase level of sertraline or other highly protein-bound drug. May increase PT, or INR may increase by 8%. Monitor patient closely; monitor PT and INR.

Drug-herb. *St. John's wort:* May cause additive effects and serotonin syndrome. Discourage use together.

EFFECTS ON LAB TEST RESULTS

● May increase ALT and AST levels.

CONTRAINDICATIONS & CAUTIONS

● Contraindicated in patients hypersensitive to drug or its components.

🚫 **Alert:** Concomitant use with linezolid or methylene blue can cause serotonin syndrome (fever, mental status changes, muscle twitching, excessive sweating, shivering or shaking, diarrhea, loss of coordination). Use drug with linezolid or methylene blue only for life-threatening or urgent conditions when the potential benefits outweigh the risks of toxicity.

● Contraindicated in patients taking pimozide or MAO inhibitors or within 14 days of MAO inhibitor therapy.

● Use cautiously in patients at risk for suicide and in those with seizure disorders, major affective disorder, or diseases or conditions that affect metabolism or hemodynamic responses.

● Use in third trimester of pregnancy may cause neonatal complications at birth. Consider the risk versus benefit of treatment during this time.

Black Box Warning Sertraline isn't approved for use in children except those with obsessive-compulsive disorder. ∎

⚠ **Overdose S&S:** Somnolence, vomiting, tachycardia, nausea, dizziness, agitation, tremor, bradycardia, bundle-branch block, coma, seizures, delirium, hallucinations, hypertension, hypotension, manic reactions, pancreatitis, prolonged QT interval, serotonin syndrome, stupor, syncope.

NURSING CONSIDERATIONS

● Give sertraline once daily, either in morning or evening, with or without food.

● Make dosage adjustments at intervals of no less than 1 week.

● Record mood changes. Monitor patient for suicidal tendencies and allow only a minimum supply of drug.

Black Box Warning Drug may increase the risk of suicidal thinking and behavior in children, adolescents, and young adults with major depressive disorder or other psychiatric disorder. ∎

🚫 **Alert:** If linezolid or methylene blue must be given, stop sertraline and monitor patient for serotonin toxicity for 2 weeks, or until 24 hours after the last dose of methylene blue or linezolid, whichever comes first.

Reactions in bold italics are *life-threatening*. Interactions may have a *rapid onset* or a *delayed onset*.

May resume selegiline 24 hours after last dose of methylene blue or linezolid.

• Don't use the oral concentrate dropper, which is made of rubber, for a patient with latex allergy.

‣ **Alert:** Combining triptans with an SSRI or an SSNRI may cause serotonin syndrome or neuroleptic malignant syndrome–like reactions. Signs and symptoms of serotonin syndrome may include restlessness, hallucinations, loss of coordination, fast heartbeat, rapid changes in blood pressure, increased body temperature, overactive reflexes, nausea, vomiting, and diarrhea. Serotonin syndrome may be more likely to occur when starting or increasing the dose of triptan, SSRI, or SSNRI.

• *Look alike–sound alike:* Don't confuse sertraline with cetirizine or Soriatane.

PATIENT TEACHING

Black Box Warning Advise families and caregivers to closely observe patient for increased suicidal thinking and behavior. ∎

‣ *Alert:* Teach patient to recognize and immediately report signs and symptoms of serotonin toxicity (fever, mental status changes, muscle twitching, excessive sweating, shivering or shaking, diarrhea, loss of coordination).

• Advise patient to use caution when performing hazardous tasks that require alertness.

• Tell patient to avoid alcohol and to consult prescriber before taking OTC drugs.

• Advise patient to mix the oral concentrate with 4 oz (½ cup) of water, ginger ale, lemon-lime soda, lemonade, or orange juice only, and to take the dose right away.

• Instruct patient to avoid stopping drug abruptly.

---

sevelamer carbonate
seh-VELL-ah-meer

Renvela

sevelamer hydrochloride
Renagel

Therapeutic class: Hypophosphatemics
Pharmacologic class: Polymeric phosphate binders
Pregnancy risk category: C

AVAILABLE FORMS
sevelamer carbonate
Oral suspension: 0.8-g, 2.4-g packets
Tablets (film-coated): 800 mg
sevelamer hydrochloride
Tablets (film-coated): 400 mg, 800 mg

INDICATIONS & DOSAGES
➤ **To control phosphorus level in chronic kidney disease patients on dialysis**
Adults not taking a phosphate binder:
Initially, 800 to 1,600 mg (one to two 800-mg tablets or two to four 400-mg tablets) P.O. with each meal, based on phosphorus level. If phosphorus level is greater than 5.5 and less than 7.5 mg/dL, start with 800 mg t.i.d. with meals. If phosphorus level is greater than or equal to 7.5 and less than 9 mg/dL, start with two 800-mg tablets t.i.d., or three 400-mg tablets t.i.d. with meals. If phosphorus level is greater than or equal to 9 mg/dL, start with 1,600 mg t.i.d. (two 800-mg tablets or four 400-mg tablets) with meals.
Adults switching from calcium acetate:
Initially, if taking one 667-mg calcium acetate tablet per meal, start with 800 mg per meal. If taking two 667-mg calcium acetate tablets per meal, start with two 800-mg tablets or three 400-mg tablets per meal. If taking three 667-mg calcium acetate tablets per meal, start with three 800-mg tablets or five 400-mg tablets per meal.
Adjust-a-dose: If phosphorus level is greater than 5.5 mg/dL, increase by one tablet per meal at 2-week intervals. If phosphorus level is 3.5 to 5.5 mg/dL, maintain current dose. If phosphorus level is less than

S

3.5 mg/dL, decrease dose by one tablet per meal.

ADMINISTRATION
P.O.
- Don't cut, crush, or allow patient to chew tablets.
- Mix powder packets with appropriate amount of water as directed. Stir mixture vigorously (it doesn't dissolve) and have patient drink entire preparation within 30 minutes.
- Give drug with meals.
- Drug may bind to other drugs and decrease their bioavailability. Give other drugs 1 hour before or 3 hours after this drug.
- Take special precautions when using antiarrhythmics or anticonvulsants with this drug.

ACTION
Inhibits intestinal phosphate absorption and decreases phosphorus levels.

Route	Onset	Peak	Duration
P.O.	Unknown	Unknown	Unknown

Half-life: Unknown.

ADVERSE REACTIONS
CNS: headache, pain, fever.
CV: hypertension, ***thrombosis.***
GI: diarrhea, dyspepsia, vomiting, nausea, constipation, flatulence.
EENT: nasopharyngitis.
Musculoskeletal: limb pain, arthralgia, back pain.
Respiratory: bronchitis, dyspnea, increased cough, upper respiratory tract infection.
Skin: pruritus.

INTERACTIONS
Drug-drug. *Ciprofloxacin:* May decrease the effectiveness of ciprofloxacin. Separate administration times by at least 4 hours.
Mycophenolate: May decrease mycophenolic acid plasma concentration, decreasing efficacy. Administer sevelamer 2 hours after mycophenolate.
Thyroid hormones (levothyroxine): May decrease effectiveness of hormones. Separate administration times by at least 4 hours. Monitor thyroid-stimulating hormone level

and patient for signs or symptoms of hypothyroidism.

EFFECTS ON LAB TEST RESULTS
None reported.

CONTRAINDICATIONS & CAUTIONS
- Contraindicated in patients hypersensitive to drug or its components and in those with hypophosphatemia or bowel obstruction.
- Use cautiously in patient with dysphagia, swallowing disorders, severe GI motility disorders, or major GI tract surgery.

NURSING CONSIDERATIONS
- Monitor calcium, bicarbonate, and chloride levels.
- Watch for symptoms of thrombosis (numbness or tingling of limbs, chest pain, shortness of breath), and notify prescriber if they occur.
- *Look alike–sound alike:* Don't confuse Renvela with Renagel.

PATIENT TEACHING
- Instruct patient to take with meals and to adhere to prescribed diet.
- ⊛ *Alert:* Inform patient that tablets must be taken whole because contents expand in water. Tell him not to cut, crush, or chew.
- Tell patient to take other drugs as directed, but they must be taken either 1 hour before or 3 hours after sevelamer.
- Inform patient about common adverse reactions. Teach patient signs and symptoms of thrombosis, such as numbness, tingling in arms or legs, or chest pain, and to report these immediately.

sildenafil citrate (oral for erectile dysfunction)
sill-DEN-ah-fill

Viagra✧

Therapeutic class: Erectile dysfunction drugs
Pharmacologic class: PDE5 inhibitors
Pregnancy risk category: B

AVAILABLE FORMS
Tablets: 25 mg, 50 mg, 100 mg

INDICATIONS & DOSAGES
➤ **Erectile dysfunction**
Adult men younger than age 65: About
1 hour before sexual activity, 50 mg P.O.,
p.r.n. Dosage range is 25 to 100 mg based
on effectiveness and tolerance. Maximum is
100 mg daily.
Elderly male patients (age 65 and older):
25 mg P.O., as needed, about 1 hour before
sexual activity. Dosage may be adjusted
based on patient response.
Adjust-a-dose: For adults with hepatic or
severe renal impairment, 25 mg P.O. about
1 hour before sexual activity. Dosage may
be adjusted based on patient response.

ADMINISTRATION
P.O.
• For most rapid absorption, give to patient
on empty stomach.

ACTION
Increases effect of nitric oxide by inhibiting
PDE5, which is responsible for degradation of cyclic guanosine monophosphate
(cGMP) in the corpus cavernosum. When
sexual stimulation causes local release of
nitric oxide, inhibition of PDE5 by sildenafil
causes increased levels of cGMP in the corpus cavernosum, resulting in smooth muscle
relaxation and inflow of blood to the corpus
cavernosum.

Route	Onset	Peak	Duration
P.O.	15–30 min	30–120 min	4 hr

Half-life: 4 hours.

ADVERSE REACTIONS
CNS: headache, *seizures,* anxiety, dizziness, somnolence, vertigo.
CV: *MI, sudden cardiac death, ventricular
arrhythmias, cerebrovascular hemorrhage,
transient ischemic attack,* hypotension,
flushing.
EENT: diplopia, temporary vision loss,
decrease or loss of hearing, tinnitus, ocular
redness or bloodshot appearance, increased
intraocular pressure, retinal vascular disease, retinal bleeding, vitreous detachment
or traction, paramacular edema, photophobia, altered color perception, blurred
vision, burning, swelling, pressure, nasal
congestion.

GI: dyspepsia, diarrhea.
GU: hematuria, prolonged erection,
priapism, UTI.
Musculoskeletal: arthralgia, back pain.
Respiratory: respiratory tract infection.
Skin: rash.
Other: flulike syndrome.

INTERACTIONS
Drug-drug. *Alpha blockers:* May cause
symptomatic hypotension. Consider dosage
reduction.
*Beta blockers, loop and potassium-sparing
diuretics:* May increase sildenafil metabolite
level. Monitor patient.
Bosentan: May decrease sildenafil level and
increase bosentan level. Monitor patient
closely for bosentan adverse reactions.
CYP450 inducers, rifampin: May reduce
sildenafil level. Monitor effect.
Delavirdine, protease inhibitors: May increase sildenafil level, increasing risk of
adverse events, including hypotension,
visual changes, and priapism. Reduce initial
sildenafil dose to 25 mg in a 48-hour period.
*Hepatic isoenzyme inhibitors (such as ci-
metidine, erythromycin, itraconazole, ketoconazole):* May reduce sildenafil clearance.
Avoid using together.
Isosorbide, nitroglycerin: May cause severe
hypotension. Use of nitrates in any form
with sildenafil is contraindicated.
Drug-food. *Grapefruit:* May increase drug
level, while delaying absorption. Advise
patient to avoid using together.
High-fat meal: May reduce absorption rate
and peak level of drug. Advise patient to
take drug on empty stomach.

EFFECTS ON LAB TEST RESULTS
None reported.

CONTRAINDICATIONS & CAUTIONS
• Contraindicated in patients hypersensitive
to drug or its components and in those
taking organic nitrates.
• Use cautiously in patients age 65 and
older; in patients with hepatic or severe
renal impairment, retinitis pigmentosa,
bleeding disorders, or active peptic ulcer
disease; in those who have suffered an MI,
a stroke, or life-threatening arrhythmia
within past 6 months; in those with history

S

of cardiac failure, coronary artery disease, uncontrolled high or low blood pressure, or anatomic deformation of the penis (such as angulation, cavernosal fibrosis, or Peyronie disease); and in those with conditions that may predispose them to priapism (such as sickle cell anemia, multiple myeloma, or leukemia).

NURSING CONSIDERATIONS

🔂 *Alert:* Systemic vasodilatory properties cause transient decreases in supine blood pressure and cardiac output (about 2 hours after ingestion).

🔂 *Alert:* Serious CV events, including MI, sudden cardiac death, ventricular arrhythmias, cerebrovascular hemorrhage, transient ischemic attack, and hypertension, may occur with drug use. Most, but not all, of these incidents involve CV risk factors. Many events occur during or shortly after sexual activity; a few occur shortly after drug use without sexual activity, and others occur hours to days after drug use and sexual activity.

• Drug isn't indicated for use in neonates, children, or women.

• *Look alike–sound alike:* Don't confuse Viagra with Allegra.

PATIENT TEACHING

• Advise patient that drug shouldn't be used with nitrates under any circumstances.

• Advise patient of potential cardiac risk of sexual activity, especially in presence of CV risk factors. Instruct patient to notify prescriber and refrain from further activity if such symptoms as chest pain, dizziness, or nausea occur when starting sexual activity.

• Warn patient that erections lasting longer than 4 hours and priapism (painful erections lasting longer than 6 hours) may occur, and tell him to seek immediate medical attention. Penile tissue damage and permanent loss of potency may result if priapism isn't treated immediately.

• Inform patient that drug doesn't protect against sexually transmitted diseases; advise patient to use protective measures such as condoms.

• Tell patient receiving HIV medications that he's at increased risk for sildenafil adverse events, including low blood pressure, visual changes, and priapism, and that he should promptly report such symptoms to his prescriber. Tell him not to exceed 25 mg of sildenafil in 48 hours.

• Instruct patient to take drug 30 minutes to 4 hours before sexual activity; maximum benefit can be expected less than 2 hours after ingestion.

• Advise patient that drug is most rapidly absorbed if taken on an empty stomach.

• Inform patient that impairment of color discrimination (blue, green) may occur and to avoid hazardous activities that rely on color discrimination.

• Instruct patient to immediately notify prescriber of vision or hearing changes.

• Advise patient that drug is effective only in presence of sexual stimulation.

• Caution patient to take drug only as prescribed.

sildenafil citrate (for pulmonary arterial hypertension)
sill-DEN-ah-fill

Revatio

Therapeutic class: Pulmonary vasodilators
Pharmacologic class: Cyclic guanosine monophosphate–specific PDE5 inhibitors
Pregnancy risk category: B

AVAILABLE FORMS
Injection: 10 mg/12.5 mL single-use vials
Oral suspension: 10 mg/mL
Tablets: 20 mg

INDICATIONS & DOSAGES
➤ **To improve exercise ability and delay clinical worsening in patients with World Health Organization group I pulmonary arterial hypertension (PAH)**
Adults: 20 mg P.O. t.i.d., 4 to 6 hours apart. Or 10 mg I.V. bolus t.i.d.

ADMINISTRATION
P.O.
• Give drug without regard for food.
• Don't give to patients taking nitrates.

I.V.

▼ Inspect solution visually for particulate matter and discoloration before administering.

▼ Don't give to patients taking nitrates.

▼ Ten-milligram I.V. dose is equivalent to 20-mg oral dose.

ACTION

Increases cyclic guanosine monophosphate level by preventing its breakdown by phosphodiesterase, prolonging smooth muscle relaxation of the pulmonary vasculature, which leads to vasodilation.

Route	Onset	Peak	Duration
P.O.	15–30 min	30–120 min	4 hr
I.V.	Unknown	Unknown	Unknown

Half-life: 4 hours.

ADVERSE REACTIONS

CNS: headache, dizziness, fever, insomnia.
CV: flushing, hypotension.
EENT: blurred vision, burning, epistaxis, impaired color discrimination, photophobia, rhinitis, sinusitis.
GI: dyspepsia, diarrhea, gastritis.
Musculoskeletal: myalgia.
Skin: erythema, flushing.

INTERACTIONS

Drug-drug. *Alpha blockers:* May cause symptomatic hypotension. Consider dosage reduction.
Amlodipine: May further reduce blood pressure. Monitor blood pressure closely.
Azole antifungals (itraconazole, ketoconazole): May increase sildenafil level and risk of adverse reactions. Monitor patient carefully.
Bosentan: May decrease sildenafil level. Monitor patient.
CYP3A4 and CYP2C9 inducers, rifampin: May reduce sildenafil level. Monitor effect.
Hepatic isoenzyme inhibitors (such as cimetidine, erythromycin): May increase sildenafil level. Avoid using together.
Isosorbide, nitroglycerin: May cause severe hypotension. Use of nitrates in any form is contraindicated during therapy.

Macrolide antibiotics (erythromycin), SSRIs (fluvoxamine), tacrolimus: May increase sildenafil level and risk of adverse reactions. Closely monitor patient and consider lower starting dose.
Protease inhibitors (ritonavir): May significantly increase sildenafil level. Don't use together.
Vitamin K antagonists: May increase risk of bleeding (primarily epistaxis). Monitor patient.
Drug-food. *Grapefruit:* May increase drug level, while delaying absorption. Discourage use together.

EFFECTS ON LAB TEST RESULTS

None reported.

CONTRAINDICATIONS & CAUTIONS

● Contraindicated in patients hypersensitive to drug or its components and in those taking organic nitrates.

● Don't use in patients with pulmonary veno-occlusive disease.

● Use cautiously in patients with resting hypotension, severe left ventricular outflow obstruction, autonomic dysfunction, and volume depletion.

● Use cautiously in elderly patients; in patients with hepatic or severe renal impairment, retinitis pigmentosa, bleeding disorders, or active peptic ulcer disease; in those who have suffered an MI, stroke, or life-threatening arrhythmia in past 6 months; in those with history of coronary artery disease causing unstable angina or of uncontrolled high or low blood pressure; in those with deformation of the penis or with conditions that may cause priapism (such as sickle cell anemia, multiple myeloma, or leukemia); and in those taking bosentan.

● It's unknown if drug appears in breast milk. Use cautiously in breast-feeding women.

● Safety and effectiveness in children haven't been established.

NURSING CONSIDERATIONS

● The serious CV events linked to this drug's use in erectile dysfunction mainly involve patients with underlying CV disease who are at increased risk for cardiac effects related to sexual activity.

S

• Patients with PAH caused by connective tissue disease are more prone to epistaxis during therapy than those with primary pulmonary hypertension.
• P.O. and I.V. doses aren't equivalent.
• I.V. use is for patients with PAH currently unable to take oral medications.
◑ **Alert:** Don't substitute Viagra for Revatio because there isn't an equivalent dose.

PATIENT TEACHING
• Warn patient that drug should never be used with nitrates, Viagra, or other PDE5 inhibitors for erectile dysfunction.
• Advise patient to rise slowly from lying down.
• Inform patient that drug can be taken with or without food.
• Warn patient that discrimination between colors, such as blue and green, may become impaired during therapy; warn him to avoid hazardous activities that rely on color discrimination.
• Instruct patient to notify prescriber of decrease or loss of hearing, tinnitus, visual changes, dizziness, or fainting.
• Caution patient to take drug only as prescribed.

silodosin
sigh-low-DOSE-in

Rapaflo

Therapeutic class: BPH drugs
Pharmacologic class: Alpha₁ blockers
Pregnancy risk category: B

AVAILABLE FORMS
Capsules: 4 mg, 8 mg

INDICATIONS & DOSAGES
➤ **To improve symptoms of BPH**
Men: 8 mg P.O once daily.
Adjust-a-dose: For patients with CrCl of 30 to 50 mL/minute, give 4 mg once daily.

ADMINISTRATION
P.O.
• Give drug once daily with a meal.

ACTION
Causes relaxation of smooth muscles in the prostate and bladder tissues by antagonizing postsynaptic alpha₁ adrenoreceptors, thereby improving urine flow and reducing signs and symptoms of BPH.

Route	Onset	Peak	Duration
P.O.	Unknown	2.6 hr	Unknown

Half-life: 5 to 21 hours.

ADVERSE REACTIONS
CNS: asthenia, dizziness, headache, insomnia.
CV: orthostatic hypotension.
EENT: nasal congestion, nasopharyngitis, rhinorrhea, sinusitis.
GI: abdominal pain, diarrhea.
GU: retrograde ejaculation.

INTERACTIONS
Drug-drug. *Alpha blockers:* May cause interactions. Avoid use together.
Antihypertensives: May cause dizziness and orthostatic hypotension. Use together cautiously and monitor patient for adverse reactions.
Moderate CYP3A4 inhibitors (such as diltiazem, erythromycin, verapamil): May increase silodosin level. Use together cautiously.
Strong CYP3A4 inhibitors (such as clarithromycin, itraconazole, ketoconazole, ritonavir): May increase silodosin level. Avoid use together if possible.
Strong P-glycoprotein inhibitors (such as cyclosporine, ketoconazole): May increase silodosin levels. Don't use together.

EFFECTS ON LAB TEST RESULTS
None reported.

CONTRAINDICATIONS & CAUTIONS
• Contraindicated in patients hypersensitive to drug or its components, in those with severe renal or hepatic impairment, and in those taking strong CYP3A4 inhibitors.
⚠ **Overdose S&S:** Orthostatic hypotension.

NURSING CONSIDERATIONS
• Because BPH and prostate cancer cause similar signs and symptoms, prostate cancer

---

Reactions in bold italics are *life-threatening*. Interactions may have a *rapid onset* or a *delayed onset*.

should be ruled out before the start of silo-dosin therapy.

• Monitor patient for orthostatic hypotension. Carefully monitor older patients for hypotension because risk of orthostatic hypotension increases with age.

• Don't use drug to treat hypertension.

• Current or previous use of an alpha blocker may predispose patient to floppy-iris syndrome during cataract surgery.

PATIENT TEACHING
• Tell patient to take silodosin with the same meal each day.

• Warn patient about possible hypotension, and explain that it may cause dizziness.

• Caution patient against driving or operating hazardous machinery until drug's effects are known.

• If patient needs cataract surgery, advise him to inform ophthalmologist that he is taking or has taken silodosin.

simethicone
sye-METH-ih-kone

Alka-Seltzer ◇, Flatulex ◇, Gas-Aid ◇, Gas Relief ◇, Gas-X ◇, Gas-X Extra Strength ◇, Genasyme ◇, Infacol† ◇, Maalox Anti-Gas Extra Strength ◇, Maalox Anti-Gas Regular Strength ◇, Mylanta Gas ◇, Mylanta Gas Relief Extra Strength ◇, Mylicon ◇, Ovol†, Ovol Drops†, Pediacol† ◇, Phazyme ◇, Phazyme-125 ◇, Phazyme-166 Maximum Strength ◇

Therapeutic class: Antiflatulents
Pharmacologic class: Polydimethyl-siloxanes
Pregnancy risk category: C

AVAILABLE FORMS
Capsules: 125 mg ◇, 180 mg ◇
Drops: 40 mg/0.6 mL ◇
Strips (orally disintegrating): 40 mg ◇, 62.5 mg ◇
Tablets: 55 mg† ◇, 60 mg ◇, 80 mg ◇, 125 mg ◇
Tablets (chewable): 40 mg ◇, 80 mg ◇, 125 mg ◇

INDICATIONS & DOSAGES
➤ **Flatulence, functional gastric bloating**
Adults and children older than age 12: 40 to 125 mg P.O. after each meal and at bedtime, up to 500 mg daily. For drops, 40 to 80 mg P.O. after each meal and at bedtime, up to 500 mg daily.
Children ages 2 to 12: 40 mg P.O. after meals and at bedtime, up to 240 mg daily.
Children younger than age 2: 20 mg P.O. after meals and at bedtime, up to 120 mg daily.

ADMINISTRATION
P.O.
• Shake drops well before giving.
• Fill the dropper to the ordered dosage level and then give slowly into the infant's mouth, toward the inner cheek.
• The dose can also be mixed with 1 ounce of cool water, infant formula, or juice.

ACTION
Disperses mucus-surrounded gas pockets in the GI tract.

Route	Onset	Peak	Duration
P.O.	Immediate	Immediate	Unknown

Half-life: Unknown.

ADVERSE REACTIONS
GI: belching, flatus.

INTERACTIONS
None significant.

EFFECTS ON LAB TEST RESULTS
None reported.

CONTRAINDICATIONS & CAUTIONS
• Contraindicated in patients hypersensitive to drug.
• For infant colic, safety is unknown.

NURSING CONSIDERATIONS
• Drug doesn't prevent gas formation.
• *Look alike–sound alike:* Don't confuse simethicone with cimetidine.

PATIENT TEACHING
• Tell patient to chew tablet before swallowing.

S

• Tell parent that drops may be mixed with 1 ounce of cool water, infant formula, or juice.
• Advise patient that changing positions often and walking will help pass flatus.

simvastatin (synvinolin)
sim-va-STAH-tin

Zocor✣

Therapeutic class: Antilipemics
Pharmacologic class: HMG-CoA reductase inhibitors
Pregnancy risk category: X

AVAILABLE FORMS
Tablets: 5 mg, 10 mg, 20 mg, 40 mg, 80 mg

INDICATIONS & DOSAGES
Adjust-a-dose (for all indications): In patients taking fibrates or niacin, maximum is 10 mg P.O. simvastatin daily. In patients taking dronedarone, diltiazem, or verapamil, maximum is 10 mg P.O. simvastatin daily. In patients taking amiodarone, amlodipine, or ranolazine, maximum is 20 mg daily. In patients with severe renal insufficiency, start with 5 mg P.O. daily.
➤ **To reduce risk of death from CV disease and CV events in patients at high risk for coronary events, to reduce total and LDL cholesterol, apolipoprotein B, and triglyceride levels and increase HDL cholesterol level in patients with primary hyperlipidemia and mixed dyslipidemia; to reduce triglyceride levels; to reduce triglyceride levels and very low-density lipoprotein cholesterol level in patients with dysbetalipoproteinemia**
Adults: Initially, 20 to 40 mg P.O. daily in evening. In patients at high risk for a coronary artery disease (CAD) event due to existing CAD, diabetes, peripheral vascular disease, or history of stroke, the recommended initial dose is 40 mg P.O. daily. Adjust dosage every 4 weeks based on patient tolerance and response. Maximum, 80 mg daily, used with caution.
➤ **To reduce total and LDL cholesterol levels in patients with homozygous familial hypercholesterolemia**

Adults: 40 mg P.O. daily in evening; or 80 mg daily in three divided doses of 20 mg in morning, 20 mg in afternoon, and 40 mg in evening.
➤ **Heterozygous familial hypercholesterolemia**
Children ages 10 to 17: Give 10 mg P.O. once daily in the evening. Maximum, 40 mg daily.

ADMINISTRATION
P.O.
• Give drug in the evening.

ACTION
Inhibits HMG-CoA reductase, an early (and rate-limiting) step in cholesterol biosynthesis.

Route	Onset	Peak	Duration
P.O.	Unknown	1–2 hr	Unknown

Half-life: 3 hours.

ADVERSE REACTIONS
CNS: asthenia, headache.
GI: abdominal pain, constipation, diarrhea, dyspepsia, flatulence, nausea, vomiting.
Respiratory: upper respiratory tract infection.

INTERACTIONS
Drug-drug. *Amiodarone, amlodipine, ranolazine:* May increase risk of myopathy and rhabdomyolysis. Don't exceed 20 mg simvastatin daily.
Azole antifungals (fluconazole, itraconazole, ketoconazole), **macrolides (azithromycin, clarithromycin, erythromycin, telithromycin):** May increase simvastatin level and adverse effects. Avoid using together or, if it can't be avoided, suspend simvastatin therapy for course of treatment.
Bile acid sequestrants (cholestyramine, colestipol): May decrease GI absorption of simvastatin. Separate administration times by at least 4 hours.
Cyclosporine, *danazol, fibrates:* May increase risk of myopathy and rhabdomyolysis. Use together is contraindicated.
Digoxin: May slightly increase digoxin level. Closely monitor digoxin levels at the start of simvastatin therapy.

---

*Dronedarone, diltiazem, **verapamil:** May increase risk of myopathy and rhabdomyolysis. Don't exceed 10 mg simvastatin daily.*
Efavirenz, rifampin: May decrease simvastatin level. Monitor effectiveness.
Hepatotoxic drugs: May increase risk for hepatotoxicity. Avoid using together.
Nefazodone, protease inhibitors (amprenavir, atazanavir, darunavir, fosamprenavir, indinavir, lopinavir–ritonavir, nelfinavir, ritonavir, saquinavir, telaprevir): May inhibit metabolism of simvastatin and increase the risk of adverse effects, including rhabdomyolysis. Use together is contraindicated.
Niacin: May increase risk of myopathy and rhabdomyolysis with niacin dose of 1 g/day or more. Chinese patients are at particular risk and shouldn't receive simvastatin 80 mg with lipid-modifying dose of niacin-containing products.
Warfarin: May slightly enhance anticoagulant effect. Monitor PT and INR when therapy starts or dose is adjusted.
Drug-herb. *Eucalyptus, jin bu huan, kava:* May increase risk of hepatotoxicity. Discourage use together.
Red yeast rice: May increase risk of adverse events or toxicity because it contains similar components to those in drugs. Discourage use together.
St. John's wort: May decrease simvastatin level. Discourage use together.
Drug-food. *Grapefruit juice:* Large amounts (greater than 1 quart/day) may increase drug levels, increasing risk of adverse effects, including myopathy and rhabdomyolysis. Discourage use together.
Drug-lifestyle. *Alcohol use:* May increase risk of hepatotoxicity. Discourage use together.

EFFECTS ON LAB TEST RESULTS
● May increase glycosylated hemoglobin (HbA$_{1c}$), fasting blood sugar, ALT, AST, and CK levels.

CONTRAINDICATIONS & CAUTIONS
● Simvastatin occasionally causes myopathy manifested as muscle pain, tenderness, or weakness, with CK more than 10 times the upper limit of normal. Myopathy sometimes takes the form of rhabdomyolysis with or without acute renal failure sec-

ondary to myoglobinuria, and rare fatalities have occurred. The risk of myopathy, including rhabdomyolysis, is dose related. Predisposing factors for myopathy include advanced age (65 and older), female gender, uncontrolled hypothyroidism, and renal impairment.
● Contraindicated in patients hypersensitive to drug and in those with active liver disease or conditions that cause unexplained persistent elevations of transaminase levels.
● Contraindicated in pregnant and breast-feeding women and in women of childbearing age.
● Contraindicated for use at its highest dosage (80 mg/day) in patients not previously prescribed simvastatin or in patients who have had prior muscle toxicity. Patients who can't reach their goal LDL cholesterol level on 40-mg dose should be switched to an alternative agent. Only patients who have tolerated the 80-mg dose without muscle toxicity for more than 12 months should continue taking 80 mg daily.
● Use cautiously in patients who consume large amounts of alcohol or have a history of liver disease.
● Rare reports of cognitive impairment (memory loss, forgetfulness, amnesia, memory impairment, confusion) have been associated with statin use. These reported symptoms are generally not serious and are reversible upon statin discontinuation, with variable times to symptom onset (1 day to years) and symptom resolution (median of 3 weeks).
● Use cautiously when treating Chinese patients with simvastatin dosages exceeding 20 mg/day administered with lipid-modifying doses of niacin-containing products (niacin 1 g/day or more) because of the increased risk of myopathy. Don't give Chinese patients simvastatin 80 mg with lipid-modifying doses of niacin-containing products. It's unknown whether this increased risk of myopathy also applies to other Asian patients.

NURSING CONSIDERATIONS
● Obtain LFT results before initiation of treatment and thereafter when clinically indicated. Obtain lipid determinations

S

after 4 weeks of therapy and periodically thereafter.
• Monitor all patients for myopathy (unexplained muscle pain, weakness, or tenderness). Periodic CK determinations may be considered in patients starting therapy or in patients whose dosage is being increased, but there's no assurance that such monitoring will prevent myopathy.
• Patient should follow a diet restricted in saturated fat and cholesterol during therapy.
• Interrupt statin therapy if patient shows signs or symptoms of serious liver injury, hyperbilirubinemia, or jaundice. Don't restart drug if another cause can't be found.
• A daily dose of 40 mg significantly reduces risk of death from CAD, nonfatal MI, stroke, and revascularization procedures.
• *Look alike–sound alike:* Don't confuse Zocor with Cozaar.

PATIENT TEACHING
• Instruct patient to take drug in the evening.
• Teach patient about proper dietary management of cholesterol and triglycerides. When appropriate, recommend weight control, exercise, and smoking cessation programs.
• Inform patient that rare instances of memory loss and confusion have occurred with statin use. These reported events were generally not serious and resolved when drug was discontinued.
• Tell patient that drug may increase blood sugar level but the CV benefits are thought to outweigh the slight increase in risk.
• Tell patient to immediately report unexplained muscle pain, tenderness, or weakness (especially if accompanied by malaise or fever) and loss of appetite, upper abdominal pain, dark-colored urine, or yellowing of skin or eyes.
◗ *Alert:* Tell woman to stop drug and notify prescriber immediately if she is or may be pregnant or if she's breast-feeding.

SAFETY ALERT!

sirolimus
sir-AH-lih-mus

Rapamune

Therapeutic class: Immunosuppressants
Pharmacologic class: Immunosuppressants
Pregnancy risk category: C

AVAILABLE FORMS
Oral solution: 1 mg/mL
Tablets: 0.5 mg, 1 mg, 2 mg

INDICATIONS & DOSAGES
➤ **With cyclosporine and corticosteroids, to prevent organ rejection in patients receiving renal transplants**
Adults and adolescents: Initially, 6 mg P.O. for patients with low to moderate immunologic risk weighing 40 kg (88 lb) or more or 3 mg/m^2 for patients weighing less than 40 kg as one-time dose as soon as possible after transplantation; then maintenance dose of 2 mg P.O. once daily for patients weighing 40 kg or more or 1 mg/m^2 P.O. once daily for patients weighing less than 40 kg. For patients with high immunologic risk, may give up to 15 mg P.O. on day 1 after transplantation, then 5 mg/day P.O. beginning on day 2 after transplantation.
    Maximum daily dose shouldn't exceed 40 mg. If a daily dose exceeds 40 mg due to a loading dose, give the loading dose over 2 days. Monitor trough concentrations at least 3 to 4 days after a loading dose.
Children age 13 and older weighing less than 40 kg (88 lb): First dose is 3 mg/m^2 P.O. as one-time dose after transplantation; then 1 mg/m^2 P.O. once daily.
Adjust-a-dose: For patients with mild to moderate hepatic impairment, reduce maintenance dose by about one-third, and by about one-half in patients with severe hepatic impairment. It isn't necessary to reduce loading dose. Two to 4 months after transplant in patients with low to moderate risk of graft rejection, taper off cyclosporine over 4 to 8 weeks. While tapering cyclosporine, adjust sirolimus dose every 1 to 2 weeks to obtain levels between 12 and

24 nanograms/mL. Base dosage adjustments on clinical status, tissue biopsies, and laboratory findings.

ADMINISTRATION
P.O.
• Follow safe-handling procedures when preparing, administering, and dispensing drug.
• Give drug consistently either with or without food.
• Patients should swallow tablets whole. Don't crush or split tablets.
• Dilute oral solution before use. After dilution, use immediately and discard oral solution syringe.
• When diluting oral solution, empty correct amount into glass or plastic (not Styrofoam) container holding at least ¼ cup (60 mL) of either water or orange juice. Don't use grapefruit juice or any other liquid. Stir vigorously and have patient drink immediately. Refill container with at least ½ cup (120 mL) of water or orange juice, stir again, and have patient drink all contents.
• A slight haze may develop during refrigeration, which doesn't affect potency of drug. If haze develops, bring to room temperature and shake until haze disappears.
• Store away from light, and refrigerate at 36° to 46° F (2° to 8° C). After opening bottle, use contents within 1 month. If needed, store bottles and pouches at room temperature (up to 77° F [25° C]) for several days. Drug may be kept in oral syringe for 24 hours at room temperature.

ACTION
Inhibits T-cell activation and proliferation that occurs in response to antigenic and cytokine stimulation. Also inhibits antibody formation.

Route	Onset	Peak	Duration
P.O.	Unknown	1–3 hr	Unknown

Half-life: About 62 hours.

ADVERSE REACTIONS
CNS: fever, headache.
CV: chest pain, edema, hypertension, peripheral edema, tachycardia, *thrombosis.*

EENT: epistaxis.
GI: abdominal pain, constipation, diarrhea, nausea, ascites.
GU: UTI, *toxic nephropathy,* dysuria, glycosuria, hematuria, hemolytic-uremic syndrome, polynephritis.
Hematologic: anemia, *thrombocytopenia, leukopenia, thrombotic thrombocytopenia purpura,* ecchymosis.
Hepatic: *hepatic artery thrombosis, hepatotoxicity.*
Metabolic: hypercholesteremia, *hyperkalemia,* hyperlipidemia, hypokalemia, hypophosphatemia, *hypoglycemia, acidosis, diabetes mellitus,* dehydration, hypercalcemia, hyperglycemia.
Musculoskeletal: arthralgia, back pain, bone necrosis, myalgia.
Respiratory: atelectasis, cough, dyspnea, upper respiratory tract infection, *interstitial lung disease, asthma,* bronchitis, *hypoxia,* lung edema, pleural effusion, pneumonia.
Skin: acne, rash, fungal dermatitis, pruritus, *melanoma, squamous cell carcinoma, basal cell carcinoma.*
Other: *sepsis;* abnormal healing, including fascial dehiscence and anastomotic disruption (wound, vascular, airway, ureteral, biliary); abscess; flu syndrome; infection; lymphadenopathy; lymphocele; hypersensitivity reactions; *angioedema;* herpes simplex; herpes zoster.

INTERACTIONS
Drug-drug. *Aminoglycosides, amphotericin B, other nephrotoxic drugs:* May increase risk of nephrotoxicity. Use with caution.
Amiodarone, bromocriptine, cimetidine, clarithromycin, clotrimazole, danazol, erythromycin, fluconazole, indinavir, itraconazole, metoclopramide, nicardipine, posaconazole, ritonavir, verapamil, voriconazole, other drugs that inhibit. CYP3A4: May increase blood levels of sirolimus. Monitor sirolimus levels closely.
Carbamazepine, phenobarbital, phenytoin, rifabutin, rifapentine, other drugs that induce CYP3A4: May decrease blood levels of sirolimus. Monitor patient closely.
Cyclosporine: May increase sirolimus level and toxicity. Give sirolimus 4 hours after cyclosporine; monitor levels and adjust dose, as needed.

S

Diltiazem: May increase sirolimus levels. Monitor sirolimus level, as needed.

HMG-CoA reductase inhibitors or fibrates: May increase risk of rhabdomyolysis with the combination of sirolimus and cyclosporine. Monitor patient closely.

Ketoconazole: May increase rate and extent of sirolimus absorption. Avoid using together.

Live-virus vaccines: May reduce vaccine effectiveness. Avoid using together.

Rifampin: May decrease sirolimus level. Alternative therapy to rifampin may be prescribed.

Drug-herb. *St. John's wort:* May decrease sirolimus levels. Discourage use together.

Drug-food. *Grapefruit juice:* May decrease drug metabolism. Discourage use together.

Drug-lifestyle. *Sun exposure:* May increase risk of skin cancer. Advise patient to avoid sunlight exposure.

EFFECTS ON LAB TEST RESULTS
● May increase BUN, creatinine, liver enzyme, cholesterol, and lipid levels. May increase or decrease phosphate, potassium, and glucose levels.
● May increase RBC count. May decrease platelet count. May increase or decrease WBC count.

CONTRAINDICATIONS & CAUTIONS
● Contraindicated in patients hypersensitive to active drug, its derivatives, or components of product.
● Use cautiously in patients with hyperlipidemia and impaired liver and renal function.
Black Box Warning Safety and effectiveness of sirolimus as immunosuppressive therapy haven't been established in liver or lung transplant patients. Use in these patients isn't recommended. ∎
⚠ *Overdose S&S:* Exaggerated adverse effects.

NURSING CONSIDERATIONS
Black Box Warning Using this drug with tacrolimus or cyclosporine may cause hepatic artery thrombosis, leading to graft loss and death in liver transplant patients. ∎
Black Box Warning Only those experienced in immunosuppressive therapy and man-

agement of renal transplant patients should prescribe drug. ∎
⟐ **Alert:** Drugs causing immunosuppression increase the risk of opportunistic infections, including activation of latent viral infections such as BK virus–associated neuropathy, which may lead to serious outcomes, including kidney graft loss.
⟐ **Alert:** This drug has been associated with angioedema; using it with ACE inhibitors increases the risk. Monitor the patient closely.
● Use drug in regimen with cyclosporine and corticosteroids; have patient take drug 4 hours after cyclosporine dose.
● Dosage adjustment more often than every 7 to 14 days may result in overdose due to the long half-life of sirolimus.
● Cyclosporine withdrawal in patients with high risk of graft rejection isn't recommended. This includes patients with Banff grade III acute rejection or vascular rejection before cyclosporine withdrawal, those who are dialysis dependent, those with serum creatinine level greater than 4.5 mg/dL, black patients, patients with retransplants or multiorgan transplants, and patients with high panel of reactive antibodies.
● After transplantation, give antimicrobial prophylaxis for *Pneumocystis jiroveci (carinii)* for 1 year and for cytomegalovirus for 3 months.
Black Box Warning Patients taking drug are more susceptible to infection and lymphoma. ∎
● Monitor renal function tests because use with cyclosporine may cause creatinine level to increase. Adjustment of immunosuppressive regimen may be needed.
● Monitor cholesterol and triglyceride levels. Treatment with lipid-lowering drugs during therapy isn't uncommon. If hyperlipidemia is detected, additional interventions, such as diet and exercise, should begin.
● Check for rhabdomyolysis.
● Monitor drug levels in patients age 13 and older who weigh less than 40 kg (88 lb), patients with hepatic impairment, those also receiving drugs that induce or inhibit CYP3A4, and patients in whom

---

Reactions in bold italics are *life-threatening*. Interactions may have a *rapid onset* or a *delayed onset*.

cyclosporine dosing is markedly reduced or stopped.

• Monitor patient for impaired or delayed wound healing, including wound dehiscence, and fluid accumulation, including edema, lymphedema, pleural effusion, ascites, and pericardial effusion.

PATIENT TEACHING
• Teach patient how to properly store, dilute, and give drug.
• Advise woman about risks during pregnancy. Tell her to use effective contraception before and during therapy and for 12 weeks after stopping therapy.
• Tell patient to take drug consistently with or without food to minimize absorption variability.
• Tell patient to take drug 4 hours after cyclosporine to avoid drug interactions.
• Advise patient to wash area with soap and water if drug solution touches skin or mucous membranes.
• Advise patient to limit ultraviolet light and sun exposure because of the increased risk of skin cancer.

SAFETY ALERT!

sitagliptin phosphate
sit-ah-GLIP-ten

Januvia◆

Therapeutic class: Antidiabetics
Pharmacologic class: DPP-4 enzyme inhibitors
Pregnancy risk category: B

AVAILABLE FORMS
Tablets: 25 mg, 50 mg, 100 mg

INDICATIONS & DOSAGES
➤ **To improve glycemic control in addition to diet and exercise in type 2 diabetes, alone or with metformin or a thiazolidinedione**
Adults: 100 mg P.O. once daily.
Adjust-a-dose: For patients with CrCl of 30 to 49 mL/minute, give 50 mg once daily; for patients with CrCl less than 30 mL/minute or ESRD with hemodialysis or peritoneal dialysis, give 25 mg once daily. Give without regard to timing of dialysis session.

ADMINISTRATION
P.O.
• Give drug without regard for food.

ACTION
Inhibits DPP-4, an enzyme that rapidly inactivates incretin hormones, which play a part in the body's regulation of glucose. By increasing and prolonging active incretin levels, the drug helps to increase insulin release and decrease circulating glucose.

Route	Onset	Peak	Duration
P.O.	Rapid	1–4 hr	Unknown

Half-life: About 12½ hours.

ADVERSE REACTIONS
CNS: headache.
EENT: nasopharyngitis.
GI: abdominal pain, nausea, diarrhea.
Metabolic: *hypoglycemia.*
Respiratory: upper respiratory tract infection.

INTERACTIONS
None significant.

EFFECTS ON LAB TEST RESULTS
• May increase creatinine level.
• May increase WBC count.

CONTRAINDICATIONS & CAUTIONS
• Contraindicated in patients with type 1 diabetes or diabetic ketoacidosis.
• Contraindicated in patients with a history of hypersensitivity to sitagliptin.
• Use cautiously in patients with moderate to severe renal insufficiency or a history of pancreatitis and in those taking other antidiabetics.
• Safety and effectiveness of drug in children haven't been evaluated.

NURSING CONSIDERATIONS
• In elderly patients and those at risk for renal insufficiency, periodically assess renal function.
• Assess renal function before start of therapy and periodically thereafter.

S

- Monitor glycosylated hemoglobin level periodically to assess long-term glycemic control.
- Management of type 2 diabetes should include diet control. Because caloric restrictions, weight loss, and exercise help improve insulin sensitivity and help make drug therapy effective, these measures are essential for proper diabetes management.
- Watch for hypoglycemia, especially in patients receiving combination therapy.
- Monitor patient for pancreatitis (persistent abdominal pain with or without vomiting). Discontinue drug if pancreatitis is suspected.
- *Look alike–sound alike:* Don't confuse sitagliptin with saxagliptin.

PATIENT TEACHING
- Tell patient that drug isn't a substitute for diet and exercise and that it's important to follow a prescribed dietary and physical activity routine and to monitor his glucose levels.
- Advise patient that acute pancreatitis has occurred with sitagliptin therapy. Instruct patient to immediately report persistent, severe abdominal pain that may radiate to the back, with or without vomiting.
- Inform patient and family members of the signs and symptoms of hyperglycemia and hypoglycemia and the steps to take if these symptoms occur.
- Provide patient with information on complications associated with diabetes and ways to assess for them.
- Tell patient to notify prescriber during periods of stress, such as fever, infection, or surgery; dosage may need adjustment.
- Tell patient drug may be taken without regard for food.

SAFETY ALERT!

sitagliptin–simvastatin
sit-ah-GLIP-ten/sim-va-STAH-tin

Juvisync

Therapeutic class: Antidiabetics–antilipemics
Pharmacologic class: DDP-4 enzyme inhibitors–HMG-CoA reductase inhibitors
Pregnancy risk category: X

AVAILABLE FORMS
Tablets: 50 mg sitagliptin and 10 mg simvastatin, 50 mg sitagliptin and 20 mg simvastatin, 50 mg sitagliptin and 40 mg simvastatin, 100 mg sitagliptin and 10 mg simvastatin, 100 mg sitagliptin and 20 mg simvastatin, 100 mg sitagliptin and 40 mg simvastatin

INDICATIONS & DOSAGES
➤ **Adjunct to diet and exercise to improve glycemic control in type 2 diabetes; adjunct to diet for hyperlipidemia, homozygous familial hypercholesterolemia; prevention of coronary events**
Adults: Initially, 100 mg sitagliptin/40 mg simvastatin P.O. once daily in evening. For patients already taking simvastatin, initiate sitagliptin–simvastatin at 100 mg sitagliptin and patient's current simvastatin dose. After initiation or dosage titration, lipid levels may be analyzed after 4 or more weeks and dosage adjusted, if needed.
Adjust-a-dose: For patients with moderate renal impairment (CrCl of 30 to less than 50 mL/minute [serum creatinine approximately 1.7 to 3 mg/dL in men or 1.5 to 2.5 mg/dL in women]), recommended starting dosage is sitagliptin 50 mg/simvastatin 40 mg once daily. For patients with moderate renal impairment already taking simvastatin (10, 20, or 40 mg daily) with or without sitagliptin 50 mg daily, sitagliptin–simvastatin may be initiated at the dose of sitagliptin 50 mg and the dose of simvastatin already being taken. No dosage adjustment is necessary for patients with mild renal impairment (CrCl of 50 mL/minute or more [serum creatinine approximately

1.7 mg/dL or less in men or 1.5 mg/dL or less in women]). Drug isn't recommended for patients with severe renal impairment or ESRD and is contraindicated in patients with active liver disease, including unexplained transaminase elevations.

ADMINISTRATION
P.O.
• Administer drug in the evening.
• Patient should swallow tablet whole and not split or crush it.
• Store at room temperature with cap tightly closed.

ACTION
Sitagliptin increases and prolongs the effects of incretin hormones, therefore increasing insulin release and decreasing glucagon levels. Simvastatin inhibits cholesterol formation by inhibiting HMG-CoA reductase, an enzyme responsible for the biosynthesis of cholesterol.

Route	Onset	Peak	Duration
P.O. (sitagliptin)	Rapid	1–4 hr	Unknown
P.O. (simvastatin)	Unknown	4–6 hr	Unknown

Half-life: Sitagliptin, 12.4 hours; simvastatin, unknown.

ADVERSE REACTIONS
CNS: headache, insomnia, vertigo.
CV: atrial fibrillation, edema.
EENT: nasopharyngitis.
GI: abdominal pain, constipation, gastritis, nausea, pancreatitis.
GU: UTI.
Metabolic: hypoglycemia, diabetes mellitus.
Musculoskeletal: myalgia.
Respiratory: upper respiratory tract infection, bronchitis, sinusitis.
Skin: eczema.

INTERACTIONS
Drug-drug. *Amiodarone, amlodipine, ranolazine:* May increase risk of myopathy and rhabdomyolysis. Maximum dosage is sitagliptin 100 mg/simvastatin 20 mg.
Bile acid sequestrants (colestipol, cholestyramine): May decrease simvastatin absorption. Separate administration times by as much as possible (give bile acid se-

questrants at least 4 hours before simvastatin).
Bosentan: May decrease simvastatin level. Closely monitor patient; adjust simvastatin dosage as needed.
Calcium channel blockers (such as diltiazem, verapamil): May increase risk of myopathy, including rhabdomyolysis. Maximum dosage is sitagliptin 100 mg/simvastatin 10 mg.
Carbamazepine: May decrease simvastatin level. Monitor patient closely.
Colchicine, lipid-lowering drugs that cause myopathy (fibrates): May increase risk of myopathy and rhabdomyolysis. Use together cautiously.
Conivaptan: May increase simvastatin level. Don't use together; restart simvastatin therapy at least 1 week after conivaptan therapy is completed.
Coumarin anticoagulants: May increase prothrombin time (PT) and INR. Determine baseline PT before initiation of sitagliptin–simvastatin therapy and recheck frequently during early therapy.
Cyclosporine, danazol, gemfibrozil: May increase risk of myopathy and rhabdomyolysis. Use together is contraindicated.
Digoxin: May increase digoxin level. Monitor digoxin level.
Diltiazem, dronedarone, verapamil: May increase risk of myopathy and rhabdomyolysis. Don't exceed simvastatin dosage of 20 mg daily.
HIV protease inhibitors, nefazodone, strong CYP3A4 inhibitors (such as clarithromycin, erythromycin, itraconazole, ketoconazole, posaconazole, telithromycin): May increase risk of myopathy and rhabdomyolysis. Use together is contraindicated. If treatment with these agents is unavoidable, temporarily stop sitagliptin–simvastatin and treat only with sitagliptin for management of glycemic control.
Insulin, sulfonylureas: May increase risk of hypoglycemia. Use cautiously together and decrease insulin or sulfonylurea dosage as appropriate.
Niacin at lipid-modifying doses: May increase risk of myopathy and rhabdomyolysis, especially in Chinese patients. Use cautiously together.

S

Nonnucleoside reverse transcriptase inhibitors (NNRTIs; delavirdine, efavirenz): Delavirdine may increase simvastatin level and risk of myopathy. Efavirenz may decrease simvastatin level. Monitor patient and LDL level closely, especially when starting or stopping NNRTIs.

Ticagrelor: May increase simvastatin level and risk of adverse reactions. Do not exceed simvastatin dosage of 40 mg daily.

Voriconazole: May increase simvastatin level. Consider decreasing simvastatin dosage during voriconazole treatment.

Drug-food. *Grapefruit juice in large quantities (greater than 1 quart daily):* May increase simvastatin plasma level. Encourage decreased juice intake (less than 1 quart/day).

Drug-herb. *St. John's wort:* May decrease simvastatin level, possibly decreasing efficacy. Avoid use together if possible.

Drug-lifestyle. *Alcohol use:* May increase risk of liver damage. Avoid excessive use.

EFFECTS ON LAB TEST RESULTS
● May increase alkaline phosphatase, creatinine, CK, gamma-glutamyltransferase, and hepatic transaminase levels.

CONTRAINDICATIONS & CAUTIONS
● Contraindicated in patients with history of serious hypersensitivity reaction (angioedema or anaphylaxis) to components of sitagliptin or simvastatin and in those with moderate to severe renal failure, end-stage renal failure, or active liver disease, including patients with unexplained persistent hepatic transaminase elevations.
● Contraindicated in women who are pregnant, may become pregnant, or are breast-feeding.
● Use cautiously in Chinese patients taking sitagliptin 100 mg/simvastatin 40 mg and niacin-containing products at lipid-lowering doses because of increased risk of myopathy. It isn't known if risk applies to other Asian patients.
● Use cautiously in elderly patients, female patients, those with uncontrolled hypothyroidism, and those with mild renal impairment because of increased risk of myopathy and rhabdomyolysis. Risk is dose-related.

NURSING CONSIDERATIONS
● Monitor renal function tests and LFTs before start of therapy and periodically thereafter if clinically indicated.
● Monitor lipid panel for 4 or more weeks after start of therapy and with dosage titration.
● Obtain periodic blood glucose and glycosylated hemoglobin (HbA$_{1c}$) testing.
● If patient is prescribed a coumarin anticoagulant, determine baseline PT before starting sitagliptin–simvastatin therapy. Then obtain PT frequently during early therapy and with sitagliptin–simvastatin dosage titration to determine if anticoagulant dosage needs adjustment.
● Monitor patient for acute pancreatitis (persistent severe abdominal pain that may radiate to the back, with or without vomiting). If present, discontinue drug immediately.
● Monitor patient for myopathy (muscle pain, tenderness, weakness, CK at least 10 times the upper limit of normal), especially after start of therapy and with dosage increase.

PATIENT TEACHING
● Advise patient about importance of adhering to low cholesterol and diabetic diet and maintaining regular physical activity.
● Inform patient that periodic blood glucose, HbA$_{1c}$, and fasting lipid panel testing will be needed.
● Teach patient how to recognize and manage hypoglycemia and hyperglycemia.
● Caution patient that medication requirements may change during periods of stress (fever, trauma, infection, or surgery) and to immediately contact health care provider if stress occurs.
● Advise patient that acute pancreatitis has occurred with sitagliptin therapy. Instruct patient to immediately report persistent, severe abdominal pain that may radiate to the back, with or without vomiting.
● Teach patient signs and symptoms of an allergic reaction (rash; hives; swelling of the face, lips, tongue, or throat; difficulty swallowing or breathing). Instruct patient to immediately discontinue drug and seek immediate medical attention if any of these occur.

• Advise patient to swallow tablets whole and not split, crush, or chew them.
• Counsel patient to inform all his health care providers that he is taking sitagliptin–simvastatin. Dosage adjustments may be needed.
• Instruct patient not to drink excessive amounts (greater than 1 quart daily) of grapefruit juice during therapy.
• Inform patient of risk of myopathy, including rhabdomyolysis. Caution patient to promptly report unexplained muscle pain, tenderness, or weakness and to discontinue sitagliptin–simvastatin immediately.
• Caution women of childbearing age to use effective birth control during therapy. If pregnancy occurs, patient should discontinue drug and inform her health care provider.
• Advise breast-feeding women not to use sitagliptin–simvastatin.

sodium bicarbonate
Neut

Therapeutic class: Antacids
Pharmacologic class: Alkalinizers
Pregnancy risk category: C

AVAILABLE FORMS
Injection: 4% (2.4 mEq/5 mL), 4.2% (5 mEq/10 mL), 5% (297.5 mEq/500 mL), 7.5% (8.92 mEq/10 mL and 44.6 mEq/ 50 mL), 8.4% (10 mEq/10 mL and 50 mEq/ 50 mL)
Powder: 30 mg/½ tsp ◇
Tablets: 325 mg ◇, 650 mg ◇

INDICATIONS & DOSAGES
➤ **Metabolic acidosis**
Adults and children: Dosage depends on blood carbon dioxide content, pH, and patient's condition; usually, 2 to 5 mEq/kg I.V. infused over 4- to 8-hour period. Or 7,800 to 15,600 mg (12 to 24 650-mg tablets) dissolved in 1 to 2 L of water and consumed over 1 hour.
➤ **Urinary alkalinization**
Adults: Initially, 3,900 mg P.O.; then 1,300 to 2,600 mg every 4 hours; dosage based on urine pH.

Children: 84 to 840 mg/kg daily in four divided doses. Titrate based on urine pH.
➤ **Antacid**
Adults and children older than age 6: 300 mg to 2 g P.O. up to q.i.d. taken with glass of water. Or 30 mg (½ tsp) oral powder in 120 mL water every 2 hours up to six doses daily for patients under age 60, or three doses daily for patients over age 60.
➤ **Cardiac arrest**
Adults and children age 2 and older: Administer according to results of arterial blood pH, partial pressure of arterial carbon dioxide, and calculated base deficit. Usual dose is 200 to 300 mEq of bicarbonate given as 7.5% or 8.4% solution. Then redetermine serum pH and bicarbonate concentration.
Children younger than age 2: 1 mEq/kg (1 mL/kg of 8.4% solution) I.V. slowly followed by 1 mEq/kg every 10 minutes of arrest. Don't give more than 8 mEq/kg I.V. total; a 4.2% solution may be preferred.
➤ **Prevention of contrast media nephrotoxicity ◆**
Adults: 154 mEq/L at 3 mL/kg/hour I.V. for 1 hour before contrast administration, followed by an infusion of 1 mL/kg/hour for 6 hours after the procedure.

ADMINISTRATION
P.O.
• Not for use with sodium-restricted diet.
• May be given without regard to meals for urinary alkalinization, 1 to 2 hours after meals as an antacid, and 2 hour apart from other medications, with a full glass of water.
• Dissolve powder in 120 mL water; dissolve granules in 120 to 180 mL cool water.
• Tablets may be swallowed whole or dissolved in water.
I.V.
▼ Drug isn't routinely used in cardiac arrest because it may produce a paradoxical acidosis from carbon dioxide production. It shouldn't be routinely given during the early stages of resuscitation unless acidosis is clearly present.
▼ The 4% form is usually used for neutralizing I.V. drugs such as erythromycin. Consult pharmacist before use.
▼ Flush I.V. line thoroughly between medications.

S

▼ **Incompatibilities:** Alcohol 5% in dextrose 5%; allopurinol; amino acids; amiodarone; amobarbital; amphotericin B; ascorbic acid injection; atropine; bupivacaine; calcium salts; carbenicillin; carboplatin; carmustine; cefotaxime; chlorpromazine; ciprofloxacin; cisatracurium; cisplatin; codeine; corticotropin; dextrose 5% in lactated Ringer's injection; diazepam; diltiazem; dobutamine; dopamine; doxapram; doxorubicin liposomal; doxycycline; epinephrine hydrochloride; fat emulsion 10%; fenoldopam; glycopyrrolate; hetastarch; hydromorphone; idarubicin; imipenem–cilastatin sodium; inamrinone; Ionosol B, D, or G with invert sugar 10%; isoproterenol; labetalol; lactated Ringer's injection; levorphanol; leucovorin calcium; lidocaine; magnesium sulfate; meperidine; meropenem; metaraminol; methylprednisolone sodium succinate; metoclopramide; midazolam; morphine sulfate; MVI-12 multivitamin; nafcillin; nalbuphine; nitrofurantoin; norepinephrine bitartrate; ondansetron; oxacillin; penicillin G potassium; pentazocine lactate; pentobarbital sodium; procaine; Ringer's injection; sargramostim; 1/6 M sodium lactate; streptomycin; succinylcholine; thiopental; ticarcillin disodium–clavulanate potassium; vancomycin; verapamil; vinca alkaloids; vitamin B complex with vitamin C. Drug inactivates catecholamines, such as norepinephrine, dobutamine, and dopamine, and it forms precipitate with calcium. Don't mix with these drugs, and flush line thoroughly.

ACTION

Restores buffering capacity of the body and neutralizes excess acid.

Route	Onset	Peak	Duration
P.O.	Unknown	Unknown	Unknown
I.V.	Immediate	Immediate	Unknown

Half-life: Unknown.

ADVERSE REACTIONS

CNS: tetany.
CV: edema.
GI: gastric distention, belching, flatulence.

Metabolic: hypokalemia, *metabolic alkalosis,* hypernatremia, hyperosmolarity with overdose.
Skin: pain and irritation at injection site.

INTERACTIONS

Drug-drug. *Anorexiants, flecainide, mecamylamine, methenamine, quinidine, sympathomimetics:* May decrease renal clearance of these drugs and increase risk of toxicity. Monitor patient closely for toxicity.
Chlorpropamide, lithium, methotrexate, salicylates, tetracycline: May increase urine alkalinization, increase renal clearance of these drugs, and decrease their effect. Monitor patient closely for drug's effect.
Enteric-coated drugs: May be released prematurely in stomach. Avoid using together.
Ketoconazole: May decrease ketoconazole absorption. Separate use by at least 2 hours.

EFFECTS ON LAB TEST RESULTS

● May increase sodium and lactate levels.
● May decrease potassium level.

CONTRAINDICATIONS & CAUTIONS

● Contraindicated in patients with metabolic or respiratory alkalosis and in those with hypocalcemia in which alkalosis may produce tetany, hypertension, seizures, or heart failure.
● Contraindicated in patients losing chloride because of vomiting or continuous GI suction and in those receiving diuretics that produce hypochloremic alkalosis. Oral drug is contraindicated for acute ingestion of strong mineral acids.
● Use with caution in patients with renal insufficiency, heart failure, or other edematous or sodium-retaining condition.
⚠ **Overdose S&S:** Alkalosis, hyperirritability, tetany.

NURSING CONSIDERATIONS

● To avoid risk of alkalosis, obtain blood pH, partial pressure of arterial oxygen, partial pressure of arterial carbon dioxide, and electrolyte levels. Tell prescriber laboratory results.

PATIENT TEACHING

● Tell patient not to take drug with milk because doing so may cause high levels

---

Reactions in bold italics are *life-threatening*. Interactions may have a *rapid onset* or a *delayed onset*.

of calcium in the blood, abnormally high alkalinity in tissues and fluids, or kidney stones.
● Instruct patient taking a prescription drug on a sodium-restricted diet to consult health care provider before taking sodium bicarbonate.
● Tell patient to stop sodium bicarbonate and contact health care provider if symptoms (acid indigestion, heartburn, sour stomach, upset stomach) last longer than 2 weeks.
● Advise pregnant or breast-feeding patient to consult health care provider before use.

sodium ferric gluconate complex
Ferrlecit

Therapeutic class: Iron supplements
Pharmacologic class: Macromolecular iron complexes–hematinics
Pregnancy risk category: B

AVAILABLE FORMS
Injection: 62.5 mg elemental iron (12.5 mg/mL) in 5-mL ampules

INDICATIONS & DOSAGES
➤ **Iron deficiency anemia in patients receiving long-term hemodialysis and supplemental erythropoietin**
Adults and children age 15 and older: 10 mL (125 mg elemental iron) I.V. over 1 hour. Most patients need minimum cumulative dose of 1 g elemental iron given over more than eight sequential dialysis treatments to achieve a favorable hemoglobin or hematocrit response.
Children age 6 and older: 1.5 mg/kg (maximum 125 mg/dose) I.V. over 1 hour during 8 consecutive hemodialysis treatments.

ADMINISTRATION
I.V.
▼ Drug contains benzyl alcohol. Don't use in neonates.
▼ For adults, dilute in 100 mL normal saline solution; for children, dilute in

25 mL normal saline solution. Give immediately over 1 hour.
▼ Alternatively, give undiluted at a rate not to exceed 1 mL/minute (12.5 mg/minute) at the end of dialysis.
▼ Life-threatening hypersensitivity reactions, such as CV collapse, cardiac arrest, bronchospasm, oral or pharyngeal edema, dyspnea, angioedema, urticaria, and pruritus—sometimes linked to pain and muscle spasm of chest or back—may occur during infusion. Have adequate supportive measures readily available. Monitor patient closely during infusion.
▼ After rapid administration, profound hypotension with flushing, light-headedness, malaise, fatigue, weakness, or severe chest, back, flank, or groin pain may occur; these symptoms aren't hypersensitivity reactions. Monitor patient closely during infusion.
▼ **Incompatibilities:** Other I.V. drugs. Don't add drug to parenteral nutrition solutions for infusion.

ACTION
Restores total body iron content, which is critical for normal hemoglobin synthesis and oxygen transport.

Route	Onset	Peak	Duration
I.V.	Unknown	Varies	Unknown

Half-life: 1 hour in healthy, iron-deficient adults.

ADVERSE REACTIONS
CNS: asthenia, headache, fatigue, malaise, dizziness, paresthesia, agitation, insomnia, somnolence, syncope, pain, chills, fever.
CV: hypotension, hypertension, tachycardia, *bradycardia,* angina, chest pain, *MI,* edema, flushing.
EENT: conjunctivitis, abnormal vision, rhinitis.
GI: nausea, vomiting, diarrhea, rectal disorder, dyspepsia, eructation, flatulence, melena, abdominal pain.
GU: UTI.
Hematologic: anemia.
Metabolic: *hyperkalemia, hypoglycemia,* hypokalemia, hypervolemia.
Musculoskeletal: myalgia, arthralgia, back pain, arm pain, cramps.

Respiratory: dyspnea, coughing, upper respiratory tract infection, pneumonia, pulmonary edema.
Skin: pruritus, increased sweating, rash, injection-site reaction.
Other: infection, rigors, flu syndrome, *sepsis, carcinoma,* hypersensitivity reactions, lymphadenopathy.

INTERACTIONS
Drug-drug. *ACE inhibitors:* May cause sensitivity reactions. Stop I.V. iron if sensitivity reactions occur.
Oral iron preparations: May reduce absorption of oral iron preparations. Avoid using together.

EFFECTS ON LAB TEST RESULTS
● May decrease glucose and hemoglobin levels. May increase or decrease potassium level.

CONTRAINDICATIONS & CAUTIONS
● Contraindicated in patients hypersensitive to drug or its components (such as benzyl alcohol) and in those with iron overload or anemias not related to iron deficiency.
● Don't use in patients with ferritin levels greater than 1,000 nanograms/mL.
● Use cautiously in elderly patients.
⚠ **Overdose S&S:** Abdominal pain, diarrhea, vomiting, pallor or cyanosis, lassitude, drowsiness, hyperventilation, CV collapse.

NURSING CONSIDERATIONS
🔆 *Alert:* Dosage is expressed in milligrams of elemental iron.
● Drug shouldn't be used in patients with iron overload, which often occurs in hemoglobinopathies and other refractory anemias.
● Monitor ferritin level, iron saturation, hemoglobin level, and hematocrit.
● In hemodialysis patients, adverse reactions may be related to dialysis itself or to chronic renal failure.
● Check with patient about other potential sources of iron, such as OTC iron preparations and iron-containing multiple vitamins with minerals.

PATIENT TEACHING
● Abdominal pain, diarrhea, vomiting, drowsiness, and rapid breathing may indicate iron poisoning. Urge patient to notify prescriber immediately.

sodium polystyrene sulfonate
pol-ee-STYE-reen

Kalexate, Kayexalate, Kionex, SPS

Therapeutic class: Potassium-removing resins
Pharmacologic class: Cation-exchange resins
Pregnancy risk category: C

AVAILABLE FORMS
Powder: 1-lb jar (3.5 g/tsp)
Suspension: 15 g/60 mL*

INDICATIONS & DOSAGES
➤ **Hyperkalemia**
Adults: 15 g P.O. daily to q.i.d. in water or sorbitol (3 to 4 mL/g of resin). Or, mix powder with appropriate medium—aqueous suspension or diet appropriate for renal failure—and instill through a nasogastric tube. Or, 30 to 50 g (120 to 200 mL) of sorbitol every 6 hours as warm emulsion deep into sigmoid colon (20 cm).

ADMINISTRATION
P.O.
● Don't heat resin; this impairs drug's effect. Mix resin only with water or sorbitol for P.O. use. Never mix with orange juice (high potassium content) to disguise taste.
● Chill oral suspension for greater palatability.
● Oral administration is preferred because drug should remain in intestine for at least 30 minutes.
● If sorbitol is given, mix with resin suspension.
● Consider giving in solid form. Resin cookie and candy recipes are available; ask pharmacist or dietitian to supply.
Rectal
● Premixed forms (SPS and others) are available. If preparing manually, mix

---

Reactions in bold italics are *life-threatening*. Interactions may have a *rapid onset* or a *delayed onset*.

polystyrene resin only with water or sorbitol for rectal use. Don't use mineral oil for P.R. administration to prevent impaction; ion exchange needs aqueous medium. Sorbitol content prevents impaction.

• Prepare P.R. dose at room temperature. Stir emulsion gently during administration.

• Use #28 French rubber tube for rectal dose; insert 20 cm into sigmoid colon. Tape tube in place. Or, consider an indwelling urinary catheter with a 30-mL balloon inflated distal to anal sphincter to aid in retention. This is especially helpful for patients with poor sphincter control. Use gravity flow. Drain returns constantly through Y-tube connection. Place patient in knee-chest position or with hips on pillow for a while if back leakage occurs.

• After P.R. administration, flush tubing with 50 to 100 mL of nonsodium fluid to ensure delivery of all drug. Flush rectum to remove resin.

• Prevent fecal impaction in elderly patients by giving resin P.R. Give cleansing enema before P.R. administration. Have patient retain enema for 6 to 10 hours if possible, but 30 to 60 minutes is acceptable.

ACTION
Exchanges sodium ions for potassium ions in the intestine: 1 g of sodium polystyrene sulfonate is exchanged for 0.5 to 1 mEq of potassium; the resin is then eliminated. Much of the exchange capacity is used for calcium, magnesium, and possibly fats and proteins.

Route	Onset	Peak	Duration
P.O., P.R.	2–12 hr	Unknown	Unknown

Half-life: Unknown.

ADVERSE REACTIONS
GI: constipation, diarrhea (with sorbitol emulsions), fecal impaction, anorexia, gastric irritation, nausea, vomiting.
Metabolic: hypokalemia, hypocalcemia, *hypomagnesemia,* sodium retention.

INTERACTIONS
Drug-drug. *Antacids and laxatives containing magnesium and calcium:* May cause systemic alkalosis and reduce potassium exchange capability. Avoid using together.

EFFECTS ON LAB TEST RESULTS
• May increase sodium level. May decrease potassium, calcium, and magnesium levels.

CONTRAINDICATIONS & CAUTIONS
• Contraindicated in patients hypersensitive to drug and in those with hypokalemia or obstructive bowel disease.

• Use cautiously in patients with severe heart failure, severe hypertension, or marked edema. Drug provides 100 mg sodium/g.

• Don't administer with products containing sorbitol because of the risk of intestinal necrosis.

NURSING CONSIDERATIONS
• Watch for constipation with oral or nasogastric administration. Give 10 to 20 mL of 70% sorbitol syrup every 2 hours, p.r.n., to produce one or two watery stools daily.

• Monitor potassium level at least once daily. Treatment may result in potassium deficiency and is usually stopped when potassium is reduced to 4 or 5 mEq/L.

• Watch for signs of hypokalemia: irritability, confusion, arrhythmias, ECG changes, severe muscle weakness or even paralysis, and digitalis toxicity in digitalized patients.

• When hyperkalemia is severe, polystyrene resin alone isn't adequate for lowering potassium. Dextrose 50% with regular insulin I.V. push may also be given.

• Watch for symptoms of other electrolyte deficiencies (magnesium, calcium) because drug is nonselective. Monitor calcium level in patients receiving sodium polystyrene therapy for more than 3 days. Supplementary calcium may be needed.

• Watch for sodium overload. Drug contains about 100 mg sodium/g. About one-third of resin's sodium is retained.

PATIENT TEACHING
• Explain use and administration of drug to patient.

• Advise patient to report adverse reactions promptly.

• Teach patient about low-potassium diet.

• Advise patient not to consume products containing sorbitol while taking this drug.

S

solifenacin succinate
sole-ah-FEN-ah-sin

VESIcare✦

Therapeutic class: Urinary antispas-
modics
Pharmacologic class: Antimuscarinics
Pregnancy risk category: C

AVAILABLE FORMS
Tablets (film-coated): 5 mg, 10 mg

INDICATIONS & DOSAGES
➤ **Overactive bladder with urinary
urgency, frequency, and urge incontinence**
Adults: 5 mg P.O. once daily. May increase
to 10 mg once daily if 5-mg dose is well
tolerated.
Adjust-a-dose: If CrCl is less than 30 mL/
minute or the patient has moderate liver
impairment (Child-Pugh class B), or if
drug is taken concurrently with CYP3A4
inhibitors, maintain the dose at 5 mg.

ADMINISTRATION
P.O.
● Give drug without regard for food.
● Drug should be swallowed whole with
liquid.

ACTION
Relaxes smooth muscle of bladder by antagonizing muscarinic receptors, relieving
symptoms of overactive bladder.

Route	Onset	Peak	Duration
P.O.	Unknown	3–8 hr	Unknown

Half-life: 2 to 3 days.

ADVERSE REACTIONS
CNS: depression, dizziness, fatigue.
CV: hypertension, leg swelling.
EENT: blurred vision, dry eyes, pharyngi-
tis.
GI: constipation, dry mouth, dyspepsia,
nausea, upper abdominal pain, vomiting.
GU: urine retention, UTI.
Respiratory: cough.
Other: influenza.

INTERACTIONS
Drug-drug. *Drugs that prolong the QT
interval:* May increase the risk of serious
cardiac arrhythmias. Monitor patient and
ECG closely.
*Potent CYP3A4 inducers (such as car-
bamazepine, phenobarbital, phenytoin,
rifampin):* May decrease solifenacin concentrations. Monitor effectiveness.
*Potent CYP3A4 inhibitors (such as keto-
conazole):* May increase solifenacin levels.
Don't exceed solifenacin dose of 5 mg daily
when used together.

EFFECTS ON LAB TEST RESULTS
None reported.

CONTRAINDICATIONS & CAUTIONS
● Contraindicated in patients hypersensitive
to drug or its components and in patients
with urine or gastric retention or uncontrolled angle-closure glaucoma. Don't use
in patients with severe hepatic impairment
(Child-Pugh class C).
● Use cautiously in patients with a history of prolonged QT interval, those being
treated for angle-closure glaucoma, and
those with bladder outflow obstruction,
decreased GI motility, renal insufficiency, or
moderate liver impairment.
⚠ *Overdose S&S:* Anticholinergic effects
(fixed and dilated pupils, blurred vision,
failure of heel-to-toe examination, tremors,
dry skin).

NURSING CONSIDERATIONS
● Assess bladder function, and monitor drug
effects.
● If patient has bladder outlet obstruction,
watch for urine retention.
● Monitor patient for decreased gastric
motility and constipation.
● Safety and effectiveness are similar in
older and younger adults, but levels and
half-life may be increased in the elderly.
● *Look alike–sound alike:* Don't confuse
Vesicare with Vesanoid.

PATIENT TEACHING
● Explain that drug may cause blurred
vision. Tell patient to use caution when
performing hazardous activities or tasks that

Reactions in bold italics are *life-threatening*. Interactions may have a *rapid onset* or a *delayed onset*.

require clear vision until effects of the drug are known.

• Discourage use of other drugs that may cause dry mouth, constipation, urine retention, or blurred vision.

• Urge patient to notify prescriber about abdominal pain or constipation that lasts 3 days or longer.

• Tell patient that drug decreases the ability to sweat normally, and advise cautious use in hot environments or during strenuous activity.

• Tell patient to swallow tablet whole with liquid.

• Inform patient that drug may be taken with or without food.

somatropin
soe-ma-TROE-pin

Genotropin, Genotropin Miniquick, Humatrope, Norditropin FlexPro, Norditropin NordiFlex, Nutropin, Nutropin AQ, Omnitrope, Saizen, Serostim, Tev-Tropin, Valtropin, Zorbtive

Therapeutic class: Growth hormones
Pharmacologic class: Anterior pituitary hormones
Pregnancy risk category: B (Genotropin, Omnitrope, Saizen, Serostim, Zorbtive); C (Humatrope, Norditropin, Nutropin, Nutropin AQ, Tev-Tropin, Valtropin)

AVAILABLE FORMS
Genotropin injection: 1.5 mg (about 4.5 international units/vial), 5.8 mg (about 17.4 international units/vial), 13.8 mg (about 41.4 international units/vial)
Genotropin Miniquick injection: 0.2 mg/vial, 0.4 mg/vial, 0.6 mg/vial, 0.8 mg/vial, 1 mg/vial, 1.2 mg/vial, 1.4 mg/vial, 1.6 mg/vial, 1.8 mg/vial, 2 mg/vial
Humatrope injection: 5 mg (about 15 international units/vial), 6 mg (18 international units/cartridge), 12 mg (36 international units/cartridge), 24 mg (72 international units/cartridge)
Norditropin injection: 5 mg/1.5 mL cartridges, 10 mg/1.5 mL cartridges, 15 mg/1.5 mL cartridges, 30 mg/3 mL cartridges

Nutropin injection: 5 mg (about 15 international units/vial), 10 mg (about 30 international units/vial)
Nutropin AQ injection: 5 mg (about 15 international units)/2-mL vial, 10 mg (about 30 international units/2-mL vial or pen, 20 mg (about 60 international units)/2-mL vial
Omnitrope injection: 1.5 mg/vial, 5.8 mg/vial, 5 mg/1.5 mL injection cartridge, 10 mg/1.5 mL injection cartridge
Saizen injection: 5 mg (about 15 international units/vial), 8.8 mg (about 26.4 international units/vial)
Serostim injection: 4 mg (about 12 international units/vial), 5 mg (about 15 international units/vial), 6 mg (about 18 international units/vial)
Tev-Tropin injection: 5 mg (15 international units/vial)
Valtropin injection: 5 mg (about 15 international units/vial)
Zorbtive injection: 8.8 mg (approximately 26.4 international units/vial)

INDICATIONS & DOSAGES
➤ **Long-term treatment of growth failure in children with inadequate secretion of endogenous growth hormone (GH)**
Children: 0.18 to 0.3 mg/kg/week Humatrope subcutaneously, divided equally and given six times weekly or once daily. Or, up to 0.3 mg/kg Nutropin or Nutropin AQ subcutaneously weekly in daily divided doses; in pubertal patients, a weekly dosage of up to 0.7 mg/kg (Nutropin or Nutropin AQ) in daily divided doses may be used. Or, 0.06 mg/kg Saizen I.M. or subcutaneously three times weekly. Or, 0.024 to 0.034 mg/kg Norditropin subcutaneously six to seven times weekly. Or, 0.16 to 0.24 mg/kg Genotropin or Omnitrope subcutaneously weekly, divided into six or seven doses. Or, up to 0.1 mg/kg Tev-Tropin subcutaneously three times weekly.
➤ **Growth failure from chronic renal insufficiency up to time of renal transplantation**
Children: Up to 0.35 mg/kg/week Nutropin or Nutropin AQ subcutaneously divided into daily doses.

S

➤ **Long-term treatment of short stature from Turner syndrome**
Children: Up to 0.375 mg/kg/week Humatrope, Nutropin, or Nutropin AQ subcutaneously, divided into equal doses given three to seven times weekly. Or, up to 0.067 mg/kg/day Norditropin subcutaneously.

➤ **Short stature in children with Noonan syndrome**
Children: Up to 0.066 mg/kg/day Norditropin subcutaneously.

➤ **Long-term treatment of growth failure in children with Prader-Willi syndrome diagnosed by genetic testing**
Children: 0.24 mg/kg Genotropin or Omnitrope subcutaneously weekly, divided into six or seven doses.

➤ **Replacement of endogenous GH in adult patients with GH deficiency**
Adults: Initially, not more than 0.006 mg/kg Humatrope, Nutropin, or Nutropin AQ subcutaneously daily. May be increased to maximum of 0.0125 mg/kg Humatrope daily. Or initially not more than 0.004 mg/kg or 0.15 to 0.3 mg Norditropin subcutaneously daily.

Nutropin or Nutropin AQ dosages may be increased to maximum of 0.025 mg/kg daily in patients younger than age 35 or 0.0125 mg/kg daily in patients older than age 35. Or, starting dosages not exceeding 0.04 mg/kg Genotropin or Omnitrope subcutaneously weekly, divided into six or seven doses, may be increased at 4- to 8-week intervals to a maximum dose of 0.08 mg/kg subcutaneously weekly, divided into six or seven doses. Initially, not more than 0.005 mg/kg Saizen daily. May increase after 4 weeks to a maximum dose of 0.01 mg/kg daily based on patient tolerance and clinical response. Norditropin may be increased to maximum of 0.016 mg/kg daily after about 6 weeks. Or increase by 0.1 to 0.2 mg/day every 1 to 2 months based on clinical response and insulin-like growth factor-1 concentration.

➤ **AIDS wasting or cachexia**
Adults and children weighing more than 55 kg (121 lb): 6 mg Serostim subcutaneously at bedtime.
Adults and children weighing 45 to 55 kg (99 to 121 lb): 5 mg Serostim subcutaneously at bedtime.

Adults and children weighing 35 to 45 kg (77 to 99 lb): 4 mg Serostim subcutaneously at bedtime.
Adults and children weighing less than 35 kg: 0.1 mg/kg/day Serostim subcutaneously at bedtime.

➤ **Long-term treatment of growth failure in children born small for gestational age (SGA) who don't catch up by age 2**
Children: 0.48 mg/kg Genotropin or Omnitrope subcutaneously weekly, divided into six or seven doses.

➤ **Short stature in children born SGA who don't catch up by age 2 to 4**
Children: Up to 0.067 mg/kg/day Norditropin or Humatrope subcutaneously.

➤ **Idiopathic short stature**
Children: Up to 0.37 mg/kg Humatrope subcutaneously weekly, divided into six or seven equal doses. Or, up to 0.47 mg/kg/week Genotropin or Omnitrope subcutaneously, divided into six or seven equal doses. Or, up to 0.3 mg/kg Nutropin subcutaneously weekly, divided into seven equal doses.

➤ **Short bowel syndrome**
Adults: 0.1 mg/kg/day Zorbtive subcutaneously daily for 4 weeks. Maximum dosage, 8 mg/day.

ADMINISTRATION
I.M.

● To prepare solution, inject supplied diluent into vial containing drug by aiming stream of liquid against wall of glass vial. Then swirl vial gently until contents are completely dissolved. Don't shake vial.

● After reconstitution, make sure solution is clear. Don't inject solution if it's cloudy or contains particles.

● For patients on hemodialysis, give drug before bedtime or 3 to 4 hours after dialysis. For long-term cycling peritoneal dialysis, give drug in the morning after completion of dialysis. For long-term ambulatory peritoneal dialysis, give drug in the evening at the time of the overnight exchange.

● Store reconstituted drug in refrigerator; use within 14 days.

● If patient develops sensitivity to diluent, reconstitute drug with sterile water for injection. When drug is reconstituted in this way, use only one reconstituted dose per vial, refrigerate solution if it isn't used immediately after reconstitution, use reconstituted dose within 24 hours, and discard unused portion.

❸ *Alert:* When administering to newborn, reconstitute with sterile water for injection.

Subcutaneous

• To prepare solution, inject supplied diluent into vial containing drug by aiming stream of liquid against wall of glass vial. Then swirl vial gently until contents are completely dissolved. Don't shake vial.

• After reconstitution, make sure solution is clear. Don't inject solution if it's cloudy or contains particles.

• For patients on hemodialysis, give drug before bedtime or 3 to 4 hours after dialysis. For long-term cycling peritoneal dialysis, give drug in the morning after completion of dialysis. For long-term ambulatory peritoneal dialysis, give drug in the evening at the time of the overnight exchange.

• Rotate injection sites.

• Store reconstituted drug in refrigerator; use within 14 days.

• If patient develops sensitivity to diluent, reconstitute drug with sterile water for injection. When drug is reconstituted in this way, use only one reconstituted dose per vial, refrigerate solution if it isn't used immediately after reconstitution, use reconstituted dose within 24 hours, and discard unused portion.

❸ *Alert:* When administering to newborn, reconstitute with sterile water for injection.

ACTION

Purified GH of recombinant DNA origin that stimulates skeletal, linear, muscle, and organ growth.

Route	Onset	Peak	Duration
I.M., subcut.	Unknown	3–5 hr	12–48 hr

Half-life: Varies by route and brand. Refer to manufacturer's drug label.

ADVERSE REACTIONS

CNS: headache, weakness, paresthesia, fatigue.
CV: mild, transient edema.
EENT: otitis media.
Hematologic: *leukemia.*
Metabolic: mild hyperglycemia, hypothyroidism.

Musculoskeletal: localized muscle pain, arthralgia, stiffness of extremities.
Respiratory: upper respiratory tract infection.
Skin: injection-site pain.
Other: antibodies to GH.

INTERACTIONS

Drug-drug. *Corticotropin, corticosteroids:* Long-term use may inhibit growth response to GH. Monitor patient for lack of effect.
Estrogen replacement: May decrease somatropin level in adult women. Increase somatropin dosage as necessary.
Insulin, oral antidiabetic agents: Somatropin may decrease insulin sensitivity. Antidiabetic agent dosage may need adjustment.

EFFECTS ON LAB TEST RESULTS

• May increase glucose, inorganic phosphorus, alkaline phosphatase, and parathyroid hormone levels.

CONTRAINDICATIONS & CAUTIONS

• Contraindicated in patients with closed epiphyses, preproliferative or severe nonproliferative diabetic retinopathy, active malignancy, or an active underlying intracranial lesion.

• For patients hypersensitive to either metacresol or glycerin, don't use supplied diluent to reconstitute Humatrope.

• Contraindicated (Genotropin only) in patients with Prader-Willi syndrome who are severely obese or have severe respiratory impairment.

• Don't begin therapy in patients with acute critical illness due to complications following open heart or abdominal surgery, trauma, or acute respiratory failure.

• Use cautiously in children with hypothyroidism and in those with GH deficiency caused by intracranial lesion.

• Use cautiously in patients with diabetes.

• May increase risk of pancreatitis. Monitor patient for persistent abdominal pain with or without vomiting.

⚠ *Overdose S&S:* Fluid retention, hypoglycemia followed by hyperglycemia, glucose intolerance, gigantism, acromegaly.

S

NURSING CONSIDERATIONS

• Frequently examine children with hypothyroidism and those whose GH deficiency is caused by an intracranial lesion for progression or recurrence of underlying disease.

❸ *Alert:* In patients with Prader-Willi syndrome who are morbidly obese and in those with a history of respiratory impairment, sleep apnea, or unidentified respiratory infection, therapy may be life-threatening. Assess patients with Prader-Willi syndrome for sleep apnea and upper airway obstruction before treatment. Interrupt treatment if signs of upper airway obstruction occur.

• Monitor patient with Prader-Willi syndrome for signs of respiratory infection.

• Monitor child's height regularly. Regular checkups, including monitoring of blood and radiologic studies, are also needed.

• Monitor patient's glucose level regularly because GH may induce a state of insulin resistance or new-onset diabetes mellitus.

• Excessive glucocorticoid therapy inhibits somatropin's growth-promoting effect. Patients with coexisting corticotropin deficiency should have their glucocorticoid replacement dosage carefully adjusted to avoid growth inhibition.

• Watch for slipped capital femoral epiphysis or progression of scoliosis in patients with rapid growth.

• Monitor results of periodic thyroid function tests for hypothyroidism; condition may need thyroid hormone treatment. Laboratory measurements of thyroid hormone may change.

• Patient should have ophthalmic examinations to monitor for intracranial hypertension before therapy (to establish baseline) and periodically thereafter.

• Only adults with GH deficiency alone or together with multiple hormone deficiencies from pituitary or hypothalamic disease, surgery, radiation, or trauma or those who were GH deficient as children and have been confirmed GH deficient as adults can take Saizen.

• *Look alike–sound alike:* Don't confuse somatropin with somatrem or sumatriptan.

PATIENT TEACHING

• Inform parents that child with endocrine disorders (including GH deficiency) may have an increased risk of slipped capital epiphyses. Tell parents to notify prescriber if they notice their child limping.

• Instruct patients with diabetes to monitor glucose level closely and report changes to prescriber.

• Instruct patient or parents in appropriate injection technique and needle disposal. Tell them to rotate injection sites.

• Stress importance of close follow-up care.

sotalol hydrochloride
SOH-ta-lol

Betapace, Betapace AF, Rylosol†, Sorine

Therapeutic class: Antiarrhythmics
Pharmacologic class: Nonselective beta blockers
Pregnancy risk category: B

AVAILABLE FORMS
Solution for injection: 15 mg/mL
Betapace
Tablets: 80 mg, 120 mg, 160 mg, 240 mg
Betapace AF
Tablets: 80 mg, 120 mg, 160 mg
Rylosol†
Tablets: 80 mg, 160 mg, 240 mg
Sorine
Tablets: 80 mg, 120 mg, 160 mg, 240 mg

INDICATIONS & DOSAGES
➤ **Documented, life-threatening ventricular arrhythmias**
Adults: Initially, 80 mg Betapace P.O. b.i.d. Increase dosage every 3 days as needed and tolerated. Most patients respond to 160 to 320 mg/day, although some patients with refractory arrhythmias need up to 640 mg/day. Or, 75 mg I.V. once daily or b.i.d. based on CrCl. After 3 days, dosage may be increased to 75 to 150 mg I.V. once daily or every 12 hours based on CrCl. For refractory life-threatening arrhythmias, dosage may be increased to 225 to 300 mg I.V. once daily or every 12 hours.

Adjust-a-dose: For oral route, if CrCl is 30 to 60 mL/minute, increase dosage interval to every 24 hours; if CrCl is 10 to 29 mL/minute, increase interval to every 36 to 48 hours; and if CrCl is less than 10 mL/minute, individualize dosage. For I.V. route, if CrCl is 40 to 59 mL/minute, give I.V. drug once daily; don't give if CrCl is less than 40 mL/minute.

➤ **To maintain normal sinus rhythm or to delay recurrence of atrial fibrillation or atrial flutter in patients with symptomatic atrial fibrillation or flutter who are currently in sinus rhythm**
Adults: 80 mg Betapace AF P.O. b.i.d. (Don't use if baseline QT interval is greater than 450 msec.) Increase dosage as needed to 120 mg P.O. b.i.d. after 3 days if the QTc interval is less than 500 msec. Maximum dose is 160 mg P.O. b.i.d. Or, 75 mg I.V. once daily or every 12 hours based on CrCl. After 3 days, dosage may be increased to 112.5 to 150 mg I.V. once daily or every 12 hours based on clearance.

Adjust-a-dose: For oral route, if CrCl is 40 to 60 mL/minute, increase dosage interval to every 24 hours; if CrCl is less than 40 mL/minute, Betapace AF is contraindicated. For I.V. route, if CrCl is 40 to 59 mL/minute, give I.V. drug once daily; don't give if CrCl is less than 40 mL/minute.

ADMINISTRATION
P.O.
• Give 1 hour before or 2 hours after antacids.
• May give without regard for food but patient should take the same way each time.
I.V.
▼ Dilute drug with normal saline solution, D_5W, or lactated Ringer solution in a volume of 120 to 300 mL to compensate for dead space in the infusion set.
▼ Use an infusion pump to administer drug at a constant rate over 5 hours.

ACTION
Depresses sinus heart rate, slows AV conduction, decreases cardiac output, and lowers systolic and diastolic blood pres-

sure. Drug also has class III antiarrhythmic properties and can prolong duration of the cardiac action potential.

Route	Onset	Peak	Duration
P.O.	Unknown	2½–4 hr	Unknown
I.V.	Unknown	Unknown	Unknown

Half-life: 12 hours.

ADVERSE REACTIONS
CNS: asthenia, headache, dizziness, weakness, fatigue, light-headedness, sleep problems.
CV: chest pain, palpitations, *bradycardia, arrhythmias, heart failure, AV block, proarrhythmic events (including polymorphic ventricular tachycardia, PVCs, ventricular fibrillation),* edema, ECG abnormalities, hypotension.
GI: nausea, vomiting, diarrhea, dyspepsia.
Metabolic: hyperglycemia.
Respiratory: dyspnea, *bronchospasm.*

INTERACTIONS
Drug-drug. *Antacids containing aluminum oxide and magnesium hydroxide:* May reduce bradycardic effect. Avoid sotalol administration within 2 hours of antacid.
Antiarrhythmics: May increase drug effects. Avoid using together.
Antihypertensives, catecholamine-depleting drugs (such as guanethidine, reserpine): May increase hypotensive effects or cause marked bradycardia. Monitor blood pressure and pulse closely.
Calcium channel blockers: May increase myocardial depression. Avoid using together.
Clonidine: May enhance rebound effect after withdrawal of clonidine. Stop sotalol several days before withdrawing clonidine.
Drugs that prolong the QT interval (class I and III antiarrhythmics, bepridil, phenothiazines, TCAs): May cause excessive QT prolongation. Monitor QT interval.
General anesthetics: May increase myocardial depression. Monitor patient closely.
Insulin, oral antidiabetics: May cause hyperglycemia and may mask signs and symptoms of hypoglycemia. Adjust dosage accordingly.

S

Macrolides and related antibiotics (azithromycin, clarithromycin, erythromycin, telithromycin): May cause additive effects or prolong the QT interval. Use with caution. Avoid use with telithromycin.

Prazosin: May increase the risk of orthostatic hypotension. Assist patient to stand slowly until effects are known.

Quinolones: May cause life-threatening arrhythmias, including torsades de pointes. Avoid using together.

Theophylline: May decrease bronchodilating effects. Avoid using together.

Drug-lifestyle. *Cocaine:* May increase cardiotoxic effects of cocaine. Don't use with cocaine-associated myocardial ischemia or infarction.

EFFECTS ON LAB TEST RESULTS
● May increase glucose level.
● May cause false-positive catecholamine level.

CONTRAINDICATIONS & CAUTIONS
● Contraindicated in patients hypersensitive to drug.
● Contraindicated in those with severe sinus node dysfunction, sinus bradycardia, second- and third-degree AV block unless patient has a pacemaker, congenital or acquired long QT-interval syndrome, cardiogenic shock, uncontrolled heart failure, CrCl of less than 40 mL/minute, serum potassium level of less than 4 mEq/L, and bronchial asthma.
● Contraindicated in patients with hypomagnesemia before correction of imbalance.
● Use cautiously in patients with renal impairment or diabetes mellitus (beta blockers may mask signs and symptoms of hypoglycemia).

⚠ *Overdose S&S:* Bradycardia, bronchospasm, heart failure, hypoglycemia, hypotension, asystole, prolongation of the QT interval, torsades de pointes, ventricular tachycardia, death.

NURSING CONSIDERATIONS
Black Box Warning Because proarrhythmic events may occur at the start of therapy and during dosage adjustments, patients should be hospitalized for a minimum of 3 days

in a facility that can provide calculations of CrCl, continuous ECG monitoring, and cardiac resuscitation. Calculate CrCl before dosing. ■

Black Box Warning The baseline QTc interval must be less than or equal to 450 msec before starting sotalol I.V. If QT interval is 500 msec or more (I.V. or P.O.), dosage or frequency must be decreased or drug discontinued. ■

● Assess patient for new or worsened symptoms of heart failure.
● Although patients receiving I.V. lidocaine may start sotalol therapy without ill effects, withdraw other antiarrhythmics before therapy begins. Sotalol therapy typically is delayed until two or three half-lives of the withdrawn drug have elapsed. After withdrawing amiodarone, give sotalol only after QT interval normalizes.
● Adjust dosage slowly, allowing 3 days between dosage increments for adequate monitoring of QT intervals and for drug levels to reach a steady-state level.

Black Box Warning Don't substitute sotalol for sotalol AF. ■

● Monitor electrolytes regularly, especially if patient is receiving diuretics. Electrolyte imbalances, such as hypokalemia or hypomagnesemia, may enhance QT-interval prolongation and increase the risk of serious arrhythmias such as torsades de pointes.
● *Look alike–sound alike:* Don't confuse sotalol with Stadol or Sudafed.

PATIENT TEACHING
● Explain to patient that he will need to be hospitalized for initiation of drug therapy.
● Stress need to take drug as prescribed, even when he is feeling well. Caution patient against stopping drug suddenly.
● Caution patient against using OTC drugs and decongestants while taking drug.
● Advise patient to take drug consistently with or without food.
● Because antacids can interfere with absorption, tell patient to take drug 2 hours before or after antacids.
● Warn patient not to double the next dose if a dose is missed.

spinosad
SPIN-oh-sad

Natroba

Therapeutic class: Scabicides–pediculicides
Pharmacologic class: Topical actinomycete bacterium derivatives
Pregnancy risk category: B

AVAILABLE FORMS
Topical solution: 0.9%*

INDICATIONS & DOSAGES
➤ **Head lice infestation**
Adults and children age 4 and older: Apply only amount needed to adequately cover scalp and hair, up to 120 mL. Leave on for 10 minutes; then thoroughly rinse off with warm water. If live lice are seen 7 days after first treatment, apply a second treatment.

ADMINISTRATION
Topical
● Store at room temperature.
● Shake well before use.
● Apply to dry scalp and hair.
● Apply to scalp first; then apply outwards toward ends of hair.
● Use timer or clock to monitor time of use; begin timing when scalp and hair are completely covered.
● Avoid contact near eyes. Rinse eyes thoroughly with water if contact occurs.
● Wash hands after application.

ACTION
Causes neuronal excitation in lice, which leads to lice paralysis and death.

Route	Onset	Peak	Duration
Topical	Unknown	Unknown	Unknown

Half-life: Unknown.

ADVERSE REACTIONS
EENT: ocular erythema.
Skin: application-site erythema or irritation.

INTERACTIONS
None significant.

EFFECTS ON LAB TEST RESULTS
None reported.

CONTRAINDICATIONS & CAUTIONS
● Contraindicated in patients hypersensitive to drug or its components.
● It isn't known if benzyl alcohol in topical solution is absorbed through the skin. Don't use for infants younger than age 6 months because of risk of systemic absorption.
● Use cautiously in pregnant and breast-feeding women because of possible absorption of benzyl alcohol. Breast-feeding women may choose to pump and discard breast milk for 8 hours (five half-lives of benzyl alcohol) after spinosad use to avoid infant ingestion of benzyl alcohol.

NURSING CONSIDERATIONS
● Use as part of overall lice-management system.
● Wash in hot water or dry-clean all used bedding and towels and recently worn clothing and hats.
● Wash personal care items, such as combs, brushes, and hair clips, in hot water.
● Use a fine-tooth comb or special nit comb to remove dead lice and nits.

PATIENT TEACHING
● Instruct patient or caregiver in use of suspension as part of an overall lice-management system.
● Tell patient not to take drug orally.
● Advise female patient to contact prescriber before using drug if she is pregnant or breast-feeding.
● Instruct caregiver that drug should be used on children only with direct adult supervision.

S

spironolactone
speer-on-oh-LAK-tone

Aldactone⬥

Therapeutic class: Diuretics
Pharmacologic class: Potassium-sparing diuretics–aldosterone receptor antagonists
Pregnancy risk category: C

AVAILABLE FORMS
Tablets: 25 mg, 50 mg, 100 mg

INDICATIONS & DOSAGES
Black Box Warning Use spironolactone only for those conditions for which it's indicated. Avoid unnecessary use. ▮
➤ **Edema due to heart failure, hepatic cirrhosis, or nephrotic syndrome**
Adults: Initially, 100 mg P.O. daily given as a single dose or in divided doses. Usual range is 25 to 200 mg P.O. daily.
➤ **Hypertension**
Adults: 50 to 100 mg P.O. daily or in divided doses. Some practitioners use a lower dosage range of 25 to 50 mg daily and add another antihypertensive to the regimen, rather than continually increasing this drug.
➤ **Diuretic-induced hypokalemia**
Adults: 25 to 100 mg P.O. daily.
➤ **To detect primary hyperaldosteronism**
Adults: 400 mg P.O. daily for 4 days (short test) or 3 to 4 weeks (long test). If hypokalemia and hypertension are corrected, a presumptive diagnosis of primary hyperaldosteronism is made.
➤ **To manage primary hyperaldosteronism**
Adults: 100 to 400 mg P.O. daily. Use lowest effective dose.
➤ **Severe heart failure (class III or IV), as adjunct to ACE inhibitor or loop diuretic, with or without cardiac glycoside**
Adults: 25 mg P.O. daily if serum potassium level is 5 mEq/L or less and serum creatinine level is 2.5 mg/dL or less. May increase to 50 mg P.O. daily as clinically indicated.
Adjust-a-dose: Patients who don't tolerate 25 mg daily may have dosage decreased to every other day.

➤ **Hirsutism ⬥**
Women: 50 to 200 mg P.O. daily.

ADMINISTRATION
P.O.
● To enhance absorption, give drug with meals.
● Give drug in morning to prevent nocturia. If second dose is needed, give it with food in early afternoon.
● Protect tablets from light.

ACTION
Antagonizes aldosterone in the distal tubules, increasing sodium and water excretion.

Route	Onset	Peak	Duration
P.O.	1–2 days	2–3 days	2–3 days

Half-life: 1¼ to 2 hours.

ADVERSE REACTIONS
CNS: headache, drowsiness, lethargy, confusion, ataxia.
GI: diarrhea, *gastric bleeding,* ulceration, cramping, gastritis, vomiting.
GU: inability to maintain erection, menstrual disturbances.
Hematologic: *agranulocytosis.*
Metabolic: *hyperkalemia,* dehydration, hyponatremia, mild acidosis.
Skin: urticaria, hirsutism, maculopapular eruptions.
Other: *anaphylaxis,* gynecomastia, breast soreness, drug fever.

INTERACTIONS
Drug-drug. *ACE inhibitors, ARBs, eplerenone:* May increase risk of severe hyperkalemia. Use together is contraindicated.
Anticoagulants: May decrease anticoagulant effects. Monitor PT and INR.
Aspirin and other salicylates: May block diuretic effect of spironolactone. Watch for diminished spironolactone response.
Digoxin: May alter digoxin clearance, increasing risk of toxicity. Monitor digoxin level.
NSAIDs, potassium-sparing diuretics, potassium supplements: May result in hyperkalemia. Avoid use together.

Reactions in bold italics are *life-threatening*. Interactions may have a *rapid onset* or a *delayed onset*.

Drug-herb. *Licorice:* May block ulcer-healing and aldosterone-like effects of herb; may increase risk of hypokalemia. Discourage use together.
Drug-food. *Potassium-rich foods, such as citrus fruits and tomatoes, salt substitutes containing potassium:* May increase risk of hyperkalemia. Urge caution.

EFFECTS ON LAB TEST RESULTS
• May increase BUN and potassium levels. May decrease sodium level.
• May decrease granulocyte count.
• May alter fluorometric determinations of plasma and urinary 17-hydroxycorticosteroid levels.

CONTRAINDICATIONS & CAUTIONS
• Contraindicated in patients hypersensitive to drug and in those with anuria, acute or progressive renal insufficiency, or hyperkalemia.
• Use cautiously in patients with fluid or electrolyte imbalances, impaired renal or hepatic function, or in pregnant women.
Black Box Warning Drug has been shown to be tumorigenic in long-term toxicity studies in rats. Avoid unnecessary use. ■
⚠ Overdose S&S: Drowsiness, confusion, rash, nausea, vomiting, dizziness, diarrhea, hyperkalemia.

NURSING CONSIDERATIONS
• Monitor electrolyte levels, fluid intake and output, weight, and blood pressure.
• Monitor elderly patients closely, who are more susceptible to excessive diuresis.
• Inform laboratory that patient is taking spironolactone because drug may interfere with tests that measure digoxin level.
• Drug is less potent than thiazide and loop diuretics and is useful as an adjunct to other diuretic therapy. Diuretic effect is delayed 2 to 3 days when used alone.
• Maximum antihypertensive response may be delayed for up to 2 weeks.
• Watch for hyperchloremic metabolic acidosis, especially in patients with hepatic cirrhosis.
• **Look alike–sound alike:** Don't confuse Aldactone with Aldactazide.

PATIENT TEACHING
• Instruct patient to take drug in morning to prevent need to urinate at night. If second dose is needed, tell him to take it with food in early afternoon.
⚠ Alert: To prevent serious hyperkalemia, warn patient to avoid excessive ingestion of potassium-rich foods (such as citrus fruits, tomatoes, bananas, dates, and apricots), salt substitutes containing potassium, and potassium supplements.
• Caution patient not to perform hazardous activities if adverse CNS reactions occur.
• Advise patient about possible breast tenderness or enlargement.

stavudine (2′ 3′-didehydro-3-deoxythymidine, d4T)
STAV-yoo-deen

Zerit

Therapeutic class: Antiretrovirals
Pharmacologic class: Nucleosides–nucleotide reverse transcriptase inhibitors
Pregnancy risk category: C

AVAILABLE FORMS
Capsules: 15 mg, 20 mg, 30 mg, 40 mg
Oral solution: 1 mg/mL

INDICATIONS & DOSAGES
➤ **HIV infection, with other antiretrovirals**
Adults weighing 60 kg (132 lb) or more: 40 mg P.O. every 12 hours.
Adults weighing less than 60 kg: 30 mg P.O. every 12 hours.
Children weighing 60 kg or more: 40 mg P.O. every 12 hours.
Children weighing 30 kg (66 lb) to 60 kg: 30 mg P.O. every 12 hours.
Neonates age 14 days and older and children weighing less than 30 kg: 1 mg/kg P.O. every 12 hours.
Neonates age 13 days and younger: 0.5 mg/kg P.O. every 12 hours.
Adjust-a-dose: For patients experiencing peripheral neuropathy, stop temporarily; then resume therapy at 50% recommended dose. Stop therapy if neuropathy recurs.

S

For patients with CrCl 26 to 50 mL/minute, adjust dosage to 20 mg (if weight exceeds 60 kg) or 15 mg (if weight is less than 60 kg) P.O. every 12 hours; if CrCl is 10 to 25 mL/minute or in adults undergoing dialysis, 20 mg (if weight exceeds 60 kg) or 15 mg (if weight is less than 60 kg) P.O. every 24 hours.

ADMINISTRATION
P.O.
● Give drug without regard for meals.
● Shake solution well before giving.
● Give drug after hemodialysis on hemodialysis treatment days.
● Discard unused solution after 30 days.

ACTION
A thymidine nucleoside analogue that prevents replication of retroviruses, including HIV, by inhibiting the enzyme reverse transcriptase and causing termination of DNA chain growth.

Route	Onset	Peak	Duration
P.O.	Unknown	1 hr	Unknown

Half-life: 1 to 2 hours.

ADVERSE REACTIONS
CNS: asthenia, fever, anxiety, headache, malaise, motor weakness, nervousness, peripheral neuropathy.
GI: abdominal pain, anorexia, diarrhea, nausea, vomiting, *pancreatitis,* constipation.
Hematologic: *neutropenia, thrombocytopenia,* anemia.
Hepatic: *hepatotoxicity,* severe hepatomegaly with steatosis.
Metabolic: *lactic acidosis,* lipodystrophy, lipoatrophy, weight loss.
Musculoskeletal: myalgia.
Respiratory: dyspnea.
Skin: diaphoresis, pruritus, rash.
Other: chills.

INTERACTIONS
Drug-drug. *Didanosine, hydroxyurea:* Coadministration may increase risk for lactic acidosis, hepatotoxicity, pancreatitis, or peripheral neuropathy. Monitor closely for adverse effects.

Doxorubicin, ribavirin: May decrease effectiveness of stavudine. Use together cautiously.
Methadone: May decrease stavudine absorption and level. Separate dosage times and monitor patient for clinical effect if drugs must be used together.
Zidovudine: May inhibit phosphorylation of stavudine. Avoid using together.

EFFECTS ON LAB TEST RESULTS
● May increase amylase, lipase, bilirubin, ALT, and AST levels. May decrease hemoglobin level.
● May decrease neutrophil and platelet count.

CONTRAINDICATIONS & CAUTIONS
● Contraindicated in patients hypersensitive to drug.
Black Box Warning Lactic acidosis and severe hepatomegaly with steatosis, including fatal cases, have been reported. ■
● Use cautiously in patients with renal impairment or history of peripheral neuropathy. Adjust dosage for CrCl of less than 50 mL/minute; adjust dosage or stop drug in patients with peripheral neuropathy.
Black Box Warning Use cautiously in pregnant women; fatal lactic acidosis may occur in pregnant women who receive stavudine and didanosine with other antiretrovirals. ■
⚠ Overdose S&S: Peripheral neuropathy, hepatotoxicity.

NURSING CONSIDERATIONS
Black Box Warning Due to increased risk of pancreatic toxicity, monitor patient for signs and symptoms of pancreatitis, especially if he takes stavudine with didanosine or hydroxyurea. If patient has pancreatitis, reinstate drug cautiously. ■
● Monitor LFT results.
☙ Alert: Motor weakness mimicking the signs and symptoms of Guillain-Barré syndrome (including respiratory failure) in HIV patients taking stavudine with other antiretrovirals may occur, especially in patients with lactic acidosis. Monitor patient for characteristics of lactic acidosis, including generalized fatigue, GI problems, tachypnea, and dyspnea. Patients with these

---

symptoms should promptly interrupt antiretroviral therapy and rapidly receive a full medical workup. Consider permanently stopping drug. Symptoms may continue or worsen when drug is stopped.

• Monitor patient for lipoatrophy and lipodystrophy, and consider the risk and benefit of treatment.

❸ *Alert:* Peripheral neuropathy may be the major dose-limiting adverse effect; it may or may not resolve after drug is stopped.

• Monitor CBC results and creatinine.

PATIENT TEACHING
• Tell patient that drug may be taken without regard to meals.

• Warn patient not to take other drugs for HIV or AIDS unless prescriber has approved them.

• Inform patient that drug doesn't cure HIV infection, that opportunistic infections and other complications of HIV infection may still occur, and that transmission of HIV to others through sexual contact or blood contamination is still possible.

• Teach patient signs and symptoms of peripheral neuropathy (pain, burning, aching, weakness, or pins and needles in the limbs), and tell him to report these immediately.

• Tell patient to report symptoms of lactic acidosis, including fatigue, GI problems, dyspnea, or tachypnea.

• Tell patient to report symptoms of pancreatitis, including abdominal pain, nausea, vomiting, weight loss, or fatty stools.

• Tell patient to monitor weight patterns and report weight loss or gain.

• Tell patient to discard unused solution after 30 days.

succinylcholine chloride (suxamethonium chloride)
SUK-seh-nil-KOH-leen

Anectine, Quelicin

Therapeutic class: Skeletal muscle relaxants
Pharmacologic class: Depolarizing neuromuscular blockers
Pregnancy risk category: C

AVAILABLE FORMS
Injection: 20 mg/mL, 100 mg/mL

INDICATIONS & DOSAGES
➤ **Adjunct to anesthesia to relax skeletal muscles for surgery and orthopedic manipulations; to facilitate intubation and assist with mechanical ventilation; to lessen muscle contractions in pharmacologically or electrically induced seizures**
Adults: 0.6 mg/kg I.V. given over 10 to 30 seconds. Dosage range is 0.3 to 1.1 mg/kg. For longer response, give 1 mg/mL solution as a continuous infusion at 0.5 to 10 mg/minute, or give an initial I.V. injection of 0.3 to 1.1 mg/kg followed by further injections of 0.04 to 0.07 mg/kg, as needed, to maintain relaxation. Or, 3 to 4 mg/kg I.M. Maximum I.M. dose is 150 mg.
Children: 1 to 2 mg/kg I.V. or 3 to 4 mg/kg I.M. Maximum I.M. dose is 150 mg.

ADMINISTRATION
I.V.
▼ Only staff skilled in airway management should use drug.
▼ Give test dose of 5 to 10 mg after patient has been anesthetized. If no respiratory depression occurs or transient depression lasts for up to 5 minutes, then patient can metabolize drug, and safe to continue. Don't give if patient develops respiratory paralysis sufficient to need endotracheal intubation. (Recovery should occur within 30 to 60 minutes.).
▼ Use within 24 hours after reconstitution.

S

▼ Store injectable form in refrigerator. Store powder form at room temperature in tightly closed container.

▼ **Incompatibilities:** Alkaline solutions, barbiturates, nafcillin, sodium bicarbonate, solutions with pH above 4.5, thiopental sodium.

I.M.
• Inject deeply, preferably high into deltoid muscle.
• Store injectable form in refrigerator. Store powder form at room temperature in tightly closed container.

ACTION

Binds with a high affinity to cholinergic receptors, prolonging depolarization of the motor end plate and ultimately producing muscle paralysis.

Route	Onset	Peak	Duration
I.V.	30–60 sec	1–2 min	4–10 min
I.M.	2–3 min	Unknown	10–30 min

Half-life: Unknown.

ADVERSE REACTIONS

CV: *arrhythmias, bradycardia, cardiac arrest,* tachycardia, hypertension, hypotension, flushing.
EENT: increased intraocular pressure.
GI: excessive salivation.
Metabolic: *hyperkalemia.*
Musculoskeletal: postoperative muscle pain, muscle fasciculation, jaw rigidity.
Respiratory: *apnea, bronchoconstriction, prolonged respiratory depression.*
Skin: rash.
Other: allergic or idiosyncratic hypersensitivity reactions, *anaphylaxis, malignant hyperthermia, rhabdomyolysis with acute renal failure.*

INTERACTIONS

Drug-drug. *Aminoglycosides, anticholinesterases (such as echothiophate, edrophonium, neostigmine, physostigmine, pyridostigmine), aprotinin, general anesthetics (such as enflurane, halothane, isoflurane), glucocorticoids, hormonal contraceptives, lidocaine, lithium, magnesium, metoclopramide, oxytocin, polymyxin antibiotics (such as colistin, polymyxin B sulfate), procainamide, quinine:* May en-

hance neuromuscular blockade, increasing skeletal muscle relaxation and potentiating effect. Use together cautiously during and after surgery.
Cardiac glycosides: May cause arrhythmias. Use together cautiously.
Cyclophosphamide, lithium, MAO inhibitors: May enhance neuromuscular blockade and prolong apnea. Use together cautiously.
Opioid analgesics: May enhance neuromuscular blockade, increasing skeletal muscle relaxation and possibly causing respiratory paralysis. Use together cautiously.
Parenteral magnesium sulfate: May enhance neuromuscular blockade, may increase skeletal muscle relaxation, and may cause respiratory paralysis. Use together cautiously, preferably at reduced doses.
Drug-herb. *Melatonin:* May potentiate blocking properties of drug. Ask patient about herbal remedy use, and recommend caution.

EFFECTS ON LAB TEST RESULTS

• May increase myoglobin and potassium levels.

CONTRAINDICATIONS & CAUTIONS

• Contraindicated in patients hypersensitive to drug and in those with abnormally low plasma pseudocholinesterase levels, angle-closure glaucoma, personal or family history of malignant hyperthermia, myopathies with elevated CK levels, acute major burns, multiple trauma, skeletal muscle denervation, upper motor neuron injury, or penetrating eye injuries.
❸ *Alert:* Drug may contain benzyl alcohol. Avoid use in neonates.
• Use cautiously in elderly or debilitated patients; in patients receiving quinidine or cardiac glycoside therapy; in patients with hepatic, renal, or pulmonary impairment; and in those with respiratory depression, severe burns or trauma, electrolyte imbalances, hyperkalemia, paraplegia, spinal CNS injury, stroke, degenerative or dystrophic neuromuscular disease, myasthenia gravis, myasthenic syndrome related to lung cancer, dehydration, thyroid disorders, collagen diseases, porphyria, fractures,

---

Reactions in bold italics are *life-threatening*. Interactions may have a *rapid onset* or a *delayed onset*.

muscle spasms, eye surgery, and pheochromocytoma. Also, use large doses cautiously in patients undergoing cesarean section.

⚠ **Overdose S&S:** Prolonged neuromuscular blockade.

NURSING CONSIDERATIONS

• Drug has no known effect on consciousness, pain threshold, or cerebration. To avoid patient distress, don't induce neuromuscular blockade before unconsciousness.

• Dosage depends on anesthetic used, individual needs, and response. Recommended dosages must be individually adjusted.

Black Box Warning Drug may cause acute rhabdomyolysis with hyperkalemia followed by ventricular arrhythmias, cardiac arrest, and death after administration to apparently healthy children who have undiagnosed skeletal muscle myopathy, most frequently Duchenne muscular dystrophy. Institute treatment for hyperkalemia when a healthy-appearing infant or child develops cardiac arrest soon after administration of succinylcholine. In children, drug should be reserved for use in emergency intubation, for instances when securing the airway is necessary, or for I.M. use when a suitable vein is inaccessible. ▪

• Children may be less sensitive to drug than adults.

• Succinylcholine is the drug of choice for procedures lasting less than 3 minutes and for orthopedic manipulations; use cautiously with fractures or dislocations.

• Monitor baseline electrolyte determinations and vital signs. Check respirations every 5 to 10 minutes during infusion.

• Monitor respirations closely until tests of muscle strength (hand grip, head lift, and ability to cough) indicate full recovery from neuromuscular blockade.

⚠ **Alert:** Don't use reversing drugs. Unlike nondepolarizing drugs, neostigmine or edrophonium may worsen neuromuscular blockade.

• Repeated or continuous infusions aren't advisable; they may cause reduced response or prolonged muscle relaxation and apnea.

• Give analgesics for pain.

• Keep airway clear. Have emergency respiratory support equipment (endotracheal equipment, ventilator, oxygen, atropine, and epinephrine) immediately available.

⚠ **Alert:** Careful dosage calculation is essential. Always verify dosage with another health care professional.

PATIENT TEACHING

• Explain all events and procedures to patient because he can still hear.

• Reassure patient that postoperative stiffness is normal and will soon subside.

---

sucralfate
soo-KRAL-fayt

Carafate⚕

Therapeutic class: Antiulcer drugs
Pharmacologic class: GI protectants
Pregnancy risk category: B

AVAILABLE FORMS
Suspension: 1 g/10 mL
Tablets: 1 g

INDICATIONS & DOSAGES
➤ **Short-term (up to 8 weeks) treatment of duodenal ulcer**
Adults: 1 g P.O. q.i.d. 1 hour before meals and at bedtime.
➤ **Maintenance therapy for duodenal ulcer**
Adults: 1 g P.O. b.i.d.

ADMINISTRATION
P.O.
• Shake suspension well before pouring.
• Following administration, flush nasogastric tube with water to ensure passage into stomach.
• Give drug on an empty stomach 1 hour before or 2 hours after meals.

ACTION
Probably adheres to and protects surface of ulcer by forming a barrier.

Route	Onset	Peak	Duration
P.O.	Unknown	Unknown	6 hr

Half-life: 6 to 20 hours.

S

ADVERSE REACTIONS
GI: constipation.

INTERACTIONS
Drug-drug. *Antacids:* May decrease binding of drug to gastroduodenal mucosa, impairing effectiveness. Separate doses by 30 minutes.
Cimetidine, digoxin, fosphenytoin, ketoconazole, phenytoin, quinidine, ranitidine, tetracycline, theophylline: May decrease absorption. Separate doses by at least 2 hours.
Ciprofloxacin, levofloxacin, moxifloxacin, ofloxacin: May decrease absorption of these drugs, reducing anti-infective response. If use together can't be avoided, give at least 6 hours apart.
Diclofenac: May decrease effectiveness of diclofenac. Monitor patient response.
Warfarin: May decrease anticoagulant effect. Monitor effectiveness and adjust dosage as necessary.

EFFECTS ON LAB TEST RESULTS
None reported.

CONTRAINDICATIONS & CAUTIONS
• Use cautiously in patients with chronic renal failure.
⚠ **Overdose S&S:** Dyspepsia, abdominal pain, nausea, vomiting.

NURSING CONSIDERATIONS
• Drug is minimally absorbed and causes few adverse reactions.
• Monitor patient for severe, persistent constipation.
• Drug is as effective as cimetidine in healing duodenal ulcer.
• Drug contains aluminum but isn't classified as an antacid. Monitor patient with renal insufficiency for aluminum toxicity.

PATIENT TEACHING
• Tell patient to take sucralfate on an empty stomach, 1 hour before each meal and at bedtime.
• Instruct patient to continue prescribed regimen to ensure complete healing. Pain and other ulcer signs and symptoms may subside within first few weeks of therapy.

• Urge patient to avoid cigarette smoking, which may increase gastric acid secretion and worsen disease.
• Antacids may be used while taking drug, but separate doses by 30 minutes.

sulfacetamide sodium 10%
sul-fah-SEE-tah-mide

Bleph-10, Cetamide

Therapeutic class: Antibiotics
Pharmacologic class: Sulfonamides
Pregnancy risk category: C

AVAILABLE FORMS
Ophthalmic ointment: 10%
Ophthalmic solution: 10%

INDICATIONS & DOSAGES
➤ **Inclusion conjunctivitis, corneal ulcers, chlamydial infection**
Adults and children age 2 months and older:
1 or 2 drops into lower conjunctival sac every 2 to 3 hours. Increase interval as condition responds. The usual duration of treatment is 7 to 10 days. Apply ½ inch of 10% ointment into conjunctival sac t.i.d. to q.i.d. and at bedtime. Ointment may be used at night along with drops during the day.
➤ **Trachoma**
Adults and children age 2 months and older:
2 drops into lower conjunctival sac every 2 hours with systemic sulfonamide or tetracycline.

ADMINISTRATION
Ophthalmic
• Store drug away from heat in tightly closed, light-resistant container.
• Apply light finger pressure on lacrimal sac for 1 minute after drops are instilled.
• Wait at least 5 to 10 minutes before instilling other eyedrops.

ACTION
Bacteriostatic; bactericidal in high concentrations. Prevents uptake of PABA, a metabolite of bacterial folic acid synthesis.

Route	Onset	Peak	Duration
Ophthalmic	Unknown	Unknown	Unknown

Half-life: Unknown.

ADVERSE REACTIONS

EENT: burning, eye itching, headache or brow pain, pain on instillation of drops, periorbital edema, photophobia, slowed corneal wound healing with ointment, bacterial and fungal corneal ulcers.

Other: overgrowth of nonsusceptible organisms, hypersensitivity reactions, *anaphylaxis.*

INTERACTIONS

Drug-drug. *Silver preparations:* May cause precipitate formation. Avoid using together.
Drug-lifestyle. *Sun exposure:* May cause photophobia. Advise patient to avoid excessive sunlight exposure.

EFFECTS ON LAB TEST RESULTS

None reported.

CONTRAINDICATIONS & CAUTIONS

● Contraindicated in patients hypersensitive to sulfonamides and children younger than age 2 months.

🔴 *Alert:* Fatalities have occurred rarely due to severe reactions to sulfonamides, including Stevens-Johnson syndrome, toxic epidermal necrolysis, fulminant hepatic necrosis, agranulocytosis, aplastic anemia, and other blood dyscrasias. Sensitizations may recur when a sulfonamide is readministered, irrespective of the route of administration. Sensitivity reactions have been reported in individuals with no prior history of sulfonamide hypersensitivity. At the first sign or symptom of hypersensitivity, rash, or other serious reaction, discontinue use.

● Contraindicated in epithelial herpes simplex keratitis, vaccinia, varicella, and many other viral diseases of the cornea and conjunctiva; in mycobacterial or fungal diseases of ocular structures; and after uncomplicated removal of a corneal foreign body (corticosteroid combinations).

● Use cautiously in patients with severe dry eye. Ointment may have a negative effect on corneal epithelial healing.

NURSING CONSIDERATIONS

● Drug is often used with oral tetracycline to treat trachoma and inclusion conjunctivitis.

● Concomitant use with topical corticosteroids may mask clinical signs and symptoms of infection and ineffective treatment. Monitor patient closely.

● *Look alike–sound alike:* Don't confuse Bleph-10 (sulfacetamide sodium) with Blephamide (sulfacetamide sodium and prednisolone acetate).

PATIENT TEACHING

● Tell patient to clean excessive discharge from eye area before application.

● Teach patient how to instill drops or apply ointment. Advise him to wash hands before and after applying ointment or solution and not to touch tip of dropper to eye or surrounding tissue.

● Instruct patient to apply light finger pressure on lacrimal sac for 1 minute after drops are instilled.

● Warn patient that eyedrops burn slightly.

● Advise patient to watch for and report signs and symptoms of sensitivity (itching lids, swelling, or constant burning).

● Tell patient to wait at least 5 to 10 minutes before instilling other eyedrops.

● Warn patient that solution may stain clothing.

● Tell patient to minimize sensitivity to sunlight by wearing sunglasses and avoiding prolonged exposure to sunlight.

● Advise patient not to use discolored solution.

● Tell patient not to share drug, washcloths, or towels with family members and to notify prescriber if anyone develops same signs or symptoms.

● Stress importance of compliance with recommended therapy.

● Advise patient to alert prescriber if no improvement occurs.

S

sulfamethoxazole–trimethoprim
sul-fa-meth-OX-a-zole–tri-meth-O-prim

Apo-Sulfatrim†, Bactrim*, Bactrim DS✧, Novo-Trimel†, Novo-Trimel DS†, Protrin DF†, Septra, Septra DS, Sulfatrim*, Trisulfa DS†

Therapeutic class: Antibiotics
Pharmacologic class: Sulfonamides–folate antagonists
Pregnancy risk category: C

AVAILABLE FORMS
Injection: trimethoprim 16 mg/mL and sulfamethoxazole 80 mg/mL in 5-mL vials *
Oral suspension: trimethoprim 40 mg and sulfamethoxazole 200 mg/5 mL*
Tablets (double-strength): trimethoprim 160 mg and sulfamethoxazole 800 mg
Tablets (single-strength): trimethoprim 80 mg and sulfamethoxazole 400 mg

INDICATIONS & DOSAGES
Adjust-a-dose (for all indications): For patients with CrCl of 15 to 30 mL/minute, reduce daily dose by 50%. Don't give to those with CrCl less than 15 mL/minute.
➤ **Shigellosis or UTIs caused by susceptible strains of *Escherichia coli*, *Proteus* (indole positive or negative), *Klebsiella*, or *Enterobacter* species**
Adults: 160 mg trimethoprim/800 mg sulfamethoxazole P.O. every 12 hours for 10 to 14 days in UTIs and for 5 days in shigellosis. If indicated, give 8 to 10 mg/kg/day I.V., based on trimethoprim component, in two to four divided doses every 6, 8, or 12 hours for 5 days for shigellosis or up to 14 days for severe UTIs. Maximum daily dose is 960 mg trimethoprim.
Children age 2 months and older: 8 mg/kg/day P.O., based on trimethoprim component, in two divided doses every 12 hours for 10 days for UTIs and 5 days for shigellosis. If indicated, give 8 to 10 mg/kg/day I.V., based on trimethoprim component, in two

to four divided doses every 6, 8, or 12 hours for up to 14 days for severe UTIs and 5 days for shigellosis. Don't exceed adult dose.
➤ **Otitis media in patients with penicillin allergy or penicillin-resistant infection**
Children age 2 months and older: 8 mg/kg/day P.O., based on trimethoprim component, in two divided doses every 12 hours for 10 days.
➤ **Chronic bronchitis, upper respiratory tract infections**
Adults: 160 mg trimethoprim/800 mg sulfamethoxazole P.O. every 12 hours for 14 days.
➤ **Traveler's diarrhea**
Adults: 160 mg trimethoprim/800 mg sulfamethoxazole P.O. b.i.d. for 5 days.
➤ **Community-acquired pneumonia ◆**
Adults: 160 mg trimethoprim/800 mg sulfamethoxazole P.O. b.i.d. for 10 to 14 days.
➤ ***Pneumocystis jiroveci (carinii)* pneumonia treatment**
Adults and children older than age 2 months: 15 to 20 mg/kg/day I.V. or P.O., based on trimethoprim component, in three or four divided doses for 14 to 21 days.
➤ ***P. jiroveci* pneumonia prophylaxis**
Adults: Trimethoprim 160 mg/ sulfamethoxazole 800 mg every 24 hours.
Children older than age 2 months: Trimethoprim 150 mg/m^2 with 750 mg/m^2 sulfamethoxazole daily in equally divided doses b.i.d., on 3 consecutive days per week.
➤ **Granuloma inguinale (donovanosis) ◆**
Adults: 160 mg trimethoprim/800 mg sulfamethoxazole b.i.d. for at least 3 weeks. Treatment should continue until all lesions have completely healed.
➤ **Methicillin-resistant *Staphylococcus aureus* osteomyelitis ◆**
Adults: 8 mg/kg/day (based on trimethoprim component) in two equally divided doses in combination with rifampin 600 mg/day for at least 8 weeks.
➤ **Methicillin-resistant *S. aureus* septic arthritis ◆**
Adults: 8 mg/kg/day (based on trimethoprim component) in two equally divided doses in combination with rifampin 600 mg/day for 3 to 4 weeks.

ADMINISTRATION

P.O.

● Before giving drug, ask patient if he's allergic to sulfa drugs.
● Obtain specimen for culture and sensitivity tests before giving. Begin therapy while awaiting results.
● Shake suspension well before using.
● Give drug with 8 ounces (240 mL) of water.

I.V.

▼ Before giving drug, ask patient if he's allergic to sulfa drugs.
▼ Obtain specimen for culture and sensitivity tests before giving. Begin therapy while awaiting results.
▼ Don't give by rapid infusion or bolus injection.
▼ Dilute each 5 mL of concentrate in 75 to 125 mL of D_5W. Don't mix with other drugs or solutions.
▼ Infuse slowly over 60 to 90 minutes.
▼ Don't refrigerate; use within 6 hours if diluted in 125 mL, within 4 hours if diluted in 100 mL, and within 2 hours if diluted in 75 mL.
▼ Discard solution if it's cloudy or crystallized.
▼ Never give drug I.M.
▼ **Incompatibilities:** Cisatracurium, fluconazole, foscarnet, linezolid, midazolam, verapamil, vinorelbine.

ACTION

Sulfamethoxazole inhibits formation of dihydrofolic acid from PABA; trimethoprim inhibits dihydrofolate reductase formation. Both decrease bacterial folic acid synthesis and are bactericidal.

Route	Onset	Peak	Duration
P.O.	Unknown	1–4 hr	Unknown
I.V.	Immediate	1–1½ hr	Unknown

Half-life: Trimethoprim, 8 to 11 hours; sulfamethoxazole, 10 to 13 hours.

ADVERSE REACTIONS

CNS: *seizures,* apathy, aseptic meningitis, ataxia, depression, fatigue, hallucinations, headache, insomnia, nervousness, tinnitus, vertigo.
CV: thrombophlebitis.

GI: *pancreatitis, pseudomembranous colitis,* diarrhea, nausea, vomiting, abdominal pain, anorexia, stomatitis.
GU: *toxic nephrosis with oliguria and anuria,* crystalluria, hematuria, interstitial nephritis.
Hematologic: *agranulocytosis, aplastic anemia, leukopenia, thrombocytopenia,* hemolytic anemia, megaloblastic anemia.
Hepatic: *hepatic necrosis,* jaundice.
Musculoskeletal: arthralgia, muscle weakness, myalgia.
Respiratory: pulmonary infiltrates.
Skin: generalized skin eruption, *erythema multiforme, Stevens-Johnson syndrome, toxic epidermal necrolysis,* exfoliative dermatitis, photosensitivity reactions, pruritus, urticaria.
Other: *anaphylaxis,* drug fever, hypersensitivity reactions, serum sickness.

INTERACTIONS

Drug-drug. *Cyclosporine:* May decrease cyclosporine level and increase nephrotoxicity risk. Avoid using together.
Digoxin: May increase digoxin level. Monitor digoxin level.
Dofetilide: May increase dofetilide level and effects. May increase risk of prolonged QT-interval syndrome and fatal ventricular arrhythmias. Avoid using together.
Methotrexate: May increase methotrexate level. Monitor methotrexate level.
Oral antidiabetics: May increase hypoglycemic effect. Monitor glucose level.
Phenytoin: May inhibit hepatic metabolism of phenytoin. Monitor phenytoin level.
Warfarin: May increase anticoagulant effect. Monitor patient for bleeding; monitor PT and INR.
Drug-herb. *Dong quai, St. John's wort:* May cause photosensitivity reactions. Advise patient to avoid excessive sunlight exposure.
Drug-lifestyle. *Sun exposure:* May cause photosensitivity reactions. Advise patient to avoid excessive sunlight exposure.

EFFECTS ON LAB TEST RESULTS

● May increase aminotransferase, bilirubin, BUN, and creatinine levels. May decrease hemoglobin level.

S

• May decrease granulocyte, platelet, and WBC counts.

CONTRAINDICATIONS & CAUTIONS
• Contraindicated in patients hypersensitive to trimethoprim or sulfonamides.
• Contraindicated in those with CrCl less than 15 mL/minute, porphyria, megaloblastic anemia from folate deficiency, or marked hepatic damage.
• Contraindicated in pregnant women at term, breast-feeding women, and infants younger than age 2 months.
• Use cautiously and in reduced dosages in patients with CrCl of 15 to 30 mL/minute, severe allergy or bronchial asthma, G6PD deficiency, or blood dyscrasia.
• May cause *Clostridium difficile*–associated diarrhea that can range from mild diarrhea to fatal colitis.
• Using sulfamethoxazole–trimethoprim with antiarrhythmics (amiodarone, bretylium, disopyramide, dofetilide, procainamide, quinidine, sotalol), arsenic trioxide, chlorpromazine, cisapride, dolasetron, droperidol, mefloquine, mesoridazine, moxifloxacin, pentamidine, pimozide, tacrolimus, thioridazine, and ziprasidone may prolong QT interval and increase the risk of life-threatening cardiac arrhythmias, including torsades de pointes.
⚠ *Overdose S&S:* Headache, drowsiness, unconsciousness, pyrexia, depression, confusion, anorexia, colic, nausea, vomiting, diarrhea, hematuria, crystalluria; blood dyscrasias and jaundice (late signs).

NURSING CONSIDERATIONS
ℹ *Alert:* Double-check dosage, which may be written as trimethoprim component.
ℹ *Alert:* "DS" product means "double strength."
• Monitor renal function test and LFT results.
• Promptly report rash, sore throat, fever, cough, mouth sores, or iris lesions—early signs and symptoms of erythema multiforme, which may progress to life-threatening Stevens-Johnson syndrome, or blood dyscrasias.
• Watch for signs and symptoms of superinfection, such as fever, chills, and increased pulse.

ℹ *Alert:* Adverse reactions—especially hypersensitivity reactions, rash, and fever—occur much more frequently in patients with AIDS.

PATIENT TEACHING
• Tell patient to take drug as prescribed, even if he feels better.
• Encourage patient to drink plenty of fluids to prevent crystalluria and kidney stone formation.
• Tell patient to report adverse reactions promptly.
• Instruct patient receiving drug I.V. to report discomfort at I.V. insertion site.
• Advise patient to avoid prolonged sun exposure, wear protective clothing, and use sunscreen.
• Instruct patient to take oral form with 8 ounces (240 mL) of water.

sulfasalazine (salazosulfapyridine, sulphasalazine)
sul-fuh-SAL-uh-zeen

Azulfidine, Azulfidine EN-tabs, Salazopyrin†, Salazopyrin EN-Tabs†

Therapeutic class: Anti-inflammatory drugs
Pharmacologic class: Sulfonamide salicylates
Pregnancy risk category: B

AVAILABLE FORMS
Oral suspension: 250 mg/5 mL
Tablets: 500 mg
Tablets (delayed-release): 500 mg

INDICATIONS & DOSAGES
➤ **Mild to moderate ulcerative colitis, adjunctive therapy in severe ulcerative colitis, prolongation of remission period between acute ulcerative colitis attacks**
Adults: Initially, 3 to 4 g P.O. daily in evenly divided doses not exceeding 8 hours apart; usual maintenance dose is 2 g P.O. daily in divided doses every 6 hours. Dosage may be started with 1 to 2 g, with gradual increase to minimize adverse effects.

Children age 6 and older: Initially, 40 to 60 mg/kg P.O. daily, divided into three to six doses; then 30 mg/kg daily in four doses. Dosage may be started at lower dose if GI intolerance occurs.

➤ **Rheumatoid arthritis in patients who have responded inadequately to salicylates or NSAIDs**

Adults (delayed-release tablets): 2 g P.O. daily in two evenly divided doses. To reduce possible GI intolerance, start at 0.5 to 1 g daily.

➤ **Polyarticular-course juvenile rheumatoid arthritis in patients who have responded inadequately to salicylates or other NSAIDs**

Children age 6 and older (delayed-release tablets): 30 to 50 mg/kg P.O. daily in two evenly divided doses. Maximum dose is 2 g daily. To reduce possible GI intolerance, start with one-quarter to one-third of planned maintenance dose and increase weekly until reaching maintenance dose at 1 month.

ADMINISTRATION
P.O.
● Give drug with food to decrease GI irritation.

ACTION
Unknown.

Route	Onset	Peak	Duration
P.O.	Unknown	3–12 hr	Unknown

Half-life: 6 to 8 hours.

ADVERSE REACTIONS
CNS: *seizures,* headache, depression, hallucinations.
GI: nausea, vomiting, diarrhea, abdominal pain, anorexia, stomatitis.
GU: *toxic nephrosis with oliguria and anuria,* crystalluria, hematuria, oligospermia, infertility.
Hematologic: *agranulocytosis, leukopenia, thrombocytopenia, aplastic anemia,* megaloblastic anemia, hemolytic anemia.
Hepatic: *hepatotoxicity,* jaundice.
Skin: generalized skin eruption, *erythema multiforme, Stevens-Johnson syndrome, epidermal necrolysis,* exfoliative dermatitis, photosensitivity reaction, urticaria, pruritus.

Other: serum sickness, drug fever, *anaphylaxis,* hypersensitivity reactions.

INTERACTIONS
Drug-drug. *Antibiotics:* May alter action of sulfasalazine by changing intestinal flora. Monitor patient closely.
Cyclosporine: May reduce cyclosporine efficacy and increase nephrotoxicity. Monitor cyclosporine level and renal function.
Digoxin: May reduce absorption of digoxin. Monitor patient closely.
Folic acid: May decrease absorption. Monitor patient closely.
Iron: May decrease levels of sulfasalazine caused by iron chelation. Monitor patient closely.
Methotrexate: May displace methotrexate from protein-binding sites and decrease renal clearance. Monitor patient for hematologic toxicity and adverse GI events, especially nausea.
Oral anticoagulants: May increase anticoagulant effect. Watch for bleeding.
Oral antidiabetics: May increase hypoglycemic effect. Monitor glucose levels.
Thiopurines (azathioprine, mercaptopurine): May increase leukopenia. Monitor WBC count closely.

EFFECTS ON LAB TEST RESULTS
● May increase ALT and AST levels. May decrease hemoglobin level.
● May decrease granulocyte, platelet, and WBC counts.

CONTRAINDICATIONS & CAUTIONS
● Contraindicated in patients hypersensitive to drug or its metabolites, in those with porphyria or intestinal and urinary obstruction, and in children younger than age 2.
● Use cautiously and in reduced doses in patients with impaired hepatic or renal function, severe allergy, bronchial asthma, or G6PD deficiency.
● Serious skin reactions, some fatal, including exfoliative dermatitis, Stevens-Johnson syndrome, and toxic epidermal necrolysis, have been reported. Patients are at highest risk for these events early in therapy, with most events occurring within the first month of treatment. Discontinue drug at the first appearance of rash or mucosal lesions.

S

⚠ **Overdose S&S:** Nausea, gastric distress, abdominal pain, drowsiness, seizures.

NURSING CONSIDERATIONS
● Therapeutic response in patients with rheumatoid arthritis may occur as soon as 4 weeks after starting therapy, but it may take up to 12 weeks in others.
● Drug may cause urine discoloration.
◊ **Alert:** Stop drug immediately and notify prescriber if patient shows signs and symptoms of hypersensitivity.
● Maintain adequate fluid intake to prevent crystalluria and stone formation.
● Obtain CBCs, including differential WBC count and LFTs, before start of treatment and every second week during first 3 months of therapy. During second 3 months, do the same tests once monthly and thereafter once every 3 months and as clinically indicated. Obtain a urinalysis with careful microscopic examination and an assessment of renal function periodically during treatment.
● Serum sulfapyridine levels greater than 50 mcg/mL appear to be associated with an increased incidence of adverse reactions.
● Observe patients with G6PD deficiency closely for signs and symptoms of hemolytic anemia.
● **Look alike–sound alike:** Don't confuse sulfasalazine with sulfisoxazole, salsalate, or sulfadiazine.

PATIENT TEACHING
● Instruct patient to take drug after eating and to space doses evenly.
● Warn patient to avoid ultraviolet light; drug may increase risk of sunburn. Advise patient to use sunscreen and wear protective clothing if outside for more than a short time and to avoid sunlamps and tanning booths.
● Advise patient that drug may produce an orange-yellow discoloration of skin and urine and may cause contact lenses to turn yellow.
● Inform patient of the possibility of adverse reactions and of the need for careful medical supervision. A sore throat, fever, pallor, purpura, or jaundice may indicate a serious blood disorder. Advise patient to contact the health care provider if any of these occur.

● Tell patient to drink plenty of water and to swallow tablets whole without crushing or chewing.
● Advise patient that he will need blood and urine tests to monitor treatment and that it's important to keep laboratory and doctor appointments.

sumatriptan succinate
sue-mah-TRIP-tan

Alsuma, Imitrex✦, Sumavel DosePro

Therapeutic class: Antimigraine drugs
Pharmacologic class: Serotonin 5-HT$_1$ receptor agonists
Pregnancy risk category: C

AVAILABLE FORMS
Injection: 4 mg/0.5 mL, 6 mg/0.5 mL prefilled syringes; 6 mg/0.5 mL vials
Nasal solution: 5 mg/0.1 mL, 20 mg/0.1 mL
Tablets: 25 mg, 50 mg, 100 mg (base)

INDICATIONS & DOSAGES
➤ **Acute migraine attacks (with or without aura)**
Adults: 6 mg subcutaneously; maximum dose is two 6-mg injections in 24 hours, separated by at least 1 hour. Or 25 to 100 mg P.O., initially. If desired response isn't achieved in 2 hours, may give second dose of 25 to 100 mg. Additional doses may be used in at least 2-hour intervals. Maximum daily oral dose, 200 mg.

For nasal spray, give 5 mg, 10 mg, or 20 mg once in one nostril; may repeat once after 2 hours, for maximum daily dose of 40 mg.
Adjust-a-dose: In patients with hepatic impairment, the maximum single oral dose shouldn't exceed 50 mg.
➤ **Cluster headache**
Adults: 6 mg subcutaneously. Maximum recommended dose is two 6-mg injections in 24 hours, separated by at least 1 hour.

Reactions in bold italics are *life-threatening*. Interactions may have a *rapid onset* or a *delayed onset*.

ADMINISTRATION

P.O.
- Give drug without regard for food.
- Give drug whole; don't crush or break tablet.

Subcutaneous
- Redness or pain at injection site should subside within 1 hour after injection.
- Use injection site with adequate skin and subcutaneous tissue thickness to accommodate length of needle.
- Use only the abdomen or thigh for needle-free injection system.

Intranasal
- Have patient blow his nose before use.
- Give medication on inhalation in one nostril, while blocking the other nostril.

ACTION

May act as an agonist at serotonin receptors on extracerebral intracranial blood vessels, which constricts the affected vessels, inhibits neuropeptide release, and reduces pain transmission in the trigeminal pathways.

Route	Onset	Peak	Duration
P.O.	30 min	90 min	Unknown
Subcut.	10 min	12 min	Unknown
Intranasal	Rapid	1–2 hr	Unknown

Half-life: About 2 hours.

ADVERSE REACTIONS

CNS: dizziness, vertigo, drowsiness, headache, anxiety, malaise, fatigue.
CV: *atrial fibrillation, ventricular fibrillation, ventricular tachycardia, coronary artery vasospasm, transient myocardial ischemia, MI,* pressure or tightness in chest.
EENT: discomfort of throat, nasal cavity or sinus, mouth, jaw, or tongue; altered vision.
GI: abdominal discomfort, dysphagia, diarrhea, nausea, vomiting, unusual or bad taste (nasal spray).
Musculoskeletal: myalgia, muscle cramps, neck pain.
Respiratory: upper respiratory tract inflammation and dyspnea (P.O.).
Skin: injection-site reaction, tingling, diaphoresis, flushing.
Other: warm or hot sensation, burning sensation, heaviness, pressure or tightness, tight feeling in head, cold sensation, numbness.

INTERACTIONS

Drug-drug. *Ergot and ergot derivatives, other 5-HT₁ agonists:* May prolong vasospastic effects. Don't use within 24 hours of sumatriptan therapy.
MAO inhibitors: May reduce sumatriptan clearance. Avoid using within 2 weeks of MAO inhibitor. Use injection cautiously and decrease sumatriptan dose.
SSRIs: May cause weakness, hyperreflexia, and incoordination. Monitor patient closely if use together can't be avoided.
Drug-herb. *Horehound:* May enhance serotonergic effects. Discourage use together.
St. John's wort: May increase serotonin levels. Use together cautiously.

EFFECTS ON LAB TEST RESULTS
- May increase liver enzyme levels.

CONTRAINDICATIONS & CAUTIONS
- Contraindicated in patients with hypersensitivity to drug or its components; those with history, symptoms, or signs of ischemic cardiac, cerebrovascular (such as stroke or transient ischemic attack), or peripheral vascular syndromes (such as ischemic bowel disease); significant underlying CV diseases, including angina pectoris, MI, and silent myocardial ischemia; uncontrolled hypertension; or severe hepatic impairment.
- Contraindicated within 24 hours of another 5-HT agonist or drug containing ergotamine and within 2 weeks of MAO inhibitor.
- Use cautiously in woman who is or may become pregnant.
- Use cautiously in patient with risk factors for coronary artery disease (CAD), such as postmenopausal women, men older than age 40, or patients with hypertension, hypercholesterolemia, obesity, diabetes, smoking, or family history of CAD.

NURSING CONSIDERATIONS
⚠ *Alert:* When giving drug to patient at risk for CAD, give first dose in presence of other medical personnel. Rarely, serious adverse cardiac effects can follow administration.
⚠ *Alert:* Combining drug with an SSRI or an SSNRI may cause serotonin syndrome. Symptoms include restlessness,

hallucinations, loss of coordination, fast heartbeat, rapid changes in blood pressure, increased body temperature, hyperreflexia, nausea, vomiting, and diarrhea. Serotonin syndrome may occur when starting or increasing the dose of drug, SSRI, or SSNRI.

• After subcutaneous injection, most patients experience relief in 1 to 2 hours.

• **Look alike–sound alike:** Don't confuse sumatriptan with somatropin.

PATIENT TEACHING

• Inform patient that drug is intended only to treat migraine attacks, not to prevent them or reduce their occurrence.

• If patient is pregnant or may become pregnant, tell her not to use drug but to discuss with prescriber the risks and benefits of using drug during pregnancy.

• Tell patient that drug may be taken any time during a migraine attack, as soon as signs or symptoms appear.

• Review information about drug's injectable form, which is available in a spring-loaded injector system for easier patient use. Make sure patient understands how to load the injector, give the injection, and dispose of used syringes.

• **Alert:** Tell patient to tell prescriber immediately about persistent or severe chest pain. Warn him to stop using drug and to call prescriber if he develops pain or tightness in the throat, wheezing, heart throbbing, rash, lumps, hives, or swollen eyelids, face, or lips.

• Teach patient to blow his nose before using nasal preparation. The patient should block other nostril while inhaling gently during administration. He should keep his head upright and breathe gently for 10 to 20 seconds after dose is given.

• Teach patient to select subcutaneous administration sites with adequate subcutaneous tissue thickness.

SAFETY ALERT!

sunitinib malate
soo-NIH-tih-nib

Sutent❤

Therapeutic class: Antineoplastics
Pharmacologic class: Protein-tyrosine kinase inhibitors
Pregnancy risk category: D

AVAILABLE FORMS
Capsules: 12.5 mg, 25 mg, 37.5 mg, 50 mg

INDICATIONS & DOSAGES
➤ **GI stromal tumor that's progressing despite imatinib therapy or because patient is intolerant of imatinib; advanced renal cell carcinoma**
Adults: 50 mg P.O. once daily for 4 weeks, followed by 2 weeks off the drug. Repeat cycle.
Adjust-a-dose: Increase or decrease dosage in 12.5-mg increments based on individual safety and tolerability. If drug must be administered with a strong CYP3A4 inhibitor such as ketoconazole, reduce dosage to a minimum of 37.5 mg/day. If drug must be administered with a CYP3A4 inducer (such as rifampin), consider increasing dosage to 87.5 mg daily; carefully monitor patient for toxicity. Refer to package insert for dosage adjustments for toxicities.
➤ **Progressive, well-differentiated pancreatic neuroendocrine tumors in patients with unresectable, locally advanced, or metastatic disease**
Adults: 37.5 mg P.O. once daily given continuously without a scheduled off-treatment period. Maximum recommended dosage is 50 mg daily.
Adjust-a-dose: Increase or decrease in increments of 12.5 mg based on patient tolerance and safety. If drug must be administered with a strong CYP3A4 inhibitor (such as ketoconazole), consider decreasing dosage to 25 mg daily. If drug must be administered with a CYP3A4 inducer (such as rifampin), consider increasing dosage to 62.5 mg daily and carefully monitor patient for toxicity. Refer to package insert for dosage adjustments for toxicities.

ADMINISTRATION

P.O.

● Give drug without regard for meals.

ACTION

A multi-kinase inhibitor targeting several receptor tyrosine kinases, which are involved in tumor growth, pathologic angiogenesis, and metastatic progression of cancer.

Route	Onset	Peak	Duration
P.O.	Rapid	6–12 hr	Unknown

Half-life: 40 to 60 hours; primary metabolite, 80 to 110 hours.

ADVERSE REACTIONS

CNS: asthenia, dizziness, fatigue, fever, headache, peripheral neuropathy.
CV: *decreased LVEF, thromboembolic events,* hypertension, peripheral edema.
EENT: increased lacrimation, periorbital edema.
GI: *GI perforation, pancreatitis,* abdominal pain, altered taste, anorexia, appetite disturbance, burning sensation in mouth, constipation, diarrhea, dyspepsia, flatulence, mucositis, nausea, oral pain, stomatitis, vomiting.
Hematologic: *bleeding, leukopenia, lymphopenia, neutropenia, thrombocytopenia,* anemia.
Metabolic: dehydration, hypernatremia, hyperuricemia, hypokalemia, *hyperkalemia,* hyponatremia, hypophosphatemia, hypothyroidism.
Musculoskeletal: arthralgia, back pain, limb pain, myalgia.
Respiratory: cough, dyspnea.
Skin: alopecia, dry skin, hair color changes, hand-foot syndrome, rash, skin discoloration, skin blistering.
Other: *adrenal insufficiency,* hypothyroidism.

INTERACTIONS

Drug-drug. *CYP3A4 inducers (such as carbamazepine, dexamethasone, phenobarbital, phenytoin, rifabutin, rifampin, rifapentine):* May decrease sunitinib level and effects. If use together can't be avoided, increase sunitinib dosage.

Strong CYP3A4 inhibitors (such as atazanavir, clarithromycin, indinavir, itraconazole, ketoconazole, nefazodone, nelfinavir, ritonavir, saquinavir, telithromycin, voriconazole): May increase sunitinib level and toxicity. If use together can't be avoided, decrease sunitinib dosage.
Drug-herb. *St. John's wort:* May cause an unpredictable decrease in drug level. Discourage use together.
Drug-food. *Grapefruit:* May increase drug level. Discourage use together.

EFFECTS ON LAB TEST RESULTS

● May increase AST, ALT, alkaline phosphatase, total and indirect bilirubin, amylase, lipase, creatinine, uric acid, and thyroid-stimulating hormone levels.
● May decrease phosphorus and hemoglobin levels and hematocrit.
● May increase or decrease potassium and sodium levels.
● May decrease RBC, neutrophil, lymphocyte, WBC, and platelet counts.

CONTRAINDICATIONS & CAUTIONS

● Contraindicated in patients hypersensitive to drug or any of its components.
● Don't use in patients with non–small cell lung cancer.
● Use cautiously in patients with electrolyte imbalance or a history of hypertension, QT-interval prolongation, concurrent antiarrhythmic use, bradycardia, MI, angina, CABG, symptomatic heart failure, stroke, transient ischemic attack, or PE.
● Using sunitinib malate with antiarrhythmics (amiodarone, bretylium, disopyramide, dofetilide, procainamide, quinidine, sotalol), arsenic trioxide, chlorpromazine, cisapride, dolasetron, droperidol, mefloquine, mesoridazine, moxifloxacin, pentamidine, pimozide, tacrolimus, thioridazine, and ziprasidone may prolong QT interval and increase the risk of life-threatening cardiac arrhythmias, including torsades de pointes.

NURSING CONSIDERATIONS

Black Box Warning Drug may cause severe, sometimes fatal, hepatotoxicity. Monitor liver function before and during each cycle of therapy. ∎

S

۞ Alert: Drug may cause CV events, including heart failure, myocardial disorders, and cardiomyopathy, which may be fatal. Monitor CV status closely.

• Obtain CBC with platelet count and serum chemistries, including phosphate level, before each treatment cycle.

• Obtain baseline evaluation of LVEF in all patients before treatment. If patient had a cardiac event in the year before treatment, check LVEF periodically.

• Interrupt therapy or decrease dose in patients with an ejection fraction less than 50% and more than 20% below baseline.

• Monitor patient's blood pressure closely. If severe hypertension occurs, notify prescriber. Treatment may need to be held until blood pressure is controlled.

• Monitor patient for signs and symptoms of heart failure, especially if he has a history of heart disease.

• If patient has seizures, he may have reversible posterior leukoencephalopathy syndrome. Signs and symptoms include hypertension, headache, decreased alertness, altered mental functioning, and vision loss. Stop treatment temporarily.

• Impaired wound healing has been reported during therapy. Temporarily interrupt therapy in patients undergoing major surgical procedures. May resume drug when health care provider determines patient has recovered.

• If patient will be undergoing surgery or suffers trauma or severe infection, assess him for adrenal insufficiency (muscle weakness, weight loss, depression, salt craving, low blood pressure).

• Provide antiemetics or antidiarrheals as needed for adverse GI effects.

• Monitor patient with renal cell carcinoma or GI stromal tumor with high tumor burden closely and treat as clinically indicated because of the risk of tumor lysis syndrome.

• Osteonecrosis of the jaw has been reported. Consider preventive dentistry before treatment with sunitinib. If possible, avoid invasive dental procedures, particularly in patients receiving I.V. bisphosphonate therapy.

۞ Alert: Drug may cause bleeding in GI tract, urinary tract, respiratory tract, and brain, which may be fatal. Monitor patient and CBC closely.

PATIENT TEACHING
• Advise patient to keep appointments for blood tests and periodic heart function evaluations.

• Tell patient about common adverse effects, such as diarrhea, nausea, vomiting, fatigue, mouth pain, and taste disturbance.

• Inform patient about changes that may occur in skin and hair, including color changes and dry, red, blistering skin of the hands and feet.

• Urge patient to tell prescriber about all prescribed and OTC drugs or herbal supplements.

• Warn patient not to consume grapefruit during therapy.

• Tell patient to notify his prescriber about unusual bleeding, trouble breathing, wheezing, severe or prolonged diarrhea or vomiting, or swelling of the hands or lower legs.

• Advise woman of childbearing potential to avoid becoming pregnant during therapy.

tacrolimus
tack-ROW-lim-us

Astagraf XL, Prograf

Therapeutic class: Immunosuppressants
Pharmacologic class: Macrolides
Pregnancy risk category: C

AVAILABLE FORMS
Capsules: 0.5 mg, 1 mg, 5 mg
Capsules (extended-release): 0.5 mg, 1 mg, 5 mg
Injection: 5 mg/mL

INDICATIONS & DOSAGES
➤ **To prevent organ rejection in allogenic liver, kidney, or heart transplant (with corticosteroids)**
Adults: For patients who can't take drug orally, give 0.03 to 0.05 mg/kg/day (liver or kidney) or 0.01 mg/kg/day (heart) I.V. as continuous infusion at least 6 hours after transplant. Switch to oral therapy as soon as possible, with first dose 8 to 12 hours after

stopping I.V. infusion. For renal transplant, give oral dose within 24 hours of transplantation after renal function has recovered. Initial P.O. dosages: For liver transplant, give 0.1 to 0.15 mg/kg daily in two divided doses every 12 hours; for kidney transplant, give 0.2 mg/kg daily (in combination with azathioprine) or 0.1 mg/kg daily (in combination with mycophenolate mofetil and interleukin-2 receptor agonist) in two divided doses every 12 hours; for heart transplant, give 0.075 mg/kg daily in two divided doses every 12 hours. Adjust dosages based on patient response.

For extended-release form (renal transplant only): When using with basiliximab induction, mycophenolate mofetil, and corticosteroids, administer initial dose of 0.15 mg/kg/day before or within 48 hours of completion of transplant procedure, but may delay until renal function has recovered. When using without basiliximab induction, give 0.1 mg/kg/day (preoperative); 0.2 mg/kg/day (postoperative). When using with mycophenolate mofetil and corticosteroids, give preoperative dose as one dose within 12 hours before reperfusion; give initial postoperative dose not less than 4 hours after preoperative dose and within 12 hours after reperfusion.

Children (liver transplant only): Initially, 0.03 to 0.05 mg/kg daily I.V. as continuous infusion; then 0.15 to 0.2 mg/kg daily P.O. on schedule similar to that of adults, adjusted as needed.

Adjust-a-dose: Give lowest recommended P.O. and I.V. dosages to patients with renal or hepatic impairment.

ADMINISTRATION
P.O.
● Give drug 1 hour before or 2 hours after a meal.
● Make sure patient swallows capsules whole and doesn't chew, divide, or crush them.
● Don't give with grapefruit juice.
I.V.
▼ Dilute drug with normal saline solution for injection or D$_5$W injection to 0.004 to 0.02 mg/mL before use.

▼ Monitor patient continuously during first 30 minutes and frequently thereafter for signs and symptoms of anaphylaxis.
▼ Store diluted infusion solution for up to 24 hours in glass or polyethylene containers. Don't store drug in a polyvinyl chloride container because of decreased stability and potential for extraction of phthalates.
▼ **Incompatibilities:** Solutions or I.V. drugs with a pH above 9, such as acyclovir and ganciclovir.

ACTION
Exact mechanism unknown. Inhibits T-cell activation, which results in immunosuppression.

Route	Onset	Peak	Duration
P.O., I.V.	Unknown	½–6 hr	Unknown

Half-life: Immediate-release: variable, 24–46 hours in healthy volunteers; 2.1–36 hours in transplant patients. Extended-release: 34.5–41 hours.

ADVERSE REACTIONS
CNS: asthenia, delirium, fever, headache, insomnia, pain, paresthesia, tremor, *coma.*
CV: peripheral edema, hypertension.
GI: abdominal pain, anorexia, ascites, constipation, diarrhea, nausea, vomiting.
GU: abnormal renal function, oliguria, UTI.
Hematologic: *thrombocytopenia,* anemia, leukocytosis.
Metabolic: hyperglycemia, *hyperkalemia,* hypokalemia, *hypomagnesemia.*
Musculoskeletal: back pain.
Respiratory: atelectasis, dyspnea, pleural effusion.
Skin: burning, photosensitivity, pruritus, rash, alopecia.

INTERACTIONS
Drug-drug. *CYP450 inducers (carbamazepine, phenobarbital, phenytoin,* **rifamycins [rifampin]):** May decrease tacrolimus level. Monitor effectiveness of tacrolimus.
CYP450 inhibitors **(azole antifungals,** *bromocriptine, cimetidine, clarithromycin, cyclosporine, danazol, diltiazem, erythromycin, methylprednisolone, metoclopramide, nicardipine, protease inhibitors [nelfinavir, ritonavir], proton pump*

T

inhibitors [lansoprazole, omeprazole], verapamil): May increase tacrolimus level. Watch for adverse effects. Dosage adjustment may be needed.

Cyclosporine: May increase risk of excess nephrotoxicity. Avoid using together.

Immunosuppressants (except adrenal corticosteroids): May oversuppress immune system. Monitor patient closely, especially during times of stress. Dosage adjustment may be needed.

Live-virus vaccines: May interfere with immune response to live-virus vaccines. Postpone routine immunizations.

Nephrotoxic drugs, such as aminoglycosides, amphotericin B, cisplatin, cyclosporine: May cause additive or synergistic effects. Monitor patient closely. Don't use tacrolimus simultaneously with cyclosporine. Stop cyclosporine at least 24 hours before starting tacrolimus.

Potassium-sparing diuretics: May cause severe hyperkalemia. Don't use together.

Sirolimus: May decrease tacrolimus level and increase risk of wound-healing complications, renal impairment, and insulin-dependent posttransplant diabetes mellitus in heart transplant patients. Avoid using together.

Ziprasidone, drugs that prolong QT interval (amiodarone, moxifloxacin): May cause cardiac arrhythmias, including torsades de pointes. Use together is contraindicated.

Drug-herb. *St. John's wort:* May decrease drug level. Discourage use together.

Drug-food. *Any food:* May inhibit drug absorption. Urge patient to take drug on empty stomach.

Grapefruit juice: May increase drug level. Discourage patient from taking together.

EFFECTS ON LAB TEST RESULTS

● May increase BUN, creatinine, and glucose levels. May decrease magnesium and hemoglobin levels.

● May increase or decrease potassium level and cause abnormal LFT values.

● May decrease WBC and platelet counts.

CONTRAINDICATIONS & CAUTIONS

● Contraindicated in patients hypersensitive to drug.

● I.V. form is contraindicated in patients hypersensitive to castor oil derivatives.

Black Box Warning Use of extended-release form in liver transplantation isn't recommended because of increased mortality rate in female liver transplant recipients. ▮

⚠ **Overdose S&S:** Exaggerated adverse effects.

NURSING CONSIDERATIONS

Black Box Warning Patient has increased risk for infections, lymphomas, and other malignant diseases. Only health care providers experienced in immunosuppressive therapy and management of organ transplant patients should prescribe this drug. Manage patients in facilities equipped and staffed with adequate laboratory and supportive medical resources. ▮

◐ **Alert:** Drugs causing immunosuppression increase the risk of opportunistic infections, including activation of latent viral infections (such as BK virus–associated neuropathy and JC virus–associated progressive multifocal leukoencephalopathy), which may lead to serious, even fatal outcomes.

◐ **Alert:** Because of risk of anaphylaxis, use injection only in patients who can't take oral form. Keep epinephrine 1:1,000 and oxygen available.

● Children with normal renal and hepatic function may need higher dosages than adults.

● Patients with hepatic or renal dysfunction should receive lowest dosage possible.

● Use with adrenocorticosteroids for all indications. For heart transplant patients, also use with azathioprine or mycophenolate mofetil.

● Don't use tacrolimus simultaneously with cyclosporine. Stop either drug at least 24 hours before initiating the other.

● Monitor patient for signs and symptoms of neurotoxicity and nephrotoxicity, especially if patient is receiving a high dose or has renal or hepatic dysfunction.

● Monitor patient for signs and symptoms of hyperkalemia, such as palpitations and muscle weakness or cramping. Obtain potassium levels regularly. Avoid potassium-sparing diuretics during drug therapy.

• Monitor patient's glucose level regularly. Also monitor patient for signs and symptoms of hyperglycemia, such as dizziness, confusion, and frequent urination. Treatment of hyperglycemia may be needed. Insulin-dependent posttransplant diabetes may occur; in some cases, it's reversible.

• African American kidney transplant patients may need higher doses of extended-release capsules to attain trough concentrations comparable to white patients.

PATIENT TEACHING
• Advise patient to check with prescriber before taking other drugs during therapy.
• Urge patient to report adverse reactions promptly.
• Tell diabetic patient that glucose levels may increase.
• Advise patient taking extended-release capsules that if a dose is missed, the dose may be taken up to 14 hours after the scheduled time (for example, for a missed 8:00 a.m. dose, take by 10:00 p.m.). Beyond the 14-hour time frame, patient should wait until the usual scheduled time the following morning to take the next regular daily dose. It isn't recommended to double the dose to make up for the missed dose.

---

tacrolimus (topical)
tack-ROW-lim-us

Protopic

Therapeutic class: Immunosuppressants
Pharmacologic class: Macrolides
Pregnancy risk category: C

AVAILABLE FORMS
Ointment: 0.03%, 0.1%

INDICATIONS & DOSAGES
➤ **Moderate to severe atopic dermatitis in patients unresponsive to other therapies or unable to use other therapies because of potential risks**
Adults: Thin layer of 0.03% or 0.1% strength applied to affected areas b.i.d. and rubbed in completely.

Children age 16 and older: Thin layer of 0.1% strength applied to affected areas b.i.d. and rubbed in completely.
Children ages 2 to 15: Thin layer of 0.03% strength applied to affected areas b.i.d. and rubbed in completely.

ADMINISTRATION
Topical
• In patients with infected atopic dermatitis, clear infections at treatment site before using drug.
• Don't use with occlusive dressings.

ACTION
Unknown. Probably acts as an immune system modulator in the skin by inhibiting T-lymphocyte activation, which causes immunosuppression. Drug also inhibits the release of mediators from mast cells and basophils in skin.

Route	Onset	Peak	Duration
Topical	Unknown	Unknown	Unknown

Half-life: Unknown.

ADVERSE REACTIONS
CNS: headache, hyperesthesia, asthenia, insomnia, fever, pain.
CV: peripheral edema.
EENT: otitis media, pharyngitis, rhinitis, sinusitis, conjunctivitis.
GI: diarrhea, vomiting, nausea, abdominal pain, gastroenteritis, dyspepsia.
GU: dysmenorrhea.
Musculoskeletal: back pain, myalgia.
Respiratory: increased cough, *asthma,* pneumonia, bronchitis.
Skin: burning, pruritus, erythema, infection, herpes simplex, eczema herpeticum, pustular rash, folliculitis, urticaria, maculopapular rash, fungal dermatitis, acne, sunburn, tingling, benign skin neoplasm, vesiculobullous rash, dry skin, varicella zoster, herpes zoster, eczema, exfoliative dermatitis, contact dermatitis.
Other: flulike symptoms, accidental injury, infection, facial edema, alcohol intolerance, periodontal abscess, cyst, allergic reaction.

INTERACTIONS
Drug-drug. *Calcium channel blockers, cimetidine, CYP3A4 inhibitors*

T

(erythromycin, itraconazole, ketocona-zole, fluconazole): May increase tacrolimus level if systemic absorption occurs. Use together cautiously.

Tacrolimus (systemic): May increase toxicity. Use together cautiously and decrease dosage as needed.

Drug-lifestyle. *Alcohol use:* May cause flushing. Discourage use together.

Sun exposure: May cause phototoxicity. Advise patient to avoid excessive sunlight or artificial ultraviolet light exposure.

EFFECTS ON LAB TEST RESULTS
None reported.

CONTRAINDICATIONS & CAUTIONS
● Contraindicated in patients hypersensitive to drug.

Black Box Warning Don't use in children younger than age 2 years. Only 0.03% ointment is indicated for children ages 2 to 15 years. ■

● Don't use in immunocompromised patients or in patients with Netherton syndrome or generalized erythroderma.

☺ Alert: Use only after other therapies have failed because of the risk of cancer.

NURSING CONSIDERATIONS
Black Box Warning Use drug only for short-term or intermittent long-term therapy. Limit application to areas of involvement with atopic dermatitis. Rare cases of malignancy have been reported. ■

● If signs and symptoms of atopic dermatitis don't improve within 6 weeks, reevaluate patient to confirm the diagnosis.

● Use of this drug may increase the risk of varicella zoster, herpes simplex virus, and eczema herpeticum.

● Consider stopping drug in patients with lymphadenopathy if cause is unknown or acute mononucleosis is diagnosed.

● Monitor all cases of lymphadenopathy until resolution.

● Local adverse effects are most common during the first few days of treatment.

PATIENT TEACHING
● Advise patient to read medication guide that comes with drug.

● Tell patient to wash hands before and after applying drug and to avoid applying drug to wet skin.

● Urge patient not to use bandages or other occlusive dressings.

● Tell patient not to bathe, shower, or swim immediately after application because doing so could wash the ointment off.

● Tell patient to stop treatment when the signs and symptoms resolve.

● Advise patient to avoid or minimize exposure to natural or artificial sunlight.

● Caution patient not to use drug for any disorder other than that for which it was prescribed.

● Encourage patient to report adverse reactions.

● Tell patient to store the ointment at room temperature.

tadalafil
tah-DAL-ah-fill

Adcirca, Cialis◊

Therapeutic class: Erectile dysfunction drugs
Pharmacologic class: PDE5 inhibitors
Pregnancy risk category: B

AVAILABLE FORMS
Tablets (film-coated): 2.5 mg, 5 mg, 10 mg, 20 mg

INDICATIONS & DOSAGES
➤ **Erectile dysfunction (Cialis)**
Adults: 10 mg P.O. as a single dose, as needed, before sexual activity. Range is 5 to 20 mg, based on effectiveness and tolerance. Maximum is one dose daily. Or 2.5 mg P.O. once daily without regard to timing of sexual activity. May increase to 5 mg P.O. daily.

Adjust-a-dose: If CrCl is 31 to 50 mL/minute, starting dosage is 5 mg once daily and maximum is 10 mg once every 48 hours. If CrCl is 30 mL/minute or less, maximum is 5 mg once every 72 hours as needed; daily use isn't recommended. Patients with mild or moderate hepatic impairment (Child-Pugh class A or B) shouldn't exceed 10 mg daily. Patients taking potent CYP450 inhibitors (such as erythromycin, itraconazole, ketoconazole, and ritonavir) shouldn't exceed one 10-mg dose every 72 hours; the once-daily dose shouldn't exceed 2.5 mg.

➤ **Pulmonary arterial hypertension (Adcirca)**

Adults: 40 mg (two 20-mg tablets) P.O. once daily. Dividing dose over course of the day isn't recommended.

Adjust-a-dose: For patients with CrCl of 31 to 80 mL/minute, start with 20 mg P.O. once daily. Increase to 40 mg once daily if tolerated. Avoid use in patients with CrCl less than 30 mL/minute. Consider starting dose of 20 mg P.O. once daily in patients with Child-Pugh class A or B. In patients receiving ritonavir for at least 1 week, start at 20 mg P.O. once daily and increase to 40 mg as tolerated. Don't use Adcirca when starting ritonavir; stop Adcirca at least 24 hours before starting ritonavir. After at least 1 week, may give 20 mg P.O. once daily and increase to 40 mg as tolerated.

➤ **BPH (Cialis)**

Adults: 5 mg P.O. once daily taken at approximately the same time every day.

Adjust-a-dose: In patients with CrCl of 30 to 50 mL/minute, starting dose is 2.5 mg P.O. daily. May increase to 5 mg P.O. daily based on individual response. Not recommended for patients with CrCl less than 30 mL/minute or in patients on hemodialysis.

➤ **BPH and erectile dysfunction**

Adults: 5 mg P.O. once daily taken at approximately the same time every day, without regard to the timing of sexual activity.

Adjust-a-dose: In patients with CrCl of 30 to 50 mL/minute, starting dose is 2.5 mg P.O. daily. May increase to 5 mg P.O. daily based on individual response. Not recommended for patients with CrCl less than 30 mL/minute or in patients on hemodialysis.

ADMINISTRATION
P.O.
● Give drug without regard for food.

ACTION
Increases cyclic guanosine monophosphate levels, prolongs smooth muscle relaxation, and promotes blood flow into the corpus cavernosum.

Route	Onset	Peak	Duration
P.O.	Immediate	½–6 hr	Unknown

Half-life: 17½ hours.

ADVERSE REACTIONS
CNS: dizziness, headache.
CV: flushing, hypertension.
EENT: decrease or loss of hearing, nasal congestion, tinnitus, nasopharyngitis.
GI: dyspepsia, abdominal pain, diarrhea, gastroesophageal reflux, gastroenteritis, nausea.
Musculoskeletal: back pain, limb pain, myalgia.
Respiratory: bronchitis, cough, upper respiratory tract infection.

INTERACTIONS
Drug-drug. *Alpha blockers:* May increase risk of hypotension. Patient should be on stable dose before starting tadalafil at lowest recommended dosage. Use with tadalafil for BPH treatment isn't recommended. Stop alpha blocker at least 1 day before starting tadalafil.
Nitrates: May enhance hypotensive effects. Use together is contraindicated.
Potent CYP450 inhibitors (such as erythromycin, itraconazole, ketoconazole, ritonavir): May increase tadalafil level. Don't exceed a 10-mg dose of Cialis every 72 hours.
Rifampin and other CYP450 inducers: May decrease tadalafil level. Monitor patient closely.
Drug-food. *Grapefruit:* May increase drug level. Discourage use together.
Drug-lifestyle. *Alcohol use:* May increase risk of headache, dizziness, orthostatic hypotension, and increased heart rate. Discourage use together.

EFFECTS ON LAB TEST RESULTS
None reported.

CONTRAINDICATIONS & CAUTIONS
● Contraindicated in patients hypersensitive to drug or its components and in those taking nitrates.
● Drug isn't recommended for patients with severe hepatic impairment (Child-Pugh class C), unstable angina, angina

T

that occurs during sexual intercourse, New York Heart Association class II or greater heart failure within past 6 months, uncontrolled arrhythmias, hypotension (lower than 90/50 mm Hg), uncontrolled hypertension (higher than 170/100 mm Hg), stroke within past 6 months, or an MI within past 90 days.

• Drug isn't recommended for patients whose cardiac status makes sexual activity inadvisable or for those with hereditary degenerative retinal disorders.

• Use cautiously in patients taking potent CYP450 inhibitors (such as erythromycin, itraconazole, ketoconazole, and ritonavir) and in patients with bleeding disorders, significant peptic ulceration, or renal or hepatic impairment.

• Use cautiously in patients with conditions predisposing them to priapism (such as sickle cell anemia, multiple myeloma, and leukemia), anatomic penis abnormalities, or left ventricular outflow obstruction.

• Use cautiously in elderly patients, who may be more sensitive to drug effects.

NURSING CONSIDERATIONS

◐ **Alert:** Sexual activity may increase cardiac risk. Evaluate patient's cardiac risk before he starts taking drug.

• Before patient starts drug, assess him for underlying causes of erectile dysfunction.

• Transient decreases in supine blood pressure may occur.

• Prolonged erections and priapism may occur.

PATIENT TEACHING

• Warn patient that taking drug with nitrates could cause a serious drop in blood pressure, which increases the risk of heart attack or stroke.

• Tell patient to seek immediate medical attention if chest pain develops after taking the drug.

• Tell patient that drug doesn't protect against sexually transmitted diseases and that he should use protective measures.

• Urge patient to seek emergency medical care if his erection lasts more than 4 hours.

• Tell patient to take drug about 60 minutes before anticipated sexual activity. Explain

that drug has no effect without sexual stimulation.

• Warn patient not to change dosage unless directed by prescriber.

• Caution patient against drinking large amounts of alcohol while taking drug.

• Instruct patient to notify prescriber of vision or hearing changes.

tafluprost
TA-floo-prost

Zioptan

Therapeutic class: Antiglaucoma drugs
Pharmacologic class: Prostaglandin analogues
Pregnancy risk category: C

AVAILABLE FORMS
Ophthalmic solution: 0.0015%

INDICATIONS & DOSAGES
➤ **Increased intraocular pressure in patients with open-angle glaucoma or ocular hypertension**
Adults: 1 drop instilled in conjunctival sac of affected eye once daily in the evening.

ADMINISTRATION
Ophthalmic
• Store drug in original pouch in refrigerator at 36° to 46° F (2° to 8° C).

• After pouch is opened, the single-use containers may be stored at room temperature (68° to 77° F [20° to 25° C]) for up to 28 days. Date pouch in space provided once it has been opened. Discard unused single units after 28 days.

• Discard single-use unit immediately after use; sterility can't be maintained.

• If patient is receiving more than one ophthalmic drug, give drugs at least 5 minutes apart.

ACTION
Exact mechanism unknown; believed to reduce intraocular pressure by increasing uveoscleral outflow.

Route	Onset	Peak	Duration
Ophthalmic	Rapid	10 min	Unknown

Half-life: Unknown.

ADVERSE REACTIONS
CNS: headache.
EENT: ocular stinging or irritation, ocular pruritus, conjunctivitis, cataract, dry eye, ocular pain, eyelash darkening, eyelash growth, blurred vision, conjunctival redness.
GU: UTI.
Respiratory: cough.
Other: common cold.

INTERACTIONS
None reported

EFFECTS ON LAB TEST RESULTS
None reported.

CONTRAINDICATIONS & CAUTIONS
• Contraindicated in patients hypersensitive to drug or its components.
• Use cautiously in patients with intraocular inflammation, aphakic eyes (lens has been removed), pseudophakic eyes (presence of artificial lens), or torn posterior lens capsule.
• Use in pregnant and breast-feeding women only if benefits outweigh risks. It's unknown if drug appears in breast milk.

NURSING CONSIDERATIONS
• Drug shouldn't be given more than once daily because more frequent administration of prostaglandin analogues may lessen the intraocular pressure–lowering effect.
• May use concomitantly with other topical ophthalmic drugs to lower intraocular pressure. If more than one topical ophthalmic drug is being used, separate administration times by at least 5 minutes.
• After opening individual unit for one or both eyes, use immediately because sterility can't be maintained. Discard remaining contents after administration.
• Drug can cause changes to pigmented tissues of the iris, periorbital tissue, and eyelashes. Pigmentation increases for as long as tafluprost is administered. After drug discontinuation, pigmentation of the iris is most likely permanent; however,

pigmentation of the periorbital tissue and eyelash changes may be reversible. Long-term effects are unknown.
• Drug may gradually change eyelashes and vellus hair in the treated eye. Changes include increased length and number of eyelashes and changes in color, thickness, and shape. Usually these changes are reversible after drug discontinuation.

PATIENT TEACHING
• Inform patient of once-daily nighttime dosing. More frequent dosing may decrease drug's effectiveness.
• Inform patient that drug comes in single-use containers and that unused portions must be discarded because containers don't contain a preservative.
• Caution patient that brown iris pigmentation may not be reversible but that eyelid skin darkening may be reversible.
• Inform patient of the possibility of eyelash and vellus hair changes, which may be reversible.
• Advise patient to immediately report new ocular conditions (such as trauma or infection), sudden decrease in visual acuity, ocular surgery, or development of ocular reactions.
• Instruct patient taking more than one topical ophthalmic drug to separate administration times by 5 minutes.
• Show patient how to store medication properly.

SAFETY ALERT!

tamoxifen citrate
ta-MOX-i-fen

APO-Tamox†, Nolvadex-D†

Therapeutic class: Antineoplastics
Pharmacologic class: Nonsteroidal antiestrogens
Pregnancy risk category: D

AVAILABLE FORMS
Tablets: 10 mg, 20 mg

T

INDICATIONS & DOSAGES

➤ **Advanced breast cancer in women and men**

Adults: 20 to 40 mg P.O. daily; divide doses of more than 20 mg/day into two doses.

➤ **Adjuvant treatment of breast cancer**

Women: 20 to 40 mg P.O. daily for 5 years; divide doses of more than 20 mg/day into two doses.

➤ **To reduce breast cancer occurrence**

High-risk women: 20 mg P.O. daily for 5 years.

➤ **Ductal carcinoma in situ (DCIS) after breast surgery and radiation**

Adults: 20 mg P.O. daily for 5 years.

➤ **Gynecomastia ◆**

Adults: 20 mg P.O. daily for 1 to 12 months.

➤ **Oligospermia ◆**

Adults: 10 mg P.O. b.i.d. for up to 18 months. Most effective when used in combination with testosterone.

ADMINISTRATION

P.O.

● Drug is a hormonal agent and is considered a potential teratogen. Follow safe-handling procedures.

● Give drug without regard to food.

ACTION

Unknown. Drug is selective estrogen-receptor modulator.

Route	Onset	Peak	Duration
P.O.	1 mo–several mo	Unknown	Several wk

Half-life: Distribution phase, 7 to 14 hours; terminal phase, more than 7 days.

ADVERSE REACTIONS

CNS: *stroke,* confusion, weakness, sleepiness, headache.

CV: fluid retention, hot flashes, *thromboembolism.*

EENT: corneal changes, cataracts, retinopathy.

GI: nausea, vomiting, diarrhea.

GU: amenorrhea, irregular menses, vaginal discharge, *endometrial cancer, uterine sarcoma,* vaginal bleeding.

Hematologic: *leukopenia, thrombocytopenia.*

Hepatic: *hepatic necrosis,* fatty liver, cholestasis.

Metabolic: hypercalcemia, weight gain or loss.

Musculoskeletal: brief worsening of pain from osseous metastases.

Respiratory: *PE.*

Skin: skin changes, rash, alopecia.

Other: temporary bone or tumor pain.

INTERACTIONS

Drug-drug. *Bromocriptine:* May elevate tamoxifen level. Monitor patient closely.

Coumarin-type anticoagulants: May significantly increase anticoagulant effect. Monitor patient, PT, and INR closely.

CYP3A4 inducers (such as rifampin): May increase tamoxifen metabolism and may lower drug levels. Monitor patient for clinical effects.

Cytotoxic drugs: May increase risk of thromboembolic events. Monitor patient.

Drug-herb. *St. John's wort:* May increase serotonin levels. Use together cautiously.

EFFECTS ON LAB TEST RESULTS

● May increase BUN, calcium, T_4, and liver enzyme levels.

● May decrease WBC and platelet counts.

CONTRAINDICATIONS & CAUTIONS

● Contraindicated in patients hypersensitive to drug.

● Contraindicated as therapy to reduce risk of breast cancer in high-risk women who also need anticoagulants or in women with history of DVT or PE.

● Use cautiously in patients with leukopenia or thrombocytopenia.

⚠ *Overdose S&S:* Tremors, hyperreflexia, unsteady gait, dizziness, seizures, prolonged QT interval.

NURSING CONSIDERATIONS

● Monitor lipid levels during long-term therapy in patients with hyperlipidemia.

● Monitor calcium level. At start of therapy, drug may compound hypercalcemia related to bone metastases.

● Women should have baseline and periodic gynecologic examinations because of a slight increased risk of endometrial cancer.

● Women should have periodic eye examinations because of increased risk of

---

Reactions in bold italics are *life-threatening*. Interactions may have a *rapid onset* or a *delayed onset*.

cataracts, retinal vein thrombosis, and retinopathy.
• Monitor CBC closely in patients with leukopenia or thrombocytopenia.
• Rule out pregnancy before therapy.
• Patient may initially experience worsening symptoms.
• Adverse reactions are usually minor and well tolerated.
• In postmenopausal women, karyopyknotic index of vaginal smears and various degrees of estrogen effect of Papanicolaou smears may vary.

Black Box Warning Women who are at high risk for breast cancer or who have DCIS and are taking drug to reduce risk may experience life-threatening endometrial cancer, uterine sarcoma, stroke, or PE. The benefits of drug outweigh its risks in women already diagnosed with breast cancer. ■

PATIENT TEACHING
• Reassure patient that acute worsening of bone pain during therapy usually indicates drug will produce good response. Give analgesics to relieve pain.
• Strongly encourage women who are taking or have taken drug to have regular gynecologic examinations because drug may increase risk of uterine cancer.
• Encourage women to have annual mammograms and breast examinations.
• Advise patient to use a barrier form of contraception because short-term therapy induces ovulation in premenopausal women.
• Instruct patient to report vaginal bleeding or changes in menstrual cycle.
• Caution women to avoid becoming pregnant during therapy and first 2 months after stopping drug. Advise consulting prescriber before becoming pregnant.
• Advise patient that breast cancer risk assessment tools are available and that she should discuss her concerns with her prescriber.
• Tell patient to report symptoms of stroke, such as headache, vision changes, confusion, difficulty speaking or walking, and weakness of face, arm, or leg, especially on one side of the body.

• Tell patients to report symptoms of PE, such as chest pain, difficulty breathing, rapid breathing, sweating, and fainting.
• Advise patient to report vision changes.

tamsulosin hydrochloride
tam-soo-LOE-sin

Flomax⌀

Therapeutic class: BPH drugs
Pharmacologic class: Alpha blockers
Pregnancy risk category: B

AVAILABLE FORMS
Capsules: 0.4 mg

INDICATIONS & DOSAGES
➤ **BPH**
Adults. 0.4 mg P.O. once daily, given 30 minutes after same meal each day. If no response after 2 to 4 weeks, increase dosage to 0.8 mg P.O. once daily.
➤ **Adjunctive treatment of ureteral stones** ◆
Adults: 0.4 mg P.O. daily for up to 6 weeks or until expulsion.

ADMINISTRATION
P.O.
• Don't crush or open capsules.
• Give drug 30 minutes after same meal each day.

ACTION
Selectively blocks alpha receptors in the prostate, leading to relaxation of smooth muscles in the bladder neck and prostate, improving urine flow and reducing symptoms of BPH.

Route	Onset	Peak	Duration
P.O.	Unknown	4–5 hr	9–15 hr

Half-life: 9 to 13 hours.

ADVERSE REACTIONS
CNS: dizziness, headache, asthenia, insomnia, somnolence, syncope, vertigo.
CV: chest pain, orthostatic hypotension.
EENT: rhinitis, amblyopia, pharyngitis, sinusitis.
GI: diarrhea, nausea.

T

GU: decreased libido, abnormal ejaculation, priapism.
Musculoskeletal: back pain.
Respiratory: increased cough.
Other: infection, tooth disorder.

INTERACTIONS
Drug-drug. *Alpha blockers:* May interact with tamsulosin. Avoid using together.
Cimetidine: May decrease tamsulosin clearance. Use together cautiously.
Warfarin: Limited studies are inconclusive. Use together cautiously.

EFFECTS ON LAB TEST RESULTS
None reported.

CONTRAINDICATIONS & CAUTIONS
• Contraindicated in patients hypersensitive to drug or its components.
• Use cautiously in patients with serious or life-threatening sulfa allergy.
⚠ *Overdose S&S:* Severe headache.

NURSING CONSIDERATIONS
• Monitor patient for decreases in blood pressure.
• Symptoms of BPH and prostate cancer are similar; rule out prostate cancer before starting therapy.
• If treatment is interrupted for several days or more, restart therapy at the 0.4-mg P.O. once-daily dose.
• *Look alike–sound alike:* Don't confuse Flomax with Fosamax or Volmax.

PATIENT TEACHING
• Instruct patient not to crush, chew, or open capsules.
• Tell patient to rise slowly from chair or bed when starting therapy and to avoid situations in which injury could occur as a result of fainting. Advise him that drug may cause sudden drop in blood pressure, especially after first dose or when changing doses.
• Inform patient about the rare, but serious, possibility of priapism.
• Instruct patient not to drive or perform hazardous tasks for 12 hours after first dose or changes in dose until response can be monitored.

• Tell patient to take drug about 30 minutes after same meal each day.
• Advise patient considering cataract surgery to inform the ophthalmologist that he is taking the drug. Floppy iris syndrome may occur during surgery.

SAFETY ALERT!

tapentadol hydrochloride
tah-PEN-tah-dol

Nucynta, Nucynta ER

Therapeutic class: Analgesics
Pharmacologic class: Centrally acting synthetic opioid analgesics
Pregnancy risk category: C
Controlled substance schedule: II

AVAILABLE FORMS
Oral solution: 20 mg/mL
Tablets: 50 mg, 75 mg, 100 mg
Tablets (extended-release): 50 mg, 100 mg, 150 mg, 200 mg, 250 mg

INDICATIONS & DOSAGES
➤ **Moderate to severe acute pain (immediate-release only)**
Adults: 50 to 100 mg P.O. every 4 to 6 hours, as needed for pain. On day 1, may give second dose in 1 hour if first dose is ineffective. Adjust subsequent dosing to maintain adequate pain control. Maximum daily dose, 700 mg on day 1; 600 mg on subsequent days.
Adjust-a-dose: For patients with moderate hepatic impairment, initially give 50 mg P.O. every 8 hours. Maximum, three doses (150 mg) in 24 hours; the interval between doses should be no less than 8 hours. Drug isn't recommended for patients with severe hepatic or renal impairment.
➤ **Severe chronic pain when continuous, around-the-clock opioid analgesia is needed for an extended period (extended-release)**
Adults: Initially, 50 mg P.O. every 12 hours. Titrate with dose increases of 50 mg no more than b.i.d. every 3 days. Therapeutic range is 100 to 250 mg P.O. b.i.d.
Adjust-a-dose: For patients with moderate hepatic impairment, initially 50 mg (extended-release) once every 24 hours.

Maximum dose is 100 mg (extended-release) once daily. Don't use for patients with severe hepatic impairment.

➤ **Neuropathic pain associated with diabetic peripheral neuropathy (extended-release)**
Adults: Initially, 50 mg P.O. every 12 hours. Titrate with dose increases of 50 mg no more than b.i.d. every 3 days. Therapeutic range is 100 to 250 mg P.O. b.i.d.
Adjust-a-dose: In patients with moderate hepatic impairment, initially give 50 mg (extended-release) once every 24 hours. Maximum dosage is 100 mg once daily. Don't use in patients with severe hepatic impairment.

ADMINISTRATION
P.O.
● Give drug with or without food.
Black Box Warning Patients must swallow extended-release tablets whole. Taking split, broken, chewed, dissolved, or crushed tablets could lead to rapid release and a potentially fatal overdose. ∎

ACTION
Unknown. Thought to work by possessing mu-opioid agonist activity and inhibiting norepinephrine reuptake in the brain.

Route	Onset	Peak	Duration
P.O.	Rapid	1¼ hr	Unknown

Half-life: 4 hours.

ADVERSE REACTIONS
CNS: abnormal dreams, anxiety, *CNS depression,* confusion, dizziness, fatigue, insomnia, lethargy, somnolence, tremor.
EENT: nasopharyngitis.
GI: constipation, decreased appetite, dry mouth, dyspepsia, nausea, vomiting.
GU: UTI.
Musculoskeletal: arthralgia.
Respiratory: *respiratory depression,* upper respiratory tract infection.
Skin: hot flushes, hyperhidrosis, pruritus, rash.

INTERACTIONS
Drug-drug. *CNS depressants (antiemetics, general anesthetics, hypnotics, opioid analgesics, phenothiazines, sedatives, tran-*

quilizers): May cause additive CNS effects. Reduce dosage of one or both drugs and monitor patient closely.
MAO inhibitors: May cause adverse CV events. Avoid use together. Avoid giving drug within 14 days of MAO inhibitor use.
MAO inhibitors, SSRIs, SSNRIs, TCAs, triptans: May cause serotonin syndrome (mental changes, tachycardia, labile blood pressure, hyperthermia, hyperreflexia, incoordination, nausea, vomiting, diarrhea). Avoid use together.
Drug-lifestyle. **Black Box Warning**
Alcohol use: May result in a potentially fatal overdose of tapentadol, if alcohol, including prescription or OTC drugs that contain alcohol, is used with extended-release form. Don't use together. ∎

EFFECTS ON LAB TEST RESULTS
None reported.

CONTRAINDICATIONS & CAUTIONS
● Contraindicated in patients with significant respiratory depression, or acute or severe bronchial asthma in unmonitored settings or when resuscitative equipment isn't available.
Black Box Warning Extended-release tapentadol must not be used as an as-needed analgesic or to treat acute or postoperative pain. ∎
Black Box Warning Schedule II opioids have the highest potential for abuse and risk of fatal overdose due to respiratory depression. ∎
● Contraindicated in patients who have or are suspected of having paralytic ileus and in those receiving MAO inhibitors or who have used MAO inhibitors within the past 14 days.
● Avoid use in patients with head injury and increased intracranial pressure.
● Use cautiously in patients with conditions accompanied by hypoxia, hypercapnia, or decreased respiratory reserve (such as asthma, COPD, cor pulmonale, severe obesity, sleep apnea syndrome, myxedema, kyphoscoliosis, CNS depression, coma, or upper airway obstruction).
● Use cautiously in patients with a history of seizures, hepatic impairment, or biliary tract

T

disease, including acute pancreatitis, and in elderly and debilitated patients.

• Safety and effectiveness during pregnancy haven't been established. Use only if the benefits to the mother outweigh the risk to the fetus.

• It isn't known if drug appears in breast milk. However, because of the risk of serious adverse reactions, breastfeeding isn't recommended.

⚠ **Overdose S&S:** CNS and respiratory depression, hypotension, bradycardia, hypothermia, shock, apnea, cardiopulmonary arrest.

NURSING CONSIDERATIONS

• Keep opioid antagonist (naloxone) available.

• Monitor vital signs, respiratory status, and level of consciousness closely, especially in elderly, cachectic, or debilitated patients and in those with chronic pulmonary disease; drug may cause hypotension and respiratory depression. If respiratory rate drops below 12 breaths/minute, hold dose and notify prescriber.

• Reassess patient's level of pain 15 to 30 minutes after giving dose.

• Avoid using drug immediately before and during labor and delivery. Monitor for respiratory depression in newborns of mothers who have been taking drug.

Black Box Warning Drug has the potential for addiction and abuse. Chewing, crushing, snorting, or injecting it can lead to overdose and death. Monitor patients for signs and symptoms of abuse or addiction. ∎

• Taper dosage gradually to prevent withdrawal symptoms (anxiety, sweating, insomnia, rigors, pain, nausea, tremors, diarrhea, upper respiratory symptoms, piloerection, and hallucinations).

• Consider dosage reduction of one or both drugs if taken with another opioid, sedative, or illicit drug because of additive effects.

• Prevent constipation with the use of stool softeners or senna preparations at the start of therapy.

• Drug may cause spasm of the sphincter of Oddi and may worsen pain in patients with biliary disease, including pancreatitis.

Black Box Warning Accidental ingestion of extended-release form may cause fatal overdose, especially in children. ∎

PATIENT TEACHING

• Instruct patient to ask for drug before pain is intense and to report episodes of breakthrough pain.

• Advise ambulatory patients to use caution when getting out of bed or walking.

• Warn patient to avoid driving and other hazardous activities that require mental alertness until drug's CNS effects are known.

• Warn patient not to crush, break, chew, or dissolve tablets.

Black Box Warning Instruct patient to keep tablets in a child-resistant container in a safe place because accidental ingestion by a child can result in death. ∎

Black Box Warning Caution patient not to consume alcohol or take drugs containing alcohol; doing so may lead to fatal overdose. ∎

• Inform patient that drug has the potential for abuse. Advise patient to protect drug from theft.

• Tell women of childbearing age to consult prescriber if pregnant or considering becoming pregnant.

• Advise breast-feeding women to choose an alternative method of feeding infants during therapy.

• Advise patient not to stop drug abruptly.

telaprevir
tel-A-pre-vir

Incivek

Therapeutic class: Antivirals
Pharmacologic class: Protease inhibitors
Pregnancy risk category: B; X when used with ribavirin

AVAILABLE FORMS
Tablets: 375 mg

INDICATIONS & DOSAGES

Adjust-a-dose (for all indications): Discontinue therapy (telaprevir, peginterferon alfa, and ribavirin) in patients with HCV-RNA levels greater than 1,000 international units/mL at treatment week 4 or 12. Discontinue peginterferon alfa and ribavirin in patients with confirmed, detectable HCV-RNA

Reactions in bold italics are *life-threatening*. Interactions may have a *rapid onset* or a *delayed onset*.

levels at treatment week 24. If peginterferon alfa or ribavirin is discontinued for any reason, telaprevir must also be discontinued.
➤ **Genotype 1 chronic hepatitis C in patients with compensated liver disease, including cirrhosis, who are treatment-naive and have had prior relapse with HCV-RNA undetectable at weeks 4 and 12**
Adults: 750 mg P.O. t.i.d., 7 to 9 hours apart, for 12 weeks in combination with peginterferon alfa and ribavirin; continue dual therapy with peginterferon alfa and ribavirin only for an additional 12 weeks for a total treatment duration of 24 weeks.
➤ **Genotype 1 chronic hepatitis C in patients with compensated liver disease, including cirrhosis, who are treatment-naive and have had prior relapse with HCV-RNA detectable (1,000 international units/mL or less) at weeks 4 and 12**
Adults: 750 mg P.O. t.i.d., 7 to 9 hours apart, for 12 weeks in combination with peginterferon alfa and ribavirin; continue dual therapy with peginterferon alfa and ribavirin only for an additional 36 weeks for a total treatment duration of 48 weeks.
➤ **Genotype 1 chronic hepatitis C in patients with compensated liver disease, including cirrhosis, who have previously been partial and null responders**
Adults: 750 mg P.O. t.i.d., 7 to 9 hours apart, for 12 weeks in combination with peginterferon alfa and ribavirin; continue dual therapy with peginterferon alfa and ribavirin only for an additional 36 weeks for a total treatment duration of 48 weeks.

ADMINISTRATION
P.O.
● Give within 30 minutes of food with 20 g fat content to increase absorption.
● Store at room temperature.

ACTION
Inhibits synthesis of proteins necessary for viral replication.

Route	Onset	Peak	Duration
P.O.	Unknown	4–5 hr	Unknown

Half-life: 9 to 11 hours.

ADVERSE REACTIONS
CNS: fatigue.
GI: dysgeusia, nausea, vomiting, hemorrhoids, anorectal discomfort, anal pruritus, diarrhea.
Hematologic: anemia, neutropenia, leukopenia, thrombocytopenia.
Skin: rash, pruritus, *Stevens-Johnson syndrome, toxic epidermal necrolysis.*

INTERACTIONS
Drug-drug. *Amlodipine, calcium channel blockers:* May increase levels of these drugs. Monitor patient closely and adjust dosage of amlodipine and calcium channel blockers as needed.
Antiarrhythmics (amiodarone, bepridil, flecainide, propafenone, quinidine): May potentially produce serious or life-threatening effects. Monitor patient closely.
Antibacterials (clarithromycin, erythromycin, telithromycin): May increase concentrations of these drugs. Monitor patient for QT-interval prolongation and torsades de pointes.
Anticonvulsants (carbamazepine, phenobarbital, phenytoin): May decrease telaprevir level and alter concentration of anticonvulsants. Monitor clinical response to telaprevir. Monitor anticonvulsant blood levels and titrate anticonvulsant drug dosage if necessary.
Antifungals (itraconazole, ketoconazole, posaconazole): May increase blood levels of antifungal and telaprevir. Don't administer high-dose (greater than 200 mg/day) itraconazole or ketoconazole. Monitor patient for QT-interval prolongation and torsades de pointes.
Benzodiazepines (alprazolam, diazepam, I.V. midazolam, lorazepam): May potentiate effects of benzodiazepines. Use cautiously together. Consider reducing benzodiazepine dosage.
Benzodiazepines (P.O. midazolam, triazolam): May cause respiratory depression and excessive sedation. Use together is contraindicated.
Colchicine: May increase colchicine toxicity. Use together only in patients with normal renal and hepatic function. If used together, reduce colchicine dosage. For

T

treatment of gout flares, give colchicine 0.6 mg P.O. for one dose, followed by 0.3 mg P.O. 1 hour later. Don't repeat dose before 3 days. For prophylaxis of gout flares, if original colchicine regimen was 0.6 mg P.O. b.i.d., decrease to 0.3 mg P.O. once a day; if original colchicine regimen was 0.6 mg once a day, decrease to 0.3 mg P.O. every other day.

Corticosteroids (inhaled): May significantly increase systemic concentrations of steroids. Weigh risks and benefits; use together cautiously.

Corticosteroids (systemic): May significantly increase systemic concentrations of steroids. Avoid use together.

Darunavir with ritonavir, efavirenz, fosamprenavir with ritonavir, lopinavir–ritonavir: May reduce effectiveness of all drugs. Avoid use together.

Desipramine, trazodone: May increase blood levels of these drugs and increase risk of adverse reactions (nausea, dizziness, hypotension, syncope). Reduce dosages of desipramine and trazodone if adverse reactions occur.

Dexamethasone: May decrease telaprevir level. Use together cautiously or consider alternative drug to dexamethasone.

Digoxin: May increase digoxin serum concentration. Monitor serum digoxin level and use lowest possible digoxin dosage.

Escitalopram: May decrease escitalopram blood level. Adjust escitalopram dosage as needed.

Estrogen hormone replacement therapy: May cause estrogen deficiency. Monitor patient for signs and symptoms of estrogen deficiency and titrate dosage as necessary.

HMG-CoA reductase inhibitors (atorvastatin, lovastatin, simvastatin): May increase risk of rhabdomyolysis. Avoid use together.

Hormonal contraceptives: May decrease effectiveness of hormonal contraceptives. Patient should use two effective, nonhormonal methods of contraception while taking telaprevir and for 2 weeks after stopping therapy.

Immunosuppressants (cyclosporine, sirolimus, tacrolimus): May cause significantly elevated concentrations of immunosuppressants. Monitor blood levels, frequently assess renal function, and monitor patient for immunosuppressant-related adverse effects. Consider dosage reductions and prolongation of dosing interval for immunosuppressants.

Methadone: May decrease methadone level. Increase methadone dosage in maintenance patients.

Rifabutin: May increase rifabutin level and decrease telaprevir level. Avoid use together.

Salmeterol: May increase risk of CV events (QT-interval prolongation, sinus tachycardia, palpitations). Avoid use together.

Sildenafil and tadalafil for pulmonary arterial hypertension: May prolong QT interval. Use together is contraindicated.

Sildenafil, tadalafil, and vardenafil for erectile dysfunction: May increase levels of these drugs. Adjust dosage of these drugs; not to exceed 25 mg in 48 hours for sildenafil, 10 mg in 72 hours for tadalafil, and 2.5 mg in 72 hours for vardenafil.

Tenofovir: May cause tenofovir toxicity. If toxicities develop, discontinue tenofovir.

Voriconazole: May alter voriconazole level unpredictably. Avoid use together.

Warfarin: May alter warfarin concentration. Monitor INR during treatment and after discontinuation of telaprevir.

Zolpidem: May decrease zolpidem level. Monitor clinical response and adjust zolpidem dosage.

Drug-herb. *St. John's wort:* May decrease telaprevir level. Avoid use together.

EFFECTS ON LAB TEST RESULTS

● May increase bilirubin and uric acid levels.

● May decrease hemoglobin level and total WBC, lymphocyte, ANC, and platelet counts.

CONTRAINDICATIONS & CAUTIONS

Black Box Warning Fatal and nonfatal serious skin reactions, including Stevens-Johnson syndrome, drug reaction with eosinophilia and systemic symptoms, and toxic epidermal necrolysis, have been reported in patients receiving telaprevir combination treatment. Fatal cases have been reported in patients with progressive rash and systemic symptoms who continued to receive telaprevir combination treatment after a serious skin reaction was identified. ■

• Contraindicated in patients hypersensitive to drug, women who are or who may become pregnant, men whose female partners are pregnant, and breast-feeding women.

• Contraindicated in patients with moderate to severe hepatic impairment (Child-Pugh class B or C), in patients with solid organ transplants, and in patients co-infected with HCV/HIV, HCV, or HBV. Also contraindicated in children.

• Telaprevir must not be administered as monotherapy and must only be prescribed with both peginterferon alfa and ribavirin.

• To prevent treatment failure, telaprevir dosage must not be reduced or therapy interrupted.

NURSING CONSIDERATIONS

Black Box Warning Immediately discontinue telaprevir, peginterferon alfa, and ribavirin if a serious skin reaction develops, including rash with systemic symptoms or a progressive severe rash, and refer patient for urgent medical care. Also consider discontinuing other medications known to be associated with serious skin reactions. ■

• Monitor HCV-RNA levels at weeks 4 and 12. Monitor CBC with differential and serum electrolyte, creatinine, uric acid, hepatic enzyme, bilirubin, and thyroid-stimulating hormone levels at weeks 2, 4, 8, and 12.

• Telaprevir must not be administered as monotherapy.

• Monitor female patients of childbearing age for pregnancy before and during therapy with telaprevir and ribavirin, and for 6 months after discontinuation of therapy.

PATIENT TEACHING

• Advise patient that telaprevir must be administered in combination with both peginterferon alfa and ribavirin. If peginterferon alfa, ribavirin, or both are discontinued, telaprevir must also be stopped.

• Warn patient that because telaprevir must be used in combination with peginterferon alfa and ribavirin, extreme care must be taken to avoid pregnancy in female patients and female partners of male patients; fetal harm and fetal death have occurred after exposure to ribavirin.

• Instruct female patient of childbearing age to use two effective, nonhormonal methods of contraception during telaprevir therapy and for 2 weeks after therapy has ended.

• Instruct patient to take telaprevir with a meal or snack that has approximately 20 grams of fat to ensure maximum absorption. Tell patient to take drug within 30 minutes of such foods as a bagel with cream cheese, ½ cup nuts, 3 tablespoons peanut butter, 1 cup ice cream, 2 ounces American or cheddar cheese, 2 ounces potato chips, or ½ cup trail mix.

Black Box Warning Warn patient that telaprevir may cause a severe, life-threatening rash. Instruct patient to seek urgent medical care if skin changes or itching develops. ■

• Caution patient not to interrupt or discontinue telaprevir treatment without notifying his health care provider because this may cause treatment failure.

• Instruct patient that the effect of telaprevir on the transmission of hepatitis C infection is unknown and that he must use and maintain appropriate precautions in case of treatment failure.

• Instruct patient that if he misses a dose of telaprevir within 4 hours of the time it is usually taken, to take the prescribed dose as soon as possible. If more than 4 hours have elapsed from the time the dose is normally taken, instruct patient to skip that dose and then resume the usual dosing schedule at his regularly scheduled time; doses should be 7 to 9 hours apart.

telavancin
tell-uh-VAN-sin

Vibativ

Therapeutic class: Antibiotics
Pharmacologic class: Lipoglycopeptides
Pregnancy risk category: C

AVAILABLE FORMS

Lyophilized powder for injection: 250-mg, 750-mg single-use vials

INDICATIONS & DOSAGES

☞ *Alert:* Drug should be used to prevent or treat bacterial infections only. Reserve use for when alternative treatments aren't suitable.

Adjust-a-dose (for all indications): For patients with CrCl of 30 to 50 mL/minute, give 7.5 mg/kg every 24 hours; if CrCl is 10 to 29 mL/minute, give 10 mg/kg every 48 hours.

➤ **Complicated skin and skin-structure infections caused by susceptible gram-positive organisms, such as** *Staphylococcus aureus,* **methicillin-resistant** *S. aureus, Streptococcus pyogenes, Streptococcus agalactiae, Streptococcus aginosus* **group, or** *Enterococcus faecalis* **(vancomycin-susceptible isolates only)**
Adults: 10 mg/kg I.V. infusion once every 24 hours for 7 to 14 days.

✷ *NEW INDICATION:* **Hospital-acquired and ventilator-associated bacterial pneumonia caused by susceptible isolates of** *S. aureus* **(including methicillin-susceptible and methicillin-resistant isolates)**
Adults: 10 mg/kg I.V. once every 24 hours for 7 to 21 days.

ADMINISTRATION

I.V.

▼ Reconstitute 250-mg vial with 15 mL sterile water for injection and 750-mg vial with 45 mL sterile water for injection. Solutions of D₅W and normal saline solution for injection also may be used. Mix thoroughly; reconstitution may take up to 20 minutes.

▼ Further dilute doses of 150 to 800 mg in 100 to 250 mL of D₅W, normal saline solution, or lactated Ringer solution before infusion. Further dilute doses less than 150 mg or greater than 800 mg to a final concentration of 0.6 to 8 mg/mL.

▼ Inspect for particulate matter before infusion.

▼ Infuse drug over 60 minutes.

▼ Reconstituted solution is stable for 4 hours at room temperature or 72 hours if refrigerated.

▼ Diluted I.V. solution is stable for 4 hours at room temperature or 72 hours if refrigerated (includes reconstituted time).

▼ **Incompatibilities:** Other I.V. drugs. If line is used for other I.V. drugs, flush with D₅W, normal saline solution, or lactated Ringer solution before and after infusion.

ACTION

Inhibits bacterial cell-wall synthesis by binding to the bacterial cell membrane and disrupting its function.

Route	Onset	Peak	Duration
I.V.	Unknown	Unknown	Unknown

Half-life: About 8 hours.

ADVERSE REACTIONS

CNS: dizziness.
GI: abdominal pain, decreased appetite, diarrhea, nausea, taste disturbance, vomiting, *Clostridium difficile–*associated diarrhea.
GU: foamy urine, new-onset or worsening renal impairment.
Skin: generalized pruritus, infusion-site pain, infusion-site erythema, rash.
Other: rigors.

INTERACTIONS

None reported.

EFFECTS ON LAB TEST RESULTS

● May falsely prolong PT, INR, PTT, and activated clotting time, and may increase factor Xa.

● May falsely affect urine qualitative dipstick protein assays and quantitative dye methods, such as pyrogallol red-molybdate.

CONTRAINDICATIONS & CAUTIONS

● Use cautiously in patients with renal impairment. Avoid use in patients with prolonged QTc interval, uncompensated heart failure, or severe left ventricular hypertrophy.

Black Box Warning Drug may cause nephrotoxicity. Monitor renal function in all patients. Use drug in patients with preexisting moderate to severe renal impairment (CrCl of 50 mL/minute or less) only when anticipated benefit outweighs potential risk. ■

Black Box Warning Women of childbearing age should have a pregnancy test before therapy. Avoid use during pregnancy

---

Reactions in bold italics are *life-threatening*. Interactions may have a *rapid onset* or a *delayed onset*.

unless the risks to the mother outweigh the potential risks to the fetus. ▪

Black Box Warning Adverse developmental outcomes observed in three animal species at clinically relevant doses raise concerns about potential adverse developmental outcomes in humans. ▪

• Register pregnant women exposed to drug in the Vibativ Pregnancy Registry by calling 1-888-658-4228.

• It isn't known if drug appears in breast milk. Use cautiously in breast-feeding women.

• Decreased efficacy has occurred among patients with moderate to severe preexisting renal impairment being treated for skin and skin-structure infections. Consider alternative drug when selecting antibacterial therapy for patients with baseline CrCl of 50 mL/minute or less.

• Safety and effectiveness in children haven't been established.

NURSING CONSIDERATIONS

• Monitor renal function before and during therapy.

☼ **Alert:** Rapid I.V. infusion may cause "red-man syndrome" (flushing of the upper body, urticaria, pruritus, or rash). Infuse over at least 60 minutes.

• If diarrhea develops, test patient for *C. difficile* infection.

• Watch for signs and symptoms of superinfection, such as continued fever, chills, and increased pulse rate.

• Reduce dosage in elderly patients who have diminished renal function.

PATIENT TEACHING

• Advise women of childbearing age to use an effective method of contraception during therapy.

• Advise women not to breast-feed while taking drug.

• Tell patient to notify prescriber if he has a history of kidney problems, heart problems (including QTc interval prolongation), or diabetes before starting drug.

• Tell patient not to skip doses or to stop treatment without notifying prescriber.

• Tell patient to notify prescriber if diarrhea develops during treatment or within 2 months of completing treatment.

telbivudine
tell-BIV-you-deen

Tyzeka, Sebivo†

Therapeutic class: Antivirals
Pharmacologic class: Nucleosides–nucleotides
Pregnancy risk category: B

AVAILABLE FORMS
Tablets: 600 mg

INDICATIONS & DOSAGES
➤ **Chronic hepatitis B**
Adults and children age 16 or older: 600 mg P.O. daily.
Adjust-a-dose: If CrCl is 30 to 49 mL/minute, give 600-mg tablet every 48 hours; if CrCl is less than 30 mL/minute and patient doesn't require dialysis, give 600-mg tablet every 72 hours. For patients with ESRD, give 600-mg tablet every 96 hours after dialysis.

ADMINISTRATION
P.O.
• Give drug without regard for meals.

ACTION
Inhibits HBV replication by interrupting DNA polymerase activity.

Route	Onset	Peak	Duration
P.O.	Immediate	1–4 hr	Unknown

Half-life: 40 to 49 hours.

ADVERSE REACTIONS
CNS: dizziness, insomnia, fatigue, headache, pyrexia.
EENT: pharyngolaryngeal pain.
GI: abdominal pain, abdominal distention, diarrhea, dyspepsia, nausea.
Hematologic: *neutropenia.*
Musculoskeletal: myalgia, arthralgia, back pain, myopathy.
Respiratory: cough.
Other: pruritus, rash.

INTERACTIONS
Drug-drug. *Drugs associated with myopathy (azole antifungals, chloroquine,*

T

corticosteroids, cyclosporine, erythromycin, fibric acid derivatives, HMG-CoA reductase inhibitors, niacin): May increase risk of myopathy. Monitor patient for muscle pain, tenderness, or weakness. Interrupt telbivudine if symptoms occur and discontinue if diagnosis is confirmed.

Drugs that alter renal function (aminoglycosides, cyclosporine, NSAIDs, tacrolimus, vancomycin): May increase risk of nephrotoxicity and cause decreased telbivudine elimination. Monitor renal function closely and adjust drug dose if necessary.

Peginterferon alfa-2a, other interferons: May increase risk and severity of peripheral neuropathy. Closely monitor patient. If symptoms occur, interrupt telbivudine and discontinue if diagnosis is confirmed.

EFFECTS ON LAB TEST RESULTS
● May increase CK, ALT, AST, lipase, creatinine, and lactate levels.
● May decrease neutrophil and platelet counts.

CONTRAINDICATIONS & CAUTIONS
● Contraindicated in patients hypersensitive to drug or its components.
● Use cautiously in those with renal impairment.
● Use cautiously in those with lamivudine-resistant hepatitis B infection.
● Give drug to pregnant women only if potential benefit outweighs fetal risk. Register patient in the Antiretroviral Pregnancy Registry by calling 1-800-258-4263 to monitor fetal outcomes.
● Drug may appear in breast milk. Don't use drug in breast-feeding women.
● Safety and effectiveness in children haven't been established.

NURSING CONSIDERATIONS
● Monitor renal function test and LFT results for liver transplant patients.
Black Box Warning The patient may develop lactic acidosis and severe hepatomegaly with steatosis during treatment. Risk factors include female gender, obesity, and concurrent antiretroviral therapy. ■
● Monitor patient for symptoms of myopathy.

Black Box Warning Stopping telbivudine may cause worsening of hepatitis B. Monitor hepatic function closely during therapy and for several months after stopping the drug. Therapy may need to be restarted. ■

PATIENT TEACHING
● Teach patient to report immediately signs and symptoms of lactic acidosis, such as weakness, muscle pain, difficulty breathing, nausea and vomiting, coldness in arms and legs, dizziness, light-headedness, and fast or irregular heartbeat.
● Advise patient not to change the dose or stop the drug because symptoms may worsen.
● Teach patient to report signs and symptoms of worsening liver disease, such as jaundice, dark urine, light-colored stool, decreased appetite, nausea, and stomach pain.
● Remind the patient that telbivudine won't cure HBV and doesn't stop the spread of HBV to others.

telithromycin
teh-lith-roh-MY-sin

Ketek

Therapeutic class: Antibiotics
Pharmacologic class: Ketolides
Pregnancy risk category: C

AVAILABLE FORMS
Tablets: 300 mg, 400 mg

INDICATIONS & DOSAGES
Adjust-a-dose (for all indications): In patients with CrCl less than 30 mL/minute, including those on dialysis, give 600 mg P.O. once daily. On dialysis days, give after session. In patients with CrCl less than 30 mL/minute and hepatic impairment, give 400 mg once daily.
➤ **Mild to moderate community-acquired pneumonia caused by** *Streptococcus pneumoniae* **(including multidrug-resistant isolates),** *Haemophilus influenzae, Moraxella catarrhalis, Chlamydophila pneumoniae,* **or** *Mycoplasma pneumoniae*

Adults: 800 mg P.O. once daily for 7 to
10 days.
➤ **Sinusitis ◆**
Adults: 800 mg P.O. once daily for 5 to
14 days or for 7 days after symptom
resolution.

ADMINISTRATION
P.O.
• Give drug with or without food.

ACTION
Inhibits bacterial protein synthesis.

Route	Onset	Peak	Duration
P.O.	Unknown	1 hr	Unknown

Half-life: 10 hours.

ADVERSE REACTIONS
CNS: dizziness, headache.
EENT: blurred vision, difficulty focusing,
diplopia.
GI: diarrhea, loose stools, nausea, taste
disturbance, vomiting.

INTERACTIONS
Drug-drug. *Antiarrhythmics (amiodarone,
bretylium, disopyramide):* May increase
risk of life-threatening cardiac arrhythmias.
Avoid using together.
Atorvastatin, lovastatin, simvastatin: May
increase levels of these drugs, increasing the
risk of myopathy. Avoid using together.
Benzodiazepines (midazolam): May
increase benzodiazepine level. Monitor
patient closely and adjust benzodiazepine
dosage.
Colchicine: May increase colchicine level.
Monitor patient for colchicine toxicity.
*CYP3A4 inducers (carbamazepine, phe-
nobarbital, phenytoin):* May decrease
telithromycin level. Avoid using together.
*CYP3A4 inhibitors (itraconazole, ketocona-
zole):* May increase telithromycin level.
Monitor patient closely.
Digoxin: May increase digoxin level. Monitor digoxin level.
*Drugs metabolized by the cytochrome P-450
system (carbamazepine, cyclosporine, hexo-
barbital, phenytoin, sirolimus, tacrolimus):*
May increase levels of these drugs, increasing or prolonging their effects. Use together
cautiously.

Ergot alkaloid derivatives such as ergotamine:
May increase the risk of ergot toxicity, char-
acterized by severe peripheral vasospasm
and dysesthesia. Avoid using together.
Metoprolol: May increase metoprolol level.
Use together cautiously.
Oral anticoagulants: May increase anticoagulant effect. Monitor PT and INR.
Pimozide: May increase pimozide level. Use
together is contraindicated.
Rifamycins: May significantly decrease
telithromycin level. Avoid using together.
Sotalol: May decrease sotalol level. Monitor
patient for lack of effect.
Theophylline: May increase theophylline
level and cause nausea and vomiting. Sepa-
rate doses by 1 hour.

EFFECTS ON LAB TEST RESULTS
• May increase AST and ALT levels.
• May increase platelet count.

CONTRAINDICATIONS & CAUTIONS
• Contraindicated in patients hypersensitive
to telithromycin or any macrolide antibiotic.
Also contraindicated in patients taking
pimozide.
Black Box Warning Contraindicated in
patients with myasthenia gravis due to
increased risk of life-threatening respiratory
failure. ∎
• Don't use in patients with congenitally
prolonged QTc interval; those with ongoing
proarrhythmic conditions, such as uncorrected hypokalemia, hypomagnesemia,
or bradycardia; or those taking class IA
antiarrhythmics, such as quinidine or procainamide, or class III antiarrhythmics such
as dofetilide.
• Use cautiously in patients with a history of
drug-induced hepatitis, jaundice, or renal or
hepatic impairment, and in breast-feeding
women.

NURSING CONSIDERATIONS
• Vision disturbances may occur, particularly in women and patients younger than
age 40. Adverse visual effects occur most
often after the first or second dose, last
several hours, and sometimes return with
later doses.

T

• Monitor patient for signs or symptoms of liver problems, including jaundice, pale stools, darkened urine, and abdominal pain.
• This drug may cause loss of consciousness. Monitor the patient closely.
• Patients with diarrhea may have pseudomembranous colitis.
• This drug may prolong the QTc interval. Rarely, an irregular heartbeat may cause the patient to faint.

PATIENT TEACHING
• Tell patient to take entire amount of drug exactly as directed, even if he feels better.
• Tell patient that drug can be taken with or without food.
• Explain that this drug may cause vision disturbances. Caution patient to avoid hazardous activities.
• Tell patient to report diarrhea or any episodes of fainting that occur while taking this drug.
• Advise patient to immediately report signs of liver problems to prescriber.

telmisartan
tell-mah-SAR-tan

Micardis✐

Therapeutic class: Antihypertensives
Pharmacologic class: Angiotensin II receptor antagonists
Pregnancy risk category: C; D in second and third trimesters

AVAILABLE FORMS
Tablets: 20 mg, 40 mg, 80 mg

INDICATIONS & DOSAGES
➤ **Hypertension (used alone or with other antihypertensives)**
Adults: 40 mg P.O. daily. Blood pressure response is dose-related over a range of 20 to 80 mg daily.
➤ **CV risk reduction in patients at high risk and unable to take ACE inhibitors**
Adults age 55 and older: 80 mg P.O. once daily.

ADMINISTRATION
P.O.
• Give drug without regard to meals.

ACTION
Blocks vasoconstricting and aldosterone-secreting effects of angiotensin II by preventing angiotensin II from binding to the angiotensin I receptor.

Route	Onset	Peak	Duration
P.O.	Unknown	30–60 min	24 hr

Half-life: 24 hours.

ADVERSE REACTIONS
CNS: dizziness, pain, fatigue, headache.
CV: chest pain, hypertension, peripheral edema.
EENT: pharyngitis, sinusitis.
GI: nausea, abdominal pain, diarrhea, dyspepsia.
GU: UTI.
Musculoskeletal: back pain, myalgia.
Respiratory: cough, upper respiratory tract infection.
Other: flulike symptoms.

INTERACTIONS
Drug-drug. *ACE inhibitors:* May affect renal function and cause acute renal failure. Monitor patient closely.
Aliskiren: Increases risk of renal impairment, hypotension, and hyperkalemia in diabetic patients. Use together is contraindicated. Also avoid coadministration in patients with moderate to severe renal impairment (GFR less than 60 mL/minute).
COX-2 inhibitors, NSAIDs: May result in worsening renal function, especially in elderly patients, volume-depleted patients, or those with coexisting renal dysfunction. Monitor renal function periodically.
Digoxin: May increase digoxin level. Monitor digoxin level closely.
Lithium: May cause reversible increase in lithium level and toxicity. Monitor lithium level and adjust lithium dose as needed.
Ramipril, ramiprilat: May increase levels of these drugs and decrease telmisartan level. Avoid use together.
Drug-herb. *Ma huang:* May decrease antihypertensive effects. Discourage use together.

Reactions in bold italics are *life-threatening*. Interactions may have a **rapid onset** or a **delayed onset**.

Drug-food. *Salt substitutes containing potassium:* May cause hyperkalemia. Discourage use together.

EFFECTS ON LAB TEST RESULTS
• May increase liver enzyme levels.
• May increase serum creatinine or BUN level.

CONTRAINDICATIONS & CAUTIONS
• Contraindicated in patients hypersensitive to drug or its components.
• Use cautiously in patients with biliary obstruction disorders or renal and hepatic insufficiency and in those with an activated renin-angiotensin system, such as volume- or sodium-depleted patients (for example, those being treated with high doses of diuretics).

Black Box Warning Use during pregnancy can cause injury and death to the developing fetus. When pregnancy is detected, stop drug as soon as possible. ▌

⚠ **Overdose S&S:** Hypotension, dizziness, tachycardia, bradycardia.

NURSING CONSIDERATIONS
• Monitor patient for hypotension after starting drug. Place patient supine if hypotension occurs, and give I.V. normal saline, if needed.
• Most of the antihypertensive effect occurs within 2 weeks. Maximal blood pressure reduction is usually reached after 4 weeks. Diuretic may be added if blood pressure isn't controlled by drug alone.
🔵 **Alert:** In patients whose renal function may depend on the activity of the renin-angiotensin-aldosterone system (such as those with severe heart failure), drug may cause oliguria or progressive azotemia and (rarely) acute renal failure or death.
• Drug isn't removed by hemodialysis. Patients undergoing dialysis may develop orthostatic hypotension. Closely monitor blood pressure.
• Monitor patients with impaired hepatic function or biliary obstruction carefully. Start telmisartan at low dose and titrate slowly.

PATIENT TEACHING
• Instruct patient to report suspected pregnancy to prescriber immediately.
• Inform women of childbearing age of the consequences of second- and third-trimester exposure to drug.
• Advise breast-feeding women about risk of adverse drug effects in infants and the need to stop either drug or breast-feeding.
• Tell patient that if he feels dizzy or has low blood pressure on standing, he should lie down, rise slowly from a lying to standing position, and climb stairs slowly.
• Tell patient that drug may be taken without regard to meals.
• Tell patient not to remove drug from blister-sealed packet until immediately before use.
• Advise patient to use NSAIDs and COX-2 inhibitors sparingly to avoid potential worsening renal function.

SAFETY ALERT!

temazepam
te-MAZ-e-pam

Restoril🔗

Therapeutic class: Hypnotics
Pharmacologic class: Benzodiazepines
Pregnancy risk category: X
Controlled substance schedule: IV

AVAILABLE FORMS
Capsules: 7.5 mg, 15 mg, 22.5 mg, 30 mg

INDICATIONS & DOSAGES
➤ **Short-term treatment (7 to 10 days) of insomnia**
Adults: 7.5 to 30 mg P.O. at bedtime.
Elderly or debilitated patients: 7.5 mg P.O. at bedtime until individualized response is determined.

ADMINISTRATION
P.O.
• Give drug 15 to 30 minutes before bedtime.
• Give drug without regard for food.

ACTION
Probably acts on the limbic system, thalamus, and hypothalamus of the CNS to produce hypnotic effects.

Route	Onset	Peak	Duration
P.O.	Unknown	1–2 hr	3–18 hr

Half-life: 8.8 hours.

ADVERSE REACTIONS
CNS: complex sleep-related behaviors, drowsiness, dizziness, lethargy, disturbed coordination, daytime sedation, confusion, nightmares, vertigo, euphoria, weakness, headache, fatigue, nervousness, anxiety, depression, minor changes in EEG patterns (usually low-voltage fast activity).
EENT: blurred vision.
GI: diarrhea, nausea, dry mouth.
Other: physical and psychological dependence.

INTERACTIONS
Drug-drug. *Antacids (aluminum hydroxide–containing):* May decrease or delay sedative effects. Monitor patient closely.
CNS depressants: May increase CNS depression. Use together cautiously.
Digoxin: May increase digoxin level. Monitor patient carefully for digoxin toxicity.
Diphenhydramine: May increase effects of both drugs. Use together cautiously.
Hormonal contraceptives: May increase temazepam clearance. Monitor patient closely.
Probenecid: May cause rapid or prolonged temazepam effects. Monitor patient for increased sedation or lethargy with concurrent use.
Theophylline: May decrease sedative effects. Monitor patient closely.
Drug-herb. *Calendula, hops, kava, lemon balm, passion flower, skullcap, valerian:* May enhance sedative effect of drug. Discourage use together.
Drug-lifestyle. *Alcohol use:* May cause additive CNS effects. Discourage use together.

EFFECTS ON LAB TEST RESULTS
• May increase LFT values.

CONTRAINDICATIONS & CAUTIONS
• Contraindicated in pregnant patients and those hypersensitive to drug or other benzodiazepines.
• Use cautiously in patients with chronic pulmonary insufficiency, impaired hepatic or renal function, severe or latent depression, suicidal tendencies, and history of drug abuse.
⚠ *Overdose S&S:* Somnolence, impaired coordination, slurred speech, confusion, coma, decreased reflexes, hypotension, seizures, respiratory depression, apnea.

NURSING CONSIDERATIONS
❸ *Alert:* Monitor patient closely. Anaphylaxis and angioedema may occur as early as the first dose (rare).
• Assess mental status before starting therapy and reduce doses in elderly patients; these patients may be more sensitive to drug's adverse CNS effects.
• Take precautions to prevent hoarding by patients who are depressed, suicidal, or drug-dependent or who have history of drug abuse.
• Don't stop drug abruptly as this may cause withdrawal symptoms (cramps, seizures, tremor, and sweating). To discontinue drug, follow a gradual dosage-tapering schedule.
• *Look alike–sound alike:* Don't confuse Restoril with Risperdal or Vistaril.

PATIENT TEACHING
❸ *Alert:* Warn patient that drug may cause allergic reactions (rare), facial swelling (rare), and complex sleep-related behaviors, such as driving, eating, and making phone calls while asleep. Advise patient to report these adverse effects.
• Tell patient to avoid alcohol during therapy.
• Caution patient to avoid performing activities that require mental alertness or physical coordination.
• Warn patient not to stop drug abruptly if taken for 1 month or longer.
• Tell patient that onset of drug's effects may take as long as 2 to 2¼ hours.

Reactions in bold italics are *life-threatening*. Interactions may have a *rapid onset* or a *delayed onset*.

SAFETY ALERT!

temozolomide
teh-moh-ZOH-loh-mide

Temodar

Therapeutic class: Antineoplastics
Pharmacologic class: Alkylating drugs
Pregnancy risk category: D

AVAILABLE FORMS
Capsules: 5 mg, 20 mg, 100 mg, 140 mg, 180 mg, 250 mg
Injection: 100 mg/vial

INDICATIONS & DOSAGES
➤ **Newly diagnosed glioblastoma in combination with radiation therapy**
Adults: Initially, 75 mg/m^2 I.V. infusion or P.O. daily for 42 days. Maintenance dose is 150 mg/m^2 I.V. infusion or P.O. on days 1 to 5 of a 28-day cycle for six cycles; may increase dose to 200 mg/m^2 for cycles two to six if common toxicity criteria (CTC) is grade 2 or less, ANC is 1.5×10^9/L or more, and platelet count is 100×10^9/L or more. If dose was increased in cycle two, maintain dose at 200 mg/m^2 for days 1 to 5 of subsequent cycles, unless toxicity occurs. If dose wasn't increased in cycle two, don't increase in subsequent cycles.
➤ **Refractory anaplastic astrocytoma**
Adults: Initially, 150 mg/m^2 I.V. infusion or P.O. daily for 5 days of a 28-day treatment cycle. May increase dose to 200 mg/m^2 for 5 days of a 28-day treatment cycle, if nadir and day 1 of next cycle ANC is 1.5×10^9/L or more and platelet count is 100×10^9/L or more.
Adjust-a-dose: For CTC grade 2, ANC 0.5 to 1.4×10^9/L, or platelet count 10 to 99×10^9/L during concurrent radiation therapy, interrupt therapy until CTC is grade 1 or less, ANC is 1.5×10^9/L or more, and platelet count is 100×10^9/L or more. For CTC grade 3, ANC less than 1×10^9/L, or platelet count less than 50×10^9/L, reduce maintenance dose by 50 mg/m^2; however, don't reduce below 100 mg/m^2. Discontinue therapy if CTC is grade 3 or 4, ANC is less than 0.5×10^9/L, or platelet count is less than 10×10^9/L.

ADMINISTRATION
● Use of gloves and safety glasses is recommended to avoid exposure due to vial or capsule breakage.
P.O.
● Give drug on an empty stomach to reduce nausea or vomiting. Bedtime administration may be advised.
● An antiemetic may be administered before or after giving drug.
● Don't open capsules or allow patient to chew them.
I.V.
▼ Preparing and giving parenteral drug may be mutagenic, teratogenic, or carcinogenic. Follow facility policy to reduce risks.
▼ Reconstitute vial with 41 mL sterile water for injection and gently swirl vial.
▼ For infusion, withdraw proper dose of solution using aseptic technique; then transfer it into an empty 250 mL PVC infusion bag. Administer by I.V. infusion over 90 minutes using an infusion pump.
▼ Discard cloudy, particulate solution.
▼ Reconstituted solution is stable at room temperature for 14 hours (including the 90-minute infusion time).
▼ **Incompatibilities:** Other I.V. diluents, medications, and additives.

ACTION
Undergoes rapid nonenzymatic conversion to a reactive compound. This compound alkalizes the cell's DNA, causing cell death.

Route	Onset	Peak	Duration
P.O., I.V.	Unknown	1 hr	7 days

Half-life: About 2 hours.

ADVERSE REACTIONS
CNS: amnesia, anxiety, confusion, depression, dizziness, fatigue, headache, hemiparesis, insomnia, memory impairment, paresthesia, paresis, *seizures,* somnolence, weakness.
CV: peripheral edema.
EENT: abnormal vision, blurred vision, diplopia, pharyngitis, sinusitis, taste perversion.
GI: abdominal pain, anorexia, constipation, diarrhea, dysphagia, nausea, stomatitis, vomiting.

T

GU: incontinence, UTI.
Hematologic: decreased hemoglobin, *leukopenia, lymphopenia, neutropenia, thrombocytopenia.*
Metabolic: adrenal hypercorticism, weight gain.
Musculoskeletal: abnormal coordination, abnormal gait, arthralgia, asthenia, back pain, myalgia.
Respiratory: cough, dyspnea, upper respiratory tract infection.
Skin: alopecia, dry skin, itching, rash.
Other: breast pain, viral infection, fever.

INTERACTIONS
Drug-drug. *Valproic acid:* May increase temozolomide drug levels. Use together cautiously.
Drug-food. *Any food:* May decrease drug absorption. Advise patient to take drug on an empty stomach.

EFFECTS ON LAB TEST RESULTS
• May decrease hemoglobin level and WBC, neutrophil, lymphocyte, and platelet counts.

CONTRAINDICATIONS & CAUTIONS
• Contraindicated in patients hypersensitive to drug, its components, or dacarbazine (because both drugs are metabolized to the same reactive compound).
• Use cautiously in patients taking other drugs that cause myelosuppression, such as carbamazepine, phenytoin, and sulfamethoxazole–trimethoprim.
• Use cautiously in patients with a history of *Pneumocystis jiroveci* (*carinii*) pneumonia, myelodysplastic syndrome, secondary malignancies, or severe renal or hepatic impairment.
• Drug can cause fetal harm when given to pregnant women. Use only when benefit to the mother outweighs risk to the fetus. Women shouldn't breast-feed while taking drug.
⚠ **Overdose S&S:** Pancytopenia, fever, multisystem organ failure, death.

NURSING CONSIDERATIONS
• Monitor vital signs and intake and output.
• Monitor CBC with differential before and after each cycle and at least weekly during therapy.

• Monitor patients, especially those receiving corticosteroids, for lymphopenia and *P. jiroveci* pneumonia.
• Oral and I.V. doses are equivalent when I.V. dose is infused over 90 minutes.
• Give antiemetic as prescribed to prevent nausea and vomiting.
• Monitor patients for signs and symptoms of another malignancy.

PATIENT TEACHING
• Tell patient to swallow capsule whole with a glass of water and not to open or chew capsule. If capsule opens accidentally, caution patient to avoid inhaling the powder or getting it on the skin or mucous membranes. If powder contacts the skin or mucous membranes, advise patient to flush the area with water immediately.
• Instruct women of childbearing age to use contraceptive measures while taking drug or if male partner is receiving therapy.
• Inform patient that common side effects include nausea, vomiting, diarrhea, constipation, and hair loss.
• Advise patient to avoid exposure to people with infections.
• Tell patient to report signs of infection (fever, sore throat, fatigue) and bleeding (easy bruising, bleeding gums, nosebleeds, tarry stools).

SAFETY ALERT!

tenecteplase
teh-NEK-ti-plaze

TNKase

Therapeutic class: Thrombolytics
Pharmacologic class: Recombinant tissue plasminogen activators
Pregnancy risk category: C

AVAILABLE FORMS
Injection: 50 mg/vial

INDICATIONS & DOSAGES
➤ **To reduce risk of death from an acute MI**
Adults weighing 90 kg (198 lb) or more: 50 mg (10 mL) by I.V. bolus over 5 seconds.

Reactions in bold italics are *life-threatening*. Interactions may have a *rapid onset* or a *delayed onset*.

Adults weighing 80 to less than 90 kg (176 to 198 lb): 45 mg (9 mL) by I.V. bolus over 5 seconds.

Adults weighing 70 to just under 80 kg (154 to 176 lb): 40 mg (8 mL) by I.V. bolus over 5 seconds.

Adults weighing 60 to just under 70 kg (132 to 154 lb): 35 mg (7 mL) by I.V. bolus over 5 seconds.

Adults weighing less than 60 kg (132 lb): 30 mg (6 mL) by I.V. bolus over 5 seconds. Maximum dose is 50 mg.

ADMINISTRATION

I.V.

▼ Use syringe prefilled with 10 mL sterile water for injection, and inject the entire contents into drug vial. Gently swirl solution once mixed. Don't shake. Visually inspect product for particulate matter before administration.

▼ Draw up the appropriate dose needed from the reconstituted vial with the syringe and discard any unused portion. Give drug immediately, or refrigerate and use within 8 hours.

▼ Give drug in a designated line. Flush dextrose-containing lines with normal saline solution before administration.

▼ Give the drug rapidly over 5 seconds.

▼ **Incompatibilities:** Solutions containing dextrose, other I.V. drugs.

ACTION

Binds to fibrin and converts plasminogen to plasmin. The specificity to fibrin decreases systemic activation of plasminogen and the resulting breakdown of circulating fibrinogen.

Route	Onset	Peak	Duration
I.V.	Immediate	Immediate	Unknown

Half-life: 90 to 130 minutes.

ADVERSE REACTIONS

CNS: *stroke, intracranial hemorrhage.*
EENT: pharyngeal bleeding, epistaxis.
GI: *GI bleeding.*
GU: hematuria.
Skin: hematoma.
Other: bleeding at puncture site.

INTERACTIONS

Drug-drug. *Anticoagulants (heparin, vitamin K antagonists), drugs that alter platelet function (aspirin, dipyridamole, glycoprotein IIb/IIIa inhibitors, NSAIDs):* May increase risk of bleeding when used before, during, or after tenecteplase use. Use together cautiously.

EFFECTS ON LAB TEST RESULTS

● May increase PT, PTT, and INR.

CONTRAINDICATIONS & CAUTIONS

● Contraindicated in patients with hypersensitivity to drug; active internal bleeding; history of stroke; intracranial or intraspinal surgery or trauma during previous 2 months; intracranial neoplasm, aneurysm, or arteriovenous malformation; severe uncontrolled hypertension; or bleeding diathesis.

● Use cautiously in patients who have had recent major surgery (such as CABG), organ biopsy, obstetric delivery, or previous puncture of noncompressible vessels.

● Use cautiously in pregnant women, patients age 75 and older, and patients with recent trauma, recent GI or GU bleeding, high risk of left ventricular thrombus, acute pericarditis, systolic blood pressure 180 mm Hg or higher or diastolic pressure 110 mm Hg or higher, severe hepatic dysfunction, hemostatic defects, subacute bacterial endocarditis, septic thrombophlebitis, diabetic hemorrhagic retinopathy, or cerebrovascular disease.

NURSING CONSIDERATIONS

● Begin therapy as soon as possible after onset of MI symptoms.

● Avoid noncompressible arterial punctures and internal jugular and subclavian venous punctures. Minimize all arterial and venous punctures during treatment.

● Avoid I.M. use.

● Give heparin but not in the same I.V. line.

● Monitor patient for bleeding. If serious bleeding occurs, stop heparin and antiplatelet drugs immediately.

🔔 *Alert:* Use exact patient weight for dosage. An overestimation in patient weight can lead to significant increase in bleeding or intracerebral hemorrhage.

● Monitor ECG for reperfusion arrhythmias.

T

• Life-threatening cholesterol embolism has been rarely reported in patients treated with thrombolytics. Signs and symptoms may include livedo reticularis (blue toe syndrome), acute renal failure, gangrenous digits, hypertension, pancreatitis, MI, cerebral infarction, spinal cord infarction, retinal artery occlusion, bowel infarction, and rhabdomyolysis.

PATIENT TEACHING

• Tell patient to report any adverse effects or excessive bleeding immediately.
• Explain use of drug to patient and family.

tenofovir disoproxil fumarate
te-NOE-fo-veer

Viread◆

Therapeutic class: Antiretrovirals
Pharmacologic class: Nucleoside–nucleotide reverse transcriptase inhibitors
Pregnancy risk category: B

AVAILABLE FORMS

Oral powder: 40 mg of tenofovir disoproxil fumarate/g (equivalent to 33 mg of tenofovir disoproxil). One level scoop delivers 1 g of powder containing tenofovir 40 mg.
Tablets: 150 mg as the fumarate salt (equivalent to 123 mg of tenofovir disoproxil), 200 mg as the fumarate salt (equivalent to 163 mg of tenofovir disoproxil), 250 mg as the fumarate salt (equivalent to 204 mg of tenofovir disoproxil), 300 mg as the fumarate salt (equivalent to 245 mg of tenofovir disoproxil)

INDICATIONS & DOSAGES

Adjust-a-dose (for all indications): For adults with CrCl of 30 to 49 mL/minute, 300 mg P.O. every 48 hours. For CrCl of 10 to 29 mL/minute, 300 mg P.O. every 72 to 96 hours. For patients receiving hemodialysis, 300 mg P.O. every 7 days or after a total of about 12 hours of hemodialysis. Give dose after session. There are no recommendations for patients with CrCl of less than 10 mL/minute not receiving hemodialysis.

➤ **HIV-1 infection, with other antiretrovirals**
Adults and children age 12 and older weighing 35 kg (77 lb) or more: 300 mg P.O. once daily. For adults weighing more than 60 kg (132 lb) who are taking didanosine concomitantly, reduce didanosine dose to 250 mg.
Children ages 2 to 11: 8 mg/kg P.O. once daily. Maximum dosage is 300 mg/day. See product insert for weight-based oral powder scoop dosing recommendations.

➤ **Chronic hepatitis B**
Adults: 300 mg P.O. once daily.
Children age 12 and older weighing 35 kg (77 lb) or more: 300 mg P.O. once daily.
Adjust-a-dose: There are no recommendations for children with renal impairment.

ADMINISTRATION

P.O.

• Give without regard to food.
• For patients receiving tenofovir and didanosine (enteric-coated form), give under fasting conditions or with a light meal (less than 400 kcal, 20% fat). Buffered form of didanosine taken with tenofovir should be given under fasting conditions.
• For patients receiving tenofovir powder, measure only with supplied dosing scoop. Mix in container with 2 to 4 ounces of soft food not requiring chewing (such as applesauce, baby food, or yogurt). Patient should ingest entire mixture immediately to avoid bitter taste. Don't administer tenofovir in a liquid because the powder may float on top of the liquid, even after stirring.

ACTION

Hydrolyzed to produce tenofovir, a nucleoside analogue of adenosine monophosphate that yields tenofovir diphosphate. Tenofovir diphosphate inhibits HIV replication.

Route	Onset	Peak	Duration
P.O.	Unknown	1–2 hr	Unknown

Half-life: 17 hours.

ADVERSE REACTIONS

CNS: asthenia, headache, pain, fever, peripheral neuropathy, insomnia, dizziness, depression, anxiety.

Reactions in bold italics are *life-threatening*. Interactions may have a *rapid onset* or a *delayed onset*.

GI: nausea, abdominal pain, dyspepsia, diarrhea, vomiting.
Hematologic: *neutropenia.*
Hepatic: hepatomegaly, *hepatitis.*
Metabolic: hyperglycemia, *lactic acidosis.*
Musculoskeletal: arthralgia, back pain, myalgia.
Skin: rash.

INTERACTIONS

Drug-drug. *Atazanavir:* May decrease atazanavir levels, causing resistance. Give both drugs with ritonavir.
Didanosine (buffered or enteric-coated form): May increase didanosine bioavailability. Monitor patient for didanosine-related adverse effects, such as bone marrow suppression, GI distress, and peripheral neuropathy. In adults weighing more than 60 kg (132 lb), reduce didanosine dosage to 250 mg when administered with tenofovir. Give under fasted conditions.
Drugs that reduce renal function or compete for renal tubular secretion (acyclovir, cidofovir, ganciclovir, valacyclovir, valganciclovir): May increase levels of tenofovir or other renally eliminated drugs. Monitor patient for adverse effects.
Lopinavir–ritonavir: May increase tenofovir-associated adverse reactions. Monitor patient carefully.

EFFECTS ON LAB TEST RESULTS

• May increase amylase, AST, ALT, CK, serum and urine glucose, creatinine, phosphate, cholesterol, and triglyceride levels.
• May decrease neutrophil count.

CONTRAINDICATIONS & CAUTIONS

• Contraindicated in patients hypersensitive to components of drug.
• Use very cautiously in patients with risk factors for liver disease or with hepatic impairment.
• Don't use tenofovir in combination with the fixed-dose combination products of efavirenz–emtricitabine–tenofovir, emtricitabine–rilpivirine–tenofovir, or emtricitabine–tenofovir because tenofovir disoproxil fumarate is a component of these products. Don't administer tenofovir with adefovir.

• Don't use triple antiretroviral therapy with abacavir, lamivudine, and tenofovir as new regimen for treatment-naive or pretreated patient with HIV infection because of high rate of early virologic resistance.
• Use in pregnant women only if benefits clearly outweigh risks.

NURSING CONSIDERATIONS

Black Box Warning Drug may cause lactic acidosis and hepatomegaly with steatosis, even fatal cases. These effects may occur without elevated transaminase levels. Risk factors include long-term antiretroviral use, obesity, and being female. Monitor all patients closely. ■
Black Box Warning Severe acute exacerbations of hepatitis have been reported in hepatitis B–infected patients after anti-hepatitis B therapy has stopped. Monitor hepatic function closely for at least several months. Resumption of therapy may be warranted. ■
• Drug may cause body fat to accumulate and be redistributed, resulting in central obesity, peripheral wasting, and buffalo hump. Monitor patient for changes in body fat.
• Drug may be linked to osteomalacia and decreased bone mineral density, increased creatinine and BUN levels, and phosphaturia. Monitor patient carefully during long-term treatment.
• Drug may lead to decreased HIV RNA level and CD4 + cell counts.
• In elderly patients, use drug cautiously because these patients may be taking other drugs and may be at higher risk for decreased renal function.
• Because of a high rate of early virologic resistance, triple antiretroviral therapy with abacavir, lamivudine, and tenofovir shouldn't be used as new regimen for treatment-naive or pretreated patient with HIV infection. Monitor patients currently controlled with this regimen and those who use this regimen with other antiretrovirals, and consider a different therapy.

PATIENT TEACHING

• Instruct patient to take drug with a meal to enhance bioavailability.

T

• Inform patient that drug doesn't cure HIV infection, that opportunistic infections and other complications of HIV infection may still occur, and that transmission of HIV to others through sexual contact or blood contamination is still possible.

• If patient takes tenofovir and didanosine (buffered or enteric-coated form), instruct him to take these drugs on an empty stomach.

• Tell patient to report adverse effects, including nausea, vomiting, diarrhea, flatulence, and headache.

---

terazosin hydrochloride
ter-AY-zoe-sin

Hytrin

Therapeutic class: Antihypertensives
Pharmacologic class: Alpha blockers
Pregnancy risk category: C

AVAILABLE FORMS
Capsules: 1 mg, 2 mg, 5 mg, 10 mg
Tablets: 1 mg, 2 mg, 5 mg, 10 mg

INDICATIONS & DOSAGES
➤ **Hypertension**
Adults: Initially, 1 mg P.O. at bedtime. Dosage may be increased gradually based on response. Usual dosage range is 1 to 5 mg daily. Maximum recommended dose is 20 mg daily.

➤ **Symptomatic BPH**
Adults: Initially, 1 mg P.O. at bedtime. Dosage may be titrated to 2, 5, or 10 mg once daily to achieve optimal response. Most patients need 10 mg daily for optimal response. Maximum recommended dosage is 20 mg/day.

➤ **Pediatric hypertension ◆**
Children ages 1 to 17: Initially, 1 mg P.O. daily. Maximum dosage is 20 mg P.O. daily.

➤ **Adjunctive therapy for symptom-producing lower ureteral tract stones (juxtavesical or ureterovesical junction) smaller than 10 mm ◆**
Adults: 2 to 5 mg P.O. daily for up to 1 month or until expulsion.

ADMINISTRATION
P.O.
• Give drug without regard for meals.

ACTION
Improves urine flow in patients with BPH by blocking alpha-adrenergic receptors in the bladder neck and prostate, relieving urethral pressure. Drug also reduces peripheral vascular resistance and blood pressure via arterial and venous dilation.

Route	Onset	Peak	Duration
P.O.	15 min	2–3 hr	24 hr

Half-life: About 12 hours.

ADVERSE REACTIONS
CNS: headache, dizziness, asthenia, first-dose syncope, nervousness, paresthesia, somnolence.
CV: peripheral edema, palpitations, orthostatic hypotension, tachycardia, atrial fibrillation.
EENT: nasal congestion, sinusitis, blurred vision.
GI: nausea.
GU: impotence, priapism.
Hematologic: *thrombocytopenia.*
Musculoskeletal: back pain, muscle pain.
Respiratory: dyspnea.

INTERACTIONS
Drug-drug. *Antihypertensives, tadalafil, vardenafil:* May cause excessive hypotension. Use together cautiously.
Drug-herb. *Butcher's broom:* May decrease drug effect. Discourage use together.
Ma huang: May decrease antihypertensive effects. Discourage use together.

EFFECTS ON LAB TEST RESULTS
• May decrease total protein and albumin levels. May decrease hemoglobin level and hematocrit.
• May decrease WBC and platelet counts.

CONTRAINDICATIONS & CAUTIONS
• Contraindicated in patients hypersensitive to drug.
⚠ *Overdose S&S:* Hypotension.

NURSING CONSIDERATIONS
• Monitor blood pressure frequently.
• **Alert:** If terazosin is stopped for several days, readjust dosage using first dosing regimen (1 mg P.O. at bedtime).

PATIENT TEACHING
• Tell patient not to stop drug suddenly, but to notify prescriber if adverse reactions occur.
• Warn patient to avoid hazardous activities that require mental alertness, such as driving or operating heavy machinery, for 12 hours after first dose.
• Tell patient that light-headedness can occur, especially during the first few days of therapy. Advise him to rise slowly to minimize this effect and to report signs and symptoms to prescriber.

---

terbinafine hydrochloride (oral)
ter-BIN-ah-fin

Lamisil

Therapeutic class: Antifungals
Pharmacologic class: Synthetic allylamine derivatives
Pregnancy risk category: B

AVAILABLE FORMS
Oral granules (packets): 125 mg, 187.5 mg
Tablets: 250 mg

INDICATIONS & DOSAGES
➤ **Fingernail and toenail onychomycosis caused by dermatophytes (tinea unguium)**
Adults: 250 mg P.O. once daily for 6 weeks for fingernail infection and 12 weeks for toenail infection.
➤ **Tinea capitis**
Adults: 250 mg P.O. once daily for 6 weeks (granules only).
Children age 4 and older: One dose of granules daily for 2 to 8 weeks based on body weight. If less than 25 kg (55 lb), give 125 mg; if 25 to 35 kg (77 lb), give 187.5 mg; if more than 35 kg, give 250 mg.

ADMINISTRATION
P.O.
• Obtain pretreatment transaminase levels for all patients taking drug. Tablets aren't recommended for patients with acute or chronic liver disease.
• Give tablets without regard for food.
• Sprinkle entire contents of granule packet on a spoonful of nonacidic food, such as pudding or mashed potatoes; don't use applesauce or fruit-based foods. Have patient swallow spoonful without chewing.

ACTION
Prevents biosynthesis of ergosterol, causing a deficiency of this essential component of fungal cell membranes.

Route	Onset	Peak	Duration
P.O.	Unknown	2 hr	Unknown

Half-life: 26 to 30 hours.

ADVERSE REACTIONS
CNS: headache.
EENT: smell disturbances, vision disturbances.
GI: taste disturbances, diarrhea, dyspepsia, abdominal pain, nausea, flatulence.
Hematologic: *neutropenia, thrombocytopenia.*
Hepatic: hepatobiliary dysfunction, including cholestatic jaundice.
Skin: *Stevens-Johnson syndrome, toxic epidermal necrolysis,* rash, pruritus, urticaria.
Other: *anaphylaxis,* hypersensitivity reactions.

INTERACTIONS
Drug-drug. *Antiarrhythmics class type 1C (flecainide) and beta blockers:* Inhibit drugs metabolized by CYP2D6 isozyme. Monitor patient carefully and decrease dosage as necessary.
Caffeine: May decrease caffeine clearance. Use cautiously together.
Cimetidine: May decrease clearance of terbinafine by one-third. Avoid using together.
Cyclosporine: May increase cyclosporine clearance. Monitor cyclosporine level.
CYP2C9, CYP3A4 enzyme inhibitors (amiodarone, fluconazole): May substantially

T

increase systemic exposure of terbinafine.
Use together cautiously.
Rifampin: Increases terbinafine clearance by
100%. Avoid use together.
SSRIs (paroxetine, venlafaxine): May
increase SSRI levels. Monitor patient
carefully and adjust SSRI dosage as necessary.

EFFECTS ON LAB TEST RESULTS
● May increase AST and ALT levels.
● May decrease neutrophil and lymphocyte
counts.

CONTRAINDICATIONS & CAUTIONS
● Contraindicated in patients hypersensitive
to drug, pregnant or breast-feeding women,
those with liver disease, and those with CrCl
of less than 50 mL/minute.
⚠ Overdose S&S: Abdominal pain, dizziness, frequent urination, headache, nausea,
rash, vomiting.

NURSING CONSIDERATIONS
☼ Alert: Rarely, patients may suffer life-
threatening liver failure.
● Monitor CBC and hepatic enzyme levels
in patients receiving drug for longer than
6 weeks. Stop drug if hepatobiliary dysfunction or cholestatic hepatitis develops.
● **Look alike–sound alike:** Don't confuse
terbinafine with terbutaline. Don't confuse
Lamisil with Lamictal.

PATIENT TEACHING
● Inform patient that successful treatment
may take 10 weeks for toenail infections and
4 weeks for fingernail infections.
● Tell patient to immediately report depression; smell, taste, or vision disturbances
(changes in the ocular lens and retina
may occur); as well as persistent nausea,
anorexia, fatigue, vomiting, right upper
quadrant pain, jaundice, dark urine, or pale
stools.
● Teach patient to sprinkle entire contents
of granule packet on spoonful of nonacidic
food, such as pudding or mashed potatoes,
and to swallow without chewing. Tell patient
not to use applesauce or fruit-based food.

terbinafine hydrochloride (topical)
ter-BIN-ah-fin

Lamisil ◊, Lamisil AT ◊

Therapeutic class: Antifungals
Pharmacologic class: Allylamine
derivatives
Pregnancy risk category: B

AVAILABLE FORMS
Cream: 1% ◊
Gel: 1% ◊
Solution: 1% ◊
Spray: 1% ◊

INDICATIONS & DOSAGES
➤ **Athlete's foot**
Adults and children age 12 and older: For
athlete's foot between the toes, apply b.i.d.
for 1 week or as directed by prescriber. For
athlete's foot on the bottom or sides of the
foot, apply b.i.d. for 2 weeks or as directed
by prescriber.
➤ **Jock itch, ringworm**
Adults and children age 12 and older:
Apply once daily for 1 week or as directed
by prescriber.

ADMINISTRATION
Topical
● Wash affected area with soap and water
and dry completely before application.
● Don't apply an occlusive dressing without
a specific order.
● This drug isn't for ophthalmic use. Avoid
contact with mucous membranes.

ACTION
Fungicidal; selectively inhibits an early
step in synthesis of sterols used by fungi for
cell-wall synthesis.

Route	Onset	Peak	Duration
Topical	Unknown	Unknown	Unknown

Half-life: About 21 hours.

ADVERSE REACTIONS
Skin: irritation, pruritus, skin exfoliation.

Reactions in bold italics are *life-threatening*. Interactions may have a *rapid onset* or a *delayed onset*.

INTERACTIONS
None significant.

EFFECTS ON LAB TEST RESULTS
None reported.

CONTRAINDICATIONS & CAUTIONS
• Contraindicated in patients hypersensitive to drug or its components and in breast-feeding women.

NURSING CONSIDERATIONS
• Observe patient for 2 to 6 weeks after therapy is complete to determine whether treatment was successful; review diagnosis if condition persists.
• Drug isn't intended for oral, ophthalmic, or vaginal use.
• *Look alike–sound alike:* Don't confuse terbinafine with terbutaline. Don't confuse Lamisil with Lamictal.

PATIENT TEACHING
• Teach patient proper use of drug. Tell him to wash affected area with soap and water and dry completely before applying.
• Advise patient to use only as directed for full recommended course, even if signs and symptoms disappear, and not to apply near eyes, mouth, or mucous membranes or to use occlusive dressings unless so directed.
• Instruct patient with athlete's foot to wear well-fitting, ventilated shoes.
• Tell patient to wash hands after applying.
• Tell patient to stop drug and contact prescriber if irritation or sensitivity develops.
• Tell patient to store drug between 41° and 86° F (5° and 30° C).

terbutaline sulfate
ter-BYOO-ta-leen

Therapeutic class: Bronchodilators
Pharmacologic class: Beta₂ agonists
Pregnancy risk category: B

AVAILABLE FORMS
Injection: 1 mg/mL
Tablets: 2.5 mg, 5 mg

INDICATIONS & DOSAGES
➤ **Bronchospasm in patients with reversible obstructive airway disease**
Adults and children age 13 and older: 0.25 mg subcutaneously. If needed, repeat in 15 to 30 minutes. Maximum, 0.5 mg in 4 hours. If patient fails to respond to second dose, consider other measures.
Adults and adolescents older than age 15: 2.5 to 5 mg P.O. t.i.d. every 6 hours while awake. Maximum, 15 mg daily.
Children ages 12 to 15: 2.5 mg P.O. t.i.d. every 6 hours while awake. Maximum, 7.5 mg daily.

ADMINISTRATION
P.O.
• Give drug without regard for food.
Subcutaneous
• Give subcutaneous injections into the side of the deltoid.
• Protect drug from light. Don't use if discolored.

ACTION
Relaxes bronchial smooth muscle by stimulating beta₂ receptors.

Route	Onset	Peak	Duration
P.O.	30 min	2–3 hr	4–8 hr
Subcut.	15 min	30 min	1½–4 hr

Half-life: Oral, 3.4 hours; subcutaneous, 5.7 hours.

ADVERSE REACTIONS
CNS: nervousness, tremor, drowsiness, dizziness, headache, weakness.
CV: palpitations, *arrhythmias,* tachycardia, flushing.
GI: vomiting, nausea, heartburn.
Metabolic: hypokalemia.
Respiratory: *paradoxical bronchospasm with prolonged use,* dyspnea.
Skin: diaphoresis.

INTERACTIONS
Drug-drug. *Cardiac glycosides, cyclopropane, halogenated inhaled anesthetics, levodopa:* May increase risk of arrhythmias. Monitor patient closely, and avoid using together with levodopa.
CNS stimulants: May increase CNS stimulation. Avoid using together.

T

MAO inhibitors: When given with sympath-omimetics, may cause severe hypertension (hypertensive crisis). Avoid using together.
Propranolol, other beta blockers: May block bronchodilating effects of terbutaline. Avoid using together.
Sympathomimetics (ephedrine): May result in additive CV effects. Monitor patient's heart rate and rhythm.

EFFECTS ON LAB TEST RESULTS
• May decrease potassium level.

CONTRAINDICATIONS & CAUTIONS
• Contraindicated in patients hypersensitive to drug or sympathomimetic amines.
Black Box Warning Don't use injectable form in pregnant women for prevention or prolonged treatment (beyond 48 to 72 hours) of preterm labor in either the hospital or outpatient setting because of the potential for serious maternal heart prob-lems and death. Oral terbutaline shouldn't be used for prevention or for any treatment of preterm labor. ∎
• Use cautiously in patient with CV disor-ders, hyperthyroidism, diabetes, or seizure disorders.
⚠ *Overdose S&S:* Seizures, angina, hyper-tension, hypotension, tachycardia, arrhyth-mias, nervousness, headache, tremors, dry mouth, palpitations, nausea, dizziness, fatigue, insomnia, hypokalemia.

NURSING CONSIDERATIONS
• Drug may reduce the sensitivity of spirometry for the diagnosis of bron-chospasm.
• Withhold drug and notify prescriber if patient's heart rate is greater than 120 beats/minute.
• Monitor patient for circulatory overload.
• *Look alike–sound alike:* Don't confuse terbutaline with tolbutamide or terbinafine.

PATIENT TEACHING
• Make sure patient and caregivers under-stand why patient needs drug.
• Remind patient to separate oral doses by 6 hours.
• Instruct patient to immediately report changes in heart rate or rhythm, which patient may experience as feeling anxious,

palpitations, or feeling that his heart is racing.

terconazole
ter-CONE-uh-zole

Terazol 3, Terazol 7

Therapeutic class: Antifungals
Pharmacologic class: Triazole deriva-tives
Pregnancy risk category: C

AVAILABLE FORMS
Vaginal cream: 0.4%, 0.8%
Vaginal suppositories: 80 mg

INDICATIONS & DOSAGES
➤ **Vulvovaginal candidiasis**
Adults: One applicatorful of cream or 1 suppository inserted into vagina at bed-time; 0.4% cream used for 7 consecutive days; 0.8% cream or 80-mg suppository for 3 consecutive days. Repeat course, if needed, after reconfirmation by smear or culture.

ADMINISTRATION
Vaginal
• Insert drug high in vagina (unless patient is pregnant).
• Store drug at room temperature.

ACTION
May increase *Candida* cell membrane per-meability.

Route	Onset	Peak	Duration
Vaginal	Unknown	Unknown	Unknown

Half-life: Unknown.

ADVERSE REACTIONS
CNS: headache, fever.
GI: abdominal pain.
GU: dysmenorrhea, genital pain, vulvovagi-nal burning.
Skin: pruritus, irritation, photosensitivity.
Other: body aches.

INTERACTIONS
None significant.

Reactions in bold italics are *life-threatening*. Interactions may have a *rapid onset* or a *delayed onset*.

EFFECTS ON LAB TEST RESULTS
None reported.

CONTRAINDICATIONS & CAUTIONS
• Contraindicated in patients hypersensitive to drug or its inactive ingredients.

NURSING CONSIDERATIONS
• Therapeutic effect of drug is unaffected by menstruation or hormonal contraceptive use.
• *Look alike–sound alike:* Don't confuse terconazole with tioconazole.

PATIENT TEACHING
• Advise patient to continue treatment during menstrual period. However, tell her not to use tampons.
• Instruct patient to insert drug high in vagina (except during pregnancy).
• Tell patient to use drug for full treatment period prescribed. Explain how to prevent reinfection.
• Instruct patient to notify prescriber and stop drug if fever, chills, other flulike signs and symptoms, or sensitivity develops.
• Caution patient to refrain from sexual intercourse during treatment.
• Tell patient that drug base may react with latex, causing decreased effectiveness of condoms and diaphragms (for up to 72 hours after treatment is completed).
• Advise patient that her partner also may need treatment if he's experiencing itching, redness, or penile discomfort.
• Instruct patient in ways to prevent future yeast infections, such as wearing loose clothing and cotton fabrics.
• Instruct patient to store drug at room temperature.

teriparatide (rDNA origin)
tehr-ih-PAHR-uh-tide

Forteo

Therapeutic class: Antiosteoporotics
Pharmacologic class: Recombinant human parathyroid hormones
Pregnancy risk category: C

AVAILABLE FORMS
Injection: 20 mcg/dose in multidose prefilled pen

INDICATIONS & DOSAGES
➤ **Osteoporosis in postmenopausal women at high risk for fracture; primary or hypogonadal osteoporosis in men at high risk for fracture; glucocorticoid induced osteoporosis in men and women**
Adults: 20 mcg subcutaneously in thigh or abdominal wall once daily.

ADMINISTRATION
Subcutaneous
• Inspect solution before giving.
• Drug is a colorless, clear liquid.
• Don't use if solid particles are present or if the solution is cloudy or colored.
• Give while patient is in a sitting position to avoid orthostatic hypotension.
• Discard the pen after the 28-day use period, even if some unused solution still remains.

ACTION
Promotes new bone formation, skeletal bone mass, and bone strength by regulating calcium and phosphorus metabolism in bones and kidneys.

Route	Onset	Peak	Duration
Subcut.	Rapid	30 min	3 hr

Half-life: 1 hour.

ADVERSE REACTIONS
CNS: asthenia, depression, dizziness, headache, insomnia, pain, syncope, vertigo.
CV: angina pectoris, hypertension, orthostatic hypotension.
EENT: pharyngitis, rhinitis.

GI: constipation, diarrhea, dyspepsia, nausea, tooth disorder, vomiting.
Metabolic: hypercalcemia.
Musculoskeletal: arthralgia, leg cramps, neck pain.
Respiratory: dyspnea, increased cough, pneumonia.
Skin: rash, sweating.

INTERACTIONS
Drug-drug. *Calcium supplements:* May increase urinary calcium excretion. Dosage may need adjustment.
Digoxin: May predispose hypercalcemic patient to digitalis toxicity. Use together cautiously.

EFFECTS ON LAB TEST RESULTS
• May increase calcium and uric acid levels. May decrease phosphorus level.
• May increase urinary calcium and phosphorus excretion.

CONTRAINDICATIONS & CAUTIONS
• Contraindicated in patients hypersensitive to teriparatide or its components.
Black Box Warning Contraindicated in patients at increased risk for osteosarcoma, such as those with Paget disease or unexplained alkaline phosphatase elevations, children and young adults with open epiphyses, and patients who have had skeletal radiation. ∎
• Contraindicated in patients with bone metastases; a history of skeletal malignancies, hypercalcemia, or metabolic bone diseases other than osteoporosis; and in patients with hypercalcemia.
• Use cautiously in patients with active or recent urolithiasis; hepatic, renal, or cardiac disease; or hypotension.
• Don't use in breast-feeding women.
⚠ *Overdose S&S:* Hypercalcemia, orthostatic hypotension, nausea, vomiting, dizziness, headache.

NURSING CONSIDERATIONS
Black Box Warning Because of the risk of osteosarcoma, give drug only to patients for whom benefits outweigh risk. ∎
• Treatment shouldn't exceed 2 years.

• If patient may have urolithiasis or hypercalciuria, measure urinary calcium excretion before treatment.
• Monitor patient for orthostatic hypotension, which may occur within 4 hours of dosing.
• Monitor calcium level. If persistent hypercalcemia develops, stop drug and evaluate possible cause.

PATIENT TEACHING
• Instruct patient on proper use and disposal of prefilled pen.
• Tell patient not to share pen with others.
• Advise patient to remain in a sitting position while taking drug to prevent orthostatic hypotension.
• Advise patient to sit or lie down if drug causes a fast heartbeat, light-headedness, or dizziness. Tell patient to report persistent or worsening symptoms.
• Urge patient to report persistent symptoms of hypercalcemia, which include nausea, vomiting, constipation, lethargy, and muscle weakness.
• Tell patient to discard pen after 28-day use period, even if some unused solution remains.

testosterone
tes-TOS-te-rone

Striant, Testopel

testosterone cypionate
Depo-Testosterone

testosterone enanthate
Delatestryl

Therapeutic class: Hormone replacements
Pharmacologic class: Androgens
Pregnancy risk category: X
Controlled substance schedule: III

AVAILABLE FORMS
testosterone
Blister packs (buccal; extended-release): 30 mg
Pellets (subcutaneous implant): 75 mg
testosterone cypionate
Injection (in oil): 100 mg/mL, 200 mg/mL

---

testosterone enanthate
Injection (in oil): 200 mg/mL

INDICATIONS & DOSAGES
➤ **Hypogonadism**
Men: 50 to 400 mg cypionate or enanthate
I.M. every 2 to 4 weeks. Or, 150 to 450 mg
(2 to 6 pellets) implanted subcutaneously
every 3 to 6 months. Or, apply 1 buccal
system (30 mg) to the gum region just above
the incisor tooth on either side of the mouth
b.i.d. (morning and evening) about 12 hours
apart. Alternate sides of the mouth with
each application.
➤ **Delayed puberty**
Men and boys: 50 to 200 mg enanthate I.M.
every 2 to 4 weeks for 4 to 6 months.
➤ **Metastatic breast cancer**
Women 1 to 5 years after menopause: 200 to
400 mg enanthate I.M. every 2 to 4 weeks.

ADMINISTRATION
I.M.
• Store I.M. preparations at room temper-
ature. If crystals appear, warm and shake
bottle to disperse them.
• Inject deep into upper outer quadrant of
gluteal muscle. Rotate injection sites; report
soreness at site.
Subcutaneous
• In most men, the pellets are implanted in
an area on the anterior abdominal wall.
Buccal
• The buccal system should be placed in the
gum region just above the incisor tooth on
either side of the mouth.
• Have the patient rotate sides of the mouth
with each administration.
• Make sure the patient doesn't chew or
swallow the buccal system.
• The buccal system should remain in place
until the next dosing. Check placement after
toothbrushing, mouthwash use, eating, and
drinking.
• To remove the system, gently slide it
downward from the gum toward the tooth.

ACTION
Stimulates target tissues to develop normally in androgen-deficient men. May have
some antiestrogen properties, making it
useful in treating certain estrogen-
dependent breast cancers.

Route	Onset	Peak	Duration
I.M.	Unknown	10–100 min	Unknown
Subcut.	Unknown	Unknown	3–6 mo
Buccal	Unknown	10–12 hr	2–4 hr

Half-life: 10 to 100 minutes.

ADVERSE REACTIONS
CNS: headache, anxiety, depression, paresthesia, sleep apnea.
CV: edema.
GI: nausea; gum or mouth irritation; bitter
taste; gum pain, tenderness, or edema; taste
perversion (with buccal application).
GU: amenorrhea, oligospermia, decreased
ejaculatory volume, priapism.
Hematologic: polycythemia, *suppression
of clotting factors.*
Hepatic: reversible jaundice, *cholestatic
hepatitis.*
Metabolic: hypernatremia, *hyperkalemia,*
hypercalcemia, hyperphosphatemia, hypercholesterolemia.
Skin: pain, induration at injection site, local
edema, acne.
Other: androgenic effects in women,
gynecomastia, hypersensitivity reactions,
hypoestrogenic effects in women, excessive hormonal effects in men, male pattern
baldness.

INTERACTIONS
Drug-drug. *Corticosteroids:* May increase
risk of edema. Use together cautiously,
especially in patients with cardiac or hepatic
disease.
Hepatotoxic drugs: May increase risk of
hepatotoxicity. Monitor liver function
closely.
Insulin, oral antidiabetics: May decrease
glucose level; may alter dosage requirements. Monitor glucose level in diabetic
patients.
Oral anticoagulants: May increase sensitivity; may alter dosage requirements. Monitor
PT and INR; decrease anticoagulant dose if
necessary.
Oxyphenbutazone: May increase
oxyphenbutazone level. Monitor patient.
Drug-food. *Licorice:* May decrease testosterone level. Avoid use.

T

EFFECTS ON LAB TEST RESULTS
• May increase sodium, potassium, phosphate, cholesterol, liver enzyme, calcium, creatinine, and serum prostate-specific antigen (PSA) levels.
• May decrease thyroxine-binding globulin, total T_4 levels, serum creatinine, and 17-ketosteroid levels.
• May increase RBC count and resin uptake of T_3 and T_4.
• May cause abnormal glucose tolerance test results.

CONTRAINDICATIONS & CAUTIONS
• Contraindicated in patients hypersensitive to drug and in those with hypercalcemia or cardiac, hepatic, or renal decompensation.
• Contraindicated in men with breast or prostate cancer and in pregnant or breast-feeding women.
• Use cautiously in elderly patients.
⚠ *Overdose S&S:* Stroke (with enanthate injection).

NURSING CONSIDERATIONS
• Unless contraindicated, use with high-calorie, high-protein diet. Give small, frequent meals to help avoid nausea.
• Don't give to women of childbearing age until pregnancy is ruled out.
• Cypionate and enanthate are long-acting solutions.
• Monitor patient's liver function, and PSA, cholesterol, and HDL levels periodically.
• Check hemoglobin and hematocrit levels periodically.
• In patients with metastatic breast cancer, hypercalcemia usually indicates progression of bone metastases. Report signs and symptoms of hypercalcemia.
• Report evidence of virilization in women. Androgenic effects include acne, edema, weight gain, increased hair growth, hoarseness, clitoral enlargement, decreased breast size, changes in libido, male pattern baldness, and oily skin or hair.
• Watch for hypoestrogenic effects in women (flushing; diaphoresis; vaginitis, including itching, drying, and burning; vaginal bleeding; menstrual irregularities).
• Watch for excessive hormonal effects in men and boys. In prepubertal boy, watch for premature epiphyseal closure, acne,

priapism, growth of body and facial hair, and phallic enlargement. In postpubertal men, watch for testicular atrophy, oligospermia, decreased ejaculatory volume, impotence, gynecomastia, and epididymitis.
• Monitor patient's weight and blood pressure routinely.
• Monitor prepubertal boys by X-ray for rate of bone maturation.
• The treatment of hypogonadal men with testosterone esters may potentiate sleep apnea. Monitor patients with risk factors such as obesity or chronic lung diseases.
🔔 *Alert:* Therapeutic response in breast cancer is usually apparent within 3 months. If disease progresses, stop drug.
• Androgens may alter results of laboratory studies during therapy and for 2 to 3 weeks after therapy ends.
• *Look alike–sound alike:* Don't confuse testosterone with testolactone.
🔔 *Alert:* Testosterone salts aren't interchangeable.

PATIENT TEACHING
• Make sure patient understands importance of using an effective nonhormonal contraceptive during therapy.
• Instruct patient to stop drug immediately and notify prescriber if pregnancy is suspected.
• Review signs and symptoms of virilization with woman, and instruct her to notify prescriber if they occur.
• Advise women to wear cotton underwear and to wash after intercourse to decrease risk of vaginitis.
• Instruct men to notify prescriber about priapism, reduced ejaculatory volume, or gynecomastia.
• Warn diabetic patient to be alert for hypoglycemia and to notify prescriber if it occurs.
• Instruct boys using testosterone for delayed puberty to have X-rays of hand and wrist obtained every 6 months during treatment.
• Tell patient to report sudden weight gain.
• Warn patient that drug shouldn't be used to enhance athletic performance.
• Instruct patient how to use the buccal system.
• Advise patient to avoid dislodging buccal system and ensure that the system is in place

---

Reactions in bold italics are *life-threatening*. Interactions may have a *rapid onset* or a *delayed onset*.

after toothbrushing, use of mouthwash, and eating or drinking.
• Tell men not to chew or swallow buccal system.

testosterone transdermal
Androderm, AndroGel, Axiron, Fortesta, Testim

Therapeutic class: Androgens
Pharmacologic class: Androgens
Pregnancy risk category: X
Controlled substance schedule: III

AVAILABLE FORMS
1% gel: 25 mg, 50 mg per unit dose; 1.25 g per pump actuation
1.62% gel: 20.25 mg per pump actuation
2% gel: 10 mg per pump actuation
Topical solution: 30 mg per metered-dose pump
Transdermal system: 2 mg/day, 4 mg/day

INDICATIONS & DOSAGES
➤ Primary or hypogonadotropic hypogonadism
Men: One or two Androderm patches applied to back, abdomen, arm, or thigh nightly for total dosage of 4 mg daily. Dose may be increased to 6 mg once daily or decreased to 2 mg once daily, depending on morning serum testosterone levels. Or, initially, 50 mg of AndroGel 1% or Testim applied every morning to shoulders, upper arms, or abdomen. Don't apply Testim to abdomen. Check testosterone level after about 2 weeks. If response is inadequate, may increase AndroGel to 75 mg daily. Then, adjust to 100 mg (either gel) if needed. Or, for AndroGel pump, 5 g (4 pumps) applied every morning to shoulders, upper arms, or abdomen. Check testosterone level after about 2 weeks. If response is inadequate, may increase to 7.5 g (6 pumps) daily or from 7.5 to 10 g (8 pumps) daily. Or, initially, 40.5 mg (2 pumps) of AndroGel 1.62% daily to upper arms or shoulders. May adjust dosage between a minimum of 20.25 mg (1 pump) and a maximum of 81 mg (4 pumps) titrated based on the predose morning serum testosterone concentration at about 14 days and

28 days after starting treatment or the last dosage adjustment. Or, initially 40 mg (4 pumps) of Fortesta once daily to the thighs in the morning. May adjust dosage between 10 mg and maximum of 70 mg based on testosterone concentration drawn 2 hours after application approximately 14 days and 35 days after start of treatment and the last dosage adjustment. Or, initially 60 mg (2 pumps) of Axiron solution, one actuation to each axilla, once daily. May adjust dosage between 30 mg (1 pump) and a maximum of 120 mg (4 pumps) based on serum testosterone concentration drawn 2 to 8 hours after application and at least 14 days after starting treatment or the last dosage adjustment.

ADMINISTRATION
Transdermal
• Wear gloves when handling patches. Fold used patches with adhesive sides together to discard.
• Apply patch nightly to clean, dry, intact skin of the back, abdomen, upper arms, or thighs only and not to the genitals or bony prominences.
Topical
• AndroGel 1.62% and AndroGel 1% and topical solution aren't interchangeable.
• Fully prime the pumps by pumping three times before first use. Discard that gel.
• Wear gloves to apply gel to clean, dry, intact skin of the shoulders, upper arms, or abdomen only and not to the genitals or bony prominences. Testim shouldn't be applied to the abdomen.
• Application in the morning is preferable. Allow application sites to dry before dressing. Cover the application sites with clothing.
• Patient should avoid swimming or washing the administration site for 2 hours after application.
• Apply Fortesta to clean, dry, intact skin of the front and inner thighs only.
• Gel contains alcohol and is flammable. Patient should avoid fire, flames, or smoking until gel has dried.
• Apply topical solution, using the applicator provided, to clean, dry, intact skin of the axilla as directed. Don't use the fingers or hand to rub the solution into the skin.

T

Patient should apply deodorants before applying the solution.

ACTION
Releases testosterone, which stimulates target tissues to develop normally in androgen-deficient men.

Route	Onset	Peak	Duration
Transdermal, topical	Unknown	2–4 hr	2 hr after removal

Half-life: 10 to 100 minutes.

ADVERSE REACTIONS
CNS: *stroke,* asthenia, depression, headache, sleep apnea.
GI: *GI bleeding.*
GU: prostatitis, prostate abnormalities, UTI.
Hepatic: *cholestatic hepatitis,* reversible jaundice.
Metabolic: hypernatremia, hyperkalemia, hypercalcemia, hyperphosphatemia, hypercholesterolemia.
Skin: pruritus, blister under patch, acne irritation, allergic contact dermatitis, burning.
Other: gynecomastia, breast tenderness, flulike syndrome.

INTERACTIONS
Drug-drug. *Corticosteroids:* May increase risk of edema. Use together cautiously, especially in patients with cardiac or hepatic disease.
Hepatotoxic drugs: May increase risk of hepatotoxicity. Monitor liver function closely.
Insulin: May alter insulin dosage requirements. Monitor glucose level.
Oral anticoagulants: May alter anticoagulant dosage requirements. Monitor PT and INR.
Oxyphenbutazone: May increase oxyphenbutazone level. Monitor patient.

EFFECTS ON LAB TEST RESULTS
● May increase sodium, potassium, phosphate, cholesterol, liver enzyme, calcium, and creatinine levels and resin uptake of T_3 and T_4. May decrease total T_4 levels.
● May increase glucose level.
● May increase RBC count.

CONTRAINDICATIONS & CAUTIONS
● Contraindicated in patients hypersensitive to drug, in women, in men with known or suspected breast or prostate cancer, and in patients with CV, renal, or hepatic disease.
● Use cautiously in elderly men.

NURSING CONSIDERATIONS
Black Box Warning Virilization in children and women can occur after secondary exposure to transdermal application sites on men. Women and children should avoid contact with application sites. ■
● Periodically assess LFT results, lipid profiles, hemoglobin level, hematocrit (with long-term use), and levels of prostatic acid phosphatase and prostate-specific antigen.
● Watch for excessive hormonal effects.

PATIENT TEACHING
● Tell patient to fully prime the AndroGel or Fortesta pump by pumping three times before first use and to discard that gel.
Black Box Warning Instruct patient to strictly adhere to recommended instructions for use. Tell patient to apply to clean, dry, intact skin as directed. ■
● Instruct patient to thoroughly wash the application site with soap and water before situations in which direct skin-to-skin contact is anticipated.
● Tell patient using patch to apply it at night.
● Tell patient using gel to apply in the morning.
Black Box Warning Tell patient to wash his hands thoroughly after using product and to cover treated area with clothing. ■
● Instruct patient that patch must be changed every 24 hours.
● For best results, advise patient not to swim or shower for at least 2 hours after applying gel. Showering or swimming at least 1 hour after applying, if done infrequently, should have minimal effects on drug absorption.
● Tell patient that if the patch falls off, it may be reapplied. If patch falls off and can't be reapplied, and it has been worn at least 12 hours, a new patch may be applied at the next application time.
● Warn diabetic patient that drug may decrease glucose level and to be alert for hypoglycemia.

• Advise patient to report persistent erections, nausea, vomiting, changes in skin color, ankle swelling, or sudden weight gain to prescriber.

• Tell patient that women and children should avoid contact with his application sites.

• Tell patient that Androderm doesn't have to be removed during sexual intercourse or while showering.

• Tell patient undergoing an MRI to alert the facility that he is using a transdermal patch.

tetracycline hydrochloride
tet-ra-SYE-kleen

Therapeutic class: Antibiotics
Pharmacologic class: Tetracyclines
Pregnancy risk category: D

AVAILABLE FORMS
Capsules: 100 mg, 250 mg, 500 mg

INDICATIONS & DOSAGES
➤ **Infections caused by susceptible gram-negative and gram-positive organisms, including** *Haemophilus ducreyi, Yersinia pestis, Campylobacter fetus, Rickettsiae* **species,** *Mycoplasma pneumoniae,* **and** *Chlamydia trachomatis;* **psittacosis; granuloma inguinale**
Adults: 1 to 2 g/day P.O. in two or four divided doses depending on the severity of infection.
Children older than age 8: 25 to 50 mg/kg P.O. daily, in divided doses every 6 hours.
➤ **Uncomplicated urethral, endocervical, or rectal infections caused by** *C. trachomatis*
Adults: 500 mg P.O. q.i.d. for at least 7 days.
➤ **Brucellosis**
Adults: 500 mg P.O. every 6 hours for 3 weeks with 1 g of streptomycin I.M. every 12 hours for first week and once daily for second week.
➤ **Uncomplicated gonorrhea in patients allergic to penicillin**
Adults: 500 mg P.O. every 6 hours for 7 days.
➤ **Syphilis in patients allergic to penicillin**

Adults and adolescents: 500 mg P.O. q.i.d. for 15 days. If infection has lasted 1 year or longer, treat for 30 days.
➤ **Acne (severe; long-term therapy)**
Adults and adolescents: Initially, 250 mg P.O. every 6 hours; then 125 to 500 mg daily or every other day.

ADMINISTRATION
P.O.
• Obtain specimen for culture and sensitivity tests before giving first dose. Begin therapy while awaiting results.
• Effectiveness is reduced when drug is given with milk or other dairy products, antacids, or iron products. For best drug absorption, give drug with a full glass of water on an empty stomach, at least 1 hour before or 2 hours after meals.
• Give drug at least 1 hour before bedtime to prevent esophageal irritation or ulceration.

ACTION
May exert bacteriostatic effect by binding to the 30S and possibly 50S ribosomal subunits of microorganisms, thus inhibiting protein synthesis. May also alter the cytoplasmic membrane of susceptible microorganisms.

Route	Onset	Peak	Duration
P.O.	Unknown	1–4 hr	Unknown

Half-life: 6 to 11 hours.

ADVERSE REACTIONS
CNS: *intracranial hypertension,* dizziness, headache.
CV: pericarditis.
EENT: sore throat.
GI: diarrhea, epigastric distress, nausea, anorexia, dysphagia, enterocolitis, esophagitis, glossitis, oral candidiasis, stomatitis, vomiting.
GU: inflammatory lesions in anogenital region.
Hematologic: *neutropenia, thrombocytopenia,* eosinophilia.
Musculoskeletal: bone growth retardation in children younger than age 8.
Skin: candidal superinfection, increased pigmentation, maculopapular and

T

erythematous rash, photosensitivity reactions, urticaria.

Other: enamel defects, hypersensitivity reactions, permanent discoloration of teeth.

INTERACTIONS

Drug-drug. *Antacids and laxatives containing aluminum, magnesium, or calcium; antidiarrheals containing kaolin, pectin, or bismuth subsalicylate:* May decrease antibiotic absorption. Give antibiotic 1 hour before or 2 hours after these drugs.

Digoxin: May increase digoxin absorption. Monitor digoxin levels and monitor patient for signs of toxicity.

Ferrous sulfate and other iron products, zinc: May decrease antibiotic absorption. Give tetracycline 2 hours before or 3 hours after these products.

Hormonal contraceptives: May decrease contraceptive effectiveness and increase risk of breakthrough bleeding. Advise patient to use nonhormonal contraceptive.

Methoxyflurane: May cause severe nephrotoxicity. Avoid using together.

Oral anticoagulants: May increase anticoagulant effects. Monitor PT and INR, and adjust anticoagulant dosage.

Penicillins: May interfere with bactericidal action of penicillins. Avoid using together.

Drug-food. *Dairy products:* May decrease antibiotic absorption. Give antibiotic 1 hour before or 2 hours after eating or drinking dairy products.

Drug-lifestyle. *Sun exposure:* May cause photosensitivity reactions. Advise patient to avoid excessive sunlight exposure.

EFFECTS ON LAB TEST RESULTS

● May increase BUN and liver enzyme levels.

● May increase eosinophil count. May decrease platelet and neutrophil counts.

CONTRAINDICATIONS & CAUTIONS

● Contraindicated in patients hypersensitive to drug or other tetracyclines.

● Some tetracyclines may contain sulfites and are contraindicated in patients with sulfite hypersensitivity.

● Use cautiously in patients with renal or hepatic impairment. Avoid using or use cautiously during last half of pregnancy

and in children younger than age 8 because drug may cause permanent discoloration of teeth, enamel defects, and bone growth retardation.

⚠ *Overdose S&S:* Dizziness, nausea, vomiting.

NURSING CONSIDERATIONS

◗ *Alert:* Check expiration date. Using outdated or deteriorated drug has been linked to severe reversible nephrotoxicity (Fanconi syndrome).

● Don't expose drug to light or heat.

● If large doses are given, therapy is prolonged, or patient is at high risk, monitor patient for signs and symptoms of superinfection.

● In patients with renal or hepatic impairment, monitor renal function tests and LFT results if drug is used.

● Check patient's tongue for signs of candidal infection. Emphasize good oral hygiene.

● Drug isn't indicated for treatment of neurosyphilis.

● Photosensitivity reactions may occur within a few minutes to several hours after sun exposure. Photosensitivity lasts after therapy ends.

PATIENT TEACHING

● Tell patient to take drug exactly as prescribed, even after he feels better, and to take entire amount prescribed.

● Tell patient to check drug's expiration date and not to use if outdated.

● Explain that effectiveness is reduced when drug is taken with milk or other dairy products, antacids, or iron products. For best drug absorption, tell patient to take each dose with a full glass of water on an empty stomach, at least 1 hour before or 2 hours after meals. Also tell him to take it at least 1 hour before bedtime to prevent esophageal irritation or ulceration.

● Warn patient to avoid direct sunlight and ultraviolet light, wear protective clothing, and use sunscreen.

● Advise patient to promptly report adverse reactions to prescriber.

Reactions in bold italics are *life-threatening*. Interactions may have a *rapid onset* or a *delayed onset*.

tetrahydrozoline hydrochloride (intranasal)
tet-rah-hi-DRAZ-oh-leen

Tyzine

Therapeutic class: Decongestants
Pharmacologic class: Sympathomimetics
Pregnancy risk category: C

AVAILABLE FORMS
Nasal solution: 0.05%, 0.1%
Nasal spray: 0.1%

INDICATIONS & DOSAGES
➤ **Nasal congestion**
Adults and children older than age 6: 2 to 4 drops or 3 to 4 sprays of 0.1% solution in each nostril no more than every 3 hours, p.r.n.
Children ages 2 to 6: Give 2 to 3 drops of 0.05% solution in each nostril no more than every 3 hours, p.r.n.

ADMINISTRATION
Intranasal
• Instill nose drops with patient in lateral head-low position.
• Give nasal spray with patient's head tilted back slightly. Wait 1 to 2 minutes between sprays.
• Rinse spray tip in hot water and dry with a clean tissue.

ACTION
Thought to cause local vasoconstriction of dilated arterioles, reducing blood flow and nasal congestion.

Route	Onset	Peak	Duration
Intranasal	Few min	Unknown	4–8 hr

Half-life: Unknown.

ADVERSE REACTIONS
EENT: rebound nasal congestion, sneezing, transient burning or stinging, mucosal dryness.

INTERACTIONS
Drug-drug. *Bromocriptine, catechol-O-methyltransferase inhibitors, such as tolcapone:* May increase the effects of these drugs. Monitor patient for increased clinical response and adverse effects.
MAO inhibitors: May cause headache, hypertension, and hyperpyrexia. Use together or within 14 days of stopping an MAO inhibitor is contraindicated.
TCAs: May decrease the effects of tetrahydrozoline. Monitor patient for clinical effect.
Drug-herb. *St. John's wort:* May increase adverse effects of herb. Discourage use together.

EFFECTS ON LAB TEST RESULTS
None reported.

CONTRAINDICATIONS & CAUTIONS
• Contraindicated in patients hypersensitive to drug and in children younger than age 2. The 0.1% solution is contraindicated in children younger than age 6.
• Contraindicated in patients being treated with MAO inhibitors or within 14 days of treatment with MAO inhibitors.
• Use cautiously in patients with hyperthyroidism, hypertension, or diabetes mellitus.
⚠ *Overdose S&S:* Hypertension, bradycardia, drowsiness, rebound hypotension, shock, profuse sweating.

NURSING CONSIDERATIONS
• Drug should be used for only 3 to 5 days.
• Overdose in young children may cause oversedation.

PATIENT TEACHING
• Teach patient how to use drug.
• Caution patient not to share drug because this could spread infection.
• Tell patient not to exceed recommended dosage and to use only as needed for 3 to 5 days.

T

tetrahydrozoline hydrochloride (ophthalmic)
tet-rah-hi-DRAZ-oh-leen

Altazine ◊, Murine Tears Plus ◊, Opti-Clear ◊, Optigene 3 ◊, Redness Reliever ◊, Visine ◊

Therapeutic class: Vasoconstrictors
Pharmacologic class: Sympathomimetics
Pregnancy risk category: NR

AVAILABLE FORMS
Ophthalmic solution: 0.05% ◊

INDICATIONS & DOSAGES
➤ **Conjunctival congestion, irritation, and allergic conditions**
Adults: Instill 1 to 2 drops in affected eye up to q.i.d., or as directed by prescriber.

ADMINISTRATION
Ophthalmic
● Apply light finger pressure on lacrimal sac for 1 minute after drops are instilled.
● Don't touch tip of dropper to any surface.

ACTION
Thought to cause vasoconstriction by local adrenergic action on the blood vessels of the conjunctiva.

Route	Onset	Peak	Duration
Ophthalmic	Few min	Unknown	1–4 hr

Half-life: Unknown.

ADVERSE REACTIONS
CNS: dizziness, drowsiness, headache, insomnia, tremor.
CV: *arrhythmias.*
EENT: eye irritation, increased intraocular pressure, keratitis, lacrimation, pupillary dilation, transient eye stinging.

INTERACTIONS
Drug-drug. *Beta blockers:* May cause more systemic adverse effects. Monitor patient for adverse systemic effects.
Guanethidine, MAO inhibitors, TCAs: May cause hypertensive crisis if tetrahydrozoline

is systemically absorbed. Avoid using together.

EFFECTS ON LAB TEST RESULTS
None reported.

CONTRAINDICATIONS & CAUTIONS
● Contraindicated in patients hypersensitive to drug or its components and in those with angle-closure glaucoma or other serious eye disease.
● Use cautiously in patients with hyperthyroidism, heart disease, hypertension, or diabetes mellitus.

NURSING CONSIDERATIONS
● Rebound congestion may occur with frequent or prolonged use.
● **Alert:** Don't confuse Visine with Visken.

PATIENT TEACHING
● Teach patient how to instill drug. Advise him to wash hands before and after instillation and to apply light finger pressure on lacrimal sac for 1 minute after drops are instilled. Warn him not to touch tip of dropper to eye or surrounding tissue.
● Warn patient not to exceed recommended dosage to avoid rebound congestion.
● Tell patient to stop drug and notify prescriber if redness or irritation persists or increases or if no relief occurs within 2 days.
● Warn patient not to share eyedrops.
● Advise patient that drug is for ophthalmic use only and shouldn't be ingested.
● Caution patient to keep drug out of the reach of small children. Children who ingest small amounts can develop bradycardia, respiratory depression, sedation, or coma and require hospitalization.

theophylline
thee-OFF-i-lin

Immediate-release liquids
Elixophyllin*

Immediate-release tablets
Theolair

Extended-release tablets
Theochron

Extended-release capsules
Theo-24

Therapeutic class: Bronchodilators
Pharmacologic class: Xanthine
derivatives
Pregnancy risk category: C

AVAILABLE FORMS
Capsules (extended-release): 100 mg,
200 mg, 300 mg, 400 mg
D_5W injection: 200 mg in 50 mL or 100 mL;
400 mg in 100 mL, 250 mL, 500 mL, or
1,000 mL; 800 mg in 500 mL or 1,000 mL
Syrup: 80 mg/15 mL*
Tablets: 125 mg, 250 mg
Tablets (extended-release): 100 mg, 200 mg,
300 mg, 400 mg, 450 mg, 600 mg

INDICATIONS & DOSAGES
Extended-release preparations shouldn't be
used to treat acute bronchospasm.
➤ **Parenteral theophylline (preferred
route) for acute bronchospasm in patients
not currently receiving theophylline**
Loading dose: 4.6 mg/kg ideal body weight
over 30 minutes; then maintenance infusion.
*Nonsmoking adults younger than age 60
and children older than age 16:* 0.4 mg/kg/
hour (maximum 900 mg daily).
Nonsmoking children ages 12 to 16:
0.5 mg/kg/hour (maximum 900 mg daily).
*Children ages 12 to 16 who smoke and
children ages 9 to 12:* 0.7 mg/kg/hour.
Children ages 1 to 9: 0.8 mg/kg/hour.
Infants ages 6 weeks to 1 year: Calculate
mg/kg/hour dosage as follows: 0.008 × (age
in weeks) + 0.21.
Neonates older than 24 days: 1.5 mg/kg
every 12 hours to achieve target theophylline concentration of 7.5 mcg/mL.

Neonates 24 days old and younger: 1 mg/kg
every 12 hours to achieve a target theophylline concentration of 7.5 mcg/mL.
Adjust-a-dose: For adults older than age
60, give 0.3 mg/kg/hour, up to a maximum
of 17 mg/hour. For adults with heart failure, cor pulmonale, liver disease, sepsis
with multiorgan failure, or shock, give
0.2 mg/kg/hour, up to a maximum infusion
rate of 17 mg/hour unless serum theophylline concentrations are monitored at
24-hour intervals. Maximum daily dose
is 400 mg.
➤ **Oral theophylline for acute bronchospasm in patients not currently
receiving theophylline**
*Adults age 60 and younger, children ages
16 and older, and children ages 1 to 15
weighing 45 kg (99 lb) or more:* 5 mg/kg
P.O., then 300 mg (immediate-release) P.O.
daily in divided doses every 6 to 8 hours for
3 days. If tolerated, increase to 400 mg P.O.
daily in divided doses every 6 to 8 hours. If
necessary, dosage may be increased after
3 days to 600 mg P.O. daily in divided doses
every 6 to 8 hours.
*Children ages 1 to 15 weighing less than
45 kg:* 5 mg/kg P.O., then 12 to 14 mg/kg
immediate-release (maximum 300 mg) P.O.
daily in divided doses every 4 to 6 hours for
3 days. If tolerated, increase to 16 mg/kg
(maximum 400 mg) P.O. daily in divided
doses every 4 to 6 hours. After 3 days, if
necessary, increase to 20 mg/kg (maximum
600 mg) P.O. daily in divided doses every 4
to 6 hours.
Adjust-a-dose: For children ages 1 to 15
with risk factors for reduced theophylline
clearance or for whom serum concentrations can't be monitored, give 5 mg/kg P.O.,
then 12 to 14 mg/kg (maximum 300 mg)
P.O. daily in divided doses every 4 to
6 hours for 3 days. If tolerated, increase
to 16 mg/kg (maximum 400 mg) P.O. daily
in divided doses every 4 to 6 hours. For
children age 16 and older and adults with
risk factors for reduced theophylline clearance or for whom serum concentrations
can't be monitored, give 5 mg/kg P.O., then
300 mg P.O. daily in divided doses every
6 to 8 hours for 3 days. If tolerated, increase
to 400 mg P.O. daily in divided doses every
6 to 8 hours.

T

➤ **Chronic bronchospasm using extended-release preparations**
Adults age 60 or younger, children age 16 and older, and children ages 6 to 15 weighing more than 45 kg: 300 mg P.O. daily in divided doses every 8 to 12 hours or 300 to 400 mg (24-hour extended-release capsule) P.O. daily for 3 days. If tolerated, increase to 400 mg P.O. in divided doses every 8 to 12 hours or 400 to 600 mg (24-hour extended-release capsule) P.O. daily. After 3 more days, if necessary, increase dose to 600 mg P.O. daily in divided doses every 8 to 12 hours. Titrate dosages greater than 600 mg according to serum blood levels.

Children ages 6 to 15 weighing less than 45 kg: 12 to 14 mg/kg (maximum 300 mg extended-release tablet) daily in divided doses every 8 to 12 hours for 3 days. If tolerated, increase to 16 mg/kg (maximum 400 mg extended-release tablet) daily in divided doses every 8 to 12 hours. After 3 more days, if necessary, increase to 20 mg/kg (maximum 600 mg extended-release tablet) daily in divided doses every 8 to 12 hours.

Adjust-a-dose: For children ages 6 to 15 with risk factors for reduced theophylline clearance or for whom serum concentrations can't be monitored, give 12 to 14 mg/kg (maximum 300 mg) daily in divided doses for 3 days. If tolerated, increase to a maximum of 16 mg/kg (maximum 400 mg) P.O. daily in divided doses every 8 to 12 hours. For children age 16 and older and adults age 60 or younger or for whom serum concentrations can't be monitored, give 300 mg P.O. daily in divided doses every 8 to 12 hours. After 3 days, if necessary, increase to maximum of 400 mg P.O. daily in divided doses every 8 to 12 hours. For adults older than age 60, the recommended maximum daily dose is 400 mg P.O. per day in divided doses every 8 to 12 hours unless symptoms continue and peak serum concentration is less than 10 mcg/mL. Administer dosages greater than 400 mg P.O. daily cautiously.

ADMINISTRATION
P.O.
● Calculate the mg/kg dose based on ideal body weight because drug distributes poorly into body fat.
● Each 0.5-mg/kg P.O. loading dose will increase drug level by 1 mcg/mL.
● Give drug with full glass of water after meals, if needed, to relieve GI symptoms, although taking with food delays absorption.
● Give drug around-the-clock, using extended-release product at bedtime.
● Don't dissolve or crush extended-release products. Small children unable to swallow these can ingest (without chewing) the contents of capsules sprinkled over soft food.
● Administer extended-release formulas in a consistent manner, either always with or always without food.

I.V.
▼ Each 0.5-mg/kg I.V. loading dose will increase drug level by 1 mcg/mL.
▼ Use commercially available infusion solution, or mix in D_5W solution.
▼ Use infusion pump for continuous infusion.
▼ **Incompatibilities:** Ascorbic acid, ceftriaxone, cimetidine, hetastarch, phenytoin.

ACTION
Inhibits phosphodiesterase, the enzyme that degrades cAMP, resulting in relaxation of smooth muscle of the bronchial airways and pulmonary blood vessels.

Route	Onset	Peak	Duration
P.O.	15–60 min	1–2 hr	Unknown
P.O. (extended)	15–60 min	4–7 hr	Unknown
I.V.	15 min	15–30 min	Unknown

Half-life: Adults, 7 to 9 hours; smokers, 4 to 5 hours; children, 3 to 5 hours; premature infants, 20 to 30 hours.

ADVERSE REACTIONS
CNS: restlessness, dizziness, insomnia, *seizures,* headache, irritability, muscle twitching.
CV: palpitations, sinus tachycardia, *arrhythmias,* extrasystoles, flushing, marked hypotension.

Reactions in bold italics are *life-threatening*. Interactions may have a *rapid onset* or a *delayed onset*.

GI: nausea, vomiting, diarrhea, epigastric pain.
Metabolic: urinary catecholamines.
Respiratory: *respiratory arrest,* tachypnea.

INTERACTIONS

Drug-drug. *Adenosine:* May decrease antiarrhythmic effect. Higher doses of adenosine may be needed.

Allopurinol, calcium channel blockers, **cimetidine,** *disulfiram, influenza virus vaccine, interferon,* **macrolides (such as erythromycin),** *methotrexate,* **mexiletine,** *oral contraceptives,* **quinolones (such as ciprofloxacin):** May decrease hepatic clearance of theophylline; may increase theophylline level. Monitor levels closely and adjust theophylline dose.

Barbiturates, nicotine, **phenytoin, rifamycins:** May enhance metabolism and decrease theophylline level; may increase phenytoin metabolism. Monitor patient for decreased therapeutic effect; monitor levels and adjust dosage.

Carbamazepine, loop diuretics: May increase or decrease theophylline level. Monitor theophylline level.

Carteolol, pindolol, propranolol, timolol: May act antagonistically, reducing the effects of one or both drugs; may reduce elimination of theophylline. Monitor theophylline level and patient closely.

Ephedrine, other sympathomimetics: May exhibit synergistic toxicity with these drugs, predisposing patient to arrhythmias or increased CNS effects. Monitor patient closely.

Lithium: May increase lithium excretion. Monitor patient closely.

Tetracyclines: May enhance the adverse effects of theophylline. Monitor patient closely.

Drug-herb. *Cacao tree:* May inhibit drug metabolism. Discourage use together.

Cayenne: May increase risk of drug toxicity. Advise patient to use together cautiously.

Ephedra: May increase risk of adverse reactions. Discourage use together.

Guarana: May cause additive CNS and CV effects. Discourage use together.

Ipriflavone: May increase risk of drug toxicity. Advise patient to use together cautiously.

St. John's wort: May decrease drug level. Discourage use together.

Drug-food. *Any food:* May cause accelerated drug release from extended-release products. Tell patient to take extended-release products on an empty stomach.

Caffeine: May decrease hepatic clearance of drug and increase drug level. Monitor patient for toxicity.

Drug-lifestyle. *Alcohol use:* Decreases theophylline clearance and increases risk of adverse reactions. Discourage use together.

Smoking: May increase elimination of drug, increasing dosage requirements. Monitor drug response and level.

EFFECTS ON LAB TEST RESULTS

● May increase free fatty acid and blood glucose levels.
● May increase uric acid, HDL, and total cholesterol levels and urinary free cortisol excretion.
● May decrease T_3 measurements.
● May falsely elevate theophylline level in the presence of acetaminophen, furosemide, phenylbutazone, probenecid, theobromine, caffeine, tea, chocolate, and cola, depending on assay used.

CONTRAINDICATIONS & CAUTIONS

● Contraindicated in patients hypersensitive to xanthine compounds (caffeine, theobromine) and in those with active peptic ulcer or poorly controlled seizure disorders.
● Use cautiously in young children, infants, neonates, elderly patients, and those with COPD, cardiac failure, cor pulmonale, renal or hepatic disease, peptic ulceration, hyperthyroidism, diabetes mellitus, glaucoma, severe hypoxemia, hypertension, compromised cardiac or circulatory function, angina, acute MI, or sulfite sensitivity.
⚠ Overdose S&S: Seizures; arrhythmias; elevated CK, myoglobin, and calcium levels; elevated leukocyte count; decreased phosphorus and magnesium levels; acute MI; urine retention in men with obstructive uropathy.

NURSING CONSIDERATIONS

● Dosage may need to be increased in cigarette smokers and in habitual

T

---

marijuana smokers because smoking causes drug to be metabolized faster.

• Monitor vital signs; measure and record fluid intake and output. Expect improved quality of pulse and respirations.

• Patients metabolize xanthines at different rates; dosage is determined by monitoring response, tolerance, pulmonary function, and drug level. Drug levels range from 10 to 20 mcg/mL; toxicity may occur at levels above 20 mcg/mL.

❸ *Alert:* Evidence of toxicity includes tachycardia, anorexia, nausea, vomiting, diarrhea, restlessness, irritability, and headache. If these signs occur, check drug level and adjust dosage, as indicated.

• *Look alike–sound alike:* Don't confuse extended-release form with immediate-release form.

• *Look alike–sound alike:* Don't confuse Theolair with Thyrolar.

PATIENT TEACHING

• Supply instructions for home care and dosage schedule.

• Warn patient not to dissolve, crush, or chew extended-release products. Small children unable to swallow these can ingest (without chewing) the contents of capsules sprinkled over soft food.

• Tell patient to relieve GI symptoms by taking oral drug with full glass of water after meals, although food in stomach delays absorption.

• Warn patient to take drug regularly, only as directed. Patients tend to want to take extra "breathing pills."

• Inform elderly patient that dizziness is common at start of therapy.

• Urge patient to tell prescriber about any other drugs taken. OTC drugs or herbal remedies may contain ephedrine or theophylline salts; excessive CNS stimulation may result.

• If a smoker quits, tell him to inform prescriber. Dosage reduction may be needed to prevent toxicity.

SAFETY ALERT!

thiotepa (TESPA, triethylenethiophosphoramide, TSPA)
thye-oh-TEE-pa

Therapeutic class: Antineoplastics
Pharmacologic class: Alkylating drugs
Pregnancy risk category: D

AVAILABLE FORMS
Injection: 15 mg/vial

INDICATIONS & DOSAGES
➤ **Breast and ovarian cancers, lymphoma, Hodgkin lymphoma**
Adults: 0.3 to 0.4 mg/kg I.V. every 1 to 4 weeks.
➤ **Bladder tumor**
Adults: 30 to 60 mg in 30 to 60 mL of normal saline solution instilled in bladder for 2 hours once weekly for 4 weeks.
➤ **Neoplastic effusions**
Adults: 0.6 to 0.8 mg/kg intracavitarily every 1 to 4 weeks.

ADMINISTRATION
I.V.
▼ Preparing and giving drug may be mutagenic, teratogenic, or carcinogenic. Follow facility policy to reduce risks.
▼ Reconstitute with 1.5 mL of sterile water for injection in 15-mg vial to yield 10 mg/mL. Don't reconstitute with other solutions.
▼ Further dilute with normal saline solution for injection. If larger volume is desired, further dilute with sodium chloride solution, D_5W, dextrose 5% in normal saline solution for injection, Ringer injection, or lactated Ringer injection.
▼ If solution appears grossly opaque or has a precipitate, discard it. Make sure solutions are clear to slightly opaque. To eliminate haze, filter solutions through a 0.22-micron filter before use.
▼ If pain occurs at insertion site, dilute drug further or use a local anesthetic to reduce pain. Make sure drug doesn't infiltrate.
▼ Use solutions within 8 hours.

Reactions in bold italics are *life-threatening*. Interactions may have a *rapid onset* or a *delayed onset*.

▼ Refrigerate and protect dry powder from direct sunlight to avoid possible drug breakdown.

▼ **Incompatibilities:** Cisplatin, filgrastim, minocycline, vinorelbine.

Intravesical

• Preparing and giving drug may be mutagenic, teratogenic, or carcinogenic. Follow facility policy to reduce risks.

• For bladder instillation, dehydrate patient 8 to 10 hours before therapy. Instill drug into bladder by catheter; ask patient to retain solution for 2 hours. If discomfort is too great with 60 mL, reduce volume to 30 mL. Reposition patient every 15 minutes for maximum area contact.

Intracavitary

• Preparing and giving drug may be mutagenic, teratogenic, or carcinogenic. Follow facility policy to reduce risks.

• For intracavitary instillation, drug may be given through the same tubing used to remove the fluid from the cavity involved.

ACTION

Cross-links strands of cellular DNA and interferes with RNA transcription, causing an imbalance of growth that leads to cell death. Not specific to cell cycle.

Route	Onset	Peak	Duration
I.V., topical	Unknown	Unknown	Unknown

Half-life: 2¼ hours.

ADVERSE REACTIONS

CNS: headache, dizziness, fatigue, weakness, fever.

EENT: blurred vision, conjunctivitis.

GI: nausea, vomiting, abdominal pain, anorexia, stomatitis.

GU: amenorrhea, decreased spermatogenesis, dysuria, increased urine levels of uric acid, urine retention, hemorrhagic cystitis (with intravesical administration).

Hematologic: *leukopenia, thrombocytopenia, neutropenia,* anemia.

Respiratory: *laryngeal edema.*

Skin: dermatitis, alopecia, injection-site pain, urticaria, rash.

Other: hypersensitivity reactions, including *anaphylaxis.*

INTERACTIONS

Drug-drug. *Anticoagulants, aspirin, NSAIDs:* May increase risk of bleeding. Avoid using together.

Live-virus vaccines: May increase risk of infection. Avoid using together.

Myelosuppressives: May increase myelosuppression. Monitor patient.

Neuromuscular blockers: May prolong muscular paralysis. Monitor patient.

Other alkylating drugs, irradiation therapy: May intensify toxicity rather than enhance therapeutic response. Avoid using together.

EFFECTS ON LAB TEST RESULTS

• May increase uric acid level. May decrease pseudocholinesterase and hemoglobin levels.

• May decrease lymphocyte, platelet, WBC, RBC, and neutrophil counts.

CONTRAINDICATIONS & CAUTIONS

• Contraindicated in patients hypersensitive to drug, in breast-feeding patients, and in those with severe bone marrow, hepatic, or renal dysfunction.

• Use in pregnant women only when benefits to mother outweigh risk of teratogenicity.

• Use cautiously in patients with mild bone marrow suppression and renal or hepatic dysfunction.

⚠ *Overdose S&S:* Hematopoietic toxicity, bleeding.

NURSING CONSIDERATIONS

• Monitor CBC weekly for at least 3 weeks after last dose.

• If patient's WBC count drops below 3,000/mm³ or if platelet count falls below 150,000/mm³, stop drug and notify prescriber. If WBC count falls below 2,000/mm³ or granulocyte count falls below 1,000/mm³, follow institutional policy for infection control in immunocompromised patients.

• Monitor uric acid level. To prevent hyperuricemia with resulting uric acid nephropathy, give allopurinol along with adequate hydration.

• Therapeutic effects are commonly accompanied by toxicity.

• To prevent bleeding, avoid all I.M. injections when platelet count is below 50,000/mm³.

T

• Give blood transfusions for cumulative anemia.

PATIENT TEACHING
• Advise patient to watch for signs and symptoms of infection (fever, sore throat, fatigue) and bleeding (easy bruising, nose-bleeds, bleeding gums, tarry stools). Tell patient to take temperature daily. Tell patient to report even mild infections.
• Instruct patient to avoid OTC products containing aspirin or NSAIDs.
• Advise women to stop breast-feeding during therapy because of risk of toxicity to infant.
• Caution women of childbearing age to consult prescriber before becoming pregnant.

tiagabine hydrochloride
tye-AG-ah-been

Gabitril Filmtabs

Therapeutic class: Anticonvulsants
Pharmacologic class: GABA enhancers
Pregnancy risk category: C

AVAILABLE FORMS
Tablets: 2 mg, 4 mg, 12 mg, 16 mg

INDICATIONS & DOSAGES
➤ **Adjunctive treatment of partial seizures in patients taking enzyme-inducing anticonvulsants (carbamazepine, phenytoin, primidone, phenobarbital)**
Adults: Initially, 4 mg P.O. once daily. Total daily dose may be increased by 4 to 8 mg at weekly intervals until clinical response or up to 56 mg daily. Give total daily dose in two to four divided doses.
Children ages 12 to 18: Initially, 4 mg P.O. once daily. Total daily dose may be increased by 4 mg at beginning of week 2 and thereafter by 4 to 8 mg per week until clinical response or up to 32 mg daily. Give total daily dose in two to four divided doses.
Adjust-a-dose: For patients with hepatic impairment, reduce first and maintenance doses or increase dosing intervals. For

patients not taking enzyme-inducing anticonvulsants, use lower doses and slower titration.

ADMINISTRATION
P.O.
• Give drug with food.

ACTION
Unknown. May act by facilitating the effects of the inhibitory neurotransmitter GABA. By binding to recognition sites linked to GABA uptake carrier, drug may make more GABA available.

Route	Onset	Peak	Duration
P.O.	Rapid	45 min	7–9 hr

Half-life: 7 to 9 hours.

ADVERSE REACTIONS
CNS: asthenia, dizziness, nervousness, somnolence, abnormal gait, agitation, ataxia, confusion, depression, difficulty with concentration and attention, difficulty with memory, emotional lability, hostility, insomnia, language problems, paresthesia, speech disorder, tremor, pain.
CV: vasodilation.
EENT: nystagmus, pharyngitis.
GI: nausea, abdominal pain, diarrhea, increased appetite, mouth ulceration, vomiting.
Musculoskeletal: generalized weakness, myasthenia.
Respiratory: increased cough.
Skin: pruritus, rash.

INTERACTIONS
Drug-drug. *Carbamazepine, phenobarbital, phenytoin:* May increase tiagabine clearance. Monitor patient closely.
CNS depressants: May enhance CNS effects. Use together cautiously.
Drug-lifestyle. *Alcohol use:* May enhance CNS effects. Discourage use together.

EFFECTS ON LAB TEST RESULTS
None reported.

CONTRAINDICATIONS & CAUTIONS
• Contraindicated in patients hypersensitive to drug or its components.

---

❸ *Alert:* Drug may cause new-onset seizures and status epilepticus in patients without a history of epilepsy. In these patients, stop drug and evaluate for underlying seizure disorder. Drug shouldn't be used for off-label uses.

● Use cautiously in patients with psychiatric symptoms.

● Use cautiously in breast-feeding women.

⚠ *Overdose S&S:* Somnolence, impaired consciousness, agitation, confusion, speech difficulty, hostility, depression, weakness, myoclonus, seizures, coma, ataxia, drowsiness, tremors, disorientation, vomiting, temporary paralysis, respiratory depression.

NURSING CONSIDERATIONS

❸ *Alert:* Closely monitor all patients taking or starting antiepileptic drugs for changes in behavior indicating worsening of suicidal thoughts or behavior or depression. Symptoms such as anxiety, agitation, hostility, mania, and hypomania may be precursors to emerging suicidality.

● Withdraw drug gradually unless safety concerns require a more rapid withdrawal because sudden withdrawal may cause more frequent seizures.

❸ *Alert:* Use of anticonvulsants, including tiagabine, may cause status epilepticus and sudden unexpected death in patients with epilepsy.

● Patients who aren't receiving at least one enzyme-inducing anticonvulsant when starting tiagabine may need lower doses or slower dosage adjustment.

● Monitor patient for cognitive and neuropsychiatric symptoms, including impaired concentration, speech or language problems, confusion, somnolence, and fatigue.

● Drug may cause moderately severe to incapacitating generalized weakness, which resolves after dosage is reduced or drug stopped.

● *Look alike–sound alike:* Don't confuse tiagabine with tizanidine; both have 4-mg starting doses.

PATIENT TEACHING

● Advise patient to take drug only as prescribed.

● Tell patient to take drug with food.

● Warn patient that drug may cause dizziness, somnolence, and other signs and symptoms of CNS depression. Advise patient to avoid driving and other potentially hazardous activities that require mental alertness until drug's CNS effects are known.

● Tell woman of childbearing age to call prescriber if she becomes pregnant or plans to become pregnant during therapy.

● Instruct woman of childbearing age to notify prescriber if she's planning to breast-feed because drug may appear in breast milk.

SAFETY ALERT!

ticagrelor
TYE-ka-GREL-or

Brilinta

Therapeutic class: Antiplatelet drugs
Pharmacologic class: P2Y$_{12}$ platelet inhibitors
Pregnancy risk category: C

AVAILABLE FORMS
Tablets: 90 mg

INDICATIONS & DOSAGES
➤ **Acute coronary syndrome (ACS)**
Adults: Initially, 180 mg P.O. as a loading dose; then a maintenance dose of 90 mg P.O. b.i.d.

ADMINISTRATION
P.O.
● Give drug without regard to food.
● Store at room temperature in the original container. Keep away from moisture and humidity.

ACTION
Inhibits platelet aggregation by reversibly interacting with the P2Y$_{12}$ adenosine diphosphate receptor.

Route	Onset	Peak	Duration
P.O.	Rapid	2 hr	8 hr

Half-life: 9 hours (active metabolite).

T

ADVERSE REACTIONS

CNS: headache, dizziness, fatigue, syncope, loss of consciousness.
CV: *bleeding,* atrial fibrillation, hypertension, hypotension, chest pain, bradyarrhythmias.
GI: nausea, diarrhea.
Musculoskeletal: back pain, noncardiac chest pain.
Respiratory: cough.

INTERACTIONS

Drug-drug. *Anticoagulants, fibrinolytics, long-term NSAIDs:* May increase risk of bleeding. Use cautiously together.
■ Black Box Warning ■ *Aspirin:* Maintenance doses of aspirin greater than 100 mg/day may decrease ticagrelor effectiveness and increase risk of bleeding. Maintenance doses of aspirin shouldn't exceed 100 mg/day. ■
CYP3A inducers (carbamazepine, dexamethasone, phenobarbital, phenytoin, rifampin): May significantly decrease ticagrelor level and therapeutic effect. Avoid use together.
CYP3A strong inhibitors (atazanavir, clarithromycin, indinavir, itraconazole, ketoconazole, nefazodone, nelfinavir, saquinavir, telithromycin, voriconazole): May significantly increase ticagrelor level and risk of adverse reactions. Avoid use together.
Digoxin: May increase digoxin level. Monitor digoxin level at start of treatment and with any changes to treatment.
Statins: May increase levels of these drugs. Don't exceed 40 mg of simvastatin or lovastatin with concurrent ticagrelor use.

EFFECTS ON LAB TEST RESULTS

● May increase uric acid and creatinine levels.

CONTRAINDICATIONS & CAUTIONS

■ Black Box Warning ■ Drug can cause serious, sometimes fatal bleeding. ■
■ Black Box Warning ■ Contraindicated in patients with history of intracranial hemorrhage or active pathologic bleeding (including peptic ulcer) because of risk of bleeding. ■
■ Black Box Warning ■ Maintenance doses of aspirin greater than 100 mg/day reduce tica-

grelor effectiveness and should be avoided. After an initial dose, give aspirin 75 to 100 mg/day. ■
■ Black Box Warning ■ Don't start ticagrelor in patients who will undergo planned urgent CABG. If possible, discontinue ticagrelor at least 5 days before any surgery. ■
● Contraindicated in patients hypersensitive to drug, in those with severe hepatic impairment, and in breast-feeding women.
● Use cautiously in patients with moderate hepatic failure, elderly patients, patients with history of a bleeding disorder, and patients who have had percutaneous invasive procedures.
● Use during pregnancy only if benefits to the mother outweigh risks to the fetus.

NURSING CONSIDERATIONS

■ Black Box Warning ■ Suspect bleeding in patients presenting with hypotension after recently undergoing coronary angiography, percutaneous coronary intervention, CABG, or other surgery while taking ticagrelor. ■
■ Black Box Warning ■ If possible, manage bleeding without discontinuing ticagrelor; premature discontinuation of treatment increases risk of MI, stent thrombosis, or death. If drug must be temporarily stopped, restart as soon as possible. ■
● Monitor patient for bleeding.
● Monitor patient for dyspnea and rule out underlying conditions that require treatment in patients with new, prolonged, or worsened difficulty breathing. Dyspnea secondary to ticagrelor therapy is usually mild to moderate, and often self-limiting with continued treatment.
● Ticagrelor can be given to patients with ACS who have already been given a loading dose of clopidogrel.

PATIENT TEACHING

■ Black Box Warning ■ Tell patient not to take more than 100 mg of aspirin per day. Warn that other OTC products may also contain aspirin. ■
● Inform patient that bleeding or bruising may occur more easily and it will take longer for the bleeding to stop. Tell patient to immediately report unexpected, prolonged, or excessive bleeding, or blood in the urine or stool.

Reactions in bold italics are *life-threatening*. Interactions may have a *rapid onset* or a *delayed onset*.

- Warn patient not to stop drug without consulting prescriber.
- Instruct patient that, before any scheduled surgery or dental appointment, he should notify all health care providers that he is taking ticagrelor. Advise patient to discuss with his original prescriber any recommendations by other providers to stop taking ticagrelor.
- Tell patient that ticagrelor may cause mild to moderate shortness of breath and to report unexpected shortness of breath, especially if it's severe.
- Advise patient that if a dose is missed to take the next dose at its scheduled time and not to take extra medication to make up for the missed dose.
- Tell female patient who is pregnant or planning to become pregnant to consult her primary health care provider before using this medication.
- Warn women taking this medication not to breast-feed.

ticarcillin disodium–clavulanate potassium
tie-kar-SIL-in and KLAV-yoo-lan-nayt

Timentin

Therapeutic class: Antibiotics
Pharmacologic class: Extended-spectrum penicillins–beta-lactamase inhibitors
Pregnancy risk category: B

AVAILABLE FORMS
Injection: 3 g ticarcillin and 100 mg clavulanic acid in 3.1-g vials
Premixed: 3.1 g/100 mL

INDICATIONS & DOSAGES
Adjust-a-dose (for all indications): If CrCl is 30 to 60 mL/minute, dosage is 2 g I.V. every 4 hours; if CrCl is 10 to 29 mL/minute, 2 g I.V. every 8 hours; if CrCl is less than 10 mL/minute, 2 g I.V. every 12 hours; if CrCl is less than 10 mL/minute and patient has hepatic dysfunction, 2 g I.V. every 24 hours. For patients receiving peritoneal dialysis or hemodialysis, give a loading dose of 3.1 g I.V. and then maintenance doses of 3.1 g I.V. every 12 hours for

patients receiving peritoneal dialysis or 2 g I.V. every 12 hours for patients receiving hemodialysis. Supplement with 3.1 g after each hemodialysis session.
➤ **Gynecologic infection**
Women weighing 60 kg (132 lb) or more: For moderate infections, 200 mg/kg (ticarcillin component) I.V. daily in divided doses every 6 hours. For severe infections, 300 mg/kg (ticarcillin component) I.V. daily in divided doses every 4 hours.
Women weighing less than 60 kg: 200 to 300 mg/kg (ticarcillin component) I.V. daily in divided doses every 4 to 6 hours.
➤ **Lower respiratory tract, urinary tract, bone and joint, intra-abdominal, or skin and skin-structure infection and septicemia caused by beta-lactamase–producing strains of bacteria or by ticarcillin-susceptible organisms**
Adults and children weighing more than 60 kg: 3.1 g (Timentin) by I.V. infusion every 4 to 6 hours.
Adults and children ages 3 months to 16 years weighing less than 60 kg: 200 mg/kg (ticarcillin component) I.V. daily in divided doses every 6 hours. For severe infections, 300 mg/kg (ticarcillin component) I.V. daily in divided doses every 4 hours.

ADMINISTRATION
I.V.
▼ Before giving, ask patient about allergic reactions to penicillin.
▼ Obtain specimen for culture and sensitivity tests. Begin therapy while awaiting results.
▼ Give drug at least 1 hour before a bacteriostatic antibiotic.
▼ Reconstitute drug with 13 mL of sterile water for injection or normal saline solution for injection. Further dilute to a maximum of 10 to 100 mg/mL (based on drug component).
▼ Infuse over 30 minutes.
▼ **Incompatibilities:** Aminoglycosides, amphotericin B, azithromycin, cisatracurium, other anti-infectives, sodium bicarbonate, topotecan, vancomycin.

T

ACTION
Inhibits cell-wall synthesis during bacterial multiplication.

Route	Onset	Peak	Duration
I.V.	Immediate	Immediate	Unknown

Half-life: 1 hour.

ADVERSE REACTIONS
CNS: *seizures,* headache, giddiness, neuromuscular excitability.
CV: phlebitis, vein irritation.
EENT: taste and smell disturbances.
GI: *pseudomembranous colitis,* diarrhea, flatulence, epigastric pain, nausea, stomatitis, vomiting.
Hematologic: *leukopenia, neutropenia, thrombocytopenia,* anemia, eosinophilia, hemolytic anemia.
Metabolic: hypernatremia, hypokalemia.
Skin: *Stevens-Johnson syndrome,* injection-site pain, pruritus, rash.
Other: *anaphylaxis,* hypersensitivity reactions, overgrowth of nonsusceptible organisms.

INTERACTIONS
Drug-drug. *Hormonal contraceptives:* May decrease contraceptive effectiveness. Advise use of another form of contraception during therapy.
Methotrexate: May increase risk of methotrexate toxicity. Monitor methotrexate concentrations twice a week for first 2 weeks.
Oral anticoagulants: May increase risk of bleeding. Monitor PT and INR.
Probenecid: May increase ticarcillin level. Probenecid may be used for this purpose.

EFFECTS ON LAB TEST RESULTS
• May increase ALT, AST, alkaline phosphatase, LDH, serum creatinine, BUN, and sodium levels. May decrease potassium and hemoglobin levels.
• May increase eosinophil count. May decrease platelet, WBC, and granulocyte counts.
• May alter results of turbidimetric tests that use sulfosalicylic acid, trichloroacetic acid, acetic acid, or nitric acid.
• May cause false-positive results on Coombs test.

CONTRAINDICATIONS & CAUTIONS
• Contraindicated in patients hypersensitive to drug or other penicillins.
• Use cautiously in patients with other drug allergies, especially to cephalosporins, because of possible cross-sensitivity and in those with impaired renal function, hemorrhagic conditions, hypokalemia, or sodium restriction. Drug contains 4.5 mEq sodium/g.
⚠ *Overdose S&S:* Neuromuscular hyperexcitability, seizures.

NURSING CONSIDERATIONS
• Check CBC and platelet counts frequently. Drug may cause thrombocytopenia.
• Monitor PT and INR in patients taking oral anticoagulants.
• Monitor potassium and sodium levels.
• If large doses are given or if therapy is prolonged, bacterial or fungal superinfection may occur, especially in elderly, debilitated, or immunosuppressed patients.

PATIENT TEACHING
• Tell patient to report adverse reactions promptly.
• Instruct patient to report discomfort at I.V. site.
• Advise patient, especially one requiring restricted salt intake, to limit salt intake during drug therapy because of drug's high sodium content.

ticlopidine hydrochloride
tye-KLOH-pih-deen

Therapeutic class: Antiplatelet drugs
Pharmacologic class: Platelet aggregation inhibitors
Pregnancy risk category: B

AVAILABLE FORMS
Tablets: 250 mg

INDICATIONS & DOSAGES
Adjust-a-dose (for all indications): For patients with renal impairment, it may be necessary to reduce dosage or discontinue drug if hemorrhage or hematopoietic problems occur.

➤ **To reduce risk of thrombotic stroke in patients who have had a stroke or stroke precursors**
Adults: 250 mg P.O. b.i.d. with meals.
➤ **Adjunct to aspirin to prevent subacute stent thrombosis in patients having coronary stent placement**
Adults: 250 mg P.O. b.i.d., combined with antiplatelet doses of aspirin. Start therapy after stent placement and continue for up to 30 days. If prescribed longer than 30 days, use is off-label.

ADMINISTRATION
P.O.
● Give drug with meals.

ACTION
Unknown. An antiplatelet that probably blocks adenosine diphosphate–induced platelet-to-fibrinogen and platelet-to-platelet binding.

Route	Onset	Peak	Duration
P.O.	Unknown	2 hr	Unknown

Half-life: About 12½ hours after single dose; 4 to 5 days after multiple doses.

ADVERSE REACTIONS
CNS: *intracranial bleeding,* dizziness, peripheral neuropathy.
GI: diarrhea, abdominal pain, anorexia, bleeding, dyspepsia, flatulence, nausea, vomiting.
GU: dark urine, hematuria.
Hematologic: *agranulocytosis, aplastic anemia, immune thrombocytopenia, neutropenia, pancytopenia.*
Skin: *thrombocytopenic purpura,* ecchymoses, pruritus, rash, urticaria.
Other: hypersensitivity reactions, postoperative bleeding.

INTERACTIONS
Drug-drug. *Antacids:* May decrease ticlopidine level. Separate doses by at least 2 hours.
Anticoagulants (enoxaparin, fondaparinux, heparin, warfarin), fibrinolytics (alteplase, drotrecogin alfa): May increase bleeding risk. Discontinue anticoagulants and fibrinolytics before starting ticlopidine.

Aspirin, NSAIDs: May increase effect of aspirin on platelets. Use together cautiously.
Cimetidine: May decrease clearance of ticlopidine and increase risk of toxicity. Avoid using together.
Digoxin: May decrease digoxin level. Monitor digoxin level.
Fosphenytoin, phenytoin: May increase phenytoin and fosphenytoin levels. Monitor patient closely.
Theophylline: May decrease theophylline clearance and risk of toxicity. Monitor patient closely and adjust theophylline dosage.
Drug-herb. *Garlic:* May increase anticoagulation. Use together cautiously.
Ginkgo biloba: May cause additive antiplatelet effects. Use caution when administering together.
Red clover: May cause bleeding. Discourage use together.

EFFECTS ON LAB TEST RESULTS
● May increase ALT, AST, alkaline phosphatase, cholesterol, and triglyceride levels.
● May decrease neutrophil, WBC, RBC, platelet, and granulocyte counts.

CONTRAINDICATIONS & CAUTIONS
● Contraindicated in patients hypersensitive to drug and in those with severe hepatic impairment, hematopoietic disorders, active pathologic bleeding from peptic ulceration, or active intracranial bleeding.
● Use cautiously and with close monitoring of CBC and WBC differentials, watching for signs and symptoms of neutropenia and agranulocytosis.
⚠ *Overdose S&S:* Increased bleeding time, increased ALT level.

NURSING CONSIDERATIONS
● Because of life-threatening adverse reactions, use drug only in patients who are allergic to, can't tolerate, or have failed aspirin therapy.
● Obtain baseline LFT results before therapy.
Black Box Warning Ticlopidine can cause life-threatening hematologic adverse reactions, including neutropenia/agranulocytosis, thrombotic thrombocytopenic purpura

T

(TTP), and aplastic anemia. Severe hematologic adverse reactions may occur within a few days of the start of therapy. During first 3 months of treatment, monitor patient for symptoms of neutropenia or TTP; discontinue drug immediately if they occur. ∎

• Determine CBC and WBC differentials prior to initiating therapy and repeat every 2 weeks until end of third month.

• Monitor LFT results and repeat if dysfunction is suspected.

• Thrombocytopenia has occurred rarely. Stop drug in patients with platelet count of 80,000/mm³ or less. If needed, give methylprednisolone 20 mg I.V. to normalize bleeding time within 2 hours.

• When used preoperatively, drug may decrease risk of graft occlusion in patients receiving CABG and reduce severity of drop in platelet count in patients receiving extracorporeal hemoperfusion during open-heart surgery.

PATIENT TEACHING

• Tell patient to take drug with meals.

• Warn patient to avoid aspirin and aspirin-containing products unless directed to by prescriber and to check with prescriber or pharmacist before taking OTC drugs.

• Explain that drug will prolong bleeding time and that patient should report unusual or prolonged bleeding. Advise patient to tell dentists and other health care providers that he takes ticlopidine.

• Stress importance of regular blood tests. Because neutropenia can result with increased risk of infection, tell patient to immediately report signs and symptoms of infection, such as fever, chills, or sore throat.

• If drug is being substituted for a fibrinolytic or anticoagulant, tell patient to stop those drugs before starting ticlopidine therapy.

• Advise patient to stop drug 10 to 14 days before undergoing elective surgery.

• Tell patient to immediately report to prescriber yellow skin or sclera, severe or persistent diarrhea, rashes, bleeding under the skin, light-colored stools, or dark urine.

tigecycline
tye-gah-SYE-klin

Tygacil

Therapeutic class: Antibiotics
Pharmacologic class: Glycylcycline antibacterials
Pregnancy risk category: D

AVAILABLE FORMS
Lyophilized powder: 50-mg vial

INDICATIONS & DOSAGES
Adjust-a-dose (for all indications): For patients with severe hepatic impairment, give initial dose of 100 mg I.V. and then 25 mg I.V. every 12 hours.

➤ **Community-acquired bacterial pneumonia**
Adults: Initially, 100 mg I.V.; then 50 mg I.V. every 12 hours for 7 to 14 days. Infuse drug over 30 to 60 minutes.

➤ **Complicated skin or skin-structure infection; complicated intra-abdominal infection**
Adults: Initially 100 mg I.V.; then 50 mg every 12 hours for 5 to 14 days. Infuse drug over 30 to 60 minutes.

ADMINISTRATION
I.V.

▼ Assess patient for tetracycline allergy before therapy.

▼ Obtain specimen for culture and sensitivity tests before first dose. Begin therapy while awaiting results.

▼ Reconstitute powder with 5.3 mL of normal saline solution or D₅W to yield 10 mg/mL. Gently swirl the vial until the powder dissolves.

▼ Immediately withdraw the dose from the vial and add it to 100 mL of normal saline solution or D₅W. The maximum concentration is 1 mg/mL.

▼ Inspect the solution for particulates and discoloration (green or black) before giving. Reconstituted solution should be yellow or orange.

▼ Immediately dilute reconstituted drug.

▼ Use a dedicated I.V. line or a Y-site, and flush the line with normal saline solution or D₅W before and after infusion.

▼ Infuse the drug over 30 to 60 minutes.

▼ Store unopened vials at room temperature in the original package. Store diluted solution at room temperature for up to 24 hours–6 hours in the vial and the remaining time in the I.V. bag; or, up to 48 hours in the I.V. bag if refrigerated.

▼ **Incompatibilities:** Amphotericin B, amphotericin B lipid complex, diazepam, esomeprazole, omeprazole.

ACTION
Inhibits protein translation in bacteria by binding to the 30S ribosomal unit.

Route	Onset	Peak	Duration
I.V.	Unknown	Unknown	Unknown

Half-life: 27 to 42 hours.

ADVERSE REACTIONS
CNS: asthenia, dizziness, fever, headache, insomnia, pain.
CV: phlebitis.
GI: diarrhea, nausea, vomiting, abdominal pain, constipation, dyspepsia, acute pancreatitis, *Clostridium difficile*–related colitis, hepatic cholestasis, jaundice.
Hematologic: *thrombocytopenia,* anemia, leukocytosis.
Metabolic: hyperglycemia, hypokalemia, hypoproteinemia.
Musculoskeletal: back pain.
Respiratory: cough, dyspnea.
Skin: local reaction, pruritus, rash, sweating.
Other: *sepsis,* abnormal healing, abscess, allergic reaction, infection.

INTERACTIONS
Drug-drug. *Hormonal contraceptives:* May decrease contraceptive's effectiveness. Advise patient to use nonhormonal form of contraception during treatment.
Warfarin: May increase risk of bleeding. Monitor INR.

EFFECTS ON LAB TEST RESULTS
● May increase alkaline phosphatase, amylase, bilirubin, BUN, creatinine, LDH, and AST and ALT levels.

● May decrease potassium, protein, calcium, sodium, and hemoglobin levels and hematocrit. May increase or decrease glucose levels.

● May increase WBC count and INR. May prolong activated PTT and PT. May decrease platelet count.

CONTRAINDICATIONS & CAUTIONS
● Contraindicated in patients hypersensitive to drug.

Black Box Warning Compared to other drugs used to treat serious infections, tigecycline has an increased mortality risk. Consider using an alternative drug when possible. ■

● Drug isn't indicated to treat diabetic foot infections, hospital-acquired pneumonia, or ventilator-assisted pneumonia.

● Use cautiously in patients with severe hepatic impairment and in those hypersensitive to tetracycline antibiotics. Also use cautiously as monotherapy in patients with complicated intra-abdominal infections caused by intestinal perforation.

● Use cautiously in breast-feeding women. Use during pregnancy only if potential benefit justifies potential risk to fetus.

⚠ *Overdose S&S:* Nausea, vomiting.

NURSING CONSIDERATIONS
● If patient develops diarrhea, monitor him closely for *C. difficile*–related colitis.

● If patient has abdominal infection caused by intestinal perforation, monitor for sepsis.

● Monitor LFTs.

● Monitor patient for symptoms of dangerous toxicities of tetracyclines, such as photosensitivity, pseudotumor cerebri, pancreatitis, and antianabolic action (increased BUN level, azotemia, acidosis, and hypophosphatemia).

PATIENT TEACHING
● Tell patient that drug is used to treat only bacterial infections, not viral.

● Tell patient to report burning or pain at the I.V. site.

● Tell woman of childbearing age to avoid becoming pregnant during treatment. Urge those who use hormonal contraception to also use an alternative contraceptive method during treatment.

T

• Advise woman to notify her health care provider if pregnancy is suspected or confirmed.

timolol maleate
tye-MOE-lol

Betimol, Istalol, Timoptic, Timoptic in Ocudose, Timoptic-XE

Therapeutic class: Antiglaucoma drugs
Pharmacologic class: Nonselective beta blockers
Pregnancy risk category: C

AVAILABLE FORMS
Ophthalmic gel-forming solution: 0.25%, 0.5%
Ophthalmic solution: 0.25%, 0.5%
Ophthalmic solution (preservative-free): 0.25%, 0.5%

INDICATIONS & DOSAGES
➤ **To reduce intraocular pressure (IOP) in ocular hypertension or open-angle glaucoma**
Adults: Initially, 1 drop of 0.25% solution in each affected eye b.i.d.; maintenance dosage is 1 drop once daily. If no response, instill 1 drop of 0.5% solution in each affected eye b.i.d. If IOP is controlled, reduce dosage to 1 drop daily. Or, 1 drop of gel-forming solution (0.25% or 0.5%) in each affected eye once daily. Or, for Istalol, initially 1 drop 0.5% solution in each affected eye once daily in the morning. If response is unsatisfactory, concomitant therapy may be considered.

ADMINISTRATION
Ophthalmic
• Don't touch tip of dropper to eye or surrounding tissue.
• Apply light finger pressure on lacrimal sac for 1 minute after instilling drug to minimize systemic absorption.
• Invert closed container of gel-forming solution and shake once before each use.
• Give other ophthalmic drugs at least 10 minutes before giving gel form of drug.

ACTION
Thought to reduce formation, and possibly increase outflow, of aqueous humor.

Route	Onset	Peak	Duration
Ophthalmic	30 min	1–2 hr	12–24 hr

Half-life: Unknown.

ADVERSE REACTIONS
CNS: syncope, confusion, depression, dizziness, fatigue, hallucinations, lethargy, headache.
CV: hypotension, *arrhythmia, bradycardia, cardiac arrest, heart block, heart failure,* worsening of angina, palpitations, slight reduction in resting heart rate, hypertension.
EENT: burning and stinging, blepharitis, conjunctivitis, decreased corneal sensitivity with long-term use, diplopia, keratitis, minor eye irritation, ptosis, visual disturbances, discharge, tearing, ocular pain, itching.
Metabolic: hyperglycemia, hyperuricemia.
Respiratory: *bronchospasm in patients with history of asthma,* dyspnea, respiratory infection.

INTERACTIONS
Drug-drug. *Calcium channel blockers, cardiac glycosides, quinidine:* May increase risk of adverse cardiac effects if large amounts of timolol are systemically absorbed. Use together cautiously.
Epinephrine: May cause a hypertensive episode, followed by bradycardia. Stop beta blocker 3 days before starting epinephrine. Monitor patient closely.
Insulin, oral antidiabetic agents: May mask symptoms of hypoglycemia (such as tachycardia) as a result of beta blockade. Use together cautiously in patients with diabetes.
Oral beta blockers: May increase ocular and systemic effects. Use together cautiously.
Prazosin: May increase risk of orthostatic hypotension in early phases of use together. Assist patient to stand slowly until effects are known.
Reserpine, other catecholamine-depleting drugs: May increase hypotensive and bradycardia-induced effects. Avoid using together.

Reactions in bold italics are *life-threatening*. Interactions may have a *rapid onset* or a *delayed onset*.

Theophylline: May act antagonistically, reducing effects of one or both drugs; may also reduce elimination of theophylline. Monitor theophylline level and patient closely.
Verapamil: May increase effects of both drugs. Monitor cardiac function closely and decrease dosages as necessary.

EFFECTS ON LAB TEST RESULTS
● May increase BUN, potassium, glucose, and uric acid levels.

CONTRAINDICATIONS & CAUTIONS
● Contraindicated in patients hypersensitive to drug and in those with bronchial asthma, sinus bradycardia, second- or third-degree AV block, cardiac failure, cardiogenic shock, or history of bronchial asthma or severe COPD.
● Use cautiously in patients with nonallergic bronchospasm, chronic bronchitis, emphysema, diabetes mellitus, hyperthyroidism, or cerebrovascular insufficiency.
⚠ *Overdose S&S:* Bradycardia, bronchospasm, dizziness, headache, shortness of breath, cardiac arrest.

NURSING CONSIDERATIONS
● Monitor diabetic patients carefully. Systemic beta-blocking effects can mask some signs and symptoms of hypoglycemia.
● Some patients may need a few weeks of treatment to stabilize pressure-lowering response. Determine IOP after 4 weeks of treatment.
● Drug can be used safely in patients with glaucoma who wear conventional polymethylmethacrylate (PMMA) hard contact lenses.
● *Look alike–sound alike:* Don't confuse timolol with atenolol. Don't confuse Timoptic with Viroptic.

PATIENT TEACHING
● Teach patient how to instill drops. Advise him to wash hands before and after instillation and to apply light finger pressure on lacrimal sac for 1 minute after drops are instilled. Warn patient not to touch tip of dropper to eye or surrounding tissue.
● Instruct patient using gel-forming solution to invert container and shake once before each use. Also tell him to use other

ophthalmic drugs at least 10 minutes before applying gel.
● Tell patient to instill drug without contact lenses in place. Lenses may be reinserted about 15 minutes after drug use.
● Drug may be absorbed systemically and produce signs and symptoms of beta blockade. Advise patient to monitor pulse rate and report slow rate to prescriber.
● Tell patient to report difficulty breathing or chest pain to prescriber.

SAFETY ALERT!

tinidazole
teh-NID-ah-zol

Tindamax

Therapeutic class: Antiprotozoals
Pharmacologic class: Antiprotozoals
Pregnancy risk category: C

AVAILABLE FORMS
Tablets: 250 mg, 500 mg

INDICATIONS & DOSAGES
Black Box Warning Use tinidazole only for the conditions for which it's indicated. ▐
Adjust-a-dose (for all indications): For patients receiving hemodialysis, give an additional dose equal to one-half the recommended dose after the hemodialysis session.
➤ **Bacterial vaginosis in nonpregnant adult women**
Adults: 2 g once daily for 2 days with food, or 1 g once daily for 5 days with food.
➤ **Trichomoniasis caused by *Trichomonas vaginalis***
Adults: 2 g P.O. as a single dose taken with food. Sexual partners should be treated at the same time with the same dose.
➤ **Giardiasis caused by *Giardia lamblia* (*G. duodenalis*)**
Adults: 2 g P.O. as a single dose taken with food.
Children age 3 and older: Give 50 mg/kg (up to 2 g) as a single dose taken with food.
➤ **Intestinal amebiasis caused by *Entamoeba histolytica***
Adults: 2 g P.O. daily for 3 days, taken with food.

T

Children age 3 and older: Give 50 mg/kg (up to 2 g) P.O. daily for 3 days, taken with food.

➤ **Amebic liver abscess (amebiasis)**
Adults: 2 g P.O. daily for 3 to 5 days, taken with food.
Children age 3 and older: Give 50 mg/kg (up to 2 g) P.O. daily for 3 to 5 days, taken with food.

ADMINISTRATION
P.O.
• Give drug with food to minimize adverse GI effects.
• For children who can't swallow pills, crush tablet into fine powder and mix with artificial cherry syrup. Suspension is stable at room temperature for 7 days. Shake well before administration.

ACTION
For *Trichomonas,* cell extracts of *Trichomonas* reduce the compound's nitro group into a free nitro radical that may be responsible for the antiprotozoal activity. Mechanism of action against *Giardia* and *Entamoeba* is unknown.

Route	Onset	Peak	Duration
P.O.	Unknown	1½ hr	Unknown

Half-life: 12 to 14 hours.

ADVERSE REACTIONS
CNS: *seizures,* dizziness, fatigue, headache, malaise, weakness.
GI: anorexia, constipation, cramps, dyspepsia, metallic taste, nausea, vomiting.

INTERACTIONS
Drug-drug. *Cyclosporine, tacrolimus:* May increase cyclosporine or tacrolimus level. Monitor closely for toxicity, including headache, nausea, vomiting, nephrotoxicity, and electrolyte abnormalities.
Disulfiram: May cause psychotic reactions and may increase abdominal cramping, nausea, vomiting, headaches, and flushing. Separate doses by 2 weeks.
Drugs that induce CYP450, such as fosphenytoin, phenobarbital, phenytoin, and rifampin: May increase tinidazole elimination. Monitor patient.

Drugs that inhibit CYP450, such as cimetidine and ketoconazole: May prolong tinidazole half-life and decrease clearance. Monitor patient.
5-FU: May decrease 5-FU clearance, increasing adverse effects without added benefit. Monitor patient for rash, nausea, vomiting, stomatitis, and leukopenia.
Fosphenytoin, phenytoin: May prolong phenytoin half-life and decrease clearance of I.V. drug. Monitor patient for toxicity.
Lithium: May increase lithium level. Monitor patient; monitor lithium and creatinine levels.
Warfarin and other oral anticoagulants: May increase anticoagulant effect. Anticoagulant dosage may need adjustment during and for up to 8 days after tinidazole therapy.
Drug-herb. *St. John's wort:* May increase or decrease drug level. Discourage use together.
Drug-lifestyle. *Use of alcohol and alcohol-containing products:* May increase abdominal cramps, nausea, vomiting, headaches, and flushing. Avoid using together and for 3 days after stopping drug.

EFFECTS ON LAB TEST RESULTS
• May increase AST, ALT, glucose, LDH, and triglyceride levels.
• May decrease WBC count.

CONTRAINDICATIONS & CAUTIONS
• Contraindicated in patients hypersensitive to drug, its component, or other nitroimidazole derivatives.
• Contraindicated in pregnant women during first trimester and in breast-feeding women until 3 days after last dose.
• Use cautiously in patients with CNS disorders, the elderly, and in those with blood dyscrasias or hepatic dysfunction.

NURSING CONSIDERATIONS
• If therapy exceeds 3 days, monitor children closely.
• Patient should take drug with food to minimize adverse GI effects.
❸ **Alert:** If abnormal neurologic signs, such as seizures or paresthesia of the arms or legs, occur, stop drug immediately.
• If candidiasis develops during therapy, the patient may need an antifungal.

Reactions in bold italics are *life-threatening*. Interactions may have a *rapid onset* or a *delayed onset*.

• Women shouldn't breast-feed during therapy and for 3 days after the last dose.
• An elderly patient may have decreased liver or kidney function or other medical conditions and may be taking other drugs that may affect dosage.

PATIENT TEACHING
• Tell patient to take drug with food.
• **Alert:** Tell patient to report to prescriber seizures and numbness in arms or legs.
• Warn patient not to drink alcohol or use alcohol-containing products while taking drug and for 3 days afterward.
• Advise woman to immediately notify her prescriber if she becomes pregnant.
• Tell woman to stop breast-feeding during therapy and for 3 days after the last dose.
• If patient is being treated for a sexually transmitted infection, explain that his sexual partners should be treated at the same time.

tiotropium bromide
tye-oh-TROH-pee-um

Spiriva

Therapeutic class: Bronchodilators
Pharmacologic class: Anticholinergics
Pregnancy risk category: C

AVAILABLE FORMS
Capsules (for inhalation): 18 mcg

INDICATIONS & DOSAGES
➤ **To reduce COPD exacerbations**
Adults: 2 oral inhalations of 1 capsule (18 mcg) once daily using HandiHaler inhalation device.
➤ **Maintenance treatment of bronchospasm in COPD, including chronic bronchitis and emphysema**
Adults: 2 oral inhalations of 1 capsule (18 mcg) once daily using the HandiHaler inhalation device.

ADMINISTRATION
Inhalational
• Give capsules only by oral inhalation with the HandiHaler device.

• Open capsule blister immediately before use.
• Capsules aren't for oral ingestion.

ACTION
Competitive, reversible inhibition of muscarinic receptors leads to bronchodilation.

Route	Onset	Peak	Duration
Inhalation	30 min	3 hr	>24 hr

Half-life: 5 to 6 days.

ADVERSE REACTIONS
CNS: depression, paresthesia.
CV: *angina pectoris,* chest pain, edema.
EENT: sinusitis, cataract, dysphonia, epistaxis, glaucoma, laryngitis, pharyngitis, rhinitis.
GI: dry mouth, abdominal pain, constipation, dyspepsia, gastroesophageal reflux, stomatitis, vomiting.
GU: UTI.
Metabolic: hypercholesterolemia, hyperglycemia.
Musculoskeletal: arthritis, leg pain, myalgia, skeletal pain.
Respiratory: upper respiratory tract infection, cough.
Skin: rash.
Other: accidental injury, allergic reaction, candidiasis, flulike syndrome, herpes zoster, infections.

INTERACTIONS
Drug-drug. *Anticholinergics:* May increase the risk of adverse reactions. Avoid using together.

EFFECTS ON LAB TEST RESULTS
• May increase cholesterol and glucose levels.

CONTRAINDICATIONS & CAUTIONS
• Contraindicated in patients hypersensitive to atropine, its derivatives, ipratropium, or any component of the product.
• Use cautiously in women who are pregnant or breast-feeding, patients with CrCl of 50 mL/minute or less, or patients with angle-closure glaucoma, prostatic hyperplasia, or bladder neck obstruction.

T

• Use cautiously in patients with severe hypersensitivity to milk protein.
⚠ **Overdose S&S:** Change in mental status, tremors, abdominal pain, severe constipation.

NURSING CONSIDERATIONS
🌓 **Alert:** Use drug for maintenance treatment of COPD, not for acute bronchospasm.
• Watch for evidence of hypersensitivity (especially angioedema) and paradoxical bronchospasm.
• **Look alike–sound alike:** Don't confuse Spiriva with Inspra.

PATIENT TEACHING
• Inform patient that drug is for maintenance treatment of COPD and not for immediate relief of breathing problems.
🌓 **Alert:** Explain that capsules are for inhalation and shouldn't be swallowed.
• Provide full instructions for the Handi-Haler device.
• Tell patient not to get powder in his eyes.
• Review signs and symptoms of hypersensitivity (especially angioedema) and paradoxical bronchospasm. Tell patient to stop the drug and contact the prescriber if they occur.
• Advise patient to report eye pain, blurred vision, visual halos, colored images, or red eyes immediately.
• Tell patient to keep capsules in sealed blisters and to remove each capsule just before use. Caution against storing capsules in the HandiHaler device.
• Instruct patient to store capsules at 77° F (25° C) and not to expose them to extreme temperatures or moisture.

tipranavir
tih-PRAN-uh-veer

Aptivus

Therapeutic class: Antiretrovirals
Pharmacologic class: Protease inhibitors
Pregnancy risk category: C

AVAILABLE FORMS
Capsules (for inhalation): 250 mg
Oral solution: 100 mg/mL

INDICATIONS & DOSAGES
➤ **HIV-1 in patients with viral replication who are highly treatment-experienced or have HIV-1 strains resistant to multiple protease inhibitors**
Adults: 500 mg P.O. b.i.d. with 200 mg of ritonavir b.i.d. Give with or without food.
Children ages 2 to 18: 14 mg/kg with ritonavir 6 mg/kg (or tipranavir 375 mg/m^2 with ritonavir 150 mg/m^2) b.i.d., not to exceed dosage of tipranavir 500 mg with ritonavir 200 mg b.i.d. For children who develop intolerance or toxicity, prescribers may consider decreasing dosage to tipranavir 12 mg/kg with ritonavir 5 mg/kg b.i.d. provided the virus isn't resistant to multiple protease inhibitors.

ADMINISTRATION
P.O.
• Give with 200 mg ritonavir and other antiretrovirals.
• Give drug with or without food.
• Do not freeze or refrigerate oral solution.
• Use within 60 days of opening capsule or oral solution bottle.

ACTION
Inhibits virus-specific processing of polyproteins in HIV-1 infected cells, preventing formation of mature virions.

Route	Onset	Peak	Duration
P.O.	Unknown	3 hr	Unknown

Half-life: 5 to 6 hours.

ADVERSE REACTIONS
CNS: dizziness, fatigue, headache, insomnia, malaise, peripheral neuropathy, pyrexia, sleep disorder, somnolence.
GI: diarrhea, *pancreatitis,* abdominal distention, abdominal pain, dyspepsia, flatulence, GERD, nausea, vomiting.
GU: renal insufficiency.
Hematologic: *neutropenia, thrombocytopenia,* anemia.
Hepatic: *hepatic failure, hepatitis.*
Metabolic: anorexia, decreased appetite, dehydration, diabetes mellitus, facial wasting, hyperglycemia, hyperlipidemia, hypertriglyceridemia, weight loss.
Musculoskeletal: muscle cramps, myalgia.
Respiratory: cough, dyspnea.

Skin: rash, acquired lipodystrophy, exanthem, lipoatrophy, lipohypertrophy, pruritus.
Other: flulike illness, hypersensitivity, reactivation of herpes simplex and varicella zoster.

INTERACTIONS

Drug-drug. *Amiodarone, bepridil, flecainide, propafenone, quinidine:* May increase levels of these drugs and risk of life-threatening arrhythmias. Avoid using together.

◑ Alert: *Atorvastatin:* May increase levels of both drugs and risk of myopathy and rhabdomyolysis. Avoid use together.

Clarithromycin: May increase levels of both drugs. If CrCl is 30 to 60 mL/minute, decrease clarithromycin dose by 50%. If CrCl is less than 30 mL/minute, decrease clarithromycin dose by 75%.

Colchicine: May increase risk of life-threatening and fatal colchicine toxicity. In patients with healthy renal and hepatic function, reduce colchicine dosage to no more than 0.3 mg b.i.d.; monitor patient carefully for colchicine-related adverse effects. Avoid coadministration in patients with hepatic or renal impairment.

Cyclosporine, sirolimus, tacrolimus: May cause unpredictable interaction. Monitor drug levels closely until they've stabilized.

Desipramine: May increase desipramine level. Decrease dose and monitor desipramine level.

Didanosine: May decrease didanosine level. Separate dosing by at least 2 hours.

Diltiazem, felodipine, nicardipine, nisoldipine, verapamil: May cause unpredictable interaction. Use together cautiously, and monitor patient closely.

Disulfiram, metronidazole: May cause disulfiram-like reaction. Use together cautiously.

Ergot derivatives (dihydroergotamine, ergonovine, ergotamine, methylergonovine): May cause acute ergot toxicity, including peripheral vasospasm and ischemia of extremities. Avoid using together.

Estrogen-based hormone therapy: May decrease estrogen level, and rash may occur. Monitor patient carefully. Advise using nonhormonal contraception.

Fluoxetine, paroxetine, sertraline: May increase levels of these drugs. Adjust dosages as needed.

Glimepiride, glipizide, glyburide, pioglitazone, repaglinide, tolbutamide: May affect glucose levels. Monitor glucose level carefully.

◑ Alert: *Lovastatin, simvastatin:* May increase risk of myopathy and rhabdomyolysis. Use together is contraindicated.

Meperidine: May increase normeperidine metabolite. Avoid using together.

Methadone: May decrease methadone level by 50%. Consider increased methadone dose.

Midazolam, triazolam: May cause prolonged or increased sedation or respiratory depression. Don't use together.

Pimozide: May cause life-threatening arrhythmias. Avoid using together.

Rifabutin: May increase rifabutin level. Decrease rifabutin dose by 75%.

Rifampin: May lead to loss of virologic response and resistance to tipranavir and other protease inhibitors. Avoid using together.

Sildenafil, tadalafil, vardenafil: May increase levels of these drugs. Use together cautiously. Tell patient not to exceed 25 mg sildenafil in 48 hours, 10 mg tadalafil every 72 hours, or 2.5 mg vardenafil every 72 hours.

Valproic acid: May reduce valproic acid plasma level. Use with caution.

Warfarin: May cause unpredictable reaction. Check INR often.

Drug-herb. *St. John's wort:* May lead to loss of virologic response and resistance to this drug and other antiretrovirals. Warn patient to avoid using together.

EFFECTS ON LAB TEST RESULTS

• May increase total cholesterol, triglyceride, blood glucose, amylase, lipase, ALT, and AST levels.
• May decrease WBC count.

CONTRAINDICATIONS & CAUTIONS

Black Box Warning Administration of tipranavir with ritonavir 200 mg has been associated with fatal and nonfatal intracranial hemorrhage, clinical hepatitis, and hepatic decompensation. ■

T

• Contraindicated in patients hypersensitive to any ingredients of the product, patients with moderate (Child-Pugh class B) and severe (Child-Pugh class C) hepatic insufficiency, and patients taking drugs that depend on CYP3A for clearance, such as amiodarone, bepridil, ergot derivatives (dihydroergotamine, ergonovine, ergotamine, methylergonovine), flecainide, midazolam, pimozide, propafenone, quinidine, and triazolam.

• Use cautiously in patients with sulfonamide allergy, diabetes, liver disease, hepatitis B or C, or hemophilia A or B.

NURSING CONSIDERATIONS

🔂 **Alert:** Don't give drug to treatment-naive patients.

• To be effective, drug must be given with 200 mg ritonavir and with other antiretrovirals.

🔂 **Alert:** Monitor patient for signs and symptoms of intracranial hemorrhage, including headache, nausea and vomiting, change in mental status, speech or balance difficulties, and seizures.

🔂 **Alert:** Obtain thorough patient drug history. Many drugs may interact with tipranavir.

• Monitor LFTs at start of treatment and often during treatment.

• Assess for evidence of hepatitis, such as fatigue, malaise, anorexia, nausea, jaundice, bilirubinemia, acholic stools, liver tenderness, and hepatomegaly.

• If patient develops signs or symptoms of hepatitis, notify prescriber.

Black Box Warning Patients with chronic hepatitis B or C are at increased risk of hepatotoxicity. ∎

• In diabetic patients, monitor glucose level closely; hyperglycemia may occur.

• Obtain baseline cholesterol and triglyceride levels at start of and periodically during therapy.

• Monitor patient for cushingoid symptoms, such as central obesity, buffalo hump, peripheral wasting, facial wasting. and breast enlargement.

• Use cautiously in elderly patients because they are more likely to have decreased organ function, multidrug therapy, and other illnesses.

PATIENT TEACHING

• Explain that drug doesn't cure HIV infection and doesn't reduce the risk of transmitting the virus to others.

🔂 **Alert:** Many drugs may interfere with this drug. Urge patient to report his use of all prescription drugs, OTC drugs, and herbal products.

• Tell patient that drug is effective only when taken with ritonavir and other antiretrovirals.

• Urge patient to stop drug and contact prescriber if he has evidence of hepatitis, such as fatigue, malaise, anorexia, nausea, jaundice, bilirubinemia, acholic stools, or liver tenderness.

• If female patient uses hormonal contraceptives, advise use of barrier contraception.

• Tell patient that redistribution or accumulation of body fat may occur.

• Advise female patient that breast-feeding isn't recommended during therapy.

SAFETY ALERT!

tirofiban hydrochloride

tye-row-FYE-ban

Aggrastat

Therapeutic class: Antiplatelet drugs
Pharmacologic class: Glycoprotein IIb/IIIa receptor antagonists
Pregnancy risk category: B

AVAILABLE FORMS

Injection (premixed bag): 50 mcg/mL in 100 mL or 250 mL

INDICATIONS & DOSAGES

➤ **Acute coronary syndrome, with heparin or aspirin, including patients who are to be managed medically and those undergoing percutaneous transluminal coronary angioplasty (PTCA) or atherectomy**
Adults: I.V. loading dose of 0.4 mcg/kg/minute for 30 minutes; then continuous I.V. infusion of 0.1 mcg/kg/minute. Continue infusion through angiography and for 12 to 24 hours after PTCA or atherectomy.
Adjust-a-dose: If CrCl is less than 30 mL/minute, use a loading dose of 0.2 mcg/kg/

minute for 30 minutes; then continuous infusion of 0.05 mcg/kg/minute. Continue infusion through angiography and for 12 to 24 hours after PTCA or atherectomy.

ADMINISTRATION

I.V.

▼ Inspect solution for particulate matter before giving, and check for leaks by squeezing the inner bag firmly. If bag leaks or particles are visible, discard solution.

▼ Avoid use of noncompressible sites (such as subclavian or jugular veins).

▼ Heparin and tirofiban may be given through the same I.V. catheter. Tirofiban may be given through the same I.V. line as dopamine, lidocaine, potassium chloride, and famotidine.

▼ Discard unused solution 24 hours after the start of infusion.

▼ Store drug at room temperature. Protect from light.

▼ **Incompatibilities:** Diazepam.

ACTION

Reversibly binds to the glycoprotein IIb/IIIa (gpIIb/IIIa) receptor on human platelets and inhibits platelet aggregation.

Route	Onset	Peak	Duration
I.V.	Immediate	Immediate	4–6 hr

Half-life: About 2 hours.

ADVERSE REACTIONS

CNS: dizziness, fever, headache.
CV: *bradycardia, coronary artery dissection,* edema, vasovagal reaction.
GI: occult bleeding, nausea.
Hematologic: bleeding, *thrombocytopenia.*
Musculoskeletal: leg pain.
Skin: sweating.
Other: bleeding at arterial access site, pelvic pain.

INTERACTIONS

Drug-drug. *Anticoagulants such as warfarin, aspirin, clopidogrel, dipyridamole, heparin, NSAIDs, thrombolytics, ticlopidine:* May increase risk of bleeding. Monitor patient closely.
Levothyroxine, omeprazole: May increase tirofiban renal clearance. Monitor patient.

EFFECTS ON LAB TEST RESULTS

● May decrease hemoglobin level and hematocrit.
● May decrease platelet count.

CONTRAINDICATIONS & CAUTIONS

● Contraindicated in patients hypersensitive to drug or its components.

● Contraindicated in those with active internal bleeding or history of bleeding diathesis within the previous 30 days and in those with history of intracranial hemorrhage, intracranial neoplasm, arteriovenous malformation, aneurysm, thrombocytopenia after previous exposure to drug, stroke within 30 days, or hemorrhagic stroke.

● Contraindicated in those with history, symptoms, or findings suggestive of aortic dissection; severe hypertension (systolic blood pressure higher than 180 mm Hg or diastolic blood pressure higher than 110 mm Hg); acute pericarditis; major surgical procedure or severe physical trauma within previous month; or concomitant use of another parenteral gpIIb/IIIa inhibitor.

● Use cautiously in patients with renal impairment and those with increased risk of bleeding, including patients with hemorrhagic retinopathy or platelet count less than $150,000/mm^3$.

● Safety and effectiveness of drug haven't been studied in patients younger than age 18.

⚠ *Overdose S&S:* Bleeding.

NURSING CONSIDERATIONS

● Monitor hemoglobin level, hematocrit, and platelet count before starting therapy, 6 hours after loading dose, and at least daily during therapy. If thrombocytopenia occurs, notify prescriber.

● Monitor aPTT before treatment and 6 hours after the start of heparin infusion.

● Give drug with aspirin and heparin.

● Monitor patient for bleeding.

⚠ *Alert:* The most common adverse effect is bleeding at the arterial access site for cardiac catheterization.

● The risk of bleeding may decrease with early sheath removal and by keeping the access site immobile. The sheath may be removed during infusion, but only after heparin has been stopped and its effects

largely reversed. Sheath hemostasis should be achieved at least 4 hours before hospital discharge.
● Minimize use of arterial and venous punctures, I.M. injections, urinary catheters, and nasotracheal and nasogastric tubes.
● Elderly patients have a higher risk of bleeding complications.
● *Look alike–sound alike:* Don't confuse Aggrastat with argatroban.

PATIENT TEACHING
● Explain that drug is a blood thinner used to prevent chest pain and heart attack.
● Explain that the benefits of the drug far outweigh the risk of serious bleeding.
● Instruct patient to report chest discomfort or other adverse effects immediately.
● Tell patient that frequent blood sampling may be needed to evaluate therapy.

tizanidine hydrochloride
tis-AN-i-deen

Zanaflex

Therapeutic class: Skeletal muscle relaxants
Pharmacologic class: Centrally acting alpha₂-adrenergic agonists
Pregnancy risk category: C

AVAILABLE FORMS
Capsules: 2 mg, 4 mg, 6 mg
Tablets: 2 mg, 4 mg

INDICATIONS & DOSAGES
Adjust-a-dose (for all indications): For patients with renal insufficiency (CrCl less than 25 mL/minute), reduce dosage. If higher dosages are needed, increase individual doses rather than frequency.
➤ **Acute and intermittent management of increased muscle tone with spasticity**
Adults: Initially, 4 mg P.O. every 6 to 8 hours, as needed, to maximum of three doses in 24 hours. Dosage can be increased gradually in 2- to 4-mg increments, reaching optimum dose over 2 to 4 weeks. Maximum, 36 mg daily.
➤ **Cerebral palsy spasticity** ◆
Children: 0.05 mg/kg P.O. daily.

ADMINISTRATION
P.O.
● Give drug consistently with or without food for same absorption rate and effect.

ACTION
Unknown. Acts as an alpha₂ agonist. May reduce spasticity by increasing presynaptic inhibition of motor neurons at the level of the spinal cord.

Route	Onset	Peak	Duration
P.O.	Unknown	1–2 hr	3–6 hr

Half-life: 2½ hours; metabolites, 20 to 40 hours.

ADVERSE REACTIONS
CNS: somnolence, sedation, asthenia, dizziness, speech disorder, dyskinesia, nervousness, hallucinations.
CV: hypotension, *bradycardia.*
EENT: amblyopia, pharyngitis, rhinitis.
GI: dry mouth, constipation, vomiting.
GU: UTI, urinary frequency.
Hepatic: hepatic injury.
Other: infection, flulike syndrome.

INTERACTIONS
Drug-drug. *Acetaminophen:* May delay acetaminophen absorption time. Monitor patient for clinical effect.
Antihypertensives, other alpha agonists (such as clonidine): May cause hypotension; monitor patient closely. Avoid using together.
Baclofen, benzodiazepines, other CNS depressants: May have additive CNS depressant effects. Avoid using together.
CYP1A2 inhibitors (amiodarone, acyclovir, cimetidine, ciprofloxacin, famotidine, fluoroquinolones, fluvoxamine, mexiletine, propafenone, ticlodipine, verapamil, zileuton): May cause significant increases in tizanidine levels. Use together should be avoided; use of ciprofloxacin or fluvoxamine with tizanidine is contraindicated.
Oral contraceptives: May decrease tizanidine clearance. Reduce tizanidine dosage.
Drug-lifestyle. *Alcohol use:* May increase CNS depression. Discourage use together.

EFFECTS ON LAB TEST RESULTS
● May increase AST and ALT levels.

Reactions in bold italics are *life-threatening*. Interactions may have a *rapid onset* or a *delayed onset*.

CONTRAINDICATIONS & CAUTIONS
• Contraindicated in patients hypersensitive to drug.
• Use of potent CYP1A2 inhibitors ciprofloxacin and fluvoxamine with tizanidine is contraindicated.
• Use cautiously in patients who are taking antihypertensives, in those with renal and hepatic impairment, in pregnant or breast-feeding women, and in elderly patients.
• Safety and effectiveness in children haven't been established.
⚠ Overdose S&S: Lethargy, somnolence, confusion, coma, bradycardia, hypotension, respiratory depression, depressed cardiac function.

NURSING CONSIDERATIONS
🔵 **Alert:** The capsules and tablets are bioequivalent only if taken on an empty stomach.
• Obtain LFT results before treatment; during treatment at 1, 3, and 6 months; and then periodically thereafter.
• May prolong QT interval and cause bradycardia and hypotension. Closely monitor vital signs, especially in patients receiving maximum recommended dosage and those taking other drugs that prolong QT interval.
🔵 **Alert:** Stop drug gradually, especially in patients taking high doses for a prolonged period. Decrease dose slowly to minimize the potential for rebound hypertension, tachycardia, and hypertonia.
• **Look alike–sound alike:** Don't confuse tizanidine with tiagabine; both have 4-mg starting doses.

PATIENT TEACHING
• Caution patient to avoid alcohol and activities that require alertness. Drug may cause drowsiness.
• Inform patient that dizziness upon standing quickly can be minimized by rising slowly and avoiding sudden position changes.
• Advise patient that tizanidine absorption varies depending on whether drug is taken with or without food and that it should always be taken the same way to reduce risk of changes in efficacy and adverse reactions.

• Instruct patient to inform the health care provider and pharmacist when any medication is added or removed from his regimen.
• Advise patient not to suddenly stop taking medication.

tobramycin
toe-bra-MYE-sin

Aktob, Tobrex

Therapeutic class: Antibiotics
Pharmacologic class: Aminoglycosides
Pregnancy risk category: B

AVAILABLE FORMS
Ophthalmic ointment: 0.3%
Ophthalmic solution: 0.3%

INDICATIONS & DOSAGES
➤ **External ocular infections by susceptible bacteria**
Adults and children age 2 months and older: In mild to moderate infections, instill 1 or 2 drops into affected eye every 4 hours, or apply 1-cm strip of ointment every 8 to 12 hours. In severe infections, instill 2 drops into infected eye every 60 minutes until condition improves; then reduce frequency. Or, apply 1-cm strip of ointment every 3 to 4 hours until condition improves; then reduce frequency to b.i.d. to t.i.d.

ADMINISTRATION
Ophthalmic
• When two different ophthalmic solutions are used, allow at least 10 minutes between instillations.
• Apply light finger pressure on lacrimal sac for 1 minute after drops are instilled.
• Apply ointment to conjunctiva. Don't let tube touch eye.

ACTION
Thought to inhibit protein synthesis; usually bactericidal.

Route	Onset	Peak	Duration
Ophthalmic	Unknown	Unknown	Unknown

Half-life: 2 to 3 hours.

T

ADVERSE REACTIONS
EENT: blurred vision (with ointment), burning or stinging on instillation, conjunctival erythema, increased lacrimation, lid itching or swelling.

INTERACTIONS
None significant.

EFFECTS ON LAB TEST RESULTS
None reported.

CONTRAINDICATIONS & CAUTIONS
• Contraindicated in patients hypersensitive to drug or other aminoglycosides.
△ **Overdose S&S:** Punctate keratitis, erythema, tearing, edema, lid itching.

NURSING CONSIDERATIONS
❸ **Alert:** Tobramycin ophthalmic solution isn't for injection.
• If topical ocular tobramycin is given with systemic tobramycin, carefully monitor levels.
• Prolonged use may result in overgrowth of nonsusceptible organisms, including fungi.
• **Look alike–sound alike:** Don't confuse tobramycin with Trobicin. Don't confuse Tobrex with TobraDex.

PATIENT TEACHING
• Tell patient to clean excessive discharge from eye area before application.
• Tell patient to remove contact lenses before using drug and not to wear contact lenses when signs or symptoms of ocular infection are present.
• Teach patient how to instill drops or apply ointment. Advise him to wash hands before and after applying and to avoid touching tip of dropper to eye or surrounding tissue.
• Instruct patient to apply light finger pressure on lacrimal sac for 1 minute after drops are instilled.
• Tell patient to wait at least 10 minutes before instilling other eyedrops.
• Advise patient to watch for itching lids, swelling, or constant burning. Tell him to stop drug and notify prescriber if these signs and symptoms develop.
• Tell patient not to share drug, washcloths, or towels with family members and to notify prescriber if anyone develops same signs or symptoms.
• Stress importance of compliance with recommended therapy.

tobramycin sulfate
toe-bra-MYE-sin

TOBI, TOBI Podhaler

Therapeutic class: Antibiotics
Pharmacologic class: Aminoglycosides
Pregnancy risk category: D

AVAILABLE FORMS
Capsules (for inhalation): 28 mg
Multidose vials (pediatric): 10 mg/mL, 40 mg/mL
Nebulizer solution (for inhalation): 300 mg/5 mL
Prefilled syringe (pediatric): 40 mg/mL
Premixed parenteral injection for infusion: 60 mg or 80 mg in normal saline solution

INDICATIONS & DOSAGES
➤ **Serious infection by sensitive strains of** *Escherichia coli, Proteus, Klebsiella, Enterobacter, Serratia, Morganella morganii, Staphylococcus aureus, Citrobacter, Pseudomonas,* **or** *Providencia*
Adults: 3 mg/kg/day I.M. or I.V. in divided doses. For life-threatening infections, give up to 5 mg/kg/day in divided doses every 6 to 8 hours; reduce to 3 mg/kg daily as soon as clinically indicated.
Children older than age 1 week: 6 to 7.5 mg/kg/day I.M. or I.V., in three or four divided doses.
Neonates younger than age 1 week or preterm infants: Up to 4 mg/kg/day I.V. or I.M. in two equal doses every 12 hours.
Adjust-a-dose: For patients with renal impairment, give loading dose of 1 mg/kg; then give decreased doses at 8-hour intervals or same dose at prolonged intervals. For hemodialysis patients, give 50% of the normal dose after dialysis and adjust according to serum concentrations. For patients with severe cystic fibrosis, initial dose is 10 mg/kg/day I.V. or I.M., in four divided doses.

➤ **To manage cystic fibrosis patients with**
Pseudomonas aeruginosa **infection**
Adults and children age 6 and older:
300 mg via nebulizer every 12 hours for
28 days. Continue cycle of 28 days on drug
and 28 days off. Or, using TOBI Podhaler
device, have patient inhale contents of four
28-mg capsules every 12 hours for 28 days,
stop therapy for 28 days, then repeat and
continue cycles of 28 days on drug and
28 days off.

➤ **Infective endocarditis caused by**
P. aeruginosa ◆
Adults: 8 mg/kg I.V. or I.M. once daily, with
maintenance peak concentrations of 15 to
20 mcg/mL and trough concentrations no
greater than 2 mcg/mL, in combination with
an extended-spectrum penicillin (such as
ticarcillin or piperacillin) or ceftazidime
or cefepime in full doses for a minimum of
6 weeks.

ADMINISTRATION

I.V.
▼ Obtain specimen for culture and sensitivity tests before giving. Begin therapy while
awaiting results.
▼ For adults, dilute in 50 to 100 mL of
normal saline solution or D_5W; use a
smaller volume for children.
▼ Keep reconstituted solution in refrigerator and use within 96 hours.
▼ Infuse over 20 to 60 minutes.
▼ After infusion, flush line with normal
saline solution or D_5W.
▼ Obtain blood for peak level 30 minutes
after infusion stops; draw blood for trough
level just before next dose. Don't collect
blood in a heparinized tube because of
incompatibility.
▼ **Incompatibilities:** Allopurinol;
amphotericin B; azithromycin; beta-
lactam antibiotics; cefepime; clindamycin;
dextrose 5% in Isolyte E, M, or P; heparin
sodium; hetastarch; indomethacin; propofol; sargramostim; solutions containing
alcohol.

I.M.
● Obtain specimen for culture and sensitivity tests before giving. Begin therapy while
awaiting results.

● Obtain blood for peak level 1 hour after
I.M. injection; draw blood for trough level
just before next dose. Don't collect blood
in a heparinized tube because of incompatibility.

Inhalational
● Obtain specimen for culture and sensitivity tests before giving. Begin therapy while
awaiting results.
● Give nebulizer solution over 10 to 15 minutes using handheld Pari LC Plus reusable
nebulizer with DeVilbiss Pulmo-Aide compressor.
● Capsules aren't for oral ingestion.
● Give capsules only by oral inhalation
using Podhaler device.
● Store capsules in blister packs at room
temperature and remove immediately before
use.
● Give doses as close to 12 hours apart as
possible. Doses shouldn't be taken less than
6 hours apart.

ACTION
Generally bactericidal. Inhibits protein
synthesis by binding directly to the 30S
ribosomal subunit.

Route	Onset	Peak	Duration
I.V.	Immediate	30 min	8 hr
I.M.	Unknown	30–60 min	8 hr
Inhalation	Unknown	Unknown	Unknown

Half-life: 2 to 3 hours.

ADVERSE REACTIONS
CNS: *seizures,* headache, lethargy, confu-
sion, disorientation, fever.
EENT: ototoxicity, hoarseness, pharyngitis.
GI: vomiting, nausea, diarrhea.
GU: *nephrotoxicity,* possible increase in
urinary excretion of casts.
Hematologic: anemia, eosinophilia,
leukopenia, thrombocytopenia, agranu-
locytosis.
Metabolic: electrolyte imbalances.
Musculoskeletal: muscle twitching.
Respiratory: *bronchospasm.*
Skin: rash, urticaria, pruritus.

T

INTERACTIONS
Drug-drug. `Black Box Warning`
Acyclovir, amphotericin B, cephalosporins, cidofovir, cisplatin, methoxyflurane, vancomycin, other aminoglycosides: May increase nephrotoxicity. Monitor renal function. ∎

Atracurium, pancuronium, rocuronium, vecuronium: May increase effects of non-depolarizing muscle relaxants, including prolonged respiratory depression. Use together only when necessary, and expect to reduce dosage of nondepolarizing muscle relaxant.

Dimenhydrinate: May mask symptoms of ototoxicity. Monitor patient's hearing.

General anesthetics: May increase neuromuscular blockade. Monitor patient for increased clinical effects.

`Black Box Warning` *I.V. loop diuretics such as furosemide:* May increase ototoxicity. Monitor patient's hearing. ∎

Parenteral penicillins: May inactivate tobramycin in vitro. Don't mix together.

EFFECTS ON LAB TEST RESULTS
● May increase AST, ALT, LDH, bilirubin, BUN, creatinine, nonprotein nitrogen, and urine urea levels. May decrease calcium, magnesium, and potassium levels.
● May increase eosinophil count. May decrease WBC and platelet counts.

CONTRAINDICATIONS & CAUTIONS
● Contraindicated in patients hypersensitive to drug or other aminoglycosides.
● Use cautiously in patients with impaired renal function or neuromuscular disorders and in elderly patients.

⚠ **Overdose S&S:** Nephrotoxicity, dizziness, tinnitus, vertigo, loss of high-tone hearing acuity, neuromuscular blockade, respiratory failure, respiratory paralysis.

NURSING CONSIDERATIONS
● Weigh patient and review renal function studies before therapy.
◑ **Alert:** Evaluate patient's hearing before and during therapy. If patient complains of tinnitus, vertigo, or hearing loss, notify prescriber.
● Don't dilute or mix with dornase alfa in a nebulizer.

● Unrefrigerated drug, which is normally slightly yellow, may darken with age. This doesn't affect product quality.
● Avoid exposing ampules to intense light.
`Black Box Warning` Peak levels over 12 mcg/mL and trough levels over 2 mcg/mL may increase the risk of toxicity. Reserve higher peak levels for cystic fibrosis patients, who need a greater lung penetration. ∎
`Black Box Warning` Due to increased risk of nephrotoxicity, monitor renal function: urine output, specific gravity, urinalysis, CrCl, and BUN and creatinine levels. Notify prescriber about signs and symptoms of decreasing renal function. ∎
`Black Box Warning` Aminoglycosides can cause fetal harm when administered to pregnant women. ∎
● Watch for signs and symptoms of superinfection, such as continued fever, chills, and increased pulse rate.
● If no response occurs in 3 to 5 days, therapy may be stopped and new specimens obtained for culture and sensitivity testing.
● *Look alike–sound alike:* Don't confuse tobramycin with Trobicin.

PATIENT TEACHING
◑ **Alert:** Explain that capsules are for inhalation only and shouldn't be swallowed.
● Provide full instructions for the Podhaler device and tell patient to always use the new Podhaler device provided with each weekly pack.
● Advise patient not to get powder in eyes.
● Tell patient to keep capsules in sealed blisters and to remove each capsule immediately before use.
● Instruct patient to store capsules at room temperature.
● Instruct patient to report adverse reactions promptly.
● Caution patient not to perform hazardous activities if adverse CNS reactions occur.
● Encourage patient to maintain adequate fluid intake.
● Teach patient how to use and maintain nebulizer.
● Tell patient using several inhaled therapies to use this drug last.

• Instruct patient not to use if the inhalation solution is cloudy or contains particles or if it has been stored at room temperature for longer than 28 days.

tocilizumab
toe-sih-LIZ-oo-mab

Actemra

Therapeutic class: Antiarthritics
Pharmacologic class: Interleukin-6 receptor inhibitors
Pregnancy risk category: C

AVAILABLE FORMS
Injection: 80 mg/4 mL, 200 mg/10 mL, 400 mg/20 mL in single-use vials

INDICATIONS & DOSAGES
Adjust-a-dose (for all indications): For patients with ANC 500 to 1000 cells/mm^3, interrupt drug until ANC is greater than 1000 cells/mm^3 and then resume drug at 4 mg/kg. May increase to 8 mg/kg if appropriate. If ANC is less than 500 cells/mm^3, discontinue drug. If platelet count is 50,000 to 100,000 cells/mm^3, interrupt drug until platelet count is greater than 100,000 cells/mm^3, and then resume drug at 4 mg/kg. May increase to 8 mg/kg if appropriate. If platelet count is less than 50,000 cells/mm^3, discontinue drug. For patients with liver enzyme levels greater than 1 to 3 times the upper limit of normal (ULN), reduce dosage to 4 mg/kg or interrupt drug until levels normalize. For liver enzyme levels greater than 3 to 5 × ULN, stop drug until levels are less than 3 × ULN and then restart at 4 mg/kg. Discontinue drug for persistent levels greater than 3 × ULN.
➤ **Systemic juvenile idiopathic arthritis (SJIA) alone or in combination with methotrexate**
Children age 2 and older weighing 30 kg (66 lb) or more: 8 mg/kg I.V. infusion over 60 minutes once every 2 weeks.
Children age 2 and older weighing less than 30 kg: 12 mg/kg I.V. infusion over 60 minutes once every 2 weeks.
Adjust-a-dose: If appropriate, concomitant methotrexate or other medications should be

dose-modified or stopped and tocilizumab dosage adjusted until the clinical situation has been evaluated. In SJIA, the decision to discontinue tocilizumab for a laboratory abnormality should be based on medical assessment of the individual patient.
➤ **As monotherapy or with methotrexate or other disease-modifying antirheumatic drugs (DMARDs), for moderately to severely active rheumatoid arthritis when response to one or more DMARDs is inadequate**
Adults: Initially, 4 mg/kg I.V. over 60 minutes every 4 weeks. May increase dosage to 8 mg/kg based on clinical response. Maximum dose is 800 mg per infusion.
✷ *NEW INDICATION:* **Polyarticular juvenile idiopathic arthritis (PJIA) alone or in combination with methotrexate**
Children age 2 and older weighing 30 kg (66 lb) or more: 8 mg/kg I.V. infusion over 60 minutes once every 4 weeks.
Children age 2 and older weighing less than 30 kg: 10 mg/kg I.V. over 60 minutes once every 4 weeks.
Adjust-a-dose: If appropriate, concomitant methotrexate or other medications should be dose-modified or stopped and tocilizumab dosage adjusted until the clinical situation has been evaluated. In PJIA, the decision to discontinue tocilizumab for a laboratory abnormality should be based on medical assessment of the individual patient.

ADMINISTRATION
I.V.
▼ Check body weight before calculating each dose.
▼ Withdraw normal saline solution from 100-mL container in volume equal to drug dose, slowly add drug to infusion bag, then gently invert bag to mix solution. Use a 50-mL infusion bag or bottle for SJIA or PJIA patients who weigh less than 30 kg (66 lb). Allow diluted solution to reach room temperature before infusing.
▼ Don't use solution if it's discolored or contains particulate matter.
▼ Store diluted solution at 36° F to 46° F (2° C to 8° C) or room temperature for up to 24 hours; protect from light.
▼ Administer infusion over 60 minutes; infusion must be administered with

infusion set. Don't administer as I.V. push
or bolus.
▼ **Incompatibilities:** Don't infuse in same
line with other I.V. drugs.

ACTION

Inhibits interleukin-6–mediated inflammatory processes by decreasing inflammatory
markers such as C-reactive protein, rheumatoid factor, and erythrocyte sedimentation
rate.

Route	Onset	Peak	Duration
I.V.	Unknown	Unknown	Unknown

Half-life: 11 to 13 days.

ADVERSE REACTIONS

CNS: dizziness, headache.
CV: hypertension.
EENT: nasopharyngitis.
GI: gastritis, mouth ulceration, upper
abdominal pain.
Hematologic: *thrombocytopenia.*
Respiratory: bronchitis, upper respiratory
tract infection.
Skin: pruritus, rash, urticaria.
Other: *antibody development, malignancy,*
infection.

INTERACTIONS

Drug-drug. *Biological DMARDs (anti-
CD20 monoclonal antibodies, interleukin-1
receptor antagonists, TNF antagonists):*
May increase risk of serious infection. Don't
use together.
Cyclosporine, theophylline, warfarin: May
decrease drug levels. Monitor levels closely
and adjust dosage as needed.
*CYP3A4 substrates (atorvastatin, lova-
statin, omeprazole, simvastatin):* May affect
levels of these drugs. Avoid use together.
Hormonal contraceptives: May decrease
effects of contraceptives. Consider nonhormonal alternatives for contraception.
Live-virus vaccines: No data are available
on secondary transmission of infection from
live-virus vaccine. Avoid using together.

EFFECTS ON LAB TEST RESULTS

• May increase ALT, AST, and lipid levels.
• May decrease platelet and neutrophil
counts.

CONTRAINDICATIONS & CAUTIONS

Black Box Warning Risks and benefits of
treatment with tocilizumab should be carefully considered before start of therapy
in patients with chronic or recurrent
infection. ■
• Don't initiate drug in patients with ANC
less than 2,000/mm^3 or platelet count less
than 100,000/mm^3, or in those with ALT or
AST level more than 1.5 × ULN.
• Contraindicated in patients hypersensitive
to drug or its components. Avoid use in
those with active infection, active hepatic
disease, or hepatic impairment.
• Use cautiously in patients who have been
exposed to tuberculosis (TB), in those with
history of chronic or recurrent infection,
serious or opportunistic infection, or underlying conditions that increase risk of
infection. Use cautiously in those who have
resided or traveled in areas with endemic TB
or mycosis.
• Use cautiously in patients at risk for GI
perforation.
• For patients older than age 65 being
treated with tocilizumab, give drug cautiously because serious infections are more
common in this population.
• Use in pregnancy only if benefit to patient
outweighs risk to fetus. It isn't known if
drug appears in breast milk. Because of risk
of serious adverse reactions, women should
stop drug or stop breast-feeding.

NURSING CONSIDERATIONS

Black Box Warning Sepsis or serious infections, including TB and bacterial, invasive
fungal, viral, and other opportunistic infections, may occur. Monitor patient closely
for signs and symptoms of infection during and after treatment. Drug may need to
be discontinued if infection occurs during
treatment. ■
Black Box Warning Patient should be
evaluated, and treated if necessary, for latent
TB before start of therapy. Monitor patient
for possible TB development during therapy,
even if he tested negative prior to therapy. ■
• Suspect GI perforation in patient with
new-onset abdominal symptoms.
• Monitor LFTs, lipid levels, and neutrophil
and platelet counts every 4 to 8 weeks during therapy.

Reactions in bold italics are *life-threatening*. Interactions may have a *rapid onset* or a *delayed onset*.

• Ensure availability of appropriate support-ive measures to treat possible hypersensitiv-ity reaction.
• Drug may increase risk of malignancy.
• Monitor patient closely for signs and symptoms of demyelinating disorders.
• Recommended immunizations (except live-virus vaccines) should be brought up-to-date before beginning therapy.

PATIENT TEACHING
🔷 *Alert:* Warn patient to seek immediate medical attention if abdominal pain or signs and symptoms of infection occur.
• Instruct patient to have TB screening before therapy.
• Advise woman to consult prescriber if she becomes pregnant or plans to breast-feed.
• Tell patient to avoid exposure to infections.
• Remind patient to contact prescriber before scheduling surgery.
• Advise patient to avoid live-virus vaccines during therapy.
• Recommend that patient use nonhormonal contraception during therapy.

✳ NEW DRUG

tofacitinib
TOE-fa-SYE-ti-nib

Xeljanz

Therapeutic class: Antirheumatics
Pharmacologic class: Janus kinase inhibitors
Pregnancy risk category: C

AVAILABLE FORMS
Tablets: 5 mg

INDICATIONS & DOSAGES
➤ **Moderately to severely active rheuma-toid arthritis in patients who have had an inadequate response or intolerance to methotrexate, as monotherapy or in combination with methotrexate or other nonbiological disease-modifying an-tirheumatic drugs (DMARDs)**
Adults: 5 mg P.O. b.i.d.
Adjust-a-dose: Reduce dosage to 5 mg once daily in patients with moderate or severe renal insufficiency or moderate hepatic impairment, in those receiving concurrent

potent CYP3A4 inhibitors (such as keto-conazole), and in those receiving a drug that moderates inhibition of CYP3A4 and acts as a potent inhibitor of CYP2C19 (such as fluconazole). Interrupt therapy if ANC is 500 to 1,000 cells/mm^3, if hemoglobin level drops more than 2 g/dL, or if hemoglobin level is less than 8 g/dL during therapy. Dis-continue drug based on confirmed lympho-cyte count of less than 500 cells/mm^3 or if confirmed ANC is less than 500 cells/mm^3.

ADMINISTRATION
P.O.
• May give with or without food.
• Store at room temperature.

ACTION
Inhibits activity of Janus kinases, preventing activation of certain intracellular activities that influence immune cell function.

Route	Onset	Peak	Duration
P.O.	Unknown	½–1 hr	Unknown

Half-life: 3 hours.

ADVERSE REACTIONS
CNS: headache, paresthesia, insomnia, fever, fatigue.
CV: hypertension, edema.
EENT: nasopharyngitis.
GI: diarrhea, abdominal pain, dyspepsia, vomiting, gastritis, nausea.
Hematologic: anemia.
Metabolic: dehydration.
Musculoskeletal: muscle and bone pain, arthralgia, tendon disorder, joint swelling.
Respiratory: upper respiratory tract infec-tion, dyspnea, cough.
Skin: rash, erythema, pruritus.
Other: infection.

INTERACTIONS
Drug-drug. **Black Box Warning** *Immuno-suppressants (corticosteroids, methotrexate):* May increase risk of serious infection. If infection occurs, discontinue tofacitinib until infection is controlled. ∎
Moderate inhibitors of CYP3A4 plus potent inhibitors of CYP2C19 (fluconazole), potent inhibitors of CYP3A4 (ketoconazole): May increase tofacitinib plasma level. Decrease tofacitinib dosage to 5 mg daily.

T

Potent immunosuppressants (abatacept, adalimumab, anakinra, azathioprine, certolizumab, cyclosporine, etanercept, golimumab, infliximab, rituximab, tacrolimus, tocilizumab): May significantly increase risk of immunosuppression and infection. Don't use together.

Potent inducers of CYP3A4 (rifampin): May decrease tofacitinib plasma level. Use together cautiously and monitor patient carefully.

EFFECTS ON LAB TEST RESULTS
● May increase creatinine, liver enzyme, and lipid levels.
● May decrease hemoglobin level.
● May increase or decrease lymphocyte count. May decrease neutrophil count.

CONTRAINDICATIONS & CAUTIONS
● Contraindicated in patients hypersensitive to drug or its components and in those with severe hepatic impairment.
● Use cautiously in patients at risk for serious infection (including those who have resided or traveled in areas of endemic tuberculosis [TB] or mycoses), those at risk for GI perforation (history of diverticulitis), and those with known malignancy.

Black Box Warning Serious infections leading to hospitalization or death, including TB and bacterial, invasive fungal, viral, and other opportunistic infections, have occurred in patients receiving tofacitinib, especially patients on concomitant immunosuppressants, such as methotrexate or corticosteroids. Weigh risk before starting therapy in patients with chronic or recurrent infection. If a serious infection develops, interrupt therapy until infection is controlled. ∎

Black Box Warning Lymphoma and other malignancies have been observed in patients treated with tofacitinib. ∎

Black Box Warning Epstein-Barr virus–associated post-transplant lymphoproliferative disorder has been increasingly observed in renal transplant patients treated with tofacitinib and concomitant immunosuppressants. ∎
● Use in pregnant women only if benefits outweigh risk to fetus. Use cautiously in breast-feeding women.

● Patients shouldn't receive live-virus vaccines during therapy.
● Prescribers must fax a copy of the prescription information and XELSOURCE Enrollment Form for each patient who receives tofacitinib to 1-866-297-3471.

NURSING CONSIDERATIONS
Black Box Warning Before therapy, patients should be tested for latent TB. If test is positive, treatment for TB should begin before start of tofacitinib therapy. Monitor all patients for active TB during treatment, even if initial latent TB test is negative. ∎
● Treat patients with latent TB with antimycobacterials before starting tofacitinib. Drug may reactivate viral infection, such as herpes zoster or hepatitis.
● Monitor patient for infection, including TB and viral reactivation. Interrupt treatment if serious infection occurs; don't restart until infection is resolved.
● Monitor lymphocyte count at baseline and every 3 months thereafter.
● Monitor neutrophil count and hemoglobin level at baseline, after 4 to 8 weeks of treatment, and every 3 months thereafter.
● Don't initiate therapy if lymphocyte count is less than 500 cells/mm^3, ANC is less than 1,000 cells/mm^3, or hemoglobin level is less than 9 g/dL.
● Monitor LFT results regularly, especially in patients with history of taking DMARDs such as methotrexate. If drug-induced liver injury is suspected, stop drug until drug cause is ruled out.
● Assess lipid levels 4 to 8 weeks after drug initiation; manage appropriately as needed.
● Monitor patients for GI perforation. Promptly evaluate patients with sudden new-onset abdominal pain or other GI signs and symptoms.

PATIENT TEACHING
● Advise patient to inform prescriber if signs and symptoms of infection, abdominal pain, or illness occurs during therapy.
● Caution patient to obtain laboratory tests (CBC, liver enzymes, lipids) regularly as directed.
● Instruct female patient to contact prescriber if she becomes pregnant or plans to become pregnant.

• Encourage female patient who becomes pregnant to enroll in the pregnancy registry at 1-877-311-8972.
• Warn patient to avoid live-virus vaccines.

tolcapone
toll-KAP-own

Tasmar

Therapeutic class: Antiparkinsonians
Pharmacologic class: Catechol-O-methyltransferase inhibitors
Pregnancy risk category: C

AVAILABLE FORMS
Tablets: 100 mg

INDICATIONS & DOSAGES
➤ **Adjunct to levodopa–carbidopa for signs and symptoms of idiopathic Parkinson disease in patients who have symptom fluctuation or haven't responded to other adjunctive treatment**
Adults: Initially, 100 mg P.O. t.i.d. with levodopa–carbidopa. Recommended daily dosage is 100 mg P.O. t.i.d. Levodopa dosage may need to be reduced by 20% to 30% to minimize risk of dyskinesias. Maximum, 600 mg daily. Stop drug if patient shows no benefit within 3 weeks.

ADMINISTRATION
P.O.
• Give drug without regard for food.
• Give first dose of the day with first daily dose of levodopa–carbidopa.

ACTION
May reversibly inhibit catechol-O-methyltransferase when given with levodopa–carbidopa, increasing levodopa bioavailability. This causes a more constant dopaminergic stimulation in the brain.

Route	Onset	Peak	Duration
P.O.	Unknown	2 hr	Unknown

Half-life: 2 to 3 hours.

ADVERSE REACTIONS
CNS: dyskinesia, sleep disorder, dystonia, excessive dreaming, somnolence, confusion, headache, hallucinations, dizziness, fever, hyperkinesia, hypertonia, fatigue, falling, syncope, balance loss, depression, tremor, speech disorder, paresthesia, agitation, irritability, mental deficiency, hyperactivity, hypokinesia.
CV: orthostatic complaints, chest pain, chest discomfort, palpitations, hypotension.
EENT: pharyngitis, tinnitus, sinus congestion.
GI: nausea, anorexia, diarrhea, vomiting, flatulence, constipation, abdominal pain, dyspepsia, dry mouth.
GU: UTI, urine discoloration, hematuria, micturition disorder, urinary incontinence, impotence.
Hepatic: *hepatotoxicity.*
Musculoskeletal: muscle cramps, stiffness, arthritis, neck pain.
Respiratory: bronchitis, dyspnea, upper respiratory tract infection.
Skin: increased sweating, rash.
Other: influenza, hyperpyrexia.

INTERACTIONS
Drug-drug. *CNS depressants:* May cause additive effects. Monitor patient closely.
Nonselective MAO inhibitors (phenelzine, tranylcypromine): May cause hypertensive crisis. Avoid using together.
SSRIs, TCAs: May increase risk of adverse effects. Use together cautiously.
Warfarin: May cause increased warfarin level. Monitor INR and adjust warfarin dosage as needed.

EFFECTS ON LAB TEST RESULTS
• May increase LFT values.

CONTRAINDICATIONS & CAUTIONS
• Contraindicated in patients hypersensitive to drug or its components and in those with history of drug-related confusion and non-traumatic rhabdomyolysis or hyperpyrexia.
Black Box Warning Tolcapone therapy shouldn't be initiated if patient exhibits clinical evidence of liver disease or two ALT or AST values greater than the upper limit of normal. Drug is contraindicated in those previously withdrawn from drug because of drug-induced hepatocellular injury. ■
Black Box Warning Use cautiously in patients with severe dyskinesia or dystonia. ■

T

• Use cautiously in patients with severe renal impairment and in breast-feeding women.

⚠ **Overdose S&S:** Nausea, vomiting, dizziness.

NURSING CONSIDERATIONS

Black Box Warning Because of risk of hepatotoxicity, stop treatment if patient shows no benefit within 3 weeks. ∎

Black Box Warning Because of fatal hepatic failure risk, use drug only in patients taking levodopa–carbidopa who don't respond to or who aren't appropriate candidates for other adjunctive therapies. If drug is discontinued because of hepatocellular injury, don't reintroduce. ∎

• Make sure patient provides written informed consent before taking drug.

Black Box Warning Monitor LFT results before starting drug, every 2 weeks for the first year of therapy, every 4 weeks for the next 6 months, and then every 8 weeks thereafter. If the dose is increased to 200 mg t.i.d., obtain liver enzyme levels before increasing dose and then resume monitoring as described. Also, discontinue treatment if ALT or AST level exceeds the upper limit of normal or if clinical signs and symptoms suggest the onset of hepatic failure. ∎

• Because drug is highly protein bound, it isn't significantly removed during dialysis.

• Monitor patient for orthostatic hypotension and syncope.

PATIENT TEACHING

• Advise patient to take drug exactly as prescribed.

Black Box Warning Teach patient to immediately report the signs and symptoms of liver injury (yellow eyes or skin, fatigue, loss of appetite, persistent nausea, itching, dark urine, or right upper abdominal tenderness). ∎

• Warn patient about risk of dizziness upon standing up quickly; tell him to stand up cautiously.

• Advise patient to avoid hazardous activities until CNS effects of drug are known.

• Tell patient that nausea may occur early in therapy.

• Inform patient that diarrhea is common, sometimes occurring 2 to 12 weeks after

therapy begins, and usually resolves when therapy stops.

• Advise patient about risk of increased problems making voluntary movements or impaired muscle tone.

• Inform patient that hallucinations may occur.

• Tell women to notify prescriber about planned, suspected, or known pregnancy.

• Inform patient that drug may be taken without regard to meals.

tolterodine tartrate
toll-TEAR-oh-deen

Detrol⃰, Detrol LA

Therapeutic class: Urinary antispasmodics
Pharmacologic class: Antimuscarinics
Pregnancy risk category: C

AVAILABLE FORMS
Capsules (extended-release): 2 mg, 4 mg
Tablets: 1 mg, 2 mg

INDICATIONS & DOSAGES
➤ **Overactive bladder in patients with symptoms of urinary frequency, urgency, or urge incontinence**
Adults: 2-mg tablet P.O. b.i.d. or 4-mg extended-release capsule P.O. daily. Dose may be reduced to 1-mg tablet P.O. b.i.d. or 2-mg extended-release capsule P.O. daily, based on patient response and tolerance.
Adjust-a-dose: For patients with significantly reduced hepatic or renal function (CrCl of 10 to 30 mL/minute) or those taking a potent CYP3A4 inhibitor, give 1-mg tablet P.O. b.i.d. or 2-mg extended-release capsule P.O. daily.

ADMINISTRATION
P.O.
• Give extended-release capsules with liquid because they must be swallowed whole.

ACTION
Relaxes smooth muscle of bladder by antagonizing muscarinic receptors, relieving symptoms of overactive bladder.

Reactions in bold italics are *life-threatening*. Interactions may have a *rapid onset* or a *delayed onset*.

Route	Onset	Peak	Duration
P.O.	Unknown	1–2 hr	Unknown
P.O. (extended-release)	Unknown	2–6 hr	Unknown

Half-life: 2 to 4 hours; about 8 hours with hepatic impairment.

ADVERSE REACTIONS

CNS: headache, fatigue, paresthesia, vertigo, dizziness, nervousness, somnolence.
CV: chest pain.
EENT: abnormal vision, xerophthalmia, pharyngitis, sinusitis.
GI: dry mouth, abdominal pain, constipation, diarrhea, dyspepsia, flatulence, nausea, vomiting.
GU: dysuria, urine retention, UTI.
Metabolic: weight gain.
Musculoskeletal: arthralgia, back pain.
Respiratory: bronchitis, coughing, upper respiratory tract infection.
Skin: dry skin.
Other: flulike syndrome, infection.

INTERACTIONS

Drug-drug. *Anticholinergics (ipratropium, tiotropium):* Coadministration may increase frequency or severity of anticholinergic adverse reactions (such as blurred vision, constipation, dry mouth, or somnolence). Monitor patient closely.
Antifungals (itraconazole, ketoconazole, miconazole), CYP3A4 inhibitors (such as clarithromycin, erythromycin): May increase tolterodine level. Don't give more than 1-mg tablet b.i.d. or 2-mg extended-release capsule daily of tolterodine if used together.
Fluoxetine: May increase tolterodine level. Monitor patient. No dosage adjustment is needed.

EFFECTS ON LAB TEST RESULTS

None reported.

CONTRAINDICATIONS & CAUTIONS

• Contraindicated in patients hypersensitive to drug or its components and in those with uncontrolled angle-closure glaucoma or urine or gastric retention.
• Use cautiously in patients with significant bladder outflow obstruction, GI obstructive disorders (such as pyloric stenosis), con-
trolled angle-closure glaucoma, myasthenia gravis, and hepatic or renal impairment.
⚠ Alert: Anaphylaxis and angioedema requiring hospitalization and emergency medical treatment have occurred with the first or subsequent doses of tolterodine. Discontinue drug and promptly initiate appropriate therapy if difficulty breathing, upper airway obstruction, or fall in blood pressure occurs.
• An additive effect of tolterodine with other drugs that prolong the QT interval cannot be excluded, which increases risk of life-threatening cardiac arrhythmias. Consider this when tolterodine is prescribed to patients with known history of QT-interval prolongation or those who are taking other drugs that prolong the QT interval, such as Class IA (procainamide, quinidine) or Class III (amiodarone, sotalol) antiarrhythmics.
⚠ Overdose S&S: Dry mouth, severe central anticholinergic effects, QT-interval prolongation.

NURSING CONSIDERATIONS

• Assess baseline bladder function and monitor therapeutic effects.
• Monitor patient for residual urine after voiding.

PATIENT TEACHING

• Tell patient that sugarless gum, hard candy, or saliva substitute may help relieve dry mouth.
• Advise patient to avoid driving or other potentially hazardous activities until effects of drug are known.
• Advise women to stop breast-feeding during therapy.
• Instruct patient to immediately report signs of infection, urine retention, GI problems, or difficulty breathing.
• Tell patient taking extended-release form to swallow capsule whole and take with liquids.

T

---

†Canada   ◊OTC   ♦Off-label use   ⌀Photoguide   *Liquid contains alcohol.

tolvaptan
tol-VAP-tan

Samsca

Therapeutic class: Antihypertensives
Pharmacologic class: Selective
vasopressin receptor antagonists
Pregnancy risk category: C

AVAILABLE FORMS
Tablets: 15 mg, 30 mg

INDICATIONS & DOSAGES
➤ **Hypervolemic and euvolemic hyponatremia (serum sodium level less than 125 mEq/L and symptomatic hyponatremia) in hospitalized patients, including those with heart failure, cirrhosis, or SIADH**
Adults: Initially, 15 mg P.O once daily. After 24 hours, may increase to 30 mg P.O. once daily, to maximum dosage of 60 mg P.O. once daily for no more than 30 days.

ADMINISTRATION
P.O.
• Give drug with or without food.
• Avoid restricting fluids during the first 24 hours of therapy.
• Patient should avoid grapefruit and grapefruit juice during therapy.

ACTION
Antagonizes the effect of vasopressin, causing an increase in urine excretion, which results in an increase in free water clearance, a decrease in urine osmolality, and ultimately an increase in serum sodium level.

Route	Onset	Peak	Duration
P.O.	2–4 hr	2–4 hr	Unknown

Half-life: 12 hours.

ADVERSE REACTIONS
CNS: asthenia, fever, *stroke.*
CV: *intracardiac thrombus, PE, ventricular fibrillation.*
EENT: dry mouth, thirst.
GI: anorexia, constipation, nausea.

GU: polyuria, urinary frequency, urethral hemorrhage, vaginal hemorrhage.
Hematologic: *disseminated intravascular coagulation.*
Metabolic: hyperglycemia, *diabetic ketoacidosis.*
Musculoskeletal: *rhabdomyolysis.*
Respiratory: *respiratory failure.*
Other: *DVT.*

INTERACTIONS
Drug-drug. *CYP3A inducers (barbiturates, carbamazepine, phenytoin, rifabutin, rifampin, rifapentin):* May decrease tolvaptan level. Avoid using together.
Moderate CYP3A inhibitors (aprepitant, diltiazem, erythromycin, fluconazole, verapamil): May increase tolvaptan level. Don't use together.
P-glycoprotein inhibitors (such as cyclosporine): May increase tolvaptan levels. Reduce tolvaptan dosage.
P-glycoprotein substrates (digoxin): May increase digoxin level. Monitor the patient, and adjust digoxin dosage as needed.
Drug-herb. *St John's wort:* May decrease drug level. Don't use together.
Drug-food. *Grapefruit juice:* May increase drug level. Don't use together.

EFFECTS ON LAB TEST RESULTS
• May increase glucose level.
• May prolong PT.

CONTRAINDICATIONS & CAUTIONS
• Contraindicated in patients with hypovolemic hyponatremia and in those who require urgent rise in serum sodium level, are anuric, or are unable to sense or appropriately respond to thirst.
• Contraindicated in patients receiving strong CYP3A inhibitors.
• Use cautiously in patients with cirrhosis and dehydration, and in those receiving hypertonic saline solution.
• Use in pregnant women only if benefit to mother outweighs risk to fetus. It isn't known if drug appears in breast milk. Patient shouldn't breast-feed during therapy.
⚠ *Overdose S&S:* Polyuria, thirst, dehydration, hypovolemia.

Reactions in bold italics are *life-threatening*. Interactions may have a *rapid onset* or a *delayed onset*.

NURSING CONSIDERATIONS

Black Box Warning Initiate and reinitiate drug in hospital setting where serum sodium level can be monitored closely. ∎

Black Box Warning Don't correct hyponatremia too rapidly (for example, more than 12 mEq/L/24 hours); doing so may cause osmotic demyelination resulting in dysarthria, mutism, dysphagia, lethargy, affective changes, spastic quadriparesis, seizures, coma, and death. Slower correction may be necessary in patients with severe malnutrition, alcoholism, or advanced liver disease. ∎

🕒 **Alert:** Drug may increase risk of irreversible and potentially fatal liver injury. Assess liver function promptly in patients reporting fatigue, anorexia, right upper abdominal discomfort, dark urine, or jaundice. If liver injury is suspected, stop drug immediately, initiate treatment, and investigate cause. Don't reinitiate drug unless cause for the observed liver injury is definitively established to be unrelated to tolvaptan treatment.

• Monitor sodium level and neurologic status regularly during therapy.

• Monitor potassium level in patients with potassium level greater than 5 mEq/L who are taking drugs known to increase potassium level.

PATIENT TEACHING

• Advise patient to promptly report difficulty speaking or swallowing, drowsiness, mood changes, trouble controlling body movement, seizures, fatigue, anorexia, right upper abdominal discomfort, dark urine, or jaundice.

• Advise patient to inform health care provider if he's taking or plans to take prescription or nonprescription drugs, because of the potential for interactions.

• Advise patient to inform health care provider if he uses strong (clarithromycin, indinavir, itraconazole, ketoconazole, nelfinavir, ritonavir, saquinavir, telithromycin) or moderate (aprepitant, diltiazem, erythromycin, fluconazole, verapamil) CYP3A inhibitors or P-gp inhibitors (cyclosporine).

• Advise patient to continue ingestion of fluid in response to thirst during therapy

and to resume fluid intake after tolvaptan is discontinued.

• Advise female patient not to breast-feed.

• Advise patient to drink when thirsty to prevent dehydration.

• Tell patient not to stop or restart the drug on his own; the drug should only be restarted in the hospital where sodium level can be monitored closely.

topiramate
toe-PIE-rah-mate

Topamax⌀, Trokendi XR

Therapeutic class: Anticonvulsants
Pharmacologic class: Sulfamate-substituted monosaccharides
Pregnancy risk category: D

AVAILABLE FORMS

Capsules, sprinkles: 15 mg, 25 mg
Capsules (extended-release): 25 mg, 50 mg, 100 mg, 200 mg
Tablets: 25 mg, 50 mg, 100 mg, 200 mg

INDICATIONS & DOSAGES

Adjust-a-dose (for all indications): For adults, if CrCl is less than 70 mL/minute, reduce dosage by 50%. For hemodialysis patients, supplemental doses may be needed to avoid rapid drops in drug level during prolonged dialysis treatment.

➤ **Initial monotherapy for partial-onset or primary generalized tonic-clonic seizures**

Adults and children age 10 or older: Recommended daily dose is 400 mg (immediate-release) P.O. in two divided doses (morning and evening). To achieve this dosage, adjust as follows: first week, 25 mg P.O. b.i.d.; second week, 50 mg P.O. b.i.d.; third week, 75 mg P.O. b.i.d.; fourth week, 100 mg P.O. b.i.d.; fifth week, 150 mg P.O. b.i.d.; and sixth week, 200 mg P.O. b.i.d. Or, using extended-release capsules, initially 25 to 50 mg P.O. daily. Increase dosage weekly by increments of 25 to 50 mg.

Children ages 2 to less than 10: During titration period, initial dosage should be 25 mg/day (immediate-release) P.O. administered nightly for the first week. Based

T

on tolerability, can increase dosage to 50 mg/day (25 mg P.O. b.i.d.) in the second week. Can increase dosage by 25 to 50 mg/day each subsequent week as tolerated. Titration to the minimum maintenance dosage should be attempted over 5 to 7 weeks of the total titration period. Based on tolerability and seizure control, additional titration to a higher dosage (up to the maximum maintenance dosage) can be attempted at 25 to 50 mg/day in weekly increments. The total daily dosage shouldn't exceed the maximum maintenance dosage for each range of body weight. Maintenance doses should be given in two equally divided P.O. doses daily. If patient weighs up to 11 kg (24 lb), the maintenance dosage range is 150 mg/day to a maximum of 250 mg/day. If patient weighs 12 to 22 kg (26 to 48 lb), the maintenance dosage range is 200 mg/day to a maximum of 300 mg/day. If patient weighs 23 to 31 kg (51 to 68 lb), the maintenance dosage range is 200 mg/day to a maximum of 350 mg/day. If patient weighs 32 to 38 kg (70 to 84 lb), the maintenance dosage range is 250 mg/day to a maximum of 350 mg/day. If patient weighs more than 38 kg (84 lb), the maintenance dosage range is 250 mg/day to a maximum of 400 mg/day.

➤ **Adjunctive treatment for partial-onset or primary generalized tonic-clonic seizures or Lennox-Gastaut syndrome**
Adults: Initially, 25 to 50 mg P.O. daily; increase gradually by 25 to 50 mg/week until an effective daily dose is reached. Adjust to recommended daily dose of 200 to 400 mg P.O. in two divided doses of immediate-release or once daily of extended-release for adults with partial seizures or 400 mg P.O. in two divided doses of immediate-release or once daily of extended-release for adults with primary generalized tonic-clonic seizures.
Children age 6 and older (extended-release): Initially, 25 mg P.O. daily at bedtime (based on range of 1 to 3 mg/kg once daily) for first week. Increase dosage at 1- or 2-week intervals by increments of 1 to 3 mg/kg once daily. Guide dosage titration by clinical outcome. Recommended daily dose is 5 to 9 mg/kg once daily.

Children ages 2 to 16 (immediate-release): Initially, 1 to 3 mg/kg P.O. daily given at bedtime for 1 week. Increase at 1- or 2-week intervals by 1 to 3 mg/kg daily in two divided doses to achieve optimal response. Recommended daily dose is 5 to 9 mg/kg, in two divided doses.

➤ **To prevent migraine headache**
Adults (immediate-release): Initially, 25 mg P.O. daily in evening for first week. Then, 25 mg P.O. b.i.d. in morning and evening for second week. For third week, 25 mg P.O. in morning and 50 mg P.O. in evening. For fourth week, 50 mg P.O. b.i.d. in morning and evening.

➤ **Bulimia nervosa ◆**
Adults: 25 mg P.O. daily for the first week; then titrate by 25 to 50 mg/week to maximum of 400 mg/day.

ADMINISTRATION
P.O.
● Give drug without regard for food.
● Crushed or broken tablets have a bitter taste.
● Immediate-release capsules may be opened and contents sprinkled on a teaspoon of soft food. Patient should swallow immediately without chewing.
● Patient should swallow extended-release capsules whole and intact. Don't sprinkle capsule contents on food or allow patient to chew or crush capsules.

ACTION
Unknown. May block a sodium channel, potentiate the activity of GABA, and inhibit kainate's ability to activate an amino acid receptor.

Route	Onset	Peak	Duration
P.O.	Unknown	2 hr	Unknown

Half-life: 21 hours.

ADVERSE REACTIONS
CNS: anxiety, asthenia, ataxia, confusion, difficulty with memory, dizziness, fatigue, nervousness, paresthesia, psychomotor slowing, somnolence, speech disorders, tremor, *generalized tonic-clonic seizures, suicide attempts,* abnormal coordination, aggressive reaction, agitation, apathy, depression, depersonalization,

difficulty with concentration, attention, or language, emotional lability, euphoria, fever, hallucination, hyperkinesia, hypertonia, hypoesthesia, hypokinesia, insomnia, malaise, mood problems, personality disorder, psychosis, stupor, vertigo.
CV: chest pain, edema, palpitations, vasodilation.
EENT: abnormal vision, diplopia, nystagmus, conjunctivitis, epistaxis, eye pain, hearing problems, pharyngitis, sinusitis, tinnitus.
GI: anorexia, nausea, abdominal pain, constipation, diarrhea, dry mouth, dyspepsia, flatulence, gastroenteritis, gingivitis, taste perversion, vomiting.
GU: amenorrhea, dysuria, dysmenorrhea, hematuria, impotence, intermenstrual bleeding, leukorrhea, menstrual disorder, menorrhagia, urinary frequency, renal calculi, urinary incontinence, UTI, vaginitis.
Hematologic: *leukopenia,* anemia.
Metabolic: decreased weight, increased weight.
Musculoskeletal: arthralgia, back or leg pain, muscle weakness, myalgia, rigors.
Respiratory: upper respiratory tract infection, bronchitis, coughing, dyspnea.
Skin: acne, alopecia, increased sweating, pruritus, rash.
Other: body odor, breast pain, decreased libido, flulike syndrome, hot flashes, lymphadenopathy.

INTERACTIONS
Drug-drug. *Carbamazepine:* May decrease topiramate level. Monitor patient.
Carbonic anhydrase inhibitors (acetazolamide, dichlorphenamide): May cause renal calculus formation. Avoid using together.
CNS depressants: May cause CNS depression and other adverse cognitive and neuropsychiatric events. Use together cautiously.
Hormonal contraceptives: May decrease effectiveness. Report changes in menstrual patterns. Advise patient to use another contraceptive method.
Phenytoin: May decrease topiramate level and increase phenytoin level. Monitor levels.

Valproic acid: May decrease valproic acid and topiramate level. Monitor patient.
Drug-lifestyle. *Alcohol use:* May cause CNS depression and other adverse cognitive and neuropsychiatric events. Discourage use together.

EFFECTS ON LAB TEST RESULTS
• May increase liver enzyme levels. May decrease bicarbonate and hemoglobin levels and hematocrit.
• May decrease WBC count.

CONTRAINDICATIONS & CAUTIONS
🛑 **Alert:** Alcohol use is contraindicated within 6 hours before and 6 hours after taking extended-release form.
• Contraindicated in patients with metabolic acidosis who are taking concomitant metformin.
• Acute myopia associated with secondary angle-closure glaucoma has been reported in adults and children receiving topiramate. Such symptoms as acute-onset decreased visual acuity or ocular pain typically occur within 1 month of therapy initiation. Discontinue drug as rapidly as possible, according to judgment of health care provider.
• Contraindicated in patients hypersensitive to drug or its components.
• Use cautiously in breast-feeding women and in those with hepatic impairment.
🛑 **Alert:** Associated with increased risk of oral clefts (cleft lip or palate) in infants born to women treated with topiramate during pregnancy. Use in pregnancy only if the potential benefit to the mother outweighs the risk to the fetus. Consider alternative medications with a lower risk of adverse outcomes for these patients.
🛑 **Alert:** Women who become pregnant while taking topiramate should register with the North American Antiepileptic Drug Pregnancy Registry at 1-888-233-2334.
• Use cautiously with other drugs that predispose patients to heat-related disorders, including other carbonic anhydrase inhibitors and anticholinergics.
⚠ **Overdose S&S:** Abdominal pain, abnormal coordination, agitation, blurred vision, seizures, depression, diplopia, dizziness, drowsiness, hypotension, lethargy, impaired

mentation, speech disturbance, stupor, severe metabolic acidosis.

NURSING CONSIDERATIONS

❸ **Alert:** Closely monitor all patients taking or starting antiepileptic drugs for changes in behavior indicating worsening of suicidal thoughts or behavior or depression. Symptoms such as anxiety, agitation, hostility, mania, and hypomania may be precursors to emerging suicidality.
• If needed, withdraw anticonvulsant (including topiramate) gradually to minimize risk of increased seizure activity.
• Monitoring topiramate level isn't necessary.
• Drug may infrequently cause oligohidrosis and hyperthermia, mainly in children. Monitor patient closely, especially in hot weather.
• Drug may cause hyperchloremic, nonanion gap metabolic acidosis from renal bicarbonate loss. Factors that may predispose patients to acidosis, such as renal disease, severe respiratory disorders, status epilepticus, diarrhea, surgery, ketogenic diet, or drugs, may add to topiramate's bicarbonate-lowering effects.
• Measure baseline and periodic bicarbonate levels. If metabolic acidosis develops and persists, consider reducing the dose, gradually stopping the drug, or offering alkali treatment.
• Drug is rapidly cleared by dialysis. A prolonged period of dialysis may cause low drug level and seizures. A supplemental dose may be needed.
• Stop drug if patient experiences acute myopia and secondary angle-closure glaucoma.
• **Look alike–sound alike:** Don't confuse Topamax with Toprol-XL, Tegretol, or Tegretol-XR.

PATIENT TEACHING

• Tell patient not to consume alcohol within 6 hours before to 6 hours after taking extended-release form.
• Instruct patient to immediately seek medical attention if blurred vision, visual disturbances, or eye pain occurs, to reduce risk of permanent vision loss.

• Advise patient to contact health care provider immediately if high or persistent fever or decreased sweating develops.
• Tell patient to use appropriate caution when engaging in activities in which loss of consciousness could result in serious danger to patient or others nearby (such as swimming, driving a car, climbing in high places). Some patients with epilepsy will continue to have unpredictable seizures and may need to avoid such activities entirely.
• Tell patient to drink plenty of fluids during therapy to minimize risk of forming kidney stones.
• Advise patient not to drive or operate hazardous machinery until CNS effects of drug are known. Drug can cause sleepiness, dizziness, confusion, and concentration problems.
• Tell women of childbearing age that drug may decrease effectiveness of hormonal contraceptives. Advise women using hormonal contraceptives to report change in menstrual patterns.
❸ **Alert:** Teach female patient of childbearing age to use effective contraceptive while taking topiramate. Tell patient to contact prescriber if she becomes pregnant or plans to become pregnant during therapy.
• Tell patient to avoid crushing or breaking tablets because of bitter taste.
• Inform patient that drug can be taken without regard to food.
• Tell patient to swallow extended-release capsules whole and intact and not to chew or crush capsules or sprinkle capsule contents on food.
• Tell patient that immediate-release capsules may either be swallowed whole or carefully opened and contents sprinkled on a teaspoonful of soft food. Tell patient to swallow immediately without chewing.

---

topotecan hydrochloride
toh-poh-TEE-ken

Hycamtin

Therapeutic class: Antineoplastics
Pharmacologic class: DNA topoisomerase inhibitors
Pregnancy risk category: D

AVAILABLE FORMS
Capsules: 0.25 mg, 1 mg
Injection: 4-mg single-dose vial (preservative-free)

INDICATIONS & DOSAGES
➤ **Relapsed small-cell lung cancer (SCLC) in patients with a prior complete or partial response who are at least 45 days from the end of first-line chemotherapy**
Adults: 2.3 mg/m^2/day P.O. once daily for 5 consecutive days. Repeat every 21 days. Round the calculated dose to the nearest 0.25 mg.
Adjust-a-dose: For patients with moderate renal impairment (CrCl 30 to 49 mL/minute), give 1.8 mg/m^2/day. Hold subsequent courses until neutrophil count is greater than 1,000 cells/mm^3, platelet count is greater than 100,000 cells/mm^3, and hemoglobin is 9 g/dL or more. Reduce the dose for subsequent courses to 0.4 mg/m^2/day for patients who experience severe neutropenia (neutrophil count less than 500 cells/mm^3 associated with fever or infection or lasting 7 days or more), neutropenia (neutrophil count 500 to 1,000 cells/mm^3 lasting beyond day 21 of the treatment course), platelet count below 25,000 cells/mm^3, or grade 3 or 4 diarrhea.
➤ **With cisplatin, stage-IVB recurrent or persistent cervical cancer unresponsive to surgery or radiation**
Adults: 0.75 mg/m^2 by I.V. infusion over 30 minutes on days 1, 2, and 3, followed by 50 mg/m^2 cisplatin by I.V. infusion on day 1. Repeat cycle every 21 days. Adjust subsequent doses of drug based on hematologic toxicities.
➤ **Metastatic carcinoma of the ovary after failure of first or subsequent chemotherapy; SCLC–sensitive disease after failure of first-line therapy**
Adults: 1.5 mg/m^2 I.V. infusion given over 30 minutes daily for 5 consecutive days, starting on day 1 of a 21-day cycle. Give a minimum of four cycles.
Adjust-a-dose: For patients with CrCl of 20 to 39 mL/minute, decrease dosage to 0.75 mg/m^2. If severe neutropenia occurs, decrease dosage by 0.25 mg/m^2 for subsequent courses or give granulocyte colony-stimulating factor (G-CSF) after subsequent course (before resorting to dosage reduction) starting from day 6 of course (24 hours after completion of topotecan administration).

ADMINISTRATION
P.O.
● Avoid direct contact with capsule contents.
● Give drug without regard to food.
● Do not crush or divide the capsules.
● If patient vomits after taking dose, do not give a replacement dose.
I.V.
▼ Protect unopened vials from light.
▼ Reconstitute each 4-mg vial with 4 mL sterile water for injection. Dilute appropriate volume of reconstituted solution in either normal saline solution or D$_5$W before giving.
▼ Lyophilized form contains no antibacterial preservative; use reconstituted product immediately.
▼ Monitor insertion site during infusion. Extravasation has been linked to mild local reactions, such as erythema and bruising.
▼ When giving topotecan with cisplatin, always give topotecan first.
▼ If stored at 68° to 77° F (20° to 25° C) and exposed to normal lighting, reconstituted drug is stable for 24 hours.
▼ **Incompatibilities:** Dexamethasone, 5-FU, mitomycin, ticarcillin disodium–clavulanate potassium.

ACTION
Interacts with topoisomerase I, inducing reversible single-strand DNA breaks. Drug binds to the topoisomerase I–DNA complex and prevents repair of these single-strand breaks.

T

Route	Onset	Peak	Duration
I.V.	Unknown	Unknown	Unknown
P.O.	Unknown	1–2 hr	Unknown

Half-life: 2 to 3 hours I.V.; 3 to 6 hours P.O.

ADVERSE REACTIONS

CNS: asthenia, fatigue, fever, headache.
GI: abdominal pain, anorexia, constipation, diarrhea, nausea, stomatitis, vomiting.
Hematologic: anemia, *leukopenia, neutropenia, thrombocytopenia.*
Hepatic: *hepatotoxicity.*
Musculoskeletal: back and skeletal pain.
Respiratory: coughing, dyspnea.
Skin: alopecia, rash.
Other: *sepsis.*

INTERACTIONS

Drug-drug. *Cisplatin, cytotoxic agents:*
May increase severity of myelosuppression.
Use together with extreme caution. Dosage reductions may be needed.
G-CSF: May prolong duration of neutropenia. If G-CSF is to be used, don't start it until day 6 of the course, 24 hours after completion of topotecan treatment.

EFFECTS ON LAB TEST RESULTS

• May increase ALT, AST, and bilirubin levels. May decrease hemoglobin level.
• May decrease WBC, platelet, and neutrophil counts.

CONTRAINDICATIONS & CAUTIONS

Black Box Warning Administer drug under the supervision of a health care provider experienced in the use of chemotherapeutic agents. Ensure that appropriate diagnostic and treatment facilities are readily available. ∎
• Contraindicated in patients hypersensitive to drug or its components and in those with severe bone marrow depression.
• Contraindicated in pregnant or breast-feeding women.
• Safety and effectiveness of drug in children haven't been established.
⚠ *Overdose S&S:* Bone marrow suppression.

NURSING CONSIDERATIONS

⦿ *Alert:* Give drug only under the supervision of a physician experienced with cancer chemotherapeutic agents.
Black Box Warning Before first course of therapy is started, patient must have baseline neutrophil count more than 1,500/mm³ and platelet count more than 100,000/mm³. ∎
Black Box Warning Perform peripheral blood counts frequently to monitor patient for bone marrow suppression, primarily neutropenia, which may be severe and result in infection and death. ∎
• Don't give subsequent courses until neutrophil count recovers to more than 1,000 cells/mm³, platelet count recovers to more than 100,000/mm³, and hemoglobin level recovers to more than 9 mg/dL (with transfusion, if needed).
• Prepare drug under vertical laminar flow hood; wear gloves and protective clothing. If drug solution contacts skin, wash immediately and thoroughly with soap and water. If mucous membranes are affected, flush areas thoroughly with water.
• Bone marrow suppression indicates toxic levels of topotecan. The nadir occurs at about 11 days. Neutropenia isn't cumulative over time.
• Duration of thrombocytopenia is about 5 days, with nadir at 15 days. The nadir for anemia is 15 days. Blood or platelet transfusions may be needed.
• WBC colony-stimulating factors may promote cell growth and decrease risk for infection.
⦿ *Alert:* Fatalities due to neutropenic colitis have been reported. Consider possibility of neutropenic colitis in patients presenting with fever, neutropenia, and a compatible pattern of abdominal pain.
⦿ *Alert:* Drug may cause interstitial lung disease, which may be fatal. Monitor patient for cough, fever, dyspnea, and hypoxia; stop drug if they occur.

PATIENT TEACHING

• Urge patient to report promptly sore throat, fever, chills, or unusual bleeding or bruising.
• Caution patient to avoid contact with people with infections.

Reactions in bold italics are *life-threatening*. Interactions may have a *rapid onset* or a *delayed onset*.

• Caution women to avoid pregnancy or breast-feeding during therapy.
• Teach patient and family about drug's adverse reactions and need for frequent monitoring of blood counts.
• Advise patient that capsules can be taken without regard to food.
• Tell patient not to chew, crush, or divide capsules; they should be swallowed whole.

torsemide
TOR-seh-mide

Demadex🖋

Therapeutic class: Diuretics
Pharmacologic class: Loop diuretics
Pregnancy risk category: B

AVAILABLE FORMS
Injection: 10 mg/mL
Tablets: 5 mg, 10 mg, 20 mg, 100 mg

INDICATIONS & DOSAGES
➤ **Diuresis in patients with heart failure**
Adults: Initially, 10 to 20 mg P.O. or I.V. once daily. If response is inadequate, double dose until desired effect is achieved. Maximum, 200 mg daily.
➤ **Diuresis in patients with chronic renal failure**
Adults: Initially, 20 mg P.O. or I.V. once daily. If response is inadequate, double dose until response is obtained. Maximum, 200 mg daily.
➤ **Diuresis in patients with hepatic cirrhosis**
Adults: Initially, 5 to 10 mg P.O. or I.V. once daily with an aldosterone antagonist or a potassium-sparing diuretic. If response is inadequate, double dose until desired effect is achieved. Maximum, 40 mg daily.
➤ **Hypertension**
Adults: Initially, 5 mg P.O. daily. Increased to 10 mg if needed and tolerated after 4 to 6 weeks. Add another antihypertensive if response is still inadequate.

ADMINISTRATION
P.O.
• To prevent nocturia, give drug in the morning.

I.V.
▼ Inspect ampules for precipitate or discoloration before use.
▼ Give by direct injection over at least 2 minutes. Rapid injection may cause ototoxicity. Don't give more than 200 mg at a time.
▼ Drug may be given as a continuous infusion.
▼ Drug remains stable for 24 hours at room temperature when mixed in D_5W, normal saline solution, or half-normal saline solution.
▼ **Incompatibilities:** Solutions with pH below 8.3. Flush line with normal saline solution before and after administration to avoid incompatibility.

ACTION
Enhances excretion of sodium, chloride, and water by acting on the ascending loop of Henle.

Route	Onset	Peak	Duration
P.O.	1 hr	1–2 hr	6–8 hr
I.V.	10 min	1 hr	6–8 hr

Half-life: 3½ hours.

ADVERSE REACTIONS
CNS: asthenia, dizziness, headache, nervousness, insomnia.
CV: ECG abnormalities, chest pain, edema, orthostatic hypotension.
EENT: rhinitis, sore throat.
GI: excessive thirst, diarrhea, constipation, nausea, dyspepsia.
GU: excessive urination, impotence.
Metabolic: electrolyte imbalances, including hypokalemia and *hypomagnesemia; dehydration;* hypochloremic alkalosis; hyperuricemia; hypercholesterolemia.
Musculoskeletal: arthralgia, myalgia.
Respiratory: cough.

INTERACTIONS
Drug-drug. *Aminoglycoside antibiotics, cisplatin:* May increase ototoxicity. Use together cautiously.
Amphotericin B, corticosteroids, metolazone: May increase risk of hypokalemia. Monitor potassium level.
Anticoagulants: May enhance anticoagulant activity. Use together cautiously.

T

Antidiabetics: May decrease hypoglycemic effect, resulting in higher glucose level. Monitor glucose level.

Chlorothiazide, chlorthalidone, hydrochloro-thiazide, indapamide, metolazone: May cause excessive diuretic response, resulting in serious electrolyte abnormalities or dehydration. Adjust doses carefully, and monitor patient closely for signs and symptoms of excessive diuretic response.

Cholestyramine: May decrease absorption of torsemide. Separate doses by at least 3 hours.

Digoxin: Electrolyte imbalance caused by diuretic may lead to digoxin-induced arrhythmia. Use together cautiously.

Lithium: May increase lithium level and cause toxicity. Use together cautiously and monitor lithium level.

NSAIDs: May decrease effects of loop diuretics. Use together cautiously.

Probenecid: May decrease diuretic effect. Avoid using together.

Salicylates: May decrease excretion, possibly leading to salicylate toxicity. Avoid using together.

Spironolactone: May decrease renal clearance of spironolactone. Use together cautiously.

Drug-herb. *Dandelion:* May interfere with drug activity. Discourage use together.

Licorice: May cause unexpected rapid potassium loss. Discourage use together.

Drug-lifestyle. *Sun exposure:* May cause photosensitivity. Advise patient to take precautions.

EFFECTS ON LAB TEST RESULTS

● May increase BUN, creatinine, cholesterol, glucose, and uric acid levels.

● May decrease potassium and magnesium levels.

CONTRAINDICATIONS & CAUTIONS

● Contraindicated in patients hypersensitive to drug or other sulfonamide derivatives and in those with anuria.

● Use cautiously in patients with hepatic disease and related cirrhosis and ascites; sudden changes in fluid and electrolyte balance may precipitate hepatic coma in these patients.

⚠ **Overdose S&S:** Dehydration, hypovolemia, hypotension, hypokalemia, hypochloremic alkalosis, hemoconcentration.

NURSING CONSIDERATIONS

● Monitor fluid intake and output, electrolyte levels, blood pressure, weight, and pulse rate during rapid diuresis and routinely with long-term use. Drug can cause profound diuresis and water and electrolyte depletion.

● Watch for signs of hypokalemia, such as muscle weakness and cramps.

● Consult prescriber and dietitian about providing a high-potassium diet or potassium supplement. Foods rich in potassium include citrus fruits, bananas, and dates.

● Monitor elderly patients, who are especially susceptible to excessive diuresis with potential for circulatory collapse and thromboembolic complications.

● **Look alike–sound alike:** Don't confuse torsemide with furosemide. Don't confuse Demadex with Denorex.

PATIENT TEACHING

● Tell patient to take drug in morning to prevent the need to urinate at night.

● Advise patient to change positions slowly to prevent dizziness and to limit alcohol intake and strenuous exercise in hot weather to prevent dizziness.

● Advise patient to immediately report ringing in ears because it may indicate toxicity.

● Tell patient to report weakness, cramping, nausea, and dizziness.

● Tell patient to check with prescriber or pharmacist before taking OTC drugs.

● Advise patient that drug may cause photosensitivity, and tell him to take precautions with sun exposure.

Reactions in bold italics are *life-threatening*. Interactions may have a *rapid onset* or a *delayed onset*.

tramadol hydrochloride
TRAM-uh-dohl

Conzip, Rybix ODT, Ultram,
Ultram ER

Therapeutic class: Analgesics
Pharmacologic class: Synthetic
centrally active analgesics
Pregnancy risk category: C

AVAILABLE FORMS
Capsules (extended-release): 100 mg,
150 mg, 200 mg, 300 mg
Tablets: 50 mg
Tablets (extended-release): 100 mg,
200 mg, 300 mg
Tablets (orally disintegrating): 50 mg

INDICATIONS & DOSAGES
➤ **Moderate to moderately severe chronic
pain**
Adults age 17 and older: Initially, 25 mg
P.O. in the morning. Adjust by 25 mg every
3 days to 100 mg/day (25 mg q.i.d.). Thereafter, adjust by 50 mg every 3 days to reach
200 mg/day (50 mg q.i.d.). Thereafter, give
50 to 100 mg P.O. every 4 to 6 hours p.r.n.
Maximum, 400 mg daily. Or, 50 to 100 mg
orally disintegrating tablets (ODTs) P.O.
every 4 to 6 hours p.r.n. Adjust by 50 mg
every 3 days to 200 mg/day (50 mg q.i.d.).
Thereafter give 50 to 100 mg P.O. every
4 to 6 hours p.r.n. Maximum dose is 400 mg
daily.
*Adults age 18 and older not taking
immediate-release tablets or ODTs:* 100 mg
extended-release form P.O. once daily.
Titrate by 100 mg every 5 days to relieve
pain. Do not exceed 300 mg/day.
Adjust-a-dose: For immediate-release form,
if CrCl is less than 30 mL/minute, increase
dose interval to every 12 hours; maximum
is 200 mg daily. For patients with cirrhosis, give 50 mg (immediate-release) every
12 hours. For patients older than age 75,
maximum is 300 mg daily in divided doses.
Don't use extended-release form in patients
with severe hepatic or renal impairment.

ADMINISTRATION
P.O.
- Give drug without regard for meals.
- Extended-release capsules and tablets
must be swallowed whole; don't break or
crush tablets.
- ODTs may be taken with or without water.
- Place ODTs on tongue until dissolved (about
1 minute). The patient shouldn't chew,
break, or split them.

ACTION
Unknown. Thought to bind to opioid receptors and inhibit reuptake of norepinephrine
and serotonin.

Route	Onset	Peak	Duration
P.O.	Unknown	2 hr	Unknown
P.O. (extended-release)	Unknown	12 hr	Unknown

Half-life: 6 to 7 hours; extended-release, 8 to
9 hours.

ADVERSE REACTIONS
CNS: dizziness, headache, somnolence,
vertigo, *seizures,* anxiety, asthenia, CNS
stimulation, confusion, coordination dis-
turbance, euphoria, malaise, nervousness,
sleep disorder.
CV: vasodilation.
EENT: visual disturbances.
GI: constipation, nausea, vomiting, abdom-
inal pain, anorexia, diarrhea, dry mouth,
dyspepsia, flatulence.
GU: menopausal symptoms, proteinuria,
urinary frequency, urine retention.
Musculoskeletal: hypertonia.
Respiratory: *respiratory depression.*
Skin: diaphoresis, pruritus, rash.

INTERACTIONS
Drug-drug. *Carbamazepine:* May increase
tramadol metabolism. Patients receiving
long-term carbamazepine therapy up to
800 mg daily may need up to twice the
recommended tramadol dose.
CNS depressants, opioids: May cause
additive effects. Use together cautiously;
tramadol dosage may need to be reduced.
*Cyclobenzaprine, MAO inhibitors, neuro-
leptics, other opioids, TCAs:* May increase
risk of seizures. Monitor patient closely.
Quinidine: May increase level of tramadol.
Monitor patient closely.

T

SSRIs: May increase risk of serotonin syndrome. Use cautiously and monitor patient for adverse effects.

Drug-lifestyle. *Alcohol, illicit drug use:* May have additive effects. Use cautiously together.

EFFECTS ON LAB TEST RESULTS
• May increase creatinine, GGT, and liver enzyme levels.
• May decrease creatinine and hemoglobin levels.

CONTRAINDICATIONS & CAUTIONS
• Contraindicated in patients hypersensitive to drug or other opioids, in patients with severe renal impairment, breast-feeding women, suicidal patients, and in those with acute intoxication from alcohol, hypnotics, centrally acting analgesics, opioids, or psychotropic drugs.
• Contraindicated in patients with significant respiratory depression or acute or severe bronchial asthma or hypercapnia in unmonitored settings or where resuscitative equipment isn't available.
⟳ Alert: Serious hypersensitivity reactions can occur, usually after the first dose. Patients with history of anaphylactic reaction to codeine and other opioids may be at increased risk.
• Use extended-release forms cautiously in elderly patients, especially those age 75 and older.
• Use cautiously in patients at risk for seizures or respiratory depression; in patients with increased intracranial pressure or head injury, acute abdominal conditions, or renal or hepatic impairment; and in patients with physical dependence on opioids.
⟳ Alert: Drug can cause life-threatening serotonin syndrome.
⟳ Alert: Use cautiously in patients taking tranquilizers or antidepressants and in those who abuse alcohol or suffer from depression or emotional disturbance because of the increased risk of suicide.
⚠ Overdose S&S: Lethargy, somnolence, stupor, coma, seizures, skeletal muscle flaccidity, respiratory depression, cool clammy skin, miosis, bradycardia, hypotension, cardiac arrest, death.

NURSING CONSIDERATIONS
• Reassess patient's level of pain at least 30 minutes after administration.
• Monitor CV and respiratory status. Withhold dose and notify prescriber if respirations are shallow or rate is below 12 breaths/minute.
• Monitor bowel and bladder function. Anticipate need for stimulant laxative.
• For better analgesic effect, give drug before onset of intense pain.
• Monitor patients at risk for seizures. Drug may reduce seizure threshold.
• In the case of an overdose, naloxone may also increase risk of seizures.
• Monitor patient for drug dependence. Drug can produce dependence similar to that of codeine and thus has potential for abuse.
• Withdrawal symptoms may occur if drug is stopped abruptly. Reduce dosage gradually.
• **Look alike–sound alike:** Don't confuse tramadol with trazodone or trandolapril.

PATIENT TEACHING
• Tell patient to take drug as prescribed and not to increase dose or dosage interval unless ordered by prescriber.
• Caution ambulatory patient to be careful when rising and walking. Warn outpatient to avoid driving and other potentially hazardous activities that require mental alertness until drug's CNS effects are known.
• Advise patient to check with prescriber before taking OTC drugs because drug interactions can occur.
• Warn patient not to stop the drug abruptly.

trandolapril
tran-DOLE-ah-pril

Mavik⬧

Therapeutic class: Antihypertensives
Pharmacologic class: ACE inhibitors
Pregnancy risk category: D

AVAILABLE FORMS
Tablets: 1 mg, 2 mg, 4 mg

INDICATIONS & DOSAGES
➤ **Hypertension**
Adults: For patients not taking a diuretic, initially 2 mg P.O. for a black patient and 1 mg P.O. for all other races, once daily. If control isn't adequate, increase dosage at intervals of at least 1 week. Maintenance doses for most patients range from 2 to 4 mg daily. Some patients taking once-daily doses of 4 mg may need b.i.d. doses. For patients also taking a diuretic, initially, 0.5 mg P.O. once daily. Subsequent dosage adjustment is based on blood pressure response.
➤ **Heart failure or ventricular dysfunction after MI**
Adults: Initially, 1 mg P.O. daily, adjusted to 4 mg P.O. daily. If patient can't tolerate 4 mg, continue at highest tolerated dose.
Adjust-a-dose: If CrCl is below 30 mL/minute or patient has hepatic cirrhosis, first dose is 0.5 mg daily.

ADMINISTRATION
P.O.
● Give drug without regard for food.
● Don't give antacid 1 hour before or up to 2 hours after dose.

ACTION
Thought to inhibit ACE, reducing angiotensin II formation, which decreases peripheral arterial resistance, decreases aldosterone secretion, reduces sodium and water retention, and lowers blood pressure. Drug is converted in the liver to the prodrug, trandolaprilat.

Route	Onset	Peak	Duration
P.O.	4 hr	4–10 hr	24 hr

Half-life: 5 to 10 hours; longer in patients with renal impairment.

ADVERSE REACTIONS
CNS: dizziness, headache, fatigue, syncope, stroke.
CV: hypotension, *bradycardia,* chest pain, intermittent claudication.
GI: *pancreatitis,* dyspepsia, diarrhea.
Hematologic: *neutropenia, leukopenia.*
Metabolic: *hyperkalemia,* hyponatremia.
Musculoskeletal: myalgia.

Respiratory: persistent, nonproductive cough; dyspnea.
Skin: rash, pruritus.

INTERACTIONS
Drug-drug. *Aldosterone blockers (eplerenone):* May increase risk of severe hyperkalemia, arrhythmias, and cardiac arrest. Monitor potassium level. Reduced dosage of aldosterone blocker may be needed to decrease potassium level.
⊙ *Alert: Aliskiren:* May increase risk of renal impairment, hypotension, and hyperkalemia in diabetic patients and those with moderate to severe renal impairment (GFR less than 60 mL/minute). Concomitant use is contraindicated in diabetic patients. Avoid concomitant use in those with moderate to severe renal impairment.
Anesthetic agents: May increase hypotension. Correct with volume expansion.
ARBs (telmisartan): May increase hyperkalemia and renal dysfunction. If coadministration can't be avoided, closely monitor renal function and potassium level.
Azathioprine: May increase risk of anemia or leukopenia. Monitor hematologic studies.
Clozapine: May increase risk of hypotension and clozapine level. Monitor blood pressure and adjust trandolapril dosage as needed.
Diuretics: May cause excessive hypotension. Stop diuretic or reduce first dosage of trandolapril.
Lithium: May increase lithium level and lithium toxicity. Avoid using together; monitor lithium level.
Loop diuretics (furosemide): May decrease diuretic effects and increase renal dysfunction. If fluid and sodium retention occur, increase diuretic dose. If renal function decreases, stop both drugs.
mTOR inhibitors (everolimus, sirolimus): May increase angioedema risk. If an interaction is suspected, stop one or both drugs.
NSAIDs: May decrease antihypertensive effects and increase risk for renal dysfunction. Monitor blood pressure and renal function. If an interaction is suspected, discontinue NSAID or use another antihypertensive.
Potassium-sparing diuretics, potassium supplements: May cause hyperkalemia. Monitor potassium level closely.

T

Drug-herb. *Capsaicin:* May cause cough. Discourage use together.
Ma huang: May decrease antihypertensive effects. Discourage use together.
Drug-food. *Salt substitutes containing potassium:* May cause hyperkalemia. Discourage use of salt substitutes.

EFFECTS ON LAB TEST RESULTS
• May increase BUN, creatinine, potassium, and liver enzyme levels. May decrease sodium level.
• May decrease neutrophil and WBC counts.

CONTRAINDICATIONS & CAUTIONS
• Contraindicated in patients hypersensitive to drug and in those with a history of angioedema related to previous treatment with an ACE inhibitor.
Black Box Warning Use during pregnancy can cause injury and death to the developing fetus. When pregnancy is detected, stop drug as soon as possible. ■
• Use cautiously in patients with impaired renal function, heart failure, or renal artery stenosis.
• Safety and effectiveness of drug in children haven't been established.
• Don't use drug in breast-feeding women.
⚠ **Overdose S&S:** Severe hypotension.

NURSING CONSIDERATIONS
• Monitor potassium level closely.
• Black patients who take ACE inhibitors as monotherapy for hypertension have a smaller reduction in blood pressure than nonblacks. Blacks should take drug with a thiazide diuretic for a more favorable response. Black patients taking ACE inhibitors have a higher incidence of angioedema than nonblacks.
• Watch for hypotension. Excessive hypotension can occur when drug is given with diuretics. If possible, stop diuretic therapy 2 to 3 days before starting trandolapril to decrease potential for excessive hypotension response. If drug doesn't adequately control blood pressure, diuretic therapy may be started again cautiously.
• Assess patient's renal function before and periodically throughout therapy.

• Other ACE inhibitors have been reported to cause agranulocytosis and neutropenia. Monitor CBC with differential before therapy, especially in patients with collagen vascular disease and impaired renal function.
⟐ *Alert:* Angioedema involving the tongue, glottis, or larynx may be fatal because of airway obstruction. Give appropriate therapy, including epinephrine 1:1,000 (0.3 to 0.5 mL) subcutaneously; have resuscitation equipment for maintaining a patent airway readily available. The risk of angioedema is higher in blacks.
• If patient develops jaundice, stop drug under prescriber's advice because, although rare, ACE inhibitors have been linked to a syndrome of cholestatic jaundice, fulminant hepatic necrosis, and death.

PATIENT TEACHING
• Instruct patient to report yellowing of skin or eyes.
• Advise patient to report fever and sore throat (signs of infection), easy bruising or bleeding; swelling of the tongue, lips, face, eyes, mucous membranes, or extremities; difficulty swallowing or breathing; hoarseness; and nonproductive, persistent cough.
• Tell patient to avoid salt substitutes during drug therapy. These products may contain potassium, which can cause high potassium level in patients taking drug.
• Tell patient that light-headedness can occur, especially during first few days of therapy. Advise him to rise slowly to minimize this effect and to report it immediately.
• Advise patient to use caution in hot weather and during exercise. Inadequate fluid intake, vomiting, diarrhea, and excessive perspiration can lead to light-headedness and fainting.
• Tell women of childbearing age to report suspected pregnancy immediately. Drug will need to be stopped.
• Advise patient planning to undergo surgery or receive anesthesia to inform prescriber that he is taking this drug.
• Tell patient drug may be taken with or without food.
• Instruct patient not to take an antacid 1 hour before or up to 2 hours after dose.

---

*Reactions in bold italics are **life-threatening**. Interactions may have a **rapid onset** or a **delayed onset**.*

trastuzumab
trass-too-ZOO-mab

Herceptin

Therapeutic class: Antineoplastics
Pharmacologic class: Monoclonal antibodies
Pregnancy risk category: D

AVAILABLE FORMS
Lyophilized powder for injection:
440 mg/vial

INDICATIONS & DOSAGES
➤ **Human epidermal growth factor receptor 2 (HER2)-overexpressing metastatic gastric or gastroesophageal junction adenocarcinoma in patients not previously treated for metastatic disease in combination with cisplatin and capecitabine or 5-FU**
Adults: Initially, 8 mg/kg I.V. over 90 minutes. Then, give 6 mg/kg I.V. over 30 to 90 minutes every 3 weeks until disease progression or intolerable toxicity develops.
➤ **Metastatic breast cancer in patients whose tumors overexpress the HER2 protein**
Adults: Loading dose of 4 mg/kg I.V. over 90 minutes. If tolerated, continue with 2 mg/kg I.V. weekly as 30-minute infusion. If patient hasn't previously received one or more chemotherapy regimens for their metastatic disease, drug is given with paclitaxel.
➤ **After surgical resection of HER2-overexpressing node-positive or node-negative breast cancer**
Adults: During treatment with paclitaxel, docetaxel, or docetaxel–carboplatin, give loading dose of 4 mg/kg I.V. over 90 minutes. Then, 2 mg/kg I.V. over 30 minutes weekly during chemotherapy for the first 12 weeks (paclitaxel or docetaxel) or 18 weeks (docetaxel–carboplatin). Continue trastuzumab 6 mg/kg I.V. over 30 to 90 minutes every 3 weeks for a total of 52 weeks.
➤ **As single agent after surgical resection of HER2-overexpressing breast**

cancer within 3 weeks of completion of multimodality, anthracycline-based chemotherapy
Adults: Initial dose, 8 mg/kg I.V. over 90 minutes. Then, 6 mg/kg I.V. over 30 to 90 minutes every 3 weeks for a total of 52 weeks.

ADMINISTRATION
I.V.
▼ Reconstitute drug in each vial with 20 mL of bacteriostatic water for injection, 1.1% benzyl alcohol preserved, as supplied, to yield a multidose solution containing 21 mg/mL. Don't shake vial during reconstitution. Make sure reconstituted preparation is colorless to pale yellow and free of particulates. Immediately after reconstitution, label vial with expiration 28 days from date of reconstitution.
▼ If patient is hypersensitive to benzyl alcohol, reconstitute drug with sterile water for injection, use immediately, and discard unused portion. Avoid use of other reconstitution diluents.
▼ Determine dose based on loading dose of 4 mg/kg or maintenance dose of 2 mg/kg. Calculate volume of 21-mg/mL solution and withdraw this amount from vial and add it to an infusion bag containing 250 mL of normal saline solution. Don't use D_5W or dextrose-containing solutions. Gently invert bag to mix solution.
▼ Don't give as I.V. push or bolus.
▼ Infuse loading dose over 90 minutes. If well tolerated, infuse maintenance doses over 30 minutes.
▼ Vials are stable at 36° to 46° F (2° to 8° C). Discard reconstituted solution after 28 days. Don't freeze drug that has been reconstituted. Store solution of drug diluted in normal saline solution for injection at 36° to 46° F (2° to 8° C) before use; it's stable for up to 24 hours.
▼ **Incompatibilities:** Other I.V. drugs or dextrose solutions.

ACTION
A recombinant DNA-derived monoclonal antibody that selectively binds to HER2, inhibiting proliferation of tumor cells that overexpress HER2.

T

Route	Onset	Peak	Duration
I.V.	Unknown	Unknown	Unknown

Half-life: Range, 1 to 32 days; mean, 5¾ days.

ADVERSE REACTIONS

CNS: asthenia, dizziness, fever, headache, insomnia, pain, depression, neuropathy, paresthesia, peripheral neuritis.
CV: peripheral edema, *heart failure,* hypotension, tachycardia.
EENT: pharyngitis, rhinitis, sinusitis.
GI: abdominal pain, anorexia, diarrhea, nausea, vomiting.
GU: UTI.
Hematologic: *leukopenia,* anemia, neutropenia.
Musculoskeletal: back pain, arthralgia, bone pain.
Respiratory: dyspnea, increased cough.
Skin: rash, acne.
Other: *anaphylaxis,* chills, flulike syndrome, infection, allergic reaction, herpes simplex.

INTERACTIONS

Drug-drug. *Anthracyclines, cyclophosphamide:* May increase cardiotoxicity. Use together very cautiously.

EFFECTS ON LAB TEST RESULTS

• May decrease hemoglobin level.
• May decrease WBC count.

CONTRAINDICATIONS & CAUTIONS

• Contraindicated in patients hypersensitive to the drug.
• Use cautiously in elderly patients, in patients hypersensitive to drug or its components, and in those with cardiac dysfunction.
• Use with extreme caution in patients with pulmonary compromise, symptomatic intrinsic pulmonary disease (such as asthma, COPD), or extensive tumor involvement of the lungs.
Black Box Warning Exposure to drug during pregnancy can result in oligohydraminos, in some cases complicated by pulmonary hypoplasia, skeletal abnormalities, and neonatal death. ∎
• Safety and effectiveness of drug in children haven't been established.

NURSING CONSIDERATIONS

Black Box Warning Before beginning therapy, patient should undergo thorough baseline cardiac assessment, including history and physical examination and methods to identify risk of cardiotoxicity. ∎
Black Box Warning Assess patient for signs and symptoms of cardiac dysfunction, especially if he is receiving drug with anthracyclines and cyclophosphamide. ∎
• Check for dyspnea, increased cough, paroxysmal nocturnal dyspnea, peripheral edema, or S₃ gallop. Treatment may be stopped in patients who develop a significant decrease in left ventricular function.
• Monitor patient receiving both drug and chemotherapy closely for cardiac dysfunction or failure, anemia, leukopenia, diarrhea, and infection.
• When used in metastatic breast cancer, drug is only indicated in tumors with HER2 protein overexpression.
Black Box Warning Drug can cause serious infusion reactions and pulmonary toxicity. Interrupt infusion if patient experiences dyspnea or clinically significant hypotension. Strongly consider discontinuation for patients who develop anaphylaxis, angioedema, pneumonitis, or acute respiratory distress syndrome. ∎
• Check for first-infusion symptom complex, commonly consisting of chills or fever. Give acetaminophen, diphenhydramine, and meperidine (with or without reducing rate of infusion). Other signs or symptoms include nausea, vomiting, pain, rigors, headache, dizziness, dyspnea, hypotension, rash, and asthenia and occur infrequently with subsequent infusions.
• *Look alike–sound alike:* Don't confuse trastuzumab with ado-trastuzumab emtansine.

PATIENT TEACHING

• Tell patient about risk of first-dose infusion-related adverse reactions.
• Urge patient to notify prescriber immediately if signs or symptoms of heart problems occur, such as shortness of breath, increased cough, or swelling in arms or legs. Tell patient that these effects can occur after infusion is complete.

- Instruct patient to report adverse effects to prescriber.
- Advise women to stop breast-feeding during drug therapy and for 6 months after last dose of drug.

travoprost
TRA-voe-prost

Travatan Z

Therapeutic class: Antiglaucoma drugs
Pharmacologic class: Prostaglandin analogues
Pregnancy risk category: C

AVAILABLE FORMS
Ophthalmic solution: 0.004%

INDICATIONS & DOSAGES
➤ **To reduce intraocular pressure (IOP) in patients with open-angle glaucoma or ocular hypertension who can't tolerate or who respond inadequately to other IOP-lowering drugs**
Adults: One drop in conjunctival sac of each affected eye once daily at bedtime.

ADMINISTRATION
Ophthalmic
- Don't touch tip of dropper to eye or surrounding tissue.
- Apply light finger pressure on lacrimal sac for 1 minute after instilling drug to minimize systemic absorption.
- If using more than one ophthalmic drug, give them at least 5 minutes apart.
- Store drug between 36° and 77° F (2° and 25° C).

ACTION
Thought to reduce IOP by increasing uveoscleral outflow.

Route	Onset	Peak	Duration
Ophthalmic	Unknown	30 min	Unknown

Half-life: 45 minutes.

ADVERSE REACTIONS
CNS: anxiety, depression, headache, pain.
CV: *bradycardia,* angina pectoris, chest pain, hypertension, hypotension.

EENT: eye discomfort, eye pain, eye pruritus, decreased visual acuity, foreign body sensation, ocular hyperemia, abnormal vision, blepharitis, blurred vision, cataract, conjunctival hyperemia, conjunctivitis, dry eye, eye disorder, iris discoloration, keratitis, lid margin crusting, photophobia, sinusitis, subconjunctival hemorrhage, tearing.
GI: dyspepsia, GI disorder.
GU: prostate disorder, urinary incontinence, UTI.
Metabolic: hypercholesterolemia.
Musculoskeletal: arthritis, back pain.
Respiratory: bronchitis.
Other: accidental injury, cold syndrome, infection.

INTERACTIONS
Drug-herb. *Areca, jaborandi, ophthalmic herbal preparations:* May increase effects. Discourage use together.

EFFECTS ON LAB TEST RESULTS
- May increase cholesterol level.

CONTRAINDICATIONS & CAUTIONS
- Contraindicated in patients hypersensitive to drug or its components; in pregnant women or women trying to become pregnant; and in those with angle-closure, inflammatory, or neovascular glaucoma.
- Use cautiously in patients with renal or hepatic impairment, active intraocular inflammation (iritis, uveitis), or risk factors for macular edema.
- Use cautiously in aphakic patients and pseudophakic patients with a torn posterior lens capsule.

NURSING CONSIDERATIONS
- Temporary or permanent increased pigmentation of the iris and eyelid may occur as well as increased pigmentation and growth of eyelashes.
- Patient should remove contact lenses before instilling drug and reinsert them 15 minutes after administration.
- If a pregnant woman or a woman attempting to become pregnant accidentally comes in contact with drug, thoroughly cleanse the exposed area with soap and water immediately.

T

• *Look alike–sound alike:* Don't confuse Travatan Z with Xalatan.

PATIENT TEACHING
• Teach patient how to instill drops, and advise him to wash hands before and after instilling solution. Warn him not to touch tip of dropper to eye or surrounding tissue.
• Advise patient to apply light finger pressure on lacrimal sac for 1 minute after instillation to minimize systemic absorption of drug.
• Tell patient to remove contact lenses before administration and explain that he can reinsert them 15 minutes afterward.
• Tell patient receiving treatment in only one eye about potential for increased iris pigmentation, eyelid darkening, and increased length, thickness, pigmentation, or number of lashes in the treated eye.
• If eye trauma or infection occurs or if eye surgery is needed, advise patient to seek medical advice before continuing to use the multidose container.
• Advise patient to immediately report eye inflammation or lid reactions.
• Tell patient to consult health care provider before using ophthalmic herbal preparations concurrently.
• If patient is using more than one ophthalmic drug, tell him to apply them at least 5 minutes apart.
• Stress importance of compliance with recommended therapy.
• If a pregnant woman or a woman attempting to become pregnant accidentally comes in contact with drug, tell her to thoroughly cleanse the exposed area with soap and water immediately.

trazodone hydrochloride
TRAYZ-oh-dohn

Oleptro

Therapeutic class: Antidepressants
Pharmacologic class: Triazolopyridine derivatives
Pregnancy risk category: C

AVAILABLE FORMS
Tablets: 50 mg, 100 mg, 150 mg, 300 mg
Tablets (extended-release): 150 mg, 300 mg

INDICATIONS & DOSAGES
➤ **Depression**
Adults: Initially, 150 mg P.O. daily in divided doses; then increased by 50 mg daily every 3 to 4 days, as needed. Dose ranges from 150 to 400 mg daily. Maximum, 600 mg daily for inpatients and 400 mg daily for outpatients. Or, 150 mg P.O. once daily (extended-release form). May increase by 75 mg/day every 3 days. Maximum dosage is 375 mg P.O. daily.
➤ **Insomnia** ◆
Adults: 50 to 100 mg P.O. daily.
➤ **Prevention of migraine** ◆
Adults: 100 mg P.O. daily.

ADMINISTRATION
P.O.
• Give drug after meals or a light snack for optimal absorption and to decrease risk of dizziness.
• Give extended-release tablets at the same time each day, preferably at bedtime, on an empty stomach.
• Extended-release tablets can be swallowed whole or broken along the score line.
• Don't crush or allow patient to chew extended-release tablets.

ACTION
Unknown. Inhibits CNS neuronal uptake of serotonin; not a tricyclic derivative.

Route	Onset	Peak	Duration
P.O.	Unknown	1–2 hr	Unknown
P.O. (extended-release)	Unknown	9 hr	Unknown

Half-life: First phase, 3 to 6 hours; second phase, 5 to 9 hours. Extended-release tablets, 10 hours.

ADVERSE REACTIONS
CNS: drowsiness, dizziness, nervousness, fatigue, confusion, tremor, weakness, hostility, anger, nightmares, vivid dreams, headache, insomnia, syncope.
CV: orthostatic hypotension, tachycardia, hypertension, shortness of breath, ECG changes.
EENT: blurred vision, tinnitus, nasal congestion.
GI: dry mouth, dysgeusia, constipation, nausea, vomiting, anorexia.
GU: urine retention, priapism possibly leading to impotence, hematuria.

Reactions in bold italics are *life-threatening*. Interactions may have a *rapid onset* or a *delayed onset*.

Hematologic: anemia.
Skin: rash, urticaria, diaphoresis.
Other: decreased libido.

INTERACTIONS

Drug-drug. *Amphetamines, buspirone, dextromethorphan, dihydroergotamine, lithium salts, meperidine, SSRIs or SSNRIs (duloxetine, venlafaxine), sumatriptan, TCAs, tramadol, tryptophan:* May increase the risk of serotonin syndrome. Avoid combining drugs that increase the availability of serotonin in the CNS; monitor patient closely if used together.
Antihypertensives: May increase hypotensive effect of trazodone. Antihypertensive dosage may need to be decreased.
Clonidine, CNS depressants: May enhance CNS depression. Avoid using together.
CYP3A4 inducers (carbamazepine): May reduce trazodone level. Monitor patient closely; may need to increase trazodone dose.
CYP3A4 inhibitors (ketoconazole): May slow the clearance of trazodone and increase trazodone level. May cause nausea, hypotension, and fainting. Consider decreasing trazodone dose.
Digoxin, phenytoin: May increase levels of these drugs. Watch for toxicity.
Linezolid, methylene blue: May cause serotonin syndrome. Use extreme caution and monitor patient closely.
MAO inhibitors: Effects unknown. Use together with extreme caution.
Protease inhibitors (amprenavir, atazanavir, fosamprenavir, indinavir, lopinavir–ritonavir, nelfinavir, ritonavir, saquinavir): May increase trazodone levels and adverse effects. Monitor patient and adjust trazodone dose, as needed.
Warfarin: May increase PT. Adjust warfarin dosage as needed.
Drug-herb. *Ginkgo biloba:* May cause sedation. Discourage use together.
St. John's wort: May cause serotonin syndrome. Discourage use together.
Drug-lifestyle. *Alcohol use:* May enhance CNS depression. Discourage use together.

EFFECTS ON LAB TEST RESULTS

● May increase ALT and AST levels. May decrease hemoglobin level.

CONTRAINDICATIONS & CAUTIONS

● Contraindicated in patients hypersensitive to drug.
Black Box Warning Trazodone isn't approved for use in children. ■
🌣 Alert: Concomitant use with linezolid or methylene blue can cause serotonin syndrome (fever, mental status changes, muscle twitching, excessive sweating, shivering or shaking, diarrhea, loss of coordination). Use drug with linezolid or methylene blue only for life-threatening or urgent conditions when the potential benefits outweigh the risks of toxicity.
● Use cautiously in patients with cardiac disease or in the initial recovery phase of MI and in patients at risk for suicide.
⚠ Overdose S&S: Priapism, respiratory arrest, seizures, ECG changes, drowsiness, vomiting.

NURSING CONSIDERATIONS

● Monitor patient for signs and symptoms of serotonin syndrome (mental status changes, tachycardia, labile blood pressure, hyperreflexia, incoordination, nausea, vomiting, diarrhea) or neuroleptic malignant syndrome (hyperthermia, muscle rigidity, rapidly fluctuating vital signs, mental status change). If these signs and symptoms occur, immediately discontinue trazodone and any other serotonergic, antidopaminergic, or antipsychotic drugs.
🌣 Alert: If linezolid or methylene blue must be given, stop trazodone and monitor patient for serotonin toxicity for 2 weeks, or until 24 hours after the last dose of methylene blue or linezolid, whichever comes first. May resume trazodone 24 hours after last dose of methylene blue or linezolid.
● Record mood changes. Monitor patient for suicidal tendencies and allow only minimum supply of drug.
Black Box Warning Drug may increase the risk of suicidal thinking and behavior in children, adolescents, and young adults ages 18 to 24, especially during the first few months of treatment, especially those with major depressive disorder or other psychiatric disorder. ■
● *Look alike–sound alike:* Don't confuse trazodone hydrochloride with tramadol hydrochloride.

T

PATIENT TEACHING

⚠ *Alert:* Tell patient to report a persistent, painful erection (priapism) right away because he may need immediate intervention.

⚠ *Alert:* Teach patient to recognize and immediately report signs and symptoms of serotonin toxicity (fever, mental status changes, muscle twitching, excessive sweating, shivering or shaking, diarrhea, loss of coordination).

• Warn patient to avoid activities that require alertness and good coordination until effects of drug are known. Drowsiness and dizziness usually subside after first few weeks.

Black Box Warning Teach caregivers how to recognize signs and symptoms of suicidal tendency or suicidal thoughts. ∎

• Tell patient to take extended-release tablets at bedtime on an empty stomach.

• Advise patient not to crush or chew extended-release tablets. Tell him that, if needed, tablets can be broken in half along the score line.

---

treprostinil sodium
tra-PROS-tin-ill

Remodulin, Tyvaso

Therapeutic class: Antihypertensives
Pharmacologic class: Vasodilators
Pregnancy risk category: B

AVAILABLE FORMS

Injection: 1 mg/mL, 2.5 mg/mL, 5 mg/mL, 10 mg/mL in 20-mL vials
Solution for inhalation: 1.74 mg/2.9-mL ampule

INDICATIONS & DOSAGES

➤ **To reduce symptoms caused by exercise in patients with New York Heart Association class II to IV pulmonary arterial hypertension (PAH)**
Adults: Initially, 1.25 nanograms/kg/minute by continuous subcutaneous infusion. If patient doesn't tolerate initial dose, reduce infusion rate to 0.625 nanogram/kg/minute. Increase by 1.25 nanograms/kg/minute each week for the first 4 weeks and then by no more than 2.5 nanograms/kg/minute each week for the remaining duration of infusion.

Experience with treprostinil dosages exceeding 40 nanograms/kg/minute is limited. May be given I.V. through a central venous catheter if subcutaneous route isn't tolerated. Or, initially, 3 breaths (18 mcg) per treatment session q.i.d., approximately 4 hours apart. Dosage should be increased by 3 breaths in 1- to 2-week intervals as tolerated to target maintenance dosage of 9 breaths (54 mcg) q.i.d. If 3 breaths aren't tolerated initially, decrease to 1 or 2 breaths and increase as tolerated.

Adjust-a-dose: For patients with mild or moderate hepatic insufficiency, initially, 0.625 nanogram/kg ideal body weight per minute by continuous I.V. infusion, and increase cautiously.

➤ **To decrease the rate of clinical deterioration in patients requiring transition from epoprostenol sodium (Flolan)**
Adults: Start treprostinil at 10% of the current epoprostenol dose; increase dose as the epoprostenol dose is reduced. Decrease epoprostenol dose in 20% increments and increase treprostinil in 20% increments, always maintaining a total dose of 110% of epoprostenol starting dose. Once epoprostenol is at 20% of starting dose and treprostinil is at 90%, decrease epoprostenol to 5% and increase treprostinil to 110%. Finally, stop epoprostenol and maintain treprostinil dose at 110% of epoprostenol starting dose plus an additional 5% to 10% as needed. Change rate based on individual patient response. Treat worsening of PAH symptoms with increases in treprostinil dose. Treat adverse effects associated with prostacyclin and prostacyclin analogues with decreases in epoprostenol dose.

ADMINISTRATION

I.V.

▼ Give I.V. through a central venous catheter only if subcutaneous route isn't tolerated.

▼ Dilute with either sterile water for injection or normal saline solution.

▼ Inspect for particulate matter and discoloration before giving.

▼ Give by continuous infusion through a surgically placed indwelling central venous catheter, using an infusion pump designed for I.V. drug delivery.

Reactions in bold italics are *life-threatening*. Interactions may have a *rapid onset* or a *delayed onset*.

▼ To avoid potential interruptions in drug delivery, make sure patient has immediate access to a backup infusion pump and infusion sets.

▼ Diluted drug is stable at room temperature for up to 48 hours.

▼ **Incompatibilities:** Other I.V. drugs.

Subcutaneous

• Preferred route is continuous subcutaneous infusion via a self-inserted subcutaneous catheter, using an infusion pump designed for subcutaneous drug delivery.

• The infusion pump should be small and lightweight; adjustable to about 0.002 mL/hour; have occlusion/no delivery, low-battery, programming-error, and motor-malfunction alarms; have delivery accuracy of ±6% or better; and be positive-pressure driven.

• The reservoir should be made of polyvinyl chloride, polypropylene, or glass.

Inhalation

• One ampule contains sufficient volume for all four treatment sessions in a single day.

• Oral inhalation is intended for use with the Optineb-ir Model ON-100/7.

• Before the first treatment of the day, empty entire ampule into medicine cup of inhalation device.

• Cap the device and store upright between treatments.

• Clean the medicine cup and discard any remaining drug at the end of the day. Clean device daily.

• Avoid skin and eye contact with treprostinil.

• Drug shouldn't be ingested orally.

• Don't mix treprostinil with other medications in the nebulizer.

• To avoid potential interruptions in drug therapy, make sure patient has access to back-up Optineb-ir device.

ACTION

Directly vasodilates pulmonary and systemic arterial vascular beds and inhibits platelet aggregation.

Route	Onset	Peak	Duration
I.V.	Unknown	Unknown	Unknown
Subcut.	Rapid	Unknown	Unknown
Inhalation	Rapid	Unknown	Unknown

Half-life: 2 to 4 hours, I.V. and subcutaneous; 4 hours, inhalation.

ADVERSE REACTIONS

CNS: dizziness, fatigue, headache.
CV: vasodilation, *right ventricular heart failure,* chest pain, edema, hypotension.
GI: diarrhea, nausea.
Musculoskeletal: jaw pain.
Respiratory: dyspnea, cough, wheezing.
Skin: infusion-site pain, infusion-site reaction, rash, flushing, pallor, pruritus.

INTERACTIONS

Drug-drug. *Anticoagulants:* May increase risk of bleeding. Monitor patient closely for bleeding.
Antihypertensives, diuretics, vasodilators: May worsen reduction in blood pressure. Monitor blood pressure.

EFFECTS ON LAB TEST RESULTS

None reported.

CONTRAINDICATIONS & CAUTIONS

• Contraindicated in patients hypersensitive to drug or structurally related compounds.

• Use cautiously in patients with hepatic or renal impairment and in elderly patients.

• Use cautiously in pregnant and breast-feeding women. Use only if clearly needed.

⚠ *Overdose S&S:* Diarrhea, flushing, headache, hypotension, nausea, vomiting.

NURSING CONSIDERATIONS

• Assess the patient's ability to accept, place, and care for a subcutaneous catheter and to use an infusion pump.

• During use, a single reservoir syringe can be given for up to 72 hours at 98.6° F (37° C).

• Don't use a single vial longer than 14 days after the initial introduction to the vial.

• Start treatment in setting where adequate monitoring and emergency care are available.

• Increase dose if patient doesn't improve or symptoms worsen, and decrease if drug

T

effects become excessive or unacceptable infusion-site symptoms develop.
• Avoid abrupt withdrawal or sudden large dose reductions because PAH symptoms may worsen.

PATIENT TEACHING
• Inform patient that he'll need to continue therapy for a prolonged period, possibly years.
• Tell patient that subsequent disease management may require I.V. therapy.
• Inform patient that many side effects, such as labored breathing, fatigue, and chest pain, may be related to the underlying disease.
• Tell patient that the most common local reactions are pain, redness, tissue hardening, and rash at the infusion site.
• Tell patient that a backup infusion pump or Optineb-ir device must be available to avoid interruption in therapy.
• Instruct patient in proper administration of inhalation solution and use and cleaning of device.

tretinoin (retinoic acid, vitamin A acid)
TRET-i-noyn

Atralin, Avita, Rejuva-A†, Renova, Retin-A, Retin-A Micro, StieVA-A†

Therapeutic class: Antiacne drugs
Pharmacologic class: Retinoids
Pregnancy risk category: C

AVAILABLE FORMS
Cream: 0.01%†, 0.02%, 0.025%, 0.0375%, 0.05%, 0.1%
Gel: 0.05%, 0.01%, 0.025%
Microsphere gel: 0.04%, 0.1%
Solution: 0.05%

INDICATIONS & DOSAGES
➤ **Acne vulgaris (except Renova)**
Adults: Clean affected area and lightly apply once daily at bedtime.
Children age 12 and older (Retin-A Micro): Clean affected area and lightly apply once daily at bedtime.

Children age 10 and older (Atralin): Clean affected area and lightly apply once daily at bedtime.
➤ **Adjunctive use in the mitigation of fine facial wrinkles in patients who use comprehensive skin care and sunlight avoidance programs (Renova)**
Adults: Apply a small, pea-sized amount (¼ inch or 5 mm in diameter) to cover the entire face lightly, once daily in the evening.

ADMINISTRATION
Topical
• Clean area thoroughly before application and avoid getting drug in eyes, mouth, or mucous membranes.

ACTION
Inhibits comedones by increasing epidermal cell mitosis and turnover.

Route	Onset	Peak	Duration
Topical	Unknown	Unknown	Unknown

Half-life: Unknown.

ADVERSE REACTIONS
Skin: feeling of warmth, slight stinging, local erythema, peeling, chapping, swelling, blistering, crusting, temporary hyperpigmentation or hypopigmentation.

INTERACTIONS
Drug-drug. *Topical drugs containing benzoyl peroxide, resorcinol, salicylic acid, or sulfur:* May increase risk of skin irritation. Avoid using together.
Topical minoxidil or photosensitizing drugs (fluoroquinolones, phenothiazines, sulfonamides, tetracyclines, thiazides): May increase risk of skin irritation. Avoid using together.
Drug-lifestyle. *Abrasive cleansers, cream depilatories, medicated cosmetics, skin preparations containing alcohol, waxes:* May increase risk of skin irritation. Discourage use together.
Sun exposure: May increase photosensitivity reaction. Advise patient to avoid excessive sunlight exposure.

EFFECTS ON LAB TEST RESULTS
None reported.

CONTRAINDICATIONS & CAUTIONS
• Contraindicated in patients hypersensitive to drug or its components and in those with sunburn.
• Use cautiously in patients with eczema.
⚠ **Overdose S&S:** Marked redness, skin peeling, skin discomfort.

NURSING CONSIDERATIONS
• Initially, drug may be applied every 2 to 3 days using a lower concentration to reduce irritation.
• Relapses typically occur within 3 to 6 weeks after therapy is stopped.
• **Look alike–sound alike:** Don't confuse tretinoin with trientine or isotretinoin.

PATIENT TEACHING
• Instruct patient to clean area thoroughly before application and to avoid getting drug in eyes, mouth, or mucous membranes.
• Tell patient to wash hands after application.
• Tell patient to wash face with mild soap no more than b.i.d. or t.i.d. Warn patient against using strong or medicated cosmetics, soaps, or other skin cleansers. Also advise him to avoid topical products containing alcohol, astringents, spices, and lime because they may interfere with drug's actions.
• Tell patient using drug for treatment of fine wrinkles to wait 20 minutes after washing face to apply drug, and to avoid washing face or applying another skin product or cosmetic for 1 hour after application.
• Tell patient that normal use of cosmetics is allowed.
• Advise patient not to stop drug if temporary worsening of inflammatory lesions occurs. If severe local irritation develops, advise patient to stop drug temporarily and notify prescriber. Dosage will be readjusted when application is resumed. Some redness and scaling are normal reactions.
• Warn patient that he may experience increased sensitivity to wind or cold temperatures.
• Instruct patient to minimize exposure to sunlight or ultraviolet rays during treatment. If he becomes sunburned, he should delay therapy until sunburn subsides. Tell patient who can't avoid exposure to sunlight to use SPF-15 sunblock and to wear protective clothing.
• Warn patient that he may have a temporary increase in lesions, which will improve in 2 to 3 weeks.

triamcinolone acetonide (injection)
trye-am-SIN-oh-lone

Kenalog-10, Kenalog-40, Trivaris

triamcinolone hexacetonide
Aristospan Intra-articular, Aristospan Intralesional

Therapeutic class: Corticosteroids
Pharmacologic class: Glucocorticoids
Pregnancy risk category: C; D (Trivaris)

AVAILABLE FORMS
triamcinolone acetonide
Injection (gel suspension): 8 mg/0.1 mL in single-use glass syringes
Injection (suspension): 10 mg/mL, 40 mg/mL
triamcinolone hexacetonide
Injection (suspension): 5 mg/mL (intralesional); 20 mg/mL (intra-articular)

INDICATIONS & DOSAGES
➤ **Severe inflammation, immunosuppression**
Adults: 60 mg acetonide I.M., then 20 to 100 mg acetonide I.M. as needed every 6 weeks, if possible. Or, 1 mg acetonide into lesions. Or, initially, 2.5 to 15 mg acetonide into joints (depending on joint size) or soft tissue; then may increase to 40 mg for larger areas. For Trivaris, doses up to 10 mg (smaller areas) and up to 40 mg (larger areas) have usually been sufficient. A local anesthetic is commonly injected with triamcinolone into the joint. For hexacetonide, up to 0.5 mg (of 5 mg/mL suspension) intralesional or sublesional injection per square inch of affected skin. Additional injections based on patient's response. Or, 2 to 20 mg (using the 20 mg/mL suspension) via intra-articular injection. Repeat every 3 to 4 weeks.

T

Children older than age 12: Initially, 60 mg acetonide I.M.; repeat with additional I.M. doses of 20 to 100 mg, as needed, at 6-week intervals, if possible.

Children ages 6 to 12: 0.03 to 0.2 mg/kg acetonide, or 1 to 6.25 mg/m² I.M. at 1- to 7-day intervals.

➤ **Inflamed cystic lesions of acne vulgaris ◆**

Adults: Inject 0.63 to 5 mg/mL into cystic lesion.

ADMINISTRATION

I.M.
• Give deep into gluteal muscle. Rotate injection sites to prevent muscle atrophy.
• Don't use 10 mg/mL strength for this route.

Intra-articular
• Strict aseptic technique is mandatory.
• Prior use of a local anesthetic may be desirable.
• Each syringe of Trivaris should only be used for a single treatment.

Intralesional
• Strict aseptic technique is mandatory.
• Inject directly into the lesion intradermally or subcutaneously.
• It is preferable to use a tuberculin syringe and small-bore needle (not smaller than 24G).

ACTION

Not clearly defined. Decreases inflammation, mainly by stabilizing leukocyte lysosomal membranes; suppresses immune response; stimulates bone marrow; and influences protein, fat, and carbohydrate metabolism.

Route	Onset	Peak	Duration
I.M., intra-articular, intralesional	Variable	Variable	Variable

Half-life: 18 to 36 hours.

ADVERSE REACTIONS

CNS: euphoria, insomnia, *pseudotumor cerebri, seizures,* headache, paresthesia, psychotic behavior, vertigo.
CV: *arrhythmias, heart failure, thromboembolism,* hypertension, edema, thrombophlebitis.

EENT: cataracts, glaucoma.
GI: *pancreatitis,* peptic ulceration, GI irritation, increased appetite, nausea, vomiting.
GU: menstrual irregularities, increased urine calcium level.
Metabolic: hypokalemia, hyperglycemia and carbohydrate intolerance, hypercholesterolemia, hypocalcemia.
Musculoskeletal: growth suppression in children, muscle weakness, osteoporosis.
Skin: hirsutism, delayed wound healing, acne, various skin eruptions.
Other: *acute adrenal insufficiency,* cushingoid state, susceptibility to infections after increased stress or abrupt withdrawal after long-term therapy.

INTERACTIONS

Drug-drug. *Antidiabetics:* May increase blood glucose level. Adjust dosage of antidiabetics as needed.
Aspirin, indomethacin, other NSAIDs: May increase risk of GI distress and bleeding. Use together cautiously.
Barbiturates, carbamazepine, fosphenytoin, phenytoin, rifampin: May decrease corticosteroid effect. Increase corticosteroid dosage.
Cyclosporine: May increase toxicity and seizures. Monitor patient closely.
Ketoconazole, macrolide antibiotics: May decrease metabolism or clearance of triamcinolone, respectively. Decrease triamcinolone dose or dosage interval if needed.
Oral anticoagulants: May alter dosage requirements. Monitor PT and INR closely.
Potassium-depleting drugs, such as thiazide diuretics and amphotericin B: May enhance potassium-wasting effects of triamcinolone. Monitor potassium level.
Salicylates: May decrease salicylate level. Monitor patient for lack of salicylate effectiveness.
Skin-test antigens: May decrease response. Postpone skin testing until after therapy.
Toxoids, vaccines: May decrease antibody response and increase risk of neurologic complications. Defer routine administration of vaccines or toxoids until corticosteroid therapy is discontinued, if possible.

Reactions in bold italics are *life-threatening*. Interactions may have a *rapid onset* or a *delayed onset*.

EFFECTS ON LAB TEST RESULTS

• May increase glucose and cholesterol levels. May decrease potassium and calcium levels.
• May decrease ^{131}I uptake and protein-bound iodine values in thyroid function tests. May alter reactions to skin tests.
• May cause false-negative results in nitro-blue tetrazolium test for systemic bacterial infections.

CONTRAINDICATIONS & CAUTIONS

• Contraindicated in patients hypersensitive to drug or its ingredients, in patients with cerebral malaria, in those with systemic fungal infections, and in those receiving immunosuppressive doses together with live-virus vaccines.
• Use cautiously in patients with recent MI, GI ulcer, renal disease, hypertension, osteoporosis, diabetes mellitus, hypothyroidism, cirrhosis, diverticulitis, nonspecific ulcerative colitis, recent intestinal anastomoses, thromboembolic disorders, seizures, myasthenia gravis, active hepatitis, lactation, heart failure, tuberculosis, ocular herpes simplex, emotional instability, or psychotic tendencies.

NURSING CONSIDERATIONS

• Determine whether patient is sensitive to other corticosteroids.
• Drug isn't used for alternate-day therapy.
• Always adjust to lowest effective dose.
• Most adverse reactions to corticosteroids are dose- or duration-dependent.
• Monitor patient's weight, blood pressure, and electrolyte levels.
• Monitor patient for cushingoid effects, such as moon face, buffalo hump, central obesity, thinning hair, hypertension, and increased susceptibility to infection.
• Watch for allergic reaction to tartrazine in patients sensitive to aspirin.
• Watch for depression or psychotic episodes, especially during high-dose therapy.
• Diabetic patient may need increased insulin dosage; monitor glucose level.
• Drug may mask or worsen infections, including latent amebiasis.
• Elderly patients may be more susceptible to osteoporosis with long-term use.

• Unless contraindicated, give low-sodium diet that's high in potassium and protein. Give potassium supplements as needed.
• Gradually reduce dosage after long-term therapy. Drug may affect patient's sleep.
• *Look alike–sound alike:* Don't confuse triamcinolone with Triaminic.

PATIENT TEACHING

• Tell patient not to stop drug abruptly or without prescriber's consent.
• Teach patient signs and symptoms of early adrenal insufficiency: fatigue, muscle weakness, joint pain, fever, anorexia, nausea, shortness of breath, dizziness, and fainting.
• Instruct patient to carry medical identification that includes prescriber's name and drug's name and dosage and indicates his need for supplemental systemic glucocorticoids during stress.
• Warn patient on long-term therapy about cushingoid effects (moon face, buffalo hump) and the need to notify prescriber about sudden weight gain and swelling.
• Tell patient to report slow healing.
• Advise patient receiving long-term therapy to consider exercise or physical therapy. Also, tell patient to ask prescriber about vitamin D or calcium supplement.
• Instruct patient to avoid exposure to infections and to notify prescriber if exposure occurs.

triamcinolone acetonide (intranasal)
trye-am-SIN-oh-lone

Nasacort AQ

Therapeutic class: Corticosteroids
Pharmacologic class: Corticosteroids
Pregnancy risk category: C

AVAILABLE FORMS
Nasal spray: 55 mcg/spray

INDICATIONS & DOSAGES
➤ **Treatment of nasal symptoms of seasonal and perennial allergic rhinitis**
Adults and children age 12 and older:
2 sprays in each nostril daily; may decrease

T

to 1 spray in each nostril daily for allergic disorders. Adjust to minimum effective dosage.

Children ages 6 to 11: 1 spray in each nostril daily. Maximum dosage is 2 sprays in each nostril daily. Adjust to minimum effective dosage.

Children ages 2 to 5: 1 spray in each nostril daily.

Adjust-a-dose: Start elderly patients at lower end of dosing range.

ADMINISTRATION
Intranasal
• Shake well before each use.
• Release 5 sprays into the air to prime before first use. Reprime with 1 spray if not used for 2 weeks or more.

ACTION
Unknown. A glucocorticoid with anti-inflammatory properties.

Route	Onset	Peak	Duration
Intranasal	Unknown	1½–4 hr	Unknown

Half-life: AQ form, about 3 hours.

ADVERSE REACTIONS
CNS: headache, fever.
EENT: nasal irritation, burning, dry mucous membranes, epistaxis, irritation, nasal and sinus congestion, otitis media, pharyngitis, rhinitis, sinusitis, sneezing, stinging, throat discomfort.
GI: dyspepsia, nausea, vomiting.
Respiratory: *asthma symptoms,* cough.

INTERACTIONS
None significant.

EFFECTS ON LAB TEST RESULTS
None reported.

CONTRAINDICATIONS & CAUTIONS
• Contraindicated in patients hypersensitive to drug or its components and in those with untreated mucosal infection.
• Use with caution, if at all, in patients with active or quiescent tuberculous infection of respiratory tract and in patients with untreated fungal, bacterial, or systemic viral infection or ocular herpes simplex.

• Use cautiously in patients already receiving systemic corticosteroids because of increased likelihood of hypothalamic-pituitary-adrenal axis suppression.
• Use cautiously in breast-feeding women and in those with recent nasal septal ulcers, nasal surgery, or trauma because drug may inhibit wound healing.
⚠ *Overdose S&S:* GI upset, nasal irritation, headache.

NURSING CONSIDERATIONS
❂ *Alert:* Excessive doses may cause signs and symptoms of hyperadrenocorticism and adrenal axis suppression; stop drug slowly.
• To decrease risk of adverse effects, individualize drug dosage and titrate to minimum effective dosage.
• Discontinue drug if symptom relief hasn't occurred after 3 weeks of treatment.
• *Look alike–sound alike:* Don't confuse triamcinolone with Triaminicin.

PATIENT TEACHING
• Urge patient to read patient instruction sheet contained in each package before using drug for first time.
• Teach patient to prime pump before first use.
• To instill, instruct patient to shake container before use, blow nose to clear nasal passages, tilt head slightly forward, and insert nozzle into nostril, pointing away from septum. Tell him to hold other nostril closed and inhale gently while spraying. Next, have patient shake container and repeat procedure in other nostril.
• Instruct patient to avoid getting aerosol in eyes. If this occurs, tell him to rinse with copious amounts of cool tap water.
• Stress importance of using drug on a regular schedule because its effectiveness depends on regular use. Warn patient not to exceed prescribed dosage because serious adverse reactions can occur.
• Tell patient to notify prescriber if signs and symptoms don't diminish or if condition worsens in 2 to 3 weeks.
• Warn patient to avoid exposure to chickenpox or measles and, if exposed, to notify prescriber.

Reactions in bold italics are *life-threatening*. Interactions may have a *rapid onset* or a *delayed onset*.

• Instruct patient to watch for and report signs and symptoms of nasal infection. Drug may need to be stopped and appropriate local therapy given.

triamcinolone acetonide (topical)
trye-am-SIN-oh-lone

Kenalog, Triderm

Therapeutic class: Corticosteroids
Pharmacologic class: Corticosteroids
Pregnancy risk category: C

AVAILABLE FORMS
Aerosol: 0.2 mg/2-second spray
Cream: 0.025%, 0.1%, 0.5%
Dental paste: 0.1%
Lotion: 0.025%, 0.1%
Ointment: 0.025%, 0.1%, 0.5%
Paste: 0.1%

INDICATIONS & DOSAGES
➤ **Inflammation and pruritus from corticosteroid-responsive dermatoses**
Adults and children: Clean area; apply aerosol, cream, lotion, or ointment sparingly b.i.d. to q.i.d. Rub in lightly. Or, 3 or 4 applications of spray daily.
➤ **Inflammation from oral lesions**
Adults and children: Apply paste at bedtime and, if needed, b.i.d. or t.i.d., preferably after meals. Apply small amount without rubbing; press to lesion in mouth until thin film develops.

ADMINISTRATION
Topical
• Gently wash skin before applying. To avoid skin damage, rub in gently, leaving a thin coat. When treating hairy sites, part hair and apply directly to lesions.
• Don't apply near eyes or in ear canal.
• When using aerosol near the face, cover patient's eyes and warn against inhaling spray. Aerosol contains alcohol and may cause irritation or burning when used on open lesions. Don't spray longer than 3 seconds or from closer than 6 inches (15 cm) to avoid freezing tissues.

• Occlusive dressings may be used in severe or resistant dermatoses.

ACTION
Unclear. Diffuses across cell membranes to form complexes with cytoplasmic receptors, showing anti-inflammatory, antipruritic, vasoconstrictive, and antiproliferative activity. Considered a medium-potency (0.025% and 0.1% cream, ointment, lotion) and high-potency (0.5% cream, ointment) drug, according to vasoconstrictive properties.

Route	Onset	Peak	Duration
Topical	Several hr	Unknown	>1 wk

Half-life: Unknown.

ADVERSE REACTIONS
GU: glycosuria.
Metabolic: hyperglycemia.
Skin: burning, pruritus, irritation, dryness, erythema, folliculitis, hypertrichosis, hypopigmentation, acneiform eruptions, perioral dermatitis, allergic contact dermatitis, maceration, secondary infection, atrophy, striae, miliaria with occlusive dressings.
Other: *hypothalamic-pituitary-adrenal (HPA) axis suppression,* Cushing syndrome.

INTERACTIONS
None significant.

EFFECTS ON LAB TEST RESULTS
• May increase glucose level.

CONTRAINDICATIONS & CAUTIONS
• Contraindicated in patients hypersensitive to drug or its components.
• Contraindicated in the presence of fungal, viral, or bacterial infections of the mouth or throat (paste).
• Don't use as monotherapy in primary bacterial infections (impetigo, paronychia, erysipelas, cellulitis, angular cheilitis), treatment of rosacea, perioral dermatitis, or acne.
• Don't use very-high-potency or high-potency agents on the face, groin, or axilla areas.
• Drug isn't for ophthalmic use.

T

• Use cautiously in pregnant or breast-feeding women.

⚠ **Overdose S&S:** Systemic effects (including reversible HPA axis suppression, Cushing syndrome, hyperglycemia, glycosuria.)

NURSING CONSIDERATIONS
• Stop drug and tell prescriber if skin infection, striae, or atrophy occur.
• If antifungal or antibiotic combined with corticosteroid fails to provide prompt improvement, stop corticosteroid until infection is controlled.
• Systemic absorption is likely with the use of occlusive dressings, prolonged treatment, or extensive body surface treatment.
• Avoid using plastic pants or tight-fitting diapers on treated areas in young children. Children may absorb larger amounts of drug and be more susceptible to systemic toxicity.

PATIENT TEACHING
• Teach patient or family member how to apply drug.
• If an occlusive dressing is ordered, advise patient to leave it in place for no longer than 12 hours each day and not to use the dressing on infected or weeping lesions.
• Tell patient to stop drug and report signs of systemic absorption, skin irritation or ulceration, hypersensitivity, infection, or lack of improvement.

triamterene–hydrochlorothiazide
try-AM-tur-een–hye-droe-klor-oh-THYE-a-zide

Dyazide, Maxzide

Therapeutic class: Antihypertensives–diuretics
Pharmacologic class: Thiazide diuretics–potassium-sparing diuretics
Pregnancy risk category: C

AVAILABLE FORMS
Capsules: triamterene 37.5 mg and hydrochlorothiazide 25 mg, triamterene 50 mg and hydrochlorothiazide 25 mg

Tablets: triamterene 37.5 mg and hydrochlorothiazide 25 mg, triamterene 75 mg and hydrochlorothiazide 50 mg

INDICATIONS & DOSAGES
➤ **Hypertension or edema in patients who develop hypokalemia on hydrochlorothiazide alone, or who require a thiazide diuretic and in whom development of hypokalemia can't be risked**
Adults: Triamterene 37.5 mg/hydrochlorothiazide 25 mg, or triamterene 50 mg/hydrochlorothiazide 25 mg P.O. once daily or b.i.d., or triamterene 75 mg/hydrochlorothiazide 50 mg P.O. once daily.

ADMINISTRATION
P.O.
• Give drug with food to minimize GI upset.
• To prevent nocturia, give drug in morning. If second dose is needed, give in early afternoon.

ACTION
Triamterene works on distal tubule to inhibit reabsorption of sodium in exchange for potassium and hydrogen; hydrochlorothiazide increases excretion of sodium, chloride, and water by inhibiting reabsorption in distal segment of the nephron.

Route	Onset	Peak	Duration
P.O. (triamterene)	2–4 hr	3 hr	7–9 hr
P.O. (hydrochlorothiazide)	2 hr	4 hr	6–12 hr

Half-life: Triamterene, unknown; hydrochlorothiazide, 5½ to 15 hours.

ADVERSE REACTIONS
CNS: weakness, fatigue, dizziness, headache, drowsiness, insomnia, depression, anxiety, vertigo, restlessness, paresthesia.
CV: arrhythmia, orthostatic hypotension, chest pain.
EENT: xanthopsia, transient blurred vision, dry mouth, sialadenitis.
GI: diarrhea, nausea, vomiting, constipation, abdominal pain, pancreatitis, change in appetite, taste alteration, anorexia, gastric irritation, cramping.

GU: erectile dysfunction, *acute renal failure,* interstitial nephritis, renal calculi.
Hematologic: *leukopenia, thrombocytopenia,* purpura, anemia, agranulocytosis.
Hepatic: jaundice, altered LFT results.
Metabolic: diabetes mellitus, hyperkalemia, hyperglycemia, glycosuria, hyperuricemia, hypokalemia, hyponatremia, metabolic acidosis, hypochloremic alkalosis.
Musculoskeletal: muscle cramps.
Respiratory: shortness of breath, *pulmonary edema.*
Skin: rash, urticaria, photosensitivity.
Other: hypersensitivity reaction, anaphylaxis.

INTERACTIONS

Drug-drug. *ACE inhibitors, potassium-containing medications (such as penicillin G potassium), potassium supplements:* May increase risk of hyperkalemia. Avoid concurrent use.
Adrenocorticotropic hormone, amphotericin B, corticosteroids: May increase electrolyte depletion, particularly potassium. Use together carefully.
Amiloride, spironolactone, triamterene-containing agents: May increase risk of hyperkalemia. Use together is contraindicated.
Antidiabetics (oral agents and insulin): May increase or decrease blood glucose level. Dosage adjustment of antidiabetic may be required.
Antigout drugs: May increase uric acid level. Increase dosage of antigout medication if indicated.
Barbiturates, opioids: May increase risk of orthostatic hypotension. Use together cautiously.
Laxatives: May increase potassium loss. Avoid use together.
Lithium: May increase lithium level, especially in patients with renal insufficiency. Avoid use together.
Methenamine: May decrease effects of methenamine due to urine alkalization. Avoid use together.
NSAIDs: May diminish antihypertensive effects and increase risk of acute renal failure. Use together cautiously.

Oral anticoagulants: May decrease anticoagulant effect. Adjust anticoagulant dosage as necessary.
Other antihypertensives: May increase risk of hypotension. Use together carefully and adjust dosage as appropriate.
Polystyrene, other exchange resins: May reduce potassium level, increase sodium retention, and increase edema. Avoid use together unless in setting of hyperkalemia.
Skeletal muscle relaxants, nondepolarizing (tubocurarine): May increase responsiveness to muscle relaxant. Avoid concurrent use.
Drug-food. *Salt substitutes with potassium:* May increase risk of hyperkalemia. Discourage use together.
Drug-lifestyle. *Alcohol use:* May increase risk of orthostatic hypotension. Discourage use together.
Sun exposure: Hydrochlorothiazide may increase risk of photosensitivity. Discourage sun exposure.

EFFECTS ON LAB TEST RESULTS

● May increase BUN, creatinine, liver enzyme, calcium, uric acid, cholesterol, and triglyceride levels.
● May decrease sodium, chloride, magnesium, and phosphate levels.
● May increase or decrease potassium or glucose level.
● May decrease protein-bound iodine level without signs of thyroid imbalance.
● May decrease leukocyte and platelet counts.
● May interfere with quinidine assays and parathyroid function tests.

CONTRAINDICATIONS & CAUTIONS

● **Black Box Warning** Abnormal elevation of serum potassium levels (5.5 mEq/L or more) can occur with all potassium-sparing diuretics and is more likely in patients with renal impairment or diabetes (even without concurrent renal impairment) and in elderly and severely ill patients. ■
● Contraindicated in patients hypersensitive to either drug or to sulfonamides; in those with preexisting hyperkalemia, anuria, acute and chronic renal insufficiency or significant renal impairment, or severe

T

hepatic disease; and in those at risk for metabolic or respiratory acidosis.

● Use with caution in patients with diabetes, impaired hepatic function, hypokalemia, hypochloremia, or other electrolyte imbalance; in those with a history of kidney stones; and in elderly patients.

● Use in pregnant woman only if benefits outweigh risks to fetus.

● Both drugs may appear in breast milk; patient should discontinue drug or discontinue breast-feeding.

⚠ *Overdose S&S:* Hyperkalemia or hypokalemia, dehydration, nausea, vomiting, weakness, hypotension, lethargy, GI irritation, coma.

NURSING CONSIDERATIONS

● ▮Black Box Warning▮ Uncorrected hyperkalemia may be fatal. Monitor potassium level at initiation of therapy, with dosage changes, and with any illness that may influence renal function. ▮

● Warning signs and symptoms of hyperkalemia include paresthesia, muscular weakness, fatigue, flaccid paralysis, bradycardia, and shock.

● Fixed-dose combinations aren't to be used for initial therapy except in patients in whom development of hyperkalemia can't be risked (patients taking cardiac glycosides and those with history of cardiac arrhythmias).

● Monitor potassium level carefully in patients using this combination; if hyperkalemia is suspected, obtain ECG and monitor levels.

● If hyperkalemia is present, stop combination and use thiazide alone.

● If potassium level is greater than 6.5 mEq/L, consider I.V. calcium chloride, sodium bicarbonate, glucose, or sodium polystyrene sulfonate; consider dialysis if no improvement.

● Monitor patient for infection (sore throat, fever) or bruising for evaluation of leukopenia or thrombocytopenia.

● Monitor patient for acute myopia and secondary angle-closure glaucoma (acute vision changes, ocular pain usually within hours to weeks of drug ingestion), especially in patient with a history of possible sulfon-

amide or penicillin allergy. Discontinue drug as soon as possible if symptoms occur.

● Monitor patient for hyperuricemia or acute gout.

● Thiazide may alter calcium and phosphate levels. Discontinue drug before testing parathyroid function.

● Monitor diabetic patients for changes in antidiabetic agent or insulin requirements. Patients with latent diabetes may become fully diabetic during therapy.

PATIENT TEACHING

● Teach patient to report light-headedness, especially during first few days of therapy.

● Warn patient to discontinue drug and notify prescriber if syncope occurs.

● Caution patient to notify prescriber if fluid loss occurs from excessive perspiration, dehydration, vomiting, or diarrhea.

● Advise patient not to use salt substitutes containing potassium.

● Instruct patient to promptly report signs and symptoms of infection (sore throat, fever) or bruising.

● Inform patient that to be effective, drug must be taken daily as prescribed, and to continue to take drug even if feeling well.

● Teach patient the warning signs and symptoms of fluid and electrolyte imbalance (decreased urine production, drowsiness, dry mouth, fast heart rate, fatigue, low blood pressure, muscular fatigue, muscle pain or cramps, restlessness, stomach disturbances, thirst, and weakness).

● Advise patient to keep follow-up appointments with prescriber in order to monitor electrolyte levels.

● Warn patient to avoid sun exposure to decrease risk of a photosensitivity skin reaction.

● Caution patient to avoid alcohol, to decrease risk of a sudden drop in blood pressure.

Reactions in bold italics are *life-threatening*. Interactions may have a *rapid onset* or a *delayed onset*.

SAFETY ALERT!

triazolam
trye-AY-zoe-lam

Halcion

Therapeutic class: Hypnotics
Pharmacologic class: Benzodiazepines
Pregnancy risk category: X
Controlled substance schedule: IV

AVAILABLE FORMS
Tablets: 0.125 mg, 0.25 mg

INDICATIONS & DOSAGES
➤ **Short-term treatment (7 to 10 days) of insomnia**
Adults: 0.125 to 0.5 mg P.O. at bedtime. Reevaluate patient if drug is used for longer than 2 to 3 weeks.
Elderly or debilitated patients: 0.125 mg P.O. at bedtime; increase, as needed, to 0.25 mg P.O. at bedtime.

ADMINISTRATION
P.O.
● Give drug without regard for food, but avoid giving with grapefruit or grapefruit juice.

ACTION
Unknown. Probably acts on the limbic system, thalamus, and hypothalamus of the CNS to produce hypnotic effects.

Route	Onset	Peak	Duration
P.O.	Unknown	1–2 hr	1½–5½ hr

Half-life: 1½ to 5½ hours.

ADVERSE REACTIONS
CNS: complex sleep-related behaviors, drowsiness, amnesia, ataxia, depression, dizziness, headache, lack of coordination, mental confusion, nervousness, physical or psychological dependence, rebound insomnia.
GI: nausea, vomiting.
Other: *anaphylaxis, angioedema.*

INTERACTIONS
Drug-drug. *Cimetidine, erythromycin, fluoxetine, fluvoxamine, isoniazid, nefazodone,* *ranitidine:* May increase triazolam level. Avoid using with azole antifungals or nefazodone. Watch for increased sedation if used with other drugs.
CNS depressants: May cause excessive CNS depression. Use together cautiously.
Diltiazem: May increase CNS depression and prolong effects of triazolam. Reduce triazolam dose.
Fluconazole, itraconazole, ketoconazole, miconazole: May increase and prolong drug level, CNS depression, and psychomotor impairment. Avoid using together.
Drug-herb. *Calendula, hops, kava, lemon balm, passion flower, skullcap, valerian:* May enhance sedative effect of drug. Discourage use together.
Drug-food. *Grapefruit:* May delay onset and increase drug effects. Discourage use together.
Drug-lifestyle. *Alcohol use:* May cause additive CNS effects. Discourage use together.
Smoking: May increase metabolism and clearance of drug. Advise patient who smokes to watch for decreased effectiveness of drug.

EFFECTS ON LAB TEST RESULTS
● May increase LFT values.

CONTRAINDICATIONS & CAUTIONS
● Contraindicated in pregnant patients and those hypersensitive to benzodiazepines.
● Use cautiously in patients with impaired hepatic or renal function, chronic pulmonary insufficiency, sleep apnea, mental depression, suicidal tendencies, or history of drug abuse.
● Use cautiously in breast-feeding women.
⚠ *Overdose S&S:* Somnolence, impaired coordination, slurred speech, confusion, coma, decreased reflexes, hypotension, seizures, respiratory depression, apnea.

NURSING CONSIDERATIONS
☝ *Alert:* Anaphylaxis and angioedema may occur as early as the first dose; monitor the patient closely.
● Assess mental status before starting therapy, and reduce doses in elderly patients; these patients may be more sensitive to drug's adverse CNS effects.

T

- Take precautions to prevent hoarding or overdosing by patients who are depressed, suicidal, or drug-dependent or who have history of drug abuse.
- Minor changes in EEG patterns (usually low-voltage fast activity) may occur during and after therapy.
- *Look alike–sound alike:* Don't confuse Halcion with Haldol or halcinonide.

PATIENT TEACHING
⚠ *Alert:* Warn patient that drug may cause allergic reactions, facial swelling, and complex sleep-related behaviors, such as driving, eating, and making phone calls while asleep. Advise patient to report these adverse effects.
- Warn patient not to take more than prescribed amount; overdose can occur at total daily dose of 2 mg (or four times highest recommended amount).
- Tell patient to avoid alcohol use while taking drug.
- Warn patient not to stop drug abruptly after taking for 2 weeks or longer.
- Caution patient to avoid performing activities that require mental alertness or physical coordination.
- Inform patient that drug doesn't tend to cause morning drowsiness.
- Tell patient that rebound insomnia may occur for 1 or 2 nights after stopping therapy.

trospium chloride
TROZ-pee-um

Sanctura, Sanctura XR

Therapeutic class: Urinary antispasmodics
Pharmacologic class: Antimuscarinics
Pregnancy risk category: C

AVAILABLE FORMS
Capsules (extended-release): 60 mg
Tablets: 20 mg

INDICATIONS & DOSAGES
➤ **Overactive bladder with symptoms of urinary urge incontinence, urgency, and frequency**

Adults younger than age 75: 20 mg P.O. b.i.d. taken on an empty stomach or at least 1 hour before a meal. Or 60 mg extended-release capsule P.O. daily in morning.
Adjust-a-dose: For adults age 75 and older, reduce dosage to 20 mg P.O. once daily based on patient tolerance. If patient's CrCl is less than 30 mL/minute, give 20 mg (immediate-release) P.O. once daily at bedtime. Extended-release form isn't recommended if CrCl is less than 30 mL/minute.

ADMINISTRATION
P.O.
- Give at least 1 hour before meals or on an empty stomach.
- Give extended-release form with water on an empty stomach at least 1 hour before meal.

ACTION
Relaxes smooth muscle of bladder by antagonizing muscarinic receptors, relieving symptoms of overactive bladder.

Route	Onset	Peak	Duration
P.O.	Unknown	5–6 hr	Unknown

Half-life: About 20 hours.

ADVERSE REACTIONS
CNS: fatigue, headache.
EENT: dry eyes.
GI: constipation, dry mouth, abdominal pain, dyspepsia, flatulence.
GU: urine retention.

INTERACTIONS
Drug-drug. *Anticholinergics:* May increase dry mouth, constipation, or other adverse effects. Monitor patient.
Digoxin, metformin, morphine, procainamide, pancuronium, tenofovir, vancomycin: May alter elimination of these drugs or trospium, increasing levels. Monitor patient closely.
Drug-food. *High-fat foods:* May significantly decrease absorption. Give drug at least 1 hour before meals or on an empty stomach.
Drug-lifestyle. *Alcohol use:* May increase drowsiness. Discourage use together.

EFFECTS ON LAB TEST RESULTS
None reported.

CONTRAINDICATIONS & CAUTIONS

• Contraindicated in patients hypersensitive to the drug or any of its ingredients and in those with or at risk for urine retention, gastric retention, or uncontrolled angle-closure glaucoma.

• Use cautiously in patients with significant bladder outflow obstruction, obstructive GI disorders, ulcerative colitis, intestinal atony, myasthenia gravis, renal insufficiency, moderate or severe hepatic impairment, or controlled angle-closure glaucoma.

⚠ **Overdose S&S:** Severe anticholinergic effects, tachycardia, mydriasis.

NURSING CONSIDERATIONS

• Assess patient to determine baseline bladder function, and monitor patient for therapeutic effects.

• Monitor patient for residual urine after voiding.

• If patient has bladder outflow obstruction, watch for evidence of urine retention.

• Monitor patient for decreased gastric motility and constipation.

• Elderly patients typically need a reduced dosage because they have an increased risk of anticholinergic effects.

PATIENT TEACHING

• Tell patient to take drug on an empty stomach or at least 1 hour before meals.

• Tell patient to take extended-release form with water in the morning on an empty stomach, at least 1 hour before a meal.

• Discourage use of other drugs that may cause dry mouth, constipation, blurred vision, or urine retention.

• Tell patient that alcohol may increase drowsiness and fatigue. Urge him to avoid excessive alcohol consumption while taking trospium.

• Explain that drug may decrease sweating and increase the risk of heatstroke when used in hot environments or during strenuous activities.

• Urge patient to avoid activities that are hazardous or require mental alertness until he knows how the drug affects him.

ulipristal acetate
UE-li-PRIS-tal

ella

Therapeutic class: Contraceptives
Pharmacologic class: Progesterone agonists–antagonists
Pregnancy risk category: X

AVAILABLE FORMS
Tablets: 30 mg

INDICATIONS & DOSAGES

➤ **Prevention of pregnancy following unprotected intercourse or a known or suspected contraceptive failure**

Women and postmenarchal adolescents: 30 mg (1 tablet) P.O. as soon as possible within 120 hours (5 days) after unprotected intercourse or a known or suspected contraceptive failure.

ADMINISTRATION

P.O.

• May give without regard for food.

• May give at any time during the menstrual cycle.

ACTION

Inhibits or delays ovulation and alters endometrium to avoid egg implantation.

Route	Onset	Peak	Duration
P.O.	1 hr	Unknown	Unknown

Half-life: 32 hours.

ADVERSE REACTIONS

CNS: headache, fatigue, dizziness.
GI: nausea, abdominal pain.
GU: dysmenorrhea, intermenstrual bleeding.
Skin: acne.

INTERACTIONS

Drug-drug. *CYP3A4 inducers (barbiturates, bosentan, carbamazepine, felbamate, griseofulvin, oxcarbazepine, phenytoin, rifampin, topiramate):* May decrease effectiveness of contraceptive. Monitor clinical response and adjust dosage if needed.

U

CYP3A4 inhibitors (itraconazole, ketoconazole): May increase serum ulipristal levels and risk of adverse reactions. Monitor clinical response and adjust dosage if needed.

Hormonal contraceptives: May decrease effectiveness of regular hormonal contraceptives if used in the same menstrual cycle. Barrier method of contraception should be used during that cycle.

Drug-herb. *St. John's wort:* May decrease effectiveness of contraceptive. Monitor efficacy.

EFFECTS ON LAB TEST RESULTS
None reported.

CONTRAINDICATIONS & CAUTIONS
• Contraindicated in patients with known or suspected pregnancy, or for use as routine contraception.
• Contraindicated in prepubescent and postmenopausal females.
• Safety and effectiveness of repeated use within the same menstrual cycle aren't known.
• Breast-feeding women shouldn't use drug.

NURSING CONSIDERATIONS
• If vomiting occurs within 3 hours of taking drug, prescriber should consider repeating dose.
• Rule out pregnancy by obtaining history and physical examination before drug administration. If pregnancy isn't ruled out, perform pregnancy test.
• Perform follow-up physical and pelvic examination if there is concern about patient's health or pregnancy status following drug administration.
• Ulipristal won't terminate existing pregnancy.
• Rule out ectopic pregnancy in those who become pregnant or complain of lower abdominal pain 3 to 5 weeks after ulipristal use.
• Fertility returns rapidly following drug administration; routine contraceptives should be initiated or continued as soon as possible.
• Drug may reduce efficacy of regular hormonal contraceptives; additional use of a barrier method is recommended for subsequent intercourse during the same menstrual cycle.

• After drug administration, menses can occur a few days earlier or later than usual. If menses is late (beyond 1 week), rule out pregnancy.
• Drug doesn't protect against HIV infection (AIDS) or other sexually transmitted infections.
• **Look alike–sound alike:** Don't confuse ulipristal with ursodiol.

PATIENT TEACHING
• Educate patient that drug isn't intended for routine use as a contraceptive, won't terminate an existing pregnancy, and should only be used once per menstrual cycle.
• Warn patient not to use ulipristal if she suspects she is pregnant or is breast-feeding because potential risks to the infant are unknown.
• Tell patient to report lower abdominal pain immediately.
• Instruct patient to resume routine contraceptives as soon as possible, and to use a barrier method during the same menstrual cycle.
• Advise patient that after drug administration, menses can occur a few days earlier or later than usual and that she should report if menses is late (beyond 1 week) because pregnancy will have to be ruled out.
• Warn patient that drug doesn't protect against HIV infection (AIDS) or other sexually transmitted infections.

ustekinumab
US-te-KIN-ue-mab

Stelara

Therapeutic class: Immune response modifiers
Pharmacologic class: Monoclonal antibodies
Pregnancy risk category: B

AVAILABLE FORMS
Injection: 45 mg/0.5 mL, 90 mg/mL single-use vials or prefilled syringes

INDICATIONS & DOSAGES
➤ **Moderate to severe plaque psoriasis in patients who are candidates for phototherapy or systemic therapy**

Reactions in bold italics are *life-threatening*. Interactions may have a *rapid onset* or a *delayed onset*.

Adults weighing more than 100 kg (220 lb):
Initially, 90 mg subcutaneously; repeat dose
in 4 weeks, followed by maintenance dose of
90 mg subcutaneously every 12 weeks.
Adults weighing 100 kg or less: Initially,
45 mg subcutaneously; repeat dose in
4 weeks, followed by maintenance dose
of 45 mg subcutaneously every 12 weeks.
➤ **Psoriatic arthritis as monotherapy or
in combination with methotrexate**
Adults: Initially, 45 mg subcutaneously;
repeat in 4 weeks. Then maintenance dose
of 45 mg subcutaneously every 12 weeks.
➤ **Psoriatic arthritis with coexistent
moderate to severe plaque psoriasis as
monotherapy or in combination with
methotrexate**
Adults weighing more than 100 kg (220 lb):
Initially, 90 mg subcutaneously: repeat
dose in 4 weeks. Then maintenance dose of
90 mg subcutaneously every 12 weeks.

ADMINISTRATION
Subcutaneous
● Before administration, inspect ustekinumab for particulate matter and discoloration. Drug is colorless to light yellow and
may contain a few small translucent or white
particles. Don't use if discolored or cloudy
or if other particulate matter is present.
🜚 *Alert:* The needle cover on the prefilled
syringe contains dry natural rubber (a
derivative of latex). Persons sensitive to
latex shouldn't handle needle cover.
● Each subcutaneous injection should be
administered at a different anatomic location
(such as upper arms, gluteal regions, thighs,
or any quadrant of abdomen) than the previous injection; drug shouldn't be administered into areas where the skin is tender,
bruised, erythematous, or indurated.
● Drug should only be administered under
the guidance and supervision of a health
care provider and to patients who will be
closely monitored and have regular follow-
up visits with a health care provider.

ACTION
Antagonizes interleukin 12 and 23 cytokines
by binding to an interleukin-specific P40
protein subunit that disrupts interleukin-
based inflammatory and immune responses.

Route	Onset	Peak	Duration
Subcut.	Unknown	7–13½ days	Unknown

Half-life: 15 to 46 days.

ADVERSE REACTIONS
CNS: depression, dizziness, fatigue,
headache.
EENT: nasopharyngitis, pharyngolaryngeal
pain.
GI: diarrhea.
Musculoskeletal: back pain, myalgia.
Respiratory: upper respiratory tract infec-
tion.
Skin: injection-site erythema, pruritus.

INTERACTIONS
Drug-drug. *CYP450 substrates (cyclosporine, warfarin):* May alter drug
concentrations. Monitor patient for clinical effects and adjust dosage as needed.
Live-virus vaccines: May transmit infection.
Use together is contraindicated.

EFFECTS ON LAB TEST RESULTS
None reported.

CONTRAINDICATIONS & CAUTIONS
🜚 *Alert:* Don't administer live-virus vaccines during or after treatment.
● Contraindicated in patients with clinically
significant hypersensitivity to drug or its
components. Hypersensitivity reactions,
including anaphylaxis and angioedema,
have been reported.
● Drug may increase risk of infections and
reactivation of latent infections, including
serious bacterial, fungal, and viral infections.
● Drug is contraindicated in patients with a
clinically important active infection. Don't
administer ustekinumab until the infection
resolves or is adequately treated. Instruct
patients to seek medical advice if signs or
symptoms suggestive of an infection occur.
Exercise caution when considering the use
of ustekinumab in patients with a chronic
infection or a history of recurrent infection.
● Don't administer to patients with active
tuberculosis (TB). Initiate treatment of latent TB before administering ustekinumab.
Consider antituberculosis therapy before
initiation of ustekinumab in patients with

U

a history of latent or active TB in which an adequate course of treatment can't be confirmed.

• Drug may increase the risk of malignancy. Safety of ustekinumab hasn't been evaluated in patients with a history of malignancy or a known malignancy.

• The rapid appearance of multiple cutaneous squamous cell carcinomas in patients with preexisting risk factors for developing nonmelanoma skin cancer has been reported.

• Drug may cause reversible posterior leukoencephalopathy syndrome (RPLS). Signs and symptoms include headache, seizures, confusion, and visual disturbances. If RPLS is suspected, discontinue drug and administer appropriate treatment.

• Drug hasn't been studied in pregnant women. Use drug during pregnancy only if the potential benefit outweighs the potential risk to the fetus.

• It isn't known whether drug appears in breast milk. Use cautiously in breastfeeding women.

NURSING CONSIDERATIONS

• Evaluate patients for TB before initiating drug. Closely monitor patients receiving drug for signs and symptoms of active TB (fever, cough, night sweats, fatigue, and unexplained weight loss) during and after treatment.

• Patients should receive all immunizations appropriate for age as recommended by current immunization guidelines before starting treatment. Patients being treated with ustekinumab shouldn't receive live-virus vaccines. Don't give bacillus Calmette-Guérin vaccines for 1 year before initiating treatment, during treatment, or for 1 year after discontinuation of treatment.

• Use caution when administering live-virus vaccines to household contacts of patient receiving drug because of the potential risk of shedding from the household contact and transmission to patient.

• Non-live-virus vaccinations received by patient during a course of ustekinumab may not elicit an immune response sufficient to prevent disease.

• Monitor patients for signs and symptoms of infection (fever, fatigue, sore throat,

erythema, pain, cough). If infection develops, withhold drug and treat infection.

• Monitor patient for signs and symptoms of RPLS.

• Monitor all patients for the appearance of nonmelanoma skin cancer. Patients older than age 60, those with a medical history of prolonged immunosuppressive therapy, and those with a history of psoralen-ultraviolet A treatment should be followed closely.

• After proper training in subcutaneous injection technique, a patient may self-inject drug if health care provider determines it's appropriate.

PATIENT TEACHING

• Instruct patient to immediately report signs or symptoms of RPLS (headache, seizures, confusion, and visual disturbances).

• Inform patient that drug may lower the ability of the immune system to fight infections. Stress importance of communicating any history of infections to the health care provider and contacting the health care provider if signs or symptoms of infection develop.

• Advise patient to seek immediate medical attention if signs or symptoms of serious allergic reactions occur.

• Instruct patient or caregiver in injection techniques. Assess their ability to inject subcutaneously to ensure proper administration. The first self-injection should be performed under the supervision of a qualified health care professional.

• Instruct patient to inject full amount of drug according to directions provided in the Medication Guide.

• Advise patient that the needle cover on the prefilled syringe contains dry natural rubber (a derivative of latex), which may cause allergic reactions in individuals sensitive to latex.

• Instruct patient or caregiver in proper technique for syringe and needle disposal (such as using a puncture-resistant container). Advise patient not to reuse needles or syringes.

• Caution patient to avoid live-virus vaccines during and after therapy.

• Warn patient that drug may increase the risk of malignancy.

Reactions in bold italics are *life-threatening*. Interactions may have a *rapid onset* or a *delayed onset*.

valacyclovir hydrochloride
val-ah-SYE-kloe-ver

Valtrex✐

Therapeutic class: Antivirals
Pharmacologic class: Nucleosides–nucleotides
Pregnancy risk category: B

AVAILABLE FORMS
Tablets: 500 mg, 1,000 mg

INDICATIONS & DOSAGES
➤ **Herpes zoster infection (shingles)**
Adults: 1 g P.O. t.i.d. for 7 days.
Adjust-a-dose: For patients with CrCl of 30 to 49 mL/minute, give 1 g P.O. every 12 hours; if clearance is 10 to 29 mL/minute, give 1 g P.O. every 24 hours; if clearance is less than 10 mL/minute, give 500 mg P.O. every 24 hours.
➤ **First episode of genital herpes**
Adults: 1 g P.O. b.i.d. for 10 days.
Adjust-a-dose: For patients with CrCl of 10 to 29 mL/minute, give 1 g P.O. every 24 hours; if clearance is less than 10 mL/minute, give 500 mg P.O. every 24 hours.
➤ **Recurrent genital herpes in immunocompetent patients**
Adults: 500 mg P.O. b.i.d. for 3 days, given at the first sign or symptom of an episode.
Adjust-a-dose: For patients with CrCl of 29 mL/minute or less, give 500 mg P.O. every 24 hours.
➤ **Long-term suppression of recurrent genital herpes**
Adults: 1 g P.O. once daily. In patients with a history of nine or fewer recurrences per year, use alternative dose of 500 mg once daily.
➤ **Patients with HIV and CD4$^+$ cell count of 100 cells/mm^3**
Adults: 500 mg P.O. b.i.d.
Adjust-a-dose: For patients with CrCl of 29 mL/minute or less, 500 mg P.O. every 24 hours (every 48 hours if patient has nine or fewer occurrences per year).
➤ **Cold sores (herpes labialis)**
Adults: 2 g P.O. every 12 hours for two doses.
Children age 12 and older: 2 g b.i.d. for 1 day taken 12 hours apart.

Adjust-a-dose: For patients with CrCl of 30 to 49 mL/minute, give 1 g every 12 hours for two doses; if clearance is 10 to 29 mL/minute, give 500 mg every 12 hours for two doses; if clearance is less than 10 mL/minute, give 500 mg as a single dose.
➤ **To reduce transmission of genital herpes in patients with history of nine or fewer occurrences per year** ◆
Adults: 500 mg P.O. daily for source partner.
➤ **Chickenpox**
Children ages 2 to 18: 20 mg/kg P.O. t.i.d. for 5 days. Maximum dose is 1 g t.i.d.
➤ **Episodic therapy of genital herpes in HIV-positive patients** ◆
Adults: 1 g P.O. b.i.d. for 5 to 10 days.
➤ **Infection prophylaxis in neutropenia (adults and adolescents weighing 40 kg [88 lb] or more)** ◆
Herpes simplex virus (HSV)-seropositive adults undergoing hematopoietic stem cell transplant (HSCT): For prevention of early reactivation regardless of donor HSV status, give 500 mg/day P.O. or 500 mg P.O. b.i.d. for highly immunosuppressed patients. Start prophylaxis at beginning of conditioning and continue until engraftment or resolution of mucositis, whichever occurs last. For prevention of late reactivation in HSCT patients, give 500 mg P.O. b.i.d. Continue therapy until 1 year after HSCT.
HSV-seropositive patients with acute leukemia undergoing induction or reinduction: 500 mg to 1 g P.O. t.i.d was used in one small trial in this patient population. The Infectious Diseases Society of America (IDSA) recommends prophylaxis but doesn't provide a dosing recommendation. The IDSA recommends beginning prophylaxis at start of induction and continuing until WBC recovery or resolution of mucositis, whichever occurs last. Prophylaxis can be extended for patients with frequent recurrences of HSV infection.
Varicella zoster virus postexposure prophylaxis for HSCT patients who develop a rash: 1 g P.O. t.i.d. Treat for 22 days after exposure.
Varicella zoster virus reactivation prophylaxis for allogeneic and autologous HSCT patients: 500 mg P.O. b.i.d. Duration of prophylaxis is 1 year. Prophylaxis may be continued beyond 1 year in allogeneic HSCT

V

patients with chronic graft-versus-host disease (GVHD) and in those receiving systemic immunosuppressants.

➤ **Infection prophylaxis in neutropenia (children weighing less than 40 kg [88 lb])** ◆

HSV-seropositive patients undergoing HSCT: For prevention of early reactivation regardless of donor HSV status, give 250 mg P.O. b.i.d. Start prophylaxis at beginning of conditioning and continue until engraftment or resolution of mucositis, whichever occurs last. For prevention of late reactivation in HSCT patients, give 250 mg P.O. b.i.d. Continue therapy until 1 year after HSCT.

Varicella zoster virus postexposure prophylaxis for HSCT recipients who develop a rash: 500 mg P.O. t.i.d. or 600 mg/m² P.O. q.i.d. Treat for 22 days after exposure.

Varicella zoster virus reactivation prophylaxis for allogenic and autologous HSCT patients: 250 mg P.O. b.i.d. Duration of prophylaxis is 1 year. Prophylaxis may be continued beyond 1 year in allogenic HSCT patients with chronic GVHD and in those receiving systemic immunosuppressants. Some experts advocate continuing prophylaxis until 6 months after discontinuation of all immunosuppressants.

ADMINISTRATION
P.O.
● Give drug without regard for meals.

ACTION
Rapidly converts to acyclovir, which in turn becomes incorporated into viral DNA, thereby terminating growth of the DNA chain; inhibits viral DNA polymerase, causing inhibition of viral replication.

Route	Onset	Peak	Duration
P.O.	30 min	Unknown	Unknown

Half-life: 2½ to 3¼ hours.

ADVERSE REACTIONS
CNS: headache, depression, dizziness.
GI: nausea, abdominal pain, diarrhea, vomiting.
GU: dysmenorrhea.
Musculoskeletal: arthralgia.

INTERACTIONS
Drug-drug. *Cimetidine, probenecid:* May reduce rate but not extent of conversion of valacyclovir to acyclovir and may decrease renal clearance of acyclovir, thus increasing acyclovir level. Monitor patient for acyclovir toxicity.

EFFECTS ON LAB TEST RESULTS
● May increase alkaline phosphatase, ALT, AST, and creatinine levels. May decrease hemoglobin level.
● May decrease platelet and WBC counts.

CONTRAINDICATIONS & CAUTIONS
● Contraindicated in patients hypersensitive to or intolerant of valacyclovir, acyclovir, or components of the formulation.
⊙ *Alert:* Drug isn't recommended for use in bone marrow or renal transplant recipients because thrombotic thrombocytopenic purpura and hemolytic-uremic syndrome may occur in these patients at doses of 8 g/day.
● Use cautiously in elderly patients, those with renal impairment, and those receiving other nephrotoxic drugs. Monitor renal function test results.
● Give drug to pregnant woman only if potential benefits outweigh fetal risk.
● If patient is breast-feeding, drug may need to be stopped.
● Safety and effectiveness in prepubertal children haven't been established.
⚠ *Overdose S&S:* Precipitation of acyclovir in renal tubules.

NURSING CONSIDERATIONS
● Safety and effectiveness of therapy beyond 6 months haven't been established.
● Start treatment for herpes zoster infection at earliest signs or symptoms. It's most effective when started within 48 hours of onset of rash.
● *Look alike–sound alike:* Don't confuse valacyclovir (Valtrex) with valganciclovir (Valcyte) or acyclovir. Don't confuse Valtrex with Keflex or Zovirax.

PATIENT TEACHING
● Inform patient that drug may be taken without regard for meals.

- Teach patient the signs and symptoms of herpes infection (rash, tingling, itching, and pain), and advise him to notify prescriber immediately if they occur. Treatment should begin as soon as possible after symptoms appear, preferably within 48 hours of the onset of zoster rash.
- Tell patient that drug isn't a cure for herpes but may decrease the length and severity of symptoms.
- Advise patient to maintain adequate hydration.

valganciclovir hydrochloride
val-gan-SYE-kloe-veer

Valcyte

Therapeutic class: Antivirals
Pharmacologic class: Nucleosides–nucleotides
Pregnancy risk category: C

AVAILABLE FORMS
Oral solution: 50 mg/mL
Tablets: 450 mg

INDICATIONS & DOSAGES
Adjust-a-dose (for all indications): For adult patients with CrCl of 40 to 59 mL/minute, induction dosage is 450 mg b.i.d.; maintenance dosage is 450 mg daily. If clearance is 25 to 39 mL/minute, induction dosage is 450 mg daily; maintenance dosage is 450 mg every 2 days. If clearance is 10 to 24 mL/minute, induction dosage is 450 mg every 2 days; maintenance dosage is 450 mg twice weekly.
➤ **To prevent CMV disease in heart, kidney, and kidney-pancreas transplantation in patients at high risk (donor CMV-seropositive or recipient CMV-seronegative)**
Adults: For patients with a heart or kidney-pancreas transplant, give 900 mg P.O. once daily starting within 10 days of transplantation until 100 days post-transplantation. For patients with a kidney transplant, give 900 mg P.O. daily starting within 10 days of transplantation until 200 days post-transplantation.

➤ **To prevent CMV disease in pediatric kidney and heart transplant patients at high risk**
Children age 4 months to 16 years: Give dose once daily starting within 10 days of transplantation until 100 days post-transplantation based on BSA and CrCl (modified Schwartz formula):

$$\text{Dose (mg)} = 7 \times \text{BSA} \times \text{CrCl}$$

Adjust-a-dose: For pediatric patients, the maximum calculated CrCl (modified Schwartz formula) to be used is 150 mL/minute/1.73 m^2, even if the calculated value is greater. The maximum pediatric dose is 900 mg, even if the calculated dose is greater.
➤ **CMV retinitis in patients with AIDS**
Adults: For active disease, give 900 mg P.O. b.i.d. with food for 21 days; maintenance dose is 900 mg P.O. daily with food. For inactive disease, give 900 mg P.O. once daily.

ADMINISTRATION
P.O.
- Give drug with food.

ACTION
Converted to the active drug ganciclovir, which inhibits replication of CMV.

Route	Onset	Peak	Duration
P.O.	Unknown	1–3 hr	Unknown

Half-life: 4 hours.

ADVERSE REACTIONS
CNS: pyrexia, tremor, headache, insomnia, peripheral neuropathy, paresthesia, tremors, *seizures,* fatigue, pain, weakness, depression, psychosis, hallucinations, confusion, agitation.
CV: hypertension, edema, peripheral edema, hypotension.
EENT: retinal detachment, pharyngitis, nasopharyngitis.
GI: diarrhea, nausea, vomiting, constipation, abdominal pain, dyspepsia, abdominal distention, ascites.
GU: UTI, renal impairment, dysuria, decreased CrCl.

V

Hematologic: *neutropenia,* anemia, *thrombocytopenia, bleeding, pancytopenia, bone marrow depression, aplastic anemia.*
Hepatic: abnormal hepatic function.
Metabolic: hyperkalemia, hypokalemia, hypomagnesemia, hyperglycemia, decreased appetite, dehydration, hypophosphatemia, hypocalcemia.
Musculoskeletal: back pain, arthralgia, muscle cramps, limb pain.
Respiratory: upper respiratory tract infection, cough, dyspnea, pleural effusion.
Skin: dermatitis, pruritus, acne.
Other: graft rejection, catheter-related infections, hypersensitivity reactions, local and systemic infections, *sepsis,* postoperative wound infection, increased wound drainage, wound dehiscence.

INTERACTIONS
Imipenem: May increase risk of seizures. Don't use together.
Mycophenolate mofetil: May increase levels of both drugs in renally impaired patients. Use together cautiously.
Nucleoside reverse transcriptase inhibitors: May cause hematologic toxicity. Consider therapy modification.
Probenecid: May decrease renal clearance of ganciclovir. Monitor patient for ganciclovir toxicity.
Tenofovir: May increase serum levels of both drugs. Monitor patient.
Drug-food. *Any food:* May increase drug absorption. Give drug with food.

EFFECTS ON LAB TEST RESULTS
• May increase creatinine level.
• May decrease hemoglobin level and hematocrit and neutrophil, platelet, RBC, and WBC counts.

CONTRAINDICATIONS & CAUTIONS
• Contraindicated in patients hypersensitive to valganciclovir or ganciclovir. Don't use in patients receiving hemodialysis.
• Drug isn't indicated for use in liver transplant patients.
• The safety and effectiveness of drug for the prevention of CMV disease in other solid organ transplant patients, such as lung transplant patients, haven't been established.

• Use cautiously in patients with cytopenias and in those who have received immunosuppressants or radiation.
⚠ *Overdose S&S:* Bone marrow depression, renal toxicity.

NURSING CONSIDERATIONS
• Adhere to dosing guidelines for valganciclovir because ganciclovir and valganciclovir aren't interchangeable and overdose may occur.
Black Box Warning Toxicities include severe leukopenia, neutropenia, anemia, pancytopenia, bone marrow depression, aplastic anemia, and thrombocytopenia. Don't use if patient's ANC is less than 500/mm^3, platelet count is less than 25,000/mm^3, or hemoglobin level is less than 8 g/dL. ∎
• Monitor CBC, platelet counts, and creatinine level or CrCl values frequently during treatment.
• Cytopenia may occur at any time during treatment and may increase with continued use. Counts usually recover 3 to 7 days after stopping drug.
• No drug interaction studies have been conducted but, because drug is converted to ganciclovir, assume that drug interactions will be similar.
Black Box Warning In animal studies, drug was carcinogenic and teratogenic and caused aspermatogenesis. ∎
• *Look alike–sound alike:* Don't confuse valganciclovir hydrochloride (Valcyte) with valacyclovir (Valtrex). Don't confuse Valcyte with Valium.

PATIENT TEACHING
• Tell patient to take drug with food.
• Tell patient to follow dosage instructions precisely. Ganciclovir capsules and valganciclovir tablets aren't interchangeable.
• Advise patient that blood tests are needed during treatment. Doses may need to be adjusted based on blood counts.
• Tell woman of childbearing potential to use contraception during treatment. Tell man to use barrier contraception during and for 90 days after treatment.
• Advise patient that ganciclovir is a carcinogen.

• Tell patient that CNS effects (seizures, ataxia, dizziness) can occur and to use care in driving or operating machinery.
• Advise patient that this drug isn't a cure for CMV retinitis and that the condition may recur. Tell patient to see an ophthalmologist at least every 4 to 6 weeks during treatment.

valproate sodium
val-PROH-ayt

Depacon

valproic acid
Depakene, Stavzor

divalproex sodium
Depakote☙, Depakote ER, Depakote Sprinkle☙, Epival ECT†

Therapeutic class: Anticonvulsants
Pharmacologic class: Carboxylic acid derivatives
Pregnancy risk category: D

AVAILABLE FORMS
valproate sodium
Injection: 100 mg/mL
Syrup: 250 mg/5 mL
valproic acid
Capsules: 250 mg
Capsules (delayed-release): 125 mg, 250 mg, 500 mg
Syrup: 200 mg/5 mL
Tablets (enteric-coated): 200 mg, 500 mg
divalproex sodium
Capsules (sprinkle): 125 mg
Tablets (delayed-release): 125 mg, 250 mg, 500 mg
Tablets (extended-release): 250 mg, 500 mg

INDICATIONS & DOSAGES
Adjust-a-dose (for all indications): For elderly patients, start at lower dosage. Increase dosage more slowly and with regular monitoring of fluid and nutritional intake, and watch for dehydration, somnolence, and other adverse reactions.
➤ **Simple and complex absence seizures, mixed seizure types (including absence seizures)**

Adults and children: Initially, 15 mg/kg P.O. or I.V. daily; then increase by 5 to 10 mg/kg daily at weekly intervals up to maximum of 60 mg/kg daily. Don't use Depakote ER in children younger than age 10.
➤ **Complex partial seizures**
Adults and children age 10 and older: 10 to 15 mg/kg Depakote or Depakote ER P.O. or valproate sodium I.V. daily; then increase by 5 to 10 mg/kg daily at weekly intervals, up to 60 mg/kg daily.
➤ **Mania**
Adults: Initially, 750 mg Depakote P.O. daily in divided doses, or 25 mg/kg Depakote ER P.O. once daily. Adjust dosage based on patient's response; maximum dose for either form is 60 mg/kg daily. Or, Stavzor 750 mg P.O. daily in divided doses. Maximum recommended dosage is 60 mg/kg/day.
➤ **To prevent migraine headache**
Adults: Initially, 250 mg delayed-release divalproex sodium P.O. b.i.d. Some patients may need up to 1,000 mg daily. Or, 500 mg Depakote ER P.O. daily for 1 week; then 1,000 mg P.O. daily. Or, Stavzor 250 mg P.O. b.i.d. Some patients may benefit from 1,000 mg/day. Maximum recommended dosage is 60 mg/kg/day.

ADMINISTRATION
P.O.
• Give drug with food or milk to reduce adverse GI effects.
• Don't mix syrup with carbonated beverages; mixture may be irritating to oral mucosa.
• Don't give syrup to patients who need sodium restriction. Check with prescriber.
• Capsules may be swallowed whole or opened and contents sprinkled on a teaspoonful of soft food. Patient should swallow immediately without chewing.
I.V.
▼ I.V. use is indicated only in patients who can't take drug orally. Switch patient to oral form as soon as feasible; effects of I.V. use for longer than 14 days are unknown.
▼ Dilute valproate sodium injection with at least 50 mL of a compatible diluent. It's physically compatible and chemically stable in D_5W, normal saline solution, and lactated Ringer solution for 24 hours.

V

▼ Infuse drug over 60 minutes at no more than 20 mg/minute and at the same frequency as oral dosage.

▼ Monitor drug level, and adjust dosage as needed.

▼ **Incompatibilities:** None reported.

ACTION

Unknown. Probably facilitates the effects of the inhibitory neurotransmitter GABA.

Route	Onset	Peak	Duration
P.O.	Unknown	15 min–4 hr	Unknown
I.V.	Unknown	1 hr	Unknown

Half-life: 6 to 16 hours.

ADVERSE REACTIONS

CNS: asthenia, dizziness, headache, insomnia, nervousness, somnolence, tremor, abnormal thinking, amnesia, ataxia, depression, emotional upset, fever.
CV: chest pain, edema, hypertension, hypotension, tachycardia.
EENT: blurred vision, diplopia, nystagmus, pharyngitis, rhinitis, tinnitus.
GI: abdominal pain, anorexia, diarrhea, dyspepsia, nausea, vomiting, *pancreatitis,* constipation, increased appetite.
Hematologic: *bone marrow suppression, hemorrhage, thrombocytopenia,* bruising, petechiae.
Hepatic: *hepatotoxicity.*
Metabolic: hyperammonemia, weight gain or loss.
Musculoskeletal: back and neck pain.
Respiratory: bronchitis, dyspnea.
Skin: alopecia, *erythema multiforme, hypersensitivity reactions, Stevens-Johnson syndrome,* rash, photosensitivity reactions, pruritus.
Other: flulike syndrome, infection.

INTERACTIONS

Drug-drug. *Aspirin, chlorpromazine, cimetidine, erythromycin, felbamate:* May cause valproic acid toxicity. Use together cautiously and monitor drug level.
Benzodiazepines, other CNS depressants: May cause excessive CNS depression. Avoid using together.
Carbamazepine: May cause carbamazepine CNS toxicity; may decrease valproic acid level and cause loss of seizure control.

Use together cautiously, if at all. Monitor patient for seizure activity and toxicity during therapy and for at least 1 month after stopping either drug.
Lamotrigine: May increase lamotrigine level; may decrease valproate level. Monitor levels closely.
Phenobarbital: May increase phenobarbital level; may increase clearance of valproate. Monitor patient closely.
Phenytoin: May increase or decrease phenytoin level; may decrease valproate level. Monitor patient closely.
Rifampin: May decrease valproate level. Monitor level of valproate.
Warfarin: May displace warfarin from binding sites. Monitor PT and INR.
Zidovudine: May decrease zidovudine clearance. Avoid using together.
Drug-lifestyle. *Alcohol use:* May cause excessive CNS depression. Discourage use together.

EFFECTS ON LAB TEST RESULTS

● May increase ammonia, ALT, AST, and bilirubin levels.

● May increase eosinophil count and bleeding time. May decrease platelet, RBC, and WBC counts.

● May cause false-positive results for urine ketone levels.

CONTRAINDICATIONS & CAUTIONS

● Contraindicated in patients hypersensitive to drug and in those with hepatic disease or significant hepatic dysfunction, and in patients with a urea cycle disorder (UCD).
Black Box Warning Avoid use in women who may become pregnant. Valproate can cause teratogenic effects, such as neural tube defects. Drug is contraindicated for use in pregnancy for the prevention of migraines. ∎
🕒 *Alert:* There is an increased risk of lower cognitive test scores in children born to mothers who took drug during pregnancy. Consider alternative medication in pregnant women unless the use of drug is essential. Women of childbearing age should use effective birth control during therapy.
● Safety and effectiveness of Depakote ER in children younger than age 10 haven't been established.

⚠ **Overdose S&S:** Somnolence, heart block, deep coma.

NURSING CONSIDERATIONS

• Obtain LFT results, platelet count, and PT and INR before starting therapy, and monitor these values periodically.

☺ **Alert:** Closely monitor all patients taking or starting antiepileptic drugs for changes in behavior indicating worsening of suicidal thoughts or behavior or depression. Symptoms such as anxiety, agitation, hostility, mania, and hypomania may be precursors to emerging suicidality.

• Adverse reactions may not be caused by valproic acid alone because it's usually used with other anticonvulsants.

• When converting adults and children age 10 and older with seizures from Depakote to Depakote ER, make sure the extended-release dose is 8% to 20% higher than the regular dose taken previously. See manufacturer's package insert for more details.

• Divalproex sodium has a lower risk of adverse GI reactions.

• Never withdraw drug suddenly because sudden withdrawal may worsen seizures. Call prescriber at once if adverse reactions develop.

Black Box Warning Fatal hepatotoxicity may follow nonspecific symptoms, such as malaise, fever, anorexia, facial edema, vomiting, weakness, and lethargy. If these symptoms occur during therapy, notify prescriber at once because patient who might be developing hepatic dysfunction must stop taking drug. Perform LFTs before initiating therapy and at frequent intervals, especially during the first 6 months. ∎

Black Box Warning Patients at high risk for hepatotoxicity include those with congenital metabolic disorders, mental retardation, or organic brain disease; those taking multiple anticonvulsants; and children younger than age 2. ∎

• Notify prescriber if tremors occur; a dosage reduction may be needed.

• Monitor drug level. Therapeutic level is commonly considered to be 50 to 100 mcg/mL.

• When converting patients from a brand-name drug to a generic drug, use caution because breakthrough seizures may occur.

☺ **Alert:** Sometimes fatal, hyperammonemic encephalopathy may occur when starting valproate therapy in patients with UCD. Evaluate patients with UCD risk factors before starting valproate therapy. Patients who develop symptoms of unexplained hyperammonemic encephalopathy during valproate therapy should stop drug, undergo prompt appropriate treatment, and be evaluated for underlying UCD.

• **Look alike–sound alike:** Don't confuse Depakote with Depakote ER or DepaKene.

PATIENT TEACHING

• Tell patient to take drug with food or milk to reduce adverse GI effects.

• Advise patient not to chew capsules; irritation of mouth and throat may result.

• Tell patient that capsules may be either swallowed whole or carefully opened and contents sprinkled on a teaspoonful of soft food. Tell patient to swallow immediately without chewing.

• Tell patient and parents that syrup shouldn't be mixed with carbonated beverages; mixture may be irritating to mouth and throat.

• Tell patient and parents to keep drug out of children's reach.

• Warn patient and parents not to stop drug therapy abruptly.

Black Box Warning Cases of life-threatening pancreatitis have been reported in children and adults receiving valproate shortly after initial use, as well as after several years of use. Warn patients and guardians that abdominal pain, nausea, vomiting, and anorexia can be symptoms of pancreatitis that require prompt medical evaluation. ∎

• Advise patient to avoid driving and other potentially hazardous activities that require mental alertness until drug's CNS effects are known.

• Instruct patient or parents to call prescriber if malaise, weakness, lethargy, facial swelling, loss of appetite, or vomiting occurs.

• Tell woman to call prescriber if she becomes pregnant or plans to become pregnant during therapy.

V

valsartan
val-SAR-tan

Diovan♦

Therapeutic class: Antihypertensives
Pharmacologic class: Angiotensin II
receptor antagonists
Pregnancy risk category: D

AVAILABLE FORMS
Tablets: 40 mg, 80 mg, 160 mg, 320 mg

INDICATIONS & DOSAGES
➤ **Hypertension (used alone or with other antihypertensives)**
Adults: Initially, 80 or 160 mg P.O. once daily. Expect to see a reduction in blood pressure in 2 to 4 weeks. If additional antihypertensive effect is needed, dose may be increased to 160 or 320 mg daily, or a diuretic may be added. (Addition of a diuretic has a greater effect than dosage increases beyond 80 mg.) Usual dosage range is 80 to 320 mg daily.
Children ages 6 to 16: Initially, 1.3 mg/kg P.O. daily. Adjust according to patient response up to 2.7 mg/kg or 160 mg daily.
➤ **New York Heart Association class II to IV heart failure**
Adults: Initially, 40 mg P.O. b.i.d.; increase as tolerated to 80 mg b.i.d., and then to target dose of 160 mg b.i.d.
➤ **To reduce CV death in stable post-MI patients with left ventricular failure or dysfunction**
Adults: 20 mg P.O. b.i.d. Initial dose may be given as soon as 12 hours after MI. Increase dose to 40 mg b.i.d. within 7 days. Increase subsequent doses, as tolerated, to target dose of 160 mg b.i.d.

ADMINISTRATION
P.O.
• Give drug without regard for food.
• Pharmacists may prepare suspension for children unable to swallow pills.
• Shake suspension at least 10 seconds before pouring. Store suspension at room temperature for 30 days or in refrigerator for 75 days.

ACTION
Blocks the binding of angiotensin II to receptor sites in vascular smooth muscle and the adrenal gland, which inhibits the pressor effects of the renin-angiotensin-aldosterone system.

Route	Onset	Peak	Duration
P.O.	2 hr	2–4 hr	24 hr

Half-life: 6 hours.

ADVERSE REACTIONS
CNS: dizziness, headache, insomnia, fatigue, vertigo.
CV: edema, hypotension, orthostatic hypotension, syncope.
EENT: rhinitis, sinusitis, pharyngitis, blurred vision.
GI: abdominal pain, diarrhea, nausea, dyspepsia.
GU: renal impairment.
Hematologic: *neutropenia.*
Metabolic: hyperkalemia.
Musculoskeletal: arthralgia, back pain.
Respiratory: upper respiratory tract infection, cough.
Other: *angioedema,* viral infection.

INTERACTIONS
Drug-drug. *ACE inhibitors:* May increase risk of renal dysfunction and hyperkalemia. Closely monitor serum potassium level and renal function.
Aliskiren: May increase risk of renal impairment, hypotension, and hyperkalemia in diabetic patients and those with moderate to severe renal impairment (GFR less than 60 mL/minute). Concomitant use is contraindicated in diabetic patients. Avoid concomitant use in those with moderate to severe renal impairment.
Lithium: May increase lithium level. Monitor lithium level and patient for toxicity.
NSAIDs: May result in deterioration of renal function in patients who are elderly or volume-depleted and in those with compromised renal function. Monitor renal function. May also decrease antihypertensive effect. Monitor blood pressure.

Potassium supplements, potassium-sparing diuretics, other angiotensin II blockers: May increase potassium level. May also increase creatinine level in heart failure patients. Avoid using together.
Trimethoprim: May increase risk of hyperkalemia, especially in elderly patients. Closely monitor serum potassium level.
Drug-herb. *Ma huang:* May decrease antihypertensive effects. Discourage use together.
Drug-food. *Salt substitutes containing potassium:* May increase potassium level. May also increase creatinine level in heart failure patients. Discourage use together.

EFFECTS ON LAB TEST RESULTS
● May increase potassium, BUN, and creatinine levels.
● May decrease neutrophil count.

CONTRAINDICATIONS & CAUTIONS
● Contraindicated in patients hypersensitive to drug.
● Contraindicated in breast-feeding women.
Black Box Warning Drugs that act directly on the renin-angiotensin system can cause injury and even death to the developing fetus. When pregnancy is detected, stop drug as soon as possible. ■
● Use cautiously in patients with renal or hepatic disease.
● Safety and effectiveness of drug haven't been established in children younger than age 6 and in children of any age with GFR less than 30 mL/minute/1.73 m^2.
⚠ *Overdose S&S:* Hypotension, tachycardia, bradycardia, decreased level of consciousness, circulatory collapse.

NURSING CONSIDERATIONS
● Watch for hypotension. Excessive hypotension can occur when drug is given with high doses of diuretics.
● Correct volume and sodium depletions before starting drug.
● Suspension has 1.6 times greater exposure than tablets. Patients may require a higher dose if switched to tablets.
● Monitor serum BUN, creatinine, and potassium levels.
● *Look alike–sound alike:* Don't confuse Diovan with Dioval, Zyban, or Darvon.

PATIENT TEACHING
● Tell women of childbearing age to notify prescriber if pregnancy occurs. Drug will need to be stopped.
● Advise patient that drug may be taken without regard for food.

vancomycin hydrochloride
van-koh-MYE-sin

Vancocin

Therapeutic class: Antibiotics
Pharmacologic class: Glycopeptides
Pregnancy risk category: C; B for capsules only

AVAILABLE FORMS
Capsules: 125 mg, 250 mg
Powder for injection: 500-mg vials, 750-mg vials, 1-g vials
Premixed: 500 mg/100 mL, 750 mg/150 mL, 1 g/200 mL

INDICATIONS & DOSAGES
Adjust-a-dose (for all indications): In renal insufficiency, adjust dosage based on degree of renal impairment, drug level, severity of infection, and susceptibility of causative organism. Initially, give 15 mg/kg, and adjust subsequent doses as needed.
➤ **Serious or severe infections when other antibiotics are ineffective or contraindicated, including those caused by methicillin-resistant *Staphylococcus aureus, S. epidermidis,* or diphtheroid organisms**
Adults: 500 mg I.V. every 6 hours or 1 g I.V. every 12 hours.
Children: 10 mg/kg I.V. every 6 hours.
Neonates and young infants: 15 mg/kg I.V. loading dose; then 10 mg/kg I.V. every 12 hours if child is younger than age 1 week or 10 mg/kg I.V. every 8 hours if older than 1 week but younger than 1 month.
Elderly patients: 15 mg/kg I.V. loading dose. Subsequent doses are based on renal function and drug levels.
➤ *Clostridium difficile*–associated diarrhea
Adults: 125 mg P.O. every 6 hours for 10 days.

V

Children: 40 mg/kg P.O. daily in divided doses every 6 hours for 7 to 10 days. Maximum daily dose is 2 g.

➤ **Staphylococcal enterocolitis**
Adults: 500 mg to 2 g P.O. in three or four divided doses daily for 7 to 10 days.
Children: 40 mg/kg P.O. daily in divided doses every 6 hours for 7 to 10 days. Maximum daily dose is 2 g.

➤ **Preoperative antimicrobial prophylaxis for GU and GI (excluding esophageal) tract procedures ◆**
Adults: 1 g I.V. slowly over 1 to 2 hours, completing infusion 30 minutes before procedure.
Children: 20 mg/kg I.V. over 1 to 2 hours, completing infusion 30 minutes before procedure.

➤ **C. difficile infection in patients with complete ileus ◆**
Adults: 500 mg in 100 mL normal saline solution given as a retention enema every 6 hours. Also give I.V. metronidazole and vancomycin by oral or nasogastric tube for 10 to 14 days.

ADMINISTRATION
P.O.
• Obtain specimen for culture and sensitivity tests before giving. Because of the emergence of vancomycin-resistant enterococci, reserve use of drug for treatment of serious infections caused by gram-positive bacteria resistant to beta-lactam anti-infectives.
🕃 *Alert:* Oral form is ineffective for systemic infections.
• Oral solution is stable for 2 weeks if refrigerated.

I.V.
▼ Obtain specimen for culture and sensitivity tests before giving. Because of the emergence of vancomycin-resistant enterococci, reserve use of drug for treatment of serious infections caused by gram-positive bacteria resistant to beta-lactam anti-infectives.
▼ This form is ineffective for pseudomembranous (*C. difficile*) diarrhea.
▼ Reconstitute 500-mg vial with 10 mL or 1-g vial with 20 mL sterile water for injection to provide a solution containing 50 mg/mL.

▼ For infusion, further dilute 500 mg in 100 mL or 1 g in 200 mL normal saline solution for injection or D₅W, and infuse over 60 minutes; if dose is greater than 1 g, infuse over 90 minutes.
🕃 *Alert:* Rapid infusion (over several minutes) has been associated with hypotension, shock and, rarely, cardiac arrest.
▼ Check site daily for phlebitis and irritation. Severe irritation and necrosis can result from extravasation.
▼ Refrigerate solution after reconstitution and use within 14 days.
▼ **Incompatibilities:** Albumin, alkaline solutions, aminophylline, amobarbital, amphotericin B, aztreonam, cephalosporins, chloramphenicol, chlorothiazide, corticosteroids, dexamethasone sodium phosphate, foscarnet, heavy metals, heparin, hydrocortisone, idarubicin, methotrexate, nafcillin, omeprazole, penicillin G potassium, pentobarbital, phenobarbital, phenytoin, piperacillin, piperacillin sodium–tazobactam sodium, sargramostim, sodium bicarbonate, ticarcillin disodium, ticarcillin disodium–clavulanate potassium, vitamin B complex with C, warfarin.

ACTION
Hinders bacterial cell-wall synthesis, damaging the bacterial plasma membrane and making the cell more vulnerable to osmotic pressure. Also interferes with RNA synthesis.

Route	Onset	Peak	Duration
P.O.	Unknown	Unknown	Unknown
I.V.	Immediate	Immediate	Unknown

Half-life: 6 hours.

ADVERSE REACTIONS
CNS: fever, pain.
CV: hypotension, thrombophlebitis at injection site.
EENT: ototoxicity, tinnitus.
GI: *pseudomembranous colitis,* nausea.
GU: *nephrotoxicity.*
Hematologic: *leukopenia, neutropenia,* eosinophilia.
Respiratory: dyspnea, wheezing.
Skin: red-man syndrome (with rapid I.V. infusion).
Other: *anaphylaxis,* chills, superinfection.

Reactions in bold italics are *life-threatening*. Interactions may have a *rapid onset* or a *delayed onset*.

INTERACTIONS
Drug-drug. *Aminoglycosides, amphotericin B, cisplatin, pentamidine:* May increase risk of nephrotoxicity and ototoxicity. Monitor renal function and hearing function tests.
Nondepolarizing muscle relaxants: May enhance neuromuscular blockade. Monitor patient closely.

EFFECTS ON LAB TEST RESULTS
• May increase BUN and creatinine levels.
• May increase eosinophil counts. May decrease neutrophil and WBC counts.

CONTRAINDICATIONS & CAUTIONS
• Contraindicated in patients hypersensitive to drug.
• Use cautiously in patients receiving other neurotoxic, nephrotoxic, or ototoxic drugs; in patients older than age 60; and in those with impaired hepatic or renal function, hearing loss, or allergies to other antibiotics.

NURSING CONSIDERATIONS
• Patients with renal dysfunction need dosage adjustment. Monitor blood levels to adjust I.V. dosage.
• Obtain hearing evaluation and renal function studies before therapy.
• Monitor patient's fluid balance and watch for oliguria and cloudy urine.
• Monitor patient carefully for red-man syndrome, which can occur if drug is infused too rapidly. Signs and symptoms include maculopapular rash on face, neck, trunk, and limbs and pruritus and hypotension caused by histamine release. If wheezing, urticaria, or pain and muscle spasm of the chest and back occur, stop infusion and notify prescriber.
• Don't give drug I.M.
• Monitor renal function (BUN, creatinine level and creatinine clearance, urinalysis, and urine output) during therapy.
• Monitor patient for signs and symptoms of superinfection.
• Have patient's hearing evaluated during prolonged therapy.
• For staphylococcal endocarditis, give for at least 4 weeks.
• *Look alike–sound alike:* Don't confuse vancomycin with clindamycin, gentamicin, or vibramycin.

PATIENT TEACHING
• Tell patient to take entire amount of drug exactly as directed, even after he feels better.
• Instruct patient receiving drug I.V. to report discomfort at I.V. insertion site.
• Tell patient to report ringing in ears.
• Tell patient to report adverse reactions to prescriber immediately.

vardenafil hydrochloride
var-DEN-ah-fill

Levitra✐, Staxyn

Therapeutic class: Erectile dysfunction drugs
Pharmacologic class: PDE5 inhibitors
Pregnancy risk category: B

AVAILABLE FORMS
Tablets (film-coated): 2.5 mg, 5 mg, 10 mg, 20 mg
Tablets (orally disintegrating): 10 mg

INDICATIONS & DOSAGES
➤ **Erectile dysfunction**
Adults: 10 mg P.O. as a single dose, as needed, 1 hour before sexual activity. Dosage range is 5 to 20 mg, based on effectiveness and tolerance. Maximum, 10 mg/day (Staxyn) or 20 mg/dose once (Levitra) daily.
Adjust-a-dose: For patients with moderate hepatic impairment (Child-Pugh class B) and patients age 65 and older, first dose of Levitra is 5 mg daily, as needed. Don't exceed 10 mg daily in patients with hepatic impairment. Don't use Staxyn in patients with moderate or severe hepatic impairment (Child-Pugh class B or C).

ADMINISTRATION
P.O.
• Give drug without regard for food.
• Don't split or crush orally disintegrating tablets.
• Place orally disintegrating tablet on the tongue to disintegrate. Have patient take without water.

ACTION

Increases cyclic guanosine monophosphate levels, prolongs smooth muscle relaxation, and promotes blood flow into the corpus cavernosum.

Route	Onset	Peak	Duration
P.O.	Immediate	30–120 min	Unknown

Half-life: 4 to 5 hours.

ADVERSE REACTIONS

CNS: headache, dizziness.
CV: flushing.
EENT: decrease or loss of hearing, tinnitus, rhinitis, sinusitis.
GI: dyspepsia, nausea.
Musculoskeletal: back pain.
Other: flulike syndrome.

INTERACTIONS

Drug-drug. *Alpha blockers:* May enhance hypotensive effects. Start concomitant treatment only if patient is stable on alpha-blocker therapy.
Antiarrhythmics of class IA (quinidine, procainamide) and class III (amiodarone, sotalol): May prolong QTc interval. Avoid using together.
Erythromycin, indinavir, itraconazole, ketoconazole, ritonavir: May increase vardenafil level. Reduce dose of vardenafil. If taken with ritonavir, reduce and extend dosage interval to once every 72 hours.
Nitrates: May enhance hypotensive effects. Use together is contraindicated.
Drug-food. *High-fat meals:* May reduce peak level of drug. Discourage use with a high-fat meal.
Drug-lifestyle. *Alcohol use:* May increase risk of hypotension and orthostasis. Discourage use together.

EFFECTS ON LAB TEST RESULTS

● May increase CK level.

CONTRAINDICATIONS & CAUTIONS

● Contraindicated in patients hypersensitive to drug or its components and in those taking nitrates.
● Contraindicated in patients with unstable angina, hypotension (systolic less than 90 mm Hg), uncontrolled hypertension (over 170/110 mm Hg), stroke, life-threatening arrhythmia, an MI within past 6 months, severe cardiac failure, severe hepatic impairment (Child-Pugh class C), ESRD requiring dialysis, congenital QTc-interval prolongation, or hereditary degenerative retinal disorders.
● Use cautiously in patients with bleeding disorders or significant peptic ulceration.
● Use cautiously in those with anatomic penis abnormalities or conditions that predispose patient to priapism (such as sickle cell anemia, multiple myeloma, or leukemia).
⚠ *Overdose S&S:* Back pain or myalgia, abnormal vision.

NURSING CONSIDERATIONS

❂ **Alert:** Sexual activity may increase cardiac risk. Evaluate patient's cardiac risk before he starts taking drug.
● Before patient starts drug, assess for underlying causes of erectile dysfunction.
● Transient decreases in supine blood pressure may occur.
● Prolonged erections and priapism may occur.

PATIENT TEACHING

● Tell patient that drug doesn't protect against sexually transmitted diseases and that he should use protective measures.
● Advise patient that drug is absorbed most rapidly if taken on an empty stomach.
● Tell patient to notify prescriber about vision or hearing changes.
● Urge patient to seek immediate medical care if erection lasts more than 4 hours.
● Tell patient to take drug 60 minutes before anticipated sexual activity. Explain that drug has no effect without sexual stimulation.
● Warn patient not to change dosage unless directed by prescriber.
● Tell patient to stop drug and seek medical attention if he experiences sudden vision loss in one or both eyes or sudden decrease in or loss of hearing.
● Tell patient not to split, crush, or chew orally disintegrating tablets.

varenicline tartrate
vah-RENN-ih-kleen

Chantix⌀

Therapeutic class: Smoking cessation aids
Pharmacologic class: Nicotinic acetylcholine receptor partial agonists
Pregnancy risk category: C

AVAILABLE FORMS
Tablets: 0.5 mg, 1 mg

INDICATIONS & DOSAGES
➤ Smoking cessation
Adults: Starting 1 week before patient stops smoking, give 0.5 mg P.O. once daily on days 1 through 3. Days 4 through 7, give 0.5 mg P.O. b.i.d. Day 8 through the end of week 12, give 1 mg P.O. b.i.d. If patient successfully stops smoking, give an additional 12-week course to help with long-term success.
Adjust-a-dose: In patient with severe renal impairment, 0.5 mg P.O. once daily. Adjust as needed to maximum of 0.5 mg b.i.d. In patient with ESRD who is undergoing dialysis, 0.5 mg once daily.

ADMINISTRATION
P.O.
● Give drug with full glass of water after a meal.

ACTION
Blocks the effects of nicotine by binding at alpha₄ beta₂ neuronal nicotinic acetylcholine receptors. Drug also provides some of nicotine's effects to ease withdrawal.

Route	Onset	Peak	Duration
P.O.	4 days	3–4 hr	24 hr

Half-life: 24 hours.

ADVERSE REACTIONS
CNS: abnormal dreams, headache, insomnia, altered attention or emotions, anxiety, asthenia, depression, dizziness, fatigue, irritability, lethargy, malaise, nightmares, restlessness, sensory disturbance, sleep disorder, somnolence.
CV: chest pain, edema, hot flush, hypertension.
EENT: altered taste, epistaxis.
GI: nausea, abdominal pain, constipation, diarrhea, dry mouth, dyspepsia, flatulence, gingivitis, vomiting.
GU: menstrual disorder, polyuria.
Metabolic: decreased appetite, increased appetite, thirst.
Musculoskeletal: arthralgia, back pain, muscle cramps, myalgia.
Respiratory: dyspnea, upper respiratory tract disorder.
Skin: rash.
Other: flulike illness.

INTERACTIONS
Drug-drug. *Cimetidine:* May decrease renal clearance of varenicline. Monitor patient closely.
Nicotine-replacement therapy: May increase nausea, vomiting, dizziness, dyspepsia, and fatigue. Monitor patient closely.

EFFECTS ON LAB TEST RESULTS
● May increase LFT values.

CONTRAINDICATIONS & CAUTIONS
⊘ **Alert:** Drug may be associated with increased risk of CV events (angina, MI, need for coronary revascularization, new diagnosis of peripheral vascular disease [PVD], or admission for a procedure to treat PVD) in patients who have CV disease. Consider risks and benefits before prescribing.
● Use cautiously in pregnant or breast-feeding women, elderly patients, and patients with severe renal impairment or pre-existing psychiatric illness.
● Not recommended for use in children younger than age 18.

NURSING CONSIDERATIONS
● Assess patient's readiness and motivation to stop smoking.
Black Box Warning Monitor patient for changes in behavior, agitation, depressed mood, hostility, suicidal ideation, suicidal behavior, and worsening of preexisting psychiatric illness and report immediately. ∎

V

• Notify prescriber if patient develops intolerable nausea; dosage reduction may be needed.

• Temporarily monitor levels of drugs—such as theophylline, warfarin, and insulin—after patient stops smoking to be sure levels are still within therapeutic range.

PATIENT TEACHING

• Provide patient with educational materials and needed counseling.

• Instruct patient to choose a date to stop smoking and to begin treatment 1 week before this date.

• Advise patient to take each dose with a full glass of water after eating.

• Teach patient to gradually increase the dose over the first week to a target of 1 mg in the morning and 1 mg in the evening.

• Explain that nausea and insomnia are common and usually temporary. Urge him to contact the prescriber if adverse effects are persistently troubling; a dosage reduction may help.

• Urge patient to continue trying to abstain from smoking if he has early lapses after successfully quitting.

• Tell patient that dosages of other drugs he takes may need adjustment when he stops smoking.

• Advise patient to use caution when driving or operating machinery until effects of the drug are known.

Black Box Warning Instruct patient and family to monitor patient for changes in behavior and mood, including agitation, depression, hostility, suicidal ideation or behavior, and worsening of preexisting psychiatric illness; stop drug and report changes to health care provider immediately. ∎

• If woman plans to become pregnant or to breast-feed, explain the risks of smoking and the risks and benefits of taking drug to aid smoking cessation.

venlafaxine hydrochloride
vin-lah-FACKS-in

Effexor XR⬦

Therapeutic class: Antidepressants
Pharmacologic class: SSNRIs
Pregnancy risk category: C

AVAILABLE FORMS
Capsules (extended-release): 37.5 mg, 75 mg, 150 mg
Tablets: 25 mg, 37.5 mg, 50 mg, 75 mg, 100 mg
Tablets (extended-release): 37.5 mg, 75 mg, 150 mg, 225 mg

INDICATIONS & DOSAGES
Adjust-a-dose (for all indications): For patients with renal impairment, reduce daily amount by 25% in patients taking immediate-release tablets. Reduce by 25% to 50% in those taking extended-release form. For those undergoing hemodialysis, withhold dose until dialysis is completed. For patients with hepatic impairment, reduce daily amount by 50%.

➤ **Depression**
Adults: Initially, 75 mg (immediate-release) P.O. daily in two or three divided doses with food. Increase as tolerated and needed by 75 mg daily every 4 days. For moderately depressed outpatients, usual maximum is 225 mg daily; in certain severely depressed patients, dose may be as high as 375 mg daily. For extended-release capsules, 75 mg P.O. daily in a single dose. For some patients, it may be desirable to start at 37.5 mg P.O. daily for 4 to 7 days before increasing to 75 mg daily. Dosage may be increased by 75 mg daily every 4 days to maximum of 225 mg daily.

➤ **Generalized anxiety disorder**
Adults: Initially, 75 mg extended-release capsule P.O. daily in a single dose. For some patients, it may be desirable to start at 37.5 mg P.O. daily for 4 to 7 days before increasing to 75 mg daily. Dosage may be increased by 75 mg daily every 4 days to maximum of 225 mg daily.

Reactions in bold italics are *life-threatening*. Interactions may have a *rapid onset* or a *delayed onset*.

➤ **Panic disorder**
Adults: Initially, 37.5 mg extended-release capsule P.O. daily for 1 week, then increase dose to 75 mg daily. If patient isn't responding, may increase dose by up to 75 mg/day in no less than weekly intervals, as needed, to a maximum dose of 225 mg daily.

➤ **Social anxiety disorder**
Adults: Initially, 75 mg extended-release capsule P.O. daily as a single dose.

➤ **Hot flashes ◆**
Adults: 12.5 mg (immediate-release) P.O. b.i.d. for 4 weeks. Or, 37.5 to 150 mg (extended-release) P.O. daily for up to 3 months.

➤ **Diabetic neuropathy ◆**
Adults: 37.5 mg P.O. daily. May increase by 75 mg each week to maximum 225 mg daily.

➤ **Premenstrual dysphoric disorder ◆**
Adults: 37.5 mg P.O. once daily or 25 mg P.O. b.i.d. during first menstrual cycle. Decrease dosage as necessary during subsequent menstrual cycles.

ADMINISTRATION
P.O.
● Give drug with food and a full glass of water.
● Give capsule whole; if patient can't swallow whole, open and sprinkle contents on spoonful of applesauce; mix and give immediately. Follow with a full glass of water.

ACTION
May increase the amount of norepinephrine, serotonin, or both in the CNS by blocking their reuptake by the presynaptic neurons.

Route	Onset	Peak	Duration
P.O.	Unknown	1–2 hr	Unknown

Half-life: 5 hours.

ADVERSE REACTIONS
CNS: asthenia, headache, somnolence, dizziness, nervousness, insomnia, ***suicidal behavior,*** anxiety, tremor, abnormal dreams, paresthesia, agitation.
CV: hypertension, tachycardia, vasodilation, chest pain.
EENT: blurred vision, mydriasis, tinnitus.
GI: nausea, constipation, dry mouth, anorexia, vomiting, diarrhea, dyspepsia, flatulence.

GU: abnormal ejaculation, impotence, urinary frequency, impaired urination.
Metabolic: weight loss, hyponatremia.
Skin: diaphoresis, rash.
Other: yawning, chills, infection.

INTERACTIONS
Drug-drug. *Lithium:* May increase lithium level and neurotoxicity. Serotonin syndrome (restlessness, hallucinations, loss of coordination, fast heartbeat, rapid changes in blood pressure, increased body temperature, hyperreflexia, nausea, vomiting, and diarrhea) may occur. Monitor patient closely.
MAO inhibitors, such as phenelzine, selegiline, tranylcypromine: May cause serotonin syndrome and signs and symptoms resembling neuroleptic malignant syndrome. Avoid using within 14 days of MAO inhibitor therapy.
Methylene blue, linezolid: May cause serotonin syndrome. Use with extreme caution and monitor patient closely.
Methylphenidate, opioid analgesics (meperidine), sibutramine, **tramadol,** *trazodone:* May cause serotonin syndrome. Monitor patient closely.
Triptans: May cause serotonin syndrome or neuroleptic malignant syndrome–like reactions. Use cautiously and with increased monitoring at the start of therapy and with dose increase.
Warfarin: May increase PT, PTT, or INR. Monitor these lab values and patient closely.
Drug-herb. *Sour date nut, St. John's wort:* May cause serotonin syndrome. Monitor patient closely.
Yohimbe: May cause additive stimulation. Urge caution.

EFFECTS ON LAB TEST RESULTS
● May cause false-positive urine immunoassay screening tests for phencyclidine and amphetamine.

CONTRAINDICATIONS & CAUTIONS
● Contraindicated in patients hypersensitive to drug or within 14 days of MAO inhibitor therapy.
Black Box Warning Venlafaxine isn't approved for use in children. ∎

V

⊙ Alert: Concomitant use with linezolid or methylene blue can cause serotonin syndrome (fever, mental status changes, muscle twitching, excessive sweating, shivering or shaking, diarrhea, loss of coordination). Use drug with linezolid or methylene blue only for life-threatening or urgent conditions when the potential benefits outweigh the risks of toxicity.

• Use cautiously in patients with renal impairment, diseases or conditions that could affect hemodynamic responses or metabolism, and in those with history of mania or seizures.

• Use in third trimester of pregnancy may be associated with neonatal complications at birth. Consider the risk versus benefit of treatment during this time.

⚠ Overdose S&S: Altered level of consciousness, tachycardia, mydriasis, seizures, vomiting, ECG changes, hypotension, liver necrosis, rhabdomyolysis, serotonin syndrome, vertigo, death.

NURSING CONSIDERATIONS

⊙ Alert: Closely monitor patients being treated for depression for signs and symptoms of clinical worsening and suicidal ideation, especially at the beginning of therapy and with dosage adjustments. Symptoms may include agitation, insomnia, anxiety, aggressiveness, or panic attacks. **Black Box Warning** Drug may increase the risk of suicidal thinking and behavior in children, adolescents, and young adults ages 18 to 24, especially during the first few months of treatment, especially those with major depressive disorder or other psychiatric disorder. ∎

⊙ Alert: If linezolid or methylene blue must be given, stop venlafaxine and monitor patient for serotonin toxicity for 2 weeks or until 24 hours after last dose of methylene blue or linezolid, whichever comes first. May resume serotonergic psychiatric drugs 24 hours after last dose of methylene blue or linezolid.

• Carefully monitor blood pressure. Drug therapy may cause sustained, dose-dependent increases in blood pressure. Greatest increases (averaging about 7 mm Hg above baseline) occur in patients taking 375 mg daily.

• Monitor patient's weight, particularly underweight, depressed patients.

⊙ Alert: Combining triptans with an SSRI or an SSNRI may cause serotonin syndrome or neuroleptic malignant syndrome–like reactions. Signs and symptoms of serotonin syndrome may include restlessness, hallucinations, loss of coordination, fast heartbeat, rapid changes in blood pressure, increased body temperature, overactive reflexes, nausea, vomiting, and diarrhea. Serotonin syndrome may be more likely to occur when starting or increasing the dose of triptan, SSRI, or SSNRI.

PATIENT TEACHING

• If medication is to be stopped, inform patient who has received drug for 6 weeks or longer that drug will be stopped gradually by tapering dosage over a 2-week period, as instructed by prescriber. Patient shouldn't abruptly stop taking the drug.

Black Box Warning Warn family members to closely monitor patient for signs of worsening condition or suicidal ideation. ∎

• Warn patient to avoid hazardous activities that require alertness and good coordination until effects of drug are known.

• Tell patient to avoid alcohol and to consult prescriber before taking other prescription or OTC drugs.

• Teach patient to recognize and immediately report signs and symptoms of serotonin toxicity (fever, mental status changes, muscle twitching, excessive sweating, shivering or shaking, diarrhea, loss of coordination).

• Advise woman of childbearing age to contact prescriber if she becomes pregnant or intends to become pregnant during therapy or if she's breast-feeding.

• Tell patient to take each dose with food and a full glass of water.

• Tell patient that if he can't swallow capsule whole, he may carefully open it and sprinkle contents on a spoonful of applesauce, mix, and take immediately. Follow with a full glass of water.

---

verapamil hydrochloride
ver-AP-a-mill

Apo-Verap†, Calan⋇, Calan SR,
Covera-HS, Novo-Veramil†,
Nu-Verap†, Verelan⋇, Verelan PM

Therapeutic class: Antihypertensives
Pharmacologic class: Calcium channel
blockers
Pregnancy risk category: C

AVAILABLE FORMS
Capsules (extended-release): 100 mg,
120 mg, 180 mg, 200 mg, 240 mg, 300 mg
Capsules (sustained-release): 120 mg,
180 mg, 240 mg, 360 mg
Injection: 2.5 mg/mL
Tablets: 40 mg, 80 mg, 120 mg
Tablets (extended-release): 120 mg,
180 mg, 240 mg
Tablets (sustained-release): 120 mg,
180 mg, 240 mg

INDICATIONS & DOSAGES
➤ **Vasospastic angina (Prinzmetal or
variant angina); unstable angina; classic
chronic, stable angina pectoris; chronic
atrial fibrillation**
Adults: Starting dose is 80 to 120 mg P.O.
t.i.d. Increase dosage at daily or weekly
intervals as needed. Some patients may
require up to 480 mg daily. Don't exceed
480 mg/day. For Covera-HS, initial dose is
180 mg/day P.O. at bedtime. Dosage range is
180 to 540 mg/day P.O. at bedtime.
➤ **To prevent paroxysmal supraventricular tachycardia**
Adults: 80 to 120 mg (immediate-release)
P.O. t.i.d. or q.i.d.
➤ **Supraventricular arrhythmias**
Adults: 0.075 to 0.15 mg/kg (5 to 10 mg)
by I.V. push over 2 minutes with ECG and
blood pressure monitoring. Repeat dose
of 0.15 mg/kg (10 mg) in 30 minutes if no
response occurs.
Children ages 1 to 15: Give 0.1 to 0.3 mg/kg
as I.V. bolus over 2 minutes; not to exceed
5 mg. Repeat dose in 30 minutes if response
is inadequate.
Children younger than age 1: Give 0.1 to
0.2 mg/kg as I.V. bolus over 2 minutes with

continuous ECG monitoring. Repeat dose in
30 minutes if no response occurs.
➤ **Digitalized patients with chronic atrial
fibrillation or flutter**
Adults: 240 to 320 mg P.O. daily, in three or
four divided doses.
➤ **Hypertension**
Adults: 240 mg extended-release tablet
(Verelan) P.O. once daily in the morning.
If response isn't adequate, may increase
by 120 mg daily (maximum, 480 mg). If
using Verelan PM, 200 mg P.O. daily at
bedtime. May increase to 300 mg at bedtime
if response is inadequate. Maximum dose
is 400 mg. If using Covera-HS, 180 mg P.O.
daily at bedtime. May increase to 240 mg
daily if response is inadequate. Subsequent
dosage adjustments may be made in 120-mg
increments up to a maximum of 480 mg
at bedtime. If using Calan SR, give 180 mg
P.O. in the morning. Evaluate weekly and
approximately 24 hours after previous
dose. May increase as follows: 240 mg each
morning, 180 mg each morning plus 180 mg
each evening, or 240 mg each morning plus
120 mg each evening; 240 mg every 12 hours.
For immediate-release, 80 mg P.O. t.i.d.

ADMINISTRATION
P.O.
• Pellet-filled capsules may be given by
carefully opening the capsule and sprinkling
the pellets on a spoonful of applesauce. This
should be swallowed immediately without
chewing, followed by a glass of cool water
to ensure that all the pellets are swallowed.
• Give long-acting forms of the drug whole;
don't crush or break tablet.
I.V.
▼ This form is contraindicated in patients
receiving I.V. beta blockers and in those
with ventricular tachycardia.
▼ Inject directly into a vein or into the tubing of a free-flowing, compatible solution,
such as D_5W, half-normal saline solution,
normal saline solution, Ringer solution, or
lactated Ringer solution.
▼ Give doses over at least 2 minutes
(3 minutes in elderly patients) to minimize
the risk of adverse reactions.
▼ Monitor ECG and blood pressure continuously.

V

▼ **Incompatibilities:** Albumin, aminophylline, amphotericin B, ampicillin sodium, sulfamethoxazole–trimethoprim, dobutamine, hydralazine, nafcillin, oxacillin, propofol, sodium bicarbonate, solutions with a pH greater than 6.

ACTION

Not clearly defined. A calcium channel blocker that inhibits calcium ion influx across cardiac and smooth-muscle cells, thus decreasing myocardial contractility and oxygen demand; it also dilates coronary arteries and arterioles.

Route	Onset	Peak	Duration
P.O.	30 min	1–2 hr	8–10 hr
P.O. (extended)	30 min	5–9 hr	24 hr
I.V.	Immediate	1–5 min	1–6 hr

Half-life: 6 to 12 hours.

ADVERSE REACTIONS

CNS: dizziness, headache, asthenia, fatigue, sleep disturbances.
CV: transient hypotension, *heart failure, bradycardia, AV block, ventricular asystole, ventricular fibrillation,* peripheral edema.
GI: constipation, nausea, diarrhea, dyspepsia.
Respiratory: dyspnea, pharyngitis, *pulmonary edema,* rhinitis, sinusitis, upper respiratory infection.
Skin: rash.

INTERACTIONS

Drug-drug. *Beta blockers, digoxin:* May increase effects of both drugs. Monitor cardiac function closely and decrease doses as needed.
Amiodarone: May cause bradycardia and decrease cardiac output. Monitor patient closely.
Antihypertensives, quinidine: May cause hypotension. Monitor blood pressure.
Carbamazepine: May increase levels of carbamazepine. Monitor patient for toxicity and adjust dosage as needed.
Cyclosporine: May increase cyclosporine level. Monitor cyclosporine level.
Disopyramide, flecainide: May cause heart failure. Avoid using together.

Dofetilide: May increase dofetilide level. Avoid using together.
HMG-CoA reductase inhibitors (atorvastatin, lovastatin, simvastatin): May elevate plasma concentrations of these drugs. If coadministration can't be avoided, administer conservative dose of the HMG-CoA reductase inhibitor.
Lithium: May decrease or increase lithium level. Monitor lithium level.
Neuromuscular blockers: May potentiate the activity of these drugs. Monitor neuromuscular function and adjust dosages of either drug as needed.
Phenytoin: May decrease effects of verapamil. Monitor patient closely and adjust dose as needed.
Rifampin: May decrease oral bioavailability of verapamil. Monitor patient for lack of effect.
Sirolimus, tacrolimus: May increase levels of these drugs. Monitor drug levels closely and adjust dosage as needed.
Theophylline: May decrease clearance of theophylline. Monitor for signs of theophylline toxicity.
Drug-herb. *Black catechu:* May cause additive effects. Discourage use together.
St. John's wort: May decrease drug level and effect. Discourage use together.
Yerba maté: May decrease clearance of herb's methylxanthines and cause toxicity. Urge caution.
Drug-food. *Grapefruit juice:* May increase drug level. Discourage use together.
Drug-lifestyle. *Alcohol use:* May enhance the effects of alcohol. Discourage use together.

EFFECTS ON LAB TEST RESULTS

● May increase ALT, AST, alkaline phosphatase, and bilirubin levels.

CONTRAINDICATIONS & CAUTIONS

● Contraindicated in patients hypersensitive to drug and in those with severe left ventricular dysfunction, cardiogenic shock, second- or third-degree AV block or sick sinus syndrome except in presence of functioning pacemaker, atrial flutter or fibrillation and accessory bypass tract syndrome, severe heart failure (unless secondary to therapy), and severe hypotension.

Reactions in bold italics are *life-threatening*. Interactions may have a *rapid onset* or a *delayed onset*.

• I.V. form is contraindicated in patients receiving I.V. beta blockers and in those with ventricular tachycardia.

• Use cautiously in elderly patients and in those with increased intracranial pressure or hepatic or renal disease.

⚠ **Overdose S&S:** Hypotension, bradycardia, arrhythmias, hyperglycemia, depressed mental status, noncardiogenic pulmonary edema, increasing AV block.

NURSING CONSIDERATIONS

• Patients receiving beta blockers should receive lower doses of this drug. Monitor these patients closely.

• When clinically advisable, have the patient perform vagal maneuvers before giving drug.

• Frequently monitor PR interval.

• Monitor blood pressure at the start of therapy and during dosage adjustments. Assist patient with walking because dizziness may occur.

• If signs and symptoms of heart failure occur, such as swelling of hands and feet and shortness of breath, notify prescriber.

• Monitor renal function test and LFT results during prolonged treatment.

• **Look alike–sound alike:** Don't confuse Verelan with Vivarin, Voltaren, or Virilon.

PATIENT TEACHING

• Instruct patient to take oral form of drug exactly as prescribed.

• Tell patient that long-acting forms shouldn't be crushed or chewed.

• Caution patient against abruptly stopping drug.

• If patient continues nitrate therapy during oral verapamil dosage adjustment, urge continued compliance. S.L. nitroglycerin may be taken, as needed, for acute chest pain.

• Encourage patient to increase fluid and fiber intake to combat constipation. Give a stool softener.

• Drug significantly inhibits alcohol elimination. Advise patient to avoid or severely limit alcohol use.

• Inform patient taking Covera-HS that the outer shell of the drug may be excreted in feces.

vigabatrin
veye-gah-BA-trin

Sabril

Therapeutic class: Anticonvulsants
Pharmacologic class: GABA transaminase inhibitors
Pregnancy risk category: C

AVAILABLE FORMS
Powder for oral solution: 500 mg
Tablets: 500 mg

INDICATIONS & DOSAGES
➤ **Refractory complex partial seizures**
Adults and children age 16 and older and children age 10 to 16 weighing more than 60 kg (132 lb): Initially, 500 mg P.O. b.i.d. May increase dosage by 500 mg weekly to maximum of 1,500 mg P.O. b.i.d.
Children age 10 to 16 weighing 60 kg or less: Initially, 250 mg P.O. b.i.d. Increase at weekly intervals to a maintenance dosage of 1,000 mg b.i.d.
Adjust-a-dose: For patients with CrCl of 51 to 80 mL/minute, reduce dosage by 25%; for CrCl of 31 to 50 mL/minute, decrease dosage by 50%; for CrCl of 11 to 30 mL/minute, decrease dosage by 75%.
➤ **Infantile spasms**
Infants and children ages 1 month to 2 years: 50 mg/kg/day P.O. given in two divided doses. Titrate in 25- to 50-mg/kg/day increments. Maximum dose is 150 mg/kg/day.

ADMINISTRATION
P.O.
• Drug may be given with or without food.
• The entire contents of the appropriate number of packets (500 mg/packet) of powder should be emptied into an empty cup, and should be dissolved in 10 mL of cold or room-temperature water per packet using the 10-mL oral syringe supplied with the medication. The concentration of the final solution is 50 mg/mL.

ACTION
Precise mechanism unknown. Thought to control seizures by inhibiting GABA

V

transaminase, the enzyme responsible for metabolizing the inhibitory neurotransmitter GABA, thereby increasing GABA levels in the CNS.

Route	Onset	Peak	Duration
P.O.	Unknown	1 hr	Unknown

Half-life: 7½ hours.

ADVERSE REACTIONS

CNS: abnormal behavior, abnormal coordination, abnormal dreams, abnormal thinking, anxiety, asthenia, attention disturbance, confusion, *seizures,* depression, dizziness, dysarthria, expressive language disorder, fatigue, fever, headache, hyperreflexia, hypoesthesia, hyporeflexia, insomnia, irritability, lethargy, malaise, memory impairment, nervousness, paresthesia, peripheral neuropathy, postictal state, sedation, sensory disturbance, sensory loss, sinus headache, somnolence, *status epilepticus,* tremor, vertigo.
CV: chest pain, peripheral edema.
EENT: asthenopia, blurred vision, diplopia, nystagmus, eye pain, nasopharyngitis, pharyngolaryngeal pain, tinnitus, toothache, visual field defect.
GI: abdominal distention, constipation, diarrhea, dyspepsia, nausea, stomach discomfort, upper abdominal pain, vomiting.
GU: dysmenorrhea, erectile dysfunction, UTI.
Metabolic: increased appetite, weight gain.
Musculoskeletal: arthralgia, back pain, contusion, extremity pain, gait disturbance, joint sprain, myalgia, muscle spasm, muscle twitching.
Respiratory: bronchitis, cough, influenza, pulmonary congestion, upper respiratory tract infection.
Skin: rash, wound secretion.
Other: thirst.

INTERACTIONS

Drug-drug. *Clonazepam:* May increase clonazepam level. Use together cautiously.
Drugs associated with serious adverse ophthalmic effects, such as retinopathy (hydroxychloroquine) or glaucoma (corticosteroids, TCAs): May increase risk of serious adverse ophthalmic effects. Avoid coadministration unless benefits clearly outweigh risks.

Phenytoin: May decrease phenytoin level, especially when drug is started or stopped. Monitor drug levels.

EFFECTS ON LAB TEST RESULTS

● May decrease hemoglobin, hematocrit, and RBC count.
● May decrease ALT and AST levels. May increase amino acid levels in urine.

CONTRAINDICATIONS & CAUTIONS

● Use cautiously in patients with a history of vision problems, abnormalities noted on magnetic resonance imaging, neurotoxicity, depression, suicidal behavior or ideation, or anemia.
● Avoid use during pregnancy unless benefit to mother outweighs risk to fetus.
● Drug appears in breast milk. Because of the risk of serious adverse effects in breast-fed infants, patient should stop either breast-feeding or drug.
● Safety and effectiveness in children younger than age 16 haven't been established.
⚠ *Overdose S&S:* Unconsciousness, coma, drowsiness, vertigo, psychosis, apnea, respiratory depression, bradycardia, agitation, irritability, confusion, headache, hypotension, abnormal behavior, increased seizure activity, status epilepticus, speech disorder.

NURSING CONSIDERATIONS

Black Box Warning Drug may cause progressive and permanent bilateral concentric visual field constriction and reduce visual acuity. Risk of visual impairment increases with use and may continue after drug is discontinued. Because of risk of permanent vision loss, drug is available only through the SHARE program. Prescribers, pharmacists, and patients must enroll by calling 1-888-45-SHARE. A visual examination should be performed before, every 3 months during, and 3 to 6 months after therapy. ∎
◑ *Alert:* Closely monitor all patients taking or starting therapy with antiepileptics for changes in behavior indicating worsening suicidal thoughts or behavior or depression. Symptoms such as anxiety, agitation, hostility, mania, and hypomania may be precursors to emerging suicidality.
● Discontinue drug if patient fails to comply with therapy.

• Discontinue drug within 3 months if patient shows no improvement.

❸ Alert: Don't withdraw drug suddenly. For adults, taper by decreasing daily dose by 1,000 mg/day weekly until discontinued. For infants and children, decrease the daily dose at a rate of 25 to 50 mg/kg every 3 to 4 days.

• Monitor patient closely for such adverse reactions as dizziness, which may lead to falls.

• Drug may cause anemia, somnolence, fatigue, peripheral neuropathy, peripheral edema, and weight gain. Monitor patient closely.

• Monitor ALT and AST levels; drug decreases levels, making these measurements unreliable for detecting early hepatic injury.

PATIENT TEACHING

• Advise patient that drug may be taken without regard to food.

• Instruct patient to read the manufacturer's medication guide before starting treatment and before each prescription refill.

• Warn patient that drug may cause dizziness and somnolence and that he should avoid driving or other hazardous activities until drug's effects are known.

• Inform patient that drug may cause vision loss and explain the importance of regular eye examinations and of immediately reporting vision changes.

• Advise patient to call prescriber and not to stop drug suddenly if adverse reactions occur.

• Tell women of childbearing age to notify prescriber if she becomes pregnant or plans to become pregnant while taking vigabatrin. If a woman becomes pregnant during therapy, encourage her to enroll in the Antiepilepsy Drug Pregnancy Registry at 1-888-233-2334.

• Inform patient who is breast-feeding that drug appears in breast milk and that she should use another method of feeding the baby.

vilazodone hydrochloride
vil-AZ-oh-dohne

Viibryd

Therapeutic class: Antidepressants
Pharmacologic class: SSRI–partial
5-HT$_{1A}$ receptor agonists
Pregnancy risk category: C

AVAILABLE FORMS
Tablets: 10 mg, 20 mg, 40 mg

INDICATIONS & DOSAGES
➤ **Major depressive disorder**
Adults: Initially,10 mg P.O. daily for 7 days, then 20 mg P.O. daily for 7 days, then 40 mg P.O. daily thereafter.

ADMINISTRATION
P.O.
• Give drug with food.
• Don't give within 14 days of starting or stopping an MAO inhibitor.

ACTION
Binds to serotonin reuptake sites and 5-HT$_{1A}$ receptors; is a partial agonist at serotonergic 5-HT$_{1A}$ receptors.

Route	Onset	Peak	Duration
P.O.	Unknown	4–5 hr	Unknown

Half-life: 25 hours.

ADVERSE REACTIONS
CNS: *suicidal thoughts or actions,* dizziness, somnolence, paresthesia, tremor, insomnia, abnormal dreams, restlessness, fatigue, jittery feeling, sedation, migraine.
CV: palpitations.
EENT: blurred vision, dry eye.
GI: diarrhea, nausea, dry mouth, vomiting, dyspepsia, flatulence, gastroenteritis, increased or decreased appetite.
GU: delayed ejaculation, erectile dysfunction, sexual dysfunction, abnormal orgasm.
Musculoskeletal: arthralgia.
Skin: hyperhidrosis, night sweats.
Other: decreased libido.

V

INTERACTIONS
Drug-drug. *Aspirin, NSAIDs, warfarin:* May increase risk of bleeding. Monitor patient closely; adjust dosages of these drugs, or discontinue them.
CNS drugs: May cause additive effects. Use together cautiously.
CYP3A4 inducers: May decrease vilazodone level. Monitor patient for efficacy.
CYP3A4 inhibitors (moderate to strong, such as erythromycin, ketoconazole): May increase vilazodone level. Reduce vilazodone dosage to 20 mg daily.
Drugs metabolized by CYP2C8 (thiazolidinedione class of antidiabetics, such as pioglitazone, rosiglitazone): May increase levels of these drugs. Monitor patient closely.
Highly protein-bound drugs (aripiprazole, diazepam, fluoxetine): May increase levels of these drugs. Monitor patient closely.
MAO inhibitors: May increase risk of serious or fatal adverse effects. Don't use concurrently with MAO inhibitor or within 14 days of starting or discontinuing an MAO inhibitor.
Serotonergics (buspirone, MAO inhibitors, SSNRIs, SSRIs, tramadol, triptans): May cause serotonin syndrome. Use together with extreme caution.
Triptans (almotriptan, sumatriptan): May increase risk of serotonin syndrome or neuroleptic malignant syndrome (NMS). Use together isn't recommended. If coadministration can't be avoided, closely monitor patient for emergence of serotonin syndrome or NMS-like signs or symptoms. If signs or symptoms occur, discontinue both drugs immediately and initiate supportive symptomatic treatment.
Drug-lifestyle. *Alcohol use:* May increase bioavailability of vilazodone. Discourage use together.

EFFECTS ON LAB TEST RESULTS
None reported.

CONTRAINDICATIONS & CAUTIONS
◆ *Alert:* Life-threatening serotonin syndrome (fever, mental status changes, muscle twitching, excessive sweating, shivering or shaking, diarrhea, loss of coordination) and NMS (hyperthermia, muscle rigidity, autonomic instability with possible rapid fluctuation of vital signs, mental status changes) have been reported with antidepressant use.
◆ *Alert:* Concomitant use with methylene blue or linezolid can cause serotonin syndrome. Use drug with methylene blue or linezolid only for life-threatening or urgent conditions when potential benefits outweigh risks of toxicity.
• Contraindicated in patients hypersensitive to drug or its inactive components and with concurrent use or within 14 days of MAO inhibitor therapy.
• Use cautiously in patients with history or family history of depression, bipolar disorder, mania, hypomania, severe hepatic dysfunction, seizure disorder, or hyponatremia and in patients taking NSAIDs, aspirin, or warfarin.
• Neonates of women who used vilazodone in the third trimester of pregnancy can develop complications upon delivery requiring prolonged hospitalization, respiratory support, and tube feeding. Complications include respiratory distress, cyanosis, apnea, seizures, temperature instability, feeding difficulty, vomiting, hypoglycemia, hypotonia, hypertonia, hyperreflexia, tremor, jitteriness, irritability, and constant crying. Pregnant women should only use this drug when potential benefits outweigh risks to the fetus.
• Drug may appear in breast milk. Use drug only when benefit to the mother outweighs risk to the infant.
⚠ *Overdose S&S:* Serotonin syndrome, lethargy, restlessness, hallucinations, disorientation.

NURSING CONSIDERATIONS
• Evaluate patients for the diagnosis of major depressive disorder according to established guidelines.
Black Box Warning Drug may increase the risk of suicidal thinking and behavior in children, adolescents, and young adults with major depressive disorder or other psychiatric disorders. Drug isn't approved for use in children. ∎

Reactions in bold italics are *life-threatening*. Interactions may have a *rapid onset* or a *delayed onset*.

• Screen patients for risk of bipolar disorder. Vilazodone isn't approved for treatment of bipolar depression. Use of an antidepressant in bipolar patients may precipitate mixed or manic episodes.

◑ *Alert:* If linezolid or methylene blue must be given concurrently with vilazodone (or other serotonergic drug), stop serotonergic drug and monitor patient for serotonin toxicity for 2 weeks (5 weeks if fluoxetine was taken) or until 24 hours after the last dose of methylene blue or linezolid, whichever comes first. May resume vilazodone 24 hours after last dose of methylene blue or linezolid.

• Evaluate patient for history of drug abuse, and watch closely for signs and symptoms of misuse or abuse (increased tolerance, drug-seeking behavior, requests for dosage increase).

• If patient had recently been taking MAO inhibitors, monitor him closely for tremor, myoclonus, diaphoresis, nausea, vomiting, flushing, dizziness, hyperthermia with features that resemble NMS, seizures, rigidity, autonomic instability with possible rapid fluctuations of vital signs, and mental status changes that include extreme agitation progressing to delirium and coma.

• Monitor patient for signs and symptoms of NMS (hyperthermia, rigidity, autonomic instability with possible rapid fluctuations of vital signs, mental status changes).

• Drug hasn't been studied in patients with severe hepatic dysfunction. Closely monitor patient with hepatic impairment for excessive fatigue or yellowing of the eyes or skin.

• Monitor patients taking aspirin, NSAIDs, or warfarin for signs and symptoms of bleeding.

• When discontinuing vilazodone, avoid abrupt discontinuation, which may cause dysphoric mood, irritability, agitation, dizziness, sensory disturbances (paresthesia, electric shock sensations), anxiety, confusion, headache, lethargy, labile emotions, insomnia, hypomania, tinnitus, and seizures. Gradually reduce dosage and monitor patient for adverse events. If withdrawal symptoms are intolerable, consider resuming the previous prescribed dosage and decreasing the dosage at a more gradual rate. Wait at least 14 days before starting an MAO inhibitor.

• Hyponatremia, which may be life-threatening, has occurred as a result of treatment with other SSRIs and SSNRIs, especially in elderly patients and in patients taking diuretics or who are otherwise volume-depleted. Discontinue vilazodone in patients with symptomatic hyponatremia and treat appropriately. Monitor patient for signs and symptoms of hyponatremia, such as headache, difficulty concentrating, memory impairment, confusion, weakness, unsteadiness, hallucinations, syncope, seizures, coma, and respiratory arrest.

PATIENT TEACHING

Black Box Warning Advise families and caregivers to closely observe patient for increased suicidal thinking and behavior. ■

◑ *Alert:* Teach patient to recognize and immediately report signs and symptoms of serotonin toxicity (fever, mental status changes, muscle twitching, excessive sweating, shivering or shaking, diarrhea, and loss of coordination) and NMS (hyperthermia, rigidity, autonomic instability with possible rapid fluctuations of vital signs, and mental status changes).

• Teach patient to take drug with food.

• Warn patient not to stop drug abruptly.

• Instruct patient to inform prescriber of all other medicines he is taking to avoid dangerous interactions.

• Tell patient to immediately seek medical attention if fever, rigidity, rapid changes in pulse rate or blood pressure, sweating, or confusion occurs.

• Counsel patient to keep all appointments for monitoring blood work and for follow-up care.

• Advise patient to use caution when driving or operating hazardous equipment until effects of drug are known; drug may impair judgment, thinking, and motor skills.

• Advise patient and caregivers to watch for signs and symptoms of the onset of manic or hypomanic episodes.

• Warn patient to avoid alcohol during drug therapy.

• Advise female patient to notify her health care provider if she becomes pregnant or intends to become pregnant during therapy. Counsel her to consult prescriber before breast-feeding.

SAFETY ALERT!

vinBLAStine sulfate (VLB)
vin-BLAS-teen

Therapeutic class: Antineoplastics
Pharmacologic class: Vinca alkaloids
Pregnancy risk category: D

AVAILABLE FORMS
Injection: 10-mg vials (lyophilized powder); 1 mg/mL in 10-mL vials

INDICATIONS & DOSAGES
Adjust-a-dose (for all indications): For patients with serum bilirubin level of 1.5 to 3 mg/dL and AST level of 60 to 180 units/L, give 50% of usual dose. For patients with serum bilirubin level of 3 to 5 mg/dL, give 25% of usual dose. For patients with serum bilirubin level greater than 5 mg/dL and AST level greater than 180 units/L, don't administer. For patients with recent exposure to radiation therapy or chemotherapy, single doses usually don't exceed 5.5 mg/m². Once a dose is determined to produce a WBC count below 3,000/mm³, give maintenance doses of one increment less than this amount at weekly intervals.
➤ **Breast or testicular cancer, Hodgkin and malignant lymphoma, choriocarcinoma, lymphosarcoma, mycosis fungoides, Kaposi sarcoma, histiocytosis**
Adults: 3.7 mg/m² I.V. weekly. May increase to maximum dose of 18.5 mg/m² I.V. weekly based on response. Don't repeat dose if WBC count is below 4,000/mm³. Increase dosage at weekly intervals in increments of 1.8 mg/m² until desired therapeutic response is obtained, WBC count decreases to 3,000/mm³, or maximum weekly dose of 18.5 mg/m² is reached.
➤ **Hodgkin disease**
Children: 6 mg/m² I.V. in combination with other chemotherapeutic drugs.
➤ **Letterer-Siwe disease (histiocytosis X)**
Children: 6.5 mg/m² I.V. as a single agent.

➤ **Testicular germ-cell carcinomas**
Children: 3 mg/m² I.V. in combination with other chemotherapeutic drugs.

ADMINISTRATION
I.V.
▼ Preparing and giving drug may be mutagenic, teratogenic, or carcinogenic. Follow institutional policy to reduce risks.
▼ Reconstitute drug in 10-mg vial with 10 mL of bacteriostatic saline solution for injection. This yields 1 mg/mL. Don't use other diluents. Protect solution from light.
▼ Inject drug directly into tubing of running I.V. line over 1 minute.
Black Box Warning Make sure catheter is properly positioned in vein. Drug is a vesicant; if extravasation occurs, stop infusion immediately and notify prescriber. The manufacturer recommends that moderate heat be applied to area of leakage. Local injection of hyaluronidase may help disperse drug. Moderate heat may be applied on and off every 2 hours for 24 hours. Drug is fatal if given intrathecally; it's for I.V. use only. ∎
▼ Drug reconstituted with diluent containing preservatives is stable for 28 days if refrigerated. Immediately discard any unused portion of solution reconstituted with diluent that doesn't contain preservatives.
▼ **Incompatibilities:** Cefepime, doxorubicin, furosemide, heparin.

ACTION
Arrests mitosis in metaphase, blocking cell division.

Route	Onset	Peak	Duration
I.V.	Unknown	Unknown	Unknown

Half-life: Initial phase, 3 minutes; second phase, 1½ hours; terminal phase, 25 hours.

ADVERSE REACTIONS
CNS: numbness, paresthesia, peripheral neuropathy and neuritis, *seizures, stroke,* depression, headache.
CV: *MI,* hypertension.
EENT: pharyngitis.
GI: anorexia, constipation, ileus, nausea, stomatitis, vomiting, abdominal pain, bleeding ulcer, diarrhea.

Reactions in bold italics are *life-threatening*. Interactions may have a *rapid onset* or a *delayed onset*.

Hematologic: anemia, *leukopenia, thrombocytopenia.*
Metabolic: weight loss, hyperuricemia.
Musculoskeletal: loss of deep tendon reflexes, muscle pain and weakness, jaw pain.
Respiratory: *acute bronchospasm,* shortness of breath.
Skin: irritation, phlebitis, cellulitis, reversible alopecia, vesiculation and necrosis with extravasation.
Other: SIADH.

INTERACTIONS
Drug-drug. *Azole antifungals, erythromycin, other drugs that inhibit cytochrome P-450 pathway:* May increase toxicity of vinblastine. Monitor patient closely for toxicity.
Mitomycin: May increase risk of bronchospasm and shortness of breath. Monitor patient's respiratory status.
Ototoxic drugs, such as platinum-containing antineoplastics: May cause temporary or permanent hearing impairment. Monitor hearing function.
Phenytoin: May decrease plasma phenytoin level. Monitor phenytoin level closely.

EFFECTS ON LAB TEST RESULTS
● May increase uric acid and bilirubin levels. May decrease hemoglobin level.
● May decrease WBC and platelet counts.

CONTRAINDICATIONS & CAUTIONS
● Contraindicated in patients with severe leukopenia or bacterial infection or in patients hypersensitive to the drug.
● Use cautiously in patients with hepatic dysfunction.
⚠ *Overdose S&S:* Exaggerated effects, neurotoxicity.

NURSING CONSIDERATIONS
● To reduce nausea, give antiemetic before drug.
● Don't give drug into a limb with compromised circulation.
🔶 *Alert:* After giving drug, be alert for development of life-threatening acute bronchospasm. If this occurs, notify prescriber immediately. Reaction is most likely to

occur in patients who are also receiving mitomycin.
● Monitor patient for stomatitis. If stomatitis occurs, stop drug and notify prescriber.
● Assess bowel activity. Give laxatives as indicated. Stool softeners may be used prophylactically.
● Don't repeat dosage more frequently than every 7 days or severe leukopenia will occur. Nadir occurs on days 4 to 10 and lasts another 7 to 14 days.
● Assess patient for numbness and tingling in hands and feet. Assess gait for early evidence of footdrop.
● Drug is less neurotoxic than vincristine.
● Stop drugs known to cause urine retention for first few days after therapy, particularly in elderly patients.
● *Look alike–sound alike:* Don't confuse vinblastine with vincristine or vinorelbine.

PATIENT TEACHING
● Tell patient to report evidence of infection (fever, sore throat, fatigue) and bleeding (easy bruising, nosebleeds, bleeding gums, tarry stools). Tell patient to take temperature daily.
● Urge patient to report pain, swelling, burning, or any unusual feeling at injection site during infusion.
● Warn patient that hair loss may occur but that it's usually temporary.
● Caution women to avoid pregnancy during therapy.
● Tell patient that pain may occur in jaw and in the organ with the tumor.

SAFETY ALERT!

vinCRIStine sulfate (VCR)
vin-KRIS-teen

Therapeutic class: Antineoplastics
Pharmacologic class: Vinca alkaloids
Pregnancy risk category: D

AVAILABLE FORMS
Injection: 1 mg/mL in 1-mL, 2-mL, 5-mL multidose vials; 1 mg/mL in 1-mL, 2-mL, 5-mL preservative-free vials

V

INDICATIONS & DOSAGES

➤ **Acute lymphoblastic and other leukemias, Hodgkin lymphoma, malignant lymphoma, neuroblastoma, rhabdomyosarcoma, Wilms tumor**
Adults: 1.4 mg/m² I.V. weekly. Typical weekly dose is 2 mg.
Children weighing more than 10 kg (22 lb): 1 to 2 mg/m² I.V. weekly.
Children weighing 10 kg and less or with BSA less than 1 m²: Initially, 0.05 mg/kg I.V. weekly. Titrate dosage as tolerated, up to 2 mg/dose.
Adjust-a-dose: For patients with direct bilirubin level of 1.5 to 3 mg/dL, reduce dose by 50%. If serum bilirubin level is 3 to less than 5 mg/dL, give 25% of usual dose. If bilirubin level is greater than 5 mg/dL, don't give drug.

ADMINISTRATION

I.V.
▼ Preparing and giving drug may be mutagenic, teratogenic, or carcinogenic. Follow institutional policy to reduce risks.
▼ Inject directly into tube of running I.V. line of normal saline solution or dextrose in water only, slowly over 1 minute.
Black Box Warning Make sure catheter is positioned correctly in vein. Drug is a vesicant; if it extravasates, stop infusion immediately and notify prescriber. Apply heat on and off every 2 hours for 24 hours. Drug is fatal if given intrathecally; it is for I.V. use only. ■
▼ If protocol requires a continuous infusion, use a central line.
▼ All vials contain 1 mg/mL solution; refrigerate them.
▼ **Incompatibilities:** Cefepime, furosemide, idarubicin, sodium bicarbonate.

ACTION

Arrests mitosis in metaphase, blocking cell division.

Route	Onset	Peak	Duration
I.V.	Unknown	Unknown	Unknown

Half-life: Initial phase, 4 minutes; second phase, 2¼ hours; terminal phase, 3½ days.

ADVERSE REACTIONS

CNS: loss of deep tendon reflexes, paresthesia, peripheral neuropathy, *coma, seizures,* ataxia, cranial nerve palsies, fever, headache, sensory loss.
CV: hypertension, hypotension.
EENT: blindness, diplopia, hoarseness, optic and extraocular neuropathy, photophobia, ptosis, visual disturbances, vocal cord paralysis.
GI: constipation, cramps, nausea, stomatitis, vomiting, *intestinal necrosis,* anorexia, diarrhea, dysphagia, ileus that mimics surgical paralytic ileus.
GU: dysuria, polyuria, SIADH, urine retention.
Hematologic: *leukopenia, thrombocytopenia,* anemia.
Metabolic: hyponatremia, weight loss.
Musculoskeletal: cramps, jaw pain, muscle weakness.
Respiratory: *acute bronchospasm,* dyspnea.
Skin: phlebitis, cellulitis at injection site, rash, reversible alopecia, severe local reaction following extravasation.

INTERACTIONS

Drug-drug. *Asparaginase:* May decrease hepatic clearance of vincristine. Use together also may result in additive neurotoxicity. Monitor patient for toxicity.
Digoxin: May decrease digoxin's effects. Monitor digoxin level.
HIV protease inhibitors (atazanavir, ritonavir): May increase pharmacologic effects of vinblastine. Monitor patient for profound neutropenia and severe neuropathy. Temporarily suspend HIV protease inhibitor or reduce vincristine dosage if significant hematologic or GI toxicity occurs.
Mitomycin: May increase frequency of bronchospasm and acute pulmonary reactions. Monitor patient's respiratory status.
Ototoxic drugs: May potentiate loss of hearing. Use together with caution.
Phenytoin: May reduce phenytoin level. Monitor phenytoin level closely.
Triazole antifungals (itraconazole, posaconazole, voriconazole): Concomitant use may increase risk of neurotoxicity. Monitor patient closely.

Reactions in bold italics are *life-threatening*. Interactions may have a *rapid onset* or a *delayed onset*.

EFFECTS ON LAB TEST RESULTS
• May decrease sodium and hemoglobin levels. May increase uric acid level.
• May decrease WBC and platelet counts.

CONTRAINDICATIONS & CAUTIONS
• Contraindicated in patients hypersensitive to drug and in those with demyelinating form of Charcot-Marie-Tooth syndrome.
• Don't give to patients who are receiving radiation therapy through ports that include the liver.
• Use cautiously in patients with hepatic dysfunction, neuromuscular disease, or infection.
⚠ Overdose S&S: Exaggerated effects, death.

NURSING CONSIDERATIONS
• Don't use the 5-mg vials for single doses.
۞ Alert: Patient also taking mitomycin has a higher risk of life-threatening bronchospasm. Monitor him after dose, and notify prescriber immediately if it occurs.
۞ Alert: Drug is considered a vesicant. If signs or symptoms of extravasation occur, stop infusion immediately and notify prescriber. Extravasation site may need to be injected with hyaluronidase.
• Watch for hyperuricemia, especially in patients with leukemia or lymphoma. Maintain hydration and give allopurinol to prevent uric acid nephropathy. Watch for toxicity.
• If SIADH develops, fluid restriction may be needed. Monitor fluid intake and output.
• Because of risk of neurotoxicity, don't give drug more often than once weekly. Children are more resistant to neurotoxicity than adults. Neurotoxicity is dose related and usually reversible.
• Elderly patients and those with underlying neurologic disease may be more susceptible to neurotoxic effects.
• Monitor patient for Achilles tendon reflex depression, numbness, tingling, footdrop or wristdrop, difficulty walking, ataxia, and slapping gait. Monitor his ability to walk on heels. Support him while walking.
• Monitor bowel function. Give stool softener, laxative, or water before giving dose. Constipation may be an early sign of neurotoxicity.

• Stop drugs known to cause urine retention, particularly in elderly patients, for first few days after therapy.
• **Look alike–sound alike:** Don't confuse vincristine with vinblastine or vinorelbine.

PATIENT TEACHING
• Advise patient to report any pain or burning at site of injection during or after administration.
• Tell patient to report evidence of infection (fever, sore throat, fatigue) and bleeding (easy bruising, nosebleeds, bleeding gums, tarry stools). Tell patient to take temperature daily.
• Warn patient that hair loss may occur, but explain that it's usually temporary.
• Caution women to avoid becoming pregnant during therapy and to consult prescriber before becoming pregnant.

SAFETY ALERT!

vinCRIStine sulfate liposome
vin-KRIS-teen

Marqibo

Therapeutic class: Antineoplastics
Pharmacologic class: Vinca alkaloids
Pregnancy risk category: D

AVAILABLE FORMS
Injection: 5 mg/31-mL single-dose vial

INDICATIONS & DOSAGES
Black Box Warning Liposomal form has different dosage recommendation than nonliposomal form. To avoid overdose, verify drug name and dose before preparation and administration. ∎
➤ **Patients with Philadelphia chromosome–negative (Ph-) acute lymphoblastic leukemia (ALL) in second or greater relapse or whose disease has progressed following two or more antileukemia therapies**
Adults: 2.25 mg/m^2 I.V. over 1 hour every 7 days.
Adjust-a-dose: For grade 3 or persistent grade 2 peripheral neuropathy, interrupt drug. Resume at 2 mg/m^2 if patient recovers

V

to grade 1 or 2; discontinue if patient remains at grade 3 or 4. For persistent grade 2 peripheral neuropathy after first dosage reduction to 2 mg/m^2, interrupt drug for up to 7 days. Resume at 1.825 mg/m^2 if patient recovers to grade 1; discontinue if neuropathy increases to grade 3 or 4. For persistent grade 2 peripheral neuropathy after second dosage reduction to 1.825 mg/m^2, interrupt drug for up to 7 days. Resume at 1.5 mg/m^2 if patient recovers to grade 1; discontinue if neuropathy increases to grade 3 or 4.

ADMINISTRATION

I.V.

Black Box Warning Drug is for I.V. use only; it's fatal if given by other routes. Death has occurred with intrathecal use. ■

▼ Drug is supplied in a single-dose kit containing vincristine sulfate 5 mg/5-mL vial plus vials of liposome injection, sodium phosphate, and assorted supplies to prepare drug.

▼ Drug will be prepared by pharmacy under aseptic technique and chemotherapy precautions.

▼ Inspect for particulate matter and discoloration before administering. Don't use if a precipitate or foreign matter is seen.

▼ Only give by secure, free-flowing venous access line. Discontinue immediately if extravasation is suspected.

▼ **Incompatibilities:** Other I.V. drugs.

ACTION

Arrests mitosis in metaphase, blocking cell division.

Route	Onset	Peak	Duration
I.V.	Unknown	Unknown	Unknown

Half-life: Unknown.

ADVERSE REACTIONS

CNS: peripheral neuropathy, motor neuropathy, mental status changes, fatigue, pain, pyrexia, insomnia, asthenia.
CV: hypotension, *cardiac arrest.*
GI: constipation, ileus, abdominal pain, nausea, diarrhea, decreased appetite.
GU: renal and urinary disorders.
Hematologic: *febrile neutropenia,* anemia, *neutropenia, thrombocytopenia.*

Musculoskeletal: muscle weakness, musculoskeletal or connective tissue disorders.
Respiratory: *respiratory distress, respiratory failure,* pneumonia.
Other: *septic shock, tumor lysis syndrome.*

INTERACTIONS

Drug-drug. *Asparaginase:* May decrease hepatic clearance of vincristine; also may result in additive neurotoxicity. Monitor patient for toxicity.
Digoxin: May decrease digoxin's effects. Monitor digoxin level.
Mitomycin: May increase risk of bronchospasm and shortness of breath. Monitor respiratory status.
Ototoxic drugs (platinum-containing antineoplastics): May cause temporary or permanent hearing impairment. Monitor hearing function.
P-glycoprotein inducers (efavirenz, nevirapine, rifampin) or inhibitors (atazanavir, atazanavir–ritonavir, ketoconazole, lopinavir–ritonavir, ritonavir, saquinavir): May alter pharmacokinetics or pharmacodynamics of vincristine. Avoid use together.
Strong CYP3A inducers (carbamazepine, dexamethasone, phenobarbital, phenytoin, rifabutin, rifampin, rifapentine): May alter blood level of inducer or vincristine. Avoid use together. If used together, monitor drug levels of CYP3A inducer closely.
Strong CYP3A inhibitors (atazanavir, clarithromycin, indinavir, itraconazole, ketoconazole, nefazodone, nelfinavir, posaconazole, ritonavir, saquinavir, telithromycin, voriconazole): May alter blood levels of inhibitor or vincristine. Avoid use together.
Drug-herb. *St. John's wort:* May alter effects of vincristine. Discourage use together.

EFFECTS ON LAB TEST RESULTS

● May increase bilirubin or AST levels.
● May decrease WBC, RBC, and platelet counts.
● May cause immunogenicity.

CONTRAINDICATIONS & CAUTIONS

● Contraindicated in patients hypersensitive to drug or its components; in those with demyelinating conditions, including Charcot-Marie-Tooth syndrome; and in pregnant and breast-feeding women.

• Use cautiously in patients with preexisting neuromuscular disorders or in combination with other neurotoxic drugs.

⚠ **Overdose S&S:** Motor neuropathy, generalized tonic-clonic seizures, elevated AST and bilirubin levels.

NURSING CONSIDERATIONS

• Monitor patient for extravasation. If extravasation occurs, stop infusion and treat per facility protocol.

• Monitor patient for constipation, bowel obstruction, and ileus. Recommend prophylactic bowel regimen, including adequate dietary fiber intake, hydration, and routine use of stool softeners such as docusate. Additional treatments, such as senna, bisacodyl, milk of magnesia, magnesium citrate, and lactulose, may be considered.

• Observe for sensory and motor neuropathies, which are common and cumulative (hypoesthesia, hyperesthesia, paresthesia, hyporeflexia, neuralgia, jaw pain, decreased vibratory sense, cranial neuropathy, ileus, burning sensation, arthralgia, myalgia, muscle spasm, orthostatic hypotension, or weakness), before and during treatment.

• Monitor complete blood count before each dose.

• Monitor patient for tumor lysis syndrome (hyperuricemia, hyperkalemia, hyperphosphatemia, hypocalcemia, and acute renal failure).

• Monitor hepatic enzyme levels.

• **Look alike–sound alike:** Don't confuse vincristine liposome with vincristine, vinblastine, or vinorelbine.

PATIENT TEACHING

• Instruct patient to notify prescriber of numbness, tingling of the feet or hands, decreased sensitivity to hot or cold, pain, difficulty picking up things, difficulty walking, pain in head or jaw, muscle spasms, dizziness with change of position, or difficulty speaking.

• Caution patient to report constipation or difficulty passing urine.

• Caution patient that drug can cause fetal harm and to use effective contraception during treatment.

• Advise female patient to inform prescriber immediately if she becomes pregnant or is breast-feeding.

• Instruct patient to immediately report fever or other signs and symptoms of infection.

SAFETY ALERT!

vinorelbine tartrate
vin-oh-REL-been

Navelbine

Therapeutic class: Antineoplastics
Pharmacologic class: Semisynthetic vinca alkaloids
Pregnancy risk category: D

AVAILABLE FORMS
Injection: 10 mg/mL, 50 mg/5 mL

INDICATIONS & DOSAGES

➤ **Alone or as adjunctive therapy with cisplatin for first-line treatment of ambulatory patients with nonresectable advanced non–small-cell lung cancer (NSCLC); alone or with cisplatin in stage IV of NSCLC; with cisplatin in stage III of NSCLC**

Adults: 30 mg/m^2 I.V. weekly as monotherapy. In combination treatment, 25 mg/m^2 I.V. weekly with cisplatin given every 4 weeks at a dose of 100 mg/m^2. Or, 30 mg/m^2 I.V. weekly in combination with cisplatin, given on days 1 and 29, then every 6 weeks at a dose of 120 mg/m^2.

Adjust-a-dose: If granulocyte count is 1,000/mm^3 to 1,499/mm^3, give 50% of dose. If less than 1,000/mm^3, dose is withheld. Repeat granulocyte count in 1 week. If three consecutive doses are withheld, discontinue drug. For patients who develop fever or sepsis while granulocytopenic or had two consecutive doses withheld due to granulocytopenia, give 75% of dose if granulocyte count is 1,500/mm^3 or more, or 37.5% if granulocyte count is 1,000 to 1,499/mm^3. If granulocyte count is less than 1,000/mm^3, don't give dose. Repeat granulocyte count in 1 week. If three consecutive doses are withheld, discontinue drug. For patients who develop hyperbilirubinemia,

V

adjust dosage as follows: If total bilirubin is 2.1 to 3 mg/dL, give 50% of starting dose; if total bilirubin is greater than 3 mg/dL, give 25% of starting dose.

ADMINISTRATION

I.V.

▼ Drug may be a contact irritant; handle and give with care. Wear gloves. Avoid inhaling vapors and allowing contact with skin or mucous membranes, especially those of the eyes. In case of contact, wash with generous amounts of water for at least 15 minutes.

▼ Dilute drug before use to 1.5 to 3 mg/mL with D₅W or normal saline solution in a syringe. Or, dilute to 0.5 to 2 mg/mL in an I.V. bag.

▼ Give drug I.V. over 6 to 10 minutes into side port of a free-flowing I.V. line that is closest to I.V. bag; then flush with 75 to 125 mL or more of D₅W or normal saline solution.

▼ Monitor site for irritation and infiltration because drug can cause localized tissue damage, necrosis, and thrombophlebitis. **Black Box Warning** Make sure catheter is properly positioned in vein. If extravasation occurs, stop drug immediately and inject remaining dose into a different vein; notify prescriber. Drug is fatal if given intrathecally; it's for I.V. use only. ■

▼ Drug may be stored for up to 24 hours at room temperature.

▼ **Incompatibilities:** Acyclovir, allopurinol, aminophylline, amphotericin B, ampicillin sodium, cefazolin, ceftriaxone, cefuroxime, 5-FU, furosemide, ganciclovir, methylprednisolone, mitomycin, piperacillin, sodium bicarbonate, thiotepa, sulfamethoxazole–trimethoprim.

ACTION

Exerts its primary antineoplastic effect by disrupting microtubule assembly, which in turn disrupts spindle formation and prevents mitosis.

Route	Onset	Peak	Duration
I.V.	Unknown	Unknown	Unknown

Half-life: About 27 to 43½ hours.

ADVERSE REACTIONS

CNS: asthenia, fatigue, peripheral neuropathy.
CV: chest pain, phlebitis.
GI: anorexia, constipation, diarrhea, nausea, stomatitis, vomiting.
Hematologic: anemia, *agranulocytosis, bone marrow suppression, granulocytopenia, thrombocytopenia, leukopenia.*
Hepatic: hyperbilirubinemia.
Musculoskeletal: arthralgia, jaw pain, loss of deep tendon reflexes, myalgia.
Respiratory: dyspnea, shortness of breath.
Skin: alopecia, injection-site pain or reaction, rash.

INTERACTIONS

Drug-drug. *Cisplatin:* May increase risk of bone marrow suppression when used with cisplatin. Monitor hematologic status closely.
Cyclosporine: May increase therapeutic and toxic effects of vinorelbine. Close clinical and laboratory monitoring is indicated.
Cytochrome P-450 inhibitors: May decrease metabolism of vinorelbine. Watch for increased adverse effects.
Mitomycin: May cause pulmonary reactions. Monitor respiratory status closely.
Paclitaxel: May increase risk of neuropathy. Monitor patient closely.
Triazole antifungals: May increase risk of neurotoxicity. Monitor patient closely.
Vaccines, live-virus: May increase risk of live-virus vaccine–induced adverse reactions. Concurrent use isn't recommended.

EFFECTS ON LAB TEST RESULTS

● May increase bilirubin level. May decrease hemoglobin level.
● May increase LFT values. May decrease granulocyte, WBC, and platelet counts.

CONTRAINDICATIONS & CAUTIONS

● Contraindicated in patients with pretreatment granulocyte count below 1,000/mm³ and in patients hypersensitive to the drug.
● Use with caution in patients whose bone marrow may have been compromised by previous exposure to radiation therapy or chemotherapy or whose bone marrow is still recovering from chemotherapy.

• Use with caution in patients with hepatic impairment.
• Safety and effectiveness in children haven't been established.
⚠ *Overdose S&S:* Paralytic ileus, stomatitis, esophagitis, bone marrow aplasia, sepsis, paresis, death.

NURSING CONSIDERATIONS

Black Box Warning Drug should be administered under the supervision of a physician experienced in the use of cancer chemotherapeutic agents. ∎

Black Box Warning Check patient's granulocyte count before giving; make sure count is $1,000/mm^3$ or higher before giving drug. ∎

• If count is lower, withhold drug and notify prescriber. Granulocyte count nadir occurs between days 7 and 10.
• In patients with hepatic impairment, monitor liver enzyme levels.
• Patient may receive injections of WBC colony-stimulating factors to promote cell growth and decrease risk of infection.
● *Alert:* Monitor deep tendon reflexes; loss may represent cumulative toxicity.
• Monitor patient closely for hypersensitivity.
• As a guide to the effects of therapy, monitor patient's peripheral blood count and bone marrow.
• *Look alike–sound alike:* Don't confuse vinorelbine with vinblastine or vincristine.

PATIENT TEACHING

• Advise patient to report any pain or burning at site of injection.
• Instruct patient not to take other drugs, including OTC preparations, until approved by prescriber.
• Tell patient to report evidence of infection (fever, sore throat, fatigue) and bleeding (easy bruising, nosebleeds, bleeding gums, tarry stools). Tell him to take temperature daily.
• Advise patient to report increased shortness of breath, cough, abdominal pain, or constipation.
• Caution women to avoid becoming pregnant during therapy.

vismodegib
VIS-moe-DEG-ib

Erivedge

Therapeutic class: Antineoplastics
Pharmacologic class: Hedgehog pathway inhibitors
Pregnancy risk category: D

AVAILABLE FORMS
Capsules: 150 mg

INDICATIONS & DOSAGES
➤ **Metastatic basal cell carcinoma; locally advanced basal cell carcinoma that has recurred following surgery or in patients who aren't candidates for surgery or radiation**
Adults: 150 mg P.O. once daily until disease progression or unacceptable toxicity.

ADMINISTRATION
P.O.
• May give with or without food.
• Store capsules at room temperature.
• Don't open, crush, or allow patient to chew capsules.
• Determine pregnancy status within 7 days before start of treatment.

ACTION
Inhibits hedgehog signaling pathway by binding to and inhibiting smoothened, a transmembrane protein involved in hedgehog signal transmission. Inhibition of this protein slows pathway for tumor growth.

Route	Onset	Peak	Duration
P.O.	Unknown	Unknown	Unknown

Half-life: 4 days with continued dosing; 12 days after one dose.

ADVERSE REACTIONS
CNS: fatigue.
GI: nausea, diarrhea, vomiting, constipation, taste perversion, absence of taste, decreased appetite.
GU: azotemia, amenorrhea.
Musculoskeletal: muscle spasms, arthralgia.

Skin: alopecia.
Other: weight loss.

INTERACTIONS
Drug-drug. *Antacids, H₂-receptor antagonists, proton pump inhibitors:* May decrease vismodegib exposure and its effects. Avoid use together.
P-glycoprotein inhibitors (macrolides such as azithromycin, clarithromycin, erythromycin): May increase vismodegib exposure and adverse effects. Avoid concurrent use.

EFFECTS ON LAB TEST RESULTS
• May increase BUN and creatinine levels.
• May decrease sodium and potassium levels.

CONTRAINDICATIONS & CAUTIONS
• Contraindicated in patients hypersensitive to drug.
Black Box Warning Contraindicated in pregnant women. Drug can cause embryo-fetal death or severe birth defects. ▪
• It's unknown if drug appears in breast milk; potentially serious reactions may occur in breast-feeding infant. A decision should be made whether patient should breast-feed during therapy.

NURSING CONSIDERATIONS
Black Box Warning Verify pregnancy status within 7 days before start of therapy. ▪
Black Box Warning Advise male and female patients of the risks to an embryo or fetus, the need for contraception, and the potential risk of drug exposure through semen. ▪
• Report exposure during pregnancy to Genentech Adverse Event Line at 1-888-835-2555.
• It's unknown if drug-induced amenorrhea is reversible.
• *Look alike–sound alike:* Don't confuse vismodegib with vemurafenib or vandetanib.

PATIENT TEACHING
Black Box Warning Exposure during pregnancy can cause embryo-fetal death or severe birth defects; counsel all patients of childbearing potential and their partners in the use of contraception during and after drug therapy. ▪

• If patient misses a dose, instruct him not to make up that dose but to resume dosing with the next scheduled dose.
• Tell patient to use highly effective contraception during therapy and for 7 months after last dose.
• Instruct patient to immediately contact health care provider if pregnancy occurs or is suspected after exposure to drug, or if patient has unprotected sex.
• Advise pregnant patient to immediately report exposure to drug and to participate in the pregnancy pharmacovigilance program by calling the Genentech Adverse Event Line at 1-888-835-2555.
• Advise women experiencing drug-induced amenorrhea that it's unknown if amenorrhea will be reversed after drug discontinuation.
• Caution patient not to donate blood or blood products while taking drug and for at least 7 months after last dose.
• Teach patient to swallow capsules whole and not to crush, chew, or open them.

---

voriconazole
vor-ah-KON-ah-zole

Vfend

Therapeutic class: Antifungals
Pharmacologic class: Synthetic triazoles
Pregnancy risk category: D

AVAILABLE FORMS
Oral suspension: 40 mg/mL (after reconstitution)
Powder for injection: 200 mg
Tablets: 50 mg, 200 mg

INDICATIONS & DOSAGES
Adjust-a-dose (for all indications): For patients with mild or moderate hepatic impairment (Child-Pugh class A or B), decrease the maintenance dosage by 50%. In patients with a CrCl of less than 50 mL/minute, use oral form instead of I.V. form to prevent accumulation of a component of the I.V. mixture. In patients also receiving phenytoin, increase maintenance dose of voriconazole to 5 mg/kg I.V. every 12 hours, or increase P.O. dose from 100 mg to 200 mg (in patients

---

weighing 40 kg or less) or from 200 mg to 400 mg (in patients weighing more than 40 kg). In patients also receiving efavirenz, increase voriconazole dosage to 400 mg P.O. every 12 hours and decrease efavirenz dosage to 300 mg P.O. every 24 hours. When treatment with voriconazole is stopped, restore initial dosage of efavirenz.

➤ **Esophageal candidiasis**
Adults and children age 12 and older weighing 40 kg (88 lb) or more: 200 mg P.O. every 12 hours. Treat for a minimum of 14 days and for at least 7 days after symptoms resolve.
Adults and children age 12 and older weighing less than 40 kg: 100 mg P.O. every 12 hours. Treat for a minimum of 14 days and for at least 7 days after symptoms resolve.

➤ **Invasive aspergillosis; serious infections caused by *Fusarium* species and *Scedosporium apiospermum* in patients intolerant of or refractory to other therapy**
Adults and children age 12 and older: Initially, 6 mg/kg I.V. every 12 hours for two doses; then maintenance dose of 4 mg/kg I.V. every 12 hours. If patient can't tolerate 4-mg dose, decrease to 3 mg/kg. Switch to P.O. form as tolerated, using the maintenance dosages shown here.
Adults and children age 12 and older weighing 40 kg or more: 200 mg P.O. every 12 hours. May increase to 300 mg P.O. every 12 hours, if needed. If unable to tolerate the 300-mg dose, reduce dose in 50-mg decrements to a minimum of 200 mg every 12 hours.
Adults and children age 12 and older weighing less than 40 kg: 100 mg P.O. every 12 hours. May increase to 150 mg P.O. every 12 hours, if needed. If unable to tolerate the 150-mg dose, reduce dose to 100 mg every 12 hours.

➤ **Candidemia in nonneutropenic patients; *Candida* infections of the kidney, abdomen, bladder wall, or wounds and disseminated skin infections**
Adults and children age 12 and older: Initially, 6 mg/kg I.V. every 12 hours for two doses, then 3 to 4 mg/kg I.V. every 12 hours for maintenance, depending on severity of the infection. If patient can't tolerate 4-mg

dose, decrease to 3 mg/kg. Switch to P.O. form as tolerated, using the maintenance dosages shown here.
Adults and children age 12 and older weighing 40 kg or more: 200 mg P.O. every 12 hours. May increase to 300 mg P.O. every 12 hours, if needed. If unable to tolerate the 300-mg dose, reduce dose in 50-mg decrements to a minimum of 200 mg every 12 hours.
Adults and children age 12 and older weighing less than 40 kg: 100 mg P.O. every 12 hours. May increase to 150 mg P.O. every 12 hours, if needed. If unable to tolerate the 150-mg dose, reduce dose to 100 mg every 12 hours.

Treat patients with candidemia for at least 14 days after symptoms resolve or after the last positive culture result, whichever is longer.

➤ **Allogenic hematopoietic stem cell transplant (HSCT) patients and select autologous HSCT patients with prolonged neutropenia and mucosal damage from intense chemotherapy, graft manipulation, or recent purine analogue treatment; patients with acute myeloid leukemia undergoing remission induction or salvage induction chemotherapy; patients with myelodysplastic syndrome receiving intensive treatment ♦**
Adults weighing more than 40 kg (88 lb): 200 mg P.O. every 12 hours. Or, 4 mg/kg I.V. every 12 hours. Begin prophylaxis at start of chemotherapy or the day of transplantation. The American Society for Blood and Marrow Transplantation (ASBMT) recommends continuing prophylaxis until engraftment (that is, 30 days) or for 7 days after ANC reaches greater than 1,000 cells/mm^3. The Infectious Diseases Society of America (IDSA) recommends antimold prophylaxis in allograft HSCT patients "through the neutropenic period and beyond," based on a demonstrated survival advantage in patients receiving prophylaxis for 75 days post-HSCT, or until cessation of immunosuppressive therapy.
Children: For those weighing 20 kg (44 lb) or more, give 100 mg P.O. or I.V. every 12 hours. For children weighing less than 20 kg, give 50 mg P.O. or I.V. every 12 hours. Begin prophylaxis at start of

V

chemotherapy or the day of transplantation. The ASBMT recommends continuing prophylaxis until engraftment (that is, 30 days) or for 7 days after ANC reaches greater than 1,000 cells/mm³. The IDSA recommends antimold prophylaxis in allograft HSCT patients "through the neutropenic period and beyond," based on a demonstrated survival advantage in patients receiving prophylaxis for 75 days post-HSCT, or until cessation of immunosuppressive therapy.

Adults weighing 40 kg (88 lb) or more with graft-versus-host disease (GVHD): 200 mg P.O. every 12 hours. Or, 4 mg/kg I.V. every 12 hours.

Children weighing 20 kg (44 lb) or more with GVHD: 100 mg P.O. or I.V. every 12 hours.

Children weighing less than 20 kg with GVHD: 50 mg P.O. or I.V. every 12 hours.

ADMINISTRATION
P.O.
● Give tablets or oral suspension at least 1 hour before or 1 hour after a meal.
● For the oral suspension, use only the dispenser provided in the medication package.
● Don't mix oral suspension with other drugs or beverages.
● Discard unused portion of suspension after 14 days.

I.V.
▼ In patients with CrCl less than 50 mL/minute, use I.V. form cautiously. Change to oral form is recommended.
▼ Reconstitute the powder with 19 mL of water for injection to obtain a volume of 20 mL of clear concentrate containing 10 mg/mL of drug. Discard the vial if a vacuum doesn't pull the diluent into the vial. Shake the vial until all the powder is dissolved. Use the reconstituted solution immediately.
▼ Further dilute the 10-mg/mL solution to 5 mg/mL or less. Follow the manufacturer's instructions for diluting.
▼ Infuse over 1 to 2 hours at 5 mg/mL or less and a maximum hourly rate of 3 mg/kg/hour.
▼ **Incompatibilities:** Blood products, electrolyte supplements, 4.2% sodium bicarbonate infusion.

ACTION
Inhibits the cytochrome P-450–dependent synthesis of ergosterol, a vital component of fungal cell membranes.

Route	Onset	Peak	Duration
P.O., I.V.	Immediate	1–2 hr	12 hr

Half-life: Depends on dose.

ADVERSE REACTIONS
CNS: fever, headache, hallucinations, dizziness.
CV: tachycardia, hypertension, hypotension, vasodilation.
EENT: abnormal vision, photophobia, chromatopsia, dry mouth.
GI: abdominal pain, nausea, vomiting, diarrhea.
Hepatic: cholestatic jaundice.
Metabolic: hypokalemia, hypomagnesemia.
Skin: rash, pruritus.
Other: chills, peripheral edema.

INTERACTIONS
Drug-drug. *Benzodiazepines, calcium channel blockers, methadone, sulfonylureas, vinca alkaloids:* May increase levels of these drugs. Adjust dosages of these drugs; monitor patient for adverse reactions.
Carbamazepine, long-acting barbiturates, rifabutin, rifampin, *ritonavir (high-dose therapy):* May decrease voriconazole level. Use together is contraindicated.
Cyclosporine, tacrolimus: May increase levels of these drugs. Adjust dosages; monitor levels.
Efavirenz: May significantly decrease voriconazole levels while significantly increasing efavirenz levels. Adjust dosage of both drugs.
Ergot alkaloids (such as ergotamine), sirolimus: May increase levels of these drugs. Use together is contraindicated.
HIV protease inhibitors (amprenavir, nelfinavir, ritonavir, saquinavir), NNRTIs (delavirdine): May increase levels of both drugs. Monitor patient for adverse reactions and toxicity.
HMG-CoA reductase inhibitors (atorvastatin, fluvastatin, lovastatin, pravastatin, rosuvastatin, simvastatin): May increase levels and adverse effects, including rhabdomyolysis, of these drugs. Monitor patient closely and

---

reduce dose of HMG-CoA reductase inhibitor as needed.

Omeprazole: May increase omeprazole level. When initiating voriconazole therapy in patients already receiving omeprazole, reduce omeprazole dose by one-half.

Oral contraceptives containing ethinyl estradiol and norethindrone: May increase levels and adverse effects of these drugs. Monitor patient closely.

Phenytoin: May decrease voriconazole level and increase phenytoin level. Increase voriconazole maintenance dose; monitor phenytoin level.

Pimozide, quinidine: May increase levels of these drugs, leading to torsades de pointes and prolonged QT interval. Use together is contraindicated.

Warfarin: May significantly increase PT. Monitor PT and other anticoagulant test results.

Drug-herb. *St. John's wort:* May increase drug level. Discourage use together.

Drug-lifestyle. *Sun exposure:* May cause photosensitivity. Advise patient to avoid excessive sunlight exposure.

EFFECTS ON LAB TEST RESULTS
- May increase alkaline phosphatase, AST, ALT, bilirubin, and creatinine levels. May decrease potassium and hemoglobin levels and hematocrit.
- May decrease platelet, WBC, and RBC counts.

CONTRAINDICATIONS & CAUTIONS
- Contraindicated in patients hypersensitive to drug or its components; in those with rare hereditary galactose intolerance, Lapp lactase deficiency, or glucose–galactose malabsorption; and in those taking carbamazepine, efavirenz, ergot alkaloid, a long-acting barbiturate, pimozide, quinidine, rifabutin, rifampin, ritonavir, or sirolimus.
- Use cautiously in patients hypersensitive to other azoles.

⚠ Overdose S&S: Photophobia.

NURSING CONSIDERATIONS
- Correct electrolyte disturbances before initiating therapy.
- Infusion reactions, including flushing, fever, sweating, tachycardia, chest tightness,

dyspnea, faintness, nausea, pruritus, and rash, may occur as soon as infusion starts. If reaction occurs, notify prescriber; infusion may need to be stopped.
- Monitor LFT results at start of and during therapy. Monitor patients who develop abnormal LFT results for more severe hepatic injury. If patient develops signs and symptoms of liver disease, drug may need to be stopped.
- If treatment lasts longer than 28 days, vision changes may occur.
- ***Look alike–sound alike:*** Don't confuse voriconazole with fluconazole.

PATIENT TEACHING
- Tell patient to take oral form at least 1 hour before or 1 hour after a meal.
- Tell patient taking the oral suspension to only use the dispenser provided with the medication pack.
- Advise patient not to mix oral suspension with other drugs or beverages.
- Tell patient to discard any unused portion of suspension after 14 days.
- Advise patient to avoid driving or operating machinery while taking drug, especially at night, because vision changes, including blurring, photophobia, and changes in color perception, may occur.
- Tell patient to avoid strong, direct sunlight during therapy.
- Advise patient to avoid becoming pregnant during therapy because of the risk of fetal harm.

SAFETY ALERT!

warfarin sodium
WAR-far-in

Coumadin🖊, Jantoven

Therapeutic class: Anticoagulants
Pharmacologic class: Coumarin derivatives
Pregnancy risk category: X

AVAILABLE FORMS
Powder for injection: 2 mg/mL
Tablets: 1 mg, 2 mg, 2.5 mg, 3 mg, 4 mg, 5 mg, 6 mg, 7.5 mg, 10 mg

W

INDICATIONS & DOSAGES

➤ **Pulmonary embolism, deep vein thrombosis, MI, rheumatic heart disease with heart valve damage, prosthetic heart valves, chronic atrial fibrillation**

Adults: 2 to 5 mg P.O. or I.V. daily for 2 to 4 days; then dosage based on daily PT and INR. Usual maintenance dosage is 2 to 10 mg P.O. or I.V. daily. Base dosages on INR target goals. Consider lower initiation and maintenance doses for Asian and elderly patients.

ADMINISTRATION
P.O.

• Draw blood to establish baseline coagulation parameters before therapy. PT and INR determinations are essential for proper control. Recommended INR range is usually 2 to 3.

• Give drug at same time daily.

I.V.

▼ Draw blood to establish baseline coagulation parameters before therapy. PT and INR determinations are essential for proper control. Recommended INR range is usually 2 to 3.

▼ I.V. form may be ordered in rare instances when oral therapy can't be given.

▼ Reconstitute powder with 2.7 mL sterile water, or as instructed in manufacturer guidelines.

▼ Give as a slow bolus injection over 1 to 2 minutes into a peripheral vein.

▼ Because onset of action is delayed, heparin sodium is often given during the first few days of treatment of embolic disease. Blood for PT and INR may be drawn at any time during continuous heparin infusion.

▼ **Incompatibilities:** Aminophylline, ammonium chloride, bretylium tosylate, ceftazidime, cimetidine, ciprofloxacin, dobutamine, esmolol, gentamicin, heparin sodium, labetalol, lactated Ringer's injection, metronidazole, promazine, Ringer's injection, vancomycin.

ACTION

Inhibits vitamin K–dependent activation of clotting factors II, VII, IX, and X, formed in the liver.

Route	Onset	Peak	Duration
P.O.	Within 24 hr	4 hr	2–5 days
I.V.	Within 24 hr	<4 hr	2–5 days

Half-life: 20 to 60 hours.

ADVERSE REACTIONS

CV: vasculitis.
GI: abdominal pain, diarrhea, flatulence, bloating, nausea, taste perversion, vomiting.
Hematologic: *hemorrhage.*
Hepatic: *hepatitis.*
Skin: alopecia, pruritus, rash, dermatitis, bullous eruptions.
Other: chills, hypersensitivity or allergic reactions, including *anaphylactic reactions* and urticaria.

INTERACTIONS

Drug-drug. *Acetaminophen:* May increase bleeding with long-term therapy (more than 2 weeks) at high doses (more than 2 g/day) of acetaminophen. Monitor patient very carefully.

Allopurinol, **amiodarone, anabolic steroids,** *anticoagulants (argatroban, bivalirudin),* **azole antifungals,** *aspirin, beta blockers (atenolol, propranolol), cephalosporins, chloramphenicol, cimetidine,* **danazol,** *diazoxide, diflunisal, disulfiram, erythromycin, ethacrynic acid, felbamate,* **fibric acids, fluoxymesterone, fluoroquinolones,** *furosemide, glucagon, HMG-CoA reductase inhibitors (fluvastatin, lovastatin, simvastatin), heparin, influenza virus vaccine, isoniazid,* **lansoprazole,** *macrolide antibiotics (azithromycin, clarithromycin, erythromycin), meclofenamate, methimazole, methyldopa, methylphenidate,* **methyltestosterone, metronidazole, nalidixic acid,** *neomycin (oral),* **NSAIDs,** *omeprazole,* **oxandrolone,** *pentoxifylline, propafenone, propoxyphene, propylthiouracil, quinidine, quinolones (ciprofloxacin, levofloxacin, norfloxacin, ofloxacin),* **salicylates,** *selective cyclo-oxygenase-2 inhibitors (celecoxib, rofecoxib, valdecoxib), SSRIs,* **sulfinpyrazone,** *sulfamethoxazole–trimethoprim,* **sulfonamides,** *tamoxifen, tetracyclines, thiazides, thrombolytics,* **thyroid drugs,** *ticlopidine, tramadol, vitamin E, valproic acid, zafirlukast:* May increase anticoagulant effect.

Reactions in bold italics are *life-threatening*. Interactions may have a *rapid onset* or a *delayed onset*.

Monitor patient carefully for bleeding. Reduce anticoagulant dosage as directed.

*Aprepitant, ascorbic acid, **barbiturates**, bosentan, carbamazepine, clozapine, corticosteroids, corticotropin, cyclosporine, dicloxacillin, ethchlorvynol, griseofulvin, haloperidol, meprobamate, mercaptopurine, nafcillin, oral contraceptives containing estrogen, protease inhibitors (indinavir, ritonavir), raloxifene, ribavirin, rifampin, spironolactone, sucralfate, thiazide diuretics, trazodone, vitamin K:* May decrease PT and INR with reduced anticoagulant effect. Monitor PT and INR carefully. Increase warfarin dosage, as needed.

Cholestyramine: May decrease response when given too closely together. Give 6 hours after oral anticoagulants.

Cyclophosphamide, phenytoin, propylthiouracil, ranitidine: May increase or decrease PT and INR. Monitor PT and INR carefully.

Sulfonylureas (oral antidiabetics): May increase hypoglycemic response. Monitor glucose levels.

Drug-herb. *Agrimony, anise, arnica flower, asafoetida, bogbean, boldo, bromelain, buchu, capsicum, celery, chamomile, clove, dandelion, danshen, devil's claw, dong quai, fenugreek, feverfew, garlic, ginger, **ginkgo**, **ginseng**, horse chestnut, horseradish, licorice, meadowsweet, motherwort, onion, papain, parsley, passion flower, quassia, red clover, Reishi mushroom, rue, sweet clover, turmeric, white willow:* May increase risk of bleeding. Discourage use together.

Coenzyme Q10, ginseng, St. John's wort: May reduce action of warfarin. Ask patient about use of herbal remedies, and advise caution.

Green tea: May decrease anticoagulant effect caused by vitamin K content of green tea. Advise patient to minimize variable consumption of green tea and other foods or nutritional supplements containing vitamin K.

Drug-food. *Cranberry juice:* May increase risk of severe bleeding. Discourage use together.

Foods, multivitamins, and other enteral products containing vitamin K: May impair anticoagulation. Tell patient to maintain consistent daily intake of foods containing vitamin K.

Drug-lifestyle. *Alcohol use:* May enhance anticoagulant effects. Tell patient to avoid large amounts of alcohol.

EFFECTS ON LAB TEST RESULTS
- May increase ALT and AST levels.
- May increase INR, PT, and PTT.
- May falsely decrease theophylline level.

CONTRAINDICATIONS & CAUTIONS
- Contraindicated in patients hypersensitive to drug and in those with bleeding from the GI, GU, or respiratory tract; aneurysm; cerebrovascular hemorrhage; severe or malignant hypertension; severe renal or hepatic disease; subacute bacterial endocarditis, pericarditis, or pericardial effusion; or blood dyscrasias or hemorrhagic tendencies.
- Contraindicated during pregnancy, threatened abortion, eclampsia, or preeclampsia, and after recent surgery involving large open areas, eye, brain, or spinal cord; recent prostatectomy; or major regional lumbar block anesthesia, spinal puncture, or diagnostic or therapeutic invasive procedures.
- Avoid using in patients with a history of warfarin-induced necrosis; in unsupervised patients with senility, alcoholism, or psychosis; or in situations in which there are inadequate laboratory facilities for coagulation testing.
- Use cautiously in patients with diverticulitis, colitis, mild or moderate hypertension, or mild or moderate hepatic or renal disease; with drainage tubes in any orifice; with regional or lumbar block anesthesia; with heparin-induced thrombocytopenia and deep venous thrombosis; or in conditions that increase risk of hemorrhage.
- Use cautiously in breast-feeding women.
- ⚠ ***Overdose S&S:*** Blood in stools or urine, excessive bruising, persistent oozing from superficial injuries, excessive menstrual bleeding, melena, petechiae.

NURSING CONSIDERATIONS
Black Box Warning Warfarin can cause major or fatal bleeding, which is more likely to occur during the starting period and with a higher dose. Regularly monitor INR in all patients. Consider more frequent

W

INR monitoring in those at high risk for bleeding. ∎

• Avoid all I.M. injections.

• Regularly inspect patient for bleeding gums, bruises on arms or legs, petechiae, nosebleeds, melena, tarry stools, hematuria, and hematemesis.

• Check for unexpected bleeding in breast-fed children of women who take this drug.

• Monitor patient for purple-toes syndrome, characterized by a dark purple or mottled color of the toes; may occur 3 to 10 weeks, or even later, after start of therapy.

❸ Alert: Withhold drug and call prescriber at once in the event of fever or rash (signs of severe adverse reactions).

• Effect can be neutralized by oral or parenteral vitamin K.

• Elderly patients and patients with renal or hepatic failure are especially sensitive to drug's effect.

• **Look alike–sound alike:** Don't confuse Coumadin with Avandia, Cardura, or Kemadrin. Don't confuse Jantoven with Janumet or Januvia.

PATIENT TEACHING

• Stress importance of complying with prescribed dosage and follow-up appointments. Tell patient to carry a card that identifies his increased risk of bleeding.

Black Box Warning Tell patient and family about measures to prevent bleeding, to watch for signs of bleeding or abnormal bruising, and to call prescriber at once if they occur. ∎

• Warn patient to avoid OTC products containing aspirin, other salicylates, or drugs that may interact with warfarin unless ordered by prescriber.

• Advise patient to consult prescriber before initiating any herbal therapy; many herbs have anticoagulant, antiplatelet, or fibrinolytic properties.

• Tell patient to consult prescriber before using miconazole vaginal cream or suppositories. Abnormal bleeding and bruising have occurred.

• Instruct female patient to notify prescriber if menstruation is heavier than usual; she may need dosage adjustment.

• Tell patient to use electric razor when shaving and to use a soft toothbrush.

• Tell patient to read food labels. Food, nutritional supplements, and multivitamins that contain vitamin K may impair anticoagulation.

• Tell patient to eat a daily, consistent diet of food and drinks containing vitamin K, because eating varied amounts may alter anticoagulant effects.

zafirlukast
zah-FUR-luh-kast

Accolate

Therapeutic class: Antiasthmatics
Pharmacologic class: Leukotriene-receptor antagonists
Pregnancy risk category: B

AVAILABLE FORMS
Tablets: 10 mg, 20 mg

INDICATIONS & DOSAGES
➤ **Prevention and long-term treatment of asthma**
Adults and children age 12 and older: 20 mg P.O. b.i.d.
Children ages 5 to 11: 10 mg P.O. b.i.d.

ADMINISTRATION
P.O.
• Give drug 1 hour before or 2 hours after meals.

ACTION
Selectively competes for leukotriene receptor sites, blocking inflammatory action.

Route	Onset	Peak	Duration
P.O.	Rapid	3 hr	Unknown

Half-life: 10 hours.

ADVERSE REACTIONS
CNS: headache, asthenia, dizziness, pain, fever.
GI: abdominal pain, diarrhea, dyspepsia, gastritis, nausea, vomiting.
Musculoskeletal: back pain, myalgia.
Other: accidental injury, infection.

Reactions in bold italics are *life-threatening*. Interactions may have a *rapid onset* or a *delayed onset*.

INTERACTIONS

Drug-drug. *Aspirin:* May increase zafirlukast level. Monitor patient for adverse effects.

Erythromycin, theophylline: May decrease zafirlukast level. Monitor patient for decreased effectiveness.

Warfarin: May increase PT. Monitor PT and INR, and adjust anticoagulant dosage.

Drug-food. *Any food:* May reduce rate and extent of drug absorption. Advise patient to take drug 1 hour before or 2 hours after a meal.

EFFECTS ON LAB TEST RESULTS

• May increase liver enzyme levels.

CONTRAINDICATIONS & CAUTIONS

• Contraindicated in patients hypersensitive to drug and in those with hepatic impairment.

• Use cautiously in elderly patients.

• Use in pregnant women only if clearly needed. Don't use in breast-feeding women.

⚠ Overdose S&S: Rash, upset stomach.

NURSING CONSIDERATIONS

❸ Alert: Reducing oral corticosteroid dose has been followed in rare cases by eosinophilia, vasculitic rash, worsening pulmonary symptoms, cardiac complications, or neuropathy, sometimes as Churg-Strauss syndrome.

• Drug isn't indicated to reverse bronchospasm in acute asthma attacks.

• Drug may cause behavior and mood changes. Monitor patient and consider discontinuing drug if neuropsychiatric symptoms develop.

• **Look alike–sound alike:** Don't confuse Accolate with Accupril or Aclovate.

PATIENT TEACHING

• Tell patient that drug is used for long-term treatment of asthma and to keep taking it even if symptoms resolve.

• Advise patient to continue taking other antiasthmatics, as prescribed.

• Instruct patient to take drug 1 hour before or 2 hours after meals.

• Warn patient that drug may cause behavior and mood changes, and to report development of these symptoms to prescriber.

• Teach patient to report rare but serious signs and symptoms of hepatic dysfunction (right upper quadrant abdominal pain, nausea, fatigue, lethargy, pruritus, jaundice, flulike symptoms, anorexia).

SAFETY ALERT!

zaleplon
ZAL-ah-plon

Sonata

Therapeutic class: Hypnotics
Pharmacologic class: Pyrazolopyrimidines
Pregnancy risk category: C
Controlled substance schedule: IV

AVAILABLE FORMS
Capsules: 5 mg, 10 mg

INDICATIONS & DOSAGES
➤ **Short-term treatment (7 to 10 days) of insomnia**

Adults: 10 mg P.O. daily at bedtime; may increase to 20 mg as needed. Low-weight adults may respond to 5-mg dose. Limit use to 7 to 10 days. Reevaluate patient if drug is used for more than 2 to 3 weeks.

Adjust-a-dose: For elderly or debilitated patients, initially, 5 mg P.O. daily at bedtime; doses of more than 10 mg aren't recommended. For patients with mild to moderate hepatic impairment or those also taking cimetidine, 5 mg P.O. daily at bedtime.

ADMINISTRATION
P.O.

• Give drug immediately before bed or after patient has gone to bed and has experienced difficulty falling asleep.

• Don't give drug after a high-fat or heavy meal.

ACTION

A hypnotic with chemical structure unrelated to benzodiazepines that interacts with the GABA–benzodiazepine receptor complex in the CNS. Modulation of this complex is thought to be responsible for sedative, anxiolytic, muscle relaxant, and anticonvulsant effects of benzodiazepines.

Z

Route	Onset	Peak	Duration
P.O.	1 hr	1 hr	3–4 hr

Half-life: 1 hour.

ADVERSE REACTIONS

CNS: complex sleep-related behaviors, headache, amnesia, anxiety, asthenia, depersonalization, depression, difficulty concentrating, dizziness, fever, hallucinations, hypertonia, hypesthesia, malaise, migraine, nervousness, paresthesia, somnolence, tremor, vertigo.
CV: chest pain, peripheral edema.
EENT: abnormal vision, conjunctivitis, ear discomfort, epistaxis, eye discomfort, hyperacusis, smell alteration.
GI: abdominal pain, anorexia, colitis, constipation, dry mouth, dyspepsia, nausea.
GU: dysmenorrhea.
Musculoskeletal: arthritis, back pain, myalgia.
Respiratory: bronchitis.
Skin: photosensitivity reactions, pruritus, rash.
Other: *anaphylaxis, angioedema.*

INTERACTIONS

Drug-drug. *Carbamazepine, phenobarbital, phenytoin, rifampin, other CYP3A4 inducers:* May reduce zaleplon bioavailability and peak level by 80%. Consider using a different hypnotic.
Cimetidine: May increase zaleplon bioavailability and peak level by 85%. Use an initial zaleplon dose of 5 mg.
CNS depressants (imipramine, thioridazine): May cause additive CNS effects. Use together cautiously.
Drug-food. *High-fat foods, heavy meals:* May prolong absorption, delaying peak drug level by about 2 hours; may delay sleep onset. Advise patient to avoid taking with meals.
Drug-lifestyle. *Alcohol use:* May increase CNS effects. Discourage use together.

EFFECTS ON LAB TEST RESULTS
None reported.

CONTRAINDICATIONS & CAUTIONS
● Contraindicated in patients with severe hepatic impairment.

● Use cautiously in elderly, depressed, or debilitated patients; in breast-feeding women; and in patients with compromised respiratory function.
⚠ *Overdose S&S:* Drowsiness, confusion, lethargy, ataxia, hypotension, respiratory depression, coma, death.

NURSING CONSIDERATIONS
● Closely monitor patients who have compromised respiratory function caused by illness or who are elderly or debilitated because they are more sensitive to respiratory depression.
● Start treatment only after carefully evaluating patient because sleep disturbances may be a symptom of an underlying physical or psychiatric disorder.
● Adverse reactions are usually dose-related. Consult prescriber about dose reduction if adverse reactions occur.
● *Look alike–sound alike:* Don't confuse zaleplon with Zelapar, Zemplar, or Zolpidem.

PATIENT TEACHING
⚠ *Alert:* Warn patient that drug may cause allergic reactions, facial swelling, and complex sleep-related behaviors, such as driving, eating, and making phone calls while asleep. Advise patient to report these adverse effects.
● Advise patient that drug works rapidly and should only be taken immediately before bedtime or after he has gone to bed and has had trouble falling asleep.
● Advise patient to take drug only if he will be able to sleep for at least 4 undisturbed hours.
● Caution patient that drowsiness, dizziness, light-headedness, and coordination problems occur most often within 1 hour after taking drug.
● Advise patient to avoid performing activities that require mental alertness until CNS adverse reactions are known.
● Advise patient to avoid alcohol use while taking drug and to notify prescriber before taking other prescription or OTC drugs.
● Tell patient not to take drug after a high-fat or heavy meal.
● Advise patient to report sleep problems that continue despite use of drug.

Reactions in bold italics are *life-threatening*. Interactions may have a *rapid onset* or a *delayed onset*.

• Notify patient that dependence can occur and that drug is recommended for short-term use only.

• Warn patient not to abruptly stop drug because of the risk of withdrawal symptoms, including unpleasant feelings, stomach and muscle cramps, vomiting, sweating, shakiness, and seizures.

• Notify patient that insomnia may recur for a few nights after stopping drug but should resolve on its own.

• Warn patient that drug may cause changes in behavior and thinking, including outgoing or aggressive behavior, loss of personal identity, confusion, strange behavior, agitation, hallucinations, worsening of depression, or suicidal thoughts. Tell patient to notify prescriber immediately if these symptoms occur.

---

zidovudine (azidothymidine, AZT, Compound S)
zid-oh-VEW-den

Novo-AZT†, Retrovir✐

Therapeutic class: Antiretrovirals
Pharmacologic class: Nucleoside–nucleotide reverse transcriptase inhibitors
Pregnancy risk category: C

AVAILABLE FORMS
Capsules: 100 mg
Injection: 10 mg/mL
Syrup: 50 mg/5 mL
Tablets: 300 mg

INDICATIONS & DOSAGES
Adjust-a-dose (for all indications): In patients with significant anemia (hemoglobin level less than 7.5 g/dL or more than 25% below baseline) or significant neutropenia (granulocyte count less than 750 cells/mm^3 or more than 50% below baseline), interrupt therapy until evidence proves marrow has recovered. In patients receiving hemodialysis or peritoneal dialysis, give 100 mg P.O. or 1 mg/kg I.V. every 6 to 8 hours. For patients with mild to moderate hepatic dysfunction or liver cirrhosis, daily dose may need to be reduced.

➤ **HIV infection, with other antiretrovirals**
Adults: 600 mg daily P.O. in divided doses with other antiretrovirals. If patient is unable to tolerate oral drug, give 1 mg/kg I.V. over 1 hour five to six times daily.
Children ages 4 weeks to less than 18 years: Do not exceed the recommended adult dose. For patients weighing 30 kg (66 lb) or more, 300 mg P.O. b.i.d. or 200 mg P.O. t.i.d. For patients weighing 9 kg to less than 30 kg (20 lb to less than 66 lb), 9 mg/kg P.O. b.i.d. or 6 mg/kg P.O. t.i.d. For patients weighing 4 kg to less than 9 kg (9 lb to less than 20 lb), 12 mg/kg P.O. b.i.d. or 8 mg/kg P.O. t.i.d.

➤ **To prevent maternal-fetal transmission of HIV**
Pregnant women at more than 14 weeks' gestation: 100 mg P.O. five times daily until the start of labor. Then, 2 mg/kg I.V. over 1 hour followed by a continuous I.V. infusion of 1 mg/kg/hour until the umbilical cord is clamped.
Neonates: 2 mg/kg P.O. every 6 hours starting within 12 hours after birth and continuing until 6 weeks old. Or, give 1.5 mg/kg via I.V. infusion over 30 minutes every 6 hours.

ADMINISTRATION
P.O.
• Drug should be taken on an empty stomach. To avoid esophageal irritation, patient should take drug with adequate fluids while sitting upright.
• Capsules shouldn't be kept in the kitchen, bathroom, or other places that may be damp or hot. Heat and moisture may cause the drug to break down and affect the intended results.

I.V.
▼ Give by this route only until oral drug can be tolerated.
▼ Remove the calculated dose from the vial; add to D_5W to achieve a concentration no greater than 4 mg/mL.
▼ Infuse drug over 1 hour at a constant rate. Avoid rapid infusion or bolus injection.
▼ Protect undiluted vials from light.
▼ Give diluted solution within 24 hours if stored at room temperature or 48 hours if refrigerated.

Z

▼ **Incompatibilities:** Biological or colloidal solutions, such as blood products or protein-containing solutions; meropenem.

ACTION

Nucleoside reverse transcriptase inhibitor that inhibits replication of HIV by blocking DNA synthesis.

Route	Onset	Peak	Duration
P.O., I.V.	Unknown	30–90 min	Unknown

Half-life: 1 hour.

ADVERSE REACTIONS

CNS: asthenia, dizziness, fever, headache, malaise, *seizures,* insomnia, paresthesia, somnolence.
GI: anorexia, nausea, vomiting, *pancreatitis,* abdominal pain, constipation, diarrhea, dyspepsia, taste perversion.
Hematologic: *agranulocytosis, severe bone marrow suppression, thrombocytopenia,* anemia.
Hepatic: hepatomegaly.
Metabolic: *lactic acidosis.*
Musculoskeletal: myalgia.
Respiratory: cough, wheezing.
Skin: rash, diaphoresis.

INTERACTIONS

Drug-drug. *Acetaminophen:* May decrease bioavailability of zidovudine. Adjust zidovudine dosage, as needed.
Atovaquone, fluconazole, methadone, probenecid, trimethoprim, valproic acid: May increase bioavailability of zidovudine. May need to adjust dosage.
Doxorubicin, ribavirin, stavudine: May have antagonistic effects. Avoid using together.
Ganciclovir, interferon alfa, other bone marrow suppressive or cytotoxic drugs: May increase hematologic toxicity of zidovudine. Use together cautiously.
Methadone: May increase zidovudine level. Monitor patient for myalgia, fever, and rash.
Phenytoin: May alter phenytoin level and decrease zidovudine clearance by 30%. Monitor patient closely.

EFFECTS ON LAB TEST RESULTS

● May increase ALT, AST, alkaline phosphatase, and LDH levels. May decrease hemoglobin level.
● May decrease granulocyte and platelet counts.

CONTRAINDICATIONS & CAUTIONS

● Contraindicated in patients hypersensitive to drug.
Black Box Warning Use cautiously and with close monitoring in patients with advanced symptomatic HIV infection and in those with severe bone marrow depression. Use of this drug has been associated with hematologic toxicity, including neutropenia and severe anemia. ∎
● Use cautiously in patients with hepatomegaly, hepatitis, or other risk factors for liver disease and in those with renal insufficiency. Monitor renal function tests and LFTs.
Black Box Warning Prolonged use has been associated with myopathy. ∎
⚠ *Overdose S&S:* Fatigue, headache, vomiting, hematologic disturbances.

NURSING CONSIDERATIONS

Black Box Warning Although rare, lactic acidosis without hypoxemia and severe hepatomegaly with steatosis may occur. Notify prescriber if patient develops unexplained tachypnea, dyspnea, or a decrease in bicarbonate level. Therapy may need to be suspended until lactic acidosis is ruled out. ∎
● Monitor blood studies every 2 weeks to detect anemia or agranulocytosis. Patients may need reduced dosage or temporary stop to therapy.
● Drug may temporarily decrease morbidity and mortality in certain patients with AIDS.
🜂 *Alert:* Drug is a potential teratogen. Follow safe-handling procedures when preparing, administering, or dispensing this drug.
● *Look alike–sound alike:* Don't confuse Retrovir with ritonavir.

PATIENT TEACHING

● Instruct patient to take drug on an empty stomach. To avoid esophageal irritation, tell patient to take drug while sitting upright and with adequate fluids.

Reactions in bold italics are *life-threatening*. Interactions may have a *rapid onset* or a *delayed onset*.

- Tell patient to take drug exactly as directed and not to share it with others.
- Remind patient to comply with the dosage schedule. Suggest ways to avoid missing doses, perhaps by using an alarm clock.
- Tell patient that dosages vary among patients and not to change his dosing instructions unless directed to do so by his prescriber.
- Warn patient not to take other drugs for AIDS unless prescriber has approved them.
- Advise patient that monotherapy isn't recommended and to discuss any questions with prescriber.
- Advise patient that blood transfusions may be needed during therapy because of drug-related anemia.
- Tell patient that his gums may bleed. Recommend good mouth care with a soft toothbrush.
- Advise pregnant, HIV-infected patient that drug therapy only reduces the risk of HIV transmission to her newborn. Long-term risks to infants are unknown.
- Tell patient not to keep capsules in the kitchen, bathroom, or other places that may be damp or hot. Heat and moisture may cause the drug to break down and affect the intended results.
- Advise health care worker considering prophylactic use after occupational exposure (such as needlestick injury) that drug's safety and effectiveness haven't been established.

ziprasidone hydrochloride
zih-PRAZ-i-done

Geodon✐

ziprasidone mesylate
Geodon

Therapeutic class: Antipsychotics
Pharmacologic class: Benzisoxazole derivatives
Pregnancy risk category: C

AVAILABLE FORMS
Capsules: 20 mg, 40 mg, 60 mg, 80 mg
I.M. injection: 20 mg/mL single-dose vials (after reconstitution)

INDICATIONS & DOSAGES
➤ Symptomatic treatment of schizophrenia
Adults: Initially, 20 mg P.O. b.i.d. with food. Dosages are highly individualized. Adjust dosage, if necessary, no more frequently than every 2 days; to allow for lowest possible doses, the interval should be several weeks to assess symptom response. Effective dosage range is usually 20 to 80 mg b.i.d. Maximum dosage is 100 mg b.i.d.
➤ Rapid control of acute agitation in schizophrenic patients
Adults: 10 to 20 mg I.M. as needed, up to a maximum dose of 40 mg daily. Doses of 10 mg may be given every 2 hours; doses of 20 mg may be given every 4 hours.
➤ Acute bipolar mania, including manic and mixed episodes, with or without psychotic features; maintenance treatment of bipolar I disorder as an adjunct to lithium or valproate
Adults: 40 mg P.O. b.i.d. with food on day 1. Increase to 60 to 80 mg P.O. b.i.d. with food on day 2; then adjust dosage based on patient response from 40 to 80 mg b.i.d. with food.

ADMINISTRATION
P.O.
- Always give drug with food for optimal effect.
I.M.
- To prepare I.M. ziprasidone, add 1.2 mL of sterile water for injection to the vial and shake vigorously until drug is completely dissolved.
- Don't mix injection with other medicinal products or solvents other than sterile water for injection.
- Inspect parenteral drug products for particulate matter and discoloration before administration.
- The effects of giving I.M. for more than 3 consecutive days are unknown. If long-term therapy of drug is necessary, switch to P.O. as soon as possible.
- Store injection at controlled room temperature, 59° to 86° F (15° to 30° C) in dry form, and protect from light. After reconstituting, it may be stored away from light for up to 24 hours at 59° to 86° F (15° to

Z

30° C) or up to 7 days refrigerated, 36° to 46° F (2° to 8° C).

ACTION

May inhibit dopamine and serotonin-2 receptors, causing reduction in schizophrenia symptoms.

Route	Onset	Peak	Duration
P.O.	1–3 days	6–8 hr	12 hr
I.M.	Unknown	1 hr	Unknown

Half-life: 2¼ to 7 hours.

ADVERSE REACTIONS

CNS: dizziness, headache, somnolence, *suicide attempt,* akathisia, dizziness, extrapyramidal symptoms, hypertonia, asthenia, dystonia (P.O.); anxiety, insomnia, agitation, cogwheel rigidity, paresthesia, personality disorder, psychosis, speech disorder (I.M.).
CV: *bradycardia, QT-interval prolongation,* orthostatic hypotension, tachycardia, chest pain (P.O.); hypertension, vasodilation (I.M.).
EENT: rhinitis, abnormal vision (P.O.).
GI: nausea, constipation, dyspepsia, diarrhea, dry mouth, anorexia, abdominal pain, *rectal hemorrhage,* vomiting, dyspepsia, tooth disorder (I.M.).
GU: dysmenorrhea, priapism (I.M.).
Metabolic: hyperglycemia.
Musculoskeletal: myalgia (P.O.), back pain (I.M.).
Respiratory: cough (P.O.).
Skin: rash (P.O.); injection-site pain, furunculosis, sweating (I.M.).
Other: flulike syndrome (I.M.).

INTERACTIONS

Drug-drug. *Antiarrhythmics (amiodarone, bretylium, disopyramide, dofetilide, procainamide, quinidine, sotalol), arsenic trioxide, dolasetron, droperidol, levomethadyl, mefloquine, pentamidine, phenothiazines, pimozide, quinolones, tacrolimus:* May increase the risk of life-threatening arrhythmias. Use together is contraindicated.
Antihypertensives: May enhance hypotensive effects. Monitor blood pressure.
Carbamazepine: May decrease ziprasidone level. May need to increase ziprasidone dose to achieve desired effect.

Drugs that decrease potassium or magnesium, such as diuretics: May increase risk of arrhythmias. Monitor potassium and magnesium levels if using these drugs together.
Itraconazole, ketoconazole: May increase ziprasidone level. May need to reduce ziprasidone dose to achieve desired effect.

EFFECTS ON LAB TEST RESULTS

None reported.

CONTRAINDICATIONS & CAUTIONS

● Contraindicated in patients hypersensitive to drug and in those with recent MI or uncompensated heart failure.
● Contraindicated in those with history of prolonged QT interval or congenital long QT syndrome and in those taking other drugs that prolong QT interval, such as dofetilide, sotalol, quinidine, other class IA and III antiarrhythmics, mesoridazine, thioridazine, chlorpromazine, droperidol, pimozide, sparfloxacin, gatifloxacin, moxifloxacin, halofantrine, mefloquine, pentamidine, arsenic trioxide, levomethadyl acetate, dolasetron mesylate, probucol, and tacrolimus.
◆ **Alert:** Neonates exposed to antipsychotics during the third trimester of pregnancy are at risk for developing extrapyramidal signs and symptoms (repetitive movements of the face and body) and withdrawal symptoms (agitation, abnormally increased or decreased muscle tone, tremors, sleepiness, severe difficulty breathing, difficulty feeding) following delivery. Use in pregnancy only if the potential benefit to the mother justifies the risk to the fetus.
P.O.
● Contraindicated in patients with a history of QT-interval prolongation or congenital long QT syndrome and in those taking other drugs that prolong QT interval.
● Use cautiously in patients with history of seizures, bradycardia, hypokalemia, or hypomagnesemia; in those with acute diarrhea; and in those with conditions that may lower the seizure threshold (such as Alzheimer dementia).
● Use cautiously in patients at risk for aspiration pneumonia.
● Don't use drug in breast-feeding women.

I.M.
- Contraindicated in schizophrenic patients already taking P.O. ziprasidone.
- Use cautiously in elderly and renally or hepatically impaired patients.

⚠ **Overdose S&S:** Sedation, slurred speech, transitory hypertension, anxiety, extrapyramidal symptoms, somnolence, tremor.

NURSING CONSIDERATIONS

Black Box Warning In elderly patients with dementia-related psychosis, drug isn't indicated for use because of increased risk of death from CV events or infection. ∎

🕘 **Alert:** Hyperglycemia may occur. Monitor patients with diabetes regularly. Patients with risk factors for diabetes should undergo fasting blood glucose testing at baseline and periodically. Monitor all patients for symptoms of hyperglycemia, including excessive hunger or thirst, frequent urination, and weakness. Hyperglycemia may be reversible when drug is stopped.

🕘 **Alert:** Monitor patient for symptoms of metabolic syndrome (significant weight gain and increased body mass index, hypertension, hyperglycemia, hypercholesterolemia, and hypertriglyceridemia).
- Stop drug in patients with a QTc interval more than 500 msec.
- Dizziness, palpitations, or syncope may be symptoms of a life-threatening arrhythmia such as torsades de pointes. Provide CV evaluation and monitoring in patients who experience these symptoms.
- Don't give to patients with electrolyte disturbances, such as hypokalemia or hypomagnesemia, because these increase the risk of arrhythmia. Monitor serum electrolyte levels periodically.

🕘 **Alert:** Patient taking an antipsychotic may develop life-threatening neuroleptic malignant syndrome (hyperpyrexia, muscle rigidity, altered mental status, and autonomic instability) or tardive dyskinesia. Assess abnormal involuntary movement before starting therapy, at dosage changes, and periodically thereafter, to monitor patient for tardive dyskinesia.
- Monitor patient for abnormal body temperature regulation, especially if he is exercising strenuously, is exposed to

extreme heat, is also receiving anticholinergics, or is subject to dehydration.
- Symptoms may not improve for 4 to 6 weeks.
- **Look alike–sound alike:** Don't confuse ziprasidone with trazodone.

PATIENT TEACHING
- Tell patient to take drug with food.
- Tell patient to immediately report to prescriber signs or symptoms of dizziness, fainting, irregular heartbeat, or relevant heart problems.
- Advise patient to report any recent episodes of diarrhea, abnormal movements, sudden fever, muscle rigidity, or change in mental status.
- Advise patient that symptoms may not improve for 4 to 6 weeks.
- Advise patient to avoid environments with high temperature and humidity.

zoledronic acid
zoh-leh-DROH-nik

Reclast, Zometa

Therapeutic class: Antiosteoporotics
Pharmacologic class: Bisphosphonates
Pregnancy risk category: D

AVAILABLE FORMS
Injection as ready-to-infuse solution:
5 mg/100 mL (Reclast), 4 mg/100 mL (Zometa)
Injection (Zometa): 4 mg/5-mL vial

INDICATIONS & DOSAGES
➤ **Hypercalcemia caused by malignancy**
Adults: 4 mg (Zometa) by I.V. infusion over at least 15 minutes. If albumin-corrected calcium level doesn't return to normal, may repeat 4 mg. Let at least 7 days pass before retreatment to allow a full response to the first dose.
Adjust-a-dose: For patients with CrCl of 50 to 60 mL/minute, give 3.5 mg. If 40 to 49 mL/minute, give 3.3 mg. If 30 to 39 mL/minute, give 3 mg. For patients with normal baseline creatinine level but an increase of 0.5 mg/dL and in those with abnormal baseline creatinine level who have an increase of

Z

1 mg/dL, withhold drug. Resume treatment only when creatinine level has returned to within 10% of baseline value. If CrCl is less than 30 mL/minute, don't give drug.

➤ **Multiple myeloma and bone metastases of solid tumors in conjunction with standard antineoplastics**

Adults: 4 mg (Zometa) I.V. infused over at least 15 minutes every 3 to 4 weeks. Treatment duration depends on type of cancer. Use for prostate cancer only after it has progressed after treatment with at least one course of hormonal therapy. Give patients an oral calcium supplement of 500 mg and a multiple vitamin containing 400 international units of vitamin D daily.

Adjust-a-dose: For patients with CrCl of 50 to 60 mL/minute, give 3.5 mg. If 40 to 49 mL/minute, give 3.3 mg. If 30 to 39 mL/minute, give 3 mg. For patients with normal baseline creatinine level but an increase of 0.5 mg/dL and in those with abnormal baseline creatinine level who have an increase of 1 mg/dL, withhold drug. Resume treatment only when creatinine level has returned to within 10% of baseline value. If CrCl is less than 30 mL/minute, don't give drug.

➤ **Paget disease of bone (osteitis deformans)**

Adults: 5 mg (Reclast) by I.V. infusion over at least 15 minutes. Give through a vented infusion line. May repeat if relapse occurs. Patient also needs 1,500 mg elemental calcium and 800 international units vitamin D daily, especially during the 2 weeks after dosing.

➤ **Treatment of osteoporosis in men; to reduce the incidence of fractures in postmenopausal women with osteoporosis and a recent low-trauma hip fracture; to treat and prevent glucocorticoid-induced osteoporosis in patients expected to be treated for at least 12 months**

Adults: 5 mg (Reclast) by I.V. infusion over no less than 15 minutes once a year.

➤ **Prevention of osteoporosis**

Postmenopausal women: 5 mg (Reclast) by I.V. infusion over no less than 15 minutes once every 2 years.

➤ **Osteopenia secondary to androgen-deprivation therapy in prostate cancer ◆**

Adults: 4 mg (Zometa) I.V. infused over 15 minutes every 3 months.

➤ **Osteopenia in estrogen-deprived breast cancer ◆**

Adults: 4 mg (Zometa) I.V. infused over 15 minutes every 6 months for up to 5 years.

ADMINISTRATION

I.V.

Zometa

▼ For patient with CrCl greater than 60 mL/minute, withdraw 5 mL to obtain 4 mg of drug and mix in 100 mL of normal saline solution or D₅W. For patient with CrCl of 60 mL/minute or less, withdraw 4.4 mL for the 3.5-mg dose, 4.1 mL for the 3.3-mg dose, or 3.8 mL for the 3-mg dose.

▼ Give as I.V. infusion over at least 15 minutes.

▼ If drug is not used immediately after reconstitution, refrigerate solution and give within 24 hours.

Reclast

▼ Reclast is infused over not less than 15 minutes given at a constant infusion rate. Give as a single I.V. solution through a separate vented infusion line.

▼ If refrigerated, allow the refrigerated solution to reach room temperature before administration.

▼ After opening, solution is stable for 24 hours at 36° to 46° F (2° to 8° C).

▼ **Incompatibilities:** Solutions containing calcium (such as lactated Ringer's solution) or other I.V. drugs.

ACTION

Inhibits bone resorption, probably by inhibiting osteoclast activity and osteoclastic resorption of mineralized bone and cartilage. Decreases calcium release induced by the stimulatory factors produced by tumors.

Route	Onset	Peak	Duration
I.V. (Zometa)	Unknown	Unknown	7–28 days
I.V. (Reclast)	Unknown	Unknown	Unknown

Half-life: Alpha is 0.23 hours; beta is 1.75 hours for early distribution. Terminal half-life is 167 hours.

ADVERSE REACTIONS

CNS: headache, anxiety, somnolence, insomnia, confusion, agitation, depression, paresthesia, hypoesthesia, fatigue, weakness, dizziness, fever, asthenia, malaise, vertigo, lethargy.

CV: hypotension, hypertension, atrial fibrillation, leg edema, chest pain.
GI: nausea, constipation, diarrhea, abdominal pain, vomiting, anorexia, dysphagia, decreased appetite, dyspepsia, abdominal distention, mucositis, stomatitis.
EENT: eye pain.
GU: *increased creatinine level,* urinary infection, moniliasis.
Hematologic: anemia, *granulocytopenia, neutropenia, thrombocytopenia, pancytopenia.*
Metabolic: decreased calcium, phosphate, and *magnesium* levels; dehydration; weight decrease.
Musculoskeletal: skeletal pain, arthralgia, myalgia, back pain, osteonecrosis of the jaw, osteoarthritis, muscle spasms, bone pain, neck pain, shoulder pain, extremity pain.
Respiratory: dyspnea, cough, pleural effusion.
Skin: alopecia, dermatitis, rash, pruritus.
Other: *progression of cancer,* rigors, infection, influenza, hyperhidrosis.

INTERACTIONS
Drug-drug. *Aminoglycosides, loop diuretics:* May have additive effects that lower calcium level. Use together cautiously, and monitor calcium level.
Nephrotoxic drugs, such as NSAIDs: Renal toxicity may be greater in patients with renal impairment. Use Reclast cautiously with other potentially nephrotoxic drugs. Monitor serum creatinine before each dose.
Thalidomide: May increase risk of renal dysfunction in patients with multiple myeloma. Use together cautiously.

EFFECTS ON LAB TEST RESULTS
• May increase creatinine level.
• May decrease calcium, phosphorus, magnesium, potassium, and hemoglobin levels and hematocrit.
• May decrease RBC, WBC, and platelet counts.

CONTRAINDICATIONS & CAUTIONS
• Contraindicated in patients hypersensitive to drug, other bisphosphonates, or any of its ingredients; in patients with hypercalcemia of malignancy whose creatinine level is more than 4.5 mg/dL; in patients with bone metastases and a creatinine level of more than 3 mg/dL; and in breast-feeding women.
❸ *Alert:* There may be an increased risk of fractures of the thigh in patients treated with bisphosphonates.
• Reclast is contraindicated in patients with hypocalcemia. Patients must be adequately supplemented with calcium and vitamin D.
❸ *Alert:* Reclast may increase risk of renal failure, especially in patients with underlying renal impairment, dehydration, and increased age. Screen patients before use and monitor carefully.
❸ *Alert:* Reclast is contraindicated in patients with CrCl less than 35 mL/minute and in patients with evidence of acute renal failure.
• Use cautiously in elderly patients and those with aspirin-sensitive asthma because other bisphosphonates have been linked to bronchoconstriction in aspirin-sensitive patients with asthma.
⚠ *Overdose S&S:* Hypocalcemia, hypophosphatemia, hypomagnesemia, renal impairment.

NURSING CONSIDERATIONS
• Reclast contains the same active ingredient found in Zometa, used for oncology indications. A patient being treated with Zometa shouldn't be treated with Reclast
• Hydrate patient adequately before giving; urine output should be about 2 L daily.
• Each vial of Zometa contains 220 mg mannitol and 24 mg sodium citrate.
❸ *Alert:* Because of the risk of decreased renal function progressing to renal failure, don't exceed 4 mg as a single dose of Zometa and always infuse over at least 15 minutes.
• Monitor calcium, phosphate, magnesium, and creatinine levels carefully. Correct decreased calcium, phosphorus, and magnesium levels using I.V. calcium gluconate, potassium and sodium phosphate, and magnesium sulfate.
• Monitor renal function closely. Patients with renal impairment may be at a greater risk for adverse reactions.
❸ *Alert:* Patients, especially those who have cancer or poor oral hygiene or who are receiving chemotherapy or corticosteroids, should have a dental examination with

Z

appropriate preventive dentistry before therapy.

● Osteonecrosis of the jaw has been reported rarely in postmenopausal osteoporosis patients treated with bisphosphonates, including zoledronic acid. All patients should have a routine oral examination before treatment and should be monitored while on therapy.

● Severe incapacitating bone, joint, and muscle pain may occur. Withhold future doses of Reclast if severe symptoms occur. When drug is stopped, symptoms may resolve partially or completely.

PATIENT TEACHING

● Review the use and administration of drug with patient and family.

● Instruct patient to report adverse effects promptly.

● Explain the importance of periodic laboratory tests to monitor therapy and renal function.

● If a woman becomes pregnant or is breastfeeding, advise her to alert prescriber.

zolmitriptan
zohl-mah-TRIP-tan

Zomig, Zomig-ZMT

Therapeutic class: Antimigraine drugs
Pharmacologic class: Serotonin 5-HT$_1$ receptor agonists
Pregnancy risk category: C

AVAILABLE FORMS
Nasal spray: 5 mg
Tablets (immediate-release): 2.5 mg, 5 mg
Tablets (orally disintegrating): 2.5 mg, 5 mg

INDICATIONS & DOSAGES
➤ **Acute migraine headaches**
Adults: Initially, 2.5 mg or less P.O. Break a 2.5-mg immediate-release tablet in half if a lower dose is needed. Increase to 5 mg per dosage, as needed. If using orally disintegrating tablets (ODTs), initially, 2.5 mg P.O. Or, 1 spray (5 mg) into nostril. If headache returns after first dose, give a second dose at least 2 hours after the first dose. Maximum dosage is 10 mg in 24 hours.

Adjust-a-dose: In patients with hepatic disease, use doses less than 2.5 mg. Don't use ODTs because they shouldn't be broken in half, or nasal spray because 5 mg is the lowest deliverable dose.

ADMINISTRATION
P.O.
● Give ODT immediately after opening.
● Don't break or crush ODT.
● ODT dissolves on tongue and is swallowed with saliva; fluid isn't needed.
Intranasal
● Don't test the spray before use.

ACTION
May act as an agonist at serotonin receptors on extracerebral intracranial blood vessels, which constricts the affected vessels, inhibits neuropeptide release, and reduces pain transmission in the trigeminal pathways.

Route	Onset	Peak	Duration
P.O.	Unknown	2 hr	3 hr
Intranasal	5 min	3 hr	Unknown

Half-life: 3 hours.

ADVERSE REACTIONS
CNS: dizziness, somnolence, vertigo, hypesthesia, paresthesia, asthenia, pain.
CV: *coronary artery vasospasm, transient myocardial ischemia, MI, ventricular tachycardia, ventricular fibrillation,* palpitations, pain; tightness, pressure, or heaviness in chest.
EENT: pain, tightness, or pressure in the neck, throat, or jaw.
GI: dry mouth, dyspepsia, dysphagia, nausea.
Musculoskeletal: myalgia, myasthenia.
Skin: sweating.
Other: warm or cold sensations.

INTERACTIONS
Drug-drug. *Cimetidine:* May double halflife of zolmitriptan. Limit maximum single dose of zolmitriptan to 2.5 mg, not to exceed 5 mg in any 24-hour period. Monitor patient closely.

Reactions in bold italics are *life-threatening*. Interactions may have a *rapid onset* or a *delayed onset*.

Ergot-containing drugs, other triptans: May cause additive effects. Avoid using within 24 hours of zolmitriptan.

Hormonal contraceptives, propranolol: May increase zolmitriptan level. Monitor patient closely.

MAO inhibitors: May increase zolmitriptan level. Avoid using within 2 weeks of MAO inhibitor.

SSRIs: May cause additive serotonin effects, resulting in weakness, hyperreflexia, or incoordination. Monitor patient closely if given together.

EFFECTS ON LAB TEST RESULTS
● May increase alkaline phosphatase and glucose levels.

CONTRAINDICATIONS & CAUTIONS
● Contraindicated in patients hypersensitive to drug or its components, pregnant or breast-feeding patients, and those with uncontrolled hypertension, hemiplegic or basilar migraine, ischemic heart disease (angina pectoris, history of MI or documented silent ischemia), symptoms of ischemic heart disease (coronary artery vasospasm, including Prinzmetal variant angina), or other significant heart disease.
● Contraindicated within 24 hours of other triptans or drugs containing ergot or within 2 weeks of stopping MAO inhibitor.
● Use cautiously in patients with liver disease and in those who may be at risk for coronary artery disease (such as postmenopausal women or men older than age 40) or those with risk factors, such as hypertension, hypercholesterolemia, obesity, diabetes, smoking, or family history.

⚠ *Overdose S&S:* Sedation.

NURSING CONSIDERATIONS
● Drug isn't intended for preventing migraines or treating hemiplegic or basilar migraines.
● Safety of drug hasn't been established for cluster headaches.

☺ *Alert:* Combining drug with an SSRI or an SSNRI may cause serotonin syndrome. Signs and symptoms may include restlessness, hallucinations, loss of coordination, fast heartbeat, rapid changes in blood pressure, increased body temperature, overactive reflexes, nausea, vomiting, and diarrhea. Serotonin syndrome may be more likely to occur when starting or increasing the dose of drug, SSRI, or SSNRI.

PATIENT TEACHING
● Tell patient that drug is intended to relieve, not prevent, signs and symptoms of migraine.
● Advise patient to take drug as prescribed and not to take a second dose unless instructed by prescriber. Tell patient if a second dose is indicated and permitted, he should take it 2 hours after first dose.
● Instruct patient to release the ODTs from the blister pack just before taking; tablet should dissolve on tongue.
● Advise patient not to break the ODTs in half.
● Advise patient to immediately report pain or tightness in the chest or throat, heart throbbing, rash, skin lumps, or swelling of the face, lips, or eyelids.
● Tell woman not to take drug if she is or may become pregnant.

SAFETY ALERT!

zolpidem tartrate
ZOL-pih-dem

Ambien✒, Ambien CR, Edluar, Intermezzo, Zolpimist

Therapeutic class: Hypnotics
Pharmacologic class: Imidazopyridines
Pregnancy risk category: C
Controlled substance schedule: IV

AVAILABLE FORMS
Oral spray: 5 mg/actuation
Tablets: 5 mg, 10 mg
Tablets (extended-release): 6.25 mg, 12.5 mg
Tablets (S.L.): 1.75 mg, 3 mg, 5 mg, 10 mg

INDICATIONS & DOSAGES
➤ **Short-term management of insomnia**
Adults: 5 or 10 mg (men) or 5 mg (women) immediate-release or 6.25 or 12.5 mg (men) or 6.25 mg (women) extended-release P.O. immediately before bedtime. Or, Intermezzo 1.75 mg (women) or 3.5 mg (men) S.L.

Z

once per night as needed for middle-of-the-night waking and difficulty returning to sleep, only if at least 4 hours of bedtime remain. Or, 10 mg Zolpimist once per night immediately before bedtime.

Adjust-a-dose: For elderly or debilitated patients and those with hepatic insufficiency, 5 mg P.O. immediately before bedtime. Or, 6.25 mg of extended-release form. Or, 1.75 mg P.O. Intermezzo if needed in men and women older than age 65. Maximum daily dose is 10 mg immediate-release and 6.25 mg extended-release.

ADMINISTRATION
P.O.
● For rapid sleep onset, drug should not be taken with or immediately after meals.
● Don't crush, break, or divide extended-release tablets.
● Place S.L. tablet under tongue to disintegrate. Patient shouldn't swallow tablet whole or take with water.
● Prime oral spray pump before first use or if the pump hasn't been used for 14 days.
● Pump spray directly over tongue. Have patient press down fully to make sure full dose is delivered.

ACTION
Although drug interacts with one of three identified GABA-benzodiazepine receptor complexes, it isn't a benzodiazepine. It exhibits hypnotic activity and minimal muscle relaxant and anticonvulsant properties.

Route	Onset	Peak	Duration
P.O.	Rapid	30–120 min	Unknown

Half-life: 2½ hours.

ADVERSE REACTIONS
CNS: headache, amnesia, change in dreams, complex sleep-related behaviors, daytime drowsiness, depression, dizziness, hangover, lethargy, light-headedness, nervousness, sleep disorder.
CV: palpitations.
EENT: pharyngitis, sinusitis.
GI: abdominal pain, constipation, diarrhea, dry mouth, dyspepsia, nausea, vomiting.
Musculoskeletal: arthralgia, myalgia.
Skin: rash.

Other: *anaphylaxis, angioedema,* back or chest pain, flulike syndrome, hypersensitivity reactions.

INTERACTIONS
Drug-drug. *CNS depressants:* May cause excessive CNS depression. Use together cautiously.
Rifampin: May decrease effects of zolpidem. Avoid using together, if possible. Consider another hypnotic.
Drug-herb. *Gotu kola, kava kava, valerian:* May increase risk of CNS depression. Avoid concomitant use.
St. John's wort: May decrease zolpidem level and effects. Avoid concomitant use.
Drug-food. *Grapefruit juice:* May decrease zolpidem metabolism. Avoid grapefruit juice.
Drug-lifestyle. *Alcohol use:* May cause excessive CNS depression. Discourage use together.

EFFECTS ON LAB TEST RESULTS
● May increase ALT and AST levels.
● May decrease radioactive iodine uptake.

CONTRAINDICATIONS & CAUTIONS
● No known contraindications.
● Use cautiously in patients with compromised respiratory status.
● Complex behaviors such as "sleep driving" (driving while not fully awake after taking a sedative-hypnotic with subsequent amnesia of the event) have been reported. These can occur with therapeutic doses, although the use of alcohol and other CNS depressants appears to increase the risk. Strongly consider discontinuing drug if patient reports such an event.
◑ **Alert:** Drug level may remain elevated the day after drug use, impairing mental alertness. Risk increases if patient sleeps for less than 7 hours, takes drug with other CNS depressants including alcohol, or takes higher than recommended dose.
◑ **Alert:** Patients taking extended-release formulation shouldn't drive or engage in other activities that require complete mental alertness the day after taking drug because drug level can remain high enough to impair these activities.

Reactions in bold italics are *life-threatening*. Interactions may have a *rapid onset* or a *delayed onset*.

⚠ **Overdose S&S:** Impaired consciousness, somnolence, coma, CV or respiratory compromise, death.

NURSING CONSIDERATIONS

❸ **Alert:** Anaphylaxis and angioedema may occur as early as the first dose. Monitor patient closely.

• Use drug only for short-term management of insomnia, usually 7 to 10 days.

• Use the smallest effective dose in all patients.

• Take precautions to prevent hoarding by patients who are depressed, suicidal, or drug-dependent, or who have a history of drug abuse.

• **Look alike–sound alike:** Don't confuse Ambien with Amen.

PATIENT TEACHING

❸ **Alert:** Warn patient that drug may cause allergic reactions, facial swelling, and complex sleep-related behaviors, such as driving, eating, and making phone calls while asleep. Advise patient to report these adverse effects.

❸ **Alert:** Tell patient that drug has the potential to cause next-day impairment, and that this risk increases if dosing instructions aren't carefully followed. Tell patient to wait for at least 8 hours after dosing before driving or engaging in other activities requiring full mental alertness. Inform patient that impairment can be present even though he may feel fully awake.

• For rapid sleep onset, instruct patient not to take drug with or immediately after meals.

• Instruct patient to take drug immediately before going to bed; onset of action is rapid.

• Tell patient to take Intermezzo in bed when he awakens in the middle of the night and has difficulty returning to sleep, and only if he has at least 4 hours of bedtime remaining.

• Tell patient to avoid alcohol use while taking drug.

• Tell patient to place the S.L. tablet under the tongue and allow the tablet to disintegrate. Tell the patient not to swallow, chew, break, or split the tablet, or take the tablet with water.

❸ **Alert:** Tell patient not to crush, chew, or divide the extended-release tablets.

• Instruct patient to prime the spray pump before first use or if the pump hasn't been used for 14 days.

• Tell patient to aim the spray directly over the tongue and press down fully to make sure the full dose is delivered.

• Caution patient to avoid performing activities that require mental alertness or physical coordination during therapy.

zonisamide
zoh-NISS-a-mide

Zonegran

Therapeutic class: Anticonvulsants
Pharmacologic class: Sulfonamides
Pregnancy risk category: C

AVAILABLE FORMS
Capsules: 25 mg, 50 mg, 100 mg

INDICATIONS & DOSAGES
➤ **Adjunctive therapy for partial seizures in adults with epilepsy**
Adults and children older than age 16:
Initially, 100 mg P.O. as a single daily dose for 2 weeks. Then, dosage may be increased to 200 mg daily for at least 2 weeks. Dosage can be increased to 300 mg and then to 400 mg P.O. daily, with the dose stable for at least 2 weeks to achieve steady state at each level. Doses can be given once daily or b.i.d., except for the daily dose of 100 mg at start of therapy. Maximum recommended dose is 600 mg daily.
Adjust-a-dose: For patients with renal or hepatic impairment, titrate dosages more slowly and monitor patients more frequently.

ADMINISTRATION
P.O.
• Give drug without regard for food.
• Don't crush or open capsule.

ACTION
May stabilize neuronal membranes and suppress neuronal hypersynchronization, which prevents seizures.

Z

Route	Onset	Peak	Duration
P.O.	Unknown	2–6 hr	Unknown

Half-life: 63 hours.

ADVERSE REACTIONS

CNS: dizziness, headache, somnolence, *seizures, status epilepticus,* agitation or irritability, anxiety, asthenia, ataxia, confusion, depression, difficulties in concentration or memory, difficulties in verbal expression, fatigue, hyperesthesia, incoordination, insomnia, mental slowing, nervousness, paresthesia, schizophrenic or schizophreniform behavior, speech disorders, tremor.

EENT: amblyopia, diplopia, pharyngitis, rhinitis, taste perversion, tinnitus, nystagmus.

GI: anorexia, abdominal pain, constipation, diarrhea, dry mouth, dyspepsia, nausea, vomiting.

GU: kidney stones.

Hematologic: ecchymoses.

Metabolic: weight loss.

Respiratory: cough.

Skin: pruritus, rash.

Other: accidental injury, flulike syndrome.

INTERACTIONS

Drug-drug. *Drugs that induce or inhibit CYP3A4:* May change zonisamide level; phenytoin, carbamazepine, phenobarbital, and valproate increase zonisamide clearance. Monitor patient closely.

EFFECTS ON LAB TEST RESULTS

• May increase BUN and creatinine levels.

CONTRAINDICATIONS & CAUTIONS

• Contraindicated in patients hypersensitive to drug or to sulfonamides.

• Contraindicated in those with GFR less than 50 mL/minute.

• Use cautiously in patients with renal and hepatic dysfunction or kidney stones.

• Use cautiously in patients with history of psychiatric symptoms.

• Use cautiously with other drugs that predispose patients to heat-related disorders, including but not limited to carbonic anhydrase inhibitors and drugs with anticholinergic activity.

• Safety and effectiveness in children younger than age 16 haven't been established; children are at increased risk for oligohidrosis and hyperthermia caused by zonisamide.

⚠ *Overdose S&S:* CNS symptoms, coma, bradycardia, hypotension, respiratory depression.

NURSING CONSIDERATIONS

❸ *Alert:* Rarely, patients receiving sulfonamides have died because of severe reactions, such as Stevens-Johnson syndrome, fulminant hepatic necrosis, aplastic anemia, otherwise unexplained rashes, and agranulocytosis. If signs and symptoms of hypersensitivity or other serious reactions occur, stop drug immediately and notify prescriber.

❸ *Alert:* Closely monitor all patients taking or starting antiepileptic drugs for changes in behavior indicating worsening of suicidal thoughts or behavior or depression. Symptoms such as anxiety, agitation, hostility, mania, and hypomania may be precursors to emerging suicidality.

• If patient develops acute renal failure or a significant sustained increase in creatinine or BUN level, stop drug and notify prescriber.

• Drug can cause metabolic acidosis, especially in those with predisposing conditions or therapies. This risk is more frequent and severe in younger patients. Measure serum bicarbonate level before starting treatment and periodically during treatment, even in the absence of symptoms.

• Don't stop drug abruptly because this may cause increased seizures or status epilepticus; reduce dosage or stop drug gradually.

• Achieving steady-state levels may take 2 weeks.

• Monitor patient for signs and symptoms of hypersensitivity.

• Increase fluid intake and urine output to help prevent kidney stones, especially in patients with predisposing factors.

• Monitor renal function periodically.

• Monitor patient for cognitive and neuropsychiatric adverse reactions, including psychomotor slowing, difficulty with

---

Reactions in bold italics are *life-threatening*. Interactions may have a *rapid onset* or a *delayed onset*.

concentration, speech or language problems (especially word-finding difficulties), somnolence or fatigue, depression, and psychosis.

PATIENT TEACHING
• Tell patient to take drug with or without food and not to bite or break capsule.
• Advise patient to call prescriber immediately if rash develops or seizures worsen.
• Tell patient to contact prescriber immediately if he develops sudden back or abdominal pain, pain when urinating, bloody or dark urine, fever, sore throat, mouth sores or easy bruising, decreased sweating, fever, depression, or speech or language problems.
• Tell patient to drink 6 to 8 glasses of water a day.
• Caution patient that this drug can cause drowsiness and not to drive or operate dangerous machinery until drug's effects are known.
• Advise patient not to stop taking drug without prescriber's approval.
• Instruct women of childbearing age to call prescriber if pregnant or breast-feeding or planning to become pregnant or breast-feed.
• Advise women of childbearing age to use contraceptives while taking drug.

Appendices

Avoiding common drug errors:
Best practices and prevention

In addition to following your institution's administration policies, you can help prevent errors in drug administration by reviewing these common errors and ways to prevent them. The Joint Commission, the Institute for Safe Medication Practices (ISMP), and the FDA also maintain resources to help improve drug safety.

Topic	Error	Best practices and prevention
Drug orders		
Pharmacy computer system	The system may not detect all unsafe orders.	• Don't rely on the pharmacy computer system to detect all unsafe orders. • Before giving a drug, understand the correct indication, dosage, and potential adverse effects. • Consult the pharmacist if there is any question, and verify the information using a current drug reference.
Confusing drug names	Many drugs have names that look alike–sound alike and may easily be mistaken one for the other.	• Be aware of the drugs your patient takes regularly, and question any deviations from his routine. • Take your time and read the label carefully. • Consult the ISMP list of look alike–sound alike drugs. • Be aware of tall man lettering, which helps differentiate similar drug names.
Abbreviations	Using dangerous abbreviations can result in giving the wrong drug or wrong dose, by the wrong route, or at the wrong time.	• Don't abbreviate drug names. • Be aware of The Joint Commission's official "Do not use" list of drug abbreviations to avoid (see *Appendix 4: Abbreviations to avoid*, page 1490). • Consult your facility's list of approved abbreviations and the ISMP's list of "Error-prone abbreviations, symbols, and dose designations" (www.ismp.org/tools/errorproneabbreviations.pdf).
Unclear order	A drug order with incomplete or unclear information can result in giving the wrong drug or wrong dose, by the wrong route, or at the wrong time.	• Keep in mind that each order should specify the correct drug name, dosage, route, and frequency of administration. • Clarify all incomplete or unclear orders with the prescriber.
Inadvertent overdose	A prescriber may write an order for a combination drug such as acetaminophen/opioid analgesic tablets without realizing the total acetaminophen dose could be toxic (exceed 4 g).	• Note the amount of acetaminophen in each combined formulation. • Be aware of pharmacy substitutions because acetaminophen amounts may vary. • Warn patients not to take additional drugs that contain acetaminophen.
Anticoagulants	Lack of standardization for drug naming, labeling, and packaging can create confusion. Dosing regimens, assay methods, narrow therapeutic ranges, complex drug interactions, and drug monitoring methods create high potential for complications.	• Keep current with the different dosing regimens, assay methods, drug interactions, monitoring methods, and reversal regimens for each anticoagulant given. • Be especially aware of the correct doses and indications for neonates and children. • Teach patients to manage their therapy appropriately.

Topic	Error	Best practices and prevention
Drug preparation		
Crushing drugs for oral or enteral administration	Crushing certain oral or enteral drugs may: • alter the drug's effects, causing overdose or other adverse reactions • result in skin irritation or other adverse reactions for the preparer • produce teratogenic effects in pregnant women.	• Use a liquid formulation instead of crushing a drug whenever possible. • Before crushing a drug, always check with the pharmacist and established references, such as the ISMP's list of "Oral dosage forms that should not be crushed" (www.ismp.org/tools/donotcrush.pdf). • See *Appendix 11: Drugs that shouldn't be crushed or chewed*, page 1509.
Solution color change or particulate matter	Unusual appearance may indicate that: • the drug has been improperly stored or manufactured • the drug has expired • the wrong drug was provided by the pharmacy.	• Closely examine all solutions before giving them, and know what their appearance should be. • If you note a color change, contact the pharmacist who dispensed the solution and report it. • Don't give a drug until verifying that the drug has been correctly labeled and that it is safe to give.
Incorrect drug storage	Incorrect storage may change a drug's physical properties or result in its being inadvertently administered.	• Follow your facility's policy for storing drugs. • Always store drugs in the appropriate container, in the appropriate place, at the appropriate temperature.
Incomplete or incorrect drug labels	Incorrect or incomplete labeling can result in giving the wrong drug, formulation, or dose.	• Never give a drug whose label is incomplete or incorrect. Notify the pharmacy immediately and obtain the correctly labeled drug. • Label all medications, medication containers, and other solutions on and off the sterile field.
Drug administration		
Using a parenteral syringe for oral or enteral drugs	Using a parenteral syringe with a luer-lock to prepare small amounts of oral or enteral drugs can result in misadministration because the drug could be accidentally injected into an I.V. line.	• Always use special oral syringes to give oral or enteral drugs. Their hubs won't support a needle and they don't have a luer-lock, so they can't be attached to I.V. lines.
Infusion pump safety problems	Problems with infusion pumps (used to deliver controlled fluids, drugs, and nutrients) can cause fluid overload or administration of inaccurate doses.	• Make sure you know how to safely operate an infusion pump. Consult your facility's policy on proper usage. • Before beginning an infusion, always verify that the pump is working properly. Make sure all alarms are functional and never bypass them. • Double-check all dosing.
Calculation errors	Dosage calculation errors can cause significant patient harm, especially with "high alert" medications, and in neonates and children.	• Be aware of medications that are considered high alert. • Write out the mg/kg or mg/m^2 dose and the calculated dose as a safeguard. • Whenever a prescriber provides a calculation, double-check it and document that the dose was verified in the medical record. • Use only approved abbreviations, and be aware of the placement of decimal points.

Topic	Error	Best practices and prevention
Herbal supplements	Because herbal supplements aren't subject to the same quality assurance standards as drugs, their labels may be misrepresented and their effects and interactions with drugs may not be well studied.	• Always assess and document all drugs and herbal supplements that the patient is taking in his medical record. • Monitor the patient carefully, and report unusual adverse reactions. • Consult a drug reference for known drug-herb interactions.

Pregnancy risk categories

The FDA has assigned a pregnancy risk category to each drug based on available clinical and preclinical information. The five categories (A, B, C, D, and X) reflect a drug's potential to cause birth defects. Although drugs should ideally be avoided during pregnancy, sometimes they're needed; this rating system permits rapid assessment of the risk-benefit ratio. Drugs in category A are generally considered safe to use in pregnancy; drugs in category X are generally contraindicated.

- A: Adequate studies in pregnant women have failed to show a risk to the fetus in the first trimester, and there is no evidence of risk in the second and third trimesters.
- B: Animal studies haven't shown a risk to the fetus, but controlled studies haven't been conducted in pregnant women; or animal studies have shown an adverse effect on the fetus, but adequate studies in pregnant women haven't shown a risk to the fetus.
- C: Animal studies have shown an adverse effect on the fetus, but adequate studies haven't been conducted in humans. The benefits from use in pregnant women may be acceptable despite potential risks.
- D: There is positive evidence of human fetal risk, but the potential benefits of use in pregnant women may warrant use of the drug despite the potential risks (such as in a life-threatening situation or a serious disease for which safer drugs can't be used or are ineffective).
- X: Studies in animals or humans show fetal abnormalities, or adverse reaction reports indicate evidence of fetal risk. The risks involved clearly outweigh potential benefits.

Controlled substance schedules

Drugs regulated under the jurisdiction of the Controlled Substances Act of 1970 are divided into the following groups or schedules:

- Schedule I (C-I): High abuse potential and no accepted medical use. Examples include heroin and LSD.
- Schedule II (C-II): High abuse potential with severe dependence liability. Examples include opioids, amphetamines, and some barbiturates.
- Schedule III (C-III): Less abuse potential than schedule II drugs and moderate dependence liability. Examples include nonbarbiturate sedatives, nonamphetamine stimulants, anabolic steroids, and limited amounts of certain opioids.
- Schedule IV (C-IV): Less abuse potential than schedule III drugs and limited dependence liability. Examples include some sedatives, anxiolytics, and nonopioid analgesics.
- Schedule V (C-V): Limited abuse potential. This category includes mainly small amounts of opioids, such as codeine, used as antitussives or antidiarrheals. Under federal law, limited quantities of certain Schedule V drugs may be purchased without a prescription directly from a pharmacist if allowed under specific state statutes. The purchaser must be at least age 18 and must furnish suitable identification. All such transactions must be recorded by the dispensing pharmacist.

Abbreviations to avoid

The Joint Commission requires every health care facility to develop a list of approved abbreviations for staff use. Certain abbreviations should be avoided because they're easily misunderstood, especially when handwritten. The Joint Commission has identified a minimum list of dangerous abbreviations, acronyms, and symbols. This do-not-use list includes the following items.

Official "Do Not Use" List[1]		
Do not use	Potential problem	Use instead
U, u (unit)	Mistaken for "O" (zero), the number "4" (four), or "cc"	Write "unit"
IU (International Unit)	Mistaken for IV (intravenous) or the number 10 (ten)	Write "International Unit"
Q.D., QD, q.d., qd (daily)	Mistaken for each other	Write "daily"
Q.O.D., QOD, q.o.d, qod (every other day)	Period after the Q mistaken for "I" and the "O" mistaken for "I"	Write "every other day"
Trailing zero (X.0 mg)* Lack of leading zero (.X mg)	Decimal point is missed	Write X mg Write 0.X mg
MS	Can mean morphine sulfate or magnesium sulfate	Write "morphine sulfate" Write "magnesium sulfate"
MSO_4 and $MgSO_4$	Confused for one another	

[1]Applies to all orders and all medication-related documentation that is handwritten (including free-text computer entry) or on pre-printed forms.

*Exception: A "trailing zero" may be used only where required to demonstrate the level of precision of the value being reported, such as for laboratory results, imaging studies that report size of lesions, or catheter/tube size. It may not be used in medication orders or other medication-related documentation.

Additional Abbreviations, Acronyms, and Symbols
(For possible future inclusion in the Official "Do Not Use" List)

Do not use	Potential problem	Use instead
> (greater than) < (less than)	Misinterpreted as the number "7" (seven) or the letter "L" Confused for one another	Write "greater than" Write "less than"
Abbreviations for drug names	Misinterpreted due to similar abbreviations for multiple drugs	Write drug names in full
Apothecary units	Unfamiliar to many practitioners Confused with metric units	Use metric units
@	Mistaken for the number "2" (two)	Write "at"
cc	Mistaken for U (units) when poorly written	Write "mL" or "ml" or "milliliters" ("mL" is preferred)
μg	Mistaken for mg (milligrams) resulting in one thousand-fold overdose	Write "mcg" or "micrograms"

© The Joint Commission, 2013. Reprinted with permission.

Pediatric drugs commonly involved in drug errors

According to the Joint Commission, the rate of medication errors for pediatric and adult inpatients is similar, but potentially harmful errors occur almost three times as frequently in children. One of the most common errors that occur in hospitalized children is administering the incorrect pediatric dosage. Here are some of the medications most commonly involved in medication errors as reported to the national voluntary medication error reporting system, MEDMARX, with their FDA-approved dosages.

Medication	Indication	Route	Usual dosage
albuterol sulfate	Bronchospasm in children with reversible obstructive airway disease	P.O. (immediate-release tablets and extended-release tablets)	• *Children older than age 12:* Initially, 2 or 4 mg (immediate-release tablets) P.O. t.i.d. or q.i.d. If patient fails to respond, may increase dosage to maximum of 8 mg P.O. q.i.d. Or, 8 mg (extended-release tablets) P.O. every 12 hours. If patient fails to respond, increase dosage cautiously to maximum of 16 mg P.O. every 12 hours. • *Children ages 6 to 12:* Initially, 2 mg (immediate-release tablets) P.O. t.i.d. or q.i.d. May increase dosage cautiously, but total daily dosage shouldn't exceed 24 mg/day (given in divided doses). Or, 4 mg (extended-release tablets) P.O. every 12 hours. If control of reversible airway isn't achieved with optimized asthma therapy, may cautiously increase dosage to maximum of 12 mg P.O. every 12 hours.
	Bronchospasm in children with reversible obstructive airway disease	P.O. (syrup)	• *Children older than age 14:* Initially, 2 mg (1 teaspoonful) or 4 mg (2 teaspoonfuls) P.O. t.i.d. or q.i.d. If patient fails to respond, dosage may be cautiously increased to maximum of 8 mg P.O. q.i.d. • *Children ages 6 to 14:* Initially, 2 mg (1 teaspoonful) P.O. t.i.d. or q.i.d. If patient fails to respond, dosage may be increased to maximum of 24 mg/day given in divided doses. • *Children ages 2 to younger than 6:* Initially, 0.1 mg/kg P.O. t.i.d. Initial dose shouldn't exceed 2 mg (1 teaspoonful) P.O. t.i.d. If patient fails to respond, may increase dosage to 0.2 mg/kg P.O. t.i.d. Maximum dosage is 4 mg (2 teaspoonfuls) P.O. t.i.d.

Medication	Indication	Route	Usual dosage
ceftriaxone sodium	Acute bacterial otitis media in children younger than age 12	I.M.	• *Children:* Give single dose of 50 mg/kg I.M. Maximum dosage is 1 g.
	Serious infections (including skin and skin-structure infections) other than meningitis	I.V. infusion over at least 30 minutes or I.M.	• *Children younger than age 12:* 50 to 75 mg/kg I.M. or I.V. in divided doses every 12 hours. Continue for at least 2 days after signs and symptoms of infection have disappeared. Usual duration of therapy is 4 to 14 days. Maximum dosage is 2 g/day.
	Meningitis	I.V. infusion over at least 30 minutes or I.M.	• *Children younger than age 12:* Initially, 100 mg/kg (not to exceed 4 g) I.M. or I.V. Thereafter, give total daily dose of 100 mg/kg/day I.M. or I.V. for 7 to 14 days. Maximum dosage is 4 g daily. Daily dose may be administered once a day or in equally divided doses every 12 hours.
dopamine	Hypotension, low cardiac output, poor perfusion of vital organs, shock	I.V. (continuous infusion)	• *Children:* Initially, 2 to 5 mcg/kg/minute I.V. in patients who are likely to respond to modest increments of heart force and renal perfusion. In more severely ill patients, begin I.V. infusion at 5 mcg/kg/minute. In more severely ill patients, increase dosage gradually, using 5- to 10-mcg/kg/minute increments, up to 20 to 50 mcg/kg/minute as needed. If doses greater than 50 mcg/kg/minute are required, check urine output frequently. Should urine flow begin to decrease in the absence of hypotension, consider reducing dopamine dosage. More than 50% of patients have been satisfactorily maintained on doses of less than 20 mcg/kg/minute. Patients treated with MAO inhibitors within 2 to 3 weeks before administration of dopamine should receive initial doses of dopamine not greater than one-tenth of usual dose.
fentanyl	To manage persistent, chronic pain only in opioid-tolerant patients (children receiving at least 60 mg/day of morphine P.O.)	Transdermal	• *Children age 2 and older:* When converting to transdermal system, base first dose on the daily dose, potency, and characteristics of the current opioid therapy; reliability of the relative potency estimates used to calculate the needed dose; degree of opioid tolerance; and patient's condition. Each patch is worn for 72 hours; dosage may be increased 3 days after first dose and then no sooner than every 6 days thereafter.
gentamicin sulfate	Serious infections caused by sensitive strains of *Pseudomonas aeruginosa, Escherichia coli, Proteus, Klebsiella, Serratia,* or *Staphylococcus*	I.V. infusion over 30 minutes to 2 hours or I.M.	• *Children:* 2 to 2.5 mg/kg I.V. or I.M. every 8 hours. • *Infants and neonates:* 2.5 mg/kg I.V. or I.M. every 8 hours. • *Premature or full-term neonates age 1 week or younger:* 2.5 mg/kg I.V. or I.M. every 12 hours.

Medication	Indication	Route	Usual dosage
heparin	Thrombosis	I.V.	• *Children:* Initially, 50 units/kg I.V., followed by continuous I.V. infusion that delivers 100 units/kg every 4 hours or 20,000 units/m²/ 24 hours.
morphine sulfate	Analgesia	I.V.	• *Children:* 50 to 100 mcg (0.05 to 0.1 mg)/kg I.V., administered very slowly. Not to exceed 10 mg/dose.
		I.M. or subcuta-neously	• *Children:* 0.1 to 0.2 mg/kg I.M. or subcutaneous-ly every 4 hours. Maximum dosage is 15 mg.
	Preanesthetic medication	I.M. or subcuta-neously	• *Children age 1 and older:* 0.1 mg/kg subcuta-neously or I.M. Maximum dosage is 10 mg.
vancomycin	Endocarditis or staphylococcal infections	I.V.	• *Children age 1 month and older:* 10 mg/kg/dose I.V. every 6 hours. Administer over at least 60 minutes.
	Endocarditis	I.V.	• *Neonates:* Initially, 15 mg/kg I.V., followed by 10 mg/kg I.V. every 12 hours for neonates in the first week of life and every 8 hours there-after up to the age of 1 month. Administer over 60 minutes. In premature infants, longer dos-ing intervals may be necessary.
	Pseudomembranous colitis or staphylococ-cal enterocolitis	P.O.	• *Children:* 40 mg/kg/day P.O. in three or four di-vided doses for 7 to 10 days. Maximum dosage is 2 g/day.

Elder care medication tips

Age-related changes can alter the way older people absorb, distribute, metabolize, and eliminate medications compared to younger adults or children. Medication dosages and routes may need adjustment to optimize the patient's response to medication and help prevent adverse reactions. Understanding how age-related factors can alter how an older patient's body uses medication will help you plan and implement your patient's medication regimen and monitor his response appropriately. The table below describes how age-related factors can change the pharmacokinetics of medications in older adults.

Pharmacokinetics	Age-related change	Effect on pharmacokinetics
Absorption	Diminished quality and quantity of digestive enzymes	⬇
	Increased gastric pH	⬆ or ⬇
	Decreased GI motility and emptying time	⬇
	Decreased GI blood flow	⬇
	Diminished number of absorbing cells	⬇
Distribution	Diminished cardiac output and reserve	⬇
	Diminished blood flow to target organs and tissues	⬇
	Decreased lean body mass	⬇
	Increased adipose tissue	⬆ or ⬇
	Decreased circulating plasma proteins	⬇
	Decreased total body water	⬇
Metabolism	Decreased liver size	⬇
	Diminished intestinal and portal vein blood flow	⬇
Excretion	Decreased GFR	⬇
	Decreased renal tubular secretion	⬇
	Decreased renal blood flow from renovascular occlusive disease, microvascular nephropathy, or heart failure	⬇

Drugs that prolong the QTc interval

Changes in a patient's heart rate can affect the QT interval of his ECG. To account for such changes, you can use a formula such as the one below. Such formulas let you determine the corrected QT (QTc) interval.

$$\frac{QT\ interval}{\sqrt{R\text{-}R\ interval}} = QTc\ interval$$

For men younger than age 55, a normal QTc interval is 350 to 430 msec; for women younger than age 55, a normal QTc interval is 350 to 450 msec.

A prolonged QTc interval may cause fatal arrhythmias, including ventricular tachycardia and torsades de pointes. The causes of a prolonged QTc interval include disorders such as hypokalemia, hypomagnesemia, renal failure, and heart failure. These drugs may also cause an abnormal QTc interval.

albuterol	droperidol	levofloxacin	quinine
amantadine	efavirenz	levomethadyl	ranolazine
amiodarone	erythromycin	lithium	rilpivirine
arformoterol	escitalopram	maprotiline	risperidone
aripiprazole	famotidine	mefloquine	salmeterol
arsenic trioxide	felbamate	mesoridazine	serotonin reuptake inhibitors
artemether–lumefantrine	fexofenadine	methadone	
	flecainide	moexipril	sotalol
asenapine	fluconazole	moxifloxacin	sparfloxacin
atomoxetine	fluoxetine	naratriptan	sulfamethoxazole
azithromycin	fluphenazine	nicardipine	sumatriptan
bedaquiline	formoterol	nilotinib	tacrolimus
celecoxib	foscarnet	octreotide	tamoxifen
chloroquine	fosphenytoin	ofloxacin	telithromycin
chlorpromazine	furosemide	ondansetron	terbutaline
citalopram	gemifloxacin	oxytocin	tetrabenazine
clarithromycin	granisetron	paliperidone	thioridazine
clindamycin	halofantrine	palonosetron	tizanidine
clozapine	haloperidol	papaverine	trazodone
cyclobenzaprine	halothane	paroxetine	TCAs
degarelix	hydroxyzine	pentamidine	trifluoperazine
diphenhydramine	ibutilide	perphenazine	trimethoprim
disopyramide	iloperidone	prednisolone	vardenafil
dofetilide	indapamide	prednisone	vasopressin
dolasetron	isoproterenol	procainamide	voriconazole
domperidone	isradipine	propafenone	vorinostat
doxorubicin	itraconazole	quetiapine	ziprasidone
dronedarone	ketoconazole	quinidine	zolmitriptan

Therapeutic drug monitoring guidelines

Drug	Laboratory test monitored	Therapeutic ranges of test
ACE inhibitors (benazepril, captopril, enalapril, enalaprilat, fosinopril, lisinopril, moexipril, quinapril, ramipril, trandolapril)	Creatinine BUN Potassium WBC with differential	0.6–1.3 mg/dL 5–20 mg/dL 3.5–5 mEq/L *****
aminoglycoside antibiotics (amikacin, gentamicin, tobramycin)	Amikacin peak Amikacin trough Creatinine Gentamicin, tobramycin peak Gentamicin, tobramycin trough	20–30 mcg/mL 1–8 mcg/mL 0.6–1.3 mg/dL 6–10 mcg/mL <2 mcg/mL
amphotericin B	BUN CBC with differential and platelets Creatinine Electrolytes (especially potassium and magnesium) Liver function	8–25 mg/dL ***** 0.6–1.3 mg/dL Potassium: 3.5–5 mEq/L Magnesium: 1.5–2.5 mEq/L Sodium: 135–145 mEq/L Chloride: 98–106 mEq/L *
antibiotics	Cultures and sensitivities WBC with differential	*****
biguanides (metformin)	CBC Creatinine Fasting glucose Glycosylated hemoglobin	***** 0.6–1.3 mg/dL 70–110 mg/dL 5.3%–7.5% of total hemoglobin
carbamazepine	BUN Carbamazepine CBC with differential Liver function Platelet count	8–25 mg/dL 6–12 mcg/mL ***** * $140–400 \times 10^3/mm^3$
clozapine	WBC with differential	*****
corticosteroids (cortisone, hydrocortisone, prednisone, prednisolone, triamcinolone, methylprednisolone, dexamethasone, betamethasone)	Electrolytes (especially potassium) Fasting glucose	Potassium: 3.5–5 mEq/L Magnesium: 1.3–2.2 mEq/L Sodium: 135–145 mEq/L Chloride: 98–106 mEq/L Calcium: 8.6–10 mg/dL 65–115 mg/dL

***** For those areas marked with asterisks, the following values can be used:

Hemoglobin: Women: 12–16 g/dL
          Men: 14–18 g/dL
Hematocrit: Women: 37%–48%
        Men: 42%–52%
RBCs: $4–5.5 \times 10^6/mm^3$
WBCs: $5–10 \times 10^3/mm^3$

Differential: Neutrophils: 45%–74%
        Bands: 0%–8%
        Lymphocytes: 16%–45%
        Monocytes: 4%–10%
        Eosinophils: 0%–7%
        Basophils: 0%–2%

Monitoring guidelines

Monitor WBC with differential before therapy, monthly during the first 3 to 6 months, then periodically for the first year. Monitor renal function and potassium level periodically.

Wait until after the third dose is given to check drug levels. Obtain blood for peak level 30 minutes after I.V. infusion ends or 60 minutes after I.M. administration. For trough levels, draw blood just before next dose. Dosage may need to be adjusted accordingly. Recheck after three doses. Monitor creatinine and BUN levels and urine output for signs of decreasing renal function. Monitor urine for increased proteins, cells, and casts.

Monitor creatinine, BUN, and electrolyte levels at least weekly during therapy. Regularly monitor blood counts and LFT results during therapy.

Monitor WBC with differential weekly during therapy. Specimen cultures and sensitivities will determine the cause of the infection and the best treatment.

Check renal function and hematologic values before starting therapy and at least annually thereafter. If the patient has impaired renal function, don't use metformin because it may cause lactic acidosis. Monitor response to therapy by periodically evaluating fasting glucose and glycosylated hemoglobin levels. A patient's home monitoring of glucose levels helps monitor compliance and response.

Monitor blood counts and platelets before therapy, monthly during the first 2 months, then yearly. LFTs, BUN, and urinalysis should be checked before and periodically during therapy.

Before starting, patient must have a baseline WBC count of at least 3,500/mm^3 and a baseline ANC of at least 2,000/mm^3. During the first 6 months of therapy, monitor patient weekly. If acceptable WBC and ANC values are maintained, reduce monitoring to every other week. After 6 months of monitoring without leukopenia, monitor every 4 weeks. WBC count and ANC must be monitored weekly for at least 4 weeks after stopping drug.

Monitor electrolyte and glucose levels regularly during long-term therapy.

(continued)

---

* For those areas marked with one asterisk, the following values can be used:
ALT: 7–56 units/L
AST: 5–40 units/L
Alkaline phosphatase: 17–142 units/L
LDH: 140–280 units/L
GGT: <40 units/L
Total bilirubin: 0.2–1 mg/dL

Drug	Laboratory test monitored	Therapeutic ranges of test
digoxin	Creatinine	0.6–1.3 mg/dL
	Digoxin	0.8–2 nanograms/mL
	Electrolytes	Potassium: 3.5–5 mEq/L
		Magnesium: 1.7–2.1 mEq/L
		Sodium: 135–145 mEq/L
		Chloride: 98–106 mEq/L
		Calcium: 8.6–10 mg/dL
erythropoietin	CBC with differential	*****
	Hematocrit	Women: 36%–48%
		Men: 42%–52%
	Platelet count	140–400 × 10^3/mm^3
	Serum ferritin	10–383 nanograms/mL
	Transferrin saturation	220–400 mg/dL
ethosuximide	CBC with differential	*****
	Ethosuximide	40–100 mcg/mL
	Liver function	*
gemfibrozil	CBC	*****
	Lipids	Total cholesterol: <200 mg/dL
		LDL: <130 mg/dL
		HDL: ≥60 mg/dL
		Triglycerides: 150 mg/dL
	Liver function	*
	Serum glucose	70–110 mg/dL
heparin	Partial thromboplastin time (PTT)	1.5–2.5 times control
	Hematocrit	*****
	Platelet count	150–450 × 10^3/mm^3
HMG-CoA reductase inhibitors (atorvastatin, fluvastatin, lovastatin, pravastatin, rosuvastatin, simvastatin)	Lipids	Total cholesterol: <200 mg/dL
		LDL: <130 mg/dL
		HDL: ≥60 mg/dL
		Triglycerides: <150 mg/dL
	Liver function	*
insulin	Fasting glucose	65–115 mg/dL
	Glycosylated hemoglobin	5.3%–7.5% of total hemoglobin
isotretinoin	CBC with differential	*****
	Liver function	*
	Lipids	Total cholesterol: <200 mg/dL
		LDL: <130 mg/dL
		HDL: ≥60 mg/dL
		Triglycerides: <150 mg/dL
	Platelet count	140–400 × 10^3/mm^3
	Pregnancy test	Negative

***** For those areas marked with asterisks, the following values can be used:

Hemoglobin: Women: 12–16 g/dL
          Men: 14–18 g/dL
Hematocrit: Women: 37%–48%
         Men: 42%–52%
RBCs: 4–5.5 × 10^6/mm^3
WBCs: 5–10 × 10^3/mm^3

Differential: Neutrophils: 45%–74%
        Bands: 0%–8%
        Lymphocytes: 16%–45%
        Monocytes: 4%–10%
        Eosinophils: 0%–7%
        Basophils: 0%–2%

Monitoring guidelines

Check digoxin levels just before the next dose or at least 6 to 8 hours after the last dose. To monitor maintenance therapy, check drug levels at least 1 to 2 weeks after therapy is initiated or changed.
Make any adjustments in therapy based on entire clinical picture, not solely on drug levels. Also, check electrolyte levels and renal function periodically during therapy.

After therapy is initiated or changed, monitor the hematocrit twice weekly for 2 to 6 weeks until they are stabilized in the target range and a maintenance dose has been determined. Monitor hematocrit regularly thereafter.

Check drug level 8 to 10 days after therapy is initiated or changed. Periodically monitor CBC with differential, LFTs, and urinalysis.

Therapy is usually withdrawn after 3 months if response is inadequate. Patient must be fasting to measure triglyceride levels. Periodically obtain blood counts during the first 12 months.

When drug is given by continuous I.V. infusion, check PTT every 4 hours in the early stages of therapy, and daily thereafter. When drug is given by deep subcutaneous injection, check PTT 4 to 6 hours after injection, and daily thereafter. Periodically during therapy, check platelet counts and hematocrit and test for occult blood in stools.

Perform LFTs at baseline, 6 to 12 weeks after therapy is initiated or changed, and about every
6 months thereafter. If adequate response isn't achieved within 6 weeks, consider changing the therapy.

A patient's home monitoring of glucose levels helps measure compliance and response.
Glycosylated hemoglobin level is a good measure of long-term control.

Use a serum or urine pregnancy test with a sensitivity of at least 25 milli-international units/mL. Perform one test before therapy and a second test during the first 5 days of the menstrual cycle before therapy begins or at least 11 days after the last unprotected act of sexual intercourse, whichever is later. Repeat pregnancy tests monthly. Obtain baseline LFTs and lipid levels; repeat every 1 to 2 weeks until a response is established (usually 4 weeks).

(continued)

* For those areas marked with one asterisk, the following values can be used:
ALT: 7–56 units/L
AST: 5–40 units/L
Alkaline phosphatase: 17–142 units/L
LDH: 140–280 units/L
GGT: <40 units/L
Total bilirubin: 0.2–1 mg/dL

Drug	Laboratory test monitored	Therapeutic ranges of test
linezolid	Amylase	35–118 international units/L
	CBC with differential	*****
	Cultures and sensitivities	
	Liver function	*
	Lipase	10–150 units/L
	Platelet count	140–400 × 10³/mm³
lithium	Creatinine	0.6–1.3 mg/dL
	CBC	*****
	Electrolytes (especially potassium and sodium)	Potassium: 3.5–5 mEq/L
		Magnesium: 1.7–2.1 mEq/L
		Sodium: 135–145 mEq/L
		Chloride: 98–106 mEq/L
	Fasting glucose	70–110 mg/dL
	Lithium	0.6–1.2 mEq/L
	Thyroid function tests	TSH: 0.2–5.4 microunits/mL
		T₃: 80–200 nanograms/dL
		T₄: 5.4–11.5 mcg/dL
methotrexate	CBC with differential	*****
	Creatinine	0.6–1.3 mg/dL
	Liver function	*
	Methotrexate	Normal elimination:
		~ 10 micromol 24 hours postdose
		~ 1 micromol 48 hours postdose
		<0.2 micromol 72 hours postdose
	Platelet count	150–450 × 10³/mm³
NNRTIs (nevirapine, delavirdine, efavirenz)	Amylase	35–118 international units/L
	CBC with differential and platelets	*****
	Liver function	*
	Lipids (efavirenz)	Total cholesterol: <200 mg/dL
		LDL: <130 mg/dL
		HDL: ≥60 mg/dL
		Triglycerides: <150 mg/dL
phenytoin	Albumin	3.6–5 g/dL
	CBC	*****
	Phenytoin	10–20 mcg/mL
procainamide	ANA titer	Negative
	CBC	*****
	Liver function	*
	N-acetylprocainamide (NAPA)	10–30 mcg/mL
	Procainamide	3–10 mcg/mL

***** For those areas marked with asterisks, the following values can be used:

Hemoglobin: Women: 12–16 g/dL
      Men: 14–18 g/dL
Hematocrit: Women: 37%–48%
      Men: 42%–52%
RBCs: 4–5.5 × 10⁶/mm³
WBCs: 5–10 × 10³/mm³

Differential: Neutrophils: 45%–74%
      Bands: 0%–8%
      Lymphocytes: 16%–45%
      Monocytes: 4%–10%
      Eosinophils: 0%–7%
      Basophils: 0%–2%

Monitoring guidelines

Obtain baseline CBC with differential and platelet count. Repeat weekly, especially if more than 2 weeks of therapy are received. Monitor LFTs and amylase and lipase levels during therapy.

Checking drug levels is crucial to the safe use of the drug. Obtain level immediately before next dose. Monitor level twice weekly until stable. Once at steady state, level should be checked weekly; when the patient is on the appropriate maintenance dose, levels should be checked every 2 or 3 months. Monitor CBC; creatinine, electrolyte, and fasting glucose levels; and thyroid function test results before therapy starts and periodically thereafter.

Monitor drug levels according to dosing protocol. Monitor CBC with differential, platelet count, and LFT and renal function test results more frequently when therapy starts or changes and when methotrexate levels may be elevated, such as when the patient is dehydrated.

Obtain baseline LFTs and monitor closely during the first 12 weeks of therapy. Continue to monitor regularly during therapy. Check CBC with differential and platelet count before therapy and periodically during therapy. Monitor lipid levels during efavirenz therapy. Monitor amylase level during efavirenz and delavirdine therapy.

Monitor drug level immediately before next dose and 7 to 10 days after therapy starts or changes. Obtain a CBC at baseline and monthly early in therapy. Watch for toxic effects at therapeutic levels. Adjust the measured level for hypoalbuminemia or renal impairment, which can increase free drug levels.

Measure drug levels 6 to 12 hours after a continuous infusion is started or immediately before the next oral dose. Combined procainamide and NAPA levels can be used as an index of toxicity when renal impairment exists. Obtain CBC, LFTs, and ANA titer periodically during longer-term therapy.

(continued)

---

* For those areas marked with one asterisk, the following values can be used:
ALT: 7–56 units/L
AST: 5–40 units/L
Alkaline phosphatase: 17–142 units/L
LDH: 140–280 units/L
GGT: <40 units/L
Total bilirubin: 0.2–1 mg/dL

Drug	Laboratory test monitored	Therapeutic ranges of test
quinidine	CBC	*****
	Creatinine	0.6–1.3 mg/dL
	Electrolytes (especially potassium)	Potassium: 3.5–5 mEq/L
		Magnesium: 1.7–2.1 mEq/L
		Sodium: 135–145 mEq/L
		Chloride: 98–106 mEq/L
	Liver function	*
	Quinidine	2–6 mcg/mL
sulfonylureas	Fasting glucose	65–115 mg/dL
	Glycosylated hemoglobin	4%–7% of total hemoglobin
theophylline	Theophylline	10–20 mcg/mL
thiazolidinediones (rosiglitazone, pioglitazone)	Fasting glucose	65–115 mg/dL
	Glycosylated hemoglobin	4%–7% of total hemoglobin
	Liver function	*
thyroid hormones	Thyroid function tests	TSH: 0.2–5.4 microunits/mL
		T_3: 80–200 nanogram/dL
		T_4: 5.4–11.5 mcg/dL
valproate sodium, valproic acid, divalproex sodium	Ammonia	15–45 mcg/dL
	Amylase	35–118 international units/L
	BUN	8–25 mg/dL
	CBC with differential	*****
	Creatinine	0.6–1.3 mg/dL
	Liver function	*
	Platelet count	$150–450 \times 10^3/mm^3$
	PTT	10–14 seconds
	Valproic acid	40–100 mcg/mL
vancomycin	Creatinine	0.6–1.3 mg/dL
	Vancomycin	20–40 mcg/mL (peak)
		5–15 mcg/mL (trough)
warfarin	INR	For an acute MI, atrial fibrillation, treatment of pulmonary embolism, prevention of systemic embolism, tissue heart valves, valvular heart disease, or prophylaxis or treatment of venous thrombosis: 2–3 For mechanical prosthetic valves or recurrent systemic embolism: 2.5–3.5

***** For those areas marked with asterisks, the following values can be used:

Hemoglobin: Women: 12–16 g/dL
        Men: 14–18 g/dL
Hematocrit: Women: 37%–48%
       Men: 42%–52%
RBCs: $4–5.5 \times 10^6/mm^3$
WBCs: $5–10 \times 10^3/mm^3$

Differential: Neutrophils: 45%–74%
      Bands: 0%–8%
      Lymphocytes: 16%–45%
      Monocytes: 4%–10%
      Eosinophils: 0%–7%
      Basophils: 0%–2%

Monitoring guidelines

Obtain levels immediately before next oral dose and 30 to 35 hours after therapy starts or changes. Periodically obtain blood counts, LFT and renal function test results, and electrolyte levels.

Monitor response to therapy by periodically evaluating fasting glucose and glycosylated hemoglobin levels. Patient should monitor glucose levels at home to help measure compliance and response.

Obtain drug levels right before next dose of sustained-release oral product and at least 2 days after therapy starts or changes.

Monitor response by evaluating fasting glucose and glycosylated hemoglobin levels. Obtain baseline LFT results, and repeat tests periodically during therapy. Don't initiate therapy with pioglitazone or rosiglitazone if ALT is more than 2.5 times the upper limit of normal.

Monitor thyroid function test results every 2 to 3 weeks until appropriate maintenance dose is determined and annually thereafter.

Monitor LFT results, ammonia level, coagulation test results, renal function test results, CBC, and platelet count at baseline and periodically during therapy. LFT results should be closely monitored during the first 6 months.

Drug levels may be checked with the third dose administered, at the earliest. Draw peak levels 1.5 to 2.5 hours after a 1-hour infusion or I.V. infusion is complete. Draw trough levels within 1 hour of the next dose administered. Renal function can be used to adjust dosing and intervals.

Check INR daily, beginning 3 days after therapy starts. Continue checking it until therapeutic goal is achieved, and monitor it periodically thereafter. Also, check level 7 days after change in dose or start of a potentially interacting therapy.

* For those areas marked with one asterisk, the following values can be used:
ALT: 7–56 units/L
AST: 5–40 units/L
Alkaline phosphatase: 17–142 units/L
LDH: 140–280 units/L
GGT: <40 units/L
Total bilirubin: 0.2–1 mg/dL

Cytochrome P-450 enzymes and common drug interactions

Cytochrome P-450 enzymes, identified by "CYP" followed by numbers and letters identifying the enzyme families and subfamilies, are found throughout the body (primarily in the liver) and are important in the metabolism of many drugs. This table lists some common drug-drug interactions based on substrates, inducers, and inhibitors that can influence drug metabolism.

CYP enzyme	Substrates
1A2	acetaminophen, aminophylline, amitriptyline, betaxolol, caffeine, chlordiazepoxide, clomipramine, clozapine, cyclobenzaprine, desipramine, diazepam, doxepin, flutamide, fluvoxamine, haloperidol, imipramine, mirtazapine, naproxen, olanzapine, pimozide, propranolol, ropinirole, tacrine, theophylline, verapamil, warfarin, zileuton, zolmitriptan
2C9	alosetron, amiodarone, amitriptyline, bosentan, carvedilol, clomipramine, dapsone, diazepam, diclofenac, flurbiprofen, fluvastatin, glimepiride, glipizide, ibuprofen, imipramine, indomethacin, losartan, mirtazapine, montelukast, naproxen, omeprazole, phenytoin, pioglitazone, ritonavir, sildenafil, tolbutamide, torsemide, vardenafil, voriconazole, warfarin, zafirlukast, zileuton
2C19	amitriptyline, carisoprodol, celecoxib, citalopram, clomipramine, cyclophosphamide, desogestrol, diazepam, doxepin, escitalopram, esomeprazole, fenofibrate, fluoxetine, glyburide, imipramine, irbesartan, lansoprazole, mephenytoin, omeprazole, pantoprazole, pentamidine, phenobarbital, phenytoin, rabeprazole, voriconazole, warfarin
2D6	amitriptyline, amphetamine, aripiprazole, atomoxetine, betaxolol, captopril, carvedilol, chlorpheniramine, chlorpromazine, clomipramine, clozapine, codeine, cyclobenzaprine, delavirdine, desipramine, dextromethorphan, donepezil, doxepin, fentanyl, flecainide, fluoxetine, fluphenazine, fluvoxamine, haloperidol, hydrocodone, imipramine, labetalol, loratadine, maprotiline, meperidine, methadone, methamphetamine, metoprolol, mexiletine, mirtazapine, morphine, nefazodone, nortriptyline, oxycodone, paroxetine, perphenazine, procainamide, propafenone, propranolol, risperidone, tamoxifen, thioridazine, timolol, tolterodine, tramadol, trazodone, venlafaxine
3A	albuterol, alfentanil, alprazolam, amiodarone, amitriptyline, amlodipine, amprenavir, aripiprazole, atazanavir, atorvastatin, bosentan, bromocriptine, buspirone, busulfan, carbamazepine, chlordiazepoxide, chlorpheniramine, citalopram, clarithromycin, clomipramine, clonazepam, clorazepate, cocaine, colchicine, corticosteroids, cyclophosphamide, cyclosporine (neural), dapsone, delavirdine, dexamethasone, diazepam, diltiazem, disopyramide, docetaxel, doxepin, doxorubicin, doxycycline, efavirenz, enalapril, eplerenone, ergotamine, erythromycin, escitalopram, esomeprazole, estrogens, ethosuximide, etoposide, felodipine, fentanyl, fexofenadine, finasteride, flurazepam, flutamide, fluvastatin, haloperidol, ifosfamide, imatinib, imipramine, indinavir, isosorbide, isradipine, itraconazole, ketamine, ketoconazole, lansoprazole, lidocaine, loratadine, losartan, lovastatin, methadone, methylprednisolone, miconazole, midazolam, mirtazapine, montelukast, nefazodone, nevirapine, nicardipine, nifedipine, nimodipine, nisoldipine, ondansetron, paclitaxel, pantoprazole, pioglitazone, pravastatin, prednisone, quinidine, quinine, rabeprazole, rifabutin, ritonavir, saquinavir, sertraline, sildenafil, simvastatin, tacrolimus, tamoxifen, teniposide, testosterone, tolterodine, trazodone, triazolam, troleandomycin, vardenafil, verapamil, vinca alkaloids, voriconazole, warfarin, zileuton, zolpidem

Inducers	Inhibitors
carbamazepine, cigarette smoking, insulin, omeprazole, phenobarbital, phenytoin, primidone, rifampin, ritonavir	atazanavir, caffeine, cimetidine, ciprofloxacin, clarithromycin, enoxacin, erythromycin, fluvoxamine, grapefruit juice, interferon, isoniazid, ketoconazole, levofloxacin, mexiletine, norethindrone, norfloxacin, omeprazole, paroxetine, tacrine, ticlopidine, zileuton
carbamazepine, phenobarbital, phenytoin, primidone, rifampin	amiodarone, atazanavir, chloramphenicol, cimetidine, delavirdine, disulfiram, fluconazole, fluoxetine, fluvastatin, fluvoxamine, isoniazid, itraconazole, ketoconazole, lovastatin, metronidazole, omeprazole, ritonavir, sertraline, sulfamethoxazole–trimethoprim, sulfinpyrazone, ticlopidine, trimethoprim, zafirlukast
carbamazepine, phenytoin, prednisone, rifampin	cimetidine, delavirdine, esomeprazole, felbamate, fluconazole, fluoxetine, fluvoxamine, ketoconazole, lansoprazole, omeprazole, sertraline, ticlopidine, topiramate
carbamazepine, dexamethasone, phenobarbital, phenytoin, primidone	amiodarone, bupropion, celecoxib, chloroquine, chlorpheniramine, cimetidine, citalopram, cocaine, delavirdine, fluoxetine, fluphenazine, fluvoxamine, haloperidol, methadone, nefazodone, paroxetine, perphenazine, propafenone, quinidine, quinine, ritonavir, rosiglitazone, sertraline, terbinafine, thioridazine, venlafaxine
barbiturates, carbamazepine, glucocorticoids, griseofulvin, nafcillin, nevirapine, oxcarbazepine, phenytoin, primidone, rifabutin, rifampin	amprenavir, atazanavir, bromocriptine, cimetidine, clarithromycin, cyclosporine (neural), danazol, delavirdine, diltiazem, erythromycin, fluconazole, fluoxetine, fluvoxamine, fosamprenavir, grapefruit juice, imatinib, indinavir, isoniazid, itraconazole, ketoconazole, metronidazole, miconazole, nefazodone, nelfinavir, nicardipine, nifedipine, norfloxacin, omeprazole, prednisone, quinidine, quinine, rifabutin, ritonavir, saquinavir, sertraline, troleandomycin, verapamil, zafirlukast

Dialyzable drugs

The amount of a drug removed by dialysis differs among patients and depends on several factors, including the patient's condition, the drug's properties, length of dialysis, dialysate used, rate of blood flow or dwell time, and purpose of dialysis. This table indicates the effect of conventional hemodialysis on selected drugs.

Drug	Level reduced by hemodialysis	Drug	Level reduced by hemodialysis
acebutolol	Yes	carvedilol	No
acetaminophen	Yes (may not influence toxicity)	cefaclor	Yes
		cefadroxil	Yes
acetazolamide	No	cefazolin	Yes
acetylcysteine	Yes	cefepime	Yes
acyclovir	Yes	cefotaxime	Yes
albuterol	No	cefotetan	Yes (only by 20%)
allopurinol	Yes	cefoxitin	Yes
alprazolam	No	cefpodoxime	Yes
amantadine	No	ceftaroline	Yes
amikacin	Yes	ceftazidime	Yes
amiodarone	No	ceftibuten	Yes
amitriptyline	No	ceftizoxime	Yes
amlodipine	No	ceftriaxone	No
amoxicillin	Yes	cefuroxime	Yes
amoxicillin–clavulanate potassium	Yes	cephalexin	Yes
		cephradine	Yes
amphotericin B	No	chloral hydrate	Yes
ampicillin	Yes	chlorambucil	No
ampicillin–sulbactam sodium	Yes	chloramphenicol	Yes (very small amount)
		chlordiazepoxide	No
apixaban	No	chlorpheniramine	Yes
aprepitant	No	chlorpromazine	No
arsenic trioxide	No	chlorthalidone	No
ascorbic acid	Yes	cimetidine	Yes
aspirin	Yes	ciprofloxacin	Yes (only by 10%)
atenolol	Yes	cisplatin	No
atorvastatin	No	clavulanic acid	Yes
atropine	No	clindamycin	No
auranofin	No	clofibrate	No
azathioprine	Yes	clonazepam	No
aztreonam	Yes	clonidine	No
bivalirudin	Yes	clorazepate	No
bumetanide	No	cloxacillin	No
bupropion	No	codeine	No
buspirone	No	colchicine	No
busulfan	Yes	cortisone	No
captopril	Yes	cyclophosphamide	Yes
carbamazepine	No	dabigatran	Yes
carbenicillin	Yes	deferoxamine	Yes
carboplatin	Yes	desloratadine	No
carisoprodol	Yes	dexamethasone	No
carmustine	No	dexlansoprazole	No

Drug	Level reduced by hemodialysis	Drug	Level reduced by hemodialysis
diazepam	No	hydroxyzine	No
diazoxide	Yes	ibuprofen	No
diclofenac	No	ifosfamide	Yes
dicloxacillin	No	imipenem	Yes
didanosine	No	imipramine	No
digoxin	No	indapamide	No
digoxin immune Fab	No	indomethacin	No
diltiazem	No	insulin	No
diphenhydramine	No	irbesartan	No
dipyridamole	No	iron dextran	No
dopamine	No	isoniazid	No
doripenem	Yes	isosorbide	Yes
doxazosin	No	isradipine	No
doxepin	No	kanamycin	Yes
doxorubicin	No	ketoconazole	No
doxycycline	No	labetalol	No
eltrombopag	No	lacosamide	Yes (by 50%)
emtricitabine	Yes	lamivudine	No
enalapril	Yes	lansoprazole	No
enoxaparin	No	lapatinib	No
epoetin alfa	No	levetiracetam	Yes
ertapenem	Yes	levocetirizine	No
erythromycin	Yes (only by 20%)	levofloxacin	No
ethacrynic acid	No	lidocaine	No
ethambutol	Yes (only by 20%)	linezolid	Yes
ethosuximide	Yes	lisinopril	Yes
famciclovir	Yes	lithium	Yes
famotidine	No	lomefloxacin	No
fenoprofen	No	lomitapide	No
filgrastim	No	lomustine	No
flecainide	No	loratadine	No
fluconazole	Yes	lorazepam	No
flucytosine	Yes	mannitol	No
fluorouracil	Yes	maraviroc	Yes
fluoxetine	No	mefenamic acid	No
flurazepam	No	meperidine	No
foscarnet	Yes	meprobamate	Yes
fosinopril	No	mercaptopurine	Yes
furosemide	No	meropenem	Yes
gabapentin	Yes	mesalamine	Yes
ganciclovir	Yes	metformin	Yes
gemcitabine	Yes	methadone	No
gemfibrozil	No	methotrexate	Yes
gemifloxacin	Yes	methyldopa	Yes
gentamicin	Yes	methylprednisolone	Yes
glipizide	No	metoclopramide	No
glyburide	No	metolazone	No
guanfacine	No	metoprolol	Yes
haloperidol	No	metronidazole	Yes
heparin	No	mexiletine	Yes
hydralazine	No	miconazole	No
hydrochlorothiazide	No	midazolam	No

Drug	Level reduced by hemodialysis	Drug	Level reduced by hemodialysis
minocycline	No	quinine	No
minoxidil	Yes	ramipril	No
misoprostol	No	ranitidine	Yes
morphine	No	rifampin	No
nabumetone	No	ritodrine	Yes
nadolol	Yes	rituximab	No
nafcillin	No	rosiglitazone	No
nalmefene	No	rufinamide	Yes (by 30%)
naltrexone	No	salsalate	Yes
naproxen	No	saxagliptin	Yes
nelfinavir	No	sertraline	No
nicardipine	No	sotalol	Yes
nifedipine	No	stavudine	Yes
nimodipine	No	streptomycin	Yes
nitazoxanide	No	sucralfate	No
nitrofurantoin	Yes	sulbactam	Yes
nitroglycerin	No	sulfamethoxazole	Yes
nitroprusside	Yes	sulfisoxazole	No
nizatidine	No	sulindac	No
norfloxacin	No	tazobactam	Yes
nortriptyline	No	telbivudine	Yes (by 23%)
octreotide	Yes	temazepam	No
ofloxacin	Yes	theophylline	Yes
olanzapine	No	ticarcillin	Yes
omeprazole	No	ticarcillin–clavulanate	Yes
oxazepam	No	timolol	No
paclitaxel	No	tirofiban	Yes
paroxetine	No	tobramycin	Yes
penicillin G	Yes	tocainide	Yes
pentamidine	No	tofacitinib	No
pentazocine	Yes	tolbutamide	No
pentobarbital	No	topiramate	Yes
perindopril	Yes	topotecan	Yes
phenobarbital	Yes	torsemide	No
phenylbutazone	No	tramadol	No
phenytoin	No	trandolapril	No
piperacillin	Yes	trazodone	No
prazosin	No	triazolam	No
prednisone	No	trimethoprim	Yes
pregabalin	Yes	valacyclovir	Yes
primidone	Yes	valganciclovir	Yes
procainamide	Yes	valproic acid	No
promethazine	No	valsartan	No
propranolol	No	vancomycin	Yes
protriptyline	No	venlafaxine	No
pseudoephedrine	No	verapamil	No
pyrazinamide	Yes	vigabatrin	Yes
pyridoxine	Yes	warfarin	No
quinapril	No	zolpidem	No
quinidine	No	zonisamide	Yes

Drugs that shouldn't be crushed or chewed

This list contains names of drugs and their respective forms that shouldn't be crushed or chewed because of their special pharmaceutical formulations or characteristics.

Aciphex (Tablet)
Actiq (Lozenge)
Actonel (Tablet)
Adalat CC (Tablet)
Adderall XR (Capsule)
AeroHist Plus (Tablet)
Afeditab CR (Tablet)
Allegra-D (Tablet)
Allfen Jr (Capsule, tablet)
Alpophen (Tablet)
Alprazolam ER (Tablet)
Altoprev (Tablet)
Ambien CR (Tablet)
Aptivus (Capsule)
Aquatab C (Tablet)
Aquatab D (Tablet)
Arthrotec (Tablet)
Asacol (Tablet)
Ascriptin A/D (Tablet)
Augmentin XR (Tablet)
Avinza (Capsule)
Avodart (Capsule)
Azulfidine EN-tabs (Tablet)
Bayer Enteric Coated (Caplet)
Bayer Low Dose Adult (Tablet)
Bayer Regular Strength (Caplet)
Bellahist-D LA (Tablet)
Biaxin XL (Tablet)
Bidhist (Tablet)
Bidhist-D (Tablet)
Biltricide (Tablet)
Biohist LA (Tablet)
Bisac-Evac (Tablet)
Bisacodyl (Tablet)
Bisa-Lax (Tablet)
Boniva (Tablet)
Bromfed-PD (Capsule)
Budeprion SR (Tablet)
Calan SR (Tablet)
Carbatrol (Capsule)
Cardene SR (Capsule)
Cardizem (Tablet)

Cardizem CD (Capsule)
Cardizem LA (Tablet)
Cardura XL (Tablet)
Cartia XT (Capsule)
Cefaclor Extended-Release (Tablet)
Ceftin (Tablet)
Cefuroxime (Tablet)
CellCept (Capsule, tablet)
Charcoal Plus (Tablet)
Chlor-Trimeton 12 Hour (Tablet)
Cipro XR (Tablet)
Claritin-D 12 Hour (Tablet)
Claritin-D 24 Hour (Capsule)
Colace (Capsule)
Colestid (Tablet)
Commit (Lozenge)
Concerta (Tablet)
Cotazym-S (Capsule)
Covera-HS (Tablet)
Creon 5, 10, 20 (Capsule)
Crixivan (Capsule)
Cymbalta (Capsule)
Cytovene (Capsule)
Cytoxan (Tablet)
Dallergy (Tablet)
Dallergy-JR (Capsule)
Deconamine SR (Capsule)
Depakene (Capsule)
Depakote (Tablet)
Depakote ER (Tablet)
Detrol LA (Capsule)
Dilacor XR (Capsule)
Dilatrate-SR (Capsule)
Dilt-CD (Capsule)
Diltia XT (Capsule)
Dilt-XR (Capsule)
Ditropan XL (Tablet)
Doxidan (Tablet)
DriHist SR (Tablet)
Drisdol (Capsule)

Drixoral Allergy Sinus (Tablet)
Drixoral Cold & Allergy (Tablet)
Drixoral Non-Drowsy (Tablet)
Droxia (Capsule)
Drysec (Tablet)
Dulcolax (Capsule, tablet)
DynaCirc CR (Tablet)
EC-Naprosyn (Tablet)
Ecotrin Adult Low Strength (Tablet)
Ecotrin Maximum Strength (Tablet)
Ecotrin Regular Strength (Tablet)
E.E.S. 400 (Tablet)
Effer-K (Tablet)
Effervescent Potassium (Tablet)
Effexor XR (Capsule)
Efidac/24 (Tablet)
Entocort EC (Capsule)
Equetro (Capsule)
Eryc (Capsule)
Ery-Tab (Tablet)
Erythrocin Stearate (Tablet)
Erythromycin Base (Tablet)
Evista (Tablet)
Feen-a-Mint (Tablet)
Feldene (Capsule)
Fentora (Tablet)
Feosol (Tablet)
Feratab (Tablet)
Fergon (Tablet)
Fero-Grad-500 (Tablet)
Ferro-Sequels (Tablet)
Flagyl ER (Tablet)
Fleet Laxative (Tablet)
Flomax (Capsule)
Focalin XR (Capsule)
Fosamax (Tablet)
Geocillin (Tablet)
Gleevec (Tablet)
Glipizide (Tablet)
Glucophage XR (Tablet)

Glucotrol XL (Tablet)
Glumetza (Tablet)
Guaifenesin/Pseudoephedrine (Tablet)
Halfprin 81 (Tablet)
Heartline (Tablet)
Hydrea (Capsule)
Imdur (Tablet)
Inderal LA (Capsule)
Indocin SR (Capsule)
InnoPran XL (Capsule)
Invega (Tablet)
Ionamin (Capsule)
Isoptin SR (Tablet)
Isordil Sublingual (Tablet)
Isosorbide Dinitrate Sublingual (Tablet)
Isosorbide SR (Tablet)
Kadian (Capsule)
Kaletra (Tablet)
Kaon-Cl 10 (Tablet)
Keppra (Tablet)
Ketek (Tablet)
Klor-Con (Tablet)
Klor-Con M (Tablet)
Klotrix (Tablet)
K-Lyte (Tablet)
K-Lyte CL (Tablet)
K-Lyte DS (Tablet)
K-Tab (Tablet)
Lescol XL (Tablet)
Levbid (Tablet)
Levsinex Timecaps (Capsule)
Lexxel (Tablet)
Lialda (Tablet)
Lipram 4500 (Capsule)
Lipram PN 10, 16, 20 (Capsule)
Lipram UL 12, 18, 20 (Capsule)
Liquibid-D 1200 (Tablet)
Liquibid-PD (Tablet)
Lithobid (Tablet)
Mestinon Timespan (Tablet)
Metadate CD (Capsule)
Metadate ER (Tablet)
Methylin ER (Tablet)
Metoprolol Succinate ER (Tablet)
Micro-K Extencaps (Capsule)
Modane (Tablet)

Morphine sulfate Extended-Release (Tablet)
Morphine sulfate and naltrexone hydrochloride Extended-release (Capsule)
Motrin (Tablet)
MS Contin (Tablet)
Mucinex (Tablet)
Mucinex DM (Tablet)
Myfortic (Tablet)
Naprelan (Tablet)
Nexium (Capsule)
Niaspan (Tablet)
Nicotinic Acid (Capsule, tablet)
Nifedical XL (Tablet)
NitroQuick (Tablet)
Nitrostat (Tablet)
Norpace CR (Capsule)
Opana ER (Tablet)
Oracea (Capsule)
Oramorph SR (Tablet)
OxyContin (Tablet)
Pancrease MT (Capsule)
Pancrecarb MS (Capsule)
Pancrelipase (Capsule)
Paxil CR (Tablet)
Pentasa (Capsule)
Plendil (Tablet)
Prevacid (Capsule)
Prevacid SoluTab (Tablet)
Prilosec (Capsule)
Prilosec OTC (Tablet)
Procardia XL (Tablet)
Propecia (Tablet)
Proquin XR (Tablet)
Proscar (Tablet)
Protonix (Tablet)
Prozac Weekly (Tablet)
QDALL (Capsule)
QDALL AR (Capsule)
Ranexa (Tablet)
Razadyne ER (Capsule)
Renagel (Tablet)
Ritalin LA (Capsule)
Ritalin-SR (Tablet)
Rythmol SR (Capsule)
Sinemet CR (Tablet)
Slo-Niacin (Tablet)

Solodyn (Tablet)
Somnote (Capsule)
Sprycel (Tablet)
Strattera (Capsule)
Sudafed 12 hour (Capsule)
Sudafed 24 hour (Capsule)
Sular (Tablet)
Symax Duotab (Tablet)
Symax SR (Tablet)
Taztia XT (Capsule)
Tegretol-XR (Tablet)
Temodar (Capsule)
Tessalon Perles (Capsule)
Theo-24 (Capsule)
Tiazac (Capsule)
Topamax (Capsule, tablet)
Toprol-XL (Tablet)
Tracleer (Tablet)
Trental (Tablet)
Tylenol Arthritis (Tablet)
Ultram ER (Tablet)
Uniphyl (Tablet)
Uroxatral (Tablet)
Valcyte (Tablet)
Verapamil SR (Tablet)
Verelan (Capsule)
Verelan PM (Capsule)
VESIcare (Tablet)
Videx EC (Capsule)
Voltaren-XR (Tablet)
VoSpire ER (Tablet)
Wellbutrin SR, XL (Tablet)
Xanax XR (Tablet)
ZORprin (Tablet)
Zyban (Tablet)

Antidotes: Indications and dosages

activated charcoal
Actidose-Aqua ◇, Actidose
with Sorbitol ◇, CharcoAid ◇,
CharcoAid 2000 ◇, Liqui-Char ◇

charcoal
Charcoal Plus DS ◇, CharcoCaps ◇

Therapeutic class: Antidotes
Pharmacologic class: Adsorbents
Pregnancy risk category: Undetermined

AVAILABLE FORMS
activated charcoal
Granules: 15 g ◇
Liquid: 12.5 g ◇*, 15 g ◇*, 25 g ◇*,
30 g ◇*, 50 g ◇*
Oral suspension: 15 g ◇, 30 g ◇
Powder: 15 g ◇, 30 g ◇, 40 g ◇, 120 g ◇,
240 g ◇
charcoal
Capsules: 260 mg ◇
Tablets: 250 mg ◇

INDICATIONS & DOSAGES
➤ **Flatulence, dyspepsia, diarrhea**
Adults and children age 3 and older: 500 to
520 mg (charcoal) P.O. after meals or at
first sign of discomfort. Repeat as needed,
up to 5 g daily.
➤ **Poisoning**
*Adults and children age 13 and older
weighing more than 32 kg (71 lb):* 50 to
60 g P.O. of drug in sorbitol base.
*Children ages 1 to 12 weighing 16 to 32 kg
(38 to 71 lb):* 25 to 30 g P.O. (sorbitol base).
Adults and children older than age 1: 5 to
60 g P.O. (aqueous base). Dosage should be
10 times by volume the amount of poison
ingested, if known. If amount of poison
ingested isn't known, a dosage of at least
20 to 30 g should be given.

deferiprone
de-FER-i-prone

Ferriprox

Therapeutic class: Chelating drugs
Pharmacologic class: Heavy metal
antagonists
Pregnancy risk category: D

AVAILABLE FORMS
Tablets: 500 mg

INDICATIONS & DOSAGES
➤ **Treatment of transfusional iron overload due to thalassemia syndromes when
current chelation therapy is inadequate**
Adults: Initially, 25 mg/kg P.O. t.i.d. for a
total of 75 mg/kg/day. May titrate to maximum dosage of 33 mg/kg t.i.d. for a total
of 99 mg/kg/day based on patient response
and therapeutic goals. Round dose to
nearest 250 mg (half tablet).

digoxin immune Fab (ovine)
di-JOX-in

DigiFab

Therapeutic class: Antidotes
Pharmacologic class: Antibody
fragments
Pregnancy risk category: C

AVAILABLE FORMS
Injection: 40-mg vial

INDICATIONS & DOSAGES
➤ **Life-threatening digoxin toxicity**
Adults and children: Base dosage on ingested
amount or level of digoxin. When calculating
amount of antidote, round up to the nearest
whole number. For digoxin tablets, calculate
number of antidote vials as follows: multiply
ingested amount by 0.8; then divide answer by
0.5. For example, if patient takes 25 tablets
of 0.25 mg digoxin, the ingested amount is
6.25 mg. Multiply 6.25 mg by 0.8 and divide
answer by 0.5 to obtain 10 vials of antidote. If

digoxin level is known, determine the number of antidote vials as follows: multiply the digoxin level in nanograms per milliliter by patient's weight in kilograms; then divide by 100. For example, if digoxin level is 4 nanograms/mL, and patient weighs 60 kg, multiply together to obtain 240. Divide answer by 100 to obtain 2.4 vials; then round up to 3 vials.

➤ **Acute toxicity or if estimated ingested amount or digoxin level is unknown**
Adults and children: Consider giving 10 vials of digoxin immune Fab and observing patient's response. Follow with another 10 vials if indicated. Dosage should be effective in most life-threatening cases in adults and children but may cause volume overload in young children.

dimercaprol
dye-mer-KAP-rawl

BAL in Oil

Therapeutic class: Chelating drugs
Pharmacologic class: Heavy metal antagonists
Pregnancy risk category: C

AVAILABLE FORMS
Injection: 100 mg/mL

INDICATIONS & DOSAGES
➤ **Severe arsenic or gold poisoning**
Adults and children: 3 mg/kg deep I.M. every 4 hours for 2 days; then q.i.d. on third day; then b.i.d. for 10 days.
➤ **Mild arsenic or gold poisoning**
Adults and children: 2.5 mg/kg deep I.M. q.i.d. for 2 days; then b.i.d. on third day; then once daily for 10 days.
➤ **Mercury poisoning**
Adults and children: Initially, 5 mg/kg deep I.M.; then 2.5 mg/kg daily or b.i.d. for 10 days.
➤ **Acute lead encephalopathy or lead level greater than 100 mcg/mL**
Adults and children: 4 mg/kg deep I.M.; then every 4 hours with edetate calcium disodium for 2 to 7 days. Use separate sites. For less severe poisoning, reduce dose to 3 mg/kg after first dose.

doxapram hydrochloride
DOCKS-a-pram

Dopram

Therapeutic class: CNS stimulants
Pharmacologic class: Analeptics
Pregnancy risk category: B

AVAILABLE FORMS
Injection: 20 mg/mL (benzyl alcohol 0.9%)

INDICATIONS & DOSAGES
➤ **Postanesthesia respiratory stimulation**
Adults: 0.5 to 1 mg/kg as a single I.V. injection (not to exceed 1.5 mg/kg) or as multiple injections every 5 minutes, total not to exceed 2 mg/kg or 3 g daily. Or, 250 mg in 250 mL of normal saline solution or D_5W infused at initial rate of 5 mg/minute I.V. until satisfactory response is achieved. Maintain at 1 to 3 mg/minute. Don't exceed total dose for infusion of 4 mg/kg or 3g daily.
➤ **Drug-induced CNS depression**
Adults: For injection, priming dose of 1 to 2 mg/kg I.V., repeated in 5 minutes and again every 1 to 2 hours until patient awakens (and if relapse occurs). Maximum daily dose is 3 g.

For infusion, priming dose of 1 to 2 mg/kg I.V., repeated in 5 minutes and again in 1 to 2 hours, if needed. If response occurs, give I.V. infusion (1 mg/mL) at 1 to 3 mg/minute until patient awakens. Don't infuse for longer than 2 hours or give more than 3 g/day. May resume I.V. infusion after rest period of 30 minutes to 2 hours, if needed.
➤ **COPD related to acute hypercapnia**
Adults: 1 to 2 mg/minute by I.V. infusion using 2 mg/mL solution. Maximum, 3 mg/minute for up to 2 hours.

edetate calcium disodium
ED-e-tate

Calcium Disodium Versenate

Therapeutic class: Chelating drugs
Pharmacologic class: Heavy metal antagonists
Pregnancy risk category: B

Black Box Warning Drug is capable of producing toxic effects that can be fatal. Never exceed the recommended daily dosage. ■

AVAILABLE FORMS
Injection: 200 mg/mL

INDICATIONS & DOSAGES
➤ **Acute lead encephalopathy or lead level greater than 70 mcg/dL**
Adults and children: Use in conjunction with dimercaprol. Consult published protocols and specialized references for dosage recommendations.
➤ **Lead poisoning without encephalopathy or asymptomatic with lead level less than 70 mcg/dL but greater than 20 mcg/dL**
Adults and children: 1 g/m^2 I.V. infused over 8 to 12 hours once daily or 1 g/m^2 I.M. daily in divided doses spaced 8 to 12 hours apart for 5 days. Or, for adults with lead nephropathy, give as follows: If serum creatinine level is 2 to 3 mg/dL, give 500 mg/m^2 every 24 hours for 5 days; if serum creatinine level is 3 to 4 mg/dL, give 500 mg/m^2 every 48 hours for three doses; if serum creatinine level is more than 4 mg/dL, give 500 mg/m^2 once weekly.

flumazenil
floo-MAZ-eh-nill

Romazicon

Therapeutic class: Antidotes
Pharmacologic class: Benzodiazepine antagonists
Pregnancy risk category: C

AVAILABLE FORMS
Injection: 0.1 mg/mL in 5-mL and 10-mL multiple-dose vials

INDICATIONS & DOSAGES
➤ **Complete or partial reversal of sedative effects of benzodiazepines after anesthesia or conscious sedation**
Adults: Initially, 0.2 mg I.V. over 15 seconds. If patient doesn't reach desired level of consciousness after 45 seconds, repeat dose. Repeat at 1-minute intervals, if needed, until cumulative dose of 1 mg has been given (first dose plus four more doses). Most patients respond after 0.6 to 1 mg of drug. In case of resedation, dosage may be repeated after 20 minutes, but never give more than 1 mg at any one time or exceed 3 mg in any 1 hour.
Children age 1 year and older: 0.01 mg/kg (up to 0.2 mg) I.V. over 15 seconds. If patient doesn't reach desired level of consciousness after 45 seconds, repeat dose. Repeat at 1-minute intervals, if needed, until cumulative dose of 0.05 mg/kg or 1 mg, whichever is lower, has been given (first dose plus four more doses).
➤ **Suspected benzodiazepine overdose**
Adults: Initially, 0.2 mg I.V. over 30 seconds. If patient doesn't reach desired level of consciousness after 30 seconds, give 0.3 mg over 30 seconds. If patient still doesn't respond adequately, give 0.5 mg over 30 seconds. Repeat 0.5-mg doses, as needed, at 1-minute intervals until cumulative dose of 3 mg has been given. Most patients with benzodiazepine overdose respond to cumulative doses between 1 and 3 mg; rarely, patients who respond partially after 3 mg may need additional doses, up to 5 mg total. If patient doesn't respond in 5 minutes after receiving 5 mg, sedation is unlikely to be caused by benzodiazepines. In case of resedation, dosage may be repeated after 20 minutes, but never give more than 1 mg at any one time or exceed 3 mg in any 1 hour.
➤ **Hepatic encephalopathy** ◆
Adults: 1 mg I.V. bolus.

glucarpidase
gloo-CAR-pi-daze

Voraxaze

Therapeutic class: Antidotes
Pharmacologic class: Recombinant
bacterial enzymes
Pregnancy risk category: C

AVAILABLE FORMS
Powder for injection: 1,000 units/vial

INDICATIONS & DOSAGES
➤ **Methotrexate toxicity (more than
1 micromole/L) in patients with delayed
methotrexate clearance due to impaired
renal function**
Adults and children age 1 month and older:
50 units/kg as a single I.V. injection over
5 minutes.

lanthanum carbonate
LAN-thah-num

Fosrenol

Therapeutic class:
Antihyperphosphatemics
Pharmacologic class: Non-calcium,
non-aluminum phosphate binders
Pregnancy risk category: C

AVAILABLE FORMS
Tablets (chewable): 500 mg, 750 mg, 1 g

INDICATIONS & DOSAGES
➤ **To reduce phosphate level in patients
with ESRD**
Adults: Initially, 250 to 500 mg P.O. t.i.d.
with meals. Adjust every 2 to 3 weeks by
750 mg daily until reaching desired phosphate level. Reducing phosphate level to
less than 6 mg/dL usually requires 1,500 to
3,000 mg daily.

naloxone hydrochloride
nal-OX-one

Therapeutic class: Antidotes
Pharmacologic class: Opioid
antagonists
Pregnancy risk category: B

AVAILABLE FORMS
Injection: 0.4 mg/mL, 1 mg/mL

INDICATIONS & DOSAGES
➤ **Known or suspected opioid-induced
respiratory depression, including that
caused by pentazocine, methadone,
nalbuphine, and butorphanol**
Adults: 0.4 to 2 mg I.V., I.M., or subcutaneously. Repeat dose every 2 to 3 minutes,
p.r.n. If patient doesn't respond after 10 mg
have been given, question diagnosis of
opioid-induced toxicity.
Children age 1 month and older:
0.01 mg/kg I.V.; then, second dose of
0.1 mg/kg I.V., if needed. If I.V. route isn't
available, drug may be given I.M. or subcutaneously in divided doses.
Neonates: 0.01 mg/kg I.V., I.M., or subcutaneously. Repeat dose every 2 to 3 minutes, p.r.n.
➤ **Postoperative opioid depression**
Adults: 0.1 to 0.2 mg I.V. every 2 to 3 minutes, p.r.n. Repeat dose within 1 to 2 hours,
if needed.
Children: 0.005 to 0.01 mg I.V. repeated
every 2 to 3 minutes, p.r.n.

phentolamine mesylate
fen-TOLE-a-meen

OraVerse, Regitine, Rogitine†

Therapeutic class: Antihypertensives
Pharmacologic class: Alpha blockers
Pregnancy risk category: C

AVAILABLE FORMS
Injection: 0.4 mg/1.7 mL, 5 mg/mL,
10 mg/mL†

INDICATIONS & DOSAGES
➤ **To aid in diagnosis of pheochromocytoma, to control or prevent hypertension before or during pheochromocytomectomy (except OraVerse)**
Adults: I.V. or I.M. diagnostic dose is 5 mg with close monitoring of blood pressure. Give 5 mg I.V. or I.M 1 to 2 hours before surgical removal of tumor. During surgery, patient may need an additional 5 mg I.V.
Children: I.V. diagnostic dose is 1 mg, and I.M. diagnostic dose is 3 mg with close monitoring of blood pressure. Give 1 mg I.V. or I.M 1 to 2 hours before surgical removal of tumor. During surgery, patient may need an additional 1 mg I.V.
➤ **To prevent dermal necrosis from norepinephrine extravasation (except OraVerse)**
Adults: Add 10 mg of phentolamine to each liter of solution containing norepinephrine; the pressor effect of norepinephrine is unaffected.
➤ **Dermal necrosis and sloughing after I.V. extravasation of norepinephrine or dopamine (except OraVerse)**
Adults: Infiltrate area with 5 to 10 mg phentolamine in 10 mL of normal saline solution. Must be done within 12 hours of extravasation.
➤ **Reversal of soft-tissue anesthesia (OraVerse only)**
Adults and children age 6 and older weighing more than 30 kg (66 lb): Dosage depends on amount of anesthetic used. Refer to package insert.

protamine sulfate
PROE-ta-meen

Therapeutic class: Antidotes
Pharmacologic class: Heparin antagonists
Pregnancy risk category: C

AVAILABLE FORMS
Injection: 10 mg/mL

INDICATIONS & DOSAGES
➤ **Heparin overdose**
Adults: Base dosage on venous blood coagulation studies; usually 1 mg neutralizes not less than 100 units of heparin. Give by slow I.V. injection over 10 minutes in doses not to exceed 50 mg. *Note:* Because heparin disappears rapidly from the circulation, the dose of protamine required also decreases rapidly with the time elapsed after I.V. injection of heparin. For example, if protamine is administered 30 minutes after heparin, one-half the usual dose may be sufficient.

succimer
SUX-i-mer

Chemet

Therapeutic class: Chelating drugs
Pharmacologic class: Heavy metal chelators
Pregnancy risk category: C

AVAILABLE FORMS
Capsules: 100 mg

INDICATIONS & DOSAGES
➤ **Lead poisoning in children with lead levels greater than 45 mcg/dl**
Children age 12 months and older: Initially, 10 mg/kg or 350 mg/m^2 P.O. every 8 hours for 5 days. Because capsules come only in 100 mg, round dose to nearest 100 mg, as appropriate (see table). Then reduce frequency of administration to every 12 hours for another 14 days.

Weight in kg (lb)	Dose (mg)
> 45 (>100)	500
35–44 (76–100)	400
24–34 (56–75)	300
16–23 (36–55)	200
8–15 (18–35)	100

Selected biologicals and blood derivatives: Indications and dosages

albumin 5%
al-BYOO-min

Albumarc, Albuminar-5, Albutein 5%, Buminate 5%, Plasbumin-5

albumin 25%
Albuminar-25, Albutein 25%, Buminate 25%, Plasbumin-25

Therapeutic class: Plasma volume expanders
Pharmacologic class: Blood derivatives
Pregnancy risk category: C

AVAILABLE FORMS
albumin 5%
Injection: 50 mg/mL in 50-mL, 250-mL, 500-mL, 1,000-mL vials
albumin 25%
Injection: 250 mg/mL in 20-mL, 50-mL, 100-mL vials

INDICATIONS & DOSAGES
➤ **Hypovolemic shock**
Adults: Initially, 500 to 750 mL of 5% solution by I.V. infusion, repeated every 30 minutes, as needed. As plasma volume approaches normal, rate of infusion of 5% solution shouldn't exceed 2 to 4 mL/minute. Dosage of 25% solution varies with patient's condition and response. As plasma volume approaches normal, rate of infusion of 25% solution shouldn't exceed 1 mL/minute.
Children: 12 to 20 mL of 5% solution/kg by I.V. infusion, repeated in 15 to 30 minutes if response is inadequate.
➤ **Burns**
Adults: 25% solution infused no faster than 2 to 3 mL/minute to maintain plasma albumin concentration at approximately 2.5 plus or minus 0.5 g/100 mL with a plasma oncotic pressure of 20 mm Hg (equal to a total plasma protein concentration of 5.2 g/100 mL). The duration of therapy is determined by the loss of protein from burned areas and in the urine.

➤ **Hypoproteinemia**
Adults: 200 to 300 mL of 25% albumin. Dosage varies with patient's condition and response. Usual daily dose is 50 to 75 g. Rate of infusion shouldn't exceed 2 mL/minute.
Children: Usual daily dosage is 25 g.

antihemophilic factor (AHF factor VIII)
an-tye-he-mo-FILL-ik

Advate, Alphanate, Helixate FS, Hemofil M, Hyate:C, Koate-DVI, Kogenate FS, Monarc-M, Monoclate-P, Recombinate, ReFacto, Xyntha

Therapeutic class: Clotting factors
Pharmacologic class: Plasma proteins
Pregnancy risk category: C

AVAILABLE FORMS
Injection: Vials, with diluent; units specified on label

INDICATIONS & DOSAGES
Drug provides hemostasis in factor VIII deficiency, hemophilia A. Specific dosage depends on patient's weight, severity of hemorrhage, and presence of inhibitors. Mild bleeding episodes require a circulating factor VIII level 20% to 30% of normal; moderate to major bleeding episodes and minor surgery, a level 30% to 50% of normal; severe bleeding or major surgery, a level 80% to 100% of normal. The following dosages provide guidelines. Refer to specific brand for actual dosage.
➤ **Control and prevention of mild bleeding in patients with hemophilia**
Adults and children: 10 international units/kg I.V. daily.
➤ **Control and prevention of moderate bleeding and minor surgery in patients with hemophilia**
Adults and children: Initially, 15 to 25 international units/kg I.V. If further therapy is

required, give a maintenance dose of 10 to 15 international units/kg every 8 to 12 hours.

➤ **Control and prevention of severe bleeding and bleeding near vital organs in patients with hemophilia**

Adults and children: Initially, 40 to 50 international units/kg I.V., then 20 to 25 international units/kg every 8 to 12 hours, as needed.

➤ **Major surgery in patients with hemophilia**

Adults and children: 50 international units/kg I.V. 1 hour before surgery, then repeat as needed 6 to 12 hours after first dose. Maintain circulating factor levels at 30% to 60% of normal for 10 to 14 days after surgery.

---

anti-inhibitor coagulant complex

Feiba VH, Feiba VH Immuno†

Therapeutic class: Clotting factors
Pharmacologic class: Plasma proteins
Pregnancy risk category: C

Black Box Warning Thrombotic and thromboembolic events have been reported during postmarketing surveillance. ∎

AVAILABLE FORMS

Injection: Number of units of factor VIII correctional activity indicated on label of vial

INDICATIONS & DOSAGES

➤ **To prevent or control hemorrhagic episodes in some patients with hemophilia A and B in whom inhibitor antibodies to antihemophilic factor have developed; to manage bleeding in patients with acquired hemophilia who have spontaneously acquired inhibitors to factor VIII, XI, and XII**

Adults and children: Drug controls hemorrhage in hemophilia A patients who have a factor VIII inhibitor level above 10 Bethesda units. Patients with a level of 5 to 10 Bethesda units may receive the drug if they have severe hemorrhage or respond poorly to factor VIII infusion.

Adults and children age 31 days and older: Dosage is highly individualized and varies among manufacturers. For Feiba VH, give 50 to 100 units/kg I.V. every 6 or 12 hours until patient shows signs of improvement. Maximum daily dose of Feiba VH is 200 units/kg.

➤ **Joint hemorrhage**

Adults and children age 31 days and older: 50 to 100 units/kg Feiba VH I.V. every 12 hours until patient's condition improves.

➤ **Mucous membrane hemorrhage**

Adults and children age 31 days and older: 50 units/kg Feiba VH I.V. every 6 hours, increasing to 100 units/kg every 6 hours if hemorrhage continues. Maximum daily dose, 200 units/kg.

➤ **Soft-tissue hemorrhage**

Adults and children age 31 days and older: 100 units/kg Feiba VH I.V. every 12 hours. Maximum daily dose, 200 units/kg.

➤ **Other severe hemorrhage**

Adults and children age 31 days and older: 100 units/kg Feiba VH I.V. every 12 hours (occasionally, every 6 hours).

---

beractant (natural lung surfactant)

ber-AK-tant

Survanta

Therapeutic class: Lung surfactants
Pharmacologic class: Bovine lung extracts
Pregnancy risk category: NR

AVAILABLE FORMS

Suspension for intratracheal instillation: 25 mg/mL

INDICATIONS & DOSAGES

➤ **To prevent respiratory distress syndrome (RDS), also known as hyaline membrane disease, in premature neonates weighing 1,250 g (2 lb, 12 oz) or less at birth, or having symptoms consistent with surfactant deficiency**

Neonates: 4 mL/kg intratracheally. Divide each dose into four quarter-doses and give each quarter-dose with infant in a different position to ensure even distribution of drug; between quarter-doses, use a hand-held resuscitation bag at 60 breaths/minute and sufficient oxygen to prevent cyanosis. Give drug as soon as possible, preferably within 15 minutes of birth. Repeat in 6 hours if respiratory distress continues. Give no more than four doses in 48 hours.

➤ **Rescue treatment of RDS in premature infants**

Neonates: 4 mL/kg intratracheally; before giving, increase ventilator rate to

60 breaths/minute with an inspiratory time of 0.5 second and a fraction of inspired oxygen of 1. Divide each dose into four quarter-doses and give each quarter-dose with infant in a different position to ensure even distribution of drug; between quarter doses, continue mechanical ventilation for at least 30 seconds or until stable. Give dose as soon as RDS is confirmed by X-ray, preferably within 8 hours of birth. Repeat in 6 hours if respiratory distress continues. Give no more than four doses in 48 hours.

calfactant
kal-FAK-tant

Infasurf

Therapeutic class: Lung surfactants
Pharmacologic class: Bovine lung extracts
Pregnancy risk category: NR

AVAILABLE FORMS
Intratracheal suspension: 35 mg phospholipids and 0.65 mg proteins/mL; 6-mL vial

INDICATIONS & DOSAGES
➤ **To prevent respiratory distress syndrome (RDS) in premature infants younger than 29 weeks' gestational age at high risk for RDS; to treat infants younger than age 72 hours who develop RDS (confirmed by clinical and radiologic findings) and need an endotracheal tube**
Neonates: 3 mL/kg of body weight at birth intratracheally, given in two aliquots of 1.5 mL/kg each, every 12 hours for a total of up to three doses.

eltrombopag
ell-trom-BOW-pag

Promacta

Therapeutic class: Hematopoietics
Pharmacologic class: Thrombopoietin receptor agonists
Pregnancy risk category: C

AVAILABLE FORMS
Tablets: 12.5 mg, 25 mg, 50 mg, 75 mg

INDICATIONS & DOSAGES
Black Box Warning Eltrombopag may cause hepatotoxicity. Consult prescribing information for specific monitoring guidelines. Only prescribers enrolled in the Promacta Cares program may prescribe eltrombopag. ∎
➤ **Thrombocytopenia associated with chronic immune thrombocytopenic purpura when response to corticosteroids, immunoglobulins, or splenectomy is inadequate**
Adults: Initially, 50 mg P.O. once daily. Adjust dosage as necessary to achieve and maintain platelet count at 50×10^9/L or greater; maximum dosage is 75 mg daily.
Adjust-a-dose: For patients of East Asian descent and those with moderate or severe hepatic impairment, reduce dosage to 25 mg P.O. once daily. For patients with platelet count less than 50,000/mm³ after at least 2 weeks of therapy, increase daily dosage by 25 mg to maximum dosage of 75 mg daily. For platelet count of 200,000 to 400,000/mm³, decrease daily dosage by 25 mg; wait 2 weeks to assess the effects, then adjust dosage as needed. For platelet count greater than 400,000/mm³, stop drug and monitor platelet count twice weekly. Restart therapy at 25 mg less than the daily dosage when platelet count is less than 150,000/mm³. When platelet count is greater than 400,000/mm³ after 2 weeks at lowest dosage, permanently discontinue drug.
➤ **Thrombocytopenia in patients with chronic hepatitis C to allow use of interferon-based therapy**
Adults: Initially, 25 mg P.O. once daily. Increase by 25-mg increments every 2 weeks as necessary to achieve target platelet count required to initiate antiviral therapy. Maximum dose is 100 mg daily.
Adjust-a-dose: During antiviral therapy, adjust dosage to avoid dose reduction of peginterferon. For patients with platelet count less than 50,000/mm³ after at least 2 weeks of therapy, increase daily dosage by 25 mg to a maximum dosage of 100 mg daily. For platelet count of 200,000 to 400,000/mm³, decrease daily dosage by 25 mg; wait 2 weeks to assess the effects, then make dosage adjustment as needed. For platelet count greater than 400,000/mm³, stop drug and monitor platelet count twice weekly. Restart therapy at 25 mg less than the daily dosage when platelet count

is less than 150,000/mm^3. If the patient was taking 25 mg once daily, restart therapy at 12.5 mg once daily. When platelet count is greater than 400,000/mm^3 after 2 weeks at the lowest dosage, permanently discontinue drug. Discontinue drug when antiviral treatment is stopped.

factor IX complex
Bebulin VH, Profilnine SD, Proplex T

factor IX (human)
AlphaNine SD, Mononine

factor IX (recombinant)
BeneFIX

Therapeutic class: Clotting factors
Pharmacologic class: Plasma proteins
Pregnancy risk category: C

AVAILABLE FORMS
Injection: Vials, with diluent; international units specified on label

INDICATIONS & DOSAGES
➤ **Factor IX deficiency (also called hemophilia B or Christmas disease), anticoagulant overdose; factor VII deficiency (Proplex T only)**
Adults and children: To calculate international units of factor IX needed, use the following equations:
Human product

| 1 international unit/kg | × | body weight in kg | × | percentage of desired increase of factor IX level |

Recombinant product

| 1.2 international units/kg | × | body weight in kg | × | percentage of desired increase of factor IX level |

Proplex T

| 0.5 international unit/kg | × | body weight in kg | × | percentage of desired increase of factor VII level |

Infusion rates vary with product and patient comfort. Dosage is highly individualized, depending on degree of deficiency, level of factor VII or IX desired, patient weight, and severity of bleeding.

hepatitis B immune globulin (human)
hep-ah-TYE-tis

HepaGam B, HyperHEP BS/D, Nabi-HB

Therapeutic class: Prophylaxis drugs
Pharmacologic class: Immune serums
Pregnancy risk category: C

AVAILABLE FORMS
Injection: 1-mL, 5-mL vials; 0.5-mL neonatal single-dose syringe; 1-mL single-dose syringe

INDICATIONS & DOSAGES
➤ **Hepatitis B exposure in high-risk patients**
Adults and children: 0.06 mL/kg (usual dose is 3 to 5 mL) I.M. as soon as possible, but within 7 days after exposure (within 14 days if sexual exposure). Repeat dose 28 days after exposure if patient doesn't elect to receive the hepatitis B vaccine.
Neonates born to hepatitis B surface antigen (HBsAg)-positive patients: 0.5 mL I.M. within 12 hours of birth.
➤ **To prevent hepatitis B recurrence following liver transplantation in HBsAg-positive liver transplant patients (HepaGam B only)**
Adults: 20,000 international units I.V. at rate of 2 mL/minute. Give first dose simultaneously with the grafting of the transplanted liver (anhepatic phase); then give daily on days 1 through 7, every 2 weeks from day 14 through 12 weeks, and monthly from month 4 onward.
Adjust-a-dose: Adjust dosage in patients who don't reach anti-HBs levels of 500 international units/L within the first week after transplantation. Give 10,000 international units I.V. until target level is reached.

plasma protein fractions
Plasmanate, Plasma-Plex, Protenate

Therapeutic class: Plasma volume expanders
Pharmacologic class: Plasma proteins
Pregnancy risk category: C

AVAILABLE FORMS
Injection: 5% (50 mg/mL) solution in 50-mL, 250-mL, 500-mL vials

INDICATIONS & DOSAGES
➤ **Shock**
Adults: Dosage varies with patient's condition and response, but usual dosage is 250 to 500 mL I.V. (12.5 to 25 g protein), usually no faster than 10 mL/minute.

SAFETY ALERT!

protein C concentrate
Ceprotin

Therapeutic class: Anticoagulants
Pharmacologic class: Protein C replacements
Pregnancy risk category: C

AVAILABLE FORMS
Vials: 500 international units, 1,000 international units

INDICATIONS & DOSAGES
Adjust-a-dose (for all indications): Dose is adjusted based on severity of protein C deficiency, plasma level of protein C, and patient's age and condition.
➤ **Venous thrombosis and purpura fulminans in patients with severe congenital protein C deficiency**
Adults, neonates, and pediatric patients: Initially for acute episodes and short-term prophylaxis, 100 to 120 international units/kg I.V.; then, 60 to 80 international units/kg I.V. every 6 hours for subsequent three doses to maintain peak protein C activity of 100%. Maintenance dose of 45 to 60 international units/kg I.V. every 6 to 12 hours to maintain trough protein C activity levels above 25%.
➤ **Long-term prevention of venous thrombosis and purpura fulminans**
Adults, neonates, and pediatric patients: 45 to 60 international units/kg I.V. every 12 hours to maintain trough protein C activity levels above 25%.

rabies immune globulin (human)
RAY-beez

HyperRAB S/D, Imogam Rabies-HT

Therapeutic class: Antibodies
Pharmacologic class: Immunoglobulins
Pregnancy risk category: C

AVAILABLE FORMS
Injection: 150 international units/mL in 2-mL, 10-mL vials

INDICATIONS & DOSAGES
➤ **Rabies exposure**
Adults and children: 20 international units/kg I.M. at time of first dose of rabies vaccine. If anatomically feasible, up to the full dose is used to infiltrate wound area; remainder is given I.M. in a different site.

Rho(D) immune globulin (human) (IGIM)
HyperRHO S/D Full Dose, HyperRHO S/D Mini-Dose, MICRhoGAM, RhoGAM

Rho(D) immune globulin intravenous (human) (IGIV)
Rhophylac, WinRho SDF

Therapeutic class: Immune globulins
Pharmacologic class: Immunoglobulins
Pregnancy risk category: C

AVAILABLE FORMS
IGIM
Injection: 300 mcg vial (standard dose); 50 mcg vial (microdose)
IGIV
Injection: 120-mcg (600 international units), 300-mcg (1,500 international units), 500-mcg (2,500 international units), 1,000-mcg (5,000 international units), 3,000-mcg (15,000 international units) vials

INDICATIONS & DOSAGES
➤ **Rh exposure after abortion, miscarriage, ectopic pregnancy, or childbirth**
Adults: Transfusion unit or blood bank determines fetal packed RBC volume entering patient's blood; one vial IGIM is given I.M.

if fetal packed RBC volume is less than 15 mL. More than one vial I.M. may be needed if severe fetomaternal hemorrhage occurs; must be given within 72 hours after delivery or miscarriage.

➤ **To prevent Rh antibody formation after abortion or miscarriage**
Adults: Consult transfusion unit or blood bank. Up to and including 12 weeks' gestation, one IGIM microdose vial I.M. will suppress immune reaction to 2.5 mL Rho(D)-positive RBCs. At 13 weeks' gestation and later, use one vial IGIM standard dose. Ideally, give within 3 hours, but may be given up to 72 hours after abortion or miscarriage.

➤ **Rh exposure after abortion, amniocentesis after 34 weeks' gestation, or other manipulations past 34 weeks' gestation with increased risk of Rh isoimmunization**
Adults: 120 mcg IGIV, given I.V. or I.M. within 72 hours of delivery, miscarriage, or manipulation.

➤ **To suppress Rh isoimmunization during pregnancy**
Adults: 300 mcg I.V. or I.M. at 28 weeks' gestation. If given early in pregnancy, give additional doses at 12-week intervals to maintain adequate levels of passively acquired anti-Rh antibodies. Then, within 72 hours of delivery, give 120 mcg WinRho or 300 mcg HyperRHO, RhoGAM, or Rhophylac I.M. or I.V. If 72 hours have elapsed, give drug as soon as possible, up to 28 days.

➤ **Incompatible blood transfusion**
Adults: 600 mcg I.V. every 8 hours or 1,200 mcg I.M. every 12 hours until total dose given. Total dose depends on volume of packed RBCs or whole blood infused. Consult blood bank or transfusion unit at once; must be given within 72 hours.

➤ **Idiopathic thrombocytopenic purpura in Rho(D) antigen–positive adults**
Adults: Initially, 50 mcg/kg I.V. as single dose or divided into two doses on separate days. If hemoglobin level is less than 10 g/dL, reduce first dose to 25 to 40 mcg/kg. Then, give 25 to 60 mcg/kg I.V. as needed to elevate platelet count with specific individually determined dosage.

romiplostim
roh-mih-PLOH-stim

Nplate

Therapeutic class: Hematopoietics
Pharmacologic class: Thrombopoietin receptor agonists
Pregnancy risk category: C

AVAILABLE FORMS
Injection: 250-mcg, 500-mcg single-use vials

INDICATIONS & DOSAGES
➤ **Thrombocytopenia in patients with chronic immune idiopathic thrombocytopenic purpura who have had an insufficient response to corticosteroids, immunoglobulins, or splenectomy**
Adults: Initially, 1 mcg/kg subcutaneously once weekly. Adjust dosage in increments of 1 mcg/kg to maintain platelet count of 50×10^9/L or higher, as needed to reduce the risk of bleeding. Maximum dosage is 10 mcg/kg weekly. If platelet count is more than 200×10^9/L for 2 consecutive weeks, reduce dosage by 1 mcg/kg. Withhold drug if platelet count exceeds 400×10^9/L. Continue to assess platelet count weekly. After platelet count has fallen to less than 200×10^9/L, resume therapy at dosage reduced by 1 mcg/kg. Discontinue if platelet count doesn't increase after 4 weeks at maximum dosage.

tetanus immune globulin (human)
BayTet, HyperTET S/D

Therapeutic class: Prophylaxis drugs
Pharmacologic class: Immunoglobulins
Pregnancy risk category: C

AVAILABLE FORMS
Injection: 250-unit vial or syringe

INDICATIONS & DOSAGES
➤ **Postexposure prevention of tetanus after injury, in patients whose immunization is incomplete or unknown**
Adults and children: 250 units deep I.M. injection.

➤ **Tetanus**
Adults and children: Single doses of 3,000 to 6,000 units I.M. have been used. Optimal dosage schedules haven't been established.

Common combination drugs: Indications and dosages

Amphetamines

Adderall
Adderall XR

Controlled Substance Schedule II

GENERIC COMPONENTS

dextroamphetamine sulfate–dextroamphetamine saccharate–amphetamine aspartate–amphetamine sulfate

Tablets

5 mg: 1.25 mg dextroamphetamine sulfate, 1.25 mg dextroamphetamine saccharate, 1.25 mg amphetamine aspartate, and 1.25 mg amphetamine sulfate

7.5 mg: 1.875 mg dextroamphetamine sulfate, 1.875 mg dextroamphetamine saccharate, 1.875 mg amphetamine aspartate, and 1.875 mg amphetamine sulfate

10 mg: 2.5 mg dextroamphetamine sulfate, 2.5 mg dextroamphetamine saccharate, 2.5 mg amphetamine aspartate, and 2.5 mg amphetamine sulfate

12.5 mg: 3.125 mg dextroamphetamine sulfate, 3.125 mg dextroamphetamine saccharate, 3.125 mg amphetamine aspartate, and 3.125 mg amphetamine sulfate

15 mg: 3.75 mg dextroamphetamine sulfate, 3.75 mg dextroamphetamine saccharate, 3.75 mg amphetamine aspartate, and 3.75 mg amphetamine sulfate

20 mg: 5 mg dextroamphetamine sulfate, 5 mg dextroamphetamine saccharate, 5 mg amphetamine aspartate, and 5 mg amphetamine sulfate

30 mg: 7.5 mg dextroamphetamine sulfate, 7.5 mg dextroamphetamine saccharate, 7.5 mg amphetamine aspartate, and 7.5 mg amphetamine sulfate

Capsules (extended-release)

5 mg: 1.25 mg dextroamphetamine sulfate, 1.25 mg dextroamphetamine saccharate, 1.25 mg amphetamine aspartate, and 1.25 mg amphetamine sulfate

10 mg: 2.5 mg dextroamphetamine sulfate, 2.5 mg dextroamphetamine saccharate, 2.5 mg amphetamine aspartate, and 2.5 mg amphetamine sulfate

15 mg: 3.75 mg dextroamphetamine sulfate, 3.75 mg dextroamphetamine saccharate, 3.75 mg amphetamine aspartate, and 3.75 mg amphetamine sulfate

20 mg: 5 mg dextroamphetamine sulfate, 5 mg dextroamphetamine saccharate, 5 mg amphetamine aspartate, and 5 mg amphetamine sulfate

25 mg: 6.25 mg dextroamphetamine sulfate, 6.25 mg dextroamphetamine saccharate, 6.25 mg amphetamine aspartate, and 6.25 mg amphetamine sulfate

30 mg: 7.5 mg dextroamphetamine sulfate, 7.5 mg dextroamphetamine saccharate, 7.5 mg amphetamine aspartate, and 7.5 mg amphetamine sulfate

DOSAGES

Narcolepsy

Adults and children over age 12: Initially, 10 mg immediate-release tablet P.O. daily. Increase by 10 mg weekly to maximum of 60 mg in 2 or 3 divided doses every 4 to 6 hours. *Children ages 6 to 12:* Initially, 5 mg immediate-release tablet P.O. daily. Increase by 5 mg weekly until optimal response achieved.

Attention deficit hyperactivity disorder

Adults: Initially, 5 mg P.O. once daily or b.i.d. May increase by 5-mg weekly. Maximum dose is 40 mg/day. Or, 10 mg extended-release capsule P.O. once daily in a.m. May increase by 10 mg weekly. Maximum dose is 30 mg/day. *Children age 6 and older:* Initially, 5 mg immediate-release tablet P.O. daily or b.i.d. Increase by 5 mg weekly until optimal response. Dosage should rarely exceed 40 mg. Or, 5 or 10 mg (ages 6 to 12) or 10 mg (ages 13 to 17) extended-release capsule P.O. daily in a.m. Increase by 5 to 10 mg weekly to a maximum dose of 30 mg. *Children ages 3 to 5:* Initially, 2.5 mg immediate-release tablet P.O. daily. Increase by 2.5 mg weekly until optimal response. Extended-release form not studied in children under age 6.

Analgesics

Duexis

GENERIC COMPONENTS

ibuprofen–famotidine

Tablets

800 mg ibuprofen and 26.6 mg famotidine

DOSAGES
Rheumatoid arthritis and osteoarthritis; to decrease risk of upper GI ulcers
Adults: 1 tablet P.O. t.i.d.

Fioricet with Codeine
Controlled Substance Schedule III
GENERIC COMPONENTS
acetaminophen–butalbital–caffeine–codeine phosphate
Capsules
325 mg acetaminophen, 50 mg butalbital, 40 mg caffeine, and 30 mg codeine phosphate
DOSAGES
Headache, mild to moderate pain
Adults: 1 to 2 capsules P.O. every 4 hours. Maximum dosage, 6 capsules in 24 hours.

Fiorinal with Codeine
Controlled Substance Schedule III
GENERIC COMPONENTS
codeine phosphate–aspirin–butalbital–caffeine
Tablets, Capsules
30 mg codeine phosphate, 325 mg aspirin, 50 mg butalbital, and 40 mg caffeine
DOSAGES
Headache, mild to moderate pain
Adults: 1 to 2 tablets or capsules P.O. every 4 hours. Maximum dosage, 6 tablets or capsules in 24 hours.

pentazocine–naloxone hydrochloride
Controlled Substance Schedule IV
GENERIC COMPONENTS
pentazocine–naloxone hydrochloride
Tablets
50 mg pentazocine and 0.5 mg naloxone hydrochloride
DOSAGES
Moderate to severe pain
Adults and children age 12 and older: 1 tablet P.O. every 3 to 4 hours. May increase to 2 tablets if necessary. Maximum dosage, 12 tablets in 24 hours.

Percodan
Controlled Substance Schedule II
GENERIC COMPONENTS
oxycodone hydrochloride–oxycodone terephthalate–aspirin

Tablets
4.5 mg oxycodone hydrochloride, 0.38 mg oxycodone terephthalate, and 325 mg aspirin
DOSAGES
Moderate to moderately severe pain
Adults: 1 tablet P.O. every 6 hours. Maximum dosage, 12 tablets in 24 hours.

Reprexain
Controlled Substance Schedule III
GENERIC COMPONENTS
hydrocodone bitartrate–ibuprofen
Tablets
2.5 mg hydrocodone bitartrate and 200 mg ibuprofen
5 mg hydrocodone bitartrate and 200 mg ibuprofen
10 mg hydrocodone bitartrate and 200 mg ibuprofen
DOSAGES
Acute pain (short-term)
Adults and children age 16 and older: 1 tablet P.O. every 6 hours. Maximum dosage, 5 tablets in 24 hours.

Ultracet ✔
GENERIC COMPONENTS
tramadol hydrochloride–acetaminophen
Tablets
37.5 mg tramadol hydrochloride and 325 mg acetaminophen
DOSAGES
Acute pain
Adults: 2 tablets P.O. every 4 to 6 hours as needed.

Vicoprofen
Controlled Substance Schedule III
GENERIC COMPONENTS
hydrocodone–ibuprofen
Tablets
7.5 mg hydrocodone and 200 mg ibuprofen
DOSAGES
Acute pain (short-term)
Adults and children age 16 and older: 1 tablet P.O. every 4 to 6 hours. Maximum dosage, 5 tablets in 24 hours.

Vimovo
GENERIC COMPONENTS
naproxen–esomeprazole
Tablets
375 mg naproxen and 20 mg esomeprazole
500 mg naproxen and 20 mg esomeprazole

DOSAGES
Osteoarthritis, rheumatoid arthritis, ankylosing spondylitis; to decrease risk of gastric ulcer development
Adults: 1 tablet P.O. b.i.d.

Antiacne drugs

Epiduo
GENERIC COMPONENTS
benzoyl peroxide–adapalene
Topical gel
2.5% benzoyl peroxide and 0.1% adapalene
DOSAGES
Adults and children age 12 and older: Apply a thin film to affected areas of the face or trunk once daily after washing.

Estrostep Fe
GENERIC COMPONENTS
norethindrone–ethinyl estradiol
norethindrone–ethinyl estradiol–ferrous fumarate
Tablets
1 mg norethindrone and 20 mcg ethinyl estradiol
1 mg norethindrone and 30 mcg ethinyl estradiol
1 mg norethindrone and 35 mcg ethinyl estradiol and 75 mg ferrous fumarate
DOSAGES
Acne vulgaris
Women older than age 15: 1 tablet P.O. daily.

Ortho Tri-Cyclen
GENERIC COMPONENTS
norgestimate–ethinyl estradiol
Tablets
0.18 mg norgestimate and 35 mcg ethinyl estradiol
0.215 mg norgestimate and 35 mcg ethinyl estradiol
0.25 mg norgestimate and 35 mcg ethinyl estradiol
DOSAGES
Acne
Women older than age 15: 1 tablet P.O. daily.

Veltin
Ziana
GENERIC COMPONENTS
clindamycin phosphate–tretinoin
Topical gel
Clindamycin phosphate 1.2% and tretinoin 0.025%

DOSAGES
Acne vulgaris
Adults and children age 12 and older: Apply pea-size amount to cover entire affected area once daily in evening. Avoid eyes, lips, and mucous membranes.

Antibacterials

erythromycin ethylsuccinate–sulfisoxazole
GENERIC COMPONENTS
erythromycin ethylsuccinate–sulfisoxazole
Granules for oral suspension
Erythromycin ethylsuccinate (equivalent of 200 mg erythromycin activity) and 600 mg sulfisoxazole per 5 mL when reconstituted according to manufacturer's directions
DOSAGES
Acute otitis media
Children age 2 months and older: 50 mg/kg/day erythromycin and 150 mg/kg/day sulfisoxazole in three or four divided doses for 10 days. Give without regard to meals. Refrigerate after reconstitution; use within 14 days.

Antidiabetics

ActoPlus Met
ActoPlus Met XR
GENERIC COMPONENTS
pioglitazone–metformin hydrochloride
Tablets
15 mg pioglitazone and 500 mg metformin hydrocloride
15 mg pioglitazone and 850 mg metformin hydrochloride
Tablets (extended-release)
15 mg pioglitazone and 1,000 mg extended-release metformin hydrochloride
30 mg pioglitazone and 1,000 mg extended-release metformin hydrochloride
DOSAGES
Adjunct to diet and exercise to improve glycemic control in adults with type 2 diabetes
Adults: 15 mg pioglitazone with 500 mg metformin or 15 mg pioglitazone with 850 mg metformin P.O. once daily or b.i.d. with food. Maximum dosage, 45 mg pioglitazone with 2,550 mg metformin per day. Or, 15 mg pioglitazone with 1,000 mg extended-release metformin or 30 mg pioglitazone with 1,000 mg extended-release metformin P.O. once daily with

evening meal. Maximum dosage of extended-release formula, 45 mg pioglitazone with 2,000 mg extended-release metformin per day.

Avandamet
GENERIC COMPONENTS
rosiglitazone–metformin
Tablets
2 mg rosiglitazone and 500 mg metformin
2 mg rosiglitazone and 1 g metformin
4 mg rosiglitazone and 500 mg metformin
4 mg rosiglitazone and 1 g metformin
DOSAGES
Adjunct to diet and exercise to improve glycemic control in adults with type 2 diabetes
Adults: 4 mg rosiglitazone with 500 mg metformin, once per day or in divided doses. Not for initial therapy; adjust using individual drugs alone, then switch to the appropriate dosage of the combination product. See package insert for details on adjusting dosage based on use of other drugs and previous dosage levels. Maximum dosage, 8 mg rosiglitazone and 2,000 mg metformin per day.

Glucovance
GENERIC COMPONENTS
glyburide–metformin
Tablets
1.25 mg glyburide and 250 mg metformin
2.5 mg glyburide and 500 mg metformin
5 mg glyburide and 500 mg metformin
DOSAGES
As initial therapy as adjunct to diet and exercise to improve glycemic control in type 2 diabetes; as secondline therapy when diet, exercise, and initial treatment with a sulfonylurea or metformin don't achieve glycemic control
Adults: 1 or 2 tablets P.O. daily or b.i.d. with meals. Maximum dosage, glyburide 20 mg and metformin 2,000 mg for treatment of type 2 diabetes, as second-line therapy.

Janumet
GENERIC COMPONENTS
sitagliptin–metformin
Tablets
50 mg sitagliptin and 500 mg metformin hydrochloride
50 mg sitagliptin and 1,000 mg metformin hydrochloride

DOSAGES
Adjunct to diet and exercise to improve glycemic control in type 2 diabetes when treatment with both sitagliptin and metformin is appropriate
Adults already on metformin: 50 mg sitagliptin P.O. b.i.d. plus the dose of metformin already being taken. For patients taking 850 mg metformin P.O. b.i.d., recommended starting dosage is 50 mg sitagliptin and 1,000 mg metformin P.O. b.i.d.
Adults not on metformin: 50 mg sitagliptin and 500 mg metformin P.O. b.i.d.

Janumet XR
GENERIC COMPONENTS
sitagliptin–metformin
Tablets (extended-release)
50 mg sitagliptin and 500 mg extended-release metformin hydrochloride
50 mg sitagliptin and 1,000 mg extended-release metformin hydrochloride
100 mg sitagliptin and 1,000 mg extended-release metformin hydrochloride
DOSAGES
Adjunct to diet and exercise to improve glycemic control in type 2 diabetes when treatment with both sitagliptin and metformin is appropriate
Adults already on metformin: 100 mg/day sitagliptin plus previously prescribed dose of metformin. For patients taking 850 mg immediate-release metformin P.O. b.i.d. or 1,000 mg metformin P.O. b.i.d., recommended starting dosage is 100 mg sitagliptin and 2,000 mg extended-release metformin P.O. once daily.
Adults not on metformin: 100 mg sitagliptin and 1,000 mg extended-release metformin P.O. once daily.

Jentadueto
GENERIC COMPONENTS
linagliptin–metformin
Tablets
2.5 mg linagliptin and 500 mg metformin hydrochloride
2.5 mg linagliptin and 850 mg metformin hydrochloride
2.5 mg linagliptin and 1,000 mg metformin hydrochloride
DOSAGES
Adjunct to diet and exercise to improve glycemic control in type 2 diabetes when

treatment with both linagliptin and metformin is appropriate
Adults already on metformin: 2.5 mg linagliptin P.O. b.i.d. plus current dose of metformin already being taken. For patients taking 1,000 mg metformin b.i.d., recommended starting dosage is 2.5 mg linagliptin and 1,000 mg metformin P.O. b.i.d.
Adults not on metformin: 2.5 mg linagliptin and 500 mg metformin P.O. b.i.d.

Kazano
GENERIC COMPONENTS
alogliptin benzoate–metformin
Tablets
12.5 mg alogliptin benzoate and 500 mg metformin
12.5 mg alogliptin benzoate and 1,000 mg metformin
DOSAGES
Adjunct to diet and exercise to improve glycemic control in type 2 diabetes
Adults: 1 tablet P.O. b.i.d. with food. Adjust dosage based on effectiveness and tolerability. Maximum daily dose, 25 mg alogliptin and 2,000 mg metformin

Metaglip
GENERIC COMPONENTS
glipizide–metformin
Tablets
2.5 mg glipizide and 250 mg metformin
2.5 mg glipizide and 500 mg metformin
5 mg glipizide and 500 mg metformin
DOSAGES
Adjunct to diet and exercise to improve glycemic control in type 2 diabetes
Adults: 1 tablet P.O. per day with a meal; adjust dose based on patient response. Maximum daily dose, 20 mg glipizide with 2,000 mg metformin.

Oseni
GENERIC COMPONENTS
alogliptin benzoate–pioglitazone hydrochloride
Tablets
12.5 mg alogliptin benzoate and 15 mg pioglitazone hydrochloride
12.5 mg alogliptin benzoate and 30 mg pioglitazone hydrochloride
12.5 mg alogliptin benzoate and 45 mg pioglitazone hydrochloride

25 mg alogliptin benzoate and 15 mg pioglitazone hydrochloride
25 mg alogliptin benzoate and 30 mg pioglitazone hydrochloride
25 mg alogliptin benzoate and 45 mg pioglitazone hydrochloride
DOSAGES
Adjunct to diet and exercise to improve glycemic control in type 2 diabetes mellitus when treatment with both alogliptin and pioglitazone is appropriate
Adults inadequately controlled on diet and exercise, inadequately controlled on metformin monotherapy, or who require additional glycemic control on alogliptin: Alogliptin 25 mg/pioglitazone 15 mg or alogliptin 25 mg/pioglitazone 30 mg P.O. once daily. May titrate to a maximum of alogliptin 25 mg/pioglitazone 45 mg once daily based on glycemic response as determined by hemoglobin A_{1c} (HbA_{1c}).
Adults who require additional glycemic control on pioglitazone: Alogliptin 25 mg/pioglitazone 15 mg, alogliptin 25 mg/pioglitazone 30 mg, or alogliptin 25 mg/pioglitazone 45 mg P.O. once daily as appropriate based on current therapy. May titrate to a maximum of alogliptin 25 mg/pioglitazone 45 mg once daily based on glycemic response as determined by HbA_{1c}.
Adults switching from alogliptin administered with pioglitazone: Initiate at the dosage of alogliptin and pioglitazone based on current therapy. May titrate to a maximum of alogliptin 25 mg/pioglitazone 45 mg once daily based on glycemic response as determined by HbA_{1c}.
Adults with congestive heart failure (New York Heart Association class I or II): Alogliptin 25 mg/pioglitazone 15 mg P.O. once daily. May titrate to a maximum of alogliptin 25 mg/pioglitazone 45 mg once daily based on glycemic response as determined by HbA_{1c}.

PrandiMet
GENERIC COMPONENTS
repaglinide–metformin
Tablets
1 mg repaglinide and 500 mg metformin
2 mg repaglinide and 500 mg metformin
DOSAGES
Adjunct to diet and exercise to improve glycemic control in type 2 diabetes
Adults: Individualize dosage based on patient's current regimen. Can be administered

b.i.d. to t.i.d. up to maximum daily dose of 10 mg repaglinide and 2,500 mg metformin.

Antigout drugs
Col-Probenecid
GENERIC COMPONENTS
probenecid–colchicine
Tablets
500 mg probenecid and 0.5 mg colchicine
DOSAGES
Gouty arthritis
Adults: 1 tablet P.O. daily for 1 week, then 1 tablet P.O. b.i.d. Adjust dosage based on symptoms and uric acid levels. Maximum dosage, 4 tablets daily.

Antihypertensives
Accuretic
Quinaretic
GENERIC COMPONENTS
quinapril–hydrochlorothiazide
Tablets
10 mg quinapril and 12.5 mg hydrochlorothiazide
20 mg quinapril and 12.5 mg hydrochlorothiazide
20 mg quinapril and 25 mg hydrochlorothiazide
DOSAGES
Hypertension
Adults: 1 tablet P.O. per day in the morning. Adjust drug using the individual products, then switch to appropriate dosage of the combination product.

Atacand HCT
GENERIC COMPONENTS
candesartan–hydrochlorothiazide
Tablets
16 mg candesartan and 12.5 mg hydrochlorothiazide
32 mg candesartan and 12.5 mg hydrochlorothiazide
32 mg candesartan and 25 mg hydrochlorothiazide
DOSAGES
Hypertension
Adults: 1 tablet P.O. daily in the morning. Adjust dosage using the individual products, then switch to appropriate dosage of the combination product.

Avalide
GENERIC COMPONENTS
irbesartan–hydrochlorothiazide
Tablets
150 mg irbesartan and 12.5 mg hydrochlorothiazide
300 mg irbesartan and 12.5 mg hydrochlorothiazide
300 mg irbesartan and 25 mg hydrochlorothiazide
DOSAGES
Hypertension
Adults: 1 tablet P.O. daily. Adjust dosage with individual products, then switch to combination product when patient's condition is stabilized. Maximum daily dose, 300 mg irbesartan and 25 mg hydrochlorothiazide.

Azor
GENERIC COMPONENTS
amlodipine–olmesartan medoxomil
Tablets
5 mg amlodipine and 20 mg olmesartan medoxomil
5 mg amlodipine and 40 mg olmesartan medoxomil
10 mg amlodipine and 20 mg olmesartan medoxomil
10 mg amlodipine and 40 mg olmesartan medoxomil
DOSAGES
Hypertension
Adults: Initially, 5 mg amlodipine with 20 mg olmesartan P.O. once daily for 1 to 2 weeks. Titrate as needed up to maximum of 10 mg amlodipine with 40 mg olmesartan once daily.

Benicar HCT ✐
GENERIC COMPONENTS
olmesartan medoxomil–hydrochlorothiazide
Tablets
20 mg olmesartan medoxomil and 12.5 mg hydrochlorothiazide
40 mg olmesartan and 12.5 mg hydrochlorothiazide
40 mg olmesartan and 25 mg hydrochlorothiazide
DOSAGES
Hypertension
Adults: 1 tablet P.O. daily in the morning. Adjust dosage using the individual products,

then switch to the combination product when patient's adjustment schedule is stable. Dosage may be titrated at 2- to 4-week intervals. Maximum dosage, 40 mg olmesartan plus 25 mg hydrochlorothiazide.

Capozide
GENERIC COMPONENTS
captopril–hydrochlorothiazide
Tablets
25 mg captopril and 15 mg hydrochlorothiazide
50 mg captopril and 15 mg hydrochlorothiazide
25 mg captopril and 25 mg hydrochlorothiazide
50 mg captopril and 25 mg hydrochlorothiazide
DOSAGES
Hypertension
Adults: 1 to 2 tablets P.O. daily, in the morning. Adjust dosage using the individual products, then switch to the combination product when patient's adjustment schedule is stable. Maximum daily dose is 150 mg captopril or 50 mg hydrochlorothiazide.

Clorpres
GENERIC COMPONENTS
chlorthalidone–clonidine hydrochloride
Tablets
15 mg chlorthalidone and 0.1 mg clonidine hydrochloride
15 mg chlorthalidone and 0.2 mg clonidine hydrochloride
15 mg chlorthalidone and 0.3 mg clonidine hydrochloride
DOSAGES
Hypertension
Adults: 1 to 2 tablets P.O. daily in the morning. Adjust dosage using the individual products, then switch to the combination product when patient's adjustment schedule is stable. Maximum dosage, 0.6 mg clonidine plus 30 mg chlorthalidone.

Corzide
GENERIC COMPONENTS
nadolol–bendroflumethiazide
Tablets
40 mg nadolol and 5 mg bendroflumethiazide
80 mg nadolol and 5 mg bendroflumethiazide

DOSAGES
Hypertension
Adults: 1 tablet P.O. daily in the morning. Adjust dosage using the individual products, then switch to the combination product when patient's adjustment schedule is stable.

Diovan HCT ✐
GENERIC COMPONENTS
valsartan–hydrochlorothiazide
Tablets
80 mg valsartan and 12.5 mg hydrochlorothiazide
160 mg valsartan and 12.5 mg hydrochlorothiazide
160 mg valsartan and 25 mg hydrochlorothiazide
320 mg valsartan and 12.5 mg hydrochlorothiazide
320 mg valsartan and 25 mg hydrochlorothiazide
DOSAGES
Hypertension
Adults: 1 tablet P.O. daily. Not for initial therapy; start using each component first. Maximum dosage, 320 mg valsartan and 25 mg hydrochlorothiazide.

Exforge
GENERIC COMPONENTS
amlodipine besylate–valsartan
Tablets
5 mg amlodipine besylate and 160 mg valsartan
5 mg amlodipine besylate and 320 mg valsartan
10 mg amlodipine besylate and 160 mg valsartan
10 mg amlodipine besylate and 320 mg valsartan
DOSAGES
Hypertension
Adults: Initially, 5 mg amlodipine with 160 mg valsartan P.O. once daily. Increase after 1 to 2 weeks to a maximum of 10 mg amlodipine with 320 mg valsartan P.O. once daily.

Exforge HCT
GENERIC COMPONENTS
amlodipine besylate–valsartan–hydrochlorothiazide
Tablets
5 mg amlodipine besylate, 160 mg valsartan, and 12.5 mg hydrochlorothiazide

10 mg amlodipine besylate, 160 mg valsartan, and 12.5 mg hydrochlorothiazide
5 mg amlodipine besylate, 160 mg valsartan, and 25 mg hydrocholorothiazide
10 mg amlodipine besylate, 160 mg valsartan, and 25 mg hydrochlorothiazide
10 mg amlodipine besylate, 320 mg valsartan, and 25 mg hydrochlorothiazide

DOSAGES
Hypertension
Adults: Give dose P.O. once daily. Dosage may be increased after 2 weeks. Maximum recommended dosage is 10 mg amlodipine, 320 mg valsartan, and 25 mg hydrochlorothiazide.

fosinopril and hydrochlorothiazide

GENERIC COMPONENTS
fosinopril–hydrochlorothiazide
Tablets
10 mg fosinopril and 12.5 mg hydrochlorothiazide
20 mg fosinopril and 12.5 mg hydrochlorothiazide

DOSAGES
Hypertension
Adults: 1 tablet P.O. per day in the morning. Adjust dosage using the individual products, then switch to appropriate combination product.

Hyzaar

GENERIC COMPONENTS
losartan–hydrochlorothiazide
Tablets
50 mg losartan and 12.5 mg hydrochlorothiazide
100 mg losartan and 12.5 mg hydrochlorothiazide
100 mg losartan and 25 mg hydrochlorothiazide

DOSAGES
Hypertension
Adults: 1 tablet P.O. daily in the morning. Not for initial therapy; start using each component and if desired effects are obtained, Hyzaar may be used. Maximum dosage, 100 mg losartan and 25 mg hydrochlorothiazide daily.

Lopressor HCT

GENERIC COMPONENTS
metoprolol–hydrochlorothiazide
Tablets
50 mg metoprolol and 25 mg hydrochlorothiazide

100 mg metoprolol and 25 mg hydrochlorothiazide

DOSAGES
Hypertension
Adults: 1 tablet P.O. per day. Adjust dosage using the individual products, then switch to appropriate combination product.

Lotensin HCT

GENERIC COMPONENTS
benazepril–hydrochlorothiazide
Tablets
5 mg benazepril and 6.25 mg hydrochlorothiazide
10 mg benazepril and 12.5 mg hydrochlorothiazide
20 mg benazepril and 12.5 mg hydrochlorothiazide
20 mg benazepril and 25 mg hydrochlorothiazide

DOSAGES
Hypertension
Adults: 1 tablet P.O. daily in the morning. Adjust dosage using the individual products, then switch to appropriate combination product.

Lotrel

GENERIC COMPONENTS
amlodipine–benazepril
Capsules
2.5 mg amlodipine and 10 mg benazepril
5 mg amlodipine and 10 mg benazepril
5 mg amlodipine and 20 mg benazepril
5 mg amlodipine and 40 mg benazepril
10 mg amlodipine and 20 mg benazepril
10 mg amlodipine and 40 mg benazepril

DOSAGES
Hypertension
Adults: 1 tablet P.O. daily in morning. Monitor for hypertension and adverse effects closely over first 2 weeks and regularly thereafter.

methyldopa and hydrochlorothiazide

GENERIC COMPONENTS
methyldopa–hydrochlorothiazide
Tablets
250 mg methyldopa and 15 mg hydrochlorothiazide
250 mg methyldopa and 25 mg hydrochlorothiazide

DOSAGES
Hypertension

Adults: 1 tablet P.O. b.i.d. or t.i.d. Adjust dosage using individual products, then switch to appropriate combination product. Maximum dosage, 3,000 mg methyldopa and 50 mg hydrochlorothiazide daily.

Micardis HCT
GENERIC COMPONENTS
telmisartan–hydrochlorothiazide
Tablets
40 mg telmisartan and 12.5 mg hydrochlorothiazide
80 mg telmisartan and 12.5 mg hydrochlorothiazide
80 mg telmisartan and 25 mg hydrochlorothiazide
DOSAGES
Hypertension
Adults: 1 tablet P.O. per day; may be adjusted up to 160 mg telmisartan and 25 mg hydrochlorothiazide, based on patient's response.

Prinzide
Zestoretic
GENERIC COMPONENTS
lisinopril–hydrochlorothiazide
Tablets
10 mg lisinopril and 12.5 mg hydrochlorothiazide
20 mg lisinopril and 12.5 mg hydrochlorothiazide
20 mg lisinopril and 25 mg hydrochlorothiazide
DOSAGES
Hypertension
Adults: 1 tablet P.O. daily in the morning. Adjust dosage using individual products, then switch to appropriate combination product. The hydrochlorothiazide dose should generally not be increased until 2 to 3 weeks have elapsed. Maximum dosage, 80 mg lisinopril and 50 mg hydrochlorothiazide daily.

propranolol and hydrochlorothiazide
GENERIC COMPONENTS
propranolol hydrochloride–hydrochlorothiazide
Tablets
40 mg propranolol hydrochloride and 25 mg hydrochlorothiazide
80 mg propranolol hydrochloride and 25 mg hydrochlorothiazide
DOSAGES
Hypertension

Adults: 1 tablet P.O. b.i.d. Adjust dosage using individual products, then switch to appropriate combination product. Maximum daily dose not to exceed 160 mg propranolol and 50 mg hydrochlorothiazide.

Tarka
GENERIC COMPONENTS
trandolapril–verapamil
Tablets
1 mg trandolapril and 240 mg verapamil
2 mg trandolapril and 180 mg verapamil
2 mg trandolapril and 240 mg verapamil
4 mg trandolapril and 240 mg verapamil
DOSAGES
Hypertension
Adults: 1 tablet P.O. per day, taken with food. Adjust dosage using the individual products, then switch to appropriate combination product. Make sure that patient swallows tablet whole. Don't cut, crush, or allow him to chew.

Tekamlo
GENERIC COMPONENTS
aliskiren hemifumarate–amlodipine besylate
Tablets
150 mg aliskiren hemifumarate and 5 mg amlodipine besylate
150 mg aliskiren hemifumarate and 10 mg amlodipine besylate
300 mg aliskiren hemifumarate and 5 mg amlodipine besylate
300 mg aliskiren hemifumarate and 10 mg amlodipine besylate
DOSAGES
Hypertension
Adults: 1 tablet P.O. daily. Initiate therapy with 150 mg aliskiren and 5 mg amlodipine. Titrate as needed after 2 to 4 weeks to maximum of 300 mg aliskiren and 10 mg amlodipine. Tekamlo may be substituted for its titrated components.

Tekturna HCT
GENERIC COMPONENTS
aliskiren hemifumarate–hydrochlorothiazide
Tablets
150 mg aliskiren hemifumarate and 12.5 mg hydrochlorothiazide
150 mg aliskiren hemifumarate and 25 mg hydrochlorothiazide
300 mg aliskiren hemifumarate and 12.5 mg hydrochlorothiazide

300 mg aliskiren hemifumarate and 25 mg hydrochlorothiazide
DOSAGES
Hypertension
Adults: 1 tablet P.O. daily. Initiate therapy with 150 mg aliskiren and 12.5 mg hydrochlorothiazide. Titrate up as needed after 2 to 4 weeks to a maximum of 300 mg aliskiren and 25 mg hydrochlorothiazide.

Tenoretic
GENERIC COMPONENTS
atenolol–chlorthalidone
Tablets
50 mg atenolol and 25 mg chlorthalidone
100 mg atenolol and 25 mg chlorthalidone
DOSAGES
Hypertension
Adults: 1 tablet P.O. daily in the morning. Adjust dosage using individual products, then switch to appropriate combination product.

Teveten HCT
GENERIC COMPONENTS
eprosartan–hydrochlorothiazide
Tablets
600 mg eprosartan and 12.5 mg hydrochlorothiazide
600 mg eprosartan and 25 mg hydrochlorothiazide
DOSAGES
Hypertension
Adults: 1 tablet P.O. each day. Establish dosage with each component alone before using the combination product; if blood pressure isn't controlled on 600 mg/25 mg tablet, 300 mg eprosartan may be added each evening.

Tribenzor
GENERIC COMPONENTS
amlodipine besylate–hydrochlorothiazide–olmesartan medoxomil
Tablets
5 mg amlodipine besylate, 12.5 mg hydrochlorothiazide, and 20 mg olmesartan medoxomil
5 mg amlodipine besylate, 12.5 mg hydrochlorothiazide, and 40 mg olmesartan medoxomil
5 mg amlodipine besylate, 25 mg hydrochlorothiazide, and 40 mg olmesartan medoxomil

10 mg amlodipine besylate, 12.5 mg hydrochlorothiazide, and 40 mg olmesartan medoxomil
10 mg amlodipine besylate, 25 mg hydrochlorothiazide, and 40 mg olmesartan medoxomil
DOSAGES
Hypertension
Adults: 1 tablet P.O. daily. Adjust dosage of individual products; then switch to appropriate combination product. May increase dosage after 2 weeks. Maximum recommended dose is 10 mg amlodipine, 25 mg hydrochlorothiazide, and 40 mg olmesartan.

Twynsta
GENERIC COMPONENTS
amlodipine besylate–telmisartan
Tablets
5 mg amlodipine besylate and 40 mg telmisartan
5 mg amlodipine besylate and 80 mg telmisartan
10 mg amlodipine besylate and 40 mg telmisartan
10 mg amlodipine besylate and 80 mg telmisartan
DOSAGES
Hypertension
Adults: 1 tablet P.O. daily. Substitute for its individually titrated components or initiate therapy with 5 mg amlodipine and 40 mg telmisartan or 5 mg amlodipine and 80 mg telmisartan. May increase dosage after at least 2 weeks to maximum dose of 10 mg amlodipine and 80 mg telmisartan.

Uniretic
GENERIC COMPONENTS
moexipril hydrochloride–hydrochlorothiazide
Tablets
7.5 mg moexipril hydrochloride and 12.5 mg hydrochlorothiazide
15 mg moexipril hydrochloride and 12.5 mg hydrochlorothiazide
15 mg moexipril hydrochloride and 25 mg hydrochlorothiazide
DOSAGES
Hypertension
Adults: Give ½ tablet to 2 tablets P.O. per day. Not for initial therapy. Adjust dose after 2 to 3 weeks to maintain appropriate blood pressure.

Vaseretic

GENERIC COMPONENTS
enalapril maleate–hydrochlorothiazide
Tablets
5 mg enalapril maleate and 12.5 mg
hydrochlorothiazide
10 mg enalapril maleate and 25 mg
hydrochlorothiazide
DOSAGES
Hypertension
Adults: 1 to 2 tablets P.O. daily in the morning.
Adjust dosage using individual products, then
switch to appropriate combination product.
Maximum dosage, 20 mg enalapril and 50 mg
hydrochlorothiazide daily.

Ziac

GENERIC COMPONENTS
bisoprolol fumarate–hydrochlorothiazide
Tablets
2.5 mg bisoprolol fumarate and 6.25 mg
hydrochlorothiazide
5 mg bisoprolol fumarate and 6.25 mg hydrochlorothiazide
10 mg bisoprolol fumarate and 6.25 mg
hydrochlorothiazide
DOSAGES
Hypertension
Adults: 1 tablet P.O. daily in morning. Initial
dose is 2.5 mg/6.25 mg tablet P.O. daily. Increase dosage in 14-day intervals; optimal antihypertensive effect may require 2 to 3 weeks.
Maximum dosage, 20 mg bisoprolol and
12.5 mg hydrochlorothiazide daily.

Antimigraine Drugs

Cafergot
Migergot

GENERIC COMPONENTS
ergotamine tartrate–caffeine
Tablets
1 mg ergotamine tartrate and 100 mg caffeine
Suppositories
2 mg ergotamine tartrate and 100 mg caffeine
DOSAGES
**Prevention and treatment of migraine
headache**
Adults: 2 tablets P.O. at the first sign of attack.
Follow with 1 tablet every 30 minutes, if needed. Maximum dose is 6 tablets per attack. Don't
exceed 10 tablets per week. Or, 1 suppository

P.R. at first sign of attack; follow with second
dose after 1 hour, if needed. Maximum dose is
2 suppositories per attack. Don't exceed 5 suppositories per week. Don't combine this drug
with ritonavir, nelfinavir, indinavir, erythromycin, clarithromycin, or troleandomycin, as serious vasospasm could occur.

Treximet

GENERIC COMPONENTS
sumatriptan succinate–naproxen sodium
Tablets
85 mg sumatriptan succinate and 500 mg
naproxen sodium
DOSAGES
Migraine headache
Adults: 1 tablet P.O. at first sign of migraine.
May follow with 1 tablet 2 hours later. Maximum dosage is 2 tablets/24 hours.

Antiplatelet drugs

Aggrenox

GENERIC COMPONENTS
dipyridamole–aspirin
Capsules
200 mg dipyridamole and 25 mg aspirin
DOSAGES
Reduce stroke risk
Adults: 1 capsule P.O. b.i.d. in the morning
and evening. Swallow capsule whole; may be
taken with or without food.

Antiretrovirals

Atripla

GENERIC COMPONENTS
efavirenz–emtricitabine–tenofovir disoproxil
fumarate
600 mg efavirenz, 200 mg emtricitabine, and
300 mg tenofovir disoproxil fumarate
DOSAGES
Treatment of HIV infection
*Adults and children older than age 12 weigh-
ing at least 40 kg (88 lb):* 1 tablet P.O. daily on
empty stomach. Dosing at bedtime may improve tolerability of nervous system symptoms.

Combivir ✐

GENERIC COMPONENTS
lamivudine–zidovudine
Tablets
150 mg lamivudine and 300 mg zidovudine

DOSAGES
Treatment of HIV infection
Adults and children weighing 30 kg (66 lb) or more: 1 tablet P.O. b.i.d.

Complera
GENERIC COMPONENTS
emtricitabine–rilpivirine–tenofovir disoproxil fumarate
Tablets
200 mg emtricitabine, 25 mg rilpivirine, and 300 mg tenofovir
DOSAGES
Treatment of HIV infection
Adults: 1 tablet P.O. once daily with a meal.

Epzicom
GENERIC COMPONENTS
abacavir sulfate–lamivudine
Tablets
600 mg abacavir and 300 mg lamivudine
DOSAGES
Treatment of HIV infection
Adults: 1 tablet P.O. daily, taken without regard to food and in combination with other antiretrovirals.

Trizivir
GENERIC COMPONENTS
abacavir sulfate–lamivudine–zidovudine
Tablets
300 mg abacavir sulfate, 150 mg lamivudine, and 300 mg zidovudine
DOSAGES
Treatment of HIV infection
Adults and adolescents weighing 40 kg (88 lb) or more: 1 tablet P.O. b.i.d., alone or with other antiretrovirals.

Truvada
GENERIC COMPONENTS
emtricitabine–tenofovir disoproxil fumarate
Tablets
200 mg emtricitabine and 300 mg tenofovir disoproxil fumarate
DOSAGES
Pre-exposure prophylaxis (adults) and treatment of HIV infection (adults and adolescents)
Adults and adolescents age 12 and older weighing more than 35 kg (70 lb): 1 tablet P.O. daily in combination with other anti-retrovirals.

Antiulcer drugs

Helidac
GENERIC COMPONENTS
bismuth subsalicylate–metronidazole–tetracycline hydrochloride
Tablets
262.4 mg bismuth subsalicylate, 250 mg metronidazole, and 500 mg tetracycline hydrochloride
DOSAGES
Active duodenal ulcers associated with *Helicobacter pylori* infection
Adults: Give each dose (2 chewable bismuth subsalicylate tablets, 1 metronidazole tablet, and 1 tetracycline capsule) P.O. q.i.d. for 14 days along with a prescribed H_2 antagonist.

Prevpac
GENERIC COMPONENTS
lansoprazole–amoxicillin–clarithromycin
Daily administration pack
Two 30-mg lansoprazole capsules, four 500-mg amoxicillin capsules, and two 500-mg clarithromycin tablets
DOSAGES
Eradication of *Helicobacter pylori* infection
Adults: Divide pack equally to take in two equal doses, morning and evening.

Pylera
GENERIC COMPONENTS
bismuth subcitrate potassium–metronidazole–tetracycline hydrochloride
Capsules
140 mg bismuth subcitrate potassium, 125 mg metronidazole, and 125 mg tetracycline hydrochloride
DOSAGES
Eradication of *Helicobacter pylori* infection; active duodenal ulcers associated with *H. pylori* infection
Adults: Give each dose (which includes all 3 capsules) P.O. q.i.d. after meals and at bedtime for 10 days with omeprazole 20 mg P.O. b.i.d. (after the morning and evening meals) for 10 days.

Benign prostatic hyperplasia drugs

Jalyn
GENERIC COMPONENTS
dutasteride–tamsulosin hydrochloride

Capsules
0.5 mg dutasteride and 0.4 mg tamsulosin hydrochloride

DOSAGES

Treatment of symptomatic benign prostatic hyperplasia

Adult men: 1 capsule P.O. daily 30 minutes after same meal each day. Capsules should be swallowed whole.

Diuretics

Aldactazide

GENERIC COMPONENTS

spironolactone–hydrochlorothiazide

Tablets

25 mg spironolactone and 25 mg hydrochlorothiazide

50 mg spironolactone and 50 mg hydrochlorothiazide

DOSAGES

Edema or hypertension

Adults: One to eight 25-mg spironolactone and 25-mg hydrochlorothiazide tablets P.O. daily. Or, one to four 50-mg spironolactone and 50-mg hydrochlorothiazide tablets P.O. daily.

amiloride and hydrochlorothiazide

GENERIC COMPONENTS

amiloride–hydrochlorothiazide

Tablets

5 mg amiloride and 50 mg hydrochlorothiazide

DOSAGES

Edema or hypertension

Adults: 1 to 2 tablets P.O. per day with meals.

Maxzide

GENERIC COMPONENTS

triamterene–hydrochlorothiazide

Tablets

37.5 mg triamterene and 25 mg hydrochlorothiazide

75 mg triamterene and 50 mg hydrochlorothiazide

DOSAGES

Edema or hypertension

Adults: 1 to 2 tablets P.O. daily.

Heart failure drugs

BiDil

GENERIC COMPONENTS

isosorbide dinitrate–hydralazine

Tablets
20 mg isosorbide dinitrate and 37.5 mg hydralazine

DOSAGES

Adjunct to standard heart failure therapy

Adults: 1 to 2 tablets P.O. t.i.d.

Lipid-lowering drugs

Advicor

GENERIC COMPONENTS

lovastatin–niacin

Tablets

20 mg lovastatin and 500 mg niacin

20 mg lovastatin and 750 mg niacin

20 mg lovastatin and 1,000 mg niacin

40 mg lovastatin and 1,000 mg niacin

DOSAGES

Treatment of hypercholesterolemia and mixed dyslipidemia

Adults: 1 tablet P.O. daily at night.

Liptruzet

GENERIC COMPONENTS

ezetimibe–atorvastatin calcium

Tablets

10 mg ezetimibe and 10 mg atorvastatin calcium

10 mg ezetimibe and 20 mg atorvastatin calcium

10 mg ezetimibe and 40 mg atorvastatin calcium

10 mg ezetimibe and 80 mg atorvastatin calcium

DOSAGES

Homozygous familial hypercholesterolemia

Adults: 10 mg ezetimibe with 40 or 80 mg atorvastatin P.O. once daily.

Primary hyperlipidemia

Adults: 10 mg ezetimibe with 10 or 20 mg atorvastatin P.O. once daily. For patients who require a larger reduction in LDL-C (more than 55%), start with 10 mg ezetimibe and 40 mg atorvastatin. After starting drug or titrating dosage, assess lipid levels within 2 or more weeks and adjust dosage accordingly. Usual dosage is 10 mg ezetimibe/10 mg atorvastatin to 10 mg ezetimibe/80 mg atorvastatin once daily.

Simcor

GENERIC COMPONENTS

niacin–simvastatin

Tablets

500 mg niacin extended-release and 20 mg simvastatin

500 mg niacin extended-release and 40 mg simvastatin

750 mg niacin extended-release and 20 mg simvastatin
1,000 mg niacin extended-release and 20 mg simvastatin
1,000 mg niacin extended-release and 40 mg simvastatin
DOSAGES
Treatment of primary hypercholesterolemia and mixed dyslipidemia or hypertriglyceridemia
Adults: For patients naive or switching from immediate-release niacin, 500 mg extended-release niacin and 20 mg simvastatin P.O. daily. Initial dose for patients already receiving extended-release niacin shouldn't exceed 2,000 mg extended-release niacin and 40 mg simvastatin. Maintenance dose ranges from 1,000 mg extended-release niacin and 20 mg simvastatin to 2,000 mg extended-release niacin and 40 mg simvastatin. Give drug at bedtime with low-fat snack.

Vytorin ℘

GENERIC COMPONENTS
ezetimibe–simvastatin
Tablets
10 mg ezetimibe with 10, 20, 40, or 80 mg simvastatin
DOSAGES
Homozygous familial hypercholesterolemia and primary hyperlipidemia
Adults: 1 tablet P.O. daily, taken in the evening in combination with a cholesterol-lowering diet and exercise. Dosage of simvastatin in the combination may be adjusted based on patient response. If given with a bile acid sequestrant, must be given at least 2 hours before or 4 hours after the bile acid sequestrant.
Children age 10 and older: 10 mg ezetimibe with 10 or 20 mg simvastatin once daily.

Menopause drugs

Activella
Femhrt

GENERIC COMPONENTS
ethinyl estradiol–norethindrone acetate
Tablets
2.5 mcg ethinyl estradiol and 0.5 mg norethindrone acetate (Femhrt)
5 mcg ethinyl estradiol and 1 mg norethindrone acetate (Femhrt)
0.5 mg ethinyl estradiol and 0.1 mg norethindrone acetate (Activella)

1 mg ethinyl estradiol and 0.5 mg norethindrone acetate (Activella)
DOSAGES
Signs and symptoms of menopause; to prevent osteoporosis
Women with intact uterus: 1 tablet P.O. daily.

Prefest

GENERIC COMPONENTS
estradiol
estradiol–norgestimate
Tablets
1 mg estradiol; 1 mg estradiol and 0.09 mg norgestimate
DOSAGES
Moderate to severe symptoms of menopause; to prevent osteoporosis
Women with intact uterus: 1 tablet P.O. per day (3 days of peach tablets: estradiol alone; followed by 3 days of white tablets: estradiol and norgestimate combination; continue cycle uninterrupted).

Premphase

GENERIC COMPONENTS
conjugated estrogens
conjugated estrogens–medroxyprogesterone
Tablets
0.625 mg conjugated estrogens; 0.625 mg conjugated estrogens and 5 mg medroxyprogesterone
DOSAGES
Moderate to severe symptoms of menopause; to prevent osteoporosis
Women with intact uterus: 1 tablet P.O. per day. Use estrogen alone on days 1 to 14 and estrogen–medroxyprogesterone tablet on days 15 to 28.

Prempro

GENERIC COMPONENTS
conjugated estrogens–medroxyprogesterone
Tablets
0.3 mg conjugated estrogens and 1.5 mg medroxyprogesterone
0.45 mg conjugated estrogens and 1.5 mg medroxyprogesterone
0.625 mg conjugated estrogens and 2.5 mg medroxyprogesterone
0.625 mg conjugated estrogens and 5 mg medroxyprogesterone

DOSAGES
Symptoms of menopause; to prevent osteoporosis
Women with intact uterus: 1 tablet P.O. per day.

Miscellaneous cardiac drugs

Caduet

GENERIC COMPONENTS
amlodipine–atorvastatin
Tablets
2.5 mg amlodipine with 10 mg, 20 mg, or 40 mg atorvastatin
5 mg amlodipine with 10 mg, 20 mg, 40 mg, or 80 mg atorvastatin
10 mg amlodipine with 10 mg, 20 mg, 40 mg, or 80 mg atorvastatin
DOSAGES
Treatment of hypertension, chronic stable angina, or suspected vasospastic angina in patients with primary hypercholesterolemia and mixed dyslipidemia or hypertriglyceridemia
Adults, boys, and postmenarchal girls age 10 and older: Determine the most effective dose for each component. Then select the most appropriate combination product.

Opioid agonists

Suboxone
Zubsolv

Controlled Substance Schedule III
GENERIC COMPONENTS
buprenorphine–naloxone
Sublingual tablets (Suboxone)
2 mg buprenorphine and 0.5 mg naloxone
8 mg buprenorphine and 2 mg naloxone
Sublingual tablets (Zubsolv)
1.4 mg buprenorphine and 0.36 mg naloxone
5.7 mg buprenorphine and 1.4 mg naloxone
Sublingual film
2 mg buprenorphine and 0.5 mg naloxone
4 mg buprenorphine and 1 mg naloxone
8 mg buprenorphine and 2 mg naloxone
12 mg buprenorphine and 3 mg naloxone
DOSAGES
Opioid dependence
Adults: Maintenance dose is based on buprenorphine. Give 12 to 16 mg (buprenorphine) S.L. tablet once daily, after induction with S.L. buprenorphine (one Zubsolv 5.7-mg buprenorphine/1.4-mg naloxone sublingual

tablet is equivalent to one 8-mg buprenorphine/2-mg naloxone tablet). Or, buprenorphine 4 to 24 mg with naloxone 1 to 6 mg S.L. film as a single daily maintenance dose after buprenorphine induction.

Psychotherapeutics

Limbitrol
Limbitrol DS

Controlled Substance Schedule IV
GENERIC COMPONENTS
chlordiazepoxide–amitriptyline
Tablets
5 mg chlordiazepoxide and 12.5 mg amitriptyline
10 mg chlordiazepoxide and 25 mg amitriptyline
DOSAGES
Severe depression
Adults: 10 mg chlordiazepoxide with 25 mg amitriptyline P.O. t.i.d. to q.i.d. up to six times daily. For patients who don't tolerate the higher doses, 5 mg chlordiazepoxide with 12.5 mg amitriptyline P.O. t.i.d. to q.i.d. Reduce dosage after initial response.

perphenazine and amitriptyline

GENERIC COMPONENTS
perphenazine–amitriptyline
Tablets
2 mg perphenazine and 10 mg amitriptyline
2 mg perphenazine and 25 mg amitriptyline
4 mg perphenazine and 10 mg amitriptyline
4 mg perphenazine and 25 mg amitriptyline
4 mg perphenazine and 50 mg amitriptyline
DOSAGES
Treatment of anxiety, agitation, or depression
Adults: 2 to 4 mg perphenazine with 10 to 50 mg amitriptyline P.O. t.i.d. to q.i.d. Reduce dosage after initial response.

Symbyax

GENERIC COMPONENTS
olanzapine–fluoxetine
Capsules
3 mg olanzapine and 25 mg fluoxetine
6 mg olanzapine and 25 mg fluoxetine
6 mg olanzapine and 50 mg fluoxetine
12 mg olanzapine and 25 mg fluoxetine
12 mg olanzapine and 50 mg fluoxetine

DOSAGES
Treatment of bipolar I disorder or depression
Adults: 1 capsule P.O. daily in the evening. Begin with 6 mg/25 mg capsule and adjust according to efficacy and tolerability.

Respiratory tract drugs

Claritin-D ◊
Claritin-D 24 Hour ◊

GENERIC COMPONENTS
loratadine–pseudoephedrine
Extended-release tablets
5 mg loratadine and 120 mg pseudoephedrine
10 mg loratadine and 240 mg pseudoephedrine
DOSAGES
Seasonal allergic rhinitis
Adults and children age 12 and older:
1 tablet P.O. every day.

Combivent

GENERIC COMPONENTS
ipratropium bromide–albuterol
Metered-dose inhaler
18 mcg ipratropium bromide and 90 mcg albuterol
DOSAGES
Bronchospasm with COPD in patients who require more than a single bronchodilator
Adults: Two inhalations q.i.d. Not for use during acute attack. Use caution with known sensitivity to atropine, soy, or peanuts.

Dulera

GENERIC COMPONENTS
mometasone furoate–formoterol fumarate dihydrate
Oral inhalation
100 mcg mometasone furoate and 5 mcg formoterol fumarate dihydrate
200 mcg mometasone furoate and 5 mcg formoterol fumarate dihydrate
DOSAGES
Asthma
Adults and children over age 12: 2 inhalations b.i.d. Starting dose based on prior asthma therapy.

Symbicort

GENERIC COMPONENTS
budesonide–formoterol fumarate dihydrate

Aerosol inhalation
80 mcg budesonide and 4.5 mcg formoterol fumarate dihydrate per actuation
160 mcg budesonide and 4.5 mcg formoterol fumarate dihydrate per actuation
DOSAGES
Asthma, COPD
Adults and children age 12 and older: 2 inhalations b.i.d.

Tussionex Pennkinetic ER
Controlled Substance Schedule III

GENERIC COMPONENTS
chlorpheniramine–hydrocodone bitartrate
Oral solution
8 mg chlorpheniramine and 10 mg hydrocodone bitartrate/5 mL
DOSAGES
Cough and upper respiratory tract infection signs and symptoms
Adults and children age 12 and older:
5 mL (8 mg chlorpheniramine and 10 mg hydrocodone) P.O. every 12 hours.
Children ages 6 to 12: 2.5 mL (chlorpheniramine 4 mg and hydrocodone 5 mg) P.O. every 12 hours.

Vaccines and toxoids: Indications and dosages

***Haemophilus* b conjugate vaccines**

***Haemophilus* b conjugate vaccine, diphtheria CRM 197 protein conjugate (HbOC)**
HibTITER

***Haemophilus* b conjugate vaccine, meningococcal protein conjugate, hepatitis B**
Comvax

***Haemophilus* b conjugate vaccine, meningococcal protein conjugate (PRP-OMP)**
PedvaxHIB

***Haemophilus* b conjugate, tetanus toxoid conjugate (PRP-T)**
ActHIB, Hiberix

Pharmacologic class: Vaccines
Pregnancy risk category: C

AVAILABLE FORMS
***Haemophilus influenzae* type b (HIB) conjugate vaccine, diphtheria CRM 197 protein conjugate**
Injection: 10 mcg of purified HIB saccharide and about 25 mcg CRM 197 protein per 0.5 mL
HIB conjugate vaccine, hepatitis B
Injection: 7.5 mcg of HIB capsular polysaccharide and 5 mcg hepatitis B surface antigen (HBsAg) per 0.5 mL
HIB conjugate vaccine, meningococcal protein conjugate
Injection: 7.5 mcg of HIB PRP and 125 mcg *N. meningitides* OMPC per 0.5 mL
HIB conjugate vaccine, tetanus toxoid conjugate
Injection: 10 mcg HIB capsular polysaccharide, and 24 mcg tetanus toxoid

INDICATIONS & DOSAGES
➤ **Immunization against HIB infection**
Conjugate vaccine, diphtheria CRM 197 protein conjugate
Infants: 0.5 mL I.M. at age 2 months. Repeat at ages 4 and 6 months. Give booster dose at age 15 months.
Previously unvaccinated children ages 15 months to 6 years: 0.5 mL I.M. Booster dose isn't needed.
Previously unvaccinated infants ages 12 to 14 months: 0.5 mL I.M. Give booster dose at age 15 months (but no sooner than 2 months after first vaccination).
Previously unvaccinated infants ages 7 to 11 months: 0.5 mL I.M. Repeat in 2 months, for a total of two doses. Give booster dose at age 15 months (but no sooner than 2 months after last vaccination).
Previously unvaccinated infants ages 2 to 6 months: 0.5 mL I.M. Repeat in 2 months and again in 4 months for total of three doses. Give booster at age 15 months.
Conjugate vaccine, hepatitis B
Infants born to HBsAg-negative mothers: 0.5 mL I.M. at ages 2, 4, and 12 to 15 months for a total of three doses. Infants who received a dose of hepatitis B vaccine at or shortly after birth can still receive the full three-dose series of Comvax.
Conjugate vaccine, meningococcal protein conjugate
Infants: 0.5 mL I.M. at age 2 months; repeat at age 4 months. Give booster dose at age 12 months.
Previously unvaccinated children ages 15 months to 6 years: 0.5 mL I.M. Booster dose isn't needed.
    Premature infants follow same schedule as full-term infants.
Previously unvaccinated infants ages 12 to 14 months: 0.5 mL I.M. Give booster dose at age 15 months (but no sooner than 2 months after first vaccination).
Previously unvaccinated infants ages 7 to 11 months: 0.5 mL I.M.; repeat in 2 months. Give booster dose at age 15 months (but no sooner than 2 months after last vaccination).

Previously unvaccinated infants ages 2 to 6 months: 0.5 mL I.M.; repeat in 2 months. Give booster dose at age 12 months.
Conjugate vaccine, tetanus toxoid conjugate
Infants: 0.5 mL I.M. at age 2 months. Repeat at ages 4 and 6 months. Give booster doses at ages 15 to 18 months.
Previously unvaccinated infants ages 7 to 11 months: 0.5 mL I.M. Repeat in 2 months, for a total of two doses. Give booster doses at ages 15 to 18 months.
Previously unvaccinated infants ages 12 to 14 months: 0.5 mL I.M. Repeat in 2 months, for a total of two doses.

diphtheria and tetanus toxoids and acellular pertussis vaccine adsorbed (DTaP)
Daptacel, Infanrix, TRIPACEL†

tetanus toxoid and reduced diphtheria toxoid and acellular pertussis vaccine adsorbed (Tdap)
ADACEL, Boostrix

Pharmacologic class: Vaccines/toxoids
Pregnancy risk category: C

AVAILABLE FORMS
DTaP
Daptacel
Injection: 15 limit flocculation (Lf) units diphtheria toxoid, 5 Lf units tetanus toxoid, and 10 mcg pertussis toxoid adsorbed per 0.5 mL
Infanrix
Injection: 25 Lf units diphtheria toxoid, 10 Lf units tetanus toxoid, and 25 mcg inactivated pertussis toxins adsorbed per 0.5 mL
Tripedia
Injection: 7 Lf units diphtheria toxoid, 5 Lf units tetanus toxoid, and 47 mcg inactivated pertussis toxins adsorbed per 0.5 mL
Tdap
Adacel
Injection: 5 Lf units tetanus toxoid, 2 Lf units diphtheria toxoid, and 2.5 mcg detoxified pertussis toxins adsorbed per 0.5 mL

Boostrix
Injection: 5 Lf units tetanus toxoid, 2.5 Lf units diphtheria toxoid, and 8 mcg inactivated pertussis toxins adsorbed per 0.5 mL

INDICATIONS & DOSAGES
➤ **Primary immunization (Daptacel, Infanrix)**
Children ages 6 weeks to 7 years: 0.5 mL I.M. 4 to 8 weeks apart for three doses (6 to 8 weeks for Daptacel) and a fourth dose at least 6 months after the third dose.
➤ **Booster immunization**
Children ages 6 weeks to 7 years: Daptacel may be given to complete the immunization series in children who have received at least one dose of whole-cell DTP vaccine.

Infanrix is indicated as a fifth dose in children ages 4 to 6 before entering school in those who received at least one dose of whole-cell DTP vaccine, unless the fourth dose was given after the fourth birthday.

If Tripedia was used for the first four doses, a fifth dose is recommended at age 4 to 6 before entering school. If the fourth dose was given after age 4, a fifth dose isn't needed.
Adults and children ages 11 to 64 (ADACEL): 0.5 mL I.M. as a single dose at least 5 years after the last DTaP vaccination.
Children and adolescents ages 10 to 18 (Boostrix): 0.5 mL I.M. as a single dose at least 5 years after the last DTaP vaccination.

diphtheria and tetanus toxoids, acellular pertussis adsorbed, hepatitis B (recombinant), and inactivated poliovirus vaccine combined
Pediarix, Pediatrix†

Pharmacologic class: Vaccines/toxoids
Pregnancy risk category: C

AVAILABLE FORMS
Injection: 0.5-mL single-dose vials and disposable, prefilled Tip-Lok syringes

INDICATIONS & DOSAGES
➤ **Active immunization**
Children ages 6 weeks to 7 years: Primary series is three 0.5-mL doses I.M. at 6- to 8-week intervals (preferably 8), usually starting at age 2 months; may start at age 6 weeks.

diphtheria and tetanus toxoids, acellular pertussis adsorbed, and inactivated poliovirus combination vaccine (DTap/IPV)
Kinrix

Pharmacologic class: Vaccines/toxoids
Pregnancy risk category: C

AVAILABLE FORMS
Injection: 25 limit flocculation (Lf) units diphtheria toxoid, 10 Lf tetanus toxoid, 25 mcg inactivated pertussis toxin (PT), 25 mcg filamentous hemagglutinin, 8 mcg pertactin, 40 D-antigen units type 1 poliovirus (Mahoney), 8 D-antigen units type 2 poliovirus (MEF-1), and 32 D-antigen units/0.5 mL type 3 poliovirus (Saukett)

INDICATIONS & DOSAGES
➤ **Active immunization against diphtheria, tetanus, pertussis, and poliomyelitis as the fifth dose in the DTaP vaccine series and the fourth dose in the IPV series in those whose previous DTaP vaccine doses have been with Infanrix (diphtheria and tetanus toxoids and acellular pertussis vaccine adsorbed) or Pediarix (diphtheria and tetanus toxoids, acellular pertussis adsorbed, hepatitis B [recombinant], and IPV vaccine combined) for first three doses and Infanrix for fourth dose**
Children ages 4 through 6: 0.5 mL I.M., preferably in the deltoid muscle of the upper arm.

diphtheria and tetanus toxoids, acellular pertussis adsorbed, inactivated poliovirus, and *Haemophilus influenzae* type b conjugate vaccine combined
Pentacel

Pharmacologic class: Vaccines/toxoids
Pregnancy risk category: C

AVAILABLE FORMS
Injection: 15 limit flocculation (Lf) diphtheria toxoid, 5 Lf tetanus toxoid, 20 mcg pertussis toxin detoxified, 20 mcg filamentous hemagglutinin, 3 mcg pertactin, 5 mcg fimbriae types 2 and 3, 40 D-antigen units type 1 inactivated poliovirus (Mahoney), 8 D-antigen units type 2 inactivated poliovirus (MEF-1), 32 D-antigen units type 3 inactivated poliovirus (Saukett), and 10 mcg lyophilized polyribosyl-ribitol-phosphate of *H. influenzae* type b bound to tetanus toxoid 24 mcg/0.5 mL

INDICATIONS & DOSAGES
➤ **Active immunization against diphtheria, tetanus, pertussis, poliomyelitis, and invasive disease caused by *H. influenzae* type b**
Children ages 6 weeks to 4 years (prior to 5th birthday): 0.5 mL I.M. Approved for administration as a four-dose series at ages 2, 4, 6, and 15 through 18 months. The first dose may be given as early as age 6 weeks.

hepatitis A vaccine, inactivated
Havrix, Vaqta

Pharmacologic class: Vaccines
Pregnancy risk category: C

AVAILABLE FORMS
Havrix
Injection: 720 enzyme-linked immunosorbent assay (ELISA) units (ELU)/0.5 mL; 1,440 ELU/mL

Vaqta
Injection: 25 units/0.5 mL, 50 units/mL

INDICATIONS & DOSAGES
➤ **Active immunization against hepatitis A virus; with immune globulin, to prevent hepatitis A in those exposed to virus or who travel to endemic areas**
Adults: 1,440 ELU Havrix or 50 units Vaqta I.M. as single dose. For booster dose, give 1,440 ELU Havrix 6 to 12 months after first dose or 50 units Vaqta I.M. 6 to 18 months after first dose. Booster is recommended for prolonged immunity.
Children ages 12 months to 18 years: 720 ELU Havrix or 25 units Vaqta I.M. as single dose. Then, give booster dose of 720 ELU Havrix 6 to 12 months after first dose or 25 units Vaqta I.M. 6 to 18 months after first dose. Booster is recommended for prolonged immunity.

---

hepatitis B vaccine, recombinant
Engerix-B, Recombivax HB, Recombivax HB Dialysis Formulation

Pharmacologic class: Vaccines
Pregnancy risk category: C

AVAILABLE FORMS
Injection: 5 mcg hepatitis B surface antigen (HBsAg)/0.5 mL (Recombivax HB, pediatric and adolescent form with or without preservative); 10 mcg HBsAg/0.5 mL (Engerix-B, pediatric and adolescent form); 10 mcg HBsAg/mL (Recombivax HB, adult form); 20 mcg HBsAg/mL (Engerix-B, adult form); 40 mcg HBsAg/mL (Recombivax HB Dialysis Formulation)

INDICATIONS & DOSAGES
➤ **Immunization against infection from all known subtypes of hepatitis B virus (HBV), primary preexposure prophylaxis against HBV, postexposure prophylaxis when given with hepatitis B immune globulin (HBIG)**
Engerix-B
Adults age 20 and older: Initially, 20 mcg I.M.; then second dose of 20 mcg I.M. after 30 days. A third dose of 20 mcg I.M. is given 6 months after the first dose.
Adjust-a-dose: For adults undergoing dialysis or receiving immunosuppressants, initially, 40 mcg I.M. (divided into two 20-mcg doses and given at different sites). Then second dose of 40 mcg I.M. in 30 days, a third dose after 2 months, and final dose of 40 mcg I.M. 6 months after first dose.
Adolescents ages 11 to 19: Initially, 10 mcg (pediatric and adolescent form) I.M.; then second dose of 10 mcg I.M. 30 days later. Give third dose of 10 mcg I.M. 6 months after first dose. Or, 20 mcg (adult form) I.M.; then second dose of 20 mcg I.M. 30 days later. Give third dose of 20 mcg I.M. 6 months after first dose.
Neonates and children up to age 10: Initially, 10 mcg I.M.; then second dose of 10 mcg I.M. 30 days later. Give third dose of 10 mcg I.M. 6 months after first dose.
Recombivax HB
Adults age 20 and older: Initially, 10 mcg I.M.; then second dose of 10 mcg I.M. after 30 days. Give third dose of 10 mcg I.M. 6 months after first dose.
    For adults undergoing dialysis, initially, 40 mcg I.M. (use dialysis form, which contains 40 mcg/mL); then second dose of 40 mcg I.M. in 30 days, and final dose of 40 mcg I.M. 6 months after first dose. A booster or revaccination may be indicated if anti-HBs titer is below 10 mIU/mL 1 to 2 months after third dose.
Infants, children, and adolescents age 19 or younger: Initially, 5 mcg I.M.; then second dose of 5 mcg I.M. after 30 days. Give third dose of 5 mcg I.M. 6 months after first dose. Or, in adolescents ages 11 to 15, give 10 mcg (1 mL adult form) I.M.; then second dose of 10 mcg 4 to 6 months later.
Infants born of HBsAg-positive mothers or mothers of unknown HbsAg status: Initially, 5 mcg I.M.; then second dose of 5 mcg I.M. after 30 days. Give third dose of 5 mcg I.M. 6 months after first dose.
Infants born of HBsAg-negative mothers: Initially, 5 mcg I.M.; then second dose of 5 mcg I.M. after 30 days. Give third dose of 5 mcg I.M. 6 months after first dose.
Note: If the mother is found to be HbsAg-positive within 7 days of delivery, also give

the infant a dose of HBIG (0.5 mL) in the opposite anterolateral thigh.

➤ **Chronic hepatitis C infection**

Engerix-B

Adults: Initially, 20 mcg I.M.; then second dose of 20 mcg I.M. after 30 days. Give third dose of 20 mcg I.M. 6 months after first dose.

human papillomavirus recombinant vaccine, bivalent
Cervarix

Pharmacologic class: Vaccines
Pregnancy risk category: B

AVAILABLE FORMS
Injection: 0.5 mL single-dose vial

INDICATIONS & DOSAGES
➤ **To prevent cervical cancer, cervical intraepithelial neoplasia (CIN) grade 2 or worse and adenocarcinoma in situ, and CIN grade 1 caused by human papillomavirus types 16 and 18**
Women and girls ages 10 to 25: 0.5 mL I.M. given as three doses according to the following schedule: 0, 1, and 6 months.

human papillomavirus recombinant vaccine, quadrivalent
Gardasil

Pharmacologic class: Virus antigens
Pregnancy risk category: B

AVAILABLE FORMS
Injection: 0.5 mL single-dose vial

INDICATIONS & DOSAGES
➤ **To prevent cervical cancer, genital warts, cervical adenocarcinoma in situ, and cervical, vulval, vaginal, and anal intraepithelial neoplasias caused by human papillomavirus types 6, 11, 16, and 18**
Women and girls ages 9 to 26: Three separate I.M. injections of 0.5 mL each. Give second injection 2 months after first, then give third injection 6 months after the first.

➤ **To prevent genital warts and anal cancer**
Men and boys ages 9 to 26: Three separate I.M. injections of 0.5 mL each. Give second injection 2 months after first, then give third injection 6 months after first.

influenza virus vaccine, live
Afluria, Fluarix, FluLaval, FluLaval Quadrivalent, Fluvirin, Fluzone, Fluzone High-Dose, Fluzone Intradermal, Fluzone Quadrivalent

Pharmacologic class: Vaccines
Pregnancy risk category: B

AVAILABLE FORMS
Injection: 0.25 mL single-dose syringes (FluLaval Quadrivalent, Fluzone Quadrivalent); 0.1 mL single-dose microinjection system (Fluzone Intradermal); 0.5 mL single-dose syringes (Afluria, Fluarix, FluLaval Quadrivalent, Fluvirin, Fluzone, Fluzone High-Dose, Fluzone Quadrivalent); 5 mL multidose vials (Afluria, FluLaval, Fluvirin, Fluzone)

INDICATIONS & DOSAGES
➤ **Active immunization to prevent disease caused by influenza A and B viruses**
Adults ages 18 to 64: 0.5 mL I.M. as a single dose or 0.1 mL intradermally as a single dose (Fluzone Intradermal).
Children age 9 and older: 0.5 mL I.M. as a single dose (Afluria, Fluarix, FluLaval Quadrivalent, Fluvirin, Fluzone, Fluzone Quadrivalent).
Children ages 3 to 8: 0.5 mL I.M. as a single dose (Afluria, Fluarix, FluLaval Quadrivalent, Fluzone, Fluzone Quadrivalent). Repeat at least 1 month later for those receiving influenza vaccine for first time or who were vaccinated for first time last season with only one dose.
Children ages 4 to 8: 0.5 mL I.M. as a single dose (Fluvirin). Repeat at least 1 month later for those receiving influenza vaccine for first time or who were vaccinated for first time last season with only one dose.
Children ages 6 months to 35 months: 0.25 mL I.M. as a single dose (Afluria, Fluzone, Fluzone Quadrivalent). Repeat at least

1 month later for those receiving influenza vaccine for first time or who were vaccinated for first time last season with only one dose.
Elderly patients (age 65 and older):
0.5 mL I.M. as a single dose (Fluzone High-Dose, Fluzone Quadrivalent).

influenza virus vaccine, live, intranasal
FluMist

Pharmacologic class: Vaccines
Pregnancy risk category: B

AVAILABLE FORMS
Intranasal spray: 0.2 mL

INDICATIONS & DOSAGES
➤ **Active immunization to prevent disease caused by influenza A and B viruses**
Adults younger than age 50 and children older than age 9: 0.2-mL intranasal dose (0.1 mL in each nostril) once each season.
Children ages 2 through 8 not previously vaccinated with FluMist: Two intranasal doses of 0.2 mL (0.1 mL in each nostril) at least 1 month apart for the first season.
Children ages 2 through 8 previously vaccinated with FluMist: 0.2-mL intranasal dose (0.1 mL in each nostril) once each season.

Japanese encephalitis virus vaccine
Ixiaro

Pharmacologic class: Vaccines
Pregnancy risk category: B

AVAILABLE FORMS
Injection: 6 mcg/0.5 mL

INDICATIONS & DOSAGES
➤ **To prevent disease caused by Japanese encephalitis virus**
Adults and children age 3 and older: Two doses of 0.5 mL I.M. 28 days apart. Complete immunization at least 1 week before exposure.
Children ages 2 months to younger than 3 years: Two doses of 0.25 mL I.M. 28 days apart.

measles, mumps, and rubella virus vaccine, live
M-M-R II

Pharmacologic class: Vaccines
Pregnancy risk category: C

AVAILABLE FORMS
Injection: Single-dose vial containing at least 1,000 tissue culture infective doses ($TCID_{50}$), 20,000 $TCID_{50}$ of mumps strain, and 1,000 $TCID_{50}$ rubella virus per 0.5-mL dose

INDICATIONS & DOSAGES
➤ **Routine immunization**
Adults: 0.5 mL subcutaneously.
Children age 12 months and older: 0.5 mL subcutaneously. A two-dose schedule is recommended, with first dose given between ages 12 and 15 months (between ages 6 and 12 months in high-risk areas) and second dose given either at ages 4 to 6 or 11 to 12.

measles, mumps, rubella, and varicella (MMRV) virus vaccine, live, attenuated
ProQuad

Pharmacologic class: Vaccines
Pregnancy risk category: C

AVAILABLE FORMS
Injection: Single-dose vial containing at least 3.00 log_{10} measles tissue culture infective doses ($TCID_{50}$), 4.30 log_{10} mumps $TCID_{50}$, 3.00 log_{10} rubella $TCID_{50}$, and at least 3.99 log_{10} varicella plaque-forming units (PFU) per 0.5-mL dose

INDICATIONS & DOSAGES
➤ **Routine immunization**
Children ages 12 months to 12 years: 0.5 mL subcutaneously. At least 1 month should elapse between a dose of a measles-containing vaccine and a dose of MMRV vaccine. If a second dose of a varicella-containing vaccine is required, at least 3 months should elapse between administration of the two doses.

meningococcal (groups A, C, Y, and W-135) polysaccharide diphtheria toxoid conjugate vaccine (MCV4)
Menactra

meningococcal polysaccharide vaccine, groups A, C, Y, and W-135 combined (MPSV4)
Menomune A/C/Y/W-135, Menveo (Men ACWY-CRM)

Pharmacologic class: Vaccines
Pregnancy risk category: C

AVAILABLE FORMS
Injection: 0.5 mL single-dose vials

INDICATIONS & DOSAGES
➤ Active immunization for the prevention of invasive meningococcal disease caused by *Neisseria meningitidis* serogroups A, C, Y, and W-135
Adults and children ages 2 to 55: 0.5 mL MCV4 I.M. as a single dose, preferably in the deltoid muscle.
Children ages 9 to 23 months: 0.5 mL MCV4 I.M. given as a two-dose series 3 months apart.
Adults and children older than age 2: 0.5 mL MPSV4 subcutaneously as a single dose, preferably in the upper-outer triceps area.
Adults and children ages 2 to 55: 0.5 mL Menveo I.M. as single dose, preferably into deltoid muscle. For children ages 2 to 5 at continued high risk for meningococcal disease, a second dose may be given 2 months after the first dose.

meningococcal (groups C and Y) and *Haemophilus* b tetanus toxoid conjugate
Menhibrix

Pharmacologic class: Vaccines
Pregnancy risk category: C

AVAILABLE FORMS
Injection: Single-dose vials containing 5 mcg *Neisseria meningitidis* C capsular polysaccharide, 5 mcg *N. meningitidis* Y capsular polysaccharide, and 2.5 mcg *Haemophilus* b capsular polysaccharide 0.5 mL

INDICATIONS & DOSAGES
➤ To prevent invasive disease caused by *N. meningitidis* serogroups C and Y and *Haemophilus influenzae* type b
Children ages 6 weeks through 18 months: 0.5 mL I.M. at age 2, 4, 6, and 12 through 15 months. May give first dose as early as age 6 weeks. May give fourth dose as late as age 18 months.

palivizumab
Synagis

Pharmacologic class: Monoclonal antibodies
Pregnancy risk category: C

AVAILABLE FORMS
Injection: 50-mg, 100-mg vials

INDICATIONS & DOSAGES
➤ Prevention of serious lower respiratory tract disease caused by respiratory syncytial virus (RSV)
High-risk infants age 24 months and younger: 15 mg/kg I.M. monthly throughout RSV season. Give first dose before commencement of RSV season.

pneumococcal vaccine, polyvalent
Pneumovax 23

13-valent conjugate vaccine
Prevnar 13

Pharmacologic class: Vaccines
Pregnancy risk category: C

AVAILABLE FORMS
Injection: 25 mcg each of 23 polysaccharide isolates/0.5 mL (Pneumovax 23); 2.2 mcg each of *Streptococcus pneumoniae* serotypes 1, 3, 4, 5, 6A, 7F, 9V, 14, 18C, 19A, 19F, and 23F saccharides and 4.4 mcg of serotype 6B saccharides (Prevnar 13)

INDICATIONS & DOSAGES
➤**Pneumococcal immunization**
Adults and children age 2 and older:
0.5 mL Pneumovax I.M. or subcutaneously.
➤**Immunization against *S. pneumoniae* and otitis media (Prevnar 13)**
Infants ages 6 weeks to 15 months: 0.5 mL I.M. for a total of four doses at ages 2, 4, 6, and 12 to 15 months.
Children ages 7 to 11 months, previously unvaccinated: 0.5 mL I.M.; three doses with at least 4 weeks between first and second doses, and 8 weeks between second and third doses.
Children ages 12 to 23 months, previously unvaccinated: Two doses of 0.5 mL I.M at least 2 months apart.
Children ages 24 months to 5 years, previously unvaccinated: 0.5 mL I.M. as a single dose.
Children ages 6 to 17: 0.5 mL I.M. as a single dose. For children previously vaccinated with PCV7, wait at least 8 weeks.
Children who have received one or more doses of Prevnar (7-valent conjugate vaccine): Complete the four-dose immunization series with 13-valent conjugate vaccine.
Children ages 15 months through 5 years who have previously received four doses of Prevnar: 0.5 mL I.M as a single dose.

---

poliovirus vaccine, inactivated (IPV)
IPOL

Pharmacologic class: Vaccines
Pregnancy risk category: C

AVAILABLE FORMS
0.5-mL prefilled syringe: Mixture of three types of poliovirus (types 1, 2, and 3) grown in tissue culture

INDICATIONS & DOSAGES
➤**Poliovirus immunization**
Unvaccinated adults: 0.5 mL subcutaneously or I.M.; give second dose 4 to 8 weeks later. Give third dose 6 to 12 months later.
Children: 0.5 mL subcutaneously or I.M. at ages 2 months and 4 months. Give third dose at ages 6 to 18 months. Give a reinforcing dose of 0.5 mL subcutaneously before entry into school at ages 4 to 6.

---

rabies vaccine, human diploid cell (HDCV)
Imovax Rabies, RabAvert

Pharmacologic class: Vaccines
Pregnancy risk category: C

AVAILABLE FORMS
I.M. injection: 2.5 international units rabies antigen/mL, in single-dose vial with diluent

INDICATIONS & DOSAGES
➤**Postexposure antirabies immunization**
Adults and children: Five 1-mL doses of HDCV I.M. Give first dose as soon as possible after exposure; give additional doses on days 3, 7, 14, and 28 after first dose. If no antibody response occurs after this primary series, booster dose is recommended.
➤**Postexposure antirabies immunization in previously immunized people**
Adults and children: 1 mL I.M. immediately and 1 mL I.M. 3 days later.
➤**Preexposure preventive immunization for persons in high-risk groups**
Adults and children: Three 1-mL injections I.M. Give first dose on day 0 (first day of therapy), second dose on day 7, and third dose on day 21 or 28.

---

rotavirus, live
Rotarix, RotaTeq

Pharmacologic class: Vaccines
Pregnancy risk category: C

AVAILABLE FORMS
Lyophilized powder for oral suspension: Rotavirus human 89-12 strain (G1P[8] type); $\geq 10^6$ cell culture infective dose per 1 mL (after reconstitution)
Oral suspension: Rotavirus outer capsid protein (2.2×10^6 infectious units of G1, 2.8×10^6 infectious units of G2, 2.2×10^6 infectious units of G3, 2×10^6 infectious units of G4, and 2.3×10^6 infectious units of rotavirus attachment protein P1A[8]) per 2 mL

INDICATIONS & DOSAGES
➤ **Prevention of rotavirus gastroenteritis**
RotaTeq
Children ages 6 to 32 weeks: 2 mL P.O.
Give second dose 4 weeks later, followed by
third dose at 10 weeks. Do not give third
dose after the patient reaches age 32 weeks.
Rotarix
Infants ages 6 to 24 weeks: Give first dose of
1 mL P.O. at age 6 weeks. Give another
1-mL dose P.O. after at least 4 weeks. The
two-dose series should be completed by age
24 weeks.

tetanus toxoid, adsorbed

tetanus toxoid, fluid

Pharmacologic class: Vaccines
Pregnancy risk category: C

AVAILABLE FORMS
tetanus toxoid, adsorbed
Injection: 5 limit flocculation (Lf) units inactivated tetanus/0.5-mL dose, in 0.5-mL
syringes and 5-mL vials
tetanus toxoid, fluid
Injection: 4 Lf units inactivated tetanus/
7.5-mL vials

INDICATIONS & DOSAGES
➤ **Primary immunization to prevent
tetanus**
Adults and children age 7 and older:
0.5 mL (adsorbed) I.M. 4 to 8 weeks apart
for two doses; then give third dose 6 to
12 months after second.
➤ **Booster dose to prevent tetanus**
Adults and children age 7 and older:
0.5 mL I.M. at 10-year intervals.
➤ **Postexposure prevention of tetanus**
Adults and children age 7 and older: For a
clean, minor wound, give emergency booster dose if more than 10 years have elapsed
since last dose. For all other wounds, give
booster dose if more than 5 years have
elapsed since last dose.

varicella virus vaccine
Varivax

Pharmacologic class: Vaccines
Pregnancy risk category: C

AVAILABLE FORMS
Injection: Single-dose vial containing
1,350 plaque-forming units of Oka/Merck
varicella virus (live)

INDICATIONS & DOSAGES
➤ **To prevent varicella zoster
(chickenpox) infections**
Adults and children age 13 and older:
0.5 mL subcutaneously; then, second
0.5-mL dose 4 to 8 weeks later.
Children ages 1 to 12: 0.5 mL subcutaneously.

zoster vaccine, live
Zostavax

Pharmacologic class: Vaccines, live
attenuated
Pregnancy risk category: C

AVAILABLE FORMS
Injection: Lyophilized vaccine of 19,400
plaque-forming units/0.65 mL

INDICATIONS & DOSAGES
➤ **Prevention of herpes zoster (shingles)**
Adults age 50 and older: 0.65 mL subcutaneously as a single dose, preferably in the
upper arm.

Vitamins and minerals: Indications and dosages

vitamin A (retinol)
Aquasol A, Palmitate-A ◇

Pregnancy risk category: A if dose is under 800 mcg retinol equivalents; C if dose exceeds 800 mcg retinol equivalents; X for Aquasol A

AVAILABLE FORMS
Capsules: 10,000 international units ◇, 15,000 international units ◇, 25,000 international units
Injection: 2-mL vials (50,000 international units/mL with 0.5% chlorobutanol, polysorbate 80, butylated hydroxyanisole, butylated hydroxytoluene)
Tablets: 5,000 international units ◇

INDICATIONS & DOSAGES
➤ **RDA**
Men and boys older than age 14: 900 mcg retinol equivalent (RE) or 3,000 international units.
Women and girls older than age 14: 700 mcg RE or 2,330 international units.
Children ages 9 to 13: 600 mcg RE or 2,000 international units.
Children ages 4 to 8: 400 mcg RE or 1,330 international units.
Children ages 1 to 3: 300 mcg RE or 1,000 international units.
Infants ages 7 to 12 months: 500 mcg RE or 1,665 international units.
Neonates and infants younger than age 6 months: 400 mcg RE or 1,330 international units.
Pregnant women ages 14 to 18: 750 mcg RE or 2,500 international units.
Pregnant women ages 19 to 50: 770 mcg RE or 2,564 international units.
Breast-feeding women ages 14 to 18: 1,200 mcg RE or 4,000 international units.
Breast-feeding women ages 19 to 50: 1,300 mcg RE or 4,330 international units.
➤ **Severe vitamin A deficiency**
Adults and children older than age 8: 100,000 international units I.M. or 100,000 to 500,000 international units P.O. for 3 days; then 50,000 international units P.O.

or I.M. daily for 2 weeks, followed by 10,000 to 20,000 international units P.O. for 2 months. Follow with adequate dietary nutrition and RE vitamin A supplements.
Children ages 1 to 8: 17,500 to 35,000 international units I.M. daily for 10 days.
Infants: 7,500 to 15,000 international units I.M. daily for 10 days.
➤ **Maintenance dose to prevent recurrence of vitamin A deficiency**
Adults and children older than age 8: 10,000 to 20,000 international units P.O. daily for 2 months.
Children ages 1 to 8: Give 5,000 to 10,000 international units P.O. daily for 2 months; then adequate dietary nutrition and RE vitamin A supplements.

vitamin B complex
cyanocobalamin (vitamin B$_{12}$)
Crysti 1000, Cyanocobalamin, Cyanoject, Cyomin, Nascobal, Rapid B-12 Energy ◇, Twelve Resin-K

hydroxocobalamin (vitamin B$_{12}$)
Hydro-Crysti-12, LA-12

Pregnancy risk category: A; C if dose exceeds RDA

AVAILABLE FORMS
cyanocobalamin
Injection: 100 mcg/mL, 1,000 mcg/mL
Intranasal spray: 500 mcg/spray
Lozenges: 50 mcg ◇, 100 mcg ◇, 250 mcg ◇, 500 mcg ◇
Tablets ◇: 25 mcg ◇, 50 mcg ◇, 100 mcg ◇, 250 mcg ◇, 500 mcg ◇, 1,000 mcg ◇, 5,000 mcg ◇
hydroxocobalamin
Injection: 1,000 mcg/mL; 2.5 g/vial

INDICATIONS & DOSAGES
➤ **RDA for cyanocobalamin**
Adults and children age 14 and older: 2.4 mcg.
Children ages 9 to 13: 1.8 mcg.

Children ages 4 to 8: 1.2 mcg.
Children ages 1 to 3: 0.9 mcg.
Infants ages 6 months to 1 year: 0.5 mcg.
*Neonates and infants younger than age
6 months:* 0.4 mcg.
Pregnant women: 2.6 mcg.
Breast-feeding women: 2.8 mcg.
➤ **Vitamin B₁₂ deficiency from inadequate diet, subtotal gastrectomy, or other condition, disorder, or disease, except malabsorption, related to pernicious anemia or other GI disease**
Adults: 30 mcg hydroxocobalamin I.M. daily for 5 to 10 days, depending on severity of deficiency. Maintenance dose is 100 to 200 mcg I.M. once monthly or 500 mcg gel intranasally once weekly. For subsequent prophylaxis, advise adequate nutrition and daily RDA vitamin B₁₂ supplements.
Children: 1 to 5 mg hydroxocobalamin in single doses of 100 mcg I.M. over 2 or more weeks, depending on severity of deficiency. Maintenance dose is 30 to 50 mcg I.M. every 4 weeks. For subsequent prophylaxis, advise adequate nutrition and daily RDA vitamin B₁₂ supplements.
➤ **Pernicious anemia or vitamin B₁₂ malabsorption**
Adults: Initially, 100 mcg cyanocobalamin I.M. or subcutaneously daily for 6 to 7 days. If response is observed, 100 mcg I.M. or subcutaneously every other day for 7 doses, then 100 mcg every 3 to 4 days for 2 to 3 weeks; then 100 mcg I.M. or subcutaneously once monthly.
➤ **Maintenance therapy for remission of pernicious anemia after I.M. vitamin B₁₂ therapy in patients without nervous system involvement; dietary deficiency, malabsorption disorders, and inadequate secretion of intrinsic factor**
Adults: Initially, 1 spray in one nostril once weekly (Nascobal). Give at least 1 hour before or after hot foods or liquids. Or 1 spray in each nostril daily. May increase to 1 spray in each nostril b.i.d. (total daily dose of 100 mcg) as needed.
➤ **Schilling test flushing dose**
Adults and children: 1,000 mcg hydroxocobalamin I.M. as single dose.
➤ **Cyanide poisoning**
Adults: Initially, 5 g hydroxocobalamin I.V. over 15 minutes. Based on patient's condition, may repeat 5 g dose I.V. over 15 minutes to 2 hours.

Coenzyme Q10
Chew Q, CoQ10, HzQ, LiQsorb,
ProNutrients CoQ10, Q-Gel, Q-Sorb,
Quin-Zyme, Vitaline CoQ10, YL
Coenzyme Q10

Pregnancy risk category: Undetermined

AVAILABLE FORMS
Capsules: 10 mg, 30 mg, 50 mg, 60 mg,
75 mg, 100 mg, 120 mg, 150 mg, 200 mg,
300 mg, 400 mg
Capsules (extended-release): 100 mg
Oral liquid: 30 mg/5 mL, 100 mg/mL,
500 mg/5 mL
Powder: 50 g
Tablets: 25 mg, 50 mg, 60 mg, 100 mg, 200 mg
Tablets (chewable): 30 mg, 50 mg, 60 mg,
100 mg, 600 mg
Tablets (dispersible): 50 mg, 90 mg
Wafers: 60 mg, 100 mg, 300 mg

INDICATIONS & DOSAGES
➤ **Dietary supplement for conditions associated with coenzyme Q10 deficiency**
Adults: 10 to 300 mg/day P.O. in one or divided doses. Higher doses (up to 3,000 mg/day) have been used.

folic acid (vitamin B₉)
Folvite

Pregnancy risk category: A

AVAILABLE FORMS
Injection: 10-mL vials (5 mg/mL with 1.5% benzyl alcohol, 5 mg/mL with 1.5% benzyl alcohol and 0.2% ethylenediaminetetraacetic acid)
Tablets: 0.4 mg◊, 0.8 mg◊, 1 mg

INDICATIONS & DOSAGES
➤ **RDA**
Adults and children age 14 and older: 400 mcg.
Children ages 9 to 13: 300 mcg.
Children ages 4 to 8: 200 mcg.
Children ages 1 to 3: 150 mcg.
Infants ages 7 months to 1 year: 80 mcg.
*Neonates and infants younger than age
6 months:* 65 mcg.

Pregnant women: 600 mcg.
Breast-feeding women: 500 mcg.
➤ **Megaloblastic or macrocytic anemia from folic acid or other nutritional deficiency, hepatic disease, alcoholism, intestinal obstruction, or excessive hemolysis**
Adults and children age 4 and older: 0.4 to 1 mg P.O., I.M., or subcutaneously daily. After anemia caused by folic acid deficiency is corrected, proper diet and RDA supplements are needed to prevent recurrence.
Children younger than age 4: Up to 0.3 mg P.O., I.M., or subcutaneously daily.
Pregnant and breast-feeding women: 0.8 mg P.O., I.M., or subcutaneously daily.
➤ **To prevent fetal neural tube defects during pregnancy ♦**
Adults: 400 to 800 mcg P.O. daily before conception through at least first 4 to 12 weeks of fetal formation. For women at high risk, recommended dosage is 4 mg daily starting up to 3 months before conception and through first 3 months of pregnancy.
➤ **To prevent megaloblastic anemia during pregnancy to prevent fetal damage**
Adults: Up to 1 mg P.O., I.M., or subcutaneously daily throughout pregnancy.

---

leucovorin calcium (citrovorum factor, folinic acid)
Fusilev

Pregnancy risk category: C

AVAILABLE FORMS
Injection: 1-mL ampule (3 mg/mL with 0.9% benzyl alcohol); 10 mg/mL in 5-mL vial; 50-mg, 100-mg, 350-mg, 500-mg vials for reconstitution (contains no preservatives)
Tablets: 5 mg, 15 mg, 25 mg

INDICATIONS & DOSAGES
➤ **Leucovorin rescue after high-dose methotrexate therapy**
Adults: 15 mg (approximately 10 mg/m^2) P.O., I.M., or I.V. every 6 hours for 10 doses starting 24 hours after start of methotrexate infusion. Continue treatment until methotrexate level is less than 5×10^{-8} M, as follows: If serum methotrexate level is approximately 10 micro-

molar at 24 hours after administration, 1 micromolar at 48 hours, and less than 0.2 micromolar at 72 hours, give 15 mg every 6 hours for 60 hours; if serum methotrexate level remains above 0.2 micromolar at 72 hours and more than 0.05 micromolar at 96 hours, continue 15 mg every 6 hours until methotrexate level is less than 0.05 micromolar; if serum methotrexate level is 50 micromolar or more at 24 hours, or 5 micromolar or more at 48 hours, or if there is a 100% increase in serum creatinine level at 24 hours, give 150 mg I.V. every 3 hours until methotrexate level is less than 1 micromolar; then 15 mg I.V. every 3 hours until methotrexate level is less than 0.5 micromolar.
➤ **Impaired methotrexate elimination or inadvertent overdose**
Adults: 10 mg/m^2 P.O., I.M., or I.V. every 6 hours until serum methotrexate level is less than 10^{-8} M. If 24-hour serum creatinine level increases 50% over baseline or if 24-hour methotrexate level is greater than 5×10^{-6} M or 48-hour level is greater than 9×10^{-7} M, increase dosage to 100 mg/m^2 I.V. every 3 hours until methotrexate level is less than 10^{-8} M.
➤ **Folate-deficient megaloblastic anemia**
Adults and children: Up to 1 mg I.M. daily. Duration of treatment depends on hematologic response.
➤ **Palliative treatment of advanced colorectal cancer**
Adults: 20 mg/m^2 I.V.; then fluorouracil 425 mg/m^2 I.V. or 200 mg/m^2 I.V. (over 3 minutes or longer) followed by fluorouracil 370 mg/m^2 daily for 5 consecutive days. Repeat at 4-week intervals for two additional courses; then at intervals of 4 to 5 weeks, if tolerated.

---

niacin (nicotinic acid, vitamin B$_3$)
Niacor, Niaspan, Slo-Niacin ◊

niacinamide ◊ (nicotinamide ◊)

Pregnancy risk category: A; C if dose exceeds RDA

AVAILABLE FORMS
niacin
Capsules (timed-release): 250 mg ◊ , 500 mg
Tablets: 50 mg ◊ , 100 mg ◊ , 250 mg ◊ , 500 mg

Tablets (extended-release): 250 mg ◇,
400 mg ◇, 500 mg ◇, 750 mg ◇, 1,000 mg ◇
niacinamide
Tablets: 50 mg ◇, 100 mg ◇, 125 mg ◇,
250 mg ◇, 500 mg ◇

INDICATIONS & DOSAGES
➤**RDA**
Adult men and boys ages 14 to 18: 16 mg.
Adult women and girls ages 14 to 18: 14 mg.
Children ages 9 to 13: 12 mg.
Children ages 4 to 8: 8 mg.
Children ages 1 to 3: 6 mg.
Infants ages 7 months to 1 year: 4 mg.
*Neonates and infants younger than age
6 months:* 2 mg.
Pregnant women: 18 mg.
Breast-feeding women: 17 mg.
➤**Pellagra**
Adults: Initially, 500 mg Niaspan P.O. daily
at bedtime. Titrate to patient response and
tolerance. Maximum dose is 2,000 mg daily.
➤**Niacin deficiency**
Adults: Up to 100 mg P.O. daily.
➤**Hyperlipidemias, especially with hy-
percholesterolemia**
Adults: 250 mg Niacor P.O. daily at bedtime.
Increase at 4- to 7-day intervals up to 1.5 to
2 g P.O. daily in two or three divided doses.
Maximum 6 g daily. Or, 1 to 2 g extended-
release tablets P.O. daily at bedtime.

paricalcitol
Zemplar

Pregnancy risk category: C

AVAILABLE FORMS
Capsules: 1 mcg, 2 mcg, 4 mcg
Injection: 2 mcg/mL, 5 mcg/mL

INDICATIONS & DOSAGES
➤**To prevent or treat secondary
hyperparathyroidism in patients with
stage 3 or 4 chronic kidney disease**
Adults: Initial dose is based on baseline intact parathyroid hormone (iPTH) levels. If
iPTH is less than or equal to 500 picograms
(pg)/mL, give 1 mcg P.O. daily or 2 mcg
P.O. three times weekly, no more often than
every other day. If iPTH is greater than 500
pg/mL, give 2 mcg P.O. daily or 4 mcg P.O.

three times weekly, no more often than
every other day. Adjust dose at 2- to 4-week
intervals, based on iPTH levels.
➤**To prevent or treat secondary
hyperparathyroidism in patients with
chronic renal failure**
Adults: 0.04 to 0.1 mcg/kg (2.8 to 7 mcg) I.V.
no more often than every other day during
dialysis. Doses as high as 0.24 mcg/kg
(16.8 mcg) may be safely given. If satisfactory response isn't observed, increase dosage
by 2 to 4 mcg at 2- to 4-week intervals.

pyridoxine hydrochloride
(vitamin B₆)
Aminoxin, Vitelle Nestrex

Pregnancy risk category: A; C if dose
exceeds RDA

AVAILABLE FORMS
Capsules: 250 mg
Injection: 100 mg/mL
Tablets: 25 mg ◇, 50 mg ◇, 100 mg ◇,
200 mg ◇, 250 mg ◇, 500 mg ◇
Tablets (enteric-coated): 200 mg ◇

INDICATIONS & DOSAGES
➤**RDA**
Adults ages 19 to 50: 1.3 mg.
Men age 51 and older: 1.7 mg.
Women age 51 and older: 1.5 mg.
Boys ages 14 to 18: 1.3 mg.
Girls ages 14 to 18: 1.2 mg.
Children ages 9 to 13: 1 mg.
Children ages 4 to 8: 0.6 mg.
Children ages 1 to 3: 0.5 mg.
Infants ages 7 months to 1 year: 0.3 mg.
*Neonates and infants younger than age
6 months:* 0.1 mg.
Pregnant women: 1.9 mg.
Breast-feeding women: 2 mg.
➤**Dietary vitamin B₆ deficiency**
Adults: 100 to 200 mg P.O. daily. Or, 10 to
20 mg I.M. or I.V. daily for several weeks;
then maintenance dose is 2 to 5 mg P.O.
daily for several weeks.
➤**Antidote for isoniazid poisoning**
Adults: 4 g I.V.; then 1 g I.M. every 30 min-
utes until amount of pyridoxine given
equals amount of isoniazid ingested.

sodium fluoride
Fluor-A-Day†, Fluoritab, Flura, Flura-Drops, Flura-Loz, Karidium, Luride, Luride Lozi-Tabs, Luride-SF Lozi-Tabs, Pediaflor, Pedi-Dent†, Pharmaflur, Pharmaflur df, Pharmaflur 1.1, Phos-Flur

sodium fluoride, topical
ACT ◇, Fluorigard ◇, Fluorinse, Gel-Kam, Gel-Tin ◇, Karigel, Karigel-N, Luride, Minute-Gel, MouthKote F/R ◇, Point-Two, Prevident, Stop Gel ◇, Thera-Flur, Thera-Flur-N

Pregnancy risk category: NR

AVAILABLE FORMS
sodium fluoride
Drops: 0.125 mg/drop, 0.25 mg/drop, 0.2 mg/mL, 0.5 mg/mL
Lozenges: 1 mg
Tablets: 1 mg
Tablets (chewable): 0.25 mg, 0.5 mg, 1 mg
sodium fluoride, topical
Gel: 0.1%, 0.5%, 1.2%, 1.23%
Gel drops: 0.5%
Rinse: 0.02% ◇, 0.04% ◇

INDICATIONS & DOSAGES
➤ **To prevent dental caries**
Adults and children older than age 6: 5 to 10 mL of rinse or thin ribbon of gel applied to teeth with toothbrush or mouth trays for at least 1 minute at bedtime.
If fluoride ion level in drinking water is less than 0.3 parts/million (ppm)
Children ages 6 to 16: 1 mg P.O. daily.
Children ages 3 to 5: 0.5 mg P.O. daily.
Infants and children ages 6 months to 2 years: 0.25 mg P.O. daily.
If fluoride ion level in drinking water is 0.3 to 0.6 ppm
Children ages 6 to 16: 0.5 mg P.O. daily.
Children ages 3 to 5: 0.25 mg P.O. daily.

thiamine hydrochloride (vitamin B$_1$)
Betaxin†, Thiamiject†, Thiamilate

Pregnancy risk category: A; C if dose exceeds RDA

AVAILABLE FORMS
Injection: 100 mg/mL
Tablets: 50 mg ◇, 100 mg ◇, 250 mg ◇, 500 mg
Tablets (enteric-coated): 20 mg ◇

INDICATIONS & DOSAGES
➤ **RDA**
Adult men: 1.2 mg.
Adult women: 1.1 mg.
Boys ages 14 to 18: 1.2 mg.
Girls ages 14 to 18: 1.2 mg.
Children ages 9 to 13: 0.9 mg.
Children ages 4 to 8: 0.6 mg.
Children ages 1 to 3: 0.5 mg.
Infants ages 7 months to 1 year: 0.3 mg.
Neonates and infants younger than age 6 months: 0.2 mg.
Pregnant women: 1.4 mg.
Breast-feeding women: 1.4 mg.
➤ **Beriberi**
Adults: Depending on severity, 10 to 20 mg I.M. t.i.d. for 2 weeks; then dietary correction and multivitamin supplement containing 5 to 10 mg thiamine daily for 1 month.
Children: 25 mg I.V. daily.
➤ **Wet beriberi with myocardial failure**
Adults and children: 10 to 20 mg I.V. t.i.d.
➤ **Wernicke encephalopathy**
Adults: Initially, 100 mg I.V.; then 50 to 100 mg I.M. daily until patient is consuming a regular balanced diet.

vitamin C (ascorbic acid)
Ascocid ◇, Ascor L 500, Cecon ◇, Dull-C ◇, Flavorcee ◇, N'ice ◇, Vicks Vitamin C Drops ◇, Vita-C ◇

Pregnancy risk category: A; C if dose exceeds RDA

AVAILABLE FORMS
Capsules: 500 mg ◇
Capsules (timed-release): 500 mg ◇, 1,000 mg ◇
Crystals: 1,000 mg/¼ tsp ◇
Injection: 500 mg/mL
Lozenges: 60 mg ◇
Oral solution: 100 mg/mL ◇
Powder: 60 mg/¼ tsp ◇, 1,060 mg/¼ tsp ◇
Tablets: 250 mg ◇, 500 mg ◇, 1,000 mg ◇, 1,500 mg ◇
Tablets (timed-release): 500 mg ◇, 1,000 mg ◇

---

†Canada   ◇ OTC   ♦ Off-label use

INDICATIONS & DOSAGES
➤ **RDA**
Men age 19 and older: 90 mg.
Women age 19 and older: 75 mg.
Boys ages 14 to 18: 75 mg.
Girls ages 14 to 18: 65 mg.
Children ages 9 to 13: 45 mg.
Children ages 4 to 8: 25 mg.
Children ages 1 to 3: 15 mg.
Infants ages 7 months to 1 year: 50 mg.
Neonates and infants up to age 6 months: 40 mg.
Pregnant women: 80 to 85 mg.
Breast-feeding women: 115 to 120 mg.
➤ **Frank and subclinical scurvy**
Adults: Depending on severity, 100 to 250 mg P.O., I.V., I.M., or subcutaneously daily; then 70 to 150 mg daily for maintenance.
Children: Depending on severity, 100 to 300 mg P.O., I.V., I.M., or subcutaneously daily; then at least 30 mg daily for maintenance.
➤ **Extensive burns, delayed fracture or wound healing, postoperative wound healing, severe febrile or chronic disease states**
Adults: 200 to 500 mg I.V., I.M., or subcutaneously daily for 7 to 10 days; 1 to 2 g daily for extensive burns.
Children: 100 to 200 mg P.O., I.V., I.M, or subcutaneously daily.

---

vitamin D
cholecalciferol (vitamin D_3)
Baby DDrops◊, Delta-D◊, Maximum-D

ergocalciferol (vitamin D_2)
Calciferol, Drisdol

Pregnancy risk category: A; C if dose exceeds RDA

AVAILABLE FORMS
cholecalciferol

Capsules: 250 mcg (10,000 international units)
Tablets: 10 mcg (400 international units), 25 mcg (1,000 international units)
ergocalciferol
Capsules: 1.25 mg (50,000 international units)
Injection: 12.5 mg (500,000 international units)/mL
Oral liquid: 200 mcg (8,000 international units)/mL in 60-mL dropper bottle ◊

INDICATIONS & DOSAGES
➤ **RDA for cholecalciferol or ergocalciferol**
Adults older than age 70: 15 mcg (600 international units).
Adults ages 51 to 70: 10 mcg (400 international units).
Infants, children, and adults up to age 50: 5 mcg (200 international units).
Pregnant or breast-feeding women: 5 mcg (200 international units).
➤ **Rickets and other vitamin D deficiency diseases**
Adults: Initially, 10,000 international units P.O. or I.M. daily; expect to increase, based on response, to maximum of 500,000 international units daily.
Children: 1,500 to 5,000 international units P.O. or I.M. daily for 2 to 4 weeks; repeat after 2 weeks, if needed. Or, give single dose of 600,000 international units. After correction of deficiency, maintenance includes adequate diet and RDA supplements.
➤ **Hypoparathyroidism**
Adults: 625 mcg to 5 mg ergocalciferol P.O. daily with calcium supplement.
Children: 1.25 to 5 mg of ergocalciferol P.O. daily with calcium supplement.
➤ **Familial hypophosphatemia**
Adults: 250 mcg to 1.5 mg P.O. daily of ergocalciferol with phosphate supplement.
Children: 1 to 2 mg P.O. daily of ergocalciferol with phosphate supplement, increased in 250- to 500-mcg increments at 3- to 4-month intervals based on response.

---

vitamin D analogue
doxercalciferol
Hectorol

Pregnancy risk category: B

AVAILABLE FORMS
Capsules: 0.5 mcg, 2.5 mcg
Injection: 2 mcg/mL

INDICATIONS & DOSAGES
➤ **Secondary hyperparathyroidism in dialysis patients with chronic kidney disease**
Adults: Initially, 10 mcg P.O. three times weekly at dialysis. Adjust dosage as needed to lower intact parathyroid hormone (iPTH)

levels to 150 to 300 picograms (pg)/mL. Increase dose by 2.5 mcg at 8-week intervals if iPTH level hasn't decreased by 50% and fails to reach target range. Maximum dose is 20 mcg P.O. three times weekly. If iPTH levels fall below 100 pg/mL, suspend drug for 1 week; then give dose of at least 2.5 mcg less than last dose. Or, 4 mcg I.V. bolus three times a week at the end of dialysis, about every other day. Adjust dose as needed to lower iPTH levels to 150 to 300 pg/mL. Dosage may be increased by 1 to 2 mcg at 8-week intervals if the iPTH level isn't decreased by 50% and fails to reach target range. Maximum dose is 18 mcg weekly. If iPTH levels go below 100 pg/mL, suspend drug for 1 week, then resume at a dose that's at least 1 mcg P.O. lower than the last dose.

➤ **Secondary hyperparathyroidism in predialysis patients with stage 3 or 4 chronic kidney disease**
Adults: 1 mcg P.O. daily. Adjust dosage as needed to lower iPTH levels to 35 to 70 pg/mL for stage 3 or 70 to 110 pg/mL for stage 4. Increase dosage at 2-week intervals by 0.5 mcg if levels are above 70 pg/mL for stage 3 or above 110 pg/mL for stage 4. If level falls below 35 pg/mL for stage 3 or 70 pg/mL for stage 4, suspend treatment for 1 week, then give dose at least 0.5 mcg lower than last dose. Maximum dose, 3.5 mcg daily.

vitamin E (tocopherols)
Aquasol E ◇

Pregnancy risk category: A

AVAILABLE FORMS
Capsules: 100 international units ◇, 200 international units ◇, 400 international units ◇, 600 international units ◇, 1,000 international units ◇
Drops: 50 international units/mL
Tablets: 100 international units ◇, 200 international units ◇, 400 international units ◇, 500 international units ◇, 600 international units ◇, 1,000 international units ◇

INDICATIONS & DOSAGES
Note: RDAs for vitamin E have been converted to α-tocopherol equivalents (α-TE). One α-TE equals 1 mg of D-α tocopherol, or 1.49 international units.

➤ **RDA**
Adults and children ages 14 to 18: 15 mg.
Children ages 9 to 13: 11 mg.
Children ages 4 to 8: 7 mg.
Children ages 1 to 3: 6 mg.
Infants ages 7 months to 1 year: 5 mg.
Neonates and infants younger than age 6 months: 4 mg.
Pregnant women: 15 mg.
Breast-feeding women: 19 mg.

vitamin K analogue phytonadione (vitamin K₁)
Mephyton, Vitamin K₁

Pregnancy risk category: C

AVAILABLE FORMS
Injection (emulsion): 2 mg/mL, 10 mg/mL
Tablets: 5 mg

INDICATIONS & DOSAGES
➤ **RDA**
Men age 19 and older: 120 mcg.
Women age 19 and older, including pregnant and breast-feeding women: 90 mcg.
Children ages 14 to 18: 75 mcg.
Children ages 9 to 13: 60 mcg.
Children ages 4 to 8: 55 mcg.
Children ages 1 to 3: 30 mcg.
Infants ages 7 months to 1 year: 2.5 mcg.
Neonates and infants younger than age 6 months: 2 mcg.

➤ **Hypoprothrombinemia caused by vitamin K malabsorption, drug therapy, or excessive vitamin A dosage**
Adults: Depending on severity, 2.5 to 25 mg P.O., I.M., or subcutaneously, repeated and increased up to 50 mg as needed.

➤ **Hypoprothrombinemia caused by effect of oral anticoagulants**
Adults: 2.5 to 10 mg P.O., I.M., or subcutaneously, based on PT and INR; repeat if needed within 12 to 48 hours after oral dose or within 6 to 8 hours after parenteral dose.

➤ **To prevent hemorrhagic disease of newborn**
Neonates: 0.5 to 1 mg I.M. within 1 hour after birth.

➤ **Hemorrhagic disease of newborn**
Neonates: 1 mg subcutaneously or I.M. Higher doses may be needed if mother has been receiving oral anticoagulants.

Nutritional supplements: Indications and dosages

amino acid infusions (crystalline)
Aminosyn, Aminosyn II, Aminosyn-PF, Clinisol, FreAmine III, Premasol, Travasol, TrophAmine

amino acid infusions (in dextrose)
Clinimix

amino acid infusions (with electrolytes)
Aminosyn, Aminosyn II, FreAmine III, ProcalAmine, Travasol

amino acid infusions (for hepatic failure)
HepatAmine, Hepatasol

amino acid infusions (for high metabolic stress)
Aminosyn-HBC, FreAmine HBC

amino acid infusions (for renal failure)
Aminosyn-RF, NephrAmine, RenAmin

Therapeutic class: Nutritional supplements
Pharmacologic class: Protein substrates
Pregnancy risk category: C

AVAILABLE FORMS
Injection: 250 mL, 500 mL, 1,000 mL, 2,000 mL
amino acid infusions (crystalline)
Aminosyn: 3.5%, 5%, 7%, 8.5%, 10%
Aminosyn II: 7%, 8.5%, 10%, 15%
Aminosyn-PF: 7%, 10%
Clinisol: 15%
FreAmine III: 8.5%, 10%
Premasol: 6%, 10%
Travasol: 10%
TrophAmine: 6%, 10%
amino acid infusions (in dextrose)
Clinimix: 2.75% in 5% dextrose, 2.75% in 10% dextrose, 2.75% in 25% dextrose, 4.25% in 5% dextrose, 4.25% in 10% dextrose, 4.25% in 20% dextrose, 4.25% in 25% dextrose, 5% in 10% dextrose, 5% in 15% dextrose, 5% in 20% dextrose, 5% in 25% dextrose, 5% in 35% dextrose
amino acid infusions (with electrolytes)
Aminosyn: 3.5%, 7%, 8.5%
Aminosyn II: 8.5%, 10%
FreAmine III: 3%, 8.5%
ProcalAmine: 3%
Travasol: 3.5%, 5.5%, 8.5%
amino acid infusions (for hepatic failure)
HepatAmine: 8%
Hepatasol: 8%
amino acid infusions (for high metabolic stress)
Aminosyn-HBC: 7%
FreAmine HBC: 6.9%
amino acid infusions (for renal failure)
Aminosyn-RF: 5.2%
NephrAmine: 5.4%
RenAmin: 6.5%

INDICATIONS & DOSAGES
➤ **Total parenteral nutrition (TPN) in patients who can't or won't eat**
Adults: 1 to 1.5 g/kg I.V. daily.
Children weighing more than 10 kg (22 lb): 20 to 25 g I.V. daily for first 10 kg; then 1 to 1.25 g/kg I.V. daily for each kilogram over 10 kg.
Children weighing less than 10 kg: 2 to 4 g/kg I.V. daily.
➤ **Nutritional support for cirrhosis, hepatitis, or hepatic encephalopathy**
Adults: 80 to 120 g of amino acids (12 to 18 g of nitrogen) I.V. daily of formulation for hepatic failure.
➤ **Nutritional support for high metabolic stress**
Adults: 1.5 g/kg I.V. daily of formulation for high metabolic stress.
➤ **Nutritional support for renal failure**
Adults: 300 to 600 mL Aminosyn-RF added to 70% dextrose I.V. daily. 250 to 500 mL NephrAmine added to 70% dextrose I.V. daily. 250 to 500 mL RenAmin I.V. daily.
Children: 0.5 to 1 g/kg/day. Individualize dosage. Maximum recommended dose is 1 g/kg/day.

dextrose (d-glucose)
DEKS-trohse

Therapeutic class: Nutritional supplements
Pharmacologic class: Carbohydrate caloric agents
Pregnancy risk category: C

AVAILABLE FORMS
Injection: 3-mL ampule (10%); 10 mL (25%); 25 mL (5%); 50 mL (5% and 50% available in vial, ampule, and Bristoject); 70-mL pin-top vial (70% for additive use only); 100 mL (5%); 150 mL (5%); 250 mL (5%, 10%); 500 mL (5%, 10%, 20%, 30%, 40%, 50%, 60%, 70%); 650 mL (38.5%); 1,000 mL (2.5%, 5%, 10%, 20%, 30%, 40%, 50%, 60%, 70%); 2,000 mL (50%, 70%)

INDICATIONS & DOSAGES
➤ **Fluid replacement and caloric supplementation in patients who can't maintain adequate oral intake or are restricted from doing so**
Adults and children: Dosage depends on fluid and caloric requirements. Use peripheral I.V. infusion of 2.5%, 5%, or 10% solution or central I.V. infusion of 20% solution for minimal fluid needs. Use a 10% to 25% solution to treat acute hypoglycemia in neonate or older infant (2 mL/kg). Use a 50% solution to treat insulin-induced hypoglycemia (20 to 50 mL). Solutions of 10%, 20%, 30%, 40%, 50%, 60%, and 70% are diluted in admixtures, usually amino acid solutions, for total parenteral nutrition given through a central vein.

fat emulsions
Intralipid 10%, Intralipid 20%, Intralipid 30%, Liposyn II 10%, Liposyn II 20%, Liposyn III 10%, Liposyn III 20%, Liposyn III 30%

Therapeutic class: Nutritional supplements
Pharmacologic class: Lipids
Pregnancy risk category: C

AVAILABLE FORMS
Injection: 50 mL (20%), 100 mL (10%, 20%), 200 mL (10%, 20%), 250 mL (10%, 20%), 500 mL (10%, 20%, 30%)

INDICATIONS & DOSAGES
Black Box Warning Deaths have occurred in preterm infants after infusion of I.V. fat emulsions. Adhere strictly to the recommended total daily dose. Hourly I.V. infusion rate should not exceed 1 g/kg in 4 hours. Monitor infant's ability to eliminate the infused fat from the circulation (such as triglyceride or plasma free fatty acid levels). The lipemia must clear between daily infusions. ■
➤ **Adjunct to total parenteral nutrition (TPN) to provide adequate source of calories**
Adults: 1 mL/minute I.V. for 15 to 30 minutes (10% emulsion) or 0.5 mL/minute I.V. for 15 to 30 minutes (20% emulsion). If no adverse reactions occur, increase rate to deliver 250 mL (Liposyn II 20%) or 500 mL (10% Liposyn; Intralipid 10% or Intralipid 20%) over the first day; don't give more than 2.5 g/kg (10%) or 3 g/kg (20%) daily. For 30% Liposyn III, initial infusion rate is the equivalent of 0.1 g fat/minute for the first 15 to 30 minutes. If no adverse reactions occur, increase infusion rate to equivalent of 0.2 g fat/minute. The admixture shouldn't contain more than 330 mL of Liposyn III 30% on first day of therapy. If patient has no adverse reactions, increase dose the next day. Daily dosage shouldn't exceed 2.5 g of fat/kg of body weight.
Children: 0.1 mL/minute for 10 to 15 minutes (10% emulsion) or 0.05 mL/minute I.V. for 10 to 15 minutes (20% emulsion). If no adverse reactions occur, increase rate to deliver 1 g/kg over 4 hours; don't give more than 3 g/kg daily. For 30% emulsion, initial infusion rate is no more than 0.01 g fat/minute for the first 10 to 15 minutes. If no adverse reactions occur, change rate to permit infusion of 0.1 g fat/kg/hour. Daily dosage shouldn't exceed 3 g of fat/kg of body weight. Fat emulsion supplies 60% of daily caloric intake; protein-carbohydrate TPN should supply remaining 40%.
Premature infants: Begin at 0.5 g fat/kg/24 hours (2.5 mL Intralipid 20%, 1.7 mL Liposyn III 30%) and may be increased in relation to the infant's ability to eliminate

fat. Maximum recommended dosage is 3 g fat/kg/24 hours.

➤**Fatty acid deficiency**
Adults and children: 8% to 10% of total caloric intake I.V.

SAFETY ALERT!

sodium chloride

Slo-Salt

Therapeutic class: Electrolyte replacements
Pharmacologic class: Sodium salts
Pregnancy risk category: C

AVAILABLE FORMS
Injection: 0.45% saline solution 25 mL, 50 mL, 150 mL, 250 mL, 500 mL, 1,000 mL; 0.9% saline solution 25 mL, 30 mL, 50 mL, 100 mL, 150 mL, 250 mL, 500 mL, 1,000 mL; 3% sodium chloride solution 500 mL; 5% sodium chloride solution 500 mL; 14.6% sodium chloride solution 250 mL; 23.4% sodium chloride solution 100 mL
Tablets: 650 mg, 1 g, 2.25 g
Tablets (slow-release): 600 mg

INDICATIONS & DOSAGES
➤**Fluid and electrolyte replacement in hyponatremia**
Adults: Dosage is individualized. Use 3% or 5% solution only with frequent electrolyte level determination and only slow I.V. Don't exceed 100 mL/hour or 400 mL/24 hours. For 0.45% solution, dose according to deficiencies, over 18 to 24 hours. For 0.9% solution, dose according to deficiencies, over 18 to 24 hours.
➤**Prevention of heat prostration**
Adults: 1 g P.O. with each glass of water, or as directed by prescriber.

Antacids: Indications and dosages

aluminum hydroxide
a-LOO-mi-num

AlternaGEL ◇, Alu-Cap ◇, Alu-Tab ◇, Amphoje ◇, Dialume ◇

Therapeutic class: Antacids
Pharmacologic class: Aluminum salts
Pregnancy risk category: Undetermined

AVAILABLE FORMS
Capsules: 400 mg ◇, 500 mg ◇
Liquid: 600 mg/5 mL ◇
Oral suspension: 320 mg/5 mL ◇, 450 mg/5mL ◇, 675 mg/5 mL ◇
Tablets: 500 mg ◇, 600 mg ◇

INDICATIONS & DOSAGES
➤ **Acid indigestion**
Adults: 500 to 1,500 mg P.O. three to six times daily between meals and at bedtime. Or, 5 to 10 mL of liquid formulation or 5 to 30 mL of oral suspension between meals and at bedtime or as directed by prescriber.

calcium carbonate
KAL-see-um

Alka-Seltzer ◇, Cal-Carb Forte ◇, Calci-Chew ◇, Calci-Mix ◇, Calel-D ◇, Cal-Gest ◇, Caltrate ◇, Chooz ◇, Maalox ◇, Mylanta ◇, Nephro Calci ◇, Os-Cal ◇, Oystercal ◇, Rolaids ◇, Trial ◇, Tums ◇

Therapeutic class: Antacids
Pharmacologic class: Calcium salts
Pregnancy risk category: C

AVAILABLE FORMS
Calcium carbonate contains 40% calcium; 20 mEq calcium per gram.
Capsules: 200 mg ◇, 1,250 mg ◇
Chewing gum: 300 mg/piece ◇, 450 mg/piece ◇, 500 mg/piece ◇
Oral suspension: 1,250 mg/5 mL

Tablets: 500 mg ◇, 600 mg ◇, 650 mg ◇, 1,000 mg ◇, 1,250 mg ◇, 1,500 mg ◇
Tablets (chewable): 260 mg ◇, 400mg ◇, 420 mg ◇, 500 mg ◇, 750 mg ◇, 850 mg ◇, 1,000 mg ◇, 1,177 mg ◇, 1,250 mg ◇

INDICATIONS & DOSAGES
➤ **Acid indigestion, calcium supplement**
Adults: 350 mg to 1.5 g P.O. or two pieces of chewing gum 1 hour after meals and at bedtime, as needed.

magnesium oxide
mag-NEE-see-um

Mag-Ox 400 ◇, Maox ◇, Uro-Mag ◇

Therapeutic class: Antacids
Pharmacologic class: Magnesium salts
Pregnancy risk category: A

AVAILABLE FORMS
Capsules: 140 mg
Tablets: 400 mg, 420 mg, 500 mg

INDICATIONS & DOSAGES
➤ **Acid indigestion**
Adults: 140 mg P.O. with water or milk after meals and at bedtime.
➤ **Oral replacement therapy in mild hypomagnesemia**
Adults: 400 to 840 mg P.O. daily. Monitor magnesium level.

Laxatives: Indications and dosages

bisacodyl
bye-suh-KOH-dil

Alophen◇, Bisac-Evac◇, Bisa-Lax◇, Caroid◇, Codulax†◇, Correctol◇, Dulcolax◇, Ex-Lax Ultra◇, Feen-a-Mint◇, Fleet Bisacodyl◇, Fleet Bisacodyl Enema◇, Fleet Laxative◇, Modane◇, Soflax EX†◇, The Magic Bullet†◇,Woman's Laxative†◇

Therapeutic class: Laxatives
Pharmacologic class: Diphenylmethane derivatives
Pregnancy risk category: C

AVAILABLE FORMS
Enema: 0.33 mg/mL ◇
Suppositories: 10 mg ◇
Tablets (enteric-coated): 5 mg ◇

INDICATIONS & DOSAGES
➤ **Chronic constipation; preparation for childbirth, surgery, or rectal or bowel examination**
Adults and children age 12 and older: 5 to 15 mg P.O. in evening or before breakfast. Or, 10 mg P.R. for evacuation before examination or surgery. Enema may be given as a single daily dose.
Children ages 6 to 11: 5 mg P.O. or P.R. (suppository) at bedtime or before breakfast. Oral dose isn't recommended if child can't swallow tablet whole. Don't give enema in children younger than age 12.

calcium polycarbophil
KAL-see-um

Equalactin◇, FiberCon◇, Fiber-Lax◇, Konsyl Fiber◇

Therapeutic class: Laxatives
Pharmacologic class: Hydrophilic drugs
Pregnancy risk category: Undetermined

AVAILABLE FORMS
Tablets: 625 mg ◇
Tablets (chewable): 625 mg ◇

INDICATIONS & DOSAGES
➤ **Constipation**
Adults and children older than age 12: 2 tablets (1,250 mg) P.O. once daily to q.i.d., p.r.n.
Children ages 6 to 12: 1 tablet (625 mg) P.O. once daily to t.i.d., p.r.n.

docusate calcium (dioctyl calcium sulfosuccinate)
DOK-yoo-sayt

Calax ◇†, Surfak ◇

docusate sodium (dioctyl sodium sulfosuccinate)
Colace ◇†, Correctol Extra Gentle ◇, Diocto ◇, Diocto S.S. ◇, Docusil ◇, Docusoft-S ◇, DOK ◇, D.O.S. ◇, DSS ◇, Dulcolax Stool Softener ◇, KS Stool Softener ◇, Laxa Basic ◇, Pedia-Lax Enemeez Mini ◇, Phillips Stool Softener ◇ Promolaxin ◇, Selax† ◇, Silace ◇, Sof-Lax ◇

Therapeutic class: Laxatives
Pharmacologic class: Surfactants
Pregnancy risk category: C

AVAILABLE FORMS
docusate calcium
Capsules: 240 mg ◇
docusate sodium
Capsules: 50 mg ◇, 100 mg ◇, 240 mg ◇, 250 mg ◇
Oral liquid: 150 mg/15 mL ◇
Oral solution: 10 mg/mL ◇, 50 mg/mL ◇
Rectal suspension: 283 mg/4 mL ◇
Syrup: 20 mg/5 mL† ◇, 50 mg/15 mL ◇, 60 mg/15 mL ◇
Tablets: 50 mg ◇, 100 mg

INDICATIONS & DOSAGES
➤ **Constipation (stool softener)**
Adults and children older than age 12: 50 to 300 mg docusate calcium or sodium P.O. daily until bowel movements are normal. Or, give enema. Administer contents of 1 bottle P.R. as a single dose.

Children ages 2 to 12: 20 to 150 mg docusate sodium P.O. daily as a single dose or in divided doses.

linaclotide
LIN-a-KLOE-tide

Linzess

Therapeutic class: Laxatives
Pharmacologic class: Guanylate cyclase-C agonists
Pregnancy risk category: X

AVAILABLE FORMS
Capsules: 145 mcg, 290 mcg

INDICATIONS & DOSAGES
➤ **Irritable bowel syndrome with consti-pation**
Adults: 290 mcg P.O. once daily on an emp-ty stomach at least 30 minutes before first meal of the day.
➤ **Chronic idiopathic constipation**
Adults: 145 mcg P.O. once daily on an emp-ty stomach at least 30 minutes before first meal of the day.

lubiprostone
loo-bee-PRAHS-tohn

Amitiza ◊ ✐

Therapeutic class: Laxatives
Pharmacologic class: Chloride channel activators
Pregnancy risk category: C

AVAILABLE FORMS
Capsules: 8 mcg, 24 mcg

INDICATIONS & DOSAGES
➤ **Chronic idiopathic constipation**
Adults: 24 mcg P.O. b.i.d. with food.
Adjust-a-dose: For patients with moderately impaired hepatic function (Child-Pugh class B), starting dose is 16 mcg b.i.d.; for those with severely impaired hepatic function (Child-Pugh class C), starting dose is 8 mcg b.i.d. May increase to full dose after appro-priate interval if tolerated and an adequate response hasn't been obtained at initial dose. Monitor patient response.

➤ **Irritable bowel syndrome with constipation**
Women age 18 and older: 8 mcg P.O. b.i.d. with food and water.
Adjust-a-dose: For patients with severely impaired hepatic function (Child-Pugh class C), starting dose is 8 mcg once daily. May increase to full dose after appropriate inter-val if tolerated and an adequate response hasn't been obtained at initial dose. Monitor patient response.
✳ *NEW INDICATION:* **Opioid-induced consti-pation in patients with chronic, non-cancer pain**
Adults: 24 mcg P.O. b.i.d. with food and water.
Adjust-a-dose: For patients with moderately impaired hepatic function (Child-Pugh class B), starting dose is 16 mcg b.i.d.; for those with severely impaired hepatic function (Child-Pugh class C), starting dose is 8 mcg b.i.d. May increase to full dose after appro-priate interval if tolerated and an adequate response hasn't been obtained at initial dose. Monitor patient response.

magnesium citrate (citrate of magnesia)
magnesium hydroxide (milk of magnesia)
Milk of Magnesia ◊ , Milk of Magnesia-Concentrated ◊ , Phillips' Milk of Magnesia ◊

magnesium sulfate ◊ (Epsom salts ◊)

Therapeutic class: Laxatives
Pharmacologic class: Magnesium salts
Pregnancy risk category: A

AVAILABLE FORMS
magnesium citrate
Oral solution: About 168 mEq magnesium/ 240 mL ◊
magnesium hydroxide
Chewable tablets: 300 mg, 600 mg
Oral suspension: 400 mg/5 mL, 800 mg/5 mL
magnesium sulfate
Granules: About 40 mEq magnesium/5 g ◊

INDICATIONS & DOSAGES
➤ **Constipation; to evacuate bowel before surgery**
Adults and children age 12 and older: 11 to 25 g magnesium citrate P.O. daily as a single or divided dose. Or, 2.4 to 4.8 g or 30 to 60 mL magnesium hydroxide P.O. (2 to 4 tablespoons at bedtime or upon arising, followed by 8 ounces of liquid) daily as a single or divided dose. Or, 10 to 30 g magnesium sulfate P.O. daily as a single or divided dose.
Children ages 6 to 11: 5.5 to 12.5 g magnesium citrate P.O. daily as a single or divided dose. Or, 1.2 to 2.4 g or 15 to 30 mL magnesium hydroxide P.O. (1 to 2 tablespoons, followed by 8 ounces of liquid) daily as a single or divided dose. Or, 5 to 10 g magnesium sulfate P.O. daily as a single or divided dose. Don't use dosage cup.
Children ages 2 to 5: 2.7 to 6.25 g magnesium citrate P.O. daily as a single or divided dose. Or, 0.4 to 1.2 g or 5 to 15 mL magnesium hydroxide P.O. (1 to 3 tsp, followed by 8 ounces of liquid) daily as a single or divided dose. Or, 2.5 to 5 g magnesium sulfate P.O. daily as a single or divided dose. Don't use dosage cup.

sodium phosphate monobasic monohydrate–sodium phosphate dibasic anhydrous
OsmoPrep

Therapeutic class: Laxatives
Pharmacologic class: Osmotic laxatives
Pregnancy risk category: C

AVAILABLE FORMS
Tablets: 1.5 g sodium phosphate (1.102 g sodium phosphate monobasic monohydrate and 0.398 g sodium phosphate dibasic anhydrous)

INDICATIONS & DOSAGES
➤ **To cleanse the bowel before colonoscopy**
Adults age 18 and older: 32 tablets taken in the following manner: The evening before the procedure, 4 tablets P.O. with 8 ounces of clear liquid every 15 minutes for a total of 20 tablets. 3 to 5 hours before the procedure, 4 tablets P.O. with at least 8 ounces of clear liquid every 15 minutes for a total of 12 tablets.

sodium phosphates
Fleet Enema ◊, Pedia-Lax ◊

Therapeutic class: Laxatives
Pharmacologic class: Acid salts
Pregnancy risk category: C

AVAILABLE FORMS
Fleet Enema: 19 g monobasic sodium phosphate monohydrate and 7 g dibasic sodium phosphate heptahydrate/118 mL ◊
Pedia-Lax: 9.5 g monobasic sodium phosphate monohydrate and 3.5 g dibasic sodium phosphate heptahydrate/59 mL ◊

INDICATIONS & DOSAGES
➤ **Constipation**
Adults and children age 12 and older: 133 mL (1 bottle) Fleet Enema P.R. as an enema once in 24 hours.
Children ages 5 to 11: 66 mL (1 bottle) Pedia-Lax P.R. as an enema once in 24 hours.
Children ages 2 to younger than 5: 33 mL (1/2 bottle) Pedia-Lax P.R. as an enema once in 24 hours.

sodium picosulfate–magnesium oxide–anhydrous citric acid
Prepopik

Therapeutic class: Laxatives
Pharmacologic class: Peristaltic stimulants–osmotic agents
Pregnancy risk category: B

AVAILABLE FORMS
Powder for oral solution (16.1 g/packet, 2 packets/dosing carton): 10 mg sodium picosulfate, 3.5 g magnesium oxide, and 12 g anhydrous citric acid

INDICATIONS & DOSAGES
➤ **Cleansing of the colon in preparation for colonoscopy**
Adults: The "split dose" method is preferred. Give first dose during the evening before colonoscopy (5 p.m. to 9 p.m.) followed by five 8-ounce drinks of clear liquids within 5 hours and before bed. Give

second dose next day, during the morning approximately 5 hours before colonoscopy. Follow dose with at least three 8-ounce drinks of clear liquids before colonoscopy; continue with clear liquids within 5 hours and up to 2 hours before colonoscopy. If "split dose" method isn't appropriate, use the "day before" method: Give first dose in the afternoon or early evening (4 p.m. to 6 p.m.) before colonoscopy followed by five 8-ounce drinks of clear liquids within 5 hours and before next dose. Give second dose approximately 6 hours later in the late evening (10 p.m. to 12 a.m.) the night before colonoscopy, followed by three 8-ounce drinks of clear liquids within 5 hours and before bed.

Less commonly used drugs: Indications and dosages

alcaftadine
al-CAFF-tuh-deen

Lastacaft

Therapeutic class: Antihistamines
Pharmacologic class: Histamine$_1$-receptor antagonists
Pregnancy risk category: B

AVAILABLE FORMS
Ophthalmic solution: 0.25% (2.5 mg/mL)

INDICATIONS & DOSAGES
➤ **Prevention of itching associated with allergic conjunctivitis**
Adults and children age 2 and older: Instill 1 drop in each eye once daily.

alglucosidase alfa
AL-gloo-KOH-sih-dase

Lumizyme, Myozyme

Therapeutic class: Metabolic agents
Pharmacologic class: Lysosomal glycogen-specific enzymes
Pregnancy risk category: B

AVAILABLE FORMS
Powder for I.V. infusion: 50 mg/vial

INDICATIONS & DOSAGES
➤ **Late (noninfantile)-onset Pompe disease (alpha-glucosidase deficiency) without evidence of cardiac hypertrophy**
Adults and children age 8 and older: 20 mg/kg by I.V. infusion over 4 hours every 2 weeks. Initial infusion rate is 1 mg/kg/ hour; may increase in stepwise manner by 2 mg/kg/hour every 30 minutes, if tolerated, to maximum rate of 7 mg/kg/hour. Obtain vital signs at each step increase. May stop or slow infusion rate temporarily if infusion reactions occur.

alprostadil (intracavernosal injection; urogenital suppository)
al-PROSS-ta-dil

Caverject, Caverject Impulse, Edex, Muse

Therapeutic class: Erectile dysfunction drugs
Pharmacologic class: Prostaglandins
Pregnancy risk category: C

AVAILABLE FORMS
Intracavernosal injection: 5 mcg/vial, 10 mcg/vial, 20 mcg/vial, 40 mcg/vial
Urogenital suppository: 125 mcg, 250 mcg, 500 mcg, 1,000 mcg

INDICATIONS & DOSAGES
➤ **Erectile dysfunction of vasculogenic, psychogenic, or mixed causes**
Injection
Men: Dosages highly individualized; initially, inject 2.5 mcg intracavernosally. If partial response occurs, give second dose of 2.5 mcg; increase by 5 to 10 mcg until patient achieves erection suitable for intercourse lasting no longer than 1 hour. If no response to first dose, increase second dose to 7.5 mcg within 1 hour; then increase by 5 to 10 mcg until patient achieves suitable erection. Patient must remain in prescriber's office until complete detumescence occurs. Don't repeat for at least 24 hours. For Edex, give 1 to 40 mcg by intracavernosal injection over 5 to 10 seconds.
Urogenital suppository
Men: Initially, 125 to 250 mcg, under supervision of prescriber. Adjust dosage as needed until response is sufficient for sexual intercourse. Maximum of two administrations in 24 hours; maximum dose is 1,000 mcg.
➤ **Erectile dysfunction of neurogenic cause (spinal cord injury)**
Men: Dosages highly individualized; initially, inject 1.25 mcg intracavernosally. If partial response occurs, give second dose of 1.25 mcg. Increase in increments of 2.5 mcg, to dose of 5 mcg; then increase in

increments of 5 mcg until patient achieves erection suitable for intercourse lasting no longer than 1 hour. If no response to first dose, give next higher dose within 1 hour. Patient must remain in prescriber's office until complete detumescence occurs. Don't repeat procedure for at least 24 hours. For Edex, give 1 to 40 mcg by intracavernosal injection over 5 to 10 seconds.

apomorphine hydrochloride
ah-poe-MORE-feen

Apokyn

Therapeutic class: Antiparkinsonians
Pharmacologic class: Nonergot-derivative dopamine agonists
Pregnancy risk category: C

AVAILABLE FORMS
Solution for injection: 10 mg/mL (contains benzyl alcohol)

INDICATIONS & DOSAGES
➤ **Intermittent hypomobility, "off" episodes caused by advanced Parkinson disease (given with an antiemetic)**
Adults: Initially, give a 0.2-mL Subcut. test dose. Measure supine and standing blood pressure every 20 minutes for first hour. If patient tolerates and responds to drug, start with 0.2 mL Subcut. as needed as outpatient. Separate doses by at least 2 hours. Increase by 0.1 mL every few days, as needed.

If initial 0.2-mL dose is ineffective but tolerated, give 0.4 mL at next "off" period, but no sooner than 2 hours after the initial test dose of 0.2 mL. Measure supine and standing blood pressure every 20 minutes for first hour. If drug is tolerated, start with 0.3 mL Subcut. as outpatient. If needed, increase by 0.1 mL every few days.

If patient doesn't tolerate 0.4-mL dose, give 0.3 mL as test dose at the next "off" period, measuring supine and standing blood pressure every 20 minutes for first hour. If drug tolerated, give 0.2 mL as outpatient. Increase by 0.1 mL every few days, as needed; doses higher than 0.4 mL usually not tolerated if 0.2 mL is starting dose.

Maximum recommended dose is usually 0.6 mL as needed. Most patients use drug

t.i.d. Experience is limited at more than five times daily or more than 2 mL daily.
Adjust-a-dose: In patients with mild to moderate renal impairment, give test and starting doses of 0.1 mL subcutaneously.

artemether–lumefantrine
art-TEM-mah-ther–loo-meh-FAN-treen

Coartem

Therapeutic class: Antimalarials
Pharmacologic class: Schizontocides
Pregnancy risk category: C

AVAILABLE FORMS
Tablets: artemether 20 mg and lumefantrine 120 mg

INDICATIONS & DOSAGES
➤ **Uncomplicated malaria caused by** *Plasmodium falciparum*
Adults and children weighing 35 kg (77 lb) or more: Initially, 4 tablets P.O., followed by 4 tablets in 8 hours, and then 4 tablets b.i.d. for the next 2 days. Total course is 24 tablets.
Children weighing 25 to 34 kg (55 to 75 lb): Initially, 3 tablets P.O., followed by 3 tablets in 8 hours, and then 3 tablets b.i.d. on each of the next 2 days. Total course is 18 tablets.
Children weighing 15 to 24 kg (33 to 53 lb): Initially, 2 tablets P.O., followed by 2 tablets in 8 hours, and then 2 tablets b.i.d. on each of the next 2 days. Total course is 12 tablets.
Children weighing 5 to 14 kg (11 to 31 lb): Initially, 1 tablet P.O., followed by 1 tablet in 8 hours, and then 1 tablet b.i.d. on each of the next 2 days. Total course is 6 tablets.

asparaginase *Erwinia chrysanthemi*
as-PAR-a-jin-ase er-WIN-ee-uh chris-AN-tha-me

Erwinaze

Therapeutic class: Antineoplastics
Pharmacologic class: Enzyme inhibitors
Pregnancy risk category: C

AVAILABLE FORMS
Powder for injection: 10,000 international units/vial

INDICATIONS & DOSAGES
➤ **Acute lymphoblastic leukemia in patients who have developed hypersensitivity to *Escherichia coli*–derived asparaginase as part of a multiagent chemotherapy regimen**
Adults and children age 2 and older: When substituting for pegaspargase, give 25,000 international units/m^2 I.M. three times a week (Monday/Wednesday/Friday) for six doses. When substituting for native *E. coli* asparaginase, give 25,000 international units/m^2 I.M. for each scheduled dose of native *E. coli* asparaginase within a treatment.

auranofin
or-RAIN-oh-fin

Ridaura

Therapeutic class: Antiarthritics
Pharmacologic class: Gold compounds
Pregnancy risk category: C

AVAILABLE FORMS
Capsules: 3 mg

INDICATIONS & DOSAGES
➤ **Rheumatoid arthritis in patients who have had an insufficient response to or are intolerant of trial doses of one or more NSAIDs**
Adults: 3 mg P.O. b.i.d. or 6 mg P.O. once daily. After 6 months, may increase to 3 mg P.O. t.i.d. If response is inadequate after 3 months of 9 mg/day, stop use.

azelaic acid
aze-eh-LAY-ik

Azelex, Finacea

Therapeutic class: Antiacne drugs
Pharmacologic class: Dicarboxylic acids
Pregnancy risk category: B

AVAILABLE FORMS
Cream: 20%
Gel: 15%

INDICATIONS & DOSAGES
➤ **Mild to moderate inflammatory acne vulgaris**

Adults and children age 12 and older:
Apply thin film of cream (Azelex) and gently but thoroughly massage into affected areas b.i.d., in morning and evening.
➤ **Mild to moderate rosacea**
Adults: Apply thin film of gel (Finacea) and gently but thoroughly massage into affected areas b.i.d., in morning and evening. Reassess if no improvement in 2 weeks.

benzyl alcohol
ben-zill AL-ko-hall

Ulesfia

Therapeutic class: Scabicides–pediculicides
Pharmacologic class: Topical alcohols
Pregnancy risk category: B

AVAILABLE FORMS
Lotion: 5%

INDICATIONS & DOSAGES
➤ **Head lice infestation**
Adults age 60 and younger and children age 6 months and older: Apply to hair and scalp until completely saturated. Allow to remain for 10 minutes; then rinse thoroughly with water. Remove dead lice and nits with fine-toothed comb. Repeat treatment after 7 days. For each treatment, administer 4 to 6 oz for hair 0″ to 2″ long, 6 to 8 oz for hair 2″ to 4″ long, 8 to 12 oz for hair 4″ to 8″ long, 12 to 24 oz for hair 8″ to 16″ long, 24 to 32 oz for hair 16″ to 22″ long, and 32 to 48 oz for hair more than 22″ long.

SAFETY ALERT!

bosutinib
boe-SUE-ti-nib

Bosulif

Therapeutic classification: Antineoplastics
Pharmacologic classification: Kinase inhibitors
Pregnancy risk category: D

AVAILABLE FORMS
Tablets: 100 mg, 500 mg

INDICATIONS & DOSAGES

➤ **Chronic myelogenous leukemia with resistance or intolerance to prior therapy**
Adults: 500 mg P.O. once daily. Consider dosage escalation to 600 mg once daily in patients who don't reach complete hematologic response by week 8 or a complete cytogenetic response by week 12, who didn't have grade 3 or higher adverse reactions, and who are currently taking 500 mg daily.
Adjust-a-dose: If liver transaminase levels increase to greater than 5 times the upper limit of normal (ULN), withhold drug until recovery to 2.5 × ULN or less and resume at 400 mg P.O. once daily. If recovery takes longer than 4 weeks, discontinue drug. Discontinue drug if transaminase elevations 3 × ULN or more occur concurrently with bilirubin elevations greater than 2 × ULN and alkaline phosphatase less than 2 × ULN. Refer to manufacturer's instructions for dosage adjustments due to other adverse reactions or myelosuppression.

SAFETY ALERT!

cabazitaxel
ka-baz-ih-TAX-el

Jevtana

Therapeutic class: Antineoplastics
Pharmacologic class: Taxoids
Pregnancy risk category: D

AVAILABLE FORMS
Injection: 60 mg/1.5 mL

INDICATIONS & DOSAGES

➤ **In combination with prednisone for hormone-refractory metastatic prostate cancer previously treated with docetaxel-containing treatment regimen**
Adults: 25 mg/m² I.V. over 1 hour every 3 weeks. Give oral prednisone 10 mg daily throughout cabazitaxel therapy. Premedicate at least 30 minutes before each dose of cabazitaxel with the following I.V. medications to reduce risk or severity of hypersensitivity: antihistamine (5 mg dexchlorpheniramine, or 25 mg diphenhydramine or equivalent antihistamine), corticosteroid (8 mg dexamethasone

or equivalent steroid), and H₂ antagonist (50 mg ranitidine or equivalent H₂ antagonist). Antiemetic prophylaxis is recommended and can be given P.O. or I.V. as needed.
Adjust-a-dose: If neutrophil count is less than 1,500 cells/mm³, withhold drug. Reduce subsequent doses of cabazitaxel to 20 mg/m² if patient has severe neutropenia (neutrophil count of less than 500 mg/mm³ for 1 week or longer) or neutropenic fever. Also reduce dosage to 20 mg/m² if patient has at least seven stools/day, is incontinent, or needs parenteral support for dehydration.

canakinumab
kan-ah-KIN-yoo-mab

Ilaris

Therapeutic class: Anti-autoimmune agents
Pharmacologic class: Monoclonal antibodies
Pregnancy risk category: C

AVAILABLE FORMS
Injection: 180-mg single-use vial

INDICATIONS & DOSAGES

➤ **Cryopyrin-associated periodic syndromes (familial cold autoinflammatory syndrome and Muckle-Wells syndrome)**
Adults and children age 4 and older weighing more than 40 kg (88 lb): 150 mg Subcut. every 8 weeks.
Adults and children age 4 and older weighing 15 to 40 kg (33 to 88 lb): 2 mg/kg subcutaneously every 8 weeks; may increase dosage to 3 mg/kg in children weighing 15 to 40 kg who have an adequate response.
➤ **Active systemic juvenile idiopathic arthritis**
Children age 2 and older weighing at least 7.5 kg (16.5 lb): 4 mg/kg Subcut. every 4 weeks. Maximum dose is 300 mg.

carfilzomib
car-FIL-zoe-mib

Kyprolis

Therapeutic class: Antineoplastics
Pharmacologic class: Proteasome inhibitors
Pregnancy risk category: D

AVAILABLE FORMS
Powder for injection: 60-mg single-use vial

INDICATIONS & DOSAGES
➤ **Multiple myeloma in patients who have experienced failure of at least two prior therapies, including bortezomib and an immunomodulator, and have shown disease progression on or within 60 days of completion of last therapy**
Adults: 20 mg/m^2 I.V. over 2 to 10 minutes on 2 consecutive days each week for 3 weeks (days 1, 2, 8, 9, 15, and 16), followed by 12-day rest period (days 17 to 28). If tolerated, may increase to 27 mg/m^2 in cycle 2 and to 27 mg/m^2 for subsequent cycles. Maximum dosage is based on BSA of 2.2 m^2. Continue treatment until disease progression or intolerable toxicities occur.
Adjust-a-dose: Adjust dosage for weight change of more than 20% from baseline. Refer to manufacturer's instructions for dosage adjustments based on toxicities.

carglumic acid
kar-GLOO-mik as-id

Carbaglu

Therapeutic class: Antihyperammonemics
Pharmacologic class: Ammonia detoxicants
Pregnancy risk category: C

AVAILABLE FORMS
Tablets: 200 mg

INDICATIONS & DOSAGES
➤ **Acute or chronic hyperammonemia in patients with N-acetylglutamate synthetase deficiency**
Adults and children: Initially, 100 to 250 mg/kg/day P.O., divided into two to four doses, immediately before meals. Round each dose to nearest 100 mg. Titrate dosage according to ammonia level and symptoms.

cetrorelix acetate
SE-troe-REL-lx

Cetrotide

Therapeutic class: Infertility drugs
Pharmacologic class: Gonadotropin-releasing hormone antagonists
Pregnancy risk category: X

AVAILABLE FORMS
Powder for injection: 0.25 mg, 3 mg

INDICATIONS & DOSAGES
➤ **To inhibit premature luteinizing-hormone surges in women undergoing controlled ovarian stimulation**
Women: 3 mg Subcut. once during early to middle follicular phase, given when estradiol level indicates an appropriate stimulation response, usually on stimulation day 7 (range, days 5 to 9). If human chorionic gonadotropin (hCG) hasn't been given within 4 days after injection, give drug 0.25 mg Subcut. once daily until day of hCG administration. Or, give 0.25-mg multiple-dose regimen Subcut. on stimulation day 5 (morning or evening) or day 6 (morning), and continue once daily until day of hCG administration.

cevimeline hydrochloride
seh-vih-MEH-leen

Evoxac

Therapeutic class: Cholinergic agonists
Pharmacologic class: Cholinergic agonists
Pregnancy risk category: C

AVAILABLE FORMS
Capsules: 30 mg

INDICATIONS & DOSAGES
➤ **Dry mouth in patients with Sjögren syndrome**
Adults: 30 mg P.O. t.i.d.

SAFETY ALERT!

chlorambucil
klor-AM-byoo-sill

Leukeran

Therapeutic class: Antineoplastics
Pharmacologic class: Nitrogen mustards
Pregnancy risk category: D

AVAILABLE FORMS
Tablets: 2 mg

INDICATIONS & DOSAGES
➤ Chronic lymphocytic leukemia; malignant lymphomas, including lymphosarcoma, giant follicular lymphoma, and Hodgkin lymphoma
Adults: For initiation of therapy or for short courses of treatment, give 0.1 to 0.2 mg/kg P.O. daily for 3 to 6 weeks (usually 4 to 10 mg daily). Maintenance dosage shouldn't exceed 0.1 mg/kg/day and may be as low as 0.03 mg/kg/day. Adjust dosage according to patient response; reduce when WBC count falls abruptly. For pulse dosing, give initial single dose of 0.4 mg/kg. Then give doses at biweekly or monthly intervals, increasing by 0.1-mg/kg increments until lymphocytosis is controlled or toxicity occurs.
Adjust-a-dose: Reduce first dose if given within 4 weeks after a full course of radiation therapy or myelosuppressive drugs, or if pretreatment WBC or platelet count is depressed from bone marrow disease. For patients with severe renal impairment, adjust dosage as follows: If CrCl is 10 to 50 mL/minute, give 75% of usual dose; if CrCl is less than 10 mL/minute, give 50% of usual dose; for patients receiving hemodialysis or peritoneal dialysis, give 50% of usual dose (no supplemental dosing is needed).

chloramphenicol sodium succinate
klor-am-FEN-i-kole

Pentamycetin†

Therapeutic class: Antibiotics
Pharmacologic class: Dichloroacetic acid derivatives
Pregnancy risk category: C

AVAILABLE FORMS
Injection: 1-g vial

INDICATIONS & DOSAGES
➤ *Haemophilus influenzae* meningitis, acute *Salmonella typhi* infection, and meningitis, bacteremia, or other severe infections caused by sensitive *Salmonella* species, rickettsia, lymphogranuloma, psittacosis, or various sensitive gram-negative organisms
Adults: 50 to 100 mg/kg I.V. daily, divided every 6 hours. Maximum dosage is 100 mg/kg daily.
Full-term infants older than age 2 weeks with normal metabolic processes: Up to 50 mg/kg I.V. daily, divided every 6 hours. May use up to 100 mg/kg/day in four divided doses for meningitis.
Preterm infants, neonates age 2 weeks and younger, and children and infants with immature metabolic processes: 25 mg/kg I.V. once daily.
Adjust-a-dose: For patients with renal or hepatic impairment, excessive blood levels may result from administration of the recommended dosage. Determine drug blood concentration at appropriate intervals and adjust dosage accordingly.

chlorthalidone
klor-THAL-i-done

Thalitone

Therapeutic class: Antihypertensives
Pharmacologic class: Thiazide diuretics
Pregnancy risk category: B

AVAILABLE FORMS
Tablets: 15 mg, 25 mg, 50 mg, 100 mg

INDICATIONS & DOSAGES
➤ Edema
Adults: 50 to 100 mg P.O. daily, or 100 mg P.O. on alternating days.
➤ Hypertension
Adults: 25 mg P.O. daily. May increase to 50 mg, then 100 mg daily as needed.

collagenase *Clostridium histolyticum*
kuh-LAJ-eh-nase
klos-TRID-ee-um
hiss-toe-LIH-teh-kum

Xiaflex

Therapeutic class: Anticollagen drugs
Pharmacologic class: Enzymes
Pregnancy risk category: B

AVAILABLE FORMS
Injection: 0.9-mg single-use vial

INDICATIONS & DOSAGES
➤ **Dupuytren' contracture with palpable cord**
Adults: 0.58 mg injected into palpable cord with contracture of metacarpophalangeal joint or proximal interphalangeal joint. May repeat up to three times per cord at 4-week intervals.

crotamiton
kroe-TAM-ih-tuhn

Eurax

Therapeutic class: Scabicides-pediculicides
Pharmacologic class: Scabicides
Pregnancy risk category: C

AVAILABLE FORMS
Cream: 10%
Lotion: 10%

INDICATIONS & DOSAGES
➤ **Parasitic infestation (scabies)**
Adults: Scrub entire body with soap and water. Remove scales or crusts. Then apply thin layer of cream over entire body, from chin down (with special attention to skin-folds, creases, interdigital spaces, and genital area). Apply second coat in 24 hours. Change clothing and bed linen the next morning. Wait another 48 hours; then wash off. If retreatment is needed, use an alternative regimen.
➤ **Itching**
Adults: Apply locally, massaging gently into affected area until completely absorbed; repeat p.r.n.

cycloSERINE
sye-kloe-SER-een

Seromycin

Therapeutic class: Antituberculotics
Pharmacologic class: Isoxazolidine derivatives, D-alanine analogues
Pregnancy risk category: C

AVAILABLE FORMS
Capsules: 250 mg

INDICATIONS & DOSAGES
➤ **Adjunctive treatment for pulmonary or extrapulmonary tuberculosis**
Adults: Initially, 250 mg P.O. every 12 hours for 2 weeks; then adjust dosage to maintain blood concentrations at less than 30 mcg/mL. Dosage shouldn't exceed 1 g daily.
➤ **Acute UTIs**
Adults: 250 mg P.O. every 12 hours for 2 weeks.

diflunisal
dye-FLOO-ni-sal

Therapeutic class: NSAIDs
Pharmacologic class: Salicylates—NSAIDs
Pregnancy risk category: C

AVAILABLE FORMS
Tablets: 500 mg

INDICATIONS & DOSAGES
➤ **Osteoarthritis, rheumatoid arthritis**
Adults: 250 to 1,000 mg P.O. daily in two divided doses, usually every 12 hours. Maximum, 1,500 mg daily.
Children age 12 and older: 250 to 1,000 mg P.O. daily in two divided doses. Maximum dose is 1,500 mg daily.
➤ **Mild to moderate pain**
Adults and children age 12 and older: 1,000 mg P.O., then 500 mg every 8 to 12 hours. A lower dosage of 500 mg P.O., then 250 mg every 8 to 12 hours may be appropriate.

dinoprostone
dye-noe-PROST-ohn

Cervidil, Prepidil, Prostin E2

Therapeutic class: Oxytocics
Pharmacologic class: Prostaglandins
Pregnancy risk category: C

AVAILABLE FORMS
Endocervical gel: 0.5 mg/application
(2.5-mL syringe)
Vaginal insert: 10 mg
Vaginal suppositories: 20 mg

INDICATIONS & DOSAGES
Black Box Warning Strictly adhere to recommended dosages. ■
➤ **To terminate second-trimester pregnancy; to evacuate uterine contents in
missed abortion, intrauterine fetal death
up to 28 weeks' gestation, or benign hydatidiform mole (vaginal suppository only)**
Women: Insert 20-mg suppository high into
posterior vaginal fornix; repeat every 3 to
5 hours until abortion is complete, for a
maximum of 2 days.
➤ **To ripen an unfavorable cervix in
pregnant woman at or near term
(endocervical gel and vaginal insert only)**
Women: Apply 0.5 mg endocervical gel intravaginally; if cervix remains unfavorable
after 6 hours, repeat dose. Don't exceed
1.5 mg (three applications) within 24 hours.
After obtaining desired response, wait 6 to
12 hours before giving I.V. oxytocin. Or,
place 10-mg vaginal insert transversely in
posterior vaginal fornix immediately after
removing insert from foil. Take insert out
when active labor begins or after 12 hours
have passed, whichever occurs first. After
insert removal, wait at least 30 minutes
before giving oxytocin.

econazole nitrate
ee-KOE-na-zole

Therapeutic class: Antifungals
Pharmacologic class: Imidazole derivatives
Pregnancy risk category: C

AVAILABLE FORMS
Cream: 1%

INDICATIONS & DOSAGES
➤ **Tinea corporis, tinea cruris, tinea
pedis, tinea versicolor**
Adults and children: Rub into affected
areas daily for at least 2 weeks (1 month
for tinea pedis).
➤ **Cutaneous candidiasis**
Adults and children: Rub into affected
areas b.i.d.

SAFETY ALERT!

eculizumab
eck-u-LIZ-uh-mob

Soliris

Therapeutic class: Hemolysis inhibitors
Pharmacologic class: Monoclonal IgG
antibodies
Pregnancy risk category: C

AVAILABLE FORMS
Injection: 10 mg/mL in 300-mg single-use
vial

INDICATIONS & DOSAGES
Black Box Warning Meningococcal vaccine is required at least 2 weeks before
administration of eculizumab. ■
➤ **Hemolysis in patients with paroxysmal
nocturnal hemoglobinuria**
Adults: 600 mg I.V. every 7 days for
4 weeks, 900 mg 7 days later, then 900 mg
every 14 days thereafter.
➤ **Atypical hemolytic-uremic syndrome**
*Adults and children weighing 40 kg (88 lb)
or more:* 900 mg I.V. weekly for 4 weeks,
then 1,200 mg at week 5, then 1,200 mg
every 2 weeks.
*Children weighing 30 kg (66 lb) to 39 kg
(86 lb):* 600 mg I.V. weekly for 2 weeks,
then 900 mg at week 3, then 900 mg every
2 weeks.
*Children weighing 20 kg (44 lb) to 29 kg
(64 lb):* 600 mg I.V. weekly for 2 weeks,
then 600 mg at week 3, then 600 mg every
2 weeks.
*Children weighing 10 kg (22 lb) to 19 kg (42
lb):* 600 mg I.V. weekly for one dose, then 300
mg at week 2, then 300 mg every 2 weeks.
Children weighing 5 kg (11 lb) to 9 kg (20 lb):
300 mg I.V. weekly for one dose, then 300 mg
at week 2, then 300 mg every 3 weeks.

enzalutamide
EN-za-LOO-ta-mide

Xtandi

Therapeutic class: Antineoplastics
Pharmacologic class: Androgen receptor inhibitors
Pregnancy risk category: X

AVAILABLE FORMS
Capsules: 40 mg

INDICATIONS & DOSAGES
➤ **Metastatic castration-resistant prostate cancer previously treated with docetaxel**
Adults: 160 mg P.O. once daily.
Adjust-a-dose: For grade 3 or 4 toxicity or an intolerable adverse effect, withhold drug for 1 week or until symptoms improve to grade 2 or less. Resume at same or reduced dosage as appropriate.

ephedrine sulfate
e-FED-rin

Therapeutic class: Vasopressors
Pharmacologic class: Adrenergics
Pregnancy risk category: C

AVAILABLE FORMS
Capsules: 25 mg

INDICATIONS & DOSAGES
➤ **Bronchodilation**
Adults and children older than age 12: 12.5 to 25 mg P.O. every 4 hours, as needed, not to exceed 150 mg in 24 hours.

exemestane
ecks-eh-MES-tayn

Aromasin

Therapeutic class: Antineoplastics
Pharmacologic class: Aromatase inhibitors
Pregnancy risk category: X

AVAILABLE FORMS
Tablets: 25 mg

INDICATIONS & DOSAGES
➤ **Advanced breast cancer in post-menopausal women whose disease has progressed after treatment with tamoxifen**
Adults: 25 mg P.O. once daily after food.
➤ **Early-stage breast cancer in post-menopausal women who have taken tamoxifen for 2 to 3 years**
Adults: 25 mg P.O. once daily after food to complete a 5-year course, unless cancer recurs or is found in the other breast.

fludrocortisone acetate
floo-droe-KOR-ti-sone

Therapeutic class: Mineralocorticoids
Pharmacologic class: Mineralocorticoids
Pregnancy risk category: C

AVAILABLE FORMS
Tablets: 0.1 mg

INDICATIONS & DOSAGES
➤ **Salt-losing adrenogenital syndrome**
Adults: 0.1 to 0.2 mg P.O. daily.
➤ **Addison disease (adrenocortical insufficiency)**
Adults: 0.1 mg P.O. daily. Usual dosage range is 0.1 mg three times weekly to 0.2 mg daily. Decrease dosage to 0.05 mg daily if transient hypertension develops.

fluorometholone
flur-oh-METH-oh-lone

FML, FML Forte

fluorometholone acetate
Flarex

Therapeutic class: Anti-inflammatory drugs (ophthalmic)
Pharmacologic class: Corticosteroids
Pregnancy risk category: C

AVAILABLE FORMS
fluorometholone
Ophthalmic ointment: 0.1%
Ophthalmic suspension: 0.1%, 0.25%
fluorometholone acetate
Ophthalmic suspension: 0.1%

INDICATIONS & DOSAGES
➤ **Inflammatory and allergic conditions of cornea, conjunctiva, sclera, or anterior uvea**
Adults and children older than age 2 (acetate form not for use in children of any age):
1 drop b.i.d. to q.i.d. or ½-inch ointment once daily to t.i.d. For first 24 to 48 hours, may increase dosing frequency to every 4 hours. For fluorometholone acetate, 1 to 2 drops q.i.d.; may give 2 drops every 2 hours during the initial 24 to 48 hours of treatment.

glucagon
GLOO-ka-gon

GlucaGen Diagnostic Kit,
GlucaGen HypoKit

Therapeutic class: Diagnostic agents
Pharmacologic class: Antihypoglycemics
Pregnancy risk category: B

AVAILABLE FORMS
Powder for injection: 1-mg (1-unit) vial

INDICATIONS & DOSAGES
➤ **Hypoglycemia**
Glucagon
Adults and children weighing more than 20 kg (44 lb) or older than age 6 to 8: 1 mg (1 unit) I.V., I.M., or Subcut.
Children weighing 20 kg or less: 0.5 mg (0.5 units) or 20 to 30 mcg/kg I.V., I.M., or Subcut.; maximum dose, 1 mg. May repeat in 15 minutes, if needed. I.V. glucose must be given if patient fails to respond.
GlucaGen
Adults and children (weighing more than 25 kg or older than age 6 to 8 when weight is unknown): 1 mL I.V., I.M., or Subcut.
Children (weighing less than 25 kg or younger than age 6 to 8 when weight is unknown): 0.5 mL I.V., I.M., or Subcut.
➤ **Diagnostic aid for radiologic examination of the GI tract**
Adults: 0.25 to 0.75 mg I.V. or 1 to 2 mg I.M. before radiologic examination.

glycerin
GLI-ser-in

Fleet Babylax ◊ , Sani-Supp ◊

Therapeutic class: Laxatives
Pharmacologic class: Trihydric alcohols
Pregnancy risk category: C

AVAILABLE FORMS
Enema (pediatric): 4 mL/applicator ◊
Suppositories: Adult, children, and infant sizes ◊

INDICATIONS & DOSAGES
➤ **Constipation**
Adults and children age 6 and older: 2 to 3 g as rectal suppository; or 5 to 15 mL as enema.

Children ages 2 to 6: 1 to 1.2 g as rectal suppository; or 2 mL as enema.

SAFETY ALERT!

goserelin acetate
GOE-se-REL-in

Zoladex

Therapeutic class: Antineoplastics
Pharmacologic class: Gonadotropin-releasing hormone analogues
Pregnancy risk category: X (endometriosis and endometrial thinning); D (breast cancer)

AVAILABLE FORMS
Implants: 3.6 mg, 10.8 mg

INDICATIONS & DOSAGES
➤ **Endometriosis, including pain relief and lesion reduction**
Women: 3.6 mg Subcut. every 28 days into the anterior abdominal wall below the navel. Maximum length of therapy is 6 months.
➤ **Endometrial thinning before endometrial ablation**
Women: 3.6 mg Subcut. into the anterior abdominal wall below the navel. Give one or two implants, 4 weeks apart.
➤ **Palliative treatment of advanced breast cancer in premenopausal and post-menopausal women**
Women: 3.6 mg Subcut. every 28 days into anterior abdominal wall below navel.

➤**Palliative treatment of advanced prostate cancer**
Men: 3.6 mg Subcut. every 28 days or 10.8 mg Subcut. every 12 weeks into anterior abdominal wall below navel.

icosapent ethyl
eye-KOE-sa-pent

Vascepa

Therapeutic class: Antilipemics
Pharmacologic class: Ethyl esters
Pregnancy risk category: C

AVAILABLE FORMS
Capsules: 1 g

INDICATIONS & DOSAGES
➤**Adjunct to diet to reduce triglyceride levels 500 mg/dL or more**
Adults: 2 g P.O. b.i.d. with food.

ivacaftor
EYE-va-KAF-tor

Kalydeco

Therapeutic class: Metabolic agents
Pharmacologic class: Cystic fibrosis transmembrane conductance regulator potentiator
Pregnancy risk category: B

AVAILABLE FORMS
Tablets: 150 mg

INDICATIONS & DOSAGES
➤**Cystic fibrosis in patients with *G551D* mutation in the cystic fibrosis transmembrane conductance regulator gene**
Adults and children age 6 and older: 150 mg P.O. every 12 hours.
Adjust-a-dose: In patients with moderate hepatic insufficiency (Child-Pugh class B), 150 mg once daily. In those with severe hepatic insufficiency (Child-Pugh class C), use cautiously at 150 mg once daily or less frequently. In those taking strong CYP3A inhibitors (ketoconazole and others), 150 mg twice a week. In those taking moderate CYP3A inhibitors (fluconazole and others), 150 mg once daily.

SAFETY ALERT!

lapatinib
lah-PAH-tih-nihb

Tykerb

Therapeutic class: Antineoplastics
Pharmacologic class: Kinase inhibitors
Pregnancy risk category: D

AVAILABLE FORMS
Tablets: 250 mg

INDICATIONS & DOSAGES
Adjust-a-dose (for all indications): In patients with decreased LVEF that is grade 2 or higher by NCI Common Terminology Criteria for Adverse Events (NCI CTCAE), or LVEF that drops below the institution's lower limit of normal due to treatment, stop drug. After 2 weeks, if patient has recovered normal LVEF and is asymptomatic, resume at reduced dosage and monitor LVEF. In patients with severe hepatic impairment (Child-Pugh class C), reduce dosage. In patients with grade 2 or higher toxicity by NCI CTCAE, withhold drug. Resume normal dosage if initial episode of toxicity improves to grade 1 or lower. If toxicity recurs, resume at reduced doses.
➤**Advanced or metastatic breast cancer with capecitabine when tumors overexpress HER2 and patient has had prior therapy, including an anthracycline, a taxane, and trastuzumab**
Adults: 1,250 mg (5 tablets) P.O. once daily as a single dose on days 1 through 21, with 2,000 mg/m^2/day capecitabine given P.O. in two doses 12 hours apart on days 1 to 14. Repeat 21-day cycle.
➤**HER2-positive, hormone receptor–positive metastatic breast cancer in postmenopausal women**
Adults: 1,500 mg P.O. once daily with letrozole 2.5 mg once daily.

liothyronine sodium (T_3)
lye-oh-THYE-roe-neen

Cytomel, Triostat

Therapeutic class: Thyroid hormone replacements
Pharmacologic class: Thyroid hormones
Pregnancy risk category: A

AVAILABLE FORMS
Injection: 10 mcg/mL in 1-mL vials*
Tablets: 5 mcg, 25 mcg, 50 mcg

INDICATIONS & DOSAGES
➤ **Congenital hypothyroidism**
Children: 5 mcg P.O. daily; increase by 5 mcg every 3 to 4 days until desired response is achieved.
➤ **Myxedema**
Adults: Initially, 5 mcg P.O. daily; increase by 5 to 10 mcg every 1 to 2 weeks until daily dose reaches 25 mcg. Then increase by 5 to 25 mcg daily every 1 to 2 weeks. Maintenance dosage is 50 to 100 mcg daily.
➤ **Myxedema coma, premyxedema coma**
Adults: Initially, 10 to 20 mcg I.V. for patients with CV disease; 25 to 50 mcg I.V. for patients who don't have CV disease. Adjust dosage based on patient's condition and response. Switch patient to oral therapy as soon as possible.
➤ **Simple (nontoxic) goiter**
Adults: Initially, 5 mcg P.O. daily; may increase by 5 to 10 mcg daily every 1 to 2 weeks until daily dose reaches 25 mcg. Then increase by 12.5 to 25 mcg daily every 1 to 2 weeks. Usual maintenance dosage is 75 mcg daily.
Patients older than age 65 and children: 5 mcg daily; increase by 5 mcg daily every 1 to 2 weeks.
➤ **Thyroid hormone replacement**
Adults: Initially, 25 mcg P.O. daily; increase by up to 25 mcg every 1 to 2 weeks until satisfactory response occurs. Usual maintenance dosage is 25 to 75 mcg daily.
➤ **T_3 suppression test to differentiate hyperthyroidism from euthyroidism**
Adults: 75 to 100 mcg P.O. daily for 7 days.

liotrix
LYE-oh-trix

Thyrolar

Therapeutic class: Thyroid hormone replacements
Pharmacologic class: Thyroid hormones
Pregnancy risk category: A

AVAILABLE FORMS
Tablets: Levothyroxine sodium 12.5 mcg and liothyronine sodium 3.1 mcg (Thyrolar-0.25); levothyroxine sodium 25 mcg and liothyronine sodium 6.25 mcg (Thyrolar-0.5); levothyroxine sodium 50 mcg and liothyronine sodium 12.5 mcg (Thyrolar-1); levothyroxine sodium 100 mcg and liothyronine sodium 25 mcg (Thyrolar-2); levothyroxine sodium 150 mcg and liothyronine sodium 37.5 mcg (Thyrolar-3)

INDICATIONS & DOSAGES
Dosages are expressed in thyroid equivalents and must be individualized to approximate the deficit in patient's thyroid secretion.
➤ **Hypothyroidism**
Adults: Initially, a single daily dose of Thyrolar-0.5. Adjust dosage by 1 tablet of Thyrolar-0.25 at 2- to 3-week intervals. Maintenance dose is 1 tablet of Thyrolar-1 or Thyrolar-2 daily. Readjust dosage within the first 4 weeks of therapy after proper clinical and laboratory evaluations of T_4 and thyroid-stimulating hormone.
Adjust-a-dose: For elderly patients and patients with long-standing myxedema with CV impairment, initial dose is 1 tablet of Thyrolar-0.25 daily. Reduce dosage if angina occurs.
➤ **Congenital hypothyroidism**
Children older than age 12: More than 18.75/75 (T_3/T_4) mcg P.O. daily.
Children ages 6 to 12: 12.5/50 (T_3/T_4) to 18.75/75 (T_3/T_4) mcg P.O. daily.
Children ages 1 to 5: 9.35/37.5 (T_3/T_4) to 12.5/50 (T_3/T_4) mcg P.O. daily.
Children ages 6 to 12 months: 6.25/25 (T_3/T_4) to 9.35/37.5 (T_3/T_4) mcg P.O. daily.
Newborns and infants from birth to 6 months: 3.1/12.5 (T_3/T_4) to 6.25/25 (T_3/T_4) mcg P.O. daily.

SAFETY ALERT!

lomustine (CCNU)
loe-MUS-teen

CeeNU

Therapeutic class: Antineoplastics
Pharmacologic class: Nitrosoureas
Pregnancy risk category: D

AVAILABLE FORMS
Capsules: 10 mg, 40 mg, 100 mg

INDICATIONS & DOSAGES
➤ **Brain tumor, Hodgkin lymphoma**
Adults and children: 100 to 130 mg/m^2 P.O. as single dose every 6 weeks. Repeat doses shouldn't be given until WBC count exceeds 4,000/mm^3 and platelet count is greater than 100,000/mm^3.
Adjust-a-dose: Reduce dosage according to degree of bone marrow suppression or when used with other myelosuppressive drugs. Reduce dosage by 30% for WBC count nadir 2,000 to 2,999/mm^3 and platelet count nadir 25,000 to 74,999/mm^3; by 50% for WBC count nadir less than 2,000/mm^3 and platelet count nadir less than 25,000/mm^3. Reduce dosage in patients with renal impairment: For CrCl of 10 to 50 mL/minute, give 75% of usual dose; for CrCl of less than 10 mL/minute, give 50% of usual dose.

loxapine succinate
LOX-a-peen

Therapeutic class: Antipsychotics
Pharmacologic class: Dibenzapine derivatives
Pregnancy risk category: NR

AVAILABLE FORMS
Capsules: 5 mg, 10 mg, 25 mg, 50 mg

INDICATIONS & DOSAGES
➤ **Psychotic disorders**
Adults: Initially, 10 mg P.O. b.i.d. In severely disturbed patients, up to 50 mg daily may be desirable. Increase dosage fairly rapidly over the first 7 to 10 days until symptoms are controlled. Usual therapeutic and maintenance range is 60 to 100 mg daily.

meloxicam
mel-OX-i-kam

Mobic

Therapeutic class: Antirheumatics
Pharmacologic class: NSAIDs
Pregnancy risk category: C; D in 3rd trimester

AVAILABLE FORMS
Oral suspension: 7.5 mg/5 mL
Tablets: 7.5 mg, 15 mg

INDICATIONS & DOSAGES
➤ **To relieve signs and symptoms of osteoarthritis or rheumatoid arthritis (RA)**
Adults: 7.5 mg P.O. once daily. May increase as needed to maximum dosage of 15 mg daily.
➤ **To relieve signs and symptoms of pauciarticular or polyarticular course juvenile RA**
Children ages 2 to 17: 0.125 mg/kg P.O. once daily to a maximum dosage of 7.5 mg daily.

menotropins
men-oh-TROE-pins

Menopur, Repronex

Therapeutic class: Ovulation stimulants
Pharmacologic class: Gonadotropins
Pregnancy risk category: X

AVAILABLE FORMS
Injection: 75 international units of luteinizing hormone and 75 international units of follicle-stimulating hormone activity per ampule

INDICATIONS & DOSAGES
➤ **Assisted reproductive technologies**
Adults: Initially, 225 units subcutaneously (Menopur, Repronex) or I.M. (Repronex only) for patients who have received gonadotropin-releasing hormone (GnRH) agonist or antagonist pituitary suppression. Adjust dosage based on ultrasound and estradiol levels not more frequently than every 2 days and not to exceed 75 to 150 units Repronex or 150 units Menopur per adjustment. Maximum daily dosage is 450 units. Use for maximum of 12 days (Repronex) or 20 days (Menopur). Then, 5,000 to 10,000 units of human chorionic gonadotropin (hCG) after adequate follicular development.
➤ **Infertility with oligo-anovulation (Repronex)**
Adults: Initially, 150 units subcutaneously or I.M. daily for 5 days in patients who have received GnRH agonist or antagonist pituitary suppression. Adjust dosage based on response; 75 to 150 units per adjustment and not more frequently than every 2 days. Maximum daily dosage is 450 units; don't use for more than 12 days. If patient

response is adequate, give 5,000 to 10,000 units of hCG. Hold hCG if estradiol level is greater than 2,000 picograms/mL.

nabumetone
nah-BYOO-meh-tone

Therapeutic class: NSAIDs
Pharmacologic class: NSAIDs
Pregnancy risk category: C; D in 3rd trimester

AVAILABLE FORMS
Tablets: 500 mg, 750 mg

INDICATIONS & DOSAGES
➤ **Rheumatoid arthritis, osteoarthritis**
Adults: Initially, 1,000 mg P.O. daily as a single dose or in two divided doses. Maximum, 2,000 mg daily.
Adjust-a-dose: For patients with moderate renal insufficiency, the maximum starting dosage shouldn't exceed 750 mg P.O. once daily; with careful monitoring, daily doses may be increased to a maximum of 1,500 mg. For patients with severe renal insufficiency, the maximum starting dosage shouldn't exceed 500 mg P.O. once daily; with careful monitoring, daily doses may be increased to a maximum of 1,000 mg.

SAFETY ALERT!

nelarabine
neh-LAR-uh-been

Arranon, Atriance†

Therapeutic class: Antineoplastics
Pharmacologic class: DNA demethylation agents; prodrugs of cytotoxic deoxyguanosine
Pregnancy risk category: D

AVAILABLE FORMS
Injection: 5 mg/mL in 50-mL vial

INDICATIONS & DOSAGES
➤ **T-cell acute lymphoblastic leukemia and T-cell lymphoblastic lymphoma in patients whose disease hasn't responded to or has relapsed after treatment with at least two chemotherapy regimens**

Adults: 1,500 mg/m² I.V. over 2 hours on days 1, 3, and 5. Repeat every 21 days.
Children: 650 mg/m² I.V. over 1 hour daily for 5 consecutive days. Repeat every 21 days.

nitazoxanide
nye-te-ZOCKS-a-nide

Alinia

Therapeutic class: Antiprotozoals
Pharmacologic class: Antiprotozoals
Pregnancy risk category: B

AVAILABLE FORMS
Oral suspension: 100 mg/5 mL
Tablets: 500 mg

INDICATIONS & DOSAGES
➤ **Diarrhea caused by *Cryptosporidium parvum* or *Giardia lamblia***
Adults and children age 12 and older: 500 mg P.O. with food every 12 hours for 3 days.
Children ages 4 to 11: 200 mg (10 mL) P.O. with food every 12 hours for 3 days.
Children ages 1 to 3: 100 mg (5 mL) P.O. with food every 12 hours for 3 days.

SAFETY ALERT!

panitumumab
pan-eh-TOO-moo-mab

Vectibix

Therapeutic class: Antineoplastics
Pharmacologic class: Monoclonal antibodies
Pregnancy risk category: C

AVAILABLE FORMS
Solution for infusion: 20 mg/mL

INDICATIONS & DOSAGES
➤ **Human epidermal growth factor receptor–expressing metastatic colorectal cancer with disease progression during or following fluoropyrimidine-, oxaliplatin-, and irinotecan-containing regimens**
Adults: 6 mg/kg I.V. infusion over 60 minutes every 14 days. For doses greater than 1,000 mg, infuse over 90 minutes.

†Canada   ◇ OTC   ✐ Photoguide   *Liquid contains alcohol

Adjust-a-dose: For patients with mild or moderate (grade 1 or 2) infusion reactions, reduce infusion rate by 50%. For patients with severe (grade 3 or 4) infusion reactions, stop drug permanently. For skin toxicities grade 3 or greater, or if considered intolerable, stop drug. If toxicity doesn't improve to grade 2 or less within 1 month, permanently stop therapy. If toxicity improves to grade 2 or less, and patient's symptoms improve after withholding two or fewer doses, restart treatment at 50% of original dose. If toxicity recurs, permanently stop drug. If toxicity doesn't recur, increase subsequent doses in increments of 25% of original dose until a 6-mg/kg dose is reached.

SAFETY ALERT!

pazopanib
paz-OH-pa-nib

Votrient

Therapeutic class: Antineoplastics
Pharmacologic class: Multi-tyrosine kinase inhibitors
Pregnancy risk category: D

AVAILABLE FORMS
Tablets: 200 mg, 400 mg

INDICATIONS & DOSAGES
➤ **Advanced renal cell carcinoma, soft-tissue sarcoma in patients who have received prior chemotherapy**
Adults: 800 mg P.O. daily at least 1 hour before or 2 hours after a meal.
Adjust-a-dose: For patients with moderate hepatic impairment, 200 mg P.O. daily. Drug isn't recommended for patients with severe hepatic impairment.

SAFETY ALERT!

pegaspargase
(PEG-L-asparaginase)
peg-AHS-per-jays

Oncaspar

Therapeutic class: Antineoplastics
Pharmacologic class: Modified L-asparaginases
Pregnancy risk category: C

AVAILABLE FORMS
Injection: 750 international units/mL

INDICATIONS & DOSAGES
➤ **As part of a multidrug chemotherapy regimen in the treatment of acute lymphoblastic leukemia, and acute lymphoblastic leukemia with hypersensitivity to asparaginase**
Adults and children older than age 1: 2,500 international units/m^2 I.V. or I.M. every 14 days.

pentoxifylline
pen-tox-IH-fi-leen

Pentoxil, Trental $\mathscr{O}$

Therapeutic class: Hemorheologic drugs
Pharmacologic class: Xanthine derivatives
Pregnancy risk category: C

AVAILABLE FORMS
Tablets (extended-release): 400 mg

INDICATIONS & DOSAGES
➤ **Intermittent claudication from chronic occlusive vascular disease**
Adults: 400 mg P.O. t.i.d. with meals. May decrease to 400 mg b.i.d. if GI and CNS adverse effects occur. If adverse effects persist, discontinue drug.
Adjust-a-dose: For CrCl of 10 to 50 mL/minute, give usual dose every 12 to 24 hours. For CrCl of less than 10 mL/minute, give usual dose every 24 hours. For patients undergoing peritoneal dialysis, give usual dose every 24 hours.

perphenazine
per-FEN-uh-zeen

Therapeutic class: Antipsychotics
Pharmacologic class: Phenothiazines
Pregnancy risk category: C

AVAILABLE FORMS
Tablets: 2 mg, 4 mg, 8 mg, 16 mg

INDICATIONS & DOSAGES
➤ **Schizophrenia in nonhospitalized patients**

Adults and children older than age 12:
Initially, 4 to 8 mg P.O. t.i.d.; reduce as soon as possible to minimum effective dose.
➤ **Schizophrenia in hospitalized patients**
Adults and children older than age 12:
Initially, 8 to 16 mg P.O. b.i.d., t.i.d., or q.i.d.; increase to 64 mg daily, as needed.
➤ **Severe nausea and vomiting**
Adults: 8 to 16 mg P.O. daily in divided doses to maximum of 24 mg.

plerixafor
pleh-RIX-uh-for

Mozobil

Therapeutic class: Hematopoietics
Pharmacologic class: CXCR4 chemokine receptor inhibitors
Pregnancy risk category: D

AVAILABLE FORMS
Injection: 24 mg/1.2 mL single-use vial

INDICATIONS & DOSAGES
➤ **To mobilize hematopoietic stem cells for collection and subsequent autologous transplantation in patients with non-Hodgkin lymphoma and multiple myeloma**
Adults: 0.24 mg/kg (actual body weight) subcutaneously once daily beginning about 11 hours before apheresis for up to 4 consecutive days. Begin treatment after patient receives 4 days of granulocyte-colony stimulating factor therapy.

SAFETY ALERT!

pralatrexate
PRAL-ah-TREX-ate

Folotyn

Therapeutic class: Antineoplastics
Pharmacologic class: Folate analogue metabolic inhibitors
Pregnancy risk category: D

AVAILABLE FORMS
Injection: 20-mg/1 mL, 40-mg/2 mL single-use vials

INDICATIONS & DOSAGES
➤ **Relapsed or refractory peripheral T-cell lymphoma**
Adults: 30 mg/m^2 I.V. push over 3 to 5 minutes weekly for 6 weeks in 7-week cycles until disease progresses or unacceptable toxicity develops.
Adjust-a-dose: For grade 2 mucositis, omit dose; after recovery to grade 1 or less, resume at prior dose. For grade 2 recurrence or grade 3 mucositis, omit dose; after recovery, resume at 20 mg/m^2. For grade 4 mucositis, discontinue therapy. For platelet count of less than 50,000/mm^3 or ANC of 500 to 1,000/mm^3 lasting 1 week, omit dose; after recovery, resume at prior dose. For platelet count of less than 50,000/mm^3 for 2 weeks, omit dose; after recovery, resume at 20 mg/m^2. For platelet count of less than 50,000/mm^3 for 3 weeks, discontinue therapy. For ANC of 500 to 1,000/mm^3 with fever or ANC of less than 500/mm^3 lasting 1 week, omit dose and give granulocyte-colony stimulating factor (G-CSF) or granulocyte-macrophage colony stimulating factor (GM-CSF) support; after recovery, continue prior dose along with G-CSF or GM-CSF support. For ANC of 500 to 1,000/mm^3 with fever or ANC of less than 500/mm^3 recurring or lasting 2 weeks, omit dose and give G-CSF or GM-CSF support; after recovery, resume at 20 mg/m^2 along with G-CSF or GM-CSF support. For ANC of 500 to 1,000/mm^3 with fever or ANC of less than 500/mm^3 lasting 3 weeks or for a second occurrence, discontinue therapy. For grade 3 toxicity, omit dose; after recovery to grade 2 or less, resume dose at 20 mg/m^2. For grade 4 toxicity, discontinue therapy.

primidone
PRI-mi-done

Mysoline

Therapeutic class: Anticonvulsants
Pharmacologic class: Barbiturate analogues
Pregnancy risk category: D

AVAILABLE FORMS
Tablets: 50 mg, 250 mg

INDICATIONS & DOSAGES
➤ **Tonic-clonic, complex partial, and simple partial seizures**
Adults and children age 8 and older: Initially, 100 to 125 mg P.O. at bedtime on days 1 to 3; then 100 to 125 mg P.O. b.i.d. on days 4 to 6; then 100 to 125 mg P.O. t.i.d. on days 7 to 9, followed by maintenance dose of 250 mg P.O. t.i.d. May increase maintenance dose to 250 mg q.i.d., if needed. May increase dosage to maximum of 2 g daily in divided doses.
Children younger than age 8: Initially, 50 mg P.O. at bedtime for 3 days; then 50 mg P.O. b.i.d. for days 4 to 6; then 100 mg P.O. b.i.d. for days 7 to 9, followed by maintenance dose of 125 to 250 mg P.O. t.i.d. or 10 to 25 mg/kg daily in divided doses.

SAFETY ALERT!

radioactive iodine (sodium iodide, 131I)
Hicon, Sodium Iodide 131I
Therapeutic

Therapeutic class:
Radiopharmaceuticals
Pharmacologic class: Antithyroid drugs
Pregnancy risk category: X

AVAILABLE FORMS
All radioactivity concentrations are determined at time of calibration.
Capsules: Radioactivity range 0.75 to 100 mCi/capsule
Concentrated oral solution: 1,000 mCi/mL
Oral solution: Radioactivity range 3.5 to 150 mCi/vial

INDICATIONS & DOSAGES
➤ **Hyperthyroidism**
Adults: Usual dosage is 4 to 10 mCi P.O. Dosage is based on estimated weight of thyroid gland and thyroid uptake. Repeat treatment after 6 weeks, based on T4 level as needed.
➤ **Thyroid cancer**
Adults: Initially, 30 to 100 mCi P.O., with subsequent doses of 100 to 200 mCi for metastases. Dosage is based on estimated malignant thyroid tissue and metastatic tissue as determined by total body scan. Repeat treatment according to clinical status.

➤ **Thyroid function evaluation**
Adults: Dosage ranges from 5 to 100 microcuries P.O. based on patient's weight and type of procedure.

SAFETY ALERT!

regorafenib
RE-goe-RAF-e-nib

Stivarga

Therapeutic class: Antineoplastics
Pharmacologic classification: Kinase inhibitors
Pregnancy risk category: D

AVAILABLE FORMS
Tablets: 40 mg

INDICATIONS & DOSAGES
➤ **Patients with metastatic colorectal cancer previously treated with fluoropyrimidine-, oxaliplatin-, and irinotecan-based chemotherapy, an anti–vascular endothelial growth factor therapy and, if KRAS wild type, an anti–epidermal growth factor receptor therapy**
Adults: 160 mg P.O. once a day for first 21 days of each 28-day cycle.
Adjust-a-dose: Refer to manufacturer's instructions for dosage modification due to adverse reactions. Discontinue drug permanently for failure to tolerate 80-mg dose; any occurrence of AST or ALT level more than 20 times the upper limit of normal (ULN); any occurrence of AST or ALT level more than 3 × ULN with concurrent bilirubin level more than 2 × ULN; recurrence of AST or ALT level more than 5 × ULN despite dosage reduction to 120 mg; any grade 4 adverse reaction.

riluzole
RILL-yoo-zole

Rilutek

Therapeutic class: Neuroprotectors
Pharmacologic class: Benzothiazoles
Pregnancy risk category: C

AVAILABLE FORMS
Tablets: 50 mg

INDICATIONS & DOSAGES
➤ **Amyotrophic lateral sclerosis**
Adults: 50 mg P.O. every 12 hours, taken on empty stomach 1 hour before or 2 hours after a meal.

SAFETY ALERT!

romidepsin
roh-mih-DEP-sin

Istodax

Therapeutic class: Antineoplastics
Pharmacologic class: Histone deacetylase inhibitors
Pregnancy risk category: D

AVAILABLE FORMS
Injection: 10-mg vial

INDICATIONS & DOSAGES
Adjust-a-dose (for all indications): For grade 2 or 3 toxicity, delay treatment until toxicity returns to baseline, grade 1, or less; then restart drug at 14 mg/m^2; for grade 4 toxicity, restart dose at 10 mg/m^2. Discontinue drug if grade 3 or 4 toxicities recur after dosage reduction. For grade 3 or 4 neutropenia or thrombocytopenia, delay treatment until ANC is at least 1.5×10^9 or platelet count is at least 75×10^9; then restart drug at 14 mg/m^2. For grade 4 febrile neutropenia or thrombocytopenia requiring platelet transfusion, delay treatment until toxicity returns to baseline, grade 1, or less; then permanently reduce dosage to 10 mg/m^2.
➤ **Cutaneous T-cell lymphoma in patients who have received at least one prior systemic therapy**
Adults: 14 mg/m^2 by I.V. infusion over 4 hours on days 1, 8, and 15 of 28-day cycle. Repeat every 28 days if effective and well tolerated.
➤ **Treatment of peripheral T-cell lymphoma in patients who have received at least one prior therapy**
Adults: 14 mg/m^2 I.V. over 4 hours on days 1, 8, and 15 of a 28-day cycle. Repeat cycle every 28 days if effective and tolerated.

rufinamide
roo-FIN-ah-mide

Banzel

Therapeutic class: Anticonvulsants
Pharmacologic class: Triazole derivatives
Pregnancy risk category: C

AVAILABLE FORMS
Suspension: 40 mg/mL
Tablets: 200 mg, 400 mg

INDICATIONS & DOSAGES
➤ **Adjunct treatment of seizures associated with Lennox-Gastaut syndrome**
Adults: Initially, 200 to 400 mg P.O. b.i.d. Increase dosage by 400 to 800 mg/day P.O. every 2 days to 3,200 mg P.O. daily in divided doses.
Children age 4 and older: Initially, 5 mg/kg P.O. b.i.d. Increase dosage by 10 mg/kg P.O. every other day to 45 mg/kg or 3,200 mg (whichever is less) P.O. daily in divided doses.
Adjust-a-dose: Dialysis clears drug by 30%; dosage adjustment may be necessary. For patients taking valproate, start rufinamide at dosages less than 400 mg/day (adults) or less than 10 mg/kg/day (children).

sapropterin dihydrochloride
SAP-roh-TEHR-in

Kuvan

Therapeutic class: Phenylalanine reducers
Pharmacologic class: Enzyme cofactors
Pregnancy risk category: C

AVAILABLE FORMS
Tablets: 100 mg

INDICATIONS & DOSAGES
➤ **Hyperphenylalaninemia caused by tetrahydrobiopterin-responsive phenylketonuria**
Adults and children age 4 and older: Initially, 10 mg/kg P.O. once daily with food. If phenylalanine level hasn't decreased from baseline after 4 weeks, increase dose to 20 mg/kg P.O. Stop treatment if patient has no response after 4 weeks at 20 mg/kg.

saquinavir mesylate
sa-KWEN-ah-veer

Invirase

Therapeutic class: Antiretrovirals
Pharmacologic class: Protease inhibitors
Pregnancy risk category: B

AVAILABLE FORMS
Capsules (hard gelatin): 200 mg
Tablets (film-coated): 500 mg

INDICATIONS & DOSAGES
➤ **Adjunctive treatment of advanced HIV infection in selected patients**
Adults and adolescents age 16 and older: 1,000 mg P.O. b.i.d. given at the same time with 100 mg ritonavir P.O. b.i.d.

SAFETY ALERT!

scopolamine (hyoscine)
skoe-POL-a-meen

Transderm-Scop

scopolamine hydrobromide (hyoscine hydrobromide)
Scopolamine Hydrobromide Injection

Therapeutic class: Antispasmodics
Pharmacologic class: Belladonna alkaloids–antimuscarinics
Pregnancy risk category: C

AVAILABLE FORMS
scopolamine
Transdermal patch: 1.5 mg/2.5 cm^2 (1 mg/72 hours)
scopolamine hydrobromide
Injection: 0.4 mg/mL

INDICATIONS & DOSAGES
Adjust-a-dose (for all indications): Elderly patients may require lower doses.
➤ **Delirium, preanesthetic sedation, and obstetric amnesia with analgesics**
Adults: 0.32 to 0.65 mg I.V., I.M., or subcutaneously 30 to 60 minutes before or with other agents at the time of anesthesia. Dilute solution with sterile water for injection before giving I.V.

Children ages 3 to 6: 0.2 to 0.3 mg I.V., I.M., or subcutaneously 30 to 60 minutes before or with other agents at the time of anesthesia. Maximum dosage, 0.3 mg. Dilute solution with sterile water for injection before giving I.V.
➤ **To prevent postoperative nausea and vomiting**
Adults: Apply 1 transdermal patch the evening before scheduled surgery. To minimize exposure to newborns, apply patch 1 hour before cesarean birth. Keep patch in place for 24 hours after surgery.
➤ **To prevent nausea and vomiting from motion sickness**
Adults: One transdermal patch, formulated to deliver 1 mg scopolamine over 3 days, applied to the skin behind the ear at least 4 hours before antiemetic is needed. Or, 0.3 to 0.65 mg hydrobromide I.V., I.M., or subcutaneously t.i.d. or q.i.d., as needed.
➤ **Sedation**
Adults: 0.6 mg I.V., I.M., or subcutaneously t.i.d. or q.i.d.

scopolamine hydrobromide
skoe-POL-a-meen

Isopto Hyoscine

Therapeutic class: Mydriatics
Pharmacologic class: Antimuscarinics–anticholinergics
Pregnancy risk category: C

AVAILABLE FORMS
Ophthalmic solution: 0.25%

INDICATIONS & DOSAGES
➤ **Cycloplegic refraction**
Adults: Instill 1 or 2 drops of 0.25% solution 1 hour before refraction.
➤ **Iritis, uveitis**
Adults: Instill 1 or 2 drops of 0.25% solution once daily to q.i.d.

sertaconazole nitrate
sir-tah-KAHN-uh-zole

Ertaczo

Therapeutic class: Antifungals
Pharmacologic class: Imidazoles
Pregnancy risk category: C

AVAILABLE FORMS
Topical cream: 2%

INDICATIONS & DOSAGES
➤ **Interdigital tinea pedis caused by** ***Trichophyton rubrum, Trichophyton*** ***mentagrophytes,*** **or** ***Epidermophyton*** ***floccosum*** **in immunocompetent patients**
Adults and children age 12 and older: Apply cream b.i.d. to affected areas between toes and healthy surrounding areas for 4 weeks.

silver sulfadiazine
sul-fa-DYE-a-zeen

Dermazin†, Flamazine†, Hydrogel Ag ◊, Silvadene, SSD, SSDAF, Thermazene

Therapeutic class: Antibacterials (topical)
Pharmacologic class: Broad-spectrum sulfonamides
Pregnancy risk category: B

AVAILABLE FORMS
Cream: 1%

INDICATIONS & DOSAGES
➤ **To prevent or treat wound infection in second- and third-degree burns**
Adults: Apply 1/16-inch ribbon of cream to clean, debrided wound daily or b.i.d. Burn areas should be covered with cream at all times. Reapply to areas from which it has been removed by patient activity.

SAFETY ALERT!

sorafenib tosylate
sohr-uh-FEN-ib

Nexavar

Therapeutic class: Antineoplastics
Pharmacologic class: Multi-kinase inhibitors
Pregnancy risk category: D

AVAILABLE FORMS
Tablets: 200 mg

INDICATIONS & DOSAGES
➤ **Advanced renal cell carcinoma, hepatocellular carcinoma**

Adults: 400 mg P.O. b.i.d. at least 1 hour before or 2 hours after eating. Continue until disease progresses or unacceptable toxicity occurs.
Adjust-a-dose: If grade 2 skin toxicity (pain and swelling with normal activities) develops, continue treatment and use topical drugs to relieve symptoms. If symptoms don't improve in 1 week or if they occur a second or third time, stop treatment until toxicity resolves to grade 0 or 1 (able to perform daily activities). Resume treatment at 400 mg daily or every other day. At fourth occurrence of grade 2 toxicity, stop treatment. If grade 3 skin toxicity (ulceration, blistering, severe, debilitating pain of hands and feet) or a second occurrence develops, stop treatment until toxicity resolves to grade 0 or 1. Resume treatment at 400 mg daily or every other day. At third occurrence of grade 3 toxicity, stop treatment.

sulfADIAZINE
sul-fa-DYE-a-zeen

Therapeutic class: Antibiotics
Pharmacologic class: Sulfonamides
Pregnancy risk category: C

AVAILABLE FORMS
Tablets: 500 mg

INDICATIONS & DOSAGES
➤ **Acute otitis media due to** ***Haemophilus*** ***influenzae*** **in combination with penicillin; chancroid; meningococcal meningitis prophylaxis or treatment;** ***H. influenzae*** **meningitis in combination with streptomycin; inclusion conjunctivitis; trachoma; nocardiosis; adjunctive therapy for chloroquine-resistant malaria; toxoplasmosis encephalitis in combination with pyrimethamine**
Adults: Initially, 2 to 4 g P.O.; then 2 to 4 g P.O. divided into three to six doses daily.
Children age 2 months and older: Initially, 75 mg/kg P.O.; then 150 mg/kg or 4 g/m^2 P.O. divided into four to six doses daily. Maximum dosage is 6 g daily.
➤ **UTI due to** ***Escherichia coli, Klebsiella*** **or** ***Enterobacter*** **species,** ***Proteus mirabilis,*** **or** ***Proteus vulgaris*** **after failure of other sulfonamides**

Adults: Initially, 2 to 4 g P.O.; then 2 to 4 g P.O. divided into three to six doses daily.
➤ **To prevent rheumatic fever**
Children weighing more than 30 kg (66 lb): 1 g P.O. daily.
Children weighing less than 30 kg: 500 mg P.O. daily.

taliglucerase alfa
TAL-i-GLOO-ser-ase

Elelyso

Therapeutic class: Metabolic agents
Pharmacologic class: Recombinant enzymes
Pregnancy risk category: B

AVAILABLE FORMS
Injection: 200 units/vial

INDICATIONS & DOSAGES
➤ **Long-term enzyme replacement in patients with confirmed type 1 Gaucher disease**
Adults: 60 units/kg I.V. infused over 60 to 120 minutes every other week. Initial rate of infusion should be 1.3 mL/minute; may increase to 2.3 mL/minute if tolerated.
Adjust-a-dose: Adjust dosage based on achievement and maintenance of therapeutic goals.

SAFETY ALERT!

temsirolimus
TEM-seer-OLE-ih-muss

Torisel

Therapeutic class: Antineoplastics
Pharmacologic class: Kinase inhibitors
Pregnancy risk category: D

AVAILABLE FORMS
I.V. solution: 25 mg/mL

INDICATIONS & DOSAGES
➤ **Advanced renal cell carcinoma**
Adults: 25 mg I.V. over 30 to 60 minutes once weekly until disease progresses or unacceptable toxicity occurs. Give diphenhydramine 25 to 50 mg I.V. 30 minutes before each dose.

Adjust-a-dose: In patients with an ANC of less than 1,000/mm^3, a platelet count of less than 75,000/mm^3, or National Cancer Institute Common Terminology Criteria for Adverse Events grade 3 or greater adverse reactions, hold dose. Once toxicities have resolved to grade 2 or less, may restart drug, with dosage reduced by 5 mg weekly to dosage no lower than 15 mg/week. With mild hepatic impairment (bilirubin level 1 to 1.5 times the upper limit of normal [ULN] or AST level greater than ULN but with bilirubin level less than or equal to the ULN), reduce dosage to 15 mg/week.

SAFETY ALERT!

teriflunomide
TER-i-FLOO-noe-mide

Aubagio

Therapeutic class: Immunomodulators
Pharmacologic class: Pyrimidine synthesis inhibitors
Pregnancy risk category: X

AVAILABLE FORMS

Tablets: 7 mg, 14 mg

INDICATIONS & DOSAGES
➤ **Relapsing forms of multiple sclerosis**
Adults: 7 or 14 mg P.O. once daily.

tetrabenazine
TEH-tra-BEN-ah-zeen

Xenazine

Therapeutic class: Antichorea drugs
Pharmacologic class: Monoamine depleters
Pregnancy risk category: C

AVAILABLE FORMS
Tablets: 12.5 mg, 25 mg

INDICATIONS & DOSAGES
➤ **Chorea associated with Huntington disease**
Adults: Initially, 12.5 mg P.O. daily in the morning. After 1 week, increase dosage to 12.5 mg P.O. b.i.d. Titrate dosage by

12.5 mg at weekly intervals, as needed. Maximum single dose, 25 mg. If dosage of 37.5 to 50 mg/day is needed, administer in 3 divided doses. Patients requiring more than 50 mg/day should be genotyped for CYP2D6 metabolism.

Adjust-a-dose: In patients who are extensive or intermediate CYP2D6 metabolizers, slowly titrate dosages above 50 mg at weekly intervals by 12.5 mg as needed and tolerated. Maximum daily dosage is 100 mg; maximum single dose, 37.5 mg. In patients who are poor CYP2D6 metabolizers, maximum daily dosage is 50 mg; maximum single dose, 25 mg.

thioridazine hydrochloride
thye-oh-RYE-da-zeen

Therapeutic class: Antipsychotics
Pharmacologic class: Phenothiazines
Pregnancy risk category: C

AVAILABLE FORMS
Tablets: 10 mg, 25 mg, 50 mg, 100 mg

INDICATIONS & DOSAGES
➤ **Schizophrenia in patients who don't respond to treatment with at least two other antipsychotic drugs**
Adults: Initially, 50 to 100 mg P.O. t.i.d.; increase gradually to 800 mg daily in divided doses, as needed. Daily maintenance doses range from 200 to 800 mg divided into two to four doses.
Children: Initially, 0.5 mg/kg P.O. daily in divided doses. Increase gradually to optimal therapeutic effect; maximum dose is 3 mg/kg daily.

thiothixene
thye-oh-THIX-een

Navane

Therapeutic class: Antipsychotics
Pharmacologic class: Thioxanthenes
Pregnancy risk category: C

AVAILABLE FORMS
Capsules: 1 mg, 2 mg, 5 mg, 10 mg

INDICATIONS & DOSAGES
➤ **Mild to moderate psychosis**
Adults and children age 12 and older: Initially, 2 mg P.O. t.i.d. Increase gradually to 15 mg daily, as needed.
➤ **Severe psychosis**
Adults and children age 12 and older: Initially, 5 mg P.O. b.i.d. Increase gradually to 20 to 30 mg daily, as needed. Maximum dose is 60 mg daily.

SAFETY ALERT!

toremifene citrate
tore-EM-ah-feen

Fareston

Therapeutic class: Antineoplastics
Pharmacologic class: Nonsteroidal antiestrogens
Pregnancy risk category: D

AVAILABLE FORMS
Tablets: 60 mg

INDICATIONS & DOSAGES
➤ **Metastatic breast cancer in postmenopausal women with estrogen receptor–positive or estrogen receptor–unknown tumors**
Adults: 60 mg P.O. once daily. Continue until disease progresses.

trifluoperazine hydrochloride
trye-floo-oh-PER-eh-zeen

Therapeutic class: Antipsychotics
Pharmacologic class: Phenothiazines
Pregnancy risk category: NR

AVAILABLE FORMS
Tablets (regular and film-coated): 1 mg, 2 mg, 5 mg, 10 mg

INDICATIONS & DOSAGES
➤ **Anxiety states**
Adults: 1 to 2 mg P.O. b.i.d. Maximum, 6 mg daily. Don't give drug for longer than 12 weeks for anxiety.

➤ **Schizophrenia, other psychotic disorders**
Adults and children older than age 12: 2 to
5 mg P.O. b.i.d., gradually increased until
therapeutic response occurs. Most patients
respond to 15 to 20 mg P.O. daily, although
some may need 40 mg daily or more.
Children ages 6 to 12: For hospitalized or
closely supervised patients, 1 mg P.O. daily
or b.i.d.; may increase gradually to 15 mg
daily, if needed.

trimethobenzamide hydrochloride
trye-meth-oh-BEN-za-mide

Tigan

Therapeutic class: Antiemetics
Pharmacologic class: Anticholinergics
Pregnancy risk category: C

AVAILABLE FORMS
Capsules: 300 mg
Injection: 100 mg/mL

INDICATIONS & DOSAGES
➤ **Nausea and vomiting**
Adults: 300 mg P.O. t.i.d. or q.i.d.; or 200 mg
I.M. When treating postoperative nausea and
vomiting, repeat I.M. dose after 1 hour.

SAFETY ALERT!

vandetanib
van-DET-a-nib

Caprelsa

Therapeutic class: Antineoplastics
Pharmacologic class: Kinase inhibitors
Pregnancy risk category: D

AVAILABLE FORMS
Tablets: 100 mg, 300 mg

INDICATIONS & DOSAGES
➤ **Symptomatic or progressive medullary
thyroid cancer in those with unresectable
locally advanced or metastatic disease**
Adults: 300 mg P.O. daily.
Adjust-a-dose: In patients with moderate to
severe renal impairment (CrCl of less than
50 mL/minute), initiate therapy at 200 mg
P.O. daily. In the event of corrected QT

interval (Fridericia [QTcF]) greater than
500 ms, interrupt therapy until QTcF
returns to less than 450 ms; then resume at
a reduced dosage. In patients with grade 3
or greater toxicity, stop drug until toxicity
resolves or improves to grade 1; resume at
reduced dosage of 200 mg, then 100 mg, if
necessary.

velaglucerase alfa
vel-uh-GLOO-ser-ase

VPRIV

Therapeutic class: Metabolic agents
Pharmacologic class: Hydrolytic
lysosomal glucocerebroside-specific
enzymes
Pregnancy risk category: B

AVAILABLE FORMS
Injection: 200 units/vial, 400 units/vial

INDICATIONS & DOSAGES
➤ **Long-term enzyme replacement in
patients with type 1 Gaucher disease**
Adults and children age 4 and older:
60 units/kg I.V. infused over 60 minutes
every other week.

SAFETY ALERT!

vemurafenib
VEM-ue-RAF-e-nib

Zelboraf

Therapeutic class: Antineoplastics
Pharmacologic class: Kinase inhibitors
Pregnancy risk category: D

AVAILABLE FORMS
Tablets: 240 mg

INDICATIONS & DOSAGES
➤ **Treatment of unresectable or
metastatic melanoma with *BRAF*^{V600E}
mutation**
Adults: Usual dosage is 960 mg P.O. b.i.d.
Adjust-a-dose: In patients with symptomatic
adverse drug reactions or prolongation of
QTc interval, refer to manufacturer's instructions for dosage adjustment.

zanamivir
zan-AM-ah-veer

Relenza

Therapeutic class: Antiretrovirals
Pharmacologic class: Selective
neuraminidase inhibitors
Pregnancy risk category: C

AVAILABLE FORMS
Powder for inhalation: 5 mg/blister

INDICATIONS & DOSAGES
➤ **Uncomplicated acute illness caused by influenza virus A and B in patients who have had symptoms for no longer than 2 days; treatment of H1N1 influenza A**
Adults and children age 7 and older: 2 oral inhalations (one 5-mg blister per inhalation for total dose of 10 mg) b.i.d. using the dry-powder inhalation device for 5 days. Give two doses on first day of treatment, allowing at least 2 hours to elapse between doses. Give subsequent doses about 12 hours apart (in the morning and evening) at about the same time each day.
➤ **Prevention of influenza in a household setting; prevention of H1N1 influenza A**
Adults and children age 5 and older: 2 oral inhalations (one 5-mg blister per inhalation for total dose of 10 mg) once daily for 10 days.
➤ **Prevention of influenza in a community setting**
Adults and adolescents ages 12 to 16: 2 oral inhalations (one 5-mg blister per inhalation for total dose of 10 mg) once daily for 28 days.

SAFETY ALERT!

ziv-aflibercept
ZIV-a-FLIB-er-sept

Zaltrap

Therapeutic class: Antineoplastics
Pharmacologic class: Vascular
endothelial growth factor inhibitors
Pregnancy risk category: C

AVAILABLE FORMS
Injection: 100 mg/4-mL (25 mg/mL),
200 mg/8-mL (25 mg/mL) single-use vials

INDICATIONS & DOSAGES
➤ **Metastatic colorectal cancer that is resistant or has progressed following an oxaliplatin-containing regimen in combination with 5-FU, leucovorin, and irinotecan (FOLFIRI)**
Adults: 4 mg/kg I.V. over 1 hour every 2 weeks, given before any component of FOLFIRI regimen on day of treatment.
Adjust-a-dose: For recurrent or severe hypertension, withhold drug until controlled; then permanently reduce dosage to 2 mg/kg. For proteinuria of 2 g/24 hours or greater, withhold drug until proteinuria is less than 2 g/24 hours; then permanently reduce dosage to 2 mg/kg. For neutropenia, delay treatment until ANC is greater than 1.5×10^9/L.b

Additional new drugs: Indications and dosages

SAFETY ALERT!

afatinib dimaleate
a-FA-ti-nib

Gilotrif

Therapeutic class: Antineoplastics
Pharmacologic class: Tyrosine kinase inhibitors
Pregnancy risk category: D

AVAILABLE FORMS
Tablets: 20 mg, 30 mg, 40 mg

INDICATIONS & DOSAGES
➤ **First-line treatment of patients with metastatic non–small-cell lung cancer whose tumors have epidermal growth factor receptor exon 19 deletions or exon 21 (*L858R*) substitution mutations as detected by an FDA-approved test**
Adults: 40 mg P.O. once a day on an empty stomach until disease progression or intolerability occurs.
Adjust-a-dose: Withhold drug for grade 3 or higher adverse reactions, diarrhea of grade 3 or more, diarrhea of grade 2 lasting for 2 or more consecutive days while patient is taking antidiarrheals, cutaneous reactions of grade 2 lasting more than 7 days or that are intolerable, or renal dysfunction of grade 2 or higher. If adverse reactions improve to grade 1, restart afatinib at a reduced dosage at 10 mg/day less than the dose at which the adverse reaction occurred. Discontinue drug for severe or intolerable adverse reactions occurring at a dose of 20 mg/day.

brinzolamide–brimonidine tartrate
brin-ZOL-ah-mide–brih-MOE-neh-dean

Simbrinza

Therapeutic class: Antiglaucoma drugs
Pharmacologic class: Carbonic anhydrase inhibitors–alpha$_2$ adrenergic receptor agonists
Pregnancy risk category: C

AVAILABLE FORMS
Ophthalmic suspension: brinzolamide 1% and brimonidine 0.2%

INDICATIONS & DOSAGES
➤ **Reduction of intraocular pressure in patients with open-angle glaucoma or ocular hypertension**
Adults and children age 2 and older: Instill 1 drop into affected eye(s) t.i.d.

SAFETY ALERT!

cabozantinib-s-malate
KA-boe-ZAN-ti-nib

Cometriq

Therapeutic class: Antineoplastics
Pharmacologic class: Tyrosine kinase inhibitors
Pregnancy risk category: D

AVAILABLE FORMS
Capsules: 20 mg, 80 mg

INDICATIONS & DOSAGES
➤ **Progressive metastatic medullary thyroid cancer**
Adults: 140 mg (one 80-mg and three 20-mg capsules) P.O. once daily. Maximum dosage is 180 mg daily.
Adjust-a-dose: Withhold drug for grade 4 hematologic adverse reactions, grade 3 or greater nonhematologic adverse reactions, or intolerable grade 2 adverse reactions. When the adverse reaction returns to baseline or is reduced to grade 1, resume drug; reduce pre-

vious 140-mg dose to 100 mg and previous 100-mg dose to 60 mg. Don't reduce previous 60-mg dose; if patient can't tolerate 60-mg dose, discontinue drug. Withhold drug in patients who develop intolerable grade 2 or grade 3-4 palmar-plantar erythrodysesthesia syndrome until improvement to grade 1. Resume at a reduced dosage. Permanently discontinue drug for development of visceral perforation or fistula formation, severe hemorrhage, serious arterial thromboembolic events (MI, cerebral infarction), or nephrotic syndrome; malignant hypertension, hypertensive crisis, or persistent uncontrolled hypertension despite optimal medical management; osteonecrosis of the jaw; or reversible posterior leukoencephalopathy syndrome.

SAFETY ALERT!

dabrafenib mesylate
da-BRAF-e-nib

Tafinlar

Therapeutic class: Antineoplastics
Pharmacologic class: Kinase inhibitors
Pregnancy risk category: D

AVAILABLE FORMS
Capsules: 50 mg, 75 mg

INDICATIONS & DOSAGES
➤ **Unresectable or metastatic melanoma with BRAF *V600E* mutation**
Adults: 150 mg P.O. b.i.d. approximately 12 hours apart, until disease progression or unacceptable toxicity occurs.
Adjust-a-dose: If temperature of 101.3° to 104° F (38.5° to 40° C) occurs, withhold drug until fever resolves; when fever resolves, resume drug at same or reduced dosage. If temperature is higher than 104° F (40° C) or is complicated by rigors, hypotension, dehydration, or renal failure, either permanently discontinue drug or withhold drug until fever reaction resolves; then resume at reduced dosage. If intolerable grade 2 adverse reactions or any grade 3 adverse reactions occur, withhold drug until adverse reaction resolves to grade 1 or less; then resume at reduced dosage. At first occurrence of any grade 4 reaction, either permanently discontinue drug or withhold drug until adverse reaction resolves to grade 1 or

less; then resume at reduced dosage. If a recurrent grade 4 adverse reaction or intolerable grade 2 or any grade 3 or 4 adverse reaction occurs with dosage of 50 mg b.i.d., discontinue drug permanently. When dosage reductions are necessary, first dosage reduction is to 100 mg b.i.d., second dosage reduction is to 75 mg b.i.d., and third dosage reduction is to 50 mg b.i.d. If patient is unable to tolerate 50 mg b.i.d., discontinue drug.

ferric carboxymaltose
FER-ik car-box-ee-MAL-tose

Injectafer

Therapeutic class: Iron supplements
Pharmacologic class: Hematinics
Pregnancy risk category: C

AVAILABLE FORMS
Injection: 50 mg/mL of elemental iron in 15-mL single-dose vial

INDICATIONS & DOSAGES
➤ **Iron deficiency anemia in patients intolerant to or who have had unsatisfactory response to oral iron and in those with non-dialysis-dependent chronic kidney disease**
Adults: For patients weighing at least 50 kg (110 lb), 750 mg I.V. on day 1; repeat dose after at least 7 days. May repeat course of therapy if anemia recurs. For patients weighing less than 50 kg, give 15 mg/kg body weight on day 1; repeat dose after at least 7 days. May repeat course of therapy if anemia recurs. Maximum cumulative dose is 1,500 mg per treatment course.

pasireotide diaspartate
PAS-i-REE-oh-tide

Signifor

Therapeutic class: Endocrine drugs
Pharmacologic class: Somatostatin analogues
Pregnancy risk category: C

AVAILABLE FORMS
Injection: 0.3 mg/mL, 0.6 mg/mL, 0.9 mg/mL glass ampules

INDICATIONS & DOSAGES

➤ **Cushing disease when pituitary surgery isn't an option or hasn't been curative**

Adults: Initially, 0.6 or 0.9 mg subcutaneously b.i.d. Titrate based on response and tolerability. If starting at 0.6 mg b.i.d., may increase to 0.9 mg b.i.d. based on response to treatment. Dosage range is 0.3 to 0.9 mg b.i.d.

Elderly patients: Use caution in dosage selection. Dosage for elderly patients usually starts at low end of dosing range, reflecting the greater frequency of decreased hepatic, renal, or cardiac function in this population.

Adjust-a-dose: May decrease dosage by 0.3 mg if adverse effects occur. Patients with moderate hepatic impairment should begin at 0.3 mg b.i.d. for a maximum dosage of 0.6 mg b.i.d. Avoid use in patients with severe hepatic impairment. If ALT level is normal at baseline but elevates to 3 to 5 times the upper limit of normal (ULN), repeat test within a week or within 48 hours if ALT level exceeds 5 × ULN. If results are confirmed, interrupt treatment and monitor serial liver enzymes. If ALT level returns to normal or near normal and cause other than pasireotide treatment is identified, resume drug cautiously.

pomalidomide
POE-ma-LID-oh-mide

Pomalyst

Therapeutic class: Immunomodulators
Pharmacologic class: Thalidomide analogues
Pregnancy risk category: X

AVAILABLE FORMS
Capsules: 1 mg, 2 mg, 3 mg, 4 mg

INDICATIONS & DOSAGES
➤ **Multiple myeloma in patients who have received at least two prior therapies, including lenalidomide and bortezomib, and have disease progression on or within 60 days of completion of last therapy**

Adults: 4 mg P.O. once daily on days 1 through 21 of repeated 28-day cycles. Continue until disease progression.

Adjust-a-dose: For ANC less than 500/mm³ or febrile neutropenia (temperature of 101.3° F [38.5° C]) or greater and ANC less than 1,000/mm³, interrupt regimen and monitor CBC weekly. Once ANC returns to 500/mm³ or greater, resume at 3 mg daily. For each subsequent reduction in ANC to less than 500/mm³, interrupt regimen; once ANC returns to 500/mm³ or greater, resume at 1 mg less than previous dose. For platelet count less than 25,000/mm³, interrupt regimen and monitor CBC weekly. Once platelet count returns to greater than 50,000/mm³, resume at 3 mg daily. For each subsequent reduction in platelets to less than 25,000/mm³, interrupt regimen as before; once platelet count returns to greater than 50,000/mm³, resume at 1 mg less than previous dose. For other grade 3 or 4 toxicities, interrupt regimen. Once toxicity has resolved to grade 2 or less, at prescriber's discretion, resume at 1 mg less than previous dose. To initiate a new cycle, neutrophil count must be 500/mm³ or greater, and platelet count must be 50,000/mm³ or greater. If toxicities occur after dosage reductions to 1 mg, discontinue drug.

raxibacumab
RAX-ee-BAK-ue-mab

Therapeutic class: Anti-infectives
Pharmacologic class: Monoclonal antibodies
Pregnancy risk category: B

AVAILABLE FORMS
Injection: 1,700 mg/34 mL (50 mg/mL) single-use vial

INDICATIONS & DOSAGES
➤ **Treatment of adults and children with inhalational anthrax due to *Bacillus anthracis* in combination with appropriate antibacterial drugs; prophylaxis of inhalational anthrax when alternative therapies aren't available or appropriate**

Adults and children weighing more than 50 kg (110 lb): 40 mg/kg I.V. as a single dose.

Children weighing more than 15 kg (33 lb) and less than 50 kg: 60 mg/kg I.V. as a single dose.

Children weighing 15 kg or less: 80 mg/kg I.V. as a single dose.

teduglutide [rDNA origin]
te-DUE-gloo-tide

Gattex

Therapeutic class: Miscellaneous GI drugs
Pharmacologic class: Glucagon-like peptide-2 analogues
Pregnancy risk category: B

AVAILABLE FORMS
Injection: 5-mg vials in 1- and 30-vial kits

INDICATIONS & DOSAGES
➤ **Short bowel syndrome in patients dependent on parenteral support**
Adults: 0.05 mg/kg body weight subcutaneously once daily.
Adjust-a-dose: Decrease dosage by 50% in patients with moderate to severe renal impairment (CrCl of less than 50 mL/minute) and in those with ESRD.

SAFETY ALERT!

trametinib dimethyl sulfoxide
tra-ME-ti-nib

Mekinist

Therapeutic class: Antineoplastics
Pharmacologic class: Kinase inhibitors
Pregnancy risk category: D

AVAILABLE FORMS
Tablets: 0.5 mg, 1 mg, 2 mg

INDICATIONS & DOSAGES
➤ **Unresectable or metastatic melanoma with BRAF *V600E* or *V600K* mutations, as detected by an FDA-approved test**
Adults: 2 mg P.O. once daily until disease progression or unacceptable toxicity occurs.
Adjust-a-dose: In patients with a grade 2 rash, reduce dosage by 0.5 mg or discontinue in patients taking 1 mg daily. For an intolerable grade 2 rash that doesn't improve within 3 weeks after dosage reduction or a grade 3 or 4 rash, withhold drug for up to 3 weeks. If rash improves within 3 weeks, resume at a dosage reduced by 0.5 mg or discontinue drug in patients taking 1 mg daily. For an intolerable grade 2 or grade 3 or 4 rash that doesn't improve within 3 weeks despite dosing interruption, permanently discontinue drug.

In patients with "asymptomatic, absolute" decrease in LVEF of 10% or greater from baseline and that is below institutional lower limits of normal (LLN) from pretreatment value, withhold drug for up to 4 weeks. If LVEF improves to normal value within 4 weeks after interruption of drug, resume at a dosage reduced by 0.5 mg or discontinue in patients taking 1 mg daily. In patients with symptomatic heart failure, an absolute decrease in LVEF of greater than 20% from baseline that is below LLN, or an absolute decrease in LVEF of 10% or greater from baseline that is below LLN that doesn't improve to normal LVEF value within 4 weeks after interruption of drug, permanently discontinue drug.

In patients with grade 2 to 3 retinal pigment epithelial detachments (RPED), withhold drug for up to 3 weeks. For grade 2 to 3 RPED that improves to grade 0 to 1 within 3 weeks, resume at a dose reduced by 0.5 mg or discontinue drug in patients taking 1 mg daily. For grade 2 to 3 RPED that doesn't improve to at least grade 1 within 3 weeks and in patients with retinal vein occlusion, permanently discontinue drug.

In patients who develop interstitial lung disease or pneumonitis, permanently discontinue drug.

In patients with other grade 3 adverse reactions, withhold drug for up to 3 weeks. If reactions improve to grade 0 to 1 within 3 weeks, reduce dosage by 0.5 mg or discontinue drug in patients taking 1 mg daily. In patients with grade 4 adverse reaction or grade 3 adverse reactions that don't improve to grade 0 to 1 within 3 weeks, permanently discontinue drug.

vortioxetine hydrobromide
VOR-tye-OX-eh-teen

Brintellix

Therapeutic class: Antidepressants
Pharmacologic class: SSRIs
Pregnancy risk category: C

AVAILABLE FORMS
Tablets (immediate-release, film-coated):
5 mg, 10 mg, 15 mg, 20 mg

INDICATIONS & DOSAGES
➤ **Major depressive disorder**
Adults: 10 mg P.O. once daily. May increase
as tolerated up to targeted dosage of 20 mg
once daily.
Adjust-a-dose: If 10 mg once daily isn't
tolerated, decrease dosage to 5 mg once daily. If discontinuing drug when patient is
taking 15 or 20 mg daily, decrease first to
10 mg daily for 1 week, then stop drug to
avoid adverse reactions.

Index

A

A-200, 1199–1200
abacavir sulfate, 55, 65–66
abacavir sulfate–lamivudine, 1533
abacavir sulfate–lamivudine–
   zidovudine, 1533
abatacept, 41–42, 66–68
abciximab, 39–40, 68–70
Abelcet, 129–131
Abenol, 74–77
Abilify, 148–152, **C4**
Abilify Discmelt, 148–152
Abilify Maintena, 148–152
abiraterone acetate, 70–71
Abraxane, 1082–1085
Absorica, 794–796
Absorption, drug, 1
   in children, 7
Abstral, 599–604
acamprosate calcium, 72–73, **C3**
acarbose, 32–33, 73–74
Accolate, 1470–1471
AccuNeb, 92–94
Accupril, 1206–1207, **C24**
Accuretic, 1527
ACE inhibitors, 1496
Aceon, 1126–1128
Acephen, 74–77
ACET, 74–77
Acetadote, 79–81
acetaminophen, 74–77
acetaminophen–butalbital–caffeine–
   codeine phosphate, 1523
Acetazolam, 77–79
acetaZOLAMIDE, 77–79
acetaZOLAMIDE sodium, 77–79
acetylcysteine, 79–81
acetylsalicylic acid, 155–158
Acid Reducer, 1221–1223
Aciphex, 1212–1213, **C24**
Aciphex Sprinkle, 1212–1213
ACT, 1551
Actemra, 1391–1393
ActHIB, 1538–1539
Actidose with Sorbitol, 1511
Actidose-Aqua, 1511
Actimmune, 777–778
Actiq, 599–604
Activase, 108–111
activated charcoal, 1511
Activella, 1535
Actonel, 1241–1243, **C25**
ActoPlus Met, 1524–1525

ActoPlus Met XR, 1524–1525
Actos, 1145–1146, **C23**
Acular, 806–807
Acular LS, 806–807
Acuvail, 806–807
acyclovir, 81–84
acyclovir sodium, 81–84
ADACEL, 1539
Adalat CC, 1007–1009
Adalat XL, 1007–1009
adalimumab, 41–42, 84–86
Adcetris, 230–232
Adcirca, 1326–1328
Adderall, 1522
Adderall XR, 1522
adefovir dipivoxil, 86–87
Adenocard, 87–89
Adenoscan, 87–89
adenosine, 28, 87–89
Adipex-P, 1131–1132
ado-trastuzumab emtansine, 89–91
Adrenaclick, 516–519
Adrenalin Chloride, 516–519
adrenaline, 516–519
Advair Diskus 100/50, 642–644
Advair Diskus 250/50, 642–644
Advair Diskus 500/50, 642–644
Advair HFA 45/21, 642–644
Advair HFA 115/21, 642–644
Advair HFA 230/21, 642–644
Advanced Eye Relief: Redness
   Maximum Relief, 990–991
Advate, 1516–1517
Adverse reactions, drug, 3–4
Advicor, 1534
Advil, 721–724
AeroSpan HFA, 622–624
afatinib dimaleate, 1586
Afeditab CR, 1007–1009
Afinitor, 583–587
Afinitor Disperz, 583–587
Afluria, 1542–1543
Afrin, 1073–1074
Aggrastat, 1384–1386
Aggrenox, 1532
AHF factor VIII, 1518–1519
A-Hydrocort, 706–709
Akarpine, 1141–1142
AKBeta, 833–834
AK-Con, 990–991
AK-Dilate, 1136–1137
Akne-mycin, 536
Aktob, 1387–1388

Ala-Cort, 709–711
Ala-Scalp, 709–711
Alavert, 873–874
Alavert Children's 873–874
Alaway, 810
Albalon, 990–991
Albumarc, 1516
albumin 5%, 1516
albumin 25%, 1516
Albuminar-5, 1516
Albuminar-25, 1516
Albutein 5%, 1516
Albutein 25%, 1516
albuterol sulfate, 92–94, 1491
alcaftadine, 1562
Aldactazide, 1534
Aldactone, 1306–1307, **C27**
Aldara, 739–740
alefacept, 52, 94–95
alendronate sodium, 95–97, **C3**
Aler-Cap, 455–456
Aler-Dryl, 455–456
Aler-Tab, 455–456
Alertec, 964–966
Aleve, 991–993
alfuzosin hydrochloride, 23–24,
   97–98, **C3**
alglucosidase alfa, 1562
Alimta, 1110–1112
Alinia, 1575
aliskiren, 36–37
aliskiren hemifumarate, 98–99
aliskiren hemifumarate–amlodipine
   besylate, 1530
aliskiren hemifumarate–
   hydrochlorothiazide, 1530–1531
Alka-Seltzer, 1283–1284, 1557
Alkeran, 900–902
Alkylating drugs, 23
All Clear, 990–991
All Day Allergy, 309–310
Allegra Allergy, 610–611
Allegra Allergy Children's, 610–611
Allegra ODT, 610–611
Allergy, drug, 3–4
Allergy Time, 315–316
Alli, 1056–1057
allopurinol, 99–101
allopurinol sodium, 99–101
almotriptan malate, 38, 101–103
alogliptin benzoate, 103–104
alogliptin benzoate–metformin,
   1526

Boldface refers to full color photographs.

Boldface refers to full color photographs.

Boldface refers to full color photographs.

Boldface refers to full color photographs.

Boldface refers to full color photographs.

Boldface refers to full color photographs.

Boldface refers to full color photographs.

Boldface refers to full color photographs.

Boldface refers to full color photographs.

Boldface refers to full color photographs.